Nursing Practice
Hospital and Home
THE ADULT

Key features

This book has been written with the reader in mind.

The **key features** (shown on the accompanying sample pages) make the test easy to read, quick to refer to and useful for revision.

Self-assessment question with answer at end of book

Running head: title of section

Table

Running head: title of chapter

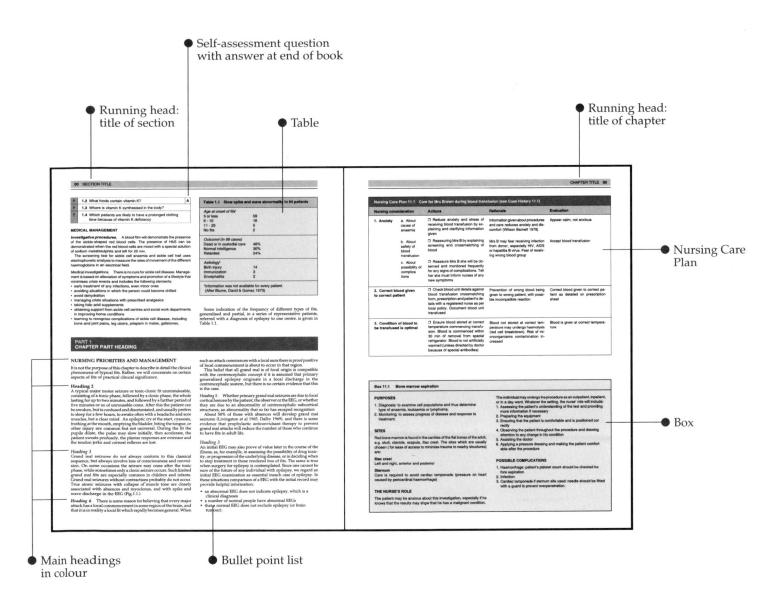

Nursing Care Plan

Box

Main headings in colour

Bullet point list

Nursing Practice

For Churchill Livingstone

Editorial Director: Mary Law
Commissioning Editor: Ellen Green
Project Development Editor: Mairi McCubbin
Copy Editor: Anne Marie Todkill
Senior Project Controller: Mark Sanderson
Design direction: Erik Bigland
Sales Promotion Executive: Hilary Brown

Nursing Practice
Hospital and Home
THE ADULT

Edited by

Margaret F. Alexander BSc PhD RGN SCM RNT FRCN
Head of Department, Nursing and Community Health,
Glasgow Caledonian University, Glasgow

Josephine N. Fawcett BSc(Hons) RGN MSc RNT
Lecturer, Department of Nursing Studies,
University of Edinburgh, Edinburgh

Phyllis J. Runciman BSc MSc MPhil RGN SCM HV RNT
Senior Lecturer, Department of Health and Nursing,
Queen Margaret College, Edinburgh

Associate Editor
Cynthia B. Edmond BA MSc GradDipEd RN RNT RM(Aust) CertAdmin(Aust) FRCNA MCNNSW
Freelance Lecturer and Clinical Nurse, Edinburgh
Formerly Lecturer, Department of Health Occupations,
University of Newcastle, New South Wales, Australia

Foreword by
Barbara Vaughan MSc RGN RCNT DipN DANS RNT
Programme Director (Nursing Developments)
King's Fund Centre, London

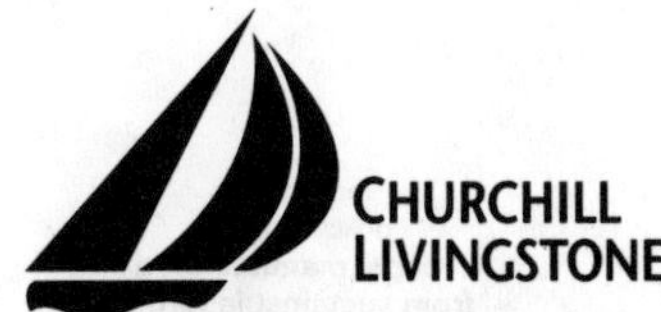

EDINBURGH LONDON MADRID MELBOURNE NEW YORK AND TOKYO 1994

CHURCHILL LIVINGSTONE
Medical Division of Pearson Professional Ltd

Distributed in the United States of America by Churchill Livingstone Inc., 650 Avenue of the Americas, New York, N.Y. 10011, and by associated companies, branches and representatives throughout the world.

First published 1994
Reprinted 1995
Reprinted 1996

ISBN 0 443 043388

British Library of Cataloguing in Publication Data
A catalogue record for this book is available from the British Library.

Library of Congress Cataloging in Publication Data
A catalogue record for this book is available from the Library of Congress.

The publisher's policy is to use **paper manufactured from sustainable forests**

Produced by Longman Singapore Publishers (Pte) Ltd
Printed in Singapore

Contents

Contributors vii

Theme advisors x

Clinical advisors xi

Foreword xiii

Preface xv

Acknowledgements xvii

About the book xviii

1 Nursing practice: an introduction 1

SECTION 1
Care of patients with common disorders

2 The cardiovascular system 9

3 The respiratory system 59

4 The gastrointestinal system, liver and biliary tract 87

5 Endocrine and metabolic disorders 133

6 Genetic disorders 187

7 The reproductive systems and the breast 211

8 The urinary system 291

9 The nervous system 325

10 The musculoskeletal system 369

11 Blood disorders 405

12 Skin disorders 443

13 Disorders of the eye 467

14 Disorders of ear, nose and throat 497

15 Disorders of the mouth 521

16 The immune system and infectious disease 543

SECTION 2
Common patient problems and related nursing care

17 Stress 575

18 Shock 597

19 Pain 615

20 Fluid and electrolyte balance 637

21 Nutrition 657

22 Temperature control 679

23 Wound healing 697

24 Continence 723

25 Sleep 743

26 Communication 757

SECTION 3
Nursing patients with special needs

27 The patient facing surgery 775

28 The patient who experiences trauma 809

29 The critically ill patient 827

30 The unconscious patient 839

31 The patient with burns 859

32 The patient with cancer 875

33 The chronically ill person 905

34 The terminally ill patient 921

35 The patient in need of rehabilitation 943

36 The older person 959

Cont'd

37 The person with dependency problems 973

38 The person with HIV/AIDS 991

Answers 1011

Appendices 1015

Appendix 1: Tests and investigations 1017

Appendix 2: Normal values 1023

Index 1027

Contributors

Erica S. Alabaster MSc RGN RNT DipN(Lond) DANS RCNT WNBCert ITEC MIFA
Nurse Teacher (Adult Branch), South East Wales Institute of Nursing and Midwifery Education, Cardiff Campus, Cardiff
33 *The chronically ill person*

Shirley Alexander DipSocRes RGN RMN SCM RNT
Formerly, Senior Nurse–Quality Development, North Tyne Health Consortium, Newcastle Upon Tyne
7 *The reproductive systems and the breast*
(Part 1 The reproductive systems)

Douglas Allan DipEd NeuroCert RGN RMN RNT
Nurse Teacher, Professional Development, Glasgow College of Nursing and Midwifery, Glasgow
9 *The nervous system*

Pat M. Ashworth MSc RGN RN FRCN
Formerly, Senior Lecturer in Nursing, University of Ulster, Northern Ireland
Editor-in-chief, Intensive and Critical Care Nursing
29 *The critically ill patient*

John Atkinson BA RGN NDNCert DipEd DNT
Scottish Office Home and Health Department Nursing Research Fellow
Honorary Lecturer, Department of Nursing and Community Health, Glasgow Caledonian University, Glasgow
38 *The person with HIV/AIDS*

Sue Bale BA RGN NDN RHV DipN
Director of Nursing Research, Wound Healing Research Unit, Department of Surgery, University of Wales College of Medicine, Cardiff
23 *Wound healing*

Teresa Barr BA SRN ONC RCNT RNT
Senior Tutor, Professional Development, Eastern Area College of Nursing Northside, Belfast, Northern Ireland
28 *The patient who experiences trauma*

Kathryn Carver MN BSc RGN NDN
Sister, Cardiothoracic Surgical Service Delivery Unit, John Radcliffe Hospital, Oxford
2 *The cardiovascular system*

Charmaine Childs BNurs MPhil PhD
Medical Research Council Trauma Group, North Western Injury Research Centre, Manchester Honorary Research Fellow, Department of Child Health, University of Manchester, Manchester
22 *Temperature control*

S. José Closs BSc(Hons) MPhil PhD RGN
Audit Coordinator, Directorate of Orthopaedic Surgery, Royal Infirmary of Edinburgh NHS Trust, Edinburgh
25 *Sleep*

David B. Cooper RMN FETC
Freelance author/lecturer and advisor on substance misuse and mental health issues
Member of the Executive Committee, Suffolk Council on Addiction, Suffolk
Chair, Alcohol Concern Workers Forum — East Anglia Region, East Anglia
37 *The person with dependency problems*

Elizabeth Craig RGN
Senior Staff Nurse, Queen Elizabeth National Spinal Injuries Unit, Southern General Hospital NHS Trust, Glasgow
9 *The nervous system*

Aileen E. Crosbie RGN HVD OHNC
Clinical Nurse Specialist, Department of Genetics, Western General Hospital NHS Trust, Edinburgh
6 *Genetic disorders*

Catherine A. Crosby BSc MSc RGN
Home Care Nurse, Prince George, British Columbia, Canada
32 *The patient with cancer*

Margaret Cutler BSc PhD CBiol FIBiol
Research Fellow and Professor, Department of Biological Sciences, Glasgow Caledonian University, Glasgow
17 *Section on 'Physiological responses to stress'*

Frances M. Davidson RSCN RGN RCNT RNT
Nurse Teacher, Lothian College of Health Studies, Livingston Site, St John's Hospital, Livingston
31 *The patient with burns*

Claire Dibbs RGN
Senior Nurse, Pfizer Clinical Research Unit, Canterbury, Kent
5 Part 1 Endocrine and metabolic disorders

Christine Docherty RGN RSCN
Senior Charge Nurse, Dermatology Unit, Ninewells Hospital, Dundee Teaching Hospitals NHS Trust, Dundee
12 *Skin disorders*

Fiona M. Duke BSc DipEd RGN RMN RNT
Nurse Teacher, Lothian College of Health Studies, Livingston Site, St John's Hospital, Livingston
11 *Blood disorders*

Cynthia B. Edmond MSc GradDipEd BA RN RNT RM(Aust.) CertAdmin(Aust.) FRCNA MCNNSW
Freelance Lecturer and Clinical Nurse, Edinburgh
Formerly Lecturer, Dept of Health Occupations, University of Newcastle, New South Wales, Australia
3 The respiratory system

E. S. Farmer PhD RGN SCM DN
Reader in Nursing and Director, Scottish Highlands Centre for Human Caring, Highland and Western Isles College of Nursing and Midwifery, Raigmore Hospital NHS Trust.
Inverness International Associate, Center for Human Caring, University of Colorado, USA
36 The older person

Ruth Gardner RGN OND SSStJ
Ophthalmic Resource Sister, West Lothian NHS Trust, Livingston
13 Disorders of the eye

Mary Gobbi MA(Ed) RGN DipNurs DipNursEd
Nurse Teacher, Southampton University College of Nursing and Midwifery, Southampton
20 Fluid and electrolyte balance
21 Nutrition

Margaret Harris MSc RGN DipN(Lond) DipSS CertEd RNT RCNT
Nurse Teacher, Continuing Education, University of Wales College of Medicine, South East Wales Institute of Nursing and Midwifery Education, Cardiff
35 The patient in need of rehabilitation

Eleanor Hayes BSc RGN SCM
Directorate Manager, Theatres, Anaesthetics and Intensive Care, The Royal Group of Hospitals and Dental Hospital HSS Trust, Belfast, Northern Ireland
18 Shock

Evelyn Howie RGN SCM
Ward Sister, Royal Infirmary of Edinburgh NHS Trust, Edinburgh
4 The gastrointestinal system, liver and biliary tract

Liz Jamieson BSc(Hons) RN ONC RNT
Clinical Lecturer, Department of Nursing and Community Health, Glasgow Caledonian University, Glasgow
10 The musculoskeletal system

Rosemary Kelly RGN SCM
Staff Nurse, West of Scotland Regional Plastic and Maxillofacial Surgery Unit, Glasgow Royal Infirmary University NHS Trust, Glasgow
15 Disorders of the mouth

Margaret Kindlen DipEd MPhil RGN SCM HV DN RNT
Unit Manager, Craigieknowes Nursing Home, Perth
34 The terminally ill patient

Vivian Leefarr BA(Hons) DipCouns RGN HV
Counsellor in General Practice, Inverness; Sister, Child Development Unit, Raigmore Hospital NHS Trust, Inverness
17 Stress

Anne Lowie RGN SCM HVD FPCert CPTD
Community Practice Teacher, Specialist Health Visitor in Genetics, Edinburgh
6 Genetic disorders

Carol MacKinnon BSc RGN NDN
Sister, Directorate of Cardiac Surgery, Royal Infirmary of Edinburgh NHS Trust, Edinburgh
2 The cardiovascular system

Janice M. McCall BA RGN RCNT
Lecturer, Department of Nursing and Community Health, Glasgow Caledonian University, Glasgow
14 Disorders of ear, nose and throat

Catherine McFarlane RN RM ONC
Business Manager, Ophthalmology, Western Infirmary, Glasgow
10 The musculoskeletal system

Rosemary McIntyre MN(Glas) RGN DipN(Lond) NDM RNT
Research Fellow, Greater Glasgow Health Board, Department of Nursing and Community Health, Glasgow Caledonian University, Glasgow
5 Part 2 Diabetes

Moira Mennie RGN HV
Prenatal Genetic Screening Coordinator, Royal Infirmary of Edinburgh NHS Trust, Edinburgh
6 Genetic disorders

Ruth Miller RGN SCM
Ward Sister, Royal Infirmary of Edinburgh NHS Trust, Edinburgh
4 The gastrointestinal system, liver and biliary tract

Maureen Morrison RGN DPSN
Ward Sister, Urology, Freeman Group of Hospitals NHS Trust, Newcastle Upon Tyne
8 The urinary system

Mary Murchie RGN SCM
Staff Nurse, Western General Hospital NHS Trust, Edinburgh
4 The gastrointestinal system, liver and biliary tract

Anne E. Murdoch RGN DipN(Lond)
Nurse/Business Manager, Neurosciences Directorate, Royal Hospitals Trust, Belfast, Northern Ireland
30 The unconscious patient

Joanna Parker BNurs RGN HVCert NDN ENB237 ENB998
Formerly Clinical Nurse Specialist, Breast Care, Royal Marsden Hospital, London
7 Part 1 The reproductive systems

Sheila E. Rodgers MSc BSc(Hons) RGN
Lecturer, Department of Nursing Studies, University of Edinburgh, Edinburgh
27 The patient facing surgery

Carmen Rose RGN DPSN
Part-time Staff Nurse, Raigmore Hospital NHS Trust, Inverness; Activities Coordinator, Cheshire House, Inverness
12 Skin disorders

Kate Seers BSc PhD RGN
Senior Research Fellow, National Institute for Nursing, John Radcliffe/Churchill NHS Trust, Oxford
19 Pain

The late **Anne Shackleton**
Formerly Sister, Gartnavel General Hospital, Glasgow
14 Disorders of ear, nose and throat

Theyaga Shandran BEd(Hons) RN RHV RNT
Nurse Teacher, Newcastle and Northumbria College of Health Studies, Newcastle Upon Tyne
8 The urinary system

Frances Smithers BSc(Hons) MBA RGN
Transplant Coordinator, Scottish Liver Transplantation Unit, Royal Infirmary of Edinburgh NHS Trust, Edinburgh
8 The urinary system

Marion C. Stewart BA MSc RGN SCM
Nursing Officer, Control of Infection, Highland Health Board, Raigmore Hospital NHS Trust, Inverness
16 The immune system and infectious disease

Margaret A. Studley CertEd RGN OND RM RCNT NT
Nurse Teacher, Continuing Education Department, Lothian College of Nursing and Midwifery, Edinburgh
13 Disorders of the eye

Jean Swaffield BSc(Hons) MSc RGN RSCN DN DNT FETC PWT
Senior Lecturer, Department of Nursing Studies, University of Glasgow, Glasgow
24 Continence

Colin Torrance BSc(Hons) PhD RSCN RGN DipLifeSci(Nurs)
Lecturer in Nursing, Mid and West Wales College of Nursing and Midwifery, University College of Swansea, Swansea
20 Fluid and electrolyte balance
21 Nutrition

Roger Watson BSc PhD RGN CBiol MIBiol
Lecturer, Department of Nursing Studies, University of Edinburgh, Edinburgh
4 Section on 'Anatomy and physiology'

Patricia Webb RGN RNT DipSocRes
Lecturer in Palliative Care, Trinity Hospice, London
26 Communication

Theme advisors

The *Theme Advisors* listed below commented on the chapters at draft stage, making suggestions from the perspective of their particular subject or 'theme': the behavioural sciences, community, health promotion or the life sciences. Their excellent work has been instrumental in achieving a consistent approach to these four major themes throughout the book.

BEHAVIOURAL SCIENCES

Beth Alder PhD CPsychol
Lecturer, Department of Management and Social Sciences, Queen Margaret College, Edinburgh

COMMUNITY

Sarah Andrews MSc RN DN CPT PGCEA
Nurse Consultant and Partner, Nursing First, Canterbury, UK; formerly Director, the Queen's Nursing Institute, London

Kathleen M, Munro BA MEd RGN SCM DN PWT RNT DNT
Senior Lecturer Curriculum Development, Course Manager, Queen Margaret College, Edinburgh

HEALTH PROMOTION

Julia Clemenson BA RGN HV HVT
Formerly Nursing Adviser, Health Education Board for Scotland, Edinburgh

Helen Mackinnon BSc MSc RGN RMN RNT
Professional Officer (Nursing), National Board for Nursing, Midwifery and Health Visiting for Scotland, Edinburgh

LIFE SCIENCES

Allan MacDonald BSc PhD
Reader, Department of Biological Sciences, Glasgow Caledonian University, Glasgow

David Scott BSc(Pharm) MSc PhD MRPharms, MIBiol, CBiol
Lecturer, Department of Biological Sciences, Glasgow Caledonian University, Glasgow

I. C. Wilkie BSc PhD
Senior Lecturer in Physiology, Department of Biological Sciences, Glasgow Caledonian University, Glasgow

Clinical advisors

The *Clinical Advisors* listed below provided advice, at draft stage, on the chapters cited after their names. Their comments and suggestions, based on their clinical expertise and knowledge, have been invaluable in providing additional depth and balance to each chapter.

David A. Alexander MA(Hons) PhD CPsychol FBPS
Senior Lecturer, Medical School, University of Aberdeen, Aberdeen; Honorary Consultant, Grampian Health Board, Aberdeen
17 *Stress*

Annie T. Altschul BA MSc RGN RMN RNT CBE FRCN
Emeritus Professor of Nursing Studies, University of Edinburgh Edinburgh
36 *The older person*

Pat Ashworth MSc RGN RM FRCN
Editor-in-Chief, Intensive and Critical Care Nursing
18 *Shock*
29 *The critically ill patient*

Chris Bulman BSc(Hons) MSc RGN PGCEA
Lecturer-Practitioner, John Radcliffe Churchill NHS Trust, Oxford, and Oxford Brookes University, Oxford
27 *The patient facing surgery*

John W. Burden BSc RGN ONC RNT
Nurse Tutor, Royal National Orthopaedic Hospital NHS Trust, Stanmore
10 *The musculoskeletal system*

E. Cameron RGN SCM DN
Diabetes Nurse Specialist, Diabetes Clinic, Glasgow Royal Infirmary NHS Trust, Glasgow
5 *Endocrine and metabolic disorders*

Elizabeth Chapman RGN
Charge Nurse, Ear, Nose and Throat Unit, Royal Infirmary of Edinburgh NHS Trust, Edinburgh
14 *Disorders of ear, nose and throat*

Doreen Couper RGN ONC
H-Grade Sister in Charge, Regional Burns Unit, Glasgow Royal Infirmary University NHS Trust, Glasgow
31 *The patient with burns*

Sally M. Davis MSc CertEd
Senior Nurse/Lecturer Practitioner, Rivermead Rehabilitation Centre, Oxford
35 *The patient in need of rehabilitation*

Sylvia E. Denton MSc RGN RHC OncCert FRCN
Senior Clinical Nurse Specialist Breast Care, Medway NHS Trust, London
7 *The reproductive systems and the breast*

Linda Downey BSc(Hons) MSc RGN NT
Tutor, Lothian College of Health Studies, Edinburgh
11 *Blood disorders*
32 *The patient with cancer*

Patricia Fathers MSc RGN OND(Hons) RM DipCNE(Edin) CertEd RNT
Nurse Teacher, Continuing Education Department, North London College of Health Studies, London
13 *Disorders of the eye*

Jean Faugier MSc RMN RNT RCNT DANS DipN DipPsych
Senior Lecturer, School of Nursing Studies, University of Manchester, Manchester
37 *The patient with dependency problems*

Patricia M. Finlay BDS FDS RCPS(Glasg)
Associate Specialist in Oral and Maxillofacial Surgery, Glasgow Royal Infirmary University NHS Trust, Glasgow; Honorary Clinical Lecturer to University of Glasgow, Glasgow
15 *Disorders of the mouth*

Madeleine Flanagan BSc(Hons) RGN DipN(Lond) ONC CertEd
Senior Lecturer, Division of Post-Registration Nursing, School of Health and Human Science, University of Hertfordshire, Hatfield
23 *Wound Healing*

Dr Morva Fordham BSc MSc PhD SRN SCM RNT
Formerly Lecturer in Nursing Studies, King's College London, University of London, London
19 *Pain*

Joan Foulkes RGN OND DipN
Research Associate, Psychology Department, University of St Andrews, St Andrews
2 *The cardiovascular system*

Annabel Froud RGN
Research Sister to Professor G M Besser, Endocrine Unit, Royal Hospitals NHS Trust, London
5 *Endocrine and metabolic disorders*

Penny Guilbert RGN DipN FETC
Senior Nurse, Clinical Genetics Service, Nottingham City Hospital, Nottingham
6 *Genetic disorders*

Mary Harkin RGN RCNT Accident & Emergency Certificate
Nurse Teacher, Nurse Education Centre, Musson House, General Hospital, Birmingham
28 The patient who experiences trauma

Phyllis Holt RGN DipN
Senior Nurse, Neurosciences, Bethlem and Maudsley NHS Trust, London
30 The unconscious patient

Christine Howden MA RGN HV
Development Officer (Stress and Relaxation), Centre for Teaching, Learning and Assessment, University of Edinburgh, Edinburgh
26 Communication

Dr T J Iveson BSc MBBS MRCP
Senior Registrar, Department of Medicine, Royal Marsden Hospital, Sutton
7 The reproductive systems and the breast

Muriel Jeffcott RGN RM
Clinical Nurse Specialist, West Midlands Regional Burns Unit, Birmingham General Hospital, Birmingham
31 The patient with burns

Enid Lewis BA SRN SCM HVCert DNCert
Finance Department, Lansdowne Hospital, Sanitorium Road, Canton, Cardiff
33 The chronically ill patient

Jean Lugton MA(Hons) MSc SRN RNT HV
Macmillan Research Associate, Department of Nursing Studies, University of Edinburgh, Edinburgh
34 The terminally ill patient

A. E. Major RGN
Nursing Officer, Neurosciences Unit; Practice Development Nurse, Surgery, Royal Hull Hospitals NHS Trust,
9 The nervous system

Anne McQueen BA MSc RGN SCM RCNT NT
Lecturer, Department of Nursing Studies, University of Edinburgh, Edinburgh
7 The reproductive systems and the breast

Kevin Morgan BSc PhD
Lecturer in Gerontology, University of Nottingham Medical School, Nottingham
25 Sleep

K. R. Paterson MB ChB FRCP
Consultant Physician – Diabetes, Diabetes Clinic, Glasgow Royal Infirmary NHS Trust, Glasgow
5 Endocrine and metabolic disorders

Norma Reed RGN CMB(Part 1)
Formerly Senior Sister, Ear Nose and Throat/Maxillofacial Theatre, Royal Infirmary of Edinburgh NHS Trust
14 Disorders of ear, nose and throat

J. A. Shepherd RGN SCM
Diabetes Nurse Specialist, Diabetes Clinic, Glasgow Royal Infirmary NHS Trust, Glasgow
5 Endocrine and metabolic disorders

Wendy Sneider SRD
Specialist Diabetes Dietitian, Diabetes Clinic, Glasgow Royal Infirmary NHS Trust, Glasgow
5 Endocrine and metabolic disorders

Diana Stewart SRM SCM HVCert DNCert FPCert
Formerly Area Continence Advisor, Argyll and Clyde Health Board, Paisley
24 Continence

Lynda Taylor RGN RM
Head of Nursing Unit, Central Public Health Laboratory, Laboratory of Hospital Infection, London
16 The immune system and infectious disease

David R. Thompson PhD RN FRCN
Clinical Reader, National Institute for Nursing, John Radcliffe/Churchill NHS Trust, Oxford
2 The cardiovascular system

Ann Townsend RGN DipN DipSocSci(Lond)
Senior Sister, Coronary Care Unit, Freeman Group of Hospitals NHS Trust, Newcastle; Co-chairperson, Nurse's Working Party, The Congress of the European Society of Cardiology, President, Association of British Cardiac Nurses
2 The cardiovascular system

Roger Watson BSc PhD RGN CBiol MIBiol
Lecturer, Department of Nursing Studies, University of Edinburgh, Edinburgh
20 Fluid and electrolyte balance
21 Nutrition
22 Temperature control

Rosemary A. Webster BSc RN
Clinical Nurse Specialist, Coronary Care Unit, Leicester General Hospital NHS Trust, Leicester
2 The cardiovascular system

Margaret M. White RGN SCM INCCDip
Services Manager, Directorate of Accident and Emergency Medicine, Royal Infirmary of Edinburgh NHS Trust, Edinburgh
28 The patient who experiences trauma

Janet Whiteway MA MCh(Oxon) FRCS(Eng)
Consultant Urological Surgeon, South Tees Acute NHS Trust, Middlesborough
8 The urinary system

Foreword

It has been said that nursing is as old as time since there always has been, and always will be, a need for the provision of care for those in need. However, the manner in which that care is offered and, to some extent, the nature of what is seen as care has shifted over the years. The advent of technology in health care throughout the twentieth century undoubtedly clouded the caring contribution. Fortunately, the humanistic value of people is slowly being recognised again, accompanied by an understanding that the diagnosis and treatment of disease is only one part of health care and that other services can be therapeutic in their own right.

Thus the 1990s are exciting times in the history of nursing. Opportunities abound for developing the way in which we offer a service to patients, and there is a growing acknowledgement that nursing itself is therapeutic and has a critical part to play in the healing process.

This new textbook, *Nursing Practice: Hospital and Home,* reflects the values, knowledge and actions which underpin modern nursing. Throughout the book, emphasis has been placed on the role of nursing in the healing process. The need to value knowledge from other disciplines has not been underestimated, but neither has it been allowed to become dominant in a text which is aimed primarily at exploring the discipline of nursing.

Changing patterns

A related aim of this text is to provide a forum for exploring new approaches to nursing. This is particularly vital now, when many of the traditional ways in which nursing work has been organised are being challenged, as is the way in which nursing is learned. In the past the emphasis was on distancing nurses from their patients: the watchwords were to remain objective and uninvolved. Now we understand that a vital part of nursing is sharing with those to whom we offer a service. Reciprocity — an acknowledgement that, while we may help patients learn about their health, they will help us learn about the human condition — is all part of the process.

The importance of the patient — his or her feelings, attitudes and beliefs — is given a welcome prominence in *Nursing Practice*. This emphasis on the 'lived experience' of the patient, brought out by means of vignettes or stories, is still fairly rare in nursing textbooks.

Nursing's interest in and appreciation for the patient's viewpoint raises issues about the knowledge base of our clinical judgements. As nurses we draw on knowledge from a wide range of other disciplines, as do all other professions concerned with service delivery. What makes the knowledge special to nursing is the unique way in which it is combined in response to the needs of patients and clients. Thus like doctors we need an understanding of the physiology of human behaviour, but our purpose in gaining this knowledge is different. For doctors it relates to the responsibility they have to diagnose and treat disease, whereas in nursing the need is to understand how disease may affect a person's ability to live independently in order to help that person to regain as much autonomy and freedom in life as is possible. In the same way a study of sociology may lead someone to a career in the formation of social policy, but for nurses it helps them to gain insight into the prevailing factors in society which may impact on an individual's ability to regain health.

The need to value knowledge from other disciplines is acknowledged throughout this new book. Section 1 uses a systems framework to introduce readers to common disorders which adult patients may face. What is, however, important is the blend of knowledge drawn from a range of different sources in order to ensure that both the disorder and the context of the disorder are clear. Thus the critical distinction between disease — the medical condition — and illness — the patient's experience — is clearly drawn (see Chapter 1). The book underscores the fact that, for nurses, the knowledge base must go well beyond an understanding of disease processes in isolation to a much wider picture of the context in which ill health may occur. There are no blueprints of the 'how' of nursing, but principles to be learned and options identified.

Being with patients

Nurses also have a special function which differs from most other health care workers in actually staying alongside people at times in their lives when they need help to manage their own health. A sound knowledge of the problems which patients face as part of many disease processes is critical in order to be able to find ways of helping them to respond to such circumstances in a meaningful way. For example, pain will manifest itself in a myriad of different ways which may be based on the past experience, cultural norms, physiological response or social expectations of any one person, and this may only be apparent to someone who journeys alongside that patient. Managing pain calls on critical nursing assessment skills as well as a breadth of interventions from which an individual package can be developed for each patient. Some will lean on analgesics for help while others may choose to consider other approaches to pain management. Yet without a knowledge of the options a nurse cannot offer choice. Section 2 of *Nursing Practice* is devoted to many of these key nursing issues, including pain, stress, continence and wound healing, to name a few.

Similar to the patient problems mentioned above, there are some situations which, by their complexity, require special attention since the skills to nurse well are so wide-ranging. It would be easy to forget, when working with patients with cancer during an acute phase, that they have to live with cancer, almost as a chronic disease, for the rest of their lives and that the fear of recurrence is very real. Similarly, chronic illness brings with it a whole set of new values since recovery, said to be the goal of many health care workers, is not possible. Responding thoughtfully to the needs of people who have to face these sorts of demands can have a significant impact on the quality of their lives. The special demands of nursing patients with special needs, such as the cancer patient or the patient with burns, are covered fully in Section 3 of this book.

Gaining knowledge

The breadth and depth of knowledge which students need to work in the diverse situations — both in hospital and in the community — which confront today's nurse are covered fully in this text. In nursing there is always opportunity to find creative ways of responding to patient need. Drawing on a range of knowledge-based options in order to bring choice into people's lives is central to nursing. This text will act as a fundamental source book to help learn these skills.

London,
1994

Barbara Vaughan

Preface

The main purpose of this book is to explore ways of knowing about nursing. It has been written during a time of fundamental change in health care. As Editors, we had certain goals:

- to reflect the changing and dynamic nature of nursing
- to move thinking away from outdated images and stereotypes and to encourage constructive reflection on practice
- to refocus the nursing perspective to encompass both hospital *and* home
- to stress the importance of the individual 'lived experience' of health and illness
- to put research firmly on the nursing agenda.

The book is the fruit of more than four years' work; the process of creating it began with a series of meetings where colleagues from nursing and other disciplines examined the changes that were occurring in nursing and debated the kinds of textbooks that would be needed in future. From these early discussions, the character, ethos and organisation of the book emerged.

The structure of the book

The book is divided into three sections, which are progressive in nature, encouraging the student to move from the broad approach of Section 1 to a more in-depth appreciation of specific nursing issues in Sections 2 and 3. There is sufficient cross-referencing to encourage students to make links and pursue lines of enquiry.

Section 1 Care of patients with common disorders

The decision to adopt the systems approach for this section was not taken lightly, given that nursing is moving away from the medical model. Our reasoning was that nurses must come to terms with medical terminology and classifications and have a thorough grounding in disease pathology in order to work effectively in the health care team and give sensitive and appropriate nursing care.

All the chapters in this section contain information on the following:

- anatomy and physiology
- pathophysiology
- medical management
- nursing priorities and management.

Only essential anatomy and physiology have been presented, as an aid to rational decision-making. There are recommendations for further reading where more detail is desired. We have been selective about the disorders chosen, concentrating on those that illustrate common presenting features and related principles of care. The nursing priorities and management section is the most important. The wording of the heading reminds the student of the need to set priorities depending on the individual's unique needs and circumstances.

Section 2 Common patient problems and related nursing care

This section presents another way of examining nursing and builds on the foundations laid in Section 1. The focus is on common patient problems, which are not merely physiological in origin but also arise from the subtle, complex interplay of social, psychological and economic factors. Some of these problems have a high profile, such as stress and pain. Others, such as nutrition and sleep, are often relatively neglected but are nevertheless very much the concern of nurses. These problems are not confined to, or only evident in, hospital care. They are part of life and may be experienced in many settings and at any time. Throughout the section, both the nurse's and the patient's perspectives have been considered and the focus is on research-based problem-solving.

Secton 3 Nursing patients with special needs

Some of the most challenging areas of nursing are explored in this section. By addressing special needs, the broad spectrum and contrasts of adult nursing are revealed. Such needs, some long term in nature, often make the greatest demands on the nurse's clinical and interpersonal skills. Section 3 challenges stereotypes and examines values and beliefs, raising awareness of the moral decision-making which underlies so much of day-to-day nursing practice.

Key features

In harmony with our commitment to exploring the different ways of knowing about nursing, certain features have been introduced throughout the book. These include interactive material; illustrations, tables and care plans, the latter written in such a way as to be useful both as an educational and as a practice tool; boxes, which include, for example, accounts of personal 'lived experience' and research abstracts; references, further reading and useful addresses.

The contributors and advisors

More than 70 nursing authors have contributed to this text. They are from all areas of nursing: hospital and community practice, education and research. We pay tribute here to their knowledge and skills and thank them for their cooperation in helping us to compile this text: the most comprehensive book yet published which is based solely on *British* nursing practice.

We owe a sincere debt of gratitude to the team of advisors who read and commented on the manuscript during its development. The **clinical advisors** were approached for their expertise in a particular field. The **theme advisors** looked at the chapters from the perspective of community, health promotion and the behavioural and physical sciences, to ensure that these themes or 'threads' were dealt with as evenly as possible throughout the text. We also received extensive advice from other colleagues, who are listed in the Acknowledgements section.

We would also like to acknowledge the valuable assistance of our Associate Editor, Mrs Cynthia Edmond, who joined the team at a crucial stage in the book's development and helped us to complete the editorial work; a daunting task, inevitably, given the size and complexity of the book.

Whether you read this book as a novice nurse, an expert practitioner, a preceptor or a teacher, it will provide a wealth of knowledge, derived from many sources: from professional nursing practice, from research and from the experiences of countless patients and clients. As Editors, we will have succeeded in our task if this book:

- encourages debate on innovations and developments in practice
- articulates the interplay between health promotion and the nursing care of those who are ill
- makes explicit the reality that people's experience of nursing is not only what takes place in the hospital ward
- emphasises and interprets nursing in the community setting
- allows the patient's voice, always anonymously, to be heard and valued.

While it is acknowledged that no single text can encompass the wealth of knowledge that underpins the practice of nursing, we believe that this text will be valuable not only for the Project 2000 student nurse but also for the established practitioner, the nurse returning to practice, and nurse educators, all of whom face the challenge of new knowledge.

Edinburgh,
1994

Margaret Alexander
Josephine (Tonks) Fawcett
Phyllis Runciman

Acknowledgements

The editors would like to extend particular thanks to the advisors listed here, who gave assistance with specific chapters:

David R. Thompson PhD RN FRCN
Clinical Reader, National Institute for Nursing, John Radcliffe/Churchill NHS Trust, Oxford
2 *The cardiovascular system*

Rosemary A. Webster BSc RN
Clinical Nurse Specialist, Coronary Care Unit, Leicester General Hospital NHS Trust, Leicester
2 *The cardiovascular system*

Jean Lowe BA RGN RNT CertEd DEM DN(Lond)
Formerly Education Officer, English National Board for Nursing, Midwifery and Health Visiting, York
4 *The gastrointestinal system, liver and biliary tract*
5 *Endocrine and metabolic disorders*

Cynthia B. Edmond MSc GradDipEd BA RN RNT RM(Aust) CertAdmin(Aust) FRCNA MCNNSW
Freelance lecturer and clinical nurse, Edinburgh; formerly Lecturer, Department of Health Occupations, University of Newcastle, New South Wales, Australia
6 *Genetic disorders*
10 *The musculoskeletal system*
13 *Disorders of the eye*

The editors would also like to thank all who provided vignettes, and all who kindly granted permission to borrow material such as illustrations and tables from existing publications, with particular thanks to **Kathleen J. W. Wilson** for the many illustrations taken from Wilson K J W 1990 Ross & Wilson: Anatomy and physiology in health and illness, 7th edn. Churchill Livingstone, Edinburgh

About the book

Readers will find it helpful to understand how information has been presented in this text:

MAIN TEXT

This has been broken up as follows:

- Colour headings—used to identify main headings and to highlight the 'Nursing Priorities and Management' sections in Section 1
- different style of type—used to present background information on 'Pathophysiology and Medical Management' in Section 1
- bullet-point lists
- Reference and Further Reading lists—at end of all chapters
- Glossary and Useful Address lists—at end of selected chapters.

DISPLAYED MATERIAL

This refers to information set off from the main text and includes:

- Boxes
- Tables
- Case Histories
- Nursing Care Plans
- Research Abstracts
- Self-assessment Questions, identified by the icon 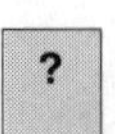 .

  Those with answers are indicated by the letter '**A**'.

- Further Reading suggestions (identified by the icon 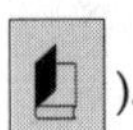).

APPENDICES

These are included at the end of the book but are referred to throughout the text:

- Tests and Investigations
- Normal Values.

FINDING INFORMATION QUICKLY

There are many features that help the reader locate topics easily:

- comprehensive index—at end of book
- section title at the top of each left-hand page
- chapter title at the top of each right-hand page
- section title pages—list the chapters in the section and give page numbers
- chapter title pages—list the main headings and give page numbers.

Readers are also referred to the **Key Features** shown on the inside front cover.

CHAPTER 1

Nursing practice: an introduction

Margaret F. Alexander Josephine N. Fawcett Phyllis J. Runciman

CHAPTER CONTENTS

The context of nursing 1

Where and how nursing is carried out 2
Where: hospital and home 2
The shift to the community 2
Government initiatives 2
How: disease and illness 2

The nurse–patient relationship 3
The image of 'the patient' 3
The nurse–patient partnership 3
The health needs of patients 3

Where and how nurses are educated 3
Where: hospital and community 3
How: the spirit of enquiry 4
How: learning through reflection 4

The aim of this book 4

References 6

Unless we are making progress in our nursing every year, every month, every week, take my word for it we are going back. (Florence Nightingale in 1914, cited in Skeet 1980, p. 100)

This book is about making progress in our profession of nursing. It is about developing ways of thinking, learning and exploring critically and creatively the nurse's role in helping individuals to maintain good health, to recover from episodes of ill-health, or to cope day by day with chronic illness. This book is also about developing greater flexibility and effectiveness in delivering nursing care in a range of 'clinical' and 'community' settings, and about responding to an evolving understanding of what 'care in the community' means.

Equally importantly, this book strives to present ill-health as a lived experience that must be understood from the patient's perspective in order for nursing care to be responsive to the concerns and priorities unique to every patient. It is about developing skills in listening and communicating that enable nurses in their interventions to acknowledge the totality of 'the person', not merely the disease of 'the patient'. It is about finding ways to provide genuinely patient-centred care.

Our overall aim as Editors has been to help the reader gain an understanding that, in all our care-giving, the whole is much more than the sum of its parts. The individual tasks we perform must be framed within a considered philosophy of care and a sensitive understanding of the patient's needs as discovered through ongoing assessment and evaluation. The wholeness of our care-giving reflects the wholeness of the patient, and expresses our partnership with the patient as we endeavour to work towards a shared goal.

To speak of the wholeness of nursing intervention is not to minimise the importance of individual aspects of care. *Every* nursing action is vital to achieving excellence in care. The poet William Blake (1757–1827) wrote that 'art and science cannot exist but in minutely organised particulars'. This book strives to illuminate many of the particulars of nursing, but in the context of the whole. It responds to the challenges of the 1990s and beyond, and the need to find a meeting-point between our professional skills and expertise and the patient's lived experience.

THE CONTEXT OF NURSING

The focus of this book is on health care in the United Kingdom. The context in which nursing takes place — the society which it serves, its values and mores — is constantly changing. Like all professions, nursing must be pro-active in bringing about, influencing, and indeed *recognising* change, since it is only by understanding and reacting creatively and intelligently to change that a profession can remain dynamic and healthy. Because of the close contact of nurses with the population, on a one-to-one basis, it can be argued that nursing must be at the forefront of change.

The need for this book arose from a number of important developments in the context of health care. These include:

- population shifts, as more and more people live to a greater age
- a growing interest in promoting and maintaining health as well as treating disease
- increasing demands from patients/clients for much greater involvement in their own health care
- a trend toward shorter hospital stays and a greater emphasis on community care
- a growing recognition of the benefits and challenges of 'home' therapy.

These developments have had a significant impact on nursing especially with regard to:

1. Where and how nursing is carried out
2. The nurse — patient relationship
3. Where and how nurses are educated.

In this chapter we will examine these three areas, since we believe that it is only by understanding the context in which nursing takes place that students can begin to appreciate the profession which they are preparing to enter. We will conclude with a brief description of the overall aims of this text. Further detail about the book's structure and features can be found in the Preface. We would urge all students and teachers to read this short chapter and the Preface before proceeding to the rest of the book.

WHERE AND HOW NURSING IS CARRIED OUT

Where: hospital and home

At present, the majority of nurses in the UK work primarily in hospital. A clear division exists between hospital and community and most of our literature and conversations about nursing refer to nurses at work 'in hospital' or 'in the community'. Our educational programmes, until the advent of Project 2000 (UKCC 1986), prepared nurses for work in one setting or the other — rarely for both.

This has now begun to change. The demarcation between hospital and community interventions is beginning to blur, and in the UK all students coming into the profession are being prepared, to some extent, to work in both settings. However our understanding of what constitutes good 'community care' is still evolving. It must be appreciated that defining the work of nurses outside the hospital involves more than finding out about the range of primary health care, social, voluntary and independent sector services that are available, and more than identifying the range of liaison and referral patterns between hospital and community. Rather, it requires us to think in new ways about the word 'community' and about the lives of people as they come into and move within the nursing and health care system. It leads us to think of the hospital as not only a 'community' in its own right — a place in which a complex set of human interrelationships and support systems operate but also an integral part of a wider community.

The shift to the community

Why is this change in the point of delivery of nursing care taking place? One major factor is early discharge. Patients are now staying in hospital for shorter and shorter periods for a number of reasons, both practical and ideological. A trend toward the use of minimally invasive techniques and new advances in treatment have shortened recovery times for many patients. New technologies have made it easier for nurses to deliver care in the home, or indeed, for patients to manage their own care with a minimum of support. And there is an increasing adherence to the belief that, wherever possible, people should be cared for in their own homes, where they can retain maximum independence and be close to their loved ones.

Therefore for most people a hospital stay may be a very brief life episode, and the 'average' person is now much more likely to draw upon health care services in the community than in a hospital setting. For others, perhaps those with chronic conditions, periodic visits to hospital will become a regular, almost routine part of life, and for a few individuals hospital itself may become home. This relaxation of the boundary between 'hospital' and 'home' has made it essential for nurses to be able to use their skills and knowledge in a range of settings.

Government initiatives

In the UK many of the major changes in community health care delivery have been the result of new governmental initiatives and legislation, such as the Community Care Act (Department of Health 1990b). One of the Government's main aims has been to break down the divisions between professional groups. Nurses in hospital and community are therefore having to find new ways of working *in partnership* with their colleagues in the National Health Service, in social services departments and in the independent sector.

Those entering nursing today will need to consider how new criteria for care, derived largely from the White Paper *Caring for People* (Department of Health 1990a), are being met in their own work settings:

- Are the right services being developed to help people to live in their own homes wherever possible and sensible?
- Is high priority being given to providing practical support for carers?
- Is there proper assessment of need and good case management?
- Are the different sectors clear about their responsibilities and is there good coordination of services?
- Is the goal of achieving better value for money in providing care being met?

As new patterns of community care develop, it will be important for nurses to listen carefully to what patients and their families have to say about the quality of care they receive (Nursing Standard 1993).

How: disease and illness

In recent years there has been an important shift in nursing practice away from the 'medical' model of care — that is, one which lays emphasis on disease — in favour of an emphasis on the *experiential* aspects of ill-health. A useful distinction can be drawn between 'illness' and 'disease'. An 'illness' is what the patient experiences; a 'disease' is a description of pathological abnormality, made from the clinician's point of view: 'Illnesses are experiences of changes in one's state of being and social function; diseases are abnormalities in the structure and function of the body organs and systems' (Eisenberg 1977). The concept of 'illness' therefore embraces all the experiential aspects of a disorder: what that patient *lives through*. Like health, illness (and, indeed, disease) is to some extent socially and culturally determined (Fitzpatrick 1982).

Nurses have now begun to appreciate their own unique role in understanding illness from the patient's point of view. Because of their close contact with patients, nurses are able to gain a good deal of insight into the 'lived experience' of coping with a disease. To give individualised and sensitive care, nurses must appreciate the meaning of an illness to the person who is experiencing it and to those who are close to him. Benner and Wrubel (1989, p. 9) state that: 'understanding the meaning of illness for the person and that person's life is a form of healing, in that such understanding can overcome the sense of alienation, loss of self understanding and loss of social integration that (may) accompany illness.'

In emphasising the importance of the 'lived experience', nursing acknowledges that no two individuals are alike. Although various patients may share a disorder in its general description and expected course, for each individual a unique subjective reality will accompany that disorder. This can be seen clearly in relation to the experience of pain: no one can *really* know how a person who is in pain actually feels (see Ch. 19 and Box 10.3, p. 400).

Increasingly, nurses are becoming aware that an understanding of the lived experience of being ill, gained from their own experience, from their interactions with patients, and from their reading of phenomenological research, can enhance their nursing practice. Benner and Wrubel (1989) state that the best nursing practitioners 'understand the differences and relationships among health, illness and disease' and recognise that 'every illness has a story'. Throughout this book, Case Histories provide excerpts from such 'stories', often told in the words of patients and their carers.

THE NURSE–PATIENT RELATIONSHIP

The image of 'the patient'

The shift toward 'community care' has far-reaching implications for many traditional views of health and illness and for the way in which the patient's role is conceptualised.

The image of the helpless person in a hospital bed — a passive recipient of paternalistic beneficence from the medical and nursing professions — is beginning to lose its validity. Patients are now becoming empowered within the health care system. They have high expectations of what that system can offer them, and demand a high level of professionalism and accountability from all practitioners. More than ever before, patients and their carers are recognising their own need for information about health, illness, treatment options and support systems. They are becoming more involved in decision-making regarding care, and expect to be given the opportunity to make *informed* choices. For patients with chronic disease, there is an increased emphasis on maintaining independence in the activities of daily living for as long as possible. These changes have placed new demands upon patients and their carers, requiring them to adopt a more participatory role and to take greater responsibility in matters related to health and health care. At the same time, the need for nurses to provide patient education and to promote healthy lifestyles has become particularly urgent.

The nurse–patient partnership

Ideally, the nurse–patient relationship is one of partnership. Nurses and other health care professionals are now trying to view health care as the product of the combined efforts of a multidisciplinary team working cooperatively with the patient and his carers. Recent policy statements such as The Patient's Charter (DOH 1991) support this view, and in their report 'A Vision for the Future — The Nursing, Midwifery and Health Visiting Contribution to Health and Health Care' the NHS Management Executive (1993) specifically identify partnership with the consumers of health care as an important goal of health care providers.

In both global and European contexts, the World Health Organization (1981, 1985) has stressed that individual and community empowerment is imperative if targets for 'Health for All' are to be achieved. The potentially significant contribution of nurses in supporting 'Health for All' is described by Salvage (1993). Christensen's (1993) research into nurse–patient partnership as a model for practice directs our attention to the quality of individual interactions between nurse and patient. Her keen and informed observations of nursing illuminate what she terms a 'passage' or 'shared journey' as nurse and patient, from their different perspectives, work their way together through a health-related experience.

The health needs of patients

It is no coincidence that the 'disease' model of care has been challenged at the same time as there has been a growth in the health and fitness movement in our society at large. As we have learned more about disease processes, we have begun to appreciate the extent to which some diseases can be prevented by adopting a healthy lifestyle.

Nurses, in particular those working in the community, have always been concerned to convey health messages to their patients. However, what has changed in recent years is the *extent* to which health promotion has become a part of what it means to be a nurse in any setting. From having been 'add-on extras', especially for nurses working in acute hospitals, health promotion and education have assumed a central place in all nursing activities. But what exactly is meant by health promotion?

We now know that promoting health is a complex process (Kelly 1990). On one level, it challenges personal beliefs and values; on another, it poses a threat to the future viability of major employers such as the tobacco industry. Health promotion relates to our day-to-day behaviour and lifestyle as well as to national taxation, changes in the law and government economic policy. As our understanding of health grows, some fascinating questions emerge. For example, why does disease develop in some healthy individuals and not in others? Or to put it another way, how is it possible that most people manage to be healthy in the face of so much disease! (Kelly & Charlton 1992). Health and ill-health are now seen to be influenced by a wide range of factors — economic, social, cultural, educational, psychological and genetic. Nurses, then, have two related functions in health promotion: to be aware of the broader concepts of health currently being debated and at the same time to be ready to respond in a very practical, everyday way to patients' growing desire for more information about how to stay healthy. In the future, nurses will undoubtedly be called on more and more to advise 'well' individuals about health, either on a one-to-one basis or by means of health promotion clinics and other advisory services.

The nurse–patient relationship changes when health rather than illness is on the agenda. Mutual respect is crucial: the patient must be recognised as an individual with the right to question and challenge. Nurses, by the very fact that they themselves are frequent consumers of health care services, are in touch with the patient's role. They too may utilise a wide spectrum of health care, using GP services, visiting pharmacies, health centres and outpatient clinics, consulting osteopaths, herbalists and aromatherapists. Like other members of the public, they become ill and need health care.

Students using this book should appreciate from the outset that their own personal perceptions and experiences as consumers of the health care system can be a useful source of insight for understanding the nursing role.

WHERE AND HOW NURSES ARE EDUCATED

Where: hospital and community

Nursing students in the UK today differ from the students of the past in two fundamental ways:

1. They are supernumerary to the NHS: that is, they are no longer salaried 'pairs of hands'
2. They are enrolled in colleges of nursing and midwifery which have links with, or may be part of, institutions of higher education.

These changes came about with the introduction of 'Project 2000', the UK scheme of nurse preparation so called because of the report from which it was derived, *Project 2000: A New Preparation for Practice* (UKCC 1986). In formulating their recommendations as to where and how the nurse of the future was to be educated, the authors of the Project 2000 report had to address some key questions:

- What were the nation's health needs likely to be in the foreseeable future?
- Would the population be healthier or not?
- Would there be a need for more care, less care, or qualitatively *different* care?
- How and where should such care be delivered?

The Project 2000 authors noted that the demand for health care would continue to rise, in particular for the elderly, the socially deprived, the unemployed, the mentally ill and people with disabilities. They concluded that nurses must be prepared, above all, to be responsive to change, since no one could predict with complete confidence the future health needs of the population.

As to where health care would be carried out, the authors of the report observed that most local health authorities were no longer thinking in terms of building more hospitals but were aiming to provide 'local', accessible and appropriate services to give support to people in their own homes and to find new forms of residential care as well as continuing to provide hospital services (UKCC 1986).

It is not surprising, therefore, that the authors of the Project 2000 report concluded that the student nurse of the future should not be solely hospital-based but be given a broad range of experience in a variety of settings:

> The registered practitioner will be competent to assess the need for care, to provide that care, to monitor and to evaluate care and to do all this in a range of institutional and non-institutional settings .... The practitioner of the future should be both a 'doer' and a 'knowledgeable doer' (UKCC 1986, p. 40).

One of the report's other recommendations — that all colleges of nursing and midwifery should quickly establish links with institutions of higher education — followed on from their conclusion that nurses must be 'educated', not 'trained'. The authors noted: 'the current system of preparation, so closely linked to service, isolates the majority of students and staff from broader fields of education' (UKCC 1986).

How: the spirit of enquiry

All Project 2000 programmes aim to produce well-informed and accountable practitioners able to respond and adapt to change. Project 2000 students are expected to be able to 'demonstrate an appreciation of research and use relevant literature and research as an aid to practice' (UKCC 1986, p. 41). The 'knowledgeable doer' will be someone who:

- bases day-to-day practice on the latest knowledge
- takes an enquiring approach to work
- uses libraries efficiently
- reads nursing and health care articles critically
- understands the contribution which research can make to practice.

The last point is important: today's Project 2000 programmes do not aim to create researchers, but rather nurses who seek out research findings in relation to their practice and who are educated in such a way that they are able to understand and, where appropriate, implement research findings.

How: learning through reflection

Underpinning many Project 2000 programmes are key educational principles; these include the active encouragement of students to take responsibility for their own learning, to question and reflect upon their practice and attitudes, and to seek out the latest knowledge. The skill of learning through reflection, like all other skills, develops with practice over time. Some of the most sensitive insights of experienced nurses come from careful, thoughtful analysis of daily work — its highs and its lows, its achievements and its frustrations.

To some extent nurses have always reflected on their work. Often they share day-to-day experiences in conversations as they relax and unwind. Working so closely with people in health and illness can be immensely satisfying but also profoundly distressing; telling the stories of the day to those who have had similar work experiences and who share the same code of patient confidentiality can be immensely therapeutic.

Much can be learned from the telling of nursing stories, which bring the practice of nursing alive and raise some important questions about giving and receiving nursing and health care. What is it like to live with a particular disability? What are the challenges and priorities in caring for someone with such a problem? Could situations such as these be prevented? How can an acceptable quality of life be achieved for such patients?

Throughout this text we have incorporated stories – vignettes – which illustrate richly, sometimes in people's own words, the lived experience of health and illness at home and in hospital.

It is vital to the progress of our profession not only that we learn to reflect upon our experience, but also that we find appropriate ways to share that experience with our colleagues and to pass our knowledge on to those who follow. One of the hallmarks of a 'profession' is its ability to draw together a body of knowledge and experience, a kind of accumulated wisdom in which all its members may share. Nurses must therefore learn to be communicators and educators, not only for their patients, but for one another and for future generations.

THE AIM OF THIS BOOK

The aim is to provide an authoritative, wholly British textbook of nursing practice for students pursuing the Adult Branch of the Project 2000 programme. It builds upon knowledge gained in the Common Foundation Programme (Kenworthy, Snowley & Gilling 1992), during which students will have been introduced to the study of certain disciplines which help to inform nursing. These include:

- sociology
- psychology
- physiology and anatomy
- health promotion and education
- ethics and morals.

This book attempts to show, in various ways, how these disciplines are related to nursing and help to inform good nursing practice. This is in line with one of the aims of the Project 2000 reforms: to put nursing students in touch with the wider academic community so that they can develop into thinking, questioning practitioners who are able to appreciate the findings and insights of other disciplines and apply them to nursing.

Primarily, the book will be used by students on the Adult Branch of Project 2000 programmes. However, some students may begin using it during their CFP as an aid to understanding clinical placements. It may also be consulted by many qualified nurses who seek to extend, deepen and update their knowledge. As our understanding of disease processes grows and as treatment options become more and more sophisticated, the conscientious practising nurse will be aware of the need to keep up to date. Novice nurses at the early stage of their education may be encouraged by the format of this book to develop a way of thinking about nursing knowledge which accepts its evolutionary nature.

The book is comprehensive in the sense that it covers all the main areas and issues of adult nursing practice. The amount of detail of necessity varies; some disorders or patient problems are dealt with extensively, while others are given only a brief mention. Space would not permit otherwise and we therefore felt it was important to include further reading suggestions so that students can pursue topics independently. We feel this is in keeping with the spirit of Project 2000 education, which promotes independent study and enquiry.

The Project 2000 report stressed the need for nursing practice to be based on up-to-date knowledge. An important feature of the present text is its inclusion of Research Abstracts and of Reference and Further Reading lists to give readers some guidance and encouragement in this pursuit of supplementary information. The Research Abstracts are intended to demonstrate the usefulness of reading research articles and reports as a way of constantly updating and re-examining practice.

The importance of referencing cannot be overstressed. No textbook for today's nurse can or should claim to provide all necessary knowledge: it can only present a distillation of current thinking. It is vital for student and qualified nurses to keep abreast of the literature relevant to their area of study or practice. Through such reading much can be learned about the process of research and about ways in which it might be implemented in practice.

Over and over again, we send our readers, irrespective of the stage at which their understanding and experience of nursing may be, or their point of development on the continuum from novice to expert nurse (Benner 1984), on a search for knowledge beyond that presented on the page which they are reading and absorbing. We encourage them, by means of self-assessment questions and by confronting them with some of the challenging dilemmas which reflect daily caring situations, to reflect on that practice, to engage in dialogue with fellow nurses or other members of the multidisciplinary health care team and to debate the issues they uncover in these reflective opportunities.

The subtitle, *Hospital and Home*, points to a central aim of the book: to provide a balanced view of nursing in different settings. This was a particular challenge both to the team of contributors who wrote the book and to ourselves as book editors, since nursing activity in the community is changing and expanding, and some aspects of nursing are only now being described and researched. We have no doubt that future editions of this book will reflect a different balance between these settings as knowledge grows and as experienced nurses working in hospital and community participate in continuing education and shared learning.

For the new entrant to nursing, Project 2000 programmes already create opportunities for more shared learning and exploration of the lived experience of patients and of caring in different settings; this book encourages that process.

Another key goal of Project 2000 education is to develop the nurse's understanding of health. Throughout this text, every opportunity has been taken to highlight opportunities for health promotion and health education that exist in everyday nursing situations.

In keeping with the aims of Project 2000, we have also highlighted ethical and moral issues in a number of chapters. Where possible, we have tried to select not only the major life-and-death issues (for example, whether or not to resuscitate a patient who arrests), but also the more everyday dilemmas faced by nurses. These dilemmas often involve truth-telling and honesty, as for example when the nurse is faced with a question such as 'Will it hurt?' or 'What is really wrong with me?'

A final comment about the book relates to the use of nursing models. The relative infrequency of the use of nursing models or conceptual frameworks reflects the state of the art in UK nursing. As nurses begin to explore innovative ways of applying models, both in hospital and in the community, models should become a more common feature of practice. A future edition may have quite a different emphasis in this regard.

Finally, we should pay tribute to the contributors — the authors of the chapters which follow this one, to whom we owe an enormous vote of thanks. Our writers, all experienced nurses, most in active practice, are experts in their fields, yet many are new to the challenge of codifying that expertise in written form. For many, articulating their knowledge and experience has seemed like undertaking an arduous journey, but so many have said to us how much they have learned from the experience, as the act of writing provided them with an opportunity to consolidate their knowledge and reflect upon current practice.

As Editors, we have likewise undertaken a long and at times daunting journey, but we too have learned a great deal about our discipline of nursing by being given the opportunity to consider, within the framework of this editorial project, the kinds of knowledge and skills that today's nurses need to meet the challenges awaiting them in their professional lives. We too, have welcomed this exercise in 'learning through reflection'.

To our readers, both entrants to the profession and those who are experienced nurses, may we say that we hope you will enjoy your journey through this text. You will all take individual routes through it, and the contents have been arranged in such a way as to allow for flexible use and to encourage you to consult other texts, research papers and journals on the way.

We feel that we will have succeeded in our task of producing a textbook for the 1990s if the reader learns never to see nursing as 'a given', but as always evolving; never to look complacently at current practice, but always to consider —or reconsider— its rationale and never to lose the gift of curiosity. The ways of thinking and learning that are implicit in the whole approach of this book are ways that are intended to encourage in the reader a love of learning, of questioning, of searching for 'latest knowledge' (Hockey 1993), which will inform nursing practice, test it and develop it in partnership with the patient and with our colleagues in the health care team. Nursing is a profession that must change and develop to meet the health care needs of the society it seeks to serve. The knowledge needed for nursing, therefore, can never be static but will also change and develop, and those who pursue such knowledge will undertake a journey which has no ending: a journey of discovery and challenge. We hope this book opens up some vistas and gives some pointers along the way towards the goal of ever better standards and quality of patient care.

REFERENCES

Benner P 1984 From novice to expert: excellence and power in clinical nursing practice. Addison-Wesley, Menlo Park
Benner P, Wrubel J 1989 The primacy of caring. Addison-Wesley, Menlo Park
Christensen J 1993 Nursing partnership: a model for nursing practice. Churchill Livingstone, Edinburgh
Department of Health 1990a Caring for people. HMSO, London
Department of Health 1990b Community care act. HMSO, London
Department of Health 1991 The patient's charter. HMSO, London
Eisenberg L 1977 Disease and illness: distinction between professional and popular ideas of sickness. Culture, Medicine and Psychiatry 1(1): 9–23
Fitzpatrick R M 1982 Social concepts of disease and illness. In: Patrick D L, Scambler G (eds) Sociology as applied to medicine. Baillière Tindall, London
Hockey L 1993 Research interview. Edinburgh
Kelly M 1990 The World Health Organization's definition of health promotion: three problems. Health Bulletin (Edinburgh) 48: 176–180
Kelly M, Charlton B G 1992 Health promotion: time for a new philosophy. The British Journal of General Practice. 42(359): 223–224
Kenworthy N, Snowley G & Gilling C 1992 Common foundation studies in nursing. Churchill Livingstone, Edinburgh
NHS Management Executive 1993 A vision for the future: the nursing, midwifery and health visiting contribution. Department of Health, Leeds
Nursing Standard 1993 Community care reforms: a guide to the changes. Nursing Standard 7(28): 18–19
Salvage J (ed) 1993 Nursing in action: strengthening nursing and midwifery to support health for all. WHO, Copenhagen
Skeet M 1980 Notes on nursing: the science and the art. Churchill Livingstone, Edinburgh
UKCC 1986 Project 2000: a new preparation for practice. UKCC, London
World Health Organization 1981 Global strategy for health for all by the year 2000. WHO, Geneva
World Health Organization 1985 Targets for health for all. WHO, Copenhagen

SECTION 1

Care of patients with common disorders

SECTION CONTENTS

2 The cardiovascular system 9

3 The respiratory system 59

4 The gastrointestinal system, liver and biliary tract 87

5 Endocrine and metabolic disorders 133

6 Genetic disorders 187

7 The reproductive systems and the breast 211

8 The urinary system 291

9 The nervous system 325

10 The musculoskeletal system 369

11 Blood disorders 405

12 Skin disorders 443

13 Disorders of the eye 467

14 Disorders of ear, nose, throat 497

15 Disorders of the mouth 521

16 The immune system and infectious disease 543

This first section of the book introduces students to people's experience of a wide range of common disorders. For ease of use, each chapter follows a similar structure.

- an introduction, which includes a discussion of **epidemiology** and current health issues
- **anatomy and physiology,** which includes references and further reading, to guide students towards more detailed information
- **key disorders,** discussed under the following headings:
  - pathophysiology
  - medical management
  - nursing priorities and management.

Nursing priorities and management, which receives the most emphasis, can be located easily as the heading has been printed in colour. The wording is intended to remind students of the value of setting priorities in response to each person's identified needs.

To help bring the material to life, many of the chapters include case histories, care plans, research abstracts and questions for self-assessment.

This section is aimed primarily, but not exclusively, at students at the beginning of the adult branch of a Project 2000 programme. It provides a solid foundation for Sections 2 and 3.

CHAPTER 2

The cardiovascular system

Kathryn Carver   Carol Mackinnon

CHAPTER CONTENTS

Introduction 9

Anatomy and physiology of the heart 10

Anatomy and physiology of the blood vessels 13

Disorders of the cardiovascular system 14
Nursing priorities and management: angina 16

Acute myocardial infarction (AMI) 22
Nursing priorities and management: thrombolytic therapy 24
Nursing priorities and management: AMI 24
Nursing priorities and management: cardiogenic shock 34

Arrhythmias 34
Nursing priorities and management: sinus arrhythmias 35
Nursing priorities and management: cardioversion 36
Nursing priorities and management: heart block 36

Expert nursing practice in ischaemic heart disease 37

Heart failure 37
Nursing priorities and management: heart failure 38

Valvular disorders 41
Nursing priorities and management: valvular disease 42

Hypertension 44
Nursing priorities and management: hypertension 46

Aortic aneurysms 47
Nursing priorities and management: aortic aneurysms 48

Peripheral vascular disease 48

Arterial disease 48
Nursing priorities and management: arterial disease 52

Venous disease 53
Nursing priorities and management: venous insufficiency 55

Glossary 57

References 57

Further reading 58

INTRODUCTION

The cardiovascular system consists of the heart and blood vessels. It is a closed circuit and is responsible for ensuring that blood flows throughout the body.

Cardiovascular disorders, being so prevalent in Western industrial societies, are likely to be encountered by all nurses, whether hospital or community based. This is particularly true now that an increasing percentage of the population is over 60 years old, an age group in which cardiovascular disorders are particularly common. Cardiovascular disease also affects the younger population group, being the main cause of premature death and handicap in the United Kingdom (Catford & Parish 1989).

There are marked regional variations in death rates from heart disease in the United Kingdom. East Anglia, the South-East and the South-West of England have the fewest deaths from heart disease; Northern Ireland and Scotland have the most (CSO 1992).

There is also a clear difference between socioeconomic groups in the prevalence of cardiovascular illness and disability, with the lowest prevalence among the professional groups and the highest among the unskilled manual group (CSO 1993).

Around half the deaths from cardiovascular disease each year in the UK are due to ischaemic heart disease (IHD), synonymous with coronary heart disease. Ischaemic heart disease is the single major cause of death in the Western world, accounting for some 150 000 deaths (roughly 26% of the total) in England and Wales (Office of Population Censuses and Surveys 1990).

The burden imposed by cardiovascular disease on the National Health Service is substantial. The annual cost of health service resources for treating coronary heart disease is approximately £500 million (Office of Health Economics 1990). Other financial costs include the economic effect of premature deaths, sickness and retirement from work. Cardiovascular disease also has an immense impact on society in human terms. Bereavement, disability, changing roles within the family and society, and fear are some examples of its consequences.

Many cardiovascular diseases take the form of progressive debilitating illness, often becoming chronic with acute episodes. Individuals have the prospect of a life-long problem. In contrast, a heart attack (myocardial infarction) is often sudden and unexpected, arousing acute distress in the individual and family as they confront a life-threatening crisis.

The government White Paper 'Health of the Nation' (Department of Health 1992) identifies ischaemic heart disease as a major cause of illness and early death and highlights the need to make significant improvements in health by making people aware of the causes of heart disease and how to avoid them (Williams 1992). Nurses, as one of the largest groups of health professionals must inevitably bear some responsibility for helping to reduce the mortality, morbidity and personal suffering caused by cardiovascular disease. Ashworth (1992) identifies ways in which nurses can intervene to contribute to such a reduction:

- facilitating lifestyle adjustment to enable people to attain and maintain a level of health compatible with their personal goals
- assisting people to modify the demands of the activities of living, to balance with their capacity to meet them
- modifying the environment to achieve for each person the optimum possible environment within available resources
- providing physical treatment and monitoring for pathophysiological conditions
- reassuring, supporting and comforting patients and their families.

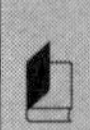

For further details of health promotion and community prevention see Catford & Parish (1989), and Williams (ed) (1992).

The following chapter is based upon a nursing framework of activities of living. This framework reflects Roper, Logan and Tierney's (1991) activities of daily living, model of nursing, which is used by many UK nurses caring for people with cardiovascular disorders. Models of nursing centred around daily activities have been criticised for being too simplistic and not placing enough emphasis on the psychosocial aspects of care. Also, the multifaceted nature of cardiovascular nursing care means that certain aspects of care cannot conveniently be fitted around these activities.

Other models such as Roy's adaptation model (1984) and Orem's self-care model (1991) have clear relevance for nursing the patient with a cardiovascular disorder and a flexible approach to the use of models is recommended (Aggleton & Chalmers 1986).

The chronic nature of a large proportion of cardiovascular disorders means that health professionals within the hospital see only parts of the spectrum of care. Much is carried out in the community by the primary health-care team, who are geared to preserving health and promoting adaptation and coping. It is therefore important that when people with cardiovascular problems are admitted to hospital, emphasis is placed on understanding their home, family and work circumstances, and on preparing them for a return to their own environment as independently as possible with any necessary support. Liaison between the hospital and community health-care teams is one approach.

ANATOMY AND PHYSIOLOGY OF THE HEART

The heart is a muscular pump that generates pressure changes resulting in the propulsion of blood around the vascular system. The right side of the heart pumps blood around the pulmonary system where gaseous exchange takes place and then on to the left side of the heart. The left side of the heart operates under much greater pressure to enable it to pump blood around the systemic circulation. The various chambers of the heart are illustrated in Figure 2.1.

The heart is composed of three layers:

1. Pericardium, a thick fibrous outer layer that protects the heart from injury and infection.
2. Myocardium, a muscular layer that varies in thickness throughout the heart. The atria, which act as filling chambers, have a thin layer of myocardium as they do not, in the fit individual, have to generate high pressures. In the ventricles the muscular layer is better developed, particularly in the left side, which is larger and thicker than in the right side, as a more forceful contraction is required to pump blood through the systemic circulation.
3. Endocardium, a thin layer of endothelium and connective tissue lines the inner chambers of the heart and coats the valves, which open and close to ensure a forward flow of blood at all times.

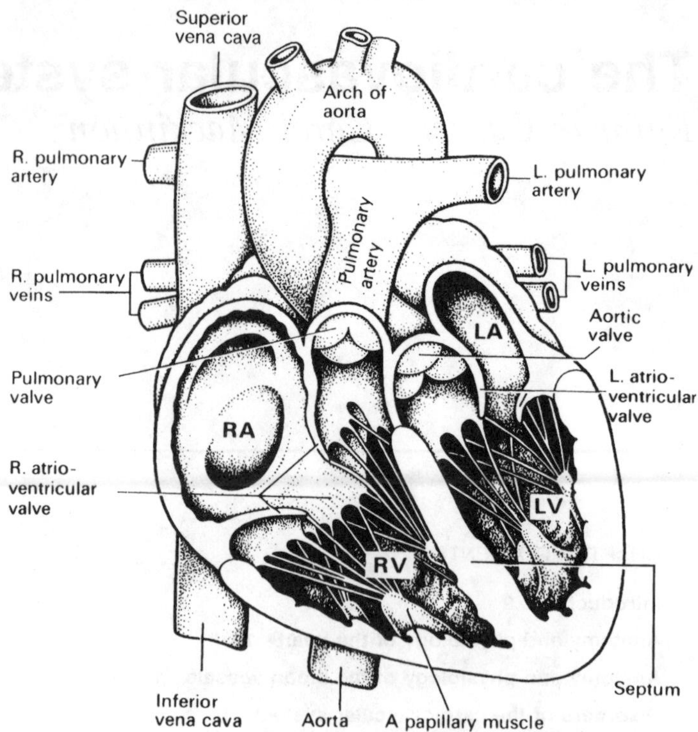

Fig. 2.1 The internal anatomy of the heart. (Reproduced with kind permission from Wilson 1990.)

Coronary blood supply

Like all major organs, the heart requires blood flow to maintain cellular activity. The myocardium cannot derive oxygen and nutrients from the blood within the chambers. It receives its blood supply from the right and left coronary arteries which arise from the aorta just beyond the aortic valve (see Fig. 2.2).

The left coronary artery runs towards the left side of the heart and divides into two major branches: the left anterior interventricular branch or left anterior descending artery (LAD) and the circumflex artery (CX). The LAD follows the anterior ventricular sulcus and supplies blood to the interventricular septum and the anterior walls of both ventricles. The CX follows the coronary sulcus and supplies blood to the lateral and posterior regions of the left atrium and left ventricle. The right coronary artery (RCA) runs to the right side of the heart and divides into two branches: the posterior interventricular artery and the marginal artery. The more important posterior interventricular artery follows the posterior interventricular sulcus to the apex of the heart and supplies blood to the posterior ventricular walls. It is near the apex of the heart that the posterior and anterior interventricular arteries merge. The marginal artery follows the coronary sulcus and supplies the right ventricle. It is the RCA that normally supplies the sinoatrial and atrioventricular node (see p. 11).

After passing through the capillary bed, the venous blood drains into the cardiac veins. These join to form the coronary sinus on the posterior surface of the heart from where venous blood drains into the right atrium.

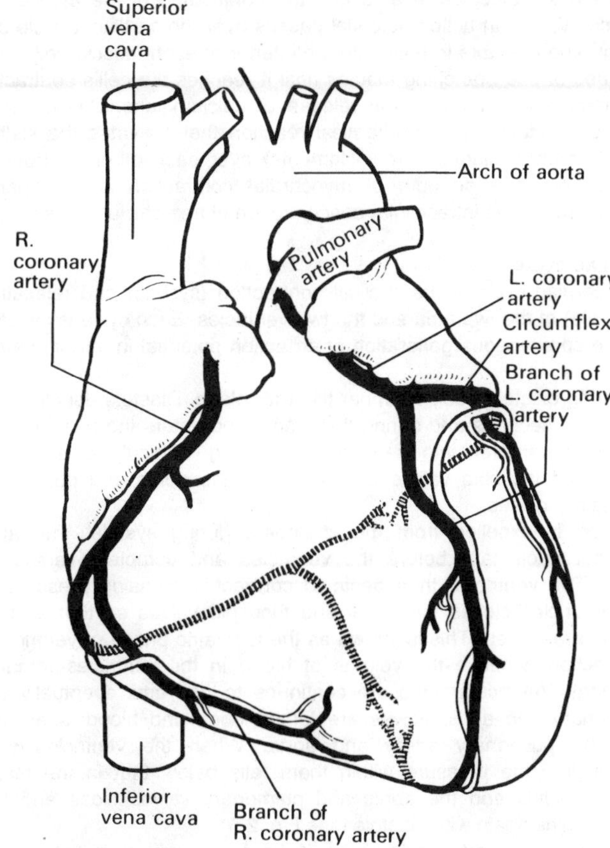

Fig. 2.2 The coronary circulation. (Reproduced with kind permission from Wilson 1990.)

Structure and function of cardiac valves

The atrioventricular valves, that is, the tricuspid and the mitral, function in a similar manner. During ventricular diastole (relaxation), they act as a funnel to promote rapid filling of the ventricles. Most of ventricular filling is passive. During ventricular systole (contraction), intraventricular pressure rises, pushing the cusps, which are restrained by the chordae tendineae, back and up towards the atria, thus preventing back flow of blood during systole. These valves can withstand high pressure, since their surface area is much greater than the orifice itself.

The semilunar valves, that is, the pulmonary and the aortic, each have three cusps. They are closed during ventricular diastole. Once ventricular contraction begins the intraventricular pressure rises and when it exceeds that in the aorta and the pulmonary artery, the semilunar valves are forced open and blood is ejected. After ventricular systole the pressure in the aorta and pulmonary artery exceeds that in the left and right ventricles, respectively. Retrograde blood flow therefore occurs due to the difference in pressure, which fills the valve cusps and snaps them home.

Pathological processes may result in valves becoming stenotic or incompetent. The term 'stenosis' means that the valve orifice has been reduced, impeding blood flow. Incompetent or insufficient refers to the fact that the cusps no longer prevent back flow of the blood to the lower pressure areas. The haemodynamic consequences of stenosis and incompetence depend upon which valve is affected.

The conducting system of the heart

It is important that the contraction of the atria and ventricles is organised to ensure that filling and emptying of the chambers is coordinated and controlled.

Cardiac cells contract and relax as a result of a stimulus response system. The heart consists of two major types of cardiac cells: myocardial cells, which are designed for contraction and automatic cells, which specialise in impulse formation.

The main bulk of the atria and ventricles consists of myocardial cells. Adjacent myocardial cells are held together by a complex system of projections known as intercalated discs with relatively low electrical resistance. These permit the movement of ions (electrically charged particles), which facilitates the propagation of action potentials from one myocardial cell to another. The main ions involved in the generation of a cardiac action potential are sodium (Na^+), potassium (K^+) and calcium (Ca^{2+}). In the normal resting state the myocardial cell is said to be polarised and due to the distribution of ions across its cell membrane, is negatively charged on the inside (intracellular) and positively charged on the outside (extracellular). When electrical activation of the cell occurs, changes in the cell membrane permeability result in movements of ions with a resulting change in electrical polarity. The membrane is now said to be depolarised and has an intracellular positive charge and an extracellular negative charge. Return to the resting state for each cell is called repolarisation and involves active pumping of ions against concentration gradients.

For further details of the cardiac action potential, consult Thompson & Webster (1992b).

As the myocardial cells are knitted closely together, the electrical stimulation of any one single cell causes the action potential to be propagated through all adjacent cells, eventually reaching the entire lattice work of the myocardium.

The automatic cells regulate the contraction of the myocardial cells by providing the initial electrical stimulation. They do not contribute significantly to the cardiac contraction itself. These cells possess three specific properties:

1. automaticity, the ability to generate action potentials, spontaneously and regularly
2. excitability, the ability to respond to electrical stimulation by generating an action potential
3. conductivity, the ability to propagate action potentials.

The electrical charge on the surface of an automatic cell leaks away until a certain threshold is reached, when spontaneous complete depolarisation occurs over the whole cell surface and spreads to adjacent cells, both automatic and myocardial. The automatic cell with the most rapid leak of charge becomes the principal pacemaking cell. Normally this is located within the sino-atrial node.

The automatic cells are found in the cardiac conducting system (see Fig. 2.3), which consists of:

- sinoatrial (SA) or sinus node
- atrioventricular (AV) junction (the AV node and bundle)
- ventricular conducting tissue (the right and left bundle branches).

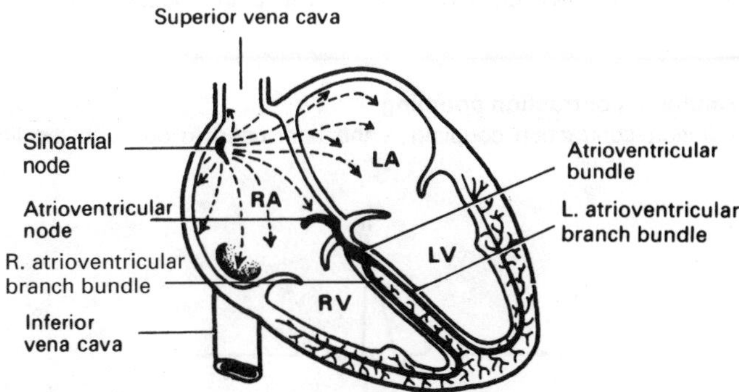

Fig. 2.3 The conducting tissues of the heart. (Reproduced with kind permission from Wilson 1990.)

Sequence of excitation

Depolarisation begins at the SA node and spreads through both atria. The activating impulse travels at a rate of about 1 m/s and reaches the most distant portion of the atria in about 0.08 seconds. The atria and ventricles remain electrically separate except via the atrioventricular (AV) junction, which allows the action potential to be conducted from the atrial to the ventricular conducting system. When the impulse reaches the AV node there is a delay of about 0.04 seconds to allow blood flow from the atria to the ventricles. After emerging from the AV node the impulse enters the rapidly conducting tissue of the bundle of His and the right and left bundle branches. The rapid spread of the impulse throughout the ventricles means that the entire ventricular mass is depolarised almost simultaneously, which is necessary for efficient contraction and pumping.

Electrocardiography

Electrocardiography is the graphic recording from the body surface of potential differences resulting from electrical currents generated in the heart. This recording may be displayed on special graph paper or on an oscilloscope (monitor) and is known as an electrocardiogram (ECG). An ECG is a graphic record of electrical changes at the skin surface plotted against time. The main value of the ECG is in the detection and interpretation of cardiac arrhythmias, diagnosis of coronary heart disease and assessment of ventricular enlargement (hypertrophy).

The sequence of electrical events produced at each heart beat has arbitrarily been labelled P, Q R S and T (see Fig. 2.4).

The P wave is associated with atrial activation. The width of the P wave represents the time necessary for the atrial activation process. Following atrial depolarisation an absence of electrical activity is noted on the ECG for a brief period, representing the passage of the impulse through the AV node. The PR interval (measured from the beginning of the P wave to the beginning of the QRS complex) is the time taken for the action potential to spread from the SA node, through the atrial muscle and the AV node, down the bundle of His and into the ventricular muscle mass.

The QR and S waves are associated with ventricular activation. The first downward deflection after the P wave is always labelled the Q wave and the R wave is the first upward deflection. If a negative deflection follows an R wave, it is labelled an S wave. The width of the QRS complex shows how long the action potential takes to spread through the ventricles.

The ST segment, a flat line between the S wave and the T wave, represents the early phase of ventricular muscle repolarisation, or recovery.

The T wave represents the actual recovery of the ventricular muscle. Occasionally, a U wave can be observed following the T wave. The origin of this wave is not well understood, but it is considered significant in a state of hypokalaemia.

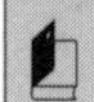

For more details on the ECG see Hampton (1992).

Excitation–contraction coupling

Excitation–contraction coupling is the term used to describe the link between the electrical events and the contraction of the myocardial muscle. When an action potential passes over the cardiac muscle cell membrane it is able to pass into the interior of each muscle cell down a series of fine branching tubules until it reaches the cell's contractile elements and stimulates the release of calcium ions. Calcium ions act as a catalyst for the chemical reaction that activates the sliding of thin muscle filaments (myofilaments) over each other to produce contraction. The strength of myocardial contraction is thus partly dependent on the intracellular concentration of free calcium ions.

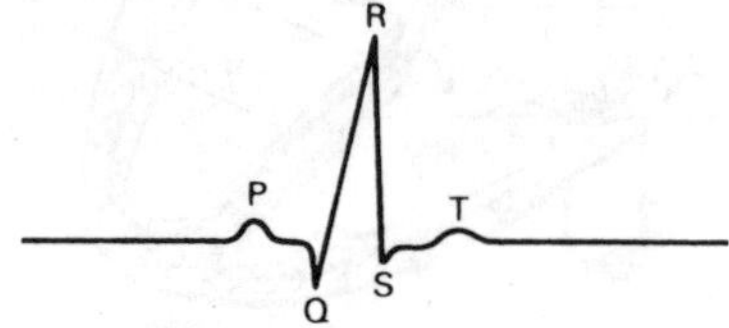

Fig. 2.4 ECG of one cardiac cycle. (Reproduced with kind permission from Boore et al 1987.)

Cardiac cycle

The cardiac cycle is the cyclical contraction (systole) and relaxation (diastole) of the two atria and the two ventricles. Each cycle is initiated by the spontaneous generation of an action potential in the sino-atrial node.

During diastole each chamber fills with blood. Diastole usually lasts about 0.4 seconds and during this time blood enters the relaxed atria and flows passively into the ventricles. During ventricular diastole, the mitral and tricuspid valves are open and the aortic and pulmonary valves are closed.

Blood is expelled from the chambers during systole. The atria contract fractionally before the ventricles and complete ventricular filling. The ventricles then begin to contract. Increasing pressure in the ventricles closes the mitral and tricuspid valves so that all four valves are closed. This is known as the isometric phase of ventricular contraction because the volume of blood in the ventricles remains constant. Ventricular pressure continues to rise until eventually the pulmonary and aortic valves are forced open and blood is ejected into the pulmonary artery and aorta. When the ventricles stop contracting, the pressure within them falls below that in the major blood vessels and the aortic and pulmonary valves close and the cycle begins again with diastole (see Fig. 2.5).

The normal heart rate is about 70 beats per minute in the resting adult with each cardiac cycle lasting about 0.8 seconds. With each ventricular contraction 65–75% of the blood in the ventricle at the end of diastole is ejected. This is usually a volume of 70–80 ml of blood and is known as the stroke volume.

Cardiac output is the volume of blood ejected from one ventricle in

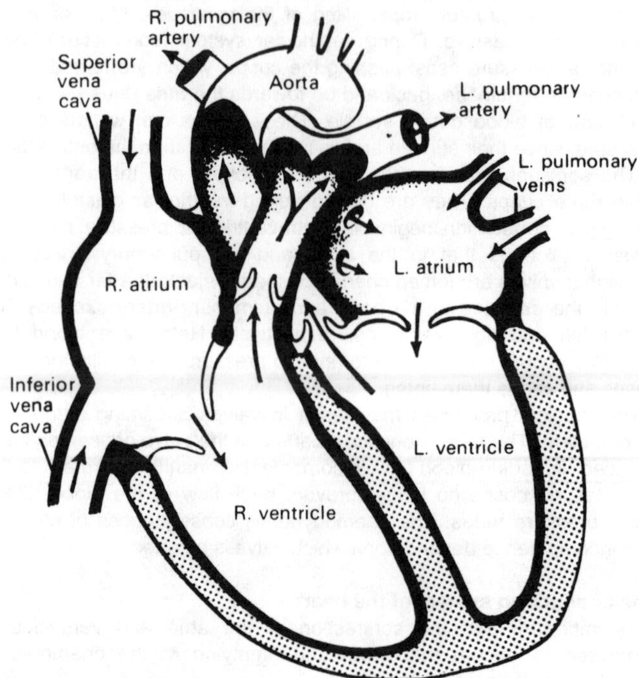

Fig. 2.5 Blood flow through the heart. (Reproduced with kind permission from Wilson 1990.)

one minute. Although cardiac output is a traditional measure of cardiac function, it differs markedly with body size. Thus, a more informative measure is the cardiac index, which is the cardiac output per minute per m^2 of body surface area. Usually it is about 3.2 litres/m^2.

The primary factors which determine cardiac output are:

1. preload, the amount of tension on the ventricular muscle fibres before they contract, determined primarily by the end-diastolic volume (EDV)
2. afterload, the resistance against which the heart must pump. Major components of afterload are:
   - blood pressure in the aorta
   - resistance in the peripheral vessels
   - the size of the aortic valve opening
   - left ventricular size
3. contractility of the heart
4. heart rate.

Within physiological limits, the volume of blood pumped out by a ventricle is the same as that entering the atrium on the same side of the heart; that is, cardiac output matches venous return. This principle is often referred to as the Frank–Starling law of the heart. This means that the heart is able to adapt to changing loads of inflowing blood from the systemic and pulmonary circulations. Within certain limits, cardiac muscle fibres contract more forcibly the more they are stretched at the start of contraction. Once the venous return increases beyond a certain limit the myocardium begins to fail. This regulation of the heart in response to the amount of blood to be pumped is known as intrinsic regulation.

?	**2.1** What are the main factors that determine cardiac output?

Regulation of cardiac function by the autonomic nervous system. The autonomic nervous system alters the rate of impulse generation by the SA node, the speed of impulse conduction, and the strength of cardiac contraction. It regulates the heart through both sympathetic and parasympathetic nerve fibres. The sympathetic fibres supply all areas of the atria and ventricles and effects on the heart include increased heart rate, increased conduction speed through the AV node, and increased force of contraction. Parasympathetic impulses are conducted to the heart via the vagus nerve and affect primarily the SA node, the AV node and the atrial muscle mass. Parasympathetic stimulation produces decreased heart rate, decreased conduction rate through the AV node and decreased force of atrial contraction.

Sympathetic and parasympathetic control of the heart occurs by reflexes coordinated in the medulla oblongata of the brain. The group of neurons in the brain that affect heart activity and the blood vessels is known as the cardiovascular centre. This cardiovascular centre receives information from various sensory receptors. Baroreceptors alter their rate of impulse generation in response to changes in blood pressure and chemoreceptors respond to changes in the chemical composition of the blood.

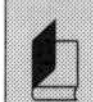

For further reading see Tortora & Grabowski (1992), p. 611.

ANATOMY AND PHYSIOLOGY OF THE BLOOD VESSELS

Systemic circulation

The systemic circulation is a high-pressure system that supplies all the tissues of the body with blood. It consists of the arteries, arterioles, capillaries, venules and veins. Blood flows through the system because of a downward pressure gradient from the aorta to the superior and inferior venae cavae. Arteries distribute oxygenated blood from the left side of the heart to the tissues and veins convey deoxygenated blood from the tissues to the right side of the heart. Adequate perfusion resulting in oxygenation and nutrition of body tissues is dependent in part upon patent and responsive blood vessels and adequate blood flow.

Arteries and arterioles

Arteries are thick-walled structures that carry blood from the heart to the tissues. The major arteries leading from the heart branch to form smaller ones, which eventually give rise to arterioles. The walls of the arteries and arterioles are divided into three layers:

- the inner layer provides a smooth surface in contact with the flowing blood
- the middle layer, the thickest, consists of elastic fibres and muscle fibres. The elasticity of the arterial wall enables it to recoil during ventricular relaxation and maintain blood flow
- the outer layer of connective tissue anchors the vessel to its surrounding structures.

There is much less elastic tissue in the arterioles than in the arteries. The middle layer of the arteriole wall consists primarily of smooth muscle which, by contraction and relaxation, controls the vessel's diameter. Arterioles regulate the pressure in the arterial system and the blood flow to the capillaries. The arterioles respond to local conditions such as a decrease in oxygen concentration or an increase in the concentration of carbon dioxide or other waste products. This ensures that a tissue that needs extra oxygen receives extra blood flow.

Arterioles will sometimes respond to changes in blood pressure. A local increase in blood pressure will cause the arterioles to constrict, to protect the smaller vessels in the tissue from increased pressure. If pressure in the arterioles suddenly decreases, the arterioles will dilate to ensure that the tissue receives sufficient blood flow for nutrition. This local regulatory mechanism is sometimes referred to as autoregulation and is an important factor in determining relatively constant blood flow despite alterations in arterial pressure. The sympathetic nervous system will also influence the diameter of the arterioles. Increased sympathetic stimulation to blood vessels usually produces constriction, whereas decreased sympathetic stimulation results in vasodilation.

Capillaries

The velocity of the blood is at its slowest in the capillaries thus allowing sufficient time for exchange of fluid between the blood and the interstitial space. Capillary walls lack muscle. They consist of a single layer of cells and have a large total surface area. Their thin walls allow efficient transport of nutrients to the cells and the removal of metabolic wastes. The density of capillary networks varies in different tissues.

Veins and venules

Capillaries join together to form larger vessels called venules, which, in turn, join to form veins. The walls of the veins are thinner and a lot less muscular than the arteries. This allows the veins to distend more, which permits storage of large volumes of blood in the veins under low pressure. Approximately 75% of total blood volume is contained in the veins. Some veins are equipped with valves to prevent the reflux of blood as it is propelled towards the heart. The sympathetic nervous system can stimulate venoconstriction, thereby reducing venous volume and increasing the general circulating blood volume. This adjustment of the total volume of the circulatory system to the amount of blood available to fill it contributes to the regulation of blood pressure.

Blood pressure

Blood pressure refers to the hydrostatic pressure exerted by the blood on the blood vessel walls and is a function of blood flow and vascular resistance. As most of the resistance to blood flow is due to the peripheral vessels, especially the arterioles, it is often described as the total peripheral resistance, as in the equation:

$$\text{mean arterial pressure} = \text{cardiac output} \times \text{total peripheral resistance.}$$

Blood pressure varies in different blood vessels. However, clinically the term 'blood pressure' refers to systemic arterial blood pressure.

Arterial blood pressure
Arterial blood pressure fluctuates throughout the cardiac cycle. The maximum pressure occurs after ventricular systole and is known as the systolic pressure. Systolic pressure is dependent on the stroke volume, the force of contraction and the stiffness of the arterial walls. The level to which arterial pressure falls before the next ventricular contraction is the minimum pressure, known as the diastolic pressure. Diastolic pressure varies according to the degree of vasoconstriction and is dependent on the level of the systolic pressure, the elasticity of the arteries and the viscosity of the blood. Alterations in heart rate will also affect diastolic pressure. A slower heart rate produces a lower diastolic pressure as there is more time for the blood to flow out of the arteries. The difference between the systolic and diastolic blood pressure is known as the 'pulse pressure'. The average pressure attempting to push the blood through the circulatory system is known as the 'mean arterial pressure'.

Blood pressure values
There is no such value as a 'normal' blood pressure as it varies both from person to person and in individuals from moment to moment, under different circumstances. Normal blood pressure is said to range from 100/60 mmHg to 150/90 mmHg. Factors such as age, sex and race influence blood pressure values. Pressure also varies with exercise, emotional reactions, sleep, digestion and time of day.

The predominant mechanisms that control arterial pressure within the 'normal' range are the autonomic nervous system and the renin–angiotensin–aldosterone system.

Baroreceptors in the aortic arch and the carotid sinus respond to changes in arterial pressure and relay impulses to the cardiovascular centre in the medulla oblongata of the brain. When the arterial pressure is increased, baroreceptor endings are stretched and relay impulses that inhibit the sympathetic outflow. This results in a decreased heart rate and arteriolar dilatation and the arterial pressure returning to its former level. If the blood pressure remains chronically high, the baroreceptors are reset at a higher level and respond as though the new level were normal.

When blood flow to the kidneys decreases, with a fall in blood pressure, renin is released. Renin is an enzyme which acts on a blood protein angiotensin I, which is then converted to angiotensin II by another enzyme. Angiotensin II produces an elevation in blood pressure by direct constriction of arterioles. Angiotensin II also directly stimulates the release of the hormone aldosterone from the adrenal cortex which leads to renal retention of sodium and water. This increases extracellular volume, which, in turn, increases the venous return to the heart, thereby raising stroke volume, cardiac output and arterial blood pressure. The kidneys respond to an increase in arterial pressure by excreting a greater volume of fluid. This decreases the extracellular fluid resulting in a lower venous return and reduced cardiac output until arterial pressure is returned towards normal.

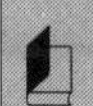
Further details of blood pressure regulation can be found in Levick (1991).

DISORDERS OF THE CARDIOVASCULAR SYSTEM

Atherosclerosis

Atherosclerosis is a complex, chronic disease of the arteries characterised by endothelial injury, the accumulation of lipids and fibrous tissue in the form of atheromatous plaques, and the thickening and hardening of the vessel walls with resultant loss of elasticity (see Figs 2.6 and 2.7). The aetiology of atherosclerosis remains unclear and although several theories have been put forward to explain its pathogenesis, it is not fully understood.

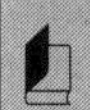
Further details of the pathogenesis of atherosclerosis can be found in Thompson & Webster (1992b).

Stress or turbulence in artery
↓
Damage to endothelial lining of vessel
↓
Platelets adhere to damaged area
↓
? lipids infiltrate at this stage → Platelets and/or endothelial cells and/or macrophages release growth stimulating factor
↓
Growth of fibrin network
↓
Migration of smooth muscle cells from media to intima or endothelium
↓
Smooth muscle cells multiply and protrude against endothelial cell lining
↓
Deposition of lipids especially cholesterol (primarily from low density lipoproteins in plasma) in and around smooth muscle
↓
Narrowing of artery, roughening of endothelial lining and loss of elasticity
↓
Continuing fibrosis and calcification

Fig. 2.6 Probable course of events in the development of atheroma. (Reproduced with kind permission from Boore et al 1987.)

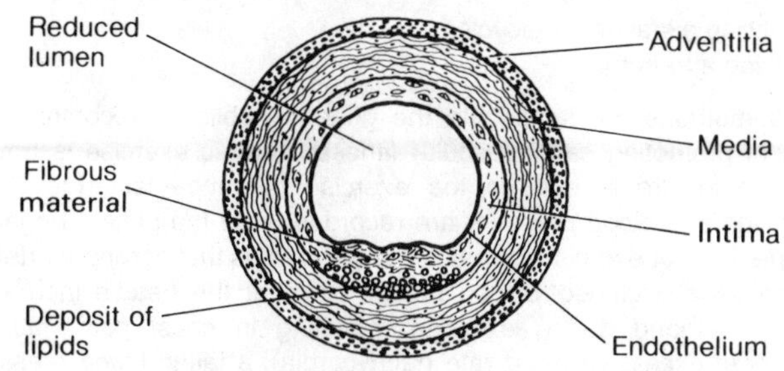

Fig. 2.7 Cross-section of an artery. (Reproduced with kind permission from Boore et al 1987.)

? **2.2** How early in life has evidence of atheromatous change in the blood vessels been found?

Atherosclerosis is responsible for most coronary artery and ischaemic heart disease and much peripheral and cerebrovascular disease. Emboli may arise as a result of pieces of dead tissue from the damaged arterial wall breaking off. With progression of the process, the lining of the vessel wall may become eaten away and, especially if the blood pressure is elevated, the vessel may become permanently dilated and weakened in the form of an aneurysm. Vessels may become blocked or stenosed or, as a result of endothelial damage and platelet adhesion, an ulcer-like site can develop, leading to thrombus formation. Thrombosis may cause complete obstruction or undergo spontaneous thrombolysis. This dynamic process occurs over a period of hours to days, preceding an acute coronary event or spontaneous resolution.

Myocardial ischaemia

Traditionally, myocardial ischaemia is defined as a condition of the heart in which there is an imbalance between oxygen supply and demand. However, such a definition excludes the removal of metabolites, particularly heat and carbon monoxide, which are an important function of myocardial blood flow.

Oxygen demand depends mainly upon heart rate, myocardial contractility and tension in the myocardial wall. Oxygen supply to the myocardium varies with coronary blood flow. The heart extracts the maximum amount of oxygen from its blood supply and is dependent upon an increased volume of blood in times of increased demand. Myocardial blood supply may be compromised by abnormalities of the vessel wall, in blood flow, or in the blood itself.

Localised myocardial ischaemia may be intermittent and have reversible effects, but it causes decreased myocardial function. Ischaemia results in acidosis and the rapid accumulation of potassium in the extracellular space. Pain is usually experienced after about a minute of myocardial ischaemia.

There are three main manifestations of ischaemic heart disease:

- angina pectoris
- acute myocardial infarction
- sudden death.

Risk factors

Epidemiological studies have sought to find associations between coronary heart disease and physical, biochemical and environmental characteristics of a population or individuals. The three predominant risk factors consistently shown to be predictors of the disease are:

- lipoproteins
- cigarette smoking
- high blood pressure.

Other main risk factors are:

- obesity
- lack of physical exercise
- a type A behaviour pattern
- diabetes mellitus
- a family history of coronary heart disease.

? **2.3** What is meant by 'Type A behaviour'? Can Type A behaviour be changed?

For further information about Type A behaviour, see Niven 1989 Health psychology. Churchill Livingstone, Edinburgh, Ch. 6.

Major geographical variations in the incidence of ischaemic heart disease are apparent. Mortality rates in the UK are very close to the top of the international league table. Scotland and Northern Ireland have the highest mortality rates and the North of England and Wales are close behind. The rates are lowest in the South-East. In the 1980s, mortality from ischaemic heart disease differed significantly between ethnic groups. Mortality was highest in men and women born in the Indian subcontinent and was also raised in Irish- and Polish-born immigrants. Risk factors need to be viewed in conjunction with each other as their effect is cumulative. Although by definition each risk factor associates positively with increased risk of coronary heart disease, it does not follow that risk factors are causal. It is also important to remember that a significant number of patients presenting with coronary heart disease do not have identifiable risk factors and that standard risk factors explain less than half the disease (Box 2.1).

? **2.4** Health promotion is defined by Downie et al (1990) as efforts to enhance positive health and prevent ill-health, through the three overlapping spheres of:

- health education
- prevention
- health protection.

The health promotion movement stresses the importance of 'empowerment'; of enabling people to make choices and to determine their own lives.
Discuss the three spheres in relation to the promotion of cardiovascular health.

? **2.5** 'Empowering' people is neither simple nor easy. What might hinder people from taking greater control over their health?

Angina pectoris

Angina pectoris is a transient, reversible episode of inadequate coronary circulation. It is a symptom and not a disease.

MEDICAL MANAGEMENT

The presentation and history vary and may mislead the practitioner initially if a thorough examination is not undertaken. History is usually of increasing discomfort over a period of time, often related to specific events. The presenting features indicate a deficiency in the oxygen supply, such as:

- Episodic pain occurring centrally in the chest, often described as 'dull', 'aching' or a 'tight band'. This may radiate to the arms,

Box 2.1 Risk factors associated with IHD

Genetic	Personal
Race	Age
Gender	Smoking
Family history.	Diet:
Medical	• obesity
Diabetes mellitus	• fat intake
Hypertension	• salt intake
Hyperlipidaemia	• fibre intake
Hypercholesterolaemia	• alcohol intake
Hypothyroidism	Lack of exercise
Gout.	Lack of relaxation
Social	Oral contraception.
Geographical location	
Living conditions	
Occupation	
Stress	
Personality type: 'Type A' behaviours.	

particularly the left arm, jaw or neck. It is often induced by exercise or emotion and is relieved by rest. The pain takes many forms (see Table 2.1). Typically, the duration of an anginal attack is 2–5 minutes.

- Breathlessness on exertion, for example, walking uphill, or in cold weather.
- Discomfort in the epigastric region after a heavy meal.

Investigations are as follows.

Electrocardiogram. The recording is invariably normal between attacks of angina, but during an episode of pain, the segment between the end of the QRS complex and the beginning of the T wave may be depressed (ST depression). The T wave may also be flattened or inverted.

Exercise tolerance test. This is a means of assessing the heart's response to increased demand. The test is based on the theory that patients with ischaemic heart disease will produce marked ST-segment depression on the ECG when exercising. The test is considered negative if there are no significant ECG abnormalities and the patient experiences no significant symptoms. The three common methods of exercise testing include:

- climbing stairs
- pedalling a stationary bicycle
- walking a treadmill.

These methods are familiar to the general public as recommended ways of promoting cardiovascular fitness. Aerobic exercise is now a common leisure pursuit. In the exercise tolerance test, the ECG, heart rate and blood pressure are recorded while the patient engages in some form of exercise (stress). The principle is that coronary arteries that may be occluded will be unable to meet the heart's increased oxygen demand during exercise, resulting in chest pain, fatigue, dyspnoea, excessive heart rate (tachycardia), a fall in blood pressure or the development of arrhythmias. The test is stopped if any of these occur, or before, at the patient's request. The patient needs to have the procedure explained in detail before the test. The term 'stress' test is best avoided as it may sound ominous and increase patient anxiety. The patient should be advised to avoid a heavy meal prior to the test and to wear loose-fitting clothes. The procedure takes about 30 minutes.

Coronary angiography. This involves the injection of contrast medium into the heart during cardiac catheterisation. The procedure shows the shape and size of the heart chambers and will pin-point any stenosis or occlusion in the coronary arteries. This test is described in Box 2.2.

Diagnosis. Angina is diagnosed by the characteristic chest pain, induced by exercise and relieved by rest. Exercise testing only confirms angina if it produces pain or ECG changes during the test. Angiography in the absence of clinical symptoms confirms the presence of myocardial ischaemia, not of angina. The differential diagnosis is very important at this stage.

The pain of angina may be confused with the pain of oesophagitis or the pain of peptic ulceration. Patients, fearing a 'heart attack', may choose to interpret the pain as 'a little indigestion'.

Treatment

The aim is:

- to restore and maintain cardiac output necessary for normal living activities
- to reduce the workload of the heart
- to bring back into balance oxygen supply and demand.

This is achieved by:

- medication to optimise cardiac function by relieving the pain of angina and improving myocardial perfusion (Table 2.2)
- reduction in activity
- reducing risk factors
- surgical intervention: percutaneous transluminal coronary angioplasty (PTCA) or coronary artery bypass graft surgery (see p. 20 and 21).

? **2.6** a. Read Case History 2.1. What is the significance of this result?
b. What other tests might be requested?
c. What are Mr B's risk factors for ischaemic heart disease?
d. How would you discuss the results of this test with Mr B?

Table 2.1 Classification of angina pectoris

Classification	Characteristics
Stable angina	Condition in which the frequency and severity of angina remains well controlled and unchanged over several months
Unstable angina	Condition in which the pain is increasing in frequency, severity and duration. Occurs with less activity or at rest
Crescendo angina	Form of angina where chance of AMI occurring within a few days is high
Angina decubitus	Pain occurring when lying down
Atypical angina	Unusual form where pain occurs at rest or long after activity has ceased. Accompanied by transient S-T segment elevation.
Printzmetals angina	Coronary artery spasm without underlying disease is often the cause
Intractable angina	Continued pain with increasing frequency, despite treatment

NURSING PRIORITIES AND MANAGEMENT: ANGINA

The major goals for the patient are to:

- prevent or minimise chest pain
- cope with the anginal pain and any other symptoms
- reduce anxiety
- be aware of the underlying nature of the disorder
- understand the prescribed care and be able to make informed decisions about future lifestyle.

Box 2.2 Cardiac catheterisation

Purpose
Cardiac catheterisation involves the insertion into one or more of the heart chambers, usually under screening, of a fine, flexible, radio-opaque catheter. The catheter is inserted via a peripheral vein or artery under sterile conditions in a cardiac catheterisation laboratory. The right and left side of the heart may be investigated separately or together. The procedure is performed to:

- visualise the heart chambers and vessels by means of a radio-opaque substance under X-ray control (angiography)
- measure pressure and record wave forms from the cavity of the heart
- obtain blood samples from the heart.

Cardiac catheterisation will always be performed on a prospective candidate for coronary artery bypass graft surgery and it is also used to evaluate the effect of thrombolytic agents. Angiography involves injecting contrast medium into the heart during cardiac catheterisation in order to pinpoint any stenosis or occlusion. It is recommended for patients with significant angina.

Procedure
Cardiac catheterisation is usually carried out under local anaesthesia, but the patient is usually asked to fast for 4–6 hours to prevent aspiration, should cardiac arrest occur. The groin area will be shaved. The procedure is performed by a cardiologist and takes about 90 minutes. The patient will be asked to wear a gown and should be prepared to lie flat on his back on a hard table during the procedure. He needs to be warned to expect a sudden burning sensation as the dye is injected into the heart. Angina may occur as a result of the catheter blocking the artery.

Following the procedure the patient may require analgesia and should be allowed to rest. A pressure dressing will be applied to the wound site, which needs to be observed for excessive bleeding. The limb needs to be kept straight for 1–2 hours to prevent turbulence of blood flow at the incision site. If the catheter is inserted via the femoral artery, the patient is advised to rest in bed for 6–8 hours to prevent flexing the hip and possible artery occlusion. The patient is usually discharged the following day.

Possible complications
Complications are uncommon but can include:

- transient cardiac arrhythmias
- perforation of the heart
- syncope
- emboli.

A reaction to the dye may produce symptoms ranging from a rash to anaphylaxis.

Table 2.2 Drugs used in angina

Drug group	*Role in angina*	*Physiological action*	*Comments*
Nitrates			
Glyceryl trinitrate (GTN)	Used for relief of angina administered as spray form or tablet under tongue to ensure rapid release into the blood stream	Venodilation with consequent reduction in preload. Also causes systemic arteriolar vasodilation with decrease in afterload	Needs to be stored correctly. Tablets lose potency over time and if exposed to light They should not be kept for more than 2 months, should be stored in an airtight container and not exposed to light.
Suscard buccal	Slow-release form of nitrate placed in the buccal cavity	As above Used for effect for 4–5 hours	
Isosorbide mononitrate	Used for prevention of angina Oral administration	As above Used as longer-term control.	Patient can develop tolerance
Beta blockers	Used in preventing angina. Administered once or twice daily Dose lower than for hypertensive patients.	Block sympathetic stimulation, so slowing heart rate and reducing oxygen demand	Need to be used with caution with patients with chronic obstructive airways disease
Calcium antagonists	Used in preventing angina	Interfere with calcium transfer across the cell membrane, causing relaxation of arteriolar smooth muscle, thus reducing afterload. Affects rate of action potential and reduces oxygen demand	
Anticoagulant therapy			
Aspirin	Small dose taken daily to protect against myocardial infarction	Aspirin prolongs the prothrombin time as well as decreasing platelet viscosity.	Small dose should not affect stomach lining

Nursing input will vary according to the type of contact a person has with health care services. Practice nurses and occupational health staff may be the main source of professional information and support for those in the community. Admission to hospital is likely to occur only if the angina is uncontrolled or further investigation is warranted.

Nursing assessment should pay particular attention to those activities that have been found to precede and precipitate attacks of angina pain and associated symptoms, so that a logical programme of prevention can be worked out with the patient, who needs to feel in control of his condition and to regain a realistic outlook for the future.

Case History 2.1

Mr B is a 55-year-old factory foreman who regards himself as being fit and well for his age. He plays badminton at the local sports club two or three times a week and enjoys taking his dog on regular rambles. He does not smoke and, being aware of factors leading to heart disease, has tried to reduce the fat intake in his diet over the past few years. His father died of a heart attack at the age of 73. Mr B's company offer regular medical checks to screen for health problems and on his last visit he underwent an exercise test. After 5 minutes of the test he felt short of breath. He was noted to have ST segment depression.

Maintaining a safe environment

The effect of angina on the person and those around him needs to be considered. The patient needs to know how to:

- prevent attacks
- manage attacks when they occur.

As the nurse will not witness many of the attacks it should be impressed on the patient that their management lies with him and his family. As much of the nursing management involves advice about potential adaptations in lifestyle, the family require the same information and support as the patient.

The individual needs to be advised to plan his daily activity around adequate rest periods. If he cannot avoid activities liable to precipitate an attack then he should rest before and after the activity. For example, a large family gathering such as a wedding can be very stressful, with socialising, a large meal to eat and a lot of preparation. As much time as possible should be spent quietly with rest periods after dressing, after the meal, etc. Explaining to other members of the family the reason for this is better than suffering an attack during the proceedings.

Taking glyceryl trinitrate (GTN) prophylactically is often the best way of managing this. Further manipulation of his environment can take place; for example, if climbing stairs induces angina and the bathroom is downstairs and the bedroom upstairs, it may help to dress in a downstairs room as climbing stairs after a hot bath is very likely to induce an attack. Advice on the practical aspects of daily routine can be given during history taking.

A change of occupation is sometimes necessary following a diagnosis of angina, for example, it would be unsafe to drive public transport vehicles. This double blow can be very difficult for the person to accept. The occupational health nurse can help as she will be aware of other areas to which he can be relocated. If retraining is required the social worker and retraining counsellors from the Department of Employment should be involved as early as possible.

Mobility

Exercise is the most common cause of an attack, and patients need to be advised to stop and rest rather than attempt to work through the pain. The patient should understand how to use GTN both to prevent and treat an attack. If the patient takes GTN prior to an activity likely to cause angina he may prevent an attack and still complete the activity. However, the patient needs to appreciate that he should not use his GTN to overexercise, but to maintain a reasonable quality of life and give him some feeling of control over his condition. He should be encouraged to keep records of the activities that induce angina. These can be reviewed with his practitioner to provide a reliable assessment of his angina and the effectiveness of therapy. Knowledge of his limitations gives the patient some feeling of control over his own life and he can then attempt to extend them by altering his daily routine.

Many of the heavier household tasks induce angina, for example, shopping, ironing and vacuuming, and often make patients feel threatened. A basket with wheels can be used to transport shopping, and other such simple measures are easily adapted into people's lifestyles. Help from other family members or domestic help in the home may be another solution.

Breathing

In some individuals angina presents as, or is accompanied by, difficulty in breathing. This is often worse in cold or windy weather. Such individuals need to be advised against walking great distances in these conditions. Smokers need to be clear about the association between ischaemic heart disease and cigarette smoking so that they can make informed decisions about stopping.

Cigarette smokers have a 2–3 times greater risk of death from ischaemic heart disease than non-smokers. The risk is greater in young adults and in those who smoke more than 20 cigarettes a day. Nicotine stimulation results in an increase in heart rate, cardiac output, blood pressure and coronary blood flow. Carbon monoxide attaches itself to the haemoglobin molecule and therefore reduces its ability to transport oxygen.

The nursing history should include information as to whether the patient has tried to give up smoking before, and if so, how he planned to stop, how long he was able to stop, what support he received and why he started smoking again. Any perceived benefits of smoking, for example stress reduction, need to be discussed and plans for stopping based on experience gained in conjunction with new information and advice given.

? **2.7** Many strategies for giving up smoking exist. Not all will suit every would-be non-smoker. What strategies can you identify? The following articles describe approaches used by a health visitor and school nurses: Gallop (1993) and McDermott (1993).

Diet and nutrition

Obese people develop cardiovascular disease more frequently than others. Obesity also denotes an increased likelihood of hypertension, hyperlipidaemia and diabetes mellitus. Total blood cholesterol levels have been shown to be associated with ischaemic heart disease mortality and morbidity (Box 2.3). However, there is a negative association between one category of lipoproteins, high-density lipoproteins (HDLs) and ischaemic heart disease (IHD), that is, the risk of the disease is lower when the concentration of HDL is raised. Early conclusions that cholesterol and saturated fat in the diet raise cholesterol and fat levels in the blood which promote atherosclerosis are now the topic of much controversy. It has been recommended that consumption of saturated fatty acids and total fat be reduced to 11% and 35%, respectively, of food energy. Dietary advice needs to take into account personal preferences, and domestic, socioeconomic and cultural factors. Alterations to general eating habits are preferable to restrictive diets. Sensible dietary advice includes:

- losing excess weight
- reducing sugar intake
- increasing fibre intake.

Eating more fish, poultry, vegetables, grains, cereals and fruit should be encouraged. Keeping within an ideal body

Box 2.3 Understanding cholesterol

Definition: a steroid found in animal fats and most body tissues, especially nervous tissue.

Cholesterol has received rather bad publicity in recent years because of the role it has been found to play in the formation of atheromatous plaques but it must be remembered that, although it is not used as an energy fuel, cholesterol is an important dietary lipid, essential in maintaining homeostatic mechanisms in the body. It is a vital constituent of cell membranes and forms the structural basis of many steroid hormones and bile salts.

The recommended daily intake of cholesterol for adults is approximately 250 mg or less. However, cholesterol is not only obtained from the diet but is synthesised in the liver, the intestinal mucosa and, to a lesser degree, other body cells. It is excreted from the body in bile salts.

Cholesterol, like fatty acids and glycerol, is insoluble in water and therefore cannot circulate freely in the bloodstream. It is transported, bound to small lipid-proteins, lipoproteins, which are essentially of high-density or low-density compositions. Low-density lipoproteins (LDLs) are responsible for transporting cholesterol to the peripheral tissue so that it is available for membrane synthesis, hormone synthesis and storage, for later use. Excessive cholesterol leads to 'dumping' of the excess in the lining of the blood vessels, for example, the coronary arteries. High-density lipoproteins (HDLs) have a different function in that they transport cholesterol from the peripheral tissue to the liver to be broken down. HDLs have been described as scavenging excess cholesterol for disposal.

High levels of total serum cholesterol have been repeatedly shown to be associated with the development of coronary artery disease and myocardial infarction. However, it is not enough merely to measure cholesterol but rather the form in which it is being transported. HDLs can be thought of as beneficial because they promote the degradation and removal of cholesterol. On the other hand, LDLs, when excessive, can lead to a potentially serious deposition of cholesterol in the artery walls.

Although it is now regarded as important to limit our dietary cholesterol, severe restriction does not lead to a correspondingly dramatic drop in plasma cholesterol. This is because, although cholesterol production is, to some extent, adjusted by a feedback mechanism such that a high dietary intake will inhibit hepatic synthesis, the liver will always produce a certain amount irrespective of the diet.

It would seem that the factor that has the most significant effect on plasma cholesterol is the amount of saturated and unsaturated fat in the diet. Saturated fats, found essentially in animal produce, stimulate the hepatic synthesis of cholesterol whilst inhibiting its removal. In contrast, unsaturated fats found in vegetable oils, enhance the excretion of cholesterol in the bile salts, thereby reducing cholesterol levels.

Other factors also appear to affect plasma cholesterol levels. Stress, coffee and smoking are thought to be implicated in increased levels of LDLs. Regular aerobic exercise has been associated with the lowering of LDLs and raising of HDLs.

If research continues to support the above findings, there are clear implications for the role of the nurse in promoting nutritional health and well-being.

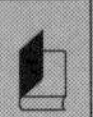
Further reading: Marieb (1989), Ch. 25.

weight range and taking suitable physical exercise are logical recommendations.

Large meals may trigger an attack of angina so small, frequent meals are preferable. It can be difficult to motivate someone to change their diet. Involving the family is very important, particularly the person primarily responsible for buying food and preparing meals.

The patient who presents to the medical services with epigastric pain may have angina, particularly if the history is vague. Diagnosis requires history-taking skills and spending time with the patient.

Alcohol intake should be discussed with the individual. In small quantities alcohol has a vasodilatory effect which is beneficial in IHD, so a small nightcap will help relax the patient and aid sleep. Heavy drinkers are, however, at risk of hepatic dysfunction.

The patient should know whether his medication should be taken before or after meals and its effect with alcohol.

Work and recreation

The person with angina has to come to terms with the progressive nature of the disease. People with limited energy reserves may put all their effort into work and find they have little left for leisure pursuits. The nurse's role is to assist the individual to assess his lifestyle and make decisions about priorities and possible changes. Those with sedentary lifestyles should be advised to take regular exercise, such as walking to work, climbing the stairs, swimming and cycling. Some apparently sedentary jobs may be mentally exhausting, which can put severe strain on the compromised myocardium and lead to an anginal attack. Planning the day is important, to allow for quiet periods, particularly before and after long meetings or heavy business lunches. For certain personality types, therapy such as relaxation techniques or yoga may help.

If a change of occupation or early retirement is the only solution, the person may resist, particularly if he is the family breadwinner.

Rest and sleep

Taking frequent naps throughout the day is often better than a longer sleep at night. The bedroom should be well ventilated but not cold or draughty (see Ch. 25).

Expressing sexuality

In some people with angina sexual intercourse can trigger an attack. This can be stressful for both the sufferer and their partner. Prophylactic use of GTN and some planning may help. The couple may have to adapt their usual position or the partner may have to take on a more dominant role. Touching and caressing may replace full intercourse while satisfying both.

This area needs delicate handling but must be addressed as the individual's perceived view on this aspect of daily living can affect all other aspects. Someone receiving β-blocker therapy may suffer from impotence and this should be explained.

An important related aspect of sexuality is role reversal, for example, if a housewife has to hand over some of her tasks and feels threatened, or where the family breadwinner is forced to give up work. This may greatly affect self esteem.

The fear of dying

People who have angina may have difficulty coming to terms with the fact that they have a progressive disease affecting their heart and most probably other parts of their body also. Angina can progress to myocardial infarction, which can cause death. This has to be discussed with the person to keep the situation in perspective. If he feels in control over some aspects of the condition to help prolong life, for example, stopping smoking, or altering his diet he will possibly cope better than the person with a strong family history over which he has no control. Encouraging the patient to discuss his fears may help him cope with them or alert the nurse to the fact that expert counselling is required.

Communication
Getting to know the person as an individual is important if appropriate support is to be given. He needs to be guided towards pinpointing aspects of lifestyle that will be affected by angina and then learning through discussion and counselling how to minimise their effect. If the person can communicate what causes pain, what relieves it, etc, management is often simplified. Anxiety will reduce the ability to communicate, particularly when in an unfamiliar environment such as the occupational health department or hospital. The use of a scoring table or a continuum for assessing and comparing attacks of angina may prove beneficial for monitoring the effect of therapy.

Personal hygiene and dressing
Here, again, the key is living within the restraints of the condition. The person should be advised against locking the bathroom door whilst in the bath so that help can reach him if necessary. Other family members must remember this and respect privacy. Spacing activities throughout the day rather than rushing to do everything first thing in the morning may minimise the occurrence of symptoms.

Constrictive clothing may induce breathlessness and chest tightness so should be avoided; however, the person should be advised to wrap up warmly in cold weather.

Elimination
Diuretic therapy may be indicated if there is a degree of cardiac failure present (p. 37). The timing of ingestion of these drugs can be controlled by the angina sufferer so that the ensuing diuresis does not disrupt daily routine.

Case History 2.2 Invasive treatment for angina

Mr B, from Case History 2.1, has now had the following investigations, all of which are normal: CXR, ECG, cardiac enzymes (p. 24) and weight. His serum lipids are high so, having had dietary advice, he has begun drug therapy to reduce these levels.

Cardiac catheterisation revealed that he had an 85% reduction of the lumen of the left coronary artery main stem. Mr B is advised that he should undergo percutaneous transluminal coronary angioplasty (PTCA). This is planned for the next day.

Straining at stool should be avoided. A healthy diet will help but the judicious use of a mild aperient may be indicated.

? **2.8** Read Case History 2.2.
a. What pre-procedure preparation is required?
b. How would you describe the procedure to the patient and his family?
c. What complications should you aim to prevent post procedure?

Nursing priorities: cardiac catheterisation
The patient will need to be fully informed about the procedure, (see Box 2.2, p. 17) its findings and their implications. Nurses need to be aware of the possible complications and place particular importance on pain relief.

Nursing priorities: percutaneous transluminal coronary angioplasty (PTCA)
This procedure is described in Box 2.4.

As the procedure is relatively new, the patient will almost certainly need to have it explained, and should be fully

Box 2.4 Percutaneous transluminal coronary angioplasty (PTCA)

Purpose
PTCA is a technique involving the introduction of a balloon catheter into the coronary artery up to the site of a coronary stenosis, where it is inflated. This process produces compression and redistribution of the lesion and a substantial increase in the size of the lumen. PTCA may be performed to relieve the symptoms of angina if medication is ineffective, or it may be performed soon after successful thrombolysis (see p. 24) to restore perfusion to the ischaemic zone.

Procedure
PTCA is carried out under local anaesthetic in a cardiac catheterisation laboratory. If the procedure is planned, the patient will be admitted to hospital the day before and asked to starve for 6–8 hours prior to the procedure. This is in case of complications necessitating by-pass surgery.

Usually, two arterial catheters are used: a guiding catheter and a dilating catheter. The guiding catheter is inserted, usually in the leg, and advanced to the coronary artery to be dilated. The dilating catheter is then inserted and manipulated into the stenotic area of the artery. Angiography is performed and heparin administered to avoid clot formation at the catheter site. When the dilation catheter is placed over the stenosis it is inflated for 5–6 seconds and then deflated. Blood flow around the balloon is assessed by angiography. Once it has been decided that maximum dilatation has been obtained, the catheters are removed.

Following this procedure, the patient is usually routinely attached to a cardiac monitor for 24 hours. Peripheral pulses are frequently checked for occlusive thrombus at the insertion site. The patient is advised to rest for 4–6 hours lying as flat as is comfortably possible to keep the leg used for catheter insertion straight in order to minimise the risk of thrombus formation at the insertion site. The introducer sheath is often left in situ for 2–3 hours, until the effects of heparin have been reduced.

The patient should be encouraged to drink extra fluid to help eliminate contrast medium.

Because of the risk of thrombosis and coronary artery spasm after angioplasty, patients are often prescribed calcium antagonists and antiplatelet agents.

Restenosis occurs in 15–30% of patients, more frequently within the first few months. Repeat angioplasty may be appropriate for some patients.

Possible complications
Complications tend to be sudden and include:

- myocardial infarction
- chest pain
- vagal reaction
- intimal injury
- bleeding at the puncture site
- occlusive thrombus at the puncture site
- coronary artery spasm
- coronary artery dissection.

aware of both the benefits and drawbacks of the procedure. The importance of notifying the nurse of any chest pain during or following PTCA should be stressed. The patient may require assistance with various activities of living whilst mobility is temporarily limited. He is likely to be fully mobile the day after the procedure and to be discharged home after 2 days. Discharge planning needs to include teaching about medication, risk-factor modification and follow-up assessment.

If the treatment was carried out as an emergency due to acute myocardial infarction, the patient must rest in bed for at least 24 hours, and can then follow the recovery and rehabilitation programme planned for him. Anginal pain often occurs when the balloon is inflated over the narrowed area, and the patient should be warned of this in advance. Nitrate therapy is used to control the pain, which lessens when the balloon is deflated and blood supply re-established.

If the patient has an elective angioplasty to prevent ischaemic tissue becoming infarcted, his stay in hospital will only last 3 days. The procedure does not dissolve the plaque but compresses the fluid portion of the atheroma back into the vessel walls, where reabsorption is thought to occur. Although often initially successful up to 30% of these stenoses will recur within 6 months. The procedure can be repeated again. At the time of the procedure complications such as sudden occlusion or dissection of the vessel may occur, requiring immediate cardiac surgery. For this reason most cardiology centres arrange for cover by cardiac surgeons before starting the procedure.

Nursing priorities: coronary artery bypass grafting (CABG)

This is now a routine operation performed on patients whose angina is severely limiting their lifestyles but whose left ventricle is functioning reasonably. It may also be carried out in an emergency on patients who have uncontrolled angina after an AMI or who have experienced complications after angioplasty.

The procedure is described in Box 2.5.

Bypass surgery is a potentially traumatic event and prior to the procedure, the nurse must address any worries or concerns that the patient may have. A visit to the operating theatre and the recovery room may help some patients. The patient needs to know that he will have his chest shaved prior to the operation and he may be asked to take a bath with antibacterial soap. An aperient may be required to reduce the likelihood of postoperative abdominal discomfort. The patient will be asked to fast prior to surgery and may benefit from a sedative to help him relax the night before.

The nurse should prepare the patient for what to expect on regaining consciousness, that is, an endotracheal tube, chest drains, intravenous infusions, arterial lines, urinary catheter, cardiac monitoring, and possibly a nasogastric tube. He can be taught breathing, coughing and leg exercises.

After the operation nursing objectives include:

- pain relief
- assistance with activities of living
- psychological support and
- preparation for discharge home.

Patients should be told to expect pain from the sternotomy for several weeks, leg swelling, and discomfort on coughing or lifting the hands above the head. Short-term anxiety and depression may occur if the person feels his recovery is slower than anticipated. The spouse and other family members will also need information and support.

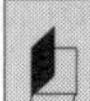
More information on recovery from coronary artery bypass grafting can be found in Wilson-Barnett & Fordham (1986).

? **2.9** In a group, discuss whether someone with persistent angina who continues to smoke warrants CABG.

? **2.10** Find out the relative costs of PTCA and CABG. What are the advantages and disadvantages of each procedure?

Box 2.5 Coronary artery bypass graft surgery (CABG)

Purpose

Coronary artery bypass graft surgery is a technique in which an occluded or stenosed section of a coronary artery is bypassed using part of a vein or artery from elsewhere in the body. Most commonly the long saphenous vein is used, although increasingly the internal mammary artery is being considered. The objectives of CABG are:

- restoration of perfusion and increased oxygenation to the ischaemic myocardium in the peri-infarction patient
- relief of angina pectoris
- improvement of functional status and quality of life
- prolongation of life.

Surgery is only feasible if the risk of the operation is less than continuing with medical therapy. The procedure tends to be offered to those who have:

- symptoms despite maximum therapy
- triple vessel disease or left main stem coronary artery stenosis
- unstable angina.

Procedure

During surgery, the heart is exposed by median sternotomy, the aorta clamped off and cardiopulmonary bypass maintained via cannulae in the atria and descending aorta. The body temperature is reduced to 32°C and cardiac arrest induced with potassium. The long saphenous vein is stripped from the patient's leg while the chest is being opened. The distal end of the bypass grafts are sutured to as many vessels as required. The aorta is then unclamped, the patient is rewarmed and normal cardiac rhythm re-established by internal defibrillation. The proximal ends of the grafts are sutured to the ascending aorta and cardiopulmonary bypass is then stopped, the cannulae are removed and the chest closed. The whole operation takes up to 4 hours.

The patient is normally cared for in an intensive care unit after the procedure and will be ventilated until he is haemodynamically stable. An arterial line and pulmonary artery flotation catheter will be used to monitor cardiac pressures for 24 hours.

The patient will usually be able to eat a solid diet on the first or second day. Activity is increased as tolerated over the first 2 days and early mobilisation is encouraged. Patients are often fit for discharge home after about a week.

Possible complications

Complications include:

- leakage at the incision site, producing discomfort and shock
- hypertension as a result of increased sympathetic activity
- hypotension as a result of reduced cardiac output following hypothermia
- pain at both the graft and incision sites
- shortness of breath due to heart failure or chest infection.

Case History 2.3

Mr B's angioplasty is unsuccessful as it has not been possible to enter the left coronary artery (LCA) and pass the balloon over the occlusion. The patient is returned to the ward after 2 hours in the cardiac catheterisation room. He is told that he can go home that evening and asked to return in 2 weeks for cardiac surgery.

? **2.11** Read Case History 2.3.

a. What information will Mr B require before discharge on the following:
   - cardiac catheterisation site
   - reasons for failure of angioplasty and what this implies
   - imminent surgery.

b. What other health professionals might you contact to provide him with information and support?

The procedures outlined above unfortunately do not stop the process of atherosclerosis; they only delay it and aim to provide the sufferer with a good quality of life for a while. All procedures can be repeated but ultimately the blood supply may become insufficient to sustain the ventricle so that cardiac failure ensues.

ACUTE MYOCARDIAL INFARCTION (AMI)

Myocardial infarction refers to the death or necrosis of a portion of myocardium as a result of reduction, interruption or cessation in blood flow.

PATHOPHYSIOLOGY

Myocardial cells require a constant supply of oxygen and nutrients in order to generate the high-energy phosphate compounds required for contraction. Generally, myocardial cells are irreversibly injured by 30–40 minutes of total ischaemia. If the lumen of an artery is blocked for about 20 minutes and blood supply by the small vessels of the surrounding collateral circulation is inadequate, myocardial infarction may develop. Surrounding the area of necrotic tissue there is usually a zone of injury. This tissue cannot contract but may be salvaged if an adequate blood supply can be quickly established. The ischaemic zone separates the zone of injury from undamaged tissue. This tissue can usually be salvaged if treatment is prompt (see Fig. 2.8).

During the first 6 hours after the onset of symptoms the affected myocardium becomes oedematous and swells. There is a shift in the distribution of sodium and potassium ions and an increased risk of arrhythmias. A summary of events following an acute myocardial infarction is shown in Table 2.3. The infarcted area is replaced by fibrous scar tissue over the course of 3–6 weeks.

The site of infarction depends on the coronary artery which has become occluded. The extent of infarction and therefore the amount of muscle involved depends on both the artery involved, the previous rate of progression of the disease and the effectiveness of the surrounding collateral circulation. About 17% of the total deaths in England and Wales each year are the result of AMI (Office of Population Censuses and Surveys 1990). In 60% of fatal myocardial infarctions, death occurs in the first hour after the attack, usually as a result of a cardiac arrhythmia. Most of these fatalities involve males. Below the age of 65 years male deaths outnumber females by a ratio of 3.6:1. Above this age, the ratio is roughly 1:1.

Myocardial infarction can occur both in people who are known to have angina, and those who are not. Pain is usually experienced about 60 seconds after the onset of ischaemia. Pain occurs in some 80% of people suffering an acute myocardial infarction but is less likely to be experienced in the elderly or those with diabetes. Pain typical of myocardial infarction often:

- occurs at rest
- awakens the individual from sleep
- is unrelieved by rest or nitrates
- lasts longer than 20 minutes
- is described as crushing, vice-like, tight or constricting in nature
- may radiate to the arms and neck.

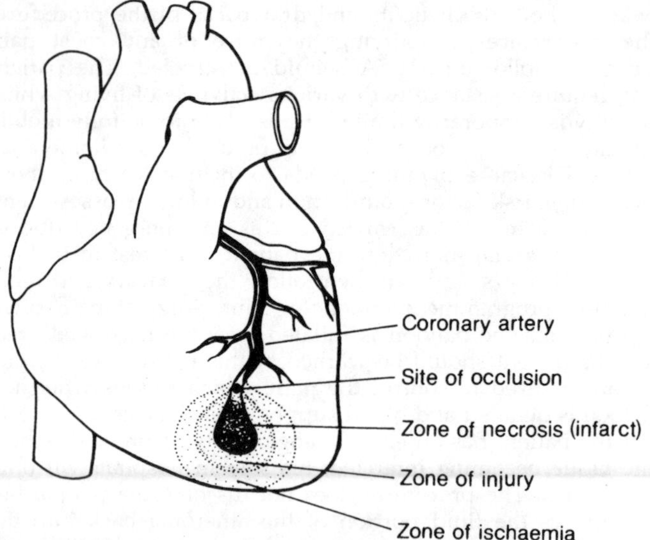

Fig. 2.8 Zones of necrosis, injury and ischaemia. (Reproduced with kind permission from Boore et al 1987.)

Table 2.3 Events following AMI (Adapted, with kind permission, from Boore et al 1987)

Length of time following AMI event	
0–6 hours	Cellular breakdown No electrical impulses conducted Necrosis occurs
24 hours	Phagocytosis occurs in the infarcted area
5 days	Area infiltrated by fibroblasts, capillaries and collagen tissue Reperfusion of capillaries
2–3 wks	Fibrosis occurs
2–3 mths	Ventricular scarring

Other signs and symptoms may include:

- shortness of breath at rest, on exertion or when lying flat
- hyperventilation as a result of anxiety
- change in cardiac rhythm or rate
- change in blood pressure
- change in level of consciousness
- increased anxiety or restlessness
- pallor
- sweaty or clammy skin
- nausea and vomiting
- cyanosis.

MEDICAL MANAGEMENT

Management strategies aim to re-establish perfusion, decrease the work of the myocardium, and prevent and eradicate life-threatening complications. Patients may be managed at home, on a general medical or elderly ward, or on a coronary care unit. Because of the high mortality outside hospital, certain areas have developed mobile coronary care units whose aim is to enable trained personnel to reach the patient as soon as possible after the onset of symptoms.

History and examination. The history provides subjective information about the presenting symptoms, previous patterns of health and illness, and the activities of living. A family history of ischaemic heart disease together with risk-factor identification and social and psychological background adds to the picture.

It may be inappropriate to obtain a full history if the patient is in pain or acutely ill. An initial assessment can be enough to set early priorities, without a full physical examination or diagnostic tests.

Clinical examination includes:

- observation of general appearance, build, body posture and facial expression
- assessment of the location, nature and severity of the pain, any relieving or aggravating factors, and attempted methods of pain relief
- observation of other signs of reduced cardiac output
- vital signs: arrhythmias are common; blood pressure may be low with reduced cardiac output or high due to pain and anxiety
- temperature: slight pyrexia is a common response to muscle damage
- auscultation, usually performed by medical staff, involves using a stethoscope to listen to the sounds the heart makes throughout the cardiac cycle, to identify heart murmurs produced by changes in the force and direction of blood flow
- palpation, usually performed by medical staff, and involving a systematic examination of the chest to feel for abnormal vibrations or pulsations.

Investigation will be as follows.

Electrocardiogram may show characteristic changes pinpointing the area of ventricle affected. Early ECGs may appear normal so a series is necessary. The classic infarct change is ST elevation (see Fig. 2.9).

Blood tests

- Cardiac enzymes. Myocardial necrosis results in the release of certain intracellular enzymes into the circulating blood. The rate and pattern of release is important (see Table 2.4).
- White cell count. This is usually elevated for the first few days following acute myocardial infarction.
- Erythrocyte sedimentation rate (ESR). This usually rises after the first few days and may remain elevated for several weeks.
- Glucose. Stress-related hyperglycaemia is common in the acute phase following infarction. Previously undetected diabetes is found in about 5% of coronary patients admitted to hospital.
- Electrolytes. It is important to know serum sodium and potassium levels as these electrolytes can have a major effect on cell excitability.
- Lipids. The important lipids in ischaemic heart disease are plasma cholesterol and triglycerides.

Chest X-ray may show evidence of pulmonary oedema or hypertrophy.

MEDICAL TREATMENT

Pain relief. IV opiates are used, usually diamorphine, together with an anti-emetic.

Limit infarct size by:

Increasing myocardial oxygen supply through:

- thrombolytic therapy (see Box 2.6)
- nitrate therapy
- supplemental oxygen therapy
- coronary artery surgery
- percutaneous transluminal coronary angioplasty (PTCA) (see p. 20).

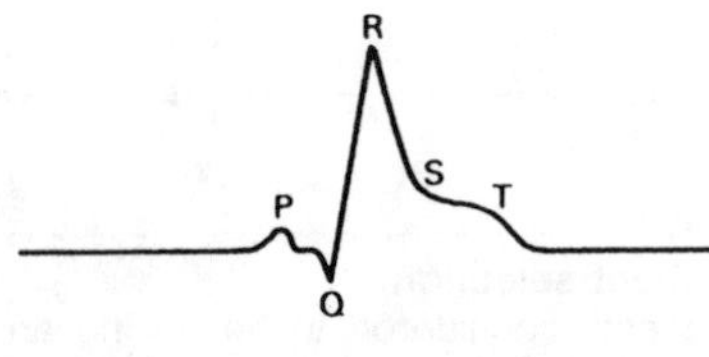

0-6 Hours post-infarction
S-T elevation

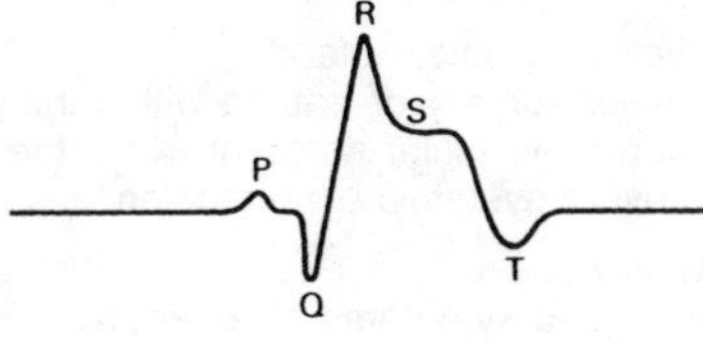

6-24 Hours post-infarction
Abnormal Q wave
S-T elevation
T wave inversion

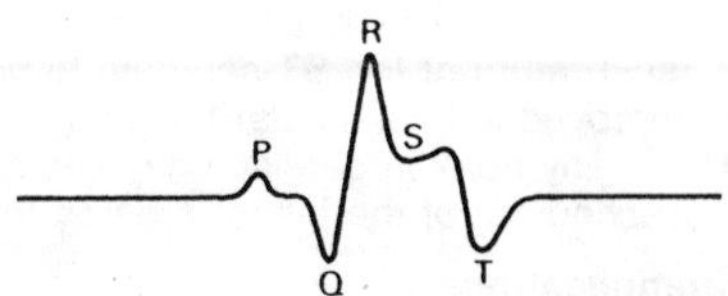

12 Hours — 14 days post-infarction
Abnormal Q wave
S-T elevation less than previously
T wave inversion

Long-term—Abnormal Q waves usually persist indefinitely but may resolve in inferior infarcts

—S-T elevation resolves in inferior infarcts in 2 weeks but persists in 40% of all infarcts and may be associated with aneurysm formation

—T wave inversion may persist or resolve

Fig. 2.9 ECG changes in myocardial infarction. (Reproduced with kind permission from Boore et al 1987.)

Table 2.4 Enzyme-level changes following AMI

Enzyme	Released into circulation		Range
	Initially	Peaks	(Normal)
Creatinine phosphokinase (CPK)	6 hr	18–36 hr	200–1000 u/ml (100 u/ml)
Serum aspartate transferase formerly glutamic oxaloacetic transaminase (SGOT)	12–24 hr	36–48 hr	> 100 u/ml (50 u/ml)
Lactic dehydrogenase (LDH)	2–3 days	7 days	

Decreasing myocardial oxygen demand through cardiac depressant drugs, for example, beta-blockers.

Prevention of complications. AMI is a very serious condition in the early stages, although the risks diminish rapidly after the first 48 hours. AMIs affect different areas of the heart and therefore put the patient at risk of various complications. Careful observation of the patient will help in the prevention or at least early treatment of these complications to prevent them becoming life threatening.

NURSING PRIORITIES AND MANAGEMENT: THROMBOLYTIC THERAPY

The nurse needs to be aware of patient selection criteria and appreciate the importance of prompt medical attention for prospective candidates for thrombolysis.

As thrombolysis is a relatively new development, the nurse should explain to the patient its benefits and potential problems. It is important that she is aware of possible complications so that she can monitor and observe appropriately.

People who have been thrombolysed receive a card, on discharge, indicating the drug they received and when. Changes in drug regimes are ongoing in response to research findings and the nurse should keep up to date with these. Thrombolysis does not have any effect on the underlying cause of thrombus formation and patients may require subsequent mechanical recanalisation with either PTCA or surgery.

For further information about the use of thrombolytic therapy, see Bradbury & Cruickshank (1993).

NURSING PRIORITIES AND MANAGEMENT: ACUTE MYOCARDIAL INFARCTION

Not all people who have had an AMI will be admitted to hospital. Studies carried out before the use of thrombolytic therapy showed that the elderly with uncomplicated acute myocardial infarctions, particularly those who lived some distance from a hospital, would be better off at home. These people will need input from their GP and community nursing services. Priorities of care and information for recovery will be based on the same principles as those for the patient admitted to hospital.

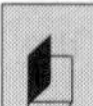

For further details of the home versus hospital debate see Thompson & Webster (1992b).

Most patients admitted to hospital are likely to benefit from admission to a coronary care unit. These units were first established in the 1960s in order to provide surveillance from skilled personnel with electrocardiographic and resuscitation facilities in a specialised setting.

Possible patient problems include:

Box 2.6 Thrombolytic therapy

Purpose
The primary aim in limiting infarct size is the rapid recanalisation of the occluded coronary artery. Occlusion is most often caused by a thrombus at the site of a ruptured atheromatous plaque. The aim of thrombolysis is to induce dissolution of the thrombus through the administration of an intravenous drug in order to establish recanalisation and provide subsequent reperfusion to the ischaemic zone. Thrombolysis is the single most important advance in coronary care since defibrillation.

Action
Optimal benefit results when the thrombolytic drug is given promptly after the onset of chest pain, although it is considered worthwhile administering the treatment up to 12 hours later. The main thrombolytic drugs currently available are:

Streptokinase, to date, the most widely tested and used, and also the cheapest. It is a bacterial protein whose administration results in a systemic lytic state, with reduced levels of circulating fibrinogen and clotting factors V and VIII. Once given, a patient cannot receive this drug again for at least 4 years.

Recombinant tissue-type plasminogen activator (tPA), a naturally occurring human protease that is fibrin specific and thus works predominantly on the clot, with less risk of systemic bleeding.

Anistreplase (APSAC). Like tPA this agent attains high concentrations at the site of the clot so that systemic effects are minimised. It also has the advantage that it can be given as a bolus over a few minutes.

Patient selection
Patients considered to be having an acute myocardial infarction, with the onset of symptoms within the previous 12 hours. Contraindications include:

- active or recent bleed
- major surgery or trauma within the previous month
- cerebrovascular accident within the previous 3 months
- severe systemic hypertension.

Reperfusion
Signs and symptoms of reperfusion may include:

- abrupt cessation of chest pain
- reperfusion arrhythmias or conduction disturbances
- rapid return of the ST-segment to normal
- improved left-ventricular function
- an early peak in cardiac enzymes as a result of enzymes being washed out of the infarct area by the reperfused artery.

Complications
These include:

- bleeding episodes (including rarely cerebral bleeds)
- reperfusion arrhythmias
- allergic reactions
- hypotension.

- pain and discomfort
- fear and anxiety
- decreased activity levels
- lack of knowledge and understanding
- misconceptions
- altered activities of living
- loss of control
- ineffective or inappropriate coping responses.

Immediate priorities

The priorities on admission to hospital include:

- cardiac monitoring (see Table 2.5)
- establishment of intravenous access
- relief of pain and anxiety
- decrease in the workload of the heart.

In the acute phase, nursing management is aimed at:

- observation for signs of complications
- rehabilitation and recovery.

Maintaining a safe environment

The nurse is responsible for her patient's safety. This involves being aware of possible complications and how they are likely to present. The temptation to respond to monitor tracings without assessing the patient needs to be avoided.

Pain control. The patient needs to be kept free from pain. Pain is a sign of ongoing myocardial ischaemia and needs to be controlled. Patients should be told of the importance of reporting pain.

Accurate pain assessment is essential to ensure that appropriate analgesia is given. Assessment scales, where patients rate their pain numerically, can be useful, as nurses have been shown to be unreliable in assessing cardiac pain (Bondestam et al 1987). Ischaemic pain can easily be confused with pain from other sources, particularly pericarditic or pleuritic pain (see Table 2.6). Opiates are the first line analgesics for ischaemic pain and diamorphine intravenously is the drug of choice. It is likely to produce beneficial effects through:

- decreasing anxiety through action on the central nervous system
- vasodilation of the peripheral circulation
- central nervous system sedation and primary analgesia through stimulation of opiate receptors.

Intravenous diamorphine reaches its peak effect within 20 minutes of administration. Undesirable effects include:

- nausea and vomiting, due to reduced gut motility, so should be given with an anti-emetic
- depressant effects on the central nervous system, so the antidote naloxone should be available
- hypotension if vasodilation occurs alongside hypovolaemia
- dry mouth and slow heart rate as a result of decreased sympathetic activity.

Table 2.5 Observing the cardiac monitor

Rate	Is it fast/slow/normal?
Rhythm	Is it irregular/regular?
'P' waves	Are they present/absent?
'QRST' complex	Is each complex preceded by a P wave? Is each complex the same?
'P-R' interval	Is it normal/prolonged?
Ectopics (extras)	Are there any extra P waves or extra QRST complexes?

Table 2.6 Characteristics of chest pain

Description	Location	Medical diagnosis
Tight like a band around the central chest. Precipitated by cold, exercise, large meals emotion. Usually relieved by rest & GTN.	Central chest Radiating to jaw, shoulders and arms usually on left side	Angina pectoris
As above but not relieved by GTN or other measures. Lasts longer & more severe	As above	Myocardial infarction
Stabbing or burning pain. Worse an deep inspiration, often relieved by bending forward.	Substernal and often affecting the trapezius muscle and upper abdominal area	Pericarditis
Sudden sharp pain, worsened by inspiration. Dyspnoea, cough, cyanosis & possible haemoptysis	Lateral very often	Pulmonary embolus
Excruciating pain 'burning' towards the spine	Intrascapular region	Dissecting aneurysm

? **2.12** In a group, discuss how the management of cardiac ischaemic pain might differ for the person cared for on a coronary care unit and someone cared for on a general medical ward.

Warn the patient to expect episodes of pain after discharge as he needs to be aware of the importance of reducing activity; how to use glyceryl trinitrate (GTN); and how to distinguish between angina and another heart attack.

GTN should be taken before doing something that produces pain. It should be taken sublingually and the person should sit down after taking it, to minimise the risk of fainting. Pain should be resolved 5–10 minutes after taking the drug. Once the pain has gone, any remaining tablet should be spat out or swallowed.

GTN can produce unpleasant side effects such as flushing and headache due to generalised vasodilation. If one tablet is ineffective, the dose can be repeated but medical help should be obtained (an ambulance is often quicker than the general practitioner) if severe pain still persists after 20 minutes. For effective use, GTN needs to be:

- stored in a cool glass container without cotton wool
- stored at a temperature not exceeding 25°C
- replaced after 8 weeks of opening the bottle.

Observation of all vital signs is aimed at early detection of complications.

Pulse. The ECG will be continually monitored on a screen. Knowledge of the normal rhythm is vital and diagnosis of arrhythmias is part of the CCU nurse's role. Deviations from the normal must be acted upon immediately. Someone who is in pain or who is anxious may be tachycardic (heart rate > 100 bpm) and these causes should be excluded.

Blood pressure. Recording the patient's blood pressure is a means of assessing how effectively blood is being pumped from the left ventricle. Frequency of recordings needs to be balanced against the patient's need for undisturbed rest. A fall in blood pressure may indicate that further damage or complications are occurring and certainly indicates reduced supply to the vital organs. The cardiac output can also be assessed by examining perfusion in the peripheries.

Temperature. Pyrexia as a response to muscle damage is normal in the first 48 hours, following which it should settle. Continued pyrexia may indicate pericarditis.

Respiration. The patient with AMI is given oxygen therapy in conjunction with analgesia on admission, to ensure oxygen uptake in the lungs is optimised. Dyspnoea may indicate hypoxia or the onset of pulmonary oedema, a serious complication. It can also be induced by anxiety. Raised anxiety levels in coronary patients admitted to hospital have been well documented, with serial measurements generally showing that anxiety is highest on admission to the coronary care unit (Thompson 1990).

To exclude anxiety from masking more serious complications the patient may benefit from the use of anxiolytics for a short period, particularly at night. Pain must also be controlled.

Ongoing care

The majority of life-threatening problems develop within the first 48 hours and after this time the patient will be transferred to the ward. Initially, he should be in the area of the ward most continuously observed by nurses, which is generally around the nurses' station. The move usually induces anxiety and the patient will be aware that the nurse–patient ratio has been reduced. Explaining that the immediate danger period is over and that he is now beginning to recover will help convey optimism to the patient and family. Ideally, the transfer can be planned well in advance and the nursing staff on the ward should take time to discuss natural fears and vulnerability.

These same feelings are likely to resurface as the time of discharge from hospital approaches and again nursing staff must prepare both the patient and the family to resume their life as an integral unit. See Nursing Care Plan 2.1.

Both in the coronary care unit and on the ward the patient needs to have within reach articles he is likely to need, for example, a glass of water, a book, or an oxygen mask. This minimises danger and inconvenience when trying to reach these articles.

Any restrictions such as not smoking and limited activity should be fully explained. Although certain activities should ideally be avoided, the patient may feel less stress if permitted a low level of involvement, for example, the business man who requires to continue working may rest more easily if he has limited contact with his secretary.

Communicating

Someone who has suffered an AMI is likely to be worried about the eventual outcome. Some people are able to express their feelings openly but others may be labelled awkward or difficult patients. The nurse should try to probe beneath outward signs such as hostility, withdrawal and denial to ensure they are not masking fear. She should keep the patient informed of his progress and how it will affect his stay in hospital. Communication skills are important to CCU nurses and answers to questions should be honest and supportive (Ashworth 1984). The hospital chaplain or the patient's own spiritual adviser may be of help in this area.

Communication must also extend to the family. They experience shock and anxiety on seeing their loved one in such an environment, and will fear for his survival. The attitude of the partner has been shown to be determined during the time the patient is in the CCU. Caplin and Sexton (1988) showed that the major stress areas during this time related to the possibility of the death of their loved one and trying not to upset the patient. High on their list of stresses was the lack of information about the patient and being kept waiting at visiting times without knowing why. The family's main need is to feel that there is hope (Norris and Grove 1986), although other needs include support from the family and health professionals and the need for information and relief from anxiety.

Stresses can be reduced if the nurse spends time with the relatives, both when they are visiting and when they are alone so that fears and worries can be expressed. Frequent and adequate information about the equipment and the patient's progress is vital. The family member whose trust is gained can be a source of information to the nurse and an ally in helping reduce anxiety in the patient. Unrestricted visiting for designated close family members is also useful in reducing anxiety.

Appropriate advice for the patient and family in hospital may include (see Research Abstract 2.1).

- explaining the structure and function of the heart as a pump, where it lies in the body, and how it works
- explaining how a heart attack occurs, narrowing of the coronary arteries, obstruction and heart muscle damage
- describing symptoms and explaining terminology
- outlining the reasons for admission and treatment
- explaining the healing process, muscle damage, swelling, scar formation and the healing period
- discussing the outlook for the future and the need to accept the illness
- describing the likely mobility level
- explaining the reasons for stopping smoking
- explaining how to recognise possible limiting factors in physical activity
- explaining the residual symptoms
- giving advice on diet, social activities and sexual life
- giving advice on resuming work
- being prepared for changes in mood, anxiety, depression, etc
- preparation of the partner and family.

Preparation for discharge

Patients and their families need to be prepared for rehabilitation and recovery. Cay (1982) identifies various issues raised by patients one month after a heart attack:

- uncertainty about what constitutes a safe level of exercise
- over-protectiveness by the family
- conflicting advice from the hospital and family doctors
- when to return to work and strenuous activity
- boredom and irritability at home
- concern over angina and breathlessness
- the reason for the heart attack
- uncertainty about informing the insurance company and Department of Social Security
- concern over the use of GTN
- the need for definite guidelines about resuming work, sexual relations, driving, drinking and leisure activities
- the need for definite guidelines about the amount of weight to lose and how to stop smoking.

Both community and hospital nurses have a role in tackling many of the above issues, so that the sufferer and family are equipped to cope with recovery and future lifestyle. There are an increasing number of coronary rehabilitation nurses who visit both in hospital and at home. The first 2 or 3 weeks at home can be the most stressful for the person and family, particularly the spouse, as they attempt to come to terms with a frightening and often unexpected event (Thompson et al 1987). Coronary rehabilitation programmes that offer individualised packages of information and support on both a one-to-one and group-session basis, in addition to a graduated

Nursing Care Plan 2.1 M is a 58-year-old company secretary who had an MI 4 days previously. She is due to be discharged from hospital in 2 days' time. The admission to hospital was sudden and unexpected and the diagnosis has come as a shock to M, her husband and their two teenage children. M's father died from an MI at the age of 59. M smokes 20 cigarettes per day. Despite the diagnosis M is talking about going back to work in 3 weeks' time and is reluctant to cancel a holiday abroad booked for 2 weeks' time.

Nursing considerations	Action	Rationale	Evaluation
1. Pain/discomfort **a) may experience recurrence of ischaemic chest pain** **b) may not know how to cope with recurrence of pain**	• Assess any pain with M, noting nature, severity, location, radiation, frequency and duration and aggravating/relieving factors • Administer appropriate analgesia: GTN for angina and evaluate effect • Minimise likelihood of ischaemic pain by advising M to space activities, rest during pain, avoid extremes of temperature and humidity, and use GTN as a prophylactic measure • Advise M about the difference between pain of angina and MI and ensure she feels confident about use of GTN and knows when to call for medical help	• It is not uncommon for patients to experience episodes of angina post-MI • Chest pain occurs as a result of metabolic changes brought about by myocardial schaemia	• Is pain free and comfortable • Feels confident about coping with further episodes of chest pain
2. Decreased activity levels	• Reinforce reasoning behind reduced activity levels and stress the need to gradually increase activity/exercise over the next few weeks • Establish previous levels of activity and discuss desired levels for recovery. Plan a programme for resumption of activity and exercise • Refer to cardiac rehabilitation programme and arrange physiotherapist to visit to discuss exercises	• Activity intolerance occurs due to imbalance between myocardial oxygen supply and demand • Pain, shortness of breath, lethargy and fear of aggravating condition may limit activity • Gradual increase in activity/exercise levels helps promote recovery, both physical and psychological	• Understands the rationale behind limited activity levels • Feels confident about gradually resuming pre-infarct activity levels and understands the importance of regular exercise
3. Lack of knowledge/ understanding	• Ensure that M and her husband understand: — the nature of ischaemic heart disease — what a heart attack is — treatment — the recovery process • Discuss risk factors, particularly smoking and hereditary aspects, and provide realistic guidelines for modifying risk factors where appropriate • Set individualised goals for activity levels during recovery and include information about — general activity — housework — leisure — return to work — driving — sexual activity • Teach M and her husband about medication • Encourage participation in outpatient cardiac rehabilitation programme • Make aware about plans for discharge, follow-up, etc	• Successful recovery depends on a gradual return to a healthy lifestyle • Reducing risk factors by modifying lifestyle may limit the recurrence of problems	• Demonstrates realistic expectations for the future and appears to have knowledge/understanding of condition, treatment and implications for the future • Feels prepared for discharge and recovery

Nursing Care Plan 2.1 ***(cont'd)***

Nursing considerations	Action	Rationale	Evaluation
4. Altered activities of living, e.g. • **breathing**	• Ensure that M is aware of the significance of shortness of breath, knows to report increased incidence to GP together with oedema, and understands her diuretic therapy	• Shortness of breath may occur due to pulmonary oedema as a result of the heart's inability to pump effectively	• Normal activities of living are maintained after discharge according to wishes and condition • M is prepared for any alterations in activities of living and feels able to cope
• **sleeping**	• Discuss the possibility that altered rest and sleep patterns may occur after discharge: advise to avoid too many visitors and encourage taking a nap in the afternoon and spacing out activities	• Anxiety, pain, alterations in activity levels may interfere with rest and sleep	
• **diet/nutrition**	• Advise about a healthy diet, stressing that meals should be enjoyed and any changes in diet need to be longterm. M isn't overweight and has normal cholesterol levels	• A healthy diet rather than a strict dietary regime is to be recommended	
• **sexuality**	• Ensure M appreciates when she can resume sexual activity	• Many post-MI patients worry that sexual activity will cause a further heart attack. In reality, this risk is extremely small	
5. Inappropriate and/or ineffective coping mechanisms	• Discuss normal coping mechanisms in a crisis	• Inappropriate coping mechanisms may impair recovery and reduce quality of life	• Appears to be confident, well adjusted and demonstrating appropriate coping responses
• **appears to be showing some signs of denying the significance of the heart attack**	• Discuss with M and her family their feelings about her condition, ways of coping and outlook for the future — correct misconceptions — offer realistic outlook — encourage sense of control • Discuss and implement stress reduction techniques, such as relaxation • Prepare for possible changes in mood states after discharge • Offer post-discharge support; refer to rehabilitation programme • Offer realistic guidelines for going abroad and returning to work	• Suffering a heart attack is likely to be a frightening experience leading to various coping responses, especially anxiety and depression, masking as denial	• Feels in control of own recovery and optimistic for the future

programme of exercises, have the potential to restore the individual to an optimum level of recovery (physical, emotional, economic and vocational) and to minimise the risk of the underlying disease progressing. It is now recommended that every major district hospital treating people with heart disease should provide such a cardiac rehabilitation service (Duddy & Parahoo 1992 and Horgan et al 1992).

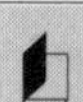

For further information on coronary rehabilitation see Wenger & Hellerstein (1992).

? **2.13** Find out about coronary rehabilitation services offered locally. What do you think are the benefits of such a programme?

Mobility

In hospital. While experiencing symptoms such as pain and dyspnoea, the patient should remain in bed, and receive analgesia and oxygen therapy. The reasons for limiting activity, and that it is only for a short period, should be explained. As symptoms resolve, then activity levels can increase.

In recent years the trend has been toward resuming activity early. This allows the person to carry out activities such as washing, using the commode and carrying out passive and active limb exercises. Periods of gentle activity should be followed by frequent rest periods and all activity should be stopped if the patient experiences pain, dyspnoea or palpitations. The ability to increase activity gradually is a positive reinforcement for recovery and the patient's family will also experience relief at seeing the patient regain independence.

By the time of discharge, usually after 5 or 6 days, the

Research Abstract 2.1 Patient education after myocardial infarction

How do you decide the content of a patient-education programme? What do you teach? Do patients feel that they need or want to know the information you provide? What do patients actually learn? When is the best time to learn?

In a study of 30 post-MI patients, Chan (1990) explored the views of patients pre- and post-discharge regarding *how important* and *how realistic* it was to learn the material presented.

It was found that most content areas, for example, anatomy and physiology, diet, medication, physical activity, psychological factors and risk factors were viewed as important for learning, pre-discharge. However, all content areas were not of equal value. Some items such as 'how the heart works' and 'what the heart looks like' were given low ratings. This might have been related to different basic levels of insight and understanding of the body and disease processes. It may not always be wise, therefore, to introduce basic concepts of normal heart function before discussing myocardial infarction. What the nurse thinks is important may not be what the patient most wants to know.

It was also found that it was more realistic for patients to learn about illness and its management during early convalescence than pre-discharge. Readiness to learn and timing of teaching are therefore as important as content of teaching. Pre-discharge, patients may be physically debilitated and psychologically stressed and less able to attend to teaching and learning. Follow-up education to reinforce and extend hospital-based education is important. Patient education pre- and post-discharge should be carefully planned and evaluated.

Chan V 1990 Content areas for cardiac teaching: patients' perceptions of the importance of teaching content after myocardial infarction. Journal of Advanced Nursing 15(10): 1139–1145

person should be fully independent in the activities of daily living.

Some centres have programmes in which the patient can chart his progress towards specific goals (see Box 2.7). In other centres, activity is increased on a much less formal basis and the nurse can point out to the patient that he is making progress. Realistic aims, both pre- and post-discharge are important.

The patient should be prepared to have good and bad days and be aware of symptoms that suggest he is doing too much, such as pain, palpitations, dyspnoea, fatigue and dizziness.

At home. Graduated physical activity should permit a return to previous daily activities over a 6–12-week period and, if applicable, return to work after about 8 weeks. The ultimate aim should be to take some exercise at least three times a week. Recommended exercise after 6–8 weeks includes walking, swimming, and cycling, for 15–20 minutes at a time.

The activity plan for convalescence needs to be based on a knowledge of the person's functional capacity, interests, previous lifestyle, needs for the future and home environment. Any inhibiting factors such as arthritis also need to be acknowledged. Many hospitals now offer formal structured exercise programmes as part of a coronary rehabilitation programme. Progressive exercise programmes may reduce cardiovascular mortality (O'Connor et al 1989). However, such programmes might not begin for 3–6 weeks after discharge and the patient needs specific advice to prepare for the first few weeks at home. For example, most patients will be able to walk 2 miles a day at the end of 4 weeks. Patients can resume driving 4 weeks after an uncomplicated myocardial infarction, although HGV drivers have to show evidence of a negative exercise test. Return to work provides increased self-satisfaction, restored self-respect and relief from financial worries, although early retirement may be a more realistic option for some. Occupational health and community nurses can support the patient and family throughout convalescence. Increased emphasis is being placed on cardiac rehabilitation

Research Abstract 2.2 Self-administration of medicines by elderly patients following discharge from a medical unit: the effect of a personal medication record card

Elderly patients are becoming increasingly dependent upon medicines for effective disease management and symptom control. The problems associated with self-administration practices among the elderly include difficulties in identifying regimes, administering medicines in the correct amount at the correct time, and problems with opening child-resistant containers. Some of these problems may be prevented by providing patients with additional information about the regime.

This study describes the benefits of providing elderly patients with complementary written information about their medication regimes. The aim of the study was to measure the effect of a Personal Medication Record Card (independent variable) — (see Fig. 2.10) on the information which an elderly patient could recall about his/her medication (dependent variables — name, purpose and physical description of the medicines; the amount and timing of each dose and the special instructions attached to the medicine). An intervention study incorporating a pre-experimental design coupled with a quasi-action research approach was used. The record card was developed with the assistance of medical, nursing and pharmacy staff from the experimental ward. Information was collected from 24 patients (61–95 years) who received the card (experimental ward) and 24 patients (62–91 years) who did not receive the card (control ward). Patients participating in the study were visited 2–5 days following discharge from hospital and a newly developed and tested interview schedule was used to elicit information about their prescribed medicines. Most of the information was coded and analysed using a computerised statistical package (SPSS-X).

Patients responded favourably to the card, using it as a memory aid, reminding them of when to take their medicines. Of equal importance was the reassurance provided by the card that they were administering their regimes correctly.

The results also highlighted differences between the groups. When each of the dependent variables was examined it was shown that patients who received the card were able to recall more information about three of the variables (the name of the medicine, the purpose of the medicine and the special instructions attached to the medicine).

Another finding was that patients had difficulty in opening child-resistant containers, foil and blister packaging, and that they adopted 'unsafe practices' to make their medicines accessible such as leaving lids off containers and transferring medicines to other bottles.

This study has demonstrated that informational care can successfully be developed as a multi-disciplinary team activity. It has also supported the role of the qualified nurse (in both institutional and community settings) in the area of information provision as many have the necessary expertise to assess the patient's ability to self-administer medicines and thereafter to plan, implement and evaluate appropriate management strategies.

Whyte L A 1992 Self-administration of medicines by elderly patients following discharge from a medical unit: the effect of a personal medication record card. Unpublished MPhil Thesis, University of Edinburgh.

Date	Name and strength	Purpose	Timings: Break-fast	Midday meal	Evening meal	Bedtime snack	As required	Special instructions
4.8.94	Atenolol 100 mg	Angina	1					Do not stop taking except on doctor's advice
4.8.94	Aspirin 75 mg	Circulation	2					Take with or after food
9.9.94	Glyceryl Trinitrate 300 mcg	Angina pain					1	Dissolve under the tongue Discard 8 weeks after opening
10.11.94	Ampicillin 250 mg	Chest infection	1	1	1	1		Take 1 hour before food Complete the course

Fig. 2.10 Sample: personal medication record card (Whyte 1992)

Box 2.7 A typical exercise programme for a patient following AMI

PHASE 1 (In the coronary care unit)

Step 1
- rest in bed. Out to chair for short periods
- 2-hourly passive range of motion exercises
- twice-daily breathing exercises
- independent with personal cleansing at bedside, i.e. wash hands and face
- use bedside commode.

Step 2
- up to sit unlimited by bedside
- walk around bed area.

PHASE 2 (In the ward area)

Step 3
- walk to bathroom/toilet
- personal cleansing in bathroom on chair.

Step 4
- unrestricted walking in ward area
- sit in day room if desired
- shower/bath unaided.

Step 5
- climb one flight of stairs
- increase exercises, e.g. use of exercise bike.

PHASE 3 (Early days at home)

Step 6 (First week at home)
- stay within own home/garden
- use the stairs 2–3 times daily
- undertake any activity that involves standing for short periods, e.g. washing-up, dusting, shaving
- keep as active as possible and walk around little and often.

Step 7 (Second week)
- walk approximately 100 yards on flat ground, increasing by approximately 10 yards daily, e.g. walk to the corner shop
- use stairs 4–5 times daily.

Step 8 (Third week)
- walk 250–300 yards; two or three times a day
- use stairs as normal
- begin to do light shopping, gardening or housework
- take a bus.

Step 9 (Fourth week onwards)
- begin to resume a normal way of life; participate in most normal daily activities, avoiding heavy gardening, moving heavy furniture, etc.
- begin to take regular exercise, e.g. swimming and walking, progressing gradually
- start driving again.

as hospital stays become shorter and the government targets cardiovascular disease (Department of Health 1992).

For further information on activity levels and exercise programmes see Thompson & Webster (1992b).

The aim for all patients is that they will be able to resume their daily lifestyle without physical symptoms, but this depends on their residual left ventricular function. An important part of the rehabilitation process is teaching the person and family how to live with these new limitations. If there is residual ischaemic tissue and angina, drug therapy will help control this (see p. 17).

Breathing
Oxygen therapy should be given alongside analgesia, to ensure maximal relief of pain. A semi-upright position also eases breathing. Smoking is not permitted if oxygen therapy is being given and the patient should be encouraged to give up this habit. Anxious people often hyperventilate and, here, deep breathing exercises may help.

Sleeping
The importance of punctuating exercise with rest periods is vital and people should be encouraged to have catnaps at home. In hospitals night sedation may help the patient settle in a strange environment with a high noise level. Interventions need to be co-ordinated to allow the patient undisturbed periods or rest. A patient who is unable to sleep at night, often becomes worried and anxious. An observant nurse can talk to the patient and help put these fears into perspective.

Fear of dying
This is a very real fear for someone who has had an AMI. Once the initial fear has subsided the patient has to come to terms with the cause of AMI and the consequences of atherosclerosis. Complications with a high mortality rate occur at two stages:

- in the first 48 hours, when cardiogenic shock and arrhythmias cause death
- 7–10 days later, due to myocardial rupture and ventricular septal defect.

Family fears of death must also be discussed. If not put

into perspective, relatives can become overprotective once the person returns home.

Diet and nutrition

In the early stages of AMI the patient may have little appetite and opiates may induce nausea. Anti-emetics should always be given in conjunction with opiates. Dietary advice needs to be tailored to the individual and will be similar to that given to those with angina pectoris.

Eliminating

Fluid balance is a vital means of assessing renal function, as 25% of cardiac output goes to the kidneys. If left ventricular function is compromised fluid intake may be restricted to prevent the onset of cardiac failure and pulmonary oedema (p. 38). Electrolyte balance must also be maintained within normal limits and any deviations from normal acted upon.

Potassium regulation is important in the cardiac patient as both low and high levels of serum potassium lead to life-threatening arrhythmias. Hypokalaemia causes ECG changes and increases the susceptibility to digoxin therapy and therefore toxicity. It can result from acidosis and diuretic therapy with insufficient potassium replacement. Hyperkalaemia in the cardiac patient also results in bradycardia and heart block, and leads to other ventricular arrhythmias. Causes include renal failure and tissue breakdown, which leads to large amounts of intracellular potassium being released into the circulation.

Sodium levels also require to be kept within normal limits. Assessment for obvious signs of fluid overload, such as oedema in the ankles and other dependent parts, and a daily weight check are also part of fluid-balance monitoring.

An increased workload is placed on the heart if there is straining at stool to aid defaecation. Aperients may be used to soften stools and attention should be paid to diet. A commode is usually easier to use than a bedpan and even someone confined to bed is likely to expend less energy using a commode than balancing on a bedpan (Winslow et al 1984).

Personal hygiene

Initially the patient with AMI will be dependent on nursing staff but this is one of the first areas where independence can quickly be regained. It is possible even in bed to wash the face and upper body and by discharge to be fully independent. It is safer not to lock the bathroom door, in case of emergency, and the family should discuss how to maintain the person's privacy while using the bathroom.

Expressing sexuality

Although discussion of this intimate aspect of life is often a difficult process, sexual counselling should be an integral part of cardiac rehabilitation (Thompson 1990). The severity of the infarction and resulting cardiac decompensation are much less important causes of sexual debility than the person's psychological state. Up to three quarters of coronary patients have been shown to reduce their sexual activity (Papadopoulos 1989). Reasons for not resuming previous levels of activity include:

- fear of chest pain or another heart attack
- feelings of depression
- partner concern about symptoms
- poor sexual advice from health professionals.

The energy levels and demands placed on the heart during sexual intercourse are comparable to walking briskly or climbing two flights of stairs. It is very rare for sexual intercourse to trigger off another heart attack and as a general guide sex can usually be resumed about 2 weeks after discharge, although touching and caressing may be comfortable for some earlier than this.

The subject of sex is best approached as a routine part of the rehabilitation of all coronary patients and their partners. The patient needs to feel at ease and the nurse needs to be well informed and prepared for questions. The aim of sexual advice is to restore the couple to approximately pre-infarction levels of sexual activity (Jones 1992).

Complications of AMI

There are a considerable number of complications of AMI, listed in Box 2.8. It is not possible to look at each in detail, however, the nurse should be able to recognise and report the following major problems, and carry out the appropriate nursing intervention.

Cardiac arrest

Cardiac arrest may be defined as the failure of the heart to pump sufficient blood to keep the brain alive. The three main mechanisms of cardiac arrest are:

- ventricular fibrillation (VF)
- ventricular asystole
- electromechanical dissociation (EMD).

Brain death usually occurs because of the failure of oxygenation of brain cells associated either with failure in ventilation or failure of the heart to pump oxygenated blood to the brain. The brain can only tolerate 4–6 minutes of anoxia. The signs of cardiac arrest are:

- abrupt loss of consciousness
- absent carotid and femoral pulses
- absent respirations.

A rapidly developing pallor often associated with cyanosis follows. Apnoea, gasping and gagging may occur.

The risk of sudden death in AMI patients is great. In 25% of cases this occurs within minutes of the onset of pain, before the patient has reached hospital. The nurse must be familiar with resuscitation procedures within the hospital but should also know how to perform basic cardio-pulmonary resuscitation (CPR) without hospital technology. If she can administer CPR in the community setting, someone's life may be saved. Training programmes in basic CPR for lay people are aimed at reducing this very high early mortality rate, as are the development of trained paramedical staff in ambulances and mobile coronary care units.

The risk of sudden death remains high for the first 24 hours, following which it rapidly diminishes. In the coronary

Box 2.8 Complications of AMI

Sudden death
Arrhythmias
Cardiac failure
Hypoxia
Hypotension
Cardiogenic shock
Papillary muscle insufficiency
Ventricular septal defect
Ventricular aneurysm
Myocardial rupture
Pulmonary embolus
Pericarditis
Deep-vein thrombosis
Post-MI syndrome
Emotional difficulty.

care unit, cardiac arrest may be anticipated; in the ward it is often diagnosed by the nurse, who finds the patient unconscious and pulseless. This is an emergency and every nurse is responsible for:

- recognising that cardiac arrest has occurred
- knowing the procedure for summoning help within the hospital
- commencing effective resuscitation.

The priorities of CPR are:

- airway
- breathing
- circulation.

The nurse is also responsible for maintaining the person's comfort and dignity, anticipating events and procedures and giving care and support to the person and relatives after the event.

Restoration of an oxygenated blood supply to the brain involves external cardiac massage and artificial ventilation. There is much controversy over whether to establish artificial ventilation or external cardiac massage first. In the known AMI patient, it seems sensible to commence external cardiac massage first as the patient was likely to have been adequately perfused up until the moment of the arrest.

External cardiac massage can only provide limited cardiac output. If the arrest is witnessed, an initial blow to the chest (precordial thump) may be attempted as this may restore the heart rhythm and takes only seconds to perform (Chamberlain 1989). Blood flow during cardiac massage is thought to occur due to increased intrathoracic pressure rather than direct heart compression. External cardiac massage involves:

- placing the patient supine on a firm surface
- placing the heel of one hand on the lower half of the patient's sternum, and the other hand on top of the first
- keeping the rescuer's arms straight and elbows locked
- kneeling level with the patient and applying firm downward pressure
- compressing the sternum at a rate of about 80–100 per minute depressing the sternum 4–5 cm.

Artificial ventilation should closely follow the commencement of external cardiac massage and involves:

- maintaining a clear airway through the removal of dentures, food, sputum, vomit or other debris
- performing the head-tilt/chin-lift or the head-tilt/jaw-thrust method to allow maximum air entry with the patient in a supine position
- inserting an airway or endotracheal tube if available
- ventilating the patient, mouth to mouth, mouth to mask or with a self expanding 'ambu' bag and pure oxygen if available
- observing for a rise and fall in the patient's chest wall.

The European Resuscitation Council (1993) recommends a cycle of 15 compressions followed by two inflations for one rescuer and 5 compressions to one inflation for two rescuers (Fig. 2.11).

Drug therapy. Ideally, all drugs used during CPR are best administered through a central line to ensure swift distribution, as circulation time is greatly reduced. Cardiopulmonary resuscitation should continue for ten cycles to allow circulation of the drug. Drug therapy for the various forms of cardiac arrest is shown in Fig. 2.11.

Defibrillation involves the delivery of a direct current (DC) shock to the heart through the chest wall. This causes depolarisation of all the myocardial cells that are able to respond to a stimulus, thereby terminating the fibrillation and allowing the normal conducting pathways to regain control of the heart. Gel pads are placed on the patient's chest, one below the right clavicle and the other over the apex of the heart in the fifth intercostal space. Precautions should be taken to ensure that floor surfaces are dry and all personnel warned that the shock is about to be delivered. The defibrillator is charged initially to 200 J and the defibrillator pads placed over the gel pads to deliver the shock (Thompson and Hopkins 1987).

Aftercare. After successful resuscitation the patient will require skilled nursing care. Full recovery can only be said to have occurred when the patient is fully conscious, with full cardiac, cerebral and renal function. The chances of achieving this are greatly enhanced if the patient is on a coronary care unit where the arrest is witnessed and treatment initiated within 2–3 minutes. Success is less likely in the street where resources are limited.

Several body systems need assessment post-arrest, including the cardiovascular, renal, respiratory and central nervous system. The patient may have been incontinent, have a sore chest and feel exhausted and somewhat embarrassed by his current state. An assessment of his level of orientation, recall, anxiety and general feelings should be made. The psychological support needed will vary. Relatives and witnesses to the arrest will also need support.

Ethical considerations. Unsuccessful resuscitation attempts do not enhance the dignity that is hoped for when we die. It can be debated that resuscitation that merely prolongs the process of dying is inappropriate. The decision not to resuscitate should involve the patient and the family, and be documented to avoid confusion. Policy also needs to be reviewed on at least a 24-hourly basis.

The joint statement of the British Medical Association and the Royal College of Nursing (1993) on cardiopulmonary resuscitation (CPR) points out, that

> Do-not-resuscitate (DNR) orders may be a potent source of misunderstanding and dissent amongst doctors, nurses and others involved in the care of patients. Many of the problems in this difficult area would be avoided if communication and explanation of the decision were improved.

?	**2.14** Read the guidelines for decision making in the joint statement. What are your local policies on CPR? How are decisions made in individual situations?

Cardiogenic shock

This is a serious degree of heart failure in which the cardiac output is not sufficient to give an adequate blood pressure to maintain perfusion. The patient develops clinical shock with low urine output, cold clammy skin and hypoxia. Lactic acid is produced in the skeletal muscle beds as the metabolism changes giving rise to a metabolic acidosis. This process is cyclical with the heart continually trying to pump harder for an ever falling stroke volume. See Ch. 18.

PATHOPHYSIOLOGY

Clinical features. In the early stages the patient may be restless and agitated, followed by mental confusion and lethargy as cerebral hypoxia increases. The skin becomes cold and clammy to touch.

Examination. There will be signs of central cyanosis. Vital recordings will reveal a rapid, thready pulse; hypotension; tachypnoea and hypothermia. Urinary output will be reduced.

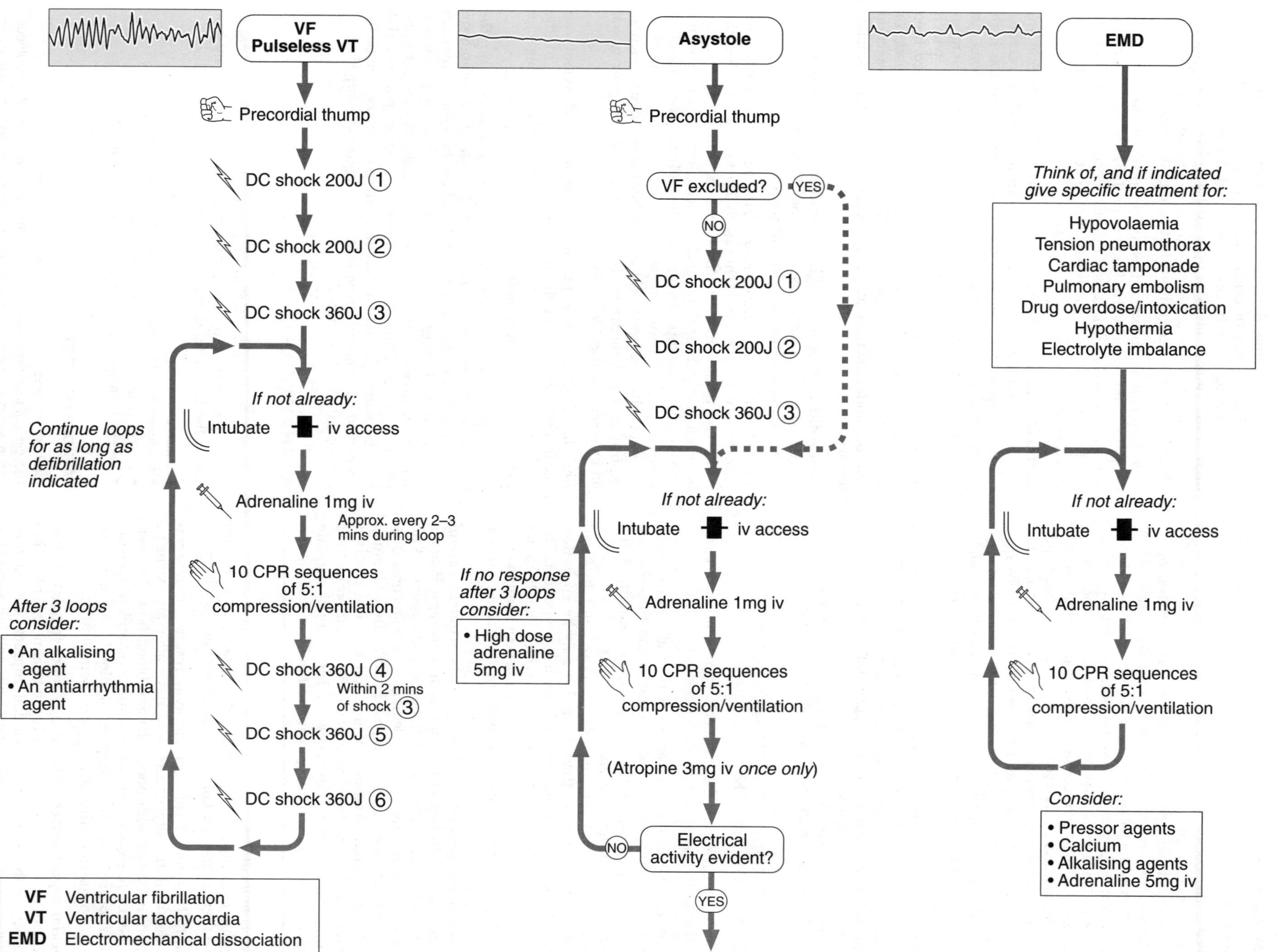

Fig. 2.11 Revised advanced resuscitation protocols. (Reproduced with kind permission from the European Resuscitation Council 1992.)

MEDICAL TREATMENT

The priorities are:

- enhance cardiac output
- restore tissue perfusion
- effect a diuresis through increased renal flow. This is achieved by drug therapy, often requiring manipulation of multiple drugs to obtain the best effect for the patient. The aim is to improve cardiac output using inotropic drugs such as adrenaline, dopamine and dobutamine. These drugs, often given via a central line, improve cardiac output by increasing contractility and often heart rate, which increase the demand on the myocardium for oxygen. Cardiac output can also be improved by using vasodilators to reduce afterload. The use of nitrates will have the additional benefit of dilating coronary arteries, so increasing the supply of oxygen to the myocardium. Diuretics are widely used in cardiac shock to induce a diuresis and maintain glomerular filtration. The patient will require urinary catheterisation to assess hourly urine output and may be haemodynamically monitored using a pulmonary artery flotation (Swan Ganz) catheter. (See Ch. 18.) If pharmacological intervention is ineffective in treating cardiogenic shock then more invasive therapy such as the intra aortic balloon pump (IABP) or ventricular assist device may be required.

The outlook for patients developing cardiogenic shock is poor and mortality is high, as the process is very difficult to reverse.

NURSING PRIORITIES AND MANAGEMENT: CARDIOGENIC SHOCK

The priority in caring for these patients is prevention or early recognition of the signs that shock is developing.

Observation. Recording and assessment of all vital signs is important. The pulse will initially be rapid and thready as a compensatory response to the falling cardiac output; in the late stages bradycardia develops.

Initially systolic and later diastolic pressure will fall. A fall in pulse pressure of more than 30 mmHg may be an indication that shock is developing in the hypertensive patient. The initial response to hypoxia is tachypnoea, which later becomes shallow and irregular. Some patients may benefit from oxygen therapy. Urine output falls as a result of the falling cardiac output.

Nursing management of these patients requires careful observation and recording of response to drug therapy. Patients are likely to become increasingly immobile and dependent on nursing care. They may also be lethargic or semiconscious. Anxiety and fear need to be recognised and addressed. Small doses of opiates may promote comfort and rest. The relatives need time spent with them to explain the condition of their loved one and how they can best help. The hospital chaplain may provide comfort for the patient and family at this time.

Medical complications

This group of complications results in reduced cardiac output because there is specific failure of one area of myocardium.

Myocardial rupture. This complication results in instantaneous death. It usually occurs 8–10 days after an extensive infarction in a heart with poor collateral blood flow. Necrosis occurs before fibrosis of the myocardium is complete, causing muscle rupture and the pumping of blood into the pericardium. Fortunately, this is a very rare complication.

Ventricular septal defect. This occurs more frequently than rupture but in some cases is amenable to treatment. The pathophysiology is the same as myocardial rupture, with a hole developing in the septum separating right and left ventricles. The right ventricle has to cope with increased pressures and blood volumes while the left ventricle suffers a fall in cardiac output. Rapid onset of cardiogenic shock may be the result. Operative repair can be undertaken but the mortality rate is high. If the patient can be supported for 2–4 weeks by aggressive medical management until the septum has become fibrosed then the surgical results are slightly better.

Papillary muscle rupture. Loss of blood supply to the muscle supporting the mitral valve leads to prolapse and malfunctioning of the valve. If acute rupture occurs then sudden death may result. Surgical repair can be attempted but, again, survival rates are low.

Ventricular aneurysm. This occurs when the infarction involves the full thickness of the myocardium. As the necrotic tissue is replaced by fibrous tissue it is subject to the high pressures in the left ventricle. This fibrous tissue balloons out to form a blood pouch, which does not contract. Blood stagnation in this pouch leads to the development of thrombi, which may embolise. If a large area of myocardium is affected then it can lead to cardiac failure; if near the papillary muscle or mitral valve then incompetence will result. Surgical resection can be undertaken successfully with some of the smaller aneurysms.

Pericarditis. This is thought to be due to an auto-immune reaction in which antigens from the damaged myocardium cause inflammation of the pericardium.

Medical and nursing management. The patient presents with pain at any time from 24 hours to up to a week after the AMI. On examination, a 'friction rub' caused by friction between the pericardium and myocardium, is often heard and is often accompanied by an unresolving post-infarction pyrexia. Medical treatment and nursing care involve treating the pain with analgesia and anti-inflammatory drugs such as aspirin and indomethacin. Reassurance that the pain is not an extension of the AMI is important.

Emboli. Embolus of a pulmonary or systemic vessel can occur after AMI. Emboli arise from clots forming in the healing myocardium or from circulatory stasis causing clot formation in the lower limbs.

Nursing care involves maintaining passive exercises on the patient, whose mobility is restricted. The use of anti-embolism stockings should be considered. It is now becoming common practice for all post-AMI patients and those with known IHD to be given aspirin, which, taken daily, is thought to be effective in reducing clot formation. In most patients this may be sufficient but in people with pulmonary emboli or known to have mural thrombi a more aggressive approach to anticoagulation is required.

ARRHYTHMIAS

The term arrhythmia is used to imply an abnormality either in electrical impulse formation or electrical impulse conduction within the heart. An arrhythmia may cause an effect by any one of the following changes:

- change in heart rate
- increase in myocardial oxygen requirement
- decrease in myocardial blood flow
- loss of synchronicity of ventricular contraction.

PATHOPHYSIOLOGY

Clinical features

The clinical manifestation of an arrhythmia depends on the ventricular rate, the conduction of the myocardium and the psychological response of the patient. Patient problems include:

- palpitations
- dizziness
- faintness
- shortness of breath
- chest pain
- headache
- reduced activity tolerance
- anxiety.

Nursing assessment needs to include the apparent effect of the arrhythmia on the patient, a history of any past experiences with the problem; a knowledge of any relevant medications or other treatments and identification of any possible precipitating factors.

In cardiac disease the normal sinus mechanism can be altered if the disease affects the heart's specialised conduction tissue. Various conditions result in specific conduction disturbances and while this chapter cannot deal with them all it will concentrate on a few of the more common ones, with which the nurse should be familiar. In interpreting heart rhythms the method used must be systematic and consider all components of the ECG complex.

Normal sinus rhythm should be recognisable to all nurses as patients attached to cardiac monitors are increasingly nursed on general wards. The nurse's priorities are to:

1. Recognise and immediately report anything abnormal.
2. Assess quickly the effect of the abnormality on the patient and take the appropriate action, which may be reassurance or resuscitation. The normal electrocardiogram and the basic rules for observing cardiac monitors discussed earlier in the chapter apply here.

Sinus arrhythmia (SA)

The SA node is under autonomic control, primarily vagal, but is influenced by sympathetic stimulation, temperature, oxygen saturation and other metabolic changes. Sinus arrhythmias are often secondary to these influences.

SA is characterised by a constant PR interval but progressive beat-to-beat change in varying R-R intervals but is otherwise a normal sinus rhythm. During expiration, the reflex discharge of the vagal nerve slows the sinus mechanism; during inspiration this influence is diminished, allowing a speeding up of the sinus rhythm.

Sinus bradycardia

This meets the requirements for sinus rhythm but the rate is less than 60 beats per minutes (bpm). It may result from increased vagal tone but also results from hypothermia, certain medications e.g. beta-blockers, raised intracranial pressure and inferior MI. Some individuals may experience sinus bradycardia when sleeping; it may be the norm in athletes.

Sinus tachycardia

This also fits the criteria for sinus rhythm but this time the rate is greater than 100 bpm. It is a direct result of decreased vagal tone and often a response to sympathetic stimulation.

NURSING PRIORITIES AND MANAGEMENT: SINUS ARRHYTHMIAS

Sinus arrhythmias tend to be observed and not treated directly. They are not life-threatening and resolution of the primary cause resolves the arrhythmia. Atropine i.v. is given for symptomatic sinus bradycardia.

Atrial arrhythmias

Atrial flutter

This is characterised by rapid and regular atrial excitation at a level above 200 bpm. The AV node is not capable of conducting atrial rates above this level. The atrial waves form a saw-tooth pattern. Ventricular deflections usually occur regularly within the atrial pattern and the block is described as a ratio, for example, 4:1, which means 4 P waves per QRS complex.

Almost always associated with organic disease, it is not a stable rhythm and progresses to atrial fibrillation.

Atrial fibrillation

When individual muscle fibres of the atria or ventricles contract independently, they are said to be 'fibrillating'. There is rapid disorganised atrial depolarisation because the atrial tissues have lost synchrony with each other. The atrial waves can occur up to 600 times per minute. Ventricular depolarisation is also irregular as a result of the variable response at the AV node but the QRS complex is normal. It occurs in congestive cardiac failure and mitral disease, and often presents with ischaemic changes in old age.

MEDICAL MANAGEMENT

Atrial fibrillation can severely compromise cardiac output as the loss of the effect of atrial systole can reduce stroke volume by up to 25%. With chronic atrial fibrillation the danger of thrombi forming in the atria and then embolising is high.

Treatment

Treatment is aimed at reducing the rapid ventricular rate. Once this is controlled, cardioversion (see Box 2.9) to revert the rhythm to

Box 2.9 Cardioversion

Purpose

The term 'cardioversion' is used to mean the delivery of a specific and predetermined amount of energy to the heart, timed (synchronised) in such a way that the shock is delivered well away from the vulnerable period of the T wave on the ECG. It is usually performed electively, with the patient lightly anaesthetised. This differs from defibrillation, which usually involves the delivery of a larger amount of electricity to a patient in ventricular fibrillation without anaesthetic, as the patient is usually unconscious. Elective cardioversion is used to treat supraventricular and ventricular arrhythmias.

Electrical treatment has the advantage that it is free from pharmacological side-effects.

Procedure

Cardioversion usually takes place at the patient's bedside. The patient is asked to remove any dentures or restrictive clothing. An ECG will be perfomed before and after the procedure, and the patient attached to a cardiac monitor throughout. Oxygen is given both before and after the procedure. A light anaesthetic is usually given and the patient asked to fast for 4–6 hours. Resuscitation equipment needs to be on hand. The defibrillator is set to the required output and the paddles placed in position on gel pads, usually placed one below the right clavicle and the other over the apex of the heart in order to depolarise an optimum mass of myocardial cells. The patient is usually awake and talking 5–10 minutes after the procedure, although nausea and vomiting are not uncommon as is a sore throat from the ET tube and chest-wall soreness due to the cardioversion. Cardioversion is often performed on a day-case basis.

sinus can be considered. This is only of benefit in the acute episode. Secondary cardioversion after digoxin therapy may precipitate ventricular fibrillation if large doses of digoxin have been used. Anticoagulation in the form of warfarin may be prescribed if thrombi are thought to be a problem.

NURSING PRIORITIES AND MANAGEMENT: CARDIOVERSION

The procedure should be fully explained to the patient so that he is aware of what to expect. The thought of an anaesthetic and an electric current being put across the heart may be frightening. Care should be taken to ensure that the floor is dry and that all personnel are warned that the shock is about to be delivered. The patient is likely to want to know the outcome of the procedure and this should be explained. Topical creams may help to ease any chest soreness.

?	**2.15** Clarify the differences between emergency defibrillation and elective cardioversion.

AV junctional arrhythmias

The AV node, unlike the SA node, normally has no pacemaking role so arrhythmias arise in the intranodal pathways or bundle of His. Impulses must travel in both directions to stimulate atrial and ventricular contraction so the position of the P wave may vary. The QRS complex is of normal configuration and duration since the normal conduction pathway is followed below the AV node.

Junctional (nodal) tachycardia is similar to sinus tachycardia. Nodal tachycardia can occur in paroxysms or sustained rates. The rate is usually around 120–200 beats per minute. The significance of the arrhythmia depends on its haemodynamic effect.

Supraventricular tachycardia. This applies to rapid arrhythmias that originate above the His bundle. Because of their rapid rate, P waves are difficult to see and are often in the previous T wave. The QRS is of normal configuration.

Medical management of supraventricular tachycardia aims to reduce the rapid ventricular rate using carotid sinus pressure or antiarrhythmic drugs e.g. amiodarone, adenosine or digoxin. If these measures are unsuccessful then cardioversion may be indicated.

Ventricular arrhythmias

In these rhythms the focus arises below the AV node.

Ventricular tachycardia. The QRS complex looks wide and bizarre. The rate is regular at around 140–200 beats per minute. It is generally caused by an irritable or ischaemic myocardium. Treatment, if the patient is symptomatic, is with immediate synchronised cardioversion and/or intravenous lignocaine. Other medication includes amiodarone and mexiletine. Persistent episodes of ventricular tachycardia may be treated with over-ride pacing or ablation therapy (where the ectopic focus or source of the arrhythmia is identified and removed).

Ventricular fibrillation. In this rhythm there are no distinguishable complexes on the screen and only an erratic baseline trace is evident. Treatment is immediate initiation of resuscitation procedures and defibrillation.

Heart block

This arrhythmia results when there is a delay in the impulse conduction from the atria to the ventricles at the AV node. It is described as:

- first degree heart block
- second degree heart block
- complete heart block.

Heart block is usually a complication of myocardial infarction.

First degree block appears as a prolonged PR interval with a mild bradycardia. It is asymptomatic and seldom requires treatment.

Second degree block appears as occasional blocking: for example, there may be alternate conducted and non-conducted atrial beats, giving twice as many P waves as QRS complexes. The patient may have no symptoms and require no treatment. If compromised, the heart block is treated pharmacologically with isoprenaline or by the insertion of a pacemaker (see Box 2.10).

Complete heart block exists when atrial and ventricular activity are unrelated. The atria and ventricles are electrically dissociated and desynchronised with a subsidiary pacemaker developing in the ventricles. Cardiac output is reduced and the patient haemodynamically compromised. The ventricles are often contracting very slowly and at less than 40 beats per minute and a pacemaker requires to be inserted immediately to restore cardiac output. The nurse's role is one of observation, reporting and patient support.

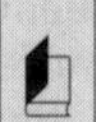

For further details of cardiac arrhythmias and the appropriate medication see Hampton (1992) and Jowett & Thompson (1989).

NURSING PRIORITIES AND MANAGEMENT: HEART BLOCK

The nursing management involves anticipating and resolving patient problems, monitoring the patient, including his response to treatment, and providing information and support.

Pacemakers

Nursing considerations include assessing pacemaker function, ensuring patient comfort and safety, preventing and dealing with complications, and teaching the patient about his condition and management. The patient needs to be prepared for the procedure, even if it is done as an emergency. (See Box 2.10.)

Following pacemaker insertion the patient should be attached to a cardiac monitor to assess whether the pacemaker is functioning properly. Cardiac output needs to be assessed frequently by recording the patient's blood pressure and asking him to report any symptoms of faintness, dizziness, chest pain or shortness of breath.

Limited mobility may make the patient more dependent on nursing care for a while. He should be aware of how long the temporary pacing is likely to continue and appreciate what is likely to happen next.

Removal of the temporary pacemaker is performed at the patient's bedside under aseptic conditions.

Permanent pacing

Nursing considerations are similar to temporary pacing, initially. Some patients will be helped by a visit from a person who already has a permanent pacemaker, and also by being given an opportunity to handle a pacemaker. The patient needs to be reassured that the pacemaker will not be damaged by day-to-day activities. He should be taught to take his own pulse and be aware of the signs of reduced cardiac output. Signs of infection, such as redness or increased soreness at the implantation site, should also be reported. The importance of follow-up appointments should be explained. It is also useful

Box 2.10 Pacemaker insertion

Purpose
Pacemakers are used to gain control over the electrical activity of the heart. They have two basic components:

- a pulse generator containing a power source and electrical circuitry
- one or two pacing leads, each with an electrode on its tip.

Pacemakers may either be temporary or permanent depending on whether the pulse generator is located externally or implanted. If pacing is planned for a short duration, an external source is used to deliver electricity to the heart via the skin. When long-term control of the heart is required, a permanent pacemaker is implanted. The two most common modes of pacing are:

- demand (ventricular inhibited), which senses intrinsic cardiac rhythm and stimulates myocardial depolarisation and contraction as necessary
- fixed rate, which fires at a predetermined rate, irrespective of intrinsic cardiac activity.

Temporary pacing
This is used to maintain cardiac output during episodes of extreme bradycardia, heart block and asystole. It may also be used for the suppression of tachyarrhythmias, which are resistant to drug therapy. It is usual for a special room to be set aside for temporary cardiac pacing, with ECG monitoring, fluoroscopy and resuscitation equipment being readily available.

Most commonly, a bipolar catheter is inserted into the subclavian vein, external jugular vein or antecubital fossa under local anaesthesia. The catheter is then passed into the right atrium and thence through the tricuspid valve and into the apex of the right ventricle where the tip of the catheter is lodged against the ventricular wall. The external end of the catheter is stitched into place at the skin surface. The bipolar catheter is stimulated by the pacemaker's external pulse generator. Verification of pacing is judged from the appearance of a pacing spike preceding the QRS complex of the ECG. Pacing 'threshold' is obtained by determining the lowest voltage needed to elicit a paced beat, ideally less than 0.5 V. The threshold needs to be checked at least every 12 hours, as it may increase over time.

Possible complications
These include arrhythmias, failure of the electrode to sense the heart's own electrical activity, failure of the electrode to generate a contraction, abdominal muscle twitching, pneumothorax, infection.

Permanent pacing
The decision to implant a permanent pacemaker is made after careful patient assessment. It is usually offered to patients with symptomatic bradycardias and heart block. The modern pacemaker is a small, metal unit weighing between 30–130 g. It is powered by a lithium battery with a life of up to 15 years. Two types of pulse generator currently available are:

- single chamber with an electrode placed either in the atrium or the ventricle
- dual chamber with electrodes situated in both chambers.

The pacemaker is usually implanted under local anaesthesia in a cardiac catheterisation laboratory. The pulse generator is implanted in a subcutaneous pocket, usually under the clavicle, axilla or abdominal wall. The procedure is usually performed on a day-case basis.

to warn people that the pacemaker may trigger off alarms at airports.

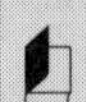
See Jowett & Thompson (1989b) for more detailed information on pacemakers.

EXPERT NURSING PRACTICE IN ISCHAEMIC HEART DISEASE

Despite extraordinary advances in medical and surgical therapy in cardiac disease, cure is often not possible. Living with heart problems and caring for people with them, presents many moral and personal dilemmas and can challenge the limits of nursing expertise.

An example of such dilemmas and of expert nursing practice in severe coronary illness is given by Benner and Wrubel (1989). They summarise the nurse's expertise as follows:

> Mary Cucci notices that Mr Jones is terrified and reflects and clarifies his feelings. She reads his body language. She notices that Mr Jones appears 'frozen' in bed. She clarifies with him that he is afraid to move because it may trigger his tachycardia again. She selects an approach that matches his own coping style, they set a goal and create a plan for his recovery. She uses humor and even dances with him as he transfers to the chair. She makes him notice his progress and monitor his abilities. She enlists the family to solicit his participation in life again. She draws on the chaplain and the psychiatric nurse specialist to augment her own care. She interprets the patient's fears and understanding to the physicians. Mr Jones has become a prisoner in his own body. His world has shrunk, and he is a classic case of the effects of being institutionalized. Illness robs one of perspective and shrinks both the familiar world and the world of possibility. Mary Cucci demonstrates expertise in world conserving and world restoring, as well as expertise in assisting someone to imagine the next step. We can learn much from such expert nursing practice on the nature of the shrinking world of illness, the personal consequences of institutionalization, and the nature of recovery.

HEART FAILURE

The term 'heart failure' is used to describe a clinical syndrome which results from an inability of the heart to provide an adequate cardiac output for the body's metabolic requirements.

The diagnosis of heart failure is not difficult to make, but discovering the underlying cause can be. Heart failure can result from primary heart disease or from non-cardiac causes (see Box 2.11). Many of these conditions are very common, particularly in the elderly. They are often found in combination, making their individual contribution to the heart

Box 2.11 Primary cardiac conditions causing heart failure

RIGHT HEART FAILURE

- pulmonary hypertension secondary to left heart failure
- congenital heart defect
- thromboembolism
- cor pulmonale
- atrial septal defect
- pulmonary venous stenosis.

LEFT HEART FAILURE

Ventricular origin
- coronary artery disease
- aortic or mitral valve disease
- congenital heart defect
- hypertension
- ventricular septal defect.

Atrial origin
- atrial myxoma
- mitral stenosis.

failure difficult to assess. Non-cardiac causes include chronic obstructive airways disease, hyperthyroidism and chronic anaemia (see Ch. 3, Ch. 5 and Ch. 11).

PATHOPHYSIOLOGY

Heart failure can involve either ventricle independently or both together. Pure left- or right-ventricular failure may not exist for long because of their dependence on each other to maintain adequate blood flow. It is useful to look at the heart as two pumps. The left ventricle can cope better with alterations in pressure. The right can cope with volume alterations.

Cardiac reserve. The function of the heart is to pump blood to the body at sufficient volume and pressure to perfuse the tissues with oxygen. The requirements of many areas are fairly constant, but the needs of the skeletal musculature vary with the level of physical activity. An increase in activity leads to an increase in cardiac output, this capacity to increase being the 'cardiac reserve'. The increase results mainly from increased heart rate and contractile force as a direct result of sympathetic nervous system (SNS) stimulation. In the patient with heart failure the cardiac reserve is used to maintain baseline cardiac function and so the ability to respond to increased activity is limited. When the baroreceptors at various points in the body sense a fall in pressure and therefore a fall in cardiac output the principal response is to increase stimulation of the SNS, followed up by a longer term response.

Myocardial dilatation. Increased stretching of the myocardial cells, which occurs with an initial inability to expel the stroke volume, increases their contractile power and induces a reflex increase in cardiac output. This compensatory mechanism becomes limited as myocardial oxygen demand increases.

Renal response. Reduced cardiac output has a depressant effect on the kidneys, which will not improve until the cardiac output returns to normal. The fall in blood pressure and sympathetic constriction of renal arterioles reduce glomerular pressure and filtration rates. Reduced blood flow through the kidneys leads to increased angiotensin production with eventual reabsorption of sodium and water. The final mechanism in the renal chain is increased secretion of aldosterone, further increasing sodium and, therefore, water reabsorption. The fluid retention in itself does not interfere with the pumping ability of the heart, but is does increase venous return. The rise in extracellular fluid and blood volume increases systemic filling pressures, so more of the cardiac reserve has to be used to maintain perfusion further reducing its ability to respond to increased physical activity.

Myocardial hypertrophy. This is the final compensatory mechanism in an attempt to increase the contractile mass. This compensation is usually of a temporary nature and at this stage the prognosis is poor.

Oedema

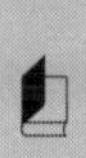

In order to understand oedema, the nurse must first understand the normal tissue fluid exchange that occurs between the capillaries and the cells to ensure that nutrients, O_2 and H_2O are delivered to the cell and waste products are removed. See Wilson (1990).

Oedema may result when anything increases the flow of fluid from the bloodstream and impairs its return. One of the most common causes is congestive cardiac failure, where the failure of the pump to move the blood volume forward results in back pressure, which raises the hydrostatic pressure such that it exceeds the colloidal pressure created by plasma proteins. As a result, the tissue fluid formed is not returned to the vascular compartment and, when excessive, cannot be effectively drained away by the lymphatic system.

In the early stages of heart failure, patients may complain of 'puffy ankles', being unable to fit comfortably into their shoes. There will also be sacral oedema. Both types are dependent oedema.

Pulmonary oedema. As systemic pressure and, therefore, afterload increase so does pressure in the left heart. Increased LVEDP results in increased pulmonary pressure and an accumulation of blood in the lungs. If the pulmonary pressure rises above 28 mmHg there is movement of fluid into the alveoli and interstitial spaces. This causes pulmonary oedema (Wilson 1989). If this occurs as an acute event it can lead to death in 30 minutes. In the congestive failure situation, it is a chronic progressive state where the reduced lung compliance and high pulmonary pressure lead to increased right-heart pressures and blood congestion on this side. This further raises pressure in the systemic circulation, making the whole process one of cyclical deterioration. As the systemic pressure rises there is movement of fluid into the tissues giving rise to peripheral oedema. This is initially gravitational but as the condition progresses the oedema becomes more widespread (see Fig. 2.12).

MEDICAL MANAGEMENT

The presentation and history will depend on which side of the heart is failing. It may present gradually, as occurs in the ageing process, or suddenly manifesting as acute pulmonary oedema:

- fatigue on exertion, dyspnoea with mild exercise and paroxysmal nocturnal dyspnoea are common early signs of failure of the left ventricle
- fatigue, awareness of fullness in the neck and abdomen, ankle swelling are early signs of failure of the right ventricle.

Features appearing in systemic examination are listed in Table 2.7.

?	**2.16** How do the features of nursing assessment relate to and complement the doctor's examination?

Investigations. The main concern is to identify the primary cause of failure, to ensure that correctable lesions are treated and contributing factors eliminated if possible.

ECG: there may be no specific abnormalities but indications of ventricular hypertrophy, heart block and acute MI may help pinpoint the aetiology of the heart failure.

Other investigations include chest X-ray, auscultation and palpation.

Treatment. The main treatment approaches are:

- oxygenation to improve myocardial contractility
- rest to reduce cardiac rate and work
- digoxin to increase myocardial contractile force and efficiency
- diuresis of excess fluid in conjunction with restricted salt intake
- correction of arrhythmias.

A combination of digitalis and diuretic therapy is the standard management of heart failure. Digoxin helps increase the strength of myocardial contraction, and slows the heart rate by increasing vagal activity. Diuretics help by reducing sodium and therefore water reabsorption in the kidneys, thus increasing fluid loss.

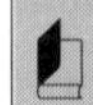

For the pharmacological aspects of management of heart failure, see Ashworth & Clarke (1992) Ch. 3.

NURSING PRIORITIES AND MANAGEMENT: HEART FAILURE

Much of the day-to-day support of this group of patients is done by the general practitioner. Nursing may not be needed until the patient requires assistance with basic daily activities when the community nursing services become involved. The individual is only hospitalised if adjustment to therapy requires

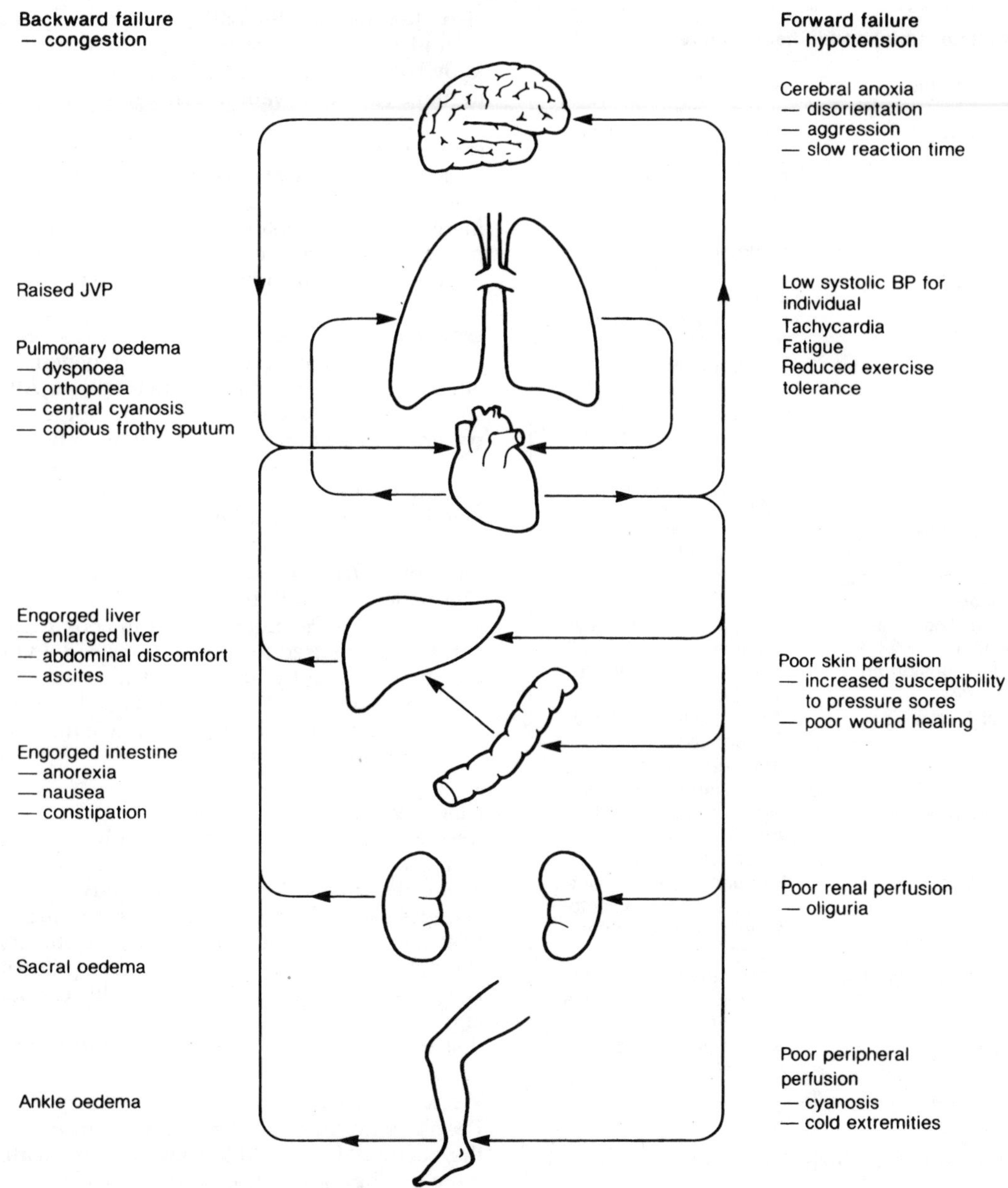

Fig. 2.12 Clinical effects of decompensatory phase of ventricular failure. (Reproduced with kind permission from Boore et al 1987.)

careful monitoring, or an episode of acute failure is exacerbating the chronic condition (Letterer et al 1992). See Table 2.7.

Ongoing concerns

Maintaining a safe environment

The prime concern is to restore haemodynamic stability, using a combination of drugs to optimise cardiac function and control fluid loss through the kidneys. The effects of this therapy should be regularly assessed and practice nurses may be involved in monitoring the patient's weight, heart rate and rhythm. People living with heart failure should be taught how to monitor their pulse and to check their ankles for signs of oedema.

In the patient admitted to hospital with an acute exacerbation of heart failure, the manipulation of medication will form a major part of therapy. Sensitive day-to-day nursing care will depend on having a sound understanding of medication and its effects.

Breathing

The patient will often describe breathlessness, especially on exertion, as the main symptom. Control of fluid balance and reducing energy demands may help to minimise the symptoms, and the patient should be encouraged to stop smoking.

Acute left ventricular failure leading to pulmonary oedema results in marked respiratory distress, agitation and production of copious frothy sputum. The priority is to reduce both the psychological and respiratory distress, using intravenous morphine, diuretics and oxygen therapy. Being with the patient and explaining what is being done in a reassuring way can allay anxiety and help the person through the alarming experience.

In hospital, the nurse is responsible for:

- ensuring that respiration is recorded regularly
- assessing the patient's subjective feelings about his breathing
- reporting acute episodes of dyspnoea
- administering oxygen therapy to help reduce anoxia

Table 2.7 Systemic examination in heart failure

System	Points to note	Rationale
CVS	Chest X-ray	Evaluation of chamber enlargement Indication of primary cardiac abnormality
	Auscultation	Arrhythmia especially AF common
	Vital signs	Venous hypertension common Observe jugular venous pressure
	Presence of oedema	Visible oedema in dependent parts, e.g. ankles, hands and sacrum, in bed-bound patients is a sign of inability to excrete sufficient water
Respiratory	Wheeze, bronchospasm	Possible increased pulmonary fluid
	Paroxysmal nocturnal dyspnoea	Evidence of poor LV compensation
	Amount and consistency of sputum	Evidence of pulmonary oedema
	Pleural effusion on right side	Often found in patients with CCF
	Chest X-ray	Recognition of oedema
GIS	Diet	Sodium control important part of controlling fluid retention
	Palpation of abdomen	Signs of hepatic and splenic engorgement Presence of ascites
GUS	Micturition	Frequency and amount of urine passed; vital to assess effect of diuretic therapy
MS	Physical activity levels	Often severely limited by reduced cardiac reserve
CNS	Mental status	Signs of cerebral hypoxia
Skin	Skin integrity	Risk of pressure sores and delayed healing

(cautiously, in the patient with chronic obstructive airways disease (COAD))
- assessing the nature and amount of sputum
- working in partnership with the physiotherapist, to apply chest physiotherapy and naso-pharyngeal suctioning to help with sputum clearance.

Sleeping
Respiratory distress is often worse at night when the patient lies flat, and paroxysmal nocturnal dyspnoea is a very frightening experience. Sleeping supported with extra pillows helps. Patients with congestive failure may not sleep for long periods. Many doze for periods during the day. Some people stay in a chair at night, instead of going to bed, because of their respiratory distress. These factors should be remembered when patients are taken to hospital. A restless patient awake in bed at 2 a.m. may get more rest if he follows his normal pattern, and is not constricted by hospital policy.

Elimination
Accurate estimation of fluid losses in conjunction with daily weights provides information on the effectiveness of diuretics; output should be in excess of 30 ml per hour. Input of fluid and sodium should be restricted. Restricting sodium intake also often reduces the patient's thirst, which is very important if fluid intake is to be restricted to around 1 litre a day. The knowledge that fluid is being restricted is almost guaranteed to make someone want to drink more. The use of loop diuretic therapy, such as frusemide, will cause loss of potassium. Potassium supplements are given and serum levels of potassium closely monitored to ensure they remain within normal limits 3.5–5.5 mmol/l (see Ch. 20). To assist in the accurate assessment of haemodynamic status a central venous catheter or pulmonary artery pressure catheter may be inserted.

Constipation must be avoided (see p. 112).

Oedema
Daily assessment of the extent of oedema will indicate the effectiveness of therapeutic intervention. All dependent areas should be assessed, including the spine and sacrum, if the patient is bed-bound. All patients with heart failure should be advised to have their legs raised above their hips when not walking. People at home should be taught how to monitor weight and the signs of oedema.

Diet and nutrition
The patient should be encouraged not to use salt at the table and to reduce the amount used in cooking. Herbs or salt substitutes can be used to add taste, instead. In hospital, a low-salt diet may be rigidly enforced, if the oedema is severe. Obese patients should also be on a reduced-calorie diet, to prevent further strain on the heart. Iron intake may need to be assessed if the person is anaemic.

Mobility
Rest is important for patients with congestive heart failure, to reduce the cardiac workload and oxygen demand. In the acute phase complete bed rest is advocated until pulmonary oedema is controlled. Activity is gradually increased until tolerated without signs of physical difficulty. A patient confined to bed or chair rest requires pillows for support, to keep his breathing comfortable. With cardiac beds, both foot and head ends can be altered, helping to relieve respiratory distress, while aiding the peripheral drainage of fluid.

Work and leisure
People with heart failure may require help to live within their activity limits and to come to terms with the fact that they have a progressive disease for which there is no cure. Many people consider they are doomed to, and a few adopt, the role of invalid and dependant. The response to gradually increased activity is assessed to calculate the patient's functional capacity. See also the section on mobility for people with AMI (p. 28).

Personal hygiene
A patient with congestive failure can usually retain independence in this area by taking certain precautions. Showers demand less energy expenditure than a bath and a seat in the shower is helpful. A common difficulty is in drying the lower half of the body because bending affects respiration, but by sitting all except the toes can be reached.

Someone with oedema will have very fragile, papery skin in the affected areas and great care must be taken not to break the skin by too much rubbing dry. Soap also has a drying effect on the skin; emulsifying oils may be better.

Communication
The importance of information being exchanged between the patient, family and health professionals cannot be overemphasised. It should be remembered that heart failure is a

progressive disease which affects many old people. The restrictions on mobility may confine these people to their home further isolating them. Community nurses, health visitors and practice nurses are increasingly involved in health assessment and screening of old people at home. Their assessment needs to take careful account of the social and psychological consequences, as well as the physical consequences of disease processes and disability. It may be possible to arrange for attendance at a day hospital, for those who wish it, or for a charity group such as Age Concern or the WRVS to provide transport to social events or day centres.

Expressing sexuality
The patient's role within the family may have to alter as the disease increasingly restricts activities. Women may have to give up some household tasks to partners or to a home help. This can further demoralise and requires tactful support from family and health professionals. Sexual activity may need to be modified if the individual's activity levels decrease or shortness of breath becomes a problem. The nurse needs to be equipped to offer realistic, non-judgmental advice.

VALVULAR DISORDERS

Most adult valvular disease is either congenital or acquired. The effects of congenital problems largely manifest themselves in childhood and so are excluded from discussion here (Frankl & Brest 1986).

The major causes of valve pathology are rheumatic heart disease (RHD), sub-acute bacterial endocarditis (SBE) and, to a lesser extent today, syphilis. Major disruption can also result from papillary muscle dysfunction following AMI or penetrating chest wounds, when onset of symptoms can be sudden and severe.

Rheumatic heart disease

Rheumatic fever (RF) is usually a childhood ailment. It is closely associated with streptococcal pharyngitis and so shows seasonal variation with a peak in colder months. In 85% of those with RF, the fever recurs within 8 years and the subsequent risk of heart disease increases with each bout. It may take up to 10 years before the signs of heart disease appear but 25% of those affected may have died by then. Of the rest, 66% go on to develop RHD. Within 20 years, almost 80% die from heart failure, cerebral embolisation and respiratory failure (Boore et al 1987).

PATHOPHYSIOLOGY

The connective tissue of heart, joints and skin respond to infection by a proliferative and exudative inflammatory response with oedema and fragmentation of collagen fibres. The arthritic pain flits from joint to joint. Fever is low grade. All layers of the heart can be affected. Endocarditis is most common, usually affecting the left side involving the mitral valve, although any valve is at risk. The valve leaflets become oedematous with small, firmly attached vegetations. In the acute stages this results in incompetence of the valve. Subsequent fibrosis deforms and thickens the leaflets and shortens the chordae tendineae, leading to stenosis with or without incompetence (Majeed 1989).

Prophylactic antibiotic cover is instituted, following the first occurrence of RF, and if this prevents recurrence then most of those who develop endocarditis will have normal hearts in the long term. Outbreaks are now more common in third world countries than they are in the west, especially within communities that are becoming progressively urbanised. Poor housing and socio-economic conditions exacerbate the problem. Prevention would have to take these factors into account to be effective. In the UK it is the elderly population that is now presenting with the effects of earlier exposure although many have no recollection of an acute episode of RF.

Subacute bacterial endocarditis (SBE)
The majority (75%) of cases are streptococcal or staphylococcal infections, although an increasing number of infective agents are being isolated, due to increasingly invasive medical techniques, such as in dental treatment or urinary investigation. Intravenous drug users also introduce bacteria to their systems by the use of contaminated needles. As well as being a cause of valvular disorder, those who have pre-existing valve disease or congenital lesions are more at risk of developing bacterial endocarditis, as the underlying structures are already damaged and the blood flow is more turbulent. Certain sites are more favoured for bacterial proliferation. When blood flows from a high-pressure to a low-pressure system via a narrow orifice, the organisms tend to gather on the low-pressure side. If a high-pressure jet or regurgitant stream is created due to, for example, valve dysfunction then satellite colonies will be seeded in the endothelial wall where the jet hits. In, for example, aortic regurgitation, blood flows back from the high-pressure aorta via the supposedly closed aortic valve to the low-pressure left ventricle. Colonisation by bacteria would most likely occur on the ventricular surface of the aortic valve. Similar patterns can be elicited for other areas of dysfunction.

The vegetations of SBE are, in contrast to those in RHD, large and friable and can aggregate to form up to 6 cm masses. This poses a double threat to the patient in that they:

- are more likely to embolise
- may cause ventricular insufficiency themselves by prolapsing into the valve orifice and obstructing flow.

Presentation may be slow and insidious, with general malaise, lethargy, intermittent, often low-grade pyrexia and joint pain. Microembolisation may manifest as splinter haemorrhages of the nail beds. If the infection has eroded tissue close to the valves where the conduction system lies, then there may be evidence of rhythm and conduction disturbances. Evidence of embolisation may be seen in renal, cerebral, pulmonary and gastrointestinal systems. Myocardial infarction may also result from septic embolisation of the coronary arteries. Heart failure secondary to valve failure varies in its severity, depending on the valve affected and acuteness of onset.

MEDICAL MANAGEMENT

Investigations. These should include ECG CXR echocardiography (Monaghan 1993). Cardiac catheterisation is also necessary in those who will be referred for surgery to assess valve function, ventricular function, and the patency of coronary arteries.

For more information on subacute bacterial endocarditis see Thompson & Webster 1992a.

MEDICAL MANAGEMENT

The aim is to improve the haemodynamics by improving any aberrant rhythm, for example, atrial fibrillation (AF) by digitalisation or cardioversion. This reduces the heart rate, allowing more time for filling the coronary arteries in the longer diastolic period. Atrial contribution to cardiac output is regained. Congestive failure is relieved by diuretics and physical demands by reduced activity. Oxygen therapy may be of use to those with pulmonary congestion. Fever should be investigated and treated appropriately. Anticoagulation may be commenced on those with evidence of previous embolisation, those in atrial fibrillation (AF) and those in low output states with left and right failure. The latter may require inotropic support to increase cardiac output and renal perfusion. Sudden onset with pulmonary oedema, for example, with papillary muscle rupture post-AMI, requires artificial ventilation, full monitoring, afterload reduction and the possible aid of an intra-aortic balloon pump (IABP) as in cardiogenic shock (see Ch. 18) to gain time prior to urgent surgery.

Those with chronic disease processes may be maintained on medication. Increasing interest is being shown in the technique of balloon valvuloplasty for stenotic valves where a catheter is introduced across the valve, the balloon is inflated and the calcified stenosis cracked and opened up.

In the mitral position the approach is across the septum while with the aortic valve the catheter is introduced retrogradely. Problems include:

- bradycardias
- profound hypotension when the balloon is inflated
- embolisation
- tamponade
- possible myocardial rupture.

The aim, to increase the functional area of the valve and therefore cardiac output, has met with some success. It may find application in the treatment of elderly, people with aortic stenosis, for whom a full operation would hold too many risks but whose life expectancy is short without it. It has the advantage of a short hospital stay and the prompt resumption of normal life, compared to an operation. An alternative would be prosthetic valve replacement (Kolvekar & Forsyth 1991).

NURSING PRIORITIES AND MANAGEMENT: VALVULAR DISEASE

Breathing

Shortness of breath, often initially on exertion, is the hallmark of progressive heart failure. Sudden valvular failure may result in an alarming onset of breathlessness. In others it is a slow progressive problem which starts with exertion and ends with breathlessness at rest. Orthopnoea (breathlessness in the supine position) may also occur and the increasing number of pillows people require is an indicator of the progression of their disease. Diuretic therapy is used to reduce fluid in the pulmonary interstitium. Sudden valve failure can be very alarming and these patients may require an urgent operation. They should be within sight of the nursing staff and have means of summoning help. An upright position, well supported by pillows, helps chest expansion. Observations should include:

- the depth, rate and pattern of respirations
- the colour of the person's mucous membranes and peripheries
- the quantity of sputum produced and its nature
- any evidence of infection.

The white frothing sputum of pulmonary oedema is characteristic of heart failure. Oxygen therapy may improve symptoms. Some people find the masks very claustrophobic and may benefit from nasal cannulae if low flow oxygen is all they require.

Breathlessness may be precipitated by alterations in heart rate, especially the irregularity of atrial fibrillation. Pulse oximeters (Coull 1992) are often used to monitor heart rate and oxygen saturation by the use of non-invasive skin probes. Their accuracy depends, in part, on the adequacy of the circulation through the skin and so are less suitable for those who have poor peripheral circulation. The probes should be moved from finger to finger regularly to avoid skin damage when circulation is poor.

Diet and nutrition

General fatigue may be the major limiting factor in maintaining adequate nutrition. Small, frequent meals may be more easily digested. They should be high in protein and carbohydrate, especially if the metabolism is raised by fever. Long-term mitral insufficiency does not allow sufficient forward flow of oxygenated blood to nourish the peripheries. The nutritional state of people with valvular disorders should be optimised, prior to surgery. Liver failure may already be a problem due to right-sided failure, which is secondary to primary left-sided heart failure. Altered function affects the liver's ability to metabolise and synthesise basic substrates of cellular construction and function.

The advice of the dietitian may be valuable. High-protein, commercially available drinks can be given to supplement the diet; however, fluid restriction can also be necessary to prevent pulmonary oedema. Fluid restriction and oxygen therapy often leave the mouth dry, and sucking ice or frozen fruit juice helps to keep the mouth as fresh as possible, while minimising fluid intake.

Personal hygiene

The ability to look after personal hygiene may be limited by fatigue and breathlessness. The district nursing team can help at home with bathing and can arrange, through the occupational therapist, to provide aids that make getting in and out of baths easier. Helping patients in this way allows nurses to assess perfusion of the peripheries. Those with fever or who experience sweating, associated with aortic insufficiency, may need more frequent attention to personal freshness.

Sleeping

It can be difficult to sleep due to shortness of breath, even when sitting upright. Each person may have to amend daily activities to allow for periods of rest. Nursing care should be similarly planned.

Mobility

Movement may be limited by the symptoms of the individual. If restricted to bed rest, deep breathing and leg exercises should be encouraged. People whose activities are limited at home might benefit from a home help or may be eligible for mobility allowance. Advice can be sought from the Social Services Department.

Local Authorities issue car stickers for the disabled, to allow greater access to public amenities in prohibited zones.

Wheelchair use. Access to public buildings is slowly improving; public planning incorporates wheelchair access and many older buildings have been adapted to cater for the less mobile. Lists of places that are suitable for access are available. Wheelchairs can be provided to allow people to tour exhibitions or to travel more easily between trains and aircraft, and most large travel organisations provide this service. Holiday brochures often specify which hotels are easily accessible. The Red Cross also hires wheelchairs and aids for limited periods.

For patients who have had surgery, mobility is regained gradually. Each person should set himself the daily goal of walking a little further. Strenuous exercise should be avoided until the sternum heals; for example, any sport involving swinging movements of the arms, such as golf, could prevent the bone edges from knitting together. Some surgeons restrict strenuous exercise for longer, since they feel too great a gradient can be developed across the prosthetic valve.

Work and recreation

Some lines of work may prove too strenuous, necessitating a change of profession. After cardiac valve surgery the patient will be unable to return to work for at least 3 months. Returning part-time is desirable, as people often tire easily at first. This can gradually be increased back to full time. Very physical work is to be avoided for about 6 months. The employer might be able to find a lighter task for these people to do initially but still involve them in the working environment. Some work is forbidden after cardiac surgery, for example, an HGV licence cannot be held. Advice from the social worker about claiming social security allowance and information about retraining schemes can be given, if appropriate. Worry about loss of income can add to the stress of undergoing major surgery.

Maintaining a safe environment

Once a prosthetic valve is in situ, the recipient should be aware of how to avoid putting the valve and himself at risk. Anticoagulation is routine for life in those with metal valves and for a shorter time for those with tissue valves. The person should understand the drugs' use and their potential risks. They should also be aware of the risk of infection and to inform other health professionals, for example dentists, that they have a prosthetic valve and take warfarin. Antibiotic cover is given for dental treatment and any other invasive investigation, for example cystoscopy.

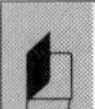

For further details on the use of anticoagulants, see Trounce (1990).

Driving post-operatively is to be avoided until the sternum heals as sudden movement, for example to avoid an accident, could disrupt sternal wire sutures, as could sudden impact to the chest. A small pillow between the seat belt and the chest can reduce friction on the wound, but does not necessarily absorb impact. Eyesight, especially of those who wear glasses, and concentration span are both affected for some weeks after cardio-pulmonary bypass.

Expressing sexuality

Many worry about sexual function after major operation but it is little mentioned. Nurses need to provide an opportunity for such issues to be discussed. Avoiding strain on the sternal suture line is the most important limitation until the bone heals, but after that resumption of relationships should not be excluded. Intimacy between couples can be maintained without full intercourse prior to this. Fear of the valve not coping under exertion should be allayed. Some surgeons do not recommend that young women with prosthetic valves become pregnant because of the increase in circulating volume and cardiac workload. However, successful pregnancies have been completed and obviously this should be as planned an event as possible. Women of child-bearing age are given tissue valves as this allows the period of anticoagulation to be relatively short. Warfarin is teratogenic, especially during the first trimester of pregnancy. Oral contraceptives also inhibit the effects of warfarin. Some may find the prospect of sharing a bed with a partner who 'ticks' off-putting, especially as increases in heart rate can be clearly heard, which can increase fears that catastrophic events will take place during intercourse. They can be reassured that the metallic noise becomes softened with time. As a last resort, tissue valves might be considered although they have a shorter life span and would require replacement within a few years.

Valve stenosis and incompetence

Aortic stenosis

PATHOPHYSIOLOGY

The left ventricle becomes progressively hypertrophied, working at a higher pressure to eject blood past the stenosed valve. The chamber size of the ventricle is reduced by the increased muscle mass which may itself contribute to outflow obstruction. This state is asymptomatic until the orifice is reduced to 0.5–0.7 cm^2 (normal 2.6–3.5 cm^2) when the patient may experience angina as oxygen supply does not meet demand.

The other major effect is syncope, as cardiac output fails to rise in response to exercise. Hypertrophy may progress to decompensation and heart failure with rising left-ventricular end-diastolic pressure (LVEDP) and pulmonary oedema. Aortic stenosis is also associated with occult GI bleeds. The reason for this is still unclear, however the problem subsides with valve replacement (Tuchek 1991).

Mitral stenosis

PATHOPHYSIOLOGY

Here, the left atrium has to eject through a resistant valve. Left atrial pressure rises, the atrium distends and eventually decompensates, with fibrous tissue interspersed between cardiac muscle. Conduction becomes aberrant and atrial fibrillation results. This decreases cardiac output as there is no atrial contribution to ventricular filling. If sinus rhythm persists, evidence of atrial hypertrophy can be seen on the ECG. Since conduction takes longer to spread across the enlarged left atria the P wave becomes broadened and bifid. Left atrial pressure rises futher with the stasis of blood within the chamber. This pressure increase is transmitted to the pulmonary vasculature, where vascular resistance rises with resultant greater right-sided afterload and possible failure. Acute elevations of pressure with exercise, for example, will precipitate pulmonary oedema. Stasis of blood allows the formation of mural thrombus within the atria. The obvious danger is that this may be dislodged and carried forward into the systemic circulation with profound ischaemic consequence for the area supplied by the vessel embolised. See Case History 2.4.

Case History 2.4 Living with mitral stenosis

K is an infant-school teacher in her early 30s. At the age of 12 she had developed rheumatic fever, thought to have resulted from a streptococcal throat infection, although it was not a common disorder and no-one else in her family had ever suffered from it. She had been in hospital for several weeks and had been left with inflammation of her mitral valve, valvulitis, which had caused a progressive narrowing, stenosis of her mitral valve, over the years. On auscultation K's mitral stenosis was identified by the characteristic diastolic murmur.

Until the age of 25, K had felt quite healthy and often wondered just why she had to have regular medical checks and be prescribed antibiotics so quickly when some minor infection occurred. However, in her late 20s she began to experience breathlessness after various activities with the children at school. She often had to sit down, feeling light-headed and developed a persistent, irritating cough. At first she dismissed it but eventually she contacted her GP. Investigations showed that K's stenosis of the mitral valve was becoming worse and that she was developing the early signs of heart failure.

As a result of K's mitral stenosis, the pressure in the left atrium, pulmonary veins and capillaries increases. The left atrium dilates, fluid may accumulate in the alveoli, the pulmonary artery pressure rises, and the right ventricle hypertrophies. Systemic effects become apparent in the form of peripheral oedema, ascites and hepatic engorgement. Atrial fibrillation can occur which may potentiate pulmonary oedema and systemic emboli.

Managing such symptoms will include the use of digoxin to control atrial fibrillation, diuretics, a low-sodium diet and anticoagulant therapy. K will have to adjust her lifestyle to accommodate her valvular disorder but she will be at home.

> ? **2.17** The continuing care of people with valvular disorders is essentially in the community. The desired outcome for someone like K, in Case History 2.4, is that:
>
> - she enjoys a full and happy life within the limitations imposed by her disorder
> - she can cope with the medications and dietary restriction
> - she maintains medical and nursing advice and support.
>
> Which members of the primary health care team will support K?
> What would their priorities be in caring for K at home?

Aortic incompetence

PATHOPHYSIOLOGY

Left-ventricular end-diastolic pressure (LVEDP) is approximately one-eighth of the concomitant aortic pressure, therefore any breach of the valve would allow large amounts of blood to flow back into the ventricle. The ventricle dilates to encompass this volume, LVEDP rises, stroke volume increases and so does systolic pressure. Diastolic pressure within the aorta is low because of regurgitation, therefore there is a wide pulse pressure, often about 190/50 mmHg. Chronic gradual aortic incompetence (AI) is well tolerated but if there is an acute onset, left-ventricular failure (LVF) quickly develops. AI also occurs when the valve annulus becomes dilated so that the cusps cannot coapt, for example in connective tissue disorders, syphilis and aortic dissection.

Mitral incompetence

PATHOPHYSIOLOGY

This allows back flow of blood to the left atrium in systole, where regurgitated blood and the normal atrial volume mix and return to the ventricle before systole. In order to cope with this increased load the ventricle hypertrophies and then dilates. Forward flow diminishes, with progressive failure of the ventricle, and with backflow into the atria at systole. Weight loss and lethargy are marked as the heart can no longer provide the nutrition the blood usually carries. The left atrium dilates and changes in conduction and rhythm occur. In an acute onset, due, for example, to papillary muscle dysfunction in acute inferior MI, sinus rhythm may persist (O'Sullivan 1992).

Tricuspid stenosis and incompetence

PATHOPHYSIOLOGY

These both result in increased right-sided pressure, with evidence of stasis and engorgement of the portal and peripheral circulations, for example, ascites, liver dysfunction and peripheral oedema. If the right atrium becomes hypertrophied due to tricuspid stenosis the P wave on the ECG will become peaked. The majority of right-sided failure is usually secondary to failure on the left; however there is an increase in bacterial endocarditis of the right heart, with the increasing use, or abuse, of intravenous drugs.

HYPERTENSION

Hypertension is difficult to define and there is controversy as to what level of pressure, systolic or diastolic, constitutes hypertension. The technique of measuring blood pressure can also vary, resulting in differences, principally in diastolic definition. The scope of the problem may well be under-estimated since the majority of people are without symptoms until target organs are affected. They then present with major consequences such as renal failure, ischaemic heart disease, cerebral emboli or infarction.

Being aware of associated predisposing factors may enable health workers to target screening towards at-risk groups, as they will be largely unaware of the problem.

Associated factors

Several factors associated with hypertension have been identified. These are:

- obesity
- sodium intake
- alcohol
- genetic factors
- smoking
- stress.

Obesity

The interaction between obesity and hypertension is not fully understood. Overweight adolescents are at significant risk of later hypertension. Those involved in health education and school nursing may play an important part in educating children about diet and exercise in general. An increased intake of sodium is consumed in general over-eating and it is thought that the sodium pump may become impaired in this group. However, this is a reversible situation and blood pressure decreases with weight loss (Rocchini et al 1988).

Sodium intake

The link between sodium and hypertension may be caused by increased sodium and water retention by kidneys faced by an increased sodium loading. Sodium is also stored in greater amounts within the arterial walls of hypertensive people. These vessels then become more responsive to substances that cause vasoconstriction. People who reduce their sodium intake also reduce their blood pressure. There is some evidence (Shore et al 1988) that the interaction of other ions could be important. Left ventricular mass is also increased in those with a high-sodium intake, and hypertrophy, often seen as the response to increased afterload, may be exacerbated (Schmieder et al 1988). High sodium intake is a feature of Western lifestyle and more isolated peoples with a lower intake have a lower incidence of hypertension; once they adopt a Western diet the incidence rises. Compliance with low-sodium diets is poor, as they are so unpalatable.

Emphasis is now laid on not adding salt after cooking and salt substitutes are widely available. There is a generally increased awareness of the contents of packaged foodstuffs; clear product labelling helps people at risk to identify substances that contain sodium. Weinberger and his co-workers (1988) highlight the problem of compliance with a modest sodium-restricted diet, with 14% of their group defaulting within 30 weeks and only 25% of the compliers achieving target sodium levels.

Alcohol

The contribution of alcohol is difficult to assess, as there is a tendency to under-report alcohol consumption due to social pressures. However, blood pressure rises with increasing intake and a reduction in intake reverses this.

Genetic factors

A family history of hypertension predisposes individuals to the same condition. Certain ethnic groups are more susceptible to the condition: the black population in the USA has a 50% greater prevalence than their white counterparts. It appears that the mean resting renal blood flow of normotensive individuals with hypertensive parents is greater than those with normotensive parents. The kidneys' ability to handle sodium is also thought to be genetically influenced.

Smoking

Nicotine promotes catecholamine release and so increases heart rate and blood pressure.

Stress
This is presumed to relate to increased sympathetic outflow (see Ch. 17). Certain occupations are associated with a higher risk of developing hypertension, for example, crane drivers and air-traffic controllers. People who work in noisy over-stimulating environments also run a higher risk of occupational stress, especially if the tasks are repetitive and monotonous.

PATHOPHYSIOLOGY

Although difficult to define in terms of elevated blood pressure, hypertension is commonly classified according to cause:

- primary or essential hypertension refers to a raised blood pressure where no cause can be found
- secondary hypertension is a result of the underlying conditions, most commonly
  - — renal disease (see Ch. 8)
  - — an adrenaline-secreting tumour, for example, phaeochromocytoma in the adrenal cortex
  - — diseases of the pituitary or adrenal glands, where there is an elevation of glucocorticoids (see Ch. 5)
  - — coarctation (narrowing) of the aorta
  - — hyperthyroidism (see Ch. 5).

Hypertension can also be classified according to severity:

- *mild*, when elevation of blood pressure is only moderate and occurs over a long period of time
- *malignant*, when there is a sudden and severe blood pressure elevation.

The malignancy does not refer to cellular changes but to the fact that this is a life-threatening condition. Whatever form of hypertension is diagnosed, the concern is always the effect of this high blood pressure:

1. on the heart, where the increased demand on its pumping capacity can lead to ventricular hypertrophy
2. on the brain, where any elevation of blood pressure could precipitate a cerebral catastrophe (see Ch. 9).

Other organs that give rise to concern are the kidneys, where the delicate function of the nephrons can be impaired by constant high pressure, and the eyes, where fine retinal vessels may rupture and significantly impair vision.

Common presenting symptoms. People who are aware that they have a condition that predisposes them to hypertension will have been alerted to this potential problem and the symptoms may be more readily appreciated. However many may be completely unaware of their hypertensive state, either having no symptoms at all or dismissing complaints such as headaches, vertigo, nosebleeds and fatigue.

MEDICAL MANAGEMENT

Examinations. The elevated blood pressure may only be noticed at some routine examination, for another reason, such as insurance cover. A single elevated reading does not justify a diagnosis of hypertension since anxiety about the examination itself may be the temporary cause, however the person should be reassessed at a later date. Examiners should also be aware of the possible contribution their own technique and instrument calibration may make to errors in estimation, for example, using inappropriately sized cuffs.

Generally, hypertension is defined by grading, with arbitrary cut-off points according to diastolic pressure, as follows:

- mild: 95–104 mmHg
- moderate 105–120 mmHg
- severe > 120 mmHg.

The higher the diastolic pressure, the greater the risk of CVA, renal failure, coronary artery disease and heart failure.

MEDICAL MANAGEMENT

Investigations include:

- blood-pressure monitoring
- chest X-ray and ECG to determine the degree of left-ventricular hypertrophy and heart failure
- full blood count, electrolytes, urea or nitrogen and creatine, to exclude secondary causes and renal effects of the disease process
- urinalysis with microscopy, 24-hour collections for creatinine clearance and vanillylmandelic acid (VMA)
- intravenous pyelogram (IVP) to assess renal perfusion.

Treatment depends largely on how elevated the blood pressure is.

Mild elevation. Advice focuses on modifying lifestyle to minimise the individual's risk factors. Regular 6-monthly follow-ups to reinforce the information and check the blood pressure may be all that is required. Practice nurses may find a developing role as counsellors as GP practice moves more towards preventative medicine.

The benefit of drug treatment for diastolic pressures under 100 mmHg is still uncertain. Over that level it is accepted for men between 45 and 65 years of age.

Moderate elevation is treated largely with thiazide diuretics or cardioselective beta blockade along with general advice on risk reduction. Some of these drugs can increase serum cholesterol and sugar levels, and so contribute to IHD (Hall and Ball 1988). If the desired level of pressure is not achieved with these agents alone, then they can be tried in combination. Long-acting preparations allow a once-daily dose, which the patient might prefer. Failing this, a third-line drug is introduced. This is often a calcium channel antagonist, which promotes vasodilation of the coronary bed and peripheries. There may be negative inotropic effects; it is also thought that they may have cardioprotective properties by reducing platelet aggregation and inhibiting atherosclerosis (Hall and Ball 1988).

Angiotensin converting enzyme (ACE) inhibitors block the conversion of angiotensin I to angiotensin II. Thus vasoconstriction is reduced and the blood pressure becomes normal. These may also reduce serum lipid levels, which may benefit those with familial hyperlipidaemia (Costa et al 1988).

If these measures fail to control pressure, or if there is severely raised diastolic pressure, the patient will be referred to specialised clinicians. Investigation for secondary causes of hypertension should ensue promptly. Tests should include assays for evidence of renal disease, primary aldosteronism, hypothyroidism and phaeochromocytoma, while urgent assessment and control of blood pressure takes place. It may be that this is a side effect of other treatment, for example, oral contraception. Only 4–5% develop overt hypertension due to oestrogen ingestion but it may take several months for it to settle. Other forms of contraception should be advised. Hypertension is also one of the signs of pre-eclampsia of pregnancy.

Overzealous treatment to achieve good blood pressure figures, rather than a good effect for the individual should be avoided. Many people with hypertension have co-existing CAD, even if asymptomatic, and since the extraction of oxygen within the coronary circulation is close to maximum at rest, lowering the blood pressure may further compromise the coronary circulation, causing myocardial ischaemia. Studies have shown an increased frequency of AMI when achieving acceptable diastolic pressures on anti-hypertensive therapy (Cruikshank 1988).

Malignant elevation. At any point in primary hypertension sudden acute elevation of pressure can occur. This malignant hypertension can rapidly become life threatening. Death can ensue from CVA, or from the cerebral oedema of hypertensive encephalopathy. Hypertension generally promotes the progression of atherosclerosis. Sudden increased pressure in vessels already compromised may lead to rupture or embolisation of existing thrombus. The importance of this depends on where the emboli occlude. Renal function is usually already impaired by renal artery sclerosis and the effects of chronic hypertension. Further occlusion of the afferent arterioles exacerbates the situation by stimulating increased renin release which, in turn, contributes to the hypertensive state. Increased pressure may result in internal haemorrhage and infarction of the kidneys.

The progress of the increasing pressure is mirrored in changes to the vessels of the optic fundi, termed hypertensive retinopathy. Once papilloedema occurs, intracranial pressure has increased and the individual may complain of blurring of vision. Prognosis at this point is poor.

Management of hypertensive crisis

The aim of medical and nursing management of this life threatening condition is a controlled reduction in blood pressure, with monitoring of other systems in order to minimise futher damage or to prevent it from occurring (O'Donnell 1990). Cerebral function should be assessed continuously. Blood pressure should be monitored, preferably by direct arterial cannulation, at least every 15 minutes to assess the efficacy of drug therapy. Cardiac demand should be reduced as much as possible by bed rest and sedation. Straining at stool should be avoided. The patient should have urinary catheterisation and frequent observation of their urine output. 24-hour urine collection should commence for excretory products of catecholamines, such as vanillyl mandelic acid (VMA), levels being twice that of normal, in the presence of adrenal tumours, such as phaeochromocytoma. The nurse should also be alert for haematuria or any other sign of blood loss. Complaints of ischaemic chest pain should be investigated and treated as already described.

Anxiolytic drugs may benefit people whose condition is exacerbated by anxiety.

NURSING PRIORITIES AND MANAGEMENT: HYPERTENSION

Where hypertension is secondary to an underlying condition, nursing priorities will reflect the needs of the primary problem. Hypertension will affect lifestyle and sense of wellbeing in many ways.

Since people with hypertension present in various ways, it is difficult to generalise about their management plans.

The experience of pain

Pain control is appropriate in those experiencing headaches or anginal pain, with or without palpitations. Oral analgesics can be prescribed to combat the headaches although the prescription may have to be tailored to the individual, to find an effective agent. This symptom may only lessen once the level of hypertension is controlled and this may motivate the patient to comply with other treatments. Angina will be approached as previously discussed and will also be helped by other treatments aimed at lowering blood pressure, for example, beta blockade.

Diet and nutrition

Dietary changes are aimed at the reduction of obesity, the control of any underlying problem such as diabetes, and the reduction of the salt content. It is best to involve the whole family, as it is less socially disruptive if everyone can continue to sit down to the same meals together. Also, the hereditary aspect of hypertension would indicate that it is in the whole family's interest to prevent the problem developing. No salt added at table, or salt substitutes, are advised (see p. 44). The nurse may be able to assist patients in interpreting labels on food products.

Moderating alcohol intake is advised. This may be difficult for some, where entertaining forms a great part of their work, however, low-alcohol wines and beers are increasingly available.

Elimination

Diuretic drugs can result in the need to pass urine at socially inconvenient times. This can often be avoided if the drugs are taken first thing in the morning, so that their effect is largely over by the time the person leaves home. Discussing the person's daily routine and flexibility in the timing of treatment, to adapt to the person's lifestyle can result in greater compliance with treatment. It is often difficult for an asymptomatic individual to realise the importance of continuing with medication, especially if there are undesirable side effects. It is often best to broach the subject of side effects before they occur and point out that there can be other treatments if this one does not suit. The individual is then less likely to stop taking his medication independently and more likely to seek futher advice (Jordan 1992, Hargrove-Huttel 1991).

Diuretics, apart from potassium-sparing varieties, promote the excretion of potassium in the urine. Low levels of K can result in muscle weakness and fatigue and cardiac arrhythmias. It is therefore important that potassium supplementation is also adhered to by those taking diuretics. Many products combine both diuretic and potassium. A list of foods rich in potassium, for example bananas, can be supplied.

Sleeping

Relaxation and rest are important. Daily routines should be examined in order to find appropriate periods for rest. Night sedation may be necessary to ensure adequate sleep, although the patient should be encouraged to maintain his own relaxation habits, for example, soaking in a warm bath. Referral to agencies that practise relaxation and stress-management techniques may be of benefit to some (see Ch. 17).

Work and leisure

Some working environments may add to the stress individuals experience. Work routines should be re-examined to see if more opportunity exists for delegation of work and for rest. Smoking may be a habit engendered by stress and reinforced by working with a group of people in similar positions. Finding other interests other than work may help the 'workaholic'. Sporting hobbies should be encouraged, as exercise will increase cardiac fitness as long as strenuous exercise is not embarked on without advice.

Breathing

Every effort should be made to stop smoking. Various approaches exist, from cigarette substitutes to hypnosis, acupuncture and sheer will-power. People should be encouraged to find their own way and, as in changing eating habits, the whole family can also be involved here.

Beta blockade, using the non-cardioselective varieties, may result in bronchospasm. This side effect could be extremely alarming if the patient were not aware of the possibility.

Expressing sexuality

Anxiety and tension between couples may lead to sexual dysfunction. Openness on the part of health professionals may help them to feel they can discuss their fears with them and with each other. Beta blockade may also cause impotence.

> ? **2.18** Health-education leaflets related to cardiovascular disease are widely available. Where do these leaflets come from? Who uses them? Do health professionals and the public find them useful? Explore these questions during your placements in community and hospital.

> See Murphy & Smith (1993), 205–215 and Kelly (1992), 1291–1296.

AORTIC ANEURYSMS

PATHOPHYSIOLOGY

The aorta is divided into three segments:

- the ascending aorta
- the arch
- the descending aorta, which consists of abdominal and thoracic portions.

Aneurysms are also classified by shape, as being:

- fusiform, involving a complete circumferential section
- saccular, which describes an outpouching from one weakened area.

Saccular aneurysms can be tied off surgically at the neck of the sack, while fusiform types require excision and replacement with a tubular graft. If the graft is required close to the aortic valve, a composite prosthetic valve and tube graft may be employed, with reimplantation of the coronary arteries if necessary.

There are several causes of aneurysm formation:

- Atherosclerotic disease is the major cause of aneurysms, especially of the descending portion, 75% being below the diaphragm. Plaque formation reduces the nutritional supply to the aortic wall, by hampering diffusion of nutrients from blood in the lumen.
- Turbulence around bifurcations
- Hypertension and medial degeneration. The medial layer of the vessel wall undergoes degenerative changes associated with ageing. Since this is the layer that, due to its elasticity, withstands the most pressure, degeneration allows the wall to dilate. This often occurs without symptoms and may be found on routine examination. The patient is often hypertensive. Increased blood pressure, especially diastolic pressure, reduces the blood flow to the medial layer which becomes ischaemic and weakened (Lekander 1986).

  Cystic medial degeneration also occurs as a consequence of connective tissue diseases, for example Marfan's and Ehlers–Danlos syndromes (Weiland & Walker 1986). These affect the ascending aorta and may cause the annulus of the aortic valve to dilate. This may result in an incompetent valve as the cusps cannot completely cover the larger area. First presentation may be as a consequence of valvular failure.
- Infection. Aneurysms due to syphilis and other infectious causes are less prevalent today; they largely affect the ascending aorta.

Abdominal aortic aneurysms (AAA)

Common presenting symptoms. The majority are without symptoms but a pulsating abdominal mass may be felt when lying in bed. Pain relates to compression of neighbouring organs. It is severe, unrelated to movement and radiates through to the low back, and possibly down into the thighs and buttocks. Presentation may be as ischaemia of end organs whose arterial supply originates within the aneurysmal section. Ischaemia may also be the result of embolisation of thrombus that gathers in the dilated portion due to sluggish blood flow and turbulence around atherosclerotic plaques. Half of the dilatations greater than 6 cm will rupture within a year, so prompt surgical management is called for. The risk of spontaneous dissection is that severe blood loss, hypotension and death will supervene. Emboli may enter the inferior vena cava and result in pulmonary infarction. Mortality in ruptured aneurysms is high. Emergency management aims to stabilise blood pressure by large volume infusion of colloid or other volume expanders, the use of military anti-shock trousers (MAST) and pharmacological support with inotropic drugs. Surgical repair should not be delayed.

MEDICAL MANAGEMENT

Investigations prior to planned surgery include X-ray, which will highlight any vessel calcification, echocardiography, ultrasound and CT scanning, all of which are non-invasive. Some centres also perform angiography, however this may precipitate embolisation. Full cardiac investigation is required since atherosclerosis is a diffuse disease. Correction of any coronary insufficiency is recommended prior to surgical non-emergency aneurysm repair, since postoperative mortality is largely due to myocardial infarction.

Thoracic aneurysms

The aetiology is similar to those in the abdomen. False thoracic aneurysms can be secondary to blunt or penetrating injury to the chest in road traffic accidents, although they are more often associated with true rupture of the aorta, from which mortality is high. Some thoracic aneurysms are stabilised by surrounding tissue for long enough to present at cardiothoracic services.

PATHOPHYSIOLOGY

Atherosclerosis affects the arch and descending thoracic aorta, while cystic medial degeneration and infections are found as causative agents in the ascending portion.

Common presenting symptoms depend on the site of occurrence. Chest X-ray shows a widened mediastinum. Dilatation causes pressure on other structures: bronchospasm may result from deviation of the trachea; secretion retention and alveolar collapse from obstruction; shortness of breath, and even haemoptysis, if erosion occurs into the left main bronchus. Obstruction of the oesophagus may present as dysphagia, while fainting may be the result of reduced cardiac output due to obstruction of the superior vena cava.

Dissecting aortic aneurysms

PATHOPHYSIOLOGY

Tears in the intima due to the forces of hypertension and the degenerative changes already discussed, allow a column of blood to enter and disrupt the media creating a false lumen. Classification is by site of the tear. In addition to previously discussed predisposing diseases there is a higher, but as yet unexplained, incidence of dissection among pregnant women.

Common presenting symptoms depend upon the site and severity of the rupture. Severe anterior chest pain can be mistaken for AMI, but it is often described as tearing in nature. Pain may migrate as the dissection progresses. Alterations of neurological function may reflect involvement of the vessels originating from the arch of the aorta. As the dissection progresses, loss of peripheral pulses and palpable blood pressure will track its course. Renal artery dissection or occlusion will result in acute renal failure, exacerbated by the effects of profound hypotension. Alterations in rhythm or degrees of heart block may result from septal disruption as a consequence of aortic valve regurgitation. Leakage into the pericardium or pleural space manifests as compression known as tamponade. The signs of cardiac tamponade are:

- hypotension
- tachycardia
- raised CVP/JVP
- oliguria
- peripheral vascular constriction
- fall in peripheral temperature.

MEDICAL MANAGEMENT

Investigations are identical to AAA.

Treatment. Operative correction is urgently required. If hypertension persists this should be controlled by the use of arterial vasodilators, intensively and invasively monitored. If hypotension and collapse has supervened then intervention is as for AAA.

NURSING PRIORITIES AND MANAGEMENT: AORTIC ANEURYSMS

Preoperative care

Although this type of aneurysm is the most life threatening any vessel may become aneurysmal.

Pain control

The pain is often described as ripping or tearing in nature. Its location varies according to the section of artery affected and may progress as a dissection progresses. Intravenous opiate is the appropriate measure but the patient may be so shocked that immediate operative procedure is of greater priority.

Anxiety and fear of dying

The prospect of surgery is extremely frightening, whether emergency or elective and this should be acknowledged by carers. Operations hold high risks, but there is often no alternative intervention. Those going for elective procedures may wish access to legal advisors. The need for spiritual care should also be recognised. There may be times when a dignified, peaceful death is more appropriate than surgery.

Maintaining a safe environment

Rupture of an aneurysmal vessel is a potentially catastrophic and largely unpredictable event. Those with known aneurysms that do not yet merit surgery should be aware of signs that indicate a progression of their disease. Control of hypertension by medication is indicated and should be adhered to (see p. 46).

Breathing

Shortness of breath may be experienced by those with aneurysms of the thoracic aorta as the vessel impinges on the trachea. This may also result in bronchospasm. Rupture of the vessel can create a fistula into the bronchus, with resulting haemoptysis. Changing the person's position to allow maximal lung expansion may help. Oxygen therapy will often be required. Bronchodilators may be of limited use as the problem is mechanical rather than irritant. Chest infection due to atelectasis as the lung is collapsed under the weight of the expanding aorta is to be expected. Since maintaining the airway is a potential problem, an airway, suction equipment, an Ambu-bag and other resuscitation equipment should be available.

Mobility and rest

Anxiety may prevent the patient from sleeping, so sedation may be helpful if the blood pressure is not adversely affected. The patient's condition can be so unstable that performing routines of care can exhaust them. Plan care so that people are left in peace for periods. Nurses sometimes have to accept that their patient's condition will not allow care that would otherwise be thought essential, for example pressure-area care. Consider the use of aids such as air-fluidised beds to dissipate pressure on what is often already poorly perfused skin.

Elimination

Since approximately 25% of cardiac output perfuses the kidneys, urine output is a useful and important reflection of cardiac function. Accurate observation and recording of fluid balance is essential.

Hygiene

Because of their poor status and poor tissue perfusion, this is an area where the patient becomes dependent on a nurse to maintain standards of personal hygiene.

Expressing sexuality

People attending electively for resection of abdominal aneurysms may be offered counselling before surgery. There can be a possibility of impotence and paraplegia postoperatively if the arterial supply to the spinal cord is interrupted. It is possible to arrange storage in sperm banks against this eventuality. These issues need to be handled with sensitivity by the nurse.

Surgical intensive care

Once the patient's condition has deteriorated and surgery is necessary the patient is completely dependent on hospital staff for circulatory support. Accurate haemodynamic assessment is essential. Careful observation and documentation of the response to drug therapy and large-volume colloid infusion is essential. This may require invasive monitoring and the specialist nursing skills of the intensive therapy unit and the patient should be moved to such a unit as soon as is feasible. This can mean journeys of several hours by road or air, a daunting prospect for patient and escorting staff, alike. It often necessitates the separation of the patient from his family at a time of great stress, so every effort should be made to ensure effective communication. The management of cardiogenic shock is covered in Chapter 18. Postoperative care is similar to that following cardiac surgery (see Nursing Care Plan 2.2).

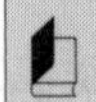
For further information read Ch. 7 'Vascular conditions requiring intensive care' in: Ashworth & Clarke (1992).

PERIPHERAL VASCULAR DISEASE

Arterial and venous peripheral disease can occur alone or together and it is important to be able to differentiate between the two (Bright & Georgi 1992).

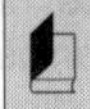
Revise the anatomy of arteries and veins of the lower limbs in Wilson (1990).

ARTERIAL DISEASE

Arterial occlusions

Like the rest of the cardiovascular system, the lower limbs may also be affected by atherosclerosis. Symptoms of impaired blood supply may be slow to appear if collateral circulation has had time to develop.

Arteriosclerosis obliterans

PATHOPHYSIOLOGY

This is the state of chronic occlusive atheroma of the arteries supplying the extremities. Turbulence at bifurcations, as occurs in larger vessels, predisposes to intimal changes. There is also a degenerative element in its development. The same process is found in the cerebral and visceral arteries. The factors influencing its development have been discussed in the section on IHD and hypertension. It is typically a disease of middle-aged to elderly men, who may be hypertensive, diabetic, have a diet high in lipids and who smoke, resulting in greater risk of atherosclerosis.

Nursing Care Plan 2.2 B is a 54-year-old unemployed welder who had an abdominal aortic aneurysm repair 36 hours previously. This was an elective operation and involved the insertion of a synthetic graft. Since the operation B has been cared for in an intensive care unit. He had artificial respiratory support on a ventilator up until 12 hours ago. A urinary catheter, nasogastric tube and central venous pressure line were inserted in theatre. B's wife and family are very concerned about his condition and his wife is spending most of the day at his bedside.

Nursing considerations	Action	Rationale	Evaluation
1. Potential problem of hypovolaemic shock	• Continue to monitor vital signs noting for: — fall in blood pressure — increase in heart rate • Observe for fall in hourly urine output • Observe for changes in mental state: restlessness, confusion • Note and report significant changes in temperature • Observe for signs of peripheral oedema and cold, pale peripheries • Observe wound site for excessive leakage • Give intravenous fluids as prescribed • Continue with central venous pressure recordings, noting and reporting trends	• Hypovolaemic shock may arise due to excessive blood loss/inadequate fluid replacement	• Stable vital signs • Urine output > 30 mls/hour • Stable neurological function
2. Possibility of developing hypertension	• Regular measurement of blood pressure • Monitor effects of any hypertensive drug therapy • Ensure that B knows to report any pain/discomfort. Assess and plan intervention, and evaluate pain relief measures • Observe wound site regularly for any sign of suture line being under stress due to increased blood pressure • Attempt to limit anxiety by providing information and support, and creating a calm, relaxed atmosphere for B and his family	• May have been hypertensive prior to operation • Systemic vascular response may increase as a result of — decreased circulatory volume — increased sympathetic tone as a stress response • To control/relieve pain and anxiety	• Vital signs within normal limits • Is pain free, comfortable and relaxed
3. Risk of infection	• Monitor temperature recordings at regular intervals • Give prophylactic antibiotics • Observe sites of intravenous and arterial access for redness/ inflammation • Observe colour and consistency of urine	• Risk of infection due to: — surgical procedure — immobility — urinary catheterisation — venous and arterial convolution	• Remains apyrexial and free from infection
4. Possibility of gastro-intestinal disturbance	• Note nature of stools, especially diarrhoea and bloody stools • Observe for increase in abdominal girth • Maintain position and patency of nasogastric tube, gradually introducing fluids orally • Ensure that B knows to report abdominal pain • Ensure B is aware of the planned time scale for resuming eating and drinking	• May develop as a result of handling the colon during surgery with resultant oedema • May develop as a result of antibiotics	• Remains free from gastro-intestinal disturbance

Nursing Care Plan 2.2 *(cont'd)*

Nursing considerations	Action	Rationale	Evaluation
5. Possibility of difficulty in breathing	• Ensure B knows to report any difficulty breathing • Observe respiratory rate and chest expansion • Offer oxygen therapy • Encourage turning 2-hourly to promote postural drainage • Encourage deep breathing and coughing • Liaise with physiotherapist regarding chest physiotherapy	• Wound may limit deep breathing • Abdominal distention may raise the diaphragm reducing breathing capacity • Signs of heart failure may suggest a rupture into the vena cava.	• Is comfortable when breathing • Displays no evidence of cyanosis or heart failure
6. Potential problem of pain/discomfort	• Ensure B knows to report any pain/discomfort • Give prescribed analgesics on a regular basis for abdominal pain at incision site • ECG if B experiences chest pain • Observe for signs associated with ischaemic pain: shortness of breath, nausea and vomiting	• May experience abdominal pain at wound site • May experience ischaemic chest pain as a result of decreased coronary artery blood flow	• Is pain free and comfortable
7. Potential problem of renal impairment	• Maintain record of fluid input and output • Record weight at the same time daily • Give intravenous fluids at the rate prescribed • Note trends in urine output in relation to blood pressure and rates of drug infusion	• May develop renal impairment as a result of embolisation; fall in blood pressure; trauma to the renal artery during surgery; or pre-operative renal ischaemia due to renal artery involvement in development of aneurysm	• Urine output > 30 mls/hr
8. Reduced mobility	• Assist to maintain desired activities of living: hygiene, personal grooming, mouth care, etc. • Place objects within reach. Offer access to radio, papers, books as requested • Liaise with physiotherapist • Formulate plan for gradually increasing mobility, beginning with sitting out of bed for short periods • Involve family members in care, if acceptable to them • Encourage frequent changes in position whilst in bed • Advise how to support wound when moving about	• Mobility is reduced as a result of monitoring equipment, intravenous lines, urinary catheter, abdominal discomfort and uncertainty as to permitted safe level of movement	• Effects of limited mobility will be minimised • Mobility levels will be gradually increased
9. Anxiety and lack of information	• Explain all treatment and expected course of hospital stay to B and his family • Encourage B's family to visit when they can promoting a welcoming and open atmosphere • Develop one-to-one relationship between nurse and B to foster open communication and individualised support and information giving • Provide realistic outlook for future and recovery	• B and his family are likely to be anxious about the outcome of the operation and the future • The ITU environment may exacerbate these feelings	• B and his family will appear to be coping effectively with the operation and recovery • B and his family will express that they feel able to cope and state that they understand the operation, treatment and plans for recovery

Table 2.8 Presenting features of arterial and venous peripheral vascular disease (Adapted from Bright and Georgi 1992.)

Assess	Arterial disease	Venous disease
Pain	Acute: sudden, severe pain, peaks rapidly Chronic: intermittent claudication; rest pain	Acute: little or no pain; tenderness along course of inflamed vein Chronic: heaviness, fullness
Impotence	May be present with aorto-iliac femoral disease	Not associated
Hair	Hair loss distal to occlusion	No hair loss
Nails	Thick, brittle	Normal
Skeletal muscle	Atrophy may be present; may have restricted limb movement	Normal
Sensation	Possible paraesthesia	Normal
Skin colour	Pallor or reactive hyperaemia (pallor when limb elevated; rubor [red] when limb dependent)	Brawny (reddish-brown); cyanotic if dependent
Skin texture	Thin, shiny, dry	Stasis dermatitis; veins may be visible; skin mottling
Skin temperature	Cool	Warm
Skin breakdown (ulcers)	Severely painful; usually on or between toes or on upper surface of foot over metatarsal heads or other bony prominences	Mildly painful, with pain relieved by leg elevation; usually in ankle area
Oedema	None or mild; usually unilateral	Typically present, usually foot to calf; may be unilateral or bilateral
Pulses	Diminished; weak; absent	Normal
Blood flow	Bruit may be present; pressure readings lower below stenosis	Normal

The result of increasing occlusion of the vessels, with medial calcification and loss of elastic fibres, is the slowing of blood flow. The blood becomes hypercoaguable. Thrombosis of the deep veins may occur, secondary to sudden arterial thrombosis. The ischaemia of surrounding tissue is evidenced by skin and muscle atrophy, loss of subcutaneous fat deposits and ischaemic neuropathy. Severe occlusion will result in gangrene, usually first seen at the toes, then extending into the foot and leg. At the boundary between viable and necrotic tissue an area of inflammation is often seen. The extent of the ischaemia will depend on how quickly occlusion developed and how extensive collateral circulation has become. Gangrene occurs when insufficient oxygen is conveyed to the tissue to sustain life. This can be exacerbated by any other superimposed demand for example, infection, when oxygen demand rises but cannot be sustained by an impaired blood flow. Diabetic patients are more prone to infected ulceration in association with gangrene (see Ch. 5). Vasoconstriction should be avoided if at all possible.

Common presenting symptoms may occur gradually or with sudden acute thrombosis, which may be the first indication of a process that has been silently progressing for some time (see Table 2.8).

Pain: intermittent claudication. This is exercise-induced pain in muscle groups distal to the occluded vessel. Its nature varies from a numb cramp to severe pain. It is a manifestation of increased oxygen demand with exercise and the subsequent accumulation of metabolic wastes. This is relieved by rest. The calf muscles are the most commonly affected but thigh and buttock muscles can also be involved, depending on the site of occlusion. The distance the individual can walk on the flat before onset of symptoms (claudication distance) is an indication of the progress of his disease. Pain may eventually occur at rest most often in the toes and foot, particularly at night when it interferes with sleep. Pain may become severe and difficult to contain when gangrene intervenes. However a degree of neuropathy reduces sensation and may make the person unaware of the progressive gangrenous changes. Any exercise that can be tolerated should be encouraged.

MEDICAL MANAGEMENT

Investigations are as follows.

Pulses should be assessed at rest in a warm room. They may remain intact until two-thirds of the lumen is occluded. Posterior tibial, popliteal and femoral pulses should be included in the examination. (Dorsalis pedis pulses are not consistently present in all people.) The volume of the pulses should be compared, as well as simple absence or presence. Many people find it difficult to differentiate between their own pulses and the patient's and increasing the examiner's rate by exercising can help in this situation. Bruits may also be heard over areas of turbulence in arteries that are still pulsating.

Colour and temperature. As occlusion develops the feet, and especially the toes, may be red in colour. This can later develop into bluish mottled areas or areas of pallor. With sudden occlusion, pallor may be marked. Elevation of legs with severe occlusion results in deathly pallor. Once legs return to the dependent position, colour normally returns. Superficial veins normally refill within 15 seconds but in these cases it may take a minute or more. In severe cases the limbs may become a cyanotic red colour (rubor). Temperature changes accompany reduced blood flow with cool pale extremities.

Chest X-rays will show calcification of the vessel wall.

Doppler ultrasound. When low-intensity sound is directed through the tissue towards a blood vessel, sound waves strike moving blood cells and are transmitted back. The frequency of the sound waves that are reflected changes in proportion to the velocity of the blood. Sound waves diminish in arterial occlusion and stenosis (Williams et al 1993).

Arteriograms are usually performed in order to assess the occlusion prior to surgery.

Other examinations include ECG, a full blood count, urea, electrolytes and blood sugar estimation.

MEDICAL MANAGEMENT

Underlying disease states, for example, diabetes and infection should be as well controlled as possible. Advice aimed at minimising symptoms and the risk of extending atherosclerosis should be given:

- modify the diet to reduce lipid intake
- avoid
  - — cigarette smoking
  - — tight clothing
  - — cold temperature

all of which lead to vasoconstriction.

- Avoid direct use of heat because of the risk of burns in a limb with decreased sensation
- promote increased blood supply by a generally warm environment and elevation of the head of the bed
- avoid maintaining a completely dependent position since the resultant oedema will further reduce circulation
- encourage exercising up to the limit of pain, partly to maintain joint and muscle function and to promote collateral circulation; by walking 3–4 times a day, ischaemic time will decrease, and pain control can also be improved by increasing blood flow; however ischaemic pain is notoriously difficult to manage and may require opiate analgesia and night sedation
- avoid trauma to the impaired limb
- avoid ill-fitting shoes; referral to a chiropodist may be required.

Following assessment, sympathectomy may be considered to increase blood flow by obliterating neural control of vasoconstriction (Forrest et al 1991).

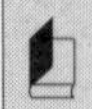

Williams, Picton & McCollum (1993), 9–12.

If the occlusion is sudden and acute and the viability of the limb is in question, then surgical intervention will be required to bypass the occlusion using either saphenous vein or prosthetic material, for example, a femoro-popliteal bypass (Whitehead 1988). Endarterectomy of the vessel may be performed first to core out the atheroma of the vessel.

Prior to surgery the patient may undergo arteriography, and should be rehydrated and have blood coagulation status assessed. There is a strong association with IHD, so full cardiac assessment is required prior to operation. If the lesion is localised and accessible, embolectomy under local anaesthesia may be sufficient to reperfuse the limb. In this procedure a catheter is inserted into the artery up to the level of the occlusion when the balloon at the end is inflated, aiming to fracture the plaque. Inflammation and re-endothelialisation occurs secondary to this. Fibrinolytic drugs can be infused at the site of the occlusion. The advantage of embolectomy is that general anaesthesia can be avoided in an elderly population; however, reocclusion occurs more frequently than with bypass grafting (Greenhalgh 1984).

Pain may become so severe and gangrene so advanced that the limb is no longer viable and amputation may become unavoidable. Bypass grafting may minimise the extent of amputation by restoring circulation, for example to a foot, but losing some of the toes. Amputation of a limb is traumatic for anyone but may be accepted as a relief from intolerable pain. It may, however, require skilled counselling before this fact can be faced by the patient and the full support of rehabilitation and limb-fitting services postoperatively.

? **2.19** Find out about the rehabilitative care for any patient who has had amputation of a lower limb and is adapting to the use of a prosthesis.

For further information on surgical or operation details, see Whitehead 1988 and Forrest, Carter & McLeod 1991, Ch. 21.

Thromboangiitis obliterans or Buergers disease

This occlusive inflammatory disease has no known pathogenesis. It manifests in a younger population than atherosclerosis, is predominant in men and is strongly associated with smoking. It is postulated that carbon monoxide has a toxic effect on the arterial wall, and nicotine has vasoconstrictive effects. In contrast to atherosclerosis, it affects small and medium vessels of the extremities. It is not a diffuse disease, affecting only segments of arteries with inflammatory lesions. Thrombosis is a secondary feature. The lumen may become occluded and the intima thickened but the medial wall structure remains intact, in contrast to atherosclerotic disease. Presentation, investigation and management differ little, however, with an emphasis on giving up smoking.

Raynaud's disease

This is a vasospastic condition, usually occurring in young women. Constriction of the arterioles associated with cold and emotional stress results in colour changes, usually in the hands. The fingers become pale and cold but pulses are intact. Cyanosis may also be a feature. Pain is not always present but function may be lost. Similar episodes of vasospasm can be found secondary to scleroderma, some neurological conditions and in some occupational groups, for example, those that use pneumatic vibrating tools. Treatment includes avoiding the situation that triggers the problem. This may mean a change in occupation, giving up smoking and keeping warm. Vasodilating drugs, including calcium channel blockers, have been tried to improve circulation as has sympathectomy.

A distinction should be made between Raynaud's phenomenon, which results in no permanent damage, and Raynaud's disease, the more advanced condition associated with permanent damage.

NURSING PRIORITIES AND MANAGEMENT: ARTERIAL DISEASE

Almost all the activities of life are affected by the distress of arterial disease.

Maintaining a safe environment

Possible loss of sensation increases the risk of trauma to tissue that has reduced ability to combat infection and to heal. The person's home and work circumstances can be considered, and hazards minimised. (See Case History 2.5.) Useful advice would include the following points:

- toe nails may be best cut by the chiropodist in case soft-tissue injury is inflicted, especially as some people with atherosclerotic disease, with or without diabetes, may also have poor sight
- caution should be exercised with electric blankets, hot-water bottles, open fires and hot baths as burns may not be felt
- cold can be damaging
- constrictive clothing, for example tight underwear, is best avoided
- sitting with crossed legs causes constriction
- remaining in one position for any length of time puts pressure on one area of tissue, allowing ischaemic changes to occur
- bed cradles can be used to support bedclothes without causing constriction.

Case History 2.5

Mrs C is 75, living alone in a large apartment. She has extensive arterial disease and is awaiting admission for femoro-popliteal artery bypass surgery. The community nurse and occupational therapist carry out a personal and environmental assessment pre-surgery. During their home visit, they note many environmental hazards that could cause accidents and lower limb damage.

? **2.20** Drawing on your experience of visiting old people at home, identify the range of possible hazards.
Think of your own home and work environment. How aware are you of actual and potential damage to your lower limbs from knocks, friction, pressure and cuts?

Health professionals try to act in the best interests of their patients but may fail to assess the situation adequately. For example, the community nurse slipped on Mrs C's rug, which was lying in the centre of the highly polished hallway floor. She promptly rolled up the rug and put it away in a cupboard.

? **2.21** How might Mrs C feel in that situation?
In fact, Mrs C quickly returned the rug to the hallway floor saying, 'Don't worry. That lovely rug was my mother's. I never set foot on it. I just walk round the edge. I'll be quite safe, but you be careful.'

Pain control
The pain of claudication is relieved by rest; however, exercise to the limit of pain is to be encouraged in the hope of developing increased perfusion and collateral circulation. Controlling ischaemic pain is essential and will often require the use of opiate analgesics, which may cause drowsiness as a side effect. Keeping warm, especially for people affected by vessel spasm, and positioning the affected limb in a dependent position from time to time are also advised. Anti-inflammatory drugs are used in diseases with an inflammatory response. Distraction techniques can also be helpful (see Ch. 19).

Eating and drinking
Excessive weight increases circulatory demand, and people with diabetes need to be particularly careful about what they eat. Dehydration contributes to the process of clot formation because of increased blood concentration, so taking plenty of liquids is recommended. A balanced diet, including the vitamins and trace elements that aid tissue healing and integrity can help to prevent aggravation of symptoms. See Ch. 23. People with hyperlipidaemia could be encouraged to follow the diet suggested for those with coronary artery disease (CAD) and may also be prescribed drugs to reduce their lipid levels.

Sleep
This is often impaired by pain. Elevating the bed-head is suggested to increase flow. See also Ch. 25.

Breathing
Smoking reduces the amount of oxygen the haemoglobin can carry and nicotine results in venous spasm. Encouraging the patient to give up therefore may produce benefits.

Mobility
Maintaining as great a degree of mobility as possible can help to prevent general stiffness of all joints, which can develop if they are under-utilised. Muscle wasting and weakness are associated problems; the patient can be encouraged to carry out a wide range of joint exercises.

Hygiene
Careful attention to hygiene helps to prevent infection, especially if the person is diabetic. After bathing, the skin should be thoroughly dried, especially between the toes. This gives the opportunity to assess the skin for any signs of ischaemia. Points to note are:

- bath water should be neither too hot nor too cold
- tight socks with elastic tops cause constriction
- clean clothing, daily, is preferred
- plastic shoes encourage sweating and maceration of the skin as water cannot evaporate.

Work
Consideration should be given as to the physical demands and environmental hazards at the person's work. Strong analgesics may also impair performance and safety.

? **2.22** Read Case History 2.6 and consider the following questions.

a. What is meant by the term gangrene?
b. Mr L was suffering from the pain of ischaemia prior to surgery. What was meant by phantom limb pain and how do you think such pain could be alleviated?
c. Can you explain, in physiological terms, why his aching legs were relieved by rest?
d. Describe the tests Mr L might have undergone to assess his arterial insufficiency?
e. How *does* smoking affect feet?
f. What vasodilatory medication might have been prescribed?
g. What was the surgery Mr L had?
h. It was clear that Mr L found it almost impossible to change his lifestyle. What role do you think hospital and community nurses can play in helping someone like Mr L?
i. Outline a plan of care for Mr L for the immediate postoperative period after an above-knee amputation of his right leg.

Discharge planning
After successful surgery, it is important to consider how vascular improvement can be maintained to ensure a reasonable quality of life and prevent further hospital admissions.

? **2.23** What kind of discharge planning would be appropriate for Mrs C (see Case History 2.5), following femoro-popliteal bypass grafting?

VENOUS DISEASE

Venous insufficiency
Venous disease results from:

- obstruction, by thrombus or thrombophlebitis
- incompetence of valves in the veins.

Some diseases, such as varicose veins, may seem trivial but contribute to day-to-day discomfort and to absence from work. Other venous diseases are associated with chronic health prob-

Case History 2.6 Peripheral vascular disease; Mr L's memories

Mr L lay back on his hospital pillow, wishing he was at home. The powerful analgesic was at last easing the pain in his gangrenous foot. Tomorrow he would have surgery that would rid him of the limb, but losing a limb had been difficult to come to terms with and what was this phantom pain he had heard so much about?

Thirty years ago Mr L had been strong and fit, fond of long country walks and watching football. His first complaint had been aching legs after his long walks but it hadn't lasted long and was easily relieved by sitting down. However the aching became a great deal worse and his walks became shorter and shorter. Fond of his food, he had gained weight and spent more of his leisure time smoking.

His GP had described his symptoms as intermittent claudication or limping. He had said it was due to impairment of the blood supply to his lower limbs and had organised several tests to confirm this. At first the treatment had seemed quite easy. Mr L had to cut down on his smoking, alter his diet to avoid rich and fatty food that could 'clog up' his arteries and avoid extremes of temperature, which would make the symptoms worse.

It had been hard to stick to his diet and give up smoking and, seeing no visible evidence of it working, he had soon given up. The ache in his legs eventually became worse, developing into excruciating pain. At night he had to sit up in bed and hang his legs down to cool them and ease the pain. The GP had given him tablets to help dilate the blood vessels but they hadn't helped and not long afterwards he had found himself facing an operation to improve the blood supply.

Mr L hadn't minded the operation too much. One of his veins had been used to bypass the occlusion in the artery of his thigh. He had thought this rather clever at the time and he had quickly felt the benefits. After the operation he had felt much more enthusiastic about changing his lifestyle. The surgeon had stressed that the success of the operation in the long term would depend on his ability to stop smoking, and he had, for a while. Friends and family had said he looked so much better but somehow it didn't last. He had lost weight but just couldn't stop smoking. He had known the pain was coming back. His toes were looking discoloured and often felt either very sensitive or numb. The skin on his right leg, particularly, was thin and dry and there had seemed to be less muscle. Once again, he had found himself in hospital, the circulation to his lower limbs being thoroughly assessed.

The night before his operation he was unable to sleep and feared both the immediate and long-term future.

lems such as venous ulcers or sudden medical emergency such as pulmonary embolus following deep vein thrombosis.

Deep vein thrombosis (DVT)

Clot formation is more likely to occur when flow is reduced within the veins. This can occur due to obstruction and stasis but is also associated with increased blood viscosity, slower flow and damage to the endothelial wall of the vessel. Hypercoagulability may be a feature of dehydration or malignant disease. It seems that there is also an imbalance between fibrinolysis and coagulation in the postoperative patient, which predisposes them to DVT. Trauma may be mechanical or chemical.

The increasing use of vascular cannulae predisposes the patient in hospital to the irritant effects of pharmacological preparations, the plastic of the cannula itself and the possibility of intimal trauma at insertion.

Stasis allows clotting factors that normally would be cleared from the circulation to remain active for longer. The effects of the muscle pumps of the leg and negative intra-thoracic pressure during inspiration normally promote venous return. Any situation that obliterates their action predisposes to stasis of the venous circulation. Immobility and the recumbent position are frequently features of the postoperative patient and the elderly. Muscle-relaxant drugs used during surgery abolish the muscle pump and breathing is under positive pressure when ventilated mechanically. Stasis is more common in the dilated portions of varicosities. Mechanical obstruction to flow can be seen in pregnancy and abdominal tumours.

The affected area will be tender, swollen and hot. Once diagnosed, treatment includes pain relief and anticoagulation, first with heparin and later with warfarin; bedrest with leg elevation will be necessary until swelling and pain subside. Bedrest may prevent the thrombus dislodging, resulting in embolisation, usually of the lungs.

However, prevention is the priority. Acute venous thrombosis has been estimated to occur in 30–60% of surgical patients (Boore et al 1987). Early ambulation, especially of the elderly postoperative patient, will help prevent stasis. Anti-embolism stockings should be worn and prophylactic subcutaneous heparin is almost a routine postoperative prescription. Avoidance of dehydration, external pressure, immobility in those at risk, as well as careful observation and use of i.v. cannulae are all part of the preventive management of this condition.

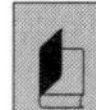

For further information on respiratory problems, see Love (1990a) 40–43 and Love (1990b) 52–55.

Chronic venous insufficiency

Of those suffering from chronic venous insufficiency, 90% have usually had episodes of DVT previously (Lofgren 1983). Pressure within the venous system remains high resulting in increased capillary pressure allowing chronic oedema to develop. The valves and elastic fibres of the vein wall are also destroyed by thrombophlebitis, aggravating the situation (Picton et al 1993). The accumulation of interstitial fluid increases pressure locally. Eczema may occur secondary to this, possibly with pruritis. Due to stasis red blood cells may be trapped and haemolysed. This manifests as areas of brown pigmentation (haemosiderin). Melanin may also be deposited. Prolonged oedema reduces the nutrition available to subcutaneous tissue which then fibroses. This induration further prevents drainage of any oedema. Ulceration may follow trauma or dermatitis of such an area. Ulcers are commonly seen around the internal malleolus and tend to reoccur in the same place, as the scar tissue is atrophic. Infection of such ulcers is common.

Prompt and correct treatment of thrombophlebitis goes a long way to prevent chronic venous insufficency. Pain is worse in the dependent position, so elevation of the limb or walking should be advised. Standing should be avoided.

Oedema is treated by elevation during bed rest. Once it is reduced support stockings should be fitted. Any infection should be isolated and treated with appropriate medication. If varicose veins contribute to ulceration they may be dealt with surgically. Chronic ulcers may have to be skin grafted. Details of the management of arterial and venous ulcers are in Ch. 23.

Varicose veins
Varicosities are long and tortuously dilated veins. They are partly due to the effects of gravity. Dilatation causes the valves to become incompetent and retrograde flow is no longer prevented. It has a genetic component: 50% of sufferers have a family history of varicosities. The hormonal changes in pregnancy also reduce venous tone while the obstruction to venous return by the gravid uterus combines to increase pregnant women's susceptibility. Simple obesity has a similar obstructive effect. Standing for prolonged periods maximises the force of gravity. Thrombophlebitis of the deep veins increases venous pressure while inflammation destroys valve tissue. This increase in pressure is transmitted to the superficial veins which, being relatively less supported by surrounding structures, dilate. Most people complain of dull aching in their legs. Trauma may result in significant blood loss and should be guarded against. Ulcers are rare. Some individuals are concerned by appearance. Elevation and support stockings may help the aching and reduce oedema.

MEDICAL MANAGEMENT

If symptoms persist, the most common management is the surgical stripping and ligation of the varicose vein. For some, the injection of a sclerosing agent would be considered.

NURSING PRIORITIES AND MANAGEMENT: VENOUS INSUFFICIENCY

Mobility
Mobility should be maintained as much as possible. Patients should be advised to elevate the legs when sitting, to increase venous return and reduce oedema and to avoid standing for long periods. After an operation for ligation of varicosities measures to prevent DVT should be considered. The patient will be advised to:

- walk a prescribed distance of perhaps 2 miles daily
- avoid standing for long periods
- always elevate the feet when sitting.

See Nursing Care Plan 2.3.

Eating and drinking
Adequate hydration and balanced nutrition assist flow and maintain vessel integrity. Some supplementation of vitamins, trace elements and iron may have to be considered in the elderly.

Maintaining a safe environment
Avoidance of trauma and infection is important, as in arterial disease. Blood loss can be severe even from venous circulation.

Working
Occupations that involve standing for long periods, for example, as a shop assistant, may present a problem. Prophylactic use of support hose by at-risk groups may be something the occupational health nurse could advise.

Pain control
Bed rest or limb elevation reduces the throbbing pain of venous insufficiency. Walking, rather than standing, is advisable. Supportive anti-embolism stockings, by aiding venous return, reduce the feeling of pressure in the legs. However they can be hot and uncomfortable. Once any oedema has reduced, the patient should be measured again, to ensure that the stockings fit properly and are still therapeutic. Similarly, swollen legs should not be squeezed into elastic stockings that have become too small. Anti-inflammatory drugs may be prescribed to settle the inflammatory process of thromboembolism.

Lifestyle issues
Women taking oral contraception run a slightly increased risk of DVT, especially if there is a family history of thrombosis. If a DVT was to develop then oral contraception would have to be discontinued and another form adopted. Pregnant women are also more prone to DVT and varicose vein formation. The cosmetic affect of these problems can prove very upsetting as wearing thick white stockings is far from attractive. Trousers and opaque coloured tights may make them more acceptable.

> The perfect compression stocking would be easy to put on, comfortable to wear, give adequate graduated compression and look fashionably sheer. Whoever succeeds in designing it will not only make a fortune but will also earn the eternal gratitude of the millions of people who need to wear support for their legs.
> (Dale & Gibson 1989 p. 550)

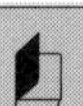
For further information, see Dale & Gibson (1990), 481–486.

Nursing Care Plan 2.3 J is a 68-year-old lady admitted to hospital 2 days previously for surgical stripping and ligation of varicose veins in her left leg. J lives alone and is concerned about how she will cope after discharge.

Nursing considerations	Action	Rationale	Evaluation
1. Pain/discomfort	• Explain normal pains/sensations likely to be felt over forthcoming days/weeks • Ensure support stockings are fitted correctly • Give analgesics to promote pain-free movement of affected extremities • Inspect bandages regularly for bleeding	• It is normal for the leg to feel painful and be very bruised. This may be a problem in the groin, particularly if the support stocking ends over a bruise • Complaints of patchy numbness are to be expected, but these disappear over a year • Sensation of pins and needles or hypersensitivity to touch in the involved extremity may indicate a temporary or permanent nerve injury as a result of surgery; the saphenous vein and saphenous nerve are in close proximity	• Ultimately, is pain free and comfortable • Feels informed about the pains/sensations to expect • Wears support stockings correctly
Cont'd			

Nursing Care Plan 2.3 *(cont'd)*

Nursing considerations	Action	Rationale	Evaluation
2. Leg needs to be supported	• Elevate leg 30° to provide adequate support for whole leg • Leg to be encased in pressure bandage from toe to groin for about a week, followed by knee level stockings for 3–4 weeks after surgery • Ensure J has adequate supply of stockings	• Long-term elastic support after discharge will promote circulation and limit likelihood of recurrence	• Is aware of the importance of supporting the leg
3. Fear/difficulty in walking	• Encourage J to walk with normal gait, offering support if necessary • Encourage short frequent walks to regain confidence and promote circulation • Give analgesics to ease movement of affected extremity • Advise to continue leg exercises after discharge	• Early ambulation needs to be encouraged to promote circulation	• Feels confident about walking and is able to walk without discomfort
4. Potential for recurrence of varicosities	• Advise J to continue to avoid activities that cause venous stress by obstructing blood flow — avoid wearing tight socks or tight girdle — avoid sitting or standing for long periods of time — avoid dangling legs (causes stasis of blood in lower leg) — avoid crossing legs at the knee for long periods whilst sitting (decreases circulation by 15%) • Elevate front of bed 15–20° at night • Avoid excessive weight gain • Wear elastic support tights • Attend outpatients follow-up visits every 6 months • Avoid knocking/damaging leg	• It is possible that varicosities may recur, therefore conservative measures learned perioperatively need to be continued	• Recurrence of varicosities will be avoided • Will feel confident about practising preventative measures
5. Coping after discharge	• Ensure that she knows what to expect after discharge • Discuss availability of support from family and neighbours after discharge; assist in coordinating these resources • Discuss feelings about wearing support bandages; arrange to talk to someone who has previously had this operation to talk through feelings • Arrange for district nurse to visit after 12–14 days to remove sutures • Advise about keeping bandage dry when washing • Ensure she is aware of outpatient follow up	• May feel isolated after support of hospital • May feel embarrassed about having to wear support stockings • May have difficulty coping with activities of living at home • Sutures are removed after 2 weeks	• Feels more confident about coping after discharge home

GLOSSARY

Arteriogram: a radio-opaque dye is injected into an artery and a series of X-rays taken to show the path of the dye in the arteries and pinpoint any obstruction to blood flow.

Echocardiogram: a non-invasive technique which uses pulses of high frequency sounds (ultrasound) emitted from a transducer to evaluate cardiac anatomy, pathology and function. The procedure involves an operator applying a lubricant to the skin surface of the chest wall and moving the transducer or probe back and forth by hand across the surface.

Electromechanical dissociation: a profound myocardial pump failure despite normal or near to normal electrical excitation. It usually occurs as a result of drugs or mechanical problems such as cardiac rupture. A failure of excitation coupling may be seen in acute myocardial infarction; the ECG trace will appear normal but there will be no recordable pulse. Cardiopulmonary resuscitation will need to be initiated. The prognosis is poor.

Embolism: the plugging of a blood vessel by material which has been carried through the larger vessels by the bloodstream. Usually due to fragments of a clot, but can be due to other factors such as a mass of air bubbles or bacteria.

Hypertrophy: increase in size which takes place in an organ as a result of an increased amount of work demanded of it.

Intra-aortic balloon pump: intra-aortic balloon counterpulsation is a mechanical means of supporting the acutely failing left ventricle. The balloon is introduced under local anaesthetic usually via the femoral artery into the descending thoracic aorta. During diastole the balloon is inflated with helium and blood is driven out of the aorta into the distributing arteries. The balloon is deflated at the end of diastole, just prior to the opening of the aortic valve reducing afterload and left ventricular work.

Thrombosis: formation of a blood clot within the blood vessels or the heart. The indirect cause is usually some damage to the smooth lining of the blood vessels brought about by inflammation or the result of atheroma.

Ventricular assist device: this is a device that provides temporary circulatory support in heart failure in order to promote optimum myocardial tissue recovery. Ventricular assist devices partially bypass either the left or right ventricle using an artificial pump that maintains systemic circulation. A median sternotomy is made, blood is diverted away from the heart, bypasses the ventricle and is returned to the patient.

REFERENCES

Aggleton P, Chalmers A 1986 Nursing models and the nursing process. Macmillan, London

Ashworth P 1984 Staff-patient communication in coronary care units. Journal of Advanced Nursing 9(1): 35–42

Ashworth P 1992 Cardiovascular problems and nursing. In: Cardiovascular intensive care nursing. P M Ashworth, C Clarke (eds) 1992 Churchill Livingstone, Edinburgh 1–19

Benner P, Wrubel J 1989 The primacy of caring: stress and coping in health and illness. Addison Wesley, California

Bondestam E, Hovgren K, Gaston-Johansson F, Jern S, Herlitz J, Holmberg S 1987 Pain assessment by patients and nurses in the early phase of acute myocardial infarction. Journal of Advanced Nursing 12(6): 677–682

Boore J R P, Champion R, Ferguson M C (eds) 1987 Nursing the physically ill adult: a textbook of medical-surgical nursing. Churchill Livingstone, Edinburgh

Bradbury M, Cruickshank J P 1993 Use of thrombolytic therapy in acute myocardial infarction. British Journal of Nursing 2(12): 619–624

Bright L D, Georgi S 1992 Peripheral vascular disease: is it arterial or venous? American Journal of Nursing 92(9): 34–47

British Medical Association and Royal College of Nursing 1993 Cardiopulmonary resuscitation: a statement from the BMA and RCN, London

Caplin M S, Sexton G L 1988 Stresses experienced by spouses of patients in a coronary care unit with myocardial infarction. Focus on Critical Care 15(5): 31–40

Catford J, Parish R 1989 Heart beat Wales: new horizons for health promotion in the community. In: Seedhouse D, Cribb A (eds) Changing ideas in health care. Wiley, New York

Cay E L 1982 Psychological problems in patients after a myocardial infarction: advances in cardiology 29: 108–112

Central Statistical Office 1992 Regional trends 27. HMSO, London

Central Statistical Office 1993 Social trends 23. HMSO, London

Chamberlain D A 1989 Guidelines for cardiopulmonary resuscitation. Advanced life support. British Medical Journal 299(6696): 446–448

Costa F V, Borghi C, Mussi A, Ambrosioni E 1988 Use of captropil to reduce serum lipids in hypertensive patients with hyperlipidaemia. American Journal of Hypertension 1(3 Pt 3): 221S–223S

Coull A 1992 Making sense of pulse oximetry. Nursing Times 88(32): 42–43

Cruikshank J M 1988 Coronary flow reserve and the J curve relation between diastolic blood pressure and MI. British Medical Journal 297(6658): 1227–1230

Dale J, Gibson B 1989 Which compression stocking? The Professional Nurse 4(11): 550–556

Department of Health 1992 Health of the nation: a strategy for health in England. HMSO, London

Duddy I, Parahoo K 1992 The evaluation of a community coronary specialist nursing service in Northern Ireland. Journal of Advanced Nursing 17(3): 288–293

European Resuscitation Council Basic Life Support Working Group 1993 Guidelines for basic life support. British Medical Journal 306(6892): 1587–1589

European Resuscitation Council Working Party 1993 Adult advanced cardiac life support: the European Resuscitation Council Guidelines 1992 Abridged. British Medical Journal 306(6892): 1589–1592

Frankl W, Brest A (eds) 1986 Valvular heart disease: comprehensive evaluation and management. Davis, Philadelphia

Gallop M 1993 Kissing the weed goodbye. Health Visitor 66(3): 97–98

Greenhalgh R M 1984 Management of risk factors in patients undergoing arterial surgery. In: Bergen J (ed) Arterial Surgery. Churchill Livingstone, Edinburgh

Guyton A C 1977 Basic human physiology: normal function and mechanism of disease. W B Saunders, Philadelphia

Hall A S, Ball S G 1988 Calcium channel antagonists, angiotensin converting enzyme inhibitors and serotonin antagonists. Current Opinion in Cardiology 4(5): 647

Hampton J 1992 The ECG made easy, 4th edn. Churchill Livingstone, Edinburgh

Hargrove-Huttel R A 1991 Arterial hypertension: a non-pharmacological approach. Advancing Clinical Care 6(1): 4–10

Horgan J, Bethell M, Carson P, Davidson C, Julian D, Mayou R A, Nagle R 1992 Working party report on cardiac rehabilitation. British Heart Journal 67: 412–419

Jones C 1992 Sexual activity after myocardial infarction. Nursing Standard 6(48): 25–28

Jordan S 1992 Reducing hypertension: drugs update. Nursing Times 88(21): 44–47

Jowett N, Thompson D R 1989 Comprehensive coronary care. Scutari Press, London

Kolvekar S, Forysth A 1991 Valvular surgery. Nursing Standard 5(32): 48–49

Lekander B J 1986 Aortic and peripheral vascular disease. In: Weeks L C (ed) Advanced cardiovascular nursing. Blackwell Scientific Publications, Boston

Letterer R A, Carew B, Reid M, Woods P 1992 Learning to live with cardiac failure. Nursing 22(5): 34–41

Levick J R 1991 An introduction to cardiovascular physiology. Butterworth, London

Lofgren E P 1983 Chronic venous insufficiency. In: Spittell J A (ed) Clinical vascular disease. F A Davies, Philadelphia

Love C 1990a Deep vein thrombosis: threat to recovery. Nursing Times 86(5): 40–43
Love C 1990b Deep vein thrombosis: methods of prevention. Nursing Times 86(6): 52–55
Majeed H A 1989 Acute rheumatic fever. Medicine International OCT 70: 2910
Monaghan M 1993 The sound revolution. Nursing Standard 7(18): 50–51
Norris L O, Grove S I C 1986 Investigation of selected psychosocial needs of family members of critically ill adult patients. Heart and Lung 15: 194–199
O'Connor G T, Buring J E, Yusuf S, Goldhaber S Z, Olmstead E M, Paffenbarger R S, Hennekens O H 1989 An overview of randomized trials of rehabilitation with exercise after myocardial infarction. Circulation 80: 234–244
O'Donnell M E 1990 Assessment of the patient with malignant hypertension. Dimensions of Critical Care Nursing 9(5): 280–286
Office of Health Economics 1990 Coronary heart disease. The Need for Action. HMSO, London
Office of Population Censuses and Surveys 1990 OPCS monitor. DH2/90/2. HMSO, London
Orem D 1991 Nursing, concepts of practice, 2nd edn. McGraw-Hill, New York
O'Sullivan C K 1992 Mitral regurgitation as a complication of MI: pathophysiology and nursing implications. Journal of Cardiovascular Nursing 6(4): 26–37
Papadopoulos C 1989 Sexual aspects of cardiovascular disease. Praeger, New York
Picton A J, Williams M, McCollum C N 1993 The use of Doppler ultrasound: venous disease. Wound Management 4: 13–15
Rocchini A P, Katch V, Anderson J, Hinderliter J, Becque D, Martin M & Marks C 1988 Blood pressure in the obese adolescent: effect of weight loss. Paediatrics 82(1): 16–23
Roper N, Logan W W & Tierney A J 1990 The elements of nursing, 3rd edn. Churchill Livingstone, Edinburgh
Roy C 1984 Introduction to nursing: an adaptation model. Prentice Hall, New Jersey
Schmieder R E, Messerli F H, Garavaglia G E & Nunez B D 1988 Dietary salt intake: a determinant of cardiac involvement in essential hypertension. Circulation 78(4): 951–956
Shore A C, Markandu N D & MacGregor G A 1988 A randomised cross over study to compare the blood pressure response to sodium loading with and without chloride in patients with essential hypertension. Journal of Hypertension 6(8): 613–617
Thompson D R 1990 Intercourse after myocardial infarction. Nursing Standard 4(43): 32–33
Thompson D R 1990 Counselling the coronary patient and partner. Scutari, London
Thompson D R, Hopkins S 1987 Making sense of defibrillation. Nursing Times 89(49): 54–55
Thompson D R, Webster R A, Cordle C J, Sutton T W 1987 Specific sources and patterns of anxiety in male patients with first myocardial infarction. British Journal of Medical Psychology 60: 343–348
Thompson D R, Webster R A 1992a Infective endocarditis. In: Cardiovascular intensive care nursing. P M Ashworth, C Clarke (eds) Churchill Livingstone, Edinburgh
Thompson D R, Webster R A 1992b Caring for the coronary patient. Butterworth Heinemann, Oxford
Tuchek M F 1991 Valvular heart disease in the older adult: a case study presentation. Nursing 4(1): 58–68
Weiland A P, Walker W E 1986 Thoracic aneurysms. Critical Care Quarterly 9(3): 20–31
Weinberger M H, Cohen S J, Miller J Z, Luft F C, Grim C E & Fineberg N S 1988 Dietary sodium restrictions as adjunctive treatment of hypertension. Journal of the American Medical Association 259(17): 2561–2565
Wenger N K, Hellerstein H K 1992 Rehabilitation of the coronary patient, 3rd edn. Churchill Livingstone, New York
Whitehead S 1988 Illustrated operation notes. Edward Arnold, London
Williams I M, Picton A J, McCollum C N 1993 The use of Doppler ultrasound: arterial disease. Wound Management 4(1): 9–12
Williams K (ed) 1992 The community prevention of coronary heart disease. HMSO, London
Wilson D D 1989 Acute pulmonary oedema: how to respond in a crisis. Nursing 19(10): 34–41
Wilson K J W 1990 Ross & Wilson Anatomy and physiology in health and illness, 7th edn. Churchill Livingstone, Edinburgh
Winslow E H, Lane L D, Gaffney F A 1984 Oxygen consumption and cardiovascular response in patients and normal adults during in bed and out of bed toileting. Journal of Cardiac Rehabilitation 4: 348–354
Wilson-Barnett J, Fordham M 1986 Recovery from surgery for ischaemic heart disease. In: Wilson-Barnett J and Fordham M (eds), Recovery from illness. Wiley, Chichester 88–102
Wynne G, Marteau T M, Johnston M, Whiteley C A, Evans T R 1987 Inability of trained nurses to perform basic life support. British Medical Journal 294: 1198–1199

FURTHER READING

Ashworth P M, Clarke C (eds) 1992 Cardiovascular intensive care nursing. Churchill Livingstone, Edinburgh
Burch K O, Todd K, Crosby F E, Ventura M R, Lohr G, Grace M L 1991 PVD: nurse–patient interventions. Journal of Vascular Nursing 9(4): 13–16
Byng P 1990 Cardiac transplantation: the patient's view. Nursing Standard 4(33): 30–31
Dale J J, Gibson B 1990 Back-up for the venous pump: compression hosiery. Professional Nurse 5(9): 481–484
Dennis B 1989 Case study: a problem of 'malignant hypertension'. Midwives Chronicle 102(1219): 266–268
Doughty C 1991 A multidisciplinary approach to cardiac rehabilitation. Nursing Standard 5(45): 13–15
Downie R S, Fyfe C, Tannahill A 1990 Health promotion, models and values. Oxford University Press, Oxford
Forrest A P, Carter D C, McLeod I B 1991 Principles and practice of surgery. Churchill Livingstone, Edinburgh Ch. 21
Gortner S R et al 1991 Self efficacy and activity level following cardiac surgery. Journal of Advanced Nursing 15(10): 1132–1138
Kelly M P 1992 Health promotion in primary care: taking account of the patient's point of view. Journal of Advanced Nursing 17(11): 1291–1296
Marieb E N 1989 Human anatomy and physiology. Benjamin Cummings, California
McCrissican D 1991 Patient education in coronary care. Nursing Standard 5(40): 37–39
McDermott J 1993 Setting up a no-smoking support group. Health Visitor 66(3): 99–100
Monaghan M 1993 The sound revolution: echocardiography. Nursing Standard 7(18): 50–51
Murphy S, Smith C 1993 Crutches, confetti or useful tools? Professionals' views on and use of health education leaflets. Health Education Research 8(2): 205–215
Niven N 1989 Health psychology. Churchill Livingstone, Edinburgh
Roper N, Logan W W & Tierney A J 1990 The elements of nursing, 3rd edn. Churchill Livingstone, Edinburgh
Scordo K A 1992 Helping your patient cope with mitral valve prolapse. Nursing 22(10): 34–39
Thomas S 1988 Thrombolysis, wallchart. Nursing Standard: March 12
Tortora G J, Grabowski S R 1992 Principles of anatomy and physiology, 7th edn. Harper & Collins, New York
Trounce J 1990 Clinical pharmacology for nurses, 13th edn. Churchill Livingstone, Edinburgh
Why H 1993 Modern management of cardiac failure. Nursing Standard 7(18): 52–54
Wood R 1990 Health promotion: information all the way. Nursing Times 86(48): 31–33

CHAPTER 3

The respiratory system

Cynthia B. Edmond

CHAPTER CONTENTS

Introduction 59

Anatomy and physiology 60

Principles of nursing management in the prevention and treatment of respiratory disorders 64

The nurse's role in disease prevention and health promotion 64
Cigarette smoking and health 66
Environmental pollution and health 67

Common respiratory disorders 67

Infections of the respiratory system 68
Nursing priorities and management: acute bronchitis and tracheobronchitis 68
Nursing priorities and management: bronchopneumonia 69
Nursing priorities and management: PAP 69
Nursing priorities and management: pulmonary tuberculosis 70

Obstructive disorders of the airways 70
Nursing priorities and management: chronic bronchitis 70
Nursing priorities and management: emphysema 71
Nursing priorities and management: asthma 74

Bronchogenic carcinoma 78
Nursing priorities and management: lobectomy 78
Nursing priorities and management: pneumonectomy 79

Respiratory emergencies 79
Nursing priorities and management: fractured ribs and flail chest 80
Nursing priorities and management: pneumothorax and haemopneumothorax 80
Nursing priorities and management: pulmonary oedema 82

Respiratory failure 82

Emergency airway management, endotracheal intubation and mechanical ventilation 82

Genetic disorders 84

Continuity of care: hospital and community 84

Conclusion 85

References 85

Useful addresses 85

Further reading 86

INTRODUCTION

The respiratory system is one of the most vital systems in the human body. In health it functions automatically and usually without our awareness. There are, however, few disease processes that do not have some disruptive effect on the respiratory system. There are also many respiratory disorders relating to environmental pollution, trauma, infection, genetic susceptibility and primary disease as well as conditions secondary to other diseases. Although causative agents differ, the aetiology of each condition follows certain common patterns. To know the anatomy and physiology of the respiratory system is to understand how respiratory disorders inevitably relate to breakdown in ventilation, gaseous exchange or pulmonary perfusion. Symptoms differ only in degree and effect and the treatment of symptoms will always have certain basic aims.

The effects of respiratory disorders range from the minor discomforts of the common cold to the distressing and life-threatening symptoms associated with respiratory failure. All are disabling to some extent to the individual and his family. As respiratory conditions and diseases cover such a broad spectrum and are common in both community and hospital settings it is essential that nurses have a broad knowledge base relating to the basic concepts of normal respiration and an understanding of the factors that can lead to respiratory dysfunction.

Research indicates that some of the more serious respiratory disorders are related to lifestyle and are actually preventable. This chapter will therefore emphasise and outline various approaches to health promotion and disease prevention and the nurse's expanding role, opportunities and challenges in this field. It will also explore some of the more common disorders and in discussing them draw out the basic principles of management for all respiratory disorders. Although the emphasis is on nursing management, implicit in all discussion is the assumption that nurses work in close collaboration with other health care professionals and in many instances are responsible for coordinating the work of the whole team.

As you read this you are most likely unaware that you are breathing quietly and effortlessly; once you become attentive to the process of breathing, however, you can voluntarily vary the depth and pace of your respirations. You can sigh, cough, or hold your breath for a time, and you can force air out through your vocal chords and sing or shout. When you go to sleep tonight you can be reasonably confident that you will continue to breathe automatically and wake up in the morning feeling refreshed and well. However, if for any reason your respiratory system broke down, this whole picture would change. Case History 3.1(A) gives some insight into a patient's perspective on an acute episode of respiratory distress.

Case History 3.1(A) C

C was brought into the casualty department one night by his wife and this is his account of his first severe asthma attack.

'Everything was getting really confused but what I remember most was that I was *really scared*. My chest was tight, like being crushed in a vice, and I couldn't breathe. I was gasping and wheezing. My heart was pounding, my head was splitting — it was a nightmare. Then there was a nurse . . . muffled sounds and tight, tight pain in my chest . . . but her voice was steady. I don't know what she said, but her voice was steady, and I passed out.

'When I did come to I was propped up and there were all kinds of strange sounds. There was something blowing cool air under my nose, a plastic bag of fluid hanging over me, breathing was hard work and I struggled to get air. I could feel the panic again. I was *exhausted* and wished that I could just give up and die. Everything went blurred again. I don't know how long I struggled through the nightmare. I think I passed out again. Next time I surfaced the tight rings around my chest were beginning to ease and I could breathe again, but, I was *so tired*!

'This was my first bad attack of asthma. Two years ago I'd started to wheeze and cough a lot and had a few bouts of feeling that I just wasn't breathing properly. My GP said I had asthma. That was a real shock, at first. At 40, I thought I'd got away with it! Dad has asthma — has had all his life — his is bad and rules his life! But I thought I was one of the lucky ones.

'Anyway, my GP gave me tablets and a puffer to use and I cut down on smoking and seemed to be able to manage. It was something you just had to learn to live with. I had a lot of other things on my mind.

'I did wonder if that change in work had anything to do with my starting to cough and wheeze. That was about 2 years ago, too, when I was made redundant from my old job. There's always a lot of dust and fumes around in this new place. I did wonder . . . . anyway I've been really run down recently, had a lot of worry, mainly, money. We've all had 'flu' as well, and now this!'

The essential elements of life support are the essential elements of respiration. Airway, breathing (ventilation) and circulation are the ABC of life support. If any one of the three is cut off or becomes dysfunctional, the others are of no use and an emergency situation exists which requires instant action if irreparable brain damage and death are to be prevented. An airway must be established and the individual's breathing and circulation restored in order to get oxygen to the vital organs and tissues.

? **3.1** What is the critical response time in CPR (cardiopulmonary resuscitation) if you are to prevent irreparable brain damage? Refer to your first aid manual and, with the guidance of your teacher, *be sure to practice CPR regularly throughout your nursing career: it is an essential procedure.*

? **3.2** As well as following up suggested reading and activities, you may find it useful to compile an information folder on essential procedures relating to respiratory care as you work your way through this chapter. It is also very important when you are in the clinical area to observe the patients who are undergoing these procedures, to note their reactions and the effects of the procedures on them, and to talk to them about how they feel. Analyse the context. Reflect on your experiences and make notes of critical incidents. Include these in your folder too. Discuss them with your preceptor or teacher.

ANATOMY AND PHYSIOLOGY

The reader is advised to review the anatomy and physiology of the respiratory system as a whole and to use a model of the thoracic cage to establish the relationship between all the structures illustrated in Figure 3.1. This section is intended as an overview of the most relevant points relating to normal respiratory function. Two texts which can be consulted in conjunction with the present discussion are suggested below.

For further information, see Wilson (1990) and Rutishauser (1994).

Physiology of respiration

A continuous supply of O_2 and the elimination of CO_2 is necessary for the survival and functioning of body cells. The respiratory system in conjunction with the red blood cells (RBCs) of the circulatory system is responsible for this vital exchange. The process of respiration involves both external and internal respiration. External respiration is oxygenation of the pulmonary capillary blood supply and elimination of CO_2 by diffusion across the alveolar and capillary membrane. Internal respiration is the exchange of O_2 and CO_2 at the cellular level and the use of O_2 and production of CO_2 in the tissues (see Fig. 3.2).

External respiration

External respiration involves ventilation, gaseous exchange and perfusion of the lungs with blood.

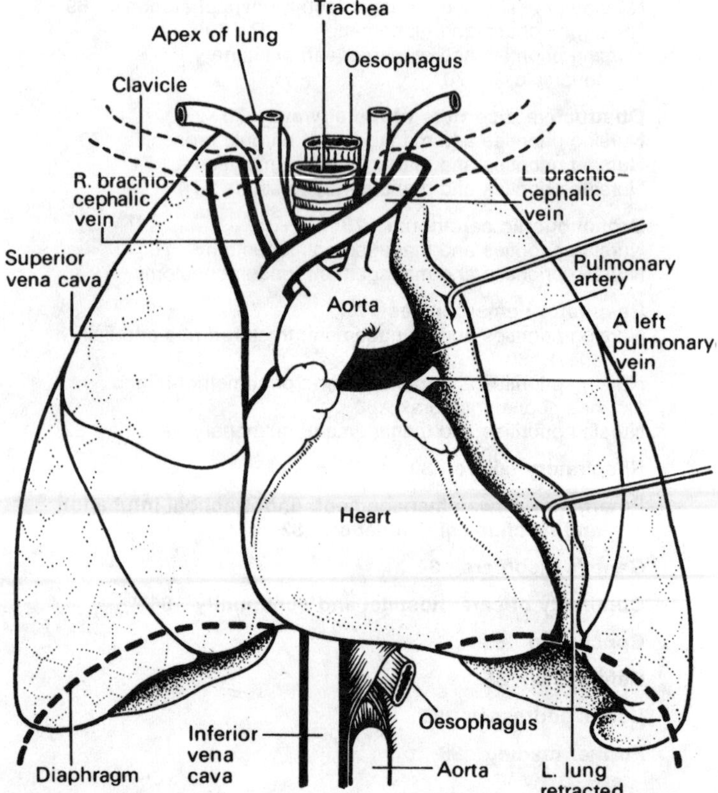

Fig. 3.1 Organs associated with the lungs. (Reproduced with permission from Wilson 1990.)

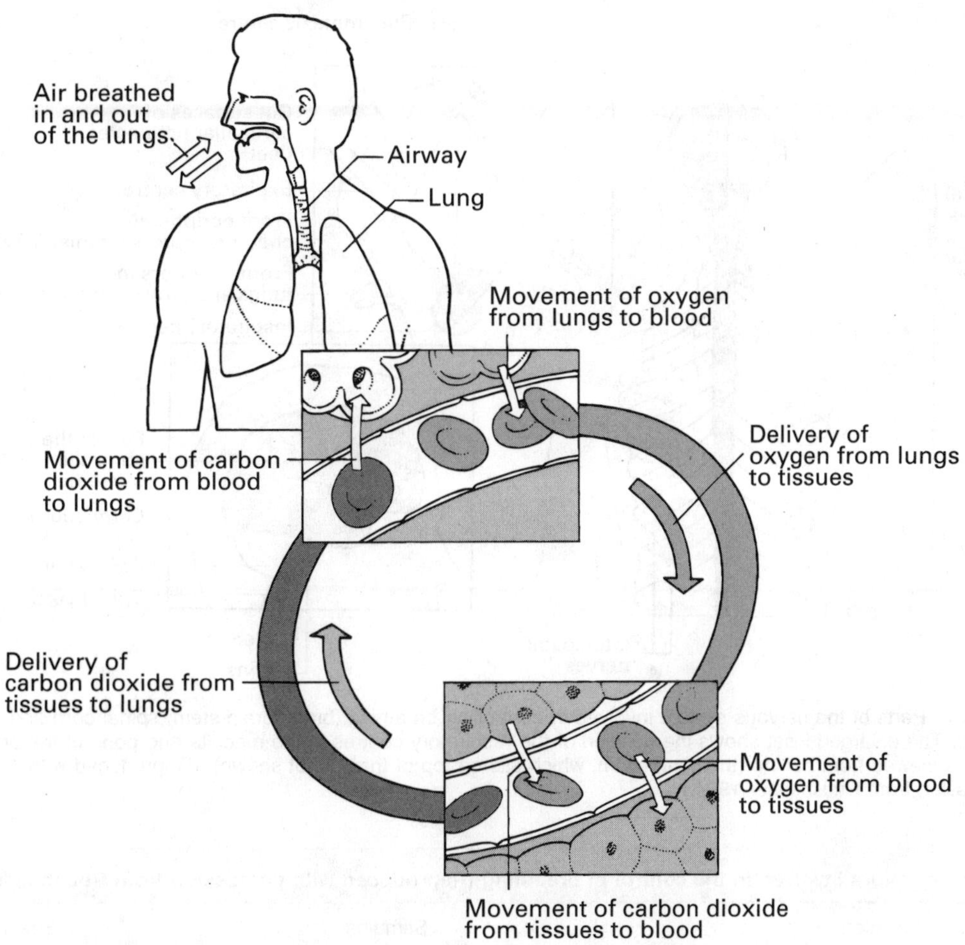

Fig. 3.2 Transport of oxygen and carbon dioxide between the lungs and the tissues. (Reproduced with permission from Rutishauser 1994.)

Ventilation is the bellows effect which moves air in and out of the lungs via the airways. This process is powered by the respiratory muscles — mainly the diaphragm and the intercostal muscles, which work together to increase and decrease the size of the thoracic cavity. They are responsive to both voluntary and involuntary central nervous system (CNS) control. The thoracic cavity is lined with parietal pleura and the lung surfaces have a covering of visceral pleura. The negative pressure and serous lubricant between the parietal and visceral pleura has the effect of 'sticking' the lungs to the thoracic wall so that they expand and contract with these ventilatory movements. In health there is only a potential space between the pleural layers.

Central control. Most of the time the involuntary system maintains the regular automatic breathing cycle and is controlled by respiratory centres in the brain (see Fig. 3.3). These centres receive information from sensory receptors throughout the respiratory system and from chemoreceptors located in the carotid arteries, aorta and medulla.

The sensory receptors in the respiratory system itself monitor local irritants and lung expansion. A cough, for example, is a reflex response to airway irritants and a natural defence mechanism to clear the airways. The chemoreceptors monitor the levels of CO_2, O_2 and H^+ in the blood and the H^+ in the CSF, and alter ventilation of the lungs to restore a normal balance of gases (see Table 3.1).

Lung volume capacity and compliance. It is important to bear in mind the basic principles relating to lung volume capacity and compliance and to recognise the significance of their measurement. They are important factors in ventilation and are often affected by respiratory disorders.

The volume of air breathed in and out and the number of breaths per minute varies from one individual to another according to age, size and activity. Normal, quiet breathing gives about 15 complete cycles per minute in the adult. Lung volume can be assessed in the following terms (see also Fig. 3.4). Assessment of air flow is summarised in Box 3.1.

1. Tidal volume (TV). This is the amount of air that passes in and out of the lungs during each cycle of quiet breathing (approximately 500 ml in the adult). Exchange of gases takes place only in the alveolar ducts and sacs. The rest of the air passages are known as 'dead space' and contain about 150 ml of air.
2. Inspiratory capacity. This is the amount of air that can be inspired with maximum effort. This consists of tidal volume plus the inspiratory reserve volume (IRV).
3. Functional residual capacity (FRC). This is the amount of air remaining in the air passages and alveoli at the end of quiet respiration. This is composed of expiratory reserve volume (ERV) and residual volume (RV). The RV prevents collapse of the alveoli and makes continuous gaseous exchange possible as the alveolar gas mix remains constant.
4. Vital capacity (VC). This is the TV plus the IRV and ERV.
5. Total lung capacity (TLC). With maximum effort the adult lungs can hold 4–6 l of air. Most of this can be forcibly expelled, leaving a RV of about 1 l.

Lung expansion and recoil. Elastic fibres in lung tissue and the surface tension of the fluid lining the alveoli give the lungs their natural recoil tendency. Ease of expansion and recoil depends on normal compliance and elasticity and on the presence of surfactant in the fluid lining the alveoli. Compliance can be reduced by the stiffening of

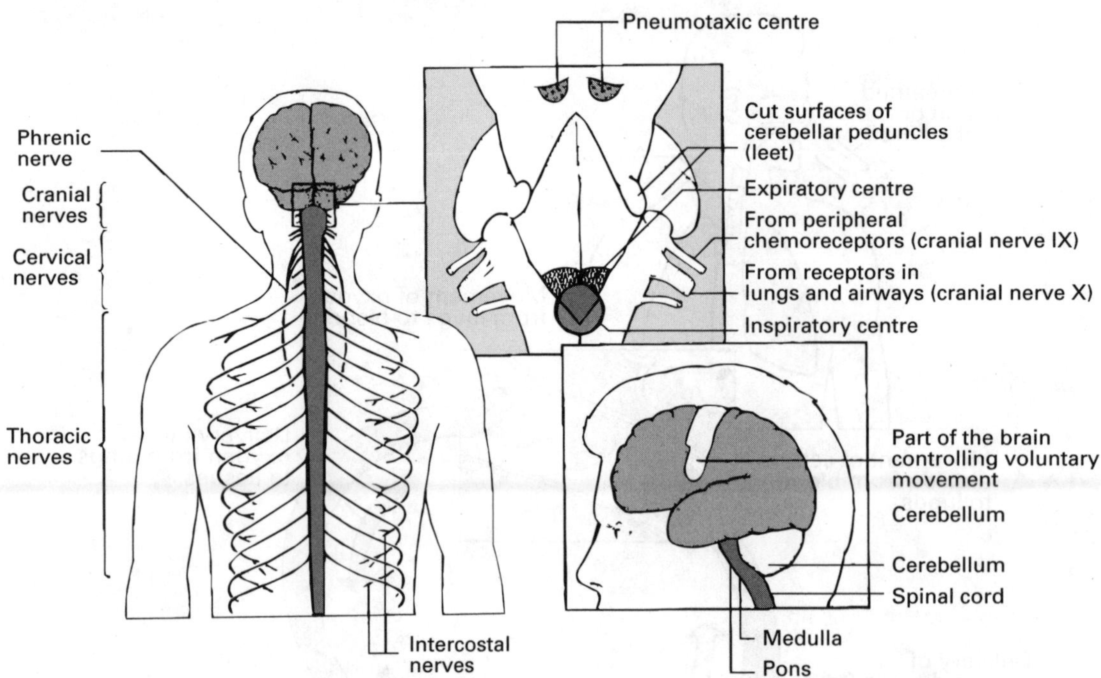

Fig. 3.3 Parts of the nervous system involved in controlling breathing: brain, brain stem, spinal cord and nerves. The enlarged inset shows the position of the respiratory centres in the medulla and pons of the brain stem as viewed from behind (the cerebellum, which sits on top of this, is not shown). (Reproduced with permission from Rutishauser 1994.)

Table 3.1 Sensory receptors involved in the control of breathing (Reproduced with permission from Rutishauser 1994)

Type	Location	Stimulus	Effect on breathing
(A) Within the respiratory system			
Irritant receptor	Airway epithelium — Nose	Inhaled particles and vapours	Sneeze
	— Trachea and bronchi		Cough
	— Bronchioles		Increased rate and depth
Stretch receptors	Airway smooth muscle	Inflation	Slowed down
J receptors	Alveolar wall	Interstitial oedema Pulmonary emboli	Rapid and shallow
Muscle spindles	Respiratory muscles (e.g. diaphragm, intercostals)	Elongation of the muscles	Made smoother and more efficient
(B) Elsewhere			
Chemoreceptors	Carotid artery Aorta	↑ CO_2 ↓ O_2 ↑ H^+ in blood	Increased rate and depth
	Brain (medulla)	↑ H^+ in CSF	

normally soft alveolar tissue due to pulmonary oedema or to the ageing process, or by extreme softening due to loss of lung tissue, as in emphysema.

Surfactant is a substance composed of lipids and cellular secretions of the alveolar epithelium which lowers the surface tension of the alveolar fluid, making it easier for the alveoli to expand. Lack of surfactant in premature infants results in alveoli that remain collapsed (atelectasis) and leads to a ventilatory problem known as infant respiratory distress syndrome. A surfactant deficiency can also occur in adults as a response to severe shock, trauma or massive blood transfusion. This leads to increasing ventilatory difficulty, with rapid, shallow breathing and ineffectual respiration — a critical condition known as adult respiratory distress syndrome (ARDS) which may require artificial ventilatory support.

Ventilation then depends on CNS control, functioning respiratory muscles, and adequate volume capacity of the lungs. Conditions which affect ventilation include some neurological diseases, diaphragmatic compression from constricting dressings or appliances, injuries to the chest wall, lungs or diaphragm, obstructive airways diseases such as asthma, space-occupying lesions, thoracic deformities and severe pain.

Gaseous exchange is the second vital component in the respiratory process. By a process of diffusion O_2 passes from the alveoli into the bloodstream and CO_2 passes from the bloodstream into the alveoli.

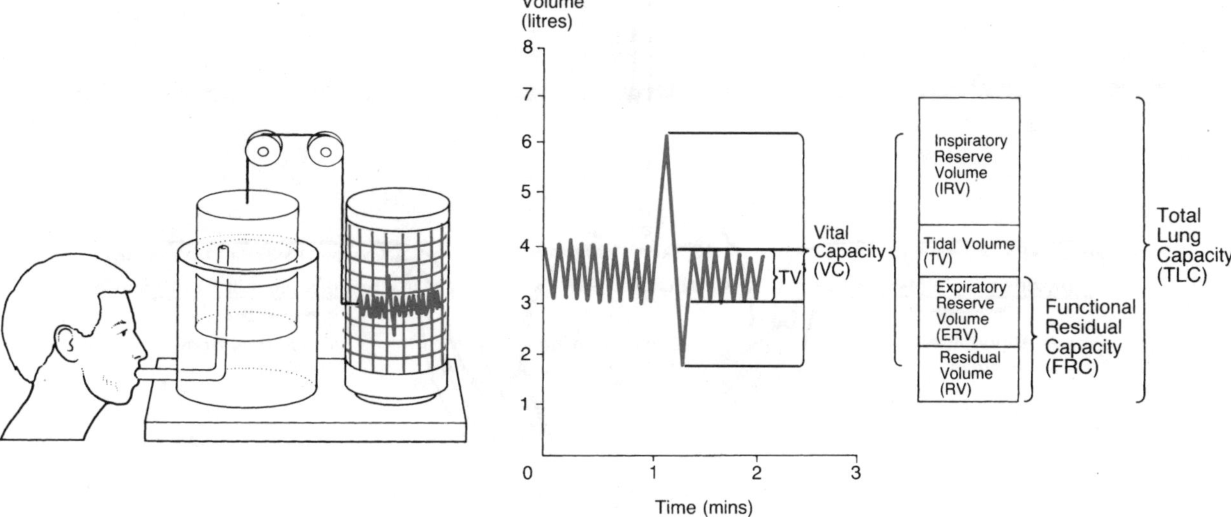

Fig. 3.4 Measurement of lung volumes by spirometry. The spirometer consists of a cylinder filled with air which is inverted into a container of water. As air is breathed in and out, the cylinder rises and falls. This movement is inscribed on the chart fixed to a slowly revolving drum. Note: the valves in the system, and the CO_2 absorbant within the spirometer, are not shown. (Reproduced with permission from Rutishauser 1994.)

This exchange is dependent on adequate perfusion by the pulmonary blood supply.

Perfusion, i.e. the volume of blood passing through the lungs, determines the amount of O_2 taken into the body and the amount of CO_2 eliminated. In health, regulatory mechanisms ensure a balance between ventilation and perfusion such that well-ventilated parts of the lung receive an adequate blood supply and blood does not pass through the pulmonary circulation without being oxygenated (termed 'shunting'). Shunting occurs where there is an area of consolidation, as in pneumonia; although there is adequate perfusion there is no ventilation.

Box 3.1 Assessment of air flow

VITAL CAPACITY

This is the sum of inspiratory reserve volume, tidal volume, and expiratory reserve volume; about 4,800 ml.

PEAK EXPIRATORY FLOW RATE (PEFR), OR PEAK FLOW

This is an expression of the maximum rate of air flow when the individual is breathing out as hard and fast as possible, starting with full lungs. The normal range is 400–600 l/min. PEFR is measured with a simple instrument called a peak flow meter. Patients with diseases such as asthma are taught to record their own peak flow at regular intervals. A fall in PEFR provides warning of bronchospasm before breathlessness occurs and therefore alerts patients to use prescribed bronchodilator drugs or to seek medical advice before the condition worsens. PEFR measures are also recorded before and after administration of bronchodilatory drugs to assess their effectiveness.

FORCED EXPIRATORY VOLUME (FEV)

This is the proportion of vital capacity that can be forcibly expelled from the lungs as measured at 1 and 3 seconds: FEV_1 and FEV_3. Normal FEV_1 is approximately 80% of the vital capacity and FEV_3 is about 100%. Where the airways are narrowed, as in asthma or in the presence of tumours, the FEVs will be lower.

? **3.3** Revise the properties of gases.

Gaseous exchange and lung perfusion. Each microscopic, grape-like alveolus is surrounded by an intimate structural network of capillaries which together provide the lungs with an enormous capacity for gaseous exchange. This exchange is smooth and uninterrupted because the composition of the alveolar air remains constant due to the tidal ebb and flow of inspired air and the residual volume (RV) which is warmed and saturated with water vapour. As indicated in Figure 3.5, the gases in the blood leaving the lungs are in equilibrium with the air in the alveoli.

See Rutishauser (1994), Ch. 7, for a detailed explanation of gaseous exchange.

The total pressure exerted in the walls of the alveoli by the mixture of gases in air is the same as atmospheric pressure (100 kPa). Each gas in the mixture exerts a part of that total pressure proportional to its concentration; this is known as its partial pressure (*P*).

Arterial blood gas (ABG) levels. As a nurse you may be involved in interpreting blood gas results, administering oxygen and monitoring respirators. A working knowledge of the properties of gases, of partial pressure and of gaseous exchange is essential. (See Table 3.2 and Fig. 3.6.)

Table 3.2 Composition of air (Reproduced with permission from Rutishauser 1994)

	Dry atmosphere		*Alveolar air (37°C)*	
	%	kPa[1]	%	kPa[1]
Oxygen	21	21	13.2	13.2
Carbon dioxide	0.04	0.04	5.3	5.3
Nitrogen[2]	79	79	75.2	75.2
Water vapour	*	*	6.3	6.3

[1] assuming barometric pressure is 100 kPa
[2] includes < 1% rare gases (argon, helium etc.)
* Amount of moisture in atmosphere depends on humidity and temperature. If moisture is present, percentage of other constituents will then be correspondingly decreased.

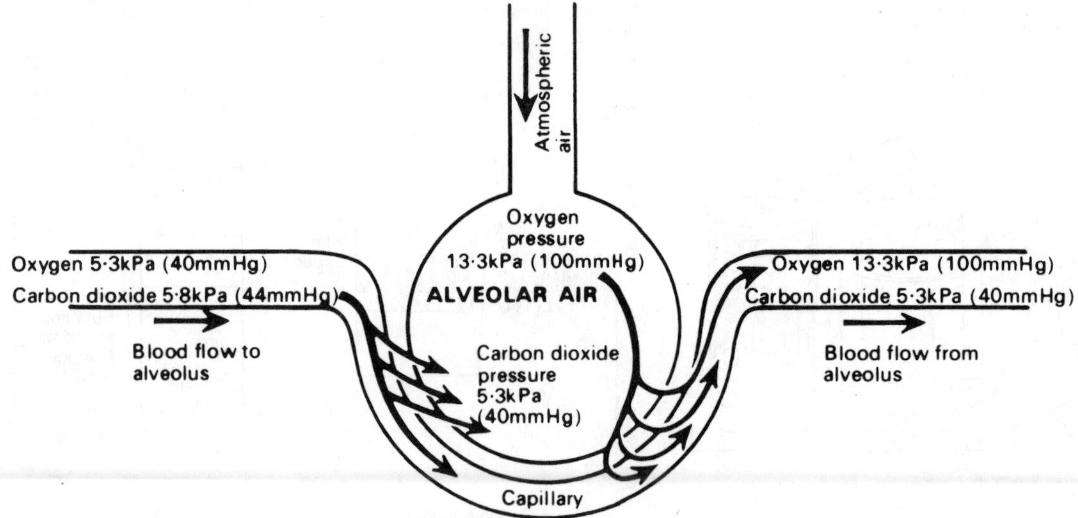

Fig. 3.5 Diagram of the interchange of gases between air in the alveoli and the blood capillaries. (Reproduced with permission from Wilson 1990.)

Internal (cellular) respiration

Cellular respiration is an essential part of the whole process of respiration.

The haemoglobin of the red blood cells (RBCs) carries O_2 to the tissues where, by the process of diffusion, gaseous exchange takes place between the arterial end of the capillaries and the tissue fluid. CO_2, which is one of the waste products of carbohydrate and fat metabolism in the cells, transfers to the venous capillary blood, where it is carried to the lungs in three ways, i.e.:

- dissolved in the blood plasma
- combined with haemoglobin
- in combination with sodium as sodium bicarbonate.

These processes are described more fully in Chapter 2.

PRINCIPLES OF NURSING MANAGEMENT IN THE PREVENTION AND TREATMENT OF RESPIRATORY DISORDERS

There are two main areas of nursing concern:

1. health promotion and disease prevention
2. developing clinical skills in order to ensure competent care.

The first concern will be addressed in relation to preventing serious respiratory diseases caused by environmental pollution and cigarette smoking; the second concern will be addressed in relation to specific respiratory disorders later in the chapter.

Conceptual framework

It is assumed that in all care planning for patients with respiratory disorders, whether in the hospital or the community, an appropriate driving philosophy and model of nursing care will be adopted. It is suggested, for example, that a modified version of Orem's (1971) philosophy of promoting independence and balancing self-care deficit with nursing compensatory intervention could be appropriate in the care of an asthma patient (see Table 3.3). For example, on admission during an acute attack of asthma (Case History 3.1A) C is unable to meet his self-care needs and requires major compensatory intervention by both medical and nursing staff. As he recovers, the deficit is less and nursing intervention (always in collaboration with other members of the health care team) moves through partly compensatory to supportive educative as he is prepared for discharge home and is more able to control his asthma and maintain a higher degree of independence. (See Case History 3.1B, p. 77 and Collaborative Care Plan 3.1, p. 77.)

THE NURSE'S ROLE IN DISEASE PREVENTION AND HEALTH PROMOTION

The importance of health promotion and disease prevention to the social and economic well-being of our society is gaining increasing recognition. This awareness has been reflected in

Table 3.3 Orem's basic nursing system (With kind permission from Orem (1971).)

Nurse action		Some characteristics of patient		Patient action
Nurse action intense	⟶	Patient unable to meet own self-care needs – state of coma – inability to make decisions Wholly compensatory system		Patient action limited
Nurse action shared	⟶	Patient has limited ability to meet self-care needs – limited knowledge – limited ability to ambulate and to perform manipulative skills Partly compensatory system	⟵	Patient action shared
Nurse action supported	⟶	Patient can accomplish self-care – has learned new self-care activities – needs limited help in decision making Supportive-educative system	⟵	Patient action intensive

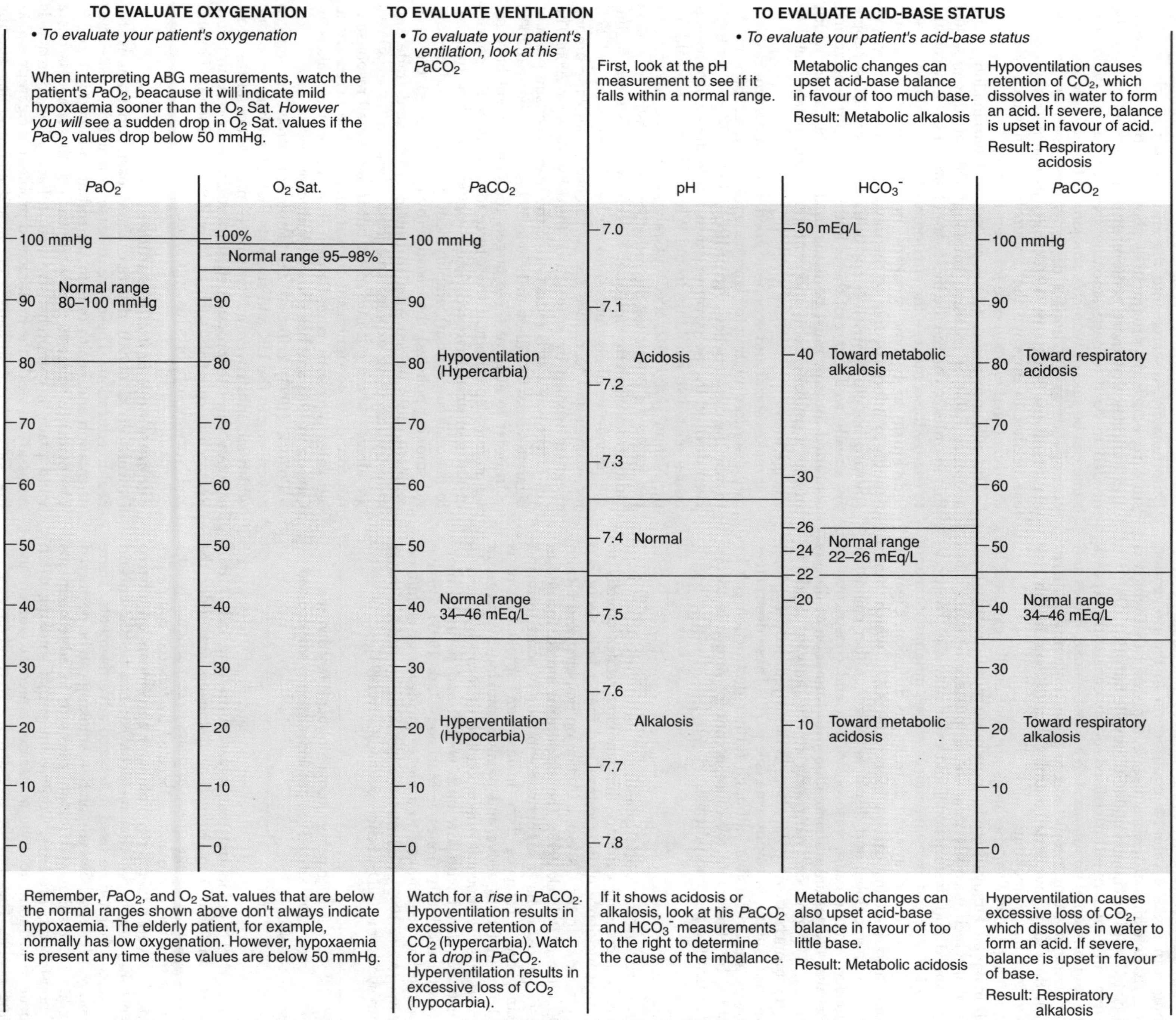

TO EVALUATE OXYGENATION		TO EVALUATE VENTILATION	TO EVALUATE ACID-BASE STATUS		
• *To evaluate your patient's oxygenation*		• *To evaluate your patient's ventilation, look at his* $PaCO_2$	• *To evaluate your patient's acid-base status*		
When interpreting ABG measurements, watch the patient's PaO_2, beacause it will indicate mild hypoxaemia sooner than the O_2 Sat. *However you will* see a sudden drop in O_2 Sat. values if the PaO_2 values drop below 50 mmHg.			First, look at the pH measurement to see if it falls within a normal range.	Metabolic changes can upset acid-base balance in favour of too much base. Result: Metabolic alkalosis	Hypoventilation causes retention of CO_2, which dissolves in water to form an acid. If severe, balance is upset in favour of acid. Result: Respiratory acidosis
PaO_2	O_2 Sat.	$PaCO_2$	pH	HCO_3^-	$PaCO_2$
100 mmHg	100%	100 mmHg	7.0	50 mEq/L	100 mmHg
	Normal range 95–98%				
90 Normal range 80–100 mmHg	90	90	7.1		90
80	80	80 Hypoventilation (Hypercarbia)	Acidosis 7.2	40 Toward metabolic alkalosis	80 Toward respiratory acidosis
70	70	70	7.3		70
60	60	60		30	60
50	50	50	7.4 Normal	26 24 Normal range 22–26 mEq/L 22	50
40	40	40 Normal range 34–46 mEq/L	7.5	20	40 Normal range 34–46 mEq/L
30	30	30	7.6		30
20	20	20 Hyperventilation (Hypocarbia)	Alkalosis	10 Toward metabolic acidosis	20 Toward respiratory alkalosis
10	10	10	7.7		10
0	0	0	7.8		0
Remember, PaO_2, and O_2 Sat. values that are below the normal ranges shown above don't always indicate hypoxaemia. The elderly patient, for example, normally has low oxygenation. However, hypoxaemia is present any time these values are below 50 mmHg.		Watch for a *rise* in $PaCO_2$. Hypoventilation results in excessive retention of CO_2 (hypercarbia). Watch for a *drop* in $PaCO_2$. Hyperventilation results in excessive loss of CO_2 (hypocarbia).	If it shows acidosis or alkalosis, look at his $PaCO_2$ and HCO_3^- measurements to the right to determine the cause of the imbalance.	Metabolic changes can also upset acid-base balance in favour of too little base. Result: Metabolic acidosis	Hyperventilation causes excessive loss of CO_2, which dissolves in water to form an acid. If severe, balance is upset in favour of base. Result: Respiratory alkalosis

Fig. 3.6 A guide to understanding a patient's arterial blood gas (ABG) measurements. (Reproduced with permission from Robinson & Russo 1983.)

recent years by the development of large-scale screening and health education programmes, and has demanded a greater involvement of nurses in this area of primary health care. With respect to respiratory disease, nurses in a range of work settings can make a valuable contribution to the prevention and early detection of serious disease, especially that which is associated with environmental and lifestyle factors.

Living in a modern industrialised society constantly exposes us to environmental pollutants such as dust, smoke, fumes and other irritants. Many people add to these contaminants, over which they may have little control, the additional health risk posed by tobacco smoking.

What happens when the lungs are continually exposed to such irritants? Firstly, there is an increase in mucus secretion. The cilia, which normally clear the air passage of mucus, become coated and dysfunctional and eventually die. The presence of irritants and excessive mucus causes inflammation and narrowing of the airways and disrupts gas diffusion. Cigarette smoke also contains carbon monoxide (CO), which binds easily to haemoglobin and displaces oxygen. Other chemicals in tobacco smoke cause vasoconstriction and constriction of the airways. Constant inflammation with formation of fibrous tissue and permanent narrowing of the airways leads to chronic bronchitis. Alveolar tissue is destroyed, reducing lung area and resulting in emphysema (see p. 70). These destructive changes are irreversible, although further destruction can be avoided by eliminating the cause: a concept simple in theory but difficult to put into practice.

Cigarette smoking and health

There is increasing evidence that smoking relates directly to the high incidence of lung cancer and that it kills about 300 people a day in the UK alone (Action on Smoking and Health 1993, cited in Pollock 1993). The 'sidestream' smoke inhaled in passive smoking has a higher concentration of some toxic and carcinogenic substances than 'mainstream' smoke. There is evidence that both active and passive smoking by pregnant women has detrimental effects on the unborn child and is clearly associated with low birth weight and perinatal mortality and morbidity (Jones & MacLeod-Clark 1993). Passive smoking has been linked to a higher incidence of childhood asthma (Azizi 1993), and maternal smoking to sudden infant death syndrome (SIDS; Schoendorf & Kiely 1993).

> ? **3.4** Look through current journals in your library and see how many articles you can find relating to smoking and health.

Pollock (1993) points out that cigarette smoking kills 1 in 4 smokers and that 5 in every 6 new smokers are under the age of 16 years. This age group appears to be particularly susceptible to advertising and is targeted by tobacco companies through covert advertising. Voluntary agreements on tobacco advertising and promotion restrict what can be shown and the images that can be used in tobacco advertisements. There are no restrictions, however, on how smoking can be portrayed in editorial, fashion and feature pages or in advertisements for non-tobacco products. Positive images of smoking often appear in fashion and style magazines aimed at women and young people. This may be considered 'covert advertising'.

> ? **3.5** Review a selection of magazines and newspapers for images of smoking.

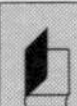

> For further information, see Amos (1993).

Unfortunately, research into the effectiveness of school anti-smoking education programmes shows disappointing results and indicates that more comprehensive interventions will be needed to curb teenage smoking (Nutbeam et al 1993). The same can be said of women's smoking, where a high incidence corresponds to the impact of material stresses on working class mothers. Blackburn (1993) suggests that new approaches are needed to improve the circumstances in which socially disadvantaged women care for their families.

The evidence points to the *contextual* determination of the addictive habit of cigarette smoking. This in turn indicates that in order to change the incidence of smoking it is necessary to change the context — the environment — which predisposes individuals to become smokers. In other words, it is not enough to inform people of the devastating consequences of smoking both to themselves and to their children. Most people are already well aware of these. Rather, a comprehensive and concerted attempt must be made to define the factors which initiate a smoking habit and contexts which sustain it and to change these.

It makes social and economic good sense to prevent respiratory disorders relating to cigarette smoking rather than simply to treat the consequences. Accordingly, in the UK policies have been devised by the government to tackle the environmental issues related to smoking. In the White Paper 'The Health of the Nation' (July 1992, cited in Graham 1993) the government put forward a policy for the reduction of mortality and morbidity from cigarette smoking. Targets were set for reducing the prevalence of cigarette smoking by 30% for men and 29% for women and to reduce the prevalence of smoking among pregnant women by at least one third by the year 2000. The key target was a 40% reduction in the overall consumption of cigarettes from 98 billion in 1990 to 59 billion by the year 2000.

In order to achieve these targets the Government have set up an interdepartmental work-force to coordinate the policies of the ministries involved. These include education (relating to national curriculum), employment (workplace and personnel smoking policies), the treasury (by tax increases), the environment (bans on smoking in public places) and trade and industry (affecting exports and jobs). Some of these policies are already being put into effect but if the overall response is not found to be significant then it may still be necessary to legislate to ensure compliance. This course was taken in Canada in 1988 and has shown significant results.

Pollock (1993) criticises the limited controls on tobacco advertising in the UK and suggests that a total ban — i.e. one which includes covert advertising — may be one of the most effective ways to produce significant drops in consumption. Research in countries such as New Zealand, Canada, Finland and Norway supports his argument.

The nurse's role in health education

Downie et al (1990) describe three basic orientations for health education. These are disease orientation, risk-factor orientation and health orientation and are outlined in Box 3.2. The evidence suggests that while each of these models has a valid place, a comprehensive and collaborative approach is necessary to tackle the multifaceted problem of cigarette smoking. Government initiatives are aimed at preventing specific diseases and eliminating risk factors while health-orientated programmes initiated by the health professions reinforce government policies by offering a more positive focus and a more satisfying outcome for the individual. It is within the health orientation model that nurses are becoming increasingly involved.

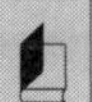
For further information, see Downie (1990).

The provision of up-to-date information is a basic necessity. Moreover, people have a right to know the facts about health-related issues. Information should be presented in an innovative and effective way; this means that nurses whose duties include health education must have accurate information, good teaching skills and adequate resources.

Midwives have a unique opportunity to be closely involved with the family in both the antenatal and postnatal period to promote the health and well-being of the newborn. Early screening and advice are essential and time spent defining specific social problems and ensuring that the family is given appropriate social referral and support is invaluable. School nurses can begin health education early in the child's school life and involve the parents. Conveying information about health to young people demands a creative approach and may involve promoting sporting and other leisure-time activities for both parent and child. Community nurses can be active in defining social needs, lobbying local councils to provide recreational and child care facilities and giving time to individuals to lessen their sense of isolation. Practice nurses can make a valuable contribution by identifying heavy smokers and emphasising to them the benefits of a positive feeling of well-being that comes even by simply cutting down on daily consumption.

For many, smoking is a coping mechanism that maintains some kind of individuality and equilibrium in everyday life. For some, a cigarette represents a well-deserved treat, or a small luxury that counters a sense of deprivation. Thus a smoker might remark: 'The only time I sit down is when I have a cigarette', or 'Having a cigarette is my only luxury.' Health professionals involved in education must also appreciate how difficult it is to break the smoking habit. Nicotine is a powerful and addictive stimulant and does have a stress-relieving effect in the short term.

Box 3.2 Orientations for health education

Downie et al (1990) describe the following orientations for health education:

1. Disease orientated education. This approach aims to prevent specific diseases. The emphasis is on measuring success in terms of progress towards target rates for morbidity and mortality
2. Risk-factor orientated education. Efforts are aimed at eliminating particular risk factors to prevent associated diseases
3. Health orientated education. The aim is to enhance positive health as well as to prevent ill-health. This orientation recognises the physical, mental and social facets of both positive and negative health and acknowledges that:
   - Provision of information is not enough. The educational process needs to be participatory, to help people clarify their values (e.g. how they see themselves and their health) and acquire and develop life skills (e.g. decision-making and assertiveness). The educator seeks to understand people's perspectives and opinions, to respect them rather than correct them or blame them for their behaviour
   - There are major constraints to freedom of choice in health-related behaviour (e.g. sociopolitical factors).

? **3.6** Design a health education programme for teenagers at school. What activities would you include? What teaching aids could you use?

Environmental pollution and health

Many industrial workplaces expose workers to pollutants such as dust, chemicals and toxic fumes. Miners of nickel, coal, cobalt and radium are exposed to fluorocarbons, which have been shown to be related to an increased incidence of serious lung disease, including carcinoma (Kidd 1989). Agricultural workers are exposed to biohazards such as grain dust, bacteria and metabolites (endotoxins), fungi and metabolites (glucans) and storage mites; they are also exposed to airborne insecticides, fungicides and pesticides and to animal parasites and debris. Epidemiological and clinical studies have identified strong associations between agricultural exposure and chronic bronchitis, asthma, hypersensitivity pneumonitis and organic dust toxic syndrome (Zejda & Dosman 1993).

Occupational and community nurses have a responsibility to educate workers and management about environmental hazards and to press for the use of protective respiratory masks and for improved working conditions. They should also encourage leisure activities that give workers an opportunity to get some fresh air and exercise.

COMMON RESPIRATORY DISORDERS

Respiratory disorders involve a breakdown in the integrity of the alveolar walls. They either cause or are caused by oedema, the presence of exudate, or by inflammation, resulting in scarring and alteration in the process of gaseous exchange. Causes of respiratory inflammation are varied and range from common diseases such as 'the flu' and colds to bronchitis, pneumonia, tuberculosis, cystic fibrosis and the opportunistic infections of AIDS and other immunosuppressive conditions. While causative factors, organisms or irritants differ, the aetiology of respiratory disorders is similar and they are in varying degrees similar in their clinical manifestations.

The incidence of emphysema and malignancy due to environmental pollutants and cigarette smoking appears to have increased significantly in recent years (Kidd 1989, Pollock 1993). Additionally the lungs are often involved in terminal or critical illness where pulmonary oedema, bronchitis, pneumonia or atelectasis (collapse of alveoli) may develop.

Common clinical manifestations of all of these disorders include varying degrees of breathlessness, cough and sputum production, dyspnoea (difficulty in breathing), tachypnoea (increased respiratory rate), cyanosis (blue discoloration of the skin), hypoxia (low O_2 concentration in the tissues) and hypercapnia (high concentration of CO_2 in arterial blood).

Wherever there is disruption of the respiratory process there is the probability that oxygen therapy will be necessary to relieve breathlessness and improve tissue perfusion (Allan 1989). See Box 3.3.

Each of the processes involved in external respiration — ventilation, gaseous exchange and circulatory perfusion — is a critical component in maintaining the life and function of body cells. Disruption in any of these processes results in respiratory disorders of varying severity.

INFECTIONS OF THE RESPIRATORY SYSTEM

Infections of the upper respiratory tract are dealt with in Chapter 14. This chapter will focus on bronchitis, pneumonia and tuberculosis.

Acute bronchitis and tracheobronchitis

Acute bronchitis is the inflammation of the mucous membranes of the bronchial tree. Tracheobronchitis, as the name implies, affects the trachea as well as the bronchi. Both conditions are associated with infections of the upper respiratory tract (see Ch. 14) but may also occur as a result of atmospheric pollutants, cigarette smoking or when some other chronic respiratory disorder already exists. It affects people of all ages and is usually only of real concern in the very young, the very old and the debilitated. A normally healthy person will usually recover quite quickly. The concern in terms of health promotion is to ensure that acute bronchitis does not develop into bronchopneumonia or that acute attacks become so frequent that the condition becomes chronic (see p. 70).

Common presenting symptoms. The individual feels generally unwell with initially a dry painful cough and a moderate pyrexia. The cough becomes increasingly productive as the inflamed mucosal cells pour out mucus and the sputum produced becomes increasingly mucopurulent. Bronchospasm can occur causing wheezing and a degree of dyspnoea.

MEDICAL MANAGEMENT

Investigative procedures. For otherwise healthy individuals, investigations are usually unnecessary. However, if there is marked mucopurulent sputum produced, a sputum culture will be taken to identify the causative organism. A chest X-ray may also be required.

Medical intervention. The treatment is aimed at relieving the symptoms. Bed rest is advocated until the pyrexia has resolved. Moist inhalations can relieve the bronchial symptoms and a high fluid intake is encouraged. Expectorants will also help relieve the congestion and antibiotic therapy will be prescribed and taken as appropriate.

NURSING PRIORITIES AND MANAGEMENT: ACUTE BRONCHITIS AND TRACHEOBRONCHITIS

The nurse's priority will be for those vulnerable individuals for whom acute bronchitis could prove serious. Over-exertion must be avoided and such patients may need support with expectoration and maintaining respiratory hygiene. Optimal nutritional and fluid intake will aid recovery and help prevent further infection.

When the individual is well enough, advice should be given as to how further attacks can be avoided. The avoidance of cigarette smoke, dusty, ill-ventilated, cold or crowded environments is encouraged but is not always easy to achieve. The advice given and the outcomes aimed for must be realistic and tailored to the lifestyle and socio-economic circumstances of the individual. An influenza vaccination may prove an effective preventative measure in particularly vulnerable individuals.

Pneumonia

Pneumonia is an infection of lung tissue and is most usefully classified according to the causative organism, which may be bacterial or viral. However, it can be further defined according to the area of lung that is involved, i.e. bronchopneumonia or lobar pneumonia.

?	3.7 What physiological advantage is gained and what adverse effects are avoided by humidifying and warming inspired gases?

Box 3.3 Oxygen (O_2) therapy

The need for O_2 therapy arises when oxygen transport to the tissues is insufficient due to breakdown in either the respiratory or the circulatory systems. Clinical signs and blood gas levels are the main indicators of degree of hypoxia. Profound hypoxaemia will cause death in minutes, whereas death from carbon dioxide (CO_2) narcosis is a more lengthy process (see Box 3.4).

The aim of O_2 therapy is to administer sufficient oxygen to maintain tissue oxygenation at a functional level and eliminate detrimental compensatory responses to hypoxaemia, and to prevent serious or irreparable damage to vital organs and tissues.

The percentage of oxygen that is to be delivered is carefully determined, either by circumstances (as in life-threatening emergencies, where 100% pure oxygen may be given initially) or by carrying out ABG measurement or percutaneous oximetry and prescribing oxygen accordingly. An oximeter is a small, clip-on, non-invasive device which can register arterial oxygen saturation through the skin.

For therapeutic purposes the range of prescription is usually between 24% and 60% of O_2. Hyperbaric oxygen (oxygen given at greater than 1 atmosphere) may be used to improve oxygen perfusion of the tissues by increasing the dissolved oxygen in the blood, as in treatment of CO poisoning or deep-sea divers' 'bends'.

In certain conditions the amount of oxygen given is determined by prior knowledge of adverse effects. For example, in patients with known COAD (see p. 71) it is dangerous to give too much oxygen, and in premature babies high oxygen saturation is known to cause blindness.

Means of giving oxygen include nasal cannulae, oxygen masks, oxygen tents, mechanical ventilators and hyperbaric oxygen chambers. Each of these devices can deliver controlled amounts of oxygen and is selected according to overall patient requirements and tolerance.

Humidification chambers attached to the oxygen equipment ensure that the oxygen is humidified before being inhaled. In mechanical ventilators it is also warmed and therefore enters the respiratory tract as vapour, fully saturated, and at body temperature.

OXYGEN TOXICITY

The lungs may be damaged if high concentrations of oxygen are given over several days. This is thought to increase alveolar permeability so that capillary walls break down and fluid and blood accumulate. Severe cases may progress to pneumonia, fibrosis, pulmonary hypertension and right-sided heart failure.

Bronchopneumonia

PATHOPHYSIOLOGY

Bronchopneumonia is characterised mainly by patchy areas of consolidated lung tissues. Causative organisms are bacterial and fungal and include staphylococci, pneumococci, streptococci, haemophilus influenzae and candida. It usually occurs in individuals weakened by other conditions and often in the very old, the very young, the unconscious, and as a result of a pre-existing disease, such as chronic bronchitis, atelectasis or carcinoma in adults, or infectious diseases in infants.

Clinical features. These vary in severity depending on the overall condition of the patient but include varying degrees of pyrexia, cough with copious purulent sputum, exhalatory râles, dyspnoea and tachypnoea. Consolidation of the lower lobes is found on auscultation.

MEDICAL MANAGEMENT

The causative organism is isolated by sputum culture and sensitivity and appropriate antibiotic therapy is commenced. The patient's general condition is improved by attention to nutrition, hydration and physiotherapy.

NURSING PRIORITIES AND MANAGEMENT: BRONCHOPNEUMONIA

The patient with bronchopneumonia will be very ill and he and his family will need a great deal of comfort and reassurance. Attention to personal hygiene and physical comfort is important. The patient should be turned or encouraged to move regularly. A sitting position where possible will make breathing easier and if oxygen is prescribed this therapy should be monitored carefully. Aids to prevent pressure sores developing should be selected judiciously (see Ch. 23).

Bronchopneumonia can be prevented in many hospitalised high-risk patients by thorough nursing assessment and meticulous nursing care.

Lobar pneumonia

PATHOPHYSIOLOGY

This is an acute bacterial infection which sometimes involves a whole lobe. It occurs mainly in young adults (usually males) but its full-blown effects are uncommon now because of the early and effective use of antibiotics. However, if left untreated lobar pneumonia can progress to further areas of consolidation as well as pleurisy, pericarditis, bacteraemia and possibly death.

Viral pneumonia: primary atypical pneumonia (PAP)

PATHOPHYSIOLOGY

In viral pneumonia the inflammatory reaction is localised within the septal walls of the alveoli and there is no exudate. This is its point of difference from other types of pneumonia and the reason why it is known as 'atypical'. There are many known and highly contagious viruses which can begin as a 'common cold' and progress to more severe respiratory tract infections — which may include PAP in susceptible individuals. These viral agents include *Mycoplasma pneumoniae*, influenza types A and B, respiratory syncytial virus (RSV), rubella and varicella, Rickettsia and echoviruses. PAP was responsible for the highly fatal influenza pandemics of the early and middle 1900s.

Clinical features. Symptoms include pyrexia, muscular pains, headaches and a dry, hacking cough. Treatment is symptomatic with attention given to general nutrition, hydration and antibiotic treatment of any intercurrent bacterial infections. The disease runs its course and, except in the weaker individual, resolution is expected. However, the patient may be left feeling weak and exhausted for some time afterwards.

NURSING PRIORITIES AND MANAGEMENT: PAP

Susceptible individuals — the aged, the debilitated and health workers at high risk of infection — should be encouraged to attend the practice nurse clinic for a course of 'flu' vaccinations in preparation for the winter months or where epidemics are forecast.

Most individuals with PAP can be treated at home. Some may need nursing advice or assistance to carry out the activities of daily living and to ensure they are properly nourished and hydrated. Individuals nursed at home can be referred back to their GP if medical treatment becomes necessary.

Tuberculosis (pulmonary)

Tuberculosis (TB) is a chronic infectious disease mainly of the lungs (pulmonary tuberculosis) but can infect other parts of the body (miliary tuberculosis). In the early part of the 20th century it was common in developed as well as developing countries. With the advent of compulsory chest X-ray, vaccination and effective drug treatment the incidence in developed countries became almost negligible. However, since the discontinuation of compulsory screening and treatment of the adult population and increased immigration from developing countries there has been a significant increase in incidence. The disease is rife in developing countries and in many is complicated by the susceptibility of AIDS victims to respiratory infections (Cayla et al 1993).

PATHOPHYSIOLOGY

Tuberculosis is a notifiable disease caused mainly by Mycobacterium tuberculosis, although Mycobacteria avium and bovis also can cause the respiratory form. The disease is characterised by two types of lesions: exudative and productive.

The exudative lesion arises from the inflammatory process in which the bacterial organism is surrounded by fluid containing polymorphonuclear leucocytes and monocytes. If the lesion fails to heal it may become necrosed and develop into a productive lesion (tubercle).

A tubercle consists of a fibrous or a soft outer cover with a core of giant cells, lymphocytes, monocytes, fibroblasts and epithelioid cells. The mycobacterium can live in the centre of this tubercle for years. The soft tubercle can rupture and spread its contents into surrounding tissue. Spread of infection is by direct contact with the infected tissue, by the bloodstream or by the lymphatics. Spread to others is by droplet infection from coughing or saliva.

Clinical features vary in severity, depending on the virulence of the organism and the susceptibility of the individual. Manifestations include: a productive cough, sometimes with blood-stained sputum; fatigue; weight loss; low-grade evening fever; night sweats and pleuritic pain. Advanced cases will manifest wheezing and râles, deviation of the trachea, pulmonary consolidation and haemoptysis (frank bleeding from the lungs).

MEDICAL MANAGEMENT

Investigative procedures. A Mantoux skin test may be performed (see below). Specimens of sputum, gastric washings, or a lymph node biopsy may be sent for bacteriology. Chest X-ray will indicate the condition of the lungs.

Medical intervention. The patient is isolated until there is complete compliance with the drug therapy (usually 2–4 weeks). Drugs used include isoniazid, rifampicin, streptomycin, ethambutol and pyrazinamide. Until the specific sensitivity is determined, the patient is usually on a rotating regime of several of these drugs because of the high probability of bacterial resistance to some combinations. Therapy will then continue with long-term treatment with at least two of the drugs. Regular clinic attendance and supervision of treatment is mandatory. Contacts are traced and tested and treated if necessary.

NURSING PRIORITIES AND MANAGEMENT: PULMONARY TUBERCULOSIS

Prevention

Prevention is based upon public health education and on screening and vaccination to protect those at risk. Nurses are actively involved in these programmes in clinics and schools.

Schoolchildren, health care workers and contacts of people identified as having TB are screened by the Mantoux skin test. This test uses a single intradermal injection of purified protein derivative (PPD). The result is read within 24–72 h. If the area of induration is 10 mm or more the test is positive, which indicates either that a past subacute infection stimulated present immunity or that present infection exists which needs treatment. In the case of past infection the result signifies that there is good immunity and vaccination is not necessary. An area of 5 mm in a person recently exposed to tuberculosis indicates that a course of prophylactic treatment should be given. A negative Mantoux test (i.e. no reaction) indicates that there is no natural immunity and the BCG (Bacille-Calmette-Guérin) vaccination is necessary.

> ? **3.8** As a student nurse you have no doubt had a Mantoux test and possibly a BCG vaccination. Visit your college or staff clinic or the practice nurse at your GP practice. Ask for the information leaflets that accompany the PPD Mantoux test and the BCG vaccine and study them.

Management of a newly diagnosed patient

This patient will be isolated for 2–4 weeks and barrier nursed (see Ch. 16, p. 555). He will need reassurance that treatment will be effective, as well as rest, diversionary therapy, good nourishment and administration of prescribed drugs. He should be encouraged to retain his independence in activities of daily living. When he is discharged home he will need minimal community nurse support and advice but must attend chest clinic check-ups regularly. All sputum must continue to be incinerated and the patient must use tissues and cover his mouth when coughing.

OBSTRUCTIVE DISORDERS OF THE AIRWAYS

'Chronic obstructive airways disease' (COAD) is a term used to describe a group of disorders which cause obstruction to airflow. Included in this group are chronic bronchitis, emphysema, asthma, and bronchiectasis. In chronic bronchitis the inflammation and constant productive cough obstructs air flow; in emphysema the overdistended alveoli with reduced permeability results in impaired gaseous exchange; in asthma there is both inflammatory reaction and bronchospasm; and in bronchiectasis there are chronic copious secretions filling the lungs. Bronchiectasis is usually a separate condition but the others often coexist and complicate each other in presenting as a set of symptoms commonly termed COAD or COPD (chronic obstructive pulmonary disease (Hahn 1987)).

Chronic bronchitis

The definition of chronic bronchitis is the presence of a persistent productive cough for at least 2 months over 2 consecutive years. It can occur in any age group but is common in middle-aged men, and amongst cigarette smokers and people exposed to high levels of environmental pollution.

PATHOPHYSIOLOGY

Chronic irritation causes hypertrophy and hyperplasia of the mucous glands of the tracheobronchial tree, which results in excessive mucus production and impaired ciliary action. The bronchi and bronchioles are usually the most severely affected and may become blocked with purulent mucus. This, together with the resultant oedema and congestion, can affect respiratory defence mechanisms and predispose to recurrent bacterial and viral infections.

Clinical features. A chronic productive cough with mucopurulent sputum may persist for years, accompanied by gradual and increasing airway resistance and functional impairment. Untreated, this will lead to increasing dyspnoea, hypoxia and hypercapnia.

MEDICAL MANAGEMENT

Management is to advise the patient to avoid the causal irritant, if this is possible, and to treat the symptoms. This may involve prescribing physiotherapy, bronchodilatory drugs, antibiotics and oxygen therapy.

NURSING PRIORITIES AND MANAGEMENT: CHRONIC BRONCHITIS

Prevention of deterioration

The patient is advised and supported in avoiding causitive agents.

When identifying patient problems and nursing priorities, it is useful to consider chronic bronchitis and emphysema together as the two conditions often coexist (Jess 1992).

Pulmonary emphysema

Pulmonary emphysema is a chronic destructive disease of the respiratory bronchioles, alveolar ducts and alveoli. It is most common in the over-40 age group and is often associated with other chronic lung disorders. There are two main types of pulmonary emphysema which may coexist and which are exacerbated by persistent and severe coughing. These are alveolar emphysema and centrilobar emphysema (see Fig. 3.7).

Alveolar emphysema

PATHOPHYSIOLOGY

In this form of emphysema the walls between adjacent alveoli break down, the alveolar ducts dilate and there is loss of interstitial elastic tissue. This results in distension of the lungs and loss of normal elastic recoil and therefore trapping and stagnation of alveolar air. As alveoli merge there is loss of surface area for gaseous exchange, and this is further reduced by loss of permeability of the stretched and damaged alveolar walls. Predisposing factors include cigarette smoking, congenital deficiency of α_1-antitrypsin (making the individual more susceptible to environmental pollutants), acute lower respiratory inflammatory conditions and chronic coughing (which puts pressure on the already stretched tissues).

> ? **3.9** Maintaining a clear airway by regular aspiration of tracheal secretions is a common nursing procedure. As a rule of thumb the procedure should not be carried out for more than 10–15 seconds at a time, with adequate periods of rest between. What is the reason for this? (Refer back to residual volume (RV) and the composition of alveolar air.)

A full description of tracheal suctioning can be found in Jamieson, McCall & Blythe (1992).

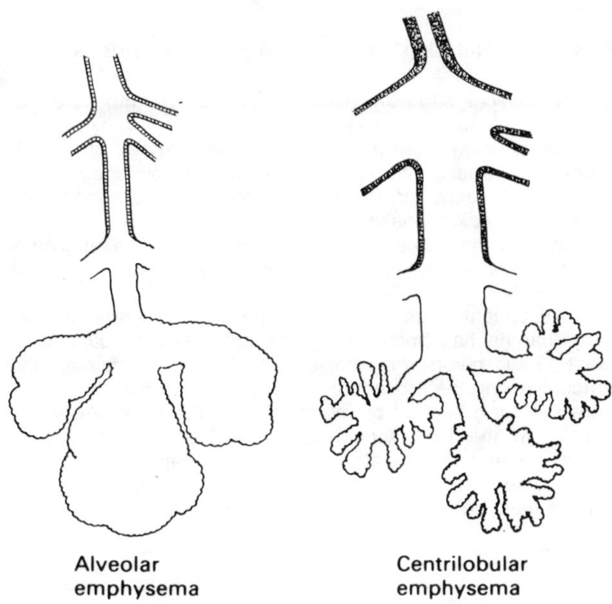

Fig. 3.7 Emphysema. (Adapted from Wilson 1990.)

Centrilobar emphysema

This type of emphysema involves irreversible dilatation of the bronchioles in the centre of the lobules, which affects airway pressure and ventilation efficiency. Predisposing conditions include recurrent bronchiolitis, pneumoconiosis and chronic bronchitis.

Clinical features. Emphysema becomes symptomatic when about one third of the lung parenchyma is affected. The patient is dyspnoeic and in advanced cases the slightest physical activity can cause severe respiratory distress and cyanosis. Ventilation is forced and exhalation is particularly lengthy and difficult. The patient learns to push the air out through pursed lips, which automatically brings the upper abdominal muscles into play and helps maintain positive pressure in the airways. The hyperinflation of the lungs makes the chest barrel-shaped and rigid and exerts pressure on thoracic structures so that neck and facial veins are distended. There is a chronic, productive cough and wheezing. Abnormal ventilation:perfusion ratios result in chronic hypoxia (low O_2 in tissues), hypercapnia (high CO_2) and polycythaemia. The clinical picture representing this is of peripheral cyanosis (due to low O_2) and facial flushing (because CO_2 is a vasodilator). Respiratory acidosis may occur in acute exacerbations of the disease, although the body may adapt its buffer system to some extent given the chronic nature of the condition.

The patient is weakened by constant respiratory effort and unable to tolerate normal basic activities of daily living. Laughing and coughing may stimulate life-threatening attacks and respiratory failure is always a possibility.

MEDICAL MANAGEMENT

Investigative procedures. History, symptoms and clinical examination are diagnostic. Pulmonary function tests (spirometry) indicate the type and extent of restricted function: reduction in all parameters indicates obstructive disease because of the prolonged exhalation time, and reduced FEV_1 and FVC (forced vital capacity) indicate restrictive disease. Blood gas analysis and chest X-ray will confirm the stage and effect of the disease and influence treatment.

Medical intervention. Oxygen is prescribed according to individual need and blood gas results (see Box 3.3). It is given in strictly controlled percentages because of the importance of the 'hypoxic drive' in COAD patients and the fact that too much oxygen can knock out this drive,

Box 3.4 Carbon dioxide narcosis (Reproduced with permission from Rutishauser 1994)

In healthy people when CO_2 levels rise the respiratory rate increases. This increase allows excess CO_2 to be blown off by the lungs. However, in chronic obstructive airways disease (COAD), where chronic ventilatory problems result in constantly high levels of arterial CO_2, this mechanism becomes blunted and eventually $P\text{CO}_2$ has no effect on the respiratory centre in the brain.

With severe CO_2 retention the respiratory drive is created by the low $P\text{CO}_2$ stimulating the carotid and aortic bodies. This is known as the *hypoxic drive*. A high concentration of O_2 will suppress this hypoxic drive and if $P\text{O}_2$ is raised even to normal, breathing becomes shallow and more and more CO_2 is retained, further depressing the respiratory centre, and a condition known as carbon dioxide narcosis develops. This is characterised by increasing drowsiness and eventual death.

The hypoxic drive must always be considered when O_2 is prescribed for patients with COAD. Usually this is not more than 24% of O_2 — slightly more than the 21% in room air — which is enough to improve oxygenation without eliminating the hypoxic drive. Prior to, and during, O_2 therapy it is essential to determine ABG levels and to prescribe O_2 accordingly. Correct percentage is ensured by using controlled flow O_2 masks and other appliances.

? **3.10** How would you explain the concept of hypoxic drive and its importance for self-treatment to a patient with COAD who is about to be sent home on O_2 therapy?

resulting in carbon dioxide narcosis and respiratory arrest (see Box 3.4). Oxygen may be required constantly both in hospital and at home.

Bronchodilator drugs and antibiotics may be prescribed. Physiotherapy is essential.

NURSING PRIORITIES AND MANAGEMENT: EMPHYSEMA

Major considerations

Reassurance and support

In advanced cases of emphysema the patient will be constantly striving for breath and will need maximum reassurance and calm support. His lifestyle will be drastically curtailed and every effort should be made to make a realistic assessment of his capabilities and need for assistance in designing his care plan. His limitations may be extreme and affect even minor activities such as eating, drinking, combing hair, brushing teeth and moving about the room. Time should be spent helping, observing and listening.

Oxygen therapy

Oxygen should be administered strictly according to the prescribed amount because of the danger of switching off this patient's hypoxic drive. It is vital that the nurse understands this and can explain it in simple terms to the patient, especially if he is to use and control his own oxygen supply at home. The patient and his family will need both verbal and written information and plenty of opportunity for discussion (see Box 3.5). A controlled percentage face mask (Ventimask) is usually used for this purpose (see Fig. 3.12).

Arterial blood gas analysis

ABG analysis is the most reliable way to monitor blood gas levels and the nurse should be prepared to follow the required

Box 3.5 Patient teaching in O_2 therapy (Reproduced with permission from Rutishauser 1994)

Increasingly, patients go home on O_2 therapy and will need information on how to get a supply of medical O_2 and how to set it up at home. The following instructions, which should accompany the patient, should be discussed fully and reinforced on every contact.

INSTRUCTIONS FOR HOME USE OF OXYGEN

- Oxygen is highly combustible. Do not use it near a fire or open flame. Post a 'NO SMOKING' sign on the cylinder and explain to relatives and friends the reason for so doing. Electrical appliances and kinetic toys that may produce a spark are also a source of danger.
- Adjust the flow meter to the flow rate the doctor prescribes and do not change it without his consent.
- Keep water in the humidifier to the correct level and change it daily.
- NOTIFY DOCTOR IF ANY OF THE FOLLOWING OCCUR:
  - you have increased difficulty breathing
  - you feel unusually restless or upset
  - your breathing gets irregular
  - you feel abnormally drowsy
  - your lips or fingernails look blue
  - you have trouble concentrating or get confused.

Do not assume that you will feel better if you take more oxygen. This may not be the case and you should consult your doctor or go to the nearest casualty department immediately.

procedure for obtaining the blood sample (see Box 3.6). A basic understanding of normal levels is also assumed (see Fig. 3.6).

The nurse must be aware that cyanosis may be a *late* sign of hypoxia and should not be relied upon as an early indicator. As a rule of thumb, cyanosis is usually noticeable when the concentration of deoxygenated haemoglobin in blood exceeds 50 g/l. The distinction between central and peripheral cyanosis is an important one. Central cyanosis is due to low oxygen content of the arterial blood (hypoxic hypoxia) and can be determined by inspecting the tongue and mucous membranes of the eye in addition to the skin. Peripheral cyanosis is due to a sluggish circulation (stagnant hypoxia) where release of oxygen from the blood is slowed down even though the arterial oxygen content may be normal, as for example in cardiac failure and shock.

Box 3.6 Monitoring arterial blood gas levels (ABGs)

In the clinical situation ABG levels can be monitored by laboratory blood gas analysis.

Blood is drawn from the radial or femoral artery, or from an established arterial line, using a heparinised syringe. Care is taken not to draw air into the syringe, which is capped and sent for immediate analysis.

Following the procedure, firm pressure must be applied to the puncture site for at least 5 min, as the artery may spurt significantly.

If the patient is on oxygen therapy it is important to make sure that he has been having the prescribed amount for at least 15 min before the sample is drawn and to maintain that amount during the procedure. If he has been on a mechanical ventilator for a session of intermittent positive pressure breathing (IPPB), the nurse should wait at least 20 min before taking a sample and 20 min after commencing ventilation or post-tracheal suctioning. The prescribed amount of oxygen or the IPPB should be noted on the laboratory request form.

? **3.11** Which kind of cyanosis would you expect to find in a patient with advanced COAD?

For further information, see Rutishauser (1994), Ch. 11.

Positioning and breathing

The patient will be more comfortable sitting up and well supported by pillows. He may find breathing easier if he leans forward on an overbed table with his elbows extended to the side. Emphysematous patients tend to take short, shallow

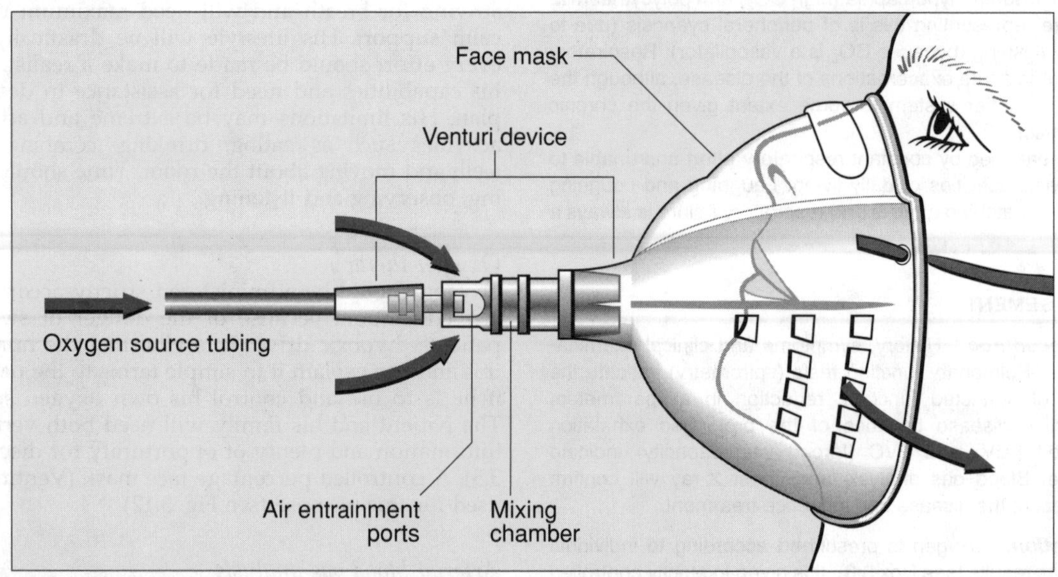

Fig. 3.8 The Ventimask. (Reproduced with kind permission from Allan 1989.)

breaths and should be taught diaphragmatic breathing to improve and slow down ventilation. Pursed-lip exhalation is helpful because it improves positive airway pressure and brings the abdominal muscles into play.

Chest physiotherapy
The physiotherapist will teach the patient deep breathing and coughing exercises and postural drainage techniques. Frappage (patterns of clapping the chest wall) may be necessary to loosen tenacious secretions. These exercises should be reinforced by nursing staff and the patient should be taught to perform them independently so that he can continue them after discharge home.

Patient education
The patient should understand the disease process and the aims of treatment. If the disease is in the early stages removal of predisposing factors such as cigarette smoking will help prevent further deterioration. If the condition is advanced he may need help to adapt to a severely compromised lifestyle and to preserve what pulmonary function he has. Ensuring that the patient obtains optimal relief from his symptoms and is given adequate psychological support will present a considerable challenge for the nurse. The whole health care team will often be involved in providing support, advice and practical help to the whole family.

Asthma

Asthma is a common chronic inflammatory condition of the airways which is characterised by bronchospasm, severe dyspnoea, wheezing, chest tightness and expiratory exertion. As a result of inflammation the airways are hyperresponsive and narrow easily in response to a wide range of provoking stimuli. Although much is known about asthma it is a complex condition about which much remains to be understood.

Broadly speaking, there are two types of bronchial asthma: extrinsic and intrinsic. The extrinsic form occurs in children and young adults who are hypersensitive to foreign proteins such as dust mites, pollens, animal dander and feathers. Familial allergic tendencies can often be traced. Intrinsic or chronic asthma occurs later in life and is often associated with chronic respiratory inflammatory disease. Although there is no history of childhood asthma there may be a family history of asthma and allergic tendencies. In many cases the role of allergens is still suspected. A large group of asthma sufferers are found to be vulnerable to stimuli of both extrinsic and intrinsic origin. There is increasing evidence that the psychsomatic element is negligible and can no longer be regarded as a major causative factor in most cases (Barnes 1993).

Studies show that asthma affects about 5% of the adult population in Britain and between 10–15% of children (Action Asthma 1990). There is presently a greater awareness of asthma and an increase in the number of people being diagnosed and treated, especially children. There is no cure for asthma as yet, although most symptoms can be controlled by drug therapy.

Recent research suggests that there is a critical trigger time early in the development of asthma when, if steroid therapy is introduced, the process can not only be controlled but 'turned off' so that the condition does not progress or recur. However, there continues to be some resistance to steroid therapy from the general public, especially in relation to treating children. This is because of the misconceived fear of side-effects, which in fact are minimal with inhaled steroids (Barnes 1993).

Morbidity remains extensive and the death rate for asthma has remained at over 2000 per annum for over a decade. This has been attributed to underdiagnosis and undertreatment (Tettersell 1993).

PATHOPHYSIOLOGY

The immunoglobulin IgE is present in small amounts in normal sera but in increased amounts in asthma suffers. In allergic extrinsic asthma the disease process involves inhalation of antigens (allergens) which are absorbed by the bronchial mucosa and trigger production of IgE antibodies. These antibodies bind to mast cells and basophils around the bronchial blood vessels. When the allergen is encountered again the antigen–antibody reaction releases histamines and bradykinin, resulting in bronchial muscle spasm, oedema and excessive secretion of thick mucus. In many cases the severity of attacks lessens with age and good treatment unless other factors are involved.

There are various theories of the pathogenesis of intrinsic asthma. Allergens may be implicated. Whatever the cause, the bronchi and bronchioles are chronically inflamed, oedematous, full of mucus and subject to bronchospasm. Air is trapped in the alveoli and expiration is difficult. The disease can be progressive and impaired ventilation can result in hypoxia, hypertension and right-sided heart failure.

Clinical features. Asthma attacks can last for minutes, hours or days (status asthmaticus). They manifest as paroxysms of severe ventilatory difficulty with rapid, laboured breathing accompanied by wheezing. Expiration is forced and prolonged due to bronchospasm, hyperinflated lungs and trapped alveolar air. This may be accompanied by a dry or a moist cough. There may be extreme anxiety, sweating, dyspnoea, orthopnoea and peripheral cyanosis with hypoxia and hypercapnia. Tachycardia is common because of anxiety and hypoxia and may be increased by bronchodilatory drugs such as salbutamol. If there is no response to treatment, exhaustion will occur rapidly and may be followed by respiratory failure.

Investigative procedures. Diagnosis is by typical clinical presentation and past history. After an attack has subsided lung function tests such as FEV_1 will be helpful in establishing the degree of impairment and in monitoring response to treatment. Prolonged FEV_1 indicates loss of elasticity of lung tissue. Chest X-rays will indicate clarity of lung fields and size of the heart. Skin sensitivity tests and history of exposure to specific allergens may help in isolating and avoiding triggering factors.

Medical intervention. Because of the complexity of asthma and concern about the continuing high incidence of mortality, a group of experts from the British Thoracic Society, the Research Unit of the Royal College of Physicians of London, the King's Fund Centre and the National Asthma Campaign drew up a comprehensive set of guidelines (a protocol) for the treatment of adult asthma. Their main concerns were that there was underuse of inhaled and oral corticosteroid treatment, underuse of objective measures of severity of asthma and inadequate supervision. This protocol is available to all GPs, A & E departments and respiratory units.

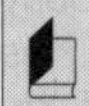
For further information, see British Thoracic Society (1993).

? **3.12** Obtain and study carefully the British Thoracic Society guidelines for the management of asthma.

The best treatment for asthma is avoidance of the cause, if this is known. In the event of an attack, initial treatment is usually with a bronchodilatory drug such as salbutamol and possibly a corticosteroid drug such as beclomethasone (an anti-inflammatory) given via a nebuliser or metered dose inhaler. First aid and home treatment can include steam inhalation to relax muscle spasm and loosen secretions. Severe cases may be treated in the A & E department, where oxygen therapy may be given in addition to nebulised or i.v. drugs. Oxygen is usually given at 4–6 l/min and by intranasal catheter because of the claustrophobic effect of oxygen face masks. ABGs will be analysed and oxygen prescribed accordingly. If the patient comes within the diagnostic category of COAD, care must be taken not to overprescribe

Box 3.7 Self-management of asthma (Reproduced with kind permission from British Thoracic Society)

1. As far as possible patients should be trained to manage their own treatment rather than be required to consult the doctor before making changes.
2. The patient should have a relevant understanding of the nature of asthma and its treatment. This would include:
   - training in the proper use of inhaled treatment and the use of a peak flow meter
   - knowledge of the difference between relieving and anti-inflammatory therapies
   - instruction to ensure recognition of signs that asthma is worsening, especially the significance of nighttime symptoms and of changes in PEF (peak expiratory flow)
3. Patients should be given adequate opportunity to express their expectations of treatment and to hear how far those expectations can be met. They should have a balanced view of the possible side-effects of the treatments.
4. Education and training of the patient are the responsibility of the doctor but can profitably be shared with specially trained health care professionals. Advice should be consistent, and repeated. It may be supported by written or audiovisual material. The patient should be acquainted with the resources of the National Asthma Campaign.
5. Patients who have required or who are likely to require a course of systemic corticosteroid treatment should be trained to initiate or increase inhaled and oral corticosteroid treatment themselves under specified pre-arranged circumstances as outlined in a self-management plan.
6. The three elements of a self-management plan are:
   - symptom, peak flow and drug usage monitoring leading to
   - the patient taking pre-arranged action according to
   - written guidance.

   Such self-management plans should be carefully discussed with the patient and written down individually or by using a National Asthma Campaign Adult Asthma Card. The plans should include information about how and where to obtain urgent medical attention.
7. Patients should regard the plan of management as subject to a process of continuing but orderly review in which they play an active part. Review of a patient's progress at a pre-arranged visit to the doctor should include review of:
   - symptoms, especially nocturnal
   - interference with normal activities (e.g. work loss)
   - the patient's own record of treatment changes
   - peak flow recordings
   - understanding of asthma
   - understanding of management
   - inhalation skills
   - the action to be taken by the patient if pre-arranged signs of deterioration develop.
8. Requests for help from a patient with asthma should be accorded the highest priority by doctors. Other health care workers should be aware that medical help may be required promptly in the event of worsening asthma.

because of possible compromise of hypoxic respiratory drive (see Box 3.5).

The majority of patients are treated by their GP and can administer their own treatment at home and avoid asthma attacks (see Box 3.7). Severe cases are referred to specialist respiratory units. Once diagnosed, if the patient does not respond to the usual prescribed treatment and he notices a significant drop in his peak flow reading or experiences increasing difficulty, he may present and self-admit to the respiratory unit where he is known or to the nearest A & E department (see Boxes 3.9 and 3.10).

Treatment outcome. It is thought that asthma deaths relate to underdiagnosis and undertreatment of the disease with 25% being underdiagnoses and 15% being undertreated (Barnes 1993). The problem is possibly compounded because treatment by GPs is usually guided by the patient's perceptions and report of their symptoms. Research indicates that, in general, patients discriminate very poorly with regard to the severity of and changes in their condition. This finding has led to a strong recommendation that the severity of the disease and efficacy of treatment can be determined only by a series of objective measurements of peak flow in addition to self-assessment of symptoms (Kendrick et al 1993).

NURSING PRIORITIES AND MANAGEMENT: ASTHMA

Major considerations

The first priority of nursing intervention is to ensure that the individual experiencing an asthma attack is seen by a doctor as soon as possible. The condition can deteriorate rapidly.

Giving psychological support

An attack of asthma is extremely frightening. The patient will be fighting for breath and is often panic stricken. It is vital for the nurse to maintain a calm and reassuring manner. The nurse with a sound knowledge base will be able to anticipate the course of the attack and the patient's reactions to it, and thus will be better equipped to help him to remain calm. The nurse should stay with the patient at all times.

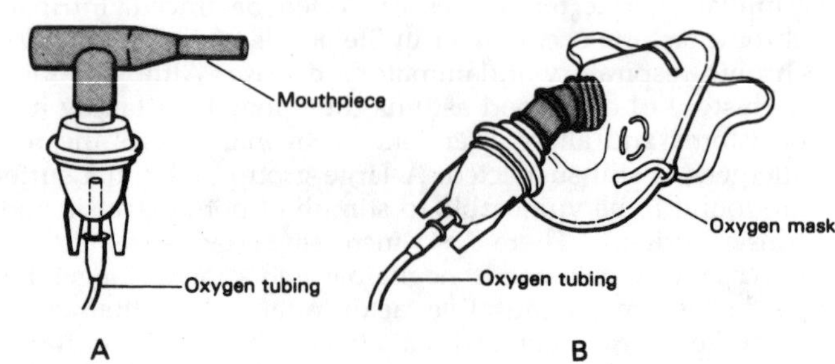

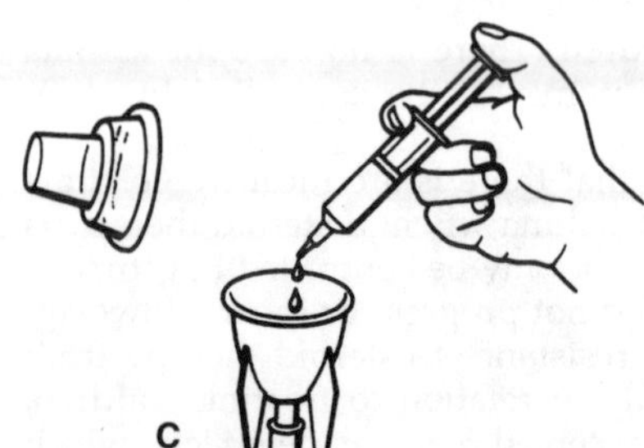

Fig. 3.9 Nebulisers. (A) Nebuliser attached to a mouthpiece. (B) Nebuliser attached to an oxygen mask. (C) Nebuliser taken apart to introduce a prepared medication. (Reproduced with permission from Jamieson et al 1992.)

Box 3.8 Assisting a patient to use a nebuliser

A nebuliser attached to a flow of oxygen or air converts a liquid into an aerosol mist. The medication is prescribed by the doctor along with 2–3 ml of normal saline. The procedure may be coordinated with chest physiotherapy and peak flow of tidal volume may be measured and recorded before and after the treatment. The equipment is assembled according to the procedure illustrated in Figure 3.9.

The medication is checked and drawn up into a syringe and diluted with the prescribed 2–3 ml of normal saline. If two medications are prescribed they should *not* be mixed together. Separate nebulisers should be used and the bronchodilator drug given first.

- The equipment and purpose of the medication is explained to the patient. The medication is put into the nebuliser, which is assembled and attached to the oxygen or air supply. If oxygen is used a 'No Smoking' sign is put up and the reason explained. Air is used instead of oxygen if the patient has COAD because of the danger of disrupting his hypoxic drive (see Box 3.5).
- Peak flow is measured if required and the best of three attempts is charted.
- The patient sits up in a comfortable position.
- The oxygen flow meter is adjusted to 5 l to ensure vaporisation of the medication.
- The nurse observes to ensure that there is a fine vapour coming from the nebuliser and encourages the patient to breathe it in through the mouthpiece if possible. If this is too difficult for him he may use an oxygen mask instead. The patient is instructed to breathe normally, taking an occasional deep breath. If the patient is on a respirator a nebuliser can be introduced into the ventilator circuit.
- The nurse should stay with the patient until all the medication is nebulised and observe his respirations. She should ask him how he feels and encourage him to cough and expectorate if he has mucus in his lungs. A clean sputum container should be ready to hand.
- Half an hour after the treatment peak flow readings are taken again and the best of three is charted.
- The procedure is documented and the equipment washed and dried and stored in the patient's locker until needed again.

Positioning and monitoring

The patient should sit up well supported by pillows or lean forward on an overbed table. Vital signs, oxygen therapy and ABGs should be monitored constantly and interpreted intelligently. The nurse should be on the alert for signs of impending respiratory failure (see p. 82).

Assisting with inhalation technique

The nurse should make sure that the patient is using his nebuliser or inhaler correctly (see Box 3.10 and Figs 3.9 and 3.10). There are different kinds of inhalation delivery systems and it is essential to follow the manufacturer's instructions specific to each type. A common cause of failed home treatment is that the patient does not use his inhaler correctly and therefore does not get his full dose of the drug (see Research Abstract 3.1). There is some debate about which kind of metered dose inhaler is best, but the weight of opinion gives preference to the breath-actuated pressurised aerosol for patients with poor inhaler technique. Between 40 and 50% of patients have poor technique which can be improved by changing from the conventional metered dose inhalers to the breath-actuated pressure inhaler and being given proper instruction in its use (Crompton 1991). Conventional inhalers use carrier substances (CFCs) to deliver the prescribed drug; these substances are suspected of causing additional bronchospasm and coughing in some patients (Engel et al 1989).

Practice nurses, community nurses and hospital nurses are in a good position to make a realistic assessment of patient capabilities and inhaler technique and to give advice accordingly. The effectiveness of received medication can be determined by measuring lung function (peak flow) before and

Research Abstract 3.1 Improvement of drug delivery with a breath-actuated pressurised aerosol (Newman et al 1991)

The metered dose inhaler is difficult to use correctly, the synchronising of actuation with inhalation being the most important problem. A breath-actuated pressurised inhaler (autohaler), designed to help patients with poor inhaler technique, was compared with a conventional metered dose inhaler in terms of aerosol deposition and bronchodilator response in a group of 18 asthmatic patients. Results from the 10 patients with good coordination and technique indicated that there was no significant difference between inhalers for them. However, the 8 patients with poor inhaler technique showed a significant improvement in amount of aerosol deposited in the lungs and bronchodilatory response when using the breath-actuated pressurised inhaler. The conclusion was that due consideration should be given to selecting the type of inhaler to fit the individual patient's needs.

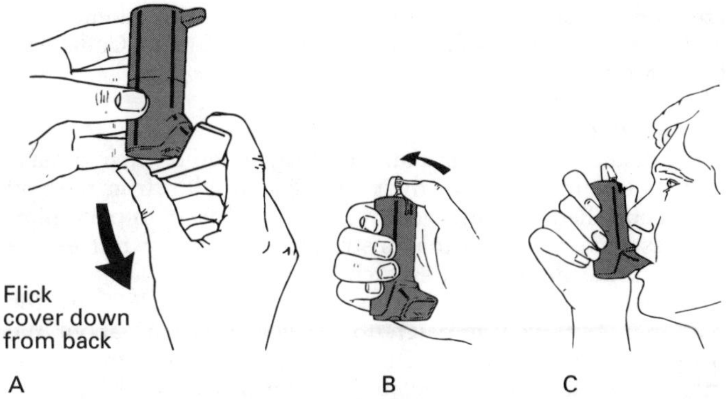

Fig. 3.10 How to use the Respolin Autohaler. (A) Remove the cover from the mouthpiece. (B) Shake the inhaler. Then hold it upright as shown and push the lever right up so that it stays in the 'on' position. (C) Breathe out normally. Put the mouthpiece in your mouth and close your lips firmly around it. Ensure that the air holes are not blocked with your hand and that the inhaler is upright. Take in a deep breath steadily through the mouthpiece. Hold your breath for up to 10 sec and then breathe out slowly. Push the lever down into the off position immediately after each puff. If you need to take a second puff, wait at least 1 min. (Reproduced with kind permission of 3M Pharmaceuticals.)

Box 3.9 Recognition and management of acute severe asthma (Reproduced with kind permission from British Thoracic Society)

The severity of an attack of acute severe asthma is often underestimated by patients, their relatives and their doctors. This is largely because of failure to make objective measurements. If not recognised and not treated appropriately such attacks can be fatal.

AIMS OF MANAGEMENT

The aims of management are:

1. To prevent death
2. To restore the patient's clinical condition and lung function to best levels as soon as possible
3. To maintain optimal function and prevent early relapse.

RECOGNITION AND ASSESSMENT OF ACUTE SEVERE ASTHMA

1. Potentially life-threatening features:
   The presence of any of the following indicates a severe attack:
   - increasing wheeze and breathlessness so that the patient is unable to complete sentences in one breath or get up from a chair or bed
   - respiratory rate ≥ 25 breaths/min
   - heart rate persistently ≥ 110 beats/min
   - peak expiratory flow (PEF) < 40% of predicted normal or of best obtainable if known (< 200 l/min where best obtainable value not known)
   - inspiratory fall in systolic blood pressure ⩾ 10 mmHg.
2. Imminently life-threatening features:
   The presence of any of the following indicates a very severe attack:
   - a silent chest on auscultation
   - cyanosis
   - bradycardia
   - exhaustion, confusion or unconsciousness.
3. Arterial blood gas markers of severity
   Arterial blood gases should always be measured in patients with acute severe asthma admitted to hospital. The following are markers of a very severe (or life-threatening) attack:
   - a normal or high arterial carbon dioxide tension ($Paco_2$) in a breathless asthmatic patient
   - severe hypoxia: arterial oxygen tension (Pao_2) < 8 kPa (60 mmHg) irrespective of oxygen therapy
   - a low pH.

There are no other investigations that are needed for immediate management.

Note on assessment of severity
Patients with a *severe* (i.e. life-threatening) attack often do not have distressing symptoms and they do not necessarily have all of the abnormalities in signs and measurements outlined above, but the presence of any of these should alert the doctor.

Peak expiratory flow (PEF)
Ideally, the results of PEF measurements are most easily interpreted when expressed as a percentage of the predicted normal value or of the previous best obtainable value on optimal treatment. In patients in whom neither of these is known decisions have to be taken based on the absolute level recorded, remembering that normal values vary with age, sex and height (older people, females and shorter people having a lower normal range). Values expressed as a percentage of the predicted normal are not useful in patients with chronically impaired lung function. Bearing in mind these qualifications, the guidelines express PEF as a percentage of predicted normal or of best. Absolute values are shown in parentheses to suggest the levels at which action should be taken in instances in which previous best values are not known.

after inhalation. Patients can be taught to do this themselves and to record the results (Case History 3.1(B) and Collaborative Care Plan 3.1).

Health education
The adequacy of asthma patients' knowledge of their disease and its treatment and of their compliance with drug therapy has been called into question by Tettersell (1993). In particular, her research indicates that instructions given by nurses are poorly understood (see Research Abstract 3.2).

A telephone information line was set up in 1990 by the National Asthma Campaign to answer questions about the disease and its treatment. This line continues to be inundated by calls for information relating to the disease and its treatment, medication, delivery systems, peak flow readings, asthma in schools and many other related topics. The calls have been from asthma sufferers themselves, from mothers of children with asthma, from relatives, and from health professionals (Crone et al 1993).

The volume of requests indicates that there is an extensive lack of knowledge and a need for clarification in every aspect of the disease and its management. This is backed up by current research (see Research Abstract 3.3). Nurses are increasingly involved in health education and will need to be well prepared to meet the specific challenges that are emerging in the field of asthma management and education.

Research Abstract 3.2 Asthma patients' knowledge in relation to compliance (Tettersell 1993)

Patient knowledge about asthma and its treatment and treatment compliance levels were assessed among 100 moderate to severe asthmatics recruited from general practice. Postal questionnaires were used. Non-compliance was found to be high, with 39% of patients omitting to take their asthma treatment as prescribed. Reasons given were 'believing the drugs not to be necessary' and 'forgetting'. Almost half the cohort admitted a reluctance to use their inhalers in public and a third stated a preference for tablets. The highest compliers were respondents who reported never receiving an explanation about the condition. The level of patient knowledge had no significant effect on compliance to drug therapy, although it did correlate with ability to manage asthma attacks. The majority of patients believed they would know how to manage an attack, but when 'scored' on actual ability only 34.4% were deemed to be safe. Less than half the patients who had had asthma explained to them reported to have understood the initial explanation. Explanations made by nurses were particularly poorly understood. Health professionals need to look to both their teaching techniques and to methods other than education in isolation as a means of improving patient compliance. Since the GP contract was introduced in April 1990, nurses working in general practice have become increasingly involved with health education as part of health promotion and chronic disease management clinics. This study highlights the need for a more comprehensive approach to patient education and more research into contextual factors involved in non-compliance.

Multidisciplinary Collaborative Care Plan 3.1 C: acute asthma

Problem focus	Date	Medical	Nursing	Patient	Physiotherapy	Social work
Transfer from ICU for stabilisation and establishment of self care treatment regime following an acute severe asthma attack.	9/2/93	• priority if called to review patient's condition	Co-ordinate team care • educative – supportive role • priority to any signs of deteriorating condition. Action STATIM • monitor vital signs and respiratory status		• ensure clear airways – deep breathing, coughing exercises, use of ancillary muscles	• problem with work environment. Assist C to change job. • advise on family benefits
Patient involvement and understanding essential in: • disease process • symptoms • management • interpretation of symptoms and PEF • specific drug actions and side effects • written self care plan and action to be taken when pre-arranged signs of deterioration evident		• select and prescribe treatment and drugs • discuss with patient and care team: — asthma disease process — treatment and action of drugs — taking and monitoring peak expiratory flow (PEF) — significance — nebuliser technique • monitor ABGs • establish individual acceptable range PEF • establish written self care plan for patient and action to be taken	• reassurance • reinforce and repeat doctor's explanations in lay terms • teach use of peak flow meter. Repeat significance of PEF readings • teach use of nebuliser and inhaler • co-ordinate physio and medication times • assist with ABGs • medications as prescribed • monitor effects • assist C to work out role in care team and express questions and concerns • contact Asthma Campaign • assist with written self care plan	• co-operate with health care team to learn more about: — asthma — treatment — management — using nebuliser/ inhaler — recording PEF and what readings signify Work out action to take at set points • ask questions — discuss results • practice use of equipment • talk to social worker and get advice on work and family problems • help to work out written self care plan • aim to control asthma and avoid further severe attacks	• co-ordinate physiotherapy with inhalation regime. Assist with nebuliser technique • discuss general fitness • teach C respiratory mechanics and exercises	• funding for Peak Flow Meter

Case History 3.1(B) C's story continued

'At the team conference just before C was discharged from hospital he made the following comments. 'I just did not realise how important it was to know about asthma — and in particular to know about how it affects me and how the medications work. I hadn't given it much thought really before this severe attack and usually just had a few more puffs with the inhaler when I thought I needed them.

'When I first came to this ward I remember how surprised I was that the other patients seemed to know so much and take such an active part in their own treatment. I thought you came into hospital to have things done to you not to learn how to do it yourself but I see now. They treated the unit a bit like a 'club'. Mostly they'd been in before and their good-natured 'advice' was a great help, especially when I got depressed about being stuck with asthma. I realised it wasn't the end of the world.

'Knowing about asthma makes me feel more in control; and now I've learnt how to use the inhaler properly and the peak-flow meter, and you've explained what my safe limits are, I shall know what to do in future. Having it all written down too, is somehow reassuring. I certainly don't want another episode like this last one so its worth taking a bit more time to understand things and look after myself. I don't intend to let asthma rule *my* life though but I will change my job and try to look after my general health more.'

Box 3.10 Home management of catastrophic, sudden, severe (brittle) asthma (Reproduced with kind permission from British Thoracic Society (1993))

This implies patients with an attack of asthma that becomes severe within minutes or a few hours — with little instability of asthma in the preceding days. Such patients are rare but are at great risk of sudden death.

1. Such patients are best handled by a mutually negotiated management plan, with involvement of the patient, the GP and the consultant. They should be under active review by a chest physician and carry a Medic-Alert bracelet or equivalent.
2. The patient must carry β2-agonist and prednisolone at all times and have duplicate supplies of emergency treatment for hand-bag, car glove compartment, office etc. Provision of a resuscitation box and oxygen cylinder in the patient's home should be considered.
3. As soon as an attack starts, the patient's management plan might be:
   a. Call for help.
   b. Inhale β2-agonist in high dose, (e.g. 20–50 puffs, or nebulised salbutamol 5 mg or terbutaline 10 mg). (If the above has been shown to be ineffective on previous occasions, a syringe pre-loaded with adrenaline (0.5 mg) 'Minijet' for subcutaneous injection may be helpful. The patient and/or relative must be shown how to use the syringe under supervision using normal saline for practice. The shelf life is limited to 6 months. No similar β2-agonist preparation is commercially available.)
   c. Swallow prednisolone 40–60 mg.
   d. Go to the nearest hospital as previously agreed with GP.
4. If such a patient is seen during an attack, the previous history may suggest direct admission to ITU.

Research Abstract 3.3 Evaluation of an instructional programme in the self-management of asthma (Byrne et al 1993)

Severe asthma can impose restrictions on personal, interpersonal and work-related goals. In this study 23 patients under the care of GPs were surveyed by interview to determine their current control over their asthma in relation to exercise and use of medication. An instructional programme was offered to them to assist in tailoring exercise to their tolerance levels and to help improve compliance with prescribed medication regimes. Findings indicated that 18 patients experienced moderate to severe restrictions when troubled by asthma. Although over 50% exercised regularly for fitness, including 7 with aerobic exercise, some chose sports they thought could provoke an asthma attack. Half took precautionary measures when exercising. All patients used bronchodilators to relieve asthma but one third did not keep their inhalers handy. The most troubled 18 lived or worked in environments where people smoked cigarettes and one third kept furry animals as pets. This study underlines the complexity of trying to help patients tailor their lifestyle to maximise their health.

BRONCHOGENIC CARCINOMA

Bronchogenic carcinoma can be of primary origin, as discussed above, or can occur as secondary metastatic spread from other primary sources.

PATHOPHYSIOLOGY

Bronchogenic carcinomas are classified according to their basic cell type, i.e. squamous cell adenocarcinoma (the most common), undifferentiated carcinoma, and large- and small-cell carcinoma. The tumour presents as a cauliflower-shaped mass which slowly infiltrates the lung parenchyma. Because this form of cancer is difficult to detect in the early stages it has a high potential for metastatic spread before being discovered.

Common presenting symptoms. The patient presents with a persistent cough of several months' duration which may be accompanied by haemoptysis (blood-stained sputum), chest pain, hoarseness and breathlessness. There may also be weight loss, anaemia, pleural effusion and bone pain. The patient will look generally unwell. (See Case History 3.2)

MEDICAL MANAGEMENT

Investigative procedures. Diagnosis is confirmed by auscultation (listening to the chest with a stethoscope), chest X-ray or CT scan and sputum cytology. A bronchoscopy (direct visualisation of the trachea and bronchi using a bronchoscope, i.e. a flexible tube with a light source) may be performed. A small piece of lung tissue (biopsy) may be taken via the bronchoscope and sent for pathology.

Medical intervention. A full explanation of the diagnosis and prognosis will be given to the patient and his family, who will be involved in decision-making regarding treatment. About 15% of primary lung tumours can be treated successfully by surgical removal. This will involve either lobectomy (removal of the affected lobe) or pneumonectomy (removal of the whole lung) followed by cytotoxic chemotherapy. Where there is invasive and metastatic spread the treatment is usually conservative, involving chemotherapy, deep X-ray, intervention to alleviate symptoms, and pain control (see Chs. 19 and 32).

NURSING PRIORITIES AND MANAGEMENT: CARE OF THE PATIENT FOLLOWING LOBECTOMY

General perioperative care is as described in Chapter 27. The reader should also review the position and function of the structures illustrated in Figure 3.1.

Specific considerations

The following points are of particular importance to postoperative management following lobectomy:

- The physiotherapist will manage the pre- and postoperative chest physiotherapy; however, the role of nursing staff in giving assistance and ensuring continuity is extremely important
- Chest surgery can be very frightening and the patient and his family will need careful explanations and constant reassurance
- In order to allow full expansion of the operated lung the patient must be nursed in a semi-upright position, well-supported with pillows, following a lower lobectomy. Following an upper lobectomy the patient must be nursed in the position requested by the surgeon
- If oxygen therapy is required it will be prescribed by the doctor. The nurse will need to monitor the equipment, the amount given, and the effect of the therapy on the patient
- There are usually two chest drains in situ, one anterior to the apex and one posterior to the base. These are attached to underwater seal drainage and pleural suction (see Fig. 3.12). Their purpose is to allow air to escape from the lobectomy space and to allow drainage of haemoserous

fluid caused by the surgical procedure. Management of underwater seal drainage is discussed in detail in Box 3.11

- The patient can sit out of bed and walk short distances while the drains are in place but care must be taken not to put traction on the tubes and to keep the drainage system below the level of the chest. Two pairs of chest drain clamps should accompany the patient at all times.

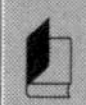
For further information, see Campbell (1993).

NURSING PRIORITIES AND MANAGEMENT: CARE OF THE PATIENT FOLLOWING PNEUMONECTOMY

Specific considerations

Postoperative positioning

It is vital to find out whether the pericardium has been opened during the operation or not. If it has been opened the patient must *not* be allowed to lie on the operated side because of the danger of herniation of the heart through the pericardium and a mediastinal shift (that is, a shifting of the heart and greater vessels into the pleural space, causing kinking of the vessels and acute circulatory failure).

Unless otherwise indicated by the surgeon, the best practice is to nurse the patient upright, well-supported by pillows.

Chest drains

Usually there are no drainage tubes in position, the main aim being for the space to fill with haemoserous fluid. This will slowly become organised into fibrous tissue and, together with contraction of the intercostal and diaphragmatic muscles and gradual slight shift of the mediastinum, will eventually fill the residual space.

However, if chest drains are in position they will be attached to an underwater seal drainage system and *double clamped.* There may be a request that the clamps be released for brief periods at given times to allow escape of excess fluid and air. If this is the case, *the nurse must stay with the patient during the unclamped period and be prepared to clamp the tubings immediately if the patient is about to cough.* Because a cough is a full inspiration followed by forced expiration, it will force air from the lung space out through the drainage tube, allowing a sudden mediastinal shift which could be fatal.

Other considerations

The knowledge that he has lost an entire lung can cause the patient to panic and to be extremely agitated. It is vital for the nurse to remain with the patient as much as possible and to maintain a calm and reassuring manner.

There may be a degree of postanaesthetic atalectasis (collapse of the alveoli) causing breathlessness. Oxygen will be given as prescribed.

Pain can be severe following this procedure and prescribed pain relief should be given promptly. It should be borne in mind that effective pain control will help to promote calm, relaxed breathing and is therefore important to the patient's recovery (see Ch. 19).

RESPIRATORY EMERGENCIES

This section begins with a brief consideration of the mechanism and early warning signs of respiratory failure. This is followed by a discussion of chest injuries and of pulmonary oedema. A brief introduction to endotracheal intubation and mechanical ventilation is also given. Pulmonary embolism, a fairly common and potentially lethal complication of surgery and trauma is discussed in Chapter 27, p. 783.

CHEST INJURIES

Fractured ribs and flail chest

PATHOPHYSIOLOGY

Any injury to the thoracic cavity has the potential to compromise respiratory function. Penetrating injuries caused by knives, bullets, fractured ribs or sharp objects can disrupt ventilatory mechanisms or pierce vital structures, resulting in collapse of the lung or abnormal collections of blood or air in the pleural cavity. Non-penetrating

Case History 3.2 Mrs M. Bronchogenic carcinoma

M was 40 years old, mother of an 18-year-old son, and two daughters aged 17 and 15. Her son was unemployed and had been involved in one or two minor skirmishes between his local gang and the police. The girls were still at school. M's husband walked out on her 8 years ago and she had supported her family as best she could on social benefits and the occasional odd job.

They lived in a high-rise housing estate in the inner-city area. She seldom went out except to get bare necessities and to window shop during the daytime. It wasn't safe for a woman at night in that part of town. She spent a lot of time in front of the television. She had smoked heavily for the past 10 years, saying it was her only luxury and that when she tried to cut down she got 'stressed out of her mind'.

Recently she had lost a lot of weight and been breathless after climbing the stairs to the flat. She had had a 'smoker's' cough for years and been prone to 'chest colds' but when she started to find breathing painful she visited her GP asking for antibiotics for her 'chest infection'.

A series of tests (chest X-ray, sputum culture and lung scan) showed that she had advanced bronchogenic carcinoma. She was immediately referred to the oncology department at the local hospital, where further tests showed that she had boney metastases (secondary cancer in the bones). Having discussed a range of options for treatment, which included chemotherapy and irradiation therapy and their side effects, she elected not to have any treatment except pain relief when the symptoms got worse.

M's symptoms and breathing difficulties quickly did get worse and her few activities were severely curtailed. She insisted on staying at home until a week before her death and she died 6 months after she had been diagnosed. Apart from her three children and an elderly mother in a nursing home, there were no other relatives to call upon.

? **3.13** Discuss the social problems contributing to M's heavy smoking habit? What additional problems were created by her early death and what impact could it have on her children? What kind of interventions are called for, and by whom? Consider the ethical dilemmas that a community nurse could be faced with in offering support and advice, remembering the fine balance between beneficence and patient autonomy and the fact that most of this life drama was played out in M's own home.

injuries caused by blunt trauma or crushing can also disrupt ventilatory mechanisms, especially if the diaphragm or other structures are ruptured or contused. Both types of injury will involve dysfunctional pain, and both will restrict surface area and gaseous exchange.

Clinical features. Signs and symptoms shared by all chest injuries include varying degrees of dyspnoea, chest pain, cyanosis, hypoxia, tachycardia and possibly haemoptysis.

MEDICAL MANAGEMENT

Investigative procedures. Diagnosis is confirmed by chest X-ray and the degree of hypoxia determined by blood gas analysis.

Medical intervention. Simple fractured ribs are usually stable and heal without intervention. Compound fractured ribs may cause a pneumothorax (see below).

When several successive ribs are fractured and become disassociated completely from the rest of the rib-cage the condition is known as flail chest and is characterised by paradoxical breathing (see Fig. 3.11).

NURSING PRIORITIES AND MANAGEMENT: FRACTURED RIBS AND FLAIL CHEST

Providing there are no complications or other serious injury the patient with fractured ribs can be nursed at home. Flail chest, however, is often associated with more serious chest trauma requiring hospital care.

The main aim of nursing care is to promote rest and control pain until the intercostal muscles have had a chance to stabilise the fractured ribs. In the case of flail chest the patient will need bedrest and probably narcotic pain relief by i.m. injection.

The patient should be advised to avoid heavy lifting or exertion until the fractures are healed.

Pneumothorax and haemopneumothorax

PATHOPHYSIOLOGY

The term 'pneumothorax' refers to the presence of air in the pleural space and 'haemopneumothorax' to the presence of blood and air in the pleural space. Both conditions cause partial or complete collapse of the lung on the affected side.

In 'tension pneumothorax' the opening into the pleural space from either the lung or the outside chest wall acts as a one-way valve and sucks air into that space during inhalation but does not allow it to escape during exhalation. Gradually there is a buildup of air in the affected side and a mediastinal shift occurs with resultant cardio-pulmonary compromise.

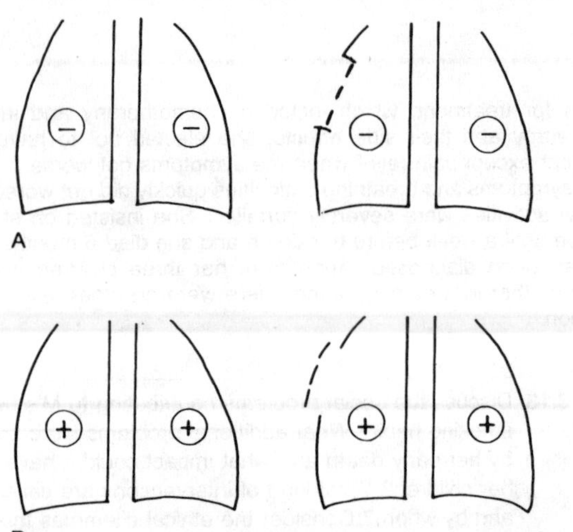

Fig. 3.11 Paradoxical breathing. (A) On inhalation, the rib-cage expands to create a negative pressure in the lungs and thus sucks in air. This negative pressure also draws in the disassociated ribs. (B) On exhalation, the rib-cage contracts to expel air from the lungs, but the resultant positive pressure also forces out the disassociated ribs. (Reproduced with permission from Game et al 1989.)

Clinical features. An open pneumothorax is characterised by the presence of an open wound and a sucking sound as air is drawn into the pleural cavity. In a closed pneumothorax air enters the space from torn lung tissue and there is little or no movement on the affected side.

MEDICAL MANAGEMENT

First aid. The patient is kept in an upright position or lying on the affected side. Penetrating foreign bodies are not removed until intensive care facilities are available, in case of massive haemorrhage or mediastinal shift. Open wounds can be covered by a clean occlusive dressing; this must be released at intervals to avoid a tension pneumothorax developing.

On admission to the accident and emergency (A & E) department the patient will have a chest X-ray. An apical intercostal chest drain will be inserted and connected to an underwater drainage system. If there is a haemopneumothorax, the patient will require a second chest drain in the basal chest wall. Narcotic analgesia will usually be necessary to manage the patient's pain and anxiety.

NURSING PRIORITIES AND MANAGEMENT: PNEUMOTHORAX AND HAEMOPNEUMOTHORAX

Specific considerations

General principles of care for the initial period will be as described in Chapter 28. Specific considerations are as follows.

Observation and monitoring

Constant vigilance must be maintained in observing for any change in respiratory status. These injuries are potentially life threatening and the patient should never be left unattended. Changes in respiratory patterns, in symptoms, and in vital signs should be monitored frequently and action taken accordingly.

Assisting with insertion of chest drain

The patient will usually be given a narcotic analgesic to relax him and relieve the pain. This will also result in slower, deeper and more effective breathing. The nurse assisting should offer simple explanations and reassurance. If possible the patient should be sat up so that he can lean his arms forward on an overbed table. This will help to expand the thoracic cavity and provide good support for the patient. The pressure needed to pierce the chest wall is unpleasant but should not be painful. The nurse assembles all the equipment. Often a complete, sterile chest drain set is kept pre-packaged in the A & E department. Before the chest drain is inserted the drainage system should be opened, connected and the drainage jar filled with sterile water to the requisite level. The whole system should be carefully checked to ensure that it is airtight. A local anaesthetic is then given at the chosen site,a small incision made, and the chest drain inserted and connected to the underwater drainage system (see Box 3.11 and Fig. 3.12).

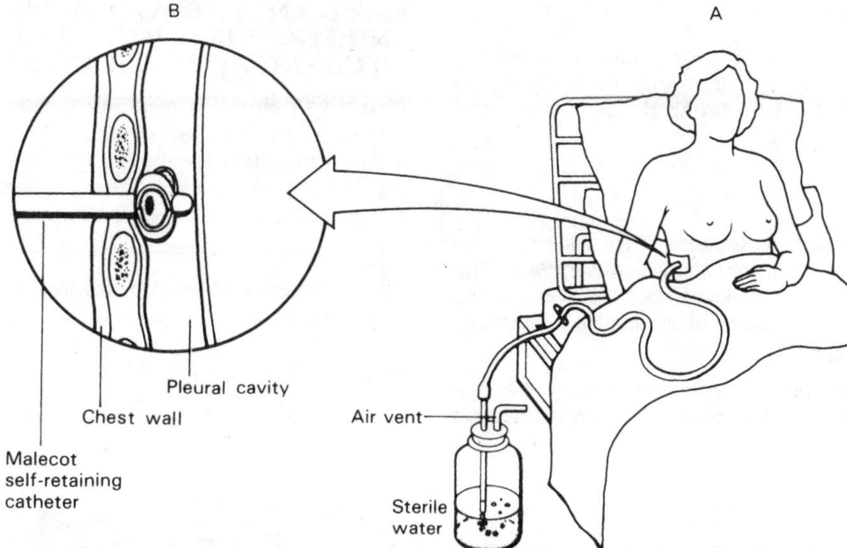

Fig. 3.12 Underwater seal chest drainage. (A) Drainage system in position. (B) Detail of the position of the catheter. (Reproduced with permission from Jamieson et al 1992.)

Assisting with removal of chest drain

This procedure must be carried out by two people, usually a doctor and an experienced nurse. A careful explanation of the procedure should be given to the patient and he should be shown how to practise the Valsalva manoeuvre (forcible exhalation against a closed glottis). Alternatively, he can be asked to take a deep breath in and hold it, as this prevents a rush of air into the puncture site and is more easily controlled than the Valsalva manoeuvre. An occlusive dressing and airtight tape must be ready to apply to the insertion site. The purse-string suture is located and the retaining suture removed. The drain is steadied, and as the patient performs the Valsalva manoeuvre the drain is quickly removed and the purse-string suture tied to close the insertion hole. The dressing and airtight tape are then applied firmly. The patient should be observed carefully following the procedure. A check X-ray may be performed.

Box 3.11 Care of underwater seal drainage

BASIC PRINCIPLES

The drainage system is sterile throughout. It is completely assembled prior to the chest drain being inserted. Connections are airtight and sealed with transparent tape to allow inspection. Water level in the drainage bottle or device is determined by hospital policy but should be at least enough to submerge the drainage tube by 2.5 cm. In the case of prepacked drainage units the manufacturer's instructions should be followed. The water acts as a valve and prevents air re-entering the pleural space. The outlet tube allows expelled air to escape. Drainage may be by gravity and respiratory movements or may be assisted by attaching a vacuum pump to the outlet tube. Single-, two- and three-bottle systems are available.

The chest drain is sutured in place and has an additional purse-string suture around the skin entry site. A sterile dressing surrounds the entry site.

NURSING MANAGEMENT

- Give a full explanation and reassurance to the patient to allay his anxiety and gain his cooperation.
- Administer pain relief as required.
- Keep the patient sitting up, well supported by pillows whilst he is in bed and encourage deep breathing and coughing exercises as discussed with the physiotherapist.
- Ensure that two pairs of chest drain clamps accompany the patient at all times in case of accidental disconnection. If the system becomes disconnected air will be drawn into the interpleural space, extending the pneumothorax.
- When clamping is necessary the clamps must not be left on for long periods as a tension pneumothorax may develop (see p. 80). The patient must never be left unattended while the tubing is clamped.
- Ensure that the drainage system is always kept below the level of the chest to prevent back-flow into the interpleural space.
- Check regularly to ensure that the system is airtight and the water level is correct.
- Note the presence of bubbling. If the tube is bubbling, air is being evacuated from the pleural space. If there are no bubbles there should be a swinging movement of fluid in the down tube which reflects the pressure changes in the pleural cavity with respiration. The amount of fluid swing should lessen as the lung re-expands. If there are no bubbles and there is no fluid swing this means either that the drainage tube is blocked or that the lung is fully expanded. Chest X-ray will confirm.
- Prevent accidental disconnection by:
  - — supporting the chest drain with adhesive tape on the chest wall, taking care to loop and not bend it
  - — securing the tubing to the bedclothes or the patient's clothes with tape and pins, taking care not to pierce the tubing
  - — stabilising the drainage jar by housing it in a special cradle on the floor.
- Maintain patency by gently lifting sections of the tubing at regular intervals to facilitate the gravitational drainage of blood and viscous fluid.
- Maintain sterility when changing the down tube and drainage bottle.
- Measure and record the amount and consistency of drainage.

PULMONARY OEDEMA

Pulmonary oedema (excess fluid in lung tissue) is associated with many conditions, including inflammatory response to infections, shock, cardiac failure, nephrotic syndrome and severe allergic reactions.

PATHOPHYSIOLOGY

The lungs are susceptible to oedema because of the minimal tissue resistance offered by the thin alveolar cells and the capillary walls. The condition is akin to drowning in that the lungs are full of water, blood and mucus. Pulmonary oedema is usually acute and life threatening, as it disrupts gaseous exchange.

Clinical features. The patient presents with a moist cough that produces copious, frothy, pink sputum. He is dyspnoeic, tachycardiac, and extremely distressed.

MEDICAL MANAGEMENT

Diagnosis is made on presenting signs and symptoms, auscultation, chest X-ray and medical history. The main principles of treatment are to remove the water from the lungs and to assist the respiratory process. Treatment consists of sitting the patient upright, giving oropharyngeal suction, diuretic therapy, narcotic analgesia, bronchodilator drugs and oxygen. In severe cases it may be necessary to intubate and mechanically ventilate the patient.

NURSING PRIORITIES AND MANAGEMENT: PULMONARY OEDEMA

As pulmonary oedema is usually associated with cardiovascular disease, specifically left ventricular failure, the principles of nursing management are discussed in Ch. 2.

RESPIRATORY FAILURE

If impending respiratory failure is recognised early then the actual state can be avoided and nurses should be alert for the following clinical signs:

- the patient appears restless and confused
- there is an increase in respiratory rate with laboured ventilatory effort and use of auxilliary respiratory muscles (sternomastoid and abdominal muscles)
- forced and abnormal movement of the diaphragm
- flaring nostrils with each breath
- pale or cyanosed and clammy skin.

Where impending respiratory failure is suspected sedation must be withheld as it will further depress respiratory function.

Arterial blood gas levels (ABGs) will confirm the diagnosis.

Respiratory failure is indicated where there is respiratory acidosis with a falling pH, pO_2 below normal and raised pCO_2. See Figure 3.6 for normal blood gas values. Untreated, the condition will worsen steadily and increasingly difficult ventilatory effort will leave the patient exhausted and hypoxic, and he will eventually become comatosed and die. However, patients with impending respiratory failure are normally intubated and mechanically ventilated and are nursed in ITU. Only then can sedation be given with safety.

In order to cut down on dead space and improve respiratory efficiency a tracheostomy (opening into the trachea) is usually performed. Refer to Ch. 14 for indications for a tracheostomy and nursing management of a patient with a tracheostomy.

EMERGENCY AIRWAY MANAGEMENT, ENDOTRACHEAL INTUBATION AND MECHANICAL VENTILATION

Nursing priorities and management

The nurse must be prepared at all times to perform emergency airway procedures and to assist in endotracheal intubation and mechanical ventilation. These procedures are reviewed in Boxes 3.12 and 3.13. See also Figures 3.13 and 3.14.

For further information, see McGarvey (1990).

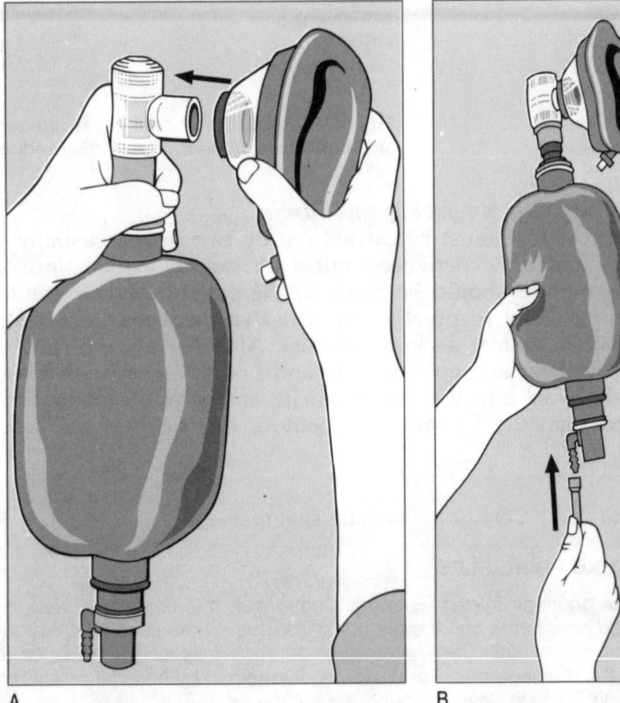

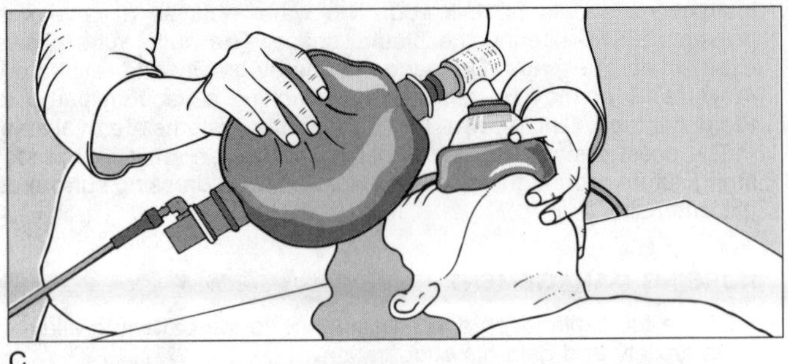

Fig. 3.13 Assembling and using the AMBU bag resuscitator. (A) The mask is attached to the bag. (B) When time permits, the resuscitator is attached to the oxygen supply. (C) The patient's neck is hyperextended and the mask placed firmly over the mouth and nose. The bag is compressed every 5 sec for an adult, delivering approx 1 l of air with each compression. Smaller-sized masks and AMBU bag are used for children with compressions every 3 sec. (Adapted with kind permission from Robinson and Russo 1983.)

Box 3.12 Endotracheal intubation and mechanical ventilation

Endotracheal intubation and mechanical ventilation are both specialist procedures and will be performed and monitored by doctors and nurses specially trained in this area. However, it is necessary for the generalist nurse to be familiar with the relevant procedures and equipment in order to be prepared to assist in emergency situations and to better understand the needs of the patient who has been intubated and ventilated during general anaesthesia.

ENDOTRACHEAL INTUBATION

Maintenance of equipment

Equipment on resuscitation trolleys and in the anaesthetic room must be checked regularly to ensure that it is complete and functional. Equipment must include a full range of sizes of both nasal and oral endotracheal (ET) tubes, at least two laryngoscopes with a supply of new batteries, universal connectors, catheter mounts, 20 ml syringes, artery forceps, Magill intubating forceps, introducers, masks, oral airways, laryngeal spray, suction, lubricant and scissors.

Assisting the anaesthetist

During induction of general anaesthesia the anaesthetist will select the tube suitable for the patient and will test and lubricate it. The nurse will ensure that suction is available and hold the prepared tube ready to hand to the anaesthetist. The patient is given a full explanation and should be continually reassured until the i.v. anaesthetic, muscle relaxant and anaesthetic gas have taken effect. The anaesthetist will visualise the vocal chords with the laryngoscope, introduce the endotracheal (ET) tube, inflate the cuff and connect the ET tube to the anaesthetic machine. The nurse may be requested to apply cricoid pressure during induction of the anaesthetic in order to prevent regurgitation of stomach contents, especially in emergency cases. Pressure is applied using the thumb and forefinger and continued until the patient is asleep and the cuff of the ET tube has been inflated (see Fig. 3.14).

Extubation

Following extubation the nurse must be alert for complaints of sore throat due to damage to the tracheal mucosa, or oedema of the larynx leading to tracheal obstruction. The nurse should raise the head of the bed unless this is contraindicated and report the symptoms to the surgical team.

MECHANICAL VENTILATION

There are many reasons why a patient may need mechanical help with respiration. Extrapulmonary causes which affect the respiratory process include:

- those which affect the respiratory control centres in the brain; e.g. CNS disease, brain contusion or haemorrhage, drug overdose or anaesthesia.
- those of neuromuscular origin which cause respiratory paralysis, e.g. Guillain-Barré syndrome, myaesthenia gravis, poliomyelitis, organic phosphate poisoning and cervical spine injury.
- those which restrict expansion of the thoracic cavity, e.g. musculoskeletal injuries such as extensive flail chest and ruptured diaphragm.

In addition, disorders which affect gaseous exchange can result in severe hypoxia. These include adult respiratory distress syndrome (ARDS), cardiac disease resulting in pulmonary oedema, smoke inhalation, and respiratory infection in a patient with chronic obstructive airways disease (COAD).

When a patient needs help to breathe he may be intubated and attached to a mechanical ventilator. The ventilator will simulate the bellows action normally provided by his diaphragm and thoracic cage and will deliver oxygen-enriched air to his lungs. The type of ventilator used will depend on the specific needs of the individual and will be prescribed by the respiratory specialist. The patient will be nursed in the intensive therapy unit (ITU) and will need specialist nursing care, the principles of which are described in Chapter 29.

? **3.14** When a patient is mechanically ventilated and in certain other instances it is necessary to flood the lungs with pure oxygen both before and after carrying out aspiration. What is the reason for this? (See Ch. 30, p. 850.).

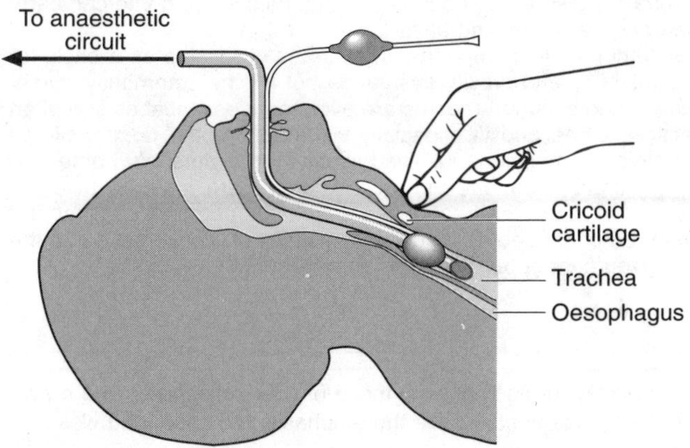

Fig. 3.14 Cuffed ET tube in situ showing position for cricoid pressure. (Adapted from McGarvey 1990.)

Box 3.13 Emergency airway management

Emergency airway management is an essential clinical procedure. The nurse must be familiar with the assembly and use of the hand-held resuscitator known as the AMBU bag and should always be aware of its location in her work area. In cases of respiratory arrest the AMBU bag will ensure more effective ventilation. The procedure for its use is as follows:

- First, clear the airway of any obstruction, mucus or vomitus. Position the patient to open the airway and insert an oral pharyngeal airway (Brook or Guedel).
- Position the face mask to seal the mouth and nose and compress the AMBU bag with the other hand every 5 seconds (see Fig. 3.13). This will deliver approximately 1 l of air with each compression. A smaller bag is used for a child. Oxygen may be attached to the AMBU bag if available.
- Should you need to aspirate mucus from the patient's airway do so via the oral pharyngeal airway. *Avoid nasotracheal suctioning where possible because this can stimulate the sensory receptors of the vagus nerve, causing disordered heart rate and rhythm — usually bradycardia (slowing).*

GENETIC DISORDERS OF THE RESPIRATORY SYSTEM

There is considerable evidence of genetic predisposition and susceptibility to some of the more common respiratory diseases such as asthma. Of the classic genetic disorders, cystic fibrosis has the most dramatic and distressing impact on the respiratory system. This is a disease which disturbs the mucus-producing glands throughout the body, particularly those of the respiratory tract. For a full description of the disease process and its nursing management see Ch. 6, p. 199.

> ? **3.15** To complete your essential procedures folder scan current nursing and medical journals and identify recent trends in nursing involvement and the delivery of health care. Can you relate these to the management of respiratory disorders?

CONTINUITY OF CARE: HOSPITAL AND COMMUNITY

Communication between hospital and community health care teams is vital for continuity and ultimate effectiveness of care and issues relating to discharge planning, accountability and ethical implications are outlined in Box 3.14.

CONCLUSION

In health we are seldom aware of the functioning of our respiratory system but disorders and diseases that affect respiration have the potential to affect every aspect of daily living. Airway, breathing and pulmonary circulation are the ABC — the essential elements — of survival.

This chapter has emphasised the importance of a thorough understanding of the anatomy and physiology of the respiratory system — particularly its physiology, for to understand the function of the system is to understand the profoundly disrupting effects that respiratory disorders can have for the individual's health and well-being. A sound knowledge base in respiratory care must inform nursing interventions in every field of practice. Whether she is working with children or adults, in a general practice or a hospital ward, in educational programmes or in an industrial setting, the nurse must be prepared to recognise and to act upon any compromise, whether chronic or acute, in respiratory function. The potential for nursing intervention will range from resuscitative procedures in an emergency to giving day-to-day advice on the prevention or management of respiratory disease.

The nursing role today encompasses both community-based primary health care and the specialised 'high-tech' skills required in acute care. Nurses are developing new interdependent and independent roles every day to meet the demands of new approaches to health care delivery. In-

Box 3.14 Principles of nursing management: dimensions of community respiratory care

Recent trends have highlighted certain basic issues involved in management of respiratory disorders in the community. These trends include early discharge home from hospital, a higher incidence of severe and chronic respiratory disorders being cared for in the home and respiratory consultants visiting patients in the community and working alongside GPs, practice nurses and clinical nurse specialists (King's Health Care 1993).

THE DISCHARGE PROCESS

Patient education

Teaching self-care and teaching relatives to assist with care should be started early during hospitalisation so that an acceptable level of proficiency is achieved before discharge and problems identified and addressed.

Liaison between hospital and home

When a patient is discharged home following acute hospital care it is vital that there is close liaison between the hospital and the community health care teams. Ideally the community nurse or another member of the multidiciplinary community care team is allocated time to visit the patient while he is still in hospital and to participate in planning for his discharge. At the very least the community nurse should have direct patient and family contact before the patient is discharged home. She may already know them and therefore be able to provide valuable input into discharge planning. The earlier this is done the better, so that arrangements can be made to have the necessary equipment and services in place.

In addition to basic aids to daily living, special equipment such as that required for oxygen therapy, inhalation and nebulisation therapy, airway suctioning, or mechanical ventilation can be installed before the patient is discharged, and patient and carers taught to manage it efficiently.

LINKING

Knowing and utilising all the statutory and voluntary support bodies that are available and appropriate to the patient and his family is crucial in ensuring effective community care.

PRACTICE PROFILE

A descriptive and statistical record, the practice profile, is compiled by each community nurse and is a vital tool in overviewing case type and frequency and workload, and in planning maximum and effective use of resources and skill mix.

DOCUMENTATION

Respiratory disorders and their management in the home can carry a fair degree of risk and hazard.

Documentation is important in all areas of nursing as a basis for accountability and quality assurance but for the community nurse, detailed and accurate records are even more essential as she often practices alone and is especially vulnerable to the complex legal and ethical dimensions involved in entering a person's home and administering treatment and advice. Great care must be taken to ensure that entry and treatment are with that person's consent and cannot be construed as intrusion or assault or, conversely, that the care given cannot be described as negligent.'

> ? **3.16** During your community placement ask your community nursing team leader to discuss her Practice Profile with you.
>
> Select two respiratory care patients from the profile and then collect as much relevant information about the type of statutory and voluntary services available for these particular patients as you can and add this to your resource folder.
>
> Compare your findings with those of your colleagues who may have had placements where the emphasis and case load was different.
>
> Suggested resource people: Local Council of Social Services Directory of Statutory and Voluntary Services. GP surgeries, local libraries, health education libraries, day hospitals, community nursing services.

creasingly, they are being employed in community and specialist clinics to screen, advise, immunise and treat patients and to promote disease prevention and health education. At the same time, technological and medical advances are demanding a higher level of clinical nursing skills.

The chapter has illustrated two of the major principles in nursing management of respiratory disorders: disease prevention and health promotion, and the active, reflective acquisition of a sound knowledge base and clinical skills. Although the emphasis has been on nursing management, the implicit assumption is always that nurses work in close collaboration with other health care professionals and, in many instances, will be responsible for coordinating the work of the whole team.

REFERENCES

Action Asthma 1990 In Tettersell M J 1993 Asthma patients' knowledge in relation to compliance with drug therapy. Journal of Advanced Nursing 18(1): 103

Allan D 1989 Making sense of oxygen delivery. Nursing Times 85(18): 40–42

Azizi B H O 1993 The effects of passive smoking on children's health: the evidence. Paper given 27th Congress of Medicine, Kuala Lumpur (Aug)

Barnes P 1993 Asthma prevention. Paper given at 27th Congress of Medicine, Kuala Lumpur (Aug)

Blackburn C 1993 Gender, class and smoking cessation work. Health Visitor 66(3): 83–85

British Thoracic Society 1993 Guidelines for the management of asthma in adults. British Thoracic Society, London

Byrne D M, Dvory J, Mackay R C, Robinson S, Faranda C & Macadam D B 1993 Evaluation of the efficacy of an instructional programme in the self-management of patients with asthma. Journal of Advanced Nursing 18(4): 637–646

Cayla J A et al 1993 Predictors of AIDS in a cohort of HIV-infected patients with pulmonary or pleural tuberculosis. Tubercle and Lung Disease 74(2): 113–119

Crompton G 1991 Turbuhaler: the essential issues. Paper given at International Symposium of Medicine, Sydney (June)

Crone S, Partridge M & McLean F 1993 Launching a national helpline. Health Visitor 66(3): 94–96

Downie R S, Fyfe C, Tannahill A 1990 Health promotion, models and values. Oxford University Press, Oxford

Engel T, Heinig J H, Malling H J, Scharling B, Nikander K & Madsen F 1989 In: Inhaler additives can cause bronchoconstriction. Corticosteroid Therapy in Asthma: Highlights of an International Symposium, Sydney Convention Centre, 14–15 June 1991, Oxford Clinical Communications, Australia

Game C, Anderson R E, Kidd J R 1989 Medical-surgical nursing: a core text. Churchill Livingstone, Edinburgh

Graham H 1993 Women's smoking: government targets and social trends. Health Visitor 66(3): 80–82

Hahn K 1987 Slow-teaching the COPD patient. Nursing 87 17(4): 34–41

Jamieson E M, McCall J M, Blythe R 1992 Guidelines for clinical nursing practices related to a nursing model, 2nd edn. Churchill Livingstone, Edinburgh

Jess L W 1992 Chronic bronchitis and emphysema: airing the differences. Nursing 92 22(3): 34–41

Jones K, MacLeod-Clark J 1993 Smoking and pregnancy: the role of health professionals. Health Visitor 66(3): 88–90

Kendrick A H, Higgs C M B, Whitfield M J & Laszlo G 1993 Accuracy of perception of severity of asthma: patients treated in general practice. British Medical Journal 307(6901): 422–424

Kidd J R 1989 In: Game C, Anderson R E, Kidd J R (eds) Medical-surgical nursing: a core text. Churchill Livingstone, Melbourne

King's Health Care 1993 Chest disease: a consultant at work in the community. In: A review of quality initiatives. King's College Hospital, London

McGarvey H 1990 Making sense of endotracheal intubation. Nursing Times 86(42): 35–37

Newman S P, Weise A W B, Talace N & Clarke S W 1991 Improvement of drug delivery with a breath actuated pressurised aerosol for patients with poor inhaler technique. Paper for 3M Health Care, Department of Thoracic Medicine, Royal Free Hospital and School of Medicine, London

Nutbeam D, Macaskill P, Smith C, Simpson J & Catford J 1993 Effectiveness of school smoking education programmes. In: Thompson J 1993 Recent papers. Health Visitor 66(3)

Orem D E 1971 Nursing: concepts of practice. McGraw-Hill, New York

Pollock D 1993 Curbing the death merchants. Health Visitor 66(3): 86–87

Robinson F, Russo P (eds) 1983 Providing respiratory care. Nursing Photobook Series. Springhouse Corporation, Springhouse, PA

Rutishauser S 1994 Physiology and anatomy: a basis for nursing and health care. Churchill Livingstone, Edinburgh

Schoendorf K C, Kiely J L 1993 Maternal smoking and sudden infant death syndrome. In: Thompson J 1993 Recent papers. Health Visitor 66(3):

Tettersell M J 1993 Asthma patients' knowledge in relation to compliance with drug therapy. Journal of Advanced Nursing 18(1): 103–113

Wilson K J 1990 Ross and Wilson anatomy and physiology in health and illness, 7th edn. Churchill Livingstone, Edinburgh

Zejda J E, Dosman J A 1993 Respiratory disorders in agriculture. Tubercle and Lung Disease 74(2): 74–83

USEFUL ADDRESSES

National Asthma Campaign Helpline
National Asthma Campaign
Providence House
Providence Place
London N1ONT
Telephone: (0345) 010203

Local Council of Social Services
Dept of Statutory and Voluntary Services
Your Town

FURTHER READING

Amos A 1993 Youth and style magazines: hooked on smoking. Health Visitor 66(3): 91–93

Badnall P, Haslop A 1987 Chronic respiratory disease: educating patients at home. Professional Nurse 2(9): 293–296

Brunner L S, Suddarth D S 1991 The Lippincott manual of medical-surgical nursing, 2nd edn. Harper & Row, London

Campbell J 1993 Making sense of underwater sealed drainage. Nursing Times 89(9): 34–36

Game C, Anderson R E, Kidd J R (eds) 1989 Medical-surgical nursing: A core text. Churchill Livingstone, Melbourne

Kendrick A H 1992 Simple measurements of lung function. Professional Nurse 6: 395–404

Lee R N F, Graydon J E, Ross E 1991 Effects of psychological well-being, physical status and social support on oxygen dependent COPE patients' level of functioning. Research in Nursing and Health 14: 323–328

McDermott J 1993 Setting up a no smoking support group. Health Visitor 66(3): 99–100

Price J 1993 Joint account. Nursing Times 89(13): 44–46

Stevenson G 1992 Infection risks in respiratory therapy. Nursing Standard 6(18): 32–34

Yeaw E M J 1992 Good lung down. American Journal of Nursing 92(3): 27–29

Williams S J 1989 Chronic respiratory illness and disability: a critical review of the psychological literature. Social Science and Medicine 28: 791–803

CHAPTER 4

The gastrointestinal system, liver and biliary tract

Ruth Miller   Evelyn Howie   Mary Murchie

Roger Watson (Section on 'Anatomy and Physiology')
Josephine N Fawcett (Additional material and advice)

CHAPTER CONTENTS

Introduction 87
Anatomy and physiology 88
DISORDERS OF THE GASTROINTESTINAL TRACT 91
Disorders of the mouth 91
Disorders of the oesophagus 91
Disorders of the stomach and duodenum 96
Disorders of the small and large intestine 101
Anorectal disorders 111
DISORDERS OF THE HEPATOBILIARY SYSTEM 113
Disorders of the liver 113
Disorders of the biliary system 120
Disorders of the pancreas 124
Disorders of the spleen 129
Glossary 130
References 130
Further reading 131
Useful addresses 131

INTRODUCTION

The study of the gastrointestinal (GI) system is essential to nursing practice, as the digestive processes are the means by which foods and liquids are digested and absorbed and then transported by the blood for cellular metabolism. Nutrition and dietary factors are integral to the care of individuals receiving treatment for diseases affecting either the digestive system itself or other systems of the body.

Because the GI system comprises a large number of organs with a range of interrelated functions, disorders can produce diverse symptoms, including pain, dysphagia, anorexia, loss of weight, heartburn, vomiting, constipation and diarrhoea.

Disorders of the GI system may be acute, presenting as life-threatening emergencies, or chronic, requiring long-term management and sometimes admission to hospital for more intensive treatment and/or surgical intervention. The specific needs of patients with GI disorders will vary, although in GI surgery there general principles of perioperative care which can be followed. Although many advances in pharmacological treatment have been made over the years, surgery is still the treatment of choice for some conditions, allowing many patients to make a complete and rapid recovery. Those patients whose condition is such that palliative surgery is the only option will require skilled nursing care in hospital and the community.

The nurse's role

The nurse working in a community or hospital setting will be able to advise individuals on how an appropriate diet can contribute to their health and well-being. The nurse is also in a good position to provide explanations of any investigations or treatments, diagnoses and prognoses, and to follow up any information given by medical colleagues. The principles of holistic care and a process of continuous assessment, planning, intervention and evaluation should be followed. This process should be flexible, allowing priorities to be changed as the patient's condition and circumstances evolve.

This chapter begins with a review of the basic anatomy and physiology of the GI tract and its related structures, describing the basic functions of that system and how the specialised organs and tissues which it comprises contribute to its effective functioning. The disorders of the GI system, liver and biliary tract that will most commonly be encountered by nurses in hospital or community settings are then described, working logically through the various components of the digestive system. A separate chapter has, however, been devoted to disorders of the mouth and its related structures, and it will be vital for nurses caring for patients undergoing surgery, terminally ill patients, and patient with GI and related disorders to appreciate the importance of giving careful attention to mouth care, as described in Chapter 15.

Many of the disorders considered in the present chapter often require surgical intervention; the reader is therefore advised to review, along with the specific information given here, the essential principles of perioperative nursing care discussed in detail in Chapter 27.

ANATOMY AND PHYSIOLOGY

The gastrointestinal or digestive tract runs from the mouth to the anal canal and includes the oesophagus, the stomach, the duodenum and the small and large intestines. The ancillary organs of digestion which are connected to, but do not form part of, the digestive tract include the liver, the pancreas and the gall bladder. For the purposes of the present chapter, the spleen will also be considered to form part of the GI system.

The digestive tract is responsible for taking in food and fluids at the mouth (ingestion), breaking up the food into pieces of a manageable size, extracting the nutritional content of the food and expelling residues and waste products from the rectum via the anus (defaecation). This section will briefly describe the structure and function of the different components of the digestive tract in order to help the reader to understand the adverse effects of diseases of this organ system.

The mouth

The anatomy of the mouth is described in detail in Chapter 15 (see p. 521 and Fig. 15.1). Here, however, it will be helpful to consider the three functions that the mouth carries out in the process of digestion: mechanically breaking down food (chewing or mastication); initiating the chemical breakdown of food (salivation); and swallowing food (deglutition) to allow it to proceed on its journey through the digestive tract.

Movement of food within the mouth is achieved mainly by the tongue, which is largely composed of skeletal muscle. The tongue is also a sensory organ, allowing the taste, texture and temperature of food and fluids to be perceived. The sensation of taste is enabled by the fungiform papillae, or taste buds, which house the relevant sensory nerve endings. The filiform papillae give the tongue a roughness which allows it to be used for manipulating semi-solid food.

Saliva is released from three pairs of glands located around the lower jaw. These are, moving anteriorly, the parotid, the submandibular and the sublingual glands. A constant stream of saliva is released into the mouth, of which the submandibular glands contribute about 70% in the absence of a food stimulus. However, the sight, smell or presence of food in the mouth will stimulate the parotid glands to make the major contribution.

Saliva is a mildly alkaline and slightly viscous fluid which serves to keep the mouth moist and clean. It is mildly antibacterial. In digestion it helps to lubricate food prior to swallowing and, since it contains the enzyme amylase, it also initiates the digestion of starch.

The final process in which the mouth participates is that of swallowing, whereby food is passed into the oesophagus. After food has been sufficiently chewed, which is partly a subjective decision and partly determined by the texture of the food ingested, it is formed into a ball (bolus) between the palate and the tongue and pushed to the back of the mouth by the tongue. The swallowing reflex is initiated by the bolus touching the oropharynx and involves the following steps: the temporary cessation of breathing; the soft palate shuts off the nasal passage; the raising of the larynx and the lowering of the epiglottis to protect the trachea; and the opening of the upper oesophageal sphincter to receive the bolus of food.

The oesophagus

The oesophagus is a hollow, muscular tube connecting the pharynx to the stomach. It exists solely to enable the passage of food between these two areas and performs no digestive or absorptive roles. In basic terms, the oesophagus is composed of three layers of tissue: an inner mucosal layer with an underlying submucosal layer; a middle muscular layer; and an outer connective tissue layer. The mucosal layer contains glands which secrete mucus for the lubrication of food as it passes down the oesophagus. The submucosal layer provides a nerve and blood supply. The muscles of the middle layer are arranged both circularly and longitudinally. The composition of this layer changes throughout the length of the oesophagus in such a way that there is more striated, or voluntary, muscle at the pharyngeal end. Towards the stomach end the muscle becomes predominantly and then entirely smooth, or involuntary.

The propulsion of food towards the stomach is achieved by peristalsis. This can be described as follows:

1. A descending wave of contraction of circular muscle narrows the lumen of the oesophagus, thereby compressing the bolus of food.
2. This is preceded by contraction of the longitudinal muscles to widen the lumen in order to receive the bolus.

Peristalsis is entirely under involuntary control. Relaxation of the lower oesophageal sphincter allows food to enter the stomach. (See Fig. 4.1.)

The stomach

Digestion continues in the stomach when the bolus of food enters through the lower oesophageal sphincter. The basic structure of the stomach is illustrated in Wilson (1990). On the inner surface of the stomach a mucosal, secretory, layer of tissue is supplied with blood vessels and lymph glands by an underlying submucosal layer. Between the mucosal layer and the outermost, peritoneal, layer lies a muscular layer composed of three layers of muscle: an inner layer of oblique fibres, a middle layer of circular fibres and an outer layer of longitudinal fibres. These layers of muscle allow increasingly stronger waves of contraction in three directions to mix the food in the stomach and allow maximum contact with gastric juice. Innervation of the stomach is from a branch of the 10th cranial (i.e. vagus) nerve, which provides parasympathetic nerve endings that stimulate the secretory cells of the stomach. The internal surface area of the stomach is increased by the arrangement of folds, or rugae, in the lining.

Cells in the mucosa of the stomach produce mucus, hydrochloric acid and pepsinogen. This mixture is referred to as 'gastric juice', and when combined with food in the stomach as 'chyme'. Hydrochloric acid helps to maintain the acidity of the stomach at about pH2. At this level of acidity the pepsinogen, an inactive precursor, is converted to pepsin, a protein-digesting enzyme which works optimally at pH2. The stomach, therefore, is mainly responsible for initiating protein digestion, although some carbohydrate digestion can continue inside a bolus of food by the action of any salivary amylase which has not yet become inactivated by the acidity of the stomach.

Release of gastric juice by the stomach mucosa is stimulated by the

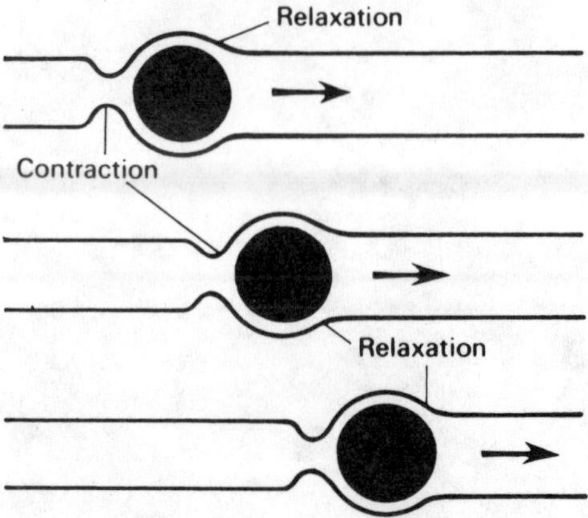

Fig. 4.1 Illustration of the movement of the bolus through the oesophagus by peristalsis. (Reproduced with kind permission from Wilson 1990.)

sight, smell and thought of food. This is known as the cephalic phase of digestion. The gastric phase of digestion begins when food reaches the stomach and continues until chyme enters the duodenum, where the intestinal phase of gastric digestion begins. The length of time taken to empty the stomach is variable and depends on the composition of the meal eaten. An average time for emptying of the stomach after a meal is about 4 h. Emptying takes place through the pyloris. The pyloric region holds about 30 ml of chyme; with each wave of contraction in the stomach about 3 ml of chyme is released into the duodenum. This process is regulated by the pyloric sphincter.

Digestion in the stomach is controlled by several factors. The presence of food in the stomach stretches the stomach wall, activating stretch receptors and stimulating the release of gastric juice. A hormone called gastrin is released by the stomach walls; this also stimulates the release of gastric juice. The presence of food substances such as protein and caffeine also stimulate gastrin release. Waves of contraction in the stomach are also increased by stretching of the stomach wall and by the presence of protein. On the other hand, low pH inhibits gastrin release. Both the cephalic and gastric phases of digestion can be inhibited by emotional factors. The stomach is essentially not involved in the process of absorption, although some water, alcohol, and certain drugs such as aspirin are absorbed in the gastric phase.

The intestinal phase of digestion begins when chyme enters the duodenum. This stimulates the release of enteric gastrin, which increases the release of gastric juice by the stomach. Despite this release of gastric juice in the intestinal phase, the main effect on gastric digestion of the entry of food into the duodenum is inhibitory. The enterogastric reflex, which is mediated via the medulla, leads to the inhibition of gastric secretion. In addition, the presence of food in the duodenum stimulates the release of three hormones, secretin, cholecystokinin and gastric inhibitory peptide, all of which inhibit gastric juice secretion and reduce gastric motility. (See Fig. 4.2.)

The small intestine

Extending from the pyloric sphincter to the ileocaecal valve, the small intestine is responsible for the completion of digestion, the absorption of nutrients, and the reabsorption of most of the water which enters the digestive tract. The duodenum, which takes up the first 25 cm or so of the small intestine, plays a key role in the process of digestion. It collects chyme from the stomach and is the site where the secretions of the gall bladder and the pancreas are mixed with chyme. These secretions enter the duodenum through the ampulla of Vater, i.e. the joining of the common bile duct and the pancreatic duct, which meets the duodenum at the duodenal papilla. The emptying of the gall bladder is regulated by the sphincter of Oddi at the duodenal papilla.

In common with the remainder of the small intestine, the duodenum has a mucosal layer, a submucosal layer, a muscular layer and a peritoneal layer. Unlike the remainder of the small intestine, however, the duodenum is relatively immobile. Its regulatory role is fulfilled when the stimulus of chyme entering the duodenum triggers the entero-gastric reflex as well as stimulating the release of gastrin, secretin, cholecystokinin and gastric inhibitory peptide. The effects of cholecystokinin and secretin on the functioning of the stomach, gall bladder and pancreas have been mentioned. Secretin also stimulates the cells of the liver to secrete bile, and cholecystokinin stimulates the release of digestive enzymes by the small intestine.

Chyme is very acidic because of its high concentration of hydrochloric acid. When it enters the duodenum it is brought to a neutral pH by the effect of alkaline bicarbonate released by the pancreas. The effect of bile is to emulsify fats in the chyme, that is, to break up fat globules into smaller particles more amenable to the effects of fat-digesting enzymes. The enzymes of pancreatic juice can then begin to digest their respective food substances in the duodenum; this action is continued as the chyme is passed down the small intestine.

The first two-fifths of the small intestine following the duodenum is called the jejunum and the remaining three-fifths the ileum. Two types of movement, segmentation and peristalsis, take place in the small intestine; these, respectively, mix and move the food along the tract.

Secretory cells of the mucosa of the small intestine release a slightly alkaline juice containing mainly water and mucus. The remaining enzymes of digestion in the GI tract are contained, immobilised, on the villi, the hair-like structures that line the small intestine. The enzymes of the small intestine complete the digestion of all components of the diet, including protein, fat, carbohydrate and nucleic acids.

Absorption takes place along the full length of the small intestine, and 90% of all the products of digestion are absorbed here. The products of digestion are amino acids and peptides from protein; fatty acids and monoglycerides from fats: hexose sugars from carbohydrates

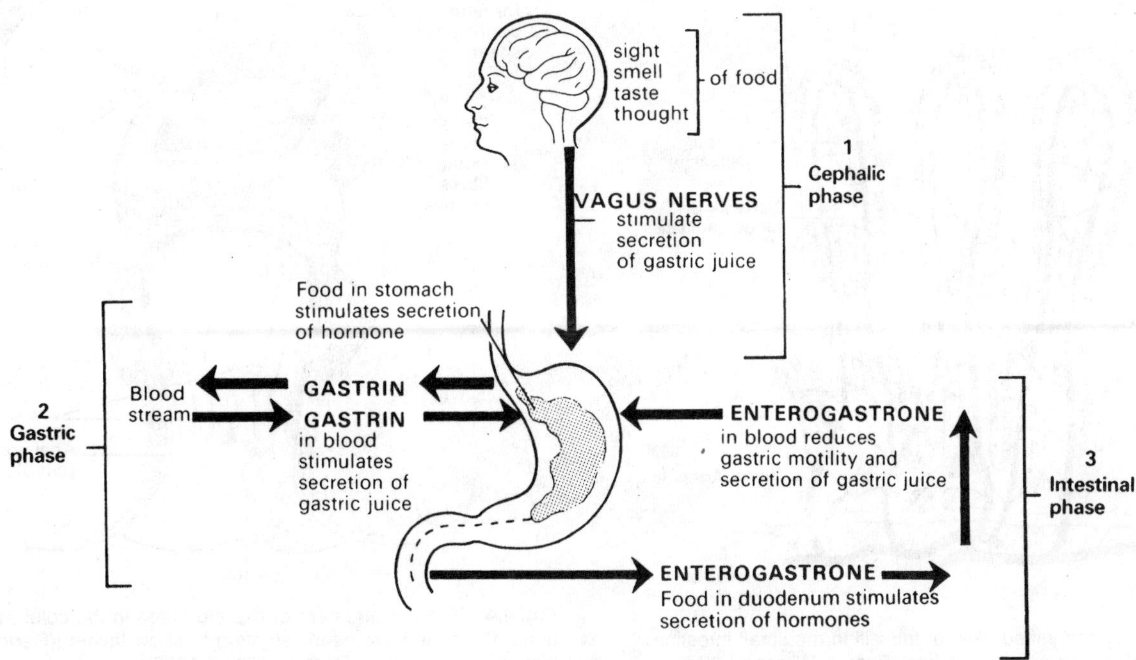

Fig. 4.2 The phases of secretion of gastric juices. (Reproduced with kind permission from Wilson 1990.)

and pentose sugars and nitrogen-containing bases from nucleic acids. About 7.5 l of water are secreted into the small intestine daily and 1.5 l ingested. As only about 1 l enters the large intestine, the major portion of the water is reabsorbed in the small intestine. Absorption takes place at the villi, which greatly increase the digestive and absorptive area of the small intestine. Each villus contains an arteriole and a venule connected by a capillary network, and a central lacteal, which is a projection of the lymphatic system. Short-chain fatty acids, amino acids and carbohydrates are absorbed directly into the bloodstream. Triglycerides, which form bodies called chylomicrons, are absorbed into the lacteals and then enter the bloodstream where the thoracic lymphatic duct empties into the left subclavian vein. (See Fig. 4.3.)

The large intestine

With most of the nutrients removed, the indigestible residue of food from the small intestine passes through the ileocaecal valve and enters the large intestine. The mesentery attaches both the small and large intestines to the rear wall of the abdomen and provides both with their blood supply.

The large intestine can be divided into four portions: the ascending, the transverse, the descending colon and pelvic or sigmoid colon. The curves joining the ascending with the transverse colon and the transverse with the descending colon are referred to as the right and left colic flexures respectively. Near the ileocaecal valve two features can be identified: the caecum, which is a pouch below the ileocaecal valve; and the appendix, which is a finger-like projection of the caecum. The descending colon leads to the sigmoid colon, which terminates in the rectum. Three muscular bands called the taeniae coli run the length of the large intestine. These maintain a slight longitudinal tension in the large intestine and give it its characteristic segmented appearance (haustration). The rectum stores food residue as faeces before expulsion via the anus. The anal canal, which opens externally at the anus, controls evacuation, and has an internal anal sphincter of smooth muscle and an external anal sphincter of skeletal muscle.

In common with the small intestine, the large intestine has mucosal, submucosal, muscular and peritoneal layers. But it differs in appearance from the small intestine in that there are no villi. The large intestine is designed mainly for the absorption of water and the lubrication of food residue as it is passed, by the mass action of food entering at the ileocaecal valve, to the rectum. Any nutrients which do enter the large intestine are broken down by commensal bacteria, causing the gases methane, hydrogen, carbon dioxide and sulphur dioxide to be produced. Food can take up to 24 h to pass through the large intestine.

When food reaches the rectum a reflex is initiated whereby stretch receptors in the wall of the rectum send signals to the brain informing it of the presence of faeces. However, the desire to expel faeces (defaecation) can be suppressed until the time and place are appropriate. When it is appropriate to defaecate the internal anal sphincter automatically relaxes and the external anal sphincter, under voluntary control, is relaxed. Intraabdominal pressure is increased as the individual breathes in and holds the breath against a closed glottis (Valsalva's manoeuvre), and faeces are expelled from the rectum via the anal canal. (See Fig. 4.4.)

The hepatobiliary system, pancreas and spleen

The liver

With the exception of the skin, the liver is the largest single organ in the body. It is located mainly in the upper right quadrant of the abdomen, just below the diaphragm, and weighs about 1.5 k. It is a compact lobular organ with large right and left lobes and two smaller caudate and quadrate lobes. Oxygenated blood is supplied to the liver by the hepatic artery, as well as by the hepatic portal vein, which carries blood containing the products of digestion from the small intestine directly to the liver. The hepatic portal system also collects blood from the lower oesophagus, the stomach, the spleen and the large intestine.

Each lobe of the liver is subdivided into functional units called lobules. In these lobules, branches of the hepatic artery, the hepatic portal vein and a bile duct run concurrently in a structure known as the portal triad. All of the blood entering the liver mixes in spaces called sinusoids and is then drained into a central vein. Bile is manufactured by liver cells, arranged as canaliculi, and these drain into the bile ducts.

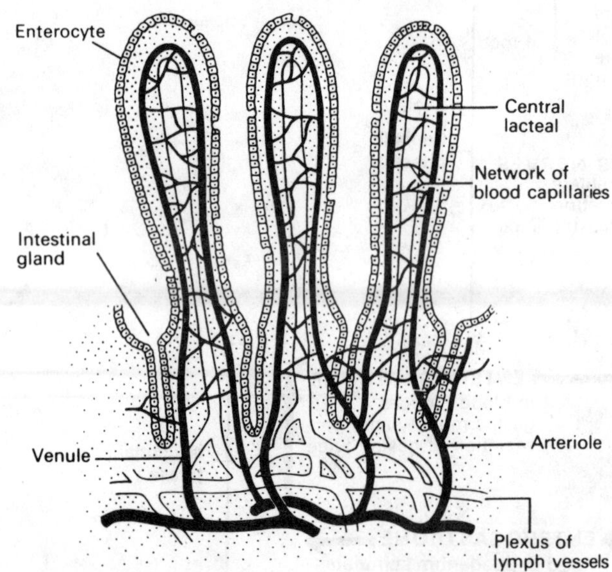

Fig. 4.3 A highly magnified view of the villi in the small intestine. (Reproduced with kind permission from Ross & Wilson 1990.)

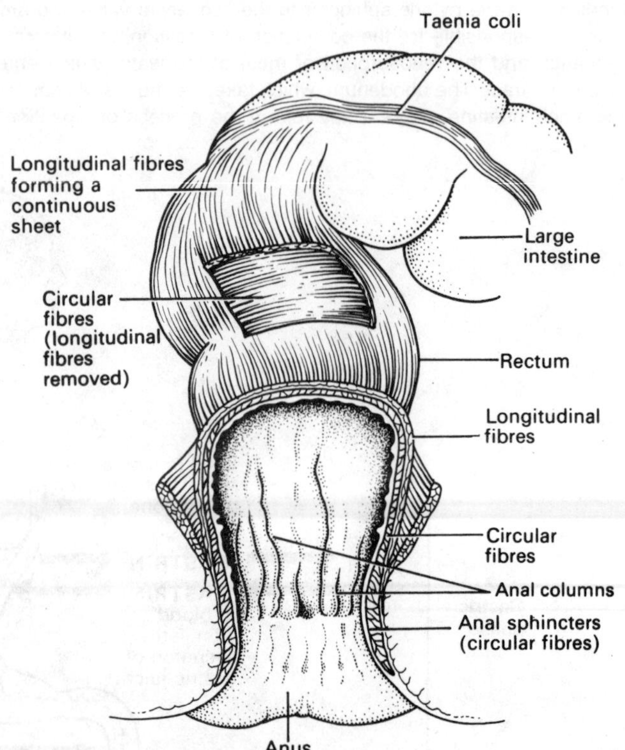

Fig. 4.4 The arrangement of muscle fibres in the colon, rectum and anus. Sections have been removed to show layers. (Reproduced with kind permission from Ross & Wilson 1990.)

A major metabolic role with respect to carbohydrates, fats and proteins is played by the liver. The liver stores some glycogen and also forms part of the monophage/macrophage system which scavenges old erythrocytes, leucocytes and bacteria.

The gallbladder

Lying underneath the liver, the gallbladder has the function of storing and concentrating bile, which is composed principally of bilirubin (derived from the breakdown of haemoglobin from erythrocytes) and of bile salts (formed from excess steroid hormones). The gallbladder is a pear-shaped sac about 10 cm long. It lacks a submucosal layer but, in common with other parts of the digestive system, has a middle muscular layer comprised of smooth muscle under vagal and hormonal control. Vagal stimulation causes the gallbladder to contract. The internal surface area of the gallbladder is increased by the presence of rugae; this promotes the reabsorption of water and a tenfold concentration of the bile which enters from the cystic duct. The liver secretes bile at a rate of about 1 l/24 h but the capacity of the gallbladder is only 30 ml. Bile ducts in the right and left lobes of the liver empty their contents into the right and left hepatic ducts, respectively, which join to form the common hepatic duct. Bile is taken by the cystic duct from the common hepatic duct to the gallbladder, where it is stored and water is reabsorbed. When the gallbladder is stimulated it contracts and the bile travels to the duodenum down the common bile duct. The release of bile is stimulated by cholecystokinin and secretin.

The pancreas

The pancreas, which lies below and behind the stomach, manufactures and releases pancreatic juice containing enzymes (including enzymes which digest protein, carbohydrate, fat and nucleic acids) and bicarbonate. These constituents of pancreatic juice are produced in the acinar cells of the pancreas.

The exocrine function of the pancreas is discrete from its endocrine function whereby insulin and glucagon are secreted into the bloodstream in response to fluctuating blood glucose levels. The exocrine secretory functions of the pancreas are under vagal and hormonal control. The initial stimulus for the release of pancreatic juice is food entering the duodenum and stimulating the release of cholecystokinin and secretin. Cholecystokinin is responsible for stimulating the release of the pancreatic enzyme portion of pancreatic juice and secretin is responsible for the release of bicarbonate. The pancreatic duct (which delivers pancreatic juice to the duodenum) and the common bile duct join at the ampulla of Vater. Release of bile and pancreatic juice into the duodenum is controlled by the sphincter of Oddi. This sphincter, a ring of smooth muscle, is relaxed by cholecystokinin.

The spleen

The spleen is composed of lymphatic tissue and lies in the upper left quadrant of the abdomen, between the stomach and the diaphragm. It is richly supplied with blood via the splenic artery. Blood flow through the spleen is slowed down by the fact that it must pass through sinuses in which the monophage/macrophage system scavenges old erythrocytes and pathogenic particles and passes the breakdown products on to the liver via the hepatic portal system.

DISORDERS OF THE GASTROINTESTINAL TRACT

DISORDERS OF THE MOUTH

Good oral hygiene and dental care are important not only for the maintenance of healthy teeth and gums, but also for the individual's general well-being. Unfortunately, dental health is not always given adequate attention, resulting in dental caries and sometimes extraction. Many adults in Britain have full or partial dentures. In the edentulous person, well-fitting dentures help to ensure that a wide range of foods can be eaten with comfort. Elderly people often struggle on with ill-fitting dentures, restricting themselves to a soft diet which lacks adequate fresh fruit, vegetables and fibre. This can have serious consequences for their overall health.

The mouth and tongue are often examined by the physician during clinical examination, as local abnormalities or indications of disease elsewhere can often be detected in this manner. For example, a dry, furred tongue can indicate the presence of a digestive problem or dehydration.

The role of the nurse with regard to the maintenance of good oral hygiene is an extremely important one, especially when the patient is unable to eat and drink normally, whether due to disease of the GI tract or when undergoing investigations or surgery (Boyle 1992). The principles of mouth care and of the treatment of a range of disorders affecting the mouth and related structures are described in detail in Chapter 15.

DISORDERS OF THE OESOPHAGUS

Because the oesophagus has a relatively narrow lumen any obstruction rapidly affects the passage of food. The two most common symptoms which are experienced by patients with diseases of the oesophagus are dysphagia and pain. The term dysphagia refers to difficulty in swallowing. This can present in varying degrees, ranging from slight and intermittent difficulty in swallowing solid food to total occlusion of the oesophagus preventing the patient even from swallowing saliva. Oesophageal pain can be extremely severe and should not be underestimated. There are three main presentations:

- a burning pain (known as 'heartburn') felt high in the epigastrium and behind the sternum. It sometimes radiates to the neck and one or both arms. It is usually due to the reflux of gastric contents
- a deep, boring, gripping pain across the front of the chest which may radiate to the back, neck or arms. It is usually due to spasm of the oesophageal muscle and is similar in nature to angina pectoris
- pain behind the sternum on swallowing, especially hot liquids. It is usually due to oesophagitis.

Oesophageal moniliasis

This condition is caused by the yeast-like fungus *Candida (Monilia) albicans*. The following groups of patients may be vulnerable to this condition:

- patients with chronic oesophageal obstruction. Oesophageal dysfunction causes stasis of saliva and food particles which predisposes to infection
- patients with immunosuppressive disorders such as diabetes mellitus, leukaemia, lymphoma, AIDS
- patients taking immunosuppressive therapy, e.g. chemotherapy or corticosteroids
- debilitated patients receiving long-term antibiotic therapy.

PATHOPHYSIOLOGY

Common presenting symptoms. These will vary according to the severity of the infection but may include dysphagia, heartburn and retrosternal pain. Candida affecting the mouth will show as white patches on the mucosa. A mild fever may be present.

MEDICAL MANAGEMENT

Diagnosis will be made using endoscopy, in which biopsies will be taken. Treatment is with antifungal oral antibiotics such as nystatin suspension, amphotericin lozenges or parenteral fluconazole.

NURSING PRIORITIES AND MANAGEMENT: OESOPHAGEAL MONILIASIS

The priority of nursing care is to minimise the dysphagia and pain experienced on eating and drinking. The patient should be given a soft diet tailored to his likes and dislikes. Supplemental drinks should also be given to ensure weight loss does not occur. Oral hygiene is, of course, extremely important. Patients who prefer to wear their dentures at all times may have to be persuaded of the benefits of removing them at night, as the presence of dentures could exacerbate the problem.

Hiatus hernia and gastro-oesophageal reflux

A hernia is the protrusion of an organ through the wall of the cavity which contains it. It may apply to any part of the body but is most commonly thought of in terms of abdominal hernias, which are discussed later in this chapter (see p. 106).

A hiatus hernia results from herniation of a portion of the stomach through the oesophageal hiatus in the diaphragm. The opening of the diaphragm normally encircles the oesophagus tightly, and therefore the stomach lies within the abdominal cavity. When the opening through which the oesophagus passes becomes enlarged, part of the stomach protrudes into the thoracic cavity.

PATHOPHYSIOLOGY

Hiatus hernias occur most frequently from middle age onwards. They are 4 times more common in women than men and are often found in association with obesity. Burkitt et al (1990) suggest that perhaps the pressure of intra-abdominal fat is a contributory factor. Such hernias can also result from a congenital abnormality presenting in early infancy. Hiatus hernias can be described as 'sliding' or 'rolling', the former being by the far the most common. In sliding hernias the oesophageal sphincter mechanism is defective, causing reflux of acid-peptic stomach contents. Many individuals with a hiatus hernia are symptomless.

Clinical features. The most important symptom is heartburn as a result of the reflux oesophagitis. It occurs after eating and can be initiated by bending over and lying down. Waterbrash (pyrosis) and a feeling of fullness are common. Dysphagia is a relatively uncommon symptom; it may be caused by reflux oesophagitis. Bleeding may also be a feature, involving a chronic, small loss leading to anaemia. This may occur in the elderly patient with reflux oesophagitis.

MEDICAL MANAGEMENT

Investigative procedures. Diagnosis is by medical history, barium swallow and meal.

Medical intervention. In mild cases, it may be sufficient simply to advise the individual to make certain lifestyle adjustments, e.g. losing weight if appropriate, taking small meals at more frequent intervals, wearing loose clothing, and avoiding bending over from the waist. Sleeping well supported by pillows is also helpful. It is essential for the individual not to smoke. Drug therapy may include antacids or acid-inhibiting drugs.

In more extreme cases surgery may be indicated to reduce the hernia and re-form the angle between the oesophagus and stomach. The procedures used are gastropexy or fundoplication (Whitehead 1988).

NURSING PRIORITIES AND MANAGEMENT: HIATUS HERNIA

Gastro-oesophageal reflux

Not all patients with hiatus hernia will experience gastro-oesophageal reflux. In many individuals, reflux occurs without associated hiatus hernia due to obesity, pregnancy or the use of drugs that may relax the gastro-oesophageal sphincter, e.g. anticholinergic drugs. Reflux can be most distressing and is often mistaken for angina. Most people are able to manage their symptoms by conservative means. For example, raising the head of the bed may be all that is needed to relieve symptoms at night. However, if reflux is chronic or severe, the inflammation of the oesophagus can lead to fibrosis and narrowing of the oesophagus, the development of dysphagia and a predisposition to malignant change (see p. 93).

Perioperative case

Preoperative preparation

Preparation for surgery will be as for elective abdominal surgery on the GI tract (see p. 781 and Nursing Care Plan 27.1, p. 788). Following careful assessment a care plan should be formulated to meet the specific needs of the patient.

Postoperative monitoring

Immediate observations include:

- blood pressure and pulse: a drop in blood pressure and a rising pulse indicate bleeding and hypovolaemic shock
- wound suture line and any drains for evidence of bleeding
- respirations: if a thoracic approach was used, underwater sealed drainage will be in situ. This is observed for good respiratory function by the swinging water level in the tube (see Ch. 3, p. 81)
- nasogastric (NG) tube aspirate for colour and amount. Aspirations are initially, hourly. Aspirated fluid volume must be recorded on the fluid balance chart
- i.v. infusion: maintained at correct flow rate
- fluid balance: all input and output must be recorded on the fluid balance chart.

Postoperative care

Adequate analgesia using opiate analgesics by syringe driver or i.m. administration must be given regularly to ensure that the patient is pain free and hence able to cooperate in deep breathing and coughing exercises to help full expansion of the lungs. Causes of postoperative pain are described in Box 27.3. Analgesics commonly used in postoperative pain control are listed in Table 27.6. The underwater sealed drain will be removed when a chest X-ray shows full lung expansion.

The i.v. infusion must be monitored to ensure that adequate fluid intake is maintained. Oral fluids are withheld for 24 h. As bowel sounds return sips of water can then be given, increasing to 30 ml of water hourly and then greater amounts as they are tolerated. The NG tube is then removed.

A soft diet and then small normal meals are introduced gradually. Before discharge home, the patient should be eating a normal diet. With good pain control, activity is encouraged as soon as possible. The patient is helped out of bed for a short time on the 1st postoperative day and encouraged to take short walks from the 2nd day.

Prior to discharge the patient should be advised to take small, regular meals, to avoid heavy lifting and to avoid smoking.

Achalasia of the oesophagus

PATHOPHYSIOLOGY

This condition is a motility disorder of the lower two-thirds of the oesophagus. It can arise at any age, but is found predominantly among individuals aged between 40 and 70. The cause is probably a failure of nerve conduction due to degeneration and loss of ganglion cells. There is lack of effective peristalsis and failure of the lower oesophageal sphincter to relax because the inhibitory nerves to the sphincter are absent or impaired. There may be ulceration of the epithelium, which may predispose the individual to the development of squamous cell carcinoma.

Clinical features are as follows:

- Dysphagia: initially intermittent, becoming constant as the disease progresses. Only soft, minced food can be swallowed
- Regurgitation of food from above the obstruction often occurs
- Many patients complain of a cough and dyspnoea after meals
- Recurrent bronchitis, bronchial spasm, and aspiration pneumonia are often seen
- Retrosternal pain which is felt initially and resolves as dilatation of the oesophagus occurs
- Weight loss which becomes pronounced as the disease progresses.

MEDICAL MANAGEMENT

Investigative procedures. Diagnosis is usually confirmed by oesphagoscopy, barium examination or intraluminal pressure readings (manometry).

Medical intervention. This condition is at present incurable. The main aim of treatment is to relieve the obstruction, and some patients are able to perfect the Valsalva manoeuvre to assist propulsion of food (Burrell 1992). Medication to relax the lower oesophagus may include calcium channel blockers and long-acting nitrates but their efficacy is uncertain. Dilatation techniques may be employed; if these prove unsuccessful surgical division of the sphincter muscles may be performed. The nursing care of the symptoms experienced is similar to that for patients with oesophageal cancer.

Carcinoma of the oesophagus

The majority of carcinomas of the oesophagus occur in the elderly. Men are affected more frequently than women. This form of cancer is extremely unpleasant and distressing. The patient will rapidly becoming emaciated due to the difficulty in eating and drinking, and skilled nursing care is essential to comfort and support the patient as he copes with these and other effects of the illness.

Several predisposing factors for oesophageal cancer have been identified:

- smoking: this form of cancer is more prevalent among individuals who smoke or chew tobacco or betal
- alcohol consumption: individuals who have had a high intake of alcohol are more likely to develop a malignant tumour. In England a high incidence of oesophageal cancer among publicans and brewers has been noted
- achalasia of the cardia, gastro-oesophageal reflux, Paterson–Kelly (Plummer–Vinson) syndrome and previous trauma are all associated with an increased risk of oesophageal cancer.

PATHOPHYSIOLOGY

Squamous cell carcinoma and adenocarcinoma form the majority of malignant oesophageal tumours, squamous cell carcinoma being the most common. In squamous cell carcinoma 10% occur in the upper oesophagus, 45% in the mid-oesophagus, and 45% in the lower end. Most adenocarcinomas occur at the lower end and the gastro-oesophageal junction. The primary tumour can spread locally up or down the oesophagus and through the wall to the trachea, bronchi, pleura, aorta and lymph vessels. Distant metastases may occur in the liver and lungs.

Common presenting symptoms. The most prominent presenting feature is dysphagia. In the initial stages, this symptom will occur only occasionally and the individual will probably not seek medical help. As the disease progresses and the tumour enlarges, dysphagia will increase and becomes a constant feature. There will be regurgitation and vomiting and pain will become intense, indicating a spread of the cancer to surrounding tissues. Because of the dysphagia the patient will be anorexic and lose weight rapidly. Many patients develop a cough due to pressure on the bronchus and a chest infection due to aspiration of oesophageal contents. Haematemesis and melaena occasionally occur as a result of an ulcerated tumour.

MEDICAL MANAGEMENT

Investigative procedures. Diagnosis is confirmed by oesophagoscopy (see Box 4.1), during which biopsies will be taken. Computerised tomography (CT scans) may be used to help identify local and metastatic spread to surrounding tissues. Bronchoscopy may be performed if the tumour is in the upper zone. This will identify if the bronchus has been invaded and will have a bearing on treatment and care. An ultrasound scan of the liver will show if there are metastases present.

Medical intervention. As the prognosis is poor, treatment is directed mainly towards the relief of symptoms. Each patient is carefully assessed as to the extent of the disease before a treatment plan is chosen and commenced. Time is also spent improving the general nutritional state of the patient by either nasogastric or parenteral feeds.

Surgical intervention will be attempted if the tumour is resectable and if there is no local spread or metastases (see Fig. 4.5).

Radiotherapy may be used if the tumour is radiosensitive, i.e. a squamous cell carcinoma. This treatment is usually used for tumours of the upper third of the oesophagus, but is also sometimes used for the relief of pain.

Atkinson or Celestin tube. The insertion of a radio-opaque tube via endoscopy in patients with tumours of the lower oesophagus may restore patency and the ability to eat at least semi-solid food (Marshall 1984). It is also sometimes used as a temporary measure to allow passage of an NG tube for feeding purposes prior to surgery or other forms of treatment.

Laser therapy can be used for a tumour at any site and as an alternative to a radio-opaque tube.

NURSING PRIORITIES AND MANAGEMENT: CARCINOMA OF THE OESOPHAGUS

The 'typical' patient with this distressing form of cancer will be miserable and emaciated, his life dominated by the symptoms of his disease and by the thought that there is no cure. However, by adopting a caring and sensitive approach, the nurse can do much to alleviate the patient's physical and emotional suffering (Belk 1983).

Box 4.1 Endoscopy in GI medicine

Endoscopy refers to the visualisation of the interior of the body cavities and hollow organs by means of a flexible fibreoptic instrument (endoscope). The use of this technique has contributed greatly to diagnosis and therapy in many areas of medical practice. For use in the gastrointestinal tract, the endoscope is variously designed to view the oesophagus, the stomach, the duodenum, the colon and the rectum. It is also possible, by a modification of the gastroduodenoscope, to visualise the pancreatic and common bile duct; this is called endoscopic retrograde cholangiopancreatography (ERCP). Although most endoscopes are flexible, a rigid instrument may be used for a sigmoidoscopy. For further information see Forrest et al 1991.

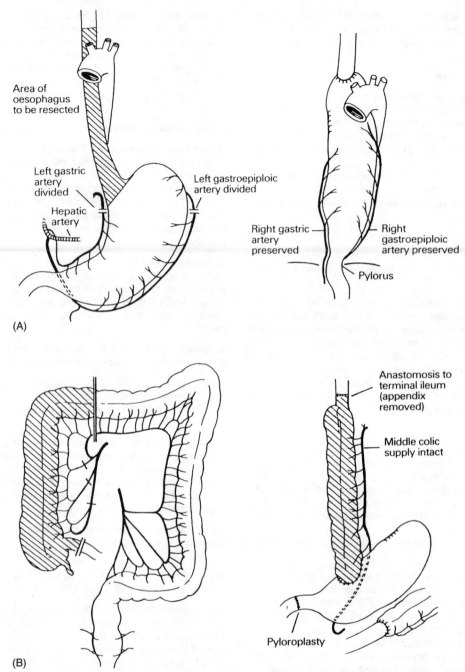

Fig. 4.5 Oesophagectomy and methods of reconstruction. (A) Replacement by stomach. (B) Replacement by colon. (Reproduced with kind permission from Forrest et al 1991.)

> ? **4.1** Mr J is a 65-year-old, newly retired accountant, with a wife and two married sons. He has recently been diagnosed as having oesophageal cancer with metastases in the bronchus and lungs. What would you consider to be the main priorities of his nursing care?

Major patient problems

Dysphagia

The first step in nursing care is to assess the extent of the dysphagia and whether the patient's nutritional intake is adequate. The patient's weight should be recorded and noted in relation to his pre-illness weight. An accurate account of daily dietary intake should be taken (the dietitian may help with this) and a description made of the consistency of the food he is able to swallow. If he can manage semi-solids, he will be able to take an adequate diet if careful thought is put into its components, e.g. large chunks of meat, 'stringy' foods such as oranges, and 'stodgy' foods such as scones should be avoided. The patient should be encouraged to take fluids with his meals and to chew foods twice as long as normal. It may be necessary to provide a liquidised diet. If the patient cannot afford to purchase a liquidiser, one can be borrowed from the Macmillan Nursing Service. The patient should be weighed weekly.

At a later stage the patient will be able to swallow liquids only and he should be supplied with a variety of nutritionally supplemented liquids. Unfortunately, most of these drinks (e.g. Build Up, Fresubin, etc.) are quite sweet and the patient may soon tire of them. However, Build Up is now also available in savoury flavours and tonic water can be added to Fresubin to give it a fresher taste.

Eventually, total dysphagia will occur. It cannot be overemphasised what a miserable condition this is. Nursing management is discussed on page 94.

In the case of a bolus obstruction it may be necessary to perform an endoscopy to relieve the obstruction. The insertion of an Atkinson tube is often used to relieve dysphagic symptoms. The oesophagus is dilated at endoscopy and the tube inserted. Following this procedure, the patient will lose the action of the gastro-oesophageal sphincter and therefore will suffer from reflux. The head of the bed should be elevated at all times and the patient should be provided with blocks to take home if necessary. He will be prescribed an H_2 blocking agent (e.g. cimetidine) to help prevent reflux oesophagitis; this should be given in syrup form. He should be encouraged to eat a semi-solid diet, to avoid lumps of meat, etc. and to chew food well. The patient should take carbonated drinks with every meal as this helps keep the tube clear.

Immediately after the insertion of an Atkinson tube the patient may suffer quite severe discomfort and it may be necessary to give him an analgesic injection, e.g. i.m. pethidine. A chest X-ray will be performed and the patient should not be allowed any food or fluid until this has been done in case of perforation.

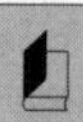
For further information, see Donahue P A (1990).

Pain

In the earlier stages, if pain is present, mild analgesics such as paracetamol given in dispersible form may be all that is necessary. As the disease advances opiates may be required. Initially, the patient may be able to swallow a morphine suspension but if total occlusion of the oesophagus occurs it may be necessary to give the morphine by injection. The most effective and convenient way of administering this is by s.c. route via, for example, a Graseby syringe driver. This delivers a constant level of pain relief and avoids peaks and troughs. The patient will be able to be at home, if circumstances allow, with a community nurse visiting daily to change the syringe. If necessary, an antiemetic such as haloperidol can also be added to the syringe driver.

Psychological distress

Time must be set aside to allow these patients to express their thoughts, fears and anger, which may be directed towards either the distressing nature of their symptoms or the poor prognosis of the disease, or perhaps both. In the final stages of the disease every effort should be made to allow the patient to die in the environment of his choice (see Ch. 34). If he wishes to be at home, a Macmillan nurse can provide the support and medical and nursing care he requires.

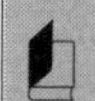
For further information, see Fletcher & Freeling (1988), Savage (1992).

Traumatic conditions of the oesophagus

Foreign bodies

Most cases of foreign bodies being lodged in the oesophagus involve children who have swallowed small items such as buttons or safety pins. Adults also occasionally swallow such items, but more frequently present with a bolus of food (usually meat).

MEDICAL MANAGEMENT

History and examination. The patient's description of what occurred and the symptoms that followed are very important in diagnosis. Symptoms may range from mild discomfort to severe pain, dysphagia and haemorrhage. Diagnosis may be made by a plain X-ray, but in the case of a bolus of food barium examination may be required.

Medical intervention. Once haemodynamic stability is ensured, the foreign body can be removed using endoscopic technique, care being taken not to cause further damage (especially if the object is sharp). If a food bolus proves to be the problem, gas producing pellets may be swallowed which can push the bolus on into the stomach.

NURSING PRIORITIES AND MANAGEMENT: FOREIGN BODIES

The patient may be very distressed and extremely anxious for the offending object to move either up or down. He may be in considerable pain, and analgesics such as i.m. pethidine may be required. Observations for signs of shock denoting perforation should be made.

Corrosive agents

Strong acids or alkalis may be swallowed accidentally or deliberately. Accidental cases usually involve children who have drunk cleaning fluids left within reach. Deliberate ingestion by an adult indicates a serious psychological disturbance requiring professional intervention and probably psychiatric referral after the initial treatment.

MEDICAL MANAGEMENT

First aid measures include ensuring a clear airway and allowing nothing to be taken orally. It is vital that the patient is *not* made to vomit, as this would only exacerbate the corrosive damage. Immediate referral to the emergency services is essential. On admission to hospital the antidote specific to the chemical will be administered but gastric lavage should be avoided.

Longer-term treatment will probably involve dilatation of the oesophagus to relieve fibrosis and stricture. Occasionally a gastrostomy tube must be inserted for feeding purposes until the oesophageal tissue has healed.

NURSING PRIORITIES AND MANAGEMENT: CORROSIVE AGENTS

The key components of care will be:

- maintenance of a clear airway
- observation for shock
- analgesics (i.m. or i.v.)
- nil by mouth
- antibiotic therapy for infection.

Observations of pulse and blood pressure should be made half-hourly until the patient's condition is stable. A raised temperature may indicate severe inflammatory changes, infection or abscess formation.

Anxiety and fear will be a major feature; the support, reassurance and understanding shown by nursing and medical staff will help to allay these feelings.

Oesophageal perforation

PATHOPHYSIOLOGY

Instrumental perforation may occur during endoscopy, especially if the oesophagus has been made friable by disease. There is an increased risk of perforation with oesophageal dilatation and the insertion of an oesophageal tube in the palliative management of patients with oesophageal carcinoma.

Spontaneous perforation may occur following a sudden increase in oesophageal pressure caused by vomiting, straining, convulsions or blunt abdominal pressure, e.g. steering wheel pressure in a car accident.

Clinical features. The individual will experience severe pain, which may be accompanied by dyspnoea, cyanosis, dysphagia and fever due to leakage into the mediastinum.

MEDICAL MANAGEMENT

Treatment will be centred on managing shock (if this has resulted), providing analgesics and prescribing antibiotic therapy. If perforation is severe surgery may well be required. Such a patient may be acutely ill and required intensive nursing support (see Ch. 29).

DISORDERS OF THE STOMACH AND DUODENUM

Disorders of the stomach and duodenum are the most common organic disorders of the GI tract. They are considered together here because disorders of one organ commonly affect the other. A recent survey revealed that only 37% of 2066 people questioned had never had symptoms of dyspepsia (Jones et al 1989). Of people presenting with more serious symptoms, 30 000 are admitted to hospital in the UK with upper gastro-intestinal haemorrhage and, of these, 3000 die (Longman 1985).

Gastritis

PATHOPHYSIOLOGY

Gastritis is an inflammatory condition of the stomach which may be acute or chronic. Acute gastritis is commonly caused by the ingestion of an irritant substance such as aspirin or an anti-inflammatory drug, or by the excessive intake of alcohol. Chronic gastritis develops over many years and is found in patients with pernicious anaemia, auto-immune disorders, chronic alcohol abuse, peptic ulceration, gastric cancer and after gastric surgery.

Common clinical features. The outstanding presenting symptom in gastritis is abdominal pain, accompanied by a feeling of distension, nausea, vomiting and anorexia. However, in chronic gastritis the patient is often asymptomatic. Where symptoms are present, these are the same as those found with acute gastritis, pain being associated with eating and often being described as 'indigestion'.

MEDICAL MANAGEMENT

Investigative procedures. Diagnosis is made endoscopically by gastric biopsy. *Helicobacter pylori* is found in the biopsy of many patients with chronic gastritis.

Medical intervention. An antacid may be prescribed to relieve discomfort and an H_2 blocker such as cimetidine prescribed to prevent histamine from stimulating the gastric parietal cells to secrete hydro-chloric acid. Most important is dietary advice, as the patient should avoid causative agents such as alcohol and highly spiced foods.

NURSING PRIORITIES AND MANAGEMENT: GASTRITIS

In a very acute stage, when vomiting is present, an antiemetic will be given and i.v. fluid replacement therapy may be necessary for a short time. Frequent mouthwashes are given and an appropriate diet gradually reintroduced. The opportunity should be taken to explore the patient's dietary habits and to promote a healthy eating pattern. This is particularly important where the problem of alcohol abuse has been identified.

Peptic ulcer

A peptic ulcer occurs in those parts of the digestive tract which are exposed to gastric secretions. Extensive research has been undertaken into peptic ulceration with a view to identifying causative factors. Despite this extensive research the definitive cause is not known, but a number of contributing factors such as diet, lifestyle, patterns of employment, social class and geographical region are now recognised.

PATHOPHYSIOLOGY

Chronic peptic ulcers penetrate through the mucosa to the muscle layers. They can damage blood vessels and cause bleeding. In the duodenum they are found immediately beyond the pylorus and in 10–15% of cases are multiple. The fibrosis can lead to pyloric stenosis, which in turn can lead to gastric outlet obstruction. Gastric ulcers are found on the lesser curvature of the stomach in 90% of cases.

Important contributing factors in the development of peptic ulcers are hypersecretion of acid and pepsin and impaired mucosal resistance. These factors are probably mediated by hereditary, environmental and dietary factors. The fact that acid and pepsin secretion is necessary for the development of a peptic ulcer is demonstrated by the fact that ulcers never develop where there is complete achlorhydria (e.g. in pernicious anaemia).

The gastric mucosa is protected by mucus and buffered by food. The duodenum is protected by its alkaline digestive juices, which neutralise the acid chyme. Should there be chronic reflux of bile and intestinal secretions into the stomach the mucosa can over time become impaired. Drugs such as aspirin and non-steroidal anti-inflammatory drugs (NSAIDs) also cause damage, resulting in localised ulceration of the mucosa.

Smoking is considered to have a causative influence in the development of peptic ulcers and is known to impair ulcer healing. There is growing evidence that cigarette smoking prevents healing of gastric and duodenal ulcers and may be a factor in contributing to their development (Edwards & Bouchier 1991).

While no definite conclusions have been reached with regard to the relationship between food and ulcer formation, some evidence exists that a diet low in fibre can contribute, as can the consumption of alcohol, tea, coffee and cola, all of which stimulate gastric secretion. Research studies have yielded conflicting evidence as to whether emotional factors such as stress and anxiety are causative factors (See Box 4.2). A further point to note is that as in chronic active gastritis, *Helicobacter pylori* is often present in the gastric mucosa biopsies of individuals with peptic ulceration.

Common presenting features. The individual with a chronic peptic ulcer will describe a pattern of episodic pain and dyspepsia. Pain is a classic symptom and is described as a burning or boring pain in the epigastrium; often the patient points directly to where the pain is felt. The pain is sometimes more diffuse or radiates through to the back.

While studies show the relationship to food and mealtimes to be variable, the person with a duodenal ulcer is more likely to feel pain and

Box 4.2 Stress ulceration

Unlike other forms of peptic ulceration, stress ulcers are superficial in nature and are often referred to as erosions, since they do not penetrate muscle layers. Although their cause is still not clear it is believed that an emotional or physical stressor can give rise to ischaemia and vasospasm of the gastric micro-circulation. This impairs the natural mucosal resistance such that acidpepsin is able to diffuse into the epithelial cells of the gastric lining. Within a clinical setting these ulcers tend to occur after major surgery, trauma, burns or severe illness and commonly present with bleeding (which may be dramatic). The recognition of such a life-threatening occurrence will be less likely if the patient has been receiving prophylactic i.v. H_2 antagonist medication. See Kalder (1985) for further information.

'hunger feelings' about 2–3 h after a meal, whereas with a gastric ulcer pain is felt about 30–60 min after a meal and is not relieved by more food. Sometimes patients admit to inducing vomiting in an attempt to relieve the pain. Persistent vomiting of large amounts indicates an obstruction to the pylorus: pyloric stenosis.

Other common features are belching and regurgitation which causes heartburn.

MEDICAL MANAGEMENT

Investigative procedures. A full medical history will be taken. Investigations may include endoscopy (often with biopsy), CT scan, barium swallow and meal, full blood count and Hb estimation.

Medical intervention. Management centres on lifestyle changes — getting adequate rest, avoiding stress, eating properly, refraining from smoking, etc. — drug therapy, and, in some cases, surgery.

Drug therapy may include:

- antacids for the relief of dyspepsia. A common side-effect of preparations based on magnesium is diarrhoea.
- H_2 receptor antagonists, e.g. cimetidine and ranitidine. These assist in healing by preventing histamine from stimulating the gastric parietal cells to secrete hydrochloric acid.
- a proton pump inhibitor (i.e. omeprazole) to inhibit the release of hydrochloric acid from the parietal cells.

Surgical intervention. Indications for surgery for peptic ulcer are as follows:

- failure of response to medical therapy
- recurrence
- development of complications, i.e. perforation, haemorrhage, pyloric stenosis
- suspicion of malignancy (gastric ulcers)
- combined duodenal and gastric ulcers (because of their poor response to medical treatment).

The aim of surgical intervention is to reduce acid and pepsin secretion. This is achieved by interrupting the vagus nerve or by resection of the gastric acid producing section of the stomach. The options for surgical intervention in peptic ulceration are summarised in Table 4.1.

NURSING PRIORITIES AND MANAGEMENT: PEPTIC ULCER

Perioperative care

Preoperative preparation (see Case History 4.1)

The patient who is to undergo an elective procedure is normally admitted one day prior to surgery. This allows time for final medical examinations to be made regarding the individual's fitness for the operation and for receiving a general anaesthetic. Blood is taken for grouping and crossmatching.

Table 4.1 Surgical procedures used in the treatment of peptic ulceration (After Whitehead 1988 and Forrest et al 1991.)

Site	Elective	Emergency
Gastric	Partial gastrectomy, or truncal vagotomy and pyloroplasty, or gastrojejunostomy	Partial gastrectomy Excision of gastric ulcer with truncal vagotomy and pyloroplasty or gastrojejunostomy Simple closure
Duodenal	Highly selective vagotomy	Simple closure with truncal vagotomy and pyloroplasty, or gastrojejunostomy
	Truncal vagotomy and pyloroplasty, or gastrojejunostomy Partial gastrectomy	

Case History 4.1 Mr R

Mr R has been diagnosed as having a duodenal ulcer with pyloric stenosis. He is 54 years old. He has lost a lot of weight over the last few months due to vomiting and does not eat much now. He is very thin and is also very anxious. He admits that he smokes 30–40 cigarettes a day and has difficulty sleeping. He has difficulty in hearing but does not use a hearing aid. His particular identified care needs are:

- relief of pain
- relief of anxiety caused by difficulty in hearing the doctor's explanations
- breathing exercises pre- and postoperatively, especially in view of his smoking
- pressure area care due to weight loss
- optimal maintenance of nutritional status
- getting adequate sleep.

A full nursing assessment is made and a care plan formulated to meet the specific needs identified as well as to fulfil standard preoperative nursing requirements (see Ch. 27). Explanations are given of the timescale for the preparation which will take place. If the patient is a smoker and has still not stopped, the importance of doing so now is explained.

Preparation of the GI tract will include:

- fasting by mouth for at least 4–6 h preoperatively (see Ch. 27, p. 784)
- rectal suppositories to clear the lower bowel may be administered.

On the morning of the operation, the patient is prepared for theatre. A nasogastric (NG) tube is passed either before transfer to theatre or following the anaesthetic.

For emergency surgery, bowel preparation is omitted, and the timescale is shortened. Careful observations are made of blood pressure and pulse in order to detect any deterioration of the patient's condition. Analgesics are given for pain relief and clear, concise explanations are given to the patient and his relatives regarding treatment.

? **4.2** In the light of Mr R's identified needs in Case History 4.1, create a plan for this patient's preoperative care in hospital.

Postoperative management

On the patient's return to the ward the nurse will monitor and/or observe the following:

- airway, blood pressure and pulse
- the NG aspirate
- bleeding and drainage of the wound
- skin colour
- the i.v. infusion and site
- urinary output.

During the first 24–48 h these observations are maintained, decreasing in frequency as haemodynamic stability is regained.

The NG tube is usually left on free drainage between aspirations to allow air to escape. The aspirate should be observed for colour and amount. Normally the aspirate diminishes and bowel sounds are heard within 24–48 h. Should large amounts of aspirate continue to be obtained, this would indicate that absorption from the stomach is not occurring; it may also indicate the onset of paralytic ileus (see Ch. 27, p. 799).

Fluids are withheld for at least 24 h, after which period, if bowel sounds have returned, sips of water may be given. Water may then be given at hourly intervals, beginning with 30 ml and gradually increasing the amount until free fluids are well tolerated. Light, easily digested food is gradually introduced.

Care should be taken that the NG tube is positioned comfortably and well supported. Nasal care is given as required. Oral hygiene is also very important and the mouth should be kept clean and moist using mouthwashes or by brushing the teeth if the patient can tolerate this.

The i.v. infusion must be maintained as prescribed to preserve fluid and electrolyte balance and prevent dehydration while oral fluids are not being taken.

> ? **4.3** What observations could the nurse make of the patient that would indicate whether adequate fluid intake is being maintained? (See Ch. 20.)

Following surgery patients should be encouraged to sit up, get out of bed and take a few steps as soon as possible. They should also be encouraged to breathe deeply and cough to clear the lungs of anaesthetic gases and excess mucus. These measures will help to prevent chest infection. Mobilisation also helps to prevent the development of deep vein thrombosis. Adequate analgesia and holding the wound firmly when the patient moves or coughs will encourage the patient to cooperate with postoperative therapy.

Dumping syndrome

Dumping syndrome is a postoperative complication of gastric surgery which occurs following eating. Symptoms are varied and may consist of epigastric fullness and discomfort, sweating, an increase in peristalsis, a feeling of faintness and sometimes diarrhoea.

These symptoms occur within 10–15 min of eating and usually settle within 30–60 min. Patients frequently have to lie down until symptoms subside. The symptoms are caused by sudden emptying of hyperosmolar solutions into the small bowel, resulting in rapid distension of the jejunal loop anastomosed to the stomach and a withdrawal of water from the circulating blood volume into the jejunum to dilute the high concentration of electrolytes and sugars.

The symptoms of dumping may be alleviated by eating smaller portions of food more frequently, reducing carbohydrate intake and avoiding fluids during meals. If symptoms persist, changes in dietary intake and further surgery may eventually be indicated.

Discharge planning

Patients who have undergone surgery in peptic ulcers are generally fit to be discharged one week after the operation. However, elderly patients and those with intercurrent disease may need a longer period in hospital. Therefore, it is important for the nurse to be fully aware of the patient's social circumstances from the time of admission so that adequate preparation for discharge can be made and potential problems anticipated. For example, will the patient need transport home? Is a home help required? Does the patient have young children? Again, communication with the patient's relatives or friends can be extremely helpful in planning for the patient's discharge.

> ? **4.4** In view of the patient profile given in Case History 4.1 what advice should be given to Mr R prior to his discharge?

It is customary to arrange an outpatient follow-up appointment so that the success of the surgery can be assessed and the patient's rehabilitation monitored. The general practitioner is always advised of the patient's surgery and discharge and of any special after-care that may be required. If continuing care of the wound is required, it will be arranged with the community nursing team.

Complications of peptic ulcer

The three major complications of peptic ulcer are:

- haemorrhage
- perforation
- pyloric stenosis.

Haemorrhage

Severe abdominal bleeding is a life-threatening emergency. Immediate measures must be taken to replace blood loss and arrest the bleeding (see Ch. 18, p. 600).

MEDICAL MANAGEMENT

Careful assessment of the extent of the bleeding is made, and fibreoptic endoscopy may be used to identify the exact site. In the first instance an i.v. infusion is commenced and blood transfusion given if the patient is shocked. I.v. cimetidine is commenced to reduce gastric secretion. Hourly drinks and a light diet are commenced when bleeding has stopped. Surgery is undertaken as an emergency if the bleeding does not cease. Elective surgery at a later date may be advised for patients who do not respond to conservative treatment.

NURSING PRIORITIES AND MANAGEMENT: ABDOMINAL HAEMORRHAGE

Major nursing considerations

Nursing and medical staff must promptly implement resuscitative techniques as necessary. Oxygen therapy should be commenced and maintained at the prescribed rate. Blood pressure, pulse and respirations should be checked and recorded frequently to assess the patient's general condition and to observe for continuing haemorrhage. Central venous pressure monitoring may also be instituted.

Any vomitus should be observed for amount and for the presence of fresh blood or a 'coffee ground' appearance. If the bleeding is severe and vomiting continuous an NG tube will be passed to determine blood loss and to prevent further vomiting. Stools should be observed for malaena.

Pain is usually severe, requiring opiate analgesic relief. The patient should be monitored for his response to analgesia (see Ch. 19, p. 624).

Urinary output must be monitored, as hypotension can affect kidney function, diminishing filtration. A urinary catheter may be passed to assist in monitoring output.

I.v. plasma protein substitutes or whole blood and plasma should be given promptly to restore circulating blood volume. Continuous monitoring must be maintained.

Efforts should be made to allay the patient's anxiety. Ongoing explanations will help to reassure him and his relatives that appropriate treatment is available and that everything possible is being done to arrest the bleeding.

When the patient's condition has stabilised, preparation for surgery can be finalised. Alternatively, if conservative treatment has been successful, surgery may be avoided.

Perforation

PATHOPHYSIOLOGY

A perforated ulcer allows the duodenal and gastric secretions to leak into the peritoneal cavity, resulting in peritonitis.

Perforation of a duodenal ulcer is 3 times more common than perforation of a gastric ulcer (Burkitt et al 1990).

Common presenting symptoms. Haemorrhage is not a constant feature and the patient may have had very few symptoms. The major presentation is the onset of severe epigastric pain, which becomes generalised abdominal pain and tenderness made worse by any movement. Therefore the patient typically stays remarkably still, as a result of which the abdomen develops a 'board-like' rigidity — a classic sign.

MEDICAL MANAGEMENT

Diagnosis is usually quite obvious but will be confirmed by plain erect X-ray of the upper abdomen. In a positive diagnosis this will show air collected under the diaphragm. If the diagnosis is uncertain barium examination may be undertaken; gastroscopy, which requires inflation of the stomach, is contraindicated. Emergency surgery is the usual course of action, either to repair the perforation or make a more extensive intervention.

NURSING PRIORITIES AND MANAGEMENT: PERFORATION

Nursing care will include the following:

- giving resuscitative therapy as necessary
- giving oxygen therapy
- monitoring blood pressure and pulse for shock
- passing an NG tube and performing aspiration to empty the stomach and prevent further peritoneal contamination
- commencing antibiotic therapy as prescribed
- giving i.v. fluids to correct electrolyte balance
- providing analgesics
- preparing the patient for surgery
- giving careful explanations and calm reassurance.

Pyloric stenosis

PATHOPHYSIOLOGY

This complication of peptic ulceration is less common than haemorrhage or perforation and most people associate the disorder with the congenital hypertrophy of the pylorus that sometimes occurs in male babies. It occurs in the first part of the duodenum and in adults is due to repeated healing and breakdown of a chronic peptic ulcer. The buildup of fibrous tissues causes the stenosis, which results in partial or complete obstruction to the gastric outlet.

Common presenting symptoms include a feeling of fullness after meals, anorexia and occasional vomiting, which progresses to an over-distended stomach full of partly digested food, and projectile vomiting.

MEDICAL MANAGEMENT

Investigative procedures. Diagnosis is by clinical examination and a barium meal.

Medical intervention. Dehydration and electrolyte imbalance, which may be severe due to the vomiting, is corrected by i.v. fluids. A daily stomach washout may be performed to clear the stomach of stale contents. Once the aspirate is clear an NG tube can be passed and repeatedly aspirated to avoid distension. Surgical intervention is usually undertaken when the patient's condition has stabilised.

For further details on the management of pyloric stenosis see Forrest et al (1991), pp. 459–460.

> ? **4.5** In light of the above details what would you consider to be the nursing priorities for a patient with pyloric stenosis in the time before surgical intervention is undertaken?

Carcinoma of the stomach

Gastric carcinomas are more common in men than women and are usually found in the 55–70-year-old age group. The highest incidence is in Japan. A diet high in carbohydrates and low in fat, fresh fruit and vegetables is thought to predispose to gastric cancer. An increased risk is associated with pernicious anaemia, chronic gastritis and following gastric surgery. The incidence is greater in individuals with blood group A.

PATHOPHYSIOLOGY

Gastric carcinomas are almost always adenocarcinomas derived from the mucus-secreting cells of the gastric glands; 60% occur at the pylorus or in the antrum, 20–30% in the body and 5–20% in the cardia. The tumour spreads along the gastric wall to the duodenum and oesophagus and through the wall to the peritoneum. Adjacent organs become infiltrated. Metastatic spread may occur locally to neighbouring organs, within the peritoneal cavity, or via the lymphatic or blood vessels to the liver, lung and bones.

Common presenting symptoms. The most common symptoms are anorexia, loss of weight and epigastric pain. Often such symptoms are either rationalised as trivial or tolerated despite the distress they cause; consequently there may be considerable delay before the patient seeks medical help. By this time, the disease may be well advanced and have spread to adjacent organs. Dysphagia indicates that the cardia of the stomach is involved. Vomiting suggests obstruction by a tumour at the gastric outlet.

MEDICAL MANAGEMENT

Investigative procedures. Diagnosis is made by medical history, clinical examination and barium meal, when a filling defect will be seen. Fibre-optic gastroscopy allows direct inspection and a biopsy to be taken.

Medical intervention. The prognosis is poor. A partial or total gastrectomy — which is either palliative or so-called curative, depending on the extent of the tumour — may be undertaken. Details of surgery are given in Whitehead 1988. Sadly, for some patients the carcinoma is so advanced that surgical intervention is inappropriate. See Figs 4.6, 4.7 and 4.8.

NURSING PRIORITIES AND MANAGEMENT: CARCINOMA OF THE STOMACH

See Chapter 27 for details of perioperative nursing priorities in abdominal surgery.

Long-term care after palliative surgery

Major patient problems

After the patient has been discharged home, it is very likely that the symptoms of the cancer will gradually increase. Skilful and sensitive nursing care will be required to help the patient to remain as comfortable and free from anxiety as possible.

Pain from the tumour, metastases and ascites (see p. 931) can be relieved by the judicious use of analgesics (usually diamorphine). This is usually given subcutaneously via a syringe driver. Such delivery gives a consistent level of analgesia and is often the key factor in enabling the patient to be pain free and to remain at home.

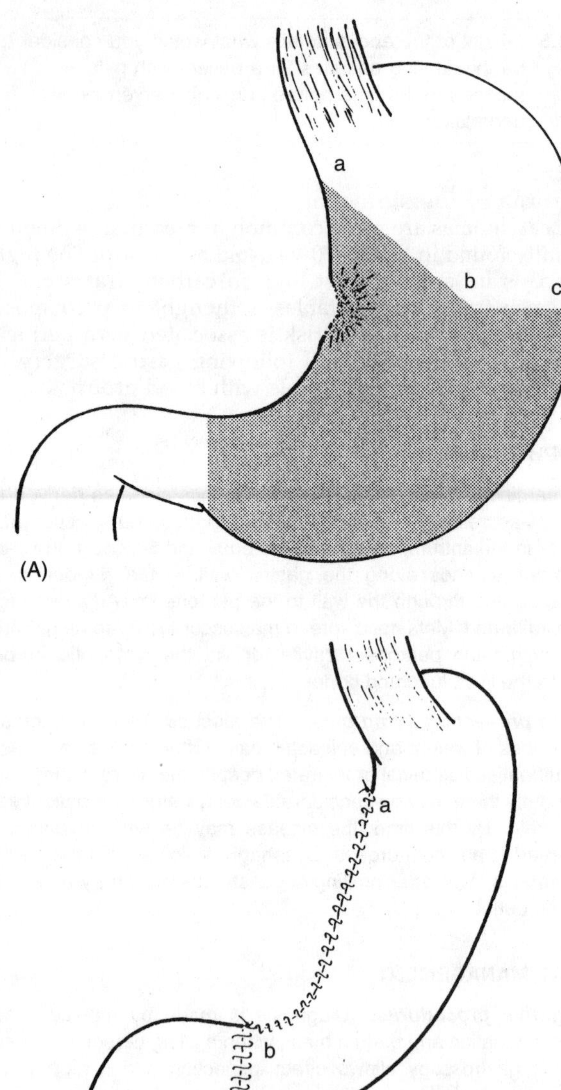

Fig. 4.6 Partial (Billroth I) gastrectomy. This procedure is used for gastric ulceration and in carcinoma of the stomach. The distal stomach with the ulcer or tumour are removed and the remnant closed to form a new inner curve and anastomosed to the duodenum. (Reproduced with kind permission from Whitehead 1988.)

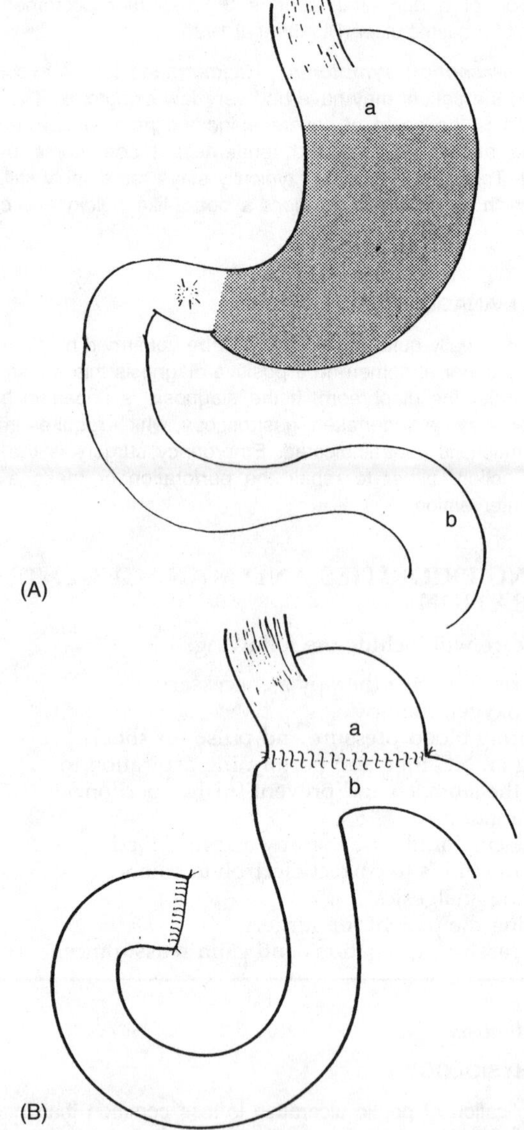

Fig. 4.7 Polya (Billroth II) gastrectomy. The distal four-fifths of the stomach is removed. After closure of the duodenal stump (often leaving the ulcer in situ), continuity is restored by anastomising the remains of the stomach (A) to the jejunum (B). (Reproduced with kind permission from Whitehead 1988.)

Dietary intake may prove a problem. Persistent nausea and vomiting may develop and be difficult to control. Regular and pre-emptive antiemetic medication can be most beneficial. Meals should be small and attractively served at times when the effect of antiemetics is at its optimal level. Nutritious drinks such as Fresubin can help supplement nutrition without extra effort on the part of the patient.

Diarrhoea and constipation can both occur. A common side-effect of opiate analgesics is constipation. Orally or rectally administered medications can help control these symptoms, as can dietary care.

Mouth infection. As in all malignant disease, candidiasis is very common. Nystatin lozenges or suspensions may be given after meals and oral hygiene and dental/denture care must be meticulously maintained (see Ch. 15, p. 528).

Ascites. For some patients there may be the added distress of ascites. Abdomin-paracentesis whereby the ascitic fluid can be drained off may be preferred to relieve the symptoms.

Psychological distress. The support of the community nursing team and perhaps the Macmillan nursing service can prove indispensible in giving the patient the confidence to remain at home rather than in hospital. The daily visits of such a nurse, as well as ensuring that the practical aspects of care are achieved, give the patient and his family the opportunity to talk about their fears and worries. The visiting nurse is in an ideal postion to monitor the well-being of the patient and his family and to recognise when plans of care should be renewed. Chapters 32 and 34 explore many ways in which a sensitive continuity of care can be achieved, whether in hospital, at home or in a hospice.

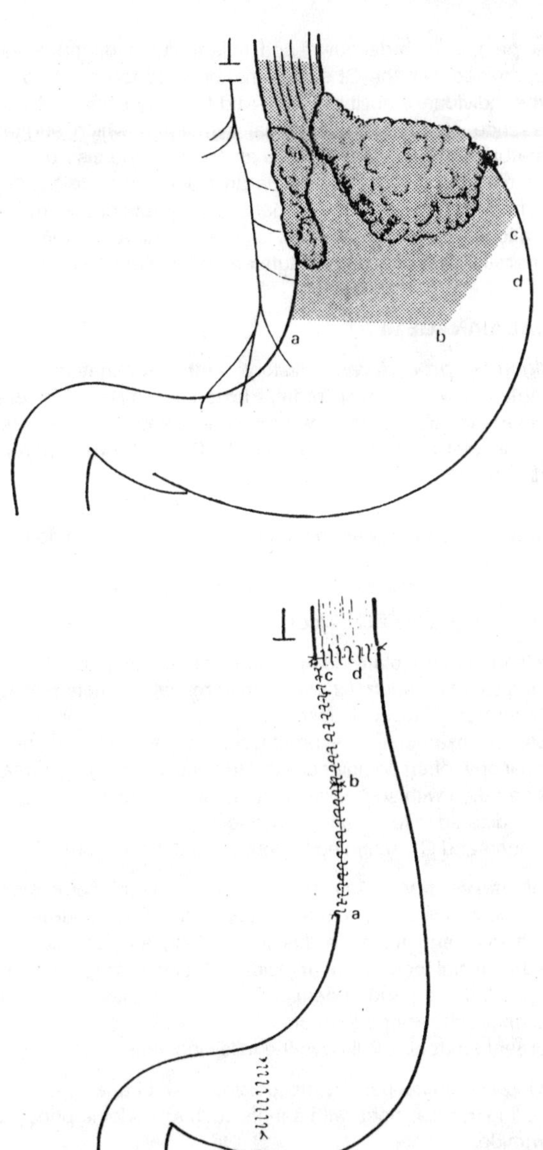

Fig. 4.8 Proximal gastrectomy. This procedure is performed for carcinoma of the cardia or body of the stomach. The proximal part of the stomach is removed with the tumour and the vagus nerve. The remnant is sutured into a tube and anastomosed to the lower oesophagus. A pyloroplasty is performed, as cutting the vagus nerve will result in pyloric sphincter paralysis. (Reproduced with kind permission from Whitehead 1988.)

DISORDERS OF THE SMALL AND LARGE INTESTINE

Unlike disorders of the upper GI tract, in which the major problem is that of ingestion of nutrients, disorders of the small and large intestine result in problems of absorption of nutrients or the transit and elimination of bowel contents. People suffering from such problems complain of varying degrees of abdominal pain and discomfort, diarrhoea and/or constipation. Often the symptoms are insidious and/or embarrassing, such that they are ignored or tolerated and not mentioned even to close relatives. Health education strategies must strive to overcome this and encourage the early reporting of symptoms before serious and perhaps irreversible changes have occurred. An example of this is the recent efforts to promote the early detection of colorectal cancer. Mant et al (1992), for example, describe a trial to predict patient compliance with faecal occult blood screening.

Malabsorption syndrome

PATHOPHYSIOLOGY

Malabsorption syndrome may result from any of the following causes:

1. Incomplete digestive processes, which may be due to:
   - damage or dysfunction of the pancreas
   - reduction or absence of bile salts to emulsify fats for absorption; this can occur in biliary obstruction, liver disease or extensive resection of the small bowel
   - excessive transit time, impairing optimal absorption; this can occur in disorders of metabolic rate, inflammatory bowel disease and even prolonged and excessive stress
2. Faulty absorption of nutrients due to:
   - damage to the absorptive surfaces, as in inflammatory bowel disease and coeliac disease
   - impaired enzyme activity, e.g. in lactose intolerance
   - resection of the absorptive surfaces, e.g. in inflammatory bowel disease.

Common presenting symptoms. Malabsorption may not be immediately or directly observable but indicative features would include loss of weight together with abdominal distension, oedema and fatty diarrhoea (steatorrhoea). There is general malaise and lack of energy which may be easiest to detect in children. In children, growth failure may also be obvious and anaemia and vitamin deficiency will be apparent.

The symptoms that tend to prompt the individual to seek medical advice are the distressing diarrhoea and general malaise. Parents will very quickly seek advice if their child fails to thrive.

MEDICAL MANAGEMENT

Investigative procedures. When a careful history and clinical examination suggest malabsorption the following diagnostic tests will be carried out to determine the cause:

- faecal fat estimation
- glucose and lactose tolerance tests
- haematological studies
- radiological and barium studies
- endoscopic examination and biopsy.

Medical intervention. The form of treatment offered will clearly depend upon the cause of the malabsorption. In coeliac disease, where there is a sensitivity to gliadin or in lactose intolerance, the advice seems simple: to avoid foods containing the offending element. However, for the person, such advice is not always easy to follow and his condition can potentially cause disruption and stress in everyday life, undermining his sense of well-being.

Where malabsorption is part of, or has resulted from, some other disorder, nutritional supplementation may be required on a temporary or permanent basis.

NURSING PRIORITIES AND MANAGEMENT: MALABSORPTION SYNDROME

Major considerations

The assessment and planning of care will necessarily focus on the problems of nutritional impairment, diarrhoea and any associated feeling of embarrassment, anger or despair. For some, pain will be a distinctive feature, in which case providing analgesia must be a priority.

A full nutritional assessment should be made (see Ch. 21) with the assistance of the dietitian. While assessing eliminatory function, efforts should be made to minimise the physical misery and embarrassment caused by diarrhoea. Attention to hygiene and the provision of soothing creams for any excoriation can make all the difference. General malaise can be helped by ensuring rest and relaxation; this is not always easy, as investigations may be many and frequent. Supporting the patient through such tests and ensuring his full understanding will help him to cope and to maintain a positive attitude.

Counselling and teaching will be a priority once the problem and treatment have been determined. This is especially important as discharge approaches and the patient begins to take responsibility for dietary modification. Support in the community can be given by the community nurse, GP and self-help groups, but probably the best support can be gained from the people closest to the patient. The involvement of family and significant friends in any teaching and health promotion programme should be encouraged.

Inflammatory bowel disease: Crohn's disease and ulcerative colitis

Inflammatory bowel disease is the term used to describe the two chronic and debilitating conditions, Crohn's disease and ulcerative colitis. Both disorders are relatively common in developed countries and commonly affect people in young adulthood. Crohn's disease (CD) appears to be increasing in prevalence, especially among children (Stapleford & Long 1990). In the UK the disease has an incidence of 5–10 per 100 000 per year and a prevalence of 50 per 100 000 (Edwards & Bouchier 1991). Harrison (1984) argues that the incidence is probably higher than perceived as many sufferers go undiagnosed. As yet no definitive cause has been found. Genetic factors, autoimmunity, diet, bacteria, allergens and stress have all been implicated and probably all play a part. It would seem that UC and CD are different manifestations of the same disease; UC, however, affects primarily the descending colon and rectum whereas CD can affect any part of the GI tract from the mouth to the anus.

PATHOPHYSIOLOGY

In UC inflammatory changes occur in the mucosa and submucosa. These changes are diffuse, with widespread superficial ulceration. In CD the inflammatory changes seem to affect isolated segments of all layers of the intestinal tract. The damaged mucosa develops granulomas, which give the bowel a cobblestoned appearance. Fibrosis and narrowing of the tract can occur and the transmural damage can lead to fistula formation whereby abnormal passageways develop between loops of the bowel.

In UC the rectum is almost always involved (proctitis) and a variable amount of the rest of the colon (the full colon can be affected). The inflammatory process affects primarily the mucosa and is continuous. Initially, there is reddening and oedema of the mucosa with bleeding points. This is followed by ulceration, which is usually superficial. In very acute disease, especially of the transverse colon, there may be gross dilatation (toxic dilatation) causing the bowel wall to become thin and rupture. In chronic disease the colon becomes shortened and narrowed. It should be noted that when Crohn's disease affects the colon or rectum, the presentation, treatment and prognosis are very similar to that of UC.

Common presenting symptoms. Whether the diagnosis is UC or CD, the presenting symptoms are very similar. Diarrhoea is pronounced, especially in UC where it is often combined with rectal bleeding. Abdominal pain is also present and is often the dominant feature in CD, where a persistant low-grade 'grumbling' pain can be quite debilitating. Tenesmus, the painful and ineffectual straining to empty the bowel, may be a feature. However, the problems that often take the patient to the doctor are general malaise, low-grade fever and weight loss. In addition there may be extraintestinal symptoms such as joint pain, skin breakdown and inflammation of the eyes which, when combined with the GI symptoms, become too much to bear and affect the individual's ability to work and to enjoy social activities. (It is the presence of the extra intestinal symptoms which suggests that inflammatory bowel disease may be an autoimmune disorder.)

Sometimes the disease is in quite an advanced state before help is sought. In such situations the symptoms may reflect the more serious complications of rectal abscesses, fissures, fistulae or even obstruction and perforation, which will constitute an abdominal emergency.

MEDICAL MANAGEMENT

Investigative procedures. History and examination suggesting inflammatory bowel disease prompt hospital admission for diagnostic tests. Haematological studies will reveal a raised WBC, a raised ESR, a raised platelet count and lowered Hb, B_{12} and zinc. There is often hypoproteinaemia.

?	**4.6** Can you explain these abnormalities in the blood picture?

Other investigations will include:

- examination of the diarrhoea for blood, fat and infective agents
- radiological and barium examination to reveal characteristic features of inflammatory bowel disease
- endoscopic examination — proctoscopy, sigmoidoscopy and colonoscopy, often combined with radionuclide imaging. Great care must be taken with such examinations, which are in fact contraindicated in fulminating disease
- ultrasound and CT scanning to determine abscess formation.

Medical intervention. As there is no real cure for inflammatory bowel disease, the aim of medical intervention is to bring about remission of active disease and maintain this for as long as possible. This may involve the initial correction of fluid and electrolyte imbalance (see Ch. 20), malnutrition and anaemia. Close observation will be made for signs of obstruction or perforation.

Treatment strategies will have the following aims:

- relieving abdominal pain by the judicious use of analgesics
- controlling the diarrhoea with agents such as codeine phosphate or loperamide
- controlling the inflammation by the use of steroid therapy and sulphasalazine — a combination of the anti-inflammatory aminosalicylic acid and the antibacterial sulphonamide. Occasionally immunosuppressive agents such as azathioprine may be employed
- Restoring nutritional and fluid and electrolyte status. In fulminating disease enteral nutrition may not be possible and total parenteral nutrition (TPN) will be required (see Ch. 21, p. 672). If enteral nutrition is possible an elemental diet free of residue may be necessary for a short while before a low-residue diet can be reintroduced. As the inflammation settles, dietary restrictions can be reduced. During any quiescent phase a 'normal' healthy diet is recommended. Such a diet should have sufficent kilocalories to restore and maintain weight, as well as being high in protein and carbohydrate and low in fat. Supplements of vitamins, iron, folic acid, zinc and potassium will usually be required.

Surgical intervention. Surgery is required in 20–30% of patients with inflammatory bowel disease but it is always preferred that any surgery be postponed for as long as possible. As a result, living with this condition can mean living with the constant anxiety that symptoms will become severe and complications arise. Surgery becomes unavoidable when:

- acute episodes fail to respond to medical treatment and there is a deterioration leading to generalised debility, malnutrition, fluid and electrolyte disturbance and anaemia
- obstruction is acute and/or fails to resolve by conservative means

- fistulae develop. These may be internal or enterocutaneous
- abscesses fail to respond to intensive treatment
- toxic megacolon occurs. (The colon hypertrophies and dilates and could rupture.)
- perforation occurs
- malignant changes are considered to be a risk.

The choice of operation will depend on the extent and severity of the disease. In UC surgery usually requires the removal of the entire large bowel. This will effect a cure but will necessitate an ileostomy formation. Great strides have been made in recent years to develop sphincter-preserving operations which avoid a stoma (Salter 1990). (See Box 4.3.) Salter (1990) discusses the possible alternatives to conventional stoma formation, recognising the undoubted impact stoma formation can have on the patient's self-concept and body image. (See also Salter 1988.)

In CD the patient may undergo more than one operation over many years, as surgery may initially be limited to resection of the affected segments of the bowel. However, because the disease affects the total GI tract, alternatives to stoma formation are not so easily achieved (Salter 1990).

NURSING PRIORITIES AND MANAGEMENT: INFLAMMATORY BOWEL DISEASE

General considerations

The nursing care of patients with inflammatory bowel disease is essentially symptomatic and must be individualised. Assessment will focus on nutritional status, pain and discomfort, eliminatory patterns, how much the person knows about the condition and how he has been coping with it. It will also be important to get to know the patient and his lifestyle, likes and dislikes, and to identify any sources of stress in daily life. For some patients developing a treatment plan will be much easier if a trusting relationship is developed with the nurse. Having a 'named nurse' can be a great comfort and support in coping with the stress of being hospitalised and undergoing a range of often exhausting investigations for which fasting and bowel preparation is required (see Case History 27.4).

Once a diagnosis of inflammatory bowel disease is confirmed, the patient will have even more stress to contend with. Time must be spent on a regular basis to help the patient to adjust and to plan positively for the future. The National Association for Colitis and Crohn's disease (NACC) can offer a great deal of support to both patients and their families (see Useful Addresses).

In addition, nursing priorities must include assessing and relieving pain; providing comfort measures that will promote rest; ensuring a high standard of personal hygiene, and providing emotional support to both the patient and family.

It is essential that privacy and ease of access to a toilet or commode is ensured, as the patient will be embarrassed and sensitive about the frequent bowel movements. The patient should be encouraged to maintain an adequate nutritional intake. Small snacks between meals will help to increase calorie intake. The provision of regular oral hygiene and antiseptic mouthwashes is essential to prevent moniliasis. The use of an oil-based barrier cream will help prevent excoriation around the anal area.

Fatigue will be a constant feature. A tactful approach when disturbing an exhausted patient in order to carry out essential care is helpful in gaining his cooperation, although he may appear unappreciative of the nursing care being carried out.

Nursing care in acute episodes

During fulminating episodes, the patient may be acutely ill. Abdominal pain can be severe and diarrhoea unremitting, and the presence of fissures, fistulae and rectal abscesses may make the symptoms worse. Dehydration and electrolyte imbalance must be corrected and nutritional status maintained by the parenteral route. The patient will be very prone to infection, and the nurse should be alert to pyrexia and tachycardia which may indicate the presence of infection. Intestinal perforation may occur without any sign other than a subtle, non-specific deterioration in the patient's condition.

Monitoring

Specific monitoring of the patient's physical condition would include:

- recording of vital signs, particularly any elevation in temperature or pulse rate or signs of impending shock
- recording fluid intake and ouput. This would include all fluid replacement, whether i.v. or oral, and all losses: urine, liquid diarrhoea and fistula loss. A drop in urine output may indicate fluid depletion. However, if TPN is necessary, signs of fluid overload could occur (see Ch. 20, p. 643).
- recording frequency and nature of diarrhoea on a stool chart.

Perioperative care

The essential principles of perioperative care are discussed in Chapter 27. In inflammatory bowel disease there are additional concerns of which the nurse must be aware. Many patients are physically debilitated and should they present with an abdominal emergency, it may not be possible to improve this state prior to surgery (see Case History 27.2). The psychological preparation for surgery that may involve stoma formation is essential even if time is limited. If optimal time is available such preparation, in which the stoma therapist plays a key role, has been shown to have a very beneficial effect in helping the patient come to terms with and manage the stoma (Watson 1983; Elcott 1988a, 1988b). (See also Box 4.4 and Nursing Care Plan 27.2.)

Stoma care

Postoperatively the nurse must maintain close observation of the stoma to ensure that it is viable and has a good blood supply. The stoma should be pink; if it darkens in colour this indicates that the blood supply is threatened. Initially the stoma will be oedematous, but should reduce over a few days.

Box 4.3 Surgical intervention in inflammatory bowel disease (Kalideen 1990, Whitehead 1988)

Sphincter-preserving operations by which an ileostomy can be avoided and continence preserved are now more commonly performed than panproctocolectomy with the formation of a permanent ileostomy. In panproctocolectomy the entire colon, rectum and anal canal are removed, and the terminal ileum formed in the right iliac fossa.

Alternatively, an ileal reservoir or pouch may be fashioned by suturing together loops of terminal ileum into the shape of a J or W. The walls of the loops are then incised to form one large cavity, and the outlet is anastomosed to the upper anal canal. This retains continence and allows elective pouch evacuation (see Kalideen 1990). Most surgeons advocate making a temporary ileostomy for the initial postoperative period, with the patient returning some 6–8 weeks later, once the reservoir has healed, for the ileostomy to be reversed and bowel continuity restored.

This procedure is not used in Crohn's disease because of the risk of disease recurrence in the reservoir. Where it can be employed, it has the advantage over ileoanal anastomoses of reducing the frequency of bowel actions.

Box 4.4 The role of the stoma nurse

Psychological preparation for ileostomy and colostomy is essential. Watson (1983) identifies the particular needs of the stoma patient as:

- the need for information
- the need to develop specific skills
- the need for emotional support.

Watson suggests that if these needs are met both preoperatively and on an ongoing basis individuals with stomas will feel independent and competent in self-care and will be more likely to continue in activities outside of the home.

The stoma therapist is a nurse certified to assist in the specialised care of patients who are undergoing stoma surgery. In the case of elective surgery she will visit the patient and his family prior to the operation to give information and support. It is essential that the patient is fully informed of the surgical options available to him so that he can give his informed consent to treatment. Clear explanations can help to ensure that the patient understands the changes in body function that will take place and help him to adjust to the accompanying alteration of body image and self-concept. The individual should be given the opportunity to voice his feelings and concerns. The individual's spouse or partner should be included in these discussions and topics such as sexuality and fertility should be covered. Referral for specialist counselling may be made as required. Part of the stoma nurse's function is to liaise with other members of the health care team in hospital and in the community to ensure that optimal care and support is given during the patient's treatment and rehabilitation.

The stoma nurse is usually involved in helping to choose the stoma site; this decision should be made after observing the patient standing, walking and sitting, rather than just lying in bed (Stockley 1982). The chosen stoma site should be marked before the patient is transferred to theatre. The various appliances which are available should be demonstrated before the operation and, if this seems appropriate to arrange, it may be helpful for an individual who has a stoma to visit the patient to talk about what it is like to cope with a stoma in day-to-day living and to reinforce the fact that general health will improve after the surgery.

Research has shown that adequate counselling and education prior to surgery has a positive effect upon the individual's ability to cope following the procedure.

A clear drainage stoma bag will be in position and allow good observation of the stoma. No discharge will be seen for 48–72 h, after which fluid faeces will become copious. If an ileostomy has been formed digestive enzymes will be present; care must be taken that the skin is protected by the correct application of the stoma bags. The stoma is formed so that it is about 3.5 cm long, thus protecting the surrounding skin. However, care is still needed to protect the skin and position the appliance with care. No pressure should be put on the stoma during care.

The patient should be reassured that the output will reduce and will become more 'paste-like' in consistency as the small intestine recovers and adjusts. The stoma nurse can demonstrate the various appliances available so that the patient has a supply of the most suitable ones prior to discharge. Initial care of the stoma is given by the nursing staff, with the patient gradually taking over under supervision and then performing care independently before going home. Continuity of care is given in the community by the primary health care team and the stoma therapist. Advice is also available from the ward staff as required.

Dietary advice should be given by the dietitian before discharge, and the patient and his family should be advised of the long recovery and adjustment time which will be required before a return to good health and a full lifestyle can be achieved.

For further information, see Kelly & Henry (1992).

?	**4.7** Arrange to accompany a stoma nurse specialist on a follow-up visit if possible.
?	**4.8** Ensure you are aware of the different stoma appliances which are available to ostomists. What are the arrangements for the supply and disposal of the appliances?
?	**4.9** As part of your community studies, find out the allowances and benefits which a person with Crohn's disease may be entitled to.

Diverticular disease

Diverticular disease presents as small hernias or out-pouchings of the mucosa through the muscular wall of the bowel. These occur predominantly in the sigmoid and descending colon. The presence of uncomplicated diverticula with minimal or no symptoms is known as diverticulosis. If inflammation occurs, causing severe symptoms, the condition is referred to as diverticulitis and if persistent will be considered a chronic inflammatory disease. However, it is often impossible to distinguish one condition from the other on radiological examination, and hence it is useful to include both active and asymptomatic disease in the term 'diverticular disease'.

It is thought that a diet low in fibre is a major factor in the development of the disease. Research has shown that people with diverticular disease have diets low in fresh fruit and vegetables, brown bread and potatoes and high in meat and milk products. It is also thought that chronic constipation and the excessive use of purgatives may cause diverticular disease by raising intraluminal pressure. Women are affected more often than men.

PATHOPHYSIOLOGY

It is thought that a low volume of colonic content leads to a reduction in the diameter of the colon. Increased luminal pressure during segmentation causes herniation of the mucosa through the muscle wall. Faeces may collect in the hernia, causing inflammation, perforation and abscess formation, the formation of fistulae into the small intestine, bladder or vagina, and peritonitis. Repeated attacks can eventually lead to obstruction.

Common presenting symptoms include intermittent grumbling, spasmodic pain in the left iliac fossa or suprapubic region. A mass may be palpable on abdominal or rectal examination. Constipation, intermittent constipation or intermittent diarrhoea are usual. The majority of patients with diverticular disease are asymptomatic but Fig. 4.9 shows the range of clinical presentations that can occur.

MEDICAL MANAGEMENT

Investigative procedures. Diagnosis is made by barium enema. Sigmoidoscopy is undertaken to exclude cancer. Colonoscopy is indicated when there is rectal bleeding or where a carcinoma is

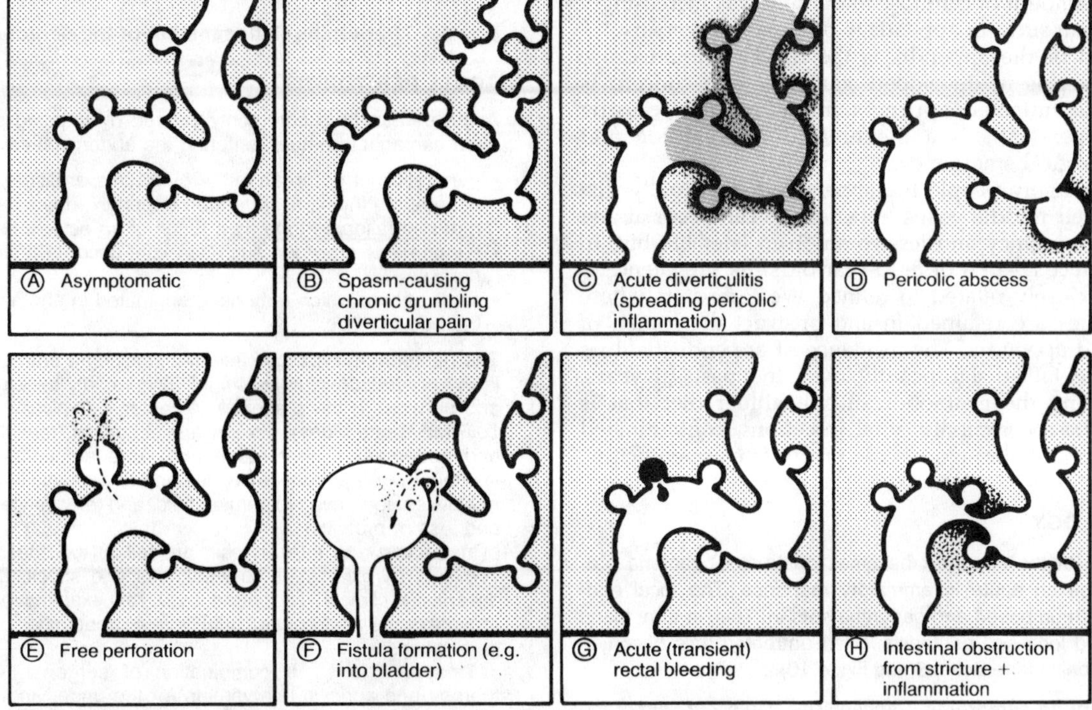

Fig. 4.9 Clinical presentations in diverticular disease. (Reproduced with permission from Burkitt et al 1990.)

suspected. Most individuals are treated in the community by their GP.

Medical intervention. The principles of treatment are to give advice on increasing dietary fibre including unprocessed bran, wholemeal bread, fruit and vegetables in the diet. The individual should also drink plenty of water. Antispasmodics such as propantheline bromide can be used. It must be emphasised that laxatives should *not* be used.

In severe exacerbations, admission to hospital may be necessary. Treatment will include broad-spectrum antibiotics if there is marked abdominal pain and pyrexia, and i.v. infusion and NG aspiration until the inflammation settles. Although many people who live with diverticular disease feel able to cope and have no difficulty in adhering to dietary advice, for about 25% of sufferers complications do occur and surgical intervention will be required. Figure 4.9 (c–h) identifies the complications that may necessitate surgery. Depending on the nature and severity of the problem, resection and temporary or permanent stoma formation may be necessary.

> ? **4.10** Possible surgical procedures for diverticular disease might include:
>
> - colectomy
> - 'Hartmann's' procedure (See Ch. 27)
> - transverse loop colostomy.
>
> An anxious elderly patient cannot remember what the surgeon actually said in describing these operations. How would you explain the nature and purpose of these procedures to the patient?

Irritable bowel syndrome

PATHOPHYSIOLOGY

Irritable bowel syndrome is thought to be due to a disturbance in normal intestinal motility with no underlying pathology. While the cause is unknown, it is thought that stress can predispose the individual to the development of the syndrome. Some patients claim that certain foods such as salad, fruit, coffee or alcohol exacerbate their symptoms.

Approximately half the patients referred to GI intestinal clinics with abdominal symptoms are diagnosed as having irritable bowel syndrome. Moreover, about a third of healthy adults experience abdominal symptoms such as those encountered in irritable bowel syndrome without consulting a doctor. The syndrome is a chronic one with periods of remission and relapse, with the individual's general health remaining generally good (Thompson & Heaton 1989).

Common presenting symptoms include altered bowel habit, diarrhoea (especially in the morning), tenesmus, and colicky abdominal pain felt in the left iliac fossa. The pain can often be relieved by passing flatus or faeces. Other signs may include gastro-oesophageal symptoms such as heartburn or belching. These symptoms may often be accompanied by other stress-related symptoms, e.g. menstrual disturbance, palpitations and urinary frequency.

MEDICAL AND NURSING MANAGEMENT

Investigations include a careful history noting details of the individual's physical symptoms, life stressors and reactions to these, and general personality. Sigmoidoscopy is always performed, and if the patient is over 40 years with a relatively short onset of symptoms a barium meal and follow-through and barium enema are performed to exclude any other cause, e.g. tumours.

After the diagnosis is confirmed, time is spent discussing the symptoms and findings and reassuring the patient that there is no underlying pathology to the condition. A high-fibre diet is recommended and the patient is offered counselling to help him to cope with stress.

Appendicitis

The appendix develops from the dependent pole of the caecum as a blind-ended tube. It has a large amount of lymphoid tissue in its walls, and is covered by the peritoneum. The appendix is described as vestigial in that it constitutes the remnant of a structure whose function is no longer required. Our ancestors required an appendix for the digestion of cellulose but as the amount of cellulose in the diet was increasingly replaced by meat, such an appendage became unnecessary.

Inflammation of the appendix is the most common cause of abdominal sepsis in developed countries. The concern is always that the inflamed appendix might rupture, causing peritonitis. Appendicitis is a life-threatening condition and constitutes a surgical emergency.

Although for many people the appendix has virtually disappeared by their middle years, appendicitis can occur at any age. It is rare in infancy and less common in later life but, in the UK, can affect 12–15% of 8–15-year-olds. Its prevalence is thought to be closely related to refined Western diets where faecalith residues are retained in and obstruct the lumen of the blind-ended appendix. The incidence of appendicitis does appear to have fallen significantly over the past 10 years, perhaps reflecting the promotion of a healthier diet that is high in fibre. Less commonly, viral infections, contaminated food and intestinal (tape) worms can precipitate appendicitis.

PATHOPHYSIOLOGY

When the lumen of the appendix becomes obstructed, bacteria proliferate and cause an acute inflammatory response. The local end-arteries become thrombosed and gangrene sets in. This, in turn, leads to perforation and localised peritonitis. If left untreated, this becomes generalised peritonitis (see Box 4.5 and Fig. 4.10).

Common presenting symptoms. Appendicitis can occur, 'out of the blue'. Many an anecdote tells of individuals who at 9 p.m. were happily enjoying an evening at the theatre or a restaurant and at 3 a.m. found themselves in a hospital bed minus their appendix.

For others, symptoms of colic and fever may 'grumble' on for some time before an acute episode occurs. In such cases, the obstruction has perhaps been partial and the inflammation transitory. These recurrent episodes can result in adhesions forming that can cause further problems (see Box 4.6).

The classic and cardinal features are usually seen in the young person and readily 'diagnosed' even by family and friends (see Case History 4.2).

?	**4.11** After reading Case History 4.2, try to answer the following questions: a. How do you account for the discomfort affecting P's right leg? b. Why would any delay in admitting P to hospital have been unwise? c. Why might P have experienced postoperative urinary retention? (See Ch. 27, p. 799.)

Box 4.5 Peritonitis (inflammation of the peritoneum)

ACUTE PERITONITIS

Acute peritonitis is commonly caused by irritating substances, often bacterial in nature, entering the abdominal cavity due to:

- perforation of an organ either by trauma or disease, e.g. a penetrating injury, a perforated appendix, duodenal ulcer, or ruptured fallopian tube as a result of an ectopic pregnancy
- gangrene of an organ such as might occur in a strangulated hernia
- septicaemia, which may have originated in another part of the body.

The peritoneum becomes inflamed, inciting a dramatic increase in the production of serous fluid. This rapidly becomes infected and purulent in the presence of bacteria, (typically *Escherichia coli* and Bacteroides). Toxins are absorbed from the inflamed and oedematous peritoneum and large amounts of fluid are lost into the peritoneal cavity, leading to paralytic ileus, abdominal distension, hypovolaemia, fluid and electrolyte imbalance and loss of protein.

Immediate and intense pain are felt at the site, followed by vomiting, pyrexia, extreme weakness and shock. Diagnosis is essentially clinical, supported by X-ray examination to detect the presence of free air, fluid levels, abdominal masses and perforations.

Treatment is by a combination of surgery, i.v. antibiotic therapy and specific intervention for the underlying cause. The peritoneal cavity may need to be opened to remove the toxic material and allow drainage of the peritoneal cavity. Supportive therapy includes: i.v. fluids to maintain fluid and electrolyte balance; NG aspiration to relieve distension; oxygen therapy; and analgesia. If the patient continues to remain pyrexial, tachycardic and in pain, an abdominal abscess should be suspected as a complication.

CHRONIC PERITONITIS

This is far less common than acute peritonitis but may occur in association with tuberculosis (see Ch. 3) or as a complication of some long-standing irritant such as peritoneal dialysis or a foreign body. Symptoms are less severe and include low-grade fever, vague pain and malaise. Treatment will essentially depend on the cause.

MEDICAL MANAGEMENT

Investigative procedures. Diagnosis is essentially clinical; following a careful history and examination, only essential investigation will be made to confirm diagnosis. If the diagnosis is in doubt, ultrasound or laparoscopic techniques may be employed.

Surgical intervention. Appendicectomy is the treatment of choice. To remove the offending appendix a small incision is made, the appendix 'delivered' and the stump sutured. The cavity will be irrigated and a drainage tube inserted if any infected material is evident.

NURSING PRIORITIES AND MANAGEMENT: APPENDICITIS

As appendicitis so often presents as an emergency, the patient may have to be prepared quickly. Every detail of safe physical preparation must be attended to but psychological support must not be considered 'a luxury we can't afford'. The skilled nurse will blend clinical and interpersonal skills to support the patient and his family in this crisis.

In the majority of cases, postoperative recovery will be uneventful and rapid. Pain relief should be ensured and vital signs monitored at frequent intervals until stability is restored (see Ch. 27, p. 796).

Complications

Should perforation and peritonitis occur (see Box 4.5) the patient may become seriously ill. Intestinal peristalsis will be halted and the risk of dehydration, electrolyte imbalance and septicaemic shock are very real. Treatment will involve the removal of the appendix and toxic material, drainage of any abscess and the administration of systemic antibiotics. Oxygen therapy will be necessary and vascular volume will be restored and maintained intravenously. An NG tube will be passed to aspirate gastric contents. Opiate analgesics will be given to ensure pain is not allowed to exacerbate an already serious situation. Fortunately, with effective and prompt intervention the mortality rate of such complications is low.

Abdominal hernia

In the discussion of hiatus hernia (see p. 92) a hernia was

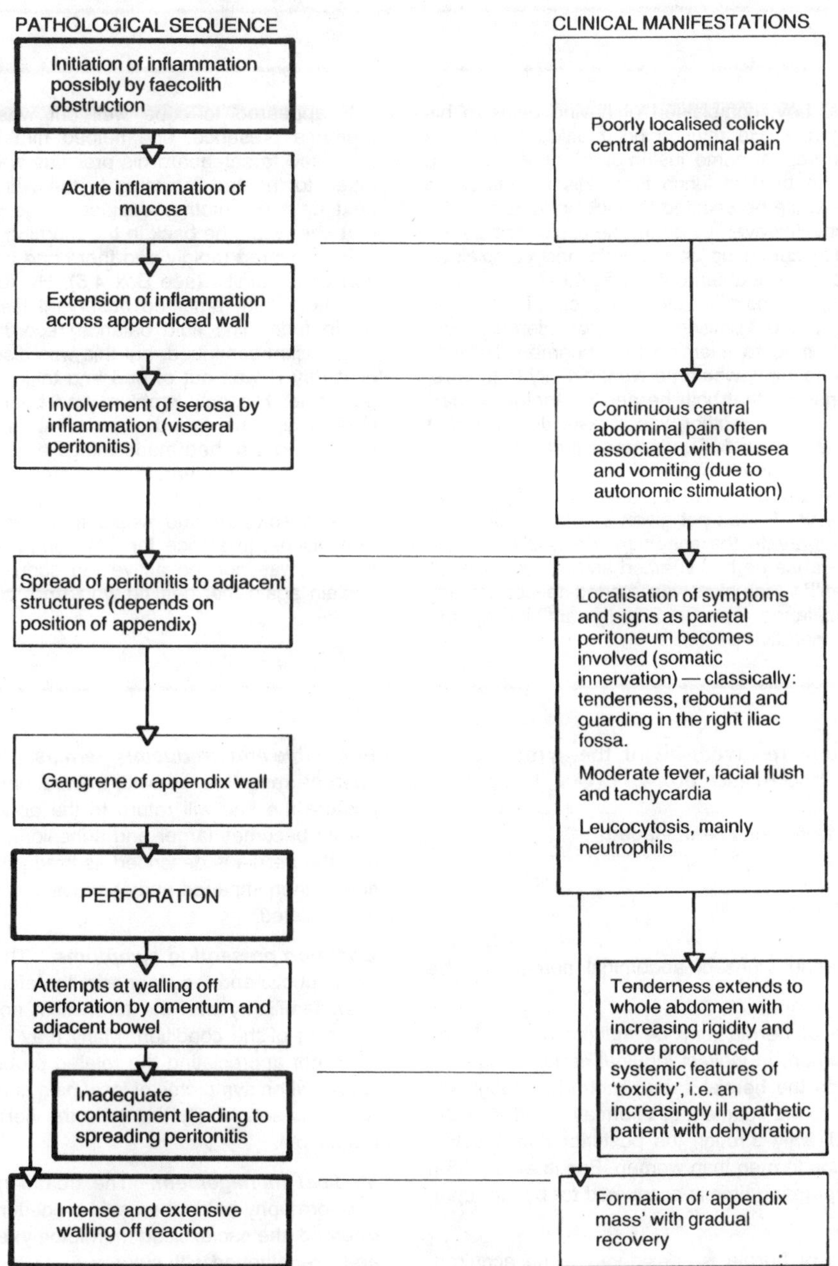

Fig. 4.10 The pathophysiology and clinical manifestations of acute appendicitis. (Reproduced with permission from Burkitt et al 1990.)

Box 4.6 Adhesions

An adhesion is the union of two surfaces that are normally separate. In the abdomen they are commonly the result of abdominal surgery, injury or inflammation. As healing occurs, fibrous scar tissue develops which may adhere to adjoining tissue, e.g. loops of bowel. These adhesions can distort tissue and by so doing impair function, e.g. the transit of intestinal contents. Adhesions may be asymptomatic but occasionally cause obstruction and require surgical division.

Such fibrous bands can also occur around pelvic organs, in the pleura, the pericardium and in damaged joints.

defined as a protrusion of an organ through the structures that normally contain it. Abdominal hernias occur where there is an acquired or congenital weakness in the muscle wall of the abdomen, allowing an outpouching of peritoneum to form a sac (see Fig. 4.11 (a+b)). Acquired weakness can occur in any condition that may result in chronically raised intra-abdominal pressure (e.g. a chronic cough, constipation, or heavy lifting) or where abdominal muscle weakness has developed (e.g. in obesity, old age, illness, or pregnancy). An untreated hernia may progress to contain peritoneal contents, typically the small or large bowel. The major concern is that, due to twisting and/or constriction at the neck of the sac, the blood supply becomes impaired at that site (see Fig. 4.11).

Case History 4.2 P

P, an active 13-year-old boy, complained of having pains in his stomach and of feeling sick. He refused his breakfast and was reluctant to go to school. Kept at home 'just in case', he was listless and vomited the soup he tried at lunch time. His friends came round after school; for a while he seemed to 'pick up' and laughter was heard from his room. However, by 8 p.m. he could localise the pain to his right side. He curled up on the sofa and complained particularly when he tried to straighten out his right leg.

His mother, suspecting appendicitis called the doctor. By the time the GP arrived, P was flushed, vomiting and in considerable pain, especially when the GP tried to examine his abdomen. He was immediately admitted to hospital, where he went directly to theatre. His designated nurse ensured that both he and his mother understood what was to happen. P's mother was relieved to know that an analgesic could now be given but understood that P's description of the pain had been important in aiding diagnosis. The reader may wish to refer to Attard et al (1992) and Jones (1992) for further debate on this issue. P was not given any bowel preparation, as it would only aggravate the condition. He had not eaten since lunch time but, because he had vomited and on examination appeared dehydrated an i.v. infusion was started to correct any fluid and electrolyte imbalance (see Ch. 20). I.v. antibiotics were administered in the perioperative period.

P appeared to cope well but was clearly comforted by his mother's presence; she helped him into his theatre gown and promised to safeguard his precious watch. Once prepared, P was taken to theatre, returning to the ward in the early hours of the next day. P's mother decided to go home, having reassured P that she would be back in the morning.

P recovered rapidly and there had been no evidence of perforation or peritonitis (see Box 4.5). He required little analgesic relief but the nurse remained observant lest he was just putting on a brave face. The fluid balance record was maintained while the i.v. infusion continued, but this was discontinued after 24 h. By the next day P was out of bed and taking a light diet and wanting to go home. His only problem had been an initial inability to pass urine which he found unpleasant and embarrassing. However, standing out of bed made things easier. The nurse running water from the tap, however, didn't impress him at all.

P was discharged on the 3rd postoperative day. His sutures were dissolvable and would therefore not need to be removed. The discharge advice for this normally active boy was to ensure that he was not too active too soon and his nurse took time to explain again that healing would not be fully complete for about 6 weeks.

Unless this is immediately resolved, all of the symptoms of intestinal obstruction will occur (see Box 4.7).

? **4.12** How would paralytic ileus be managed?

PATHOPHYSIOLOGY

The most commonly occurring types of abdominal hernia may be described as follows.

Inguinal hernia. This type of hernia may be indirect or direct, the former being the more common. In indirect inguinal hernia congenital abdominal weakness causes the hernial sac to protrude through the inguinal ring and follow the round ligament or spermatic cord. A direct inguinal hernia protrudes directly through the posterior ring. Inguinal hernias are far more common in men than women. Burkitt et al (1989) comment that 12% of UK operating time is accounted for by the repair of inguinal hernias.

Femoral hernia. This type of hernia is considered to be acquired, resulting from herniation through the femoral canal. This canal is wider in women, making such herniation more commonly a female complaint. Femoral hernias also have a greater risk of complications.

Umbilical hernia. Many infants are born with an umbilical hernia. This normally disappears in the first year of life without surgical repair. Acquired umbilical hernias can develop in overweight individuals or in those with abdominal ascites (see p. 116).

Incisional hernia. Following abdominal surgery, the incision site is a point of potential weakness. This becomes a problem if the patient experiences postoperative problems such as impaired healing (especially if drainage of the wound has been required), abdominal distension or generalised debility.

? **4.13** It is often difficult to picture the anatomical features of inguinal or femoral hernias. Review again normal abdominal anatomy with the help of your physiology textbook and take time to understand for yourself how hernias develop.

Reducible and irreducible hernias. In the early stages a hernia may often be reducible, i.e. with manual palpation or a change to standing posture the sac will return to the abdominal cavity. However as the hernia becomes larger and adhesions form, this becomes impossible and the hernia is described as irreducible or incarcerated. If the blood flow is then impaired and obstruction occurs the hernia is described as strangulated.

Common presenting symptoms. The term hernia is usually familiar to the public and the diagnosis, therefore, is often of no surprise. However, familiarity with the term must not be confused with full understanding of the condition. Many may live with the condition for some time, not appreciating the related problems that could occur. Often it is only when symptoms of local pain and tenderness occur that medical advice is sought. By that time the hernia will probably have become irreducible.

Medical management. The treatment of choice is surgical repair, herniorrhaphy being the usual procedure. The abdominal contents are returned, the sac excised (herniotomy) and the abdominal wall repaired and strengthened with sutures.

If surgery is contraindicated, a supporting truss may be worn to keep the hernia reduced and the patient free of symptoms. However, this option is not ideal. Surgery under epidural or local anaesthetic for those patients with chronic respiratory or cardiac problems has greatly improved patient outcome and obviated the need for many people to wear a truss.

Strangulation of a hernia

This life-threatening complication presents with all of the symptoms of intestinal obstruction, i.e. vomiting, severe abdominal pain, distension and absolute constipation. The patient rapidly becomes shocked, dehydrated and pyrexial. Diagnosis is made by history and clinical examination. A plain X-ray may identify the location and the associated distended loops of bowel. Rapid preparation for surgery will be necessary and definitive therapy will include oxygen, opiate analgesia, i.v. correction of fluid and electrolyte balance, NG aspiration and antibiotic administration. Surgery may well necessitate resection of the affected bowel and intensive nursing care will probably be required in the early postoperative period.

When such an occurrence is unexpected, relatives will find it

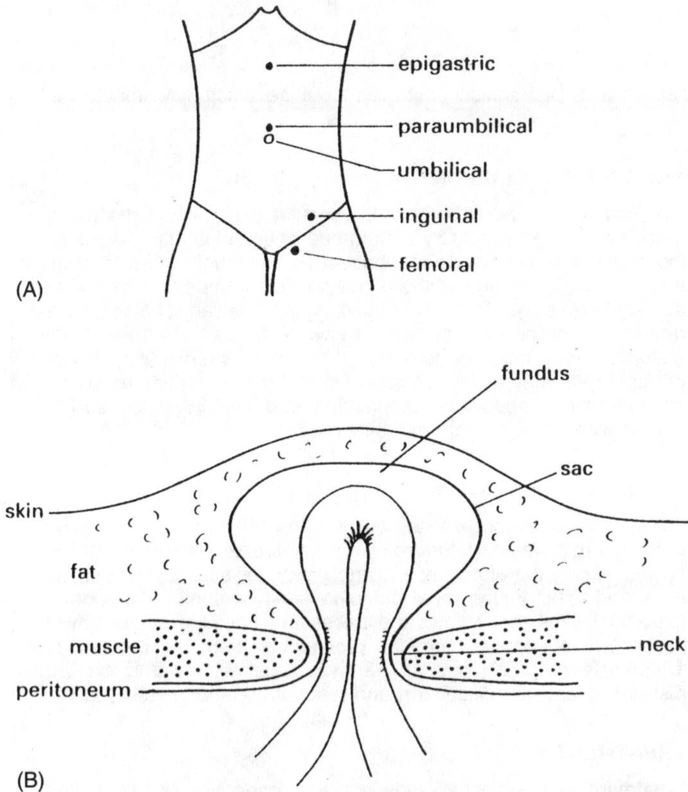

Fig. 4.11 **(A)** Common abdominal wall hernias. **(B)** The principles of the anatomy are the same in each case, although there are obviously individual differences. There is a protrusion of the peritoneum through a natural gap or weakness in the muscle wall of the abdomen. This gap narrows the sac of peritoneum into a neck before it opens out into the fundus. The sac may or may not contain some of the contents of the peritoneal cavity, e.g. omentum, small bowel. (Reproduced with kind permission from Whitehead 1988.)

especially hard to cope and will need regular contact with nursing staff for information, explanation and support. The patient is often too ill to appreciate more than simple, gentle communications.

NURSING PRIORITIES AND MANAGEMENT: ABDOMINAL HERNIA

Perioperative care

Ideally, the surgery will be elective and the patient fit. Care must be taken to ensure the patient is not suffering from a chest complaint, allergy or severe smoker's cough. In such situations, surgery should be postponed, as postoperative coughing could threaten the integrity of the repair. Smoking is always discouraged, even if for only the perioperative period, and the physiotherapist and nurse should teach the patient how to support the wound and flex the hip on the affected side should coughing or sneezing occur. Postoperative recovery is usually uneventful and mobilisation should be encouraged as soon as possible. Potential problems that must be recognised are urinary retention, infection of the wound, and pain (particularly scrotal pain when inguinal herniorrhaphy has been peformed). A scrotal support used in conjunction with analgesics usually eases the symptoms.

?	**4.14** What specific nursing care is required if the patient has had his hernia repaired under epidural anaesthetic?

Hernia repair should never be considered lightly. Often surgery is more complicated than anticipated and the patient may experience considerable postoperative pain and temporary loss of peristalsis. If this is the case, postoperative recovery will necessarily take a little longer (see Ch. 27).

Discharge advice

Time must be taken to ensure that the patient and his family understand the precautions that must be taken to ensure optimal recovery and well-being. Although activity is encouraged, lifting or straining must be avoided. Elderly men may be troubled by an enlarged prostate gland and may strain to pass urine. (One operation may well lead to another.) Equally, coughs, colds and known allergens, and constipation — that is anything that might raise intra-abdominal pressure during the weeks of healing — should be avoided if at all possible. The time allocated to give advice and support prior to discharge presents an ideal opportunity for general health promotion (e.g. on smoking, diet and alcohol) and, in the vulnerable patient, for a sensitive reappraisal of home circumstances and community support.

Colorectal cancer

Neoplasms, both benign and malignant, can occur in the large bowel. The concern with benign neoplasms such as polyps is that if they are extensive, large and of prolonged duration there is a propensity for malignant change to occur. As a result, if polyps are diagnosed they are usually removed surgically. Malignant tumours of the large bowel — colorectal cancer — is second only to cancer of the lung in causing death from malignant disease in Western society. Although it affects all age groups, it is uncommon under the age of 40.

Cancer can affect any part of the large bowel but is most common in the rectum and sigmoid colon (Forrest et al 1991). It affects men and women equally but rectal carcinoma is more common in men and colonic carcinoma more common in women.

The exact cause of colorectal cancer is unclear. As it is virtually unknown in third world rural communities, its association with the Western diet is increasingly accepted. The work of Burkitt (1971) relating low-fibre diets to disease has proved very influential. Certainly, a low-residue diet prolongs transit time, thus allowing any potential carcinogen increased contact with the intestinal mucosa. Colorectal cancer is also associated with other disorders of the bowel, e.g. ulcerative colitis, adenomatous polyps and, significantly, the hereditary disorder known as familial polyposis.

PATHOPHYSIOLOGY

The tumours arise from the epithelial cells of glandular tissue — adenocarcinomas. As they grow they progressively obstruct the bowel by extending into the lumen or spreading circumferentially to form a ring-like stricture (see Box 4.8). Metastatic spread is by direct infiltration of local tissues and organs, lymphatically or via the portal circulation.

Common presenting symptoms. Unfortunately, patients tend not to present until the disease is at an advanced stage. The symptoms are subtle, gradual and easily ignored or explained away. Symptoms will vary somewhat according to the site of the tumour but will essentially involve an alteration in bowel habit. Constipation alternating with diarrhoea is the common concern, combined with rectal bleeding and excess mucus in the stool. Pain is not a common feature and, perhaps

Box 4.7 Intestinal obstruction

Intestinal obstruction occurs when the normal transit of intestinal contents is impeded due to mechanical obstruction, vascular occlusion or impaired innervation. Obstruction may be partial or complete.

MECHANICAL OBSTRUCTION

Intraluminal causes:

- Neoplasms
- Strictures
- Foreign bodies
- Faeces
- Intussusception: a telescoping of one part of the bowel into another part.

Extramural causes:

- Adhesions
- Strangulated hernia
- Volvulus: twisting of the bowel (See Roberts 1992 for information.)
- Neoplasms outwith the intestinal tract.

When the obstruction occurs, the affected intestine becomes distended with GI secretions. (As much as 8 l is formed each day.) As the fluid accumulates, the pressure rises and the bowel responds by attempting to propel the contents forward. This serves only to increase secretions; eventually, the increase in pressure increases capillary permeability and fluid is forced out into the peritoneal cavity. The distension may cause respiratory embarrassment. Severe abdominal colic is experienced. If the obstruction is in the small bowel, vomiting occurs. Obstruction in the large bowel results in distension with air and faeces, and the eventual increase in pressure results in necrosis and the threat of perforation. The outcome of unresolved obstruction will be electrolyte imbalance, hypovolaemia and possibly peritonitis.

VASCULAR OCCLUSION

Obstruction may occur if there is vascular occlusion of the major mesenteric blood supply by a thrombus or embolus. It is the resulting ischaemia that leads to obstruction. Although there is pain, there is no distension. As the condition deteriorates, the pain may actually decrease. If undiagnosed, gangrene and bacteraemia develop as toxins from the lumen invade the peritoneum and are absorbed into the bloodstream. If surgical intervention is not prompt death may result. It should also be noted that any mechanical obstruction such as strangulation that impairs blood supply carries with it a significant mortality risk.

IMPAIRED INNERVATION: PARALYTIC ILEUS

Paralytic ileus will occur when trauma, inflammation or pain in the thoracolumbar region interferes with the normal innervation of the bowel. It can therefore be a complication of such conditions as back and chest injury, renal pathology and peritonitis. Temporary (paralytic) ileus that follows the necessary handling of the bowel in certain abdominal surgical procedures usually resolves in 12–48 h (see Ch. 27, p. 799). Paralytic ileus will result in marked distension, causing discomfort and respiratory embarrassment.

TREATMENT

Treatment will essentially involve the correction of fluid and electrolyte imbalance, the relief of the distension and pain and surgical intervention to address the cause.

due to this, medical advice is often not sought until either the patient is very anaemic and debilitated or the symptoms associated with obstruction are marked.

MEDICAL MANAGEMENT

Investigation procedures. Many patients will present with a palpable mass that can be detected on abdominal or rectal examination. Specific investigations to confirm diagnosis will include barium studies, sigmoidoscopy, colonoscopy and biopsies. CT and ultrasound scans will be necessary to seek metastases, particularly in the lung and liver. For the latter, liver function tests will also be carried out.

Staging. The staging of the carcinoma is based on histological examination of a resected specimen (see Ch. 32). For colorectal cancer the Dukes staging is most widely used. At its simplest this describes four stages:

- A: the tumour is confined to the bowel mucosa and submucosa
- B: the tumour has invaded the muscle wall to extracolonic tissue but there is no lymph node involvement
- C: lymph node metastases are present
- D: distant metastases or severe local or nodal spread makes surgical 'cure' impossible.

Medical intervention. Surgical removal of the tumour is the only effective management. The type and extent of surgery will depend on the site of the tumour. It may be possible for resection and end-to-end anastomosis to be performed, (see, for example, Fig. 4.12) but often stoma formation is necessary on a temporary or permanent basis. The reader is also referred to Forrest et al (1991), p. 508–512, for further detail.

? **4.15** Turn to Chapter 27 and read Case History 27.2. Mrs B represents a common clinical reality. She had felt unwilling to talk about her symptoms, hoping they were just haemorrhoids. Ultimately she required emergency intervention and a stoma formation for which she was totally unprepared. Can you think (or discuss as a group) how such a situation might have been prevented?

NURSING PRIORITIES AND MANAGEMENT: COLORECTAL CANCER

Major considerations

Giving psychological support

The realisation that seemingly minor ailments are actually symptoms of cancer is most stressful for any individual. From the moment a patient is referred, as an outpatient or inpatient, a sensitive and tactful approach is of paramount importance. This is not easy: Wilkinson (1992) suggests that many nurses still feel ill-equipped in terms of their ability to communicate effectively with cancer patients. Psychological care needs to include the family and significant others in order to develop a trusting relationship. The beneficial effect of spending time to allow fears to be expressed and explanations and support to be given cannot be overstated.

Perioperative care

The principles of perioperative nursing care are given in Chapter 27. If surgery is to include stoma formation, this will

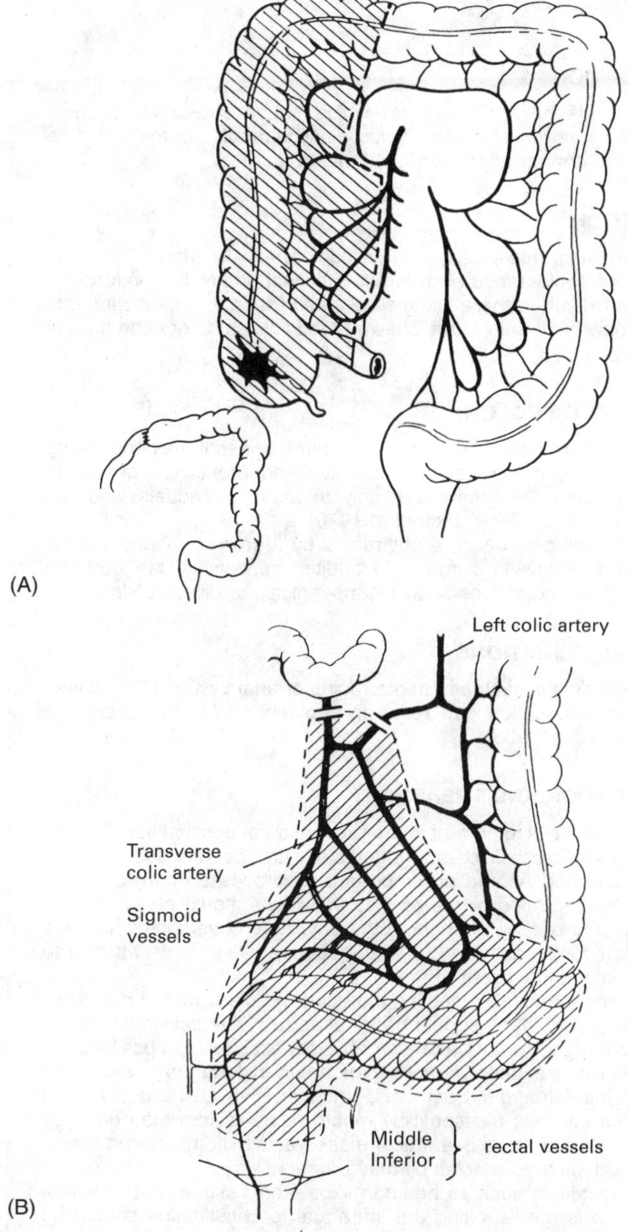

Fig. 4.12 (A) Right hemicolectomy for carcinoma of the caecum. (B) Anterior resection of rectum for carcinoma of the middle third of the rectum. (Reproduced with kind permission from Forrest et al 1991.)

present a further source of stress. A cooperative team approach by the diverse health care professionals involved will greatly assist the patient's physical and psychological recovery and adjustment to what may prove to be major and perhaps only palliative surgery. For the specific input of the stoma therapist, see Box 4.3.

Discharge planning

For those patients for whom cure is not a possibility, planning for discharge and home care should aim to maximise the patient's independence and quality of life for as long as possible. This requires the coordination and integration of hospital and community services, and a respect for the wishes of both the patient and his family. The reader is referred to Case History 32.4 for a more detailed examination of this issue.

Health promotion

Great efforts are being made to detect colorectal cancer early, when its prognosis is so much more favourable. Factors that are being addressed include fostering awareness of early warning signs and counselling those people who might be especially at risk. Preventive measures also include providing advice concerning diet and health screening.

ANORECTAL DISORDERS

Anorectal conditions such as haemorrhoids, abscesses, fissures, fistulae and sinuses are relatively common and always distressing, but are often tolerated for many months or even years before professional help and advice are sought.

Haemorrhoids

PATHOPHYSIOLOGY

Haemorrhoids, commonly called 'piles', are generally considered to be varices of the superior haemorrhoidal veins as a result of congestion of the venous plexus. It would seem that, yet again, a lack of dietary fibre is the most important predisposing factor (see Box 4.8). The resulting chronic constipation and straining during bowel movements raises intra-abdominal pressure, leading to venous plexus engorgement. The bulging mucosa is dragged down and as the condition worsens the haemorrhoids prolapse into the anal canal. Other conditions that can lead to or aggravate the congestion are pregnancy (where the development of haemorrhoids is often neglected), tumours and cardiac failure.

Haemorrhoids may be internal or external. Internal haemorrhoids are classified according to the degree to which they prolapse into the anal canal. External haemorrhoids occur outside the anal canal and are less common.

Common presenting symptoms. Commonly the patient complains of 'fresh' blood in his bowel movements, which at first may be thought to be due simply to the passing of constipated motions. The experience of prolapse, at first transient, becomes increasingly frequent and is associated with pain, the discharge of mucus and pruritis. Often such symptoms have been managed by over-the-counter (OTC) remedies such as creams to reduce the itching and pain but it is not common for the patient to be aware of the significance of changing his diet (Hope 1993). Should the haemorrhoidal vessels thrombose, pain is always severe and it may be only at that stage that the patient seeks help.

MEDICAL MANAGEMENT

Investigative procedures. History and examination will be carefully carried out to exclude other pathologies, particularly a carcinoma. Rectal examination, proctoscopy and sigmoidoscopy will confirm the diagnosis.

Medical intervention. If the haemorrhoids are identified in their early stages, management requires no more than attention to the patient's diet and, perhaps, a bulk laxative. If the constipation is corrected, the problem will usually resolve but the patient must understand this and feel confident in his ability to alter his diet. The practice nurse can play an important part in patient education and in arranging a follow-up visit to monitor the patient's well-being.

Surgical intervention. The following surgical treatments may be used to resolve haemorrhoids that do not respond to conservative management:

1. Injection. For haemorrhoids in the early stages injection of the haemorrhoidal veins with an irritant solution provokes fibrosis and atrophy with minimal discomfort
2. Band ligation. Bands are applied to the mucosa-covered

Box 4.8 Constipation

Constipation may be defined as difficult and infrequent defaecation. The following factors can contribute to the development of constipation.

DIET

A diet which is low in fibre and bulk predisposes to small faecal bulk. A low fluid intake also contributes to small bulk. Small bulk predisposes the GI tract to reduced peristaltic action and slow passage of contents along the colon. Epidemiological studies indicate that low-fibre diets contribute to many of the GI diseases found in the Western world, such as diverticulosis, appendicitis and haemorrhoids.

EXERCISE

Lack of exercise contributes to reduced peristalsis due to reduced muscle tone of the bowel and abdominal muscles. Individuals who take less exercise include the elderly and those who are ill or have a physical disability. Hospital patients are in general restricted in their mobility given their environment and their medical condition, and often investigations and treatment predispose patients to constipation.

ELIMINATION HABITS

Neglect to empty the rectum when the stimulation caused by faeces in the rectum (the 'call to stool') is ignored results in constipation; if this occurs repeatedly, faecal impaction can result. Watery diarrhoea, caused by the breakdown of faecal material proximal to the hard impacted mass, can bypass the mass. Impacted faeces can press on the urethra and cause retention of urine. (See also Ch. 24.)

SOCIOECONOMIC FACTORS

Nutritional and dietary intake is determined by eating patterns formed in childhood and influenced by familial and social norms and by income levels. A low income can result in the exclusion of fresh fruit and vegetables, which can be relatively expensive, from the diet. Low-income families and elderly people living alone may have to make difficult choices in spending their limited resources on food, heating and clothing. Lack of transport or reduced mobility can also limit shopping expeditions and therefore the choice of foods. The elderly person living alone may be less likely to cook nutritious meals for a number of reasons, e.g. lack of motivation, poor appetite, and limited mobility.

MEDICATION

Many drugs have side-effects which cause constipation; these include ganglion-blocking drugs, psychotropic drugs, muscle relaxants, and morphine and its derivatives.

DENTITION

Poor dentition makes chewing difficult, especially where there has been dental clearance and dentures do not fit well or comfortably. This can result in the avoidance of fresh fruit and vegetables, and an emphasis on soft, easily chewed foods which do not add fibre to the diet.

MOTILITY OF COLON

A reduction of muscle tone can result in the faecal mass not being propelled along the colon. Peristalsis and propulsion of faeces is increased after meals, but only in those individuals who are physically active (Holdstock et al 1970).

The bowel may become obstructed by a growth, a hernia, or by adhesions following surgery. In addition, spasticity can occur in inflammatory conditions such as appendicitis or diverticulitis.

RECTAL CONDITIONS

Local conditions such as haemorrhoids or anal fissure which cause pain on defaecation can result in avoidance of defaecation with eventual constipation.

PREVENTION AND TREATMENT

Dietary advice is important in the prevention of constipation. Wholemeal bread, fresh fruit and vegetables, and cereals such as porridge oats and Allbran are important. Unprocessed bran can also be added to soups or stews. The individual should be advised to drink plenty of fluid throughout the day. Elderly persons who have urinary incontinence tend to take inadequate fluid in an attempt to avoid being incontinent of urine.

The importance of emptying the bowel regularly and of not ignoring the 'call to stool' should be emphasised. The individual should be encouraged to take as much physical exercise as possible.

The initial treatment of constipation can include the use of laxatives. Bulk-forming preparations such as Fybogel and stimulant laxatives such as bisacodyl by mouth or by rectum may be used initially. Where there is a faecal mass, rectally administered faecal softeners such as arachis oil may be necessary.

Any condition such as haemorrhoids, anal fissure, or diverticulosis which is predisposing the individual to constipation should be treated.

haemorrhoidal pedicle, constricting the vessels, which then eventually shrink

3. Infrared coagulation. Infrared radiation is applied in pulses to the haemorrhoid by means of a fibreoptic probe. This causes coagulation and shrinkage
4. Haemorrhoidectomy. The above interventions are the most commonly used and can be carried out on an outpatient basis. If however the haemorrhoids are not amenable to such therapies haemorrhoidectomy to ligate and excise the haemorrhoids may be required. If thrombosis has occurred, this procedure will be required immediately.

NURSING PRIORITIES AND MANAGEMENT: HAEMORRHOIDS

General considerations

Whether it is the cause or the effect it is most important that difficulty with defaecation is effectively corrected. Measures to achieve this include:

- increasing dietary fibre
- maintaining a high fluid intake (2–3 l each day)
- prescribing a stool softener to facilitate water and fat absorption into the faeces
- ensuring sufficient activity.

In addition, nursing priorities must include measures to alleviate pain and itching, to ensure good personal hygiene, to provide appropriate privacy in a hospital setting, and to prevent infection.

Preoperative preparation (see Box 4.9)

If surgery is required, the aim of nursing care in the preoperative period is to control the patient's acute symptoms and to ensure that he feels comfortable and free from any distress when defaecating. One of the major postoperative fears in any form of anorectal surgery is the pain that might be experienced upon the first bowel movement. Time is well spent explaining postoperative care and how any pain and discomfort will be relieved or minimised. The patient is very often comforted merely by the fact that the nurse understands his fears and has the knowledge and skill to help him to manage the problem.

Postoperative care (See Box 4.9.)

Care priorities in the postoperative period include:

- the relief of pain and promotion of comfort
- the prevention of postoperative haemorrhage
- the prevention of postoperative urinary retention
- the prevention of infection
- the promotion of optimal faecal elimination
- patient education prior to discharge vis-à-vis lifestyle and diet.

?	**4.16** Anaesthesia and pain may inhibit urination in the early postoperative period. What support and interventions might be considered?
?	**4.17** What would be the key points in any pre-discharge advice and support given to a patient following anorectal surgery?

Other common anorectal disorders

Fissure in ano

PATHOPHYSIOLOGY

This is a tear in the lining of the lower anal canal. Pain is experienced only on defaecation. The cause of a primary fissure is uncertain, but it often follows an episode of constipation and the forceful passage of a hard stool. It is commonly a complication of Crohn's disease.

Common presenting symptoms. The main symptom is extreme pain on defaecation which persists for some hours. Rectal bleeding may be seen on defaecation.

MEDICAL MANAGEMENT

Anal fissures can heal spontaneously with the local application of creams or suppositories. Constipation is treated and then avoided by a high residue diet. Surgical treatment is a lateral internal sphincterectomy.

Fistula in ano

PATHOPHYSIOLOGY

A fistula is an opening between two epithelial surfaces. The cause is uncertain, but it may be associated with an infection which produces an abscess which then tracks. Fistulas are associated with Crohn's disease.

Common presenting symptoms. Commonly an abscess is present, as well as pain, rectal discharge and excoriation of skin, and pruritis.

MEDICAL MANAGEMENT

The fistula is laid open and heals gradually by granulation over some weeks.

Pilonidal sinus

PATHOPHYSIOLOGY

This is a sinus which contains hair and occurs in the natal cleft. The hair curls and penetrates the skin, causing irritation. Secondary infection is common, which can lead to a pilonidal abscess.

Common presenting symptoms. The individual will experience pain which is throbbing in nature. The site will be tender to the touch if an abscess is present. A discharge is often the first sign that a sinus is present.

MEDICAL MANAGEMENT

Antibiotic therapy is given prior to surgery if an infection is present, followed by excision of the sinus opening when the infection has cleared.

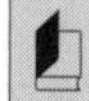

For further information, see Norris (1991).

Box 4.9 Principles of nursing care for patients undergoing perianal surgery

PREOPERATIVE PREPARATION

- Ensure the patient's privacy to reduce embarrassment
- Give analgesics for the acute pain which is often present
- Provide bowel preparation. This may include the administration of suppositories or an enema to clear the rectum. Some surgeons prefer not to give any bowel preparation prior to haemorrhoidectomy so that evacuation of the bowel after surgery can occur more quickly

POST-OPERATIVE CARE

- Observe for haemorrhage during the first 24 h by monitoring vital signs and checking the anal area
- Give analgesics as this area can be very painful after surgery
- Observe for a pack; this is removed on the 1st postoperative day after a bath. Analgesics are required as removal of the pack is very painful. The bath water must not be too hot as vasodilation coupled with pain could result in marked hypotension
- Assess the patient for urinary retention
- Assess for return of bowel movement
- Administer a bulk-forming aperient as initially prescribed to facilitate easier bowel evacuation. Analgesics may be required prior to the first bowel movement
- Give the patient a bath after the bowels have opened to keep the area clean and to relieve discomfort
- Advise the patient on avoiding constipation

DISORDERS OF THE HEPATOBILIARY SYSTEM

DISORDERS OF THE LIVER

The liver can be affected by a large number of diseases, some of which are more commonly encountered than others. Because of the large number of functions which the liver performs, both specific and non-specific clinical features are seen.

Manifestations of liver disease

Non-specific symptoms such as anorexia, nausea, lethargy, malaise and vomiting are common. Weight loss also occurs in chronic liver disease, notably in malignant disease.

Specific features include enlargement of the liver, liver failure, portal hypertension with associated ascites and splenomegaly, and oesophageal varices. Jaundice, pruritis and pain are common.

Jaundice (hyperbilirubinaemia)

Jaundice is the clinical term for the typical yellow appearance of the skin and mucous membranes in liver disease. It is caused by bilirubin and is detectable when the serum bilirubin exceeds 50 mmol/l. Jaundice may be classified according to the pathological mechanisms which cause the hyperbilirubinaemia:

1. *Haemolytic (prehepatic) jaundice:* results from an increased rate of red blood cell destruction
2. *Hepatocellular (hepatic) jaundice:* results from an inability of the liver to transport bilirubin, as a result of cellular destruction
3. *Cholestatic (post-hepatic) jaundice:* caused by a failure of bile flow. This is commonly referred to as obstructive jaundice. Normally, bilirubin is excreted from the liver in the bile. The cause of excretion failure may be obstruction in the liver ducts from cirrhosis or malignancy. Large duct obstruction outside the liver may be caused by gallstones or cancer of the head of pancreas.

Pruritis

Pruritis, i.e. itching of the skin, may be caused by bile salt deposition. It is a feature of cholestasis and occurs most often in primary biliary cirrhosis or where a large duct obstruction has occurred. Not all patients with jaundice complain of pruritis and not all patients with pruritis are icteric (jaundiced).

Pain

The liver itself has no sensory nerve innervation and so any pain experienced by the patient is from involvement or stretching of the highly sensitive liver capsule. Pain occurs in inflammatory conditions such as hepatitis, although it is unlikely to be severe. It will occur in malignant disease, in which case it can range from mild discomfort to extremely severe pain.

Hepatitis

Hepatitis denotes inflammation of the liver which may be acute or chronic. It is usually viral in origin or a response to certain drugs (see Box 4.10). All types of hepatitis will cause the same symptoms, although in each type severity can vary enormously. Specific viruses which have been identified as causing different forms of hepatitis are as follows:

- Common viruses:
  - hepatitis A
  - hepatitis B
  - hepatitis C
  - hepatitis non-A, non-B
  - hepatitis D (delta)
  - hepatitis E
- Uncommon viruses:
  - Epstein–Barr (EB) virus
  - cytomegalovirus (CMV)
  - measles.

Box 4.10 Drug-induced hepatitis

Hepatitis may be caused by any drug but the more common culprits include analgesics such as paracetamol taken in excess, psychotropic drugs such as the phenothiazines, antibiotics such as erythromycin and anaesthetics such as halothane. Any patient with hepatitis should be questioned regarding drugs taken recently, including those taken without medical advice, and including herbal remedies.

In most incidences of any drug-induced hepatitis the biopsy shows changes as for viral hepatitis. However, some drugs will *also* cause fatty changes in the liver cells.

Hepatitis A

PATHOPHYSIOLOGY

Hepatitis A is an acute condition of which a chronic form does not occur. It is usually a mild illness, often occurring in epidemics in communities such as schools, prisons, army camps and mental institutions. It is transmitted by the faecal–oral route. The incubation period is 2–4 weeks, with faeces being the most important infective material. They become infectious 2–3 weeks prior to the onset of the clinical illness and remain so for 2 weeks thereafter. Blood and urine can rarely be infectious. People who are homosexual are at great risk of hepatitis A due to oral–anal contact.

Patients with Hepatitis A are usually only mildly unwell and are rarely admitted to hospital.

MEDICAL MANAGEMENT

Investigative procedures. The diagnosis of hepatitis A virus (HAV) depends on the presence of antibodies to HAV in the patient's blood. The presence of anti HAV IgM denotes recent or current infection. It is present from 1 week of onset of the clinical illness and disappears after approximately 3 months. The presence of anti HAV IgG denotes an old infection and can persist for many years.

Medical and nursing intervention. If hospitalisation is required, the patient is usually independent and therefore risk of infection is low. However, if a patient has diarrhoea and requires nursing assistance, the following precautions should be taken:

- plastic gloves and aprons to be used for all procedures
- linen and disposable wipes, etc. to be disposed of as per local policy
- thorough hand-washing after patient contact.

Immune serum globulin i.m. can prevent hepatitis A if given within a few days of exposure. It will also prevent infection for 2–3 months in those visiting endemic areas.

Hepatitis B

PATHOPHYSIOLOGY

Hepatitis B can cause acute or chronic infection. The virus is transmitted by the parenteral route. Patients receiving blood or blood products and i.v. drug abusers who share needles are greatly at risk. Tattooing can also cause spread of the virus. The virus is also present in body fluids such as saliva, urine and semen and therefore the disease can be spread by close personal contact, e.g. sexual intercourse (especially homosexually) and in areas of overcrowding, poverty and poor sanitation. The disease can also be transmitted from mother to baby either at or soon after birth. Faeces will not transmit infection provided they are free of blood. The incubation period is approximately 2–6 months.

MEDICAL MANAGEMENT

Investigative procedures. The most important test in the diagnosis of hepatitis B Virus (HBV) is for the hepatitis B surface antigen (HBsAg) in the blood. This appears from one to several weeks before the onset of the clinical illness and disappears 1–12 weeks later. However, this may not be present in patients who either clear the virus from the blood quickly or who present late. It is therefore also necessary to look for antibodies to the hepatitis core antigen (anti HB_c). The presence of anti HB_c IgM denotes acute HBV; anti HB_c IgG denotes chronic HBV.

Medical and nursing intervention. There is great risk to medical and nursing staff when dealing with blood, blood products, body fluids and open wounds, e.g. venepuncture sites, skin lesions, and ulcers on injection sites in i.v. drug abusers. Care should also be taken in areas where the patient is unknown, e.g. casualty departments. All precautions should be taken as per individual hospital policies, and hospital staff should be vaccinated against hepatitis B virus infection.

Hepatitis B immune globulin i.m. can prevent hepatitis B if given within a few days of a high-risk exposure (e.g. a 'sharps' injury). Vaccination provides good long-term immunity but booster doses are needed every 3–5 years.

> ? **4.18** A staff member sustains a 'sharps' injury. What procedure should be followed and how can the individual be prevented from developing hepatitis?

Other hepatitis viruses

Hepatitis C virus can now be diagnosed by finding an antibody (anti HCV) in the blood. The tests currently available are best at identifying chronic HCV infection, and screening tests currently need to be confirmed when positive by more sophisticated tests, as false positive results occur.

Non-A, non-B hepatitis viruses. The ability to diagnose hepatitis A and B viruses has led to the recognition that there are other viruses which cause hepatitis. These are referred to as non-A, non-B (NANB) viruses. The responsible viruses have until recently been entirely unknown but now one such virus causing about 80% of post-transfusion hepatitis as well as sporadically occurring hepatitis in the community has been recognised and named hepatitis C virus (HCV).

Hepatitis D (delta) virus. The delta virus occurs either simultaneously with an acute hepatitis B infection or as an added infection in a chronic hepatitis B carrier. It never occurs when the B virus is not present. It is diagnosed by the presence of anti-delta (anti-HD) in the blood.

Hepatitis E. This form of hepatitis resembles hepatitis A in incubation and in faecal–oral spread. It mainly causes water-borne epidemics in developing countries.

Acute hepatitis

PATHOPHYSIOLOGY

Clinical features. Acute hepatitis produces a wide range of features. The degree of severity ranges from that experienced by an asymptomatic, anicteric patient who is coincidentally found to have abnormal liver function tests denoting a hepatitis to that suffered by a patient with fulminant hepatic failure leading to death. The latter, however, is fortunately rare (1 in 1000) and most patients have generalised symptoms as listed below:

1. Prodromal illness. Flu-like symptoms lasting 2–7 days in HAV, slightly longer in HBV. Symptoms include headache, low-grade fever (37.5–38.5°C), nasal congestion, sore throat, anorexia, lethargy, mild upper abdominal pain or discomfort (right hypochondrium), arthralgia and arthritis.
2. The icteric phase. Prodromal symptoms usually disappear. Jaundice, of varying intensity, occurs but rarely causes plasma bilirubin to be above 200 μmol/l.
3. The convalescent phase. Occurs approximately 2 weeks after onset of jaundice. Jaundice lessens and eventually disappears. Other symptoms resolve.

Postviral syndrome. It is recognised that hepatitis is a common cause of a postviral syndrome in which despite liver function tests returning to normal lethargy persists for some months. Patients need to be reassured firmly as many feel that they have developed chronic liver disease.

MEDICAL AND NURSING MANAGEMENT

There is no specific treatment for acute hepatitis but advice can be given to help the patient cope with his illness. Drugs thought to have caused the hepatitis should be stopped, and no other drugs should be taken without medical advice. Whilst strict bedrest is not necessary, it is advisable for the patient to rest as much as possible and to avoid strenuous exercise. The patient may have an intolerance to fatty foods. A well-balanced, high calorie diet should be encouraged. Simple hygiene measures, such as strict handwashing, should be undertaken in the home to reduce the risk to others of infection.

Fulminant hepatic failure

PATHOPHYSIOLOGY

This is a rare condition which results in sudden massive necrosis of liver cells and severe impairment of hepatic function. The most common causes are drug-induced hepatitis and viral hepatitis, all other causes being extremely rare.

Clinical features. The patient develops encephalopathy; confusion leads to stupor and progresses rapidly to coma. Jaundice and fetor hepaticus are present and ascites may develop later. Abnormal neurological signs, cerebral oedema, hypoglycaemia, circulatory and renal failure and coagulation defects develop.

MEDICAL MANAGEMENT

The medical management of fulminant hepatic failure is supportive care of the above symptoms and management of complications such as infection. Liver transplant should be considered if early improvement does not occur so that patients can be transferred to a transplant centre before severe coma occurs.

The prognosis is extremely poor, with the survival rate being approximately 10% once deep coma has occurred. However, patients who do survive recover normal hepatic structure and function. Liver transplantation allows 50–60% of patients to survive.

The nursing care of these patients is highly specialised and is of paramount importance to the patient's recovery. For this reason, patients with fulminant hepatic failure should, if possible, be nursed in a specialist liver unit.

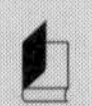
For further information, see Shearman & Finlayson (1989).

Chronic hepatitis

Hepatitis is referred to as chronic when 6 months after the onset of the illness the patient still has clinical symptoms or abnormal liver function tests. Two main forms of chronic hepatitis occur: chronic persistent hepatitis and chronic active hepatitis. A liver biopsy is necessary to determine which one is present.

Chronic persistent hepatitis

PATHOPHYSIOLOGY

This is a mild illness most often caused by one of the hepatitis viruses (not HAV). There is chronic inflammatory infiltration confined to the portal triads. There is no progression and the lobular architecture is always preserved.

Common presenting symptoms. The patient may be asymptomatic and the disease discovered only on routine testing of liver function following an acute hepatitis. A raised serum transaminase is the most likely abnormality. Patients may complain of general malaise, fatigue, anorexia, intolerance of fatty foods and alcohol, and indigestion.

MEDICAL MANAGEMENT

Although there is no specific treatment for this condition the prognosis is very good. Patients should be reassured that there is no permanent damage to their liver and that it is not necessary to restrict their diet or physical activity. In general it is thought best to avoid alcohol for 6 months, after which time it can be recommenced in moderation. These patients do not require hospital admission, except for their liver biopsy.

Chronic active hepatitis

PATHOPHYSIOLOGY

This is a more severe illness in which there is heavy infiltration of the portal triads with chronic inflammation damaging the surrounding periportal liver parenchyma. There is destruction of the lobular architecture and cirrhosis develops. It may be caused by:

- hepatitis viruses B and C.
- autoimmune antibodies. This occurs most often in females 20–40 years old.
- drugs, e.g. nitrofurantoin and isoniazid. This is uncommon but important, as withdrawing the drug is curative provided cirrhosis has not occurred.
- Wilson's disease (see p. 130).
- alpha-antitrypsin deficiency.

Clinical features. The patient will complain of fatigue, anorexia, arthralgia and arthritis. He will be mildly jaundiced with pale stools and dark urine and he may have acne or other rashes. Those with autoimmune chronic active hepatitis are more often female and may have a Cushingoid appearance, hirsutism and cutaneous striae on the abdomen and thighs. On examination the liver and spleen will be found to be enlarged and spider telangiectasis will be present. Most patients go on to develop cirrhosis, leading to portal hypertension (see p. 117), ascites and hepatic encephalopathy.

MEDICAL MANAGEMENT

If the patient feels unwell he should be encouraged to rest and to take a light but well-balanced diet. If the disease has been shown to be an autoimmune disorder the patient is prescribed prednisolone; if necessary, azathioprine may be added later. These drugs are given for their anti-inflammatory and immunosuppressive effects.

If the disease is drug-induced the offending drug is withdrawn. If hepatitis B or C is the causal agent a trial of interferon may be offered. If the condition has arisen from Wilson's disease the patient will be prescribed penicillamine.

NURSING PRIORITIES AND MANAGEMENT: ACUTE AND CHRONIC HEPATITIS

Unless the patient develops cirrhosis and its complications, it is unlikely that he will be admitted to hospital. For nursing management of complications (i.e. hepatic encephalopathy, ascites and GI haemorrhage from oesophageal varices) see page 118. Patients with HBV infection will need advice on preventing the spread of the virus, especially by sexual activity. Family members in close contact and regular sexual partners should be vaccinated, and newborns of infected women should be given hepatitis B immune globulin and vaccine to prevent what is likely to be chronic infection. Hepatitis C virus patients receive similar advice on spread, although sexual transmission is less likely.

Alcoholic hepatitis

PATHOPHYSIOLOGY

Clinical features. This condition usually follows years of alcohol abuse and often a recent prolonged bout of heavy drinking. The patient will complain of anorexia, vomiting, lethargy, diarrhoea and upper abdominal pain. A fever will be present and the patient will appear generally unwell and malnourished. Signs of chronic liver disease may be present, i.e. ascites and oedema, encephalopathy, jaundice and spider telangiectasis. GI bleeding may occur from erosions, peptic ulceration or bleeding tendencies.

The diagnosis is made from an accurate picture of the patient's alcohol intake (often obtained from relatives and friends), liver function tests and liver biopsy if the patient's clotting time allows.

Cirrhosis of the liver

Cirrhosis or scarring of the liver is a chronic condition. It is irreversible and advances slowly over a variable timespan. The most common cause is alcohol abuse.

PATHOPHYSIOLOGY

Prolonged low-grade inflammation causes progressive scarring and destruction of the liver cells. The remaining liver cells proliferate to form nodules; this results in the liver becoming irregular and distorted in shape. The blood vessels are also destroyed. The resistance to the flow of blood increases, which in turn leads to portal hypertension (see p. 117). The major complications of cirrhosis result from the hepatocellular failure and portal hypertension. These are: ascites, GI bleeding, renal dysfunction, carcinoma, and hepatic encephalopathy.

Common presenting features. As the disease progresses, the patient feels increasingly fatigued and lethargic. Anorexia, nausea and weight loss are common. Jaundice, bruising, spider telangiectasis and finger clubbing are also seen. Endocrine abnormalities such as gynaecomastia and impotence in males and amenorrhoea and infertility in females can also develop.

Hepatic encephalopathy is a chronic and recurrent feature in cirrhosis, probably due to neurotoxins which the damaged liver cannot destroy and which interfere with normal cerebral functioning.

MEDICAL MANAGEMENT

The aim of treatment is the removal of any identifiable cause such as alcohol abuse and the management of the major symptoms and complications. Liver transplantation is considered when earlier treatment fails. Considerable counselling and support may be required to eliminate an alcohol problem and improve nutrition.

The medical and nursing management of the major complications of cirrhosis of the liver — ascites, portal hypertension, oesophageal varices and hepatic encephalopathy — are considered in more detail below.

Ascites

Ascites is the abnormal accumulation of serous fluid within the peritoneal cavity. It results from a combination of the following factors:

- raised portal pressure
- increased lymphatic pressure in the liver
- low plasma protein — albumin
- sodium retention.

Box 4.11 gives further details on pathophysiology.

MEDICAL MANAGEMENT

The main components of treatment are: restriction of sodium intake, restriction of fluid intake, administration of diuretics, and abdominal paracentesis (see Box 4.12).

Box 4.11 Ascites

The term ascites refers to a marked increase in the volume of fluid in the peritoneal cavity. This is usually due to an underlying disease in which the total body fluid is increased, such as cardiac failure, cirrhosis or nephrotic syndrome, or to a local disease in the peritoneum, such as malignancy or an infection such as tuberculosis.

In health, serous fluid is continually produced in the peritoneal cavity and is sufficient to provide lubrication only, but ascites occurs when fluid enters the peritoneal cavity more quickly than it can be returned to the circulation by the capillaries and lymphatics. Fluid normally leaves a capillary at its arteriolar end and returns at its venous end, but, in cirrhosis, portal hypertension and hypoalbuminaemia combine to reduce the re-entry of peritoneal fluid at the venous end. The presence of ascites in liver disease is a poor prognostic sign as it implies poor liver function and portal hypertension.

Severe ascites can cause great discomfort: dyspnoea, anorexia and the ability to eat only small meals, inhibited mobility and discomfort when lying in bed or sitting upright in a chair. If pain occurs it is often felt in the back. Many of the symptoms correspond to the discomfort of full-term pregnancy! Increased intra-abdominal pressure also leads to hernias, especially at the umbilicus.

Ascitic fluid in cirrhosis is usually straw-coloured. Blood-stained ascites indicates malignant disease; bile staining indicates a communication with the biliary system, and cloudy fluid denotes infection. Chylous ascites, which has a milky appearance, is caused by lymphatic obstruction.

Box 4.12 Abdominal paracentesis

In intractable ascites, i.e. when sodium restrictions and diuretic therapy have little effect, it is possible to drain the fluid from the peritoneal cavity by means of a catheter inserted through the abdominal wall. This procedure is known as abdominal paracentesis. Such patients are already hypoproteinaemic and the sudden loss of fluid and protein by paracentesis is likely to lead to a shift of both from the rest of the body into the abdominal cavity, sometimes with consequent hypovolaemia, shock and even death. The protein is therefore replaced at the time of paracentesis by an infusion of salt-poor albumin. The patient's blood pressure should be monitored closely and the fluid drained no more quickly than at a rate of approximately 2 l/h. Strict aseptic technique should be used when inserting the catheter to avoid introducing infection leading to bacterial peritonitis. This procedure requires cooperation from the patient to lie relatively still in bed while the catheter is in situ over several hours. He will require help from the nursing staff to remain comfortable over this period. Any leakage on removal of the catheter can be collected in a drainable bag, e.g. a stoma bag, until the puncture site heals (usually within 48 h).

NURSING PRIORITIES AND MANAGEMENT: ASCITES

Major nursing considerations

The main aims of nursing care are as follows:

- to promote bedrest in the position most comfortable for the patient. The legs should be elevated to help reduce peripheral oedema
- to provide pressure area care. This is vital because of the oedema and the patient's likely reluctance and difficulty in moving
- to encourage mobility in order to prevent deep vein thrombosis
- to encourage the patient to eat a diet very low in salt. Daily sodium intake must be restricted to 60 mmol and to 40 mmol in severe ascites
- to ensure that the patient manages the restriction in fluid intake and understands why it is necessary. It is important to help the patient to 'pace' the fluid intake throughout the day
- to administer diuretics as prescribed. Spironolactone is the drug of choice because of its potassium-sparing properties. Fluid loss is measured by weighing the patient at the same time each day in the same clothes.
- pain may be mild and responsive to non-opioid analgesics. However, in malignant disease it can be severe and difficult to control. Strong analgesics and small doses of prednisolone are used to control this severe pain.

Portal hypertension

PATHOPHYSIOLOGY

Portal hypertension occurs when there is an obstruction in the intrahepatic or extrahepatic circulation. Hepatic cirrhosis accounts for over 90% of cases of intrahepatic hypertension in this country. Extrahepatic portal hypertension is less common. In adults it is usually due to thrombosis (as occurs in polycythaemia rubra vera), local inflammation or sepsis (as in pancreatitis), or invasion by malignant tumours.

Common clinical features. The cardinal signs of portal hypertension are splenomegaly, hypersplenism and a portal–systemic collateral circulation. These collateral vessels bleed easily, the result of which is the development of varicosities of the lower oesophageal and gastric veins. The patient most often presents with massive GI haemorrhage from these oesophageal and gastric varices (see p. 118).

MEDICAL MANAGEMENT

Investigative procedure. Diagnosis is by medical history, palpation of the abdomen, and ultrasound when splenomegaly is demonstrated. Angiography of the portal venous system will determine the cause and site of the obstruction. Endoscopy will demonstrate gastro-oesophageal varices. Hyperplenism will cause thrombocytopenia and leucopenia. Anaemia may also be present.

Medical intervention. The presenting symptoms are treated. Bleeding from oesophageal varices is treated by blood transfusion, and by sclerotherapy, which is performed at the initial endoscopy and repeated at 1–4 weekly intervals. Balloon tamponade and drugs such as vasopressin are used only to stop active bleeding until sclerotherapy is performed.

Sclerotherapy is a treatment for oesophageal varices involving the injection of an irritant solution. This causes thrombosis and obliteration of the varicosed vein.

Banding has been introduced recently for the long-term treatment of varices as it has fewer complications than sclerotherapy.

Splenectomy is particularly valuable where there is a regional portal hypertension due to obstruction in the splenic vein.

Transjugular intrahepatic portosystemic shunting (TIPS). More recently, as a result of great advances in radiological techniques, a method has been developed whereby a connecting track can be created between the portal vein and the hepatic vein. The procedure is performed under local anaesthetic and offers an alternative to sclerotherapy.

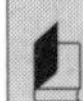
For further information, see Thomas (1992).

NURSING PRIORITIES AND MANAGEMENT

Oesophageal varices

If the patient is vomiting profusely from bleeding oesophageal varices a high-flow suction catheter should be available for intermittent suction and maintenance of a clear airway.

Blood pressure and pulse should be observed ¼-hourly and signs of hypovolaemic shock observed for (see Ch. 18).

I.v. fluids and a blood transfusion should be maintained and an accurate record of all fluid intake and output is made.

A urinary catheter is passed and urine output measured hourly during the acute phase, as under-perfusion of the kidneys due to shock can cause renal impairment.

The patient is fasted prior to transfer to theatre for endoscopy and sclerotherapy. Standard preparation is followed and on return to the ward, a clear airway and nil by mouth must be maintained until sensation and the ability to swallow have returned; the nurse must also be sure that there has been no recurrence of bleeding.

Because of the experience of either vomiting blood or passing melaena, the patient will be extremely anxious. A calm approach and clear explanations of treatment and care will be essential in order to help relieve the natural fears that extensive bleeding causes.

Should the bleeding not be arrested by the sclerotherapy a gastric or esophageal tamponade is used to stop the bleeding by balloon tamponade, i.e. compression.

Anxiety and agitation can be relieved by small i.v. doses of a benzodiazepine sedative such as midazolam. As patients with liver disease are very sensitive to sedatives, the benzodiazepine antagonist flumazenil should be immediately available. Antiemetics such as metoclopramide should be given if the patient is nauseated and retching, as this increases the pressure in the varices and could cause further haemorrhage.

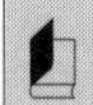
For further information, see Dewar (1985).

Hepatic encephalopathy

In encephalopathy, the priorities of care are to maintain a safe environment and to prevent further complications. The patient may be drowsy and a little unsteady when walking, or he may be fully unconsious. Care must therefore be responsive to the patient's level of function. For the very drowsy or comatose patient a protein-restricted diet will be necessary to reduce nitrogenous waste, which cannot be dealt with by the liver and will therefore accumulate. A good fluid intake is essential to prevent dehydration, and an i.v. infusion should be administered if necessary. If lactulose is being administered for its osmotic laxative effect, bowel activity should be observed and the lactulose dosage adjusted accordingly. Lactulose reduces the pH in the colon, which inhibits ammonia absorption and alters colonic bacterial metabolism so that less ammonia is produced and more nitrogen is excreted in the stool. (See Nursing Care Plan 4.1.)

Cancer of the liver

Tumours of the liver can be either primary or secondary growths. The liver is the most common site for metastatic spread and patients often present with symptoms from the secondary rather than the primary lesion.

Primary tumours

Hepatocellular carcinoma is the principal primary tumour. As it occurs predominantly in males it is thought that hormonal factors may be significant. Although hepatocellular cancer is uncommon in Europe and North America it is so common in other areas such as Africa and south east Asia as to be one of the most common cancers in the world. Chronic hepatitis B and C virus infections are the main cause of the cancers in high incidence areas. Hepatocellular carcinomas also occur in haemochromatosis and alcoholic cirrhosis of the liver.

PATHOPHYSIOLOGY

The tumour is highly vascular and occurs most frequently in the right lobe. It invades the hepatic and portal vein. The obstruction to these vessels results in portal hypertension. There may be local spread to the peritoneum or metastatic spread to the lungs or lymphatic system.

MEDICAL MANAGEMENT

Investigative procedures. A very high serum alphafetoprotein (AFP > 200 ku) is diagnostic. Ultrasound with fine-needle aspiration or biopsy at laparoscopy is performed to obtain cells for histological examination. Ultrasound, CT scan and angiography are needed to define the extent of liver involvement and venous invasion prior to a decision being taken on treatment.

Medical intervention. The first objective is to see whether the tumour is localised sufficiently in the liver to be resected surgically (see Box 4.13). Unfortunately, surgery is usually impossible, either because liver involvement is too extensive or because metastasis to other organs has occurred. Some patients may benefit from chemotherapy or chemo-embolisation of the vessels supplying the tumour (or both), but as these treatments can have unpleasant side-effects they are often reserved for patients with hepatic symptoms (see Box 4.14). Radiotherapy is of no value. Medical therapy also aims to relieve symptoms such as pain or ascites.

Secondary tumours

These are the most common malignant liver tumours and can originate from a primary growth in any part of the body.

PATHOPHYSIOLOGY

Multiple deposits are usually found, and may be sited anywhere in the liver. The histology of the cells may indicate the primary site; however, the cancer cells may be anaplastic, giving no indication of their origin.

Clinical features are as for primary malignant tumours, with signs of associated cirrhosis. Pain is often the most common symptom for which the patient seeks medical help. The abdomen will become distended due to the enlarged liver, peritoneal invasion and ascites. The patient will have difficulty in bending and is usually anorexic. Jaundice may be present. Weight loss is usually marked.

MEDICAL MANAGEMENT

Diagnosis is by fine-needle aspiration under ultrasound imaging to obtain cells for histology. If the primary site is unknown and causing no symptoms, but there are metastatic deposits in the liver, the patient is not subjected to investigations to locate the primary tumour, as outcome is determined by the spread to the liver.

Treatment must generally be restricted to symptom control, although occasionally a localised metastasis from the colon can be resected.

NURSING PRIORITIES AND MANAGEMENT: CANCER OF THE LIVER

Major patient problems

Nursing management is aimed at symptom control as well as providing the emotional support patients require when facing a terminal illness. Time should be spent with the patient so that he has the opportunity to express his thoughts, fears and anger. As the prognosis of this form of cancer is so poor,

Nursing Care Plan 4.1 Care plan for elderly man with liver failure due to alcoholic cirrhosis

Problem (actual/potential)	Reason	Nursing action
1. Anxiety, anger and fear	due to: lack of knowledge, fear of the unknown and perhaps denial of the reality of his condition.	Encourage fears to be expressed and questions to be asked. Explain all procedures and maintain a non-judgemental approach. Confidence will be restored and he will feel better able to cope.
2. Loss of self concept: • **body image** • **role performance** • **self identity** • **self esteem (McLane 1987)**	due to: physical alteration resulting from jaundice, ascites and weight loss. Loss of libido, impotence and gynaecomastia due to retention of oestrogens normally broken down in the liver.	• restore optimal liver function • provide a trusting relationship • refer to a specialist counsellor as appropriate
3. Pain and discomfort	due to: • the enlarged liver that stretches the liver capsule (the liver itself has no sensory nerve innervation) • biliary obstruction secondary to the cirrhosis gastritis due to alcohol abuse • oedema, ascites, bowel disturbance, dyspepsia and itching	Relieve pain and discomfort via: • comfort measures such as positioning, gentle movement and distraction techniques • medication for pruritis — sodium bicarbonate baths — calamine lotion — cholestyramine which binds the bile — salts in the intestines — anti-histamines • analgesics, used with caution to avoid hepatotoxic effects
4. Insomnia	due to: pain, anxiety, dyspnoea induced by ascites, itching and the strange environment	• relieve pain, anxiety, dyspnoea and itching (see above) • provide optimal peace and quiet when appropriate
5. Nutritional impairment: anorexia, anaemia and weight loss	due to: the inability of the liver to perform its metabolic functions and the reduction in production of bile. Iron, Vit B12 and red blood cells are reduced. Foetor hepaticus (a bad taste in the mouth and bad breath)	• a diet high in calories — protein* to restore plasma proteins — glucose, thought to aid liver cell recovery • supplements e.g. vitamins and iron • low salt to reduce oedema • controlled fat intake according to degree of jaundice • small tempting meals • oral hygiene • monitoring of weight * — if ammonia levels rise and features of encephalopathy present, protein reduced to 20 gm per day If anaemia becomes severe a blood transfusion and oxygen therapy may be required.
6. Fluid and electrolyte imbalance and impaired tissue perfusion	due to: • reduced arterial flow, portal hypertension, ascites • salt retention due to loss of detoxification of aldosterone and the triggering of the renin-angiotension mechanism	• reduce salt intake to no added salt (NAS) or less as necessary • fluid restriction (1–1.5 litres per day) if hyponatraemia develops • gentle use of diuretics • paracentesis if necessary
7. Infection	due to: loss of Kupffer cell function and lymphocyte production and exacerbated by nutritional, circulatory and respiratory impairment	• hygiene maintained at a high standard. Strict asepsis with any invasive techniques. Regular monitoring of vital signs • chest physiotherapy as appropriate • infection screening as appropriate • antibiotics if necessary but used with caution
8. Impaired skin integrity	due to: oedema, loss of protein, jaundice, weight loss and bleeding tendency (See problem 11)	• regular relief of pressure • sensitive care of the skin, nails and when shaving • use of emollients • optimal positioning and repositioning

Nursing Care Plan 4.1 *(Cont'd)*

Problem (actual/potential)	Reason	Nursing action
9. Immobility	due to: malaise, weakness, ascites, dyspnoea and perhaps confusion	• ensure optimal activity and rest. Provide companionship • relieve symptoms as described
10. Impaired detoxification of natural and medicinal substances	due to: liver cell damage	• careful and tactful enforcement of abstinence from alcohol • vigilance with all medications
11. Tendency to bleed that might be insidious or dramatic leading to hypovolaemic shock	due to: • portal hypertension and development of oesophageal varices • gastritis • loss of clotting factors • inadequate absorption of Vitamin K • reduced reserves of blood in the liver	• regular monitoring of vital signs • monitoring of any vomit for blood, fresh or digested • skin and mucous membranes observed for bruises or bleeding • give Vitamin K as necessary • manage hypovolaemic shock (see p. 600)
12. Encephalopathy **• lethargy** **• flapping tremor (asterixis)** **• irrational behaviour** **• aggression** **• loss of ability to perform daily duties**	due to: inability of the liver to convert ammonia to urea. Ammonia levels rise to such a level that cerebral cell damage occurs due to nitrogenous neurotoxins NB 1 a GI bleed constitutes a 'high protein meal' and will exacerbate encephalopathy 2 infection will exacerbate encephalopathy by inducing a catabolic state 3 hypoxia will exacerbate encephalopathy	• careful monitoring of behaviour and ability to communicate effectively • observe for precipitating factors, e.g. 1, 2 or 3 Management of encephalopathy: • reduce protein intake • give rectal and colonic washouts, if necessary, to remove blood from bowel • give oral Lactulose an osmotic laxative, to reduce ammonia by acidification of bowel environment and to help evacuate bowel contents; and/or ... • give oral Neomycin (poorly absorbed from the gut) to reduce intestinal floral • monitor level of consciousness (L.O.C.) • Ensure safety and comfort

Box 4.13 Surgical resection of liver tumours

Resection of liver tumours constitutes major surgery. In some cases complete removal of the tumour may be possible, depending on the site and size of the tumour and on liver function. Resection is contraindicated in patients with extensive liver cirrhosis.

Because the liver has a good capacity to regenerate, following small hepatic lobectomy the prognosis is relatively good if all of the tumour has been resected. More extensive resections carry a higher mortality rate.

The nursing management of a patient following major liver surgery is intensive and should be carried out in a specialist unit.

Box 4.14 Hepatic artery ligation and tumour embolisation

Hepatic artery ligation may give worthwhile palliation in patients with hepatocellular carcinoma. Following ligation tumour necrosis occurs. This treatment is contraindicated in patients with portal vein obstruction and cirrhosis because of the ensuing massive hepatic necrosis.

Tumour embolisation may also provide worthwhile palliation. During hepatic angiography a gelatin sponge is injected into the branches of the hepatic artery, causing tumour infarction.

Chemotherapy may also be used; if so, the drug is delivered directly into the tumour to avoid systemic side-effects.

this patient may be left with a very short time to put his affairs in order and to prepare himself and his loved ones for his impending death. His family and friends will also need support from nursing and medical staff.

Initially, the patient may be able to attend to his own needs, and may also be able to return home. However, repeated admission may be necessary for abdominal paracentesis (see Box 4.12). As his disease advances he will become progressively more dependent on nurses and/or relatives for care. Due to extreme weight loss much attention is required in maintaining intact pressure areas and oral hygiene should be given regularly in the hope of preventing moniliasis. At this point the patient and his family may appreciate the privacy of a single room, but this should not be undertaken without prior discussion with them.

DISORDERS OF THE BILIARY SYSTEM

? **4.19** With the help of your physiology textbook, review the structure and function of the biliary system.

Cholelithiasis

Cholelithiasis (the presence of gallstones) is the commonest disorder of the biliary tree. It is more prevalent among women than men and its incidence appears to be increasing. In developed countries at least 20% of women over 40 will develop gallstones. Until about 20 years ago the most likely person to develop gallstones was an obese woman in her forties with fair skin ('fair, fat, female and forty'). This categorisation is now considered outdated as, for unknown reasons, gallstones are now affecting people at a much younger age.

PATHOPHYSIOLOGY

Gallstones are formed from the constituents of bile salts. They occur in three main types:

- mixed stones (mainly cholesterol): 75%
- pure cholesterol stones (a 'solitaire' that fills the gallbladder): 10%
- pigmented stones ('jack stones', black and shiny): 2–3%.

Stones vary in size and shape, and may be solitary or multiple. Their colour can vary from yellow to dark brown.

Biliary colic

Gallstones can be asymptomatic but more often they cause biliary colic or an acute or chronic cholecystitis. Cholecystitis can also, less commonly, be caused by trauma and, even more rarely, by tumours.

PATHOPHYSIOLOGY

Biliary colic is caused by a transient obstruction of the gallbladder from an impacted stone.

Common presenting symptoms. The patient complains of a sudden onset of severe gripping pain in the right hypochondrium which often radiates to the back. It can be associated with nausea and vomiting. The pain may vary in intensity and can last for several hours. The pain will ease when the stone either passes into the common bile duct or falls back into the gallbladder.

MEDICAL MANAGEMENT

The patient will recover quickly but repeated bouts of colic are common. Following investigations a cholecystectomy may be performed.

Acute cholecystitis

PATHOPHYSIOLOGY

It is thought that in this condition gallstones irritate the mucous membrane of the gallbladder, which then becomes inflamed.

Common presenting symptoms. The patient presents with an acute illness which is severe in nature. He may be in shock due to pain and vomiting.

A mass may be felt and Murphy's sign (a catching of the breath at the height of inspiration when the gallbladder is palpated) is usually positive. The pain will be severe in the right hypochondrium and may radiate to the right shoulder tip.

Tenderness and guarding of the whole abdomen may be present and the patient may not tolerate examination. Sweating and pallor may be present.

Pyrexia and tachycardia will be present due to infection. Jaundice may be present if there is obstruction of the common bile duct; in this case the patient will have a history of pale stools and dark urine. A history of fatty intolerance may also be given; the pain often starts following a fatty meal.

MEDICAL MANAGEMENT

Investigative procedures. Tests that may be used to establish a diagnosis are as follows:

- plain abdominal X-ray
- ultrasound
- oral cholecystogram
- intravenous cholangiogram
- ERCP (endoscopic retrograde cholangiopancreatography).

Ultrasound is now the main investigative procedure for patients with suspected gallstones. It is non-invasive, causes minimal discomfort to the patient and can be used on both jaundiced and non-jaundiced patients. It can identify stones in the gallbladder, thickening of the gallbladder wall and intra- and extrahepatic duct dilatation. It can be done quickly and is relatively inexpensive.

Medical intervention. The treatment of gallstones is usually by surgical removal of the gallbladder with or without exploration of the common bile duct. Some surgeons prefer to wait for about 6 weeks following an acute attack, i.e. until the inflammation has fully resolved, before performing a cholecystectomy. However, it has become accepted practice to operate within 72 h of onset of the attack, since provided this is done under antibiotic cover complications are minimal and the patient's stay in hospital will be much shorter. Moreover, with an 'early' cholecystectomy the patient is not at risk of further attacks of acute cholecystitis while waiting for elective surgery. Removal of gallstones can also be performed by ERCP and sphincterotomy. In more specialised centres surgeons are now performing laparoscopic cholecystectomy.

Laparoscopic cholecystectomy. The advantages to the patient of this procedure are:

- reduced stay in hospital
- early mobilisation with lower risk of complications
- minor nature of surgical wounds
- reduced need for opiate analgesia
- speedy return to normal life.

The procedure is performed with the patient under general anaesthetic. The surgeon passes a laparoscope into the abdomen at the umbilicus. He then insufflates the abdomen with CO_2 to allow clear visualisation of the gallbladder.

Three more incisions are made in the region of the right hypochondrium to allow instruments to be manipulated. The cystic artery is identified and ligated. The cystic duct is identified, at which stage an intraoperative cholangiogram can be done to check for stones in the common bile duct. If stones are present these can be reduced immediately.

By careful dissection the gallbladder is then removed from the liver bed. It is brought to the undersurface of the umbilicus, where the stones are extracted and the gallbladder removed.

All stab wounds are then sutured. On return from theatre, immediate nursing care is as for any routine general anaesthetic.

Free fluids can be given when the patient has fully recovered from the general anaesthetic. Normal diet is commenced the following day. Most patients are discharged on the 2nd or 3rd postoperative day.

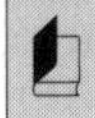

For further information, see Johnson (1993).

NURSING PRIORITIES AND MANAGEMENT: ACUTE CHOLECYSTITIS

Immediate concerns

Patients experiencing an acute opisode of cholecystitis will be severely ill and will be referred to hospital as quickly as possible after being seen by their GP. The priorities of care while the attack is being managed before surgical intervention include the following:

- administration of an i.m. opiate analgesic at frequent intervals. Pethidine 100 mg is the drug of choice. Morphine can cause spasm at the sphincter of Oddi, but when it is used it is very effective
- hourly recording of vital signs until the patient's condition stabilises
- fasting the patient and commencing i.v. fluids
- careful monitoring of fluid and electrolyte balance

- i.v. administration of a broad-spectrum antibiotic
- if vomiting is persistent an NG tube may be passed and an antiemetic given.

Major patient problems

The patient will be restless due to the pain and will be unable to make himself comfortable. He should be nursed in bed in the most comfortable position for him and given regular analgesics. Fear of pain and the unknown increases pain (see Ch. 19). It is therefore vital to explain what is happening and to assure the patient that his condition can be treated. When the patient's condition is stable he should be introduced to his surroundings and given information about the ward, visiting times, mealtimes, etc.

Once the acute phase has passed fluids can be given and foods gradually reintroduced. The i.v. infusion may be discontinued when the patient can manage an adequate oral intake. I.v. antibiotics are usually given for 5 days and then discontinued.

Sweating can be a problem and frequent washes and changes of bedclothes may be necessary to keep the patient comfortable. Oral hygiene should be maintained as necessary.

While the patient is in bed he should be encouraged to change his position at frequent intervals to alleviate pressure. He should be taught gentle leg exercises to prevent deep venous thrombosis. If he can tolerate taking deep breaths to avoid pulmonary complications he should be encouraged to do so. Smoking should be discouraged.

Perioperative care

Cholecystectomy is carried out on patients with acute cholecystitis to relieve symptoms and prevent complications. In chronic cholecystitis the patient's general condition must be taken into account, particularly if he is elderly or suffering from other medical conditions which may increase the risks of surgery. Exploration of the common bile duct will be undertaken if there is evidence of stones in the common bile ducts, biliary colic, jaundice or dilatation of the bile ducts.

Nursing care following an open cholecystectomy

In this procedure the surgeon approaches the gallbladder through a subcostal paramedian or midline incision. An intraoperative cholangiogram is performed to identify any stones in the common bile duct. If stones are present, the surgeon will explore the duct, remove the stones, insert a T-tube and bring the long leg of the tube out through a stab wound in the abdominal wall and then connect it to a drainage bag. It is vital that this tube is not removed accidentally (see Box 4.15). A T-tube cholangiogram is done 8–10 days postoperatively to ensure patency of the duct prior to removal. If the ducts are stone free the tube will be removed following instructions from the surgeon. (See Fig. 4.13.)

Immediate postoperative care is as for any major abdominal surgery requiring general anaesthesia. Adequate analgesia is vital so that the patient can perform deep breathing and coughing exercises to prevent atelectasis and pneumonia. In most cases the anaesthetist will perform an intercostal nerve block and top it up at regular intervals so that the patient is pain free. This can be supplemented with i.m. or i.v. analgesia given regularly over the first 24–48 h. The nurse should check at regular intervals that the incision site and surrounding area are numb to ensure the intercostal nerve block is working effectively. The patient should be raised in an upright position and encouraged to do his breathing exercises to prevent pulmonary complications.

There is usually a wound drain inserted to the gallbladder bed. Careful observation of the colour and amount of blood draining postoperatively is vital. Excessive drainage of bright red blood must be reported immediately to the surgeon. This drain is usually removed 24–48 h postoperatively.

Other considerations. The patient may be commenced on fluids gradually after the first 24 h (30–60 ml/h). If this is tolerated free fluids may be commenced. Diet is gradually increased over the next 3 days. An NG tube is not used unless the patient shows signs of paralytic ileus. In this case the patient should be fasted, an NG tube passed and the stomach kept empty.

Sutures are removed 7–10 days postoperatively unless, as has become more common, a subcutaneous suture is used, in which case there will be no need to remove it. If the wound is dry and clean, the dressing can be removed 24–48 h postoperatively and the wound left exposed.

Depending on the patient's fitness and age, he can usually be discharged in 6–10 days. Discharge plans will need to be discussed with relatives or carers. The patient must be instructed to do no heavy lifting for 4–6 weeks to avoid wound herniation. Normal diet is allowed but if the patient is unable to tolerate fats these should be avoided. In an uncomplicated recovery the patient should be fit to return to work 4–6 weeks later. A detailed discharge summary will be sent to the GP, who will then certify when the patient is fit for work. A follow-up appointment will be given for 4 weeks after discharge so that the surgeon can make sure that the outcome is satisfactory. (See Case History 4.3.)

Box 4.15 Management of a T-tube

A T-tube is inserted into the common bile duct following exploration. This tube is necessary as a 'safety valve' because following surgery the duct will become inflamed and oedematous, blocking the flow of bile into the duodenum. Approximately 300–500 ml of bile should drain in the first 24 h. This amount will gradually decrease over the next 8–10 days as the patency of the duct returns. An accurate recording of the amount of bile must be made. The presence of insufficient or excessive bile must be reported. When there is a sudden cessation of bile drainage, a kinked or compressed tube must be suspected.

It is also important to support the bile drainage bag at all times to prevent traction on the tube and accidental removal. An aseptic technique must be used when emptying or changing the bag. Daily cleaning of the skin at the drain site is necessary and the nurse should check for bile leakage from around the tube, inflammation, or excoriation of the skin. Any excess tubing should be coiled and taped to the abdomen. Prior to removal a T-tube choliangiogram will be done to check the patency of the bile duct and the flow of bile into the duodenum. If the duct is patent the tube is removed. If there are residual stones in the duct the T-tube is left in situ. These residual stones may pass spontaneously into the duodenum; otherwise it will be necessary to remove them under X-ray vision.

Prior to performing a T-tube cholangiogram some surgeons ask for the T-tube to be clamped for 24 h. This procedure is, however, becoming less common. If there is any complaint of abdominal pain whilst the tube is clamped it must be respected and the clamp removed immediately.

The patient will require analgesia 30 min before the tube is removed. The skin suture is removed and a firm steady pressure applied to the tube. The nurse should observe the amount of bile leakage following removal and apply a sterile dressing. Observation of the patient for any signs of biliary peritonitis should be made for 24 h.

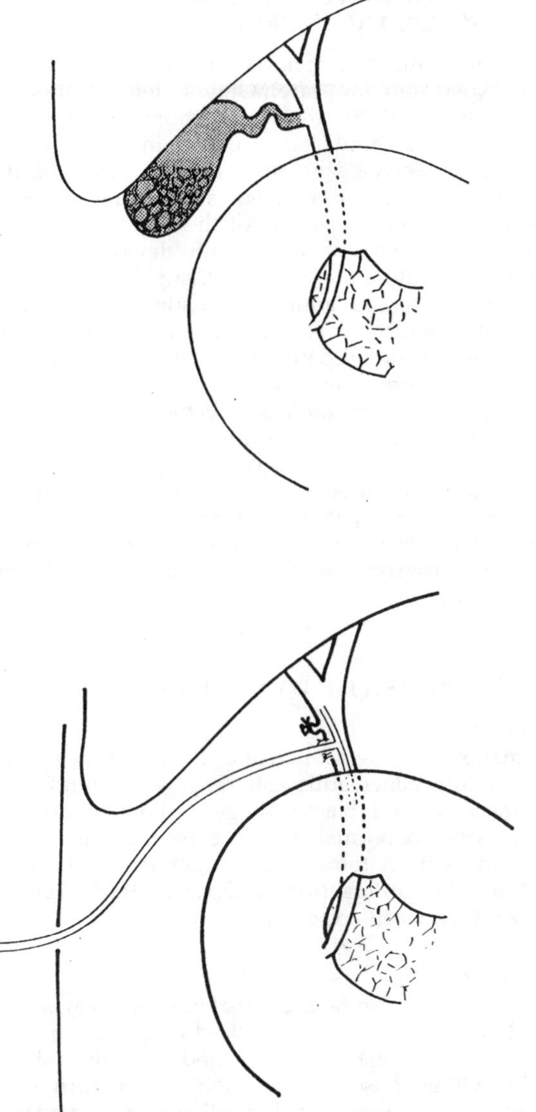

Fig. 4.13 The T-tube in the common bile duct. (Reproduced with kind permission from Whitehead 1988.)

Chronic cholecystitis

PATHOPHYSIOLOGY

Chronic cholecystitis is caused by the presence of stones in the gallbladder. In this condition the gallbladder wall becomes thickened and fibrosed.

Common presenting symptoms. The patient may present with biliary colic but more often complains of pain in the right upper quadrant of the abdomen, often following a big meal. There will be a history of fat intolerance, flatulence and heartburn. Abdominal distension may also be a problem following meals.

The pain is less severe than in acute cholecystitis and patients often put up with their symptoms for years before seeking medical advice.

MEDICAL MANAGEMENT

Investigative procedures. Tests and investigations are as for acute cholecystitis.

Medical intervention. Usually the diseased gallbladder is removed, either by an open cholecystectomy or, more commonly now, by a laparoscopic cholecystectomy. If, for whatever reason, surgery is inadvisable, medication to dissolve the stones, i.e. chenodeoxycholic acid (e.g. Chendol) may be prescribed. The application of this drug is, however, limited.

Case History 4.3 Mrs G

Mrs G had suffered from episodes of cholecystitis and biliary colic for many months before she finally went to her GP. She was a busy mother of three and, as she recounted at a later date, 'There really was no time to be going to the doctor. Besides, the pain always went eventually, especially if my husband rubbed my back up between the shoulder blades.'

Eventually, when she felt so ill that she was forced to stay in bed, she 'gave in'.

The investigations and surgery passed uneventfully in surgical terms, as she had been quite well and free from symptoms at the time of admission. Unlike her sister in London, she had had an open cholecystectomy. It was the first time she had had an operation and, although she thought the nurses were wonderful and had explained everything, she later remarked that 'No one ever tells you just how awful the first day after the operation really is.'

Within 10 days, Mrs G was at home once more, delighted that at least her sutures were dissolvable ones. She knew that she must not do too much lifting and that although she should have a normal diet, she should avoid fatty foods as they might make her feel 'squeamish'. 'It's like only having weak washing-up liquid to deal with greasy dishes instead of good concentrated liquid,' she explained to a friend.

Three weeks after discharge, she visited the doctor. She was quite distressed and reported the following problems: 'I keep having episodes of diarrhoea and I'm so tired. No one said who was going to do the hoovering or put the shopping away in those high cupboards. The family think I'm back to normal because the wound is healed but I am so tired still. Everything is an effort.'

 For further information, see Smith (1992).

Choledocholithiasis

Stones in the bile duct occur in about 10–15% of patients with gallstones.

PATHOPHYSIOLOGY

Common presenting symptoms. Colicky pain occurs if the stones impede the flow of bile through the sphincter of Oddi. Impaction of a stone at the sphincter will cause jaundice. The patient will have pale, fatty stools and dark urine. Some stones will clear spontaneously following passage into the small intestine.

If the stone becomes impacted, the bile duct will become dilated. Infection can cause cholangitis with rigors, severe pain and jaundice. Acute pancreatitis may develop due to obstruction of the sphincter of Oddi and reflux of bile salts into the pancreatic ducts (see p. 124).

MEDICAL MANAGEMENT

Investigative procedures are as for acute and chronic cholecystitis.

Medical intervention. Removal of the stones via ERCP and sphincterotomy to allow the stones to pass freely into the small intestine will be carried out.

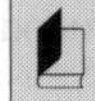 For further information, see Howard (1989).

Tumours of the biliary tract

Cancer of the gallbladder

PATHOPHYSIOLOGY

This is a rare cancer and is nearly always related to gallstones. It is more common in females than in males. Signs and symptoms are consistent with those for gallstones and a history of persistent obstructive jaundice may be present. A mass may be palpable. In most cases surgery is not a chosen treatment and survival rates are poor.

Cancer of the bile duct (cholangiocarcinoma)

PATHOPHYSIOLOGY

The cause of bile duct cancer is unknown. It is more common in the elderly, and men are affected more than women. It is a rare cancer but its incidence appears to be increasing. Patients with ulcerative colitis have a high incidence of cholangiocarcinoma which is aggressive in nature. Tumours can arise from the intra- or extrahepatic ducts. Direct spread and metastases are present in at least half of the cases that go for surgery. The main areas of spread are the portal vein, hepatic artery, pancreas, duodenum and gallbladder.

MEDICAL MANAGEMENT

Medical intervention. As cancer of the bile ducts carries a poor prognosis treatment is usually in the form of palliative therapy. Jaundice is a very distressing symptom and if this is not treated the patient may die from liver failure.

For some patients palliation can be achieved by the insertion of a stent tube, either by ERCP or by percutaneous transhepatic techniques. In a few cases where the tumour is at the lower end of the common bile duct a radical resection in the form of a Whipple resection may be possible (see Fig. 4.14). This is major surgery and should be considered only if the tumour is localised and there is a good chance of success, and if the patient is fit for major surgery.

Tumours of the upper biliary tract are resectable only in about 10% of cases. Following resection of the tumour a Roux loop of jejunum is anastomosed to the biliary tract or, in some cases, the left hepatic duct. A hepaticojejunostomy then restores the continuity of the small intestine. A hepaticojejunostomy can also be performed to bypass the tumour and achieve palliation. Radiotherapy and chemotherapy have not been shown to improve survival.

NURSING PRIORITIES AND MANAGEMENT: CHOLANGIOCARCINOMA

The patient with a diagnosis of cholangiocarcinoma will require expert nursing care. Only a few of these patients will be considered for major resection; following resection these individuals should be cared for in a high dependency ward or an intensive care unit. In some cases the patient is prepared for major resection but at the time of surgery it is discovered that only a bypass of the tumour may be carried out safely. These patients are usually devastated by this turn of events and require a great deal of support.

Following palliation jaundice will subside and the patient's appetite will improve. For a few months the patient may feel so well that he becomes unrealistic about the prognosis. Few patients survive more than a year following palliation. Following resection the outlook is better.

Expert family support is necessary. It is important to take an honest approach and to give explanations to the patient and his family as they request it. It will be necessary to spend time with the patient and his relatives to answer their questions and offer support. Close communication with the GP is also necessary so that community care can be provided when necessary.

DISORDERS OF THE PANCREAS

Pancreatitis

Inflammation of the pancreatic gland may be acute or chronic. Acute pancreatitis can range from mild oedema to severe necrosis and haemorrhage. Following an attack the gland returns to normal. Chronic pancreatitis is associated with permanent anatomical and functional abnormality. The patient usually suffers from relapsing attacks with relative good health between episodes.

Acute pancreatitis

Acute pancreatitis can be life threatening and carries a mortality of about 10%. It can affect all adult groups. In the UK its two main causes are gallstones and excessive alcohol consumption. Other causes are infection, trauma, drugs (e.g. steroids), hyperparathyroidism, hyperlipaemia, pancreatic cancer and investigation procedures (ERCP, angiography).

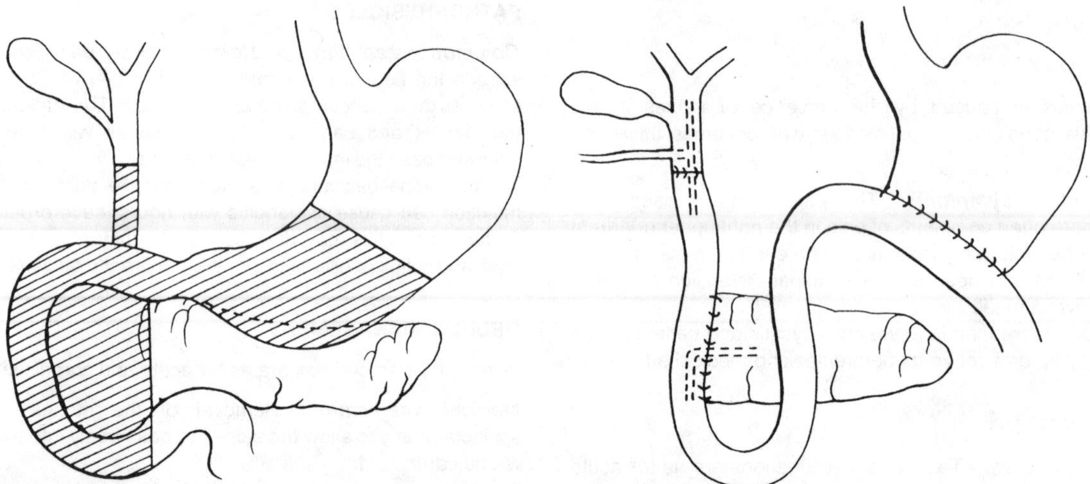

Fig. 4.14 Whipple's procedure. This extensive procedure involves resection of the head of the pancreas, the duodenum and the antrum of the stomach, as well as removal of the gallbladder. Reconstruction is carried out with choledochojejunostomy, pancreatojejunostomy and gastrojejunostomy. This is a major operation which carries a relatively high mortality rate. Leakage from the anastomosis, abscess formation and fistula are the main complications. (Reproduced with kind permission from Forrest et al 1991.)

PATHOPHYSIOLOGY

The pancreatic enzymes trypsin and lipase, which are normally activated in the duodenum, are prematurely activated within the pancreas, causing autodigestion of the gland. This autodigestion leads to varying degrees of oedema, haemorrhage, necrosis, abscess and cyst formation in and around the pancreas. Spasm of the sphincter of Oddi with reflux of duodenal contents into the pancreatic duct is thought to be an important factor in this enzyme activation. Gallstones and alcohol are two contributing factors to spasm. Passage of stones down the common bile duct may also promote reflux of infected bile along the pancreatic duct when these ducts form a common channel to the ampulla of Vater.

Activated enzymes such as trypsinogen and chymotrypsinogen, phospholipase, elastase and catalase are responsible for increased capillary permeability. This permits large volumes of fluid to escape into the peritoneal and retroperitoneal cavity, causing damage to the surrounding tissue. This severe loss of circulating fluid leads to hypovolaemic shock and predisposes the individual to acute renal failure, which may result from local intravascular coagulation in the renal vascular bed. Development of pulmonary oedema with left-sided pleural effusion may result from release of toxins. The release of lipase causes fat necrosis in the omentum and areas adjacent to the pancreas. Calcium soaps become sequestered in areas of fatty necrosis, which may result in the development of hypocalcaemia.

MEDICAL MANAGEMENT

History and examination. The patient usually presents with epigastric pain of acute onset radiating to the back, associated with nausea and vomiting. He may have a history of biliary tract disease or alcohol abuse.

Acute pancreatitis is often associated with severe shock. There may be signs of dehydration with rapid pulse and respiration, hypotension and pyrexia. Marked abdominal tenderness is usually present in the upper abdomen, which may look distended. Bruising around the umbilicus (Cullen's sign) and in the loin region (Grey Turner's sign) are rare late manifestations of acute pancreatitis.

Investigative procedures include blood analysis, urinalysis, X-ray ultrasound and CT scan, as follows:

- A serum amylase of above 1000 iu/l in the past 48 h is strongly suggestive of acute pancreatitis. Normal levels are 100–300 iu/l. Urinary amylase can remain elevated for 10–14 days.
- Plain X-ray films of the abdomen can reveal distended loops of small bowel with paralytic ileus. Chest X-ray may reveal left-sided pleural effusion.
- Urea and electrolyte levels are important indicators of the state of hydration and are necessary for the correct management of the patient.
- A raised white blood cell count (9000–20 000 μl) reveals an active inflammatory process.
- Hyperglycaemia and glycosuria are often present but are transient.
- Arterial blood gases may reveal severe hypoxia.
- Abdominal ultrasound and CT scan are used to detect the presence of peripancreatic collections and pancreatic necrosis.

Treatment. Acute pancreatitis is usually managed conservatively; for mild attacks, treatment is generally symptomatic. The principles of management are as follows:

1. Pain relief. This is usually provided in the form of opiate analgesics. Morphine and pethidine can cause some spasm at the sphincter of Oddi, but they are frequently prescribed and are effective (Forrest et al 1991).
2. Correction of shock. If haemorrhagic pancreatitis is diagnosed shock is treated by the administration of large volumes of crystalloids, plasma, dextran or blood in order to maintain circulatory blood volume and adequate urine output. Oxygen therapy is essential to correct the associated hypoxia. Hypoxaemia may develop insidiously such that respiratory failure (ARDS) can develop. Arterial blood gases are closely monitored in case ventilatory support is required. (See Chs 18, 29, and 2.)
3. Suppression of pancreatic function. The patient is fasted to decrease stimulation of pancreatic enzymes and an NG tube is passed if the patient is persistently vomiting.
4. Controlling infection. When there is evidence of infection a broad-spectrum antibiotic is prescribed. For the majority of patients this supportive treatment will settle the acute attack and surgical treatment will not be necessary. If there is any doubt about the diagnosis a laparotomy may need to be performed to exclude other causes of peritonitis, such as perforated peptic ulcer and mesenteric ischaemia.
5. Monitoring blood glucose levels. This must be performed as secondary diabetes can sometimes develop, requiring insulin therapy.
6. Monitoring cardiac status. This will be required if electrolyte derangement is such as to cause potentially lethal dysrhythmias.

Surgical intervention. At an early stage in management the presence of gallstones as a cause of the acute attack are excluded by ultrasound scanning. Cholecystectomy during the course of the patient's admission is now advocated to avoid recurrent problems following discharge. Patients with stone pancreatitis can usually be identified by their slow clinical progress and by the use of various clinical and biochemical prognosis factors.

Early ERCP may demonstrate the presence of stones in the common bile duct which can be extracted by a small balloon catheter or basket following sphincterotomy. The complication of peripancreatic necrosis or abscess can be detected by radiological imaging (see Appendix 1). Most patients will require necrosectomy (i.e. the removal of necrotic tissues) and drainage at laparotomy. It may be wise to place a gastrostomy and jejunostomy tube at this time, as recovery is slow and the patient may require prolonged nutritional support (see Ch. 21).

NURSING PRIORITIES AND MANAGEMENT: ACUTE PANCREATITIS

Major considerations (see Case History 4.4)

The care of patients with acute pancreatitis will vary according to the severity of the attack. Some individuals present with vague abdominal pain which resolves quickly. More often, patients present with severe epigastric pain, often radiating to the back, and with vomiting and shock. It should be borne in mind that the severity of the attack is not always easily judged by an initial assessment and that these patients therefore require close observation.

Priorities of nursing care are:

- to relieve pain and promote comfort (See Nursing Care Plan 4.2)
- to monitor vital functions
- to restore and maintain haemodynamic status, i.e. to restore volume deficit, correct electrolyte imbalance and correct impaired gaseous exchange
- to restore and maintain adequate nutrition
- to prevent or minimise potential complications (see Box 4.16)
- to prevent the development of pressure sores

Case History 4.4 (See Nursing Care Plan 4.2)

Mr N, aged 36, is admitted with a history of sudden, central abdominal pain which is only partially relieved by sitting forward and hugging his knees. He describes the pain as 'boring through his back'. His skin is pale and clammy and his respirations rapid and shallow, his pulse is rapid and there is marked hypotension. Mr N is clearly in an advancing state of shock. In addition, he is nauseated and repeated vomiting has led to increasing dehydration, exacerbating his shocked state.

Nursing Care Plan 4.2 Care of a patient with acute pancreatitis (See Case History 4.4): The management of pain.

Nursing consideration	Action	Rationale	Desired outcome
1. *Pain* Mr N has severe and potentially excruciating pain due to autodigestion of the pancreas, the 'chemical burn' of pancreatic exudate, inflammation, and distention caused by an adynamic bowel.	• Rapidly assess and then monitor verbal and non-verbal evidence of pain, noting factors that either aggravate or ease the pain.	To assist in achieving effective pain relief.	Mr N's pain is relieved, as evidenced by the verbal communication, body relaxation and corresponding changes in vital signs.
	• Give the prescribed analgesic. (Pethidine is the drug of choice.)	Although all opiates may cause some spasm of the sphincter of Oddi, pethidine has proved very effective (Forrest et al 1991). As analgesia is achieved smaller doses and less frequent doses may be given.	
	• Give other adjuvant medication, e.g. antibiotic therapy, sedative agents, H_2 antagonists, anti-emetics.	Such agents may be used to help control the acute attack and associated symptoms, particularly pain.	
	• Pass an NG tube and aspirate stomach contents.	This will relieve the pain associated with distention and minimise pancreatic stimulation	
	• Position Mr N as comfortably as possible, minimising any unnecessary activity.	Pain will be minimised, as will Mr N's metabolic rate and pancreatic activity.	

Box 4.16 Complications of acute pancreatitis

PANCREATIC PSEUDOCYST

This condition develops in about 10% of patients following acute pancreatitis or an exacerbation of chronic pancreatitis. A pseudocyst is a sac containing pancreatic juice, debris and blood within a lining of inflammatory tissue, directly connecting with a pancreatic duct. Small pseudocysts are often asymptomatic but large cysts can compress surrounding structures, often causing pain, nausea, vomiting and, occasionally, obstructive jaundice. A raised serum amylase will be present. Ultrasound scan can be used in diagnosis and monitoring. Surgery is necessary if the cyst is symptomatic, since there is a danger that it may rupture or precipitate haemorrhage. Surgery consists of drainage of the pseudocyst into the stomach (cyst gastrostomy) or duodenum (cyst duodenostomy).

PANCREATIC ABSCESS

This is a more serious complication of acute pancreatitis. The patient is usually very ill, with pyrexia, a raised white blood cell count, and tachycardia. Early diagnosis by CT scanning and the use of aggressive surgical intervention have improved mortality rates. Surgery consists of extensive drainage and debridement of infected tissues. Multiple large drains are used to drain the abscess cavity. Peritoneal lavage with normal saline 0.9% warmed to body temperature can be used to irrigate the cavity. Adequate nutrition following surgery is vital. Most surgeons establish a feeding jejunostomy and gastrostomy tube during surgery.

PANCREATIC NECROSIS

This complication is a major cause of death in acute pancreatitis. Early diagnosis is essential. The patient often fails to improve with conservative management. A persistent pyrexia, raised white blood cell count, tachycardia, hypotension and poor respiratory function are ominous signs. At laparotomy necrotic tissue is removed, peritoneal lavage is carried out and the pancreatic bed adequately drained. A feeding jejunostomy and gastrostomy tube are inserted.

In some cases the surgeon may opt to leave the wound open to allow for open packing of the wound and minimise the need for repeated laparatomies to deal with recurrent intra-abdominal sepsis.

DUODENAL ILEUS

Duo to persistent pancreatic inflammation duodenal ileus may persist. Nutritional status will need to be maintained either by parenteral means or by jejunostomy feeding. A gastroenterostomy may need to be performed.

HAEMORRHAGE

Severe bleeding may occur from gastric or duodenal ulceration. Prophylactic i.v. cimetidine is given to patients with acute pancreatitis. On rare occasions haemorrhage may occur into a pseudocyst or by erosion of a blood vessel by the inflammatory process.

- to maintain the NG tube if present and provide frequent mouthwashes and oral hygiene
- to monitor blood sugar level in order to detect secondary diabetes
- to support the patient in maintaining personal hygiene
- to help the patient to mobilise as early as possible.

As the patient's general condition improves clear oral fluids can be introduced, gradually progressing to a light diet.

An episode of pancreatitis can be a very traumatic time for both the patient and his family, who may have been unaware of the important functions that the pancreas performs. It is important to explain the rationale of all procedures and investigations carefully to alleviate anxiety. Showing the patient diagrams can be very helpful. The patient may be very worried about his work, family and financial situation, and a visit from the social worker may be of value. Patients with alcohol-associated acute pancreatitis may with their consent be referred for counselling to address their dependency problem (see Ch. 37).

It is important to reduce the noise level on the hospital ward to a minimum to allow patients to get adequate sleep (see Ch. 25). It may be advisable to give some form of night sedation. Restricting visits by family and friends to short periods during the day will reduce the strain on the patient during visiting hours. Communication with the family is of course vital. On the patient's admission to the ward the nurse should introduce herself to his relatives and give a full explanation of what has occurred. Medical staff should be available to give regular updates on the patient's condition.

Further considerations

When the acute episode has resolved, and if gallstones are present, an early elective cholecystectomy with possible exploration of the common bile duct will be undertaken.

If the attack has been due to alcohol, the patient must be advised prior to discharge to abstain totally or risk a life-threatening recurrence. Advice regarding return to work is important. The patient often feels tired and it is often advisable for the patient not to return to work for perhaps 4–6 weeks. The patient will be reviewed in the outpatient clinic initially at 3–4 weeks. A detailed account of the patient's management will be sent to the GP so that continuity of care can be maintained.

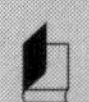

For further information, see Moorhouse et al (1988).

Chronic pancreatitis

Chronic pancreatitis is a relatively rare condition in the UK but its incidence is increasing due to the increase in alcohol consumption.

However, the mechanism by which alcohol damages the pancreas is poorly understood.

PATHOPHYSIOLOGY

Chronic pancreatitis leads to permanent damage of the gland with replacement by fibrotic tissue and calcification. The ducts become narrowed and the flow of pancreatic juice is obstructed. The cells slowly stop secreting pancreatic juice. The obstructed ducts can give rise to recurrent attacks of pancreatitis lasting a few days.

Common presenting symptoms. The patient usually presents with a history of severe epigastric pain, often radiating to the back. The pain is often eased by bending forward. Nausea and vomiting may also be present. A history of recent alcohol abuse may be given.

? **4.20** Why might bending forward ease the pain in chronic pancreatitis?

Weight loss is common, and may be due to the pain or to malnutrition associated with alcohol. Malabsorption is also present as a result of pancreatic insufficiency. The stool may be pale and offensive and difficult to flush away. This is often a distressing feature for the patient.

Diabetes mellitus develops in about ⅓ of these patients and may require treatment. Transient jaundice may be present due to inflammation of the head of the pancreas, which obstructs the common bile duct. The presence of jaundice may be upsetting for some people, who feel 'dirty' or 'old' due to the discoloration of the skin and the marked yellowness of the sclera.

MEDICAL MANAGEMENT

Investigative procedures. Clinical assessment is as follows:

- plain abdominal X-ray may show speckled calcification of the pancreas
- ultrasound scan and CT scan may show an enlarged, swollen gland
- ERCP is performed to outline the pancreatic duct if surgery is contemplated
- faecal fat estimation may reveal malabsorption
- fasting blood sugars are assessed and a glucose tolerance test may be necessary.

Medical intervention. Management of chronic pancreatitis is mainly symptomatic. The patient should be advised to stop drinking alcohol and may need professional counselling to this end. Replacement of pancreatic enzymes with a commercial preparation may help alleviate the steatorrhoea and reduce pain. Good control of diabetes will be necessary.

Pain control can be difficult, since some of these patients are addicted to opiates. Help from a pain control specialist is valuable. In a small number of patients in whom severe pain persists surgery will be indicated. It may be necessary to resect the head of the gland (Whipple's procedure; see Fig. 4.14) or the body and tail (distal pancreatectomy). Adequate drainage of the duct (pancreato-jejunostomy) may be undertaken where ERCP shows the pancreatic duct to be dilated. A total pancreatectomy is rarely undertaken due to the consequent permanent diabetes and exocrine insufficiency.

NURSING PRIORITIES AND MANAGEMENT: CHRONIC PANCREATITIS

Nursing management of an acute attack in relapsing pancreatitis is similar to that for acute pancreatitis.

Major patient problems

Pain

Pain is often constant in nature, radiating through to the back. It is often described as being like a sharp knife twisting in the gut and presents a major challenge to pain control. Assisting the patient into a comfortable position often helps. The patient may find that bending forward while leaning on a bed table helps. The use of a heat pad to the back may give some relief. The use of non-steroidal anti-inflammatory drugs (NSAIDs) such as diclofenac sodium (Voltarol) in suppository form can be of value. It may be necessary to seek advice from a pain specialist.

Alcohol dependency

Alcohol abuse is the most common cause of chronic pancreatitis. Total abstinence will help resolve the pain. If the patient has had a recent 'binge', sudden withdrawal may precipitate delirium tremens. Mild sedation is frequently used to prevent this. Expert help may be necessary to assist the patient to overcome his alcohol problem.

Patient education is vital in view of the progressive destruction of the gland by this disease. Family life is usually already disrupted by the patient's alcohol abuse, and help from a social worker will be useful in assisting the patient and his family to cope with the situation. Good liaison with the GP is important so that support can be continued in the community. Caring for these patients can present a professional and personal challenge to members of the multidisciplinary team, who may feel inclined to blame the patient for his illness.

Malnutrition

The patient's nutritional intake must be assessed. The patient is weighed and a well-balanced diet low in fat is given once the acute attack has resolved. Pancreatic enzyme supplements can be prescribed and taken prior to meals to aid absorption of nutrients. This should also alleviate the steatorrhoea. Concurrent administration of an H_2 receptor antagonist may improve the efficacy of these supplements.

Cancer of the pancreas

Tumours of the pancreas can arise from exocrine or endocrine tissue. Benign tumours are very rare. Insulinoma arises from the islet cells and results in oversecretion of insulin, causing hypoglycaemia. Gastrinomas also arise from the islet of Langerhans cells, secreting gastrin and giving rise to Zollinger–Ellison syndrome. Adenocarcinoma is by far the most common malignant tumour of the exocrine pancreas.

The cause of pancreatic cancer is unknown but smoking and a high-fat, high-protein diet are thought to increase the risk. It is twice as common in men as in women and its incidence is increasing. It is the fourth most common cause of cancer deaths in men in the UK and the sixth most common in women. It mainly affects individuals aged 50–70 years.

PATHOPHYSIOLOGY

Adenocarcinoma of the pancreas arises from the ductal tissue and is more commonly located in the head of the gland. Lesions frequently obstruct the pancreatic duct, causing chronic pancreatitis. The carcinoma can also obstruct the bile duct, giving rise to obstructive jaundice. Cancer of the pancreas carries a poor prognosis because the disease has often spread to nearby organs by the time a diagnosis is made. Surgical resection has not been shown to improve the rate of survival. However, cancer of the duodenum, lower bile duct and periampullary regions often present earlier with obstructive jaundice, and surgical resection offers a much better prognosis.

Common presenting symptoms. Jaundice is often the symptom with which the patient first presents to his GP. The urine is dark in colour, the stool pale and fatty and the skin and sclera have a yellowish tinge. Severe itch can be a very distressing symptom.

Severe weight loss and anorexia are associated with vague epigastric pain, often radiating to the back. Initially pain is intermittent but gradually becomes constant and severe.

MEDICAL MANAGEMENT

Investigative procedures are as follows:

- Blood is taken for liver function tests and to check for the presence of a coagulation defect
- An ultrasound scan will detect a dilated biliary tree and exclude the presence of gallstones
- A CT scan may demonstrate a pancreatic mass, local invasion by tumour, or metastases
- Pancreatic tissue may be obtained for cytology by using CT scan or ultrasound-guided fine-needle aspiration
- ERCP can be used to define the site of obstruction and obtain biopsies.

Medical intervention. Relief of obstructive jaundice and pain control are all that can be offered to the majority of patients with pancreatic cancer. ERCP with stenting of the biliary tree can relieve obstructive jaundice and may reduce the necessity for surgical intervention. Chemotherapy has been used but appears to have little effect. Surgery is usually palliative but jaundice may be relieved by cholecystojejunostomy or choledochojejunostomy.

In a minority of cases pancreatoduodenal resection (Whipple's procedure) may be worthwhile if the tumour is less than 2 cm in diameter and confined to the head of the pancreas (see Fig. 4.14).

NURSING PRIORITIES AND MANAGEMENT: CANCER OF THE PANCREAS

The patient with a diagnosis of pancreatic cancer requires expert nursing care. Investigative procedures are extensive and surgery in the majority of cases only offers palliation. The nurse has a very important role in helping the patient and his family to cope during this very difficult time.

Major patient problems

Anxiety

Patients with pancreatic cancer are usually very anxious. They may have no previous history of illness and often deny the diagnosis. They are often the breadwinner in the family and may even be coming up for retirement. They may have difficulty coming to terms with the diagnosis and are often angry and withdrawn, especially with close family members. Relatives often feel shut out and helpless. The nurse can help by offering support and advice to both the patient and his family, who should be encouraged to discuss the illness and its implications.

Extensive discussion with the patient and his relatives prior to surgery is necessary. Some patients are prepared for a Whipple's procedure but at surgery it is found that the disease is more extensive than expected and a bypass is all that can be safely attempted. This is devastating for the patient and his family who will have built up hopes for recovery.

Pain

Pain is often persistent, particularly when the disease is at an advanced stage. Oral opiates may be given and titrated to the patient's specific needs. An oral laxative will also be given to prevent constipation.

As the disease advances pain may become more difficult to control. An epidural catheter may be implanted to deliver morphine on a continuous basis or a coeliac plexus nerve block may be considered.

Close monitoring of the effectiveness of pain control is essential to ensure that the best possible quality of life can be maintained for the patient (see Ch. 19). If the patient is discharged to home, liaison with the primary health care team is essential to ensure that full continuity of care is achieved. As the condition of the patient deteriorates, a decision will be taken as to the best care option available (see Ch. 34).

Jaundice

Jaundice (see p. 114) is usually persistent and accompanied by severe pruritis. The itching is usually all over the body and the patient often scratches until the skin bleeds. He may be so distressed by it that he thinks it will drive him mad. Every effort should be made to relieve itching. Antihistamines are used but they can cause sedation. A twice daily bath with added sodium bicarbonate is very effective. Calamine lotion applied locally may help. Night sedation is important as itching is often worse at night.

Following ERCP and stenting, the jaundice and itch will subside over 7–10 days. The patient will feel much better as soon as the itch disappears and as the jaundice fades.

Anorexia and weight loss

Poor appetite and subsequent weight loss are further distressing aspects of the disease. Meals should be small and attractively presented. Liaison with the dietitian is necessary. High-protein drinks between meals may be tolerated well. If weight loss is severe, special care should be taken to prevent the development of pressure sores. Malaise associated with anorexia and weight loss will increase the patient's dependency; nurses and other carers will need to offer more and more assistance with many aspects of daily living.

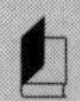

For further information, see Spross et al 1988.

DISORDERS OF THE SPLEEN

Trauma

The spleen is highly vascular and is one of the organs most frequently damaged by abdominal trauma. In 20% of patients who present with splenic injury, associated rib fractures are found on X-ray examination. The spleen is particularly susceptible to injury when pathologically enlarged.

PATHOPHYSIOLOGY

Injury to the spleen can result in rupture, evulsion from its pedicle or tearing beneath the capsule, with possible formation of a subcapsular haematoma.

Delayed rupture of the spleen occurs in about 5% of patients and is thought to be caused by haematoma bursting through the capsule wall. This usually occurs within 2 weeks of injury, but in a few cases can be delayed for months or even years.

Common presenting symptoms. Rupture and evulsion of the spleen cause immediate intraperitoneal bleeding. As blood spreads throughout the peritoneal cavity, signs of haemorrhage and hypovolaemic shock may develop. Patients generally present as an acute abdominal emergency.

The patient experiences abdominal pain with particular tenderness in the left upper quadrant. Referred pain is often felt in the left shoulder tip. Bruising to the abdomen may or may not be evident.

MEDICAL MANAGEMENT

Surgical intervention. Injury to the spleen is an indication for splenectomy, provided the organ cannot be conserved. The tendency is now to conserve splenic tissue if at all possible by suturing capsular tears or by performing a partial splenectomy. This is because of the risk of systemic infection following splenectomy. Another method used following injury is to wrap the spleen in an absorbable haemostatic mesh.

NURSING PRIORITIES AND MANAGEMENT: TRAUMA

General considerations

The patient may be in a distressed and anxious state and reassurance should be given by the nurse. Holding the patient's hand and offering encouragement may help to relieve some of the patient's anxiety, whilst measures should be taken by medical and nursing staff to establish and administer i.v. fluids along with blood and blood products as required. Oxygen therapy is commenced to raise the circulating levels and a urinary catheter inserted to assess renal function. Blood pressure, pulse and respirations should be closely monitored and any changes reported quickly. An NG tube is passed to empty the stomach contents and prevent aspiration. Analgesia to relieve pain should be given and its effect monitored.

Relatives should be kept informed of what is happening and comfort and support given during this stressful and worrying time.

Perioperative care

Any clotting defect which may be present is rectified and, once the patient's condition has stabilised, he is prepared for surgery. Close observation of the patient is required throughout this period. If at all possible, it is helpful to allow close relatives to see the patient before surgery as this may relieve a little of both their and the patient's anxiety. Postoperative care is as for abdominal surgery requiring general anaesthesia (see Nursing Care Plan 27.3 and 27.4).

Non-acute presentation

Not all patients present with splenic injury in such a dramatic way. If a diagnosis is difficult to establish and splenic injury is suspected vigilant and careful observation of the patient is vital.

The patient will be admitted to hospital for close observation, which includes frequent monitoring of blood pressure, pulse and respiration. Any pain experienced by the patient should be monitored, noting its site, type and duration. Whether the pain is increasing or decreasing may be relevant. Analgesia may initially be withheld as it may mask the true situation. The patient will be fasted during this period of observation and should be given frequent oral hygiene.

Any change in the patient's condition should be reported immediately as, following rupture, temporary improvement in the patient's condition may precede sudden deterioration.

Hypersplenism

Hypersplenism is a syndrome consisting of splenomegaly and pancytopenia. The bone marrow is normal and no autoimmune disease is present.

PATHOPHYSIOLOGY

Primary hypersplenism is due to hypertrophy of the spleen as a response to the need to destroy abnormal blood cells. Secondary hypersplenism occurs when inappropriate cell destruction is secondary to splenic enlargement; this condition may complicate inflammatory disorders such as rheumatic fever and malaria.

In portal hypertension, splenic congestion frequently leads to splenomegaly and hypersplenism. Other conditions causing splenic enlargement are haemolytic anaemias, idiopathic thrombocytopenic purpura, myelofibrosis and lymphomas. Tumours, cysts and splenic abscesses are rarely found.

Clinical features. The effects of hypersplenism include expansion of the blood volume to fill the increased vascular spaces. There is increased pooling of blood in the cells with excessive destruction, possibly induced by metabolic damage as the cells are packed tightly together in the enlarged spleen. Increased amounts of urobilinogen are present in the urine. Blood analysis will show anaemia, leucopenia and thrombocytopenia, and marrow turnover will be increased.

Splenectomy may be undertaken in many of these conditions, although removal of a grossly enlarged spleen carries an appreciable risk. Close liaison is necessary between the haematologist and the surgeon.

NURSING PRIORITIES AND MANAGEMENT: HYPERSPLENISM

Perioperative care

In preparation for elective splenectomy a full assessment of the patient's blood count and coagulation status must be made. In the presence of any bleeding tendency a transfusion of blood or platelets may be administered. In patients with thrombocytopenia, platelets should be made available for use to cover the intra- and postoperative phase.

Some surgeons advocate the use of anti-pneumococcal vaccine in an attempt to prevent or minimise chest infection postoperatively.

Preparation for surgery is as for abdominal surgery requiring general anaesthesia. An NG tube is passed because of handling of the stomach during surgery and the subsequent risk of aspiration of stomach contents.

In the postoperative period the physiotherapist plays an important role in the care of these patients because of the increased risk of collapse of the left lower lobe of the lung. The nurse must encourage the patient to perform deep breathing exercises and aid expectoration between physiotherapy sessions.

Some doctors advise the administration of low-dose heparin in all patients undergoing splenectomy as there will be a transient increase in platelet and leucocyte levels. The nurse must therefore be aware of the importance of passive exercises whilst the patient is on bedrest and encourage movement and early ambulation. Another complication which can follow splenectomy is pancreatitis caused by the handling and bruising of the tail of the pancreas during surgery. Therefore the nurse must be alert to any change in the patient's condition, especially any increase or change in the nature of the pain experienced.

Due to the loss of lymphoid tissue, there is an increased risk of infection. As most infections occurs within 3 years of splenectomy, some surgeons advise the use of prophylactic penicillin for this period or even longer. This cover is mandatory when the patient is a child.

GLOSSARY

Achalasia. A failure of the smooth muscle of the GI tract to relax. The cause is unknown but occurs due to degeneration of the ganglionic cells. The failure is most notable in the lower oesophagus which fails to relax with swallowing.

Cholangiocarcinoma. Cancer of the bile ducts.

Choledocolithiasis. Stones in the bile ducts.

Hepatomegaly. The enlargement of the liver becoming palpable below the costal margin.

Melaena. Black tarry stools due to the presence of partly digested blood from further up in the digestive tract. Melaena is not apparent in an adult unless 500 ml of blood has entered the gut.

Neoplasm. Any new and abnormal growth, a tumour. Neoplasms may be benign or malignant.

Paterson-Kelly/Plummer Vinson syndrome. A combination of dysphagia, glossitis and nutritional iron deficiency anaemia. Dysphagia is caused by a fibrous web in the post-cricoid region of the oesophagus. Oral iron therapy usually leads to complete recovery.

Pancytopenia. The abnormal suppression of all the cellular elements of the blood: red cells, white cells and platelets.

Pruritis. Itching that may result from many skin and systemic disorders. In liver disease the cause of the itching is unclear, although the deposition of bile salts is implicated.

Pseudocyst. An abnormal dilated space which resembles a cyst but has no epithelial lining, e.g. pancreatic pseudocyst where the sac contains pancreatic enzymes, debris and blood within a lining of inflammatory tissue.

Sclerotherapy. The injection of an irritant substance into varicose veins, which causes thrombophlebitis and encourages obliteration and subsequent scarring of the tissue.

Spider telangiectasis. A localised collection of distended blood capillaries arising from a central point, thereby resembling a spider's web.

Wilson's disease. An inborn defect of copper metabolism that results in free copper being deposited in the liver causing jaundice and cirrhosis. Deposits can also occur in the brain resulting in intellectual impairment. The condition is treated with Penicillamine, a derivative of penicillin, which chelates (binds) the copper in order to remove excess from the body.

REFERENCES

Attard A R, Corlett M J, Kidner N J, Leslie A P & Fraser I A 1992 Safety of early pain relief for acute abdominal pain. British Medical Journal 305(6853): 554–556

Belk D 1983 Carcinoma of the oesophagus. Nursing Times 79(43): 56–59

Boyle S 1992 Assessing mouth care. Nursing Times 88(15): 44–46

Burkitt D P 1971 Epidemiology of cancer of the colon and rectum. Cancer 28: 3–13

Burkitt H G, Quick C R G, Gatt D 1990 Essential surgery: problems, diagnosis and management. Churchill Livingstone, Edinburgh

Burrell L O 1992 Adult nursing in hospital and community settings. Appleton & Lange, Connecticut

Edwards C R W, Bouchier I A D (eds) 1991 Davidson's principles and practice of medicine, 16th edn. Churchill Livingstone, Edinburgh

Elcott C 1988a Stoma care: identified patient problems. Nursing Times 84(8): 57–60 (March 2)

Elcott C 1988b Stoma care: taking a holistic approach. Nursing Times 84(9)

Forrest A P M, Carter D C, McLeod I B 1991 Principles and practice of surgery, 2nd edn. Churchill Livingstone, Edinburgh

Hatchett R 1991 Exploring a medical phenomemon: hepatic encephalopathy. Nursing 4(37): 26–29 and 4(38): 32–34

Harrison R J 1984 Textbook of medicine. Hodder & Stoughton, London

Holdstock D J, Misciewicz J J, Smith T, Rowlands E N 1970 Propulsion (mass movements) in the human colon and its relationship to meals and somatic activity. Gut 11: 91–99

Hope J 1993 The counter revolution. BBC Good Health (March): 36–38

Jones P F 1992 Early analgesia for acute abdominal pain. British Medical Journal 305(6860): 1020–1021

Jones R, Lydeard S 1989 Prevalence of symptoms of dyspepsia in the community. British Medical Journal 298: 30–32

Kalideen D 1990 A realistic alternative to ileostomy. Nursing 14(19)

Langman M J S 1985 Upper gastro-intestinal bleeding: the trials of trials. Gut 26: 217–220

Mant D, Fuller A, Northover J, Astrop P 1992 Patient compliance with colorectal cancer screening in general practice. British Journal of General Practice (January): 18–20

Marshall C 1984 Celestin tube — oesophageal cancer, a major complication of which was dysphagia. Nursing Mirror 159(4): 50–51

McLane A M (ed) 1987 Classification of nursing diagnoses: proceedings of the seventh conference. Mosby, St Louis

Salter M 1988 Altered body image: the nurse's role. Scutari, London

Salter M 1990 Current trends in stoma care. Nursing Standard 4(22): 22–24

Shearman D J C, Finlayson N, Carter D C (eds) 1989 Diseases of the gastrointestinal tract and liver, 2nd edn. Churchill Livingstone, Edinburgh

Stapleford P, Long S 1990 Crohn's disease in children. Nursing Standard 4(48): 25–27

Stockley A 1982 Stoma care services: in hospital. In Jeker K F & Todd I P (eds) Stomas. Saunders, London, 373–376

Thompson W G, Heaton K W 1989 Irritable bowel syndrome. In:

Shearman D J C, Finlayson N, Carter D C (eds) Diseases of the gastrointestinal tract and liver, 2nd edn. Churchill Livingstone, Edinburgh
Wade 1989 A stoma is for life: a study of stoma care nurses and their patients. Scutari Press, London, p. 20
Watson P G 1983 The effects of short term postoperative counselling on cancer/ostomy patients. Cancer Nursing 6(2): 21–29
Whitehead S 1988 Illustrated operation notes. Edward Arnold, London
Wilkinson S 1992 Confessions and challenges. Nursing Times 88(35): 24–28
Wilson K J W (ed) 1990 Ross & Wilson anatomy and physiology in health and illness, 7th edn. Churchill Livingstone, Edinburgh

FURTHER READING

Burkitt D P 1982 Don't forget the fibre in your diet. Dunitz, London
Dewar B J 1985 Management of oesophageal varices. Nursing Times 81(22): 32–35
Donahue P A 1990 When it's hard to swallow: feeding techniques for dysphagia management. Journal of Gerontological Nursing 16(4): 6–9, 41–42
Fletcher C, Freeling P 1988 Talking and listening to patients: a modern approach. Nuffield Provincial Trust, London
Forrest A P M, Carter D C, MacLeod I B 1991 Principles and practice of surgery, 2nd edn. Churchill Livingstone, Edinburgh
Hayward J C 1975 Information: a prescription against pain. Royal College of Nursing, London
Health Education Authority 1989 Can you avoid cancer: a guide to reducing your risks. HEA, London
Howard V 1989 Making sense of endoscopic retrograde cholangiopancreatography. Nursing Times 85(9): 49–51
Johnson P 1993 Laparoscopic cholecystectomy. Nursing Standard 7(22): 26–29
Kalder P K 1985 Stress ulcers. Critical Care Nursing Currents 3(3): 13
Kelly M P, Henry T 1992 A thirst for practical knowledge: stoma patients' opinions of the services they receive. Professional Nurse 3: 350–356
Moorhouse P J, Geissler A C & Doenges M E 1988 Acute pancreatitis. Journal of Emergency Nursing 14(6): 387–391
Norris H T 1991 (ed) Pathology of the colon, small intestine and anus, 2nd edn. Churchill Livingstone, Edinburgh
Roberts M K 1992 Assessing and treating volvulus. Nursing 92 22(2): 56–57
Savage J 1992 Advice to take home. Nursing Times 88(38): 24–27
Shearman D J C, Finlayson N, Carter D (eds) 1989 Diseases of the gastrointestinal tract and liver, 2nd edn. Churchill Livingstone, Edinburgh
Smith S 1992 Tiresome healing. Nursing Times 88(36): 24–28
Spross J A, Manolatos A, Thorpe M 1988 Pancreatic cancer: nursing challenges. Seminars in Oncology Nursing 4(4): 274–284
Thomas S 1992 A new development in radiology: TIPS. Nursing Standard 7(2): 25–28

USEFUL ADDRESSES

British Colostomy Association
15 Station Road
Reading RG11 11LG

Ileostomy Association
Amblehurst House
Blackscotch Lane
Mansfield, Notts
NG18 4PF

National Association for Colitus and Crohn's Disease (NACC)
98A London Road
St Alban's
Herefordshire AL1 1NY

CHAPTER 5

Endocrine and metabolic disorders

Claire Dibbs (Part 1 Endocrine and metabolic disorders)
Rosemary McIntyre (Part 2 Diabetes)

CHAPTER CONTENTS

PART 1
ENDOCRINE AND METABOLIC DISORDERS 133

Introduction 133

Anatomy and physiology 134

DISORDERS OF THE ENDOCRINE SYSTEM 137
Eating disorders 137
Hypersecretion of the anterior pituitary hormones 139
Hypersecretion of adrenocorticotrophic hormone 140
Hyposecretion of the anterior pituitary hormones 140
Disorders of vasopressin (ADH) secretion 142
Disorders of the thyroid gland 144
Disorders of the parathyroid glands 146
Disorders of the adrenal glands 147
Disorders of sexual differentiation 152

References 153

Further reading 153

PART 2 DIABETES 154

Introduction 155

Anatomy and physiology 155

Primary diabetes mellitus 156

Impaired glucose tolerance (IGT) 159

Secondary diabetes mellitus 159

MANAGEMENT STRATEGIES IN DIABETES MELLITUS 159
Achieving and maintaining normoglycaemia 159
Dietary therapy 160
Insulin therapy 161

Monitoring response to therapy 164
Methods 164

Preventing and detecting diabetes-associated complications 165

Acute metabolic complications of diabetes 165
Chronic complications of diabetes mellitus 173

Facilitating self care through education 178

Promoting psychological and social adjustment 179

Conclusion 181

References 182

Further reading 183

Additional resources and useful addresses 184

PART 1
ENDOCRINE AND METABOLIC DISORDERS

INTRODUCTION

Endocrinology is the study of hormones (or chemical messengers) secreted by endocrine cells and neurones. These hormones maintain homeostasis by acting on and coordinating activity within target organs or tissues.

Endocrinology is a relatively new and rapidly growing field. Considerable progress is being made, with important implications for other areas of medicine, e.g. neuroendocrinology, which in turn has important applications within psychiatry.

Apart from diabetes mellitus and thyroid disorders, endocrine problems are not common. Many endocrine disorders are rarely seen and may be difficult to diagnose; as a result patients may be referred by their general practitioner or local hospital to specialist centres for the often complicated and exhaustive tests necessary for diagnosis. For the patient this has the advantage of offering highly specialised care and treatment. It also means however, that relatively few nurses have the opportunity to treat and care for people with these disorders.

However, given the wide-ranging effects of endocrine dysfunction, it is important that all nurses have a general understanding of endocrinology. Endocrine diseases can affect every system of the body, causing disfigurement and a change in body image or even posing a threat to life. These disorders can seriously affect the patient's psychological outlook, either as a direct result of the illness or by virtue of the individual's reaction to it.

It is well documented that individuals react differently to being ill. Some view their situation as a challenge; others see it as a punishment, or react with anger, or try to apportion blame. Anger may be directed at family members or at nursing and medical staff (Sinclair & Fawcett 1991). This situation may be exacerbated by an unstable mental state, mood swings, depression, or frank psychosis, which may in fact be sequelae of the disorder. The nurse must be aware of this possibility and react accordingly, offering support and understanding to the patient and his relatives. Explanations that the underlying illness may be influencing the patient's mood may help him and his relatives to cope.

As the tests and investigations required to diagnose some of the rarer endocrine conditions are often long and exhausting, clear explanations are essential so that the patient understands the need for the tests and the procedures that will be followed. This will help to reduce anxiety and increase the patient's confidence in the health care team.

ANATOMY AND PHYSIOLOGY

Hormones

The endocrine system is one of the two major control systems of the body, the other being the nervous system. While the nervous system mediates its activity by means of nerves directly supplying the organs and structures it relates to, the endocrine system operates by a system of hormones which are secreted into the bloodstream for transport to their respective target organs.

?	**5.1** Name the endocrine glands and identify their anatomical position (see Fig. 5.1).

Action

Although the hormones are carried to every cell in the body they affect only those cells or organs on which they have an excitatory or inhibitory action. This system allows an individual to respond to changes in his environment and is important in controlling growth and development, sexual maturation and homeostasis.

Many hormones are bound to proteins within the circulation. It is generally thought that only unbound or free hormones are biologically active, and that binding serves as a buffer against very rapid changes in plasma levels of a hormone. This principle is important to the interpretation of many tests of endocrine function.

Control

Most hormone systems are controlled by a feedback system which ensures that hormone levels, whilst fluctuating, remain within a mean. Figure 5.2 represents how negative feedback operates in the hypothalamo-pituitary-thyroid axis.

Pattern of secretion

Hormone secretion is either continuous or intermittent. An example of the former is the secretion of thyroxine by the thyroid gland, in which hormone levels over a day, month or year show very little variation.

Intermittent secretion is seen in three forms: circadian, menstrual, and pulsatile. Other factors which affect hormone secretion include stress, disease, trauma, surgery or emotional upset. As in any complex regulatory system it is likely that disequilibrium in endocrine function will have important consequences. Disorders of the endocrine system may be categorised most simply as those involving overproduction (hypersecretion) or those involving underproduction (hyposecretion).

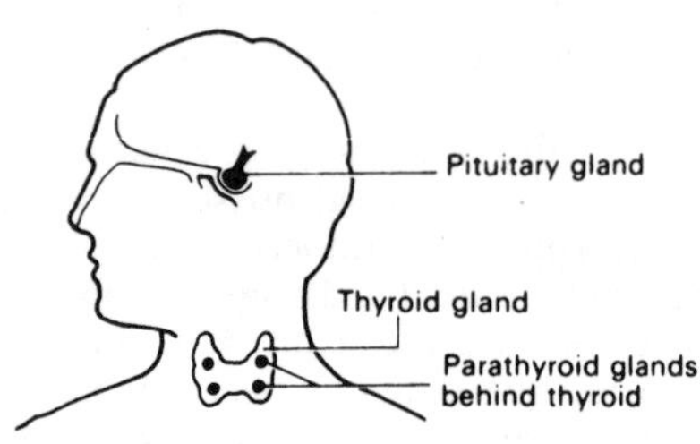

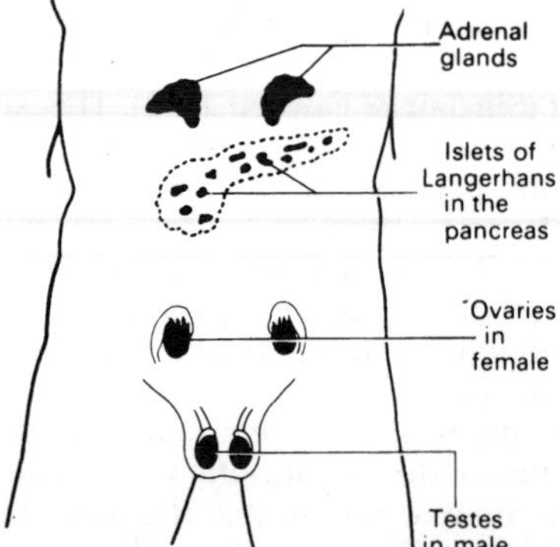

Fig. 5.1 The endocrine glands and their location in the body. (Reproduced with permission from Wilson 1990.)

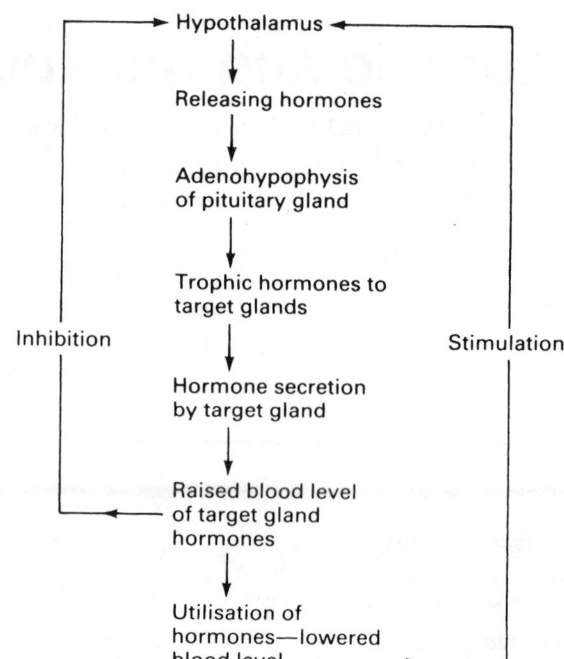

Fig. 5.2 Negative feedback regulation of the secretion of anterior pituitary hormones. (Reproduced with permission from Wilson 1990.)

The hypothalamus and the pituitary gland

The existence of the pituitary gland has been known of for at least 2000 years. It lies immediately below the hypothalamus in the pituitary fossa. It is connected to the hypothalamus by the pituitary stalk and consists of two lobes (anterior and posterior) which function independently of each other (see Fig. 5.3). In the developing fetus the anterior lobe is formed from Rathkes' pouch, which grows upwards and becomes separated from the oropharynx to become the adenohypophysis. The posterior lobe is a downgrowth from the forebrain, which becomes the neurohypophysis. The posterior pituitary contains nerve fibres which grow into it from the hypothalamus via the pituitary stalk. The hormones secreted by the pituitary gland, together with their action, are listed in Table 5.1.

The hypothalamus is part of the floor of the third ventricle of the brain. It is an area of specialised cells or nuclei which produce hormones. These hormones regulate pituitary function and act as releasing factors for the anterior pituitary hormones (see Table 5.2, Fig. 5.4). The hypothalamus also controls many centres for functions such as appetite, thirst, temperature regulation, sexual activity, sleeping and waking.

The pituitary stalk carries blood to both lobes of the pituitary in a portal system by which the hypothalamic releasing or inhibitory hormones are carried to the anterior pituitary. The tropic hormones produced in the anterior pituitary stimulate the peripheral endocrine glands. The posterior pituitary acts as a reservoir for vasopressin (ADH) and oxytocin.

The optic chiasma sits just above the pituitary fossa. Therefore an expanding lesion from the pituitary or the hypothalamus may result in a defect in the visual fields because of pressure of the optic nerve or optic chiasma.

Hypersecretion or hyposecretion of hormones, or local effects of a tumour will disturb the balance of the system.

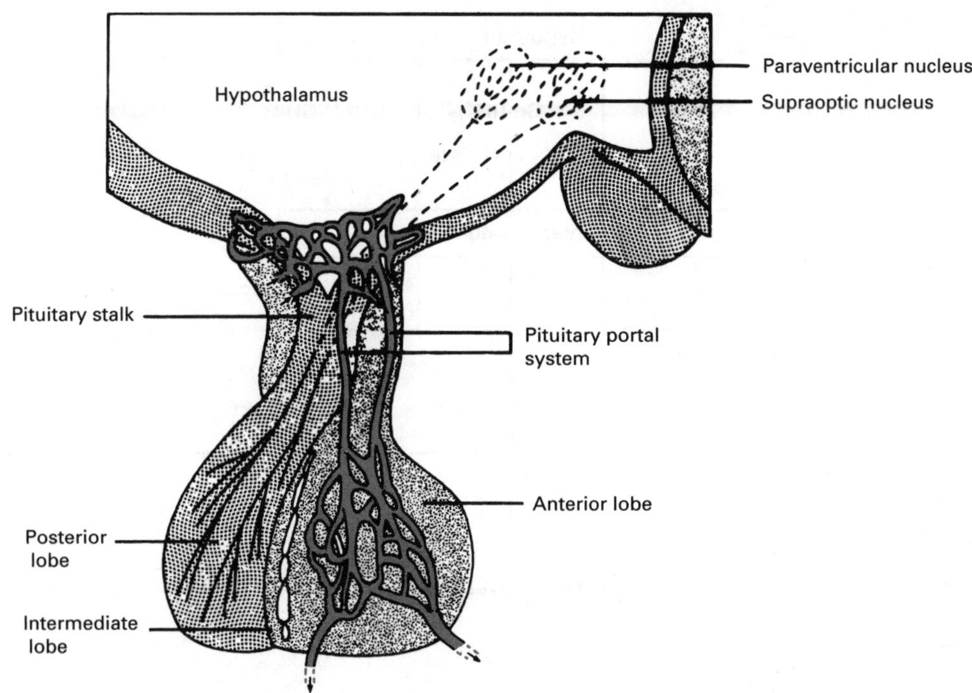

Fig. 5.3 Position of the pituitary and its associated structures. (Reproduced with permission from Wilson 1990.)

Table 5.1 Hormones of the pituitary gland and their action

Hormone	Action
Anterior lobe	
Growth hormone (GH)	Pulsatile release; does not have a single target gland but acts on a variety of tissues, e.g. bone, viscera and soft tissues. Is particularly important in children to stimulate growth. Action in adults uncertain
Prolactin (PRL)	Main action is to stimulate lactation in females, also stimulates corpus luteum to secrete progesterone
Adrenocorticotropic hormone (ACTH)	Secreted under circadian rhythm. Stimulates the adrenal cortex to secrete corticosteroids
Luteinising hormone (LH)	Promotes ovulation; stimulates formation of the corpus luteum
Follicle-stimulating hormone (FSH)	Stimulates the production of sex hormones and contributes to regulation of the menstrual cycle in women. In women, stimulates the production of ovarian follicles and secretion of oestrogen; in men, promotes the production of spermatozoa
Thyrotropic-stimulating hormone (TSH)	Stimulates the thyroid to release thyroxine
Posterior lobe	
Vasopressin; also called antidiuretic hormone (ADH)	Controls water homeostasis in the body by regulating water reabsorption from the renal tissues
Oxytocin	Induces uterine contraction during labour and ejection of milk from breasts postpartum

Table 5.2 Hypothalamic regulatory hormones (Reproduced with kind permission from Hubbard & Mechan (1987))

Hypothalamic hormone	Target pituitary hormone
Growth hormone releasing hormone (GHRH)	Growth hormone
Growth hormone inhibiting hormone (somatostatin) (GHIH)	
Thyrotropin-releasing hormone (TRH)	Thyrotropin
Gonadotropin-releasing hormone (GnRH)	Luteinising hormone *and* Follicle-stimulating hormone
or Luteinising hormone releasing hormone (LHRH)	Luteinising hormone
and Follicle-stimulating hormone releasing hormone (FSHRH)	Follicle-stimulating hormone
Corticotropin-releasing hormone (CRH)	Corticotropin
Prolactin-releasing hormone (PRH)	Prolactin
Prolactin-inhibiting hormone (PIH)	Prolactin

The thyroid gland

The thyroid gland produces the hormones tri-iodothyronine (T_3) and thyroxine (T_4). As these control metabolism overactivity or underactivity will have significant effects.

The thyroid sits anteriorly to the larynx and is attached to the thyroid cartilages and the trachea. It consists of two lobes connected by an isthmus (see Fig. 5.5). Structures which lie in close proximity include the oesophagus, the parathyroid glands, the recurrent laryngeal nerves and the carotid artery. These may all be affected by enlargement of the gland.

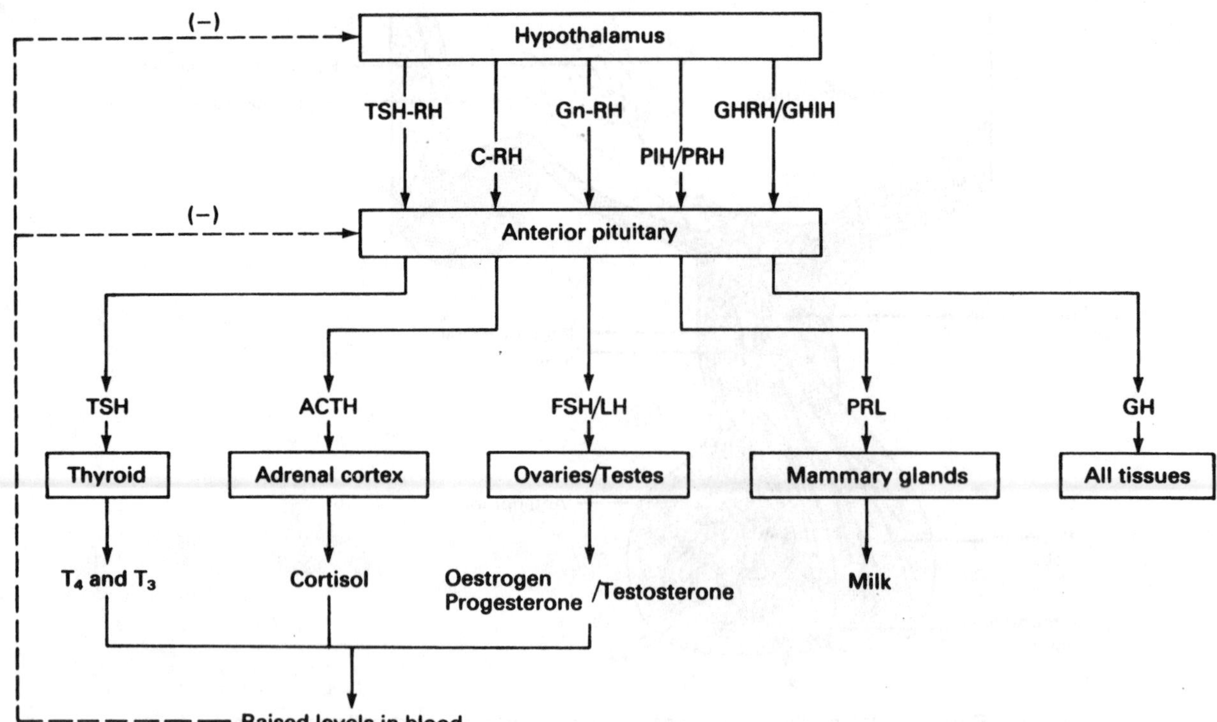

Fig. 5.4 Relationships between the hypothalamus, anterior pituitary and target organs. (Reproduced with kind permission from Hubbard & Mechan 1987.)

The thyroid receives a rich blood supply from the superior thyroid arteries, which branch from the external carotid arteries, and by the superior and inferior thyroid arteries, which branch from the subclavian arteries. Each lobe is filled with hollow vesicles called follicles, which produce and store the thyroid hormones as thyroglobulin. Between the follicles is parafollicular material, which secretes the hormone calcitonin; this together with parathormone from the parathyroid glands is involved in the metabolism of calcium.

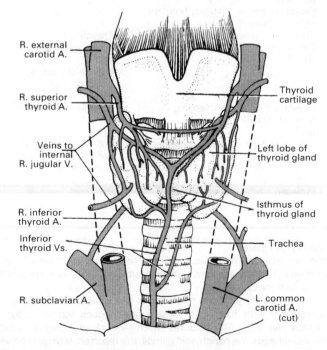

Fig. 5.5 The thyroid gland and associated structures. (Reproduced with permission from Wilson 1990.)

The thyroid hormones are synthesised from within the gland. This synthesis is dependent on the availability of iodine in the diet. Dietary iodine is absorbed from the small intestine, changed to iodide and transported in the blood to the thyroid gland, where it is taken up by the thyroid cells.

More T_4 than T_3 is produced but T_4 is converted in some tissues to the more biologically active T_3. Over 99% of all thyroid hormone is bound to plasma proteins by thyroid-binding globulins. Only the free hormone is available for use by the tissues.

?	**5.2** Describe how the thyroid hormones T_3 and T_4 are controlled (see Fig. 5.2).

The parathyroid glands

The parathyroid glands are situated on the posterior lobes of the thyroid gland. They are usually 4 in number; however, more than 4 glands occur in up to 6% of normal individuals. This has been attributed to division of the glands during development. The blood supply is from the inferior and superior thyroid arteries.

The glands secrete parathormone (or PTH), which is the most important hormone involved in calcium metabolism. Parathormone maintains plasma calcium levels within normal limits. It acts predominantly on the kidney tubules to increase reabsorption of calcium but also increases gut absorption of calcium and mobilises it from bone. Calcium levels of plasma will therefore rise, and this in turn suppresses PTH secretion; conversely, a fall in plasma calcium will stimulate the secretion of the hormone. In most instances raised levels of calcium in the plasma are caused by hyperparathyroidism and malignancy.

Vitamin D and calcitonin are also involved in calcium metabolism (see Box 5.1).

The adrenal glands

The adrenal glands have a composite origin. The cortex (the outer part) has the same embryonic site or origin as the gonads. The medulla (the

Box 5.1 Vitamin D and calcitonin in calcium metabolism

Vitamin D is found in two forms: cholecalciferol (vitamin D_3), which is formed predominantly in the skin by the action of sunlight, and ergocalciferol (vitamin D_2), which is synthetic and added to food. It is the skin-synthesised form which is of greatest importance and is perhaps best considered as a hormone.

Vitamin D is biologically inactive; only when it is metabolised by the liver (to form mildly active 25-hydroxycholecalciferol) and the kidney (to form very active 1.25-dihydroxycholecalciferol) does it have any action on calcium metabolism. The active metabolite increases calcium absorption from the gut and is essential for bone formation.

If 1.25-dihydroxycholecalciferol is present in excess it causes increased resorption of calcium from bone leading to hypercalcaemia. The kidney is able to detect rising levels and ceases production of the active form, producing an inactive form until the levels drop.

Bone is constantly being reformed by deposition and resorption of calcium. Calcitonin reduces the resorption of calcium from bone. Local stress, such as weight-bearing, is important in this process. Prolonged inactivity or immobility can result in calcium being lost from bone, while exercise increases bone formation and remodelling.

inner part) is derived from neural crest cells which have migrated from the developing neural tube and have become enclosed within the cortex. The secretions and therefore the actions of the two separate parts of the glands are quite different and will be discussed separately.

The adrenal glands are situated on the upper part of the kidneys. They are highly vascular and derive their blood supply from the renal artery, the phrenic artery and directly from the aorta; they are drained by the suprarenal veins (see Fig. 5.6).

The adrenal cortex

The adrenal cortex produces three types of hormone, collectively termed corticosteroids:

- mineralocorticoids
- glucocorticoids
- gonadotropins (sex hormones).

Mineralocorticoids. The most important of the mineralocorticoids is aldosterone, which is the most potent regulator of sodium and potassium and hence of the acid/base balance of the body. Aldosterone acts on the distal convoluted tubules of the kidney and stimulates the cells to reabsorb or conserve sodium.

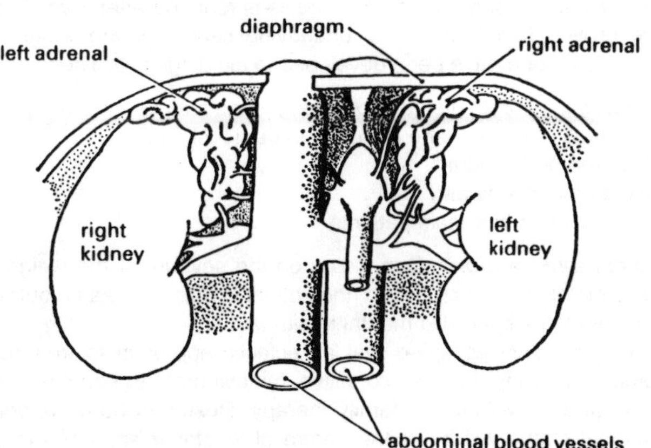

Fig. 5.6 The adrenal gland. (Reproduced with kind permission from Edwards 1986.)

Glucocorticoids such as cortiso (the principle glucocorticoid), cortisone and hydrocortisone have varied and wide-ranging actions, many of which are not yet understood. They are essential to life and in their absence blood sugar falls, blood pressure and blood volume falls, sodium excretion increases and muscle contractibility decreases. Death ensues due to low blood volume and myocardial weakness and shock. If present in excessive amounts an opposite set of changes occurs. Blood volume expands, blood pressure rises, potassium falls, glycogen storage is increased, blood sugar levels rise, connective tissue is reduced in quality and strength and immunity is impaired. Wound healing and the process of inflammation is also inhibited.

It appears that glucocorticoid effects are concerned with intermediary metabolism, inflammation, immunity and connective tissue healing (see Fig. 5.7).

Gonadotropins. The adrenal glands, in addition to the gonads, produce male sex hormones. The effects are typical in the male, but in the female excessive production may have a virilising effect.

The adrenal medulla

Adrenaline, noradrenaline and dopamine (the catecholamines) are secreted by the adrenal medulla. Of adrenomedullary secretion 80% is adrenaline, most noradrenaline and dopamine being secreted by neurones and functioning as neurotransmitters.

In normal secretion, adrenaline probably has some effect on mean blood pressure as, although it increases systolic pressure, it decreases diastolic pressure.

When secreted under the control of the sympathetic nervous system (see Ch. 9, p. 336) it causes tachycardia, decreased gut motility and the closure of sphincters in the gut, pupil dilation, bronchodilation and piloerection.

Noradrenaline raises both diastolic and systolic blood pressure but has less effect on gut motility and does not produce bronchodilation.

The difference between the effects of adrenaline and noradrenaline are partly explained by the presence of receptors on the surface of effector cells (i.e. those cells on which adrenaline and noradrenaline have their effect). These are termed alpha and beta adrenoreceptors. Noradrenaline is most active at α-adrenergic receptors and adrenaline at β-adrenergic receptors. In addition, most cardiac receptors are termed B1, to distinguish them from bronchodilator B2 adrenoreceptors.

Gonads

The gonads, ovaries in the female and testes in the male, are described in Chapters 7 and 8.

DISORDERS OF THE ENDOCRINE SYSTEM

EATING DISORDERS

Recent studies into the role of the hypothalamus have highlighted the influence it has on appetite control. It is now almost certain that the hypothalamus has a function relating to some eating disorders. Conversely, eating disorders themselves have an effect on the endocrine system.

Prader-Willi syndrome

This syndrome of hypothalamic dysfunction presents with the patient being extremely obese, with an uncontrollable appetite. Affected individuals have a learning disability and are infertile. They will eat inappropriate things in vast quantities (hyperphagia).

Anorexia nervosa

Anorexia nervosa is an eating disorder characterised by self-inflicted starvation and a relentless pursuit of thinness (Bruch 1973).

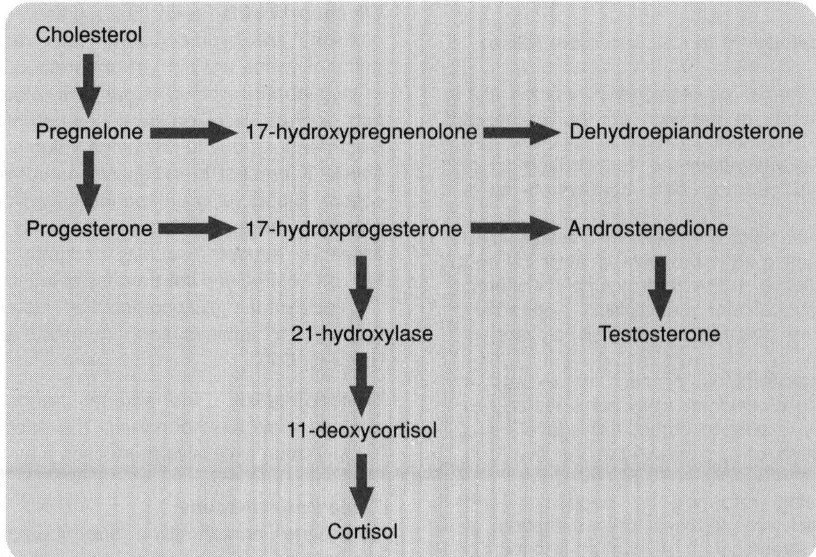

Fig. 5.7 Simplified schematisation of cortisol synthesis. (Adapted from O'Riordan et al 1982.)

Epidemiology

Anorexia nervosa is a condition which is seen in all social classes and in both sexes. However, epidemiological findings are that only 5–10% of cases occur in males and that there is a higher prevalence in social classes 1 and 2 (Edwards & Bouchier 1991). Bruch (1973) indicates that anorexic individuals tend to be young girls who come from highly successful families in which the parents hold expectations of high achievement by their children. One study by Szukler et al (1986) reported the results of 138 cases of anorexia nervosa in north-east Scotland over the period 1965–1982. A highly significant increase in the number of cases was found: 4.06 per 100 000 of the population for the years 1978–1982, with a social class bias in favour of upper and middle classes.

Aetiology

Contributory factors in the development of anorexia nervosa include:

- family background and the dynamics within the family
- the onset of puberty and psychosexual development in which there is denial and avoidance of sexuality marked by the development of the breasts and change of shape of hips and thighs
- sociocultural expectations, reflected by the emphasis on slimness in our society, and by the expectations that females will excel in a competitive vocational world as well as in traditional feminine roles (Garner et al 1983).

PATHOPHYSIOLOGY

There is a complex relationship between nutritional, endocrine and psychological factors in this condition. Disorders in nutritional status result from prolonged insufficient intake of carbohydrates, fats, and other nutrients. Metabolic disturbances (e.g. hypokalaemia) can occur following self-induced vomiting or the continual use of laxatives.

Clinical features. Endocrine dysfunction appears to relate to weight loss and affects the hypothalamo-pituitary-gonadal axis. Blood tests reveal low circulating levels of LH, FSH and oestradiol. Injections of gonadotropin hormone stimulate a rise in these, indicating that hypothalamic function is affected and the pituitary response is intact. Amenorrhoea occurs as a result of this disturbance, secondary to the loss of body fat. The individual's metabolic rate slows down, resulting in hypotension, bradycardia, reduced core body temperature and cold extremities.

Individuals with anorexia nervosa often have underlying depression. It would seem that their psychological symptoms are aggravated by the undernutrition, and some professionals argue that patients are more receptive to psychological help when they are better nourished. The characteristic mental state involves a denial of the illness, a failure to recognise the need for treatment and a need to exercise control over eating behaviour. The individual will have a distorted body image and insist that her cachectic body appears obese.

Common presenting symptoms. Most frequently, the anorexia will have been present for some months before the individual is persuaded to see her GP. A determination to lose weight coupled with the desire to change the shape of the body is typical, as is the denial of any problem or illness. The individual will claim to 'feel fat' even when she is obviously underweight or emaciated. In women, amenorrhoea typically beginning 3–6 months from the start of weight loss will be found.

MEDICAL MANAGEMENT

History and investigation. Diagnosis is reached after investigations have proved that there is no underlying cause for the weight loss. Objective criteria have been developed to aid diagnosis. These include:

- a determination to diet and lose weight and maintain the weight loss
- a change of body shape to one of extreme thinness
- distorted body image
- avoidance of sexuality
- amenorrhoea in female patients.

Medical intervention. Depending on the severity of the weight loss and its effect on general health, the patient is managed as an outpatient or inpatient in a specialist mental health unit.

It is commonly accepted that an eclectic approach to treatment is useful. This may involve cognitive–behavioural approaches, social reality, and individual and family therapy. Restoring body weight and nutritional status will be at the centre of whatever approach is used. If the weight loss has led to physiological life-threatening conditions such as hypokalaemia or renal failure, it may be necessary to correct fluid and electrolyte imbalance by i.v. fluids and to improve nutritional status by parenteral or nasogastric feeding for as short a time as possible. (Given the invasive nature of these procedures, they can be psychologically damaging for the individual.)

A multidisciplinary team approach in which dietitians, occupational therapists, medical staff and nurses work together with the anorexic individual in an agreed and consistent framework is essential.

NURSING PRIORITIES AND MANAGEMENT: ANOREXIA NERVOSA

Major considerations

The main aims of nursing care for individuals with anorexia nervosa are:

- to establish a good relationship with the patient
- to restore body weight and nutritional status
- to establish a good eating pattern and the enjoyment of mealtimes
- to eliminate self-induced vomiting and the use of laxatives
- to help the individual to acquire a positive self-image.

Because of her condition, the individual will often present strong arguments as to why she cannot eat and will resort to devious methods to avoid taking in calories. Visits to the toilet after eating (to vomit or to dispose of food not eaten) are observed for and prevented. It is important that mealtimes are handled in a relaxed manner; realistic goals should be set and agreed to by the patient with regard to foods to be eaten and weight gain. A written contract can help to create a climate of trust and help prevent manipulation of staff and parents.

As goals are met and maintained, short stays with the family can be arranged. If these visits are successful, plans can be made for discharge home. Continued support and monitoring of the individual's nutritional and weight status is essential, as relapse is common among anorexics.

Bulimia nervosa

Bulimia nervosa is an eating disorder characterised by episodes of binge eating, self-induced vomiting and the use of laxatives. While in both anorexia and bulimia there is an exaggerated concern with weight and body shape, these are separate conditions. Further reading on both subjects is suggested at the end of the chapter (see p. 153).

HYPERSECRETION OF THE ANTERIOR PITUITARY HORMONES

Acromegaly

Aetiology

Hypersecretion of growth hormone (GH) causes gigantism and acromegaly. If excessive secretion occurs before fusion of the bony epiphyses, this is termed gigantism. It is extremely rare. Acromegaly caused by excess secretion of GH after fusion of the epiphyses is seen in about 40 per million of the population. Gigantism probably constitutes only 1% of this number.

A distinction must be made between those who are constitutionally tall, i.e. individuals who have two tall parents, and gigantism. Individuals with pituitary disease can easily grow in excess of 7′ tall and some to over 8′.

PATHOPHYSIOLOGY

Clinical features. Acromegaly can remain undetected for years, as its onset is insidious. It causes enlargement of all systems and structures of the body except the nervous system. The effects of the disorder include:

- enlargement of bones and soft tissues, seen especially as an overgrowth of the supraorbital ridge, a broadening of the nose, prognathism and interdental separation
- enlargement of the hands and feet, resulting in the need for larger gloves, rings and shoes
- osteoarthritis (commonly)
- weight gain
- cardiomegaly
- hypertension
- excessive sweating
- hyperprolactinaemia with menstrual disturbances and amenorrhoea in women
- loss of libido
- diabetes mellitus (in 25% of patients due to insulin resistance as a result of high GH levels)
- enlarged pituitary fossa.

Common presenting symptoms. The patient will present with a number of symptoms. Most commonly, the enlargement of the individuals hands and feet and his changed appearance will have been noticed and commented on by relatives and friends. Other problems for which the patient will initially seek help may be related to osteoarthritis or cardiovascular problems. In women, amenorrhoea may prompt a visit to the GP. Changes in the field of vision may have been noticed. Often old photographs of the individual can be useful to the doctor in reaching a provisional diagnosis.

MEDICAL MANAGEMENT

Investigative procedures. Diagnosis can be confirmed following clinical examination and tests of pituitary function. On clinical examination, all or some of the features listed above will be evident. Skull X-rays may show an enlarged pituitary fossa. Measurement of GH levels will show uniformly elevated levels throughout the day, which do not suppress to undetectable levels following glucose administration (as in normal individuals). Further tests of pituitary function may be carried out in specialist centres to confirm the diagnosis and establish whether the normal pituitary is compromised.

Medical intervention. In untreated acromegaly, mortality is nearly doubled in comparison with the normal population. Therefore early treatment is recommended. The aim of treatment is to relieve symptoms and resolve the associated metabolic abnormalities, e.g. diabetes mellitus.

Treatment may take the form of surgery, radiotherapy or drug therapy. Hypophysectomy via the transsphenoidal route, which has a low morbidity and mortality, is the surgical procedure most commonly used. Drug therapy using oral bromocriptine has been shown to reduce tumour size as well as lowering GH levels. Octreotide, a relatively new drug, is a synthetic compound which mimics the hypothalamic hormone somatostatin (growth hormone release-inhibiting hormone, GHRIH). Octreotide has to be given by regular s.c. injection or by continuous s.c. infusion.

Usually, surgery and radiotherapy are used in conjunction, as tumour regrowth often occurs following surgery alone. Drug therapy is then used to control residual excess GH secretion, as radiotherapy only lowers GH levels gradually. In patients too old or unfit for surgery, drug therapy alone may be used. Hypopituitarism may occur as a result of either treatment.

NURSING PRIORITIES AND MANAGEMENT: ACROMEGALY

Major considerations

Giving psychological support

Change in body image is an important feature of this disorder. Most probably the individual will have considerable difficulty in coming to terms with his changed appearance and will be anxious about the investigations he must undergo and the treatment that may be required.

It is important to create a relaxed environment and to reduce anxiety by spending time with the patient and his family, explaining the reasons for his changed appearance, the effect of therapy and the expected treatment outcome.

The patient and his family will be reassured to hear that biomedical cure will eventually be followed by complete normalisation of appearance. However, although some symptoms such as sweating may be cured almost immediately, others (especially bony changes) may take years to resolve.

Some patients benefit from meeting an individual who has been treated successfully; nursing staff should determine if this might be arranged. The personal experience of one former female patient — her shoe size was reduced by 2 sizes in 6 months — is the kind of success story which could boost the morale of a newly diagnosed patient.

Perioperative care

The reader is referred to Chapter 27 for principles of preoperative preparation and postoperative care, and to Chapter 23 for information on wound healing. Specific postoperative observations would include neurological monitoring, with special care being taken to observe for leakage of cerebrospinal fluid from the nose. The patient is nursed well supported on pillows to ensure that an upright position is maintained.

Recovery is usually rapid and the patient discharged home on the 4th or 5th postoperative day.

> ? **5.3** Miss W, aged 45 years, has been diagnosed as having acromegaly. She has undergone transsphenoidal hypophysectomy for the removal of a GH-producing adenoma.
> Identify the specific or potential problems and devise a plan to meet her care needs. What long term treatment and care will she require? (See Nursing Care Plan 5.1.)

PROLACTIN HYPERSECRETION

Aetiology

It is now known that prolactin is the commonest hormone to be secreted by pituitary tumours and that tiny prolactinomas, which may be as small as 2–3 mm in diameter occur frequently (Edwards 1986). However, a wide variety of drugs and diseases can cause high prolactin levels. Before carrying out extensive investigations for pituitary disease it is important to exclude physiological causes such as hypothyroidism and to take a detailed drug history. Drugs in the dopamine receptor blocking group such as chlorpromazine and metoclopramide elevate prolactin levels.

PATHOPHYSIOLOGY

Hyperprolactinaemia in women causes galactorrhoea and amenorrhoea; lack of ovulation due to prolactin interfering with LH and FSH acting on the ovary results in infertility (Edwards 1986). In men the galactorrhoea is not so pronounced, but there is a decreased sperm count and infertility.

Common presenting symptoms in women include amenorrhoea, infertility, hirsuties and acne. Common presenting features in men are impotence, infertility and gynaecomastia.

MEDICAL MANAGEMENT

Investigation procedures. When other causes of the presenting symptoms have been excluded, prolactin levels should be measured in the unstressed patient. This involves placing a cannula in the arm and taking a blood sample 30 min later. The patient should not smoke or drink tea or coffee in this period. If the prolactin levels are raised a lateral skull X-ray should be taken. If this shows a large pituitary fossa, tests of other pituitary functions should be carried out to see if other pituitary hormones are affected (see Cushing's disease, p. 148). Visual field tests may also be carried out to exclude pressure on the optic chiasma. High resolution CT scanning and magnetic resonance imaging will usually show even a small tumour. Prolactinomas are almost always benign.

Medical intervention. The aim of treatment is to lower the excessive levels of hormone, to reduce the tumour size and to restore to normal levels deficiencies that may have resulted from the presence of the tumour. Reduction of tumour size and lowering of hormone levels may be achieved by drug therapy alone. Prolactinomas respond well to bromocriptine. Surgery is usually not performed until the tumour has been reduced in size. Surgery is carried out via the transsphenoidal route.

HYPERSECRETION OF ADRENOCORTICOTROPHIC HORMONE

This is termed 'Cushing's disease' and is found when an excess of glucocorticoid secretions is stimulated by an ACTH-producing adenoma of the pituitary. It will be discussed under 'Disorders of the adrenal cortex'.

NURSING PRIORITIES AND MANAGEMENT: PROLACTIN HYPERSECRETION

Specific nursing care is aimed at ensuring that the medication regimes are followed correctly in order to avoid side-effects. Blood pressure is observed, bearing in mind that a postural drop may occur. Bromocriptine can be poorly tolerated in many people. There should be a slow increase in dosage, the first doses being given during food and on retiring to prevent the common symptoms of postural hypotension and gastric irritation. The dosage can then be built up gradually to 2.5 mg 3 times a day. A new formulation of depot injection is reported to be effective and to reduce gastric side-effects.

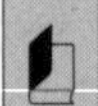
See Besser & Cudworth (1990).

HYPOSECRETION OF THE ANTERIOR PITUITARY HORMONES

Hypopituitarism

The term hypopituitarism refers to partial or total deficiency of anterior pituitary hormone secretion. It may be associated with pathological processes which destroy the pituitary itself or with disturbance of the hypothalamic control of the pituitary. Total failure of all hormone production is termed panhypopituitarism.

Aetiology

Hypopituitarism is most commonly caused by the presence of a pituitary tumour. These are frequently benign. Pituitary carcinoma is very rare indeed. Benign microadenomas having no clinical effects are surprisingly common and found in up to 25% of people at postmortem.

PATHOPHYSIOLOGY

Pituitary tumours can vary greatly in size and may extend outside the pituitary fossa to compress surrounding structures. They are generally classified as functioning or non-functioning, depending on whether they produce a hormone, e.g. GH or prolactin.

Nursing Care Plan 5.1 Postoperative care for a patient who has undergone partial thyroidectomy

Nursing considerations	Action	Rationale	Outcome/further action
1. Compromise of airway as a result of anaesthesia and surgery to neck area	Patient should be sat in an upright position with plenty of support for the neck. Oxygen may be ordered for 1–2 h after surgery	Support of the head will reduce strain on the suture line and improve the comfort of the patient, who may be very anxious about moving the neck	The airway will remain clear and strain on the suture line will be minimal
2. Risk of haemorrhage following surgery	Half-hourly observation of blood pressure and pulse, watching for signs of irregular or laboured breathing or stridor. Clip removers should be kept by the bed for up to 24 hours after surgery	A rise in pulse and a fall in blood pressure can indicate haemorrhage, which should be reported. If respiratory embarrassment occurs due to haemorrhage the clips must be removed to allow the blood compressing the trachea to escape. The wound should be covered with saline-soaked gauze and the patient returned to theatre immediately	Early detection of possible haemorrhage should prevent a crisis from developing and allow bleeding to be stopped sooner rather than later
3. Risk of tetany due to accidental removal of the parathyroid glands	Close observation for tetany including tingling of fingers and toes. A positive Chvostek's sign (facial asymmetry on tapping of cheek) or Trousseau's sign (inflation of blood pressure cuff causes spasm of hand)	Sudden drop in calcium levels can lead to tetany resulting in airway obstruction and if left untreated fitting and death	Early indications of lowered calcium levels should be reported allowing treatment in the form of i.v. calcium gluconate to be given
4. Risk of thyroid crisis (This is now rare due to improved postoperative preparation of the patient about to undergo thyroid surgery. It is a life-threatening situation)	Observation of pulse, blood pressure, temperature and respiratory rate should be made half-hourly, reducing as recovery allows	As a result of trauma to the thyroid, enormous amounts of the thyroid hormones are released into the bloodstream, causing tachycardia, a rise in blood pressure and hyperpyrexia (up to 41°C). The patient appears very restless and irritable. Death may result from heart failure	Once thyroid crisis has been diagnosed, treatment must be commenced immediately with i.v. betablockers (propranolol in high doses) carbimazole, steroid therapy (hydrocortisone 100 mg/ i.m.)
5. Risk of damage to laryngeal nerve	Observe for breathing difficulties, noisy breathing, stridor, swallowing difficulties and hoarseness, and report problems	Damage to the recurrent laryngeal nerve can result in vocal cord spasm and paralysis of larynx leading to respiratory obstruction	If damage occurs, tracheostomy is usually necessary initially. The damaged nerve should recover in a few weeks. Inhalation of nitrous oxide may help in the acute period to relieve the spasm

Common presenting symptoms. Symptoms caused by local compression may arise but the individual usually presents with signs associated with pituitary hormone deficiency. The precise symptoms will vary in accordance with the particular hormone that is deficient (see Table 5.3).

MEDICAL MANAGEMENT

Investigative procedures. Diagnostic investigations include field of vision testing and biochemical investigation to determine the severity and degree of pituitary failure and to distinguish between isolated hormone failure and complete anterior failure. Skull X-rays, CT scanning and magnetic resonance imaging (MRI) are also carried out.

Medical intervention. The choice of treatment will depend on the diagnosis of the cause of the pituitary failure and will aim to relieve the clinical effects and symptoms which the patient experiences. Treatment may involve surgery, radiotherapy and drug therapy to replace the deficient hormones (see Table 5.4).

NURSING PRIORITIES AND MANAGEMENT: HYPOPITUITARISM

Major considerations

Giving information

Effective nursing intervention depends upon the establishment of a good nurse-patient relationship in a friendly environment. As the effects of hypopituitarism can be widespread, causing diverse physical and psychological changes which can be difficult to understand, it is important to ensure that all of the patient's questions are answered in terms which are understood. Open and frank discussion about changes in body image and sexuality are essential to the individual concerned. The nurse should be aware that short stature is not always caused by a simple deficiency in the production of GH. Other factors may come into play, requiring different investigations and treatment approaches. (See Box 5.2 and Table 5.5.)

Clear ongoing explanations of the extensive and possibly uncomfortable investigations will help to relieve the patient's

Table 5.3 Symptoms associated with anterior pituitary hormone hyposecretion

Deficiency	Symptoms
LHFSH	Men: • Poor libido and impotence • Infertility • Small soft testicles • Loss of secondary sexual hair Women: • Amenorrhoea • Infertility • Dyspareunia • Breast atrophy • Loss of secondary sexual hair
TSH	Children: • Growth retardation Adults: • Decreased energy • Constipation • Sensitivity to cold • Dry skin • Weight gain
ACTH	All: • Weakness • Tiredness • Dizziness on standing • Pallor • Hypoglycaemia
GH	Children: • Growth retardation • Short stature Adults: • Uncertain significance.

Table 5.4 Hormone replacement therapy (Reproduced with kind permission from Besser & Cudworth 1990.)

Deficient hormone	Replacement	Check
Anterior pituitary		
Women		
LH	Ethinyloestradiol	Libido and
FSH	Medroxyprogesterone	symptoms of deficiency
Men		
LH	Testosterone	Libido and potency
FSH		
Children		
GH	Growth hormone	Growth chart
ACTH	Hydrocortisone	Cortisol levels throughout the day
TSH	Thyroxine	T_3 and T_4 levels
Posterior pituitary		
ADH	Desmopressin	Plasma and urine osmolality

* For men and women, the only treatment of associated infertility entails regular injections of the deficient pituitary hormones (mainly FSH in the form of Pergonal or Metrodin) or, if the defect is hypothalamic, hourly parenteral injection of a gonadotropin-releasing hormone via an implanted pump.

Box 5.2 Growth hormone deficiency and short stature

Normal growth results from a number of interacting factors; therefore short stature cannot be attributed simply to underproduction of GH from the pituitary.

From childhood into adulthood, growth relies on both extrinsic and intrinsic factors such as the height of the individual's parents, dietary intake and absorption, emotional or psychological problems, endocrine conditions such as hypothyroidism, and skeletal disorders or other congenital abnormalities (see Table 5.5).

All children should be measured before commencing school in pre-school clinics and during school attendance in order to determine their pattern of growth. Most children fall within a statistically derived height–distance curve: a child thought to be shorter than average should have his height measured at regular intervals so that his growth velocity can be calculated. In those children who are failing to grow a diagnosis will need to be made in order to commence the appropriate therapy.

anxiety. The presence of a nurse familiar to the patient during these investigations can be reassuring.

As the prospect of neurosurgery or radiotherapy is frightening for most people, careful preoperative preparation must include an explanation of procedures, the nature of immediate postoperative care and the expected outcome for the long term. Reminding the patient that his symptoms will be relieved by surgery, radiotherapy and hormone replacement therapy will be of considerable psychological benefit.

Supporting the patient in ongoing drug therapy

Replacement of gonadotropins is reasonably straightforward, requiring a once daily tablet or a monthly injection. Synthetic GH is administered by injection. The child and his parents will be taught how to carry this out at home, where supervision and support will be given by the community health team.

Hydrocortisone is given to those who need ACTH replacement. The dose can be variable and cortisol levels should be checked frequently. The omission of even one dose may have serious consequences. Such patients should be advised to carry a steroid card and to wear a Medic-Alert bracelet at all times.

Thyroid replacement is given as an oral medication. As the half-life of thyroxine is very long, the occasional missed dose is not critical.

Replacement of deficient hormones should alleviate symptoms, allowing the patient to lead a normal life within the community. It is essential that the individual feels free to contact the appropriate doctor or specialist unit at any time to discuss his condition or any related anxieties. As pituitary disease is a life-long condition that will require ongoing monitoring, hospital attendance may be frequent. It helps if visits and tests are coordinated so that they can be kept to a minimum; at the same time, advice and support must be given promptly when required so that the patient can lead as normal a life as possible.

DISORDERS OF VASOPRESSIN (ADH) SECRETION

All the conditions caused by disorders of ADH (anti-diuretic hormone) secretion or activity are uncommon. These disorders include:

- inappropriate/excessive secretion
- deficiency of hypothalamic secretion of ADH
- nephrogenic diabetes insipidus: a condition in which the renal tubules are insensitive to the action of ADH.

Table 5.5 Types of short stature: features, diagnosis and management

Type	Description	Investigations	Management
Disproportionate short stature	Short limbs and backs, e.g. hypochondroplasia	Full skeletal survey with interpretation by a specialist	Until recently, little could be done for the classic 'dwarf'. Recently, experimentation in bone lengthening has been successful in increasing height by up to 15 cm
Systemic causes of growth delay	In systemic disease, there is often delayed skeletal maturation, e.g. Crohn's disease, asthma, dietary deficiency	These causes should all be eliminated by routine investigation, including jejunal biopsy if Crohn's is suspected	Once treated, the short child with systemic disease should catch up and reach his normal growth potential
Psychological and emotional deprivation	This is commonly recognised in infancy. Behavioural abnormalities may be displayed. Short stature and delay in maturity may result	Detailed investigations may not be necessary if emotional disturbance can be identified	Support for the family including counselling for the parents may be necessary and could require cooperation from the child's school, etc. In the ward environment an observant nurse may well identify interaction difficulties and should always be aware of the child who has been non-accidentally injured, whose parents may be seeking help from outside agencies
Hormone deficiency	Important hormones required for growth are thyroid hormone, growth hormone (GH) and sex hormones. The child may display characteristic features of deficiency of these	Investigations include skeletal X-ray (to determine bone age) and testing of the hypothalamo – pituitary axis to check GH secretion	Replacement of the deficient hormone may be required to promote growth. GH is given by injection three times a week
Laron dwarfism	This occurs when GH is produced but due to receptor failure the child cannot respond to it	On testing GH levels are normal, even high, but the child appears very small	The child does not respond to GH. Both the child and family require sensitive handling and emotional support as the child will remain small as he moves into adulthood. He will usually be of normal intellect
Pseudohypoparathyroidism	The child has a short stature and round face, is obese, has short metacarpals, and is below normal intelligence	X-rays show subcutaneous calcification. It is caused by the patient having resistance to the action of parathyroid hormone. PTH levels will be high and calcium levels low	High doses of vitamin D treat the condition
Cushing's syndrome	Typical Cushing's appearance	This is extremely rare. Investigations as for Cushing's syndrome in adults will be undertaken	The treatment is the same as for adults
Constitutional growth delay	The child appears small and in proportion with no unusual features	Hand and wrist X-ray shows retarded bone development. GH levels and hyperthalamo-pituitary tests are normal	Once the child reaches puberty and experiences the associated growth spurt that accompanies it the eventual height will be within the normal range

Causes include pituitary tumours, infection, surgery, trauma, renal disease and some drugs.

Diabetes insipidus

PATHOPHYSIOLOGY

Clinical features. Deficiency of vasopressin (ADH) leads to polyuria, nocturia and a compensatory polydipsia. Urine output may reach 10–15 litres or more per day, leading to severe dehydration if the individual's thirst mechanism is impaired or if his fluid intake is restricted in any way.

MEDICAL MANAGEMENT

Investigative procedures. Diagnosis may be made by single paired urine and plasma osmolality, obviating the need for the more stressful and prolonged water depletion test. Plasma osmolality will show high concentration and urine will be dilute.

Medical intervention. Treatment is by the administration of synthetic vasopressin (desmopressin or DDAVP) 10–20 μg 1–3 times daily by the intranasal route; it is best given at night initially. It can also be given i.m. or s.c. at 1/10 of the dose.

NURSING PRIORITIES AND MANAGEMENT: VASOPRESSIN SECRETION

Major considerations

The nurse's interventions will include accurate recording of fluid intake and output with the full cooperation and participation of the patient. It is essential for the patient to have easy access to toilet facilities. Samples of urine should be kept for osmolality assessment.

The nurse will also be involved in administration of medicines and education of the patient with regard to self-administration of medicines, continued measurement of fluid balance, and regular weight recording. Most patients rapidly become aware if the therapy is no longer working and will contact their GP or the specialist physician supervising their care.

Syndrome of inappropriate anti-diuretic hormone (SIADH)

The causes of SIADH are many, but include oat cell carcinomas, pneumonia, TB, meningitis, head injury, porphyria and some chemotherapeutic agents such as vincristine.

PATHOPHYSIOLOGY

Clinical features. SIADH usually presents with vagueness, confusion, nausea and irritability and if not corrected leads to fits and coma. It is caused by an excess of ADH and leads to hyponatraemia as a result of dilution. Biochemical investigation will reveal low plasma sodium, low plasma osmolality and high urine osmolality. Blood pressure, serum potassuim levels, kidney function and adrenal function will be normal.

MEDICAL MANAGEMENT

Medical intervention may include:

- fluid restriction to 500–1000 ml/day
- treatment of the underlying cause
- administration of demeclocycline to inhibit the action of AVP on the renal tubules
- administration of hypertonic saline infusions (in severe cases).

DISORDERS OF THE THYROID GLAND

Simple goitre

A goitre is an enlargement of the thyroid gland. It can occur without over- or underactivity of the gland. If the goitre is large, it may exert pressure on surrounding structures, causing respiratory distress or dysphagia.

Hyperthyroidism

Hyperthyroidism (or thyrotoxicosis) and diabetes mellitus are the most prevalent of the endocrine diseases. (Diabetes mellitus is discussed in detail in Part 2 of this chapter.) The most common cause of hyperthyroidism is intrinsic thyroid disease; pituitary causes are extremely rare. Hyperthyroidism is a condition in which there are high levels of circulating thyroid hormones. It predominantly affects females aged between 30 and 50 years, but can occur at any age in either sex.

Graves' disease

Graves' disease is the most common form of hyperthyroidism. It is an autoimmune disorder, associated with a diffuse enlargement (or goitre) of the gland, in which antibodies behave like TSH, stimulating thyroid hormone production. Graves' disease tends to run in families and may be associated with ophthalmic features, i.e. retro-orbital inflammation leading to periorbital oedema.

Toxic multinodular goitre

This type of goitre is characterised by an asymmetrical nodular thyroid enlargement. It tends to occur in an older age group than Graves' disease.

Toxic adenoma (solitary nodule)

This type of tumour constitutes about 5% of thyroid disease. In these cases a thyroid nodule may act autonomously and produce excess levels of thyroid hormone, leading to suppression of the normal thyroid.

PATHOPHYSIOLOGY

In hyperthyroidism high levels of circulating thyroid hormones stimulate cell metabolism, resulting in a high metabolic rate. TSH secretion is suppressed. The cardiovascular system is affected, and tachycardia and atrial fibrillation are common. The individual suffers weight loss despite having an increased appetite. He will complain of general fatigue, although he may become more active and find that he is unable to rest for long. The individual may become exophthalmic due to periorbital oedema causing lid retraction and limited upward gaze. If the eyelids are unable to close, corneal ulceration can occur.

Common presenting symptoms. The patient will have noticed a variety of symptoms, notably increased irritability, inability to relax and sleep, heat intolerance with excessive sweating, weight loss despite an increased appetite, and perhaps a feeling of shakiness and a fine tremor of the hands. Eye changes may be present. An enlargement of the gland may have been noticed; if it is pressing on the trachea, there may be some breathlessness.

MEDICAL MANAGEMENT

Investigative procedures. Clinical examination will confirm the tachycardia and fibrillation, enlarged thyroid, and ophthalmic signs. The skin will be hot and moist and a fine tremor of the outstretched hands may be discernible. Diagnosis is confirmed by elevated serum T_4.

Medical intervention. The three approaches to treatment in hyperthyroidism are:

- anti-thyroid drug therapy
- surgery
- radioactive iodine therapy.

Drug therapy. Antithyroid drugs (carbimazole 30–40 mg daily or propylthiouracil 300–600 mg daily) are prescribed to inhibit the synthesis of thyroid hormones. The patient will continue to take the drug until a euthyroid state (i.e. normal thyroid function) is achieved, after which the serum T4 and the drug dose are monitored to ensure that the patient remains euthyroid and to avoid over- or under medication. Treatment usually continues for some months, with monitoring by the patient's GP and regular outpatient visits. The patient is warned to report unexplained fever or a sore throat, as the major side-effect of antithyroid drugs is agranulocytosis, which occurs in roughly 1:1000 patients.

Symptomatic control of tachycardia is obtained by administration of beta blockers such as propranolol until thyroid hormone levels are normal.

Surgical intervention. Partial thyroidectomy is performed only after drug therapy has produced a euthyroid state. In some centres, the patient is given potassium iodide for 1–2 weeks before surgery in order to reduce the vascularity of the gland and reduce the risk of postoperative haemorrhage.

About 75% of patients are cured by surgery. Partial thyroidectomy is also a useful treatment for patients with large or unsightly goitres.

Complications of partial thyroidectomy include: postoperative haemorrhage, recurrent laryngeal nerve palsy, hypocalcaemia, and hypothyroidism.

Radioactive iodine therapy. Iodine-131 (^{131}I), if given to the patient, is usually administered as a single capsule on an outpatient basis. The patient is advised to avoid eating for 3–4 h after administration to allow adequate absorption of the iodine; he is also advised to drink at least 2 l of fluid over the next 24 h and to pass urine frequently in order to excrete free circulating radioactive iodine as rapidly as possible.

Patients present a radiation hazard for approximately 1 week following this treatment. In some centres, anything more than a minimal dose requires that the patient is admitted for a few days until he is no longer significantly radioactive. This type of therapy is used when surgery is not appropriate but is not usually offered to women of childbearing age.

NURSING PRIORITIES AND MANAGEMENT: HYPERTHYROIDISM

Major nursing considerations

Preoperative preparation (see also Ch. 27)
The patient is admitted to hospital 1–2 days prior to surgery. Although euthyroid, the patient may well be over-anxious about surgery, and a quiet area of the ward should be reserved for these patients.

Blood pressure and pulse are monitored to ensure that the patient is euthyroid, and deep breathing exercises should be taught and practised. The nurse should also demonstrate the postoperative positioning and support of the head and neck to prevent strain on the sutures.

Postoperative care (see also Ch. 27)
Features of postoperative nursing care specific to patients who have undergone partial thyroidectomy are described in Nursing Care Plan 5.1.

Carcinoma of the thyroid gland

Carcinoma of the thyroid gland is rare, comprising around 1% of all cancers. In the UK, it causes approximately 400 deaths per annum, compared with 35 000 from carcinoma of the lung. It is 3 times more common in females than males and, apart from anaplastic carcinoma, tends to occur in a much younger age group (20–40 years) than most other malignancies.

The five type of thyroid carcinomas are:

- papillary
- follicular
- anaplastic
- lymphomatous
- medullary cell.

PATHOPHYSIOLOGY

Papillary or follicular carcinomas usually present with a rapidly growing lump which can cause hoarseness or difficulty in swallowing. Papillary carcinoma may prove fatal as a result of lymphatic spread to the trachea. Metastases commonly involve the brain, liver, lungs and bones and are more common with follicular carcinomas.

Common presenting symptoms. Often the patient will have noticed a small nodule or swelling in the neck. He may be euthyroid, or he may have symptoms associated with either hyper- or hypothyroidism.

MEDICAL MANAGEMENT

Investigative procedures. Tests of thyroid function (T_3, T_4, and TSH levels) are carried out and are followed by radiological examination of the neck. Needle biopsy and aspiration may be used to give a firm diagnosis and differentiate between the types. Isotope scanning will generally appear as 'cold' on scanning, but only 10% of such cold nodules are malignant. Many are cysts, and operative exploration may be avoided if aspiration cytology is convincingly normal.

Medical intervention. The treatment of choice is near-total thyroidectomy. This is usually followed by a large dose of ^{131}I to isolate any thyroid remnant. Any tissue showing radio-iodine uptake subsequently must be assumed to be recurrent disease, and further ^{131}I may be therapeutically taken up by the tumour tissue. The thyroidectomy is performed first on the principle that only when normal thyroid tissue has been removed will malignant tissue take up the ^{131}I in a concentration high enough to cause destruction.

Follow-up is important and will usually be carried out at 6-monthly intervals initially. During this time, replacement of thyroid hormone will be with T_3 (this has a shorter half-life than T_4 and allows scanning to be repeated with ^{131}I). Any local recurrence will be treated with a further dose of ^{131}I and scanning repeated.

With early treatment, thyroid carcinoma has a relatively good prognosis.

NURSING PRIORITIES AND MANAGEMENT: CARCINOMA OF THE THYROID GLAND

Major considerations

Caring for the patient receiving ^{131}I therapy
The patient and his family should be given clear explanations regarding the effect of ^{131}I, the reasons for being nursed alone with restricted access for staff and visitors, and procedures to follow in the handling of body fluids. It should be explained to the patient that he cannot be discharged until his radiation level is safe.

Immediately prior to administration of the dose, TSH may be given to increase the uptake. Measures should be taken to prevent constipation, as this inhibits the excretion of radioactive material. A high fluid intake should be encouraged to promote a good urinary output. Bedpans should be designated for the patient's exclusive use. All body fluids will be highly radioactive following ^{131}I administration and the patient should be encouraged to bath or shower regularly to remove contaminated perspiration.

The patient should be nursed in a single room with a minimum of equipment in it. Film badges should be worn at all times by staff members to indicate radiation exposure. Duties should be coordinated so that each staff member spends a minimum amount of time with the patient.

As with all endocrine disease, prompt treatment should result in complete alleviation of all signs and symptoms; the patient should be reassured to this end whilst undergoing treatment. Follow-up after treatment is essential. Nursing staff should encourage the patient to attend outpatient or GP clinics as advised. Patients should be reassured that, particularly with localised disease from a papillary carcinoma, the probability of 'cure' is extremely high.

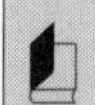
Pritchard & Mallett (1993) pp. 271–279.

Hypothyroidism

The term 'hypothyroidism' refers to low levels of circulating thyroid hormones. Underactivity of the thyroid gland may be primary, resulting from disease of the thyroid, or secondary, due to pituitary failure.

Aetiology
Primary hypothyroidism as a result of autoimmune disease is the commonest cause of thyroid underactivity. It is often termed 'Hashimoto's thyroiditis', and is often associated with other autoimmune disease. It is 6 times more common in women than in men.

Hypothyroidism (myxoedema) may also be caused by previous treatment for thyrotoxicosis by means of surgery or radioactive iodine.

Iodine deficiency is another cause of hypothyroidism and is due to insufficient dietary intake of iodine. This leads to reduced thyroid hormone production. Goitre is a common feature of this condition. Endemic hypothyroidism is occasionally seen in areas where iodine levels in the water supply are low (usually inland areas far from the sea). This was once a problem in Derbyshire. It is still seen in some areas such as the Andes, and the Alpine areas of Europe, the Himalayas, and some parts of central Africa.

Congenital hypothyroidism occurs in approximately 1 in 4000 live births and usually results from congenital absence of the thyroid gland; it can also be caused by certain genetic enzyme defects.

PATHOPHYSIOLOGY

Congenital hypothyroidism results in cretinism; if it is not detected and treated early, the child will not develop fully either mentally or physically. Most centres now screen for hypothyroidism in neonates.

In primary hypothyroidism (myxoedema), serum T_4 is low and levels of TSH high. The effect on the cardiovascular system results in low blood pressure, bradycardia, and cardiomegaly. The metabolic rate is low, resulting in lethargy, weight gain, and sensitivity to cold.

Common presenting symptoms. The onset of myxoedema is slow and insidious. Because the affected individual is often elderly, it may be accepted as a normal part of ageing for some considerable time before a medical opinion is sought. The individual may report sensitivity to cold, weight gain, a general slowing down of body functions, lethargy, depression, and an inability to 'think quickly'. His face will be puffy in appearance and his hair sparse, coarse and brittle. He may also notice an unattractive thickening of the skin.

In severe hypothyroidism, the patient may be admitted in a coma and initially thought to be suffering from hypothermia. This represents a medical emergency in which intensive treatment and care are essential.

Diagnosis of hypothyroidism is confirmed by low plasma levels of T_4 and raised TSH levels.

MEDICAL MANAGEMENT

Medical intervention. Hypothyroidism is treated with replacement doses of thyroid hormone (thyroxine) commencing with a low dose and increasing to 150 mg daily. To ensure that the patient is euthyroid, both T4 and TSH levels should be checked.

NURSING PRIORITIES AND MANAGEMENT: HYPOTHYROIDISM

It is usual to treat patients on an ongoing basis in the community. The community nursing team should follow up medical treatment and explanations and ensure that the patient understands the reasons for the thyroxine replacement therapy and the importance of attending for regular checks to ensure that he becomes and remains euthyroid.

DISORDERS OF THE PARATHYROID GLANDS

The parathyroid glands secrete parathormone (PTH) which, together with Vitamin D and calcitonin, plays an important role in calcium metabolism.

Hypercalcaemia

PATHOPHYSIOLOGY

In most instances, raised levels of calcium in the plasma are caused by hyperparathyroidism and malignancy (see Box 5.3). Mild hypercalcaemia, which is often symptomless, occurs in about 1 in 1000 of the population. Even mild symptoms can lead to an early diagnosis, thanks to advanced chemical analysis technniques; this means that it is now extremely rare to see the severe renal and bone problems associated with hypercalcaemia that occurred in the past.

Box 5.3 Causes of hypercalcaemia

Common:
- malignancy
- primary hyperparathyroidism.

Rarer:
- Addison's disease
- milk alkaline syndrome
- sarcoidosis
- thyrotoxicosis
- vitamin D poisoning

Very rare:
- immobility
- phaeochromocytoma
- thiazide diuretics
- tuberculosis

Common presenting symptoms. Patients may present with symptoms of malignancy or of hypercalcaemia. Possible signs and symptoms include:

- constipation
- depression
- drowsiness, coma
- excessive calcium intake
- malaise
- nausea, vomiting
- nocturia
- polydipsia, polyuria
- psychosis
- weakness.

MEDICAL MANAGEMENT

Investigation procedures. Diagnosis is made on the basis of medical history, clinical examination and tests to ascertain the cause. When malignancy is the cause, signs of this will be evident.

Medical intervention. Hypercalcaemia caused by malignancy is usually seen only in advanced carcinoma when bony metastases have occurred. If possible it should be treated as it may improve the quality of the patient's life. Adequate hydration is of great importance and in itself is often enough to relieve the symptoms of the hypercalcaemia. Other treatments include oral phosphate and steroid therapy. However, recent studies have established that the Biphosphonate drugs (pamidronate, etidronate) are highly effective in lowering malignant hypercalcaemia, although the best routes of administration are still under investigation.

Primary hyperparathyroidism

This condition is caused by the overproduction of PTH by the parathyroid glands. It affects 3 times more women than men, and its incidence increases with age. It is usually idiopathic.

MEDICAL MANAGEMENT

Medical intervention. Surgery is indicated for the management of hypercalcaemia due to high PTH secretion, as no long-term drug therapy is available. However, asymptomatic hypercalcaemia is treated conservatively and monitored in the GP surgery or outpatient department.

Following parathyroidectomy, hypocalcaemia of either a transient or permanent nature may ensue. This should be treated promptly to prevent tetany occurring. If severe hypocalcaemia occurs, i.v. calcium gluconate (10 ml of 10%) should be given immediately. Vitamin D and oral calcium supplements will be required. Calcium levels should be monitored closely until they have stabilised.

NURSING PRIORITIES AND MANAGEMENT: PRIMARY HYPERPARATHYROIDISM

Major considerations

The investigations required to make a diagnosis of hypercalcaemia may sometimes require hospital admission, particularly if the hypercalcaemia is severe and/or is thought to be malignant. The patient will probably have been unwell for some time and will be feeling very tired and weak on admission.

Careful explanations of the investigations and treatment are required. It is particularly important for the accuracy of the urine tests that the urine collections are completed properly. It is essential that clear explanations regarding this are made so that the patient can cooperate fully and with understanding.

If surgery is undertaken the perioperative care is the same as for thyroidectomy. In addition, regular assessment for impending hypocalcaemia is made (see Box 5.4).

Secondary and tertiary hyperparathyroidism

Secondary hyperparathyroidism occurs due to disease causing hypocalcaemia, e.g. in vitamin D deficiency or in renal disease. The parathyroid glands strive to keep the calcium levels up, while calcium remains normal or is frankly low. Rarely, this leads to permanent hypercalcaemia, termed tertiary hyperparathyroidism. This is often seen in patients with renal failure.

Hypocalcaemia

This is a rarer biochemical abnormality than hypercalcaemia. It is most commonly caused by renal failure but also occurs transiently, following surgery to the neck. As an idiopathic condition it is often associated with other autoimmune features. It may also be due to severe vitamin D deficiency.

Rickets and osteomalacia

These are diseases of calcium and phosphorus metabolism resulting from a deficiency in vitamin D intake and synthesis.

Box 5.4 Detecting increased neuromuscular irritability (tetany) due to hypocalcaemia

Positive Chvostek's sign

The nurse can test for this sign by tapping the person's facial nerve about 2 cm anterior to the ear lobe. If hypocalcaemia (or hypomagnesaemia) is present, unilateral twitching of facial muscles, especially around the mouth, may be observed.

Positive Trousseau's sign

This may be observed when the blood pressure is taken on a person with a low calcium level which as yet is not producing observable effects. The sphygmomanometer cuff is inflated around the person's arm and pressure increased to above systolic pressure for 2–3 minutes. The constrictive effect of the inflated blood pressure cuff exacerbates the hypocalcaemia in the limb distal to the cuff. During blood pressure recording or shortly after, muscular contraction or twitching will be noticed in the limb concerned.

Vitamin D deficiency during growth produces rickets in the growing skeleton. In childhood, rickets produces soft, painful bones which are readily bent; this is seen especially in the weight-bearing bones and may give rise to gross deformities. In the adult, osteomalacia is the result; symptoms are generally diffuse bone pain and myopathy.

Rickets does not now occur commonly in the endogenous population of Great Britain due to better nutrition and, possibly to a reduction in industrial pollution which allows more sunlight through. It is, however, sometimes seen in the Asian community in Britain, particularly in individuals with an increased vitamin D requirement, e.g. babies, children and pregnant women. The exact explanation for its prevalence is not clear. It may be associated with inability to synthesise vitamin D, as it occurs predominantly in people who eat a strict vegetarian diet.

Vitamin D replacement is the treatment and prophylaxis the aim in known vulnerable groups.

DISORDERS OF THE ADRENAL GLANDS

Dysfunction of the adrenal medulla

The main effect of the catecholamines (adrenaline, noradrenaline and dopamine) which are secreted by the adrenal medulla is on the cardiovascular system, the central nervous system, and on carbohydrate and lipid metabolism. Together, adrenaline and noradrenaline prepare the body for the 'fight or flight' response.

Phaeochromocytoma

Phaeochromocytoma is a rare condition occurring in about 1 in 10 000 of the population and 1 in 1000 cases of hypertension. It is a condition in which a tumour of the adrenal medulla produces excessive adrenaline and noradrenaline. The tumour is small, with about 10% being multiple tumours, and 10% being malignant.

PATHOPHYSIOLOGY

Clinical features. The tumour produces the clinical effects of excessive catecholamine secretion. Hypertension and hypertensive retinopathy are common.

Common presenting symptoms. The patient may present with anxiety, palpitations, and panic attacks. Throbbing headaches, sweating and pallor are also common. There may be a history of high blood pressure.

MEDICAL MANAGEMENT

Investigation procedures. A careful history and clinical examination may lead the physician to suspect a phaeochromocytoma. Investigations include 24-h urine collections for catecholamines or their major metabolite, vanillylmandelic acid (VMA). Normal levels of catecholamine secretion virtually exclude a diagnosis of phaeochromocytoma. Abdominal X-rays and a CT scan may show a tumour of the medulla.

Medical intervention. Treatment includes surgical removal of the tumour or treatment by β-adrenoreceptor blocking drugs (propanolol).

NURSING PRIORITIES AND MANAGEMENT: PHAEOCHROMOCYTOMA

Major considerations

The first priority of care is to limit anxiety as much as possible and to nurse the patient in a quiet, non-stressful environment. Clear, concise explanations of the reasons for the symptoms will help to relieve the anxiety.

Observations of blood pressure and pulse should be

recorded 4-hourly, and any sweating or flushing noted. Antihypertensive drug therapy must be maintained, as the risk of postoperative hypotensive collapse is reduced by adequate preparation with adrenoreceptor blocking drugs.

A care plan should be devised such that the patient can be as independent as possible in self-care tasks. Preoperative preparation is as for general abdominal surgery (see Ch. 27). Specific postoperative care includes ½-hourly recording of blood pressure to observe for immediate postoperative hypotensive collapse brought on by the reduced blood volume characteristic of chronic vasoconstriction. Specialist drugs such as sodium nitroprusside should be available to control blood pressure as required.

Disorders of the adrenal cortex

Cushing's syndrome

Cushing's syndrome is caused by the excessive and inappropriate circulation of glucocorticoids. It is most commonly seen in the therapeutic administration of synthetic steroids. Spontaneous causes of Cushing's syndrome are extremely rare. The major causes of Cushing's syndrome, excluding iatrogenic causes, are:

1. Pituitary dependent disease (Cushing's disease) (60% of cases)
2. Ectopic ACTH production (20%)
3. Adrenal adenoma (10%)
4. Adrenal carcinoma (5%)
5. Alcohol induced (1.5%).

PATHOPHYSIOLOGY

Clinical features. Increased plasma cortisol levels lead to wide-ranging clinical effects on most systems of the body, i.e. altered fat and carbohydrate metabolism, diabetes mellitus and obesity, wasting of muscles, retention of sodium leading to hypertension, oedema, compromise of the immune system, and osteoporosis. Other effects include thinning of the skin with bruising or purpura, hirsutism and oligomenorrhoea in women and impotence in men. (See also Table 5.6.)

Common presenting symptoms. Because of the wide-ranging clinical effects of Cushing's syndrome, the patient can present with varying symptoms. Frequently, the patient will complain of infections which will not resolve, weight gain, bruising and discoloration of the skin.

Table 5.6 Signs and symptoms of Cushing's syndrome

Symptoms or sign	Aetiology
Muscle wasting which can be demonstrated by the patient being unable to stand from a squatting position	Catabolic effect of the steroids
Osteoporosis which can be so severe as to result in spontaneous fracture of vertebrae or ribs	Protein loss from the skeletal matrix
Skin thinning and purple striae, plethora, easy bruising and purpura. Poor wound healing	Atrophy of the elastic lamina allows disruption of the dermis so capillaries can be seen below the surface. Weakening of the capillaries leads to easy bruising (often without trauma)
Oedema	Weakening of the capillaries.
Immunocompromisation	The lymphocytes are destroyed, lowering ability to fight infection. Signs of infection, e.g. swelling and redness, are masked
Obesity and 'buffalo hump' (pad of fat across shoulders)	Altered metabolism of fat. Fat is laid down over the trunk. Lipid levels may be raised
Hypertension	Sodium-retaining properties of glucocorticoids
Diabetes mellitus	Alteration in the normal metabolism of carbohydrate and the increased conversion of protein to carbohydrate
Depression, euphoria and frank psychosis	Unknown
Change in libido, impotence, oligomenorrhoea and infertility	Due to the general hormone imbalance that is occurring
Excess hair growth, hair loss (particularly of the male pattern type in women	This is seen in Cushing's but is not solely due to cortisol overproduction

MEDICAL MANAGEMENT

Investigative procedures. Diagnosis is confirmed by radiological and biochemical investigations (see Table 5.7). The differential diagnosis between pituitary disease, ectopic ACTH production and adrenal hypersecretion is important to establish as the treatment and management of these three causes will vary considerably.

Medical intervention. Drug therapy and surgery are the main forms of treatment.

Metyrapone is commonly used to lower cortisol levels. An alternative approach is to completely remove intrinsic cortisol and supplement levels with an oral steroid.

Transsphenoidal surgery is the treatment of choice for removal of an ACTH-producing tumour of the pituitary. An alternative approach under investigation at present is to administer ketoconazole.

Surgery for removal of a benign adenoma offers a good chance of cure, but adrenal carcinoma carries a poor prognosis. The drug mitotane (o 'p' DDD) is adrenolytic.

Following adrenalectomy the patient will require life-long hydrocortisone and mineralocorticoid replacement therapy. The patient must always wear a Medic-Alert bracelet and carry a steroid card. He should be informed of the dangers of hypocortisolaemia, which is a life-threatening condition.

Management of ectopic ACTH syndrome. This condition most often occurs in patients with an oat cell carcinoma of the lung. The neoplastic cells themselves produce ACTH and give rise to Cushing's syndrome. Care is as for malignant disease (see Ch. 32), taking into account the additional complications of Cushing's syndrome.

There is another subgroup of patients with ectopic ACTH production from less malignant tumours (the so-called carcinoid tumours) who present with a more classical Cushing's syndrome and who may survive for many years with appropriate chemotherapy.

NURSING PRIORITIES AND MANAGEMENT: CUSHING'S SYNDROME

Major considerations

The main aim of nursing care is to relieve the symptoms of the disease. On admission, a full nursing history is taken and the patient's needs thoroughly assessed to provide a basis for a care plan. A major consideration will be the psychological impact of the illness, for example as related to a change in body image. Providing clear ongoing explanations of the hormonal changes that the patient is experiencing and the investigations and subsequent treatment that he will undergo will go a long way toward providing psychological support.

Table 5.7 Radiological and biochemical tests for differential diagnosis of Cushing's syndrome

Test	Findings indicative of Cushing's syndrome
Radiological	
Adrenal CT scan	Adrenal adenomas and carcinomas are usually large and detectable in a CT scan
Skull X-ray	It is difficult to detect these often small pituitary tumours; 90% of X-rays are normal
CT head and pituitary fossa MRI scan	High resolution scanning and increasingly sophisticated techniques often allow an enlarged pituitary to be detected
Chest X-ray	May show a bronchial carcinoma which may be a source of ectopic ACTH production
Venous catheterisation	This technique may be of value in confirming by blood sampling a pituitary origin of ACTH production and blood sampling as well as locating an ectopic source
Biochemical	
Dexamethasone suppression test	Under the principle that as a result of the feedback system high levels of steroids will switch off ACTH production and therefore steroid production, failure of suppression indicates Cushing's syndrome and at a higher dose may indicate pituitary disease. Ectopic ACTH production is not suppressed with a low or a high dose
Circadian rhythms	Patients with Cushing's syndrome may lose the normal variation in levels of cortisol. These should be measured at 9 h, and at 24 h when the patient is sleeping and not warned. The patient should have been in hospital for at least 48 h before commencement of this test
Insulin tolerance test	This test, in which a dose of i.v. insulin is given, demonstrates that the normal rise in cortisol levels to hypoglycaemia is absent and will differentiate between true Cushing's, depression and alcohol-induced pseudo-Cushing's. It is performed mainly in specialist centres as a high level of supervision is required, and certain baseline measurements of pituitary function and confirmation of a normal ECG are recommended to ensure the patient's safety
Glucose tolerance test	This test will indicate that glucose metabolism is impaired; indeed, most people with Cushing's syndrome show a diabetic tendency
Urine collection	24-hour urinary collections are performed and should show an elevation in excreted steroids. Accuracy in this test is difficult to achieve as it relies on the patient managing a complete, uncontaminated 24-hour collection.

? **5.4** Recall the physical symptoms which commonly occur in Cushing's syndrome. Identify the potential care needs that the patient will have and formulate a care plan responsive to those needs (See Case History 5.1 and Nursing Care Plan 5.2.)

Ongoing follow-up after discharge from hospital is essential. Initially, 3-monthly checks will be carried out, gradually reducing to an annual check. If adrenalectomy or pituitary surgery has been performed precautions will need to be taken regarding hydrocortisone replacement; this must be explained in detail. An information leaflet can be useful as a reference for the patient when at home.

Addison's disease

Addison's disease is a rare condition in which there is total destruction of the adrenal cortex resulting in failure of cortisol secretion. It may occur at any age, and is more common in females. Autoimmune adrenalitis is the most common cause in the developed world. Adrenal destruction by adrenalytic drugs such as mitotane (o'p'DDD), malignant disease or malignancy are rare causes.

PATHOPHYSIOLOGY

Clinical features. High levels of ACTH result in pigmentation of the skin and mucous membranes. Glucocorticoid, sex steroid and mineralocorticoid production is reduced. Plasma levels of proteins are low, and plasma levels of potassium are high, with serum urea being elevated due to volume depletion.

Common presenting symptoms. The onset of the disease is usually insidious, often starting with a feeling of general malaise and weakness. The discolouring of the skin will have been noticed, especially in the palmar creases and on the inside of the lips and cheeks. Some patients present as medical emergencies with Addisonian crisis, in which there is hypotensive collapse, abdominal pain and fever.

MEDICAL MANAGEMENT

Investigative procedures. Diagnosis is by clinical examination and blood tests to confirm high levels of ACTH and low levels of cortisol.

In the short Synacthen test a dose of 250 µg of tetrosactrin (synthetic ACTH) is given i.v. or i.m.; blood samples for plasma cortisol taken at 30 and 60 min after its administration will show a failure of the adrenal glands to respond to the stimulus of the parenteral ACTH.

Medical intervention. Treatment is by long-term replacement doses of mineralocorticoid and glucocorticoid. This should lead to an improvement in the patient's well-being. Levels of hydrocortisone should be checked regularly to ensure the dose is correct. Mineralocorticoid replacement with fludrocortisone should be checked by regular blood pressure readings (which should show no postural hypotension) and by measurement of plasma renin.

Addisonian crisis. Adrenal crisis is a life-threatening event. It occurs in such situations as injury infections, anaesthesia and surgical procedures where, unlike in the healthy individual, the stress response does not occur. The absence of the cortisol surge to a major stressor results in a severely shocked patient. Addisonian crisis requires immediate intervention. This treatment is aimed at restoring steroid, sodium, and glucose levels to within normal range by i.v. administration of 100 mg hydrocortisone, and i.v. infusion of normal saline given quickly with dextrose if glucose levels are low. Hydrocortisone is then given i.v. or i.m. 6-hourly until the patient is stable, following which the steroid replacements can be given orally and mineralocorticoid introduced.

NURSING PRIORITIES AND MANAGEMENT: ADDISON'S DISEASE

Major considerations

Careful observation of temperature, pulse, and standing and lying blood pressure should be made. A raised temperature will indicate signs of infection which the patient may not be able to fight effectively. Any postural drop in blood pressure should be reported immediately.

The steroid replacement therapy should be administered with the patient's involvement so that he will have a full

Case History 5.1

J was a 20-year-old woman admitted to the unit following transfer from her local hospital with a history of weight gain, hirsuties, acne on her back and face, pain and increasing weakness in her limbs, amenorrhoea and depression.

She was transferred in a wheelchair, being unable to walk at this point. Her parents and her fiancé accompanied her.

Once J was settled into the unit, clinical examination showed her to have centripetal obesity, severe acne, marked facial hair and some loss of occipital hair. She had severe pitting oedema of her ankles and had been amenorrhoeal for 6 months. Purple striae were present on her abdomen and thighs, and bruising was noticeable on her shins. She was unable to stand from the squatting position, indicating marked proximal myopathy. She was tearful and anxious and complained of a poor sleep pattern and waking at about 4 a.m. Observations showed her to be hypertensive at 170/110 mmHg; pulse and temperature were normal. J had some photographs of herself taken at her engagement party some 4 months before, showing a pretty, very slim, smiling young woman.

She was helped to settle into the unit and her nurse sat with her and explained the investigations that were to be performed. As many of these involved multiple venepunctures she was reassured that a local anaesthetic cream would be applied. (It is inadvisable to leave cannulae in situ as the risk of infection in someone who is immunocompromised is great.)

On the first day blood tests showed that J's baseline cortisol levels were well above the normal range. Her haemoglobin, liver function and urea and electrolytes were measured, as well as her sex hormone levels and thyroid function. A measurement of ACTH was made and found to be extremely high. Skull and chest X-rays were performed.

An insulin tolerance test showed elevated cortisol levels throughout with no response to hypoglycaemia. A glucose tolerance test showed elevated glucose levels throughout; glycosuria was present 1 h post glucose load. This had not resolved at 2 h, indicating a diabetic tendency.

On the 3rd and 4th day blood was taken at 9.00 h, 18.00 h and 24.00 h and repeated the next night, the midnight samples being taken when J was asleep. This was to establish her circadian rhythm; the results showed that the levels of ACTH and cortisol did not fall at night and remained high throughout the day.

The finding that both the ACTH levels and the cortisol levels were high indicated that the high cortisol levels were being driven by ACTH. The source of the ACTH had to be established.

During this time J was seen by a psychiatrist, who established that she was depressed but not suicidal. She was constantly kept informed of the results of her tests and the implications of the results by the medical staff; further explanations were given by her nurse. A CT scan the following day showed an enlarged pituitary gland.

On the basis of this it was decided that petrosal sinus sampling would be performed and samples taken for ACTH and cortisol after a catheter had been inserted into the right groin. The procedure was explained to J and her consent obtained. Her right groin was shaved and she was fasted overnight. Samples were taken at various points, including the petrosal sinuses (the point nearest the pituitary gland on both the left and right sides). No sedation is permitted prior to this test as it interferes with the results and so extremely detailed explanation of the procedure was required to gain J's confidence and understanding. She was accompanied by her nurse, who remained with her throughout the procedure. When assayed, the results showed a higher level of ACTH on the left side of the pituitary.

Once a source had been found for the excess ACTH J could now be started on drug therapy to control her symptoms. She was started on metyrapone 500 mg tds and her cortisol levels checked daily to ensure she did not become hypocortisolaemic.

After review of her results and X-rays it was suggested that to try to remove the pituitary tumours would be the best treatment option. After discussion with J her consent for the operation was obtained. It was explained to her and her fiancé that there was a possibility that she may become deficient in all pituitary hormones following the surgery, including those which would affect her fertility. In this eventuality hormone replacement could be given.

A small adenoma was removed from the left side of her pituitary gland. On return from theatre J was nursed on the neurosurgical ward initially. Hydrocortisone injections were given (100 mg every 6 h for 48 h) to ensure that if the tumour had been removed J's cortisol levels would not fall too rapidly and predispose her to an Addisonian crisis. J returned to the endocrine unit looking rather bruised around the eyes and wearing a nasal bolster but otherwise well. Nursing staff continued to monitor her lying and standing blood pressure. Temperature and pulse were checked 4-hourly, and nasal discharge was observed and tested for signs of CSF leak.

Three days postoperatively J's hydrocortisone was withdrawn. A measurement of her 9.00 h cortisol and ACTH was taken the next day. Her cortisol level was very low and correspondingly J felt weak and light-headed. Her blood pressure showed a postural drop. The next morning the exercise was repeated and the results were the same. J was losing weight around her face and her ankle oedema was reduced. She said she felt very positive for the first time in months and was sleeping well. On the afternoon of the 4th postoperative day she became weak and dizzy and felt nauseated. Her blood pressure was measured and found to be low. She was laid down and the doctor informed. It was felt that an Addisonian crisis was impending and so a blood sample was taken for cortisol measurement and J was commenced on oral prednisolone. Some days later all of J's hormone levels were checked and as she felt well on her replacement therapy she was discharged home to the care of her family. It was arranged for her to return to the ward in 12 weeks' time.

By the time J returned for this visit, she had lost an enormous amount of weight, was walking unaided, had lost most of her facial hair and had started menstruating. Her steroid therapy was stopped and close observation maintained to observe for impending adrenal crisis. A blood test 48 h later indicated that her cortisol levels were in the normal range. It was decided to repeat all the pituitary function tests done prior to the surgery. These showed all hormones to be in the normal range and responses to hypoglycaemia, as demonstrated by the insulin tolerance test to be intact. This showed that the pituitary had recovered its normal function. J was discharged home with a regular, follow-up inpatient appointment every 12 weeks to ensure that all was well.

Some months after, the nurses received an invitation to J's wedding and one year later J was the very proud mother of a baby daughter.

knowledge of drug dosage and timing and techniques for self-administration before discharge.

The patient should be issued with a steroid card and advised to carry this and to wear a Medic-Alert bracelet on his wrist or ankle at all times.

An ampoule of hydrocortisone 100 mg should be kept at home in case of serious illness or trauma, and the GP or community nurse called to administer it. It may also be of value to teach a member of the family to administer this.

It is vital that the patient has a thorough understanding of his condition and the signs associated with complications. This will help to restore the patient's confidence and enable him to return to a full and active life.

Nursing Care Plan 5.2 Care of a patient with Cushing's syndrome

Nursing considerations	Action	Rationale	Expected outcome
1. Pain from fractured vertebrae or ribs as a result of osteoporosis	❒ Provide immediate pain relief. Administer as prescribed, noting their efficacy ❒ Handle and position patient carefully	Pain will cause the patient discomfort and will increase anxiety. Pain relief will reduce this. Fractured ribs will cause shallow breathing and will increase chances of chest infection. Gentle handling will reduce distress and prevent further fractures	The patient should be pain free and comfortable and his anxiety reduced
2. Infection as a result of immunocompromisation	❒ Make 4-hourly recordings of temperature, pulse and blood pressure. Report any variation from the normal range immediately	Death from overwhelming infection can occur. Signs of infection will be masked so infection may be advanced before signs are seen	Any infection will be identified early and correct treatment commenced
3. Damage to skin as a result of skin thinning and oedema or poor wound healing	❒ If the patient is immobile he will require care of pressure areas to prevent tissue damage. Legs will need to be elevated to relieve the oedema and any wounds will require scrupulous aseptic technique when dressed	Tissue will be rapidly broken down and slow to heal, so preventive measures are essential. Susceptibility to infection requires precautions to prevent introduction of infection	Further tissue damage will be prevented and any present source of infection healed as rapidly as possible
4. Hypertension	❒ Record blood pressure readings 4-hourly after 10 min lying flat and 1 min standing. Report levels beyond the normal range or postural deficit	Increasing blood pressure may lead to stroke or heart failure and if persistently high will need to be treated with drugs. Postural deficit will indicate a problem with sodium excretion or retention	Blood pressure levels will remain within acceptable limits
5. Diabetes mellitus as a result of abnormal carbohydrate metabolism	❒ Record pre- and postprandial blood sugar levels and perform daily urinalysis	Persistently high blood sugars will lead to the complications of diabetes mellitus and may need to be treated with insulin	Blood sugar levels will remain within the normal range
6. Psychosis and mental disorder	❒ The patient's psychological status must be ascertained early on. A psychiatric opinion should be obtained. Mood swings and bizarre behaviour should be reported. The patient may be so disturbed as to require 24 h psychiatric nurse observation	The psychological state of the patient may change rapidly and the patient must be closely observed for this. Some patients can become suicidal	The patient will not be a danger to himself or others and his safety is maintained at all times

? **5.5** With a colleague, undertake a role play exercise by acting out the education of the patient regarding steroid therapy. Formulate an information sheet which could be given to patients prior to discharge.

? **5.6** Check at your local hospital what advice is available for patients with Addison's disease. From what source do patients obtain the Medic-Alert bracelet? Are these patients exempt from prescription charges?

CONGENITAL ADRENAL HYPERPLASIA (CAH)

This is a condition caused by a deficiency in one of the enzymes involved in cortisol synthesis. It is an inherited disorder and is thought to occur in about 1 in 5000 of the population in Europe.

PATHOPHYSIOLOGY

To understand CAH it is necessary to understand the biosynthesis of steroids. If, as can be inferred from Figure 7 the enzyme 21-hydroxylase is absent (to take the most common deficiency as an example), cortisol will not be produced in sufficient quantity. By means of the negative feedback system, ACTH production will be increased to stimulate the production of cortisol. This in turn will lead to hypertrophy of the adrenal cortex and elevated levels of 17-hydroxyprogesterone, androstenedione and testosterone — the hormones occurring before the enzyme block. This will result ultimately in virilisation.

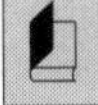
Sheppard & Franklyn 1988 *Clinical Endocrinology and Diabetes*

Common presenting symptoms. If severe, CAH presents at birth with sexual ambiguity. In the female the high level of androgens present cause clitoral hypertrophy and fusion of the labial folds. The syndrome may not be recognised in the male. Internal genitalia may develop normally. If a diagnosis is not made at birth a genotypical female may be labelled male. Furthermore, the individual may go into adrenal crisis and die if not treated with corticosteroids.

Other problems which may occur because of the excessive circulating sex hormones are primary amenorrhoea in girls, precocious puberty, and short stature due to premature fusion of the bony epiphyses.

MEDICAL MANAGEMENT

Investigations include blood tests to confirm high levels of ACTH and 17-hydroxyprogesterone. Replacement of the glucocorticoid is usually given in the form of prednisolone to suppress the ACTH production and thereby reduce the overstimulation of the adrenals. Other corticosteroids may be used.

NURSING PRIORITIES AND MANAGEMENT: CAH

General considerations

Information should be given to the individual regarding steroid replacement therapy (details of which can be read under Hypopituitarism, p. 142). Nursing care should concentrate on the psychological support which will be required, especially if the diagnosis is late.

The psychosocial implications of CAH are considerable, and formal counselling and psychotherapy should be made available. In female patients some of the effects of virilisation are not reversible with drug therapy; plastic surgical repair may therefore be necessary. This is particularly important as the patient approaches adulthood, as sexual intercourse may be rendered difficult, painful or impossible.

DISORDERS OF SEXUAL DIFFERENTIATION

In normal development gonadal and phenotypic sex follow an orderly process of development determined by chromosomal sex at the moment of conception.

During the early stages of fetal life the gonad has the potential to developing female or male characteristics. In the presence of another X chromosome (i.e. 46, XX) or the absence of another chromosome (i.e. 45, XO), development will follow the female pattern. The presence of two X chromosomes is, however, necessary for normal ovarian function.

By the second month of fetal development the genital organs are undifferentiated duct systems termed the Müllerian and Wolffian ducts. In the normal female, as development progresses the Wolffian system regresses and the Müllerian system develops to form the fallopian tubes, the uterus and the upper vagina. The external genitalia undergo little change.

In the male, the Müllerian system regresses and the Wolffian system develops to form the testes, vas deferens, prostate and seminiferous tubules. The genital tubercle present in both systems forms the clitoris in the female and the penis in the male.

There is evidence to suggest that the normal development of a male child is hormone-dependent. It appears that testosterone inhibits the regression of the Wolffian duct and stimulates its development into the male sexual structures. In contrast to this, the ovary is not affected by hormones in utero.

Abnormalities of sexual differentiation may present with abnormal genitalia at birth, growth disturbance in childhood or abnormal secondary sexual development.

Abnormalities of gonadal development

True hermaphroditism (i.e. the presence of male and female sexual characteristics in the same individual) is extremely rare. It occurs when both the Müllerian and Wolffian systems continue to develop. Ovotestes may exist or an ovary on one side and a testis on the other.

Chromosomal abnormalities

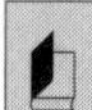

Sheppard & Franklyn 1988 *Clinical Endocrinology and Diabetes*

Chromosomal abnormalities affecting sexual differentiation may briefly be described as follows:

1. Klinefelter's syndrome. In a description of this disorder and discussion of nursing considerations see Chapter 6, p. 198.
2. Turner's syndrome. This has an incidence of 1 in 2500. Most cases have a 45, XO karyotype although some have what is known as a mosaic form (see Ch. 6) e.g. XO/XX. Affected individuals are of short stature with a 'webneck', and may have widely spaced nipples and peripheral oedema. The ovaries are atrophic and serum LH and FSH levels are elevated.
3. Kallman's syndrome. There is a normal karyotype but a deficiency of gonadotropins. This condition is sometimes termed hypogonadotropic hypogonadism. Typically the individual has a partial defect in the sense of smell. Normal function can be resumed with replacement of LH and FSH. Fertility is possible.
4. Testicular feminisation. This is a syndrome of androgen resistance. The karyotype is male (i.e. 46, XY) and testes are present but because of tissue resistance to circulating androgens at puberty, breast tissue develops although pubic hair does not. Due to tissue insensitivity the regression of the Müllerian system occurs but the Wolffian system does not develop and a blind-ended vagina results. The gonads may become malignant and are usually removed at the onset of adult life.

NURSING PRIORITIES AND MANAGEMENT: DISORDERS OF SEXUAL DIFFERENTIATION

Whilst disorders of the gonads are rarely life-threatening or require admission to hospital, their psychological implications for the individual and his family cannot be over-emphasised.

The role of the nurse in the investigation and treatment of these conditions is to offer psychological support to the individual concerned in an environment which is both relaxed and supportive.

Counselling on an informal and formal basis is essential for the individual during investigations, when complete privacy must be ensured. Feelings of inadequacy regarding sexuality and low self-esteem are common. An approach which demonstrates empathy with the individual helps to create a positive image during the initial examinations, investigations and subsequent treatment.

REFERENCES

Besser G M, Cudworth A G 1990 Clinical endocrinology. Lippincott, Philadelphia

Bruch H 1973 Eating disorders. Basic Books, New York

Edwards C R W (ed) 1986 Endocrinology. Integrated clinical science. Heinemann Medical, London

Edwards C R W & Bouchier I A 1991 Davidson's principles and practice of medicine. Churchill Livingstone, Edinburgh

Garner et al 1983 An overview of sociocultural factors in the development of anorexia nervosa. In: Darby P L, Garfinkel P E, Garner D M, Coscins D C (eds) Anorexia nervosa: recent developments in research. Alan Liss, New York, pp. 65–82

Hubbard J L, Mechan D J 1987 Physiology for health care. Churchill Livingstone, Edinburgh

O'Riordan J L H, Malan P G, Gould R P 1988 Essentials of endocrinology. Blackwell Scientific, Oxford

Sinclair H C, Fawcett J N 1991 Altschul's psychology for nurses, 7th edn. Bailliére Tindall, London

Szmukler et al 1986 Anorexia nervosa and bulimic disorders: current perspectives. Journal of Psychiatric Research. Pergamon Press

Wilson K J W (ed) 1990 Ross & Wilson anatomy and physiology in health and illness, 7th edn. Churchill Livingstone, Edinburgh

FURTHER READING

Agana-Defensor R, Proch M 1992 Pheochromocytoma: a clinical review. Clinical Issues in Critical Care Nursing 3(2): 309–18

Bayliss R I S, Tunbridge W M G 1991 Thyroid disease: the facts, 2nd edn. Oxford University Press, Oxford

Besser G M & Cudworth A G 1990 Clinical endocrinology. Lippincott, Philadelphia

Behi R 1989 Treatment and care of thyroid problems. Nursing (Oxford) 3(41): 4–6

Bryant S O, Kopeski L M 1986 Psychiatric nursing assessment of the eating disorder client. Topics in Clinical Nursing 8(1): 57–66

Chambers J K 1987 Metabolic bone disorders: imbalances of calcium and phosphorus. Nursing Clinics of North America 22(4): 861–872

Crowther J H 1992 The etiology of bulimia nervosa. Hemisphere, London

DeRubertis F R 1985 Hypocalcemia: etiology and management. Hospital Medicine 21(3): 88–90, 95–7, 100

Epstein C D 1991 Fluid volume deficit for the adrenal crisis patient. Dimensions of Critical Care Nursing 10(4): 210–7

Francis B 1990 Hypothyroidism. Advancing Clinical Care 5(2): 29–30

Hall R, Besser M (eds) 1989 Fundamentals of clinical endocrinology, 4th edn. Churchill Livingstone, Edinburgh

Goldberger J, Goldberger S 1989 Iatrogenic thyroid dysfunction: a case study. Hospital Practice 24(9): 30, 35

Graves L 1990 Disorders of calcium, phosphorus and magnesium. Critical Care Nursing Quarterly 13(3): 3–13

Halloran T H 1990 Nursing responsibilities in endocrine emergencies. Critical Care Nursing Quarterly 13(3): 74–81

Hardcastle W 1989 Management of Addison's disease. Nursing (Oxford) 3(41): 7–9

Kessler C A 1992 An overview of endocrine function and dysfunction. Clinical Issues in Critical Care Nursing 3(2): 289–99

Kessler C M 1988 Protecting the adrenalectomy patient. Nursing 18(12): 64L

Kiecolt-Glaser J, Dixon K 1984 Postadolescent onset male anorexia. Journal of Psychosocial Nursing and Mental Health Services 22(1): 10–3, 17–20

Moroney J 1991 Living with anorexia and bulimia. Manchester University Press, Manchester

Motton C, Litwack K 1989 Practical points in the care of patients following transsphenoidal surgery. Journal of Post Anaesthesia Nursing 4(2): 109–11

Nalbach D A, Carson M A 1991 Prolactinoma: a review and case study. Critical Care Nurse 11(9): 48–9, 52–7

Nusbaum J G, Drever E 1990 Inpatient survey of nursing care measures for treatment of patients with anorexia nervosa. Issues in Mental Health Nursing 11(2): 175–84

Pritchard A P & Mallet J (eds) 1993 Manual of clinical nursing procedures, 3rd edn. Harper & Row, London

Reasner C A 1990 Adrenal disorders. Critical Care Nursing Quarterly 13(3): 67–73

Rice V 1991 Hypercalcemia. Canadian Intravenous Nurses Association Journal 7(1): 6–8

Sheehy S B 1985 Metabolic and endocrine emergencies. Journal of Emergency Nursing 11(1): 49–52

Sheppard M C, Franklyn J A (eds) 1988 Clinical endocrinology and diabetes. Churchill Livingstone, Edinburgh

Smith J E 1990 Pregnancy complicated by thyroid disease. Journal of Nurse-Midwifery 35(3): 143–9

Walker M 1990 Women in therapy and counselling: out of the shadows. Ch. 7: Eating disorders; women, food and the world. Open University Press, Milton Keynes

Walpert N 1990 An orderly look at calcium metabolism disorders. Nursing 20(7): 60–4

Walworth J 1990 Parathyroidectomy: maintaining calcium homeostasis. Todays O R Nurse 12(4): 20–24, 31–33

Yeomans A C 1990 Assessment and management of hypothyroidism. Nurse Practitioner 15(11): 8, 11–2

Yucha C, Blakeman N 1991 Pheochromocytoma: the great mimic. Cancer Nursing 14(3): 136–40

PART 2
DIABETES

Rosemary McIntyre

CHAPTER CONTENTS

Introduction 155

Anatomy and physiology 155
The pancreas 155
Blood glucose regulation 155

Primary diabetes mellitus 156
Insulin-dependent diabetes mellitus (IDDM) 157
Non–insulin-dependent diabetes mellitus (NIDDM) 158

Impaired glucose tolerance (IGT) 159

Secondary diabetes mellitus 159

MANAGEMENT STRATEGIES IN DIABETES MELLITUS 159

Achieving and maintaining normoglycaemia 159
Dietary therapy 160
Diet combined with medication 160

Oral hypoglycaemic therapy 160

Insulin therapy 161
Types of insulin 161
Administering insulin 162

MONITORING RESPONSE TO THERAPY 164
Methods 164
Urinalysis 164
Blood glucose monitoring 164
Glycosylated protein estimation 165
Body weight monitoring 165

PREVENTING AND DETECTING DIABETES-ASSOCIATED COMPLICATIONS 165

Acute metabolic complications of diabetes 165
Nursing priorities and management of DKA 167
Nursing priorities and management of HHNK 170
Nursing priorities and management of hypoglycaemia 172

Chronic complications of diabetes mellitus 173
Nursing priorities and management of diabetic nephropathy 174
Nursing priorities and management of diabetic neuropathy 175
The diabetic foot 175
Infection 177
Summary 177

FACILITATING SELF CARE THROUGH EDUCATION 178

Assessment 178
Planning a teaching programme 178

PROMOTING PSYCHOLOGICAL AND SOCIAL ADJUSTMENT 179

The emotional impact of diabetes mellitus 179
Relationships 179
Lifestyle implications 181

Conclusion 181

References 182

Further reading 183

Additional resources and useful addresses 184

INTRODUCTION

The World Health Organization (WHO) describes diabetes mellitus as a chronic elevation of blood glucose (hyperglycaemia), in which the high concentrations of blood glucose and other biochemical abnormalities result from deficient production or action of insulin, a hormone that controls glucose, fat and amino acid metabolism (WHO 1985, p. 9). In the UK 1–2% of the population have been diagnosed as suffering from diabetes, but only around 25% of these will require lifelong treatment with insulin. The remainder have their disorder treated by either dietary adjustment alone (23%) or in combination with oral hypoglycaemic medication (37%).

Diabetes classification

Various classifications exist for diabetes mellitus, none of which is entirely satisfactory. In the past, the patient's age at diag-nosis was the main classification criterion. Accordingly, dia-betes was described as being either of 'juvenile onset' or 'maturity onset'. Specific diagnostic and treatment characteristics were ascribed to each type. This classification proved to be somewhat rigid and misleading and has now become obsolete (Bodansky 1989, Paton 1989, Reckless 1985).

The classification system now recommended by WHO (1985) recognises three main types of diabetes:

- primary diabetes
- secondary diabetes
- impaired glucose tolerance.

Primary diabetes can be subdivided into two broad groups:

- insulin-dependent diabetes mellitus (IDDM)
- non–insulin-dependent diabetes mellitus (NIDDM).

The terms 'Type I' and 'Type II' diabetes are often used synonymously with IDDM and NIDDM respectively.

Secondary diabetes may also be described as 'Type III' diabetes. Here, hyperglycaemia arises as a result of other disease processes or due to the effects of medication.

Impaired glucose tolerance: a new diagnostic title agreed by WHO for a subgroup of people with 'borderline' diabetes mellitus.

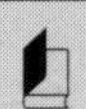

For information on diabetes in childhood and on gestational diabetes see Kinson and Nattrass 1984, Ch. 6.

ANATOMY AND PHYSIOLOGY

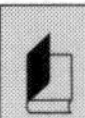

For a detailed study of normal anatomy and physiology the reader is referred to Wilson 1990, p. 185.

The pancreas

The pancreas combines both exocrine and endocrine functions. Exocrine tissue is responsible for the secretion of enzymes which are transported in ducts to the duodenum, where they play a vital role in the digestion of food (see p. 91). The endocrine function of the pancreas is concerned with the secretion of hormones. Clusters of endocrine tissue, the islets of Langerhans, are found scattered throughout the pancreas. There are two principal types of cells contained within the islets: beta cells (β cells), which secrete insulin, and alpha cells (α cells), which secrete glucagon. Each has a role in the regulation of blood glucose.

Blood glucose regulation

Within a 24-hour period the healthy human being will alternate between the 'fed state' and the 'fasting state' several times. In the two hours following a meal the blood glucose will tend to rise as absorption of nutrients takes place. This is termed the postprandial or fed state. Once absorption has peaked, blood glucose levels will tend to fall and will not rise again until the next meal is taken. This is termed the preprandial or fasting state. In health these fluctuations are very slight.

Insulin and glucagon are principally (but not exclusively) responsible for blood glucose regulation.

Insulin

Insulin, which could be described as an anabolic hormone, is secreted in response to a rising blood glucose level. Its functions are:

- to facilitate glucose uptake by the cells
- to promote glycogenesis, i.e. the conversion of glucose to glycogen for storage in the liver and skeletal muscle
- to promote protein synthesis
- to promote conversion of glucose to triglycerides for ultimate storage as body fat.

All of these functions have the effect of preventing an abnormal rise in blood glucose (hyperglycaemia) during the postprandial period (see Fig. 5.8). Insulin secretion is highest in the fed state and lowest in the fasting state.

Glucagon

Glucagon could be described as a catabolic hormone. It is secreted in response to a falling blood glucose level and has the following functions:

- to promote the conversion of stored glycogen to glucose (glycogenolysis) and its release from the liver
- to promote fat and protein breakdown in order to provide an alternative source of glucose (lipolysis and gluconeogenesis)
- to influence the generation of ketone bodies (ketogenesis). In total or near total insulin lack these weak acids are produced as a result of the chemical processes involved in fat breakdown.

The actions of glucagon and the other stress (counter-regulatory) hormones are all geared towards preventing an abnormal fall in blood glucose (hypoglycaemia). Glucagon secretion is highest in the 'fasting state' and lowest in the 'fed state'.

?	**5.7** Imagine that one hour ago you finished a three-course meal. What hormonal response would you expect from the islet cells in the pancreas right now?

Other influences on blood glucose regulation

The anterior pituitary secretes two hormones of significance to blood glucose regulation, as follows:

- *somatotrophin* (*growth hormone*). This hormone tends to raise blood glucose and is therefore described as diabetogenic in action and anti-insulin in effect. It influences blood glucose in two main ways:
  - — by promoting glycogen-to-glucose conversion (glycogenolysis)
  - — by inhibiting muscle glycogen storage.
- *adrenocorticotrophic hormone* (ACTH). This hormone stimulates the adrenal cortex to release cortisol (see below). A negative feedback mechanism operates in response to the circulating levels of cortisol in the blood.

The adrenal cortex secretes a group of hormones known as glucocorticoids, the most significant of which is cortisol. Cortisol is

Table 5.8 Insulin and its actions

Action of insulin on	Site of action	Consequences of insulin deficiency/stress hormone excess	
Carbohydrate metabolism			
Promotes glycogen storage	Liver	Impaired glycogen storage	Hyperglycaemia
Inhibits glycogen breakdown	Liver	Glycogen breakdown enhanced	
Inhibits gluconeogenesis	Liver	Gluconeogenesis enhanced	
Promotes cellular glucose uptake	Muscle/fat cells	Impaired cellular uptake of glucose	
Protein metabolism			
Promotes protein synthesis	Muscle	Impaired protein synthesis	Wasting
Inhibits protein breakdown	Muscle	Protein breakdown	
Fat metabolism			
Promotes fat synthesis	Liver	Impaired fat storage	Ketosis, Weight loss
Promotes triglyceride storage	Fat cells	Triglyceride breakdown	
Inhibits triglyceride breakdown	Fat cells		

Source: Adapted from Kinson and Nattrass, 1984.

released in a diurnal rhythm such that secretion is higher in the mornings and lower in the evenings (see p. 137).

Like glucagon, cortisol is a catabolic hormone. Secretion is increased during periods of physical or psychological stress when its effect is to raise the blood glucose level in an effort to meet the additional metabolic demands posed by the stressed state. Cortisol causes stored glycogen to be converted to glucose and promotes the breakdown of fat (lipolysis) and protein (gluconeogenesis), thus providing an alternative source of glucose to meet the energy needs of the cells.

The adrenal medulla secretes adrenaline and noradrenaline, which together are known as catecholamines. These 'fight-or-flight' hormones are catabolic in their action. In response to stress they place the body and brain in a state of 'high alert', causing blood glucose to rise as glycogen stores are released and fat/protein breakdown occurs. This increases the amount of available glucose and helps prepare the body to meet increased energy demands (see p. 137).

The liver and skeletal muscle. About 60% of absorbed nutrients are laid down as reserves in order to meet energy demands during fasting. Under the influence of insulin the liver and, to a lesser extent, skeletal muscle can store glucose in the form of glycogen. The liver is also involved in protein and fat synthesis for subsequent storage.

During fasting, or in response to stress, glucagon (and other stress hormones) will promote the release of liver and muscle glycogen in the form of glucose. The liver also contributes to the chemical processes of gluconeogenesis by which body stores of fat and protein are converted to glucose (see Fig. 5.8).

PRIMARY DIABETES MELLITUS

In primary diabetes mellitus hyperglycaemia and glycosuria occur in the absence of other known contributory disease or medication. The fault in primary diabetes is to be found in the

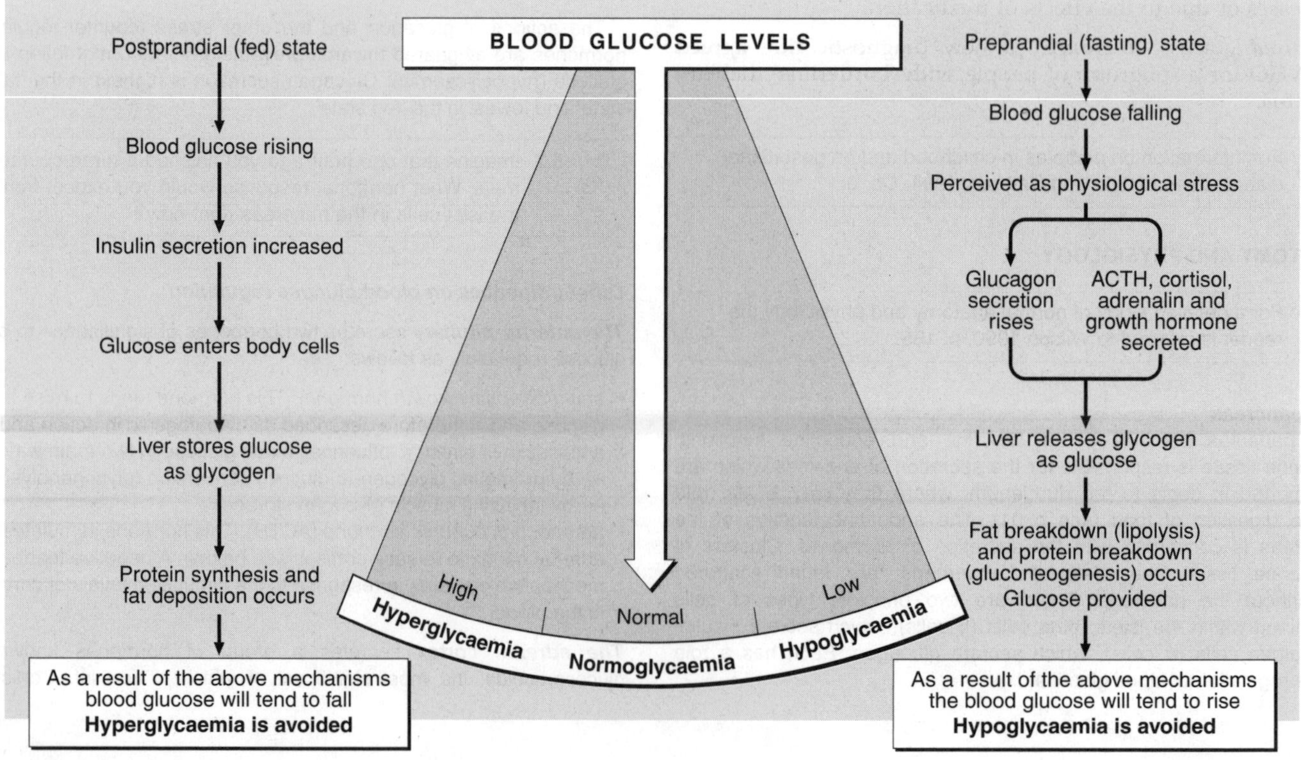

Fig. 5.8 The regulation of blood glucose in health.

pancreas, where the β cells fail to secrete sufficient insulin to meet the metabolic needs of the body. The disorder has two distinct modes of presentation. As there are clear differences in aetiology and pathophysiology each will be considered separately.

Insulin-dependent diabetes mellitus (IDDM)

Aetiology

The cause of insulin-dependent diabetes mellitus is thought to include a genetic susceptibility (see Box 5.5) which probably combines with immunological factors to cause destruction of insulin-producing pancreatic β cells. The precise triggering factor is as yet unknown. In IDDM insulin secretion is totally (or almost totally) absent and as a result lifelong treatment with insulin is required.

The precise cause of damage to the pancreatic β cells remains uncertain. Some interest has been shown in viral factors, coxsackie and mumps viruses having been implicated. Seasonal differences have been reported. It is known that an increased number of patients are diagnosed with IDDM during the winter months; this may lend further support to the viral aetiology theory (Drury 1986, Kinson & Nattrass 1984).

PATHOPHYSIOLOGY

Whatever the underlying cause of IDDM it seems likely that islet cell destruction is the underlying problem. This is a gradual process with progressive loss of β cell mass. Presentation can be abrupt, in response to a physical or psychological stress such as illness, trauma, surgery, pregnancy or bereavement. In such cases the additional metabolic demands posed by the stressed state can no longer be met by the failing pancreas and symptoms of diabetes appear. Occasionally when the crisis has passed there will again be enough insulin to meet the cells' needs and insulin can be temporarily stopped. Unfortunately, this 'honeymoon period' is short lived. As β cell mass continues to wane symptoms will reappear, necessitating lifelong treatment with insulin.

The effects of lack of insulin. The signs, symptoms and clinical features of insulin-dependent diabetes mellitus can best be explained in terms of the effects of insulin lack, as described in the following. (Clinical features are given in italic.)

1. In the face of insulin lack body cells are unable to obtain glucose for metabolism
2. Glucose which is unable to enter cells accumulates in the blood, causing an abnormally high blood glucose level — *hyperglycaemia*.
3. Increased amounts of glucose are filtered at the glomeruli. The capacity of the kidneys to reabsorb glucose (the renal threshold for glucose) is exceeded and glucose appears in the urine — *glycosuria*.
4. Glucose is highly osmotic, i.e. it attracts and holds water to itself. As glucose is lost in the urine large volumes of water are lost with it — *polyuria*.
5. As fluid loss continues the patient will begin to experience symptoms of dehydration, the most common of which is copious drinking in response to severe thirst — *polydipsia*.
6. The cells' requirements for glucose are not being met. The response is an increased secretion of glucagon and other stress hormones.
7. Under the influence of these hormones specific mechanisms come into play:
   - glycogen is converted to glucose and is released by the liver (glycogenolysis)
   - glucose is produced from the breakdown of body fat and protein (gluconeogenesis)
   - the patients' appetite may increase (polyphagia)
8. These efforts to meet the demands of the cells for glucose have the combined effect of raising the blood glucose even higher
9. *Weight loss* occurs due to the depletion of body fat and protein stores. This, together with cell deprivation of glucose and fluid/electrolyte imbalance, causes *muscle weakness* and *exhaustion*.
10. In the absence of insulin, fat breakdown results in the production and accumulation of ketone bodies (β-hydroxybutyric acid, acetoacetic acid and acetone). This leads to *ketonaemia* and *ketonuria*. Additionally, acetone excreted by the lungs gives a characteristic sweet, 'pear drop' odour to the breath.
11. Ketone bodies are weak acids which release free hydrogen ions to cause the serious condition of *metabolic acidosis* to develop.
12. Excess acidity of the blood causes a respiratory response. The patient *hyperventilates*, i.e. respirations become faster and deeper *(Kussmaul's respirations)*, which is a very useful way of removing H^+ from the blood (see p. 166).
13. Uncontrolled lipolysis, gluconeogenesis, ketogenesis and glycogenolysis combine to raise the blood glucose level still further, increase osmotic diuresis, and exacerbate dehydration and metabolic acidosis. This is a life-threatening situation known as *diabetic ketoacidosis* (DKA; see p. 165).
14. As a result of these profound biochemical disturbances the patient may experience *nausea* and *vomiting* and *colicky abdominal pain*.
15. Unless a diagnosis is reached and urgent medical treatment is established the patient will progress to *coma* and then ultimately to death.

Onset and progress of the disease. Although the onset of IDDM (Type 1 diabetes) is classically described as relatively abrupt, symptoms can develop over a period of days or weeks. Once symptoms do appear the disease will usually have a rapid progression. However, there will be variations in severity, some patients being much more acutely ill than others at the time of diagnosis.

The patient with IDDM may visit his general practitioner (GP) complaining of thirst, an increase in the amount of urine

Box 5.5 Insulin-dependent diabetes mellitus: the genetic link

An increased risk of developing IDDM is likely if a first degree relative such as a parent or sibling also has the disease. Of insulin-dependent patients 20% have a close relative with diabetes, as compared with 3% of the non-diabetic population (Shaw 1986).

A genetic susceptibility has been traced to the DR3 and DR4 genes in the human leucocyte antigen (HLA) located on chromosome 6. Studies have revealed that in identical twins identified as HLA-DR3 'types' and in whom one suffers from IDDM there is a high incidence of diabetes mellitus affecting the second twin. The HLA-DR3 group also show persistent islet cell antibodies, indicating that a genetic and an immunological (possibly autoimmune) susceptibility probably coexist. Within the general population it has been found that autoimmune disorders occur more frequently in people identified as HLA-DR3 types (see Ch. 16).

Twins identified as HLA-DR4 types have fewer autoimmune symptoms and rarely show islet cell antibodies. In this group it is less common for the second twin to be affected by IDDM. Given the identical genetic endowment shared by the twins, this may suggest that the genetic tendency is mediated by environmental influences (Haire-Joshu et al 1986, Bodansky 1989, Jones 1987; see also Ch. 6).

The HLA tissue-typing system referred to above is the one used to match potential organ donors with recipients. This helps to minimise the risk of rejection by the recipient's immune system.

passed and weight loss. He may also complain of feeling exhausted. The GP is likely to have the patient's urine tested for glucose and ketones. Blood glucose will also be measured. The presence of ketonuria and hyperglycaemia combined with symptoms of polyuria and thirst will usually be sufficient evidence upon which to refer the patient to a diabetes consultant. In hospital, following a full assessment, treatment can be commenced and the patient's response to therapy closely monitored. (See, p. 164 for diagnostic and monitoring tests.) Although most patients are referred to hospital, admission is not automatic. Some newly diagnosed patients with IDDM are managed as outpatients under the care of community staff.

The members of the diabetes care team in the hospital and community will have specialist knowledge about diabetes management. The central objective of care will be to help the patient acquire the knowledge and skills needed to resume an independent lifestyle. The patient will usually be asked to attend the diabetic outpatients clinic at specified intervals, although the GP and the community nursing staff will be principally responsible for ongoing care, treatment supervision and evaluation of progress.

Powell (1991b) describes the increasingly popular 'shared care' approach to diabetes management by which the patient's regular care and review is carried out by the GP and community nursing staff, supplemented by visits to the hospital for detection of complications annually or when difficult problems present.

Many patients with IDDM are much more acutely ill at the time of diagnosis. Often these patients have an intercurrent illness such as a severe infection. Onset can be so rapid that the patient may have progressed to full-blown DKA and may be drowsy or unconscious when the GP is first contacted. This extremely serious situation will require urgent hospital admission and intensive medical and nursing intervention.

Non–insulin-dependent diabetes mellitus (NIDDM)

Aetiology

The aetiology of NIDDM (Type II diabetes mellitus) is also unclear but it seems likely that several factors combine to cause susceptibility to the disease. Although these factors are not fully understood they differ from those thought to cause IDDM.

Genetic predisposition. Despite the fact that no HLA markers have been found for NIDDM there is undoubtedly a genetic component in its aetiology. An abnormality on the insulin gene found on chromosome 11 has been suggested as a cause but whatever the exact mechanism it seems that genetic factors are more important in NIDDM than they are in IDDM (Jones 1987). In studies of identical twins with IDDM both twins were found to be affected in 50% of the pairs. In identical twins with NIDDM it was found to be more than 90% certain that the second twin would at some stage develop the disease if it had appeared in the first twin (Haire-Joshu et al 1986, Paton 1989).

There is one unusual form of Type II diabetes which has a clearly established autosomal dominant form of inheritance. It is non–insulin-dependent, commonly develops in those under 30, and is given the rather anomalous title of 'maturity onset diabetes of the young' (MODY). (See Jones 1987, Paton 1989, Reckless 1985.)

Age. The incidence of NIDDM rises significantly with increasing age. Glucose metabolism is known to become less efficient from the third or fourth decade of life onwards and this deterioration accelerates in people over 60 years of age. Whilst this alteration in glucose tolerance may not in itself be pathological, when compounded by other factors (see below) it can contribute to the onset of symptoms of diabetes.

Insulin resistance. In NIDDM tissue sensitivity to insulin declines. The result is that hyperglycaemia can occur even when the circulating levels of insulin are normal or raised. Several reasons have been suggested for the development of insulin resistance; these include obesity (fat cells have fewer insulin receptors), the effects of ageing, and the presence of anti-insulin antibodies in the blood. Whatever the cause the result is the inefficient use of available insulin.

β cell deficiency. Up to 70% of patients with NIDDM show β cell deficit. The effect of this deficit is often that the initial postprandial surge in insulin is lost (Jones 1987).

Obesity. Obesity is known to cause insulin resistance in body cells. However, only a minority of obese people develop NIDDM and only around 60% of people with the disorder are obese.

Ethnic and environmental factors. There are wide geographical variations in the incidence of Type II diabetes. In western Europe and in the USA 1–2% of the population develop NIDDM but in certain circumscribed societies incidences of up to 40% have been reported, e.g. among the Pima Indians of North America and the Nauru Islanders of the Pacific. These remarkably high prevalences are probably due to the exposure of genetically isolated, diabetes-predisposed populations to influences such as a 'Westernised' diet and reduced physical activity. This can also be illustrated in the high rates of diabetes found in Japanese people who have migrated to Hawaii when compared with those who remain in Japan (Paton 1989).

PATHOPHYSIOLOGY

NIDDM usually presents in those over the age of 40 and most commonly in people over 60. Typically the patient is overweight.

The signs, symptoms and clinical features of NIDDM are much less severe than those of IDDM and are due to the effects of hyperglycaemia arising from a *relative* deficiency of insulin. In NIDDM there is still some insulin being secreted; as a result, ketogenesis is inhibited and, as the hyperglycaemia is less severe, dehydration is also much less common.

The effects of a relative lack of insulin are as follows.

1. Hyperglycaemia-related symptoms. Polyuria, nocturia and thirst may develop gradually. The patient, who is often obese, may initially be gratified to note that weight loss is occurring.
2. Genital or oral fungal infections. Candidal infections are common and result in the distressing symptoms of pruritus vulvae in the female and balanitis in the male. The sugar-rich urine around the genitalia appears to provide the yeast with favourable conditions in which to multiply. Staphylococcal skin infections, commonly resulting in boils and abscesses, may provide the initial stimulus for the patient to visit the GP.
3. Non-specific symptoms such as tiredness and lethargy are also frequently reported. The cause is uncertain but may be due to altered fluid and electrolyte balance. Visual disturbance may occasionally be reported, as hyperglycaemia can affect the optic lens.

Symptom-related complications. At the time the patient first seeks medical attention evidence of vascular and neurological complications such as proteinuria, sexual dysfunction, retinopathy and peripheral neuropathy may already have developed. Such patients have probably had asymptomatic diabetes with persistent hyperglycaemia for several years prior to diagnosis.

Onset and progress of the disease. NIDDM may present in several ways. A diagnosis will usually be made on the evidence of glycosuria and a fasting or random blood glucose of more than 8 mmol/l and 11 mmol/l respectively. Ketonuria is not a feature, as in NIDDM ketogenesis is inhibited by the presence of even small amounts of insulin.

Asymptomatic glycosuria may be discovered as an incidental finding, e.g. during a routine medical examination. Such a finding would normally prompt capillary or venous blood glucose analysis. Only if the results were equivocal would an oral glucose tolerance test be necessary to confirm the diagnosis.

IMPAIRED GLUCOSE TOLERANCE (IGT)

It is not clear why some people may have blood glucose results at or just above the upper limit of 'normal'. Borderline results in the absence of symptoms may not necessarily be judged abnormal. For example, since glucose tolerance is known to decline with age and obesity such factors would be considered in the overall assessment. To help determine to which category the patient should be assigned an oral glucose tolerance test may be carried out (see Table 5.9).

It is known that some people with IGT will go on to develop diabetes mellitus and that they may have a greater risk of developing atherosclerosis.

Onset and progress of the disease. Although it is clearly desirable that people should be spared the negative consequences of being inappropriately labelled (see Ch. 33, p. 906) as 'diabetic' (see Further Reading, p. 184) they should nonetheless have access to regular medical screening and should be offered information about the prevention of atherosclerosis and its consequences. These health promotion functions will normally be carried out by the GP and community nursing staff although in some areas the patient may also be asked to attend a diabetic clinic periodically.

IGT has implications for women who are planning to conceive. Current evidence suggests that it is important to correct hyperglycaemia prior to conception to reduce the risk of fetal abnormality (Tindall et al 1986). Preconception advice should be made available and the patient's blood glucose brought within normal limits before she conceives and closely monitored throughout her pregnancy. Care of this kind may be provided at a combined 'diabetic-obstetric' clinic.

SECONDARY DIABETES MELLITUS

PATHOPHYSIOLOGY

In primary diabetes the fault is to be found in the islets of Langerhans where β cell output of insulin is either absent or is insufficient to meet the needs of the cells. In contrast, hyperglycaemia in secondary diabetes occurs as a side-effect of certain drugs or secondary to disease processes other than diabetes which may either originate within or outside of the pancreas (Reckless 1985).

Some drugs, notably steroids, have a diabetogenic effect. The thiazide group of diuretics have been known to worsen established diabetes and in some elderly patients may actually hasten the onset of the disease. Excess secretion or administration of glucocorticoids, aldosterone, catecholamines or growth hormone will have a diabetogenic effect and can result in hyperglycaemia. Diabetes may therefore be a feature of Cushing's syndrome, Cushing's disease, phaeochromocytoma, primary aldosteronism and acromegaly (see Ch. 5, Part 1).

Pancreatitis and carcinoma of the pancreas may greatly reduce the number of functioning β cells and result in impaired insulin secretion. Chronic hepatic disease will have considerable consequences for carbohydrate, protein and fat metabolism. Glycogenesis and glycogenolysis may both be impaired and consequently hyperglycaemia and hypoglycaemia frequently feature in chronic disorders of the liver (see Ch. 4). Chronic renal failure can cause impaired glucose tolerance and insulin resistance, although the underlying mechanism by which this occurs is unclear.

Finally, there are a few rare genetic disorders which give rise to secondary diabetes. Friedreich's ataxia, an inherited disorder of balance and movement, is one example. Another is a condition which has an autosomal character and is referred to by the acronym DIDMOAD as it incorporates diabetes insipidus, diabetes mellitus, optic atrophy and deafness.

Onset and progress of the disease. Secondary diabetes is characterised by hyperglycaemia with glycosuria. Associated features such as thirst and polyuria may be experienced, and in hepatic disease the patient may also experience *hypoglycaemic* episodes, with symptoms such as trembling, sweating and clouding of consciousness. The underlying disease process will influence the nature and severity of the symptoms. Urinalysis and blood glucose will be monitored and dietary adjustment may be prescribed; this may be combined with oral hypoglycaemic medication or insulin therapy.

Table 5.9 Diagnostic glucose concentrations

Diagnosis	Venous whole blood (mmol/l)	Capillary whole blood (mmol/l)
Diabetes mellitus		
Fasting	> 7.0	> 7.0
2 hours post prandial	> 10.0	> 11.0
Impaired glucose tolerance		
Fasting	< 7.0	< 7.0
2 hours post prandial	> 7.0–<10.0	> 8.0–<11.0

In the absence of diabetic symptoms abnormality in both 2-hour postprandial and fasting blood sugar is required to establish the diagnosis of diabetes mellitus.

MANAGEMENT STRATEGIES IN DIABETES MELLITUS

Diabetes management requires a multidisciplinary approach. For those patients who are not acutely ill at the time of diagnosis management may be provided entirely within the community setting. However, many patients are more acutely ill at the time of onset and require hospital care to allow close monitoring of the effects of early treatment.

The professionals in the diabetes care team will share common goals for care, each contributing expertise in accordance with the patient's individual needs. It is, however, worth remembering that the patient is the most important member of the diabetes care team, whose full participation is necessary to the achievement of the following aims:

1. To achieve and maintain normoglycaemia
2. To monitor response to therapy
3. To prevent and detect diabetes-associated complications
4. To facilitate self-care through education
5. To promote social and psychological adjustment.

ACHIEVING AND MAINTAINING NORMOGLYCAEMIA

There are three main therapeutic approaches to this management, namely:

- dietary therapy
- oral hypoglycaemic therapy
- insulin therapy.

DIETARY THERAPY

Dietary modification is an important management strategy, whether used alone or combined with other therapies. Once the diagnosis of diabetes mellitus has been confirmed the patient is usually referred to a dietitian, who is often a diabetes specialist. The dietitian will assess the patient's calorific and nutritional needs, taking into account such factors as age, sex, lifestyle, religious or ethnic influences and current dietary habits. Establishing and maintaining links with the dietitian will help to promote a well-informed, positive and flexible approach to diabetes management.

The patient should be helped to understand how diet can influence current and future well-being. For some obese patients with NIDDM dietary therapy alone may bring the disorder under control. An individually formulated reduced calorie diet which is low in fat and refined carbohydrate and high in fibre will usually be recommended. Such a diet should have the effect of slowing down the rate of glucose absorption and reducing obesity. As a result the demand for insulin should be reduced and cell sensitivity to insulin improved.

Soluble fibre as found in peas, beans and lentils appears to have a beneficial effect on both blood glucose and blood cholesterol. The insoluble fibre found in cereals, wholegrain bread, and fresh fruit and vegetables provides energy, helps to avoid constipation and, especially if combined with a low salt diet, helps to reduce diabetes-associated cardiovascular risk (Simpson 1985).

Diet combined with medication

When dietary modification is combined with oral hypoglycaemic or insulin therapy, the patient will need additional education so that carbohydrate intake can be distributed fairly evenly throughout the day. It is particularly important that he knows that food must be taken *following* insulin or oral hypoglycaemic drugs to avoid a dangerous fall in blood glucose (hypoglycaemia).

Learning the carbohydrate 'value' of common foods can make it easier for the patient on insulin to spread carbohydrate intake over the day. The 'exchange system' may be used whereby the patient is given a list of foods with their carbohydrate value worked out in units of 10 g. A patient with a daily allowance of 150 or 200 g, for example, can quickly learn to divide this into 10, 20, 30 or 40 g portions throughout the day, thus enjoying a fair degree of choice and flexibility whilst still adhering to the prescribed diet.

The glycaemic index of food

This may also be considered in formulating dietary allowances. It is known that different carbohydrate-rich foods affect the blood glucose in different ways. Glucose has been given a glycaemic index of 100 and other carbohydrate foods are measured against this to reveal their relative potential to raise blood glucose. Pulses and bran have a low glycaemic index and are therefore recommended for diabetic diets whilst refined sugars have a very high glycaemic index and are therefore not advised except when a sharp rise in blood glucose is desired, e.g. to treat hypoglycaemia (Simpson 1985, Tredger 1989).

Team approach to dietary therapy

Although the dietitian is the key professional in dietary management it often falls to the hospital or community nurse to offer advice. Although standardised diet sheets have given way to a more individualised approach, some patients find it useful to have some form of checklist to guide them in their decisions. The British Diabetic Association (BDA) provides useful guidelines relating to diet in diabetes (see Useful Addresses, p. 184).

'Diabetic' foods can be rather expensive and are not actually necessary. Indeed, it may be worth bearing in mind that the type of diet recommended for people with diabetes could equally be commended to the general population. Such a diet is nutritious, promotes health and well-being and helps to prevent obesity, high blood pressure and heart disease (see Box 5.6).

ORAL HYPOGLYCAEMIC THERAPY

Oral hypoglycaemic medication can be effective only if β cells are capable of secreting some insulin. This form of therapy is therefore used exclusively for patients with NIDDM. In IDDM the underlying problem is total (or near-total) insulin lack and insulin replacement therapy is the only suitable treatment.

Day (1991) recommends that in the absence of persistent symptoms dietary treatment should continue for at least 3 months before drug therapy is commenced. Oral hypoglycaemic therapy would then be reserved for patients with NIDDM who have persistent hyperglycaemia despite a period of dietary adjustment.

Oral hypoglycaemic agents belong to two main groups, as described in the following (see Table 5.10).

The sulphonylureas

This is the most common group.

Mode of action. These drugs enhance insulin secretion and

Box 5.6 Recommendations for people with diabetes

(Nutrition Sub-Committee of the BDA's Professional Advisory Committee 1990)

BDA recommendations on diet: summary

- Include more complex carbohydrates in diet
- Reduce total fat intake
- Include less fat from animal sources in diet
- Balance the distribution and timing of carbohydrates with medication
- Follow a high fibre/low fat diet to assist weight loss
- Reduce sodium intake
- Consume alcohol only in modest amounts
- Avoid specialist diabetic products: they are unnecessary and can be misused
- Obtain individualised dietary advice.

The best carbohydrates for a diabetic diet

- Wholegrain or fibre-enriched breakfast cereals
- Wholemeal flour and bread
- Wholewheat pasta
- Brown rice
- Dried/baked beans and pulses
- Fruit
- Vegetables
- Biscuits and snack bars made with fibre-rich ingredients.

Table 5.10 Oral hypoglycaemic agents (Adapted from Kinson & Nattrass 1984, with kind permission.)

Sulphonylureas	*Trade names*
Chlorpropamide	Diabenese, Melitase, Glymese
Glibenclamide	Daonil, Semi-daonil, Euglucon Glutril
Gliclazide	Diamicron
Glipizide	Glibenese, Minodiab
Gliquidone	Glurenorm
Tolazamide	Tolanase
Tolbutamide	Rastinon, Pramidex
Sulphonylurea-related	
Acetohexamide	Dimelor
Glymidine	Gondafon
Biguanides	
Metformin	Glucophage

utilisation by causing the β cells to be more responsive to blood glucose levels. They may also increase the number and sensitivity of insulin receptors on fat and muscle cells.

Side-effects are uncommon but include weight gain, hypoglycaemia, mild digestive disturbance and skin rash. Facial flushing following alcohol ingestion can occur with chlorpropamide. As sulphonylureas lower blood glucose it is important that the patient and his carers are aware of the risks of hypoglycaemia. The medication should be taken with or just before food. The relationship between exercise, medication and diet will form an important part of the patient teaching programme (see p. 178).

The biguanides

These are less popular as they are more liable to cause side-effects. Only one, metformin, is in regular use in the UK.

Mode of action. The way in which the biguanides work is unclear but is thought to involve reduced glucose absorption in the gut and inhibition of gluconeogenesis in the liver. Some improvement in cell sensitivity to insulin has also been claimed (Kinson & Nattrass 1984). Metformin tends to be used to treat obese patients who show persistent hyperglycaemia despite treatment with diet alone or with diet combined with one of the sulphonylureas.

Side-effects. Medication-induced hypoglycaemia is very uncommon with biguanide therapy but vitamin B_{12} malabsorption and gastrointestinal upsets such as anorexia, nausea and diarrhoea are common. Lactic acidosis is a rare but very serious side-effect.

INSULIN THERAPY

Insulin therapy is essential to maintain life, and will be required throughout life, for all patients with insulin-dependent diabetes mellitus (IDDM). Insulin cannot be given orally as its protein structure would be inactivated by digestive enzymes. Parenteral administration will therefore be necessary and normally takes the form of subcutaneous (s.c.) injection.

Patients with NIDDM may become 'insulin requiring' during periods of stress or illness or when other therapeutic approaches cease to control their symptoms. This does not change the classification of their disorder, despite the (often temporary) requirement for insulin.

The objectives of insulin therapy are:

- to maintain blood glucose within normal limits
- to relieve hyperglycaemia-associated symptoms
- to correct metabolic/biochemical disturbances
- to prevent diabetes-associated complications.

Types of insulin

Until fairly recently all insulin preparations were derived from animal sources, mainly beef and pork. Genetic engineering and other advanced techniques have resulted in the production of bio-synthetic human insulin and purified or highly purified pork and beef insulin. As patients tend to develop antibodies to non-purified animal insulin these developments have been welcomed. It should, however, be noted that the highly purified preparations are more expensive (Home 1985). See Box 5.7.

Duration of action

There are many insulin preparations on the market. These may be categorised as short-acting, intermediate-acting or long-acting (see Fig. 5.9).

Short-acting insulins (soluble or neutral) are clear solutions. They have a rapid onset of action and when injected subcutaneously their maximal effect occurs in 2–4 h but can last up to 12 h.

Short-acting insulin may be prescribed in the following ways:

- once daily: given in the morning in combination with a long-acting insulin

Box 5.7 Human insulin

Current evidence suggests that fewer insulin antibodies develop in patients treated with purified pork or human insulins than with unpurified beef or pork insulin. The development of insulin antibodies is thought to result in reduced sensitivity to the actions of insulin, leading over time to increased dose requirements (Armitage et al 1988, Wiles 1988). As a result newly diagnosed patients are now routinely commenced on the purer 'human' insulins and it has become fairly common practice to change patients over from animal to human insulin.

For most patients the changeover has been trouble free but sadly there have been exceptions. Sadler (1991) describes patients' anxieties and adverse responses following changeover to human insulin. Concerns about disrupting previously good glycaemic control have been expressed: generally speaking, human insulins are more rapidly absorbed and in some patients this may lead to hypoglycaemic episodes. Altered awareness, with loss of the usual warning signs of hypoglycaemia has also been reported (Brooks & Boss 1989, Drug and Therapeutics Bulletin 1989).

Fisher (1991) recommends a 10% reduction in the daily insulin dosage when changing from animal to human insulin and close monitoring of blood glucose to allow further adjustments to be made during the changeover period. Patients may understandably feel anxious about a change in treatment. It is important that the patient is given the opportunity to discuss the pros and cons of changing to a different type of insulin with his doctor or diabetes nurse specialist before making a decision.

Despite the increased cost involved it is likely that newly diagnosed patients will be commenced on human insulin and thus avoid the problems of changeover which some patients with established diabetes have experienced (Jervell 1985).

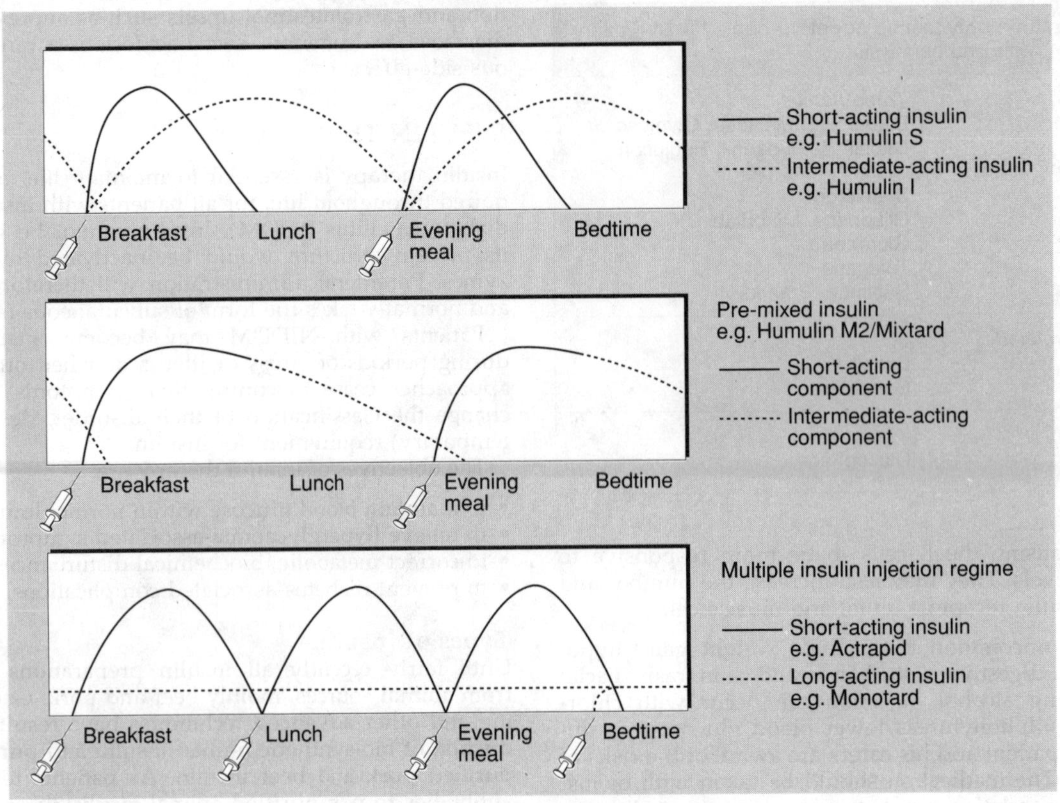

Fig. 5.9 Duration of action for short-, intermediate- and long-acting insulins.

- twice daily: given in the morning and evening in combination with an intermediate-acting insulin
- by multiple injection regime: 3 or 4 injections of short-acting insulin given about 30 min prior to each meal. This is usually combined with a single daily dose of long-acting insulin given at bedtime for overnight release
- by continuous s.c. infusion using an insulin pump (for selected patients judged likely to benefit from this form of therapy)
- intravenously: during acute metabolic emergencies when immediate insulin effect is required e.g. in diabetic ketoacidosis (DKA).

Intermediate- and long-acting insulins are cloudy. Their onset of effect is delayed for 1–2 h. The intermediate-acting insulins achieve maximum effect in 4–6 h and have a duration of action of 12–16 h. Long-acting insulins have their maximum effect in 8–12 h and a duration of action of up to 36 h.

Intermediate-acting insulins come in two main forms:

- *Isophane* insulin comes as a suspension of insulin with protamine. This is a useful type of insulin to use in combination with short-acting insulin. It provides a stable solution in which each insulin retains its own pharmacological properties even when mixed and stored in the same syringe.
- *Lente* insulins are complexed with zinc in two forms: amorphous 30% and crystalline 70%. The zinc binds the insulin and as a result onset of action is delayed and duration extended.

Long-acting insulin suspensions have a greatly extended period of action and can therefore be given once daily.

> ? **5.8** Using the British National Formulary (BNF), Home (1985) or current pharmacology text (e.g. Trounce 1990) draw up a table which illustrates examples from rapid-, medium- and long-acting insulins and indicate the species (source), onset and duration of action.

Administering insulin

The aim in administering insulin therapy is to achieve the best possible control of blood glucose without causing distressing hypoglycaemia. Ideally, the treatment should mimic the physiological response to normal variations in blood glucose.

In the healthy person 30–40 i.u. of insulin are secreted by the pancreas each day. During the fasting state there is a continual but low secretion of insulin. Following meals a surge in blood glucose results in increased insulin secretion (Bodington 1988).

Frequency

To mimic normal blood glucose fluctuations, a single injection of insulin with a 24-h period of action such as Human Ultratard (insulin zinc suspension crystalline) could be given once daily in combination with quick-acting insulin with a short (2–4 h) duration of action such as Human Actrapid (neutral insulin injection) before each meal. This multi-injection system has considerable advantages, not least of which are patient autonomy and flexibility of mealtimes. Patients using this system usually carry a precharged pen-type injection device such as the NovoPen or the B-D Pen. This allows administration of insulin to be discreet and adaptable to the day-to-day changes in the patient's activity levels, eating pattern and lifestyle. This system is most effective with patients who are able to closely monitor blood glucose and to adjust diet and insulin accordingly and does not, therefore, suit everyone. For many patients, twice-daily injections remain the favoured regime, whereas some, especially elderly patients, who have perhaps been required to progress to insulin from diet and/or oral therapy will be more willing to accept once-daily injections.

Mixing insulin

It is not advisable to mix zinc-based insulins and soluble insulins in a syringe for later use, as free zinc in the suspension can bind to the soluble insulin, extending the onset and duration of action. The injection should be given just after preparation. This problem does not arise with isophane insulins as they do not contain zinc (see Fig. 5.10).

> ? **5.9** What effect might such contamination have on the onset, effect and duration of action of the clear insulin and on the patient's blood glucose level?

Pre-mixed insulin. Various fixed ratios of short- to intermediate-acting insulins are available. Pre-mixed solutions are available for use with either syringe or pen injection devices. Pre-mixed preparations are popular but it is still common practice for insulin mixtures to be prepared by the patient or carer where fine adjustment of the dosage of each type of insulin is required.

Dosage will be carefully worked out and adjusted on an individual basis, taking account of blood glucose levels, ketonuria, lifestyle, and growth and development needs. The very real risk of hypoglycaemia needs to be addressed. Insulin must be. followed by food within 15 to 30 minutes of administration if a serious fall in blood glucose is to be avoided. The patient and his carers will need information about how they can achieve a balance of food, exercise and insulin to avoid detrimental swings in blood glucose.

Injection sites

Insulin is given by s.c. injection. The most common sites for injection are the upper arms, the upper thighs, the abdominal wall and the buttocks. Overuse of one site can lead to local tissue reaction resulting in loss of sensitivity and impaired absorption of insulin. For this reason 'site rotation' is advised (see Fig. 5.11).

Injection technique

Cleansing the skin is not considered advisable as the spirit stings, dries, and toughens the skin. Koivistov & Felig (1978) found that although cleansing the skin prior to injecting insulin did reduce the bacterial count, it was not necessary in order to prevent infection. To reduce discomfort, some patients find it helps to stretch or, alternatively, gently pinch up a mound of skin before injection. The latter is preferred in that it is more likely to ensure s.c. administration. The syringe should be held like a dart and the needle inserted straight into the subcutaneous tissue. Insulin syringes currently in use in the UK have short, fine needles attached, thus avoiding the penetration of muscle. The insulin should be injected steadily over 3–5 seconds and the needle withdrawn smoothly. If slight leakage or bleeding occurs, gentle pressure can be applied using a clean cottonwool ball. Teaching the newly diagnosed insulin-dependent patient how to give himself insulin is a significant part of diabetes education (see p. 178). For some patients, learning this skill is the most difficult part of adjusting to the diagnosis.

The care setting. The insulin-dependent patient may be managed in the primary care setting provided adequate supervision and support can be given to the patient and his family during the early stages of treatment. It is still common for initial stabilisation on insulin to take place within the hospital setting and for outpatient attendance to be advised to allow for regular screening for diabetes-related complications. If ketoacidosis or dehydration are present management in hospital will be essential.

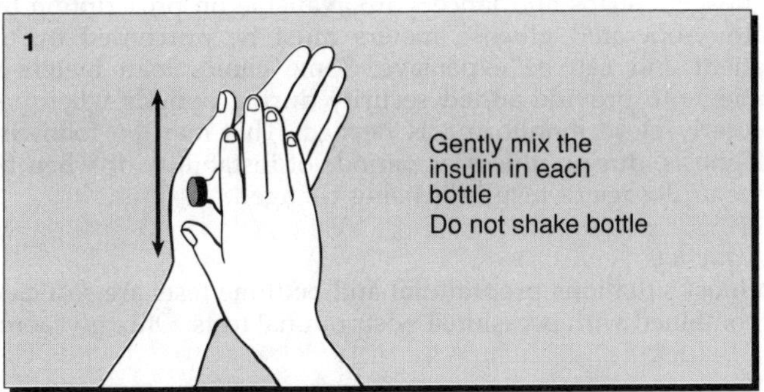
1
Gently mix the insulin in each bottle
Do not shake bottle

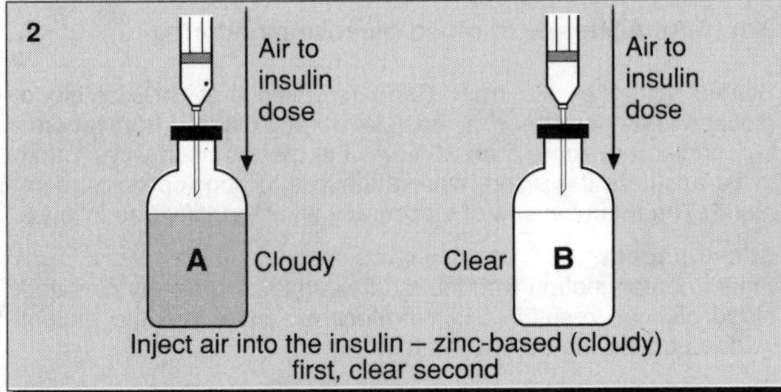

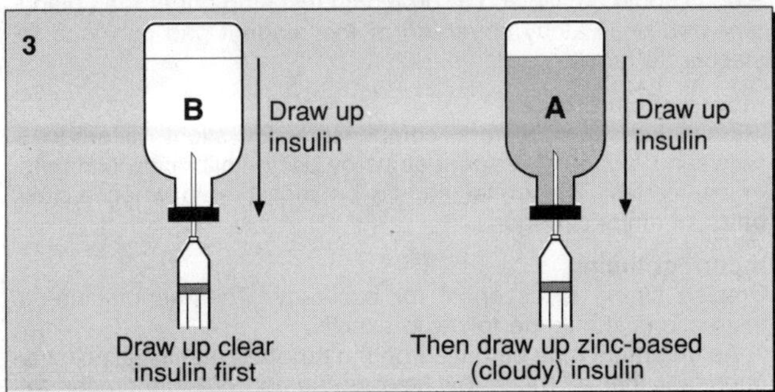

Fig. 5.10 Mixing clear and zinc-based (cloudy) insulin. This technique avoids 'contaminating' the clear (rapid-acting) insulin with zinc-based (cloudy) insulin and thus extending the onset and duration of action.

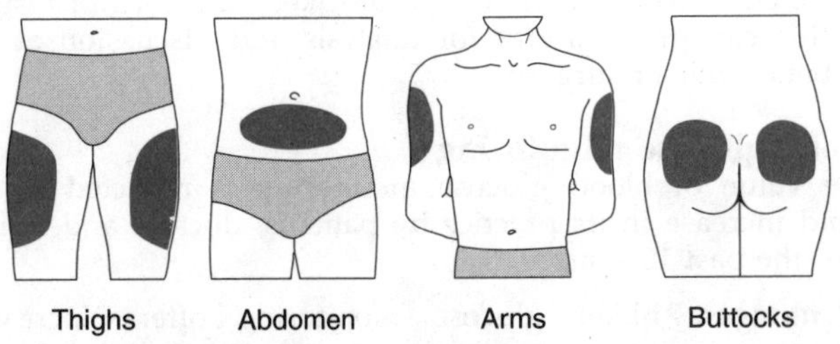

Fig. 5.11 Suitable injection sites for insulin. Repeated injections in the same area may cause pitting or lumpiness of the skin.

MONITORING RESPONSE TO THERAPY

METHODS

The methods used for monitoring glycaemic control include:

- urinalysis
- blood glucose monitoring
- glycosylated proteins estimation
- body weight monitoring.

Urinalysis

Urine tests are performed to detect the presence of glucose and ketones. (In order to screen for possible renal complications of diabetes mellitus urine may also be tested for protein). Urine testing is simple, inexpensive, non-invasive, easy to teach and generally acceptable to patients. It is still regarded as a fairly useful monitoring device for those patients for whom strict glycaemic control is not critical, e.g. patients with NIDDM who are managed by diet alone (Hindley 1989).

Urine testing does, however, have limitations. It requires a degree of manual dexterity, adequate vision (including colour vision), and urinary continence. It also requires the ability to interpret and act upon results.

It should also be remembered that urinalysis can provide only retrospective information about blood glucose, as filtration of glucose in the glomerulus may have occurred some hours prior to the urine being voided. Urinalysis is therefore not very reliable unless it is supplemented by other techniques such as blood glucose monitoring (Walford 1989).

Equipment

Chemically impregnated dip-sticks (e.g. Diastix) are the usual means of testing for glucose and, where necessary, for ketones. It should be noted that dip-sticks for testing urine glucose levels may be rendered insensitive by the presence of heavy ketonuria. As result some centres still prefer urine glucose to be checked using Clinitest tablets, believing them to be more accurate. The manufacturer's instructions for use and storage of urine-testing materials must be followed precisely in order for reliable results to be obtained.

Interpretation

The absence of glycosuria merely indicates a blood glucose level below the renal threshold for glucose, which in most people is around 10 mmol/l. Urinalysis cannot therefore detect hypoglycaemia. For this reason some physicians and diabetes nurse specialists recommend that elderly patients on oral hypoglycaemic therapy show occasional slight traces of glycosuria; but no more than 0.25%. This reassures the patient and the staff that an overdosage of oral hypoglycaemic medication is not being given.

Recording

Urinalysis results should be accurately recorded on the appropriate chart. The patient should also keep a record of results, as this can prove useful for analysis and discussion at the diabetic clinic or surgery.

Blood glucose monitoring

The value of blood glucose monitoring is reflected in the rapid increase in its practice by patients, doctors and nurses over the past 10 years.

Advantages. Blood glucose monitoring offers increased patient involvement in diabetes management and helps to improve day-to-day glycaemic control. The patient can enjoy greater flexibility at mealtimes and can participate safely in strenuous exercise. Blood glucose monitoring can also give warning of impending metabolic crisis and guide subsequent intervention.

Disadvantages

Blood glucose monitoring requires a fair degree of manual dexterity, visual acuity, cognitive ability and motivation. It is invasive and some patients find it uncomfortable and unacceptable. It is also more expensive than urinalysis and can potentially provide inaccurate information due to errors in technique (see Box 5.8). In the current climate of concern over blood-borne infection such as hepatitis B and AIDS, protective gloves must be worn by staff performing this procedure.

Equipment

This includes:

- finger-pricking devices for obtaining a capillary blood sample
- reagent strips impregnated with chemicals that change colour according to the glucose content in the blood
- meters that employ micro-technology to provide an accurate reading and visual display of the capillary blood glucose.

Reagent strips and lancets are available on prescription but battery-operated glucose meters must be purchased by the patient and can be expensive. Some clinics loan meters to patients to provide added security during periods when particularly close monitoring is needed. This may be following diagnosis, during illness or periods of instability, or when the type or dosage of insulin is being changed.

Frequency

In most situations preprandial and bedtime tests are sufficient if combined with occasional postprandial tests. Once glycaemic

Box. 5.8 Accuracy of blood glucose monitoring

Studies (cited by Rayman 1989) revealed that 50% of blood glucose tests performed by hospital nurses differed from laboratory findings by more than 20%. As the meters used were found to be accurate the errors were attributed to poor operator technique. The main causes of inaccuracy were identified as follows:

Sticky fingers
Finger contamination with foodstuffs can lead to falsely elevated blood glucose results. It is therefore essential that the patient washes his hands before the test.

Smeared test strips
Blood should be allowed to *drop* onto test strip rather than being *smeared* on. Patchy coverage of the reagent pad can lead to inaccurate results.

Incorrect calibration
Manufacturers of meters compensate for slight differences between batches of reagent strips by using calibration numbers or bar codes. The meter should be recalibrated when a new batch of strips is begun.

Incorrect timing
Precise timing is essential for accuracy. The manufacturer's instructions should be followed exactly.

As treatment may be based on the reported results it is clearly important that all those involved in carrying out this procedure should be adequately instructed and observed by an experienced supervisor who can correct any faults in technique. Only then should a nurse (or patient) be deemed competent to carry out and record blood glucose results.

control is established the frequency of monitoring should be reviewed. During periods of metabolic crisis blood glucose monitoring may be carried out hourly (Rayman 1989).

Method
The patient should wash his hands with warm soapy water before the test is carried out. A drop of blood of sufficient size should be obtained and the procedure detailed in the manufacturer's directions should be followed precisely (Hindley 1989). If a nurse is conducting the test she should wear gloves.

Blood glucose monitoring provides a simple and, if performed correctly, reliable method of monitoring glycaemic control. A suitable system of recording results must be devised. Some meters can store results on memory but for the most part a written record should be kept for analysis. The nurse or patient carrying out the procedure should know the levels above and below which specific actions should be taken (Craddock 1989).

Glycosylated protein estimation

Glucose in solution binds to protein by a process of glycosylation. The rate at which proteins bind glucose is directly related to the current glucose concentration in the blood. The blood proteins in which glycosylation is most readily measured are haemoglobin, albumen and fructosamine. The *normal ranges* for glycosylated haemoglobin, albumen and fructosamine vary according to the laboratory technique used. Reference ranges should therefore be provided by the laboratory undertaking the test.

Advantages
Measurement of glycosylated proteins provides an independent check of other measures of glycaemic control. It also provides a tool to assess the effects of interventions such as diet, drugs or education.

Disadvantages
Anything which interferes with normal haemoglobin levels (such as haemorrhage or anaemia) could potentially distort glycosylated haemoglobin results. Similarly, conditions which influence serum albumen levels such as renal or hepatic disease may result in problems in interpreting glycated albumen results.

Body weight monitoring

Weight is not a sensitive indicator of glycaemic control. However, the negative significance of rapid weight loss accompanied by thirst, glycosuria and ketonuria should be recognised. Similarly, it is a positive sign if the patient's weight is stable and within an acceptable range. Body weight therefore forms part of the overall monitoring picture.

In NIDDM it is often seen as a priority to help the patient lose weight. Obesity increases insulin resistance and therefore correction of obesity can increase the sensitivity of cells to insulin. Weight reduction alone may bring the blood glucose down within normal limits.

Associated problems
Social attitudes can lead to overweight people feeling stigmatised. As a result, guilt or low self-esteem may affect the patient's response to dietary advice. It is important that nurses involved in monitoring the patient's weight in the home, clinic or hospital adopt a sensitive approach. Public weighing and castigation of patients for lack of 'success' have no place in diabetes care. Punitive attitudes only confirm guilt feelings in the patient, further lowering self-esteem (Walford 1989, Gatling 1989).

Equipment and procedure
Scales should be checked regularly for accuracy. If possible the patient should be weighed at the same time of day and as far as possible while wearing clothing of comparable weight.

Frequency
For hospital inpatients weekly weighing should be adequate. Routine weighing at each outpatients clinic appointment is probably advisable. Frequency of self-weighing by patient at home will depend upon the patient's discretion, the advice offered and the goals which have been set. On the whole, weighing more frequently than once a week is neither psychologically desirable nor valuable as a monitoring tool.

PREVENTING AND DETECTING DIABETES-ASSOCIATED COMPLICATIONS

ACUTE METABOLIC COMPLICATIONS OF DIABETES

The acute complications arising from diabetes are:

- diabetic ketoacidosis (DKA)
- hyperglycaemic hyperosmolar non-ketotic coma (HHNK)
- hypoglycaemia (insulin reaction/coma).

Diabetic ketoacidosis (DKA)

This condition could be defined as uncontrolled hyperglycaemia accompanied by dehydration and acidosis.

Epidemiology
Although relatively uncommon, DKA accounts for around 14% of all diabetes-related hospital admissions. Before the discovery of insulin, DKA was invariably fatal. Even today it carries a significant threat to life, especially in elderly patients. Lower mortality rates from DKA are recorded in specialist diabetes centres, presumably due to the improved management offered by medical and nursing staff with specific skills and knowledge in diabetes care (Conaglen & Sonksen 1985).

Aetiology
Around 30% of patients admitted with DKA have previously undiagnosed diabetes. In patients with established diabetes, DKA can be precipitated by infection, myocardial infarction, stroke or trauma as these cause increased stress hormone secretion. Stress hormones raise the blood glucose and increase insulin requirements. DKA may therefore be caused by an inadequate dosage of insulin being taken during periods of illness or other major stress, or by insulin being omitted altogether.

In 10–15% of admissions with DKA the underlying cause of the crisis remains undiscovered. Fluctuations in diabetes control are common during adolescence and this is reflected in the number of young people admitted to hospital with DKA.

?	**5.10** Consider why diabetes may be unstable during adolescence.

PATHOPHYSIOLOGY

The symptoms of DKA occur as a consequence of the combined effect of insulin lack and increased secretion of catabolic hormones. As a result, two major biochemical derangements occur simultaneously:

1. Accelerated gluconeogenesis and glycogenolysis cause

Box 5.9 The development of diabetic ketoacidosis (DKA)

The key precipitating factors are inadequate supply of insulin and increased demand for insulin, often in combination. These are often triggered by:

- infection (especially respiratory, urinary or abscesses)
- trauma or surgery
- severe illness, e.g. myocardial infarction or cerebrovascular accident
- failure to take sufficient insulin.

As a result of reduced insulin and increased stress hormone levels, the following will occur:
cells will be unable to utilise glucose; glycogen will be converted to glucose, protein broken down to provide glucose (gluconeogenesis) and fat broken down (lipolysis), releasing ketone bodies. The combined effects of these events are:

- hyperglycaemia and hyperketonaemia
- osmotic diuresis
- fluid and electrolyte disruption
- catabolism/wasting
- acidosis.

As a result the patient will exhibit the following symptoms, signs and clinical features:

Symptoms	Signs and clinical features
• polyuria	• hyperglycaemia and glycosuria
• polydipsia	• polyuria progressing to oliguria
• lethargy/weakness	• ketonuria
• nausea/vomiting	• ketone breath (sweet fruity odour)
• abdominal colic	• weight loss
• muscle cramps	• hypokalaemia
	• hypotension and tachycardia
	• acidaemia
	• rapid, deep (Kussmaul's) respirations
	• evidence of intercurrent infection/illness
	• skin flushed and warm
	• hypothermia *may* develop
	• drowsiness progressing to coma

hyperglycaemia, which in turn results in osmotic diuresis, electrolyte disruption and dehydration

2. Increased fat breakdown (lipolysis) results in the formation of ketone bodies which are weak acids and cause metabolic acidosis (see Box 5.9).

? **5.11** Explain the pathophysiological basis for the signs, symptoms and clinical features of diabetic ketoacidosis. See Gill & Alberti (1985a) and Conaglen & Sonksen (1985).

MEDICAL MANAGEMENT

Reversing the hyperglycaemia. Rapid-acting insulin is administered to lower blood glucose. Initially, approximately 6 i.u./h is given via i.v. infusion pump (0.1 i.u./kg/h). The insulin dose will later be varied in accordance with the blood glucose level. If blood glucose does not fall within 2 h the insulin dose may be increased.

Capillary blood glucose should be checked hourly. Venous blood glucose and plasma potassium (K^+) is measured 2 hourly.

Rehydrating. Sodium chloride (NaC1) 0.9% is given by rapid i.v. infusion: e.g., 1–2 litres may be given over the first h then 1 litre hourly for 2–5 h. The rate is then adjusted according to the patient's state of hydration. When blood glucose falls below 15 mmol/l i.v. dextrose 5–10% is introduced.

Replacing potassium. Derangements in plasma potassium can vary. Hyperkalaemia may be evident in the very early stages due to severe acidosis but once rehydration is under way hypokalaemia is usual and may be severe. Intravenous potassium chloride (KCl) is prescribed in accordance with the blood biochemistry. Initially 10–30 mmol/h may be administered within the i.v. fluids. Ideally this should be by a regulated infusion delivery system.

Monitoring. The patient will be closely monitored for the following:

Hyperglycaemia. Capillary blood glucose is measured hourly and venous blood glucose 2 hourly.

Dehydration. Blood urea, electrolytes and plasma osmolality are checked 2 hourly.

Response to fluid and K^+ replacement. Central venous pressure (CVP) or capillary pulmonary wedge pressure (PCWP), blood pressure and pulse are measured hourly as a guide to blood volume. A 12-lead ECG is performed and continuous cardiac monitor commenced to detect cardiac arrythmias associated with serum potassium lack or excess (see p. 34).

Acidosis. Arterial or venous blood gases and hydrogen ion (H^+) concentration are checked 1–2 hourly.

Underlying infection. A chest X-ray is performed. Blood cultures, urine and sputum specimens and a throat swab are sent to microbiology. Temperature, pulse and respiration are recorded hourly.

Ketosis and renal function. Urine is tested for glucose, ketones, protein, urea and electrolytes. In addition, urine volumes may be measured hourly.

Additional therapy which can be used in the treatment of DKA includes:

Sodium bicarbonate. This is not routinely used as it may exacerbate tissue hypoxia and hypokalaemia. As overcorrection may result in alkalosis, sodium bicarbonate is usually reserved for the treatment of very severe acidosis where the pH is below 7.0 and hydrogen ion concentration exceeds 100 mmol/l (Gill & Alberti 1989b; see also Ch. 20, p. 648).

Broad-spectrum antibiotics. These may be given if infection is suspected and as a prophylaxis against supervening infection.

Anticoagulants. Low-dose heparin 5000 i.u. s.c. twice daily may be given (especially if the patient is elderly or is deeply comatosed) to reduce the risks of circulatory complications of dehydration and immobility.

Oxygen therapy. This will be administered in accordance with blood gas results.

Nasogastric aspiration will be performed to protect the airway if the patient is vomiting, drowsy or unconscious.

Urinary catheterisation. Urine volume is measured hourly as severe dehydration carries a risk of acute renal failure.

Space blanket. This may be used if the patient is hypothermic due to the vasodilatory response to acidosis.

Subsequent medical management of DKA will address the following concerns:

Insulin. When blood glucose is below 15 mmol/l it is common to change the i.v. prescription to a regime which combines glucose, potassium and insulin (GKI 'cocktail'). A typical cocktail would consist of 500 ml 10% dextrose plus 20 units of soluble insulin plus 20 mmol of potassium chloride (KCl) given via regulated infusion 4 hourly.

Fluid and electrolytes. If the patient is still dehydrated, or severely hyponatraemic, further i.v. sodium chloride 0.9% can be given in combination with the GKI cocktail. Plasma electrolytes, osmolality and glucose levels will be checked 4–6 hourly. Capillary blood glucose is monitored (visually or by meter) 2 hourly. The GKI cocktail and infusion rate will be adjusted in accordance with blood glucose and other biochemical results. When the patient is deemed to be clinically and biochemically stable s.c. insulin and an oral diet are resumed; i.v. GKI insulin is discontinued 1 h after the first s.c. injection of insulin.

Prevention. Once the patient is stable, every effort is made to discover its cause and, if possible, to prevent recurrences. For many patients, however, the experience of DKA is what first makes them aware that they have diabetes mellitus.

NURSING PRIORITIES AND MANAGEMENT OF DKA

Each patient admitted with DKA will have unique problems and needs. The biochemical disruption of DKA is profound and life-threatening and priorities for nursing care will be strongly influenced by the prescribed medical therapy and the need for complex monitoring. Whilst the nurse must draw upon her technical skills in such a situation it is vitally important that she remembers to care for the patient as a *person*.

Immediate priorities

The newly admitted patient with DKA is vulnerable in a variety of ways. The nurse should be sensitive to this vulnerability and try to accommodate individual needs when planning and implementing care.

Case History 5.2 and Nursing Care Plan 5.3 provide an example of how a patient may present in DKA and how nursing priorities may be met following admission and until consciousness is regained. It should be pointed out, however, that not all patients presenting with DKA will be unconscious. Individuals with long-standing diabetes mellitus can usually recognise the signs and symptoms of impending ketoacidosis and will seek medical help at a much earlier stage in its development.

Further considerations

When the patient is alert and able to respond the focus of care will change. The nurse will work with the patient, the dietitian and the medical staff to stabilise blood glucose and to monitor the effects of therapy.

The subsequent care of the patient in hyperglycaemic crisis, whether due to DKA or HHNK will be similar in many respects and is described on page 171.

Hyperglycaemic hyperosmolar non-ketotic coma (HHNK)

This term refers to uncontrolled hyperglycaemia and dehydration in the absence of ketonaemia.

Epidemiology

HHNK is less common than DKA. It occurs in people with NIDDM and as such tends to affect an older age group. Mortality rates ranging from 40–70% have been reported (Gill & Alberti 1985c).

Aetiology

Severe physical or psychological stress such as cerebrovascular accident (CVA), myocardial infarction, trauma or bereavement can precipitate HHNK (as in DKA). Thiazide diuretic therapy has also been found to precipitate HHNK in some people.

Dietary indiscretion such as a marked increase in refined carbohydrate intake (perhaps over Christmas or a holiday period) may account for the onset of HHNK. Some patients give a history of drinking large volumes of sugar-containing drinks in an effort to quench an ever-increasing thirst.

In 50% of patients the cause of this metabolic disturbance will remain unknown.

PATHOPHYSIOLOGY

HHNK may develop gradually over a period of 2–15 days. This can be contrasted with DKA, in which severe symptoms develop in 0.5–3 days (Gill & Alberti 1985a). The more insidious onset in HHNK is probably due to the patient being less obviously 'ill' in the absence of ketosis. The signs and symptoms are similar to those found in DKA, with these notable exceptions:

- ketonuria is absent or slight
- severe weight loss is unusual
- in the absence of the serious symptoms of ketosis, the blood glucose may be even higher than in DKA before the patient feels ill and seeks medical attention
- blood glucose range is 20–150 mmol/l, with a mean of 55 mmol/l (Simpson 1989)
- response to dehydration can be more marked due to the degree of hyperglycaemia and to age-associated intolerance to fluid and electrolyte disruption
- symptoms associated with ketonaemia/acidosis will not be in evidence.

> ? **5.12** Given the above differences draw up a list of signs, symptoms and clinical features of HHNK. Compare this to the list given for DKA and discuss the reasons for the differences.

The features of HHNK may be further described as follows:

Hyperglycaemia can be severe but develops gradually. Although some insulin is still being secreted there is a relative insulin deficiency and the blood glucose continues to rise. The severe hyperglycaemia in

Case History 5.2 R (see Nursing Care Plan 5.3)

R is a lively 18 year old and the eldest of three children. At present she lives with her family but she is soon to leave home to undertake a secretarial course at a college some 30 miles away.

R and her two brothers have recently suffered a bad bout of flu. The boys are now fully fit but R is far from well. She has been passing a lot of urine and is constantly thirsty. She has lost weight and has recently been complaining of feeling tired all the time.

This morning she is very drowsy. Her skin feels hot and dry and she looks flushed. She has vomited several times and has complained of abdominal pain and cramps in her limbs. Her breath has a peculiar sweet smell and her mouth is very dry.

Her parents are alarmed and have called the GP to request an urgent visit. Alerted by the 'acetone' breath, her symptoms, and the history of recent illness, the GP checks R's capillary blood glucose and finds it to be 44 mmol/1. R is too sleepy to produce a urine specimen to check for ketones but the doctor is in little doubt about the diagnosis.

An ambulance is summoned and R and her parents are taken to hospital. The ward is alerted to expect an unconscious patient with diabetic ketoacidosis (DKA).

On admission R is acutely ill and has complex care requirements. A nurse who has the appropriate levels of knowledge and skill is assigned to care for her. She has prepared for R's admission and will subsequently assess her nursing needs and plan and evaluate her care.

Nursing Care Plan 5.3 Nursing care for R, a patient with DKA, first 24 h post admission (see Case History 5.2)

Nursing considerations	Action	Rationale	Evaluation
Impaired consciousness	❒ Position and support R in semi-prone or lateral position	To prevent asphyxia and prevent aspiration of secretion/vomitus	Skin colour and respirations are normal
	❒ Keep artificial airway in position until voluntarily expelled		
	❒ Perform oropharangeal suction if secretions audible		
	❒ Provide nasogastric (NG) aspiration (due to unconscious state and recent vomiting)		
	❒ Continuously monitor colour and breathing		Risk factors eliminated
	❒ Administer oxygen as prescribed, ensuring that fire safety rules are observed	To correct hypoxia and prevent O_2 combustion	Blood gases improving
	❒ Monitor neurological status hourly. Record report findings	To detect improvement/deterioration in conscious level	R is progressively more responsive
Hyperglycaemia and ketonaemia	❒ Administer prescribed rapid-acting insulin i.v. by infusion pump	To correct hyperglycaemia and ketonaemia	Trends indicate blood glucose returning to within the normal range
	❒ Monitor capillary blood glucose hourly; record/report findings	To evaluate response to insulin therapy and prevent hypoglycaemia	
Fluid deficit/replacement	❒ Administer i.v. fluids as prescribed. Observe venepuncture site for redness, swelling or extravasation. Record all fluids in fluid balance chart	To correct hypovolaemia	No discomfort or swelling of venepuncture site
	❒ Monitor CVP, BP, breathing, temperature; observe neck veins, skin colour and urine volumes	To monitor effects of fluid replacement	Vital signs are returning to within their normal ranges
	❒ Catheterisation usually prescribed if unconsciousness persists and if patient is oliguric	To monitor renal function and detect renal insufficiency (urine < 30 ml/h)	Urine volume > 30 ml/h
	❒ Test urine hourly for ketones; record results		Ketonuria diminishing
Electrolyte imbalance/ replacement	❒ Observe effects of potassium replacement; provide continuous cardiac monitoring	Overzealous K^+ replacement can cause ventricular fibrillation leading to cardiac arrest	
	❒ Report tall peaked 'T' wave (indicates hyperkalaemia)		K^+ should be 3.5–5 mmol/l
	❒ Report flattened or inverted 'T' wave (indicates hypokalaemia)	Persistent hypokalaemia due to inadequate K^+ replacement can result in heart block, which may lead to cardiac arrest	Cardiac monitor should display normal tracing
	❒ REPORT ECG CHANGES PROMPTLY (See Ch. 2, p. 25.)		
Probable current infection/ potential risk of infection	❒ Collect throat swab, catheter specimen of urine and when consciousness returns a specimen of sputum. Monitor TPR. Doctor will collect a specimen for blood culture	To detect/monitor current infection	Specimen analysis Blood culture results and TPR normal
	❒ Administer prescribed antibiotics and note/report side-effects	To safely administer therapy	
	❒ Reduce risks of infection by high standards of nursing care (e.g. personal and catheter hygiene)	To prevent hospital-acquired infection	Patient infection free

Nursing Care Plan 5.3 *(cont'd)*

Nursing considerations	Action	Rationale	Evaluation
Inability to meet or communicate comfort needs	❒ Ensure bed is smooth, cool and crease-free. Provide regular position change and use of pressure-relieving aids to protect skin. Ensure careful positioning of limbs	To promote general comfort	Skin unblemished and free from discomfort
	❒ Wash, rinse and dry skin: observe for signs of pressure	To protect skin from damage	
	❒ Clean oral cavity 2 hourly. Lubricate lips. Clean nostrils and apply lubricant	To prevent oral and nasal discomfort and drying due to O_2 and the effects of dehydration and nasogastric tube	Oral/nasal mucosa intact
	❒ Keep hair groomed in preferred style. Use R's own nightwear. Maintain privacy throughout	To maintain R's individuality	Patient feels/looks comfortable
Fear and shock as consciousness returns and diagnosis becomes apparent	❒ Display calm, empathic manner. Provide *brief*, clear explanations of reason for hospital admission and current care and treatment	To convey positive attitudes To provide relevant information	R appears less acutely distressed
	❒ Provide access to parents and family		
	❒ Encourage patient to verbalise concerns and express emotions	To recognise R's rights as an individual	R is able to express her needs
	❒ Avoid bombarding R with information at this stage		
	❒ Show sensitivity to the emotional needs of this vulnerable young patient		
R's parents are anxious and shocked due to their daughter's hospitalisation and diagnosis	❒ Provide a comfortable, private waiting area for parents	To provide essential information to answer immediate concerns	Parents are reassured and able to meet with and support their daughter
	❒ Explain (briefly at this stage) what has happened to their daughter		
	❒ Encourage/accept verbalisation of fears and expression of emotions		
	❒ Provide access to R and to medical staff	To establish a trusting relationship, facilitate early educational interventions and offer support to the family.	Parents immediate needs have been met; they appear to feel supported
	❒ Supply information about the ward/hospital (booklets etc)		
	❒ When parents feel able to cooperate complete admission documentation and patient profile		
	❒ Assure parents of access to nursing staff to answer their questions as they occur		
	❒ Arrange a visit from the diabetic nurse specialist at a mutually suitable time		

HHNK is due to the combined effects of cellular resistance to insulin and the generation of glucose by stress hormone driven glycogenolysis and gluconeogenesis.

Hyperosmolarity. Normal plasma osmolality is around 285–295 mmol/kg. This is calculated using a formula which takes account of the sodium, potassium, urea and glucose levels in the blood. Hyperglycaemia accounts for much of the hyperosmolar state in HHNK. The high blood glucose will exert an osmotic pull and as a result fluid is drawn out of the cells into the circulation. Initially this will cause an increase in the glomerular filtration rate and large volumes of fluid will be lost by osmotic diuresis. As a result the patient will develop polyuria, thirst, dehydration and hypovolaemia.

Hypernatraemia. The normal range for plasma sodium (Na^+) is 135–145 mmol/l. In HHNK Na^+ may be raised above this level. Hypernatraemia can develop in response to a reduction in circulatory volume: in order to conserve a falling blood volume aldosterone is secreted by the adrenal cortex, causing the kidney to retain sodium and excrete potassium (see p. 599).

By the time the patient comes to medical attention the period of osmotic diuresis has usually passed and dehydration has developed. As a result the glomerular filtration rate falls, oliguria develops and blood urea rises. The combined effect of fluid loss, raised sodium levels, high blood glucose and raised plasma urea, is that the blood becomes highly 'concentrated', i.e. hyperosmolar (hyperosmotic).

Non-ketosis. The production of ketones (ketogenesis) will be inhibited by the presence of insulin. Insulin also enables the small amount of ketones which result from lipolysis to be metabolised, thus preventing their accumulation in the blood.

Impaired level of consciousness. This occurs due to the effects of dehydration (hyperosmolality) on brain cells impairing cerebral function and leading ultimately to coma.

MEDICAL MANAGEMENT OF HHNK

This follows a similar approach to that of DKA, with some important differences, and centres on the following concerns.

Rehydration. The fluid deficit is vast and can be as much as 8–12 l. Replacement must, however, be approached with a degree of caution, given the risks associated with over-vigorous fluid replacement to which elderly patients are especially vulnerable.

- Sodium chloride 0.9% (normal saline) is given if plasma Na^+ levels are either not yet known or are lower than 145 mmol/l.
- If plasma sodium is higher than 145 mmol/l then half-strength normal saline (0.45% NaCl) may be given. This approach is controversial in view of the risks it carries. Rapid reduction in plasma osmolality can result in fluid moving from the vascular compartment into the cells, causing cerebral oedema and hypovolaemia (Simpson 1989, Gill & Alberti 1985c).

Replacement of potassium. As potassium levels are so variable and unpredictable in HHNK, extreme care is required during replacement to monitor cardiac effects. Continuous cardiac monitoring is strongly recommended.

Insulin therapy. As in DKA, a dose of 6 units h of soluble insulin is given until the blood glucose falls below 15 mmol/l, after which a GKI 'cocktail' is given.

Anticoagulant therapy. A major cause of death in HHNK is thrombosis (often cerebral), which is presumed to result from dehydration and hyperosmolality. Heparin 5000 units s.c. may be given twice daily although some physicians prefer full i.v. heparinisation as a means of preventing intravascular coagulation.

All other therapy and monitoring is as for ketoacidosis.

NURSING PRIORITIES AND MANAGEMENT IN HHNK

Aspects of medical management which have implications for the planning of nursing care include:

- i.v. infusion (fluid replacement)
- i.v. insulin (by infusion pump)
- heparin (s.c. or by i.v. infusion pump)
- central venous pressure (CVP) monitoring
- cardiac monitoring
- urinary catheterisation
- oxygen therapy
- nasogastric aspiration (if patient is unconscious).

Immediate priorities

These interventions will need appropriate attention to ensure the safety and comfort of the patient. In addition, the patient is likely to be vulnerable due to impaired level of consciousness, dehydration, electrolyte imbalance, the hazards of immobility and diabetes-associated risk factors. Nursing interventions will therefore include the following:

Monitoring consciousness level

In patients with HHNK the level of consciousness is of particular importance as there is a risk of cerebral thrombosis due to the combined effects of immobility, dehydration and diabetes-associated atherosclerosis (see Chs. 9 and 30).

Another reason for vigilance is that the patient may be prescribed an i.v. infusion of half-strength normal saline aimed at reducing hyperosmolality. As explained above, if the fall in plasma osmolality is too rapid, cerebral oedema can develop, raising intracranial pressure. The nurse should therefore promptly report any evidence of deterioration in the patient's neurological function (see p. 341).

Monitoring dehydration and electrolyte balance

The nurse should observe for the following warning signs.

Evidence of persistent hypovolaemia. Hourly monitoring is usual. The nurse should report hypotension, a rapid thready pulse, CVP reading lower than 5 cm H_2O, and urine volume less than 30 ml/h. Measures to raise blood volume and blood pressure will probably be prescribed. This can include rapid infusion of i.v. fluids or plasma. Such treatment will require close monitoring in order to detect circulatory overload (see below).

Evidence of fluid overload. The nurse should *promptly* report a rising CVP, especially if this is accompanied by breathlessness, moist breath sounds, distended neck veins and a full pulse. These may indicate fluid replacement has been too vigorous, causing overexpansion of the circulatory volume and placing strain on the left ventricle (see p. 611).

Evidence of electrolyte disruption. Changes in pulse rate and rhythm should be reported promptly, along with ECG changes associated with hypokalaemia and hyperkalaemia (see Nursing Care Plan 5.1) to allow adjustment to therapy to be prescribed and to prevent life-threatening cardiac dysrhythmias developing.

Monitoring response to insulin

Capillary blood glucose will be measured hourly to assess the response to i.v. insulin and to prevent overcorrection leading to hypoglycaemia. Accurate measurement and recording of blood glucose will provide the basis for adjusting insulin dosage.

Preventing complications

Many patients with HHNK are elderly and are especially vulnerable to the effects of hospitalisation and the complications of immobility. Maintenance of comfort and hygiene, including oral care, are of great importance.

Diabetes can cause impairment in circulation and sensation, placing the skin at particular risk. Avoidance of skin damage is therefore a priority. The patient's position should be frequently altered, suitable pressure-relieving devices should be used and the skin, clothing and bedding should be kept cool, clean and dry.

Care is required when lifting, moving or positioning the patient to avoid damage to skin, muscles or joints. Particular attention should be paid to avoiding damage to the heels. Due to vascular and neurological changes, the feet of people with diabetes require particular attention to avoid serious complications (see p. 177).

Atherosclerosis is common in patients with diabetes, thus placing them at particular risk of vascular complications. Passive limb exercises whilst the patient is unconscious, and active limb movements when he is able to cooperate will help prevent venous stasis, which may result in deep vein thrombosis and pulmonary embolism. The nurse and the physiotherapist will both be involved in encouraging limb exercises.

Breathing exercises are also important as elderly bedfast patients are at considerable risk of developing chest infections. Moreover, elderly people, and in particular those with diabetes, are less able to resist infection and tend to recover less quickly than younger non-diabetic people.

Monitoring the patient for pyrexia or other evidence of infection will allow prompt intervention. It is also important to ensure that the care environment and the standards of nursing care provided are such that infection risks are minimised.

Providing psychological support

The experience of a hyperglycaemic crisis can cause great distress not only to the patient but also to his family and close friends. Adopting a warm, empathic approach and accepting the fears of the patient and his family is important if trust and rapport are to be established. The nurse should provide essential information using brief, clear explanations. Access to medical staff and information about the ward or hospital should be provided.

Further considerations in DKA and HHNK

When the patient is deemed to be clinically and biochemically stable on the basis of observation, bedside monitoring and laboratory tests, ongoing care is planned to address the patient's changing needs. If urine volumes are satisfactory the urinary catheter is removed. The nasogastric tube is removed and oral fluids are offered. Diet is introduced under the guidance of the dietitian. When oral intake is adequate and blood urea and electrolyte levels are within normal limits the i.v. fluids will usually be discontinued.

Subcutaneous insulin

This will replace the i.v. insulin. Prescribing insulin is the responsibility of the physician but the nurse will be closely involved in monitoring patient response by frequent estimation of blood glucose. The nurse may also be required to adjust the insulin dosage within guidelines laid down in the written prescription.

Oral hypoglycaemic therapy

If possible, the patient is re-established on oral hypoglycaemic therapy. However, some patients may need to continue insulin therapy for some time before changing back to oral medication. Others may need to make a permanent change to insulin therapy in order to achieve better control of blood glucose levels.

Restoration of self-care

The physician, diabetes nurse specialist, dietitian and ward nurses will initiate the process of preparing the patient to assume responsibility for self-care, but the major contribution will be made by the GP and the community nursing staff once the patient returns home.

Patient education

The newly diagnosed patient will require information about how a balance between activity, food and medication can be achieved with the help of frequent blood glucose monitoring. This is especially important for patients with IDDM.

Once the crisis has passed perhaps the most important aspect of care is to prevent further episodes of DKA or HHNK. This involves identifying events which led up to the crisis and analysing with the patient where action may have been taken to avert the crisis or obtain help at an earlier stage. Glycated protein estimation can provide useful information about glycaemic control over the preceding weeks, as can the patient's record book containing blood glucose and urinalysis results.

It is all too easy to be wise in retrospect. It is therefore not helpful to blame the patient; to do so would be to lose the benefits of a potentially valuable teaching situation.

Emotional support

If severe underlying emotional distress or disturbance has precipitated the metabolic crisis then the patient's difficulties may need to be sensitively explored. In accordance with the patient's wishes, appropriate counselling facilities may be provided. The newly diagnosed patient will require emotional support as he prepares to meet the immediate practical demands imposed by his disorder.

Hypoglycaemia (insulin reaction/coma)

Hypoglycaemia is a condition in which blood glucose is lower than the normal fasting range of 3.5 mmol/l. In reality, symptoms of hypoglycaemia rarely occur until the blood glucose falls below 3 mmol/l.

Epidemiology

Hypoglycaemia is the most common complication of insulin therapy and is a rare but serious complication of oral sulphonylurea therapy. It can also feature in secondary diabetes, e.g. in patients with certain liver diseases. Of diabetic patients 30% experience a hypoglycaemic coma at least once; 10% are affected each year and 3% suffer severe recurrent coma. The overall mortality rate in hypoglycaemic coma is 1 in 500 (Gale 1985).

Aetiology

There are three main causes of hypoglycaemia (see Box 5.10):

- excess insulin
- insufficient food
- unusual exercise/activity.

PATHOPHYSIOLOGY

People tend to respond idiosyncratically to falling blood glucose.

Box 5.10 Hypoglycaemia: classification and causes

Classification
- Asymptomatic: biochemical hypoglycaemia without symptoms
- Mild: easily recognised and corrected by the patient
- Severe: patient conscious but requiring help from others
- Comatose: cerebral function severely affected by glucose lack

Causes
- Too much insulin
- Wrong type of insulin
- Inappropriate combination of insulins
- Excess dosage of oral sulphonylureas
- Delayed or missed meal
- More than usual amount of exercise
- alcohol ingestion, especially when hungry
- stress, such as hypothermia

Symptoms will often be absent until the blood glucose is lower than 3 mmol/l. In long-standing diabetes mellitus the sensitivity of response to hypoglycaemia can become blunted, and the patient may remain asymptomatic even when the blood glucose falls below 2 mmol/l (although at this level some signs may be obvious to others).

Onset and progression. Symptoms may develop over a very short period of time — usually 5–15 min. This can be contrasted with DKA and HHNK, both of which have a much more insidious onset.

Endocrine/autonomic response. Glucagon and other stress hormones (including adrenaline) are secreted in response to falling blood sugar. These hormones potentiate the effects of the sympathetic nervous system to cause the following symptoms:

- full, bounding pulse
- palpitations
- sweating and trembling
- 'butterflies' in the stomach
- hunger pangs (sometimes).

Central nervous system response. As brain cells are unable to use alternatives to glucose for metabolism, a fall below the normal blood sugar will cause symptoms of cerebral dysfunction (neuroglycopenic symptoms) such as:

- headache
- lack of concentration
- dizziness
- unsteady gait
- slurred speech
- tingling around the lips.

In addition, observers may notice abnormalities such as:

- irrational behaviour
- muscle twitching/seizures
- automatism
- extreme drowsiness or coma.

Some of these symptoms and signs could, with disastrous consequences, be mistakenly attributed by others to excess intake of alcohol.

Loss of sensitivity to symptoms. Recently diagnosed patients tend to rely on endocrine/autonomic symptoms such as sweating, tremor and palpitations to alert them to a fall in blood glucose. However, after some years patients may become less sensitive to these responses and come to rely on central nervous system (neuroglycopenic) signs such as visual blurring and dizziness to alert them to impending hypoglycaemia. Symptoms can also be masked by:

- Neuropathic changes. As the patient's ability to perceive the neurological early warning symptoms of hypoglycaemia may be impaired by diabetic neuropathies, progression to irrational behaviour, automatism and coma can occur.
- Alcohol can mask symptoms and lead others to mistake hypoglycaemia for intoxication.
- Ageing. In older people hypoglycaemia can develop rather more insidiously and the symptoms can be mistaken for failing mental function.
- Time of day. Nocturnal hypoglycaemia most often occurs between 03.00 h and 05.00 h and may pass unnoticed although symptoms such as night sweats, restlessness, stertorous breathing and headaches on wakening may give the patient an indication of its occurrence.

Other types of hypoglycaemia are:

- Rebound hyperglycaemia, which can occur in response to stress hormone release (the Somogyi phenomenon; Gale 1985)
- Sulphonylurea hypoglycaemia: chlorpropamide and glibenclamide, even at normal therapeutic doses, have been implicated in severe, prolonged hypoglycaemic coma. This risk is increased in elderly people. This form of hypoglycaemia has a higher mortality rate than insulin-induced hypoglycaemia.

MEDICAL MANAGEMENT

Treatment of hypoglycaemia is simple and the effects dramatic and gratifying. Nevertheless, the risks posed by hypoglycaemic coma and the importance of early detection and intervention must be stressed.

Hypoglycaemia can be treated with oral carbohydrate, s.c. or i.m. glucagon, or i.v. glucose — depending on the stage and severity of the hypoglycaemia.

The conscious patient should be given rapidly absorbed glucose together with a more gradually absorbed form of carbohydrate, e.g. Dextrosol tablets followed by a glass of milk or fruit juice and a biscuit or sandwich. If a meal has been missed this should be taken at the earliest opportunity.

The confused or drowsy patient. If he is too drowsy to safely eat or drink the patient can be given glucagon 1 mg by s.c. injection. This will have the effect of raising the blood glucose. Relatives can be taught how to administer glucagon.

The unconscious patient. Medical help should always be sought for the unconscious patient, although if hypoglycaemia is known to be the problem glucagon should be given whilst the doctor is awaited and the patient should be placed in the recovery position until consciousness returns. *Nothing should be given orally whilst the patient is unconscious.*

If glucagon is unavailable, or fails to bring a response within 10–15 min, 30–50 ml of 50% glucose may be injected i.v. by the doctor. This treatment will usually raise the blood glucose enough for the patient to regain consciousness. When unconsciousness persists hospital admission will be necessary.

The hospitalised patient with hypoglycaemic coma. A specimen of blood will be taken for estimation of blood glucose. Continuous i.v. infusion of 10–20% dextrose to be commenced and the patient's response monitored by frequent measurement of capillary blood glucose.

Unfortunately, 1–2% of hospitalised patients fail to respond promptly to therapy. For these patients other causes of coma such as alcohol or drug overdose, hypothermia or cerebral haemorrhage should be excluded. As cerebral oedema can accompany prolonged hypoglycaemia, an i.v infusion of mannitol (a hyperosmotic fluid) may be given. If coma persists beyond 24 h, full recovery of mental function is unlikely (Gale 1985).

NURSING PRIORITIES AND MANAGEMENT OF HYPOGLYCAEMIA

In hypoglycaemic coma the period of extreme vulnerability tends to be short. Nevertheless, the nurse must take the patient's vulnerabilities into account in her nursing interventions by:

- ensuring the patient's safety and comfort
- monitoring the patient's consciousness level
- administering prescribed therapy
- monitoring capillary blood glucose
- investigating the cause of the hypoglycaemic coma
- providing information and encouragement for the patient to help improve diabetes control.

Metabolic complications of diabetes vary in cause, severity and outcome. All indicate a lack of stability of diabetes control which requires investigation and possibly subsequent modification of treatment or lifestyle.

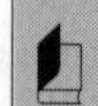

For a detailed account of the causes and management of hypoglycaemia, see Macheca (1993).

CHRONIC COMPLICATIONS OF DIABETES MELLITUS

This section will consider chronic complications of diabetes mellitus which result in pathological changes in large blood vessels (macroangiopathies), small blood vessels (microangiopathies) and nerves (neuropathies).

Although the exact mechanisms underlying pathological changes in the vascular and nervous systems of diabetic individuals are uncertain, it is thought that these changes may occur as a consequence of persistent hyperglycaemia (see for example Wales 1989). Conclusive evidence which unequivocally links poor blood glucose control to chronic complications of diabetes remains elusive. It is hoped that some of the pivotal questions may be answered when the findings of a large-scale longitudinal study, the Diabetes Control and Complications Trial (DCCT), currently in progress in the UK, are published (Pugliese et al 1991).

Detailed management of specific diabetes-related complications will not be provided in this chapter. All are dealt with fully elsewhere in this volume. The reader is therefore urged to consult the relevant chapters for detailed coverage of these disorders.

Atherosclerosis

Epidemiology

Although atherosclerosis is not peculiar to diabetes it is known that myocardial infarction, cerebrovascular accident (CVA) and gangrene are relatively frequent and are major causes of death in people with diabetes. Atherosclerosis develops at a much younger age in people with diabetes than in non-diabetic individuals; this is most noticeable in females.

Both types of diabetes carry increased risk, but those with NIDDM show the strongest tendency to develop atheroma. This is probably due to age-related factors and perhaps also to the effects of long-standing asymptomatic hyperglycaemia prior to diagnosis. In IDDM microvascular disease such as retinopathy usually precedes evidence of atherosclerosis.

Aetiology

In diabetes blood lipids and clotting factors may be elevated (Donnelly 1992). The ability to break down fibrin can also be impaired. Blood platelets tend to be stickier and platelet aggregation is often increased. All of these factors favour the development of atherosclerosis (Viinikka 1985). Factors such as obesity, hypertension and smoking, although not specific to diabetes, may further increase the risk (Kinson & Nattrass 1984).

Onset and progress of the disease

The development and vascular distribution of atherosclerosis in diabetes is similar to that found in non-diabetic people, the exception being the more severe peripheral arterial involvement which may affect the lower limbs of some people with diabetes.

Cardiovascular disease

When compared to the general population, people with diabetes, aged 25–40 years show a 10–20-fold increase in mortality from cardiovascular disease. Those over 50 years old are 2–3 times more likely to die from myocardial infarction than their non-diabetic counterparts (Jarrett 1985).

Atherosclerosis of the coronary vessels can impair oxygen delivery to the myocardium, resulting in angina pectoris or myocardial infarction. Due to the effects of autonomic neuropathy the patient may develop a cardiac arrythmia and may have a 'silent' (painless) myocardial infarction.

Cerebrovascular disease

Strokes are about twice as common in people with diabetes when compared to the general population. Hypertension is probably the most important causative factor; those factors which contribute to the development of atherosclerosis are also important.

Retinopathy

Diabetic retinopathy is the most common acquired cause of blindness in adults aged 30–65 years of age in the UK. Of registered blind diabetic patients 92% are over 50 years of age. Retinopathy results from changes in the small blood vessels of the retina (retinal microangiopathy) and can be classified as:

- background (non-proliferative) retinopathy
- maculopathy
- proliferative retinopathy.

Background retinopathy

Background retinopathy rarely causes a major threat to vision unless the macula is affected. In the early stages of retinopathy the capillaries of the retina become more permeable. This can cause fluid exudation (hard exudates) into the vitreous humor. Retinal veins may swell at localised spots, giving the appearance of 'beading'. Microaneurysms can develop; these can rupture, causing small bleeds. Arteriolar occlusions may appear as 'cotton wool spots' on the retina. More spots occur in rapidly developing retinopathy or where there is coexisting hypertension. Evidence of venous bleeding and cotton wool spots suggests progression to preproliferative retinopathy.

Maculopathy

Maculopathy can cause significant visual loss. In this condition, oedema, haemorrhages and exudates are concentrated on the macular area of the retina.

Proliferative retinopathy

Microvascular disease of the retina can result in areas of hypoxia. This will give rise to the compensatory development of new blood vessels (neovascularisation) which grow forward from the retina to invade the vitreous body. These new vessels are fragile and poorly supported; consequently, haemorrhages into the vitreous body are common. Progressive traction on the retina can result in retinal detachment. Proliferative retinopathy and retinal detachment will seriously threaten vision.

MEDICAL MANAGEMENT

The main priorities in the treatment of diabetic retinopathy are to reduce the risk of haemorrhage and to limit new vessel growth into the vitreous body. Photocoagulation by means of laser technology can be used to treat all forms of retinopathy. Treatment should be considered in all patients with visual potential (Ehlers & Bulow 1980, Hamilton 1985, Hamilton & Ubig 1991; see also Ch. 13, pp. 493–494).

Screening. Annual ophthalmoscopic examination is strongly advised. Where glycaemic control is poor, more frequent eye examinations may be recommended.

Retinal photography can be carried out annually and it is now possible to do this using non-mydriatic retinal cameras which allow the retina to be photographed without prior dilatation of the pupil. The British Diabetic Association (BDA) has already sponsored 10 mobile units to carry out photographic screening for retinopathy (Lovelock 1990).

Prevention. The patient should be aware of the presumed link between poor blood glucose control and retinopathy and of the importance of promptly reporting changes in vision. A full eye examination is recommended at least once yearly, either by an ophthalmologist or an optician. As eye tests for patients with diabetes are free of charge the optician should be made aware that the patient has diabetes. The risks of retinopathy increase if the patient is hypertensive. The benefits of following medical advice and treatment with regard to blood pressure regulation should therefore be explained.

Other eye disorders

Although retinopathy poses the main threat to vision in diabetes there is also an increased risk that the patient will develop cataracts and glaucoma. The reasons why this should be so are not entirely clear. It is possible that glycosylation of protein in the optic lens can cause the opacities of cataract (Hamilton & Ubig 1991). The management of cataracts and glaucoma are described in full in Chapter 13.

Sadly, many patients with diabetes do ultimately suffer partial or total blindness. Maintaining independence in relation to diabetes management and general self-care will present quite a challenge. Jones (1986) describes various devices which can enable the blind or partially sighted patient to draw up and administer insulin and to monitor blood glucose. These include 'click-count' syringes, the dial-a-dose NovoPen and B-D Pen, insulin cartridges and even a 'talking' blood glucose meter.

The nurse caring for the blind diabetic patient should work with him to seek out ways of reducing his dependence on others. The BDA and the Royal National Institute for the Blind (RNIB) can provide invaluable up-to-date information about the help currently available for blind diabetic patients.

Diabetic nephropathy

An estimated 20–30% of patients diagnosed as having diabetes before the age of 30 die from diabetic nephropathy. It has also been estimated that each year in the UK between 600 and 1000 diabetic people die from renal failure (Watkins 1985).

AETIOLOGY AND PATHOPHYSIOLOGY

The kidneys of people with diabetes are vulnerable with respect to the following:

1. Microvascular changes. Damage to the capillaries in the glomeruli can occur. The basement membrane initially thickens and in the later stages nodules of glycoprotein are deposited in the glomerular capsule. As a result the filtering capacity of the glomeruli is reduced.
2. Macrovascular changes. Atheromatous changes in renal vessels can lead to poor renal perfusion which will ultimately impair renal function.
3. Hypertension. A common feature in diabetes, hypertension can contribute to kidney damage and, conversely, can also result *from* kidney damage.
4. Urinary tract infection. This can occur for several reasons:
   - diabetes-associated predisposition to infection
   - damaged renal tissue vulnerable to infection
   - the need for catheterisation during metabolic crisis
   - atonic bladder associated with autonomic neuropathy, causing urinary stasis and ascending urinary tract infection.

Screening

Proteinuria. This is the clinical hallmark of diabetic renal disease. Urine testing for albumin should be undertaken at each clinic visit and at least once a year for all patients with diabetes. A positive dip-stick test for albuminuria suggests the need for more detailed biochemical analysis to provide quantitative information about the extent of protein loss from the kidney. Many centres still collect, or ask the patient to collect, urine over a 24-hour period to measure total protein excretion.

Microalbuminuria. For several years before albuminuria becomes detectable, microalbuminuria may be present, indicating early pathological changes within the kidneys. Testing kits are available to detect microalbuminuria in the clinic or GP surgery. If a positive result is obtained, laboratory methods which quantify microalbuminuria are then used (Doyle 1991, Marshall 1991).

Blood/urine biochemistry. Estimation of plasma and urine urea, creatinine, electrolytes and osmolality can be undertaken. Serum albumin will also usually be measured if albuminuria or oedema are present.

Blood pressure. All patients with proteinuria should have their blood pressure measured at every clinic or surgery visit. Many patients with evidence of proteinuria are in their 30s or 40s. A diastolic pressure above 95 mmHg should be reported, as it is likely that a decision will be taken to commence antihypertensive therapy (Watkins 1985).

MEDICAL MANAGEMENT

Diabetic renal disease is treated in the same way as renal disease in the non-diabetic population. The reader is referred to Chapter 8 for detailed coverage of early, advanced and end-stage renal failure. Only diabetes-related points will be mentioned in the short sections which follow.

Treatment choices for the patient in end-stage renal failure include haemodialysis, continuous ambulatory peritoneal dialysis (CAPD) or renal transplant using live or cadaver donors.

Renal transplantation using a live donor offers the best treatment for suitable patients. Careful selection of patients is important, given that other major diabetes-related complications usually coexist with the renal disease. Virtually all patients with end-stage renal failure have retinopathy and 20–30% are blind. Retinopathy alone would not militate against active treatment by dialysis or renal transplantation. However, it would be unlikely for renal transplant or dialysis to be considered in the presence of severe cardiovascular disease, cerebrovascular disease, infected neuropathic foot ulcers or advanced autonomic neuropathies causing postural hypotension or bladder paresis (Watkins 1985).

Blood glucose control

Insulin requirements. These can be difficult to predict. To enable insulin dosage adjustments to be made, frequent blood glucose monitoring will be required. Multiple injections using a pen injection device or continuous s.c. infusion may be advised to enable adjustments to be made more readily.

Oral hypoglycaemics. Due to the danger of lactic acidosis, metformin (a biguanide) should not be used for patients with renal impairment. Chlorpropamide (a sulphonylurea) should also be avoided as it is mainly excreted by the kidneys and in renal failure the drug can accumulate in the blood, causing serious hypoglycaemia. It may be necessary for some patients in renal failure whose diabetes was previously controlled by oral medication to be changed to insulin therapy.

NURSING PRIORITIES AND MANAGEMENT OF DIABETIC NEPHROPATHY

When renal function is impaired, diabetes control should be closely monitored by regular blood glucose measurement and urinalysis. Measurement and recording of fluid intake and output and body weight may be required to monitor renal function. Dietary and fluid restrictions may be imposed due to renal impairment. The patient and his family should be made aware of the vital importance of these measures.

Specific aspects of nursing care in renal failure can be found in Trusler 1992.

Prevention of renal failure

By identifying early renal impairment by screening for microalbuminuria, making efforts to improve diabetes control and detecting and treating hypertension it may be possible to prevent or delay the progression of renal disease (Gunnar Westberg 1980). Medical and nursing staff should exercise extreme care in the introduction and subsequent care of urinary catheters in order to prevent infection. Prompt treatment of any established urinary tract infection will normally be required to minimise damage.

5.13 Suggest three approaches which may be used in end-stage renal failure and discuss the potential lifestyle implications of each form of treatment.

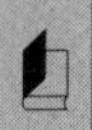

For further information on renal disease in diabetes mellitus see Conway & Davis (1987), Hoops (1990), Roberto (1990) and Trusler (1992).

Diabetic neuropathy

Aetiology

Although the cause of diabetic neuropathy is uncertain its incidence is known to rise in line with the duration of diabetes and with increasing age. A popular theory is that nerve damage occurs as a result of the accumulation of metabolites of glucose (such as sorbitol) causing osmotic swelling and subsequent damage to the nerve cell. Primary microvascular disease may also be implicated by virtue of reduced oxygen delivery to the nerve cells (Bovington 1983).

PATHOPHYSIOLOGY

Structural damage occurs affecting the nerve cells and fibres and causing segmental areas of demyelination to appear, thus impairing conduction of the nerve impulses (Kinson & Nattrass 1984). The types of neuropathy which may occur are as follows:

Peripheral neuropathies. These principally affect the lower extremities and play a major part in the aetiology of diabetic foot problems. They can affect either sensory or motor nerves and the patient's symptoms will reflect this.

Polyneuropathy. This term refers to widespread neuropathic changes affecting many nerves. Again, the lower extremities are often affected (peripheral polyneuropathy).

Mononeuropathies. It is possible for a single nerve to display evidence of damage. An example of mononeuropathy is the ptosis (drooping eyelid) and diplopia which can occur as a result of 3rd cranial nerve damage (see Table 5.11).

Autonomic neuropathies. Damage can also develop within the autonomic nervous system, causing a wide range of symptoms in many different sites. Sexual impotence, atonic bladder and silent myocardial infarction are examples of conditions associated with autonomic neuropathy (see Table 5.11).

Prevention

Whether or not diabetic neuropathy can be prevented is a contentious issue. Most experts agree that neuropathies seem to be more prevalent and more severe in poorly controlled diabetes. This may suggest that if the blood sugar is kept within the normal range and other sensible measures such as avoiding smoking are employed then the risk of neuropathy developing may be reduced. However, once neuropathies have developed the damage can not be reversed and means must be sought to help the patient deal with the particular problems which the neuropathy presents.

MEDICAL MANAGEMENT

Diabetic neuropathy can affect virtually any part of the body. Management, which is essentially symptomatic, may involve the interdisciplinary efforts of the diabetes care team. A variety of treatment approaches may be adopted, including medication, surgery and physiotherapy.

NURSING PRIORITIES AND MANAGEMENT OF DIABETIC NEUROPATHY

Devising ways to meet the particular comfort needs of the patient will be a central focus for nursing care. Reducing the risk of accidental tissue damage arising from severe sensory impairment will also be a priority.

Neuropathies can seriously interfere with lifestyle and with emotional well-being. An example of this would be diabetes-related sexual impotence. This can be devastating for both the patient and his partner. Nurses in particular can strive to improve their sensitivity to the verbal and non-verbal cues which may indicate the patient's concerns in this area.

The patient and partner may wish to consult a professional counsellor. Bancroft (1989) emphasises that not all diabetic impotence is irreversible and that even when it cannot be reversed it is possible to offer treatment or counselling. Gingell & Desai (1987) and Morrison (1988) provide clear accounts of diabetic impotence and its management.

The diabetic foot (see Table 5.12)

Disorders of the foot in diabetes can occur as a result of neuropathic and vascular changes. Generally, these two complications coexist, namely:

- neuropathic ulcers
- neuropathic arthropathy.

Neuropathic ulcers

Painless neuropathic ulcers can develop from chemical, thermal or mechanical injury. Forces applied to the foot can result in callus formation. As a result of sensory impairment, the patient is usually unaware of the developing callosity. Mechanical forces continue to be applied to the damaged area, resulting in inflammation, abscess formation and, eventually, ulceration.

MEDICAL MANAGEMENT OF NEUROPATHIC ULCERS

An infected ulcer in the foot requires urgent medical attention. Bedrest or the use of non–weight-bearing crutches is usually prescribed. A wound swab will be taken to identify infective microorganisms and to allow appropriate antibiotic therapy to be commenced. It may be necessary to undertake surgical debridement and drainage of pus. A serious complication of neuropathic ulcer is necrotising anaerobic infection and gangrene.

Once the acute situation has resolved it will be necessary to ensure redistribution of the weight-bearing forces on the vulnerable foot by specially constructed shoes or moulded insoles. If recurrence of neuropathic ulceration is to be avoided regular follow-up by a chiropodist will be required. The patient will also need supplementary information and advice on foot care.

Table 5.11 Diabetic neuropathy

Type of neuropathy	Body system/part affected	Symptoms/signs	Special points
Peripheral neuropathies			
Polyneuropathies:			
• Sensory	The lower extremities are the most frequently affected area	Reduced sensation: numbness, heaviness, insensitivity to heat, cold, and pressure Increased sensation: tingling, burning, pain (worse at night)	Serious risk of tissue damage as a result of heat, cold or pressure
• Motor — Amyotrophy — Muscle wasting	Muscles of the pelvic girdle Muscles of the hands and feet	Severe muscle wasting and pain Loss of strength in hand grip Changes in walking pattern Pressure points altered Painless foot ulcers can develop	Physiotherapy Aids to assist hand grip Chiropody Adapted footwear Care of the feet
Neuropathic arthropathy	Joints in the feet; 'Charcot's joints'	See 'The Diabetic Foot', p. 175	
Mononeuropathies:			
• Sensory	Femoral, sciatic, radial or ulnar nerve 3rd cranial nerve	Acute pain with sudden onset. Weakness and paralysis Ptosis: drooping of the upper eyelid	Provide pain relief Improve diabetes control Refer to an ophthalmologist
• Motor	3rd, 4th and 6th cranial nerves	Squint: diplopia	
Autonomic neuropathies	Cardiovascular system: • heart and blood vessels • vasomotor centre	Postural hypotension Tachycardia at rest Painless myocardial infarction Reduced perspiration in lower extremitites Increased perspiration in upper extremities	Symptoms such as syncope, dizziness and sweating; can be confused with hypoglycaemia
	Gastrointestinal system • stomach	Diabetic gastroparesis (delayed emptying) Nausea, anorexia Feeling of fullness	Altered absorption rate of nutrients can affect diabetes control
	• bowel	Constipation Nocturnal diarrhoea	Adjust diet
	Urinary system: • bladder	Loss of sensation Incomplete emptying Retention of urine Atonic bladder Sphincter incompetence	Urinary stasis creates risk of infection which may lead to renal damage
	Reproductive system • male genitalia	Sexual impotence Retrograde ejaculation Infertility	Neuropathic, vascular and psychological factors usually coexist

Table 5.12 Clinical signs in the diabetic foot (Reproduced with kind permission from Kinson & Nattrass 1984.)

	Ischaemia	Neuropathy
Pain	Considerable	Relatively free
Deformity	Nil	May be present
Skin	Thin Rubor on dependency Blanches on elevation	Often callus formation Normal colour
Temperature	Feels cold	Feels normal
Subcutaneous tissues	Atrophic	Normal
Peripheral pulses	Absent	Present

Neuropathic arthropathy (Charcot's joints)

A trivial injury such as that caused by tripping or bumping into something can lead to the development of a hot, red, and swollen (yet usually painless) joint in the foot. Gradually the joint structure is destroyed and major deformities of the foot result. The metatarsal and tarsal joints are the most commonly affected. The extent of the joint destruction can be discovered by the use of X-rays and bone scans.

MEDICAL MANAGEMENT OF CHARCOT'S JOINT

Rest, antibiotics and non-steroidal anti-inflammatory drugs (NSAIDs) such as indomethacin may be prescribed. Adapted footwear will usually be prescribed once ambulation is possible. Prevention of further joint damage will be attempted by education and by arranging supervision by a chiropodist.

Ischaemia
The ischaemic foot results from atherosclerotic changes in the distal vessels of the legs. Poor delivery of oxygen leads first to pain in the calf and foot during walking (claudication). Later, when blood flow is further impaired, pain will be experienced during rest. Localised pressure can result in ulceration; this can be complicated by secondary infection and gangrene. The foot feels cold and foot pulses may be absent. Colour changes occur in the skin and pain can be severe and unremitting.

MEDICAL MANAGEMENT OF THE ISCHAEMIC FOOT

This can include reducing oxygen demands of the tissues by rest and by cooling the area. Antibiotics to treat infection and analgesia for pain will be prescribed. Vascular reconstructive surgery may be attempted (see Ch. 2). In severe cases, where the pain is intolerable, or where sepsis is life-threatening, a major amputation may need to be considered (Edmonds 1985).

Prevention of foot problems
The diabetic foot is vulnerable on several counts. Sensory impairment can result in accidental injury remaining undetected until catastrophic damage has occurred. Vascular insufficiency deprives distal cells of their metabolic requirements, causing devitalisation of the tissue. Finally, healing of established injury may be delayed and the tendency to infection is increased. These factors can result in major complications such as gangrene developing from relatively minor injuries. The key to preventing serious diabetes-related complications in the lower limbs lies in education both for professionals and for patients. Patients may benefit from the advice given in Box 5.11. See also Research Abstract 5.1, page 181.

Infection
Infection can be viewed as a precipitating or as a complicating factor in diabetes mellitus. In established diabetes it can precipitate a metabolic crisis; in undiagnosed diabetes, it can herald the onset of symptoms.

Stress hormones such as ACTH, cortisol and catecholamines will be released in response to severe infection. These hormones will raise the blood glucose by the processes of glycogenolysis and gluconeogenesis. The resulting increase in insulin demand will present a challenge to an already malfunctioning pancreas and as a result metabolic crisis may ensue. Infection contributes to approximately 25% of deaths associated with ketoacidosis (Wheat 1980).

Infection as a complicating factor
Evidence on whether diabetic people are more prone to developing infection than non-diabetic people is somewhat conflicting. It has been suggested that people with diabetes have normal immune systems but have an impairment in their 'first line' defences against infection, i.e. bacteriocidal activity linked to the inflammatory response and phagocytosis. The action of neutrophils is impaired in the presence of an abnormally high blood glucose. High blood glucose also presents a favourable environment for bacteria, allowing them to survive longer and to reach pathogenic levels (Bagdade et al 1974, Wheat 1980).

Poor blood glucose control does seem to be linked to increased infection rates. In addition, host defences against infection may be further compromised by microvascular and neuropathic changes associated with diabetes. A good example of this is the diabetic foot.

?	**5.14** Why would microvascular and/or neuropathic changes cause an increased susceptibility to infection?
?	**5.15** Consult the above, or other, references and identify the most common infections which affect people with diabetes. Discuss why this should be so. Discuss ways in which the risks arising from impaired host defences against infection can be accommodated when providing care and information for a newly diagnosed 60-year-old female diabetic patient. (Read Donahue-Porter 1985.)

Summary
Chronic complications of diabetes can have important implications for the planning of nursing care. Whether the patient is at home or in hospital the nurse should carefully assess his nursing needs, giving special consideration to risks associated with impaired circulation and sensation, increased risk of infection, and delayed healing (see Ch. 23). Recognition of these risk factors will enable care to accommodate the patient's particular vulnerabilities and will help ensure that suitable educational support is provided.

Box 5.11 Measures to protect the feet in diabetes

General measures
- Do not smoke.
- Take a healthy diet with lots of fibre and not too much fat.
- Try to keep body weight within normal limits.
- Exercise. Try to keep active. This will help the circulation.
- Get blood pressure and blood fats checked regularly.

Footwear
- Try to get shoes which don't pinch anywhere and which allow all toes to move freely. Break in new shoes very gradually.
- Ensure that socks or stockings fit comfortably. Change them daily.
- Change footwear as soon as possible if wet.
- Avoid walking barefoot; wear slippers and beach shoes to prevent injury.

Foot care
- Bathe feet daily using lukewarm (not hot) water and soap.
- Pat feet dry gently; pay special attention to the area between the toes.
- Apply a lanolin-based moisturising cream daily to avoid dryness and keep the skin supple.
- Avoid exposing feet to excess heat or cold.
- Avoid sunburn to the feet and legs.
- Cut nails straight across while they are still soft from bathing.
- Inspect feet daily for blisters, corns, calluses, cracks or redness. (A mirror can help in seeing the underside of the foot.)
- If a minor cut or abrasion does occur, wash thoroughly and cover with a clean dressing. See your doctor if the cut has not healed in 48 hours.
- Your chiropodist should be consulted for treatment of ingrown toenails, corns, calluses or verrucae. (No home remedies, please.)
- A doctor or nurse should be consulted if foot problems such as tingling, numbness, swelling, pain or loss of feeling develop.
- Remember: most people with diabetes never have any trouble with their feet. Take reasonable care of your feet and they will reward you by lasting a lifetime!

FACILITATING SELF CARE THROUGH EDUCATION

In some hospital and community settings the overall coordination of patient teaching is undertaken by the diabetic nurse specialist working closely with the specialist dietitian and the patient's physician. In many cases, however, the care of diabetic patients will be undertaken by community and hospital nurses who are not specialists as such in diabetes care. All such nurses may be required to undertake a teaching role and must therefore ensure that their own knowledge base is adequate.

Assessment

Before embarking on a teaching programme the nurse must determine the needs of the patient and his family for information and plan teaching strategies that will make the learning experience pleasant and effective (Ley 1988). By establishing a rapport with the patient and family the nurse will be better able to assess the patient's needs in relation to:

- current level of knowledge about diabetes
- understanding about the reasons for prescribed treatment
- knowledge and skills required for self-care
- emotional response to the diagnosis
- social support from family and friends
- barriers to learning, e.g. sensory loss, mobility and manipulation problems, language difficulties, reading and writing difficulties and intellectual impairment.

Planning a teaching programme

Personnel

Any member of the diabetes care team may be involved in teaching the patient and his family about diabetes. However, it is likely that the main responsibility for patient teaching will rest with the nursing staff and, in particular, with the diabetes nurse specialist.

Materials and methods

An impressive array of informative and attractive booklets are available, mainly sponsored by manufacturers and written by diabetes health care professionals. These provide visual back-up for teaching and discussion sessions. Video programmes can sometimes be provided for patients to view individually or in groups. The British Diabetic Association (BDA) is a good source of educational materials (see Useful Addresses, p. 184).

Teaching sessions

Sessions should be short and information presented in small, easily assimilated and integrated sections with teaching points categorised into lists. Ordering presentation so that the most important point is always raised first can help the patient to prioritise information. Being direct and specific will aid retention, as will using simple words and brief sentences. Before going onto a new topic, the instructor can use sensitive questioning to check the patient's recall and understanding of the material already covered (Ley 1988).

Staff members should be consistent in the information which they provide. Adopting a friendly manner and taking time to talk about non-medical matters can relax the patient and set the scene for a more productive session. It is important to consider the age group for which teaching materials have been designed in order to avoid giving offence.

The programme

The teaching programme should be tailored to suit the patient's individual needs but is likely to include some of the following topics:

- defining diabetes mellitus
- medication in diabetes mellitus:
  - — oral hypoglycaemics
  - — insulin therapy
    - why insulin?
    - types of insulin
    - storage and administration of insulin
    - safe disposal of equipment
- the Diet – Insulin – Exercise balance (see Box 5.12)
- monitoring blood glucose and urinary glucose
- recognising hypoglycaemia and hyperglycaemia
- avoiding complications
- health screening
- safe disposal of equipment.

? **5.16** J is 15 years old and has insulin-dependent diabetes. He plays football for the school team, enjoys discos and goes swimming once a week. Discuss with your colleagues how a short teaching session might be prepared to help J understand the significance of exercise to overall diabetes control, personal well-being and the prevention of chronic complications. (See Additional Resources, p. 184 for educational material.)

Box 5.12 Exercise in diabetes

A clear understanding of the role of exercise in blood glucose control is essential for every diabetic patient. The nurse must find a way of explaining this role that is appropriate to the learning needs of individual patients. The analogy of 'fuel intake' (food) and 'energy output' (activity/exercise) is often useful for the purposes of illustration.

What happens during exercise?

When energy output is low the demand for fuel in the form of glucose is also low. However, during bursts of activity the demand for glucose will rise. The rate at which glucose is taken up by the cells is influenced by medication (insulin or tablets). If available supplies of glucose are depleted and are not replaced the patient's blood glucose will fall (hypoglycaemia).

Avoiding exercise-induced hypoglycaemia

The person on insulin therapy should be advised to monitor blood glucose before and after strenuous exercise and to take in extra carbohydrate to avoid hypoglycaemia caused by exercise or unusual activity. A quickly absorbable form of glucose such as Dextrosol tablets (or a chocolate bar) may be used to augment diet and prevent an abrupt fall in blood glucose. Another less commonly employed strategy to avoid exercise-induced hypoglycaemia is for insulin dosage to be slightly reduced prior to planned and prolonged strenuous activity. Blood glucose will then be monitored to gauge the effects of the insulin reduction.

Patients on oral sulphonylurea therapy may, less frequently, also experience exercise-induced hypoglycaemia and consequently may need to adjust their carbohydrate intake to meet the additional energy demands imposed by the exercise.

> For further information see Marks (1983).

PROMOTING PSYCHOLOGICAL AND SOCIAL ADJUSTMENT

The emotional impact of diabetes mellitus

When diabetes is first diagnosed the patient and his family are presented with a challenge on two distinct but equally important levels.

First, they are faced with the practicalities of 'learning a whole new science', for that is how some patients describe grappling with terminology and treatment. The significance of 'hypos', 'hypers', ketones, carbohydrate exchanges, insulin injections, urine testing and blood glucose monitoring all need to be understood and new and complex skills must be mastered.

Secondly, the patient has to absorb the emotional impact of being diagnosed with a chronic illness that will not go away. The patient may experience a variety of emotions. Self-image can be affected as the patient absorbs the new 'diabetic self'. One patient described this as feeling 'vulnerable and mortal', summing up her initial response to the diagnosis in this way: 'Since I was given the result it seemed as if my whole personality had changed. I wasn't the same as everyone else. I was a diabetic!' (Bow 1989).

Guilt reactions are not unusual. Patients may blame themselves (unjustifiably) for bringing on the disease. This is especially true of overweight patients with NIDDM and of parents of youngsters with IDDM (McCabe 1989).

The newly diagnosed patient with diabetes can experience a sense of loss akin to grief. Feelings of numbness, denial, anger and depression are common. A previously untrammelled lifestyle may have to be replaced by a life of enforced order. One patient describes the depression which she experienced after being diagnosed and suggests that telling a patient who is depressed about her diabetes to pull herself together is as unreasonable as telling her to make her own insulin (Kelsall 1989/90). Cox (1990), Shillitoe (1988) and Maclean & Orem (1988, Ch. 3) give detailed accounts of how the diagnosis of diabetes mellitus can affect the patient and his family.

However, it should be noted that not all patients react in a wholly negative way to their diagnosis. Maclean & Orem (1988) cite several examples of patients who have enjoyed an enhanced self-image and who appear to have experienced personal growth as they successfully rose to the challenges presented by diabetes.

How an individual will cope with a diagnosis of diabetes will be influenced by a variety of personal and social factors but perhaps most importantly by how he perceives and evaluates problems (see Ch. 17). This in turn will be influenced by his attitudes and beliefs with regard to illness. We may consider these attitudes with reference to the following concepts:

- locus of control
- the health belief model.

Locus of control

Many people believe that they exert a good degree of control over what happens to them and that by their own actions they can influence events. Those who take this view might be said to have an 'internal' locus of control and tend to be highly self-directing and self-motivated. This can have implications for treatment compliance and for self-care. Such people will tend to seek out information and will strive to master difficult tasks. Such patients are often quick to achieve and maintain stability of blood glucose control in the early post-diagnostic period.

Patients with an 'external' locus of control believe that events happen due to circumstances which are beyond their control. They view themselves as passive victims rather than active agents. Such patients may experience problems in achieving good control of blood glucose in the early stabilisation period and, accordingly, relatively frequent hospital admissions.

Some studies suggest that, in the long term, patients with an external locus of control can maintain good diabetes control, as they will be inclined to adhere rigidly to instructions. In contrast, patients with an internal locus of control, having achieved control of their diabetes, are more likely to experiment with and manipulate their treatment independently, knowing and accepting the risks to stability which this degree of self-direction may bring (Kelleher 1988, Shillitoe 1988).

Health beliefs and compliance

The health belief model (see Fig. 5.12) provides one means of examining the issue of patient compliance with medical therapy in diabetes mellitus (Becker et al 1979). Kelleher (1988) reports non-compliance rates in diabetes treatment ranging between 30 and 60% and links these rates to health beliefs. Those who regard their diabetes as 'serious' are more likely to comply with a treatment regimen, whereas non-compliance is more often found in people who do not regard their diabetes as serious or who, having weighed up the personal cost, view the loss of lifestyle choices as too high a price to pay for good control of blood glucose.

It is well known that behaviour in the present is relatively insensitive to the threat of long-term consequences. Additionally, one cannot be certain that by providing information health care professionals will ensure treatment compliance. Cognitive dissonance (Festinger 1957) is an accepted phenomenon. Few users of alcohol or tobacco, for example, would deny knowledge of the risks involved but many consciously elect to exercise their freedom of choice with regard to actual behaviour. Similarly, patients with diabetes, even if well informed, may consciously decide not to comply with diabetes treatment.

By contrast, some people with diabetes become engaged in a battle for perfection in blood glucose control and come to regard any evidence of imbalance as a personal failure. Such individuals may find that guilt plays an increasingly significant role in their lives. Maclean & Orem (1988) caution health care professionals against being 'over-authoritarian' with newly diagnosed patients. They argue that such an approach can lead to self-critical, obsessive behaviour which could become socially and emotionally crippling.

> ? **5.17** What may lead you to decide whether a patient has an external or an internal locus of control or what his 'health beliefs' are? What relevance may such judgements have for the ways in which you provide care and information for the patient? (Read from the following authors' Weinman (1987), Rosenstock (1988), Oberle (1991) and Woolridge (1992).

Relationships

Family relationships

If the family unit was previously stable, diabetes is unlikely to have an adverse effect on family relationships. Indeed, patients who enjoy good social support from their families show enhanced stability, suggesting that the family can be a positive

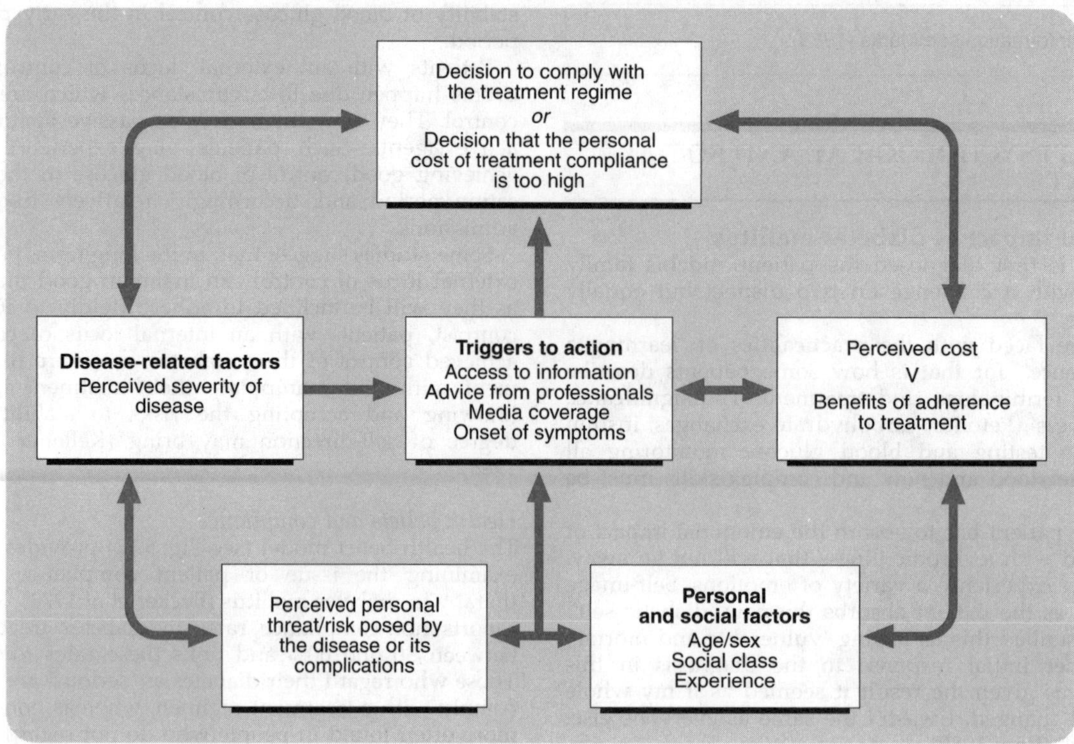

Fig. 5.12 The health belief model, summarised.

agent in the battle for glycaemic control (Maclean & Orem 1988).

However, the very nature of diabetes, with its attendant rules and restrictions, may allow the disorder to be used by family members or the patient as a means of manipulation or self-assertion. This rather unhealthy state of affairs is more likely to occur where family relationships were difficult prior to the diagnosis of diabetes.

Sexual relationships

Although embarking on a sexual relationship is anxiety-provoking for many people it raises particular concerns for people with diabetes. Uncertainty may be felt about when, and if, to tell the other person about the diabetes. Practical issues such as what to do if a 'hypo' develops when out on a date (or, even worse, during lovemaking) may cause real worry. Having to explain such things as set eating and injection times or dietary restrictions may cause embarrassment and may be seen as interfering with the spontaneity of a budding relationship.

A comprehensive overview of research into diabetes-related sexual problems and an account of various management strategies is provided by Bancroft (1989).

Family planning

People with diabetes can have healthy, happy families just like anyone else. Prospective parents may worry about passing on their diabetes to the baby. Genetic counselling may be offered to enable the couple to make an informed decision. Detailed discussion of genetic and other pregnancy-associated risks is provided by Shaw (1986).

Pre-conception. Where the woman has diabetes it would be ideal for the couple to be seen by both a physician and an obstetrician (Brudenell 1985). With the help of home blood glucose monitoring, strict blood glucose control should be achieved before conception and maintained right throughout the pregnancy. Estimation of glycated proteins can provide the health care professionals with objective evidence of the quality of glycaemic control (Tindall et al 1986).

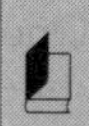
See Kinson & Nattrass (1984) for more detailed coverage of pregnancy in diabetes and for discussion of gestational diabetes.

Contraception. General advice may be offered by nurses and doctors in both community and hospital settings. The family planning clinic may also offer advice. If oral contraceptives are used it is important to monitor blood and urine glucose more frequently than usual, as some of these drugs alter glycaemic control. Risks to the vascular system associated with oral contraception should be discussed, especially with women over 35 years of age and with those who smoke (Hillson 1987).

Social relationships

Patients with diabetes quite naturally resist being singled out and labelled. This can create real difficulties. On the one hand, coping with diabetes means that the individual may have to rely on others should a crisis occur. On the other hand, the person with diabetes may resent being treated differently from others. The patient's adjustment within his social milieu will involve a complex interplay of personal and social factors; the degree of success will vary considerably from person to person.

Access to counselling should be provided for those people who are experiencing relationship difficulties arising from their diabetes.

? **5.18** What do you understand by the term 'labelling'? Why do you think people with diabetes may be concerned about being labelled?

See Bruhn 1991, Maclean & Orem 1988 Chs 3 & 4, Stockwell 1972 and World Health Organization 1985 pp. 73–76.

Lifestyle implications

Employment

In view of the risk of hypoglycaemia, people with insulin-dependent diabetes are barred from vocational driving, airline piloting, deep sea diving, and from working on offshore oil rigs, at heights, or near dangerous moving machinery. Diabetes would also exclude an applicant from joining the UK armed forces or the police.

Driving

The driver vehicle licensing centre in Swansea (DVLC) must, by law, be informed when a driver is diagnosed as having diabetes mellitus. Normally a licence for a diabetic driver will be renewed, free of charge, every three years until the driver reaches the age of 70 and then yearly thereafter. A medical practitioner may be required to advise on the stability of the driver's diabetes control prior to relicensing.

Since 1990 patients who have diet-controlled diabetes are entitled to hold an unrestricted car driving licence.

Insurance

The British Diabetic Association (BDA) have their own insurance broker who can advise on any insurance-related matter (see Box 5.13).

Travel

Altered mealtimes, crossed time zones, and dietary and climatic changes may all have an effect on diabetes stability. Blood glucose monitoring is an excellent way of keeping tabs on diabetes control. All the requirements for medication and monitoring should be carried in hand luggage as suitcases may get lost in transit and insulin can freeze in the baggage hold during air travel (Hillson 1989).

Eating out

Flexible insulin therapy and home blood glucose monitoring (HBGM) has simplified eating out for diabetic people. Most restaurant menus offer enough variety and choice to allow customers with diabetes to enjoy, without worry, the social benefits of having a meal with friends. For those who enjoy fast foods a guide has been produced (Lilly Diabetes Care 1985).

Box 5.13 The British Diabetic Association (BDA)

The BDA is a charitable organisation which raises money for diabetes research and provides information and advice for people with diabetes and professionals involved in their care. As well as being a national organisation it has local branches throughout the UK. Different sections cater for particular groups, e.g. teenagers. The BDA offers help and advice on a wide variety of topics such as monitoring and treatment approaches, insurance, holidays and travelling abroad.

Full members of the BDA receive the bimonthly journal, *Balance*, free of charge. This is an excellent publication which provides a forum for diabetic people and their families to exchange ideas and keep up-to-date with current progress in diabetes management. *Balance* is also produced on audiotape for visually impaired subscribers.

Smoking

People with diabetes are at greater risk than others of developing vascular and neuropathic disorders. Smoking would compound these risks. The health care team should try to discourage smoking and should discuss the availability of resources to provide support whilst the patient is trying to give up smoking. However, it must be accepted that the patient has freedom of choice and may against advice decide to continue to smoke.

Identification

The patient should be encouraged to carry a card or wear a Medic Alert pendant to identify him and give details of the type of diabetes he has and its management.

CONCLUSION

Research in diabetes care has reached an exciting stage. Work is progressing in the field of pancreatic gland or islet cell transplantation although the perfection of these techniques still eludes researchers (Ostman et al 1985). Aside from the problem of immunological rejection there is doubt as to how long transplanted islet cells would continue to work before they too ceased to secrete insulin (Hallett 1990, O'Toole 1990).

Genetic engineering has produced purer insulins (Jervell 1985) and microtechnology is making insulin therapy and blood glucose monitoring easier and more acceptable to patients. There is hope that current treatment approaches in controlling blood glucose will be rewarded by fewer, or at least less severe, chronic complications (Hanssen et al 1985). More sophisticated screening methods and better treatments are reducing the incidence of diabetes-related complications, notably blindness (Ehlers & Bulow 1980).

The ultimate hope is that diabetes will at some future date be preventable. Researchers continue to seek definitive answers to the questions surrounding aetiological factors with a view to finding ways of manipulating these factors to prevent the disease developing.

Recent trends in health care provision

The political and economic climate in the UK over the last decade has given rise to significant changes in the structure and function of the primary care team and has shifted the focus of health care toward the community setting. These changes are reflected in trends in diabetes care (Powell 1991 a–b). The growth in the number of practice nurses has made

Research abstract 5.1 (SHHD 1987)

The Working Group on the Management of Diabetes reports that there is evidence that about 50% of cases of amputation and of peripheral vascular disease requiring hospitalisation could have been prevented with better foot care and improved diabetes control. A number of studies were cited in this report. One study (Runyan 1975) revealed that nurses specially trained to examine the diabetic foot and to offer patients information and advice on foot care had brought about a significant reduction in the number of diabetic patients requiring amputation. This clearly highlights the potential influence of nurses in helping to maintain the integrity of the diabetic patient's limbs.

Scottish Home and Health Department (SHHD) 1987 Report of the working group on the management of diabetes. HMSO, London it possible for some GPs to run their own clinics for diabetic patients. In some areas community dietitians and chiropodists are available for consultation in the health centres where clinics are run.

Community nurses and health visitors may find themselves to an increasing extent taking high-quality diabetes care right into the patient's home. Effective hospital–community liaison will become especially important to ensure continuity for the patient in 'shared care'.

Whatever the care setting it is important that the patient has access to facilities for estimation of glycated haemoglobin and microalbuminuria and for screening for retinopathy and foot-threatening neuropathic or vascular disease. It seems likely that integrated hospital and community care will offer the best use of resources for diabetes screening. However, dealing with severe metabolic crisis such as DKA will remain the province of the hospital.

Continuing education for all members of the diabetes care team must be a priority. Diabetes specialist nurses could make a significant contribution in the education of their colleagues. Nursing care in diabetes should have a firm research base. Nurses require a clear understanding of the scientific aspects of the disorder and its management if safe care is to be provided. Diabetes care is, however, more than mere science. Providing the support which will enable the patient to move away from the despondency and fear which frequently accompany diagnosis towards independence and autonomy is surely the art of nursing care in diabetes mellitus.

REFERENCES

Armitage M, Caughey E M, Brooks A et al 1988 Insulin resistance and insulin antibodies; fact or hallowed fiction. Practical Diabetes 5(5): 200–202

Bagdade J D, Root R K, Bulger R J, Seattle M D 1974 Impaired leucocyte function in patients with poorly controlled diabetes. Diabetes 23(1): 9–15

Balance 1990 Driving and diabetes. 'News Section' Balance 116: 53

Bancroft J 1989 Human sexuality and its problems. Churchill Livingstone, Edinburgh, ch 11, pp 552–562

Becker M H, Maiman L A, Kirsct J P et al 1979 Patients' perceptions and compliance. In: Shillitoe R W 1988 (ed) Psychology and diabetes. Chapman & Hall, London, p 197

Bodansky H J 1989 The natural history of type one (insulin-dependent) diabetes. Practical Diabetes. 6(1): 7–9

Bodington M 1988 Practical aspects of insulin treatment. Practical Diabetes 5(1): 19–20

Bovington M M 1983 Neurologic complications in diabetes mellitus. Nursing Clinics of North America 18(4): 735–747

Bow M 1989 One drop = 12.5. Balance 113: 52–53

Brooks A P, Boss A H 1989 Safe changeover to Human Protaphane from porcine Semitard M C insulin. Practical Diabetes 6(2): 74–75

Brudenell M 1985 Diabetic pregnancy. Medicine International 13 2(13): 566–571

Connor H 1987 Alcohol and diabetes: what should we tell our patients? Practical Diabetes 4(July/August): 159–162

Conaglen J V, Sonksen P H 1985 Diabetic ketoacidosis. Medicine International 2(13): 546–548

Cox S 1990a How I coped emotionally with diabetes in my family. Diabetic Nursing 1(4): 7–8

Craddock S 1989 Blood glucose monitoring: Why test? Diabetic Nursing 1(2): 5–6

Day J 1991b Improving self management. (Symposium) The Practitioner 235 (October): 775–779

Donnelly D 1992 Insulin resistance and blood pressure. British Journal of Hospital Medicine 47(1): 9–11

Doyle A 1991 Microalbuminuria in diabetic patients. Nursing Times 87(28): 43

Drug and Therapeutics Bulletin 1989 Consumers Association 27(6): 21–24

Drury R 1986 Seasonal variation in incidence rates of juvenile onset, insulin-dependent diabetes. Practical Diabetes 3(4): 209–211

Edmonds M 1985 The diabetic foot. Medicine International 2(13): 551–553

Ehlers N, Bulow N 1980 Ocular complications in diabetes and their treatment. Acta Endocrinologica 94 Supplement 238: 59–66

Festinger L 1957 A theory of cognitive dissonance. Stanford University Press, Stanford CA

Fisher M 1991 Care of insulin dependent diabetes. (Symposium) The Practitioner 235(October): 783–785

Gale E 1985 Hypoglycaemia in diabetes. Medicine International 2(13): 549–551

Gatling W 1989 Home monitoring of diabetes: urine testing. Practical Diabetes 6(3): 100–101

Gill G V, Alberti K G M M 1985a Diabetic ketoacidosis: biochemical background and presentation. Practical Diabetes 2(1): 15–19

Gill G V, Alberti K G M M 1985b Management of ketoacidosis. Practical Diabetes 2(2): 12–16

Gill G V, Alberti K G M M 1985c Hyperosmolar non-ketotic coma. Practical Diabetes 2(3): 30–35

Gingell J C, Desai 1987 Investigation of impotence with particular reference to the diabetic. Practical Diabetes 4(6): 257–260

Greenwood R H, Robinson N 1989 The employment of diabetics. Practical Diabetes 6(4): 148–149

Gunnar Westberg N 1980 Diabetic nephropathy. Pathogenesis and treatment. Acta Endocrinologica 94 Supplement 238: 85–101

Haire-Joshu D, Flaven K, Clutter W 1986 Contrasting type I and type II diabetes. American Journal of Nursing 86(11): 1240–1243

Hallett L 1990 The quest for a cure. Balance 118: 52–53

Hamilton A M 1985 Retinopathy: clinical assessment and management. Medicine International 2(13): 556–560

Hamilton H, Ubig M 1991 The eye in diabetes. The Practitioner (Symposium) 235: 780–782

Hanssen K, Dahl-Jorgensen K, Brinchman-Hansen O, Aker diabetes group 1985 The influence of strict control on diabetic complications. Acta Endocrinologica 110 Supplement 272: 57–60

Hillson R 1987 Diabetes: a beyond the basics guide. Macdonald, London, chs 6 & 7

Hillson R 1989 Travelling with diabetes. Practical Diabetes 6(4): 151–153

Hindley P 1989 Monitoring diabetes at home: what the patient needs to know and the equipment necessary. Practical Diabetes 6(2): 59–61

Home P 1985 Management of diabetes with insulin. Medicine International 2(13): 538–541

Jarrett J 1985 The natural history and prognosis of diabetes. Medicine International 2(13): 530–532

Jervell J 1985 Role of human insulin in the treatment of diabetes. Acta Endocrinologica 110 Supplement 272: 61–64

Jones D B 1987 Aetiology of diabetes. Update 35(10): 1012–1014

Jones J M 1986 Practical aids for visually handicapped diabetics. Practical Diabetes 3(5): 263

Kelleher D 1988 Diabetes. The experience of illness series. Routledge, London, chs 2, 4 & 5

Kelsall L 1989/90 Understanding anxiety. Balance 114: 28–29

Kinson J, Nattrass M 1984 Caring for the diabetic patient. Churchill Livingstone, Edinburgh

Koivistov V L, Felig P 1978 Is skin preparation necessary before insulin injection? Lancet vol i: 1072–1073

Ley P 1988 Communicating with patients: improving communication, satisfaction and compliance. Croom Helm, London, ch 2

Lilly Diabetes Care 1985 Fast food CHO/calories checklist. Eli Lilly, Basingstoke

Lovelock L 1990 A day in the life of: mobile eye screening technician. Balance 116: 26–27

McCabe M 1989 'He couldn't be.' Balance 113: 52–53

Maclean H, Orem B 1988 Living with diabetes: personal stories and strategies. University of Toronto Press, Toronto, ch 3
Marshall S 1991 Microalbuminuria. Diabetes Nursing 2(3): 13–14
Morrison H 1988 Diabetic impotence. Nursing Times 84(32): 35–37
Nutrition Sub-committee of the BDA's Professional Advisory Committee (1990) Dietary recommendations for people with diabetes: an update for the 1990s. BDA, London
Ostman J, Lundgren G, Tyden G et al 1986 Pancreatic transplantation in diabetes mellitus: present status. Acta Endocrinologica 5 110 Supplement 272: 65–71
O'Toole L 1990 Why islet transplants? Balance 118: 52–55
Paton R C 1989 The natural history of type two diabetes. Practical Diabetes 6(1): 10–13
Powell J 1991a Mini clinics in general practice. The Practitioner 235: 766–772
Powell J 1991b Shared care. The Practitioner 235(October): 761–762
Pugliese G, Tilton R G, Williamson J R 1991 Glucose induced metabolic imbalances in the pathogenesis of diabetic vascular disease. Diabetes/Metabolism Reviews 7(1): 35–49
Pyke D 1990 Driving heavy goods vehicles and diabetes. Balance 119(August/September): 76
Rayman G 1989 Hospital inpatient monitoring of diabetes. Practical Diabetes 6(2): 62–64
Reckless J P D 1985 What is diabetes? Practical Diabetes 2(1): 8–11
Rosenstock 1974 The health belief model and preventative health behaviour. Health Education Monographs 2: 354–386
Rowe E 1989 Diabetes and driving. Practical Diabetes 6(4): 154–155
Runyan J W 1975 Comparison of outcome of the nurse's extended role. In: SHHD 1987 Report of the working group on the management of diabetes. HMSO, Edinburgh Appendix 2, p 75
Sadler C 1991 A change for the worse, Nursing Times 87(28): 16–17
Scottish Home and Health Department (SHHD) 1987 Report of the working group on the management of diabetes. HMSO, Edinburgh, ch 3
Shaw K M 1986 Should diabetics have children? Practical Diabetes 3(6): 313
Shillitoe R W 1988 Psychology and diabetes: psychosocial factors in management and control. Croom Helm, London, ch 7
Simpson H C R 1985 General aspects of fibre in the diet. Practical Diabetes 2(1): 21–24
Simpson H C R 1989 Hyperglycaemic hyperosmolar non-ketotic coma: a half or full blooded solution? Practical Diabetes 6(2): 66–68
Tindall H, Stickland M, Wales J K 1986 Improved results for diabetic pregnancies after pre-pregnancy counselling. Practical Diabetes 3(5): 250–251
Trounce J 1990 Clinical pharmacology for nurses, 13th edn. Churchill Livingstone, Edinburgh
Tredger J 1989 Diet in the treatment of diabetes mellitus. Nursing (London) 3(41): 20–21
Viinikki L 1985 Platelet function and thrombus in diabetes. Acta Endocrinologica 110 Supplement 272: 31–34
Wales J K 1989 The natural history of diabetes mellitus. Practical Diabetes 6(1): 4–5
Walford S 1989 Monitoring in the diabetic clinic. Practical Diabetes 6(2): 56–57
Watkins P J 1985 Diagnosis and treatment of diabetic nephropathy. Medicine International 2(13): 554–555
Wheat J L 1980 Infection and diabetes mellitus. Diabetes Care 3(1): 187–197
Wiles P G 1988 Insulin antibodies; something or nothing? Practical Diabetes 5(5): 196
World Health Organization 1980 Expert committee on diabetes mellitus, 2nd Report. WHO, Geneva
World Health Organization 1985 Diabetes mellitus: technical report series 727. WHO, Geneva

FURTHER READING

Diabetes — causes and management
Andreani D, Di Mario U, Pozzilli P 1991 Prediction, prevention and early intervention in insulin-dependent diabetes. Diabetes/Metabolism Reviews 7(1): 61–77
Daly H, Clarke P, Field J 1988 Diabetes care: a problem solving approach. Heinemann, London
Hill R D 1981 Diabetes health care: a guide to the provision of health care services. Chapman & Hall, London
Kilvert A 1987 Starting treatment in a newly diagnosed patient. Practical Diabetes 4(6): 262–263
Kinson J, Nattrass M 1984 Caring for the diabetic patient. Churchill Livingstone, Edinburgh
Lernmark A 1985 Causes of insulin dependent diabetes. Medicine International 2(13): 535–537
Leslie R D G 1985 Causes of non-insulin dependent diabetes. Medicine International 2(11): 533–534
Macheca M K K 1993 Diabetic hypoglycaemia: how to keep the threat at bay. American Journal of Nursing 93(4): 46–30
Oberle K 1991 A decade of research in locus of control: what have we learned? Journal of Advanced Nursing 16(7): 800–806
Pelkonen R, Koivisto V, Mustajoki P 1985 Comparison of insulin regimens in the therapy of type 1 diabetes. Acta Endocrinologica 110 Supplement 272: 49–55
Reading S 1986 What is diabetes? The Professional Nurse 1(12): 333–335
Sonksen P, Fox C, Judd S 1991 The comprehensive diabetes reference book for the 1990s. Class Publishing, London
Stowers J M 1985 General management of diabetes in adults. Medicine International 2(13): 542
Wilson K J W 1990 Ross & Wilson anatomy and physiology in health and illness, 7th edn. Churchill Livingstone, Edinburgh
Thomas L 1988 Diabetes mellitus. Nursing Standard 2(24): 31–33

Foot care
Burden A C, Samanta A, Jones R 1986 Setting up an advanced foot clinic in a district general hospital. Practical Diabetes 3(5): 262–263
Foster A 1987 Examination of the diabetic foot. Practical Diabetes 4(3): 105–107
Thurston R 1984 Foot lesions in diabetics: predisposing factors. Nursing Times 80(34): 44–46

Monitoring/education
Bodansky H J 1986 Tales from the diabetic clinic, or Why some patients do not bring a record book to the clinic. Practical Diabetes 3(5): 247–248
Callahan M 1988 Why you should teach your diabetic patients to chart. Nursing (Springhouse) 18(3): 48–50
Mallows C 1986 The training of nurses in the care of diabetics. Practical Diabetes 3(5): 230–231
Manning L 1988 Patient's knowledge of diabetes: an area for concern. Health Education Journal 4: 153
Marks C 1983 Teaching the diabetic patient. In: Wilson-Barnett J (ed) Patient teaching: recent advances in nursing. Churchill Livingstone, Edinburgh
Reading S 1986 Blood glucose monitoring: a tool in diabetic control. Professional Nurse 2(1): 9–11
Reading S 1986 Blood glucose monitoring: teaching effective techniques. Professional Nurse 2(2): 55–57
Rosseter P 1989 Self monitoring of diabetes at home and abroad: a patient's viewpoint. Practical Diabetes 6(3): 108–109
Wales J K 1989 Knowledge is power. Practical Diabetes 6(4): 147

Infection
Donohue-Porter P 1985 Insulin-dependent diabetes mellitus: educating the diabetic person regarding diabetes and infections. Nursing Clinics of North America 20(1): 191–198

Health belief model
Rosenstock I M, Strecher V J, Becker M H 1988 Social learning theory and the health belief model. Health Education Quarterly 15(2): 175–183
Weinman J 1987 Beliefs and behaviour in health and illness. Nursing 3(18): 658–660
Woolridge et al 1992 The relationship between health beliefs,

adherence and metabolic control of diabetes. Diabetes Educator 118(6): 495–500

Labelling

Bruhn J G 1991 Nouns that cut: the negative effects of labelling by allied health professionals. Journal of Allied Health 20(4): 229–231

Maclean H, Orem B 1988 Living with diabetes: personal stories and strategies. University of Toronto Press, Toronto, ch 4

Sinclair, Fawcett 1991 Altschul's psychology for nurses, 7th edn. Nursing Aids Series, Baillière Tindall, London, p 271

Stockwell F 1972 The unpopular patient. Royal College of Nurses and the Dept of Health and Social Services, London

World Health Organization 1985 Diabetes mellitus. Technical Report Series 727. WHO, Geneva pp 73–76

Surgery

Bovington M M, Spies M E, Troy P J 1983 Management of the patient with diabetes mellitus during surgery or illness. Nursing Clinics of North America 18(4): 661–671

Saltiel-Berzin R 1992 Managing a surgical patient who has diabetes. Nursing 92 22(4): 34–42

Hernandez C M G 1987 Surgery and diabetes: minimizing the risks. American Journal of Nursing 87(6): 788–792

Wound healing

Norris S O, Provo B, Stotts N A 1990 Physiology of wound healing and risk factors that impede the healing process. Clinical Issues in Critical Care Nursing 1(3): 545–552

Renal failure

Conway P M, Davis C P 1987 The diabetic transplant patient: nursing considerations. ANNA Journal 14(6): 379–383

Hoops S 1990 Renal and retinal complications in insulin-dependent diabetes mellitus: the art of changing the outcome. Diabetes Educator 16(3): 221–233

Roberto P L 1990 Diabetic nephropathy: causes, complications and considerations. Nursing Clinics of North America 2(1): 55–66

Trusler L A 1992 Management of the patient receiving simultaneous kidney-pancreas transplantation. Critical Care Nursing Clinics of North America 4(1): 89–95

Psycho-social aspects

Shillitoe R W, Miles D W 1989 Diabetes mellitus. In: Broome A (ed) Health psychology: processes and application. Chapman Hall, London, ch 11

ADDITIONAL RESOURCES AND USEFUL ADDRESSES

Sources of information

General Practitioner Information Pack
Directory of Diabetes Specialist Nurses
Both available free of charge from
British Diabetic Association
10 Queen Anne Street
London WIM OBD
Tel: (071) 323 1531

Diabetes — Clinical Information Folder
Royal College of General Practitioners
14 Princes Gate
Hyde Park, London SW7
Tel: (071) 581 3232

The Diabetes Handbook
Non-insulin Dependent Diabetes
Insulin Dependent Diabetes
Both by Dr John L Day
Available from the BDA

Magazines & journals

Practical Diabetes: The journal for the diabetes health team
The Newbourne Group
Home & Law Publishing Ltd
Greater London House
Hampstead Road
London NWI 7QQ
Tel: 071 388 3171

Diabetes Update
Published twice a year by the BDA and mailed free on request.

Diabetes in the News (3–4 issues per year)
Published by Paragon
Publications for Counsellor on behalf of Ames
Division Miles Ltd
For inclusion on mailing list write to:
The Editor, DITN
PO Box 277
Penn, Bucks HP10 8DB

Balance
Published by BDA (bi-monthly)
Mailed free of charge to members of The British
Diabetic Association

Diabetic Nursing — The Journal for all Nurses
involved in Diabetes Care

Media Medica, The Newbourne Group
I North Pallant, Chichester
West Sussex PO19 ITL
Sponsored by: Boehringer Mannheim UK

Sources of educational material, etc.

Becton Dickinson UK Ltd
Between Towns Road
Cowley
Oxford OX4 3LY

General information on diet, living with diabetes etc.

The British Diabetic Association
10 Queen Anne Street
London WIM OBD
Tel: 071 323 1531

Measurement of insulin and injection technique

Diabetes Care Division
Becton Dickinson (UK) Ltd
Between Towns Road
Cowley, Oxford OX4 3LY
Tel: (0865) 777722

Insulin and mode of action

Eli Lilly & Co Ltd
Dextra Court
Chapel Hill
Basingstoke, Hants
Tel: (0256) 473241

Novo Nordisk Pharmaceuticals Ltd
Novo-Nordisk House
Broadfield Park
Brighton Road
Pease Pottage
Crawley, West Sussex RHII 9RT
Tel: (0293) 613555

Blood & urine glucose monitoring

Ames Division
Miles Laboratories Ltd
Stoke Court
Stoke Poges
Slough SL2 4LY
Tel: (0753) 645151

Boehringer Mannheim U.K.
Boehringer Mannheim House
Bell Lane
Lewes, East Sussex BN7 ILG
Tel: (0273) 480444

Oral hypoglycaemics
Servier Laboratories Ltd
Fulmer Hall
Windmill Road
Fulmer
Slough SL3 6HH
Tel: (0753) 662744

Lipha Pharmaceuticals
Harrier House
High Street
Yiewsley
West Drayton
Middx UB7 7QG
Tel: (0895) 449331

Footcare
Customer Services Department
Scholl (UK) Ltd
475 Capability Green
Luton
Beds LUI 3LU
Tel: (0582) 482929

CHAPTER 6

Genetic disorders

Aileen Crosbie Anne Lowie Moira Mennie

CHAPTER CONTENTS

Introduction 187

The mechanics of genetic inheritance 188

Genetic modification and gene therapy 189

Categories of genetic disorders 191
Chromosomal anomalies 191
Single gene or Mendelian disorders 191
Multifactorial or polygenic disorders 192

Testing for genetic disorders 192
Prenatal testing 193

The genetic counselling process 194
The referral stage 194
The genetic counselling team 194
The role of the specialist genetic nurse 194
Special components of genetic counselling 195
The counselling procedure 196
The psychological impact of diagnosis 197

CLASSIC GENETIC DISORDERS AND THEIR MANAGEMENT 198

Klinefelter syndrome 198
Nursing priorities and management 198

Down's syndrome 199
Nursing priorities and management 199

Cystic fibrosis 199
Nursing priorities and management 201

Haemophilia A 202
Nursing priorities and management 204

Myotonic dystrophy 205
Nursing priorities and management 206

Huntington's disease 207
Nursing priorities and management 208

Conclusion 209

References 210

Further reading 210

Useful addresses 210

INTRODUCTION

Genetics is the study of genes and their relationship to hereditary characteristics. Genes are units of deoxyribonucleic acid (DNA) found in the chromosomes within the nuclei of living cells. They carry coded information which influences not only physical and psychological characteristics such as eye colour and temperament but also susceptibility to many major life-threatening diseases.

The aims of this chapter are:

- to provide a basic outline of the mechanics of genetic inheritance
- to raise awareness of genetic influence in common diseases
- to describe several classic but rare genetic disorders
- to outline nursing roles in health promotion, genetic counselling and genetic disorder management
- to highlight the future potential of genetic modification, gene therapy and genetic engineering and to raise awareness of the ethical issues that these techniques imply.

A Working Party for the British Medical Association (BMA) reported that genetic and genetically influenced disease affected 1 in 20 people by age 25 and possibly 2 in 3 people in their lifetime (BMA 1992). It also predicted that recent and rapidly evolving advances in genetic science have made possible an era of genetically informed health care, disease modification and genetic engineering that will have major implications for medical management and nursing involvement.

Because of the wide range of genetic influences in health and disease, nurses in most areas of practice will have occasion to apply their understanding of genetics. In the community, nurses are involved in screening for and recognising inherited traits and in providing counselling to promote optimum levels of health. Inheritance of a predisposition to common diseases such as heart disease, cancer, diabetes and asthma is much more complex than that of the classic genetic disorders and has a much higher incidence. Environmental and other triggering factors will determine whether a predisposition manifests in actual disease. Nurses must therefore promote an awareness and modification of these environmental factors in order to help their clients avert the full-blown consequences of their genetic makeup.

Nurses in the fields of mental handicap, psychiatry, community and health visiting may be involved with families in which there is an existing classic genetic disorder. Nurses in hospital wards, in particular midwives and those working in gynaecology units, will be involved with patients who have miscarried or terminated a pregnancy or who have infertility problems. And nurses in acute and long-term care will be involved with the management of the more distressing classic diseases.

Within the specialised field of genetics there is the more focused role of the nurse specialist, who works within the multidisciplinary team and is involved in non-directive counselling, diagnosis and support of individuals and families in whom classic genetic disorder occurs.

THE MECHANICS OF GENETIC INHERITANCE

Chromosomes

Each human cell contains 46 chromosomes within its nucleus, with the exception of the gametes (sex cells), which contain 23. Of the 46 chromosomes 23 come from one parent and 23 from the other parent. These chromosomes are paired, giving 22 pairs identified as autosomes 1–22 and one pair of sex chromosomes, either XX for females or XY for males.

By staining, photographing and arranging according to size the chromosomes extracted from a cell can be organised into a karyotype. A normal female karyotype would be reported as 46, XX and a normal male karyotype as 46, XY (see Fig. 6.1). Chromosomal abnormalities can be identified by this method.

Cell division

To understand the mechanisms of genetic inheritance it is necessary to be familiar with the basic processes of cell division, i.e. mitosis and meiosis.

Mitosis is the normal process of cell division for growth and replacement whereby two replica daughter cells, each with 46 chromosomes carrying identical hereditary information, are derived from a parent cell.

Meiosis is the process of cell division which results in the production of gametes (ova or spermatozoa), each of which has half the original number of chromosomes found in somatic cells, i.e. 23. New pairings are established when gametes come together at fertilisation. Reshuffling of chromosomal material results in the individual differences seen in offsprings whilst familial genetic patterns are still maintained. If meiosis is not successful, one gamete may end up with an abnormal number of chromosomes or with malformed chromosomes. The results of this are seen in the classic chromosome disorders.

Chromosomal defects affect 7.7% of all conceptions. Most are spontaneously miscarried — the majority early in pregnancy. The remainder result in various manifestations of genetic abnormality. One example of this is Down's syndrome, in which the infant has 47 chromosomes, the extra one matching the 21st pair (see p. 199).

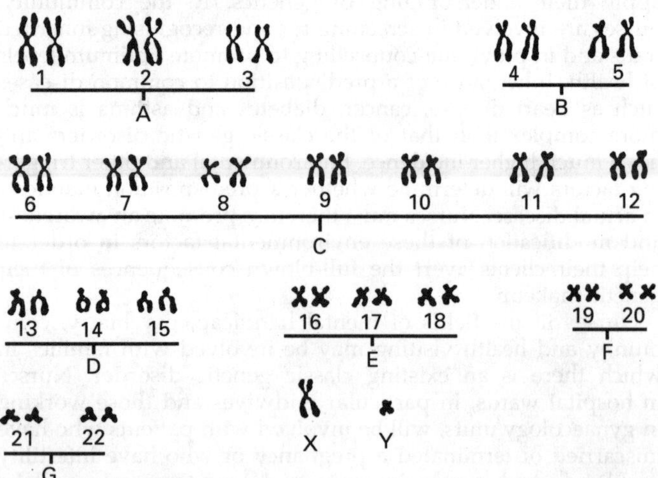

Fig. 6.1 Karyotype of a normal male.

DNA and RNA

In 1944, chromosomal nucleic acid was shown to be the carrier of genetic information. Two main types are recognised: DNA (deoxyribonucleic acid) and RNA (ribonucleic acid).

A molecule of DNA is composed of two nucleotide chains which are spiralled round one another to form a double helix. Genes are carried in this DNA. In humans the total length of DNA in a set of 46 chromosomes is 3000 million base pairs. If stretched out this would be 1.74 m in length. The average gene contains perhaps 2000 base pairs. If the total length of DNA were stretched out from Glasgow to London, a distance of 400 miles, then each gene would take up approximately 12 inches.

Genes

Genes are units of DNA which carry coded hereditary information and are carried on the chromosomes. As chromosomes are paired, each pair carries two copies of each gene (with the exception of the genes on sex chromosomes in males). Each gene is located at a specific point on a chromosome known as its locus.

Genes at the same locus on homologous chromosomes are called alleles. If the two alleles at a locus are identical, the individual is said to be homozygous at that locus. If the two alleles are non-identical, then the individual is said to be heterozygous at that locus (see Fig. 6.2).

With the exception of identical twins, each individual carries unique sequences, or patterns, of minisatellite DNA throughout their genome. These genetic patterns can be recorded by a technique known as DNA fingerprinting and can be useful in identifying individuals, as for example in forensic medicine or paternity testing (see Box 6.1).

There are at least two kinds of genes: structural genes which specify protein synthesis, and genes that act as 'switches' to turn the process on and off and maintain homeostasis.

The coded information carried by the structural genes is translated with the help of RNA into specific proteins. The RNA becomes a mobile copy of the corresponding encoded blueprint in the DNA (messenger RNA, or mRNA). Some of these proteins are enzymes that catalyse specific chemical reactions. Others form part of the structure of body cells and tissues. Together they determine appearance and behaviour. Molecular biology has been able to describe the process of enzyme movement and matching of chemical bases along the

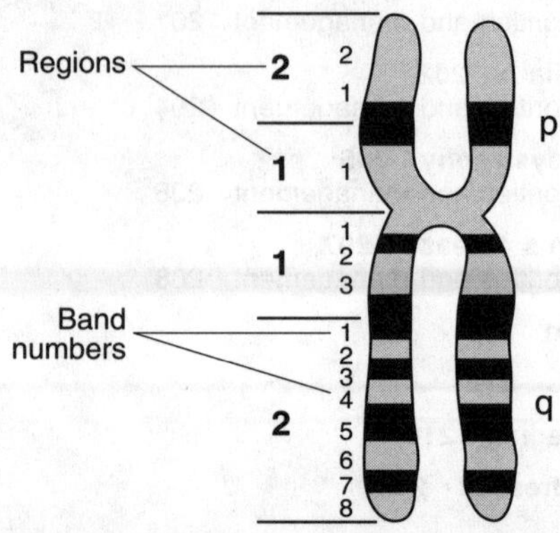

Fig. 6.2 The X chromosome: regions and bands. Each chromosome has a narrow waist called the centromere and a long and a short arm. The short arm is labelled p (from the French *petit*) and the long arm is labelled q. The tip of each arm is called a telomere. Chromosomes can be divided for reporting purposes into numbered chromosome regions, with region 1 closest to the centromere. Each region is further divided into bands.

Box 6.1 DNA fingerprinting

Paternity testing has been revolutionised by the technique known as DNA fingerprinting. Throughout the human genome there are repeats of short sequences (tandem repeats) called minisatellite DNA. They have no known function but are valuable tools for genetic analysis. After DNA digestion with a restriction enzyme and electrophoresis, a DNA minisatellite probe will identify multiple DNA fragments from many chromosomal regions. The number and size of these fragments is unique to an individual (except for identical twins). In other words, one can generate a unique genetic fingerprint specific only to that individual. Each band is inherited from one parent and therefore a putative father can be either excluded or positively identified. DNA can be extracted from dried blood stains or semen; for this reason this technique has had important implications for forensic medicine.

coding strand of the DNA double helix which is involved in translating genetic codes into mRNA for protein synthesis.

In spite of rapid progress and massive breakthroughs in recent years, the position of only 4% of human genes has been located and only a few of the 4000 recognised genetic disorders have been traced to malfunctioning genes. The Human Genome Project (HGP), a world-wide effort of coordinated research based in the USA, aims eventually to map all the 100 000 or so genes on the human chromosomes and to determine the DNA sequence of around 3 billion base pairs.

See Greener 1993.

GENETIC MODIFICATION AND GENE THERAPY

Techniques have been perfected for targeting and cutting out fragments of DNA containing one or more genes from one organism and joining them artificially to another. This results in what is known as recombinant DNA (rDNA). By modifying genes it is possible to alter the proteins they produce and thereby the structure or chemical function of the organism.

The importance of genetic coding for specific proteins can be illustrated by the two following examples. In the genetically determined condition of phenylketonuria (PKU) the absence of gene coding for the enzyme that converts the amino acid phenylalanine to tyrosine results in an accumulation of phenylalanine in the blood of newborn babies which affects the brain, causing mental retardation. Many babies are now tested routinely in the UK on the 5th day of life for high levels of phenylalanine in the blood as, when detected early, PKU can be prevented by a diet free from phenylalanine.

A second illustration relating to the importance of genetic coding for specific proteins is provided in current research on Huntington's disease (Huntington's chorea). See Research Abstract 6.1.

Research Abstract 6.1 Discovery of a gene for Huntington's disease

British and American researchers have recently identified the defect on a particular gene which is thought to be responsible for Huntington's disease. This is a progressive disease with onset in middle age and involves gradual death of nerve cells manifesting in uncontrolled physical movements and dementia. It affects about 3000 people in Britain. The gene itself codes for a protein found in the brain and now named 'Huntingtin'. The defect identified in mutations relates to a more numerous repetition of three bases (the letters of the genetic code) in a DNA molecule on chromosome 4 in people with Huntington's disease. This pattern is likened to a stutter whereby the sequence is repeated between 42 and 86 times; in healthy people the sequence is repeated between 11 and 34 times. Having identified the gene it will now be possible to test 'at risk' individuals to see if they have inherited the mutation. Understanding why this sequence repetition leads to degeneration of the brain and what the specific action of the Huntingtin protein is may also eventually lead to a cure (Connor 1993).

Applications of genetic modification

For many years innocuous bacteria and viruses have been used as the work-horses of molecular biology to ferry genetic material from one species to another or to grow genetically determined proteins. For example, the hormone insulin used in the treatment of diabetes and once extracted from the pancreas of pigs and cows is now manufactured by growing bacteria into which a human insulin gene has been inserted. Interferons used in the treatment of some forms of cancer and the human luteinising hormone used in the treatment of infertility are other examples of the use of genetic modification in pharmaceuticals. Gene modification also has important applications in agriculture, where it can be used to improve strains of livestock and plants, introducing desirable characteristics such as resilience against disease.

In addition to these beneficial applications, genetic biotechnology has the potential to do great harm. We need only consider the destructive potential of genetically engineered microbes and biological aberrations that can be produced in large numbers and loosed either accidentally or intentionally with devastating effect, as in biological warfare.

Human gene therapy

There are two major kinds of human gene therapy. The first is in treatment of somatic cells whereby offending genes can be deleted, genetic defects corrected or missing genes introduced. This therapy affects only the individual being treated and has been judged by controlling committees as acceptable practice in most cases. In this type of therapy a missing gene can be transferred to a recipient from a healthy donor's cell, as demonstrated by a recent breakthrough in gene therapy whereby the missing ADA (adenosine deaminase) gene was transferred using an innocuous virus as the vector (see Fig. 6.3).

The second type of gene therapy is germ-line therapy; this involves genetic modification of the embryo and carries potential for aberrations which would become part of every nucleated cell and be passed on to future generations. Germ-line gene therapy has been declared unacceptable because of its unforeseeable long-term consequences, the ethical implications of research on human embryos and the prohibition on human cloning.

Eugenics, the science of 'improving' the human race by either encouraging individuals deemed to be superior to reproduce or attempting to prevent individuals with characteristics considered to be undesirable from reproducing is a subject of perennial controversy. This ideal has informed many sociopolitical movements of the 20th century (most notably Nazism) with tragic effect. As genetic science rapidly advances its potential applications within eugenic thinking must continue to be scrutinised.

Ethical considerations

Genetic modification and gene therapy is subject to strict guidelines and controls by governmental and scientific bodies.

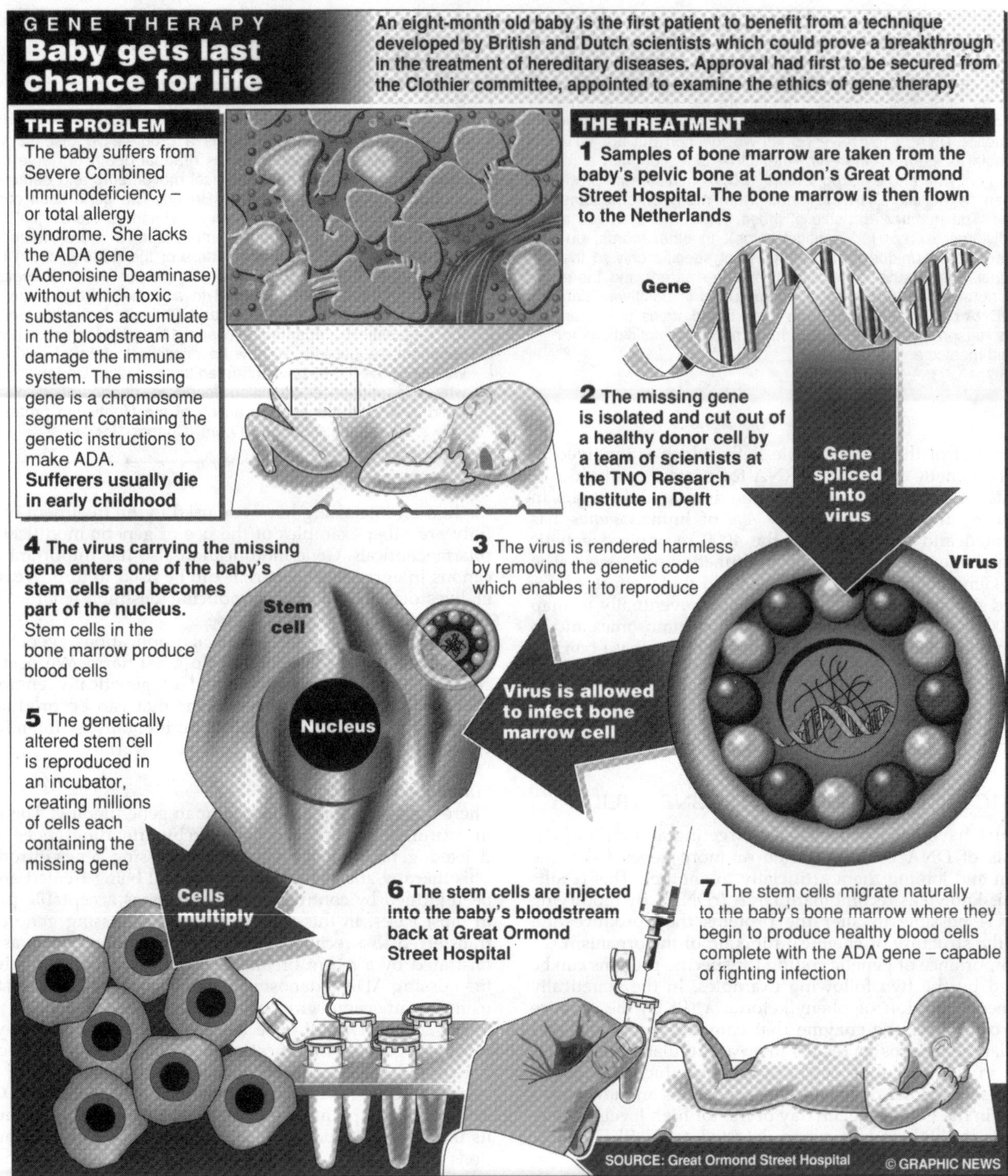

GENE THERAPY
Baby gets last chance for life
An eight-month old baby is the first patient to benefit from a technique developed by British and Dutch scientists which could prove a breakthrough in the treatment of hereditary diseases. Approval had first to be secured from the Clothier committee, appointed to examine the ethics of gene therapy
THE PROBLEM
The baby suffers from Severe Combined Immunodeficiency – or total allergy syndrome. She lacks the ADA gene (Adenoisine Deaminase) without which toxic substances accumulate in the bloodstream and damage the immune system. The missing gene is a chromosome segment containing the genetic instructions to make ADA.
Sufferers usually die in early childhood
THE TREATMENT
1 Samples of bone marrow are taken from the baby's pelvic bone at London's Great Ormond Street Hospital. The bone marrow is then flown to the Netherlands
Gene
2 The missing gene is isolated and cut out of a healthy donor cell by a team of scientists at the TNO Research Institute in Delft
Gene spliced into virus
3 The virus is rendered harmless by removing the genetic code which enables it to reproduce
Virus
4 The virus carrying the missing gene enters one of the baby's stem cells and becomes part of the nucleus.
Stem cells in the bone marrow produce blood cells
Stem cell
Nucleus
Virus is allowed to infect bone marrow cell
5 The genetically altered stem cell is reproduced in an incubator, creating millions of cells each containing the missing gene
Cells multiply
6 The stem cells are injected into the baby's bloodstream back at Great Ormond Street Hospital
7 The stem cells migrate naturally to the baby's bone marrow where they begin to produce healthy blood cells complete with the ADA gene – capable of fighting infection
SOURCE: Great Ormond Street Hospital
© GRAPHIC NEWS

Fig. 6.3 A recent advance in gene transfer technique applied to the treatment of severe combined immunodeficiency. (Reproduced with kind permission, © Graphic News.)

The principles of regulating new technologies are established in the international forum by the United Nations and by international scientific bodies. The EC has also issued a number of directives to be translated into national legislation for the control of biotechnology. Britain also has a medical ethics committee — the Clothier committee — to monitor the ethical implications of the application of genetic technology in specific cases.

Additionally, a recent British Medical Association (BMA) investigating committee recommended that 'the regulation of genetic modification should be conducted in an open, democratically accountable and representative fashion' in order to ensure that the public are fully informed and as an additional safeguard to community interest. It also stipulated that genetic screening should always be accompanied by non-directive counselling (BMA 1992, p. 234).

 British Medical Association (1992).

CATEGORIES OF GENETIC DISORDERS

The three main categories of genetic disorders are:

- chromosomal anomalies
- single gene or Mendelian disorders
- multifactorial or polygenic disorders.

Chromosomal anomalies

Autosomal variations

Numerical autosomal variations. Abnormalities can arise if during meiosis non-disjunction takes place and both of one pair of chromosomes pass to one gamete and the other gamete does not get a copy of that chromosome. If fertilisation takes place the zygote will then have either three copies of the chromosome (trisomy) or only one copy (monosomy).

Autosomal deletions and translocations. Structural variations arise if a piece of a chromosome breaks off and attaches itself to another chromosome. This will result in the gamete either having part of a chromosome missing (a deletion) or having a rearrangement (a translocation).

A balanced translocation causes no abnormality because no chromosomal material is gained or lost. However, there will be a higher risk that when the individual has a child an unbalanced form will arise, causing spontaneous abortion, or a syndrome of multiple physical and mental handicap.

Chromosomal abnormalities are often found in spontaneously aborted fetuses. The risk of a couple having a second affected child with a chromosomal abnormality is usually regarded as low, but if one of the parents is found to carry a balanced translocation that risk is greatly increased. This occurs, however, in only 5% of chromosomal abnormalities. The risk to relatives of having an affected child is even lower unless there is a familial history of translocation. In this situation all relatives could have their chromosomes checked for the abnormality if they so wish.

Sex chromosome variations

Although the psychological implications of the diagnosis of a sex chromosome anomaly are profound, the problems caused by these abnormalities tend to be less severe than those resulting from autosomal abnormalities. Consequently, a significant number of people may have a sex chromosome anomaly without being aware of it. We now know that numerical abnormalities of the sex chromosomes are not as uncommon as was once believed.

A diagnosis is often made during routine maternal age-related screening by amniocentesis, and as some of these disorders cause infertility they may be detected for the first time at infertility clinics.

Some of these disorders result in retarded or excessive growth, in which case diagnosis may be made at a paediatric growth clinic or endocrine clinic. It is rare for sex chromosome abnormalities to recur in a family, even in the offspring of affected fertile individuals.

Serious mental retardation has not been found and long-term information on prognosis and achievements is becoming available. A slightly lower mean IQ has, however, been demonstrated, as has an increase in learning difficulties. The latter are usually correctable with remedial help at school. Should more than one extra sex chromosome be present mental handicap or physical abnormality is more likely.

Mosaicism occurs when an individual has two different cell lines resulting in a certain percentage of abnormal cells, the remainder of the cells being normal. This may result from somatic mutation.

Single gene or Mendelian disorders

These disorders are caused by a defect in one of our approximately 100 000 genes. The risk of offspring being affected is usually high and can be calculated if the mode of inheritance and a detailed family history (including a family tree or pedigree) is known. A risk factor can also be given for other members of the family.

The inheritance of single-gene disorders can be:

- autosomal dominant
- autosomal recessive
- X-linked.

Autosomal dominant inheritance

Autosomal dominant conditions are caused by a defect in a dominant gene on one of the 44 autosomes. One gene on a pair of autosomes will be normal while the corresponding gene on the other of the autosome pair will be defective. If the defective gene is dominant it will overrule the normal gene. As a result, the individual will both carry the condition and suffer from it.

Those who have the defective dominant gene will have a 1 in 2 chance of passing it on to their offspring. This is because during meiosis only one of each pair of chromosomes will pass to each ovum or sperm. Whether the disease is transmitted from the parent will depend on whether the ovum or sperm contains the chromosome with the normal gene or the chromosome with the defective gene.

It is important to note that this amounts to a 50% probability in each pregnancy. Chance has no memory. If there are two children it is not inevitable that one will be affected and the other will not. It could be that both have the disorder, both are free of it, or one will have it and one will not.

As the defect is on an autosome rather than a sex chromosome the sex of the individual is of no consequence to inheritance. A child of either sex can inherit the disorder; if he or she does, again the chance of passing it on to a child of either sex will be 50%.

If an individual is proved beyond doubt not to have the disorder, and therefore not to have the defective gene, he or she will not pass on the disease. However, a defective gene can skip a generation and reappear. This is known as 'reduced penetrance' or 'non-penetrance'. Furthermore, defective genes may sometimes show a range of expressions, from very severe to barely detectable. This is known as 'variable expressivity'. Non-penetrance and variable expressivity are complicating features in diseases inherited as autosomal dominants.

Once the defective gene responsible for causing a condition has been located and identified, it becomes possible to perform direct gene testing on a blood sample to confirm a diagnosis. This eliminates the element of doubt which can be present when diagnosis relies on the presence or absence of varying signs and symptoms. Unfortunately, only a few of the genes responsible for classic genetic disorders have been located so far.

The age of onset of dominantly inherited conditions can also be variable. With some conditions symptoms may not appear until young adulthood or middle age. Examples of these are myotonic dystrophy and Huntington's disease.

A defective gene can be caused by a new mutation; that is, the genetic anomaly causing the defect may occur for the first time in an individual rather than being passed down by a parent.

Autosomal recessive inheritance

Autosomal recessive conditions are caused by a defect in a recessive gene on an autosome. An individual can have a copy of a defective gene on one of a pair of autosomes and a corresponding normal gene on the other of the pair. As the defective gene in this case is recessive, the normal gene will overrule the defective gene. As a result, the individual will carry the disorder but will not suffer from it. It is unlikely that he or she will be aware of this situation.

However, a problem may arise if two parents who carry the same recessive gene defect have offspring. It is possible for both parents to pass on to the child the defective recessive gene. In this case, the child will have two copies of the defective gene and no normal gene to compensate for it. The child will in this case suffer from the condition.

When both parents carry the same defective recessive gene there is a 1 in 4 risk in each pregnancy that the child will suffer from the disorder. Again, chance has no memory. There is unlikely to be a family history of the condition and often the parents will become aware that they are carriers only after the birth of a child affected with a recessive genetic disorder.

Consanguinity, including interfamily marriage such as between cousins, increases the risk of a recessive disorder; this is because both parents could have inherited the defective gene from a common ancestor. However, the overall increase in risk to the offspring of parents who are first cousins is moderately low, i.e. 3% above the risk to the general population.

Some recessive defects are more common in certain ethnic groups; examples are thalassaemia, sickle-cell disease and Tay-Sachs disease.

Many recessive disorders are severe. These include complex malformation syndromes and recognised inborn errors of metabolism.

X-linked recessive inheritance

X-linked recessive disorders are caused by a defect in a recessive gene on the X chromosome. If a female has a recessive gene defect on an X chromosome she will have a corresponding normal gene on her other X chromosome. This will overrule the defective gene such that she will be a carrier of the disease but is unlikely to suffer from it. Manifesting carriers have occasionally been reported but are not common.

In order to be male a boy must get a Y chromosome from his father. If a carrier female passes on her X chromosome with the defective gene to a son, his Y chromosome will have no corresponding gene to compensate for it and consequently he will suffer from the disease associated with the chromosomal defect.

If a carrier female passes on her X chromosome with the normal gene to a son there will be no defect and no disease.

In order to be female a girl must get an X chromosome from her father. If a carrier female passes on her X chromosome with the defective gene to a daughter, the X chromosome from her father with the normal gene will overrule the defective gene, but she will still be a carrier like her mother.

If a carrier female passes on her X chromosome with the normal gene to her daughter there will be no defect to be transmitted to the next generation.

The risk to the offspring of a female carrier of an X-linked recessive condition is therefore 50% of being affected by the disease (in males) and 50% of being carriers (in females). Thus the woman has an overall risk of 1 in 4 of having an affected child.

In the case of an affected male with an X-linked condition, all of his daughters will be carriers and all of his sons will neither be affected nor carry the disease unless the mother is a carrier.

New mutations arise where the defect occurs for the first time in the affected boy. If there is definite proof that this is the case there will be no risk to the boy's brothers of being affected or to his sisters of being carriers. His daughters will be carriers and his sons will not suffer from or carry the disease.

If the mother of an affected boy is known to be a carrier it is possible that her female relatives may also be carriers with similar risks of passing on the defective gene.

X-linked dominant disorders and Y-linked disorders have been described but are rare.

Multifactorial or polygenic disorders

In many disorders genetic and environmental factors combine to give rise to disease. Risks of recurrence of these disorders within a family are generally regarded as being moderately low, the greatest risk being to first- and second-degree relatives (approx. 1%). Empirical risks may be used when estimating recurrence. It is rare for third-degree relatives to have a recurrence risk of over 1%.

When environmental factors are known (e.g. diet, smoking and exercise in coronary heart disease) these can be modified with beneficial effect. However, this approach is not possible as yet for the majority of multifactorial disorders.

Factors which increase the risk of multifactorial disorders in relatives are:

- the genetic component of the disease
- the closeness of the relationship to the affected person
- the presence of the disorder in more than one family member
- the severity of the condition in the affected person
- the presence of the disorder in a person not of the sex usually affected.

It is of interest to note that intelligence is regarded as a multifactorial trait. Common disorders which are considered to be multifactorial in origin include:

- asthma
- coronary artery disease
- congenital heart disease
- diabetes
- essential hypertension
- schizophrenia
- cleft lip and palate
- neural tube defects.

TESTING FOR GENETIC DISORDERS

Categories of testing

Testing for genetic disorders can be divided into four main categories:

1. Prenatal testing. This is used to predict whether a fetus is either affected by a genetic disorder or is carrying a defective gene which will cause it to become affected by a genetic disorder.

2. Diagnostic testing. This is used to find out whether or not an individual has a particular genetic disorder and often relies on the presence or absence of signs and symptoms. The type of testing necessary will be determined by the kind of defect likely to be found. Relatives of those affected by genetic conditions often have to be assessed in this way to ascertain whether they have the same condition in a different form and are at risk of passing it on.

3. Pre-symptomatic or predictive testing. This is used to predict whether or not an individual at risk of inheriting a genetic disorder has inherited the defective gene before he or she shows any signs or symptoms of the disorder itself. The

benefits of presymptomatic testing are clear where treatment is available to prevent the occurrence of the disease. However, when no treatment can be prescribed to prevent, cure or alleviate the disease much thought has to be given to the matter and the recommended protocol must be strictly adhered to. Some of those at risk of progressive debilitating genetic diseases prefer to know what lies in store for them so that they can make appropriate decisions regarding careers, pregnancy, housing, lifestyle, etc.

4. Carrier testing. This is used to find out whether an individual carries a particular defective autosomal recessive gene. It has mainly been used for conditions known to be a high risk within certain ethnic groups. However, it can also be used for close relatives of couples who have a child with a recessive condition if there is a test available which will detect the carrier of that particular condition. As more recessive genes become isolated and testing becomes simpler and more routine, carrier testing for the more common recessive conditions such as cystic fibrosis may become widely available in some form.

Techniques for genetic testing

There is no broad-based test which can be used to screen for all genetic disorders at once. Indeed, for many disorders there is at present no test available. Where a test is available it is a specific test for a specific disorder, and in some cases the test will indicate a greatly increased or decreased *likelihood* of inheriting or carrying a disorder rather than confirming or eliminating the presence of a disorder.

The main techniques used in testing for genetic disorders are:

- biochemical tests
- chromosomal analysis or karyotyping (see Fig. 6.1)
- clinical examination
- DNA studies (see Box 6.2)
- radiography
- ultrasonography
- direct gene testing.

Table 6.1 lists the commonly used sources of tissue for chromosomal analysis.

Prenatal testing

A woman's chance of having a baby with an abnormality recognisable at birth is 1 in 40. This risk excludes those genetic disorders not recognisable at birth, e.g. familial adenomatous polyposis, Huntington's disease, familial hypercholesterolaemia, as well as the more familiar conditions such as neural tube defects or Down's syndrome. The aim of prenatal diagnosis is that of prevention by early detection and intervention.

Box 6.2 Predictive testing using DNA technology

Small blood samples (20 ml) are obtained from the at-risk individuals being tested and as many close relatives as possible. At a minimum the affected and unaffected parent and one affected sibling, or the affected parent and an 'escapee' sibling would be needed, although this would rarely be enough to work on. In the absence of these individuals, other relatives might be sufficient for establishinig the linkage. The more close relatives available the higher the probability that the test will be informative. Leucocytes are isolated from the blood and the DNA is then cut into fragments using several restriction enzymes. The resulting fragments are placed in a solution containing a specific fragment of DNA (the 'probe' or 'marker'), which binds to its complement on the fragments. The probe or marker is radioactively labelled, and so allows the pattern of cleavage of the DNA to be visualised using X-ray film. There are a finite number of cleavage patterns, 6 being most frequently found. The pattern which links the altered gene differs among families. Based on pedigree analysis, we can often determine which pattern is inherited along with the altered gene.

Table 6.1 Commonly used sources of tissue in human chromosome studies

Source	Cell	Application
Blood	T-lymphocytes	Routine analysis
Skin	Fibroblasts	Suspected mosaicism
Bone marrow	White cells, etc.	Leukaemia
Amniotic fluid	Shed epithelial cells	16–20 week fetus
Chorionic villi	Trophoblast	8–12 week fetus
Buccal smear	Shed epithelial cells	Sex chromatin

Methods of prenatal diagnosis

Diagnostic ultrasound. Various abnormalities can be detected using high-resolution ultrasound imaging. Ultrasound scanning to detect congenital abnormalities begins between 16 and 18 weeks' gestation with follow-up scans carried out at 3 to 4 week intervals.

Conditions detectable by ultrasound scanning include:

- skeletal abnormalities, e.g. severe short-limbed dwarfism, osteogenesis imperfecta
- major organ malformations, e.g. severe congenital heart disease, renal agenesis
- polyhydramnios (excess amniotic fluid)
- oligohydramnios (decreased amniotic fluid)
- hydrops (abnormal accumulation of serous fluid in a body cavity or tissues).

Amniocentesis. During pregnancy fetal cells slough off into the amniotic fluid. It is possible to withdraw a sample of amniotic fluid between 16 and 20 weeks' gestation and culture and test the fetal cells for chromosomal abnormalities. Alphafetoprotein (AFP) levels can be measured to detect neural tube defects such as spina bifida. Amniocentesis has the potential to diagnose around 200 genetic disorders. The risk of spontaneous abortion after the procedure is estimated to be less than 1%.

Conditions detectable by amniocentesis include:

- open neural tube defects: indicated by amniotic fluid AFP
- chromosomal disorders: using karyotyping
- inherited diseases: using biochemical and DNA studies.

Chorionic villus sampling (CVS). This is carried out between 8 and 11 weeks of pregnancy, and is thus termed first-trimester prenatal diagnosis. Essentially, this test provides the same diagnostic information as amniocentesis; however, it is not suitable for diagnosing all genetic disorders. For example, neural tube defects cannot be detected by this means.

Under ultrasound guidance, a catheter is inserted through the cervical os to the placental insertion site. Villi are aspirated and the cells are analysed.

Conditions detectable by CVS are chromosomal disorders (using karyotyping) and inherited diseases (using DNA studies).

Transabdominal CVS can be done at any stage of pregnancy, providing the placenta is in an accessible position. Some pregnancies are more suitable for transcervical and some for transabdominal sampling. Both techniques are practised at many centres. Depending upon the type of analysis, results may be available almost immediately. The risk of spontaneous abortion after CVS is estimated to be 2–4%.

Fetal blood sampling is used for diagnosis of haemoglobinopathies and of coagulation disorders (e.g. haemophilia) when DNA diagnosis is not possible. Under ultrasound guidance a special sampling needle is passed transabdominally. A fetal vessel near the umbilical cord insertion is punctured and fetal blood is withdrawn. This procedure is carried out at 18 weeks' gestation.

> ? **6.1** A family history reveals a high incidence of heart disease in a particular client's family. Although he has no signs of heart disease at this point in time it is possible that he may have inherited a genetic predisposition. He also has several relevant environmental risk factors: he is overweight, smokes heavily and takes little exercise. What might you predict his chances to be of developing serious heart disease? What specific action could you as a nurse take to promote his health and prevent serious disease developing?

THE GENETIC COUNSELLING PROCESS

The referral stage

Suspected genetic disease

Nurses, because of their many roles in the community, in midwifery, in mental handicap and psychiatric nursing, and in acute hospital settings, are in a strategic position to detect disease patterns and risk factors. In their many interactions with patients and their families, nurses may have occasion to suspect the possibility of the occurrence of classic genetic disease within a family. The following indications should alert the nurse that referral to specialist services for genetic counselling may be appropriate:

- family history of classic genetic disease
- newly diagnosed genetic disorder
- woman over age 40 seeking advice on pregnancy and fetal abnormalities
- cousin relationships
- ethnic groups with a high incidence of a particular disorder
- presence of dysmorphic features such as small head with large forehead, fish mouth, protruding tongue, slant eyes with epicanthal folds or low-set ears
- unexplained mental retardation
- unexplained stillbirth
- recurrent miscarriages
- primary infertility
- ambiguous sexual development
- female with short stature
- leukaemia
- family history of structural chromosomal abnormality.

Once a need for specialist genetic counselling has been identified, appropriate referral should be organised in consultation with other members of the health care team. Where family members express concern or the need for more information it may be appropriate to refer them also.

Known genetic disease

General practitioners and specialist consultants will be aware of the genetic components of diseases encountered in their own practice and will where indicated raise the matter of genetic inheritance with an adult patient or with the parents of an affected child. They will, however, be concerned mainly with diagnosis and illness management. Ideally, the doctor actively treating the patient will introduce the aspect of genetics and then refer him on for genetic counselling to a genetic unit which can allocate the large amount of time necessary to cover this aspect adequately and to follow up other family members who may be at risk of contracting the illness or passing it on to their offspring.

The patient for whom a genetic counselling referral has been suggested may not understand what this means and why it is necessary. An initial response may be concern that he or she will be given a directive as to the pattern of any future reproduction. An important part of the nurse's role is to allay this fear.

The genetic counselling team

Most genetic units provide a regional service which covers a wide range of disorders and serves a large geographical area. The staff in these units include:

- clinical geneticists
- genetic nurse specialists or health visitors
- scientists
- laboratory staff
- secretarial staff.

The main aspects of the team's work are:

- making diagnoses
- estimating risks
- giving information
- exploring options
- giving support.

There is little done in the way of physical care of individuals by any of the staff in genetic departments.

The medical staff will be most involved in the accurate diagnosis of a condition but the genetic nurse may be in a better position to explain to the individual why tests are necessary and what they will involve. Her help in this way can allay a great deal of unnecessary anxiety.

The scientific and medical staff will estimate the risk to the patient or his relatives of contracting the disease and/or passing it on to their children.

The secretary in the genetic unit has an important part to play in collating and storing background information on patients and in liaising with the Medical Records Officer to obtain details. (Permission must be given by the individual concerned for medical records to be obtained.) The secretary also coordinates appointments and may deal directly with patients who are at a critical point in their lives.

The role of the specialist genetic nurse

Information-gathering

A thorough assessment including a full family history (indicating recurrent patterns of disease) and noting the presence of risk factors in the individual's environment is an essential part of the counselling process. A family tree giving a diagrammatic representation of familial relationships over several generations can be useful in demonstrating a pattern of inheritance of family traits and recurrent diseases. Points to remember when drawing up a family tree are listed in Box 6.3. Symbols used to indicate key information in family trees are shown in Figure 6.4.

Education

The specialist genetic nurse may be asked to speak about genetic issues to students and qualified nurses and to other professionals in a formal classroom setting or on a one-to-one basis with a colleague involved with a patient with a genetic

Box 6.3 Drawing up a family tree

1. Always take details from both sides of the family.
2. Go back at least three generations.
3. Record dates of birth rather than ages if possible.
4. Record those who have died, plus cause and age of death.
5. Ask specifically about infant deaths, stillbirths and miscarriages.
6. Ask directly about consanguinity (marriage between relatives, e.g. cousins).
7. Record maiden name of women.
8. Check that the father of an individual really is the person you would expect him to be. Assume nothing. Mistaken paternity presents a serious problem.

condition who asks for specific information. The specialist nurse may also be requested to research and pass on information about rare genetic conditions to colleagues and students, as she will have access to textbooks, journals and to individual experts in given fields not always available to others. The specialist genetic nurse will also, of course, have an important role in giving the patient information about the nature of his disorder and the mechanics of genetic transmission. For example, during a routine procedure such as taking a blood sample the patient may ask questions or refer to his worries and concerns. This provides the nurse with an opportunity to give information and reassurance and to clarify issues that may be troubling the patient.

Counselling

Genetic counselling is non-directive. Individuals are not told what they should do. They are presented with information in a way they understand and encouraged to explore in detail all the paths open to them. Options that may be relevant to an individual or family members include:

- limitation of size of family by contraception
- delaying a decision until more facts are available
- sterilisation, male or female
- ascertainment of carrier status
- prediagnostic testing
- prenatal sexing in X-linked disorders
- antenatal diagnosis
- selective termination of pregnancy
- adoption
- fostering
- artificial insemination
- in vitro fertilisation.

It should be borne in mind that a risk that seems overwhelmingly high to some couples may be acceptable to others in a similar situation.

When a difficult decision such as whether to terminate an established pregnancy has to be made it is helpful to the individuals concerned if the nurse makes it clear that she will support them whatever decision is made and that it is of no consequence to her personally or professionally what that decision is. Often in these circumstances couples are inundated with advice offered by others who, for various reasons, seek to influence their decision. It will come as a relief that the only decision the genetic nurse is interested in is the decision of the couple themselves.

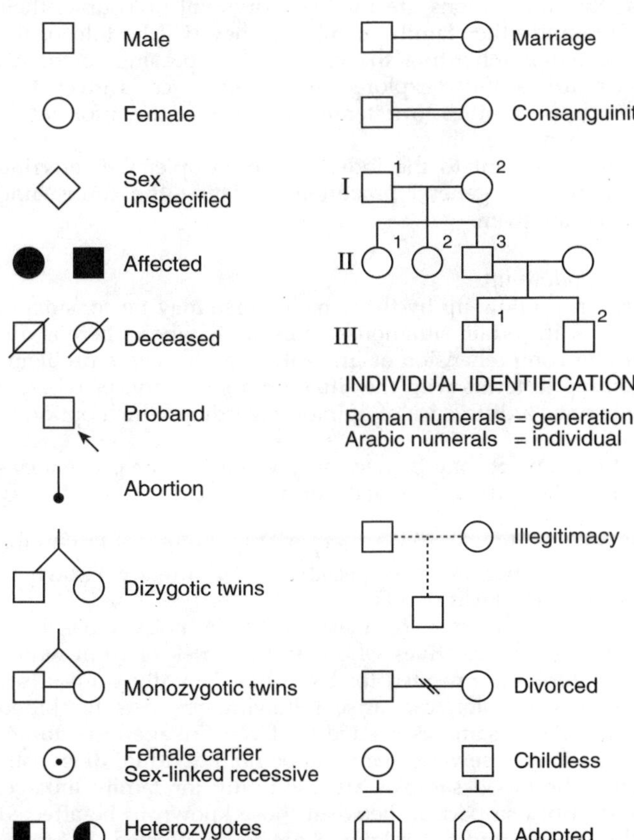

Fig. 6.4 Symbols used in family trees for genetic assessment.

Record-keeping

As always in nursing, accurate record-keeping is of supreme importance. In genetic units records are kept literally for generations. The specialist genetic nurse is also likely to be involved in maintaining genetic registers of inherited diseases.

Policy-making

As a specialist in a rapidly developing field, the genetic nurse may also become involved in policy-making at a local and national level. The National Association of Genetic Nurses and Social Workers has a growing membership who represent those working in this speciality and whose advice is sought about ethical policy decisions regarding genetic services.

Special components of genetic counselling

The work of the genetic counselling team has many interrelated aspects which require a high level of clinical expertise, excellent communication skills, and scrupulous professionalism in the handling of confidential information. Some of these special components of genetic counselling may be outlined as follows:

- Maintaining a detailed specialist knowledge of genetic conditions and keeping abreast of advances in research. Worldwide cooperation in the study of these rare conditions has contributed greatly to the advancement of knowledge. Research findings can lead to changes in the understanding of a disease and its inheritance patterns which may alter risk calculation.
- Recognising disease patterns within a family illustrating a particular mode of inheritance. This may point to health implications for the wider family, e.g. a risk of polyposis coli and hypercholesterolaemia.
- Calculating risks to family members. Not only is the presenting patient given genetic counselling but consideration is given to each member of the wider family, e.g. siblings, parents' siblings and offspring of these individuals. This is

most important in conditions such as Huntington's disease, where healthy relatives may be at risk of becoming affected by the same disease process.

- Allocating sufficient time to consider all implications of a disease or disease risk for lifestyle, family planning, and so on. Usually more than one consultation is offered; for some families, contact is maintained over a period of years — indeed, throughout generations.
- Linking family pedigrees. Identifying those at risk of a disorder in a family and of linking different branches of the same kinship is an important component of the work of the genetic counselling team. Confidentiality regarding individuals' diagnoses, attendance at clinics or any other information is very strictly maintained.
- Storing family information throughout generations. Strict control is maintained over access to genetic disease registers. Maintenance of these registers allows all individuals on a register to be contacted if new tests or treatments become available and enables family members to be offered genetic counselling at an appropriate age via their parents.

The counselling procedure

The genetic counselling procedure comprises four phases:

1. preparation for genetic counselling
2. pre-clinic visit or appointment
3. counselling appointments
4. family follow-up.

Each of these phases will now be considered in turn.

Preparation for genetic counselling

This initial phase takes the form of a departmental meeting in which all the necessary information is gathered to provide the basic core of data which enables diagnosis, prognosis, and an assessment of likely recurrence of the disorder to be made. This phase also provides an opportunity for the team to make a preliminary assessment of the emotional state of those referred, their expectations of genetic counselling, and their possible reaction to the information that will be given to them. In addition, a sensitive appraisal can be made of the family's level of knowledge, their educational, socioeconomic and cultural background, and their religious beliefs, all of which have a direct bearing on the counselling approach.

It may also be possible to fit an individual into a family tree already known to the genetic unit or to tie a family into a kinship which has been previously studied in detail.

The practicalities of deciding which nurse will be responsible for the intake visit, whether this visit should be conducted at home or at the clinic, and which clinical geneticist will be involved will be attended to.

The pre-clinic visit or appointment

A home visit will be made by the specialist genetic nurse. This is best made by prior appointment, and it is essential that the reasons for the visit are clearly stated to the person who has been referred. If a child has been referred, a letter should be addressed to both parents. The letter should explain that the client has been referred to the genetic department by his or her doctor and that the specialist nurse will visit the client at home at a particular date and time to draw up a family tree and ask about the condition in the family. A telephone number should be given for the person to contact the nurse if the date or time is inconvenient, or if the whole idea of a home visit is unacceptable. Discretion is important, as other family members may not have been told about the request for counselling. If necessary, the interview may take place at the clinic prior to the appointment with the doctor.

In order to confirm the diagnosis of the condition and to assess the mode of inheritance, it is necessary to obtain details about other family members who may be similarly affected (see Box 6.3 and Fig. 6.4). Information about one relative should never be given to another relative without the knowledge and consent of the former.

It is of benefit to ask at the home visit what has been explained to the patient or family about the condition. This will confirm that they have either a good or poor understanding of the basic facts about it.

The counselling appointments

The first session. If the nurse who visited at home to obtain the family information is present to greet the family or individual at the clinic it is usually much appreciated and helps to build on the relationship already established. It can also be helpful if she is present during the consultation should there be difficulty in comprehension due to problems with intellect, anxiety, accompanying children or a language barrier.

The clinical geneticist will usually check the family history with the patient, making amendments or additions as necessary. On completion of the data-gathering process, questions of an open-ended style can be used to ascertain the clients' experience and understanding of the disorder.

Physical examinations may be necessary to confirm or negate diagnosis. Laboratory tests or other diagnostic procedures may be requested and consultation with medical specialists in other fields may be necessary to obtain sufficient information for accurate diagnosis and estimation of risks.

The second session. A second counselling appointment is offered when the diagnosis has been ascertained, or when it becomes clear that it cannot be confirmed. It is then that the information-giving aspects of genetic counselling can begin. The clinician explains how the diagnosis was determined and what the implications are for the individual or couple, their children and other family members. They will be told of the risk of either inheriting the condition or passing it on. All aspects are carefully explored and reassurance is given that further opportunities to reiterate and explore the information will be made available.

Letters are sent to the individual or couple, the referring doctor and the general practitioner relating the counselling information given.

Family follow-up

Short-term follow-up by the genetic nurse may be considered necessary in certain situations, for example where there is difficulty in comprehension or unresolved grief, where problems in coming to terms with the situation are evident, or where a couple have a difference of opinion regarding which option to follow.

Future contact may be necessary when further pregnancies are embarked upon, especially in high-risk disorders. It may be that antenatal testing is offered and found to be acceptable. At times like this the couple may find it reassuring to talk the situation through with a specialist nurse already known to them (see Case History 6.1).

Family contact may result when an individual has been asked to contact relatives who may be at risk or from whom blood samples are needed for DNA-based family studies (see Box 6.2). Confusion can arise following requests for blood samples. Those samples needed for DNA linkage tests do not get 'tested' themselves. There will be no individual diagnostic results. The blood samples are used only for family linkage, as a kind of comparison between those known to be affected by the disease and those known not to be affected. However it can be very difficult for the individuals concerned to grasp why they will not get a result from their own test.

Case History 6.1 S and P

S is 30 years old. She and her husband have been trying to conceive a child for the past 5 years of an 8-year marriage. After undergoing infertility investigations, S conceives. She is booked to have her baby at her local maternity hospital. At the booking clinic she receives a package of leaflets explaining various screening tests available to her during her pregnancy. S opts for shared antenatal care between her GP and obstetrician. During the 16th week of her pregnancy her GP takes a blood sample for a maternal serum alphafetoprotein (MSAFP) test. One week later he tells her that the test result shows that her MSAFP is elevated. A repeat blood sample is taken and she is reassured that this will probably be normal.

The result of the second test shows that her MSAFP is still elevated. Her GP then explains that this may indicate that her baby is at risk of an open neural tube defect. He explains that further tests can help clarify the situation and that he has arranged an appointment for her to see and discuss the situation with her obstetrician. He suggests that P accompany her.

The obstetrician explains that there are two methods, which may be used in combination, of further screening the fetus to exclude an open neural tube defect: ultrasonography and amniocentesis. He advises S and P that initially an ultrasound scan is indicated and on the basis of this result he will talk to them again.

The scan is immediately carried out and reveals that the fetus has anencephaly.

S and P are seen immediately by the obstetrician, who gently but frankly explains the results of the scan and the options open to them. They understand that they have a choice of terminating the pregnancy or allowing nature to take its course, knowing that the infant cannot survive. The obstetrician leaves them to discuss this with one another in private. A midwife who specialises in the care of couples undergoing prenatal diagnosis and who is a trained counsellor is close at hand to offer practical comfort and information on how a termination would be carried out, how long it would take, and the intensity of discomfort that would be experienced. The hospital's methods of inducing labour and procedures for delivery are discussed.

Although there are no legal requirements to cremate or bury a baby born dead before 28 weeks it is explained to the couple that they could if they wish have a funeral and/or a burial service. The hospital chaplain is available to discuss any aspects of religious or personal beliefs S and P have and the arrangements that could be made. S and P find that knowing the plan of care for their infant from beginning to end helps them to come to a decision with regard to continuing or ending the pregnancy.

S and P decide that terminating their long-awaited and much-wanted pregnancy is for them the only acceptable option.

Long-term or indeed lifelong follow-up by a genetic nurse specialist may be indicated in some circumstances.

The psychological impact of diagnosis

When an individual is given a diagnosis of genetic disease his or her life is changed unalterably. For the person shown to have a particular disorder the expectation of a reasonably long and healthy life may be replaced by the terrifying prospect of progressive disability and premature death. For a parent, the anticipation of a child's day-to-day struggle to remain active or even simply survive may seem too much to bear. For a young couple whose hopes for parenthood have been dashed, the future may suddenly seem empty. Any genetic illness will affect each member of a family in a different way; for many, the diagnosis will require that extremely difficult and painful decisions concerning family planning are made. Each person's reaction will be unique, even though his or her situation will not be new to the professional. It is essential for the nurse to set aside time for each client to express his or her feelings of disbelief, anger, grief, or even hopelessness.

The following list indicates the kinds of feelings and worries that are experienced by many individuals who have received a diagnosis related to a genetic disease. But while such reactions may be anticipated, they must not be *presumed*. In her assessments, the nurse must ensure that each patient's priorities and concerns have been properly understood and that in due course they are sensitively and honestly addressed.

- Being diagnosed as having a progressive illness: 'How bad will I get?'; 'Will I be able to keep working?'; 'Will I live to see my children grow up?'; 'Will my children have it too?'
- Being told that one is a carrier of a defective gene or a balanced chromosome translocation: 'It is my fault.'; 'I feel I have caused my child to be like this.'
- Being told one's parent has a tragic illness such as Huntington's disease or cerebellar ataxia: 'Will I end up exactly the same?'; 'Are my children going to get this disease too?'
- A stillbirth or neonatal death: The hopes and aspirations of the future lie buried with the child. Friends and relatives do not know what to say to the couple and find it difficult to cope with the situation.
- The diagnosis of a mentally and/or physically handicapped child: 'Will nothing make him the child we hoped for?'; 'Will he ever go to normal school or even walk, talk and dress himself?'; 'What if another child is affected too?'
- An elective mid-trimester termination of pregnancy for fetal abnormality. The pregnancy which has been terminated was a wanted baby and the so-called mini labour endured is little different from normal labour, except there is no baby at the end of it to make up for all the suffering. The foetus has no name and there is not the comforting ritual of a funeral.

The psychological implications of termination of pregnancy

The last circumstance listed above is the one faced by the couple described in Case History 6.1. We might consider a little more closely the emotional and psychological needs of a couple in this situation to illustrate how the nurse, as an impartial professional, can provide invaluable support.

Every couple faces their own unique situation. Professionals become familiar with these situations, but for the couple it is a lonely and sad episode with an inevitably unhappy end. A couple's particular circumstances determine their own special needs. Furthermore, a couple is composed of two individuals whose reactions and needs may vary. Most couples, however, have the following basic needs:

- to be able to trust in those caring for them
- to have time to reflect upon their loss
- to be supported in coming to terms with feelings of guilt
- to be allowed to remember
- to assimilate the events.

Trust. A couple will be more reassured if they feel they can trust those professionals caring for them and their unborn child. Facts should always be given frankly and honestly. Empathy is a comfort: the nurse should not be afraid to show her feelings. She should ask the couple what they feel are their own special needs at each stage of the episode and work with them to devise a care plan which meets their physical, emotional and spiritual needs, and those of their unborn child.

Reflection upon loss. Couples need to reflect upon what the loss of their baby means to them individually and as a couple. Couples will work through their loss in their own way: by tears, silence, anger, and perhaps hostility. Some may prefer to be alone with their grief but many have a profound need to talk through their experience and to explore what this baby meant to them. Was this a long-awaited pregnancy? Was it unplanned? Did they know beforehand there was a risk to their infant? Have they arrived at this juncture unaware and shocked? What were their plans and aspirations for this child?

Feelings of guilt. The couple should be encouraged to re-examine any mistaken ideas they may have about their infant's disorder. If the fetal disorder was due to teratogenic effects (e.g. drugs or viral infection) the parents should be allowed to examine the circumstances of how this occurred. They should be helped to find out what kind of social support network is available to them. Is there someone who can give emotional support at home? Is there a local self-help group which gives ongoing support to those who have experienced termination of pregnancy as a result of fetal abnormality?

A licence to remember. Creating memories is now recognised as making a therapeutic contribution to the grieving process. The couple can be encouraged to accept tangible evidence of their experience, e.g. sonograms or fetal monitor strips. Some may decline the offer initially, only to request the same later.

If a couple lose a baby late in pregnancy they should be invited to see and/or hold their baby. The midwife can hold the baby first, allowing the parents to adapt to the situation. Some couples may wish to see the abnormality and others not. The couple should always be asked what they feel their special needs are.

Assimilation of the events. Putting the events into order is a normal and very necessary process for any couple in coming to terms with their grief. Every story needs a beginning, a middle, and an end. Talking through the sequence of events is an enormously therapeutic exercise for many, and those undertaking the support of couples in the days and months after termination of pregnancy need to recognise and positively encourage this healing process. Years afterwards, the story will continue to be retold. If we give couples the right support at the right time, it can be remembered and related by two individuals who are emotionally healed.

CLASSIC GENETIC DISORDERS AND THEIR MANAGEMENT

Although there are over 4000 described classic genetic disorders even the more common are comparatively rare. Nevertheless, their occurrence, or fear of their occurrence, can have devastating effects on the individuals concerned and their families. The aim of the following sections is to illustrate the principles of nursing management in this very complex and specialised area of care by focusing on six of these disorders, namely:

- Klinefelter syndrome
- Down's syndrome
- cystic fibrosis
- haemophilia A
- myotonic dystrophy
- Huntington's disease.

KLINEFELTER SYNDROME

Klinefelter syndrome occurs in approximately 1 in 1000 newborn males. It arises from abnormalities of the sex chromosomes, occurring in an individual who possesses at least two X chromosomes and a Y chromosome (i.e. their sex chromosome constitution is XXY). A few on chromosome analysis are found to be XXXY or XXXXY. Because the male determining gene is on the Y chromosome, individuals with Klinefelter syndrome develop male characteristics. About 10% of individuals with Klinefelter syndrome are mosaics. This means that some cells in the body are XY and other cells are XXY.

PATHOPHYSIOLOGY

Clinical features. In infancy and childhood, there are no obvious clinical features of Klinefelter syndrome, so unless the chromosomes are examined for some other reason, most males are not recognised until puberty. Many are not diagnosed until they seek treatment for infertility (see Case History 6.2). Although male in appearance, individuals with Klinefelter syndrome have abnormalities of the testes and distinctive physical traits which become apparent at puberty. They tend to be taller than normal, this resulting from abnormally long legs. The penis is frequently of normal size or may be slightly reduced. On examination, the testes are found to be small. Many individuals with this disorder manifest signs of breast enlargement and very often facial and pubic hair is scant. A patient with Klinefelter syndrome will often tell you he only needs to shave once or twice a week.

Almost all Klinefelter sufferers are sterile, although there are reported cases of individuals who have fathered children. Their sterility, however, affects neither libido nor sexual activity, erection and ejaculation being quite normal. Many individuals lead perfectly normal married lives. A very small percentage of Klinefelter syndrome patients manifest mild mental retardation.

MEDICAL MANAGEMENT

The sterility associated with Klinefelter syndrome is not treatable. Hormone treatments are sometimes prescribed to enhance male traits: they increase penis size and reduce breast enlargement.

NURSING PRIORITIES AND MANAGEMENT: KLINEFELTER SYNDROME

Major considerations

Giving psychological support

The diagnosis of a chromosome abnormality can be psychologically damaging. When an abnormality of the nature of Klinefelter syndrome is detected the affected individual's self-concept may change as he no longer sees himself as being 'normal'.

Case History 6.2 D

At the age of 30 years, D married for the second time. His first marriage had not produced any children and had, after 6 years, ended in divorce. After a year living on his own, D met M. They dated for almost a year before deciding to marry. They planned to start a family immediately. Both D and M were in excellent health and they had no reason to believe that starting a pregnancy would be difficult. However, after a year of trying to conceive M visited her general practitioner for advice. The GP took a careful history and suggested she refer D and M to the infertility clinic at their local hospital. This is how D discovered he suffered from a chromosome abnormality called Klinefelter syndrome.

For younger patients the implications of the diagnosis for future fatherhood may be difficult to accept. The parents of the patient may be involved and suffer considerable distress. They often have feelings of guilt, and mourn the grandchildren they cannot have. Counselling and support will be necessary.

For men who have already married and who planned to have children, the diagnosis and identified infertility can cause marital strain. Helping a couple to understand the necessary grieving process is important.

Giving information
As it is possible for the personality of the Klinefelter male to be more reticent, it can be necessary for information on the syndrome and appropriate treatment options to be given even if it is not requested.

Gynaecomastia
Should cosmetic mastectomy be indicated for any of the small number of affected males, considerable tact and diplomacy will be needed in preoperative discussion of the operation and also during routine pre- and postoperative nursing care.

Infertility
Following the diagnosis of infertility, the individual will need time to mourn his inability to father a child. Recovery may be aided by the knowledge that other options for parenting may be possible, i.e. adoption, fostering, artificial insemination by a donor. Each of these options requires careful consideration and counselling by workers trained in these specialities. What is acceptable for one couple may not suit another. Some may opt for childlessness.

Case History 6.3 B and R

B studied hard at university to become a dentist. She specialised in maxillofacial surgery and then entered private practice. She met and married R when she was 37 years old. Despite having a busy career and an active social life, B was keen to have a baby. Because of her age she thought she would first consult her doctor. B's GP assured her that there was no reason why she should not have a healthy pregnancy, but there was one problem: at B's age she had an increased risk of having a baby with a chromosome abnormality such as Down's syndrome. 'I think', said her GP, 'you would be better advised of the risks and the various options open to you and R by our clinical geneticist.'

B and R met the clinical geneticist 3 weeks later and listened carefully to her explanation of the potential problem of a pregnancy resulting in a chromosome abnormality at B's age. The geneticist then explained that they could consider prenatal testing to check the baby's chromosomes, and described the procedures and timing for chorionic villus sampling and amniocentesis (see p. 193).

B and R discussed the possibility of prenatal testing, should B become pregnant. Indeed, B was successful in becoming pregnant, and at 9 weeks of pregnancy she underwent CVS. The tissue sample was sent to the genetics laboratory for analysis.

Two weeks later, B and R met the obstetrician to discuss the results of the karyotype. 'The chromosomes all look normal,' she said. 'Would you like to know if the baby is a girl or a boy?' B looked at R, and they both shook their heads. They had already decided to continue the rest of the pregnancy in as normal a way as possible.

DOWN'S SYNDROME

This is a chromosomal abnormality in which the infant has 47 chromosomes instead of the normal 46. The extra chromosome matches the 21st pair. At the age of 20 years a woman's chance of having a Down's syndrome baby is about 1 in 2000. By age 30 the chance increases to 1 in 800. At the age of 37 years the risk is around 1 in 175.

PATHOPHYSIOLOGY

Clinical features. Characteristics include a small head with flat occiput and large anterior fontanelle, a short, broad neck, slanting eyes with epicanthal folds, a fish mouth with protruding tongue, a deep palmar crease (simian crease) and possibly the presence of cardiac and intestinal anomalies. Although each infant may not have all of these physical characteristics all affected infants are mentally retarded.

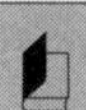
See Beischer & Mackay (1988).

NURSING PRIORITIES AND MANAGEMENT: DOWN'S SYNDROME

A couple undergoing prenatal testing for Down's syndrome will require education, counselling and emotional support, especially during the CVS procedure and whilst awaiting karyotype results. Case History 6.3 gives some insight into the kind of intervention that would be required during the diagnostic period.

CYSTIC FIBROSIS

Cystic fibrosis (CF) is a single-gene, autosomal recessive disorder which disturbs the mucus-producing glands throughout the body, leading to respiratory problems, incomplete digestion, and abnormal sweating. In the UK it affects 1 in 2500 newborns and about 1 in 25 individuals carry a gene for cystic fibrosis.

There is no known cure for CF and left untreated a child will die at a young age from severe lung infection. Over the past several decades the treatment for CF has steadily improved, and today, many live to the age of 20 years. Despite the improvement in treatment, however, affected individuals continue to suffer from numerous medical problems requiring exhaustive and expensive therapy.

PATHOPHYSIOLOGY

In CF there is a defect in the passage of sodium and chloride ions in and out of the epithelial cells of a number of organs. This in turn affects fluid secretion in various glands.

Clinical features. The air passages of people with CF secrete large amounts of thick, sticky mucus. The mucus plugs up the small airways and creates an ideal environment for bacterial infection in the respiratory tract. In the intestine a thick, abnormal mucus is also produced. Among other effects the mucus clogs the ducts leading from the pancreas to the intestine. Food is incompletely digested; weight loss occurs despite a good appetite, and fatty, bulky, foul-smelling stools are passed. The pancreas regresses and may be completely destroyed. The sweat glands also malfunction, secreting too much chloride and sodium in the sweat.

Most males with CF are infertile, as a result of an abnormality of the epididymis and vas deferens which end in blind channels instead of leading through to the urethra. In the female, fertility can be impaired because thick cervical mucus impedes the passage of spermatozoa. Delayed secondary sexual development is an almost universal finding in adolescents.

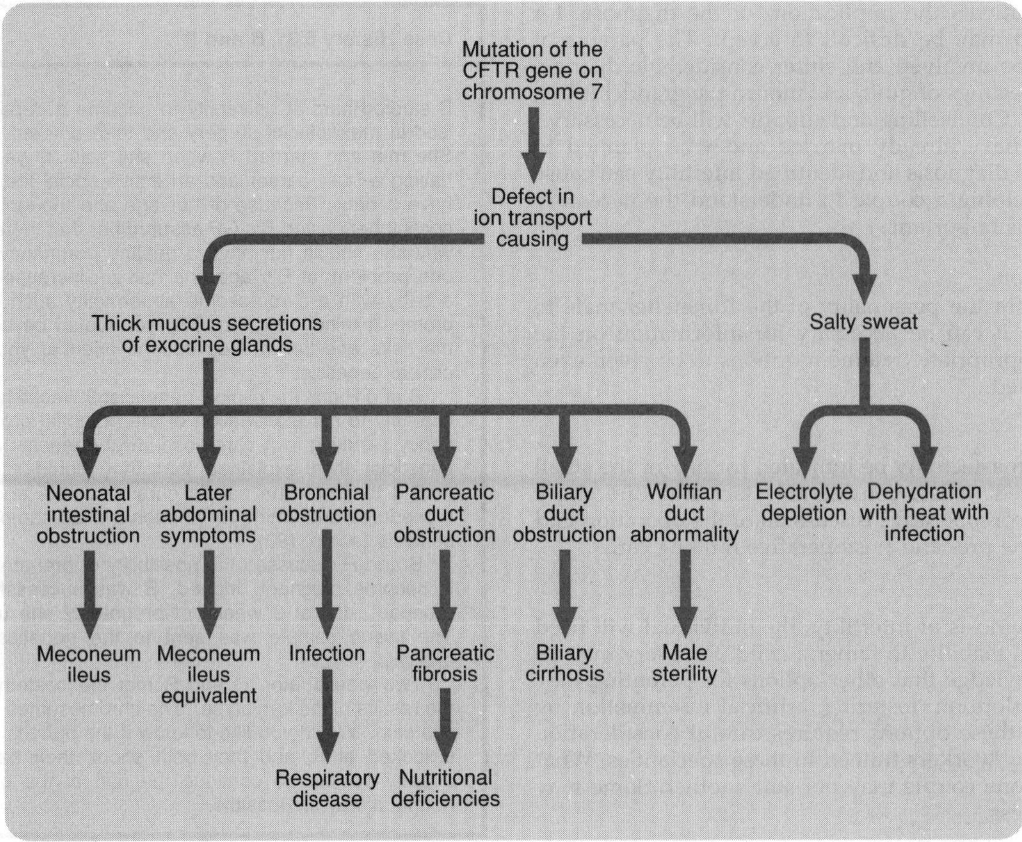

Fig. 6.5 Clinical consequences of cystic fibrosis.

Geneticists recently isolated the gene responsible for cystic fibrosis on chromosome 7. The gene has been labelled the 'cystic fibrosis transmembrane regulator' gene (CFTR).

The clinical consequences of CF are outlined in Figure 6.5.

MEDICAL MANAGEMENT

Investigative procedures. The diagnosis will have been suggested by one or more of the symptoms already described. Until the CFTR gene was identified, testing to determine levels of salt and chloride in the sweat was the single most important method for diagnosing CF. A sweat salt abnormality is present from birth and affects almost 100% of affected individuals and persists throughout life.

Other supporting evidence is based on X-ray examination and sputum cultures. There may also be evidence of pancreatic insufficiency or recurrent respiratory infection. In some cases there will already be a positive family history of CF.

Genetic diagnosis. At the time of writing, at least 60 different mutations are known which can occur within the CFTR gene to cause the disease CF. One very common mutation is found in 75% of the affected UK population. This mutation, along with a number of others, allows us to detect most affected individuals by analysing their DNA. At present most suspected CF cases are diagnosed by a combination of sweat test and genetic testing.

Prognosis. Many patients with CF are now reaching adulthood. The mean age of survival is 20 years. Some still die as young children, but increasingly affected individuals are surviving into their 30s. Patients suffering from chronic respiratory disease may eventually develop secondary heart disease.

Surgical intervention. Heart–lung transplant is a relatively new development in the management of CF patients. Although this has brought renewed hope for CF sufferers, it may also cause new problems as a direct result of the surgery or from tissue rejection. Moreover, there are psychosocial problems which can be difficult to foresee. The idea of a heart–lung transplant should be introduced very sensitively, as consenting to this procedure is a very grave decision. Who should make it? Patients, relatives and professionals may have differing viewpoints and conflicting emotions (see Case History 6.4).

Aims of treatment. The overall aim of management is to help an affected individual reach adulthood leading as normal a life as possible, with minimal dependency. The ultimate individual aim is self-advocacy and from the time of diagnosis this concept should be instilled in the parents and in turn in the child and adolescent. These aims are attained by a multidisciplinary team whose skills, along with close cooperation between the parents, patient and family, are put into action from the time of diagnosis. Regional CF treatment centres lead the way in management.

The treatment programme. On a normal clinic visit the patient is weighed, lung function tests are carried out and sputum is sent for culture and sensitivity. At regular intervals chest X-ray is carried out and blood taken for biochemistry and haematology. A standard form is used to record findings, including details of physical examination. Aspects of dietary regimes and physiotherapy techniques are checked and specific problems requiring detailed involvement of particular team members are identified.

Improved survival of affected individuals is largely due to effective antibiotic treatment against staphyloccocal and pseudomonal infections. Centres vary in their policies for antibiotic therapy, some believing in continuous treatment and others using large doses of antibiotics only when infection occurs. Once *Pseudomonas aeruginosa* colonises the lungs, it is almost impossible to eradicate and results in deterioration of lung function.

Case History 6.4 The individuals with CF

J thought about a heart–lung transplant for over a year but elected not to attend for assessment at the transplant centre. She eventually chose to discontinue active treatment because she wished to avoid coping with a protracted terminal illness. J died in relative peace and dignity in her local hospital within a short time.

A was keen to find out if he was a suitable candidate for transplant and was very pleased to be accepted and placed on the waiting list. Everything in the family centred around waiting for the moment when the buzzer to call him to the transplant unit would burst into sound. 'I won't let you down, Mum. I'll keep alive until they find a donor,' he promised solemnly. Alas, A ran out of time and was unable to keep his promise.

S was one of the lucky few. He underwent a heart–lung transplant and experienced the added bonus of giving his own heart to save someone else. S can do all sorts of things now, just like his schoolmates. But for how long? Will signs of rejection show up when next he attends for follow-up, or in a few years, or never? His parents alternate between happiness and despair, but never have complete relief.

To reduce the length of stay in hospital, parents and older children are taught to administer their own antibiotic drugs intravenously so that treatment initiated in the clinic or hospital can be completed at home. An implantable venous reservoir has greatly improved home i.v. treatment and compliance. Nebulised antibiotics have been shown to be effective, but require a special compressor and nebuliser system.

Pancreatic enzyme supplements are taken at regular intervals throughout each meal. The average adult needs at least 5 such tablets per meal. Small snacks between meals require a lower dose of tablets.

Genetic screening. For an individual to have CF, he or she must inherit 2 copies of the mutated gene, one from each parent (see Fig. 6.6). The parents are called carriers or heterozygotes. They have a CF gene on one chromosome 7 and a normal gene on the other chromosome 7. CF is a recessive disease: carriers have no symptoms of the disease, as the normal gene compensates fully for the CF gene (see p. 200).

Until recently only couples who had already had an affected child knew they were carriers. Now by a simple blood test or mouthwash sample it is possible to tell in 85% of individuals whether they carry a CF gene. If both partners of a couple are found to be carriers they can avail themselves of prenatal diagnosis. Pilot screening programmes designed to test individuals in the general population have commenced in selected centres around the UK. Two approaches are currently being tried. The first screens pregnant women in an antenatal booking clinic. The partner of a woman identified as a carrier can then be offered screening. The second approach is to offer screening through GP practices to men and women of childbearing age. The latter has the advantage of screening prior to pregnancy. Trials are currently run within strict research protocols and the psychological aspects of such screening are being carefully monitored.

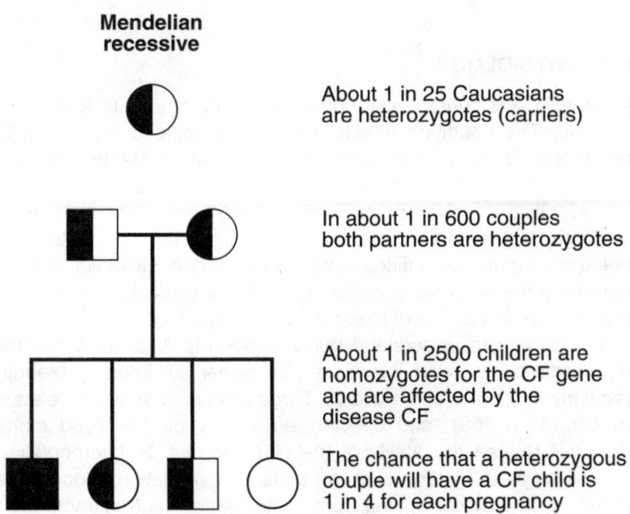

Mendelian recessive
About 1 in 25 Caucasians are heterozygotes (carriers)
In about 1 in 600 couples both partners are heterozygotes
About 1 in 2500 children are homozygotes for the CF gene and are affected by the disease CF
The chance that a heterozygous couple will have a CF child is 1 in 4 for each pregnancy

Fig. 6.6 Genetic inheritance of cystic fibrosis.

NURSING PRIORITIES AND MANAGEMENT: CYSTIC FIBROSIS

Life-threatening concerns

Cystic fibrosis is a long-term, life-threatening disorder. Because it is a multisystem disorder there are a number of essential areas of management.

Respiratory infection

Recurrent lower respiratory tract infections, which become persistent, result in damage to the lungs and impaired lung function.

Physiotherapy is an essential part of the management of the respiratory tract. Keeping the airways clear of mucus and allowing maximum entry of air requires that chest physiotherapy be carried out at least twice daily at home and 3–4 times daily in hospital. Postural drainage, in which the patient is placed in each of 5 positions and treated by percussion allows gravity to assist in the clearance of each lung segment (see Fig. 6.7). The patient assumes each position for about 3 minutes. Breathing exercises adopting the forced expiratory technique (FET) is fundamental to these sessions. Children from the age of 3 years are taught how to carry out this exercise (see Box 6.4). Much time is spent with parents and children educating them in physiotherapy techniques, as this is probably the most important element in the treatment programme.

Nutritional management. Research programmes show that CF patients require 25–50% more than the normal daily food allowance. This is because a significant amount of nutritional intake is lost in frequent, bulky, greasy stools. Extra energy is also needed to combat chest infections. Moreover, studies have shown that individuals with CF have a higher resting energy requirement. Pancreatic enzyme preparations are now so effective that fat absorption can be expected to reach 80–90% of normal. Three daily meals are required and supplemental snacks are usually required to bring the energy level up to the desired level. Fat-soluble vitamin supplements are given to compensate for loss in the stools.

Exercise. This is an extremely important element of CF management. It has been shown that regular exercise increases the efficiency of the lungs, heart and circulation. Furthermore, it improves the general physique and self-esteem. These activities must complement, not replace, physiotherapy. Salt depletion can occur in hot weather and as a result of strenuous exercise. Symptoms of weakness, cramps, vomiting and collapse with low blood pressure may occur. Prevention by drinking a salt and glucose solution before exercise in very hot weather or taking Slow Sodium tablets should be recommended.

Psychosocial considerations

Patients, parents and siblings are often profoundly affected by

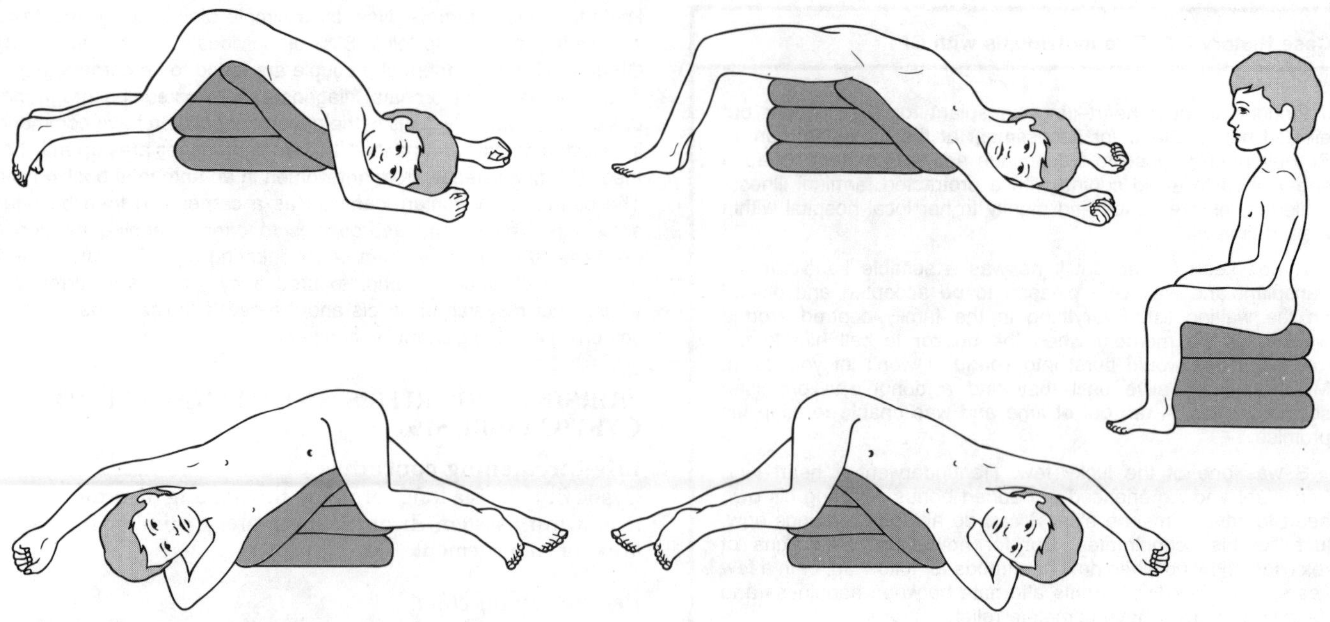

Fig. 6.7 Postural drainage techniques used in the treatment of cystic fibrosis.

Box 6.4 The forced expiration technique (FET)

1. Patient takes a medium inspiration (not a deep one)
2. Patient gives a forced and slightly prolonged expiration (called a huff)
3. Patient coughs, and can expel more sputum than coughing alone allows
4. Patient should alternate this with gentle diaphragmatic breathing.

the psychosocial and emotional stresses of living with CF. The hospital or community nurse is frequently in an ideal position to recognise that psychological problems exist, and to plan and implement measures to assist the patient and his family. Case History 6.5 describes some of the difficulties that might be faced by a teenage boy with CF, and how the sensitive intervention of a specialist nurse might help.

Affected, young, female adults have similar problems to those described in Case History 6.5. They develop much later than their peers and although they can reproduce, unlike their male counterparts, pregnancy carries risks and is a time for close cooperation between the CF multidisciplinary team and the obstetrician. The increased cardiac output and changes in pulmonary function associated with normal pregnancy can cause problems for a CF female sufferer. The mechanical reduction in lung volume as the growing uterus encroaches on the thorax further reduces pulmonary function. Moreover, the woman with CF must also reflect upon the impact upon her children of her shortened life expectancy. Progression of the disease may prevent her from carrying out day-to-day care of her child. Those who become pregnant require increased supervision as more physiotherapy is needed and antibiotic therapy must be carefully selected.

Outlook for the future

Identification of the CFTR gene is already leading to a clearer understanding of the variability of clinical manifestations of CF. In time we should gain a clearer understanding of the role of the CFTR gene in the control of ion transport. The ultimate aim is, however, treatment. The possible introduction by aerosol inhalation of normal CFTR genes into the stem cells of the lungs of CF patients is but one idea already suggested. Whatever the future, the identification of the CF gene gives hope for a greater understanding of the disease and more effective treatment.

HAEMOPHILIA A

Haemophilia is a condition recognised as early as Biblical times, when rabbis allowed infant males exemption from circumcision if two or more of their brothers had bled to death from the procedure. It is well known for its royal connection: Queen Victoria was a carrier and passed the condition on to at least 10 of her male descendants. The haemophilias are a group of inherited disorders of blood coagulation. There are 3 main types: haemophilia A, or classic haemophilia, haemophilia B or Christmas disease, and von Willebrand's disease.

PATHOPHYSIOLOGY

Haemophilia A is characterised by a deficiency or total lack of clotting factor VIII. The condition affects 1 in 10 000 male births in the UK. Haemophilia B is a less common condition characterised by a deficiency of clotting factor IX (Christmas factor). Haemophilia A and B are identical in all respects except that haemophilia A is treated with Factor VIII and haemophilia B with Factor IX. Von Willebrand's disease is as common a disease as haemophilia A. However, bleeding occurs from the mucosal surfaces such as the gastrointestinal tract. It results from a defect of a different nature in Factor VIII.

It is important to understand that haemophilia A is not a condition that manifests in overt bleeding but rather in internal bleeding, particularly into joints and muscles. Blood clots as a series of reactions (see Ch. 11, p. 409), and deficiencies in any of the blood clotting factors will reduce the ability of the blood to clot. In haemophilia A, the initial steps in clotting such as platelet aggregation, blood vessel contraction, and blood clotting from contact with tissue extracts are all normal. If a patient with haemophilia A has a tooth removed or undergoes surgery he does not bleed abnormally at the time: bleeding

Case History 6.5 G

G is a small, thin, red-haired 16-year-old in his 4th year at high school. He is judged to be academically average by his headmaster. G is a particularly keen cyclist and is a member of the school cycling team. He was diagnosed as having CF when he was 3 years old. Since that time his care has been shared by his GP, the local hospital and the Regional Cystic Fibrosis Centre. G attends the centre every 3 months. At these visits he is due a chest X-ray. Then lung function tests are carried out and blood is taken for analysis. The physiotherapist checks G's breathing exercises and postural drainage and FET technique. He then sees the dietitian, who checks his height and weight and discusses his diet and pancreatic enzyme and vitamin supplements. The chest physician in charge of the centre also examines G, who has been admitted 4 times in the past 2 years for intensive i.v. antibiotic therapy for pseudomonas respiratory infection. On these occasions G was successfully treated with the antibiotic ciprofloxacin.

Today, G is going to talk to the specialist nurse, who is going to suggest that she introduce G to a careers guidance officer. She knows G well and has already submitted a report to the careers office. G has had periods of absence from school when his condition necessitated hospital admission. Some teaching was given while he was in hospital and he has had extra tuition at home. His father helps him with his physiotherapy and has a close relationship with his son.

The specialist nurse knows from discussions with G's parents that G is quite sensitive about his illness. Firstly, he is smaller and thinner than his schoolmates. He weighs 50 kg and is currently 5' 4" tall. His friends have entered puberty at the normal time, but G has no sign of secondary sex characteristics. Naturally, he is self-conscious about this, particularly when using the communal shower and changing rooms at school. Reassurance from the consultant and his parents that he will catch up with his peers, probably continuing to grow after they have stopped, is small consolation.

For a time G had shown signs of depression, and had entered a period of non-compliance in his physiotherapy, diet and pancreatic enzyme supplements. It was then that G's parents had contacted the centre and asked the specialist nurse to visit. She was in the process of setting up a group for CF teenagers from within her own and a neighbouring region. The object of the group was to meet socially and discuss any issues which the group or a particular teenager or young adult wanted to discuss. Reluctantly, G went along to the first meeting. He met several people he had seen before at the CF centre but there were some unfamiliar faces. The meeting opened with one young man volunteering to describe an average day in his life:

> The moment I get up I start my treatment. I start with nebulised Ventolin so that I can do my physio without wheezing and feeling my chest tight. Then comes the physio followed by the nebuliser with my antibiotics. After that I have breakfast and swallow my pancreatin capsules. I take the capsules to school with me to take with my lunch and any snacks. I stay on 2 nights a week after school for games. Most of the time I can manage, although periodically I have to give up because of wheezing. I hope to sit my O levels this year, and I am having extra tuition because I got behind last year with my studies due to numerous hospital admissions for i.v. therapy. The moment I arrive home it is a repeat of the morning's treatment routine. Sometimes I feel very despondent and wonder if it is all worthwhile. My best friend at school wants us to go along to the local disco, but I don't suppose any girl will look twice at me. I am smaller than all the other lads my age and I feel very self-conscious.

This was exactly how G felt about having CF and he felt greatly comforted by hearing this young man put into words his own frustrations at this stage in his life.

starts after several hours or days with the formation of soft, jelly-like clots, and poor healing.

Individuals affected by haemophilia A vary in their levels of Factor VIII. It is now known that a number of different mutations or alterations can occur to a gene on the long arm of the X chromosome to cause haemophilia A.

Common presenting symptoms. Factor VIII levels are reduced at birth, but patients rarely present with bleeding in the neonatal period. In infancy accidental bruising or bleeding as the primary dentition erupts may be an early indication. It is usually when the baby starts to crawl and injures himself that signs first appear. Mild cases may show a tendency to bruise but fail to come to medical attention unless a surgical procedure is undergone. Severely affected infants will bleed spontaneously. Abnormal bruising as a result of a coagulation disorder should be kept in mind as a differential diagnosis in cases of suspected non-accidental injury.

In childhood, the severely affected most commonly present with haemarthrosis and haematomas. Milder cases may not present until they participate in the more vigorous activities of later childhood, or undergo dental extraction. In adulthood, mildly affected adults usually present with bleeding due to other pathological lesions such as a peptic ulcer, or with prolonged bleeding following major trauma or surgery. The most common presenting clinical features of the condition are listed in Box 6.5.

Prognosis. Thirty years ago many sufferers from haemophilia A died prematurely from uncontrollable bleeding. Since 1967 the therapeutic use of cryoprecipitate, a plasma concentrate rich in Factor VIII, has allowed sufferers to enjoy a near-normal lifespan. Due to the inadvertent use of contaminated blood and blood products between 1979 and 1984, many haemophiliacs have been infected with the human immunodeficiency virus (HIV).

Box 6.5 Presenting clinical features of haemophilia A

NEWBORN

- Cephalohaematoma
- Bleeding from umbilicus
- Intramuscular haematoma, e.g. at injection site

INFANCY

- Circumcision: excessive bleeding from
- Primary dentition: bleeding from gums
- Crawling: subcutaneous haematoma

EARLY CHILDHOOD

- Haemarthrosis
- Haematomas
- Spontaneous bleeds: severe cases
- Neurological signs from nerve compression (rare)
- Gastrointestinal bleeding (rare)

LATER CHILDHOOD

- Haemarthrosis (bleeding into joints)
- Haematomas
- Intracranial bleeding
- Prolonged bleeding: dental extractions, surgical operations

ADULTHOOD

- Prolonged/spontaneous bleeding: major trauma, minor trauma (severe cases), surgery, peptic ulcer, haematuria

MEDICAL MANAGEMENT

Diagnosis. The diagnosis of haemophilia A is made by specific assay which identifies Factor VIII deficiency.

Treatment consists of increasing plasma levels of Factor VIII to 20–30% of normal, so that clotting of an uncontrolled bleed occurs. Freeze-dried Factor VIII concentrate is reconstituted with sterile water, warmed to body temperature, and given by slow i.v. injection through a butterfly infusion set. The dose is calculated according to body weight, assumed plasma volume and the severity of the bleed. Freeze-dried Factor VIII concentrate should be stored at 4°C.

Genetic screening. Because haemophilia A is an X-linked recessive disease, affected males have inherited only one copy of the haemophilia gene, as they possess only a single X chromosome. Females, on the other hand, would have to inherit two copies of the gene, one from each parent, in order to have the disease. Consequently almost all haemophiliacs are male. Females can be carriers, possessing a single haemophilia gene along with a normal gene for clotting factor VIII. Carriers are normal, although they may experience slower clotting. If a female is a carrier, half of her sons on average will have the disease, and half her daughters will be carriers (see Fig. 6.8). If an affected male has children, all of his daughters will be carriers but none of his sons will be affected. Approximately 30% of cases occur as new or spontaneous mutations with no family history of the disease.

Prenatal diagnosis can be carried out by CVS (see p. 193), by which it is possible to say whether a male fetus has inherited his mother's defective X chromosome or her normal X chromosome.

NURSING PRIORITIES AND MANAGEMENT: HAEMOPHILIA A

The management of haemophilia A can be divided into two phases:

1. The recognition and treatment of acute haemorrhagic episodes
2. Chronic care, with attention directed toward taking preventive measures against bleeding, optimising conditions under which treatment is given, and managing the long-term musculoskeletal complications of the disease.

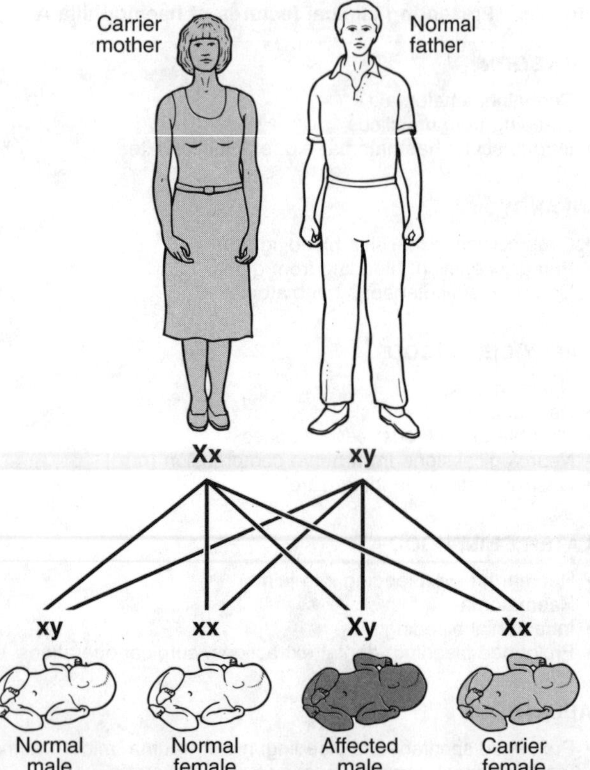

Fig. 6.8 Genetic inheritance of haemophilia A.

The Haemophilia Centre

In the UK, management of haemophilia patients is organised around regional haemophilia centres. The overall aims of these centres are summarised in Box 6.6.

A multidisciplinary approach is fundamental to the care of haemophilia patients and their families. The team is led by a consultant haematologist and the day-to-day organisation and delivery of the service is carried out by a specialist nurse. Indeed, it is she that the patient or family will contact the moment they suspect a bleed. The centre provides a 24-hour emergency service as prompt treatment of a bleed is essential. At the centre, patients are also regularly seen for liver and renal function tests, and for hepatitis antigen and HIV screening.

Major nursing considerations

Management of a bleeding episode

The moment the patient suspects a bleed he or a relative will contact the haemophilia centre Sister. The patient attends as an outpatient and is seen and examined by one of the doctors. The required dose of Factor VIII is prescribed and administered by the sister or nurse. The patient is allowed to go home with instructions to rest the affected limb and to attend the centre for review the next day if the bleed has not resolved. If necessary the affected limb may be splinted or supported in a sling. The patient is then referred to the physiotherapist. If a patient is on home treatment and is experiencing a major bleeding episode he may be advised to administer more Factor VIII some hours later.

Management of major bleeding episodes

A large dose of Factor VIII is given initially. Pre- and post-Factor VIII levels will be taken by the nurse. The patient is admitted to the ward for complete bed-rest. Major bleeds are extremely painful episodes and if necessary i.v. diamorphine is given to control the pain. Factor VIII will be given morning and evening with pre- and post-Factor VIII levels taken each morning to ensure that the correct level is being maintained. Positioning of the patient will be important to his comfort. Use of a bed cradle and support of the affected limb with an inflatable downie or pillow, as well as observation for foot drop, are basic nursing measures. When the acute bleed has subsided it is important to enlist the help of the physiotherapist to commence gentle mobilising exercises.

There are a number of fundamentally important points to remember about acute bleeding episodes:

Box 6.6 Aims of the Haemophilia Centre

- To provide a 24-hour clinical service
- To coordinate special services
- To act as a resource/reference centre for GPs, employers, schools, dentists, and community services
- To advise on problems and to undertake specialised or general surgery
- To provide additional services, e.g. carrier detection and prenatal diagnosis
- To maintain links with local schools, employment agencies, and social and voluntary services

- Always believe the patient when he tells you he has developed a bleed, or that one is starting.
- Notify the haemophilia centre Sister immediately, as it is essential that the patient receives prompt treatment. This can prevent a small bleed from becoming a large one and save the patient much pain.
- No procedure should ever be carried out on a haemophiliac patient before he has been given Factor VIII; this applies to X-ray, endoscopy, bronchoscopy, physiotherapy, a bath or getting in and out of bed.

Long-term management

All patients with haemophilia should be registered with a haemophilia centre. They should carry a special medical card giving details of their disorder, their blood group, antibodies and abnormalities. The card should give the name of the director and the address of the centre.

Patients should attend the haemophilia centre regularly for assessment, as this is central to preventive care. Regular dental care is very important to prevent tooth decay and extraction. Intramuscular injections should never be administered to a haemophiliac patient. Aspirin or aspirin-containing drugs should never be given. Severely affected patients should avoid forceful nose-blowing, coughing or straining at stool. If necessary, a stool softener should be prescribed. Physical activity should be encouraged with proper safety measures. Non-contact sports such as swimming, gymnastics, golf or hiking are suitable pursuits.

Giving psychological support to the patient and his family is an important function of the haemophilia centre team, especially the nursing staff, who may ask for input from the local community nursing staff working in the patient's locality. Throughout the patient's life, ongoing education and support is fundamental to the management of the condition.

Home treatment

If a patient is willing to learn to treat himself (or if a parent or partner wishes to learn) the Sister at the haemophilia centre will teach venepuncture and administration of Factor VIII. Each patient requires access to a refrigerator and a suitable area for preparing his treatment. He must also have good veins.

Once competence in administering his treatment is achieved the patient is supplied with a home treatment kit containing all the required equipment. All bleeds must be recorded on the record sheet, and this returned to the haemophilia Sister for documentation. All needles and syringes and empty Factor VIII bottles are also returned for safe disposal. Should a patient have difficulty resolving a bleed he must come to the centre and seek advice, or be seen by a doctor. The same applies if he experiences any allergic reaction. A major advantage of home treatment is that it can be given promptly, at the earliest sign of a bleed, saving the patient pain, joint damage and hospitalisation. Moreover, it helps the patient to feel more in control of his own treatment and less dependent upon hospital staff. This in turn raises his self-esteem. Prompt treatment will also reduce time taken from work or school.

Outlook for the future

The problem of blood-borne viruses

Freeze-dried Factor VIII originates from several thousand blood donors and consequently carries a high risk of exposing the patient to blood-borne viruses. Hepatitis is likely to prove a major cause of death in haemophiliacs over the next few years. While most who have been exposed to the hepatitis B virus show antibodies and are immune, a small proportion show persistent antigenaemia and are at risk of developing progressive liver disease. Patients who show abnormal liver function tests have mostly been infected by hepatitis C.

Shortly after the AIDS virus was identified in the early 1980s, haemophilia patients in the USA were noted to have an increased incidence of the disease. Subsequently, HIV antibody testing of sera from haemophiliacs was carried out in the UK in 1985. Since then, clotting factor concentrates have been heat-treated or treated with chemicals to destroy the virus. Researchers continue to investigate ways of inactivating blood-borne viruses.

Synthetic Factor VIII. Since commercial concentrates of Factor VIII became available almost 20 years ago, the treatment of haemophilia A has altered dramatically. Despite the improved ease and effectiveness of treatment, transfusion complications have increased. The cloning of the factor VIII gene has led to the production of genetically engineered factor VIII. This synthetic Factor VIII is structurally similar to plasma-derived Factor VIII and has a similar half-life. Trials in patients with haemophilia A are being undertaken. With continued improvements in the expression and isolation of genetically engineered factor VIII, this product will become cheaper to produce and will eventually become available to all patients. The problem of hepatitis and HIV in haemophilia patients may thus be resolved in the future. Finally, the ability to express the Factor VIII gene in mammalian cells may lead eventually to gene-insertion therapy in patients with haemophilia A.

MYOTONIC DYSTROPHY

Myotonic dystrophy is a progressive neuromuscular disease. By myotonia is meant a particular type of muscular stiffness in which the muscle contracts normally but is unable to relax normally. By dystrophy is meant weakening and wasting of the muscles.

The muscles particularly involved are:

- the facial muscles
- the sternomastoid muscles
- the distal limb muscles.

Involvement of other body systems is common. Associated problems may include:

- cataracts
- hormonal problems
- cardiac problems
- gastrointestinal tract involvement
- learning difficulties (in children).

The age of onset of this autosomal dominant disorder is variable. However, the majority of those who have the myotonic dystrophy gene will show some symptoms by the time they reach adult life. It is important to be aware that it can also occur in neonates and young children. These cases are usually the offspring of an affected mother.

There is great variation in severity: some people with the myotonic dystrophy gene can be so mildly affected that they are unaware of it, while others have major problems.

As inheritance is autosomal dominant, an affected individual of either sex has a 50% risk of passing the gene on to a child of either sex (see p. 191).

Other forms of progressive muscular dystrophies include:

- Duchenne muscular dystrophy: the severe, childhood, X-linked recessive form
- Becker muscular dystrophy: the less severe, adult, X-linked recessive form
- facioscapulohumeral dystrophy: a less severe autosomal dominant form.

Prevalence
Myotonic dystrophy is no longer thought to be a rare disorder and is regarded as the most frequently occurring muscular dystrophy of adult life. Precise figures are not easy to find and are likely to be underestimates because of the variation of expression.

New mutations are thought to be rare. It should be assumed that all cases have been transmitted unless there is positive evidence to the contrary.

PATHOPHYSIOLOGY

Characteristic changes in the muscle tissue of those affected with myotonic dystrophy can be seen on microscopic examination. It is likely that a defect in the muscle cell membrane is responsible for both the muscle wasting and the myotonia.

Electrical studies show a specific disturbance leading to failure of muscle relaxation. This seems also to point to the muscle cell membrane as the site of the problem.

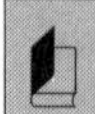 Harper 1989

MEDICAL MANAGEMENT

Tests and investigations used to diagnose myotonic dystrophy and its associated effects on body systems are as follows.

Physical examination will demonstrate the presence of muscle weakness. Patients are asked to grip an object firmly and then let go. If myotonia is present there will be a delay of several seconds in relaxation of the muscle. Percussion of the tongue may show a persistent furrow.

Slit lamp examination is an important aid in the differentiation of atypical cases of myotonic dystrophy and in its detection in asymptomatic patients. The lens opacities have a characteristic refractile, multicoloured appearance when viewed through a slit lamp (see Ch. 13, p. 471).

Electroretinography is a sensitive method of detecting retinal changes when cataract obscures an ophthalmoscopic view.

Electrocardiography will detect cardiac abnormalities such as arrhythmias, conduction defects and varying degrees of heart block.

Electromyography is mandatory before an individual can be considered to be unaffected, although it is not essential for diagnosis in most patients with obvious myotonia.

Genetic screening. The gene responsible for myotonic dystrophy was recently identified. It lies on the long arm of chromosome 19 and has an interesting feature, a sequence of three bases, CTG, that is repeated a variable number of times in different individuals. Normal people may have between 5 and 37 copies of the repeat. Patients with myotonic dystrophy have between 50 and several thousand copies. This resembles the abnormal gene found in Huntington's disease (see Research Abstract 6.1). However, in myotonic dystrophy the copy number of the repeat is much greater than in Huntington's. Furthermore, there is a rough correlation between copy number and the severity of the disorder, so that repeats of several thousands are found in infants with congenital myotonic dystrophy.

NURSING PRIORITIES AND MANAGEMENT: MYOTONIC DYSTROPHY

Major considerations

Management of complications
It is important that any medical problems are diagnosed early and treated appropriately to prevent them getting worse and to avoid further complications. This has to be stressed both to those at risk and those already affected. The severe degree of apathy which is characteristic of myotonic dystrophy can be a major obstacle to overcome and can be responsible for low attendance rates and lack of compliance with treatment.

Myotonic dystrophy affects a number of body systems and thus requires careful management both in day-to-day living and when particular medical problems arise. The nurse should be aware of the following points:

- Breathing exercises may help combat the tendency to hypoventilation found in many patients with myotonic dystrophy. Postural drainage (see Fig. 6.7) will reduce the effect of bronchial aspiration of food and secretions.
- Below-knee calipers and toestrings or plastic moulded splints may help control foot drop.
- Beta-adrenergic blockers and verapamil have been used to control cardiac arrhythmia. (Adrenaline and related bronchodilator agents should be avoided because of the risk of arrhythmias.)
- Cardiac pacemakers are inserted when there is evidence of conduction defects.
- Cataract surgery will be necessary for the majority of those with myotonic dystrophy. The existence of severe muscle disease or cardiac involvement should be taken into account when planning the anaesthetic.
- Problems with anaesthesia usually arise because the surgeons and anaesthetists are unaware that the patient has a neuromuscular disorder. The wearing of a bracelet to alert people in case of accidents requiring surgery may save lives.
- Special obstetric care is necessary during pregnancy and delivery.
- A high-fibre diet will help to alleviate constipation. Laxatives may be necessary but liquid paraffin should be avoided because of the risk of bronchial aspiration.
- Sternomastoid weakness makes the use of headrests in cars imperative.

Giving psychological support
The diagnosis of a hereditary, slowly progressive muscle disorder of varying severity with associated abnormalities of other body systems can have a profound psychological effect upon a family.

It must be difficult to live with myotonic dystrophy not only for those affected, who have little energy, little motivation, and can find daily living an overwhelming effort, but also for their partners or offspring. To live with someone who has an expressionless face, a monotonous voice, a marked lack of enthusiasm and who keeps falling asleep must put a great strain on a relationship. The sympathy and understanding necessary for both partners may be in short supply.

Patient education
It is very likely that several members within a kinship will be shown to have the myotonic dystrophy gene. Explanations will be sought for variations in the severity of the condition and for the apparently unrelated associated medical problems encountered. Although medical staff will relate the initial information to the family, many clients will come to the nurse for further explanation, advice and reassurance.

When giving information to family members care must be taken to avoid causing needless anxiety by giving the impression that everyone with the myotonic dystrophy gene will experience every complication mentioned in textbooks or information leaflets. Sudden death is not inevitable, only a few of those affected will require wheelchairs, and removal of cataracts to restore sight is now a routine procedure with a high success rate.

In some areas the Muscular Dystrophy Group, a charitable organisation, supplies a Family Care Officer — often a nurse but sometimes an occupational therapist or social worker — to act in an advisory capacity on behalf of families with various forms of muscular dystrophy. She will have built up a wealth of knowledge about muscle conditions, including myotonic dystrophy, which she can pass on to community nurses and health visitors who are involved with families with this condition.

HUNTINGTON'S DISEASE

Huntington's disease (HD), or Huntington's chorea, is a devastating neurological disorder, initially appearing in middle age, which leads to progressive motor disturbance, psychological manifestations, and intellectual deterioration. The incidence of this condition in the UK is approximately 1 per 10 000 of the population. Huntington's disease is caused by an autosomal dominant gene. It was first described in 1872 by George Huntington, of a family of New England physicians who witnessed the disease through successive generations of a number of their patients.

PATHOPHYSIOLOGY

The motor disturbance in HD is due to premature death of the cells in the basal ganglia, and the psychological and intellectual deterioration to death of cells in the frontal lobes of the cerebral cortex. In some cases, the brain stem and the spinal cord are also affected. Indeed, in advanced cases the weight of the whole brain may decrease by as much as 20–30%. Postmortem studies have revealed that levels of many neurotransmitters are abnormal; although these alterations are probably secondary to the neuronal degradation, it is thought they may contribute to the symptoms of the disorder.

Common presenting symptoms. A patient may present with any of the features listed in Box 6.7. Frequently, relatives will divulge that they were aware of personality changes long before physical symptoms became apparent.

Abnormality of movement is the most prominent feature of the disease. Although mild in the beginning, the occasional grimace, shrug or body twist, hesitation in speech or irregular trunk movement, which patients in these early stages can often control, progress to ill-sustained and jerky movement of the limbs. The speech becomes slurred and stumbling, and spasmodic inspiration may cause it to be, at times, explosive. The patient's gait is distinctive, as he walks on the heels with a wide base. Negotiating furniture or obstacles in a confined space becomes difficult. Sudden lurching can cause falls. Chewing is difficult and swallowing is frequently affected. Choking and aspiration can be a risk.

Intellectual impairment is slowly progressive. Some individuals maintain a degree of mental clarity to the end, and others show a profound dementia in the final stages. Physical activity may be maintained late into the disease; other individuals develop an almost total inertia.

Prognosis. On average, death occurs in an individual 17 years after the onset of symptoms, usually from one of the following: heart failure, pneumonia, infection, choking, or accidental injury.

MEDICAL MANAGEMENT

History and examination. For most people with the disorder the first signs appear between the ages of 30 and 45, but a few individuals experience symptoms in childhood and in others the disease is not obvious until old age. There is frequently a family history of the illness through many generations. Virtually all affected individuals inherit the gene from one of their parents.

The symptoms of HD appear slowly and subtly; where there is no obvious family history, diagnosis in the early stages is difficult and the condition may be confused with other disorders. An early sign is a marked change in personality. The affected person may become depressed and be hard to get along with; he may be obstinate and moody and exhibit erratic or inappropriate behaviours. Because these are changes which have many potential causes, HD can go unrecognised until more obvious classical symptoms are manifest.

The diagnosis can be made clinically by careful history and full neurological examination. A diagnostic protocol specifically designed for diagnosing this disorder should be used. In typical cases with a family history the diagnosis may be obvious. A cranial CT scan may show frontal horn enlargement due to caudate atrophy; however, there will be phases in the natural history of the disorder when a CT scan will be normal. The only conclusive diagnostic tool is a postmortem examination in which specific neuropathological changes show atrophy of the small neurones in the caudate and putamen and of the large neurones in the globus pallidus. Indeed, where a diagnosis has not been confirmed, or when there is scanty or absent family history, the sensitive subject of autopsy studies is best raised prior to a patient's death. Relatives can be prepared and the necessary forms signed and kept with the family GP or pathologist concerned. This may be the only means whereby an accurate diagnosis can be made and subsequent appropriate counselling offered to the patient's family.

Tests and investigations. Until recently, there has been no means of determining which family members have inherited the disorder.

Box 6.7 Presenting features of Huntington's disease

ABNORMALITIES OF MOVEMENT

- mild fidgetiness
- slight unsteadiness of gait
- occasional grimace
- problems of fine movement, e.g. handwriting
- occasional shrug or body twist

PERSONALITY OR BEHAVIOURAL DISTURBANCE

- mood swings
- decreased communication
- lethargy
- irritability
- outbursts of temper
- obsessional behaviour
- dependency
- lack of sexual inhibition
- aggression

INTELLECTUAL IMPAIRMENT

- loss of concentration
- poor organisational ability
- memory loss

SPEECH DIFFICULTIES

- mild slurring
- impaired flow of speech

Those who carry the abnormal gene and who will develop the disease are indistinguishable physically from those who do not. However, in 1983 geneticists established that the gene causing HD is located near the end of the short arm of chromosome 4; this was determined using DNA analysis and the largest known family with HD, consisting of over 7000 individuals, including 100 with the disease, living in Venezuela. Several genetic markers close to the HD gene were isolated, allowing predictive testing of those who carry the disease gene. Recently the HD gene itself was isolated (see Research Abstract 6.1). The hope now is that this will lead to a better understanding of the disease process and eventually make an effective treatment possible.

Medical intervention. There is no treatment as yet which can halt or alter the progression of the disease. There are drugs which can alleviate some of the symptoms, but these should be prescribed only when of benefit to the patient, not to alleviate the anxieties relatives may have about the abnormal movements. Tetrabenazine or reserpine can be prescribed to lessen the choreiform movements. The patient's motor signs should be regularly assessed to evaluate optimal drug levels, as overmedication can cause motor restlessness, which can be mistaken for involuntary movements. Antidepressant therapy may be prescribed. Although psychotherapy aimed at alleviating tension, stress and anxiety can be beneficial, it is seldom offered.

Genetic screening. Using DNA markers linked to the HD gene on chromosome 4, it is possible to carry out predictive testing on individuals at a high risk of having inherited the HD gene. Having information about whether one will develop the disease in later life may be useful in planning for the future and in deciding whether to have children.

Pilot studies which provide predictive testing are being conducted in selective genetic centres around the UK. These programmes are embedded in structured protocols of genetic and psychiatric counselling, aimed at preparing individuals and their families for good or bad news (see Case History 6.6). Those who are reassured they are free of the disease will be greatly relieved, but for those who receive a positive test result, the news can be devastating both for themselves and for their family. There are also many legal and social questions surrounding predictive testing, such as whether a positive diagnosis will affect employment and insurability. The outcome of the pilot trials will determine the future of this type of diagnosis.

NURSING PRIORITIES AND MANAGEMENT: HUNTINGTON'S DISEASE

Life-threatening concerns

Suicide

Undoubtedly the most devastating aspects of HD are its mental and emotional features. Depression is common among HD sufferers. Studies show suicide rates among affected individuals in the early stages of the disease, among those newly diagnosed, are up to 14 times higher than rates among the general population.

As nurses we should strive to enhance the quality of the patient's life, thereby enhancing the quality of life for family members and others close to the patient. The emphasis must be on living, not dying. Adopting a positive attitude and encouraging the patient and others to do likewise is fundamental to the nursing care of the HD patient and his family.

Choking

Swallowing can become a significant problem in some patients as the disease progresses. Inhalation of food and liquid can cause lung infections, aspiration pneumonia, or a fatal choking episode. Patients at risk benefit from regular chest physiotherapy. Nurses should observe for signs of difficulty in chewing and swallowing. Excessive nasal secretions, saliva, or regurgitation of material through the nose or mouth are indicative of swallowing difficulties. Nurses should be prepared to perform the Heimlich manoeuvre should choking occur.

Major patient problems

Weight loss

Constant involuntary movements cause calories to be burned up faster and increase appetite. Coupled with difficulty in swallowing, this can result in loss of weight.

Communication. Communication skills are frequently diminished in HD sufferers. The nurse should remember that emotion affects speech and that an HD patient may be silent due to feelings of isolation, embarrassment due to difficulty in speaking, lack of encouragement, or depression. As the disease progresses an inability to communicate a basic need can understandably result in frustrated outbursts of aggression. Gestures and signs used to communicate can also be affected, and control of the muscles involved in speech production can be lost.

There is much the nurse can do to assist in the management of speech and communication problems. Firstly, she should always give the patient her undivided attention by sitting opposite at the same level to encourage eye contact. She should try to allocate time to converse with the patient in a relaxed atmosphere free from distractions such as a TV or radio. It is best to keep to one topic at a time and to be concise. The nurse should ask open-ended questions to encourage the patient to express feelings, opinions or ideas. If she has difficulty comprehending, she should repeat part of the sentence, for even one or two words that have been understood will encourage continued communication. A conversation should not be prolonged, of course, against the patient's wishes; his inclinations should be respected.

Nurses working with patients with HD can help them to overcome some speech and communication problems by teaching a few simple strategies. The patient should face the individual he wishes to speak to and check that he has his attention by saying his name or touching him. The patient should try to speak slowly, moving his lips and tongue slowly and deliberately. Pausing and taking a breath helps to prevent words running together. The patient can be encouraged to practise words and phrases that he finds difficult, and to practise deep breathing and simple facial and tongue exercises. In the later stages of the disease, before communication becomes too difficult, a communication system can be devised. Cards with words or pictures of familiar objects which the

Case History 6.6 J

J is 33 years old. Her father suffers from HD and is cared for in a hospital for the chronically ill. Her younger sister, P, has minimal clinical signs of the disease; her diagnosis has been confirmed by CT scan. J has been referred for genetic counselling by her general practitioner. She feels that the uncertainty of being at risk for HD is very much worse than knowing her HD status and she requests predictive testing. Blood samples are obtained from her affected father and sister, and from her unaffected mother. Preliminary laboratory analysis of these samples show that it will be possible to say with 95% accuracy whether J has inherited the HD gene from her father. J attends the genetic department for several counselling sessions, of which one includes a full psychiatric assessment. Only then is a blood sample taken for analysis.

patient can respond to by hitting the card with his hand, blinking, or grunting will help to express basic needs and wants. Finally, it is essential for the nurse to remember that patients can understand even if they are unable to communicate. Staff should not isolate them further by ceasing to communicate with them.

Progressive intellectual impairment
Intellectual impairment varies enormously among HD sufferers. Lack of concentration, difficulty in thinking clearly, and lapses in short-term memory are common features. The patient should wear an identification bracelet giving his name and telephone number and with the phrase 'memory impaired' inscribed on it. The nurse should take time to reorientate the patient after awakening. Music and music therapy have been shown to promote relaxation in HD patients.

Loss of self-image
Patients should be up and dressed every day unless they are unwell for some other reason. The Kirkton Huntington's chorea chair accommodates these patients comfortably. It is a manually operated, reclining chair which is well padded and very stable. Try to enhance a positive patient self-image by encouraging independence. Do this by setting new goals within the patient's capability. Even though this capability will steadily decline, instilling a sense of achievement at any level of function is still worthwhile for patient and carers alike. Provide patients, family members, friends, and nursing and medical colleagues the opportunity to express their emotions regarding this devastating disease.

Other considerations

General care
The nurse should bear in mind the following considerations in daily patient care:

1. Mouthcare. Assist the HD patient to regularly clean his teeth. Preserving dentition will contribute to the patient's well-being (see Ch. 15, p. 525).
2. Skin care. Providing weight loss is not severe and injury is prevented, pressure sores should not present a problem. Nevertheless, the use of soft sheets and bedding and padding the sides and head of the bed provide safeguards against abrasion and injury. Keep the patient's skin clean and use skin lotion regularly.
3. Bathing. Many HD patients love a bath. They find it relaxing and consequently it reduces involuntary movements. A Parker bath designed to prevent the patient slipping too far into the water is more comfortable and secure. Always devote time to this procedure.
4. Incontinence. Try to note when the patient is wet and work out a regime for toileting (see Ch. 24).
5. Clothing. Loose-fitting clothes which can be easily put on and taken off are advisable (e.g. track suits, wrap-around skirts).

Outlook for the future

Cooperation within the international scientific community has resulted in the isolation of the HD gene. Almost certainly, its discovery will lead to an understanding of the basic genetic defect associated with the inability to synthesise the Huntingtin enzyme. Eventually it will be possible to compose a picture of how the normal functioning gene acts on the brain and in turn why the brain becomes disordered as it does in HD. Huntington's disease is becoming more widely known and is attracting more interest. Nevertheless, much needs to be done to improve medical care and welfare support for HD patients and their families. The Huntington's Disease Association gives support to families and professionals through their publications and by providing practical advice and help. The Association now has local Family Support Officers (usually nurses) in an increasing number of areas.

CONCLUSION

Although scientific knowledge in itself is neutral, its use often poses ethical and moral problems. Nowhere is this more evident than in the field of human genetics, where every advance has an enormous potential for both positive and negative applications. Recognition of the destructive potential of genetic engineering has prompted the imposition of increasingly strict controls over biotechnology and genetic research.

This chapter has presented an outline of current developments in genetics and molecular biology and has indicated the complexity of nursing involvement in the field of genetic counselling and in the care of patients with genetic disorders. Although progress is rapid and recent applications of molecular technology have indicated the potential for genetically informed health care, there is much work to be done before the aims of the HGP can be achieved. It is therefore essential that nurses keep themselves well informed in this subject, as in all others.

Nursing involvement in every branch of health care demands an awareness of genetic influences in health and disease, especially as public awareness grows and clients look for informed professional discussion on a wide range of related topics.

A brief overview of some of the main achievements in genetic science indicates its scope and potential:

- production of drugs and chemicals which can be used in the treatment of disease
- research leading to a better understanding of both common diseases and their genetic component and of the rare classic genetic disorders
- prenatal diagnosis of parental carriers of genetic disorders
- methods for early detection of genetic disorders in utero so that prospective parents have the choice of termination or acceptance of pregnancy
- sex selection
- genetic screening to detect correctable genetic deficiencies, e.g. PKU
- DNA fingerprinting
- testing for the presence of late-onset genetic disorders, e.g. Huntington's chorea
- gene therapy which involves modification of cells in order to either treat or exclude a genetic disease
- genetically engineered microbes and biological aberrations that can be used in mass environmental or human destruction.

Discussion of a few of the classic genetic disorders has emphasised the importance of nursing intervention. This intervention ranges from the non-directive counselling and supportive role of the genetic nurse specialist to that of nurses in every branch of nursing, who will be involved in recognition, treatment, referral and support of individuals and their families in order to promote optimal levels of health.

? **6.2** Refer to the list of achievements in genetic science above and decide which involve major ethical issues. Discuss these with your colleagues.

REFERENCES

British Medical Association 1992 Our genetic future: the science and ethics of genetic technology. Oxford University Press, Oxford

Connor J M & Ferguson-Smith M A 1991 Essential medical genetics. Blackwell Scientific, Oxford

Connor S 1993 Gene found for Huntington's chorea. News. British Medical Journal April 306(6882): 878

Harper P 1988 Practical genetic counselling. Wright, London

Harper P 1989 Myotonic dystrophy. W.B. Saunders, London

Kingston H 1989 ABC of clinical genetics. British Medical Journal, London

FURTHER READING

Aronstam A 1990 Haemophilia update. Update (April): 713

Baraitser M & Winter R 1988 A colour atlas of clinical genetics. Wolfe Medical Publications, London

Barber R 1978 Huntington's chorea: nursing care study. Nursing Times (July 13): 1165–1167

Beischer N A, MacKay E V 1988 Obstetrics and the newborn, 2nd edn. Saunders, London

Clark A 1991 Is non-directive genetic counselling possible? The Lancet (Oct 19) 338

Cohen F L 1984 Clinical genetics in nursing practice. Lippincott, Philadelphia, Ch. 4

Connor J M, Ferguson-Smith M A 1987 Essential medical genetics, 2nd edn. Blackwell Scientific, Oxford

Farnish S 1988 A developing role in genetic counselling. Journal of Medical Genetics 25: 392–395

Geoghegan J 1982 Huntington's chorea: community care study. Nursing Times (June 30): 1098–1101

Greener M 1993 Gene therapy: the dawn of a revolution. Professional Nurse Sept 8(12): 784–787

Guilbert P & Cheater F 1990 Health visitors awareness and perception of clinical genetic services. Journal of Medical Genetics 27: 508–511

Harper P 1989 Myotonic dystrophy. W.B. Saunders, London

Harper P S, Walker D A, Tyler A, Newcombe R G, Davies K 1979 Huntington's chorea: the basis for long-term prevention. Lancet 2(8138): 346–349

Jones P 1984 Living with haemophilia. Haemophilia Society, London

Kessler S 1988 Invited essay: The psychological aspects of genetic counselling preselection — a family coping strategy in Huntington's disease. American Journal of Medical Genetics 31: 617–621

Molleman E 1987 Social and psychological aspects of haemophilia. Patient Education and Counselling (October): 175

USEFUL ADDRESSES

Association of Cystic Fibrosis Adults (UK)
Alexandra House
5 Blyth Road
Bromley
Kent BR1 3RS

Down's Syndrome Association
153–155 Mitcham Road
Tooting, London
SW17 9BG

Haemophilia Society
123 Westminster Bridge Road
London SE1 7HR

Huntington's Disease Association
Muscular Dystrophy Group of Great Britain and Northern Ireland
35 Macaulay Road
London SW4 OQP

The Muscular Dystrophy Group
7–11 Prescott Place
London SW4 6BS

National Association of Genetic Nurses and Social Workers
Clinical Genetics Department
Box 134, Level One
Addenbrooke's Hospital
Cambridge CB2 2QQ

CHAPTER 7

The reproductive systems and the breast

Shirley Alexander (Part 1 The reproductive systems)
Joanna Parker (Part 2 The breast)

CHAPTER CONTENTS

PART 1
THE REPRODUCTIVE SYSTEMS 211
Introduction 211
Anatomy and physiology of the female reproductive system 211
Disorders of the menopause 217
Disorders of menstruation 218
Disorders of the male reproductive organs 227
Disorders of the female reproductive system 234
Gynaecological cancer 234
Benign tumours of the uterus 244
Benign tumours of the ovary 245
Ectopic pregnancy 246
Displacements of the uterus 247
Family planning services 249
Abortion 249
Childlessness 254
Embryo research 259
Glossary 260
References 260

PART 2
THE BREAST 263
Introduction 263
Anatomy and physiology of the breast 265
MALIGNANT DISORDERS OF THE BREAST AND THEIR SEQUELAE 266
Breast cancer 266
Metastatic breast cancer 276
Breast reconstruction 278
Lymphoedema in breast cancer 280
Malignant fungating breast tumours 282
BENIGN BREAST DISORDERS 287
Benign mammary dysplasia 287
Breast infections 288
Gynaecomastia 288
References 289
Further reading 289
Useful addresses 290

Part 1
THE REPRODUCTIVE SYSTEMS

INTRODUCTION

Human reproduction is a complex area, affected by inherited physical development, general health, personality characteristics of individuals, the country lived in, the influence of religion, social values, lifestyle, environmental hazards and the impact of public policies.

Some countries have major concerns about overpopulation and individuals may be urged to exert control over the number of children they have. Most women have little difficulty in becoming pregnant, but a minority of couples experience problems of infertility. Collaborative laboratory and surgical developments in techniques offer diagnostic investigations, conventional therapies, and, for some, in vitro fertilisation (IVF). Conversely, many young couples choose to remain childless, using contraception.

Human sexual behaviour is often publicly discussed by the media, highlighting the need for safe practice to protect from sexually transmitted diseases, particularly the serious threat of HIV infection. Unwanted pregnancies, and the rights of men, women and unborn children are all debated. The continuing problem of cancer, the potential for early detection through screening and the provision of necessary medical treatments are important.

This chapter seeks to present the functioning of the female reproductive system, to address disorders of the reproductive organs.

NB *The anatomy and physiology of the male reproductive system appears in Chapter 8.*

ANATOMY AND PHYSIOLOGY OF THE FEMALE REPRODUCTIVE SYSTEM

The primary function of the reproductive system is the propagation or continuation of the human species. Sexual drive and anticipated pleasure help to meet the reproductive need. The female reproductive system is structured to produce gametes (ova or eggs), to receive the penis of the male reproductive system during sexual intercourse, and facilitate the passage of sperm. It accommodates and promotes the growth of the embryo before birth and it feeds the new-born infant.

These complex functions are maintained by the following structures:

- *The internal organs,*
  - — the ovaries
  - — the uterus
  - — the uterine (fallopian) tubes (or oviducts)

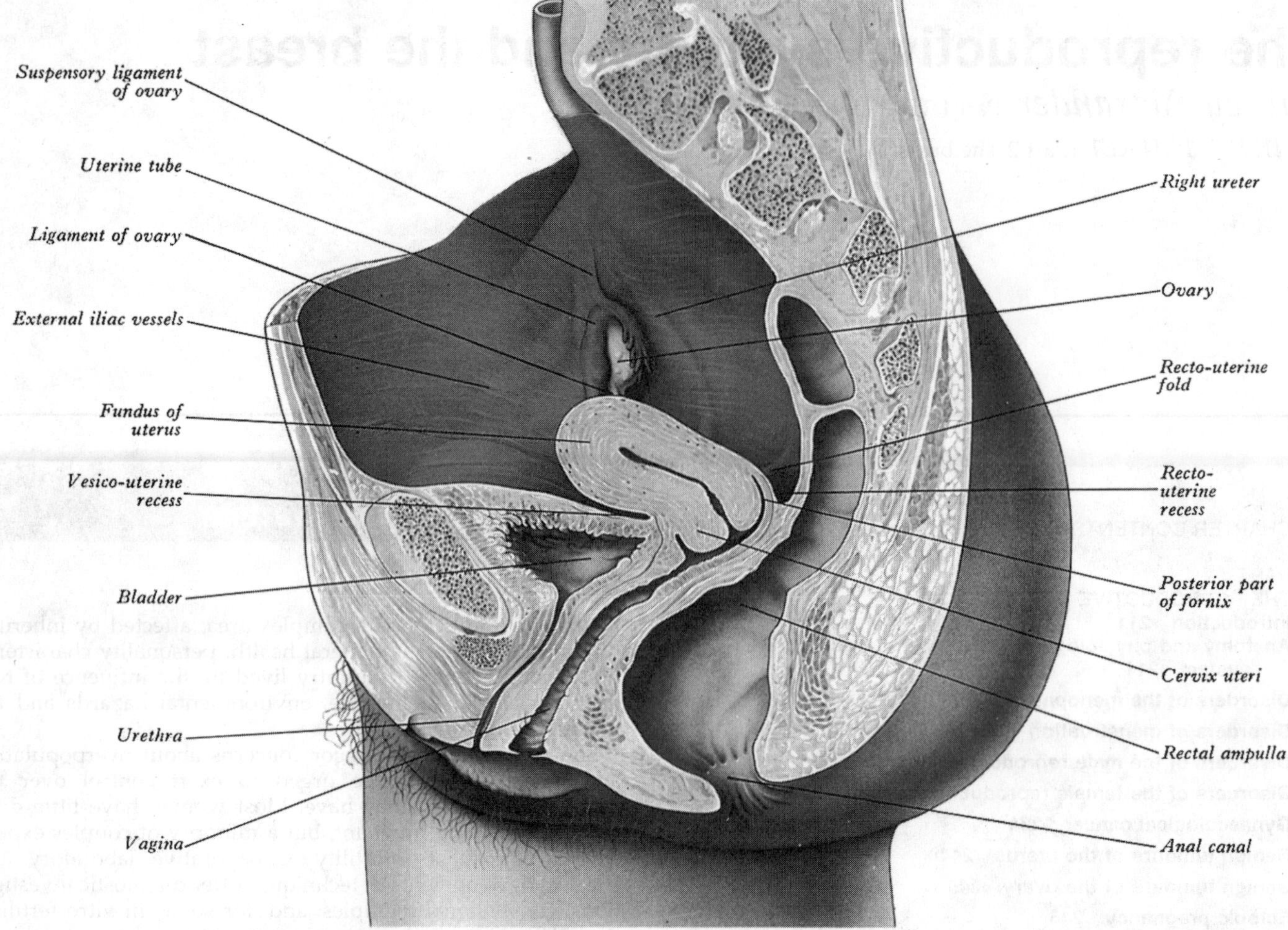

Fig. 7.1 The relationships of the female reproductive organs: sagittal section. (Reproduced with kind permission from Wilson (1990).)

— the vagina.

• *The external organs,*

— the vulva

— the mammary glands or breasts.

See Figures 7.1 and 7.2.

The male reproductive organs are described in Ch. 8.

The ovaries

All women have two ovaries, which are the size and shape of large almonds, one on either side of the uterus.

The surface of the ovary consists of a single layer of germinal epithelium. It surrounds the connective tissue that forms the stroma of the ovarian cortex and medulla.

The ovarian follicles develop in the cortex. A woman is born with approximately 100 000 follicles, although the number of follicles may reduce to approximately 30 000 by adolescence. Each follicle contains an immature ovum known as an oocyte.

The medulla, in the centre of the ovary, consists of fibrous connective tissue, blood vessels and nerves.

The production of ova and hormones

The ovary has two functions:

1. ovum production
2. internal secretion of hormones.

The ovarian cycle begins at around 12–13 years of age. Follicles begin to mature under the influence of the follicle stimulating hormone (FSH) and luteinising hormone (LH), released by the anterior pituitary gland. During the cycle, follicles can pass through five stages:

1. primary follicle: each oocyte is surrounded by a thin layer of epithelial cells
2. developing follicle: the follicular epithelium proliferates, the oocyte moves to a side position, and a fluid-filled cavity develops with the epithelium
3. mature (Graafian) follicle: the follicle reaches its maximum size
4. corpus luteum: formed after ovulation
5. corpus albicans (scar tissue).

See Figure 7.3.

The maturing follicle is surrounded by a layer of ovarian tissue, known as the theca. Several follicles may develop together but only one will mature fully, while the others regress. The mature follicle ruptures at the surface of the ovary and discharges the immature ovum and fluid into the peritoneal cavity. This is the process called 'ovulation'.

Wafting movements of the finger-like ends of the uterine tubes assist the transfer of the ovum into the tube (oviduct). It is thought that fertilisation of the ovum usually occurs in the ampulla of the uterine tube.

The ruptured follicle contracts around leaked blood after discharging the ovum. The epithelial cells (granulosa) multiply and form the corpus luteum. It synthesises steroid sex hormones for at least 8–10 days. If the ovum is not fertilised the corpus luteum degenerates, stops its hormone production, and forms scar tissue called the 'corpus albicans' near the surface of the ovary.

If the ovum is fertilised the corpus luteum continues to develop,

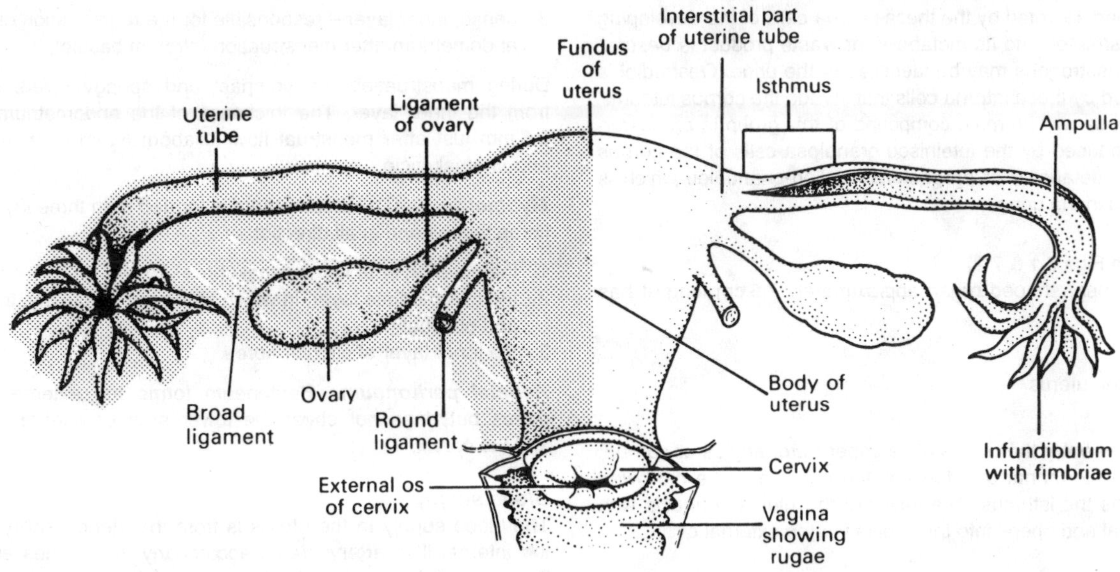

Fig. 7.2 The organs of the female reproductive system and attachments. (Reproduced with kind permission from Wilson (1990).)

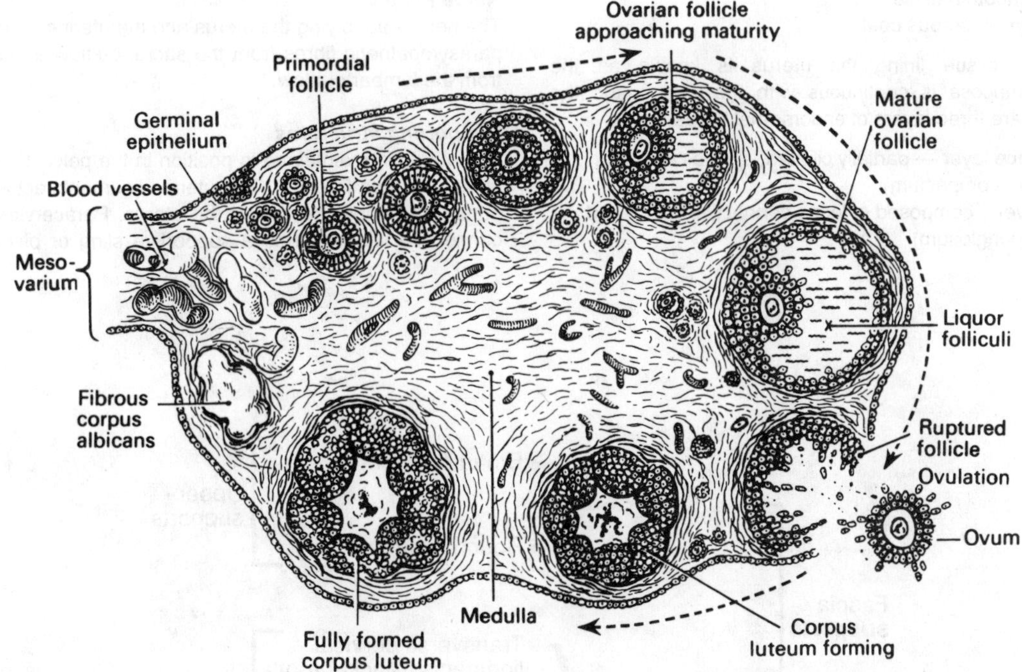

Fig. 7.3 Sequence of development of the ovarian cycle. (Reproduced with kind permission from Wilson (1990).)

increasing its size and hormone production for about 2 months, the period of implantation and development of the fertilised ovum in the uterus.

The secretion of hormones

The production of sex hormones is influenced by the hypothalamus of the brain. The hypothalamus produces gonadotrophin-releasing hormones, which stimulate the anterior pituitary gland to release follicle stimulating hormone (FSH) and luteinising hormone (LH).

During the monthly cycle the hypothalamus produces a regulatory factor called gonadotrophin-releasing factor (GnRF). This influences the release of follicle-stimulating hormone (FSH) and luteinising hormone (LH) from the anterior lobe of the pituitary gland, for their effect on the ovary. FSH stimulates the initial development of ovarian follicles and their secretion of oestrogen. LH stimulates further development of the ovarian follicles, initiates ovulation and incites production of ovarian hormones.

FSH and LH act on the ovary and control the secretion of two types of ovarian steroid hormones.

1. The oestrogens. Oestrogens are responsible for the development and maintenance of the female reproductive structures. The oestrogens have three main functions:
   1. development and maintenance of female reproductive structures
   2. control of fluid and electrolyte balance
   3. increase of protein anabolism.

The compound secreted by the theca interna cells of the developing follicle is *oestradiol*, and its metabolite or waste product is *oestriol.* Many other oestrogens may be identified in the urine. Oestradiol is also produced by theca interna cells that invade the corpus luteum.

2. The progestogens. The main compound of this group is *progesterone.* It is produced by the luteinised granulosa cells of the corpus luteum. The metabolite of progesterone is pregnanediol, which is also excreted in the urine.

The uterus (see Figs 7.1 & 7.2)
The uterus is a pear-shaped organ approximately 7.5 cm long. It has three parts:

1. the fundus
2. the body of the uterus
3. the cervix.

The uterine tubes enter the uterus at its upper outer angles or cornua. The body of the uterus narrows towards the cervix and the narrowed area is known as the isthmus. The cavity of the uterus connects with the cervical canal and opens into the vagina via the external os.

Structure
The uterus has three coats:

1. endometrium — mucous coat
2. myometrium — smooth muscle
3. parietal peritoneum — serous coat.

Endometrium. The tissue lining the uterus is known as the endometrium. This mucosa is continuous with the vagina and the uterine tubes. There are three layers of endometrial tissues:

1. the compact surface layer — partially ciliated, simple columnar epithelium (stratum compactum)
2. spongy middle layer – composed of loose connective tissue and glands (stratum spongiosum)
3. dense, inner layer – responsible for the regeneration of the endometrium after menstruation (stratum basale).

During menstruation the compact and spongy layers slough away from the inner layer. The thickness of the endometrium varies from 0.5 mm just after menstrual flow to about 5 mm near the end of the endometrial cycle.

Myometrium. The myometrium is formed from three layers of muscle fibres that extend in all directions:

1. the outer layer of longitudinal fibres
2. the intermediate layer, in which fibres run irregularly, transversely and obliquely
3. the inner layer of circular fibres.

Parietal peritoneum. Peritoneum forms the external coat of the uterus but does not cover the lower anterior quarter of the uterus and the cervix.

Blood supply
The blood supply to the uterus is from the uterine artery, a branch of the internal iliac artery. Veins accompany the arteries and drain into the internal iliac veins. Tortuous arterial vessels enter the layers of the uterine wall and divide up into capillaries between endometrial glands.

Nerve supply
The nerves supplying the uterus and the uterine tubes are formed from parasympathetic fibres from the sacral outflow and sympathetic fibres from the lumbar outflow.

Supporting structures
The uterus is maintained in position in the pelvis by fascia and muscle structures (see Fig. 7.4). The uterine ligaments act as 'guy ropes' supporting the upper section of the uterus. Paracervical tissue, fatty and connective tissue, forms a supportive sling or pivot about which the

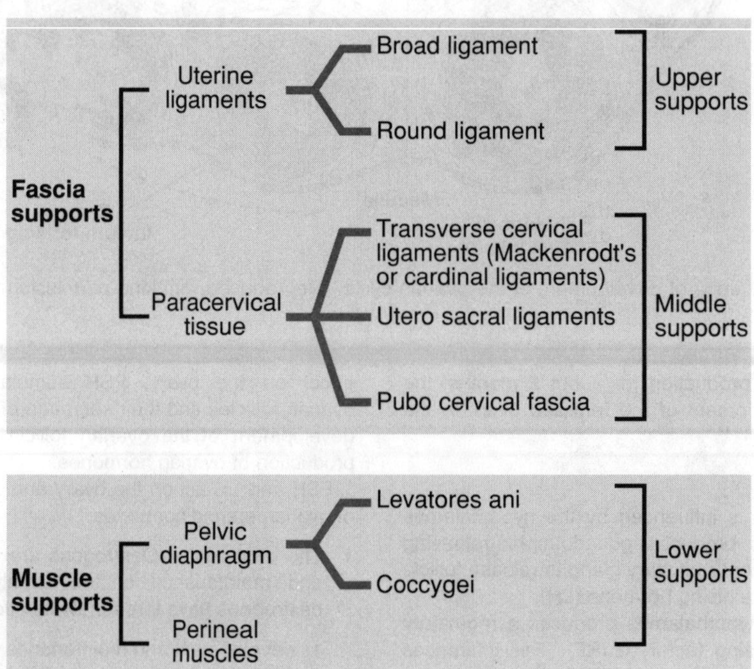

Fig. 7.4 The supports of the uterus.

uterus can rotate either backwards or forwards. This gives the uterus mobility anteriorly and posteriorly. Lateral and downward movement is limited by the muscles of the pelvic floor.

The axis of the vagina is considered to be a straight line that is related to the axis of the cervix. When the cervical axis is hinged anterior to the vaginal axis the uterus is 'anteverted' (see Fig. 7.5). This is the normal position of the uterus.

When the cervical axis is hinged backwards to lie posterior to the vaginal axis then the uterus is 'retroverted'. This can be a normal position for the uterus to occupy provided that the retroversion is mobile, and not fixed.

Functions

The functions of the uterus are:

- Menstruation — sloughing off of compact and spongy layers of endometrium attended by bleeding from torn vessels
- Maintenance of pregnancy — an embryo implants itself in the endometrium and takes all its nourishment throughout fetal life
- Initiation of labour — develops powerful, rhythmic contractions of the muscular wall for the birth of the infant.

The uterine tubes (fallopian tubes or oviducts)

The uterine tubes convey ova from the ovary to the uterus and carry sperm cells upwards to meet them. Fertilisation takes place in the uterine tube. The tube ends in tapering, finger-like projections of mucous membrane known as 'fimbriae'. These are freely mobile but are positioned close to the ovaries at the times of ovulation.

Each tube is a muscular channel lined with mucous membrane. The middle coat is muscular and the outer coat is of serous tissue. The mucous membrane layer is lined with columnar epithelium, mainly of ciliated cells that extend to the fimbriae. Their function is to produce ciliary current, which transports ova from the ovaries into the tube. Secretory cells are also present in the tubes but the action of their secretions is not fully understood, although they may be of importance where there are problems of infertility. The mucous membrane forms complicated longitudinal folds in the tubes. The transportation of ova occurs by a combination of ciliary and peristaltic action.

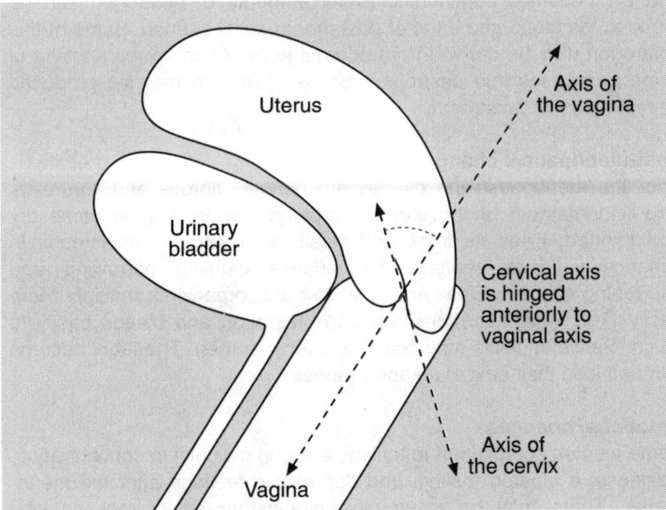

Fig. 7.5 The anteverted position of the uterus.

The vagina

The vagina is a fibromuscular channel extending from the cervix to the labia, thereby connecting the external and internal reproductive organs. It is capable of great distension and is composed mainly of smooth muscle with a lining of mucous membrane arranged in folds or rugae. In the virginal state, a fold of mucous membrane, the hymen, forms a border around the external opening of the vagina, partially closing the outlet.

Functions

The vagina functions to:

- receive the semen from the man
- serve as the lower part of the birth canal
- act as an excretory duct for uterine secretions and the menstrual flow.

The vulva

The vulva are the structures that form the female external genital organs, and consist of:

- the mons pubis
- the labia majora
- the labia minora
- the clitoris
- the urinary orifice (urethral)
- the vaginal orifice
- Bartholin's glands.

The endometrial cycle

The ovarian cycle and the endometrial cycle together constitute the menstrual cycle. The endometrial cycle is driven by the hormonal events of the ovarian cycle and can be divided into four phases:

- the menstrual phase
- the proliferative phase (follicular or pre-ovulatory)
- the secretory phase (luteal or post-ovulatory)
- the ischaemic phase.

The menstrual phase

Menstruation is believed to be caused by low levels of progesterone and oestrogens causing vasospasm of spiral arteries to the endometrium. The menstrual phase is a period of 3–6 days and is characterised by bleeding from the uterus. 50–60 ml of blood is lost at each menstrual period. Necrotic parts of the compact and spongy layers of endometrium slough away leaving a thin, bleeding area of tissue. By the third day of menstruation new epithelial cell growth has begun to cover the disorganised basal layer of endometrium. By the fifth day epithelium covers the whole surface.

The proliferative phase

The proliferative phase begins whilst bleeding is still continuing. It is a time of regrowth of endometrium under the control of oestradiol from the maturing follicle. The growth of epithelium, glands, blood vessels and connective tissue produce thickening of the endometrium. This phase extends to the fourteenth or fifteenth day of the cycle, when the peak of proliferation is reached.

The secretory phase

Soon after ovulation, glycoprotein secretory granules appear in the endometrium and can be seen, with an electron microscope, as large, clear vacuoles developing under the nuclei. Progesterone produced by the corpus luteum promotes the secretory phase. The endometrial glands become enlarged, the arteries coil, connective tissue hypertrophies, and tissues rich in glycogen become oedematous. The endometrium is now 5–6 mm in depth, 7–8 days following ovulation, in a state of readiness to implant a fertilised ovum. If implantation occurs the corpus luteum continues to produce progesterone and maintains the pregnancy. (See Fig. 7.6.)

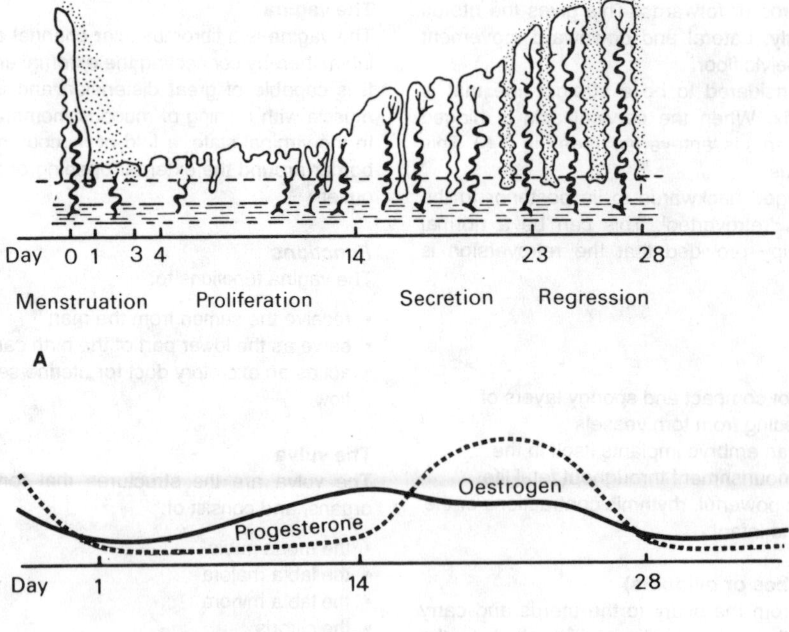

Fig. 7.6 The hormonal control of the menstrual cycle. (Reproduced with kind permission from Wilson 1990)

The ischaemic phase

In the absence of implantation, the corpus luteum degenerates and oestrogen and progesterone production declines. A leucocytic infiltration of the endometrium takes place, the stroma starts to disintegrate, oedema disappears and the endometrium shrinks. Vasoconstriction occurs. There is lack of nourishment to the endometrium and it begins to slough and separate and menstruation begins again, 14 (+/–1) days after ovulation. This time relationship is constant. Fluctuations in the length of the cycle occur in the *pre*-ovulatory phase, as follicles may not mature at the same rate each month. Thus there may be variation in the time of onset of menstruation. Most women establish an average pattern that is normal for each, although many young women have irregular patterns.

The menarche

A girl first menstruates, or reaches the menarche, within the age range of 9–16 years. Good nutrition and increased sexual awareness within the social environment may influence early sexual maturity and menstruation.

Some oestrogen synthesis stimulates early physical sexual changes to occur some time before the first menstruation. There may be follicular growth and some oestrogen withdrawal bleeding to give the early periods of the first few months. These periods are anovular, ovulation having not yet occurred. Such periods are painless. More discomfort may be experienced with the menstruation that follows ovulation.

A rise in basal temperature is a guide to whether ovulation has occurred, but it is not infallible.

Variation in menstrual cycle length occurs in response to significant life events. Excitement, stress, anxiety, or change of environment can delay the maturing of a follicle, ovulation, and menstruation. Travel through different time zones is known to disturb the menstrual pattern.

The climacteric and menopause

The climacteric refers to the time between the activity of the ovaries starting to diminish until menstruation ceases, and it may extend over 10 years. The mean age for cessation of periods is 51 years (Jaszman 1976). The date of the last menstrual period is the menopause, and is the defined end of female reproductive life.

When talking to someone about the climacteric, the normality of the stage of development needs to be emphasised. However, the need to maintain a positive outlook and to continue with activities should be encouraged. Some women regret their loss of fertility and perceive changes as the beginning of old age.

Gradual ovarian decline

Ovarian function begins to diminish from the age of 35 years. There is a general weakening of oestrogen and progesterone production. Ovarian cycles may become anovular many years before the menopause occurs. However, women between the ages of 40 and 45 years remain likely to become pregnant as regular ovulation may continue.

The ovaries begin to atrophy. The secretion of gonadotrophins FSH and LH becomes continuous. Small amounts of oestrogen can be found in the blood and urine of post-menopausal women. Some of this oestrogen may be derived from adrenal activity and the conversion of some androgens into oestrogen. Some oestrogen may be produced by residual ovarian stroma.

Post-menopausal changes

After the menopause the ovaries are densely fibrous and shrunken. The endometrium of the uterus atrophies, the vagina becomes dry and thinned, loses its folds and elasticity. There is an increase in connective tissue beneath the mucosa causing narrowing and shortening of the vagina. Acidity is lost and organisms multiply more easily. The vagina is more prone to ulceration and bleeds easily to touch. Senile vaginitis may occur in elderly women. The labia become thin and lose their sexual responsiveness.

Emotional changes

Some women complain of irritability, anxiety, difficulty in concentration, dizziness, a bloated feeling, and depressive feelings after the menopause. There may be many psychological or social reasons why women may feel emotionally disturbed.

It is difficult to establish a causal relationship between oestrogen deficiency and the emotional behaviour of women but the metabolic products of oestrogen, the catecholestrogens may have a secondary regulatory role in neurotransmitter activities that influence mood and feelings of well-being (Notelovitz 1986).

Hot flash/flush patterns

The 'hot flash' or 'hot flush' is regarded by many as the only true sign of the menopause. The woman may subjectively experience a sensation of extreme warmth which is quickly followed by flushing of the face and chest. This is caused by dilation of the blood vessels to the skin and an increased blood flow. The flush is usually accompanied by sweating, palpitations, dizziness and nausea. Shivering is often reported after the flush, probably due to compensatory constriction of the blood vessels. Hot flushes and sweats are embarrassing and uncontrollable and are experienced by 75% of women, many of whom receive no special treatment.

Although research has varied findings regarding any relationship between low levels of oestrogens and hot flushes, the relationship is reinforced by the improvement in symptoms with oestrogen therapy. Symptoms recurred when patients were given placebos in blind cross-over studies (Notelovitz 1986). (See Box 7.1.)

Uterine bleeding patterns

The climacteric is characterised by irregular menstruation. Periods may become scanty, or bleeding may be heavy. The menstrual cycle shortens, associated with a decrease in oestradiol secretion. As this continues LH levels rise, then menstrual cycles lengthen.

Anovulatory cycles result in oestrogen-withdrawal bleeding patterns, irregular cycles with intermittent and prolonged spotting (low oestrogen profile) or prolonged amenorrhoea followed by sudden, profuse bleeding (high oestrogen profile).

DISORDERS OF THE MENOPAUSE

Osteoporosis and atherosclerosis

Some of the consequences of decreased oestrogen formation are that it is known to play a significant part in the development of osteoporosis, myocardial infarction, angina and stroke. Gynaecologists may not always anticipate or recognise the conditions, as patients are usually in the care of physicians or orthopaedic specialists.

Box 7.1 Hot flush changes

A technique has been standardised for the continuous recording of skin temperature and conductance. Meldrum et al (1979) showed the first change was an increase in perspiration (conductance), followed by a rise in finger temperature and then a decrease in the central core (ear drum) temperature.

The mean temperature increase during the flush was 2.7°C and lasted an average 3.1 minutes. The subjective 'flash' was usually noted a minute before and ended a minute after the temperature rise, and lasted an average 2.6 minutes.

Consistently correlated with patients' subjective feelings was change in:

- conductance — 98%
- skin — 82%
- core temperature — 81%.

There was a marked increase in the blood flow of the hand, with the onset of symptoms. This was sustained for 3–4 minutes, with return to control level 6 minutes after symptoms abated. The blood pressure was unaltered during the flush. It was suggested that the flush occurred because of a downward setting of the hypothalamic temperature-regulating centre. The reason for change was unknown.

Caucasian and oriental women are more at risk of developing these conditions. Contributory factors include:

- inherited factors
- sedentary lifestyle
- low calcium intake
- cigarette smoking
- excessive salt intake
- excessive stress
- high protein
- alcohol
- fibre
- caffeine intake.

Decreased oestrogen levels have been shown to result in accelerated loss of bone (Nagant de Deux chaisnes 1983). Oestrogens determine the sensitivity of bone to parathyroid hormone and increase calcium absorption from the gut. People who lose bone mass rapidly have also been shown to have lower progesterone than those who lose bone slowly.

It is important for conditions of osteopenia (reduced bone mass) to be recognised early as it can be reversed. By the time osteoporosis is recognised, bone mass is reduced to the point of fractures occurring and the condition is irreversible.

Bone loss after the menopause may be related to failure to achieve maximum skeletal mass in early adulthood which becomes aggravated by oestrogen deprivation.

The incidence of hip fractures is between 70–80 per 100 000 women per year, in the UK. This makes the prevention of osteoporosis an urgent medical problem for many thousands of women.

Medical and nursing treatment of post-menopausal changes

As no other mammal shows loss of fertility with ageing, gynaecologists consider the climacteric to be an unnatural state that has arisen because women now live longer, and that women should therefore be helped to overcome this state counteracting their oestrogen deficiency.

Unpleasant symptoms, such as headaches, poor quality sleep, hot flushes or heavy bleeding at times of menstruation, that are severe enough for them to visit their doctor, are experienced by 25% of menopausal women. Some GPs prescribe hormone replacement therapy (HRT) directly; others refer women to menopause clinics, which have become established in many hospitals throughout the UK. A gynaecologist will assess the need for treatment, and a clinical nurse specialist may be available to provide information and counselling.

Non-oestrogen replacement therapy. Non-oestrogen drugs have been tested for their effect on hot flushes. Such drugs potentially carry less risk of cancer of the breast or endometrium than may be developed from oestrogen therapy. Drugs used include ethamsylate, principally for the treatment of heavy menstrual bleeding, propranolol, naproxen and, most effectively, progestogens such as norethisterone.

Oestrogen replacement therapy. Although oestrogen deficiency may not be the triggering cause of hot flushes, studies show that their incidence could be significantly reduced by oestrogen treatment (Coope et al, 1975 and Campbell & Whitehead, 1977).

Oestrogen may be administered orally, vaginally, through the skin by means of skin patches, or by subcutaneous implant. Orally, the oestrogen passes through the liver before entering the general circulation. The other routes avoid the liver, and potentially reduce risk of disturbed liver functioning.

Oestrogen is known to increase the risk of cancer in oestrogen-sensitive organs such as the endometrium and the breast, so modern therapies now combine oestrogen with progestogen. (See Research Abstract 7.1.)

Research Abstract 7.1 Study of treatment of hot flushes with oestrogen

A 4-month and a 12-month crossover study of women with hot flushes (Campbell & Whitehead 1977) found a statistically significant reduction in hot flushes during oestrogen therapy using Premarin 1.25 mg, compared to a placebo. The studies confirmed the powerful therapeutic response in those who received the placebo first but invariably the switch from oestrogen to placebo caused a rapid return of flushing.

Campbell S & Whitehead M I 1977 Oestrogen therapy and the menopausal syndrome. In: Greenblatt R & Studd J (eds) 1977 The menopause: clinics in obstetrics in obstetrics and gynaecology. W B Saunders, London

Hormone replacement therapy (HRT). Currently, long-term hormone replacement therapy is prescribed as a combination drug that includes both oestrogen and progestogen. The progestogen restores or prolongs monthly bleeding in postmenopausal women, which protects the endometrium from potentially carcinomatous change. Research evidence of causal links between hormone replacement and tumour formation is controversial. A general approach to HRT is now taken by GPs. (See Research Abstract 7.2.)

Short-term therapy is justifiable for specific menopause symptoms such as hot flushes and atrophic vaginitis, for as long as treatment is required.

Long-term therapy is needed by women under 40 years of age who have experienced a premature menopause, perhaps following hysterectomy and removal of ovaries, and those diagnosed at risk of osteoporosis with low bone mineral content at the time of the menopause.

Research Abstract 7.2 Transdermal administration of oestrogen/progestogen hormone replacement therapy

Sixteen symptomatic, postmenopausal patients (median age 54.1 years) applied oestradiol transdermal therapeutic system (TTS) 50 mg per day for 14 days, by the application of patches to the buttocks. They were then given two combined norethisterone acetate–oestradiol patches (approximately 50 mg of oestradiol and 0.2–0.3 mg of norethisterone) daily for a further 14 days. The treatment was repeated for five cycles. All but one of the patients had regular withdrawal bleeding.

Fourteen patients had endometrial biopsy samples taken during the fifth treatment cycle. No sample showed proliferative or hyperplastic features.

The patients also underwent metabolic studies. The effects of transdermal norethisterone acetate on postmenopausal symptoms of hot flushes, night sweats, and vaginal dryness, and on lipid metabolism and psychological status, were determined by comparing effects in the oestrogen-only phase and in the combined phase. The effects were very mild. Three patients experienced skin irritation.

The findings show that transdermal progestogen, at a lower dosage, can be successfully administered in hormone replacement therapy to prevent endometrial proliferation while minimising the adverse effects that may be seen with oral administration.

A small number of patients participated in this preliminary study. Caution is therefore needed in drawing broad conclusions.

Whitehead M I, Fraser D, Schenkel L, Crook J & Stevenson J C 1990 Transdermal administration of oestrogen/progestogen hormone replacement therapy. Lancet 335: 310–312

Informed request. Whilst not recommending HRT for all postmenopausal women, it is not justifiable to withhold treatment from a fully informed patient who requests it, as there are virtually no contra-indications to therapy. HRT will only be fully evaluated after a further two decades of use (Purdie 1990).

Menopause clinics. Many hospitals now provide menopause clinics that are staffed by a gynaecologist with a special interest in the management of problems associated with the menopause. Specially trained nurses and paramedical personnel contribute to the overall assessment and care of those attending the clinics and keep the costs of the service at a reasonable level.

Treatments can be more easily controlled and supervised within such a clinic; protocols are established; dietetic and diagnostic facilities are more available; and screening, general health and patient-education programmes can be introduced.

NURSING PRIORITIES AND MANAGEMENT: THE MENOPAUSE

The role of the nurse involves the development of trust within the nurse–patient relationship. The educative and supportive aspects of the self-care nursing model (Orem 1991) are useful. The nurse needs to:

- establish by open questioning what the patient is most worried about
- use a counselling approach to respond to patient's expression of feelings
- provide information about self-help in overcoming hot flushes and sweating by discussing
  - — wearing cotton, rather than nylon, loose clothing, and short sleeves rather than long
  - — reducing the layers of clothing worn
  - — avoiding wearing of bra or pantie-girdle
  - — reducing layers of bedding, or using a duvet with a low tog rating
  - — sleeping with a bedroom window open
  - — keeping living and working areas at a lower air temperature
  - — taking cool showers, twice a day rather than a hot bath
  - — minimising alcohol intake, hot curries, and foods containing ginger
  - — using self relaxation techniques
- give dietary information to encourage selecting low-fat, calcium-rich foods
  - — explain physiological links to vascular conditions, and the maintenance of bone mineral content
- check the patient's usual physical exercise pattern; reinforce the need for regular exercise, stressing the importance of the pull of muscle on bone for bone formation and health
- discuss the possible side effects of HRT
- explain the need for self-examination of breasts and teach the technique
- provide opportunities for questions
- check the patient's understanding of the information given by encouraging feedback
- give the patient a copy of the HEA (HEB in Scotland) leaflets on 'The Menopause'
- give the patient the name and telephone number of a person to contact in the event of any problem occurring.

DISORDERS OF MENSTRUATION

Gynaecology means the study of woman. It includes evaluating normal and abnormal functions and the treatment of disorders.

Amenorrhoea

Amenorrhoea means the absence of menstruation or the failure to commence menstruation.

During the menstrual life of the woman if two period cycles or more are missed then amenorrhoea may be said to exist. This often means that the woman may wait until menstruation has been absent for a year before seeking investigation. Secondary sexual development is usually complete in girls by the age of 16 years and menstruation is the last sign to appear. A delay in the onset of menstruation may be a cause of concern. There may be an anatomical fault or some disturbance in hormonal secretions.

Primary amenorrhoea is where a woman has never menstruated at any age.

Secondary amenorrhoea refers to the cessation of periods after menstruation has begun.

Physiological amenorrhoea

PHYSIOLOGY

Inheritance, race, climate and general nutrition influence when menstruation begins. The potential for maturation of ovarian tissue is in place before birth.

After puberty, full regulation of ovarian activities by the hypothalamic and pituitary gland functioning is achieved and menstrual cycles are established, but exactly when is unpredictable.

MEDICAL MANAGEMENT

A parent may take a teenage girl to see her GP because of concern over delay in the onset of menstruation. The daughter may compare her own late development with that of a sister or her peers at school and may feel abnormal. The doctor may undertake a general physical examination to be able to reassure the patient that other secondary sex characteristics are already present and that the onset of menstruation will follow in due course. Advice can be given about reducing anxiety, which may delay the onset of menstruation.

If secondary sex characteristics or menstruation fail to develop, the doctor will refer the young woman to a consultant gynaecologist and endocrinologist, for a programme of investigations.

During pregnancy

PHYSIOLOGY

After ovulation has occurred, the lining cells of the ovarian follicle are stimulated by LH to develop the corpus luteum, which produces progesterone that, in turn, stimulates the endometrium and its secretory glands into a state of readiness to receive the fertilised ovum from the uterine tube. When the fertilised ovum becomes embedded in the wall of the uterus it produces the hormone human chorionic gonadotrophin (HCG). This hormone enables the corpus luteum to continue its production of progesterone for 3–4 months until the placenta grows and produces its own progesterone and oestrogen. The presence of the growing foetus and the continued production of progesterone prevents the loss of endometrium and the menstrual flow.

MEDICAL MANAGEMENT

The doctor usually confirms a pregnancy by vaginal examination and abdominal palpation. The uterus is found to be increased in size. HCG levels in the urine provide a positive diagnosis when a test for pregnancy is completed in the clinic or laboratory.

During lactation

PHYSIOLOGY

Mothers who are totally breast feeding a baby would not ovulate or menstruate during the first 6 months after the birth. Total nipple stimulation is needed and is important for suppression of ovarian function. Breast feeding therefore exerts a measure of birth control, but only intensive, exclusive breast feeding will produce a failure rate below 2%.

The suckling stimulus to the nipple leads to a neurohormonal reflex production of prolactin by the anterior pituitary gland. It is the maintenance of high circulating levels of prolactin that inhibits gonadotrophin hormone release and prevents ovulation and menstruation. A poor state of nutrition in the mother is also known to inhibit ovulation particularly in developing countries (Lunn et al 1980, 1981; Lunn 1992).

Suppression of the ovaries declines where supplements comprise more than 50% of the diet of the baby who is breast feeding. The incidence of ovulation and the risk of pregnancy then rise rapidly.

Hartmann (1991) states that fertility may return as early as 2 weeks after birth in some women who are fully breastfeeding their infants.

MEDICAL MANAGEMENT

The doctor or health visitor will recommend a barrier method such as the condom or cap during the breast-feeding period, rather than the contraceptive pill.

After the menopause

The menopause occurs on the date of the woman's final menstrual period and may not be fully acknowledged until a year without periods has passed. Most women pass this milestone without regrets and without unpleasant physical symptoms.

MEDICAL MANAGEMENT

Medical intervention is required only if the woman experiences physical discomforts such as hot flushes, headaches or sweating. The possible treatments are described earlier in this chapter.

Pathological amenorrhoea

Uterine lesions, congenital abnormalities

PATHOPHYSIOLOGY

The uterus may exist only as a nodule of fibromuscular tissue at the top of the vagina, causing primary, permanent amenorrhoea.

Congenital absence of uterus and vagina may occur, although ovaries and secondary sex characteristics have developed.

Primary deficiency of endometrium. A diagnostic test can be performed by giving ethinyl oestradiol 0.05 mg by mouth, twice a day for 21 days. If withdrawal bleeding occurs within 7–10 days then there is not a failure of endometrium but probably failure of stimulation by the ovaries.

If there is no bleeding, an endometrium problem exists. It may be absent, deficient or unable to be stimulated by oestrogen. In this case, the amenorrhoea is entirely of uterine origin.

Ovarian lesions

Failure of normal development is a rare condition of the ovary. Chromosomal abnormalities such as Turner's syndrome, may occur.

PATHOPHYSIOLOGY

Turner's syndrome is a condition that results from the absence of one female chromosome. The chromosome complement is written as 45XO. The woman is reported to be 'chromatin negative'. The condition shows infantile development of the genitalia, absence of breasts, short stature and a webbed neck. Congenital cardiac lesions may be associated with it.

MEDICAL MANAGEMENT

Treatment is to induce sexual maturation by administering oestrogen. Ethinyl oestradiol, 0.01 mg twice daily, in 3-week cycles is given for several months, then norethisterone is added for the last 10 days of each cycle.

Arrhenoblastoma

PATHOPHYSIOLOGY

Arrhenoblastoma is a masculinising tumour of the ovary, which may cause amenorrhoea because of the high production of androgenic hormones. Most ovarian tumours, even if they are bilateral, do not usually destroy all active ovarian tissue and so would not usually cause amenorrhoea.

MEDICAL MANAGEMENT

Surgical removal of the ovary is the treatment for this condition.

Surgical removal of both ovaries, bilateral oophorectomy, which may be associated with the removal of the uterus and fallopian tubes, will result in amenorrhoea.

Effects of irradiation. Irradiation of the ovaries directly for the treatment of tumour, or indirect irradiation from treatment of other pelvic organs, bladder or rectum may cause amenorrhoea. Accidental irradiation may occur in women whose work exposes them to radiation sources.

Pituitary disorders

See also Chapter 5.

Deficiency of gonadotrophin secretion may occur without there being deficiencies of other trophic hormones. No cause may be found but it is often associated with emotional responses.

Infantilism may result from congenital failure of the pituitary gland, which results in dwarfism, lack of sexual development and amenorrhoea. Follicle stimulating hormone (FSH) is absent or low. Oestrogens may be undetectable in the urine.

Frohlich syndrome is a disturbance of the hypothalamus, which results in underdevelopment of genital tissues, amenorrhoea, obesity, hirsutism and retardation of mental responses.

Ischaemic necrosis of pituitary tissue may result from thrombosis of pituitary vessels following profound shock and anaemia, often due to severe post-partum haemorrhage. The production of trophic hormones ceases or is reduced. The condition is characterised by lethargy, weight gain, reduced metabolic rate, hypotension and amenorrhoea. Hormone therapy gives some psychological benefit only, by withdrawal bleeding effects.

New growths of the pituitary cause acromegaly, and amenorrhoea, with signs of Cushing's syndrome due to effects on the suprarenal glands.

Other endocrine disorders

Adrenogenital syndrome results from overactivity of the adrenal cortex due to the presence of a tumour or hyperplasia. Excessive production of androgens occurs, giving signs of virilism: a deepening voice, hirsuteness, an enlarged clitoris and the development of acne and amenorrhoea.

Cushing's syndrome is caused by hyperplasia of the adrenal cortex, which leads to an excess of glucocorticoids, stimulating the conversion of protein into carbohydrate. Obesity, glycosuria, hypertension, increased androgen activity and amenorrhoea from regressive changes in the genital organs are the main features of the condition.

The following disorders may also be accompanied by amenorrhoea:

- Addison's disease
- myxoedema
- thyrotoxicosis
- diabetes mellitus.

Emotional stress

PATHOPHYSIOLOGY

Emotional disturbance is likely to affect menstrual function through the hypothalamic–pituitary axis. The hypothalamus controls the output of gonadotrophins from the pituitary gland. Emotional distress caused by some traumatic event, receiving bad news, being involved in a major disaster such as a bombing incident or earthquake, may contribute to amenorrhoea.

If a woman has sexual intercourse without contraception, the fear of becoming pregnant may itself cause temporary amenorrhoea.

MEDICAL MANAGEMENT

Following discussion with the doctor, it is expected that the patient will understand and be reassured about the effects of stress on menstruation. When she makes a positive adjustment to the critical event that has preceded the problem, physical and mental relaxation will promote a spontaneous return of menstruation.

Anorexia nervosa

See also Chapter 5.

PATHOPHYSIOLOGY

Anorexia nervosa is a psychiatric illness characterised by extreme weight loss and dislike for foods, particularly carbohydrates. It occurs most commonly in adolescent girls and is associated with dieting routines and distortion of body image. There is failure in hypothalamic stimulation of luteinising hormone release. Amenorrhoea occurs.

MEDICAL MANAGEMENT

Patient management may initially be carried out by a physician who has been investigating the patient's weight loss but, when a diagnosis is made, care is usually maintained by a psychiatrist. A behavioural therapy programme is negotiated with the patient to ensure an improvement in food intake, whilst a cognitive therapist may assist her to think more rationally and improve her feelings of self-esteem and body image. Positive physical and psychological changes can promote a return to menstruation.

Psychotic illness

PATHOPHYSIOLOGY

Psychotic illness may be a cause of amenorrhoea. The person with a schizophrenic reaction may not menstruate for many months or years.

Crisis life events may contribute to disturbances in the activity of neurotransmitter catecholamines in the brain. The chemistry of the hypothalamic–pituitary axis may be disrupted, resulting in amenorrhoea.

MEDICAL MANAGEMENT

The psychiatrist would check that a pregnancy has not developed in the patient with a psychotic reaction. A reliable source of information will be needed, whether the patient herself or her partner. A laboratory pregnancy test may be necessary. The acute symptoms of the patient's illness may be treated by neuroleptic drugs or psychotherapeutic intervention. A return of the normal menstruation pattern would be expected when the body chemistry becomes more stable.

Severe general illness

PATHOPHYSIOLOGY

The stress of severe illness may induce ineffective functioning in multiple body organs and may temporarily suppress menstrual function. Stress, as experienced in refugee or prisoner-of-war camps, where it is associated with malnutrition, minimal protein and vitamin intake, will lead to amenorrhoea.

MEDICAL MANAGEMENT

The amenorrhoea is secondary to the general illness. Thus the particular illness condition must be treated before the amenorrhoea can be relieved. The influences of emotional and physical stress are complex and sometimes assisting the patient to relax and lower anxiety levels may promote menstruation before the general illness is fully relieved.

NURSING PRIORITIES AND MANAGEMENT: AMENORRHOEA

The nurse may be caring for a patient in any of the hospital specialities or in the community and the nursing management of amenorrhoea will be similar.

Nursing assessment

As part of routine assessment of the patient the nurse should ask about the date of the last menstrual period, and whether any problems are experienced with menstruation.

As the patient shares information, the nurse should be able to establish how the patient feels about the amenorrhoea that is described and how anxious she feels, using a scale of 0–8 (0 = no anxiety, 8 = most severe anxiety). The patient may not regard amenorrhoea as a problem. The nurse should ask whether the patient has any knowledge of the reason for the absence of menstruation.

Care planning

In negotiation with the patient, the nurse should plan time to give her information about the absence of menstruation. This can perhaps be associated with potential worries about the illness condition.

The patient's level of anxiety should be documented in the plan. The nurse may wish to emphasise the need to induce self-relaxation, and must be able to teach a simple relaxation exercise. Relaxation exercise audiotapes may be available from the physiotherapy department, occupational therapy or the department of clinical psychology.

Evaluation of care

The patient's long-term goal of 'a return of the menstrual period' may not be achievable within the early weeks of care and should be modified to include a short-term realistic target. Nurse and patient should negotiate a goal statement, for example, 'Julie will explain that her anxiety is reduced to 0–2 on an anxiety rating scale of 0–8'.

This goal should be evaluated daily, to check on the response to self-relaxation activity during the first 2 days of care. The patient may need more help from the nurse before she can relax fully when alone. New target times for evaluation of goal achievement will then need to be set. Therapeutic weekly evaluations may be needed until anxiety is greatly reduced.

The patient should be asked to let the nurse know if she does begin to menstruate during her stay. Achievement of such a long-term goal may occur due to medical treatments, particularly if hormonal or anxiolytic sedative drugs have been prescribed.

Cryptomenorrhoea

This is a condition of concealed menstruation.

PATHOPHYSIOLOGY

Menstrual fluid is retained in the body where there is an obstruction to the outflow. There is an accumulation of blood in the vagina (haematocolpos), which distends it. The whole pelvis may become congested, with blood in the uterine tubes (haemosalpinx), and displacement of pelvic structures. There is usually a congenital cause with incomplete canalisation of the lower end of the Mullerian cords, with intact hymen. There may be a complete absence of the vagina or cervical stenosis after cautery to the cervix or amputation of the cervix.

MEDICAL MANAGEMENT

The condition is relieved by drainage.

NURSING PRIORITIES AND MANAGEMENT: CRYPTOMENORRHOEA

Assessment

The patient is expected as an emergency admission to hospital, and an early transfer to the operating theatre. The nurse assessing the patient on admission will encounter the following symptoms:

- pelvic pain
- potential retention of urine from pressure on the urethra by distended pelvic structures
- anxiety about the condition, the strange environment and unknown procedures
- a need for safe-preoperative preparation.

Care planning

If time allows before transfer to the operating theatre, the relief of the patient's pain will be a priority, according to medical prescription.

A comforting, positive attitude of open regard shown by the nurse may help the patient feel less anxious. Giving information will prepare the patient for the procedures to be expected before surgery and in the first 24 hours after the operation. See Chapter 27.

A urethral catheter may be introduced unless there is an obstruction of the urethra. An empty bladder facilitates the work of the surgeon and reduces risk of injury to the bladder.

Post-operative care

This will ensure the patient's safe recovery from anaesthesia and that pain is fully relieved. The patient's vaginal blood loss will be observed and documented.

The patient should quickly recover, without any complications of anaesthesia or surgery.

Full information should be given about the surgery completed and expectations for future progress.

Evaluation of care

The patient should quickly achieve outcomes of:

- being free from pain
- minimal blood loss, reducing daily
- being free from nausea or vomiting
- return to self-care activities within 24 hours
- no hospital-acquired infection
- be able to explain, before discharge, the action to be taken if the condition recurs
- be discharged within 4 days or less, with an outpatient clinic appointment for 1 month's time.

If these outcomes are not achieved then discharge will be delayed whilst care is modified, until the patient's condition improves.

Abnormal uterine bleeding

Abnormal uterine bleeding is described according to the rhythm or pattern of the blood loss-episodes:

Menorrhagia which refers to heavy or profuse menstrual bleeding. The flow of blood occurs at normal intervals but is increased in amount or duration; menorrhagia is the most commonly used term

Polymenorrhoea which describes menstrual periods that occur with a frequency of less than 21 days

Polymenorrhagia refers to periods that are both heavy and frequent

Metrorrhagia describes irregular or unusual bleeding from the uterus between periods

Dysfunctional uterine bleeding is the descriptive diagnosis used when no organic cause for the abnormal bleeding can be identified.

When abnormal uterine bleeding occurs, the passing of blood clots from the uterus is significant. The menstrual flow is greater than normal if the usual anti-clotting agents released by the endometrium are not able to control the volume or rate of flow of the blood.

Menorrhagia

PATHOPHYSIOLOGY

Hormonal imbalance from any variation in the pattern of oestrogen and progesterone secretion, usually of endocrine origin with over-secretion of gonadotrophins. Emotional stress may result in excesses of these hormones being produced.

Ovarian lesions are of two types.

Polycystic growths may disturb the normal production of ovarian hormones and excessive endometrial growth occurs.

Immature follicles may fail to result in ovulation. The corpus luteum fails to form so progesterone cannot be produced. Oestrogen levels continue to rise and there is a proliferation of the endometrium.

Uterine lesions consist of the following types.

Fibroids increase the surface area of the endometrium that bleeds with greater flow. The myoma may prolong the flow by restricting or disturbing contractions.

Polyps increase the surface area of endometrium.

Adenomyosis interferes with contractions by infiltrating the myometrium with endometrial cells.

Multiparity. Someone who has had several normal pregnancies, may have loss of tone in the uterine muscle fibres. These may be replaced by fibrous tissue which will interfere in the normal contractions.

Developmental disorders, such as a bicornuate, septate, or duplicated uterus, may impede contractions.

Endometriosis, a condition in which ectopic endometrium develops. Endometrial tissue may be found in the muscle wall or in scattered areas of the pelvic cavity. An increased blood supply to the uterus results.

Tumour formation will increase blood supply and bleeding.

Intrauterine contraceptive devices cause some irritation of the endometrium and the uterus attempts to rid itself of the foreign body. Excessive bleeding may be problematic during the first 3 months after insertion.

Fallopian tubal ligation involves some alteration in the course of blood vessels that increases uterine blood supply. Following the operation menstruation is usually heavier and may lead to the need for hysterectomy in some women.

MEDICAL MANAGEMENT

Medical examination seeks evidence of stress, worry or tension in the patient and will try to establish whether bleeding is a problem of quantity, rhythm, or both. Pelvic examination may reveal tenderness, masses, or irregularities. If no pelvic abnormality is found, then a provisional diagnosis of dysfunctional uterine bleeding is made.

Investigations. Special investigation is made of haemoglobin level and full blood count to assess any anaemia present. An examination is carried out under anaesthetic (EUA) and a diagnostic curettage is performed to show the endometrial response to hormones and to exclude carcinoma. The curettage may identify uterine polyps. An estimation of urinary gonadotrophins, oestrogens and progestogens as indicators of hormonal activity may be completed.

Treatment. Depending upon the amount of blood lost it may be necessary to nurse the patient in bed and to administer an anxiolytic sedative drug as prescribed to encourage relaxation and reduce stress responses. Any anaemia identified would be corrected as appropriate. The dilatation and curettage investigation may in itself relieve the problem. Hormone therapy may be given. Progesterone may be prescribed to seek a balance with oestrogens and reduce excessive endometrial growth. One of the combined contraceptive pills may be given to suppress hormone production. Norethisterone 10–20 mg daily for 10 days, from the 15th day of the cycle. Progestogen administration will modify flow in heavy, but regular, cycles and acts as a haemostatic in dysfunctional uterine haemorrhage.

Where hormone therapy is unsuitable and large fibroids or endometriosis exists, then a hysterectomy is performed. Alternatively, in a myomectomy, the fibroids may be shelled out of the myometrium, particularly to preserve the uterus for child-bearing in a younger woman.

Metrorrhagia

PATHOPHYSIOLOGY

Lowered oestrogen level may occur just prior to the formation of the corpus luteum, resulting in vaginal blood spotting at the time of ovulation.

Changes in the cervix, for example, inflammation, erosion, polyps or carcinoma may cause slight bleeding, especially after intercourse or vaginal examination.

Changes in the vagina, for example, inflammation, ulceration and atrophy may cause bleeding.

New growth. Endometrial carcinoma is a major cause of irregular bleeding.

Complications of an early pregnancy. As an ovum settles into the endometrium slight bleeding may occur. This loss may be repeated during several months of the pregnancy. Haemorrhage might also occur due to an abnormal positioning of the placenta, known as 'placenta praevia'.

MEDICAL MANAGEMENT

Investigations. A visual examination of the vagina and cervix with a lighted vaginal speculum is usually an early investigation. A more detailed examination is possible with binocular magnifying microscopy, using the colposcope apparatus and completing the colposcopy examination. Magnification of the cervix allows for early diagnosis of cervical neoplasia through observation of the epithelial vascular pattern, surface contour and colour, which change with the neoplastic process. In 95% of patients, pre-malignant intra-epithelial neoplasia is visible only through the colposcope.

Punch biopsies are taken for histological examination. The cytology laboratory examination of tissue complements the colposcopy observations. The Papanicolaou smear test is a routine investigation to evaluate changes in cells shed or scraped from the cervix. A high vaginal swab of secretions will allow the identification of bacterial infection, fungal or parasitic infestations. The dilatation and curettage operation will provide evidence to support any further investigations that may be necessary.

Treatment. Infections of the reproductive tract will be treated with the broad spectrum antibiotic to which the organism is sensitive. Infestation with vaginal thrush, candidiasis, is relieved by nystatin pessaries. Trichomonas vaginalis is treated with metronidazole (Flagyl).

In ovulation spotting, small quantities of oestrogen may be given for 6–7 days, 3 days before ovulation.

Any malignant changes that are identified are usually treated by surgical excision, following which radiotherapy or cytotoxic drug treatment may be advised.

Dysmenorrhoea

Dysmenorrhoea is pain associated with menstruation. Most women experience some discomfort at the time of menstruation. Before the start of the period, the breasts may feel larger and ache, there may also be feelings of abdominal distension, constipation may be a problem, and the woman may feel unwell. The symptoms may persist for 1–2 days and are relieved or replaced by the symptoms of backache, frequency of passing urine and loose bowel action, with the onset of menstruation.

For some women, the first hours or the first day is most painful. Dragging sensations from the umbilical area down to the groins and thighs may be experienced, or the pain may be severe, colicky, or spasmodic in nature across the abdomen and back. The pain may be so distracting that it may reduce the woman's capacity to follow her usual daily activities. Dysmenorrhoea is a major contributing factor to absenteeism amongst schoolgirls and working women.

Two types of dysmenorrhoea are described:

Primary dysmenorrhoea (spasmodic) is due to physiological activities of the menstruation, with muscle contraction.

Secondary dysmenorrhoea (congestive) is associated with organic pelvic disease.

Primary dysmenorrhoea

This is seen in girls in their late teens and early twenties. At first they may have anovulatory, pain-free menstruation. Later, when ovulation becomes established they experience pain 24 hours before the flow begins.

The pain is of the severe colic type over the lower abdomen and back, and lasts for at least 12 hours. Nausea and diarrhoea may accompany the acute phase and the girl looks pale and drawn with a tense facial expression.

PATHOPHYSIOLOGY

It is usually necessary to assess the general health of the patient and problems associated with environment, parental pressures, and her attitude and beliefs about menstruation and sexual matters. Misconceptions about the physical changes of menstruation and the way they should be managed may underlie painful periods (Brown & Woods 1984, Smithson 1992). See also Research Abstract 7.3.

In the days prior to menstruation there is a build-up of progesterone and a raised level of prostaglandins in the endometrium. As menstruation begins, the progesterone level is lowered and arterioles in the uterus go into spasm. Muscle ischaemia results and can produce uterine pain similar to that of angina.

Muscular incoordination may be the result of improper functioning of the autonomic nervous system. This may cause spasm of muscles of the uterine isthmus and of the internal os.

Rarely, dysmenorrhoea may be due to an obstruction to the flow of blood due to a clot being lodged in the cervix. Primary dysmenorrhoea is due to excess prostaglandin (F2); the circulating prostaglandin may also cause nausea, vomiting, diarrhoea or faintness. (See Research Abstract 7.3.)

MEDICAL MANAGEMENT

Detailed interviews are needed with the girl and her mother, separately and together. In this way shared and different attitudes to the subject can be identified and problems defined. Vaginal or rectal examinations will be carried out.

Efforts are made to educate the girl and her mother, as necessary, about normal menstrual function. It is important to test their understanding by giving them opportunities for feedback about attitudes and old wives' tales. It must be understood that fear will exaggerate pain. Non-habit-forming analgesics are advised, particularly aspirin, which reduces prostaglandin synthesis. A period of rest, and applying warmth to the abdomen or back may be helpful. The need to rest should not be used as an excuse for avoiding school or work. Regular exercise, the avoidance of constipation and the prevention of anxiety and tension are emphasised.

A series of exercises to stretch the ligaments that support the uterus in the pelvis may relieve menstrual pain. Attention should be paid to maintaining good posture. Antispasmodic drugs such as hyoscine butylbromide may help with colicky pain. The contraceptive pill may be taken for 6 months to suppress ovulation. This relieves pain for that period and, when normal cycles return, the pain should be less. Progesterone alone may be given to the young girl whose skeletal growth is incomplete. Progesterone from day 5 to day 25 will relax the arteriole spasm in the myometrium without inhibiting ovulation. It is thus also useful for those with pain who wish to become pregnant.

Dilatation and curettage may be performed to relieve cervical

Research Abstract 7.3 Knowledge and attitudes about female health among girls

Questionnaires were completed by 74 girls between the ages of 11 and 17 years regarding their knowledge of personal health and attitudes towards issues of contraception and sexually transmitted diseases. Before the study, 47 girls had begun menstruating. The average age of menarche was 12 years.

Negative feelings towards menstruation were expressed by the majority of girls who had not yet started their periods. These feelings stemmed from lack of knowledge, anxiety about peer group attitudes, and fear of the 'pains' that were expected as an inevitable part of menstruation. Similar negative feelings were also expressed by the girls who had started their periods. They also mentioned 'loss of freedom' during periods and the 'messiness' of menstruation. Nine positive responses towards menstruation were recorded and associated with growing up. Knowledge about the menstrual cycle and the hormones involved varied but in a number of cases appeared limited. There was evidence that myths about menstruation still exist, they were told 'not to run about a lot, or do sport'. The research findings do not support the belief that the menarche is a positive event and that adolescents perceive menstruation as normal. The negative views of those who had begun menstruating focused mainly on pain and inconvenience. It is questioned whether negative attitudes result from the experience of pain or whether pain is a result of women's negative attitudes. Nurses should be aware of the perceptions, anxieties, and special health education requirements of teenage girls.

Smithson A 1992 Girls will be women. Nursing Times 88(6): 46–48 spasm or obstruction but is not advised as a routine intervention in dysmenorrhoea, due to the risk of incompetence of the cervix. A pregnancy and vaginal delivery of the baby may improve or cure primary dysmenorrhoea.

NURSING PRIORITIES AND MANAGEMENT: PRIMARY DYSMENORRHOEA

Assessment

The nurse will enquire about any difficulties with menstrual periods, if this information is relevant to the illness condition or planned procedures. The date of the last menstrual period should be documented. The patient's own description of the nature of her painful periods should be recorded, and any observations she makes about her physical and emotional symptoms on particular days of the cycle. Any medication used for pain relief or contraception, and its effectiveness, should be noted. Dietary habits and usual ways of taking exercise are also relevant. Gentle questioning of the patient as to whether she has any special worries or has recently experienced any stressful events may provide information helpful for planning care.

Asking the patient about the possible reasons for her pain when menstruating should give the nurse insight into the patient's need for information about normal functioning and alternative ways of coping with pain.

Planning care

The recorded date of the last menstrual period, and the time the patient will be receiving nursing care will guide whether 'pain anticipated with next menstrual period on . . .' should feature as a potential problem in the care plan. This should be negotiated with the patient, who may not regard it as a problem for inclusion in the plan. She may prefer to remain independent in her personal care, if her general condition allows it.

The stress of hospital admission or the illness condition may induce menstruation at an earlier date than expected and when the patient is more highly dependent. The nurse may then have to write up appropriate interventions to ensure the patient is 'pain-free' or 'pain is reduced to a tolerable level'. The patient's preferred methods of pain relief should guide the nursing actions planned.

The patient's need for health education should feature in the plan of care. An outline teaching plan should be completed in preparation for the patient's discharge, for example:

Problem. The need for information about factors that influence the pain of menstruation.

Goal. The patient will be able to explain, in her own words, possible changes she is able to make, that may reduce the pain and discomfort of menstruation, before discharge.

Nursing intervention

- Give a simple explanation of the functioning of hormones in the menstrual cycle, and the effects of excessive prostaglandins. Use diagrams.
- Discuss the beneficial effects of a diet adequate in fibre, vitamins and polyunsaturated fats, and low in sodium chloride.
- Compare the patient's present level of physical exercise with that of a more beneficial programme. Explain the effects of exercise and good posture in stimulating the function of all organs, and stimulating the release of pain-relieving endorphins.
- Teach a simple relaxation exercise. Ask the patient to practise the exercise regularly. Explain the effects of muscular relaxation in counteracting anxiety or tension and muscle spasm. Refer to massage and local heat application.
- Discuss the use of drugs that reduce the development of prostaglandins, particularly any drug prescribed for the patient.
- Ask the patient to explain, in her own words, some of the changes she would like to make in future. Reinforce the patient's understanding and resolve, and check whether she needs further explanations.

Evaluation

A pain rating scale 0–5, (0 = No pain, 5 = Intolerable pain) should be used to evaluate the goal of reduced pain. If the goal is not achieved it may be necessary for the doctor to change the analgesic prescribed. Relaxation exercises should be used whilst the effects of analgesia are awaited. The pain the patient is experiencing whilst menstruating in hospital may be aggravated by the illness causing admission. There may be many factors in the care plan that are interdependent and need to be reviewed when setting further goals.

The achievement of the patient's goals will be her first step in a change of lifestyle. Further support and encouragement may be given by her mother, a friend, partner, a school or practice nurse or the GP.

Secondary dysmenorrhoea

PATHOPHYSIOLOGY

Secondary dysmenorrhoea is experienced in later menstrual life by women in their mid-20s after previous years of painless menstruation. The condition is usually associated with some pelvic pathology, although anxiety or depression can be aggravating factors.

Adenomyosis. A state of increased tension in the uterine muscles, due to the accumulating of blood in the cystic spaces.

Fixed retroversion of the uterus can cause severe pain, especially if associated with a low-grade pelvic infection.

Partial stenosis of the cervix, following cautery or cone biopsy.

Endometriosis interferes with normal rhythmic contractions of the uterus.

Pelvic congestion, due to increased blood supply to the uterus, and menorrhagia.

Pelvic inflammation, particularly salpingitis, might contribute to pain.

Fibromyomata and polyps interfere with the normal rhythmic contractions of the uterus and cause muscular spasms as the uterus attempts to empty itself of the abnormal tissue.

MEDICAL MANAGEMENT

Examination. A detailed history of the problem is recorded and a full physical examination is completed. The woman usually complains of a dragging pain in the lower abdomen, pelvic area, breasts and accompanied by headache. The pain occurs some days before the menstrual flow and may continue throughout the period. The doctor seeks information about possible abnormal uterine bleeding, pain on sexual intercourse (dyspareunia), pruritis and premenstrual tension.

Treatment. Medical treatment may involve examination under anaesthetic, and dilation of the cervix and curettage of endometrium. A laparoscopy may be performed when endometriosis is suspected. The presence of fibroids or polyps will result in surgical removal. Pelvic inflammation would be treated by antibiotics. An analgesic drug will be prescribed that is suitable for inhibiting prostaglandin synthesis. See the glossary of drugs at the end of the chapter.

NURSING PRIORITIES AND MANAGEMENT: SECONDARY DYSMENORRHOEA

The nursing care of the patient with secondary dysmenorrhoea will be dependent on the problems the patient would wish to be included in the plan. A woman in her mid-20s may be anxious about a young family at home and worried about whether her partner will be able to cope with his work, the children, and the chores, as well as visiting the hospital. The nurse may need to spend time with both the mother and her partner, together and separately, to establish whether any community support is needed until the woman is able to continue with her responsibilities at home. The nurse must be alert to the potential needs of the patient's children and may need to contact the health visitor about the family.

Actual or potential pain episodes will certainly emerge as a problem on assessment. Goals and interventions will be similar to those described for primary dysmenorrhoea, particularly education for the maintenance of personal health.

Preoperative and postoperative care planning will be needed if surgical procedures are planned. The nurse will have a major role to play in establishing effective communication with the patient to convey all the details of examinations and surgical procedures to be expected. The nurse needs to be able to promote trust, and develop a warm relationship with the patient, so that she can counteract the patient's fears about explaining personal details. The patient should be encouraged to express her feelings and thoughts and the nurse should be alert to the need for the patient to gain new knowledge to cope better with her physical sexual needs.

Opportunities for counselling and teaching should feature in the care plan. At the time of discharge the patient's future prospects for an improved pattern of menstrual cycles should appear much improved.

Premenstrual syndrome

Premenstrual syndrome (PMS) is a group of recurring symptoms that occur 2–12 days prior to menstruation, affecting the latter half of the cycle and subsiding soon after the menstrual flow begins. They are luteal phase symptoms and by definition are not present for longer than 16 days. There is a symptom-free week following menstruation. It is a universal syndrome seen in all races, with only subtle differences occurring. Prevalence reports range from 5% to 97%. Differences occur in the definition of the syndrome used by those gathering data.

The following degrees of severity are experienced:

- 3–10% of women are free from physical or psychological symptoms
- 50% of women experience mild symptoms that are tolerable
- 35% have moderate-to-severe symptoms that make the woman seek treatment
- 5–10% have severely debilitating symptoms that disrupt their lives.

Premenstrual syndrome most commonly occurs after the birth of a first child, but it may occur from puberty onwards.

Researchers have described different groupings of somatic and psychological symptoms that may affect women with PMS. The timing of symptoms is more important than their specific character. The somatic symptoms are convincingly linked to the menstrual cycle. Abraham (1981) subdivides symptoms as follows:

- nervous tension, mood swings, irritability and anxiety
- weight gain, swelling of extremities, breast tenderness, abdominal bloating and pelvic pain
- headache, craving for sweets, increased appetite, heart pounding, fatigue and dizziness or fainting
- depression, forgetfulness, confusion, crying and insomnia.

More than 150 symptoms have been linked to PMS, half of them psychological and half physical, and groups may overlap. There may be serious social disturbance within the family, at school or at work. The woman may already have been seeking help from her GP and have experienced recurring symptoms for at least six previous menstrual cycles before the diagnosis is made. There may be disturbed body image and low self-esteem. The condition occurs in the woman in her 30s, at a time when her responsibilities and stress factors may be high and her tolerance diminishes. Women taking the combined contraceptive pill do not usually complain of PMS.

PATHOPHYSIOLOGY

There appears to be an exaggeration of normal physiological changes when oestrogen and progesterone are together in the circulation. The underlying endocrinology and biochemistry of PMS is poorly understood and controversial; there are frequent discrepancies between the subjective reports of women and the objective reports of research investigators. PMS is concluded to be a multifactorial psychoneuro–endocrine disorder.

The range of theories of PMS refer to imbalances, excesses or deficiency states and resulting physical changes; see Box 7.2.

Fluid retention or redistribution. Since the 1930s it has been suggested that PMS might be related to hormones responsible for fluid retention, but research studies can only suggest that there may be a redistribution of body fluids in intracellular and extracellular compartments. They have failed to demonstrate a pattern of fluid retention in most PMS patients.

Prostaglandins are produced in response to changing levels of

Box 7.2 Theories related to PMS

Imbalance
- oestrogen/progesterone
- prostaglandins.

Excess
- aldosterone
- angiotensin II
- oestrogen
- androgen
- antidiuretic hormone
- endorphin
- prolactin.

Deficiency
- progesterone
- androgen
- essential fatty acid
- blood glucose
- magnesium
- endorphin
- zinc
- vitamin B6.

Physical changes
- sodium and water retention
- abnormal water distribution
- leakage of albumen/tissue fluid
- allergy related to progesterone
- dietary abnormality
- serotonin or aspartine neurotransmitter disturbance.

oestrogen and progesterone. They exert sedative effects on the central nervous system and affect both aldosterone and ADH activity. If premenstrual changes are influenced by prostaglandins it may be the balance between the prostaglandins that is of greatest importance.

Hypoglycaemia. Research studies have shown abnormalities of glucose metabolism in the luteal phase of the menstrual cycle and concluded that exaggerated glucose swings during the luteal phase might account for premenstrual hypoglycaemic symptoms. However, it has been concluded that there is not a causal relationship with PMS, but perhaps some concurrence between it and glucose metabolism (Reid et al 1986).

Vitamin B6 (pyridoxine) deficiency is involved in the production of brain biogenic amines. It increases inhibitory amines such as dopamine and serotonin, and also acts as a co-enzyme in converting excitatory amino acids to corresponding inhibitory amino acids, with sedative effects. Several PMS behavioural symptoms represent an excitatory state of the central nervous system and Vitamin B6 can reduce the excitatory biogenic amines. However, there is little scientific data to support the theoretical assumption that Vitamin B6 relieves PMS symptoms.

Progesterone withdrawal. Although many researchers have suggested that PMS is the result of unopposed oestrogen effects, due to deficiency of progesterone production, many PMS patients have been shown to have adequate corpus luteum functioning. This suggests that it is the rate of fall of progesterone level during the late luteal phase that is causative in PMS rather than a deficiency state.

Endorphin withdrawal. Endorphins are a group of substances which are endogenous opioid peptides. They appear to be important in the physiology of pain and mood change. Data on endorphins has been derived from indirect studies involving the use of naloxone, a morphine-antagonist.

In a study of the Rhesus monkey direct measurement of beta-endorphin concentration in the portal-hypophyseal blood revealed that endorphin levels are high during the mid-luteal phase of the cycle and undetectable at the onset of menstruation (Wehrenberg et al 1982).

The direct effects of beta-endorphin have been studied in psychiatric disorders. In small numbers of depressed patients the administration of beta-endorphin was shown to improve mood, increase energy and decrease anxiety. Two patients became markedly excited and over-active (Kline et al 1977, Angst et al 1979). (See Research Abstract 7.4.)

The endorphin theory is said to be one of the most credible for PMS but the theory has not yet been proven although the Chuong results add supportive evidence. O'Brien (1987) suggests that PMS is probably related to ovarian function that, in turn, is linked to gonadotrophins, which may well be dependent on endorphin function. The relationship between such changes and their mechanisms in producing the symptoms of PMS are a long way from being fully understood.

Research Abstract 7.4 Beta-endorphins in premenstrual syndrome

In a study by Chuong and colleagues (1985) 20 symptomatic and 20 control patients were studied for levels of several peptides, including beta-endorphin, on days 7 and 25 of the menstrual cycle. There were no significant differences between the two groups in the follicular phase of the study. In the control patients beta-endorphins were higher in the luteal or premenstrual phase than in the follicular phase, but in the symptomatic PMS patients, the beta-endorphin levels fell in the luteal phase.

The difference between PMS patients and controls during the luteal phase was significantly different.

Chuong C J, Coulam C B, Kao P C, Bergstahl E J & Go V L W 1985 Neuropeptide levels in premenstrual syndrome. Fertility and Sterility 44(6): 760–765

MEDICAL MANAGEMENT

Multiple theories are available about the origins of premenstrual syndrome, and many therapeutic regimes have been prescribed for suffering patients. It is unlikely that a single cause or treatment will be found. The focus is on identifying and controlling individual symptom clusters. Drug treatments are used cautiously. Many research studies have shown marked placebo effects of 40–60% in PMS sufferers. The patient–doctor relationship is thought to be an important influence on some women, who may be relieved that their condition is being taken seriously. Knowing that many other women also suffer is helpful and anticipation that some symptoms may improve, may relieve some tension.

Examination. Accurate diagnosis of PMS is necessary and the patient may be treated by her GP or be referred to a PMS clinic. Other medical, psychiatric and gynaecological conditions must be excluded or be identified as co-existing with PMS. A general physical examination of the patient is completed. Painful breasts make many women worried that they have cancer. Breast cancer must be excluded as hormone-dependent cancers may be stimulated by therapy.

A patient with pelvic pain may have an inflammatory condition, or endometriosis, that needs further investigation. Some patients may have a depressive illness, as well as PMS. This may be referred to as secondary PMS; the depressive symptoms persist through what is expected to be a symptom-free week in the cycle.

Estimations of oestrogen, progesterone, prolactin, gonadotrophin or electrolytes are not usually helpful in making a diagnosis of PMS. However, if there is research taking place in the PMS clinic patients may be asked to give blood specimens as part of a series of investigations and treatments. Although research results are inconclusive about hormonal factors in PMS, hormonal treatments are still used and patients expect to receive hormone therapy.

Treatment is likely to be as follows.

An integrated programme approach. Patients are asked to record personal experiences in mood, behaviour, thinking patterns, and physical discomforts daily, in a diary, for at least 3 months. Symptom clusters and symptom free times can be thus easily identified.

Whilst the diary recordings are taking place the patients are asked to:

- begin taking regular exercise
- avoid coffee, tea and chocolate
- take a diet that is low in sugars and high in lean proteins
- take vitamin supplements B6, E1 and the mineral, magnesium
- chart their weight, daily
- avoid alcohol and smoking.

Evening primrose oil may be recommended but it is expensive.

Many patients experience symptom relief with this programme. They may, themselves, recognise factors that aggravate or trigger symptoms. They learn to cope and live with their condition and may not report back to the clinic or need further treatment. Knowing that professional help remains available to them gives confidence.

Drug treatments used in PMS depend partly on the preference of the doctor providing care and the particular cluster of symptoms experienced by the patient. Many women who have already tried 'over the counter' remedies, expect or request hormonal treatment. The patient needs to know that the doctor may not find the right medication at first.

Hormonal treatment of PMS is as follows.

- Some doctors continue to use progesterone or progestogen for all PMS symptoms. The drug may be given orally, by injection, by suppository, in the combined contraceptive pill, or by means of an implant.
- The drug danazol, which inhibits pituitary gonadotrophin secretion, is prescribed selectively for some patients, particularly those with severe breast pain. Danazol completely suppresses the menstrual cycle and reduces breast tenderness, but varying degrees of

improvement in other symptoms have been documented. Patients are advised to use alternative, non-hormonal contraceptive methods. The major disadvantage of danazol is that high doses cause masculinisation. Acne, hirsutism, clitoral hypertrophy, reduction of breast size, and deepening of the voice have been reported. Treatments at low dosage, not greater than 400 mg daily, usually relieve PMS symptoms without the masculinisation effects. Other minor side effects such as nausea, dizziness and rashes are troublesome to certain patients, who need to discontinue treatment.

- Analogues of gonadotrophin-releasing hormone (GnRH), such as buserelin, if given continuously and in high doses, will inhibit the release of gonadotrophins, and so suppress follicular development, ovulation and the endocrine changes of the cycle.

  GnRH analogue may be administered by nasal inhalation or as a depot preparation. Muse et al (1984) treated eight patients with clear-cut PMS symptoms. Controlled suppression of the cycle was achieved and nearly all symptoms were greatly reduced. A temporary, reversible 'medical oophorectomy' is produced by this treatment. The treatment is expensive. GnRH analogue can only be used as a short-term therapy, otherwise post-menopausal symptoms will develop.
- Bromocryptine is a stimulant of dopamine receptors in the brain and also inhibits the release of prolactin by the pituitary. The role of prolactin in PMS is poorly understood but bromocryptine has been shown to be effective in the treatment of breast symptoms. Sondheimer et al (1988) suggest that some patients are helped simply by reassurance that the breast symptoms are not cancer but are normal fluctuations in breast activity.

Diuretic treatment. In women who have a measured weight increase the diuretic, spironolactone, may be prescribed. This drug has an adrenocortical and anti-androgen action. Some investigators have found the drug useful for symptoms of depressed mood.

Analgesic treatment. Where pain is a primary symptom the anti-inflammatory analgesic, and prostaglandin inhibitor, mefenamic acid may be helpful to the patient but research as to how many PMS symptoms this drug will relieve is contradictory. There is agreement that the drug is of benefit for some PMS symptoms.

Psychological support. Supportive psychotherapy and techniques that improve coping skills and stress management should be part of the care programme. Patients have found self-help groups of benefit. Relaxation exercises undertaken together, and assertiveness training may be part of the total programme. People who experience secondary PMS, whereby their unhappy mood and agitated behaviours persist throughout their cycles, may need the clinical help of a psychiatrist. Rational emotive therapy and antidepressant medication may be necessary to relieve symptoms.

NURSING PRIORITIES AND MANAGEMENT: PMS

Personal assessment

The nurse may encounter many women who experience PMS symptoms that have not been discussed with their doctors. Nurses have opportunities to provide such friends or patients with information that may enable them to modify their lifestyles. Suggesting daily recording of physical changes, discomforts, and emotional feelings and behaviour can help with personal assessment.

Care planning

A supportive–educative approach should be used. Information given by the nurse should provide a balanced view of what the woman can do independently, to select possible changes that she can put into effect. The nurse should discuss options with particular care to avoid causing any financial embarrassment to the woman who may have little money to spare from her family budget for vitamin supplements or evening primrose oil. Useful advice includes the following:

- the value of physical exercise as a stimulant to the circulatory system and improved functioning of all bodily organs; congestion may be relieved, concentration and sleep should improve, and feelings of wellbeing may increase
- the need to reduce fat, sugar, salt, coffee and tea consumption
- the benefits of eating fresh fruit and vegetables
- reducing smoking and alcohol intake
- avoiding stressful situations to reduce tension and feelings of frustration, particularly at trigger times in the cycle
- relaxation exercises
- massage carried out by a partner, nurse, or therapist
- a counselling approach by the nurse
- support in making preferred choices about the individual programme
- information about the nature of any drugs prescribed for the patient, their action and possible side-effects
- information about self-help groups
- referral to a health visitor, if the patient needs continuing support at home.

Evaluation

The patient should be guided into self-evaluation of progress during the week when she is usually symptom free. Any measures taken will be recalled and any physical or emotional changes that the patient has recorded in the daily diary will be noted. These can be related, where possible, to the actions the patient has taken, and conclusions drawn. Some symptoms may have greatly improved, but there may be no feeling of improvement in other areas. The patient must be congratulated on her personal achievements, as appropriate, and encouraged to sustain any changes in lifestyle that are thought to have influenced the changes.

Where unresolved problems remain, the exposure to each planned action should be reviewed and the action modified or adapted for a further interval. Evidence of a sustained unhappy mood or other severe symptoms, should be referred to the GP or PMS clinic doctor. The patient may need the added interventions of a psychiatrist or psychotherapist. With support and medication if necessary most women are able to achieve some measure of improvement.

DISORDERS OF THE MALE REPRODUCTIVE ORGANS

NB *The anatomy and physiology of the male reproductive system is described in Chapter 8.*

MALDESCENT OF THE TESTES (CRYPTORCHIDISM)

PATHOPHYSIOLOGY

Cryptorchidism is a condition in which one or both testes have not descended into the scrotum before birth. It is a common condition seen in approximately 1% of boys after their first year and may be self-correcting or require surgery in the form of orchidopexy. Normal descent keeps the testes cooler in the scrotum, and avoids the germ cell degeneration that is possible in the higher temperature of the abdomen, and which carries a risk of malignancy. Three different grades of maldescent are described:

1. A retractile testicle is normally found in the scrotum but on stimulation is pulled up into the superficial inguinal pouch by an active cremaster muscle

2. An ectopic testicle is prevented by tissue structures from descending from the inguinal canal into the scrotum
3. An undescended testicle is possibly abnormal: it remains in the abdomen and fails to enter the inguinal canal and pass into the scrotum.

MEDICAL MANAGEMENT

Medical intervention. The aim of treatment is to promote normal function of the testicle. Treatment should be completed by the boy's 8th year, before the testicle starts functioning. The testicle may migrate spontaneously, or hormone treatment may be prescribed to stimulate migration. Otherwise, an orchidopexy is performed to bring down the testicle and anchor it in a pocket of skin on the thigh or by means of a suture to the thigh. The suture is removed after 7–10 days postoperatively. A further operation is needed to free the testicle from the skin pocket.

More extensive surgery may be needed with actual removal of the abnormal testicle and repair of an inguinal hernia if this has occurred. There is a high risk of malignancy if the testes are left in the abdomen.

NURSING PRIORITIES AND MANAGEMENT: MALDESCENT OF THE TESTES

General considerations

Pre- and postoperative care is routine, with particular emphasis on hygiene and wound care. The nurse should fill in any gaps in the patient's understanding of his condition and the operation performed. The patient who is still a child may feel embarrassed in expressing his need for information, and the nurse must judge where to begin and end with a health education programme. The facts of sexual life may need to be explained to the child with a parent present, or the parent may prefer to be the one to give the child the information. In some cases the nurse may find it more relevant to focus on the parent's need for education, information and advice.

Torsion of the testes

Testicular torsion is an acutely painful condition caused by the twisting of the testis on its spermatic cord. It may occur spontaneously or as the result of strenuous exertion. It commonly occurs in adolescents aged 12–18 years, but can occur in adults as well. This condition is classified as a surgical emergency requiring immediate treatment.

PATHOPHYSIOLOGY

Testicular torsion results when an abnormality of the tunica vaginalis allows increased mobility of the testis and axial rotation of the spermatic cord above. The resulting ischaemia can lead to cell damage and infection within about 6 h.

Extravaginal torsion, a rare form, can occur in utero or in the newborn. In this case the testis is not painful but on examination is found to be a firm, large mass in the scrotum.

Common presenting symptoms. The patient will present with sudden onset of acute pain in the groin, often radiating to the scrotum and abdomen. Exercise may be the precipitating factor, but the onset of pain can also occur at rest. Nausea and vomiting are common. The patient may give a history of previous, less severe episodes which resolved spontaneously.

Examination of the testis may be hampered by the severity of the pain. The affected testis will be elevated but abnomality of mobility ('bellclapper' deformity) may be present in the other testis.

MEDICAL MANAGEMENT

Medical intervention. Treatment is by immediate surgical intervention to relieve the torsion and secure testicular fixation. However, if the torsion is detected at an earlier stage, it may be possible by external manipulation to gently rotate the twisted testis in the appropriate direction. This may immediately resolve the emergency, but the testes should later be surgically secured to prevent recurrence.

NURSING PRIORITIES AND MANAGEMENT: TORSION OF THE TESTES

General considerations

The patient will normally be young and fit and his stay in hospital brief. Although the surgery is not considered major, the acute onset of pain and the nature of the problem may give rise to considerable anxiety and perhaps embarrassment. Giving the patient adequate information will help to relieve anxiety and promote recovery. He should be informed that analgesics can be given immediately, and that the acute pain will go away once the operation has been performed.

The patient's stay in hospital will normally be 24 h. Postoperatively, the patient will have a small inguinal wound and perhaps some scrotal swelling. He will normally be able to return to school or work in about 2 weeks, at which point he should feel comfortable walking and sitting. Lifting, heavy work and sports involving running, jumping or stretching should be avoided for about 6 weeks. An athletic support should always be worn when sports activities are resumed.

The patient who has received treatment in good time should also be reassured that blood supply to the testes was not interrupted to the degree that any impairment to sexual function or fertility will result.

> ? **7.1** Write a care plan for a patient following surgery for fixation of testes. Consider what problems the patient might have. The care plan should include:
>
> - checking the wound for oozing, swelling and infection
> - ensuring the wearing of a scrotal support to prevent swelling
> - relieving pain by bedrest and analgesia
> - ensuring that the patient passes urine within a specific time postoperatively (it may take him up to 24 h)
> - checking temperature, pulse and blood pressure
> - informing the patient when he may eat and drink again
> - giving discharge advice.

HYDROCELE

PATHOPHYSIOLOGY

A hydrocele is a collection of serous fluid in the membranous sac (the tunica vaginalis) that surrounds the testes. It may occur spontaneously without any cause, or it may be secondary to an acute or chronic inflammatory condition of the testis or epididymis. The hydrocele usually occurs on one side only, is painless, and can swell to a considerable size. It may accompany a condition that causes oedema of tissues, such as congestive heart failure or nephrotic syndrome.

Clinical features. A red glow on transillumination characterises the presence of fluid within the scrotal sac (Hanno & Wien 1987). Palpation of the scrotal sac will distinguish the hydrocele from fluid arising from other parts of the scrotum. As hydrocele can form around a testicular tumour, the possibility of cancer should be excluded.

Common presenting symptoms. Hydrocele is usually asymptomatic, but an increase in scrotal size and associated discomfort will often prompt the patient to seek advice. The embarrassment caused by the swelling may be such that the individual curtails social activities, swimming, sunshine holidays and sexual relations.

MEDICAL MANAGEMENT

Medical intervention. The condition may be reducible by wearing of a scrotal support, but it is often necessary to introduce a fine trochar and cannula to drain off the fluid. Bleeding and infection are common as complications, and recurrence at 6–15 weeks is common.

VARICOCELE

PATHOPHYSIOLOGY

A varicocele is a varicose state of the veins draining the testes which may cause enlargement of the spermatic cord. Palpation of the scrotum will reveal a mass of enlarged and tortuous veins. The condition most commonly occurs in men aged 15–30 years, and sometimes resolves without intervention when there is regular sexual intercourse. A persistent varicocele may induce a raised temperature within the scrotum due to the increased blood supply and contribute to a subfertile state.

MEDICAL MANAGEMENT

Medical intervention may be conservative or surgical. The patient who complains of a dragging discomfort in the scrotum may find that this is relieved by the wearing of a scrotal support. If the condition is more severe, ligation of the veins may be needed. A small length of vein may be removed.

TESTICULAR CANCER

Testicular cancer is an uncommon condition accounting for 1–2% of all cancers in men and fewer than 0.5% of all cancer deaths in men (Henderson et al 1983). It is, however, the most common tumour in men aged 29–35 years. In the last 50 years the condition has become more common among white racial groups but has remained only one third as common among black racial groups. Its incidence is highest in Scandinavian countries and lowest in Asian and African countries. In Denmark testicular cancer accounts for 6.7% of all cancers. In Japan it accounts for 0.8%. The value of screening programmes for testicular cancer remains a matter for debate (see Research Abstract 7.5).

Two factors, cryptorchidism (undescended testicle) and exogenous oestrogens are associated with an increased incidence of testicular cancer. White races have 3 times the risk of cryptorchidism than black races, and this condition carries a 3–14-fold risk of testicular cancer.

Exogenous oestrogens are used by women in birth control pills or in medication to prevent miscarriage. It has been hypothesised that the use of these however can predispose subsequent male children to testicular cancer. There is high usage of contraceptive pills in the United States and in Scandinavian countries.

Research Abstract 7.5 Testicular cancer screening

A report of a working party of the Royal College of Physicians (1991) concluded that as testicular self-examination has never been evaluated and because chemotherapy now achieves cure rates of 90% or more, even in advanced cases of testicular cancer, screening is probably unnecessary. Moreover, because there is no identifiable pre-invasive stage, screening can not reduce the incidence but might even increase it by over-diagnosis of borderline tumours. Thus screening for testicular cancer is not indicated.

Royal College of Physicians 1991 Report on preventive medicine. Royal College of Physicians, London

PATHOPHYSIOLOGY

The cell types of testicular cancer are classified in terms of embryonal tissue rather than adult testes tissue. Almost all the cancers arise from the primordial germ cell, the multipotent cell found in the yolk sac of the embryo. This multipotent cell will have many varieties of cell types as offspring, and a primary testicular tumour may have a wide variety of cell types. The normal cells of the testis have high proliferative potential and can become malignant under the influence of an abnormal environment.

Testicular cancers are grouped as:

1. Originating from germinal tissue (97%):
   - seminoma (typical, anaplastic or spermocytic)
   - non-seminomatous:
     — embryonal
     — teratocarcinoma
     — teratoma
     — choriocarcinoma
2. Arising from stromal tissue (3%):
   - interstitial cell tumour
   - gonadal stromal tumour.

Germinal testicular cancer

Clinical features. The germinal cancer types may develop from a single cell or a multifocus. The malignant growth is fairly rapid in one testis. Metastases may occur by extension locally or via the lymphatics to the retroperitoneal lymph nodes. Lymph node invasion may cause displacement of the ureters or kidneys. The ureters may be obstructed. By direct extension the tumour may invade the epididymis, extend up the spermatic cord, or extend through the tunica vaginalis to the scrotum. A late manifestation of the disease may be spread to the lung, liver, adrenal gland, or bone.

Common presenting symptoms. The first sign of testicular tumour is painless enlargement of the testicle. This may be discovered by accident or by self-examination (see Box 7.3). A dragging sensation may be felt in the scrotum from the weight of the tumour. There is usually a lack of pain on palpation of the testis. Any painless lump in the testis that does not respond promptly to antibiotics should be thought of as cancer until proven otherwise. Metastases may cause lumbar pain and abdominal or supraclavicular lymph node masses. Pain may be caused by a cough or any obstruction.

MEDICAL MANAGEMENT

Investigative procedures. Laboratory studies of serum alpha-fetoprotein (AFP) and serum beta human chorionic gonadotrophin (HCG) help in the diagnosis of germ cell cancer as tumour markers. AFP is high in aggressive non-seminomatous tumours. HCG is elevated in 30% of seminomas. These markers corroborate diagnosis but are also useful in monitoring treatment. Chest X-ray, chest CT scan, tomography, lymphangiography, abdominal CT scan, abdominal ultrasonography, and intravenous pyelography (see Ch. 8, p. 297) may all be used diagnostically.

Medical intervention will be surgical with adjuvant radiotherapy and chemotherapy.

Surgical intervention. A high radical inguinal orchidectomy is performed. The testis, epididymis, a portion of the vas and parts of the gonadal lymphatics and blood vessels are removed. The remaining testis will undergo hyperplasia and produces enough testosterone to maintain sexual capacity, male characteristics and libido. The semen, however, may be of poor quality. Ejaculatory ability may be altered.

Radiotherapy. Further to surgery, radiotherapy is recommended for lymph node areas. Fatigue, bone marrow depression, and diarrhoea may be experienced as side-effects. There may be scatter radiation to the other testicle despite the use of a protective shell. Sperm recovery is slow, variable and dose-related.

Box 7.3 Teaching testicular self-examination

The nurse can make a valuable contribution to health promotion by teaching testicular self-examination. An effective teaching plan will explain the reasons for self-examination of the testes, the best time to perform self-examination, the steps to follow in self-examination, and the types of abnormality that should be reported to a doctor.

TEACHING PLAN

1. Enquire about any previous information the patient may have gained about examination of the testes
2. Respond to what the patient says about the topic and build on that knowledge. Give the patient the opportunity to ask questions and seek clarification regularly
3. Use a simple diagram of the scrotum and testes to describe the structures involved
4. Explain that it is necessary to be aware of the normal condition of the testes so that any later change can be recognised at an early stage
5. Advise that the best time to perform self-examination is immediately after taking a shower or bath, when the body tissues are warm, the scrotum is relaxed, and the testes easy to feel
6. Emphasise the need to look at the scrotum for its colour, texture, any change in shape, or any swelling that may be noticeable
7. Instruct the patient that it is necessary to hold the scrotum in the palm of the hand and to examine each testicle by rolling the testis between his thumb and fingers:
   - Each testicle should feel smooth and be about the size of a small hen's egg
   - The epididymis, which lies behind each testicle, should also be felt, and should feel soft and slightly spongy to the touch.
   - The spermatic cords, which extend upwards from the epididymis, should feel like round, firm tubes
8. Explain that any abnormality in the shape of the testicle and any lump or swelling should be investigated by a doctor irrespective of how trivial it may seem
9. Check that the patient knows why he is completing the self-examination. Help the patient to understand that a cancerous lump can now be successfully treated.

Chemotherapy. A number of cytotoxic drugs are used as an adjunct to surgery and radiotherapy. Cyclophosphamide and chlorambucil may be used with vincristine and actinomycin D in cyclical treatments, every 2 months for 1 year and every 3 months for the 2nd year. Where there is extended disease vinblastine and bleomycin are the drugs of choice. If the disease is disseminated the drug cisplatin may be added to the previous two. Toxicity and sepsis are high and the cisplatin has nephrotoxic effects.

In non-seminomas the survival rate is high. Tumour markers are used to judge chemotherapy effects.

NURSING PRIORITIES AND MANAGEMENT: TESTICULAR CANCER

General considerations

The preoperative and postoperative needs of the patient having a testis removed are similar to those of other patients requiring major surgery (see Ch. 27). The need for information, relief of anxiety, pain relief and protection from wound infection are primary. The young adult patient with insight into his cancer condition will undoubtedly be worried about the future, the course of the illness, his family responsibilities and his career.

Postoperatively the patient will require a short period of fully compensatory care whilst recovering from the anaesthetic. A short period of partially assisted care will follow. In the long term the patient will need planned educative and supportive care. See Case History 7.1.

Case History 7.1 Mr W

Mr W is 32 years of age. He is married and has two young daughters aged 2 and 4. His wife looks after the children well but has always been very dependent on him for organising the family and helping with domestic chores and the shopping. They have usually enjoyed an average social life, babysitters permitting. Mr W works as a computer engineer. He likes to leave work promptly so that his wife isn't left too long on her own at home. She has had episodes when she has become reliant on alcohol, particularly when she is worried about the children.

? **7.2** Mr W had his left testis removed 48 h ago. He has extensive lymphatic gland metastases. The medical plan includes radiotherapy and chemotherapy over the coming months.
Consider the circumstances of the family described in Case History 7.1.

a. Identify Mr W's needs for education and support.
b. Prepare a teaching plan.
c. List the ways in which you as the nurse can provide support for Mr W during the postoperative period.
d. Explain the ways that Mr W can continue to be supported after discharge from hospital.
e. Identify the needs of the family in the short and long term.

For further information, see Bassett (1993) and Standford (1988).

VASECTOMY

MEDICAL MANAGEMENT

Preoperative counselling. Couples who have used a range of birth control methods over the years may decide that permanent sterilisation by surgical means would now be preferable. Before such a decision is taken the couple should meet with their GP or family planning counsellor to discuss their needs and circumstances and their reasons for considering sterilisation as a birth control method. The counsellor should provide information about both female and male sterilisation and the risks, side-effects and failure rates of the procedures available. The long-term effects and prospects for reversal of the sterilisation should be explained. The couple should also be encouraged to consider the implications of a breakdown of their marriage or partnership, or the loss by death of one of the couple or of their children.

A man contemplating vasectomy may have particular anxieties about the effect of the procedure on his masculinity and sex drive. He must be assured that as the testes will not be removed his hormone production, virility and sex drive will be unaffected. The nature of the operation should be explained with the aid of a simple diagram, and it may help to liken the ejaculation fluid that will remain to 'a river without

Box 7.4 Information for the patient undergoing vasectomy

Every patient undergoing vasectomy should be given an information leaflet containing the following information.

- The type of anaesthesia that will be given (i.e. general or local)
- The operation will be completed via the scrotal sac
- Between 1–5 cm of vas will be removed on each side
- A dressing will be applied to the wound and a scrotal support will be applied and should be worn for 2 weeks
- Some swelling and bruising will occur around the operation site. This may extend down over the thighs or up towards the umbilicus
- Some pain will be experienced, but this can be relieved by paracetamol or codeine tablets
- Skin sutures will dissolve spontaneously within approximately one week of the operation
- Strenuous exercise should be avoided for 2 days
- The patient will not become infertile immediately after the operation due to sperm being stored upstream from the operation. Therefore, he must continue to take contraceptive precautions until 2 successive sperm samples are proved to be free of sperm
- Normal sexual intercourse can take place from the 3rd postoperative day. As the operation site may be tender the individual may prefer to wait longer than this
- At least 12 ejaculations should have occurred before the first semen test to clear sperm. A second semen test will be completed 2 weeks later. In a small proportion of cases sperm persists in the seminal fluid for many months
- There is a 0.5–1.0% failure rate associated with the operation:
  - — the ends of a vas may join up again early or late after operation
  - — the surgeon may have removed some structure that was not the vas
  - — some men have anatomical abnormalities such as a double vas, that was not fully removed
- Reappearance of fertility after 2 negative semen tests may mean tests were not accurately completed or the ends of a vas have reunited
- Severe, prolonged pain may indicate some slow seepage of blood into tissues from a small blood vessel. A haematoma may have formed, causing the scrotum to swell. Rest in bed should ease the condition. Otherwise the site may need to be drained at the clinic
- The wound may become infected, in which case the GP will prescribe antibiotics
- There is a reasonable chance that the operation can be reversed should this be desired. Reversibility cannot be guaranteed, however, and a return to the previous level of fertility may never again be achieved.

any fish'. It should also be explained that unused sperm will be broken down and reabsorbed. Further information that the patient will require is summarised in Box 7.4.

The surgical procedure. Vasectomy is the ligation or division of the vasa differentia, the genital ducts that store and transport sperm to the urethra in the process of ejaculation (see Ch. 8, p. 296), and is performed under either general or local anaesthetic. The vas is palpated in the upper scrotum and an incision of 1 cm is made over the vas. The fascia around the vas is incised and the vas drawn out and ligated in two places.

The vas is then simply divided or a small segment is excised (see Fig. 7.7). One end of the vas is enclosed again in the fascia envelope. The other end of the vas is repositioned outside the fascia. Alternatively, the cut ends of the vas may first be cauterised, or the cut ends looped back on themselves. The skin is closed with absorbable sutures and the procedure is repeated on the opposite side. The possibility for reversal of the operation is retained.

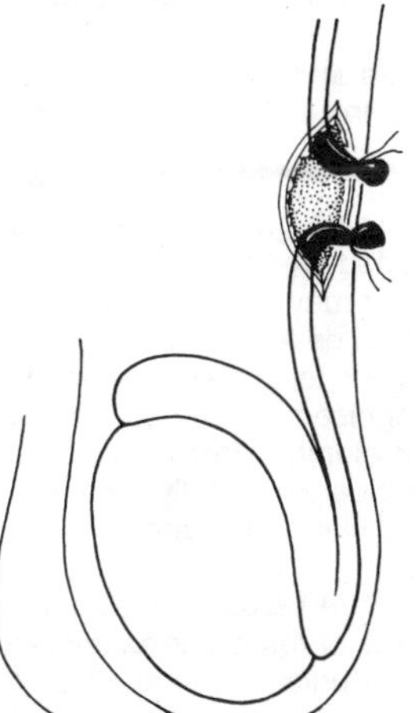

Fig. 7.7 The vas divided.

Outcome. The majority of men express their satisfaction with the vasectomy operation and would recommend it to others if asked. They usually consider it to have been minor surgery and to have caused no ill effects. They approach sexual intercourse with greater relaxation and increased enjoyment.

A minority experience regret after the operation, feeling that their sexual drive and performance have been reduced. Others who have taken new partners or remarried may regret being unable to have another child within the new relationship. A new wife who has no child may feel deprived and frustrated.

Reversal. An increasing number of men are requesting reversal of their vasectomies. Surgeons are now attaining 70–90% success rates with such reversals, which are technically feasible, but the pregnancy rate achieved is disappointingly low: only one third of the reversed vasectomies lead to pregnancy. This low rate may be due to the formation of sperm antibodies.

Surgeons in China have been successful in inserting a plug of polyurethane material into the vas rather than removing a section by vasectomy. The plugs can later be removed without surgery, reversing the sterilisation.

NURSING PRIORITIES AND MANAGEMENT: VASECTOMY

General considerations

The nurse working in a day care facility may be jointly responsible with the surgeon for ensuring that the individual undergoing vasectomy and his partner understand what the procedure will entail and what its anticipated results will be.

Postoperatively, the nurse on the ward or in the GP surgery may be involved in pain management and wound care. The nurse will have an important contribution to make in instructing the patient in postoperative self-care and in informing him about procedures for follow-up and assess-

Box 7.5 Inflammatory conditions of the male reproductive organs

BALANITIS AND BALANOPOSTHITIS

The term balanitis refers to inflammation of the glans penis. The term balanoposthitis refers to inflammation of the prepuce or foreskin as well as the glans penis. Both conditions are the result of bacterial infection. They are painful, irritating and produce a discharge. They may be associated with inadequate hygiene and phimosis. A swab from the inflamed area is sent for pathological culture and sensitivity tests. Specific antibiotic therapy can be prescribed. Local treatment will involve bathing the affected areas with normal saline to relieve discomfort.

EPIDIDYMO-ORCHITIS

In this condition infection and inflammation of the testis and epididymis occur together. It may be caused by prostatitis, a urinary tract infection, or by a sexually transmitted disease. The testes are swollen, tender and painful. The patient is pyrexial and suffers from aches and pains. He may experience nausea and vomiting. Bedrest, extra fluids, analgesics and antibiotics are necessary. Cold packs applied locally to the scrotum and the wearing of a scrotal support will help to relieve discomfort and swelling.

ORCHITIS

This condition is most often caused by mumps occurring after puberty. It may result in atrophy of the testes and sterility. Males who have not had mumps in childhood should try to avoid contact with the disease. Early administration of gammaglobulin may reduce the severity of mumps in those who have been exposed to it.

PROSTATITIS

This is an acute or chronic inflammation of the prostate gland and is usually bacterial in origin. Urgency, frequency and pain with micturition are experienced. Acute retention of urine, cystitis, low back pain, chills and haematuria may occur. The prostate gland is enlarged and tender when examined. Mid-stream urine specimens are sent to the laboratory for culture and sensitivity. Antibiotics, analgesics and a high fluid intake are prescribed. The condition is liable to recur.

ment. She should also alert him to the possible complications or problems that should be reported (see Box 7.5).

Postoperative care

Although information will have been provided preoperatively many men are concerned about the development of scrotal swelling and haematoma in the postoperative period. Scrotal support, rest and analgesia are necessary for general comfort and to improve the condition over time.

Any bleeding from the wounds may be relieved by the use of butterfly sutures to pull the wound edges together.

Psychological after-effects of vasectomy should be few if preoperative counselling and information-giving has been adequate. Some men complain of an adverse effect on sexual performance after vasectomy, but are usually those who have had similar difficulties before surgery.

Some long-term physical complications of vasectomy have been suggested but have not been supported by research. For example, Petitti et al (1982) found no evidence of increased cardiovascular disease after vasectomy. There is some question, however, whether there is an association between vasectomy and the development of testicular tumours (see Research Abstract 7.6).

The nurse should take the opportunity to check whether the patient understands how to self-examine the testes for the development of a lump (see Box 7.4). When the principles are understood the patient should accept the need to complete a self-examination at appropriate intervals. However, it would be inappropriate to associate the risk of tumour with vasectomy until more research data is available.

Occupational health nurses can take a significant role in promoting testicular self-examination in the working male population, the majority of whom seldom need to visit their general practitioner.

Impotence

Impotence, the persistent inability to obtain an erection sufficient for sexual intercourse, is suffered by about 10% of the male population due to organic causes. The total number of men who suffer from impotence is, however, not known.

PATHOPHYSIOLOGY

Impotence may be a primary or secondary condition. The term 'primary impotence' implies that the patient has never had an erection. This is rare and is usually associated with gross abnormality of the penis or hormone deficiency from childhood. Secondary impotence is much more common and may be due to psychological or organic factors, or to a combination of both.

Most men will occasionally fail to gain or maintain an erection. This can be attributed to stress, overwork, or some other reason and would not be considered impotence.

Causes of impotence. Psychological factors causing secondary impotence have been categorised by Kolodny et al (1979) as follows:

1. Developmental:
   - maternal or paternal factors
   - conflict in parent/child relationship
   - severe negative family attitude to sex
   - traumatic childhood sexual experience

Research Abstract 7.6 Vasectomy and testicular tumours

In the past 10 years an increased incidence of testicular cancer has been recorded in Scotland. Vasectomy has become a more popular form of contraception, and a retrospective research study by Cale et al (1990) has suggested that there may be an association between vasectomy and subsequent testicular tumours. It is queried whether some immunological and pathophysiological effects may occur following vasectomy, or whether such tumours in fact developed before vasectomy.

The importance of testicular examinations before and after vasectomy is recognised. Men should be screened by an examination at 12 to 18 months after vasectomy. A large prospective research study is needed to fully establish whether vasectomy contributes to testicular malignancy.

Cale A J R et al 1990 Does vasectomy accelerate testicular tumour? Importance of testicular examinations before and after vasectomy. British Medical Journal 300: 370

- gender identity conflict
- traumatic first coital experience
- homosexuality

2. Affective:
   - anxiety about performance
   - guilt
   - depression
   - poor self-esteem
   - hypochondria
   - mania
   - fear of causing pregnancy
   - fear of venereal disease
3. Interpersonal:
   - poor communication
   - hostility towards partner
   - distrust of partner
   - lack of physical attraction to partner
   - sex role conflict
   - divergent sexual preference, or sex value systems, e.g. time, place, type
4. Cognitive:
   - sexual ignorance
   - acceptance of cultural myths
   - performance demands
5. Miscellaneous:
   - premature ejaculation
   - isolated episode of erectile failure
   - iatrogenic influences.

Organic causes of secondary impotence include:

- poor arterial inflow caused by atherosclerosis and aneurysm
- venous leaks between the corpora and venous system
- neurological diseases
- endocrine dysfunction
- drugs, including antihypertensives, narcotics, and alcohol
- major surgery: cystectomy (see p. 314); radical prostatectomy (see Ch. 8, p. 312).

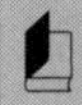

For further information, see Morrison (1988).

MEDICAL MANAGEMENT

Tests and investigations. Therapy will depend upon diagnosis of the underlying cause of the impotence. Investigations include (Hanno & Wein 1987):

- a full history of psychological and organic disorders, with particular reference to erectile function
- physical assessment, including examination of penis, testes, prostate and seminal vesicles; neurological examination; vascular examination
- blood screen for evidence of endocrine imbalance, diabetes mellitus, renal failure
- assessment of penile blood flow by Doppler studies and angiography
- psychological testing.

Medical intervention. Options for treatment are as follows.

Local injection. A local injection at the base of the penis using the α-adrenergic receptor blocking agents, papaverine or a combination or papaverine and phentolamine can cause an erection. The action is by vasodilatation and vasocongestion within the spongy tissue of the penis. An erection can be maintained for a period of about 30 min. Patients can be taught to self-inject at home. Complications include fibrosis at the base of the penis and priapism requiring emergency hospital treatment.

Penile prosthesis. There are various types of penile prosthesis available. The semi-rigid prosthesis consists of two semi-rigid silicone-covered rods cut to size. These are inserted into the shaft of the penis, in the corpora cavernosa, giving a permanent erection which is firm enough to allow the patient to have intercourse.

Infection at the site of the prosthesis and rejection may occur. The evident erection may cause the patient embarrassment and restrict the wearing of swimming trunks or tight trousers. This may on occasion prove unacceptable to both the patient and his partner.

Revascularisation of the penis. This is a new advance in surgery and can help patients who have arterial problems. It involves anastomosing an abdominal artery to the penile vein to improve the blood supply. Although not considered major surgery, it does leave the patient with a fairly large abdominal scar. Infection may be a postoperative problem. This procedure has the advantage of restoring normality, but its success rate is only about 50%. Some patients may still require a penile prosthesis.

Vacuum suction machine. These machines have been available for some time from sex shops and magazines but have only recently been recognized as a valuable treatment for patients with impotence. The machine produces a partial vacuum around the penis, causing it to engorge. An elastic band is then placed around the base of the penis to maintain the erection for a maximum of 15 min. The advantage of this treatment is that the patient can control the erection, but the duration of the erection is limited by the ischaemic effect of the tourniquet.

Psychotherapy. Impotence judged to be psychological in origin may be helped by psychotherapy for the patient and his partner.

NURSING PRIORITIES AND MANAGEMENT: IMPOTENCE

Major patient problems

Psychological considerations

A man who realises that he has become impotent is likely to be shocked and dismayed. He may be reluctant to talk about the problem, even to his partner. This can become a very complex matter, not only for the individual but for his partner and family. Failure to accept or understand the problem can lead to the breakup of a marriage or partnership. Moreover, organic causes of impotence such as multiple sclerosis, diabetes, and circulatory problems may have already caused the patient to change his lifestyle and placed the family under stress.

The patient may be very reluctant to open up to a doctor or nurse. He may present to his GP ostensibly with another problem, only managing with difficulty to mention his real concern. Occasionally it is at an outpatient appointment such as a diabetic clinic that the subject is brought up.

Medical and nursing staff must treat the patient with empathy and sensitivity. While the condition is not life-threatening and may not be considered urgent, once the patient presents he will want something done quickly.

Practical considerations for the patient receiving a penile implant

The nurse should ensure that the patient is given sufficient information about the procedure and the recovery period. He should be told that his hospital stay will be 4–7 days, and that while there will be some pain regular analgesics will be given. Catheterisation will be required for at least 24 h. Complete bedrest will not be required, but it will be important for the patient not to spend too much time walking around or sitting in a chair for the first few days. He will need to wear a scrotal support for a few weeks, to help prevent swelling and to minimise discomfort.

The consultant will discuss with the patient how soon the prosthesis may be used, but it is likely that he will recommend that it not be used until after the first outpatient appointment in 6 weeks. Sutures will not normally require removal, but will dissolve on their own. It is helpful to assure the patient that visitors or other patients on the ward will not know what procedure he is undergoing unless he tells them himself. Nor will other people know that he has a prosthesis, although it may be necessary to avoid wearing tight trousers or swimming trunks.

OTHER DISORDERS

Inflammatory disorders of the male reproductive organs are briefly described in Box 7.5. Disorders especially affecting the prostate, the urethra and urinary function, are described in Chapter 8.

DISORDERS OF THE FEMALE REPRODUCTIVE SYSTEM

Gynaecological cancer

Cancer is a state of overgrowth of tissue that is the result of disorganised cell division. Normal mechanisms limit tissue cell reproduction according to the replacement needs of the body. In some circumstances the restraining mechanism of a cell may be faulty. The cell is then able to multiply without restriction or concern for balancing body requirements.

The organs of the female reproductive system are susceptible to benign or malignant overgrowths of tissues. The property of cancerous growth may be conferred on a cell of the ovary, the body of the uterus, the cervix or the vulva.

Carcinoma of the cervix

The cervical tissue is at particular risk of carcinomatous change. There are approximately 2000 deaths in England and Wales from carcinoma of the cervix each year. Approximately 4000 cases are registered each year. The mortality rate for the UK was 8 per 100 000 of the female population in 1991, which shows a small decrease over the past 20 years (HMSO 1993). The cancer is preceded by a pre-invasive condition that can be simply and effectively treated if identified by cervical cytological screening. In more than 90% of cases cell abnormality can be detected by screening. Cancer of the cervix occurs most often in women between 30 and 50 years of age.

PATHOPHYSIOLOGY

The cancer does not develop in the original squamous or columnar epithelium of the cervix, but develops exclusively within a special type of stratified squamous epithelium which replaces columnar epithelium. The columnar epithelium is usually found in the cervical canal (endocervix) but may extend to the outer surface of the cervix (ectocervix) as far as the vaginal fornix.

The process of change is known as squamous metaplasia. Squamous metaplasia can be:

- a normal, though irreversible, change from columnar cells to squamous cells
- an atypical metaplasia or dysplasia that has a neoplastic potential providing an environment for malignancy.

A specific segment of DNA (the fundamental genetic material of all cells), known as an 'oncogena', has been identified as giving a cell its cancer potential.

Adolescence, the time of menstruation, the first pregnancy, and the prenatal period are times of maximum cellular activity in the cervix, when the tissues are more sensitive to a carcinogen that has been sexually transmitted and more prone to genetic mutation. The relationship between cervical squamous precancer and sexual intercourse appears to be conclusive since the condition is virtually unknown in celibate women. There is some aspect of the act of intercourse that may make the cervical epithelium more susceptible to the introduction of a mutagen.

Epidemiological observations indicate that the age of onset of intercourse and the number of sexual partners influence the development of cervical precancer and cancer (Lewis & Chamberlain 1990). The condition is also more common in lower socioeconomic groups.

The more sexual partners the woman has had, the more likely she is to be exposed to the unknown carcinogen(s). Two viruses have been proposed as possible carcinogens:

- the human papilloma virus (HPV) (Baird 1983, Wagner et al 1984)
- the herpes simplex virus type 2 (Cabral et al 1983, Park et al 1983, Smith 1983).

A direct causal relationship has yet to be proved. The HPV Types 16 and 18 have been classified as high risk. HPV is considered to be the most likely of the two viruses to be carcinogenic but either or both viruses may be involved.

Studies of the role of the male sexual partner suggest the possible transmission of viruses but also refer to the possible carcinogenic effect of human sperm. It is suggested that the basic proteins of histone and protamine fraction of the sperm heads may act as carcinogens. Some men may be high-risk sexual partners (French et al 1982).

Evidence suggests that women who smoke are at increased risk of developing cancer of the cervix (Berggren & Sjostedt 1983, Clarke & Hilditch 1983, Trevathan et al 1983).

The risk and causative factors in cervical cancer may combine to induce the disease process. Factors currently considered to be important are listed in Box 7.6. These factors may change as research continues.

Carcinoma of the cervix is now classified as a preventable disease if certain examinations are undertaken regularly by women. Cervical cancer that is identified in the pre-invasive stage is curable.

Box 7.6 Risk factors and possible causes of carcinoma of the cervix (Reproduced with kind permission from Shingleton & Orr (1987))

Risk factors
Early intercourse (before 17 years of age)
Multiple sexual partners
Early pregnancy
Living in an urban environment
Low socioeconomic status
Smoking
Immunosuppression
Use of oral contraception
Previous abnormal smear
Failure to participate in screening
Nutritional deficits — Vitamins A, C, folic acid
High-risk male partner
In-utero diethylstilboestrol exposure.

Possible causes
Human papilloma virus
Herpes simplex virus
Sperm from high-risk tissue-type male
Smoking
In-utero exposure to diethylstilboestrol
Immune deficiency.

MEDICAL MANAGEMENT

History and examination. The earliest knowledge that a woman may gain of a malignant change in the cervix may be from a report on a cervical smear test. A clear vaginal discharge may occur in the early stages, whereas later the discharge may be bloodstained or may have a bad odour. Irregular vaginal bleeding may be associated with prolonged menstruation, occur between periods, follow sexual intercourse, or be post-menopausal. Pain may be experienced when metastases are present or if there is nerve involvement.

Where there is advanced disease, venous or lymphatic obstruction may lead to extensive oedema. Blocked ureters may result in renal failure, and the spread of growth may lead to fistula formation between the vagina and rectum, or the vagina and the urinary bladder. Incontinence will be unavoidable. Massive haemorrhage may occur and death may be related to kidney failure or intestinal complications.

Investigations. The following procedures may be completed:

- Papanicolaou smear test
- colposcopy and biopsy
- Schiller test
- histological examination of smears and tissue specimens.

Papanicolaou (Pap) smear test. Women are advised to have a Papanicolaou cervical smear test usually at 1–2 year intervals. The death rate from carcinoma of cervix has decreased in countries with comprehensive cervical screening programmes. A dramatic decrease is recorded in Iceland where 100% of women participated in screening. A 50–75% decrease in mortality is usually reported amongst participating women.

Screening should be available to women from the time sexual activity begins through to 69 years of age.

The cells identified from the cervical smears are classified as shown in Box 7.7. This information is supplemented as appropriate with the histological grade of pre-invasive disease CIN1, CIN2 or CIN3. (See Box 7.8.)

Women are often asked to have an inconclusive smear test repeated to clarify the diagnosis. Women are encouraged to have cervical smear tests during the child-bearing years and in the post-menopausal years up to the age of 60, or later if hormone replacement therapy continues to place the woman in a high-risk category.

Box 7.7 Papanicolaou smear test results in graded classes

Class 1: cells are normal in appearance
Class 2: abnormal cells are present but are not malignant; the patient may have suffered from vaginal inflammation
Class 3: abnormal cells are present and are suggestive of malignancy
Class 4: abnormal cells are present and appear to be malignant
Class 5: abnormal cells are present and definitely malignant.

Box 7.8 Histology of cervical intraepithelial neoplasia (CIN)

Current terminology for cervical intraepithelial neoplasia describes three grades of change as part of a continuum of pre-invasive disease:

CIN 1 corresponds to mild dysplasia
CIN 2 corresponds to moderate dysplasia
CIN 3 corresponds to severe dysplasia and carcinoma in situ.

Schiller test. Iodine 3.5% is used to stain normal cells of the cervix. Abnormal cells will not pick up the colour because they do not contain glycogen. A section of tissue is taken for histology.

Colposcopy and biopsy. Every women who has an abnormal smear test result should be examined with the colposcope but the high incidence of cervical cell abnormalities makes this an unrealistic expectation. Colposcopy is recommended immediately for all women with a smear that suggests CIN2 or CIN3.

The area of the cervix where the columnar epithelium of the cervical canal and endocervix meets the squamous epithelium of the ectocervix is known as the 'transformation zone'.

Acetic acid or iodine is applied to the transformation zone and the area is carefully examined with the colposcope. Several biopsies are taken from the abnormal areas in the transformation zone. Histological examination of the biopsies will confirm the diagnosis of pre-invasive disease. If the transformation zone cannot be completely visualised because it extends too high in the cervical canal a cone biopsy is performed for diagnosis.

A diagnostic biopsy method may be that of punch biopsy or low-voltage diathermy loop excision biopsy. The punch biopsy tends to crush the sampled tissue and may not include stroma which may lead to missing invasive disease. The diathermy loop excision method produces tissue samples of better size and has better control of bleeding.

MEDICAL MANAGEMENT

Conservative treatment. Pre-invasive cancer of the cervix that can be fully visualised within the transformation zone can be treated by destruction of the entire transformation zone down to a depth of 6 mm. This depth will ensure the destruction of diseased crypts and glands, without destroying normal tissue. Accurate assessment of depth is difficult. Conservative treatment is important to the woman who has not yet started a family and needs to avoid developing an incompetent cervix to prevent loss of a future pregnancy.

The following destructive treatment methods may be used.

Cryotherapy. Cryonecrosis is produced by crystallisation of intracellular water using nitrous oxide or carbon dioxide. Freeze–thaw–freeze techniques produce the best results. Little or no analgesia is required. There is some concern about the adequacy of the technique. Cure rates have been reported between 27 and 96%. (Charles & Savage 1980).

Electrocoagulation diathermy. Temperatures of over 700°C are used to induce tissue destruction to at least 7 mm of depth. The procedure is painful and is carried out under general anaesthesia. Bleeding and discharge may occur in the postoperative period. A high success rate is achieved: 88–97% (Woodman et al 1985).

Cold coagulation. A thermasound heated to 120°C is applied for 20-second treatments to five areas of the surface of the cervix. The procedure is completed under local anaesthesetic and a cure rate of 94% is reported (Gordon & Duncan 1991).

Laser vaporisation. The carbon dioxide laser may be applied to the cervix to ablate the pre-invasive cancer by causing intracellular water to boil, create steam, and explode cells. The laser power may be pulsed or be continuous in use. The depth of tissue destruction can be controlled. The procedure can be performed under local anaesthetic. Post-operatively primary or secondary haemorrhage may occur. A 94% success rate is reported (Baggish et al 1989).

Cone biopsy. When a transformation zone is not fully visible for colposcopy then an excisional method of treating the pre-invasive cancer has to be used. A cone or cylinder of tissue is removed, either by laser or by the scalpel in the traditional way, after the application of Lugol's iodine to the tissues. The entire transformation zone is excised, which provides a large specimen for histological examination and allows confirmation that all diseased tissue has been removed or that the disease was more extensive than originally diagnosed.

The procedure may be complicated by secondary haemorrhage, infection or cervical stenosis or incompetence. Uterine perforation and pelvic abscess have been known to occur.

Large loop excision of the transformation zone (LLETZ) may be achieved by low-voltage diathermy as an alternative to cone biopsy. It is performed under colposcopic guidance. The wire loop is introduced into the cervix and taken slowly across the cervix, enveloping the transformation zone. Slow movement facilitates a clean cut with the wire, with minimum coagulation. The transformation zone may be removed in one or several pieces. The procedure is performed under local anaesthetic. Vaginal bleeding and discharge usually occurs for 2 weeks. Severe secondary haemorrhage may occasionally occur.

NURSING PRIORITIES AND MANAGEMENT: PRE-INVASIVE CANCER OF THE CERVIX

The patient with pre-invasive cancer is treated as an out-patient or a day case. Diagnosis, treatment and follow-up are completed in separate visits to a colposcopy clinic.

Information about appointments and details of cervical smears, colposcopy procedure and possible treatment of the condition is usually sent to the patient in advance of attendance at the clinic. An appointment for colposcopy is given to correspond with the middle of the menstrual cycle, which is a favourable time for the procedure. The nurse will need to reinforce the information given when the patient attends the clinic, to ensure that the patient understands the procedures planned and the expected outcome.

Opportunities need to be provided for patients to express any concerns that they have. Anxiety levels amongst women presenting for colposcopy have been found to be higher than those of women going for surgery. They were as concerned about the procedure as much as about their illness condition (Marteau et al 1990). The nurse can positively seek to reduce the anxiety level of the patient to an acceptable level for her. Sensitive approaches are required to help the patient to express her feelings and think rationally about the future after treatment.

When the patient feels more calm, other information can be given as it is more likely to be retained. The nurse has to tell the person to expect vaginal discharge and some bleeding after the treatment, and what to do if bleeding becomes suddenly very heavy or if she suspects she has an infection. The opportunity for health promotion regarding possible smoking can be taken.

Arrangements for a follow-up cervical smear test are discussed as part of the pre-discharge routine, as well as the need for future annual check-ups.

Invasive carcinoma of the cervix

PATHOPHYSIOLOGY

Commonly carcinoma develops from the vaginal surface of the cervix and less often from the cervical canal. It may form an ulcer on the cervix or become a fungating cauliflower-type growth and is of the squamous cell type. Adenocarcinoma of the cervix develops in the glands of the endocervix and accounts for 10% of cervical cancer. Tissues become eroded and infected, forming an unpleasant vaginal discharge.

The carcinoma spreads by direct infiltration of surrounding tissues and via lymphatic vessels. Blood-borne metastases in more distant organs occur less often. The prognosis for cervical cancer relates to the extent of the growth at the time of diagnosis rather than the histological type of the cancer.

The international classification of carcinoma of the cervix is shown in Box 7.9.

Box 7.9 International classification of carcinoma of the cervix

Stage O:	pre-invasive carcinoma, also known as carcinoma in situ CIN3
Stage IA:	micro-invasive carcinoma; less than 5 mm in depth
Stage IB:	neoplasm confined to the cervix
Stage IIA:	neoplasm has infiltrated adjacent parametric tissue or upper vagina; if the carcinoma is endocervical then it has extended up into the uterus in this stage
Stage IIB:	tumour extending to the parametrium but not to the pelvic wall
Stage IIIA:	lower third of the vagina is involved or the parametrium
Stage IIIB:	involves lymph nodes as far as the pelvic wall, or there are isolated metastases in the pelvis, often obstructing a ureter
Stage IVA:	spread of growth to adjacent organs
Stage IVB:	spread to distant organs.

MEDICAL MANAGEMENT

History and examination. A woman may have no particular symptoms at the time a cervical smear result confirms that cancer of the cervix exists. On the other hand, she may visit the doctor because of irregular vaginal bleeding, perhaps associated with sexual intercourse, micturition or defaecation. An ulcerated area or an overgrowth of tissue on the cervix may be directly visible to the doctor on examination using a vaginal speculum.

The vaginal discharge becomes more continuous, a thin blood-stained loss may change to a thicker, brown, offensive discharge, or heavier bleeding episodes. Lower abdominal pain develops and the growth increases in size and spread and exerts pressure on supporting structures. Very severe lower back and sciatic pain may occur and lymphatic nodes adhere to the sacral plexus. Pressure on the pudendal nerve and blood vessels causes obstruction to the venous return and oedema of the legs.

Incontinence of urine and faeces may occur as the bladder and rectum are inflated with growth or react to radiation side effects. Ureters may become blocked and renal failure may ensue.

Investigations. A number of investigations are completed before any treatment is planned to establish the spread or otherwise of the disease. A chest X-ray and intravenous pyelogram are completed to gain information of obstruction of the flow of urine from the kidneys which indicates involvement of the parametrium. Some doctors perform a cystoscopy as a routine. A lymphangiogram and a CT scan will assist with identification of disease spread to lymph nodes.

MEDICAL MANAGEMENT

Surgery. When the carcinoma is confined to the cervix, resection of the malignant tissue is necessary. This may be achieved by laser beam therapy, cone biopsy of the endocervical tissue, or amputation of the cervix. Where there is extension of the growth up into the uterus then the operation of hysterectomy and removal of pelvic lymph nodes will be necessary.

Radical surgery may be planned for some patients who are at earlier stages of the disease and are more generally fit. This surgery may be combined with radiotherapy as tumours of the cervix are particularly radiosensitive. Care is planned by the surgeon and radiotherapist, jointly. The Wertheim–Bonney–Meigs operation involves removal of the uterus, cervix, the upper third of the vagina, pelvic cellular tissue lateral to the uterus and vagina, and the uterosacral and cardinal ligaments. The lymphatic glands in the obturator fossae and along the external and internal iliac vessels are removed. The ovaries are preserved in premenopausal women.

To facilitate the excision of the cervix, vagina and supporting ligaments the ureters are dissected free during the operation. Post-operatively there may be a breakdown of the ureteric anastomosis leading to a urinary fistula. It is known for the autonomic nerve supply to the bladder to be disturbed resulting in incomplete bladder emptying as a complication.

Pelvic exenteration. Where there is extensive recurrent disease an anterior pelvic exenteration may be performed, involving removal of all the reproductive organs and the urinary bladder. The ureters are implanted into an artificial bladder fashioned from a loop of ileum. If the rectum is also removed a terminal colostomy is formed. This extremely radical surgery may be combined with cytotoxic drug therapy using cisplatin and other chemotherapeutic agents.

Radiotherapy. Stages III and IV of carcinoma of cervix are usually inoperable. Palliative irradiation therapy is then indicated. Radiotherapy is initially to reduce the size of tumour, inhibit its growth, and reduce its blood supply before surgical removal by hysterectomy. Caesium 137 rods may be inserted under general anaesthetic into the uterine cavity and vaginal vault to provide a radiation dose to the whole pelvis. The treatment will reduce the blood supply to the growth and exert a lethal effect on the cancer cells. Hysterectomy may be performed after local irradiation by caesium or standard supervoltage techniques. Cytotoxic drug treatments are used as necessary, in combination with other therapies. The surgeon may fashion a ureteric transplant or a colostomy that will provide more physical comfort for the patient in the later phase of the illness.

Radiation may also be administered via sophisticated machinery such as the Cathetron, which can pass high-intensity radiocobalt radiation from a protected store along ducts to applicators already positioned in the uterus and vagina. The patient is treated in a protected room, reducing radiation risks to others.

The dose of radiation necessary to kill the tumour cells may leave a very low level of protection for healthy tissue cells. Short- or long-term radiation reactions may be induced by therapy. The bladder and rectal tissue may become swollen, inflamed, friable or fibrosed and there is a risk of the development of a fistula. The patient may become distressed by urinary problems or diarrhoea. Symptoms are relieved as they occur. Minor surgical repair operations may be necessary. The patient's general comfort is of prime importance.

MEDICAL MANAGEMENT

Examination. The patient with carcinoma of the cervix requires a general physical examination and a thorough pelvic examination. Haematological and blood chemistry, and nutritional studies will be completed. An examination under anaesthetic (EUA) is carried out at the time of cone biopsy or the insertion of radio-isotopes. The EUA increases the accuracy of identifying the stage of development of the growth. It allows better examination of the upper vagina and improved palpation of the abdomen, pelvis, and enlarged pelvic, inguinal, and para-aortic lymph nodes. Fine needle aspiration of nodes under sonar or computer tomography guidance may be performed to delineate the spread of the cancer. The information gained is used to confirm, modify or extend treatment plans.

Serum markers. Tumour-derived and tumour-associated markers in the plasma of patients with carcinoma of the cervix continue to be studied and reported on in the medical literature (Shingleton and Orr 1987). Individual marker levels may be used at the assessment stage, in the planning of treatment, when monitoring the response to treatment, and in the follow-up years of care. Marker measurement values tend to increase with the stage of disease and decrease with effective treatment. Initial levels before treatment may be an aid to prognosis. The following are examples of serum markers that may be studied:

Carcinoembryonic antigen (CEA). Squamous cell carcinoma and adenocarcinoma have significantly different capacities for CEA release (Kjorstad & Orjasaester 1984).

Plasma *histaminase* falls during radiotherapy with a value that is inversely proportional to the radiation response (Birdi et al 1984).

Tumour associated antigen (TA-4) provides a means for monitoring squamous cell tumours (Maruo et al 1985).

Immunosuppressive acid protein (IPA). It is reported that patients with recurrent cervical cancer had elevated IPA, whilst 83% of patients previously treated but without evidence of recurrence, did not have elevated levels (Sawada et al 1984).

NURSING PRIORITIES AND MANAGEMENT: HYSTERECTOMY

Preoperative care

Assessment

The patient who is to have a hysterectomy for carcinoma of the cervix will be admitted to the ward with enough time to allow for necessary medical investigative procedures to be carried out before the operation. She is likely to be physically fairly independent of the nurse for her personal care but will need to be familiarised to the new surroundings of the ward.

The assessment process will identify the patient's individual problems and needs for nursing assistance and support. She will be invited to share details of her menstrual history, the events leading up to the admission, her last menstrual period date, and the current degree of vaginal blood loss or discharge. The patient who has previously been prescribed an oral contraceptive drug will have been advised to discontinue the contraceptive pill and use an alternative barrier method for 6 weeks prior to the operation to reduce the risk of development of a thrombus during surgery or the post-operative period. The nurse will need to check that this advice has been followed.

A particular guideline for assessment may be available to the nurse in the ward to prompt the recording of gynaecological details. A nurse who is inexperienced in the specialty may find that the nursing model used for assessment may not easily prompt her to seek the necessary information.

Identification of actual and potential problems

The summary of patient problems at the end of assessment will differ, reflecting the stage of the cervical carcinoma. Problems of distressful pain in the back or abdomen, poor appetite and weight loss, as described in the medical history section earlier in this chapter, are associated with later stages of the disease. The patient may identify few actual problems herself but may agree with the nurse that she has some special needs at this time that will be part of her care plan.

Anxiety

In anticipating hysterectomy the woman may experience considerable anxiety that is related to surviving the operation and the illness condition. A change in body image may occur, a sense of loss and some alteration in sexuality and sexual identity may be feared. The woman's loving relationship with her partner may appear to be threatened by the surgery, particularly if her child-bearing potential is lost. Anxiety may also be focused on the family that remain at home; how will the children and her partner cope whilst she is in hospital? She may have financial worries and concerns about how her illness will affect her ability to work and support the family in future. A gentle approach by the nurse may help her to speak about her main worries. Being able to talk about her feelings at the time of assessment may be the first stage of making a positive adjustment in reducing anxiety. The nurse will be able to plan to utilise opportunities to help the patient manage her anxiety during the hospital period. Part of the process to reduce anxiety will involve the giving of information to increase her understanding of all procedures and her personal progress.

The need for information

In preparation for surgery the patient needs information about the events that are to be expected leading up to the operation and during the recovery period. The benefits of planned information-giving preoperatively, based on nursing research findings is described in Chapter 27. Opportunity must be given for the patient to ask questions and to express fears.

She will need to know about how pain will be relieved. She will have her own patient-controlled analgesia system (PCA) or epidural analgesia. Time is taken to explain that sexual relations with her partner will still be possible after hysterectomy and refashioning of the vagina. An information booklet that explains the operation and the internal changes that will have occurred from surgery and answers many questions about the future should be provided for the patient to read at her leisure. This provides a permanent reminder of what she may have been told and reinforces her understanding.

The surgeon will advise when sexual intercourse may be resumed. She will benefit from knowing that a sexual climax will again be achievable even though the womb has been lost through surgery. The nurse can explain that the pleasurable sexual experience is achieved from the stimulation of the external clitoris within the vulva and the psychological stimulation of the penis in the vagina. She may already be knowledgeable of these functions but will be pleased to know that the experience should not change. It is helpful if the patient's partner or friend can be included in the information-giving session. The patient may then approach surgery more calmly and confidently, and recover with minimal physical or emotional problems. See Research Abstract 7.7.

The need for exercise and mobilising skills

Patients will have limited mobility in the first 48 hours after a hysterectomy. There will be a risk of venous stasis and pressure-sore development. People should be encouraged to practise foot and leg exercises before the day of the operation, so that they understand how to carry out the exercises whilst resting in bed after surgery. If appropriate, use of the contraceptive pill, with its potential risk of deep vein thrombosis, will already have been discontinued and a short course of intra-adipose heparin given as prophylactic medication. People will also benefit from experiencing how it feels to be moved and lifted by nurses and a mechanical hoist, and will know what they can do to assist the process. This should help reduce apprehension about being moved at a time when dependent and in some pain. A visit by the physiotherapist will complement the work of the nurse but will also include deep-breathing and coughing exercises to be used after the operation. Smokers will be asked to discontinue.

Protection from hazards

The person preparing for and undergoing hysterectomy needs to be safeguarded from misidentification and wrong operation. The patient must wear an identification bracelet at all times and this must be strictly checked at strategic times in the immediate preoperative period. The nurse responsible for planning care writes specific instructions for maintaining patient safety. Many hospitals and NHS Trusts use a preoperative checklist or protocol for every patient preparing for surgery. Such protocols have been agreed by ward nurses, anaesthetic and theatre staff and reflect the quality standard of patient safety to be achieved. Instructions to use the preoperative checklist are recorded in the patient's care plan.

The doctor is responsible for fully informing the patient about the operation planned and is required to gain the patient's informed consent in writing. The nurse preparing the patient checks that the consent form has been signed before completing the other major surgery pre-operative procedures which are described in detail in Chapter 27. The patient will wear anti-embolism stockings to counteract venous stasis during the operation period. A premedication is given as prescribed. The patient relaxes in bed until she leaves the ward escorted by her nurse who completes a safe transfer to the operating theatre suite staff.

Research Abstract 7.7 A study of self-concept and social support after hysterectomy

Webb & Wilson-Barnett (1983) studied depression, self-concept and sexual life in 128 women during recovery from hysterectomy as part of a nursing study. At the time of operation, 103 were pre-menopausal and 102 were sexually active. The women were interviewed 1 week and 4 months after the hysterectomy.

The results showed that women felt physically and emotionally much better, were less tired and irritable, had gone back to work, and had resumed leisure and social activities. Responses showed that:

- 94% were happy to have no more periods
- 84% were glad they could no longer become pregnant
- 90% of those who were sexually active said their sex life was now as good as, or even better than, previously
- 92% were glad they had the operation.

The small numbers who gave 'negative' replies to these questions were still not completely recovered and gave this as the reason for their answers. They referred to physical complications of wound, urinary, or vaginal infections which delayed recuperation rather than the psychological problems suggested in medical studies.

In studying the social support of these women results showed:

- 70% had been told 'old wives' tales' of pessimistic outcomes; 11% felt there was some truth in them after their own experiences
- 23% of partners (N = 103) had been given no extra help in the home.

The greatest area of dissatisfaction was of information from doctors and nurses. Women would have liked guidance on what they could do, how they might feel as they progressed and what symptoms or complications could occur.

The Roy adaptation nursing model was used in the care of a patient following hysterectomy (Webb 1988).

Webb C & Wilson-Barnett J 1983 Self concept, social support and hysterectomy. International Journal of Nursing Studies 20(2): 97–107

Postoperative care

The patient's individual needs and actual problems will transfer from a preoperative care plan to a postoperative care plan but a major new focus will be that of maintaining a safe internal and external environment for the patient. There are a number of potential problems the nurse is aware of that will feature in the care plan and will have been explained to the patient preoperatively. The general care of a patient following major abdominal surgery is as described in Chapter 27 and in Nursing Care Plan 7.1.

Carcinoma of the body of the uterus

Carcinoma of the body of the uterus is more common with advancing age; three quarters of sufferers are post-menopausal. The condition is associated with infertility, hormone replacement therapy, diabetes mellitus, obesity and hypertension. An excess of oestrogen is common to all the risk factors. Carcinoma of the body of the uterus is less common than carcinoma of the cervix. There are 3500 cases reported annually. As women are living longer, the present rate is expected to increase.

Nursing Care Plan 7.1 Care of a patient, following a hysterectomy

Potential problems	Expected patient outcomes	Nursing care	Rationale
Irregularity in vital signs	❐ Pulse and BP measurements are within acceptable limits for the patient. ❐ Blood loss through wound or drainage tubes is minimal in any 24 hours.	Record BP and pulse: _________ Inspect wound/drains with above. Observe for any pv loss. Record temperature: __________	Haemorrhage due to loss of haemostasis at operation site would result in hypovolaemia, requiring blood transfusion. Fine drainage tube is in position in wound. Pyrexia may occur due to infection in chest, urinary tract, wound or veins.
Body fluid imbalance	❐ No sign of dehydration or fluid overload. ❐ Patient is adequately hydrated. ❐ Signs of fluid overload are detected from fluid balance record.	Maintain intravenous therapy as prescribed. Observe IV puncture site for signs of infection or fluid being given extravenously. Record fluid intake and output. Dress cannula site with: _______ Change giving set: __________	Major surgery depletes body potassium, sodium, and water levels. Fluid and electrolyte replacement is needed by the intravenous route.
Patient to have nil by mouth	❐ Peristalsis returns within 48 hours.	Patient to be given no fluid or food by the oral route until prescribed by doctor. Record any bowel activity.	Peristaltic movement of the intestines stops when abdomen is opened and gut is handled. Food and fluid, if taken, could not be digested. Bowel sounds heard when peristalsis returns. Patient passes gas.
Urinary bladder is drained by a self-retaining catheter (suprapubic or transurethral). Risk of bladder dysfunction after catheter removal. Risk of urinary tract infection.	❐ Urine drains freely to minimise pressure on operation sites. ❐ Urine is clear and has low bacterial count.	Observe and record urinary output. Obtain catheter specimen of urine: __________ for laboratory culture and sensitivity. Complete catheter toilet: _______ Remove catheter on: _________	During the radical hysterectomy the ureter is either partially dissected to allow resection of the medical portion of the cardinal ligament, or the ureter is more extensively dissected to sever the cardinal ligament at the pelvic sidewall. There may be oedema and bruising of posterior urethral wall. Diminished bladder sensation, reduced bladder compliance and stress incontinence may occur. Urinary tract infection is a risk with a catheter in the urinary bladder.
Possibility of patient becoming distressed or uncomfortable due to postoperative pain.	❐ Patient expresses verbally or by body language that pain has decreased to an acceptable level on a pain scale of 1 = LOW to 5 = HIGH.	Remind the patient of the availability of analgesia. Reposition the patient as necessary for comfort. Give analgesia as prescribed *or* supervise the patient-controlled analgesia system (PCA). Ask patient if analgesia is adequate using pain scale 1 = LOW to 5 = HIGH.	Patients have different pain tolerance levels. It may not be possible to keep the patient pain-free at all times. A degree of pain control that is acceptable to the patient should be planned.

Nursing Care Plan 7.1 ***(Cont'd)***

Potential problems	Expected patient outcomes	Nursing care	Rationale
Limited mobility with risk of: • **venous stasis** • **pressure sores**	❒ No limb tenderness, pain, swelling or redness during hospital stay. ❒ Moves safely within limits allowed. ❒ Pressure areas remain intact.	Supervise limb exercises whilst patient in bed, to be performed ____ hourly. Move patient to relieve pressure over bony prominences: 2 hourly. Anti-embolism stockings to be worn until ______. Mobilisation programme: ____________ ____________	The patient who is immobilised by major surgery and confinement to bed may experience reduced muscular stimulation to the venous system. The blood flow in the veins of the limbs is slowed down, increasing the potential for blood clot formation, inflammation of the vein and surrounding tissues (phlebitis and cellulitis) with accompanying swelling and pain and possible embolism. Body pressure exerted over pressure areas for more than 2 hours will result in compromising the blood supply to the tissues and the development of pressure sores. Exercising of limb muscles and the wearing of anti-embolism stockings are preventative measures that reduce risk. Measures to relieve pressure over pressure areas are effective in preserving skin and other tissue integrity.
Needs information or new skills in readiness for discharge	❒ With information/instruction/ practice will be able to function independently in: ____________ ____________ by discharge on: ________	Patient preparation: ________ ____________ ____________ ____________ ____________	Depending upon progress during the hospital stay the patient will need an individualised predischarge programme. Advice and counselling in areas of the activities of living may be needed. Personal care including wound management, the importance of exercise and restricting of lifting activity should be related to the surgical removal of ligaments and supporting structures in the pelvis and the slow healing of abdominal muscle and other tissues. The patient may be discharged with a suprapubic catheter in situ. Practice will be needed in the management of the closed drainage system. The patient may have the support of a community nurse when at home to complement self-care. The patient will need to know what to do if problems occur, who to contact: GP or hospital. The patient should be encouraged to ask questions and talk about any concerns. Information about a local group of the Hysterectomy Association should be provided should the patient feel in need of support and social contact. Medical staff will need to give specific instructions about when sexual intercourse may be resumed and what follow-up surveillance will be maintained in the observation for recurrence of disease; 20-year follow-up may be achieved.

PATHOPHYSIOLOGY

The columnar epithelium that covers the surface of the endometrium and forms the lining of the glands, gives origin to the carcinoma of the body of the uterus. The growth is usually an adenocarcinoma. In a small number of cases of adenocarcinoma there may be a squamous metaplasia. This squamous element may be benign or malignant.

Endometrial carcinoma develops in an atrophic senile uterus. The lesion penetrates the endometrium, it spreads laterally and grows slowly. With time it penetrates the myometrium deeply, reaches the peritoneal covering and the lymphatic glands become involved. Secondary deposits may affect pelvic and aortic lymph nodes and the ovary. Metastases to the lung, bone, liver or brain may be late, blood-borne complications. See Box 7.10.

MEDICAL MANAGEMENT

History and examination. From the age of 45 years a woman expects changes in the menstrual cycle related to the menopause. The early signs of carcinoma of the uterus may be difficult to distinguish from the changes of the climacteric. Unexpected or irregular vaginal bleeding are significant signs. Bleeding that is too heavy, occurs too often, or happens after cessation of periods at the menopause needs to be investigated. Low abdominal pain may be a late experience for the woman with uterine carcinoma. The vaginal discharge may be clear or brown with an offensive odour.

Investigations. A routine cervical smear test may yield the first evidence of malignant endometrial cells. Diagnosis is usually concluded following curettage of the endometrium and histological identification of malignant cells from curettings or an endometrial biopsy.

MEDICAL MANAGEMENT

Total hysterectomy. Cancer of the uterus is usually treated by total hysterectomy, surgical removal of uterus and cervix with bilateral salpingo-oophorectomy, that is, removal of fallopian tubes and ovaries. The abdominal or vaginal surgical approach may be used. A vaginal hysterectomy is suitable if the uterus is small and not distended with bulky tumour.

Extended hysterectomy. An extended hysterectomy would include removal of pelvic lymph nodes. Surgical treatment may be combined with radiotherapy to the pelvic wall. Alternatively, the uterine tumour may be irradiated to shrink it and deplete its blood supply before surgery. Postoperative radiotherapy may be given either as external beam only or in combination with vault caesium.

Cytotoxic and hormonal drug treatments. Cytotoxic drugs may be used as early as possible following surgery to counteract metastatic seeding. Carcinoma of the endometrium is often sensitive to hormone therapy. High doses of medroxyprogesterone acetate (Depo-Provera) or hydroxyprogesterone caproate (Delalutin) may suppress the progress of the disease in advanced cases and limit metastatic activity. The 5-year survival rates for women treated for early cancer of the uterus are 60–70%.

Box 7.10 International classification of endometrial cancer

Stage 0: carcinoma with no stromal invasion
Stage I: carcinoma confined to the body of the uterus; the cancer is also graded according to histological type

Grade 1 — well-differentiated adenocarcinoma
Grade 2 — moderately differentiated adenocarcinoma with partly solid areas
Grade 3 — predominantly solid or entirely undifferentiated carcinoma

Stage II: the carcinoma involves the cervix as well as the corpus
Stage III: the carcinoma has extended outside the uterus, but not outside the pelvis
Stage IV: the carcinoma has involved the bladder or the rectum or has been extended outside the pelvis.

NURSING PRIORITIES AND MANAGEMENT: CARCINOMA OF THE UTERUS

The nursing care of the patient with cancer of the uterus involves pre- and postoperative care for hysterectomy. Care will be individualised but will be similar to that for the hysterectomy for the patient with carcinoma of the cervix, previously described in this chapter.

Total or extended hysterectomy does not involve dissection of the ureters, as involved in radical hysterectomy, so the patient should have less difficulty with recovery of bladder function postoperatively, as there will be no disturbance of the nerve supply or any bladder wound involved. A self-retaining urethral catheter may be used in the first few days, to avoid distending the urinary bladder and exerting pressure on the posterior urethral wall, which may be swollen and bruised.

A haematoma may form in the vault of the vagina as a complication of the vaginal hysterectomy. This will result in prolonged abdominal discomfort, raised body temperature, and a sustained feeling of being unwell for the patient until the haematoma is diagnosed and drained as a medical procedure.

The patient will need information about her progress at regular intervals in the postoperative period. Of particular concern may be the need to have cytotoxic drug therapy at an early, vulnerable stage after the major surgery. The patient may feel greatly debilitated by the side effects of nausea and vomiting. Psychological support from the nurse should help the patient view the chemotherapy as the final safety-net stage of the treatment process. Positive improvements should be seen within 3 months of treatment being completed.

Medical follow-up will be essential to monitor progress and identify early signs of recurrence of disease.

Malignant disease of the ovary

Ovarian cancer is more common in Western countries than in Japan or in some African countries. It is suggested that there is some nutritional variation and a social class difference, in that the disease is more common in the better-nourished and the upper social groups. A relationship is said to exist between multiple ovulation in women in well-nourished communities, and the incidence of cancer of the ovary. The condition is common in infertile women and in women who have not taken a sexual partner. A previous problem of endometriosis of the ovary is linked to malignant change. The peak incidence is between 40–65 years of age.

PATHOPHYSIOLOGY

Both a primary and secondary focus are equally common. The malignant tumour may occur unilaterally or bilaterally. Carcinoma of the body of the uterus may directly spread to the ovary, although this is less common with carcinoma of the cervix or vagina. The pylorus, sigmoid colon, rectum, gall bladder, breast and kidney are very possible sites of primary growth. The lymphatic channels and the blood vessels facilitate the spread of the disease of the ovary. See Box 7.11.

The ovarian cancer is histologically classified according to the type of cell from which it originates. The most common source of ovarian malignant growth is surface epithelium, which is formed from embryonic mesothelium. Three types of tumour may develop:

- serous (tubal)

Box 7.11 International classification of ovarian cancer

Stage I: disease limited to one or both ovaries
Stage II: growth extending beyond the ovaries but confined within the pelvis
Stage III: growth with widespread intraperitoneal metastases
Stage IV: cases with other distant metastases and/or parenchymal liver involvement.

- endometrioid (endometrial)
- mucinous (endocervical).

Serous papilliferous carcinoma. The malignant serous tumour is the commonest type of primary ovarian cancer and often affects both ovaries. The growth penetrates the capsule of the ovary and projects on the outside surface. Tumour cells are disseminated into the peritoneal cavity to form multiple seedling metastases. In most cases there is rapid spread in the peritoneal cavity. The peritoneum secretes excessive amounts of fluid into the abdominal cavity.

Serous papilliferous cystadenoma. The cysts of this serous new growth contain many papillary processes and are lined with a single layer of cubical epithelium on a vascular connective tissue base. The epithelium resembles that of the fallopian tube, the cells being ciliated.

Mucinous cystadenoma. Mucinous tumours are formed from columnar epithelium, similar tissue to that of the endocervix. The tumours are described as multilocular because they consist of several cysts clustered together and separated from each other by a septum. The cysts have mainly fibrous tissue walls and contain viscid mucin, a glycoprotein. This is usually the largest type of ovarian tumour that may be associated with a benign teratoma.

A mucinous cystadenoma may rupture spontaneously or may be damaged during surgery, spilling epithelial cells on to the peritoneum where seeding and further growth takes place with secretion of mucin that may form a jelly-like mass in the abdominal cavity.

Mucinous carcinoma. Approximately 10% of ovarian cancer is classified as mucinous and 5% of mucinous cysts are found to be malignant (Lewis & Chamberlain 1989). Many of these tumours tend to be identified at an early stage of growth, which gives a better prognosis for the patient.

Endometrioid carcinoma. Endometrioid carcinoma of the ovary histologically resembles adenocarcinoma of the endometrium of the uterus. The tumour tissue consists of tubular gland cells, as found in the endometrium, and may be secondary to uterine disease or it may be a primary ovarian growth that co-exists with cancer in the body of the uterus.

Germ cell tumours. Similar tumours may arise in the germ cells of either sex. They may be benign or malignant. Benign conditions are very common, whilst malignancy is rare. The commonest type of germ cell tumour is the dermoid cyst or cystic teratoma. Dermoid cysts, which are discussed in more detail later in the chapter, usually occur in the ovary but are very rare in the testis. The malignant teratoma is more common in the testis.

Amongst the malignant germ cell tumours, the highest incidence is of the dysgerminoma that histologically resembles a seminoma of the testis. It shows large round cells separated by fibrous septa and is highly malignant, perforating its capsule and spreading cells into the blood and lymphatics.

MEDICAL MANAGEMENT

History and examination. Ovarian cancer is insidious in its growth and the woman may be quite free from discomfort or suspicion until the disease has reached an advanced stage. It is possible that 50% of women with the condition will be inoperable at the time of first surgical investigation. The late symptoms that appear are related to increased pressure in the abdominal-venous channels causing oedema in the legs and pain from pressure on nerves to the legs. Metastatic growth in the peritoneum will contribute to extensive ascites, abdominal pain, frequency of micturition, nausea, vomiting, emaciation, and breathlessness. A thrombosis may form in an iliac vein or in the inferior vena cava. If growth has spread to other organs then other symptoms may occur such as obstruction of the small bowel or the colon.

Investigation. A full pelvic examination is necessary, with palpation of the ovaries. X-rays of the pelvis and vertebrae may show bony metastases. Ultrasonic scanning may help in diagnosis. A Papanicolaou smear test may show ovarian malignant cells in a specimen taken from the posterior fornix of the vagina. An intravenous pyelogram may be performed to assess the degree of involvement of the urinary system. A ureter may become obstructed and hydronephrosis may occur. A laparoscopy is performed at the diagnostic stage of investigations. Ovarian tumours are always surgically removed. It is important that the ovary and peritoneal cavity should be fully assessed to define the spread of the disease.

Treatment. In the event of malignant disease of the ovary being diagnosed, both ovaries need to be removed and total hysterectomy is completed. The tumour may involve the peritoneum or other organs, and as much malignant tissue as possible will be removed. A cytotoxic agent such as Thiotepa may be instilled into the abdominal cavity. Chemotherapy with agents such as cisplatin, doxorubicin, methotrexate or taxol, or supervoltage radiotherapy is necessary after surgery although most malignant ovarian tumours are resistant to irradiation. In advanced states palliative treatment only may be possible. Paracentesis abdominis procedures may be performed to relieve the pain and respiratory distress caused by the ascites. Hospital admissions are arranged as needed. This allows patients to live their last months with their families more comfortably.

NURSING PRIORITIES AND MANAGEMENT: OVARIAN CANCER

The patient with ovarian cancer will need full support from the nurse. The anxieties of investigations, diagnosis, and the physical effects of hysterectomy and cytotoxic drug therapy will need to be anticipated and managed in all aspects as described earlier in the Chapter. The patient may make a full recovery quite quickly or, if secondary disease remains, may be debilitated for longer. She may or may not be aware of the seriousness of the cancer condition. Full details of the illness may have been given or may have been withheld in her best interests. The nurse will work towards helping the patient to make physical and emotional adjustments. Attention will be given to relief from pain, nausea and vomiting after surgery and chemotherapy. As physical problems are relieved, the patient may cope better emotionally but time is needed to adjust to the sad news of the terminal condition. If a warm relationship has been developed with the nurse at the acute stage of treatment, it will sustain the patient who needs to return to the ward to continue with cytotoxic drug therapy or for palliative paracentesis. The patient may choose to spend her last days of illness at home with her family and support of the community nursing service or in the familiar surroundings of the ward with family and staff that are known to her and able to cope with her needs.

Hydatidiform mole (vesicular mole)

Aetiology. The hydatidiform mole is a form of chromosomal disorder where there is abnormal proliferation of the fertilised ovum, the trophoblast, that settles into the endometrium of the uterus. There is hydropic degeneration of the chorionic villi. The chromosomal pattern is 46, XX, but all the chromosomal material is derived from the sperm, which doubles its chromosomes and takes over the ovum. No fetus develops.

PATHOPHYSIOLOGY

A hydatidiform mole is a benign tumour mass of chorionic cells in the uterus, which exists as though it were a developing pregnancy. Ovarian follicles are enlarged and there is an increase in blood and urine levels of chorionic gonadotrophin (HCG). The uterus increases in size, sometimes faster than in a pregnancy. The villi of the trophoblast become swollen and the villi or vesicles cluster together like a bunch of grapes.

MEDICAL MANAGEMENT

History and examination. A woman may visit her doctor because she is uncertain about her vaginal discharge of fresh or altered blood, which does not seem like normal menstruation. She may have noticed that some jelly-like mole vesicles have been expelled. She may be feeling unwell with some nausea and vomiting that resembles early pregnancy. Pelvic pain is not usually a problem but the doctor will complete a general physical examination and vaginal examination. The uterus may be increased in size. A 'blighted ovum' might be suspected but the watery vesicles of the mole, if identified or reported, will alert the doctor to the condition.

Investigations. A series of pregnancy tests will be completed. Pregnancy tests are positive, although there is no fetus present. The urine is diluted 1:10, 1:100 and 1:1000.

A positive pregnancy test in 1:100 dilution of urine is strongly suggestive of the mole. The diagnosis is confirmed and ultrasound investigation and the finding of high levels of HCG in urine or serum. Choriocarcinoma is a serious complication following hydatidiform mole in 1 in 30 cases.

Treatment. The uterus may be stimulated to contract by administration of oxytocin to expel the mole, or it is evacuated vaginally by suction apparatus. The uterus is in a soft, delicate state and is gently curetted to prevent perforation. A hysterectomy may be advised for a woman who has had family or is past child-bearing age. Thorough follow-up of the patient is necessary if hysterectomy has not been performed. At weekly or two-weekly intervals for two years there must be measurement of urinary output of HCG by radioimmunoassay.

COMPLICATIONS

A rising level of HCG with negative curettings of the uterine cavity suggests that the mole has become invasive of the muscle of the uterus and may even erode through the uterine wall, and deposits of molar tissue may be found in other parts of the body, in the peritoneum or in the lungs, and may cause death.

Choriocarcinoma

PATHOPHYSIOLOGY

Choriocarcinoma of the uterine wall, in 50% of cases, occurs after hydatidiform mole. The malignant condition may appear to arise spontaneously from the ovary but it is more likely to be associated with other neoplastic tissues, such as a teratoma. It may follow a normal pregnancy, an abortion or an ectopic pregnancy.

Diagnosis is difficult, but confirmed by HCG estimations in urine and plasma. The tissues contain malignant syncytioblast and cytotrophoblast cells.

MEDICAL MANAGEMENT

History and examination. The patient may have experienced persistent vaginal bleeding after evacuation of a hydatidiform mole or after a termination of pregnancy. Follow-up arrangements after mole removal are usually stringent and early signs of development of the malignant tumour should become obvious, but there are greater risks in other cases if a woman delays visiting the GP.

The uterus becomes ulcerated and causes an offensive, blood-stained vaginal discharge. Metastatic spread of the cancer is speedy and extensive; the brain, lung, liver and other organs may be involved. Early deterioration to death is expected if the condition is not treated early.

Investigations. The tumour produces large amounts of HCG, which is used as a tumour marker. Urine and venous blood specimens are tested. Persistently raised HCG levels are diagnostic. Uterine curettings provide histological evidence that also confirms diagnosis and excludes a very rare ovarian teratoma. HCG levels are also used to monitor the response to therapy.

Treatment. Choriocarcinoma is a rare, highly malignant tumour but is also highly sensitive to single-agent chemotherapy. If the tumour is confined to the uterus then intensive cytotoxic drug treatment is given using the drug methotrexate, toxic to the decidua, with almost 100% successful results. Folinic acid is given to protect the bone marrow. Special facilities are needed to protect patients who have a lowered resistance to infection because of diminished white blood cells in the circulation.

If there is metastatic disease them methotrexate may be combined with other cytotoxic agents. The drugs induce marked side effects during the treatment period and cardiac toxicity may occur. Early detection and treatment of the condition is advised, the disease being known to be curable even after systemic spread. 80% of patients may make a complete recovery if the disease is identified within 6 months of onset. Good prognosis metastatic disease is associated with HCG titre levels of less than 40 000 miu/ml before chemotherapy. HCG levels above 40 000 miu/ml give a poor prognosis.

Some women may need a hysterectomy before treatment is complete but, as the condition occurs in child-bearing years, conservation of the uterus is of concern.

Women may wish to become pregnant after a lapse of 2 years from recovery.

NURSING PRIORITIES AND MANAGEMENT: HYDATIDIFORM MOLE

Nursing care following evacuation of hydatidiform mole will be similar to that following curettage of the uterus. Recovery from anaesthetic should be speedy and the patient will become self-caring very soon after returning to the ward. The nurse will wish to check on the level of blood loss from the vagina, which should be minimal within 24 hours, diminishing quickly. Persistent bleeding should be reported to the medical officer.

Minimal abdominal discomfort should be experienced by the patient. A mild analgesic will be prescribed, if necessary. If a patient experiences more severe pain she should be closely observed and have vital signs recorded. Intensive curetting of the uterus might, in rare cases, result in perforation of the uterus and even damage to the bowel. Any cause for concern should be reported to the medical officer.

A series of postoperative urine and blood specimens will need to be obtained to estimate HCG levels. Specimens may need to be sent to one of the specialised centres in the UK, where there is greater experience in assessing the significance of the HCG levels and reporting results. In the event of persistently high levels of HCG being found, a diagnosis of choriocarcinoma would require transfer of the patient to the specialised centre for the specialised chemotherapy.

The patient being transferred will be very anxious about her condition, having to face up to the seriousness of her illness and the urgency of treatment. The nurse will plan to reinforce the information already given to the patient by the doctor by emphasising the positive aspects of the care to be expected and the expertise of the staff in the specialised centre. Time must be made to help the patient talk about any worries that she has, accepting any emotion released, and facilitating any special wishes she may have. Her partner will be fully involved in the events and will wish to accompany her to the treatment centre.

Intensive nursing care will be planned for the patient at the specialised centre. Special facilities are available for reverse barrier nursing of the patient to protect her from infection as chemotherapy progresses and her immune system is suppressed. Physical, psychological, and social aspects of nursing care will be of primary concern. Many weeks of treatment may be involved before recovery is achieved and the patient returns to normal family life. Follow-up and further HCG monitoring will be essential.

BENIGN TUMOURS OF THE UTERUS

Endometrial polyps

Polyps are benign neoplasms of the endometrium of the uterus. They may develop from an overgrowth of endometrial glands and stroma. The polyp may produce a stalk and may descend towards the vulva. A single polyp or multiple polyps may occur commonly in women of any age group. Vaginal bleeding may be slight but occurs between menstrual periods or following coitus. The polyp is removed from the uterus by twisting it off at its stalk, or by curettage of the endometrium. Recurrent multiple polyps may undergo malignant change. Histological examination of all polyps is routine.

Fibromyomata

Myomas or fibroid tumours of the muscle of the uterus occur in women between 35 years of age and the onset of the menopause. The growth of the fibroids is stimulated by ovarian hormones, particularly oestrogens. Women who have not borne children and women of African origin are more liable to develop such tumours, although they are very common in all racial groups, affecting approximately 20% of women in the pre-menopausal age group.

PATHOPHYSIOLOGY

The fibroid is spherical in shape and firm in consistency, and may achieve varying levels of growth. Some fibroids are small, and some may be large enough to fill the abdominal cavity. The tumour is encapsulated and the capsule contains the blood vessels supplying the tumour. As it grows, the centre of the tumour becomes less vascular and liable to degenerative change.

Multiple fibroids are likely to be found in the uterus and give it an irregular shape (see Fig. 7.8). The fibroids may cause displacement of the uterus and uterine vessels.

MEDICAL MANAGEMENT

History and examination. Menstruation becomes heavier and is prolonged when there are fibroids in the uterus. If the tumours are submucous then menstruation may become irregular and there may be bleeding between periods, but this is not common. Uterine pain may result as the uterus strongly contracts to attempt expulsion of the fibroid. Pressure upon pelvic nerves may cause back or leg pain, or pressure upon pelvic organs may lead to:

- frequency of micturition
- retention of urine

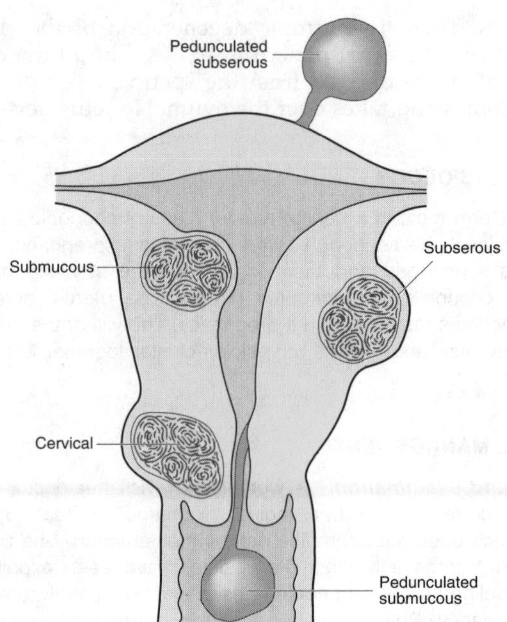

Fig. 7.8 Common sites of fibromyomata in the uterus.

- obstruction of the gastrointestinal system
- oedema of a leg.

A fibroid may become infected and necrotic, causing a purulent vaginal discharge.

The most noticeable change that the woman may talk about is that of increasing girth of the abdomen. Rapid increase in the size of the abdomen may indicate that malignant change has taken place in the fibroid. Polycythaemia is associated with uterine fibroids, but is a rare condition.

On abdominal and vaginal examination the uterus is usually found to be symmetrically enlarged. The uterus feels harder than it does in pregnancy, unless there is some degeneration of the fibroid(s), as occurs after the menopause. The uterus may feel nodular due to the presence of multiple tumours. The lower part of a tumour may be felt through the cervix and the difference between fibroid and carcinoma of cervix may be difficult to ascertain.

Investigations. Pelvic X-ray and ultrasound scan may assist with diagnosis of fibroids. Diagnostic curettage may be performed to exclude endometrial carcinoma. An examination under anaesthetic is helpful in diagnosis. Carcinoma of the bowel may have to be excluded if a hard mass of tumour exists. A sigmoidoscopy or barium enema may be performed.

Treatment. Small fibroids may not be treated and any symptoms should disappear with the menopause. In a woman who desires a future pregnancy it may be suitable to shell out the fibroids from the myometrium, by myomectomy operation. An older woman may best be treated by hysterectomy. Small fibroids may be removed by vaginal hysterectomy. Any anaemia experienced by the patient is rectified by blood transfusion before surgery.

Fibroids and pregnancy

A woman with a fibroid in the uterus may become pregnant. The pregnancy may be maintained but with increased risks to the foetus. The endometrium may fail to develop adequately to support the foetus, the placenta may be weakly attached, and the pregnancy may be aborted. The fibroid may cause retroversion of the uterus (see page 248), which will complicate the early developmental stages of the pregnancy and possibly result in abortion. The fibroid may begin to degenerate due to an obstructed venous blood supply and haemorrhage may occur into the fibroid, giving it a red discoloration. In pregnancy the uterus increases in size and moves upwards out of the pelvis, but the fibroid may remain in the pelvis and obstruct labour and the normal delivery of the infant. Caesarean section will be necessary for the birth.

Fibroids may disturb the normal contraction of the uterus after the delivery of the child. The placenta may fail to separate and cause post-partum haemorrhage. The fibroids may become involved in a puerperal uterine infection and complicate the recovery of the mother.

NURSING PRIORITIES AND MANAGEMENT: FIBROMYOMATA

Nursing care will be prioritised depending upon the type of surgery completed. The maintenance of a safe environment will be important after myomectomy. The recording of pulse rate and blood pressure, postoperatively, together with observation of the patient's vaginal blood loss will confirm an uneventful recovery or excessive bleeding from the operation site.

Care following hysterectomy will be similar to that described earlier in the chapter but the patient will not have the worry of having a malignant disease that may continue to cause problems. Fibromyomata may recur however in some women.

BENIGN TUMOURS OF THE OVARY

Benign cystic teratoma or dermoid cyst

The dermoid cyst may develop in women of all ages. It occurs as 25% of all ovarian tumours. There is a 3% possibility of the cyst becoming malignant.

PATHOPHYSIOLOGY

The dermoid cyst is believed to be developed from the aberrant division of an unfertilised oocyte, but the cause is not known (Lewis & Chamberlain 1989).

It is formed from accumulated sebaceous material from the glands of the neoplasm. It is a thick-walled cyst, whitish-yellow in colour, lined with skin, hair follicles, hair, and sweat glands. Teeth may be found emerging from primitive sockets and bone cartilage, lung and intestinal epithelium can be identified within the cyst.

MEDICAL MANAGEMENT

History and examination. The patient may visit her GP because of abdominal pain and is given an abdominal and vaginal examination. She is referred to a gynaecologist for assessment.

Pain may be caused to the patient by peritoneal irritation from the cyst. Peritonitis may result from rupture of the cyst contents into the abdomen. The cyst may become infected if salpingitis, appendicitis, or diverticulitis are present. Dense adhesions may occur between an infected cyst and the peritoneum or bowel. Torsion or twisting of the pedicle or stalk of the cyst may develop and this may reduce the blood supply, particularly the venous return, to the cyst and cause pain. Malignant change may occur in any of the primitive tissues of the cyst.

Investigations. A Papanicolau cervical smear test may be completed at the time of vaginal examination by the GP. Any malignant cells present might be associated with an ovarian cancer. An ultrasound scan may be requested to identify the ovarian cyst.

Treatment. Surgery will be undertaken by laparoscopy or laparotomy.

The extent of surgery undertaken will vary according to the age of the woman. In the younger woman with child-bearing years ahead of her, the benign cyst alone may be shelled out of the ovary, leaving the normal ovarian tissue to continue functioning. Both ovaries will be assessed as the cysts are often bilateral.

In the woman who already has a family or is over the age of 50 years, the ovary would be removed. In the event of malignancy of the dermoid cyst, both ovaries and the uterus would be removed. Involvement of the peritoneum in the spread of malignancy would necessitate the installation of a cytotoxic agency such as thiotepa into the abdominal cavity at the time of surgery.

NURSING PRIORITIES AND MANAGEMENT: DERMOID CYST

Nursing care will depend upon the extent of the surgery undertaken and has already been described in the section on ovarian cancer, p. 242.

Salpingitis

Infection of the fallopian tubes is known as salpingitis and it usually affects both tubes at the same time. It may be an ascending infection from the vagina, cervix or uterus. It may occur directly from appendicitis, a pelvic abscess, or bowel inflammatory disease such as diverticulitis. The ovaries may also be involved in the inflammatory process. Salpingitis may be part of generalised pelvic inflammatory disease (PID).

Acute salpingitis may follow childbirth, abortion, and diagnostic or operative procedures involving the uterus, or the insertion of intrauterine devices.

PATHOPHYSIOLOGY

Ascending infection of the fallopian tubes through the vagina, cervix, and uterus is most commonly caused by the organism chlamydia trachomatis. More than one infecting agent may be involved. Gonococcal infection, which is sexually transmitted may be the cause. Streptococci and staphylococci organisms are associated with salpingitis following abortion, childbirth, or the insertion of an intrauterine device. These causes are more rare and may reflect reactivation of pre-existing disease. Intestinal tract commensals, escherichia coli or streptococcus faecalis may be involved if the infection is linked to appendicitis or bowel infection. The blood-borne tubercle bacillus may unobtrusively inflame the reproductive organs.

The fallopian tubes become engorged and swollen, possibly being filled with a seropurulent exudate. Epithelium cells are shed, damaging the delicate ciliated, transporting function of the tubes.

MEDICAL MANAGEMENT

History and examination. Salpingitis may be identified for the first time at laparoscopic surgery, the tubes being observed as red, oedematous, distended and blocked. Adhesions may form between the fallopian tubes and other pelvic structures and peritonitis may be evident.

The patient experiences a generalised feeling of being unwell, with:

- raised body temperature and associated sweating
- nausea
- vomiting
- aching joints
- severe pelvic and abdominal pain
- dyspareunia.

Abdominal and vaginal examinations identify tenderness over the cornua of the uterus. Vaginal discharge may not be observable if the salpingitis has been from lymphatic spread and the muscle of the fallopian tube is mainly involved in the inflammatory process.

Infection spread via the mucous membrane of the genital tract will affect the lumen of the fallopian tube, creating a purulent, foul discharge that is drained through the vagina. Scar tissue may form, causing narrowing or closure of the fallopian tube and the severe complication of sterility may result.

Adhesions may form between the inflamed tubes and the peritoneum. Peritonitis may occur if pus leaks out of the tubes into the peritoneal cavity. Rarely, a pelvic abscess may form in the rectovaginal pouch or abscesses may form on the ovaries.

Investigations. High vaginal or cervical swabs of discharge are pathologically investigated. Throat, urethral, and rectal swabs may be taken. During surgery, exudates from the fallopian tubes, or the pouch of Douglas may be obtained. Causative organisms are identified by cell culture or antigen detection, using immunofluorescence or enzyme immunoassay. Examination for specific antibody may assist in diagnosis. The drug sensitivities of organisms are established.

Treatment. Appropriate antibiotic therapy is administered at the earliest opportunity. Analgesic drugs will be necessary to induce some physical comfort for the patient. The pain problem will be assessed to estimate the most suitable drug to use. Paracetamol, pentazocine or pethidine may be used at different levels of pain severity. Diagnosis may be confirmed by laparoscopy.

The patient appreciates rest in bed in the acute phase of the illness, and an upright position in bed is considered helpful to promote simple downward drainage within the abdominal cavity towards the utero-colonic pouch of Douglas and reducing the possible spread of infection to the structures nearer to the diaphragm. The salpingitis may follow a chronic course and surgical removal of fallopian tubes, ovaries and uterus may be necessary.

NURSING PRIORITIES AND MANAGEMENT: SALPINGITIS

Nursing care will prioritise measures to relieve the patient's pain, pyrexia and its associated sweating, nausea, vomiting and potential dehydration. Analgesia is given as prescribed together with the antibiotic drugs. Increased amounts of fluid, 3–4 litres in 24 hours, will need to be taken by mouth or intravenously if vomiting is a problem. When the patient's pain is more tolerable she will appreciate a tepid sponging and a change of linen as a general comfort measure and to reduce body temperature. An electric fan at the bedside and a reduced room temperature should be helpful. The patient needs to understand her condition and the doctor will usually explain the extent of the problem and the treatment given. Information will need to be shared with her about the risk of infertility that follows salpingitis. The possibility of an ectopic pregnancy occurring must be raised with her. A counselling approach is taken, and prevention of further infection is a focus.

ECTOPIC PREGNANCY

A pregnancy that develops outside the uterus is referred to as an 'ectopic' pregnancy. It is possible for a pregnancy to develop in the pouch of Douglas, in the omentum, the broad ligament, or in the ovary. The most common site for an ectopic pregnancy is the fallopian tube and this results in the term tubal pregnancy being interchangeable with the term ectopic pregnancy.

Chronic salpingitis is the most common condition associated with a tubal pregnancy. At greater risk of an ectopic pregnancy are women who:

- have experienced an abortion
- wear an intrauterine contraceptive device
- are of older child-bearing age
- have given birth to many children.

PATHOPHYSIOLOGY

A fallopian tube may fail in its usual function of transporting a fertilised ovum to the uterus, and the ovum will then implant itself in the tube. This delayed passage or obstruction of the ovum may be due to damage to the ciliated epithelium, a deficiency in peristaltic movement, a developmental abnormality, or adhesions from an earlier inflammation. The trophoblast erodes through the epithelium and connective tissue, and embeds itself in the muscle wall of the tube, where the pregnancy develops and erodes into blood vessels, causing bleeding around the embryo and into the muscle wall. Increased tension in the tube may lead to rupture.

MEDICAL MANAGEMENT

History and examination. The woman experiences the early indications of being pregnant: amenorrhoea, breast changes, early-morning sickness and frequency of micturition. Amenorrhoea may not occur in one-third of women with a tubal pregnancy and this may result in delayed diagnosis.

The trophoblast slowly erodes the tubal wall, which results in gradual or sudden rupture of the tube before the 10th week of gestation. The woman complains of spasms of abdominal pain that are not too severe at first. Shoulder pain may be complained of, and is referred pain from the diaphragm, which is irritated by blood in the abdominal cavity.

Tubal rupture causes severe localised pain, which is followed by intense, more generalised abdominal pain. The products of conception are expelled into the peritoneal cavity and there is haemorrhage from the tubal placental site. Uterine bleeding may occur at this time. The patient is in a state of shock, with rapid, feeble pulse rate, lowered blood pressure, sighing respirations and pallor. An acute abdominal emergency exists. Diagnosis of the condition is difficult because similar symptoms and signs may occur in other abdominal emergencies such as perforation of a peptic ulcer or torsion of an ovarian tumour.

Investigations consist of the following.

Pregnancy tests. Standard immunological pregnancy tests are not helpful as a tubal pregnancy may not produce enough HCG to give a positive result. Estimation of the β sub unit of HCG in the serum is of greater value. Absence of β HCG eliminates diagnosis of pregnancy. A level of 6000 miu/l suggests a normal pregnancy in the uterus, a level below 6000 miu/l suggests a tubal pregnancy or a missed abortion.

Ultrasound scanning. By the 6th or 7th week of pregnancy a gestational sac can be identified within the uterus on ultrasound scanning. From the 6th week onwards it may be possible to show a gestation sac and fetal cardiac echoes outside the normal uterus, directly confirming an ectopic pregnancy.

Laparoscopy. Direct vision of the fallopian tubes by the use of laparoscope allows diagnosis of an ectopic pregnancy when there is uncertainty in clinical diagnosis. Laparoscopy involves giving the patient a general anaesthetic which should be avoided if there is the possibility that a pregnancy exists in the uterus. The use of HCG estimations and ultrasound scanning may reduce the need for patients to have a laparoscopy.

Treatment. An ectopic pregnancy always requires urgent surgical intervention. The damaged tube is usually removed. An unruptured ectopic pregnancy may be removed from a linear incision in the tube, ensuring conservation.

A ruptured ectopic pregnancy quickly produces a state of hypovolaemia in the patient and a blood transfusion is necessary. This will sustain the patient through surgery and partially relieve the hypotensive symptoms. Immediate surgery is essential even though the patient is in a poor physical condition. Improvement is speedy once the intraperitoneal bleeding is controlled.

The ruptured fallopian tube is removed but the ovary is conserved if possible. Recovery after salpingectomy is usually rapid and uncomplicated. Prompt surgery ensures a low mortality rate from a ruptured ectopic pregnancy. A woman who has suffered one ectopic pregnancy is at risk of developing a similar pregnancy in the second fallopian tube. It is usual for the patient to be encouraged to be optimistic about the future and having a normal pregnancy by means of the remaining fallopian tube.

NURSING PRIORITIES AND MANAGEMENT: ECTOPIC PREGNANCY

Preoperative care

Risk of hypovolaemia

The nurse assesses and monitors the patient's physical state intensively from the time of admission to the ward. There are life-threatening concerns as the patient is at risk of hypovolaemic shock and cardiac arrest if the tubal pregnancy ruptures. Vital signs are recorded quarter-hourly. Problems of increased pulse rate, lowered blood pressure and the patient's pain experience are communicated to the doctor. A state of readiness is maintained to resuscitate the patient if necessary.

Pain

Pain is a major problem for the patient. It may be moderate but may become intense and intolerable if the pregnancy ruptures through the tube, with bleeding and spillage of gestational sac fluid into the peritoneal cavity. Analgesia is given as prescribed.

Preparation for general anaesthesia

Emergency surgery will be planned. Fasting from food and fluid by mouth prior to laparotomy will be as described in Chapter 27.

Anxiety and the need for information. The patient may be fearful about the operation to come and distressed about losing a pregnancy. She will need information about the surgery and postoperative care, and needs to be encouraged to talk about any worries she may have. It is possible that she may be too weak to talk and the nurse endeavours to communicate her understanding of how she feels to the patient. The nurse may indicate that she will talk with the patient some time after the operation, and that she will accompany her to the operating theatre and be responsible for her care when she returns to the ward.

Postoperative care

Postoperative care will be individualised according to patient need. Her condition will begin to stabilise as soon as the ectopic pregnancy is removed and bleeding is controlled. Her main problems will be similar to those of other patients who have abdominal surgery when organs and the peritoneum have been handled by the surgeon, and tissues have been cut through, as follows.

Identify any change in vital signs. The nurse monitors pulse rate, blood pressure and body temperature. Wound, drainage tube, and blood loss from the vagina are observed for more than minimal drainage. Primary or secondary haemorrhage are risks. Wound dehiscence may occur. Any causes for concern will be shared with the doctor.

Postoperative pain. The level of pain is assessed using a pain scale (1 = low, 5 = high). Analgesia is administered as prescribed to reduce pain to a tolerable level.

Postanaesthetic nausea. This problem may be prevented or treated by giving an anti-emetic drug with analgesia as prescribed.

Body fluid and electrolyte imbalance. Intravenous fluid and electrolyte replacement therapy is administered as prescribed, until oral intake is resumed. Fluid intake and output is recorded.

Venous stasis and pressure-area damage. The patient is actively encouraged to exercise her legs, hourly, whilst confined to bed. Assistance is given to change the patient's position every 2 hours to protect pressure areas. A programme of early mobilisation will be introduced.

Personal care. Whilst IVT is in situ, assistance will be given to maintain her preferred standard of personal care until fully mobile.

Loss and grieving. Time is planned for counselling the patient. She needs to talk about her feelings and express emotion freely. Information should be shared about the possibility of future pregnancies. Details of local support groups for those who suffer loss should be given.

Further considerations

Support

A woman who is suffering a second ectopic pregnancy will become infertile. She may become emotionally distressed at any time during her hospital stay and may show the behaviour associated with a crisis of loss or a grief reaction. She will need support whilst expressing her feelings of regret and possibly guilt. Both the nurse and the patient's partner may be helpful in assisting the woman to be realistic about future options and limitations. Some reorganisation of the woman's life will emerge as she accepts her inevitable situation.

Special services

Patients are now asking about possibilities such as in-vitro fertilisation (IVF) and embryo transfer into the uterus (ET) due to the publicity gained by test-tube babies. Nurses need to know about such special services and policies within their own units, so that they are informed and can respond to the patient with appropriate caution and discretion and refer enquiries to the patient's doctor.

DISPLACEMENTS OF THE UTERUS

The basic criterion of uterine normality is mobility rather than position. The cervix is laterally anchored but the fundus is free to move widely in an anterio–posterior position. If the long axis of the endometrial cavity is hinged forwards in relation to the cervical canal, then the body of the uterus is *anteflexed* in relation to the cervix.

Similarly, if the long axis of the endometrial cavity is hinged backwards in relation to the axis of the cervical canal, then the body of the uterus is *retroflexed* in relation to the cervix (see Fig. 7.9).

Careful assessment of the position of the uterus is necessary to prevent perforation of the uterus during diagnostic or therapeutic curettage.

Cervico–vaginal prolapse

The cervix can become prolapsed and elongated by the opposing forces of pull of the transverse and utero-sacral ligaments against prolapsed vaginal walls. The cervix prolapses but the uterus stays in the pelvis.

Anterior vaginal wall prolapse

Cystocele. The upper part of the vaginal wall prolapses due to underlying failure of the fascia and the bladder base descends.

Urethrocele. The lower part of the vaginal wall prolapses and the urethra descends. This is caused by stretching of the

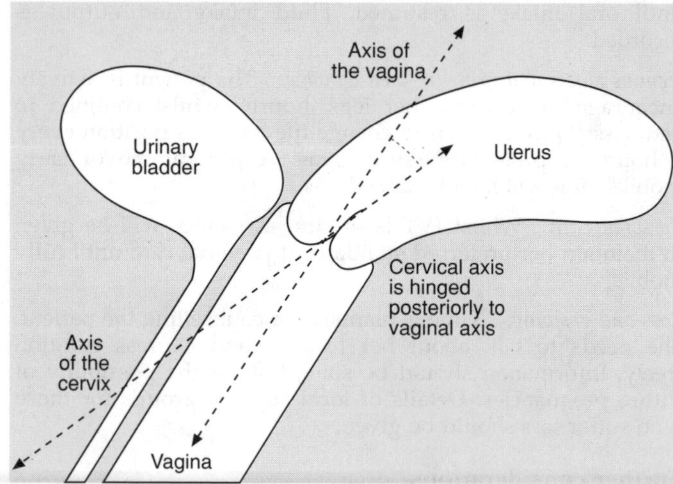

Fig. 7.9 The retroverted uterus.

urogenital diaphragm, which holds the urethra to the pubic bone.

Posterior vaginal wall prolapse

Rectocele. If the prolapse is at the level of the middle third of the vagina, the retrovaginal septum is involved and the rectum prolapses with the vaginal wall.

If the **lowest** part of the vaginal wall prolapses, the perineal body is involved rather than the rectum.

Enterocele. If the upper part of the posterior vaginal wall prolapses, the pouch of Douglas is elongated and the small bowel or omentum may descend.

Both anterior and posterior vaginal walls may be involved in the prolapse. When a cystocele is present bladder emptying tends to be incomplete, causing hypertrophy of the bladder. The uterus may become distorted, leading to reflux of urine and, ultimately, hydronephrosis. Urinary tract infection is inevitable and this contributes to hypertension and raised blood urea levels in women with prolapse.

Utero–vaginal prolapse

Procidentia. When the ligaments and muscles supporting the uterus and vagina become ineffective, the genital tract descends, prolapses, or herniates through the gap between the muscles of the pelvic floor. The uterus descends in the axis of the vagina taking the vaginal wall with it. This prolapse is essentially a post-menopausal condition.

Three degrees of procidentia are described.

First degree. The cervix is still within the vagina.

Second degree. The cervix appears outside the vulva. It becomes congested and ulcerated.

Third degree. The uterus and vagina are completely prolapsed and lie outside the vulva. Rectal prolapse may also occur. This is sometimes called complete 'procidentia' or 'vault prolapse'.

The vaginal rugae are smoothed out, the epithelium becomes thickened and keratinised. The uterus becomes dry, sore, swollen, inflamed, congested, and ulcerated from contact with clothing.

Contributing factors

- stretching of muscle and fibrous tissue from repeated child-bearing. It is suggested that it is due to the action of progesterone relaxing muscle during pregnancy
- injury to the muscles of the pelvic floor during childbirth
- constitutional predisposition to stretching of ligaments with the long-term maintenance of an upright, erect body position that strains the transverse ligaments that are the chief support of the uterus
- increased intra-abdominal pressure, as experienced by obese women with a chronic cough, or those engaged in heavy industrial work.

MEDICAL MANAGEMENT

History and examination. The woman is likely to be overweight and suffer from backache. She is aware of feelings of the internal organs coming down at a time when she is in an upright position. This is relieved by lying down or resting. Pelvic venous congestion occurs and the abdomen contents exert pressure on the inadequate, weakened pelvic floor. There is frequency of micturition, incomplete bladder emptying and the residual urine is a focus for infection. Stress incontinence may be a major problem for some women. There may be difficulty in voiding urine and in defaecation. The cystocele or rectocele may have to be supported or pushed upwards vaginally before urine can be passed or the bowel evacuated. Physical movements become difficult and uncomfortable.

Severe prolapse may be diagnosed by inspecting the vulva with the patient lying on her back and straining downwards. A vaginal speculum is used to directly view the prolapse of the anterior vaginal wall and any rectocele or enterocele formed by a prolapsed posterior vaginal wall. A rectal examination is needed to confirm the latter type of displacement. The degree of uterine prolapse is usually assessed before surgery when the patient is anaesthetised. Volsella forceps can be attached to the cervix, which is pulled downwards to show the prolapse level.

Investigation. Apart from an examination under anaesthetic, no routine procedures are necessary to assist with diagnosis of uterine displacement. Preoperative assessment will usually involve a full blood count, a dipstick urinalysis, and a midstream specimen of urine is obtained for culture and sensitivity. Other procedures, such as a chest X-ray, ECG, or blood chemistry estimation, may be necessary to assess the patient's general medical fitness for surgery.

Treatment. Surgical treatment is curative for prolapse but a small number of women may be unfit for surgery due to great age or poor physical condition. The uterus may be supported by the use of a pessary, which may have the disadvantage of acting as a foreign body in the vagina and causing an inflammatory reaction. Pessaries made from polyethylene or flexible vinyl cause fewer problems. Vaginal douching may be needed to remove accumulated secretions and reduce the incidence of infection. A complete uterine prolapse will usually be treated by hysterectomy.

Surgery to conserve the uterus. If there is only a first-degree descent of the uterus or if the woman prefers to retain her uterus, although prolapsed, then the Manchester (Fothergill) operation is performed. This involves partial amputation of the elongated cervix and the joining of the cut transverse cervical ligaments to the stump of the cervix. The shortened ligaments antevert and elevate the uterus. The vaginal walls are repaired as necessary.

Repair of utero–vaginal prolapse. Reconstruction of the pelvic floor involves restoring the pelvic aperture to its previous competent state. This is achieved by bringing together skeletal muscle between the anus, vagina and bladder, and approximating the medial borders of the pubo-coccygeus muscles. It is said that supporting structures are not destroyed in childbirth, but they may be torn apart, separated and overstretched. These structures are identified at operation and they are reconstructed. An elongated cervix may be amputated. The fascia supporting the bladder and bladder neck is tightened across the mid-line. The parametrial tissues supporting the uterus are shortened to raise the uterus to its normal position.

Repair of cystocele is known as anterior colporrhaphy, which includes supporting the urethra and urethrovesical junction. A rectocele is repaired by a posterior colpoperineorrhaphy, which includes the repair of the perineal body. Bladder, perineum and vulva have an excellent capacity for repair, related to a rich blood supply and good venous drainage. Surgery is usually very successful.

NURSING PRIORITIES AND MANAGEMENT: DISPLACEMENTS OF THE UTERUS

Preoperative care

Pre-operative assessment and care of patients for gynaecological operations has been fully described earlier in the chapter. Care is always individualised according to needs, but some problems and interventions are similar.

Information

Needs exist for information about procedures before and after the operation, to increase patient understanding and cooperation, and reduce anxiety and risk of venous stasis.

Potential embarrassment. Someone admitted for repair of prolapse may experience embarrassment in having to identify that she has a problem of stress incontinence that requires her to wear some form of protection. The nurse will ensure that her special requirements are met discreetly.

Evacuating the lower bowel before surgery. According to the surgeon's requirements, the patient will be given two rectal suppositories or an evacuant enema on the evening before the operation day.

Preparing the operation site. As required by the surgical protocol, an antiseptic vaginal douche is completed to reduce the numbers of bacteria inhabiting the area and inhibit their multiplication. This should allow healing of the vaginal wounds without infection.

Postoperative care

Risk of strain on internal suture lines from a full bladder. An in-dwelling catheter will be needed. A continuous urinary drainage system is maintained. Precautions are taken to prevent introducing infection when collecting specimens or changing drainage bags.

Loss of bladder tone is possible after catheter removal. A test catheterisation procedure is completed after the patient has passed urine once daily to assess the level of urine retained in the bladder. A residual urine of less than 60 ml is satisfactory.

Risk of wound infection. A perineal toilet is completed twice daily to minimise the risk of infection.

Constipation will potentially cause strain on the repaired posterior vaginal wall. A stool-softening agent, as prescribed, is administered to promote easy bowel actions.

Strain on healing ligaments and muscles. The patient is advised to avoid jarring or lifting activities for 2 months.

Pre-discharge counselling. An opportunity is created for the patient to explain her feelings and any worries about her level of recovery from surgery, bladder functioning, future return to sexual activity and work. An appointment is given for a medical follow-up in the outpatients department. The patient is given the name of the nurse to contact in the ward if she needs further advice.

FAMILY PLANNING SERVICES

Birth control was considered 'social' medicine prior to 1950 and responsibility for family planning advice was established within the Family Planning Association (FPA) and its clinics. The National Health Service Reorganisation Act of 1973 made provision for free family planning advice within the National Health Service. The FPA clinics and domiciliary services were merged into the NHS in 1974, when a completely free contraceptive service became available at clinics and hospitals and was extended into primary care in July 1975.

Free contraceptive services are now available from general practitioners, family planning clinics in hospitals and the community, and from voluntary organisations such as the FPA and Brook Advisory Centres. The voluntary groups receive grants from central government or from purchasing health authorities.

All contraceptive supplies are available free of charge from family planning clinics, and GPs provide prescriptions, except for condoms. Male and female sterilisation is available free in NHS hospitals. Vasectomies may be performed in some large family planning clinics and by some GPs in the surgery. Item-of-service payments are made to GPs and hospital staff.

Post-natally, midwives, health visitors and GPs routinely discuss birth control methods with the new mother. This is invaluable in reminding women of their fertility and the possibility of another early pregnancy if precautions are not taken when resuming sexual activities.

Discontinued attendance

Most women who discontinue attending the GP or Family Planning Clinic do so because they have changed their birth control method, rather than being dissatisfied with the service (Allen 1981). Women over 30 years of age may have chosen sterilisation or their partners chosen vasectomy surgery for a permanent form of birth control. Others may be abandoning contraception because the time is favourable for them to begin a family.

The contraceptive needs of young people

The sexuality of teenagers and young adults is not always acknowledged by society. Unplanned teenage pregnancy and abortion rates have increased. Provision of extra contraceptive services for young people after puberty, under 16 years and up to 20 years of age, is controversial and has been given a low priority. With more recent concern about AIDS and HIV transmission, young people have been specially targeted for health education and advice about their sexual behaviour. The value of using the condom for personal protection has made it the second most-popular method of birth control amongst young people. The most popular method remains the combined pill of progestogen and low oestrogen, because of its high contraceptive protection and ease of use.

ABORTION

The term 'abortion' refers to the premature delivery of a non-viable fetus, spontaneously or by induction. Debate surrounds the issue of 'non-viability'. A fetus is considered viable or capable of survival from the 24th week of pregnancy. This viability is recognised and safeguarded in the Infant Life (Preservation) Act 1929 and its amendment under the Human Fertilisation and Embryology Act 1990. It has been proposed that the fetus should be deemed viable as early as 18–20 weeks because of the possibility that life-support equipment can maintain the vital functions of such a small fetus. It has been argued that technological advances in medicine have the potential for saving the life of an infant as light as 500 g in body weight.

Abortion may be discussed in terms of:

- the level of certainty of the abortion occurring
  — threatened

— inevitable
— missed
— induced.

- the cause or relative incidence of the abortion
  — spontaneous
  — habitual.
- the degree of success in expulsion of the products of the pregnancy
  — incomplete
  — complete.

Threatened abortion

PATHOPHYSIOLOGY

An abortion is presumed to threaten when a woman known to be pregnant develops vaginal bleeding during the first 24 weeks of pregnancy. Some lower abdominal pain related to uterine muscle contractions may be experienced at the time bleeding occurs, but some women feel no pain. The blood loss may be brown or red.

It is not unusual for a show of blood to coincide with the woman's regular date of menstruation. This type of bleeding is due to the fertilised ovum becoming more deeply implanted in the uterine wall. There is little risk of loss of the pregnancy if the bleeding settles quickly. See Figure 7.10(A).

MEDICAL MANAGEMENT

History and examination. The presence of bleeding, slight uterine contractions, and a closed cervical os established by medical examination assist in identifying threatened abortion. 70–80% can be expected to continue to full-term pregnancies and give birth to a healthy infant.

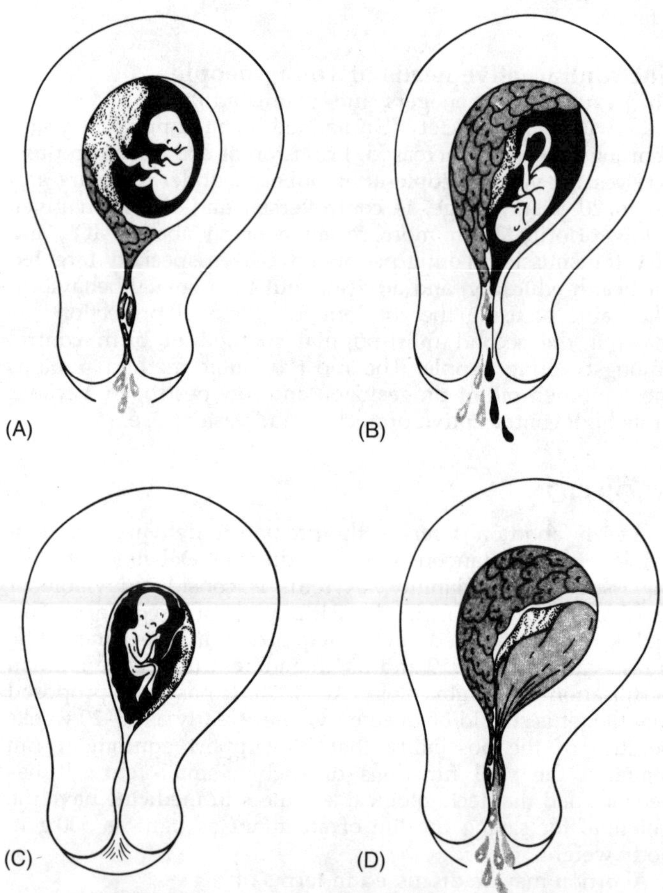

Fig. 7.10 The types of abortion that may be seen. (A) Threatened abortion. (B) Inevitable abortion. (C) Missed abortion. (D) Incomplete abortion.

Treatment. Whilst the woman is continuing to lose blood vaginally, rest in bed is prescribed to ensure the best possible adjustments can be made within the uterus, and to allow a better blood flow to the uterus. Bed rest is usually maintained as long as the blood loss is bright red. One week of bed rest may result in considerable improvement for the patient.

NURSING PRIORITIES AND MANAGEMENT: THREATENED ABORTION

The patient will be very concerned about the possible loss of the pregnancy. This may result in tearfulness, anxiety, irritability and feelings of frustration. The immediate- and long-term future may be feared. The patient may be apprehensive of pain and uncertain of what she may expect. Small doses of anxiolytic-sedative drugs and progesterone may be prescribed to sustain the pregnancy.

Nursing care will be planned with the goal of reducing anxiety and inducing relaxation in the patient. Vaginal bleeding will be observed and quantified. The patient's experience of abdominal discomfort or pain will be assessed and recorded. The supportive, counselling contact time with the nurse will be appreciated by the patient and her partner. When talking with the patient and partner both doctor and nurse will usually refer to a possible 'miscarriage' of the pregnancy rather than use the term 'abortion'.

Inevitable abortion

PATHOPHYSIOLOGY

Inevitable abortions occur in 20% of all pregnancies. An abortion becomes inevitable, with no possibility of saving the pregnancy, when there are:

- vaginal blood loss
- strong uterine contractions
- pain
- dilation of the cervix

Contractions will increase, the fetal sac membranes will rupture and the uterine contents move through the cervical os. Part, or all, of the products of conception will be voided from the uterus. See Fig. 7.10(B).

MEDICAL MANAGEMENT

The patient may be distressed by the experience of pain from strong contractions of the uterus, the sight of the fetus, and the anguish of losing a pregnancy to which she had become emotionally attached. Pain relief by analgesic drugs may be necessary.

The aborting process will involve some blood loss that will need to be evaluated. Estimation of blood loss and assessment of pulse rate, blood-pressure readings, and appearance of the patient will indicate whether a state of shock is developing. Blood-replacement therapy may become essential. The fetus that has been expelled is retained and examined to assess whether the fetal sac and contents are intact or whether remnants of placenta or membranes are retained. Ergometrine maleate 125–500 μg will be given intramuscularly or intravenously, according to blood loss. This drug will induce strong contraction of the uterine muscle, which will exert and sustain pressure on the multiple open-ended blood vessels to the placenta bed in the wall of the uterus. Thus, bleeding will be controlled until the uterus itself reduces size gradually.

If any of the products of conception are thought to have been retained then the doctor will wish to complete a dilatation and curettage procedure.

NURSING PRIORITIES AND MANAGEMENT: INEVITABLE ABORTION

Assessments of vaginal blood loss may need to be maintained

for a further period of 12 hours in the event of further heavy bleeding when the effects of ergometrine diminish and uterine muscle relaxes, blood vessels open up and bleeding and blood clots continue as problems. Further doses of ergometrine, in tablet form, may then be prescribed to control the bleeding and expel the clots of blood. The blood clots will cause further pain for the patient until they are finally voided from the vagina.

The patient is likely to experience considerable physical and emotional distress and will need the nurse to be readily available to support, reassure, comfort and assist her through the voiding of the fetus and in the recovery period. The patient will need to have the opportunity to talk about her feelings of loss. It may be that she has already had a previous miscarriage and will also be recalling that experience as part of her grieving process. The patient's sadness may be sustained for many months after the abortion occurs. To plan some continued support, the nurse in hospital can refer the patient to the community midwife, who is able to provide bereavement counselling until resolution of the grief reaction takes place.

Missed abortion

PATHOPHYSIOLOGY

The term 'missed abortion' describes the intrauterine death of a fetus that has not been expelled. The size of the uterus fails to increase over a 2-month period, and the expected signs of a normally developing pregnancy will be missing. The death of the fetus may occur at any week of gestation. Some placental tissue survives to produce progesterone and prevent expulsion. (See Fig. 7.10(C).)

MEDICAL MANAGEMENT

History and examination. The woman may have experienced movements of the fetus in the uterus but later reports that she has not felt the baby kicking for some time. The doctor will no longer be able to hear the fetal heart beat on auscultation of the abdomen. The uterus may seem to have increased in size but this is due to increased fluid level in the uterus, known as 'hydramnios'. The patient may state that she feels empty and has lost her feelings of being pregnant, and her worst feelings are confirmed. She is asked to record on a chart any sensation she has of the baby moving or kicking.

Investigations. An ultrasound scan of the uterus and a cardiotocograph reading will assess the status of the fetus and the position of the placenta.

Treatment. The diagnosis of a missed abortion will require the doctor to decide whether to wait for the fetus to be aborted spontaneously as a natural labour response, or to evacuate the uterus immediately after diagnosis. The doctor may prefer to let nature take its course and wait for labour to begin.

His decision may relate to concern for the patient who has already had to adjust to the loss of the pregnancy and may be further distressed by brooding about the dead baby and imagining the structural changes that might be going on within her. This may cause anxiety and depression.

A risk exists, with missed abortion, that hypofibrinogenaemia will occur. One-third of patients may develop defective blood coagulation due to lowering of fibrinogen levels. Death of the fetus leads to major utilisation of clotting factors at the placental site, and this reduces clotting factors in the woman's blood. Disseminated intravascular coagulation is the mechanism that is said to bring about the change in the woman's systemic circulation from the release of thromboplastins at the site of the damaged placental tissue.

The missed abortion may be evacuated from the uterus by vacuum extraction under general anaesthetic if the pregnancy was less than 12 weeks. Otherwise, induction of labour by use of drugs such as an anti-progesterone or prostaglandin, used alone or together, would be appropriate.

NURSING PRIORITIES AND MANAGEMENT: MISSED ABORTION

The nursing care of the patient with a missed abortion will focus on the patient's need for information about her condition and planned treatment, whilst responding to the sense of loss and sadness that has replaced the joy of pregnancy and anticipated childbirth. A counselling approach will be necessary to provide the patient with opportunities to express her needs and feelings freely.

If a general anaesthetic and evacuation of uterus is planned, the patient will need the usual pre-anaesthetic care in terms of fasting, taking a shower, and precautions against misidentification and maintenance of personal safety. Following surgery, a short period of fully compensatory care will include observation of vaginal blood loss, and recording of temperature, pulse rate and blood pressure.

If the products of conception are to be evacuated by inducing labour with drug treatments, the patient may be given a drug dose of mifepristone whilst an outpatient and will be admitted to hospital 36–48 hours later. Then a drug such as misoprostol is administered in divided doses. The products of pregnancy can expect to be expelled 4 hours later. The nurse must be readily available to observe the patient's temperature, pulse and blood pressure regularly, and assess her individual need for pain relief. The patient may experience drug side effects of nausea, vomiting or diarrhoea but these can be expected to be transitory rather than prolonged. The very presence of the nurse can be comforting to the patient and reduce feelings of being alone and isolated whilst treatment progresses.

The way in which individual patients cope emotionally is unpredictable, but the nurse can anticipate that any patient will feel sad and angry about the lost pregnancy. Follow-up counselling can be arranged by the nurse with the community midwife or health visitor, when the woman's level of adjustment can be assessed.

Spontaneous abortion

PATHOPHYSIOLOGY

A spontaneous abortion is a response to a naturally occurring phenomenon such as hormone deficiency, a genetic malformation in the fetus, incompetence of the cervix or psychological factors. Dependent, anxious women and independent, career-type women with mixed feelings about the female role of mother have been found to be more liable to spontaneous abortion.

Of all pregnancies, 10–20% are estimated to end in spontaneous abortion and some women may not be aware that they have aborted a blighted ovum. Of the embryos lost in the first 3 months of pregnancy, 50–60% have been shown to be genetically abnormal in research studies. Congenital abnormalities of the reproductive tract or long-standing medical problems may be an unfavourable influence on the pregnancy. Abortions in the early weeks of the second trimester of pregnancy are often found to be due to an incompetent cervix that responds to the increasing weight of the fetus. The cervical os dilates, the membranes rupture and the pregnancy is lost.

MEDICAL MANAGEMENT

To counteract recurrence of abortion it is necessary to identify the pregnancy and the incompetence of cervix at an early stage. It is possible to use Shirodker's procedure of surgically closing the internal os by a purse-string suture to increase the resistance of the cervix until the pregnancy reaches full term. When the patient goes into labour then the suture is removed for delivery to occur.

NURSING PRIORITIES AND MANAGEMENT: SPONTANEOUS ABORTION

The physical care of the patient with a spontaneous abortion is similar to that of the patient with an inevitable abortion. The patient will be distressed by the loss of the pregnancy and will need psychological support from the nurse. A counselling approach to communication will encourage expression of feelings and further need. Continued support should be arranged by referral to the community midwife.

Recurrent abortion

Recurrent abortion refers to a spontaneous abortion that occurs in three or more successive pregnancies. Many factors may contribute to recurrent abortions.

PATHOPHYSIOLOGY

Genetic, hormonal, anatomical, infectious and immunological factors have been implicated in the causation of recurrent abortion. In explaining immunological factors, Taylor and Faulk (1981) suggested that:

- couples share more HLA antigens than usual
- women lack inhibitors of cell-mediated immunity usually produced during pregnancy
- human trophoblast membranes have discrete antigens that could form the basis for a maternal immune reaction against the fetus, and they lack transplantation antigens
- having many shared HLA antigens from the husband and wife may result in an embryo that does not stimulate maternal protecting or blocking factors culminating in rejection of the blastocyst.

MEDICAL MANAGEMENT

Patients with immunological problems have been treated with leucocyte transfusions with successful results. Identified hormonal deficiencies are treated by replacement hormones, thyroid preparations and progesterone. Vaginal suppositories of progesterone 25 mg, twice daily, beginning 3 days after ovulation are given and continued throughout the luteal phase, until the 10th week of gestation. At this time the placenta should be sufficient to maintain the pregnancy. There is a 91% success rate for hormonal treatments.

The administration of antibiotic drugs is routine, where culture and sensitivity of organisms is known. Otherwise drugs of the tetracycline group are given empirically to offset an infective focus that might disrupt the pregnancy. Reconstruction surgery has achieved considerable success in treating structural abnormalities of the uterus and eventual successful pregnancies.

NURSING PRIORITIES AND MANAGEMENT: RECURRENT ABORTION

Physical and psychological care is paramount at the time that the abortion occurs. Sensitivity in responding to the woman's needs is central. Potential for future assisted maintenance of the pregnancy will be fully discussed by the doctor and reinforced by the nurse. The patient who is anxious can be helped to learn relaxation techniques that may be used for self-induction of relaxation as an everyday activity, and one that can be practised in future pregnancies.

Incomplete abortion

An incomplete abortion is one in which only part of the products of conception are expelled from the uterus (see Fig. 7.10(D)).

PATHOPHYSIOLOGY

Portions of placenta and membranes are retained, some bleeding continues and could possibly be heavy.

MEDICAL MANAGEMENT

The residual products may be voided spontaneously by the patient but usually a dilatation and curettage is required to clear away the retained remnants of the pregnancy. Ergometrine 500 µg is administered intravenously to control uterine bleeding. Heavy blood loss will necessitate blood replacement by transfusion.

NURSING PRIORITIES AND MANAGEMENT: INCOMPLETE ABORTION

The patient may experience continuous abdominal pain whilst the uterus retains products of conception. Nursing care involves the administration of analgesia as prescribed to reduce the discomfort which will possibly continue until the curettage is complete. On admission to hospital, the patient will continue to have a vaginal blood loss that will need to be observed. Heavy, continuous blood loss may reduce the patient's circulating blood volume, with the patient showing signs of shock. Recording of the pulse rate and blood pressure half hourly, will facilitate early recognition of shock and prompt correction of the condition by transfusion.

The patient will be worried about her condition and the operation planned and will feel very upset about the miscarriage. Adjustment to the loss will be gradual over time. Counselling time spent with the nurse may help to begin the adjustment process, and continuity may be gained by follow-up support of the community midwife or health visitor.

THE ABORTION ACT 1967 AND 1990 AMENDMENTS

In the United Kingdom, the Abortion Act 1967 became operative in 1968 and applies to England, Wales and Scotland but not Northern Ireland. The Act permits the termination of pregnancy by a registered practitioner subject to certain conditions. Notification of a termination must be made on a prescribed form to the Chief Medical Officer of the Department of Health within seven days of the termination. The Human Fertilisation and Embryology Act 1990 has amended the Abortion Act 1967 reducing the viability of the fetus to 24 weeks.

Conditions of the Act and statutory grounds

A legally induced abortion must be:

- performed by a registered medical practitioner
- performed, except in an emergency, in a National Health Service Hospital or in a place for the time being approved for the purpose of the Act, and
- certified by two registered medical practitioners as necessary on any of the grounds:
  - — the continuance of the pregnancy would involve risk to the life of the pregnant woman greater than if the pregnancy were terminated
  - — the continuance of the pregnancy would involve risk of injury to the physical or mental health of the

pregnant woman greater than if the pregnancy were terminated
— the continuance of the pregnancy would involve risk of injury to the physical or mental health of any existing child(ren) in the family of the pregnant woman greater than if the pregnancy were terminated
— there is a substantial risk that if the child were born it would suffer from such physical or mental abnormalities as to be seriously handicapped
- or in emergency, certified by the operating practitioner as immediately necessary:
  — to save the life of the pregnant woman, or
  — to prevent grave permanent injury to the physical or mental health of the pregnant woman.

The Conscience Clause of the Abortion Act (1967)

The Act states that no person shall be under any legal obligation to participate in any treatment authorised by the Act to which he has a conscientious objection unless the treatment is necessary to save the life, or prevent grave permanent injury to the physical or mental health of a pregnant woman.

The conscience clause does not only apply to members of a particular religion or faith. In England and Wales, a person must prove his conscientious objection in the event of any legal proceedings. The clause also makes it explicit that the conscientious objector is not exempt from participation in the emergency care of the patient should such a situation arise.

Voluntary termination of pregnancy

An unwanted pregnancy creates anguish and acute difficulties for a woman. She may experience feelings of conflict about both wanting and rejecting the pregnancy. She may fear having to explain to her family and so admit to sexual activities and her incompetence in contraceptive methods. Family standards of behaviour and religious beliefs may appear to be violated both by the pregnancy and by the possibility of an abortion. The woman may feel very alone, may have perhaps only one person to confide in, may be indecisive and be under pressure from a partner who rejects the pregnancy. The conditions of the Abortion Act require decision making to be completed early in the pregnancy.

Counselling of the pregnant woman

In many hospitals the woman who requests a termination of pregnancy is referred to the Assessment and Counselling Service. The social worker seeks to understand what the pregnancy and termination mean to the woman, identifies any contraindications to termination, and provides evidence for the final decision making and the best solution.

It is valuable to see couples together for counselling. Adolescent girls are often accompanied by parents who are angry and rejecting of their daughter's pregnancy. The risk is then that the girl passively acts in accordance with the parents' wishes. The counsellor would usually see them together and separately.

Counselling clarifies the woman's conflicting feelings about the pregnancy and strengthens her capacity to face up to her responsibilities. She may be more confident in making a decision in an unpressured atmosphere. The counsellor may have established that contraindications to the termination exist or that the request for termination be supported. In either case the information is made available to the gynaecologist. The counselling service ensures that adequate assessment and advice are provided for the woman who seeks a termination. It is suggested that in this way she will experience less regret, guilt or long-term psychological problems.

MEDICAL MANAGEMENT

Vacuum aspiration (suction curettage) is the most commonly used abortion method for early termination of pregnancy. It may be performed with a general anaesthetic or a paracervical nerve block with lignocaine hydrochloride 0.5%. The cervix is dilated, a flexible cannula is inserted and the contents of the uterus are aspirated by suction. The uterus is then curetted to ensure total removal of the products of conception and reduce haemorrhage and the possibility of infection. Ergometrine 0.5 mg is administered to promote contraction and involution of the uterus.

Dilatation and evacuation of contents. Abortion that is induced in the second trimester of pregnancy may be completed by dilatation of the cervix with graduated size of dilator. A curette is introduced into the uterus and the products of conception and the superficial layer of endometrium are curetted or scraped from the walls of the uterus. Ergometrine 0.5 mg is administered and few side-effects to the procedure are expected.

Intra-amniotic injection. The instillation of prostaglandins or other substances into the amniotic sac to induce labour and expulsion of the feotus may be used between the 14th and 20th week of the pregnancy. The procedure stimulates the uterus to contract and causes fetal death before delivery. It is a more prolonged procedure, causes more side-effects, and is more traumatic to the patient than other methods.

NURSING PRIORITIES AND MANAGEMENT

Assessment of needs

In many units a qualified nurse undertakes the nursing care of the patient presenting for a termination of pregnancy, rather than the student nurse becoming involved in a potentially stressful event. The procedure may be completed on an outpatient basis or the patient may be admitted a day earlier. There is only a short time available for the nurse to build a relationship with the patient whilst documentation is completed. The usual appraisal of the patient's needs will be made and information must be given as to what procedures are to occur before and after surgery. Every effort must be made to show acceptance of the woman and understanding of the difficulties she has been experiencing. Opportunities must be created for her to express her feelings as she wishes and the nurse should be available to listen. A consent form is signed for the termination and consent for anaesthetic is given. Blood tests such as haemoglobin and haematocrit, ABO grouping and the Rhesus factor are necessary precautions prior to the procedure.

Planning postoperative care

Attention to vital signs related to bleeding and abdominal cramping pain must be observed by the nurse. Inspection of vulval pads will indicate the degree of blood loss which is usually slight but normally not more than moderate. Heavy bleeding will usually require further administration of ergometrine to sustain the contraction of the uterus and to evacuate blood clots. Pyrexia may indicate the onset of infection. Mild analgesics may be ordered to relieve cramping pain and also to use their antipyretic properties.

The patient is advised to avoid the use of tampons, douching, strenuous activities, or sexual intercourse for a couple of weeks. The patient's contraception methods are reviewed with her so that any changes needed are understood, and appropriate decisions made. A follow-up outpatient examination is completed 2 to 3 weeks after the abortion; this excludes the possibility of a failed abortion, an ectopic pregnancy, or other complications. It allows for an assessment of the patient's acceptance of and comfort with her decision to terminate. Relief is often expressed; sadness, regret and depression may be of short duration, or be prolonged. The patient's relationship with her sexual partner may be discussed. It may be strengthened or weakened by the abortion experience. The woman may be helped by referral to a post abortion support group if there is one active in the area.

Complications of abortion

- Pelvic infection: the endiometrium and fallopian tubes may be inflamed in conditions known respectively as 'endometritis' and 'salpingitis'.
- Perforation of the uterus: accidental during insertion of cannula or use of curette.
- Haemorrhage: more than 300 ml.
- Laceration of cervix, cervical incompetence and recurrent abortion.
- Ectopic pregnancy: related to previous salpingitis.
- Incomplete removal of uterine contents.
- Hydatidiform mole.
- Delayed menstruation.
- A viable fetus may be delivered.
- Women who have had abortions induced may be more liable to subsequent pregnancy loss and premature births.
- Infertility.

With improved services the numbers of complications to abortion can be greatly reduced. Effective networks of outpatient facilities with good access to avoid delays in take up of services and reduced travel for women in need should be the aim of authorities responsible for service provision.

CHILDLESSNESS

Childlessness is a reality in 15% of all marriages. There are 400 000 marriages each year in the UK and most couples have some expectation of producing children in their reproductive life. Couples may choose not to have offspring in the early years of a relationship but later may experience difficulty in conceiving. It is usually the woman who first questions her own physical capacity to become pregnant and will seek medical advice and submit to multiple investigations. It is known that only in one-third of cases is the woman totally responsible for the subfertility. In one third of couples the man has the problem, and in the remaining third both the man and the woman contribute some causative factor (see Tables 7.1 and 7.2).

The provision of general facilities for investigation and treatment of subfertility and to assist in conception are well established at the endocrinology and gynaecological surgery level in the National Health Service but the specialist in vitro fertilisation services have been slow to develop. Currently many patients receive help from their GPs, who prescribe the drugs required to support the subfertility treatment programmes offered by infertility centres. Up to 0.5% of women are referred to specialist gynaecological services each year. The need for subfertility services is expected to grow due to the trend toward later first pregnancies and an increasing number of remarriages. Demand is increased due to raised public awareness of treatment possibilities (Effective Health Care Consortium 1992).

PATHOPHYSIOLOGY

Childlessness is deliberately maintained in women who use birth control methods such as the contraceptive pill. This is regarded as voluntary childlessness.

Sterility refers to an absolute factor preventing procreation in either the man or woman. The condition may be induced by ligation and separation of the fallopian tubes or by vasectomy.

Subfertility refers to childlessness that continues following 2 years of involuntary failure to conceive, during which there has been sexual intercourse, and without the use of contraceptive agents. The time taken to conceive increases with age.

The prevalence of subfertility in women of child-bearing age is 9–14%. Of these, 70% have not conceived before (primary subfertility) and 30% have conceived, but not achieved childbirth, or the birth of more than one child (secondary subfertility).

The principal causes of subfertility are shown in Tables 7.1 and 7.2. A proportion of couples will have more than one cause of subfertility. As diagnostic testing becomes more accurate the proportion of unexplained subfertility may decrease. The contribution of psychological factors to prolonged subfertility is not yet clearly established by research. A small proportion of subfertility may be preventable, particularly some tubal damage associated with sexually transmitted diseases.

MEDICAL MANAGEMENT OF SUBFERTILITY

The diagnosis and management of subfertility is complex. The numbers of tests and investigations that the couple may need to have completed are high and often stressful (see Tables 7.1 and 7.2).

Female subfertility

Failure to ovulate is linked with the functioning of hormones from the hypothalamus, pituitary and ovary (HPO axis). Treatments seek to remedy problems arising from imbalances in this axis and have been shown to restore fertility to near normal levels.

Clomiphene citrate, an anti-oestrogen, stimulates gonadotrophin release by inhibiting the negative feedback of gonadal steroids on the hypothalamus. It induces ovulation in patients with secondary amenorrhoea. If there is no evidence of corpus luteum development, a single injection of chorionic gonadotrophin (HCG) may be given 7 days after the clomiphene: 50 mgms daily for 5 days. Women may continue with this drug treatment for up to 9 months.

Ovarian hyperstimulation may lead to multiple pregnancies but risks may be avoided by the pulsatile administration of GnRH when medically indicated.

Where tubal factors are causative of the subfertility tubal surgery may be advised but this depends upon the nature, site and severity of the condition of the tube, the presence and extent of adhesions, and the skills of the surgeon. Diagnostic procedures will include laparoscopy and hysterosalpingography for full assessment of the condition. The most common site for tubal damage is the distal end of the fallopian tube (80%). Birth rates after surgery are 20–30% (Singhal et al 1991). Surgery for occlusion of the proximal end of the tube has a live birth rate of 40–60% (Patton et al 1987, Marana & Quagliarello 1988).

The success rate for reversal of sterilisation varies from 50 to 80%. Results are dependent upon the technique used for sterilisation and the patients selected for surgery (Gomel 1980, Wallach et al 1983, Xue and Fa 1989).

The relationship between endometriosis and subfertility is unclear. Many women with the condition conceive successfully without intervention. Drug treatments and surgery have been shown in several randomly controlled trials as not effective in increasing fertility, whereas IVF-ET and GIFT have shown increased pregnancy and maternity rates (Effective Health Care Report 1992). Assisted conception techniques are treatments of choice in endometriosis in the future, and similarly have been shown to be appropriate for unexplained subfertility.

Male subfertility

Male-factor subfertility is diagnosed by semen analysis. Numbers, shape and motility of sperm can be assessed. IVF has value in

Table 7.1 Infertility: summary of causes, investigations and treatment in women

Causes	Investigations	Treatment
1. *Disorders of ovulation* Stein-Leventhal Syndrome. Failure of one or both pituitary gonadotrophins (trauma or vascular disorder). Failure of hypothalamic releasing factor (stress, anorexia nervosa). Primary ovarian failure. Tumours of ovary. Cysts of ovary. Endometrial hyperplasia (causing upset ovarian function). XO karyotype. Drugs — post-pill amenorrhoea, phenothiazines, tricyclic antidepressants. Adrenal dysfunction. Thyroid, hyper and hypothyroidism.	1. History. 2. Examination (bimanual). 3. Skull X-ray 4. Endometrial biopsy, histology and culture 5. Plasma progesterone level. 6. Urinary oestrogens level. 7. Ovarian biopsy. 8. Cervical mucus specimen (can be used as a parameter of ovulation). 9. Full blood count and ESR (erythrocyte sedimentation rate). 10. Thyroid function tests. 11. Chromosome studies.	1. Clomiphene. 2. Bromocriptene — for raised prolactin only. 3. LH releasing hormone (LHRH) by pump injection. 4. Pergonal and human chorionic gonadotrophin (HCG). 5. Buserelin with human menopausal gonadotrophin (HMG) is useful for those with polycystic ovaries. 6. Surgical wedge resection of ovary under laparoscopy. May be effective when drug treatment failed. 7. GIFT — gamete intrafallopian transfer.
2. *Disorders of fallopian tubes* Congenital absence. Blocked due to infection — Tuberculosis Recurrent appendicitis Gonococcal infection Septic abortion. Hydrosalpinx. Disturbance of tubal secretions.	1. History. 2. Examination. 3. Hysterosalpingography. 4. Laparoscopy. 5. Biopsy of fallopian tube. 6. Hormone studies (no oestrogen surge).	1. Salpingolysis. 2. Salpingostomy. 3. Tubal reconstruction — by microscopy. 4. Tubal excision and transplantation. 5. Oral oestrogens. 6. IVF and ET — in vitro fertilisation and embryo transfer.
3. *Endometrium lining of the uterus* Not prepared due to disorder of ovulation. Endometriosis. Endometritis. Fibroids. Endometrial hyperplasia. Endocervicitis.	1. History. 2. Examination (bimanual). 3. Hysterosalpingogram. 4. Endometrial biopsy. 5. Evidence of discharge.	1. Treatment of disorders of ovulation. 2. Dilatation and curettage. 3. Myomectomy. 4. Endometriosis IVF-ET/GIFT.
4. *Factors in the cervical mucus* Hostile mucus. Cervical mucus not prepared due to deficiency of oestrogen as a result of disorders of ovulation. Sperm antibodies in cervical mucus.	1. Post-coital test. 2. Mucus/sperm match test. 3. Spinnbarkheit test. 4. Fern test. 5. Sperm invasion test.	1. Deficient oestrogen — clomiphene. 2. Ethinyl oestradiol (0.01 u daily for a three day period before ovulation). 3. Refrain from intercourse for a set period, or use condom during intercourse. At the end of this time, there may be a decrease in antibodies.
5. *Psychosexual problems* Frigidity. Vaginismus. Stress-affecting hypothalamic function. Decreased sexual libido.	1. History and interview.	1. Psychological referral. 2. Use of vaginal dilators.
6. *Others* Congenital abnormalities. (for example — bicornate uterus). Obesity. Retroverted uterus. Hirsutism and virilism (disorders of ovarian or adrenal function, also by certain drugs).	1. Examination. 2. Hysterosalpingogram.	1. Lose weight. 2. Ventro-suspension surgery. 3. Surgical restructuring of genital organs as possible.

demonstrating the capacity of sperm to fertilise the egg where subfertility is suspected. If male antibodies to spermatozoa are produced, prednisolone has been shown to be effective as an immunosuppressant (Hendry et al 1990). Other drug treatments such as clomiphene citrate have been shown to be ineffective (Sokol et al 1988). Assisted conception techniques can be effective using partner sperm (Hull et al 1992).

Intrauterine insemination by donor sperm may be chosen by a couple when the partner has proof of his permanent infertility. The process is very successful.

Provision of information and counselling

The stressful nature of investigations and treatment of subfertility and the psychological impact of the condition on

Table 7.2 Subfertility: summary of causes, investigations and treatment in men

Causes	Investigations	Treatment
1. *Testes* Congenital absence of both. Kleinfelter's syndrome. Cryptorchidism. Trauma. Testicular failure — i. torsion ii. infections iii. unrestricted pituitary output.	1. History. 2. Examination. 3. Testicular biopsy. 4. Urinary gonadotrophins. 5. Chromosome investigations.	1. Cryptorchidism should be detected early in school career and requires surgical intervention. 2. Hormone therapy.
2. *Vas deferens and epididymis* Congenital absence of both. Blockage due to infections — partial — complete — Venereal disease. Vasitis Epididymitis.	1. History. 2. Vasogram. 3. Semen analysis. 4. Post-coital test.	1. No treatment for congenital absence. 2. Vaso-epididymostomy. 3. Microsurgery — removal of blocked section of vas.
3. *Spermatozoa* *Oligospermia* (less than 20 million 1 ml). Varicocele. Hernia. Physical exhaustion and overwork. *Aspermia* Factors in 1 and 2. Endocrine abnormalities, failure of pituitary, adrenal and thyroid glands.	1. History. 2. Examination — consistency of testicles, presence/absence of varicocele. 3. Semen analysis. 4. Post-coital test. 5. Seminal plasma analysis for fructose content and its glycerol phospherol choline. 6. Interstitial cell stimulating hormone, follicle stimulating hormone and testosterone levels. 7. Testicular biopsy. 8. Thyroid tests. 9. Urine analysis — gonadotrophins, ketosteroids. 10. Vasogram.	1. Surgical treatment of varicocele or hernia. 2. Moderation with alcohol, tobacco and work. 3. Wearing loose underpants. 4. Intrauterine insemination by donor. 5. Vaso-epididymostomy. 6. Assisted conception techniques using partner sperm.
4. *Semen volume* Too low — sperms fail to contact cervical os. Too high — over dilution. Quality.	1. Semen analysis. 2. Post-coital test.	1. Pooling of two or more semen samples and intrauterine insemination by partner. 2. High doses of gonadotrophins. 3. Split ejaculate and intrauterine insemination by partner.
5. *Agglutination of spermatozoa* Sperm auto-antibodies. Hostile mucus. Sperm antibodies in cervical mucus (penetrate the mucus but become agglutinated and immobilised and die).	1. Seminal fluid analysis. 2. Rosette formation of head to head clumping, or a wheatsheaf formation of tail to tail clumping in seminal fluid. 3. No sperm invasion is seen.	1. It may be possible to wash the antibodies off these sperm and then, after centrifuging, produce a concentrated specimen; they can be inseminated directly into the cervix. 2. Corticosteroid therapy.
6. *Ejaculatory disorders* Hypospadias. Epispadias. Retrograde ejaculation.	1. History 2. Examination.	1. Collection of semen and artificial insemination by partner. 2. Surgical treatment.
7. *Sexual problems* Impotence. Premature ejaculation. Stress. Decreased sexual libido.	1. History. 2. Interview.	1. Psychological referral. 2. Help regain self confidence. 3. Apply local anaesthetic to penis before coitus. Treatment for premature ejaculation. 4. Mono-amine oxidase inhibitor drugs.
8. *Others* Poor general health. Febrile illness. Emotional shock. Acute allergic response.	1. History. 2. Examination. 3. Erythrocyte sedimentation rate.	1. Full recovery ensues naturally.

couples require an information-providing service that is sensitive to their needs. They will wish to know about the nature of investigations, the implications of and alternatives to treatment. Emotional support and therapeutic counselling will need to be easily available. The guidelines of the Human Fertilisation and Embryology Authority (HFEA) require centres licensed for IVF-ET and donor insemination to give information to all couples about the implications of treatment and to provide access to independent counselling services for those who wish to be treated.

In vitro fertilisation and embryo transfer (IVF-ET)

The work of Edwards & Steptoe in 1978 led to the birth of the first human infant after conception in vitro. Over 2000 babies worldwide have since been born by the IVF method. New developments continue to be made. One significant advance is the use of ovarian stimulants to promote follicle ripening, now used by all clinics. See Box 7.12.

MEDICAL MANAGEMENT

Treatment. Two main treatment methods have emerged.

Clomiphene citrate plus gonadotrophins. Human menopausal gonadotrophin (hMG) and human chorionic gonadotrophin (hCG). Clomiphene citrate is a non-steroidal anti-oestrogen that allows FSH and LH levels to rise.

Gonadotrophins alone. Pure follicle stimulating hormone (FSH) alone, or together with human menopausal gonadotrophin (hMG), is used to stimulate the follicles, and human chorionic gonadotrophin (hCG) is required for final maturation of the follicles.

Harvesting eggs for IVF. Eggs (oocytes) for fertilisation can be recovered from mature ovarian follicles by:

- laparoscopy and needle aspiration
- ultrasound scanner-guided follicle needle puncture and aspiration.

The laparoscopy method involves a general anaesthetic whilst the ultrasound method is completed with local anaesthetic.

The ultrasound guided follicle puncture is performed by inserting the needle via the urinary bladder (transvesical) or vagina (transvaginal), whilst using an ultrasound transducer.

Early research studies between laparoscopic and ultrasound-guided follicular punctures and clinical pregnancy rates have shown no statistical differences between the two methods (Wikland & Hamberger 1984, Feichtinger & Kemeter 1984, Belaish-Allart et al 1985).

Box 7.12 Indications for selection into IVF programmes

- husband and wife are generally healthy
- ovaries are accessible
- the uterus is functioning normally
- menstrual function is normal or correctable
- age preferred below 40 years but a flexible individual approach is taken
- the couple have an uncorrected problem that is
  - — tubal
  - — inadequate sperm for normal reproduction
  - — endometriosis
  - — cervical hostility
  - — immunological
  - — anovulation
  - — undiagnosed by available methods.

Laboratory procedures. There must be close proximity between the operating theatre and the embryology laboratory for maximum efficiency and effectiveness. There must also be ease of communication between the surgeon and the embryologist; direct verbal and visual contact is needed. Theatre time is usually booked in advance, with 24 hours' notice, but sometimes egg recovery may need to be done at short notice because of the patient's endogenous LH surge. Approximately half an hour before the woman's eggs are to be recovered, semen is collected by her husband.

A number of eggs will have been recovered from the patient and all the eggs will be fertilised and potentially become embryos. It is becoming usual to replace up to three embryos into the uterus of the patient.

Embryo replacement is a delicate procedure that does not necessarily result in successful implantation and pregnancy. The incidence of pregnancy increases with the number of embryos replaced. Some IVF units replace up to five embryos. This not only increases the chance of pregnancy but also multi-pregnancy that is associated with high risk, premature infants being born. Combined World Data presented at the Third World Congress of IVF in 1984 showed that 15.6% of women initiated pregnancy following embryo replacements. The pregnancy rate was related to the number of embryos replaced, and was as high as 23.8% when four embryos were replaced. There was a miscarriage rate of 29.9%. It is considered that the miscarriage rate is related to ovarian stimulation rather than the IVF procedure itself (Cohen J. 1986).

On discharge from hospital the patient is given instructions to send samples of urine to the unit on the 8th and 11th day after replacement so that pregnancy tests can be completed. She is also asked to notify the unit if menstruation occurs so that she can be advised about future treatment and her records can be maintained. If her pregnancy is confirmed and results in childbirth then the unit will wish to share the details and celebrate the success.

Treatment of low powered sperm in IVF-ET

New treatments involve manipulating ovum and sperm together to improve penetration of the ovum by sperm of poor motility. A deliberate injection of a single sperm into an ovum can be achieved using a sophisticated microscope and special instruments. The human embryos so formed have led to successful pregnancies for a few women. The work remains experimental as problems exist in the process of selecting a healthy sperm. A risk of manipulating an unhealthy sperm into an ovum exists, and a child with disability might result.

Prenatal analysis of DNA for genetic abnormality

Prenatal diagnosis of genetic abnormalities is now possible by analysing DNA for a known gene defect. A single cell is removed from a 4–16 cell embryo. Information can become available within a few hours and soon enough to allow the embryo to be implanted when it is known to be healthy. Diseases such as cystic fibrosis and duchenne muscular dystrophy can thus be avoided. Some women have already been treated in this way but long-term information is needed on whether the loss of a single cell from an embryo is likely to have any adverse effect.

NURSING PRIORITIES AND MANAGEMENT: IVF

The patient admitted to an IVF unit will have lived with her state of known sub-fertility for some years and will have experienced, with her husband, many tests, investigations and surgical interventions before being offered the opportunity to seek pregnancy by the IVF method. The couple will recognise that IVF is the treatment of last resort and that success is not guaranteed.

Pre-laparoscopy care

Reducing anxiety

Anxiety will be experienced as the treatment cycle is approached with great hope but the further risk of failure will always be present, causing emotional conflict.

The nurse will need to prepare a plan of care that will minimise the stress level and help the patient to relax. High stress levels are well known to disturb hormone levels and their activity. Planned counselling sessions may be needed to allow the patient to express any concerns. Similarly, information-giving sessions will need to be planned.

The use of slides and video tapes can be invaluable supplements for group work when the special needs of individuals can be identified and met within the supportive group or when another quiet opportunity presents itself or is planned.

The patient will become very knowledgeable about the detailed steps of the programme but may still have questions that need to be answered. She will need truthful information about results of hormonal assays, the number of eggs available for recovery, and the progress of the embryos. A system of open communication is important to the support of the patient, whether favourable or disappointing.

Self care in the follicular stage

The nurse, as always, should facilitate the patient's orientation to the comfortable surroundings of the IVF unit. The patient is not ill and her role in maintaining self care can be explained. She will need to learn how to collect her urine and record the time and amount passed. Verbal instructions can be complemented by a written explanation in the toilet area. A patient whose first language is not English will need written instructions in her own language.

Blood and urine samples will be required for laboratory testing. Ovarian stimulants are given according to the individual patient's needs. Some patients have difficulty in understanding that there are differences in need between individual women. The nurse's explanations can alleviate concerns that may be expressed.

Preparation for egg cell recovery

The procedure of ultrasound scanning will be explained in terms of checking the number of follicles maturing and their stage of development. Once the estimated time of ovulation is known, preparation for theatre begins. Blood is taken for haemoglobin estimation. Skin is prepared according to the policy of the unit; some surgeons still prefer that the pubic area is shaved prior to laparoscopy and oocyte recovery. Fasting arrangements are maintained according to protocol; 6 hours' maximum fasting from food and drinks is usual. No premedication drugs are prescribed to avoid compromise of the patient's physiological balance and that of the ripened follicles.

The patient is likely to be excited at this time in anticipation of a successful harvesting of eggs. The nurse should encourage the patient to relax and be calm in approach to the transfer to theatre. Via laparoscopy, each mature follicle is carefully aspirated of its egg, which is immediately passed to the laboratory for examination. When the egg is identified, the next follicle is aspirated and so on, until all mature follicles are emptied.

Post-laparoscopy care

Recovery from the laparoscopy is rapid. Rest in bed for a maximum of 8 hours is usually necessary to avoid referred pain in the shoulder from retention of residual gas in the abdomen. Mild analgesia such as paracetamol may be prescribed for relief of pain. The patient is keen to know whether the laparoscopy was successful and how many eggs were recovered.

Unfortunately, it sometimes happens that ovulation time has been misjudged and the follicles have already ruptured prior to laparoscopy, or some eggs recovered are too immature to be viable. During the laparoscopy a problem may have arisen whereby adhesions are obscuring the ovarian tissue and the procedure fails.

A counselling, sensitive approach is taken by the nurse in giving news of the failure of the procedure. The surgeon concerned may prefer to explain his difficulties to the patient and her partner. The nurse may have to repeat the information for the patient together with possible details of re-entry into the programme later.

Preparation for embryo transfer

When a patient's eggs have been successfully recovered there is a 2–3 days' wait whilst the eggs are matured in vitro, if this is necessary, and then are fertilised with the specially prepared semen of her partner. As the fertilised eggs divide and develop they are closely observed in the laboratory for their readiness for transfer back into the patient's uterus. Failures may also occur at this delicate laboratory stage and is a further worrying time for the patient.

As soon as a positive decision is made for embryo transfer the patient takes a shower and dresses in clean night clothes. A bath is avoided to ensure there is no water in the vagina. The bed is prepared with clean linen and taken to the theatre.

The patient is positioned on the bed according to the surgeon's preference. Previously surgeons usually used the knee–chest position for the patient with a normally anteverted uterus and lithotomy for the retroverted uterus but, more recently, the lithotomy position has been used for all patients with no ill-effects to the embryo.

Once the fertilised egg is successfully introduced into the uterus the mother is moved gently up the bed in a position of easy adjustment from that in which the embryo transfer was achieved. A face down position, lying on the back, or a lateral position may be utilised for the next 2 hours of undisturbed rest, still with the head of the bed tilted downwards.

After this time has passed the head of the bed is returned to a normal position. The patient can eat and drink before settling quietly to sleep for the night.

The patient should spend the next day quietly, avoiding strenuous activity. Discharge usually takes place 36 hours after embryo transfer with the mother anticipating a positive pregnancy outcome.

?	**7.3** Think about how the patient feels if failure occurs at any of the stages of the IVF treatment programme.
?	**7.4** Write down the patient's possible thoughts about failure: • during the follicular stage • at the oocyte recovery stage • at the embryo development stage in the laboratory • after embryo transfer into the uterus.
?	**7.5** Write down a few sentences of what you might say to the patient at each of the above stages.
?	**7.6** Discuss with your mentor whether what you have written down could be used as a guide to communication with the patient with allowances made for differences between patients and their partners.

Gamete intrafallopian transfer (GIFT)

GIFT is a more recent treatment than IVF. Its results in pro-

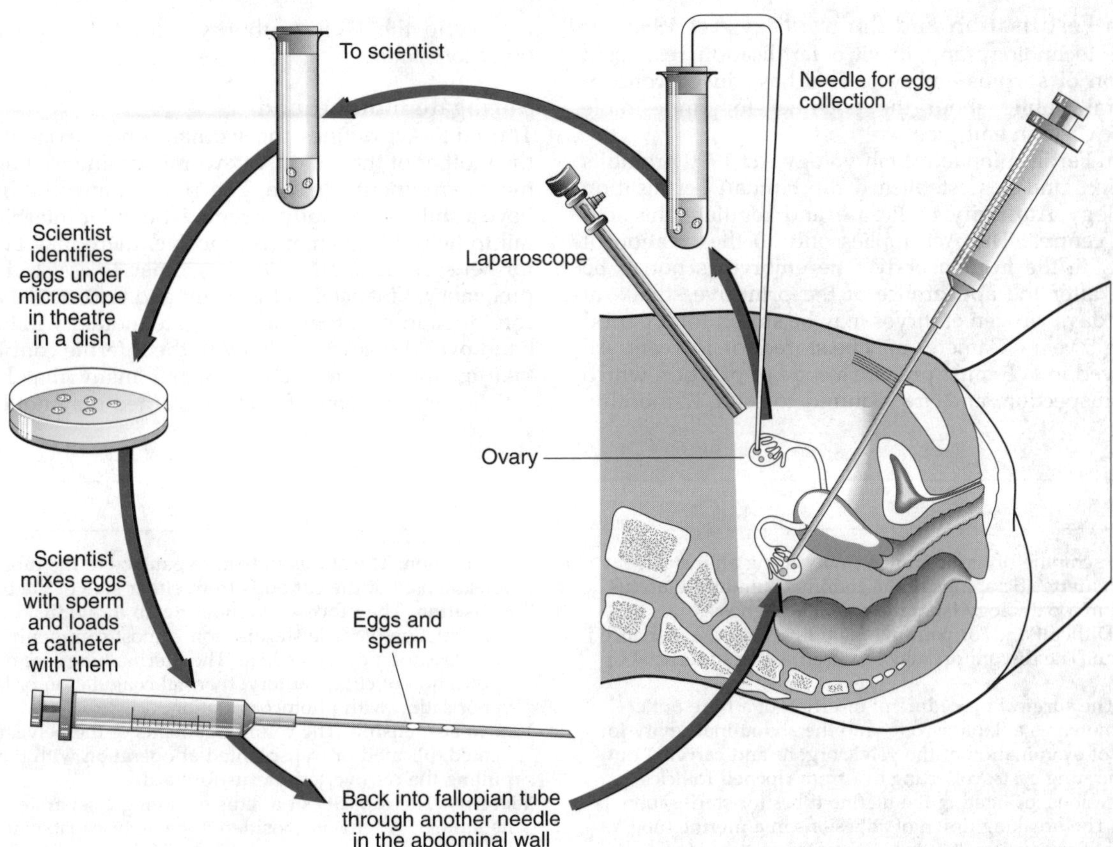

Fig. 7.11 The GIFT treatment.

moting a pregnancy and infant are not much better than those of IVF.

However, the procedure does not require expensive laboratory facilities and can be carried out in hospitals that do not have IVF facilities.

GIFT is usually carried out when there is no obvious reason for subfertility. The technique involves giving follicle-stimulating drugs to ripen several eggs. Laparoscopy is performed and a number of eggs are removed from the ovary. The eggs are then mixed with the freshly donated sperm and transferred into the fimbriated ends of both uterine tubes (see Fig. 7.11). The eggs then have the opportunity to become fertilised in the woman's own fluids in the natural environment.

Counselling

Nurses working in hospital or the community must be prepared themselves to always use their counselling skills with clients who are wanting to enter, or are involved in, or have terminated a programme of subfertility treatment. The community midwife may participate in the care of a client who has lost a pregnancy, or is currently pregnant and looking forward to childbirth. The woman's health visitor will also have a role in counselling following the loss of a pregnancy or an infant after subfertility treatment. See Case History 7.2. Couples may continue to need to talk about their feelings of inadequacy or failure and to be allowed to grieve for their losses as if they have experienced a bereavement.

EMBRYO RESEARCH

The main aim of the human embryo research has been the prevention of genetically transferred diseases. New risks to the health of the unborn child are not welcome. Embryo research improves the understanding and management of genetic diseases; animals do not have the same birth defects as humans.

Preimplantation diagnosis on embryos is possible by removing and examining a single cell, although it is not known whether this cell removal might cause a defect in the child. The treatment offers hope to those who carry genetic defects that affect the well-being of the child.

Further embryo research may help with the understanding of miscarriage of pregnancies that involve 100 000 women per year, with consequent effects on health and future fertility. Further understanding of the way embryos implant might shed more light on contraception, miscarriages and ectopic pregnancies. It is also expected that embryo research could improve understanding and treatment of cancer by the study of 'oncogenes' that control cell division and growth.

Case History 7.2 K

K achieved a pregnancy during her programme of subfertility treatments. Unfortunately, she aborted a twin-boy pregnancy, and was devastated by the loss. She returned to the programme and became a mother with the birth of quadruplets: three girls and a boy. Unfortunately the boy subsequently died. K visits the unit with her lovely girls in a triple buggy but still grieves over the boys. She has asked to re-enter the programme because she still wants a boy. K has been referred to an independent counsellor.

The Human Fertilisation and Embryology Act 1990

Reproductive technology and in vitro fertilisation results in the production of surplus embryos. This has caused concern to the general public about the potential for undesirable experimental work on embryos.

The Human Fertilisation and Embryology Act 1990 prohibits certain practices and has established the Human Fertilisation and Embryology Authority to license and regulate the activities of IVF centres. The Act applies only to the creation of embryos outside the human body. The embryo is not to be kept or used after the appearance of the primitive streak, at the end of 14 days. Frozen embryos may be stored for a period not exceeding 5 years. Gametes may be stored for 10 years. All centres involved in IVF must prepare a code of practice, which is subject to inspection, and are required to send 12-monthly reports to the HFE Authority. The Act has a conscientious objection clause.

Surrogate motherhood

The HFE Act defines the woman who carries the embryo as the mother of the child. Any womb leasing, surrogacy arrangements are unenforceable. The right of any childless couple to have a child is generally accepted, but after infertility treatments fail to help the woman to conceive, there may be less support for her seeking another fertile woman to assist in developing a pregnancy. Financial inducement and contractual arrangements cannot guarantee that the surrogate mother will be prepared to hand over the newborn baby to the infertile couple. The media take an interest in such cases but many that have positive, satisfactory outcomes for all concerned may not be reported.

GLOSSARY

Curettage. The scraping of tissue from a cavity using an instrument known as a 'curette'. Scrapings of the endometrium of the uterus are analysed in a pathology laboratory to aid diagnosis.

Dyspareunia. Difficult and/or painful sexual intercourse experienced by the woman. The discomfort may be described as superficial or deep.

Laparoscopy. The surgical procedure of insertion of a fibre optic endoscope known as a 'laparascope' into the abdominal cavity for the purpose of examination of the pelvic organs and carrying out biopsies, aspirating cysts, collecting ova from ripened follicles, dividing adhesions, or ligating the uterine tubes for sterilisation.

Salpingolysis. The breaking down of adhesions in a uterine tube.

Salpingostomy. The surgical opening of the uterine tubes for reparative procedures following inflammatory disease or sterilisation. The aim is to restore patency to the tubes by anastomoses of the cut ends from either side of the blockage.

Sterilisation. The process of rendering an individual incapable of reproduction. Female sterilisation is most commonly carried out via a laparoscopy procedure. The uterine tubes are occluded by the application of clips, cautery, thermal coagulation or laser vaporisation with photocoagulation.

Ventro-suspension. The round ligaments of the pelvis may be folded, ligated, plicated or transplanted at operation with the aim of pulling the retroverted uterus forward.

Viability. The capacity of a fetus for living a separate existence from its mother. A fetus is considered viable or capable of survival from the 24th week of pregnancy. This viability is recognised and safeguarded in the Human Fertilisation and Embryology Act 1990.

REFERENCES

Abraham G E 1981 Premenstrual tension: current problems in obstetrics and gynaecology. In: O'Brien P M S 1987 Premenstrual syndrome. Blackwell Scientific Publications, London, pp. 1–39

Allen I 1981 Family planning, sterilisation and abortion services. Policy Studies Institute, London

Angst J, Autenrieth V, Brem F, Koukkon M, Meyer J, Stassen H H, Storch U 1979 Preliminary results of treatment with beta-endorphin in depression. In: Usdin E, Burney W E, Kline N S (eds) 1979 Endorphins in mental health research. Oxford University Press, New York, p. 518

Baggish M S, Dorsey J H, Adelson M 1989 A ten year experience treating cervical intraepithelial neoplasia with the CO_2 laser. American Journal Obstetrics Gynaecology 161: 60–68

Baird P J 1983 Serological evidence for the association of papillomavirus and cervical neoplasia. Lancet (ii): 17–18. In: Shingleton H M and Orr J W (eds) 1987 Cancer of the cervix: diagnosis and treatment. Churchill Livingstone, Edinburgh, p. 21

Bassett C 1993 Pay attention to the testes. Practice Nurse 5(14): 957–958

Belaish-Allart J C, Hazout A, Guillet Rosso F, Glissant M, Testart J, Frydman R 1985 Various techniques for oocyte recovery in an in vitro fertilisation and embryo transfer program. Journal In Vitro Fertilisation Embryo Transfer 2: 99–104

Berggren G, Sjostedt S 1983 Preinvasive carcinoma of the cervix uteri and smoking. Acta Obstetrica Gynaecologica Scandinavica 62: 593–598. In: Shingleton H M, Orr J W (eds) 1987 Cancer of the cervix: diagnosis and treatment. Churchill Livingstone, Edinburgh, p. 13

Birdi A, Gupta S, Gambhir S S 1984 Plasma histaminase activity in carcinoma of the cervix: its clinical significance. Journal of Surgical Oncology 25: 296–299. In: Shingleton H M, Orr J W (eds) 1987 Cancer of the cervix: diagnosis and treatment. Churchill Livingstone, Edinburgh, Ch. 4, p. 116

Boore J 1978 A prescription for recovery. Royal College of Nurses, London

Brown M A, Woods N F 1984 Correlates of dysmenorrhoea: a challenge to past stereotypes. Journal of Obstetric, Gynaecological and Neonatal Nursing, 13(4): 259–266. In: Smithson A 1992 Girls will be women. Nursing Times 88(6): 46–48

Cabral G A, Fry D, Marciano-Cabral F, Lumpkin C, Mercer L, Goplerud D 1983 A herpes virus antigen in human premalignant and malignant cervical biopsies and explants. American Journal of Obstetrics and Gynaecology, 145: 79–86. In: Shingleton H M and Orr J W (eds) 1987 Cancer of the cervix: diagnosis and treatment. Churchill Livingstone, Edinburgh, p. 21

Campbell S, Whitehead M I 1977 Oestrogen therapy and the menopausal syndrome. In: Greenblatt R, Studd J (eds) 1977 The menopause: clinics in obstetrics and gynaecology. W B Saunders, London, pp. 31–47

Central Statistical Office 1992 Selected causes of death: by sex, 1951 and 1990. Cancer: cervix. Social Trends (22) 7.5 and 7.27: p. 124 and 135. Government Statistical Service HMSO, London

Charles E H, Savage E W 1980 Cryosurgical treatment of intra-epithelial neoplasia: a review of the literature. Obstetric Gynaecological Survey, 1980 35: 359–548. In: Studd J (ed) 1993 Progress in obstetrics and gynaecology. Churchill Livingstone, Edinburgh, Vol 10, Ch. 20: 362

Clarke E A, Hilditch S 1983 Problems in determining the incidence of cervical cancer. Canadian Medical Association Journal, 129: 1271–1273. In: Shingleton H M, Orr J W (eds) 1987 Cancer of the cervix: diagnosis and treatment. Churchill Livingstone, Edinburgh, p. 13

Coope J, Thomson J M, Poller L 1975 Effects of 'natural oestrogen' replacement therapy on menopausal symptoms and blood clotting. British Medical Journal 4: 139–143. In: Greenblatt R B, Studd J 1977 The menopause: clinics in obstetrics and gynaecology, 4(1): 31

Cohen J 1986 Pregnancy, abortion and birth after in vitro fertilisation. In: Fishel S, Symonds E M 1986 In vitro fertilisation. IRL Press, pp. 135–146

Chuong C J, Coulam C B, Kao P C, Bergstalh E J, Go V L W 1985 Neuropeptide levels in premenstrual syndrome. Fertility and Sterility 44(6): 760–765

Dickson A, Henriques N 1986 Hysterectomy, the positive recovery plan. Mackays, Chatham

Edwards R G, Steptoe P C 1983 Current status of in vitro fertilisation and implantation of human embryos. Lancet (ii): 1265–1269

Effective Health Care Consortium 1992 The management of subfertility. Effective Health Care, August (3). University of Leeds

Feichtinger W, Kemeter D 1984 Laparascopic or ultrasonically guided follicle aspiration for in vitro fertilisation. Journal In Vitro Fertilisation Embryo Transfer 1: 244–249

French P W, Coppleson M, Reid B L, Singer A 1982 III Etiology: role of sperm basic proteins as carcinogens in cervical cancer. In: Hafez E S E, Smith J P (eds) Carcinoma of the cervix: biology and diagnosis. Martinus Nijhoff, The Hague, 123–127. In: Shingleton H M, Orr J W (eds) 1987 Cancer of the cervix: diagnosis and treatment. Churchill Livingstone, Edinburgh, p. 22

Gomel V 1980 Microsurgical reversal of female sterilisation: a reappraisal. Fertility and Sterility 33: 587

Gordon H K, Duncan I D 1991 Effective destruction of cervical intra-epithelial neoplasia (CIN) 3 at 100°C using the Semur cold coagulator: 14 years' experience. British Journal Obstetric Gynaecology 98: 14–20. In: Studd J (ed) 1993 Progress in obstetrics and gynaecology. Churchill Livingstone, Edinburgh (10) Ch. 20: 363

Hartmann P E 1991 The breast and breastfeeding. In: Philipp E, Setchell M (eds) 1991 Scientific foundations of obstetrics and gynaecology, 4th edn. Butterworth Heinemann, London 33: 388

Hayward J 1975 Information: a prescription against pain. Royal College of Nurses, London

Hendry W F, Hughes L, Scammell G 1990 Comparison of prednisolone and placebo in sub fertile men with antibodies to spermatazoa. Lancet 1990 335: 85–88

HMSO 1990 Family planning clinics: methods of contraception recommended or chosen. Social Trends 20: 48, Table 2.29

Hull M G R, Eddowes H A, Fahy U, Abuzeid M I, Mills M S, Cahill D J et al 1992 Expectations of assisted conception for infertility. British Medical Journal 1992 304: 1465–1469

Human Fertilisation and Embryology Act 1990 HMSO, London

Jaszman L J B 1976 Epidemiology of the climacteric syndrome. In: Cambell S (ed) 1976 The management of the menopause and post-menopausal years. Baltimore University Park Press, pp. 11–23

Kjorstad J E, Orjasaester H 1984 The prognostic value of CEA determinations in the plasma of patients with squamous cell cancer of the cervix. Gynaecologic Oncology 19: 284–289. In: Shingleton H M, Orr J W (eds) Cancer of the cervix: diagnosis and treatment. Churchill Livingstone, Edinburgh Ch. 4: 116

Kline N S, Lehmann H E, Lajtha A, Luski E, Cooper T 1977 Beta-endorphin-induced changes in schizophrenic and depressed patients. Archives of General Psychiatry 34: 1111–1113

Kolodny R G, Masters W H, Johnston V E 1979 Textbook of human sexuality for nurses. Little Brown, Boston

Lewis T L T, Chamberlain G V P (eds) 1989 Gynaecology by ten teachers, 15th edn. Edward Arnold, London

Lunn P G, Prentice A M, Austin S, Whitehead R G 1980 Influence of maternal diet on plasma-prolactin levels during lactation. Lancet (i): 623. In: Philipp E E, Barnes J, Newton M (eds) 1986 Scientific foundations of obstetrics and gynaecology, 3rd edn. Heinemann, London, p. 299

Lunn P G, Watkinson M, Prentice A M, Morrell P, Austin S, Whitehead R G 1981 Maternal nutrition and lactational amenorrhoea. Lancet (i): 1428. In: Philipp E E, Barnes J, Newton M (eds) 1986 Scientific foundations of obstetrics and gynaecology, 3rd edn. Heinemann, London, p. 299

Lunn P G 1992 Breast feeding patterns, maternal milk output and lactational infecundity. Journal of Biosocial Science 1992 July 24 (3): 317–324

Marana R, Quagliarello J 1988 Proximal tubul occlusion: microsurgery versus IVF: a review. International Journal of Fertility 1988, 33: 338–340

Marteau T M, Walker P, Giles G, Smail M 1990 Anxieties in women undergoing colposcopy. British Journal Obstetric Gynaecology 97: 859–861. In: Studd J (ed) 1993 Progress in Obstetrics and Gynaecology. Churchill Livingstone, Edinburgh, p. 372

Maruo T, Shibata K, Kimura A, Hoshina M, Mochizuki M 1985 Tumour associated antigen, TA-4, in the monitoring of the effects of therapy for squamous cell carcinoma of the uterine cervix: serial determinations and tissue localization. Cancer 56: 302–308. In: Shingleton H M, Orr J W (eds) 1987 Cancer of the cervix: diagnosis and treatment. Churchill Livingstone, Edinburgh, p. 116

Meldrum D K, Shamonki I M, Frumar A M 1979 Elevations in skin temperature of the finger as an objective index of post menopause hot flashes: standardization of technique. American Journal Obstetric Gynaecology, pp. 135–713

Monaghan J M 1986 Bonney's gynaecological surgery. Baillière Tindall, London

Morrison H 1988 Diabetic impotence. Nursing Times 84(32): 35–37

Muse K, Cetel N, Futterman L, Yen S 1984 The premenstrual syndrome. Effects of 'medical ovariectomy'. New England Journal of Medicine 311: 1345–1349. In: O'Brien P M S 1987 Premenstrual syndrome. Blackwell Scientific, Oxford, p. 173

Nagant de Deuxchaisnes C 1983 The pathogenesis and treatment of involutional osteoporosis. In: Dixon A St J et al (eds) Osteoporosis: a multidisciplinary problem. Royal Society of Medicine, Academic Press, London, pp. 292–333

Notelovitz M 1986 Menopause and climacteric. In: Philipp E E, Barnes J, Newton M 1986 Obstetrics and Gynaecology, 3rd edn. Heinemann, London, p. 201

O'Brien P M S 1987 Premenstrual syndrome. Blackwell Scientific Publications, London, p. 115

Orem D 1991 Nursing: concepts of practice, 4th edn. McGraw Hill, New York

Park M, Kitchener H C, MacNab J C 1983 Detection of herpes simplex virus type-2: DNA restriction fragments in human cervical carcinoma tissue. EMBO Journal 2: 1029–1034. In: Shingleton H M, Orr J W (eds) 1987 Cancer of the cervix: diagnosis and treatment. Churchill Livingstone, Edinburgh, p. 21

Patton P E, Williams T J, Coulam C B 1987 Microsurgical reconstruction of the proximal oviduct. Fertility and Sterility 47: 35–39

Petitti D B, Klein R, Kipp H et al 1982 Physiologic measures in men with and without vasectomies. Fertility and Sterility 37: 438–440. In: Hendry W F 1989 Vasectomy and vasectomy reversal. In: Filshie M, Guillebaud J (eds) 1989 Butterworth-Heinemann, p. 297

Purdie D W 1990 Hormone replacement therapy and prevention of osteoporosis. In: Bonnar J (ed) 1990 Recent advances in obstetrics and gynaecology, 16. Churchill Livingstone, Edinburgh, pp. 235–251

Reid R L, Greenaway-Coate A, Hahn P M 1986 Oral glucose tolerance during the menstrual cycle in normal women and women with alleged premenstrual 'hypoglycaemic' attacks: effects of nazalone. Journal Clinical Endocrinology Metabolism 62: 1167

Royal College of Physicians 1991 Report on preventive medicine. Royal College of Physicians, London

Sawada M, Okudaira Y, Matsui Y 1984 Immunosuppressive acidic protein in patients with gynecologic cancer. Cancer 54: 652–656. In: Shingleton H M, Orr J W (eds) 1987 Cancer of the cervix: diagnosis and treatment. Churchill Livingstone, Edinburgh, p. 117

Shingleton H M, Orr J W (eds) 1987 Cancer of the cervix: diagnosis and treatment. Churchill Livingstone, Edinburgh, pp. 61–62

Singhal V, Li T C, Cooke I D 1991 An analysis of factors influencing the outcome of 232 consecutive tubal microsurgery cases. British Journal of Obstetrics and Gynaecology 98: 628–636

Smith J W 1983 Herpes simplex virus: An expanding relationship to human cancer. Journal of Reproductive Medicine 28: 116–122. In: Shingleton H M, Orr J W (eds) 1987 Cancer of the cervix: diagnosis and treatment. Churchill Livingstone, Edinburgh, p. 21

Smithson A 1992 Girls will be women. Nursing Times 88(6): 46–48

Sokol R Z, Petersen G, Steiner B S, Swerdloff R S, Bustillo M A 1988 A controlled comparison of the efficacy of clomiphene citrate in male infertility. Fertility and Sterility 49: 865–870

Sondheimer S J, Freeman E, Rickels K 1988 Gynaecologic PMS program: hormonal influences on symptom manifestation. In: Gise L H, Kase N G, Berkowitz (eds) 1988 The premenstrual syndromes. Churchill Livingstone, New York, p. 69

Standford J R 1988 Testicular cancer. Nursing 26: 957–960
Taylor C, Faulk W P 1981 Prevention of recurrent abortion with leucocyte transfusions. Lancet ii: 68. In: De Cherney A, Polan M L 1984 Evaluation and management of habitual abortion. British Journal of Hospital Medicine 31(4): 261–262 and 266–268
Trevathan E, Layde P, Webster L A, Adams J B, Benigno B B, Ory H 1983 Cigarette smoking and dysplasia and carcinoma in situ of the uterine cervix. Journal of the American Medical Association 250: 499–502. In: Shingleton H M, Orr J W (eds) 1987 Cancer of the cervix: diagnosis and treatment, Churchill Livingstone, Edinburgh p. 13
Wagner D, Ikenerg H, Boehm N, Gissman L 1984 Identification of human papilloma virus in cervical swabs by deoxyribonucleic acid in situ hybridization. Obstetrics and Gynaecology 64: 767–772. In: Shingleton H M, Orr J W (eds) 1987 Cancer of the cervix: diagnosis and treatment. Churchill Livingstone, Edinburgh, p. 21
Wallach E E, Manara L R, Eisenberg E 1983 Experience with 143 cases of tubal surgery. Fertility and Sterility, 39: 609–617
Webb C, Wilson-Barnett J 1983 Self concept, social support and hysterectomy. International Journal of Nursing Studies (20) 2: 97–107
Webb C (ed) 1988 Women's health. Midwifery and gynaecological nursing. Edward Arnold, London, pp. 140–147
Wehrenberg W B, Wardlaw S L, Franz A G, Ferin M 1982 Beta-endorphin in hypophyseal-portal blood: variations throughout the menstrual cycle. Endocrinology iii: 879–881
Whitehead M I, Fraser D, Schenkel L, Crook D, Stevenson J C 1990 Transdermal administration of oestrogen/progestogen hormone replacement therapy. Lancet 335: 310–312
Wilkland M, Hamberger L 1984 Ultrasound as a diagnostic and operative tool for in vitro fertilisation and embryo replacement programs. Journal of In Vitro Fertility and Embryo Transfer 1: 213–216
Woodman C B J, Jordan J A, Mylotte M J, Gustafeson R, Wade-Evans T 1985 The management of cervical intra-epithelial neoplasia by coagulation electrodiathermy. British Journal of Obstetrics and Gynaecology 10: 362
Xue P, Fa Y 1989 Microsurgical reversal of female sterilisation. Journal of Reproductive Medicine 34: 451–455

PART 2
THE BREAST

INTRODUCTION

The breast is the human organ of lactation which develops in puberty to enable a mother to feed her offspring. In Western society the breasts are strongly associated femininity and sexuality as well as with motherhood. The images of femininity presented in advertising and other media use the breast as a symbol of sexual desirability and promote an idealised beauty which few women can attain. It is not surprising that breast disease often has profound implications not only for a woman's physical health but also for her social and familial roles, body image and self-confidence. Women who suffer any alteration or disfigurement of the breast often experience enxiety, depression and loss of sexual satisfaction. This chapter will therefore begin by considering the significance of diseases of the breast for a woman's psychological well-being. Patient education will then be discussed in relation to promoting breast health and the early detection of disease; the importance of involving the patient and her family in making informed treatment choices and in carrrying out subsequent self-care will also be discussed.

The anatomy and physiology of the healthy breast will be discussed before the most common disorders of the breast and their treatment are described in detail. Breast cancer and related health-care issues such as breast reconstruction and the management of lymphoedema will be given particular attention, as breast cancers are among the most common malignant conditions among women in the United Kingdom. Consideration will also be given to measures for the prevention or early detection of breast cancer.

Finally, benign disorders of the breast — mammary dysplasia, fibroademomas and breast infections — will be considered more briefly. In addition, the rare condition of gynaecomastia will be described in view of its important psychological implications for the individual.

The psychological impact of breast disease

Nurses have a particularly important role to play in supporting patients through the traumatic experience of breast disease. Although many women with breast cancer, for example, will face similar problems, no two individuals will respond to their diagnosis and treatment in exactly the same way. As this chapter will stress, ongoing assessment is the key to providing psychological and emotional support that is genuinely responsive to each woman's needs and priorities.

For most women a diagnosis of breast cancer is devastating. In addition to facing the possibility that they may eventually die of the disease, they may have to cope with the prospect of mutilating surgery to a part of the body associated with femininity, sexuality and motherhood. Most women with breast cancer will have discovered a lump during self-examination or by accident. Symptoms of acute anxiety, panic, palpitations, tachycardia, loss of concentration and insomnia may be experienced in the period when a medical opinion is sought and a diagnosis awaited. Some women describe this time as the most agonising period of their illness. For some women, the fear of cancer or its treatment is so great that they deny the presence of a lump or delay seeking medical help.

Some of this fear may be based on misconceptions about the nature of cancer treatments. It is therefore important for nurses, especially those in community practice, to dispel myths about cancer therapy, to raise awareness of the success rate of breast cancer treatment, and to emphasise the importance of early detection.

Some women who undergo surgery for breast cancer initially experience euphoria that the cancer has been removed. Others deny the removal of their breast, or find themselves unable to talk about it or to look at the scar.

Much research has been carried out into the psychosocial sequelae of breast surgery. Maguire et al (1978) found that 38% of women experience anxiety, depression or sexual problems in the first year after a mastectomy. Morris et al (1977) found similar incidences of anxiety and depression. It was thought that this was related mainly to the altered body image of mastectomy, but Fallowfield et al (1985) found that women who had a lumpectomy and radiotherapy had levels of anxiety and depression similar to those experienced by women who had undergone mastectomy (see Research Abstract 7.8). Meyer & Aspegren (1989) also found that levels of anxiety and depression were similar between these two groups but that breast conservation seemed to help to preserve a woman's female identity and her acceptance of her body image.

Following diagnosis and surgery a period of adjustment occurs which is characterised by fluctuating emotions. Northouse (1989) found that following mastectomy the major concern for most women and their partners surrounded issues of survival, in particular the extent of the cancer and the possibility of recurrence. Patients may also be worried about changes in lifestyle, treatment regimes, and altered appearance.

For the majority of women who have undergone breast surgery, anxiety will show signs of reducing after about 3 months and the activities of normal life will be resumed. Some women, however, will continue to experience great anxiety, show signs of depression, withdraw from social contact or have sexual problems. These women are likely to benefit from more in-depth counselling and psychological support. Nurses, particularly those in the community and in outpatient departments, should recognise emotional problems and where necessary suggest a referral to a psychiatrist or psychologist via a GP or hospital medical staff.

Patient education

Research has shown that many patients find that information

Research Abstract 7.8

In a study by Fallowfield et al (1985) 101 women being treated for early breast cancer (stages T0, T1, T2, N0, N1, and M0) were assessed for psychiatric morbidity, sexual functioning and social adjustment. Of the group 53 were treated by mastectomy and 48 by lumpectomy and radiotherapy.

The study found that 33% of the women following mastectomy and 38% following lumpectomy experienced anxiety and/or depression; 38% in each group reported reduced sexual interest.

Reasons given for anxiety and depression varied between the two subgroups. Both were worried by the diagnosis and prognosis of breast cancer. The women who had undergone lumpectomy were concerned about the recurrence of cancer in the breast operated on and were worried about radiotherapy and its after-effects. They were also more commonly worried that they had opted for the wrong procedure. The women who had undergone mastectomy voiced more concern about the effect of surgery on their appearance and personal relationships.

This study suggests that women who undergo lumpectomy and radiotherapy do not experience less psychosocial distress than those who undergo mastectomy and therefore require as much support and counselling as those who undergo more extensive surgery.

Fallowfield L J, Baum M, Maguire G P 1986 Effects of breast conservation on psychological morbidity associated with diagnosis and treatment of early breast cancer. British Medical Journal 293: 1331–1335 helps them to make sense of their situation, and hence to feel more in control, less vulnerable and less anxious (Boore 1978). Information may also help to reduce the pain and complications experienced postoperatively (Hayward 1975). Most women have some general knowledge of breast cancer, but will not be familiar with the details of the tests or treatments they are to undergo. Many will in fact have misconceptions about breast cancer and its prognosis.

The nurse must bear in mind, however, that the amount of information each woman wants about her disease or a proposed treatment will vary. As too much information is likely to cause confusion and anxiety, it is important for the nurse to find out what each individual wants to know, and to clarify what has been understood. It is also important to remember that in times of stress information is more difficult to assimilate. It is therefore often necessary for the nurse to repeat information.

If the nurse feels unable to answer any questions she should find someone who can, or arrange a further consultation with medical staff. The nurse may be able to facilitate communication by helping the patient to articulate her concerns and by clarifying concepts or terminology unfamiliar to the patient.

Areas of information that are likely to be relevant include:

- How breast cancer is and *is not* caused, e.g. it is not caused by a knock on the breast
- The aim of treatment, and what outcome may realistically be expected
- The nature and likely cosmetic effect of any proposed surgery. The nurse should ensure that the patient understands what the operation involves and the likely pre- and postoperative experiences, including the presence of wound drains, intravenous infusions, pain, scarring, and any possible short- or long-term complications. Photographs or diagrams may be useful to demonstrate likely scarring or alteration in breast shape or size
- The possibility of breast reconstructive surgery if all, or a large part, of the breast is removed
- If axillary lymph node removal is advised, the effects of removal and the postoperative exercises necessary to ensure the return of full shoulder movement (see p. 282)
- Staging tests that will need to be performed prior to or following surgery
- The availability of prostheses, where this is appropriate.

Information given verbally may be reinforced in written form. Booklets on breast surgery and breast cancer can be obtained from BACUP, the Breast Care and Mastectomy Association (BCMA) or The Royal Marsden Hospital, if local literature is not available (see Useful Addresses, p. 290). These publications can also be useful for family and friends to read.

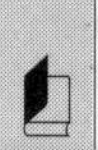

Women who wish to have more in-depth knowledge may find Baum (1988) useful. This book is written for the informed lay public. Admission booklets providing information about the hospital, its facilities and visiting hours are also helpful.

The issue of informed consent

The patient's rights

In order to give informed consent to an operation or treatment a patient must be told what the procedure or therapy entails and its consequences, and must *understand* the information that she is given.

A woman who is diagnosed as having breast cancer has the right to be told of all the possible medical options and to decide which, if any, of these options she will take. She may wish to seek a second opinion from another specialist, and to gather information to help her make a decision as to which is the best treatment for her.

The increasing recognition of the patient's right to informed consent has led to the virtual abolition of the all-in-one procedure of excision biopsy of a breast lump for frozen section pathology followed immediately by mastectomy if cancer is found.

The nurse's role

The issue of informed consent is an important one for all nurses who aim to give truly patient-centred care. Doctors have the responsibility for obtaining informed consent, but nurses can help to ensure that this occurs by asking patients to state what they understand is to happen to them, and by providing any additional information that is desired. Often patients feel very vulnerable when consulting a doctor and a nurse may act as advocate by representing the patient or support her in meetings with the doctor. Where a nurse feels she does not have the necessary information or communication skills, she may be able to contact a specialist breast care nurse, now employed by many hospitals to support women from the time of breast cancer diagnosis.

Explaining the choices

For many women with breast cancer the consultant will be able to give two treatment options which are equally promising, e.g. a mastectomy, or a wide excision of the tumour and axillary dissection followed by radiotherapy. In order for the woman to make a decision, she needs to understand what each operation or treatment involves, and any side-effects which may result.

Most women find the thought of losing a breast very distressing and will prefer a wide excision of the cancer or a segmentectomy if this is a safe option. However, mastectomy may be a better choice in some instances. The King's Fund consensus statement on Breast Cancer (King's Fund Forum 1986) reads:

> for tumours which are multi-focal, or involve a large portion of the breast, mastectomy will often be the best surgical treatment. Mastectomy may also be preferred by some women with small tumours to reduce the risks of local recurrence, and the need for adjuvant radiotherapy.

A tumour which is multi-focal (i.e. occurs in several areas of the breast) or is centrally sited cannot safely be removed by conservative surgery as the risk of local recurrence will be unacceptably high. The cosmetic result of removing a large tumour from a small breast would be so poor that a mastectomy is likely to be more acceptable; however, only the individual woman can know how she feels about this. Some women feel that by keeping their breast they would be constantly anxious about a recurrence of the cancer and so opt for a mastectomy for greater peace of mind.

Many women facing breast surgery are not aware of the possibility of reconstructive surgery. In part this reflects the lack of facilities in many areas to undertake such surgery. The long waiting lists at centres where breast reconstructions are done may cause professionals to hesitate in disclosing the possibility of this surgery. Nonetheless, in fairness to the patient all options should be explained so that she can decide whether breast reconstruction is right for her in light of the benefits and the possible complications.

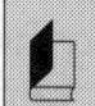

See Faulder (1985).

The role of the clinical nurse specialist in breast care

The role of the clinical nurse specialist in breast care has developed largely in response to the recognition that women with breast cancer benefit from the support and expertise of nurses specialising in this area (Watson et al 1988, Maguire et al 1980). However, it must be stressed that the clinical nurse specialist provides an additional service to that provided by hospital and community nursing staff, and not an alternative to that service. The clinical nurse specialist functions as a resource for patients, their families and nurses.

Ideally, the clinical involvement of the nurse specialist with the patient will begin at the time of diagnosis prior to hospital admission. This may involve meeting patients in screening assessment units, and requires the cooperation of outpatient nurses and doctors in informing her of new patients. Many specialist nurses follow a limited intervention strategy of seeing patients in hospital before and after their surgery, and visiting them once or twice at home in the first 4 months after surgery to assess how they are coping. Where problems arise, referral for more in-depth psychological support can be made, but the nurse is likely to continue her involvement with the patient and her family.

The nurse specialist also provides a contact point for patients and their family should they require advice or support at any time. She will also resume contact with patients should metastatic breast cancer develop. Many breast care nurse specialists also provide prosthetic and lymphoedema services.

ANATOMY AND PHYSIOLOGY OF THE BREAST

Structure of the breast

The breast is often described as a modified sweat gland. It is made up of glandular, fatty and fibrous tissue and is covered by skin. Men and women have breast tissue but in the male it remains rudimentary and does not develop in puberty.

The glandular tissue of each breast is divided into 12–20 lobes or segments (see Fig. 7.12). Each is made up of hundreds of lobules which are activated during pregnancy to produce milk. They are connected by ducts which join to form lactiferous ducts and then the ampullae beneath the areola, which function as a reservoir before ending in around ten openings in the nipple. Breast tissue is supported by Cooper's ligaments, which may contract when affected by tumour causing dimpling of the skin. With age and weight these ligaments stretch, causing the breasts to droop.

The nipple contains smooth muscle and becomes erect when stimulated, allowing a baby to suck more easily. It is surrounded by the areola, on the surface of which are Montgomery's tubercles. These lubricate the nipple during feeding.

Blood and lymph vessels

The breast is highly vascularised. It is supplied by thoracic branches of the axillary arteries laterally, and by branches of the internal mammary artery medially. Venous drainage follows arterial supply, and the lymphatic vessels follow the main ducts outwards and then branch out to the regional lymph nodes. Most drainage is via the axillary lymph nodes, proceeding from there to the supraclavicular lymph nodes. Drainage from the medial part of the breast is via the internal mammary nodes which lie beneath the ribs and lateral to the sternum.

Nerve supply

Branches of the 4th, 5th and 6th thoracic nerves containing sympathetic fibres supply the breast. Many sensory nerve endings exist around the nipple; when touched, these cause reflex erection and, after childbirth, the release of milk.

Associated muscles (see Fig. 7.13)

Behind the breast overlying the ribcage is the pectoralis major muscle. This large triangular muscle, which attaches to the clavicle, sternum and upper 6 costal cartilages is used to adduct the arm. Behind the pectoralis major lies the pectoralis minor. This muscle attaches to the 3rd, 4th and 5th ribs and the front of the scapula. Its function is to stabilise the shoulder girdle, serratus anterior and the latissimus dorsi muscle from the base and back of the axilla respectively. These and their nerve supply are important considerations when axillary surgery is performed.

Normal breast changes

The breasts constantly change as a normal consequence of ageing. Natural changes also occur with menstruation, pregnancy and lactation.

Puberty

A girl's breasts will begin to develop at puberty under the influence of hormones from the pituitary gland and ovaries, until the glandular

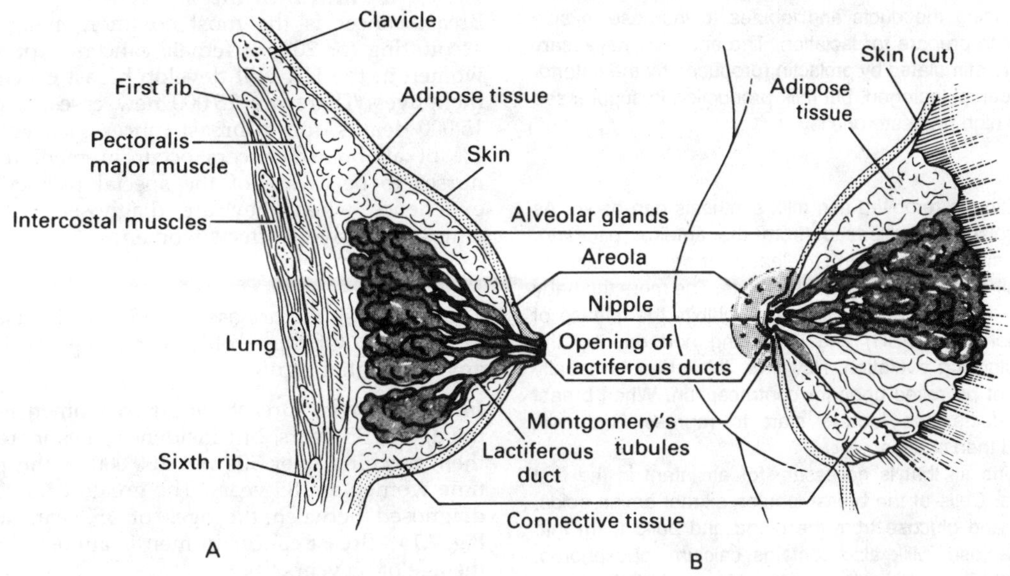

Fig. 7.12 Lateral cross-section of the breast.

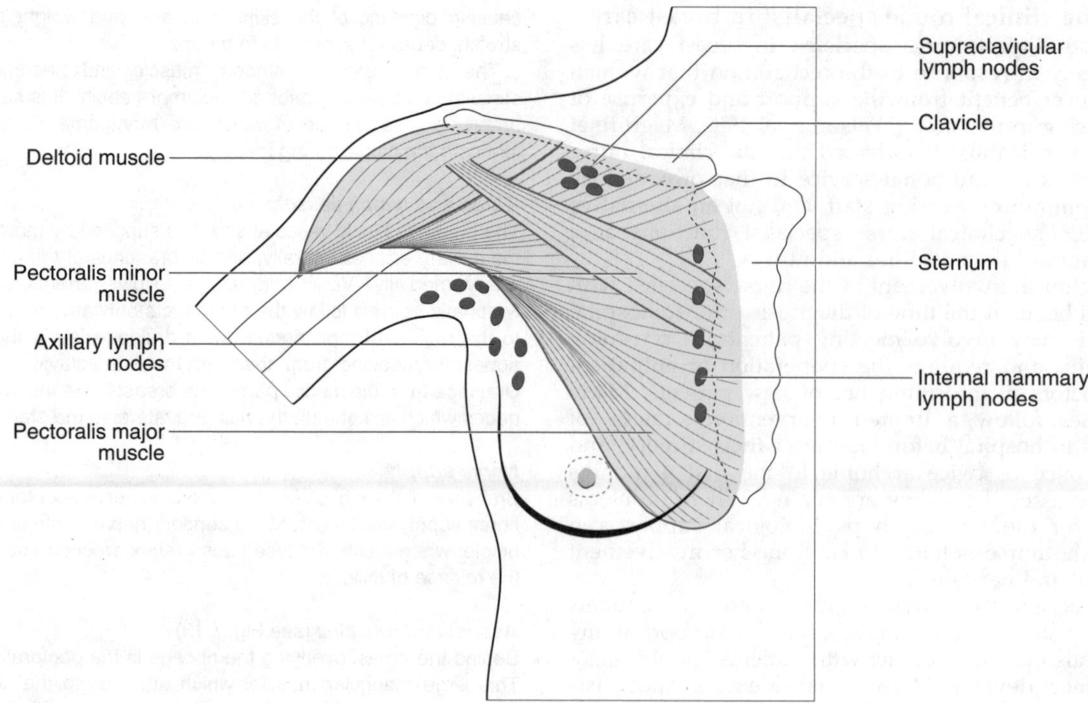

Fig. 7.13 The breast and associated structures.

tissue is mature. These hormones cause many changes during each menstrual cycle, some of which a woman is likely to be aware of.

Menstruation

At the start of each monthly cycle blood oestrogen levels rise, causing the breast ducts and lobules to enlarge. After ovulation the corpus luteum produces progesterone, which regulates breast changes. At this time tenderness and heaviness may be noticed. If pregnancy does not occur the hormone levels fall, the ducts and lobules regress, and the breasts lose their tenderness and swollen feeling. This usually precedes the onset of menstruation.

Pregnancy

If pregnancy does occur the levels of oestrogen and progesterone continue to rise, causing the ducts and lobules to increase in size and number in order to prepare for lactation. The enzymes necessary for milk production are stimulated by prolactin (produced by the anterior pituitary) and by placental lactogen, but milk production is suppressed during pregnancy by high progesterone levels.

Milk production

After birth this inhibition is removed and milk synthesis can begin. As the baby sucks, prolactin is released (from the anterior pituitary), initiating milk synthesis, and oxytocin is released (from the posterior pituitary), causing milk to be emptied from the ducts. The more the baby sucks, the more milk is produced. Sucking also inhibits the release of follicle-stimulating hormone (FSH) and luteinising hormone by the pituitary gland, so blocking ovulation. However, this effect is usually short-lived and cannot be relied upon for contraception. When breast feeding stops the ducts and lobules start to regress, and milk production slows and then ceases.

Breast milk contains all that is necessary for an infant in the first few months of its life. Cells of the breast lobules extract amino acids, fatty acids, glycerol and glucose from the blood and build them into proteins, fats and lactose. Milk also contains calcium, phosphorus, vitamins A, B, C and D, and small amounts of iron, but the exact composition depends on the mother's dietary intake.

Menopause

As a woman approaches the menopause, changes in ovarian function and hence in hormone levels cause glandular breast tissue to atrophy. This is replaced by fatty tissue so the breasts become softer, less lumpy, and consequently easier to examine and assess by mammography.

MALIGNANT DISORDERS OF THE BREAST AND THEIR SEQUELAE

BREAST CANCER

Incidence and mortality

Breast cancer is the most common malignancy in women, accounting for 20% of female cancers. Approximately 1 in 12 women in the UK will develop breast cancer at some time in their lives. There are 25 000 new cases of breast cancer and 15 000 deaths due to breast cancer each year. Approximately 1% of all breast cancers occur in men. It is important for nurses to be aware of the special problems that men may experience when they are diagnosed with a disease that almost exclusively affects women.

Risk factors

The main risk factors associated with breast cancer are listed in Box 7.13. Of these, only increasing age is known to be of any substantial significance.

Increasing age. Breast cancer in women is very rare below the age of 35 years, but incidence rates increase steadily from then, reaching over 300 per 100 000 of the population by the time women are 85 years. The greatest number of women are diagnosed between the ages of 45 years and 75 years (see Fig. 7.14). Breast cancer in men is almost always seen beyond the age of 65 years.

Geography. England and Wales have the highest mortality

Box 7.13 Factors increasing the risk of developing breast cancer

- Early menarche
- Family history of breast cancer
- First child after age 30
- Geographical location (e.g. UK has higher mortality than Japan)
- Late menopause
- Nulliparity (no pregnancies)
- Social class (Class I has highest risk)

Other possible factors under evaluation:

- High alcohol intake
- High-fat diet
- Stress

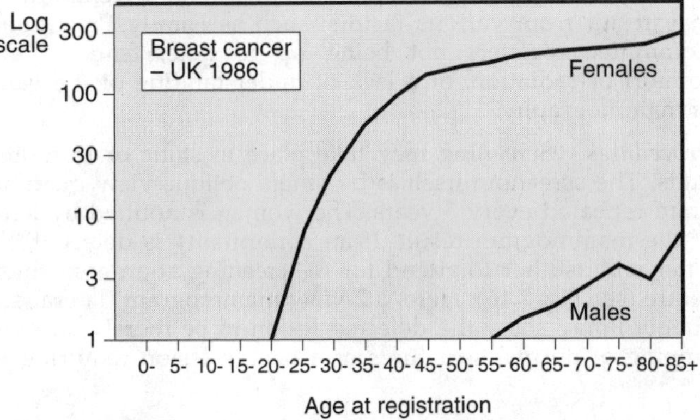

Fig. 7.14 Incidence rates of breast cancer in the UK, 1986. Breast cancer is the most common type of cancer in women. (Reproduced with kind permission from Cancer Research Campaign 1991.)

figures for breast cancer in the world, followed by Scotland, Northern Ireland, the Netherlands and the United States of America (DHSS 1986). Generally, incidence in Western Europe, North America and Australia are much higher than in Asia and Africa. Japanese women have low rates of breast cancer, but incidence rates are seen to rise by the second generation among Japanese-Americans. This suggests that environmental and social risk factors may exist.

Diet. Populations with a high rate of breast cancer generally have a diet high in fat. Obesity has also been found to be associated with a slightly increased risk of breast cancer. However, a clear link between diet and the risk of breast cancer has not been established.

Social class. Breast cancer is slightly more common amongst women in social class 1, suggesting that breast cancer is a disease of affluent societies.

Hormone-related factors. Women who have their first child after the age of 35, those who experience early menarche, and those who have a late menopause are all found to have a slightly increased rate of breast cancer. This has led to the belief that the hormone oestrogen may be implicated in the development of breast cancer. In recent years there has been much speculation as to the effects of the contraceptive pill and hormone replacement therapy on the incidence of breast cancer. Studies do not give a clear picture. A recent study by the UK National Case-Control Study Group (1989) suggests that long-term use of a high-oestrogen pill may significantly increase a woman's risk of developing breast cancer. Much more research is needed, particularly as today's contraceptive pills contain lower levels of oestrogen or none at all.

Family history. Women with a first-degree maternal relative (i.e. mother, grandmother, sister, aunt) who has developed breast cancer have an increased risk of developing the disease, particularly if the relative developed breast cancer premenopausally. The risk is greater when 2 or more relatives have had the disease.

Prevention

Over the last 30 years advances in treatments for breast cancer have failed to significantly reduce mortality from the disease. Research has been unable to identify clear causative factors that would enable the institution of a primary prevention programme. However, we know that if women are diagnosed at an early stage in their disease, treatment is likely to be more effective (see Fig. 7.15). Therefore, taking measures to detect breast cancer early would appear to be the best way of reducing breast cancer mortality.

Breast self-examination

In recent years there has been much debate as to the value of monthly breast self examination in the diagnosis of early breast cancer. Research has so far been unable to demonstrate that it alters survival from the disease. However, a woman who examines her breasts regularly is more likely to notice any changes. This encourages diagnosis when a cancer is small, so enabling a wider choice of surgical treatment options to be offered. It also allows an individual to participate in her own health care.

A woman should examine her breasts once each month, just after menstruation (e.g. day 8 of her cycle). At this time the breasts will be least lumpy and easiest to examine. If no longer menstruating, the woman should examine her breasts on the same day each month. Breasts are normally lumpy and so each woman will need to become used to how they

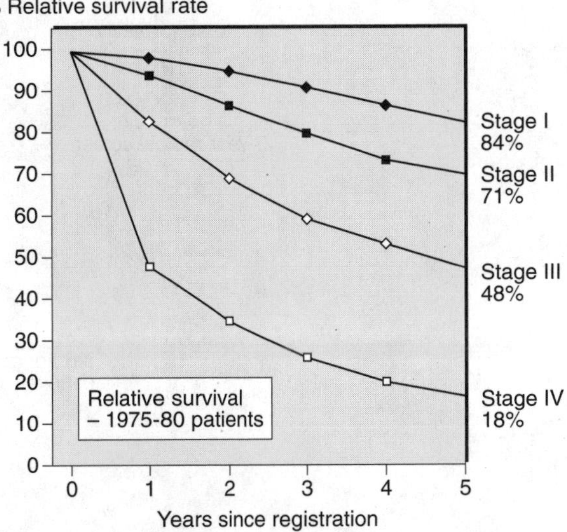

Fig. 7.15 Relative survival percentages for women with breast cancer. Statistics indicate that around 64% of British women diagnosed with breast cancer will be alive 5 years later. However, it should be remembered that breast cancer is frequently a slow-growing disease which may recur locally or in distant metastases anything up to 20 years later.

feel, and to identify her ribs, which are often mistaken for lumps.

To carry out self-examination the woman should sit in front of a mirror and lift her arms above her head, noticing the shape and size of her breasts and any changes from the previous month. She should examine her skin for dimpling and the nipple for discharge, crusting and any inversion.

Lying flat on a bed with one arm behind her head, she should then examine every area of her breast using the flat of her fingers of the opposite hand. Breast tissue is very extensive, running from the clavicle to the costal margin and the sternum to the axilla; breast examination should therefore cover all these areas systematically. Usually a hollow is noticed beneath each nipple. The upper outer quadrant of each breast will feel firmer as there is much breast tissue located there.

The axilla should be examined by bringing the arm back almost to her side and using the fingers of the opposite hand to feel deep into the armpit. If any lumps, thickening or other changes are noticed the woman should contact her GP immediately for an examination and advice.

Leaflets are very useful in teaching breast self-examination, but are not as effective as demonstrative teaching. Leaflets and videos can be obtained from several sources (see Useful Addresses, p. 290).

Breast cancer screening

In 1986 the Forrest Report (DHSS 1986) recommended the introduction of a National Breast Screening programme. Screening units are now in operation around the country, inviting women between 50 and 64 years to attend for screening using mammography, i.e. X-ray examination of the breast.

The aim of breast cancer screening by means of mammography is to detect breast cancer at an earlier stage than is possible by clinical examination or breast self-examination, i.e. before a lump is palpable in the breast. In particular, it is hoped that more women will be detected with pre-invasive (in situ) cancer before the cancer cells have shown any evidence of spreading. Some studies have suggested that screening using mammography can reduce breast cancer mortality by 30% in women over the age of 50 years (Shapiro et al 1982, Tabar et al 1985).

With good technique and reading, mammography will pick up 85–90% of all breast cancers in the breasts examined. It is most effective in postmenopausal women in whom breast tissue has been largely replaced by fat. For young women, in whom breast tissue is more dense and detection of abnormalities therefore more difficult, mammography is frequently used in conjunction with breast ultrasound.

The success of the national screening programme will depend on a high uptake of the service. The Tabar et al (1985) study in Sweden had an uptake rate of 70%; this will have to be matched in the UK if the hoped-for 30% reduction in mortality is to be achieved. Poor attendance at screening units may result from various factors, such as Family Practitioner Committee registers not being up to date, fears of discomfort or radiation, or a lack of understanding of the value of mammography.

Procedures. Screening may take place in static or in mobile units. The screening itself is by single oblique-view mammogram repeated every 3 years. The woman is notified by letter of the mammogram result. If an abnormality is detected, the letter will ask her to attend for re-screening at an assessment centre (see Fig. 7.16). Here, a 2-view mammogram (lateral and oblique) may show the detected lesion to be merely an overlapping of normal structures or a benign lesion requiring no

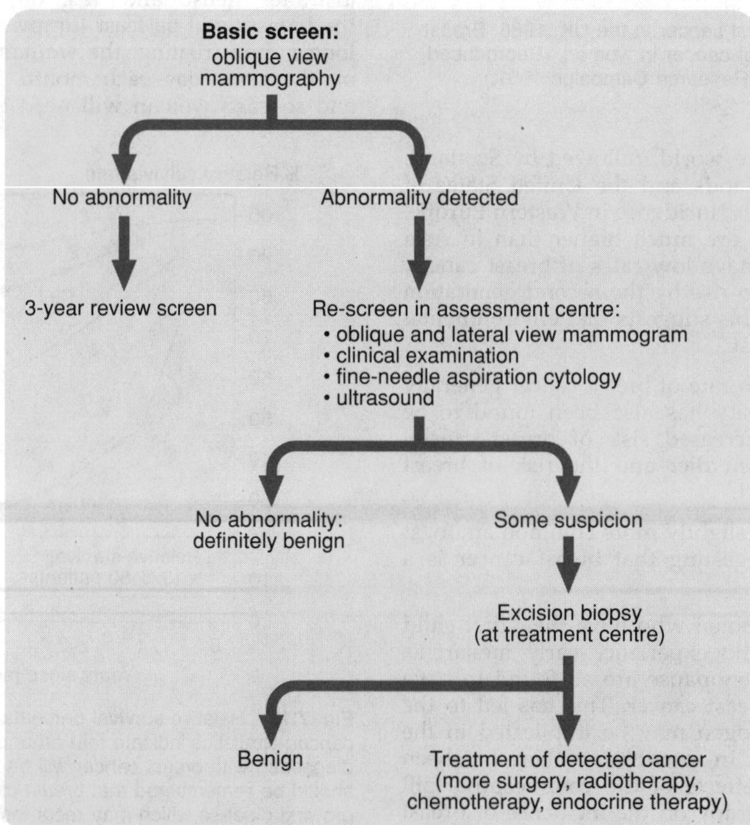

Fig. 7.16 Flow diagram of breast cancer screening procedure.

intervention. However, in some instances further assessment using fine-needle aspiration cytology or ultrasound will be indicated.

Psychological considerations. Most women who present for breast screening are asymptomatic, apparently healthy people, who, on the whole, come to be reassured that all is well. Inevitably, however, screening reminds the individual that breast cancer is a potential threat. It is therefore important that within the screening programme efforts are made to reduce anxiety where possible. It is particularly important that results are sent quickly. If the first screening is a positive experience the woman will be more likely to attend 3 years later, and may urge her friends to do the same.

Some screening units are considering the benefit of using 2-view mammography to increase the accuracy of the films and reduce the numbers of false positives (i.e. normal structures appearing as abnormalities), and thus reduce the needless anxiety caused by unnecessary recall letters.

The nurse's role. The Forrest report (DHSS 1986) recommended that trained nurses should be available to support women who are undergoing screening, and stressed particularly the role of specialist nurses with an in-depth knowledge of breast disease and its treatment and some training in counselling in supporting women recalled to assessment centres following the detection of an apparent abnormality.

However, all nurses have a role in health education and should take every appropriate opportunity to raise women's awareness of the availability and benefits of screening programmes. Community nurses in particular can encourage women to attend for screening, and can answer queries or discuss worries about breast screening as part of their general health promotion on an individual basis, or through group discussion, e.g. in Well Woman clinics.

PATHOPHYSIOLOGY

Common presenting symptoms (see Table 7.3). Discovery of a non-tender, hard, usually irregular lump or thickening in the breast is the most common presentation of breast cancer. Increasingly, it is also diagnosed after a mass or microcalcifications are seen on a mammogram during routine breast screening.

Table 7.3 Signs and symptoms of breast cancer

Sign/symptom	Comment
Breast lump	Usually hard and irregular
Change in breast size or shape	
Impalpable mammographic abnormality	Mass/microcalcifications
Pain	Sometimes
Skin dimpling	Retraction of Cooper ligaments
Peau d'orange	Thickening and oedema of skin
Nipple discharge	Usually blood-stained
Nipple retraction	Due to disease in main ducts
Nipple crusting	Usually Paget's disease of nipple
Dilation of superficial veins	Result of partial obstruction of veins by tumour
Palpable axillary lymph nodes	Usually in advanced cancer
Ulceration of skin	Usually in advanced cancer

Pain is not usually a presenting feature, but sometimes a sharp, pricking pain is the first symptom experienced. McKinna (1983) found 20% of women with breast cancer had some breast discomfort on presentation. A change in breast size or shape may be noticed. Signs of inflammation and tissue oedema may also be present, and superficial veins may dilate and become more visible if partially obstructed by a tumour. If the tumour is advanced at the time of presentation, it may be fixed to the muscles beneath the breast. There may also be large palpable axillary lymph nodes, or ulceration of the tumour through the skin causing an infected, weeping, malodorous wound. Oedema of the arm will result if the cancer in the axilla is blocking the drainage of blood and lymph from the arm.

Histology. Breast cancers may be classified according to the type of tissue from which they arise and their appearance under the microscope. The histological type of a cancer is often relevant to the choice of treatment.

Carcinomas arising from the epithelial cells of ducts are known as ductal carcinomas, and account for approximately 70–75% of all breast cancers. Comedo, medullary, colloidal and tubular carcinomas are all types of breast cancers arising from ductal tissue. They more often arise in one area of the breast but can be multifocal; they are rarely bilateral. Cancers arising from cells of the breast lobules are known as lobular carcinomas. These account for around 15% of breast cancers and are more commonly multifocal and bilateral than are ductal carcinomas.

In Paget's disease of the nipple malignant cells are found in the epidermis of the nipple and are usually associated with small multifocal areas of ductal cancer behind the nipple and deep in the breast. Other breast cancer types such as squamous cell or inflammatory carcinomas are less common. Sarcomas and lymphomas may also arise in the breast and, rarely, secondary cancer tumours.

Breast cancers may also be classified as non-invasive (located only in the ducts or lobules, i.e. 'in situ') or invasive (having spread into surrounding fatty or connective tissue). This distinction has a bearing on prognosis and treatment. Ductal carcinoma in situ represents a very early stage of breast cancer which is often seen as microcalcifications on a mammogram. It cannot be predicted when, or if, non-invasive breast cancer will become invasive.

Cellular differentiation, i.e. the degree to which cancer cells resemble their tissue of origin, is another important histological factor in determining prognosis. Cells are described as poorly, moderately, or well differentiated. Poorly differentiated cancers tend to be more aggressive, to metastasise at an earlier stage (see p. 276) and hence to carry a worse prognosis.

More detailed information on the histology of breast cancers is given in Page & Anderson (1981).

MEDICAL MANAGEMENT

Investigative procedures. Once a breast abnormality has been detected, further diagnostic investigation will be carried out following referral to a specialist. This may involve:

- clinical examination of the breast
- mammography (see p. 268)
- ultrasound to distinguish solid from cystic lesions
- fine-needle aspiration to drain cysts and to obtain samples for cytological study
- biopsy.

Fine-needle aspiration cytology of the breast. In this procedure a syringe with a small-bore needle is inserted into the breast mass and suction is applied. The contents are withdrawn, placed on a slide, and sent to the laboratory for cytological studies. Where a mass is found to be a cyst and a large amount of fluid is aspirated it is usually discarded, unless it is found to be blood-stained, in which case a sample will be sent for examination.

Cytological results will be graded C0–C5. C0 represents an insufficient specimen, C1 and C2 benign cells, C3 and C4 suspicious of carcinoma and C5 carcinoma. Fine-needle aspiration cytology is a useful diagnostic tool but is not conclusive on its own. A benign result may simply indicate that the needle missed the target; where other signs are suspicious a biopsy will still be recommended.

Biopsy. On the basis of the investigations listed above a decision is made as to whether a biopsy should be performed to confirm diagnosis. Biopsy may be of the following types:

1. Trucut biopsy: removal of a core of tissue using a special large-bore needle. Often undertaken in the outpatient department with a local anaesthetic
2. Excision biopsy: excision of the lump excised in its entirety, usually with general anaesthesia, requiring a one- or two-day hospital stay
3. Localisation biopsy: where a mammographic abnormality has been detected but there is no associated palpable mass, a wire may be inserted into the abnormal area under X-ray or ultrasound control. This ensures that the surgeon removes the right area, which will be X-rayed again once removed from the body.

Medical intervention. The choice of treatment in breast cancer will depend on several factors, including:

- the size, position and type of the tumour (see Box 7.14)
- the spread of the disease
- the woman's general health
- the woman's priorities and wishes.

Surgical intervention. Surgery is still considered to be the most effective treatment for early breast cancer. Formerly, radical mastectomy was the treatment of choice, but for many women less extensive surgery followed by radiotherapy can be just as successful (Veronesi et al 1981, Fisher et al 1989, Veronesi et al 1990).

Surgical procedures that may be used are as follows:

1. Lumpectomy. Removal of the breast lump with very little surrounding tissue. May be equivalent to an excision biopsy.
2. Wide local excision. Removal of the abnormal areas together with a 1–2 cm margin of apparently normal tissue to reduce the possibility of incompletely excising the cancer. When the pathologist indicates that excision may be incomplete, re-excision is usually recommended. The amount of tissue removed in this operation can be considerable.
3. Partial or segmental mastectomy or quadrantectomy. Removal of a portion of the breast. Invariably the breast is left smaller and its contour changed.
4. Radical or Halsted's mastectomy. This is rarely used today and involves the removal of the pectoralis major and minor muscles, as well as the breast tissue and overlying skin, the nipple and the axillary lymph nodes. A long, oblique scar remains. The axillary skin fold is usually removed and the chest wall can sometimes appear concave, with the ribs prominent.
5. Modified radical or Patey mastectomy. Removal of all the breast tissue, overlying skin and the nipple. The pectoralis major and minor remain, covering the ribs, and the axillary skin fold remains intact. The scar is oblique but less extensive than with a radical mastectomy.
6. Simple mastectomy. Removal of the breast tissue and overlying skin and nipple; all muscles are left intact and the scar is horizontal.
7. Axillary dissection. Usually performed with any of the above operations to determine whether the cancer has spread to the lymph glands. The presence of cancer in these glands indicates that micrometastatic spread is likely and hence adjuvant drug therapy is indicated. Where possible, axillary dissection removing some or all of the lymph glands will be undertaken through the same incision as that made for the breast surgery.

Box 7.14 Staging of breast cancer tumours

Stage I	Tumour <2 cm, not fixed, no axillary node involvement
Stage II	Tumour <5 cm, with/without axillary node involvement
Stage IIIa	Tumour >5 cm or fixed axillary node involvement
Stage IIIb	Any tumour with supraclavicular node involvement, fixation to the chest wall, inflammation, ulceration
Stage IV	Any size tumour and presence of distant metastatic disease

If a woman presents with a large breast cancer, the only safe surgical option will be a mastectomy. Some doctors may offer an alternative of taking drug treatment to try to shrink the tumour. When the maximum response to the drug seems to have been achieved radiotherapy may be given. If any tumour remains, limited surgery may then be performed to remove it. This provides a further option for women who cannot tolerate the thought of a mastectomy, or for those whose health precludes an operation.

Radiotherapy. This form of treatment is usually advised following a wide local excision or partial mastectomy to reduce the risk of cancer recurrence in the remaining tissue. If axillary lymph nodes are not all removed and are found to contain cancer they are also commonly irradiated. The supraclavicular region may in some cases also be irradiated. Radiotherapy is not usually considered necessary following a mastectomy.

A total of 50–60 Gy of external radiotherapy is usually given to the breast over a period of 5–6 weeks 3–5 times a week. The radiotherapy is given at different angles to protect the delicate lung tissue from receiving high doses of radiation. The only common side-effects are redness and soreness of the treated area, and a general tiredness towards the end of the treatment period.

Alternatively, radiotherapy may be administered wholly or partly by iridium wire implants. The patient must be isolated for around 5 days until the radioactive wires are removed. The main advantage of this method is its ability to deliver high doses of radiotherapy to the area from which the tumour was removed. Radiotherapy is discussed in more detail in Chapter 32.

Chemotherapy. When breast cancer is present in the axillary lymph nodes the chance of a woman developing distant metastases is high. Systemic drug therapies circulating to all areas of the body have been shown to reduce the chance of metastases developing, and so to increase the length of time before metastases become apparent.

Premenopausal women who have positive axillary lymph nodes are likely to benefit from cytotoxic chemotherapy. Two commonly used regimes are CMF (cyclophosphamide, methotrexate, 5-fluouracil) and MMM (mitozantrone, methotrexate, Mitomycin C). Six courses over a period of 6 months are usually given requiring attendance at the outpatient department twice a month.

Administration is by slow i.v. injection, but cyclophosphamide may be given as tablets for 14 days. More detailed information on chemotherapy and its management is given in Chapter 32. The common side-effects of chemotherapy in breast cancer are listed in Table 7.6.

Endocrine therapies. Many breast cancers are thought to be stimulated by female sex hormones, particularly oestrogen. Endocrine therapies act by interfering with the synthesis of oestrogen or preventing it from exerting an effect on cells.

The drug tamoxifen, which competes with oestrogen receptors in the cytoplasm of the cell and so blocks oestrogen from stimulating cancer cell growth, has been found to be effective in many women with breast cancer but generally is more effective in women who are postmenopausal and have high levels of oestrogen receptors. Because of its low toxicity, it is given to all postmenopausal women as an adjuvant therapy, regardless of cancer involvement in the lymph nodes.

Its use in preventing breast cancer in women with a strong family history of breast cancer is also being evaluated.

Premenopausal women whose axillary lymph glands are free of cancer have traditionally not received adjuvant drug therapy. However, some doctors are now advising adjuvant chemotherapy or endocrine therapy, as recent studies have indicated that these might have a preventive effect for some women (Early Breast Cancer Trialists' Collaborative Group 1988). Luteinising hormone releasing hormone (LHRH) inhibitors are also being evaluated at present and may offer less toxic adjuvant endocrine therapies for premenopausal women in the future.

?	**7.7** When is a woman likely to be advised that a mastectomy would be the best treatment for her?

NURSING PRIORITIES AND MANAGEMENT: BREAST CANCER

The pre-treatment phase

The period prior to admission to hospital is usually characterised by anxiety and uncertainty. Diagnosis often cannot be confirmed before biopsy and so the patient's hope that everything will be all right will be mixed with fears of cancer and its treatment. Nursing intervention at this time will focus on assessing the patient's situation, helping her to cope with anxiety, providing education and psychological support and assisting her in making informed choices with regard to treatment options.

Assessment

There may be limited time available for assessment at this stage, but where possible the nurse should try to identify the following:

- the woman's reaction, and that of her family, to the diagnosis or potential diagnosis of breast cancer
- the major fears and concerns of the woman and her family
- the woman's feelings about body image changes that may result from any proposed surgery.
- The woman's knowledge of breast cancer and cancer generally; how much information she has been given by medical staff; how much she has understood; and how much she wants to know.
- The kind and degree of support available to the woman through family and friends. Northouse (1989) found that patients and their partners who reported high levels of social support also reported fewer adjustment difficulties after surgery. Husbands consistently reported that they received less support than their wives from friends, nurses and doctors.
- Concurrent stressors e.g. recent bereavements, divorce, financial difficulties.
- Previous anxiety / depression. Morris (1977) found that such women are more likely to re-experience anxiety / depression following diagnosis and treatment.

The treatment phase

Assessment

On the patient's admission to hospital the nurse should undertake a more comprehensive assessment including medical history, family history and a full physical and psychological assessment. In particular the factors relevant in the pre-treatment phase should be reassessed to determine if the woman's needs and concerns have changed. Particular note should be made of preoperative shoulder function if axillary surgery is to be performed.

Preoperative preparation

The reader is referred to Chapter 27 for a detailed discussion of clinical consideration in preoperative care.

Giving psychological support

The nurse should give each patient the opportunity to discuss her fears, but must respect her wishes if she prefers not to disclose her feelings. Where possible a quiet, private room should be set aside for patients to spend some time in solitude, or to talk privately with a nurse, doctor or family member.

Relaxation tapes or gentle massage, particularly of the neck, shoulders, back or face can be comforting at a time when the patient may feel isolated and insecure. A relaxed but professional atmosphere on the ward will also help, as will allowing women to remain in their day clothes, open visiting and permitting patients to go out for meals or a walk.

Patient education

The nurse must ensure that the woman knows what operation she is to undergo and that she has been given as much information about this as she wishes. Where deficits exist the nurse should try to provide information or refer the woman back to the medical staff for further discussion.

The preoperative routine should be explained, including the approximate time of surgery and the timing and type of premedication to be administered.

The patient should be told that she will have drainage tubes in situ on return from theatre (usually one to the breast and one to the axilla to prevent the collection of blood and serous fluid beneath the suture line). She should know that she can pick them up and walk around with them, and that it is difficult to dislodge them as they are sutured in place.

Anyone undergoing axillary dissection should be warned that she will experience discomfort on moving her arm postoperatively for a few weeks. The nurse should stress the importance of postoperative exercises and, where possible, should refer the patient to a physiotherapist who can assess shoulder function preoperatively and teach exercises that can be used following surgery.

The possibility of a saline or blood i.v. infusion should also be explained so that the patient does not become alarmed at finding one in place.

Patients often find it helpful to be told of the expected appearance of the surgical scar. Wound size and position, and the type of suturing to be used can be mentioned. Drawings and photographs may be helpful aids. It is important to warn the patient that because the breast is so vascular, bruising and swelling are expected postoperatively; she should be reminded of this when she first looks at the scar.

Postoperative care

The nursing care of patients following surgical intervention is discussed in detail in Chapter 27. The following discussion will focus on considerations particularly relevant to breast surgery. The reader is also referred to Nursing Care Plan 7.2.

Wound management (see also Ch. 23). The size and position of the wound will depend on the operation performed. Generally, a low-suction drain is placed beneath the breast wound and another to the axillary region to reduce the likelihood of haematoma or seroma. The drains and the wound dressing should initially be frequently observed for signs of excessive blood loss; undue blood loss should be reported to medical staff immediately.

The wound drains will remain in situ 2–5 days until the wound drainage is minimal. The nurse should ensure that the drains are suctioned and patent and should record drainage

Nursing Care Plan 7.2 Care for a woman who has undergone a mastectomy

Nursing considerations	Action	Rationale	Expected outcome
1. Potential problem of wound complications (infection, haematoma, seroma) and delayed wound healing January 10	❒ Check drains half-hourly for blood loss. Change drainage bottles daily and record volume of drainage	Haemorrhage may occur, compromising patient's health, and may necessitate return to theatre	Prevention of infection where possible and early detection of problems and promotion of wound healing
	❒ Observe wound for signs of infection (erythema, oedema, heat, pain, discharge)	Infection may delay wound healing and compromise general health. Medical treatment may be needed to control infection	There will be no signs of infection or bleeding
	❒ 4-hourly temperature and pulse	Increased temperature and pulse may indicate infection	
	❒ Aseptic dressing change only when absolutely necessary	Wound will heal more quickly if undisturbed, providing drainage is not excessive and there is no infection	
	❒ Assess nutritional intake and encourage balanced diet with plenty of vitamin C and protein	Vitamin C and protein are particularly important in wound healing	Patient will eat a balanced diet while in hospital
	❒ Assess amount of sleep and rest patient has had postoperatively. Where inadequate consider anxiety reduction, pain control, night sedation to promote rest	Adequate sleep and rest are important in promoting wound healing	She will have at least 6 hours' sleep each night and report feeling stronger each day

Evaluation

January 11
Returned from theatre 12.30 h. All vital signs stable, now checked 4-hourly. Wound drainage 40 ml in last 4 h. Wound covered by Tegaderm dressing

January 12
Slight pyrexia of 37.4°C, but no other sign of infection. Wound discharge was 100 ml in 24 h. (Axilla 60 ml/breast 40 ml.) Not sleeping well at night but managed to sleep a little today and does not wish for night sedation to be given.

January 13
Apyrexial and wound drainage reduced to 40 ml in 24 h. Slept better last night.

January 14
Both wound drains removed today and wound dressing replaced. Wound is moist close to axilla and has oozed a little serous fluid but temperature remains normal.

January 15
Wound still a little moist close to axilla. Going home today so discussed signs of infection and advised visit to GP if they occur. Also advised that a seroma could form in axilla and to contact ward if this happens and arrange for an aspiration. Patient stated that she was worried about anything happening to her wound but particularly that it would open up but said she was reassured following our discussion.

DISCHARGED

Nursing considerations	Action	Rationale	Expected outcome
2. Anxiety/distress due to altered body image as a result of mastectomy and diagnosis of cancer (Salter 1988)	❒ Give patient time and opportunity to express and explore feelings concerning cancer diagnosis and breast loss	Expression of feelings may help patient to clarify how she feels and relieve anxiety	Some anxiety will be alleviated
12 January	❒ Encourage patient to discuss feelings with partner where appropriate	Partner may then be more easily able to understand and support and give reassurance that she is still attractive	Patient will have more acceptance of changed body image
	❒ Give information about scarring, e.g. bruising, sutures, position (photos shown pre-op may help)	May help to have realistic expectations of wound and know that bruising etc. will fade	

Nursing Care Plan 7.2 *(cont'd)*

Nursing considerations	Action	Rationale	Expected outcome
	❒ Offer to remain with patient when she first looks at wound, assess reaction and give support in discussing feelings afterwards	Moral support may help patient to sum up courage to look at the wound	Patient will be able to look at scar before discharge
	❒ Fit temporary prosthesis after removal of the drains and show how to use. Show silicone prosthesis if desired and make fitting appointment	A prosthesis may increase a woman's confidence to face the outside world and regain a healthy body image	Patient will be able to fit temporary prosthesis into bra before discharge
	❒ Discuss possibility of breast reconstruction if not previously mentioned	Breast reconstruction is known to be helpful for some women in coping with breast loss. Woman herself is best one to judge value for her	Patient will understand types of reconstruction possible
	❒ Refer to specialist nurse if one exists	Specialist nurses have been shown to aid rehabilitation and may lower anxiety and depression postoperatively	
	❒ Offer written information on breast cancer, prostheses, clothing, etc.	Practical help may increase a woman's confidence to take up her usual social activities and feel she is still the same as ever	
	❒ Ask if she would like voluntary visitor to be put in touch and arrange if desired	Some women find others who have had similar operations a great help and encouragement	

Evaluation

January

Stated that she is very frightened that cancer may recur in the future. Her friend died 2 years ago from breast cancer metastases and this fills her with fear.

Temporary prosthesis fitted today and appointment made for 6 weeks after the wound drains removed. Mrs X also looked at her scar for the first time. She found it was better than she imagined. She has asked that the nurse stay with her tomorrow whilst she shows her husband before she goes home.

Mrs X showed her husband the scar today. He also told her it was much better than he had imagined and that having her was much more important than her having two breasts. Breast reconstruction was mentioned again but Mrs X is sure she will not want this. To be followed up by clinical nurse specialist who saw her again today and gave her a booklet from the Breast Care and Mastectomy Association.

Nursing considerations	Action	Rationale	Expected outcome
3. Difficulty moving arm due to discomfort following axillary dissection 11 January	❒ Refer to physiotherapist ❒ Analgesia before physiotherapy ❒ Encourage to practice arm exercises 4 x day	Shoulder exercises are known to reduce the problems of reduced shoulder functioning that can result after an axillary dissection	To achieve and maintain full shoulder movement in 4 weeks and prevent 'frozen shoulder'.
	❒ Give written information sheets to reinforce what exercises to do and when	Written information will reinforce that given verbally and serve as a reminder after discharge home from hospital	Will be able to demonstrate physiotherapy exercises and perform 4 x each day
4. Pain 10 January	❒ Regular analgesics initially post-op. Assess effectiveness. Particularly important prior to physiotherapy	Regular analgesics more likely to be effective than PRN medication	Patient will report that pain is under control
	❒ Use pillow to support arm on affected side post-op	Pillow provides a soft, comfortable support and encourages drainage of fluid back from arm	
	❒ Consider relaxation techniques and massage to relieve tension	Tension is known to increase experience of pain	

Nursing Care Plan 7.2 *(cont'd)*

Evaluation

January 14
Seen by physiotherapist and commenced exercises. Patient says that she is able to move arm quite freely without much discomfort.

January 15
Has been practising arm exercises but a little more uncomfortable today and requested paracetamol prior to exercises this afternoon. She said this helped.

January 10
Omnopan had been given in recovery but Mrs X has declined any further analgesia since returning to the ward.

January 11
Particularly uncomfortable when moving her arm. Had declined analgesia this morning but was persuaded that regular paracetamol for 2 or 3 days will not harm her but will help her move her arm, which is important.

January 14
Much more comfortable today and has again refused analgesia.

January 15
Requested analgesia prior to exercises today as arm feeling stiff and sore.

Nursing considerations	Action	Rationale	Expected outcome
5. Potential problem of lymphoedema of the arm, postoperatively or at some time in the future January 11	❒ Explain what lymphoedema is, how it is caused and when it may occur ❒ Explain signs of lymphoedema and encourage to report to doctor as soon as it occurs	Information will help the patient to understand the pathological basis of lymphoedema and encourage early detection of lymphoedema should it occur	Risk of lymphoedema occurring will be reduced The patient will understand what lymphoedema is, and what to do if it occurs
	❒ Discuss hand and arm care:		She will be able to recount how to look after her hand and arm.
	• avoid lifting heavy objects with affected arm • avoid injections, blood tests, blood pressure recordings in affected arm • use gardening gloves when gardening, kitchen gloves with abrasive cleaners, thimbles when sewing • clean any cut on hand or arm very thoroughly and apply antiseptic. If any signs of infection appear see GP for antibiotics • use depilatory creams to remove hair under arm, rather than a razor • Elevate arm whenever possible, particularly initially after surgery • Use a gentle moisturising cream on arm if skin is dry to prevent cracking	Following removal of or obliteration of lymph nodes by surgery or radiotherapy, there is an increased risk of infection in the arm. These precautions reduce the risk of infection, and also the risk of infection precipitating lymphoedema	
	❒ Encourage arm and shoulder exercises	Exercise is thought to reduce the possibility of lymphoedema occurring	

Evaluation

January 14
Long discussion in preparation for discharge. Her friend had lymphoedema so she is very concerned this shouldn't happen to her. Very keen to have advice on hand and arm care and given leaflet about this. Stressed that she can contact clinical nurse specialist at any time if she is concerned that her arm is swollen.

volume. Removal of the drains can be uncomfortable and should be preceded by oral analgesia.

The wound should also be observed for signs of infection, i.e. redness, swelling, pain, and discharge. Temperature and pulse should be monitored 4-hourly and a raised temperature brought to the attention of the medical staff.

Wound dressings should be changed only if wound exudate is saturating the dressing. Unnecessary dressing changes reduce the rate of wound healing and increase the risk of infection. Frequently a transparent wound dressing (which allows for ready observation of signs of infection) may be left in situ until the sutures are removed from the wound at 10–14 days.

The nurse must also consider other factors such as nutritional intake, medication, stress, and concurrent illness such as diabetes which affect the rate of wound healing and resistance to infection (see Ch. 23).

Alleviating discomfort. Pain from the wound will always be experienced to some degree, but frequently pain on shoulder movement is more of a problem. Pain is sometimes more intense a day or so after the operation, when the initial numbness has faded. Every patient should be encouraged to take analgesics regularly for the first 48 h but many women find that the wound is less painful than they had expected and require oral analgesics infrequently beyond this period. It should be stressed, in any event, that it is preferable to have analgesics and continue arm exercises than to avoid the exercises and take no analgesics.

The experience of pain is affected by many factors such as anxiety and emotional distress (see Ch. 19); these must be considered by the nurse in her efforts to promote the patient's comfort after surgery. Massage may by reducing muscle tension help to reduce pain; at the same time, the use of touch may promote a feeling of self-acceptance within a woman who feels vulnerable after losing her breast.

Women who have had a mastectomy may experience phantom breast and nipple sensations at some point following surgery. This may be very distressing and requires the nurse to reassure her that this will not continue for long.

Promotion of shoulder movement. Women who have undergone surgery involving dissection of the axillary lymph nodes are at risk of developing problems with shoulder movement. This risk is greater if radiotherapy to the axilla is also given (Atkins et al 1972). Postoperative exercises will help to ensure that a full range of shoulder movement is attained within 4 weeks following surgery.

Ideally, exercises should be taught by a physiotherapist. The nurse must know what they involve, however, so that she can encourage the patient to practise them. Written information is very helpful to remind the patient of what exercises should be performed and how often. Generally, gentle exercises are begun on the second or third postoperative day and gradually increased in extent and frequency as drainage from the wound diminishes.

Preparing the patient for discharge

Looking at a mastectomy scar for the first time is often very difficult and may confirm a woman's fears about breast loss and intensify her grief. However, others find the scar neater and less distressing than imagined. Women who have lumpectomies may have a similar range of reactions.

The nurse should encourage a woman to look at her scar before she goes home, as this represents a significant step in rehabilitation. The patient must never be forced to do so, however.

Rehabilitation proceeds at different rates, but the nurse should warn each woman that it may take several months before she feels that her energy has returned to normal. Persistent fatigue may cause frustration and may give rise to anxiety that the cancer has returned. Fatigue is more likely if chemotherapy or radiotherapy are to be given postoperatively, but where it is profound, depression should also be considered as a possible contributing factor.

Most women can begin driving again in 2–3 weeks, providing they feel confident and their arm movement is not too uncomfortable. Light household duties can be undertaken when the woman feels well enough, usually 2–3 weeks postoperatively, and return to work at around 6 weeks. This will of course depend on the extent of the surgery and on the type of work.

Pain and discomfort from the wound will steadily reduce, but some discomfort often remains for 2–3 months. Paraesthesia around the scar and axilla may fade over several months, but some may always remain.

Swelling of the breast tissue or axilla following surgery will also occur, and may take 2–3 months to fully resolve. Some women believe that the large lump they can feel is cancer that has suddenly grown after surgery. Prior explanation of this and the possibility of seroma formation is likely to reduce any anxiety.

Lymphoedema is a possible long-term complication that can occur in anyone who has axillary surgery or radiotherapy. The women should be advised to contact their GP or hospital if they notice any swelling, and not to leave it until it becomes a problem. Lymphoedema following breast surgery is discussed on pages 280–282.

Prior to discharge any woman who has had a mastectomy or a large lumpectomy should be given a temporary prosthesis, shown how to position it in her bra and alter its shape, and should be told how to wash it (see Box 7.15).

?	**7.8** Simpson's (1985) survey of prosthetic services suggested that in many areas these were inadequate and did not meet the needs of women with breast cancer. What services are available in your area? Are they adequate, in your view?
?	**7.9** Prepare a 10-minute teaching session for your ward colleagues or fellow students on the subject of breast prostheses. Include what types are available and why they are important for the patient.

Adjuvant therapy

Information on adjuvant radiotherapy and drug therapies should be given as relevant in verbal and written form. The patient should understand why adjuvant treatment has been advised, for what period and at what intervals it will be administered, and what the side-effects may be.

Radiotherapy. The common side-effects of adjuvant radiotherapy in breast cancer are listed in Table 7.4. The nurse should also give advice on skin care for women undergoing radiotherapy.

Chemotherapy. The patient should be reassured that the CMF and MMM chemotherapy regimes used in breast cancer (see p. 270) tend to have milder side-effects than those used in the treatment of other cancers and can therefore usually be managed through the outpatient department.

Nausea is commonly experienced but is normally mild and can be controlled by antiemetics. Vomiting is rare. Complete alopecia is also rare, although the hair may thin and become drier and of poorer quality. Gentle shampoos should be used, and perms and the use of heated rollers and tongs should be avoided.

Box 7.15 Breast prostheses

The fitting of a breast prosthesis is an integral part of the rehabilitation of a woman who has had a mastectomy or partial mastectomy. The aim of the prosthesis is to match as closely as possible the woman's other breast in terms of size, shape, weight and feel, so that she may look normal and feel confident in clothing. This is important in helping her to resume her normal social activities and regain a healthy body image.

TEMPORARY PROSTHESES

A temporary prosthesis is fitted as soon as the wound drains have been removed and is worn until a permanent prosthesis can be fitted. It is soft, light and washable, and can be pinned securely into the cup of a bra. If a bra cannot be worn because of discomfort, the prosthesis can be pinned into a camisole or slip. The woman may find that wearing loose clothing helps to achieve an even appearance. However, it is important that the nurse spends time fitting this prosthesis well, as it is with this that the woman will first face the outside world again.

PERMANENT PROSTHESES

A permanent prosthesis is usually fitted 5 weeks after surgery or 2 weeks after the completion of radiotherapy, when the wound is well healed. Every woman should be given a fitting appointment prior to leaving hospital. The fitting may be undertaken by a specialist nurse, surgical appliance officer, or visiting prosthesis company fitter. A private room with a full-length mirror is necessary and it is essential that each woman is treated with respect and sensitivity.

Today most permanent prostheses are made of silicone gel which feels soft and comfortable next to the skin and takes on the body's temperature. Many shapes and sizes are available; it should be possible for all women to be fitted with a prosthesis that gives a balanced appearance in a bra. Partial prostheses are available for women who have breast conservation. Silicone prostheses last for 2–3 years generally but a woman is entitled to a replacement whenever it begins to show signs of wear and tear, or if she loses or gains weight or changes shape.

Special 'mastectomy bras' are not necessary, but the bra does need to be supportive and of the correct cup size, covering all of the tissue of the remaining breast. It is helpful if the nurse can give basic advice about bras and instruct a woman where she may be fitted for a bra locally, if her previous bras are now inappropriate. Volunteer organisations such as the Breast Care Mastectomy Association give helpful advice about bras, swimwear and other clothing (see Useful Addresses, p. 290).

Bone marrow depression occurs with all cytotoxic drugs but it is rare for neutropenia to be severe or for septicaemia to result. Nevertheless, every patient should be advised about good oral hygiene and the avoidance of obvious sources of infection.

Fatigue is the most common problem. Generally it is worst in the middle of a month's cycle, when blood counts are at their lowest level.

Menstruation is usually affected, with periods becoming irregular or stopping. Menopausal symptoms, e.g. hot flushes, may be experienced, but if the woman is in her early 30s, menstruation has a 90% chance of returning after chemotherapy finishes. Women in their early 40s are much more likely to go into early menopause.

Endocrine therapy. Adjuvant tamoxifen is very widely given in view of its relatively few side-effects and its proven efficacy. However, premenopausal women will usually experience menopausal symptoms. Gastric upsets are uncommon but may occur, particularly if the tamoxifen tablets are not taken with food. Very occasionally thrombocytopenia is a problem; the individual should be advised to report increased bruising.

Many women complain about an increase in weight, particularly around the abdomen, soon after starting the tablets. This may be due in part to fluid retention and in part to a reduction in physical activity following surgery.

Table 7.4 Possible side-effects of adjuvant radiotherapy used in the treatment of breast cancer

Side-effect	Comment
Redness and soreness of the area treated	More common in fair-skinned people
General tiredness	Especially toward the end of the 6-week treatment period
Photosensitivity	See Ch. 12; sun barrier creams should be worn for a year after therapy
Moist desquamation	Now rare because of the fractionation of radiotherapy
Nausea	Rare; radiotherapy affects only the area to which it is administered
Breast becomes firmer to the touch	Long-term effect due to fibrosis of tissue
Narrowing or blockage of lymph vessels	Increases risk of lymphoedema

METASTATIC BREAST CANCER

Metastatic disease is sometimes obvious at the time of diagnosis but more commonly occurs months or many years later. Women in whom axillary lymph nodes are involved at the time of diagnosis are known to be at a high risk of developing metastases at a later date. The rate at which breast cancer grows and metastasises to other areas of the body varies. It is therefore difficult to assess the long-term prognosis of an individual woman, or to say if, and when, she is cured of the disease. It is estimated that two-thirds of women who present with a breast lump already have metastatic spread. Often this is in the form of micrometastases which are too small to be detected by scans or other investigations. However, distant micrometastases are more likely to be present if the axillary lymph nodes are found to contain cancer at the time of diagnosis. The prognosis is better if axillary lymph nodes are tumour-free at the time of treatment.

PATHOPHYSIOLOGY

Spread of breast cancer is by direct invasion into the surrounding tissue, and via the lymphatic and arteriovenous systems to distant areas. If untreated, local invasion will cause ulceration, fixation to the chest wall, and oedema of the arm. It may also erode blood vessels, causing haemorrhage, and invade the ribs or lungs and pleura, causing pleural effusion. Invasion of the brachial plexus can cause severe pain with functional and sensory loss in the arm. Invasion of the cutaneous nerves causes irritation and burning pain in the affected area. Because such aggressive local disease is not necessarily accompanied by metastatic spread, a woman may survive for many years with these problems.

Table 7.5 Common problems caused by metastatic disease in patients with breast cancer

Site of disease	Problem	Treatment
Bone	Bone pain	Non-steroidal anti-inflammatory drugs, opiates, radiotherapy to site, chemotherapy
	Hypercalcaemia	Emergency: hydration, diphosphanates, chemotherapy
	Spinal cord compression	Emergency: chemotherapy, radiotherapy and steroids
Bone marrow	Pancytopenia	Supportive blood + platelet transfusions. Chemotherapy (may cause further problems)
Lung/pleura	Pleural effusion	Pleural aspiration +/– pleurodesis
	Reduced expansion/shortness of breath with persistent cough	Low-dose morphine, codeine suppressant. Chemotherapy/endocrine therapy
Liver	Liver pain	Opiates, steroids, chemotherapy
	Ascites	Paracentesis, chemotherapy
Skin	Ulceration/fungation Pain/irritation	Radiotherapy, chemotherapy, endocrine therapy, dressings, analgesia, Tegretol/flecamide. For nerve pain, steroids and anti-inflammatory drugs
Brain/CNS	Confusion, headaches, nausea, vomiting, altered behaviour, convulsions	Emergency: radiotherapy and steroids Intrathecal methotrexate
mediastinum	Superior vena cava obstruction	Emergency radiotherapy and steroids
Axilla/ supraclavicular fossa	Lymphoedema Brachial plexus pain and paraesthesia/ paralysis of arm	Chemotherapy, endocrine therapy, radiotherapy; Carbamazepine/Flecainide for nerve pain

Spread of breast cancer to distant sites is a common occurrence, but may not become apparent for months or many years after the initial diagnosis and treatment. Metastases can occur anywhere and do not follow a systematic course. However, metastatic spread may be first discernible in the axillary and then supraclavicular lymph nodes, following the pattern of lymphatic drainage from the breast. The most common sites of metastases are the bones, lungs, liver and brain. Less frequently, they occur in the ovaries and mediastinum and, rarely, in the stomach, oesophagus and intestine. The problems most commonly caused by metastasised breast cancer are listed in Table 7.5.

MEDICAL MANAGEMENT

Surgery rarely has a part to play in the management of metastatic breast cancer. Chemotherapy and endocrine therapy are the treatments of choice, given their systemic effectiveness. Radiotherapy plays an important role in the relief of bone pain and in the oncological emergencies of spinal cord compression, cerebral metastases and superior vena cava obstruction, where tumour pressure must be reduced quickly. In these contingencies, steroids are used in conjunction with radiotherapy to reduce the oedema in tissues surrounding the tumour and hence relieve pressure further.

The menopausal status of the patient, the site of the metastatic spread, and the apparent aggressiveness of the tumour will determine which drug therapies are considered most appropriate.

Chemotherapy. Disease which appears to be advancing rapidly or involves the liver is most likely to be treated by chemotherapy. The regimes CMF or MMM (see p. 270) are most commonly used if they have not previously been given as an adjuvant therapy. Side-effects are described in Table 7.6. Adriamycin or VAC (vincristine, Adriamycin and cyclophosphamide) are also quite commonly used but tend to have more toxic effects than CMF/MMM, with more nausea, vomiting, hair loss and bone marrow depression.

Endocrine therapy. Disease which is progressing more slowly may respond to endocrine therapies. These work more slowly but have fewer side-effects. Endocrine agents which may be used include:

1. Tamoxifen (see p. 270). This can be used in pre- and postmenopausal women.
2. Luteinising hormone releasing hormone (LHRH) analogues (e.g. Zoladex), which interfere with the production of luteinising hormone and thence oestrogen. Side-effects are the symptoms of menopause, e.g. amenorrhoea and hot flushes. These drugs are administered by i.m. injection every month.
3. Aminoglutethimide. This drug inhibits the synthesis of aromatase, an enzyme needed to convert androgens produced by the adrenal glands to oestrogen. It has the same effect as an adrenalectomy and hence hydrocortisone replacement must be given with it to prevent an Addisonian crisis (see Ch. 5, p. 149). Allergic rashes are common but usually resolve if treatment continues. This drug is given only to postmenopausal women. New aromatase inhibitors

Table 7.6 Common side-effects of chemotherapy regimes used in the treatment of metastatic breast cancer

Side-effect	Comment
Lethargy	All drugs to some degree, but especially Adriamycin, VAC (vincristine, Adriamycin, cyclophosphamide)
Anorexia/altered taste	Very rarely vomiting with CMF/MMM
Nausea + vomiting	More common with Adriamycin
Mouth ulceration	Particularly methotrexate
Diarrhoea	Rarely, but more commonly with 5-fluorouracil
Bone marrow depression	Greater where Adriamycin used
Alopecia	CMF/MMM: little. (Adriamycin: complete, but scalp cooling may reduce this)
Red urine	Adriamycin
Green urine	Mitozantrone
Reactivation of radiotherapy sites	Adriamycin
Nail pigmentation	Adriamycin

are being developed which eliminate the need for hydrocortisone replacement.

4. Provera. This is a progestogen drug usually used as a third-line treatment when others have failed. Side-effects include an increase in appetite and euphoria; this can be helpful if a patient is depressed, nauseated and has lost her appetite. At other times weight gain is a problem as well as fluid retention and the steroid 'moon face'.

NURSING PRIORITIES AND MANAGEMENT: METASTATIC BREAST CANCER

Major nursing considerations

Assessment

Nursing assessment should address the physical, psychological and social impact of the disease, with particular consideration of the patient's own perception of these problems. The difficulties faced by the patient are likely to be determined in part by the site or sites to which the breast cancer has spread, but it should be remembered that medical priorities will not necessarily match the personal priorities of the patient.

The reaction of the patient and her family to the news of progressive disease should be sensitively explored, and the nurse should assess how well they are coping. For many the diagnosis of metastatic disease is just as devastating as the original diagnosis of breast cancer; indeed, it can have an even greater impact as the realisation dawns that treatment is now aimed at controlling rather than curing the illness. The patient and her family may once again experience shock, anger, denial, depression and despair as they try to come to terms with the implications of the diagnosis. (See Case History 7.3.)

Even where cure is no longer possible, the philosophy of rehabilitation will remain at the centre of care, so that the highest quality of life can be maintained for as long as possible.

Palliative care

For a fuller discussion of the various aspects of long-term and palliative care that will be relevant to the patient with metastatic breast cancer, the reader is referred to Chapter 32 and Chapter 35. The important contribution of the nurse in controlling and managing symptoms such as pain, nausea and vomiting, fatigue, sexual problems, anxiety and shortness of breath is described in the following chapters: Chapter 19; Chapter 34; and Chapter 3.

Case History 7.3 Mrs J

Mrs J is a 54-year-old married woman with two adult children. She has a part-time job in a school, but spends a large part of each day looking after her elderly mother, who is disabled with rheumatoid arthritis and is unable to move around.

Mrs J was diagnosed as having cancer of the right breast 4 years ago. This was treated by a wide excision of the tumour with axillary clearance. Adjuvant radiotherapy was also given. At this time 4 axillary nodes were found to contain cancer, and Mrs J was prescribed tamoxifen 20 mg, which she has been taking ever since. She was well until a month ago, when she began to experience pain in her back; this has since increased in intensity. On admission to hospital a bone scan revealed extensive metastatic cancer in her lumbar spine, and a chest X-ray showed pulmonary metastases. Doctors have advised a course of CMF chemotherapy, to which she has agreed, but she is 'devastated' by the news of cancer recurrence and is extremely frightened by the thought of chemotherapy. Her other major concern is how she will manage to continue to look after her mother.

? **7.10** Consider the following questions with reference to Case History 7.3

a. Mrs J has extensive metastatic disease of her lumbar vertebrae. What implications does this have for nursing care?
b. What side-effects is Mrs J likely to experience with CMF chemotherapy?
c. What information should the nurse give to Mrs J to prepare her for her first course of chemotherapy?
d. Discuss other ways in which the nurse can help to allay Mrs J's anxiety about chemotherapy.

BREAST RECONSTRUCTION

Breast reconstruction may be achieved by several surgical methods but frequently includes the insertion of silicone or saline breast implants. It may be undertaken when women feel their breasts are too small, where one breast has failed to develop at puberty, or following breast cancer surgery, which has removed part or all of a woman's breast. However, only the latter will be considered here.

The aim of breast reconstruction following breast cancer surgery is to create a breast form which resembles the woman's other breast as closely as possible in terms of size, shape and consistency. Complete symmetry when naked is not possible to achieve but any differences should be slight when wearing a bra.

The King's Fund Forum (1986) consensus committee statement on breast cancer treatments suggested that 'The possibility of reconstructive surgery should be discussed with all women in whom a significant loss of breast tissue will be necessary'. Breast reconstruction may help to reduce the psychological or emotional problems experienced by women after surgery or it may enable a woman to undergo a mastectomy which she would have otherwise found intolerable (Dean et al 1983).

Only uncontrolled metastatic breast cancer is considered an absolute contraindication in breast reconstruction. The presence of bone metastases should not prohibit a woman from having reconstructive surgery if she perceives that this will improve her quality of life and she is generally well enough to undergo surgery.

MEDICAL MANAGEMENT

Routine surgical preparation involving blood tests, chest X-rays and ECGs will be undertaken prior to surgery.

Several surgical techniques can be used to achieve breast reconstruction. The most common are:

Submuscular implant. This involves inserting an implant beneath the muscle overlying the chest wall. Generally this can be done only where the remaining breast is small and droops very little.

Tissue expansion. An inflatable silicone bag is inserted beneath the muscle overlying the chest wall and gradually inflated with sterile saline over a period of several weeks via a valve and connecting tube which lie just beneath the skin. The aim of this is to slowly stretch the skin until the tissue expander is larger than the other breast. It is left expanded for 3 months and then removed in a second operation. An implant of a matching size is then inserted.

Double lumen implants that do not require removal are now being used. Tissue expansion methods are generally used where the skin of the chest wall is of good quality but inadequate quantity.

Myocutaneous flap. This involves transposing part of the latissimus dorsi muscle and overlying skin from the back, or the rectus abdominus muscle and overlying skin from the abdomen, to the chest wall. If necessary, an implant can then be placed behind this. Oval scarring on the breast form results as well as scarring on the abdomen or back.

These methods are generally used where a larger breast form is desired, following a radical mastectomy in which all chest wall muscle has been removed, or where radiotherapy has been given to the chest wall, causing the skin to lose its elasticity.

Reduction mammoplasty. Surgery to the remaining breast may be advised if it is very large or pendulous in order to achieve as much symmetry as possible. Scarring following this procedure may be extensive and nipple sensation may be lost; these effects must be discussed with the woman beforehand.

Nipple areola reconstruction. Sometimes the surgeon is able to do a subcutaneous mastectomy and leave the nipple intact. More often the nipple is not saved because of fear of cancer being present there. If this is so a nipple areola reconstruction can be undertaken. Generally, this is done around 3 months after the initial reconstruction. The nipple may be created from the skin overlying the reconstruction, saved from the other nipple or a graft taken from the labia. The areola is usually created from an upper inner thigh skin graft. Some women do not want to undergo further surgery and opt for adhesive silicone nipples.

Breast augmentation following partial mastectomy. This is usually carried out, if desired, at the time of the original surgery as it is more difficult after radiotherapy has been given. The implant is inserted into the area where tissue has been removed to reduce any alteration in breast size and shape and hence problems associated with altered body image.

Potential postoperative complications

Seroma/haematoma formation. This is more likely to occur after an immediate reconstruction than if reconstruction is delayed. Serous fluid and blood may build up behind the implant in spite of the presence of wound drains, increasing discomfort and the risk of infection. Aspiration may be necessary and, occasionally, removal of the prosthesis.

Wound infection. If wound infection occurs antibiotics will be prescribed. If the infection fails to respond to these it may be necessary to remove the prosthesis and attempt insertion after a 3-month recovery period. To try to avoid infection prophylactic antibiotics may be prescribed at the time of surgery.

Necrosis. This uncommon problem occurs where blood perfusion of the skin flap is inadequate and some of the tissue dies. It is more likely to occur when myocutaneous flaps are used.

Potential long-term complications

Capsular contracture. A fibrous band of tissue forms around the implant and, over time, will contract. If this contracture is severe the implant will become hard to the touch, uncomfortable and cause the reconstructed breast to change in shape. Manual compression under local anaesthetic may break the capsule; the only alternative is to remove the implant and scar tissue and insert a replacement prosthesis. The incidence of capsular contracture requiring removal is difficult to ascertain but is likely to be around 15%. There is some evidence that new textured implants result in a lower incidence of capsular contracture (Coleman et al 1991).

Abdominal herniation. This infrequent problem may follow a rectus abdominus myocutaneous flap reconstruction. The weakness in the abdominal wall resulting from this surgery is strengthened by the insertion of surgical mesh to reduce the possibility of herniation.

NURSING PRIORITIES AND MANAGEMENT: BREAST RECONSTRUCTION

Preoperative considerations

Assessment

Nursing assessment prior to breast reconstruction should address the following points:

1. The woman's reasons for wanting a breast reconstruction. These may include wanting to eliminate the need for an external prosthesis, a desire to improve self-confidence and self-esteem or to 'feel more whole', and a desire to have greater freedom in choosing clothing (Clifford 1979, Goldberg et al 1984).
2. Expectations of breast reconstruction. A woman who has realistic expectations is more likely to be satisfied with the overall result of her reconstruction. Expectations for both physical appearance and quality of life should be assessed.
3. The woman's knowledge of breast reconstruction and her understanding of what the surgeon has told her about the procedure and possible complications.

Giving information

The nurse has an important role in promoting realistic expectations of breast reconstruction. Showing photographs of breast reconstructions is one way of helping women to imagine what it will be like. Photographs that show the effect of the reconstruction unclothed, in a bra, and in clothing are useful, but photographs should not show only the very best results.

It may also help to arrange for the patient to talk to another woman who has also undergone a reconstruction, preferably by a similar method. The Breast Care and Mastectomy Association may be able to put the patient in touch with someone in her area if no one is known to the nurse or consultant. Some women may also like to see an implant.

Giving psychological support

The woman who is undergoing breast reconstruction at the same time as her breast cancer surgery will be dealing with her recent diagnosis of cancer as well as with the idea of reconstruction. It may be particularly difficult for her to come to a decision about reconstruction at this time and so it should be made clear to her that refusing an immediate reconstruction does not prohibit surgery at a later date. She should be given adequate opportunity to air her feelings and concerns.

Women considering a delayed reconstruction frequently have second thoughts about undergoing further surgery. The nurse can help by taking time to clarify with the patient her worries and concerns and her desire for reconstruction. Concurrent stresses and the woman's family situation should also be assessed and discussed, as these may influence how she feels about undergoing reconstruction and how she will cope postoperatively.

Postoperative considerations

Wound management

The aims and principles of wound management are described in detail in Chapter 23. The following points are of particular relevance to wound healing following breast reconstruction.

The nurse should observe the wound for signs of haematoma, seroma, infection or necrosis. Wound drainage should be observed and the volume recorded every 30 min for the first 2 h after return from theatre and then at gradually increasing intervals. Circulatory perfusion of skin flaps should be checked with the same frequency. The skin flap should be gently prodded using a blunt instrument or finger; it should go white and then quickly return to a pink colour once the pressure is released. This is particularly important where a myocutaneous flap has been used in reconstruction and where tissue expansion is placing the wound under some tension. Where the colour slowly returns, the flap looks blue, or feels cold to the touch the doctor should be informed in case it is necessary to take the patient back to theatre.

Temperature and pulse should be recorded 4-hourly. Dressings should be changed only if they become saturated with wound exudate or if it becomes essential to view the wound. Frequently, pressure dressings are applied in theatre and remain in place for 1–3 days. When these are removed, transparent dressings such as Tegaderm or OpSite are useful. Subcutaneous sutures are normally used and remain in situ for 10–14 days unless they are of the dissolvable variety. Discomfort from wounds will vary. Immediate reconstructions involving the removal of axillary lymph glands and/or abdominal myocutaneous flap procedures will be the most uncomfortable. Opiate analgesics may be required by i.v. injection or continuous infusion pump for the first 2 days; after this time, oral analgesics are usually sufficient. Promoting comfort will increase rest and sleep and so encourage healing and general rehabilitation.

Patient education

Postoperative exercises should be taught, preferably by a physiotherapist, to all patients who have undergone breast reconstruction. Some surgeons prefer shoulder movement to be restricted to 90° flexion and abduction for 2–3 weeks, particularly if the scar is very tight or if they fear movement of the implant. Because the silicone implant is usually placed behind muscle, as the muscle contracts tightening or discomfort may be experienced. This should disappear as the muscle accommodates the implant.

Advice about bras is commonly sought. Some support is likely to increase comfort, but underwired bras should usually be avoided for the first few months. Surgical breast supports may be recommended for a few weeks, whilst sport or dance bras which give firm support without bra cups may be the best option. A partial prosthesis will need to be fitted to obtain a symmetrical appearance during tissue expansion and sometimes following reconstruction.

Giving psychological support

Although having a reconstruction after a mastectomy may help a woman to cope and foster rehabilitation, research indicates that many women do mourn the loss of their breast and suffer from anxiety and depression following surgery (Dean et al 1983, Meyer & Ringberg 1986). The nurse should not assume that a woman who has had an immediate reconstruction will have no problems related to a changed body image.

Women undergoing tissue expansion often experience frustration at the length of time the process takes to complete reconstruction. Some find it difficult to cope with an inequality in breast size and shape during this time (Goin & Goin 1988). Acknowledgement of these feelings, adequate opportunity to discuss them, and access to counselling may help the woman to cope.

When complications do occur and an implant has to be removed, the individual may suffer further psychological distress. A wait of about 3 months is generally required before another implant can be inserted; during this time the woman will have to cope with another alteration in body image. Anxiety, depression and feelings of anger or despair may result. Some women may decide that they do not wish to undergo a further attempt at reconstruction. The nurse should support the patient whatever her decision and give her the opportunity to express her feelings.

LYMPHOEDEMA IN BREAST CANCER

Lymphoedema is the accumulation of a high protein fluid in the interstitial spaces between cells in the tissue of a limb or other area. It is the result of a defective mechanism of lymph drainage due to tissue fibrosis, disease, or a congenital disorder.

Approximately 25% of women with breast cancer will develop some degree of lymphoedema characterised by a swollen arm, often with some swelling of the adjacent chest and back. This condition can cause considerable physical and psychological distress.

PATHOPHYSIOLOGY

All women with breast cancer who have axillary surgery to remove some or all of their lymph glands, or those who receive radiotherapy to the axillary region, are at risk of developing lymphoedema of the limb on the affected side. Scarring from these treatments will result in the closure or narrowing of many lymph vessels and so reduce the efficiency of lymphatic drainage from the arm. For most women the drainage remains adequate, and collateral vessels may develop to increase the pathways for drainage. However, lymphoedema may develop weeks, months or years after surgery or radiotherapy, sometimes following an infection or injury, but often without an obvious reason. It may remain mild, or gradually progress until the arm is so heavy that it is difficult to lift and impossible to use. Over time, fibrosis within the tissue of the arm may occur, causing hardness. There is also a higher risk of infection and cellulitis, as the high-protein fluid is an ideal breeding-ground for bacteria.

Disease within the axillary area which causes an obstruction to lymph flow will also cause lymphoedema. This may be seen when cancer has recurred, or when a woman presents with an advanced carcinoma of the breast. Signs of venous obstruction are sometimes seen: these are commonly a pink colouring of the arm and distended veins visible on the upper arm and chest wall.

Brachial plexus nerve damage is less frequently seen, but may also result from radiation fibrosis or cancer infiltration of the nerve plexus, causing weakness, paraesthesia or nerve pain.

MEDICAL MANAGEMENT

Medical intervention. Options for medical management are at present limited. The choice of treatment depends on whether the lymphoedema has been caused by fibrosis or by axillary disease. Assessment may include CT scanning and colour Doppler ultrasound to determine the amount of scarring, venous obstruction or disease present.

Attempts to reduce the size and weight of the arm by surgically removing a large amount of tissue have had very little success and have frequently caused further problems with infection, swelling and pain as well as extensive scarring.

Diuretics have a part to play only if generalised fluid retention is exacerbating the lymphoedema. Where venous obstruction is due to a thrombosis anticoagulation, therapy with warfarin may be used.

In the case of axillary disease surgery to remove as much of the cancer as possible may be of use by reducing the obstruction of lymph and venous flow. However, chemotherapy or endocrine therapies, which have the advantage of not causing the same disruption to normal structures as surgery, are more likely to be used.

Pain relief. Analgesics ranging from paracetamol to opiates will be used as required. If, however, the pain is due to brachial plexus damage by disease or radiotherapy, it is unlikely to respond adequately to opiates and may be best treated by steroids, non-steroidal anti-inflammatory drugs and carbamazepine.

Cellulitis. The risk of infection in a swollen limb is high. Even a small cut may provide an entry point for infection and result in severe cellulitis requiring treatment by antibiotics. If cellulitis is recurrent patients are often given a prescription to have on hand so that they can obtain an antibiotic as soon as infection occurs.

NURSING PRIORITIES AND MANAGEMENT: LYMPHOEDEMA

Major considerations

Treatment effectiveness is measured in terms of the reduction in size and weight of the arm, and for most people this is possible. However, sometimes all that can be done is to increase the softness and movement of the arm, and to reduce the discomfort, but these improvements can represent a substantial increase in the quality of the life of the patient.

Assessment

Nursing interventions must be preceded by an assessment to identify the physical and psychosocial needs of the individual patient.

Physical assessment should address the following areas:

- medical history, particularly of any surgery or radiotherapy, disease in the axilla
- the condition of the skin of the arm: colouring, presence of cuts/infection, previous cellulitis
- the size of the arm. Both arms should be measured at regular specified intervals so that a comparison can be made and the severity of the oedema estimated to form a baseline for treatment
- the duration of the oedema and any precipitating or aggravating factors
- presence of oedema in the adjacent tissue of the chest wall
- any previous treatment for lymphoedema
- the type and severity of any discomfort experienced
- the individual's range of shoulder movement and ability to use the arm in activities of daily living.

Psychosocial assessment should include:

- how the lymphoedema has affected the woman's self-esteem and body image
- how the lymphoedema has altered the woman's life-style, work, and social role and how she feels about this
- whether the swelling has affected the type of clothing she can wear.

Nursing interventions

The aim of nursing interventions in the management of lymphoedema are:

- to reduce arm size
- to improve the use of the arm
- to improve the comfort of the arm
- to improve the shape of the arm.

All treatments involve compression of the limb to try to push more fluid back into the vessels that exist. The main treatment methods as related to the degree of severity of the lymphoedema are as follows:

1. Mild oedema: compression sleeve
2. Moderate oedema: compression sleeve, and sometimes a compression pump used 1–2 h/day
3. Severe oedema, or if there is lymphorrhoea: compression bandaging for 2–3 weeks; after this time the patient wears a compression sleeve.

Whatever the degree of oedema, the woman should be given advice on arm care and on the therapeutic use of arm exercises and massage (see p. 282). It is very important to explain clearly the aim of each treatment regime and to promote a realistic expectation of outcome. Although therapy is aimed at control rather than cure, the patient who is given sufficient information and encouraged to participate in treatment is likely to take a more positive attitude toward her situation.

Compression sleeves are at the centre of treatment for lymphoedema. Several specialised ready-made varieties are available e.g. Medi, Pan-Med, Sigva. Compression needs to be fairly strong (around 40 mmHg) if it is to be effective. Supports such as Tubigrip are not adequate.

Sleeves may be difficult to put on but should be supportive and comfortable. They should be worn all day but not at night, and should not be allowed to form creases, as this will cause ridging in the swollen tissue. The sleeve will need to be worn over many months, during which time the patient must be monitored regularly to assess the effect. The patient should be warned that progress will be slow.

If the oedema is mild it may be possible for the arm to return to its normal size. At this point the sleeve may be removed, but the patient should be reminded that the oedema may return, in which case the sleeve should be reapplied.

Compression pumps such as Flowtron and Lymphopress are composed of inflatable sleeves attached to an electric pump which inflates and deflates the sleeves intermittently. The degree of pressure can be varied.

Some patients find a compression pump helpful as an addition to a compression sleeve. A pump should be used for 2 hours a day and a compression sleeve the rest of the time. If a pump is used alone, any reduction in size is usually lost within a few hours, although it may keep the arm soft and prevent tissue fibrosis.

Pumps are normally used when there is a moderate degree of arm swelling which is not responding to a compression sleeve alone. Ideally, the patient should borrow a pump from the hospital to use at home, but where this is not possible treatment on an outpatient or inpatient basis may be arranged.

Compression pumps are contraindicated if the patient has cardiac failure or lung disease (such as pulmonary oedema) where fluid from the arm may increase pressure on these organs, or where there is cellulitis or axillary vein thrombosis. Pumps should be used with caution if there is axillary disease or brachial plexus nerve damage. In both these situations pain may be intensified so the pump should initially be used at a very low pressure, beginning at approximately 30 mmHg and gradually building up to a maximum of 60 mmHg.

Compression bandaging. For women with severe lymphoedema, lymphorrhoea, skin problems or difficulty using a sleeve compression bandaging is the treatment of choice. Low-stretch bandages are used to bandage the fingers and hand before the arm is encased. The pressure applied should be graduated, more being applied at the lower end of the limb.

The bandages should be reapplied daily; due to the large size of the arm and of the bandages required, this often needs to be undertaken on an inpatient basis. Although expensive, this also provides an opportunity for the provision of physiotherapy, occupational therapy and psychological support. How-ever, community nurses practised in this technique could undertake compression bandaging in the patient's home. This is particularly helpful for those who have advanced disease and are unwell. Bandaging of a large arm may provide great comfort and relief from pain even if there is no hope of reducing arm size.

Although this bandaging technique is not difficult once learned, it does require practice and guidance.

Regnard, Badger & Mortimer (1988) may be useful to nurses wishing to start bandaging for lymphoedema patients.

Patient education

Massage. This has long been used in the European continent to treat lymphoedema but is only now being recognised in Britain. The type of massage used is light, aiming to stimulate the lymphatic vessels in the skin. Deeper massage would cause increased blood flow to the muscles; this would cause more fluid to accumulate in the tissues and would thus be counterproductive.

The patient can be shown how to massage the affected limb and adjacent part of the chest and back, where some degree of swelling may also occur. Indeed, massage is really the only way of treating oedema in the tissues of the chest and back. Using the hand or an electric massager the chest and back are massaged by applying *light* pressure in a direction away from the arm. Next, the arm should be massaged starting at the top of the arm and working down the arm — but always applying pressure upwards.

It is a good idea to show relatives how to perform therapeutic massage.

Exercise. Muscle contraction exercises and shoulder exercises should be taught to improve and maintain movement, and to encourage the return of lymph and venous fluid in the arm. Appropriate exercises include:

- clenching and relaxing the hand
- full circular movement of the wrist
- extension and flexion of the elbow joint
- clasping hands in front of the body and raising the arms, held straight, above the head.

A combination of these exercises should be performed for 5 minutes 4 times a day.

Self-care. Patients should be given advice on how to care for their arm, to reduce the risk of infection and to avoid straining the arm. (Infection and straining are both likely to increase swelling.) Ideally, this advice should be given to all women undergoing surgery or radiotherapy involving the axilla; this will help to prevent lymphoedema occurring and encourage early detection where it does occur.

MALIGNANT FUNGATING BREAST TUMOURS

Breast cancer is the most common cancer to cause ulceration. The result can be an unpleasant, weeping, malodorous, infected wound which is psychologically very difficult to cope with. Women often express feelings of disgust and revulsion and curtail social activities because of their embarrassment. An altered body image may lead to anxiety, depression and sexual problems.

Nurses have an important role to play in supporting women with fungating tumours; by rising to the challenge of wound management and controlling symptoms such as odour and excessive wound exudate they can help to improve the quality of life for these women. Frequently it is the community nurse who has the greatest involvement with these women and their families. (See Case History 7.4.)

Case History 7.4 Mrs S

Mrs S has been referred by her GP to the community nurse for management of a large ulcerating left breast carcinoma and for psychological support. She is 65 years old and a retired civil servant. She lives with her husband in a large house which they own. She visited her GP ostensibly to have her blood pressure checked but broke down in tears and told him that she had had a breast lump for 3 years. She hadn't told anyone, including her husband, because she 'feared the worst'. Now the lump was smelly and oozing and she could no longer hide it from her husband, who made her visit the GP.

On visiting Mrs S for the first time, the nurse finds a withdrawn and depressed lady who has stopped going out. She is embarrassed to show the nurse her breast, which is a large ulcerating mass with nodules extending to the surrounding tissue on the chest wall. The wound is malodorous, with a large amount of necrotic tissue and a profuse discharge. Mrs S has been covering it with gauze pads but has not cleaned it for some time, as she cannot bear to look at it.

Mrs S describes her husband as supportive and loving, but she will not allow him near her any more because she feels that she is 'disgusting'. She has taken to sleeping in a separate room and avoiding him when she can.

The nurse is able to speak very briefly to Mr S, who appears caring but very anxious about his wife's condition. He is not allowed by his wife to be present during her discussion with the nurse.

PATHOPHYSIOLOGY

Ulceration occurs when breast cancer infiltrates the epithelium and causes a breakdown of the skin. The resulting wound may be superficial or deep; it may affect a small area of the breast or may be very extensive, involving all of the chest wall. Frequently, as a tumour grows its blood supply becomes inadequate, causing central tissue death and necrosis. When such a tumour ulcerates a large necrotic mass is revealed, providing an ideal environment for infection to develop. This in turn will increase exudate and cause odour.

As the disease progresses ulceration becomes more extensive and may erode blood vessels, causing haemorrhage. The severity of bleeding will depend on the size of the blood vessel. Capillary bleeding causing a slow loss of blood is commonly seen but blood loss may be life-threatening if a large vessel is eroded.

Tumour involvement of the cutaneous nerves can cause pain and irritation. There is often tenderness due to inflammation in the surrounding tissues. Whilst many women have remarkably little pain from these wounds, some have severe pain.

MEDICAL MANAGEMENT

Medical treatment will depend on the extent and position of the tumour and on what therapy for breast cancer, if any, the woman has previously had. Management may be considered in terms of treatments to try to control the disease and interventions aimed at symptom control.

Treatments for disease control are as follows.

Surgery. For women who have an ulcerating tumour that appears confined to the breast region it may be possible to surgically remove the tumour by performing a mastectomy. Where the tumour extends to the chest wall or a large area of skin, the surgery will be more extensive and surgical closure will require a skin graft or the use of a muscle and skin flap from the abdomen or back. These have been successfully used in some women to increase their quality of life, but careful discussion with the patient beforehand is important to ensure that she understands what the surgery entails, what benefits can be expected and what risks are involved. If the woman's general health is reasonable and she has a life expectancy of more than a few months, she may feel that this approach is the best for her even if recovery is protracted.

Radiotherapy can be used with great success in controlling some breast tumours. Complete remissions are occasionally seen, but more commonly radiotherapy achieves a reduction in tumour size and in the wound symptoms.

Chemotherapy and endocrine therapy may also be used sometimes in combination with radiotherapy. Systemic drug therapies have the added advantage of treating disease elsewhere in the body as well as in the breast.

Symptom control measures are as follows.

Analgesics may frequently need to be provided to alleviate constant pain or to make dressing changes more comfortable. The choice of analgesia will depend on the type and severity of the pain (see Ch. 19).

Antibiotics may be required in the fight against infection.

Supportive transfusion may be indicated where blood loss has caused anaemia.

Surgical debridement may be very useful in removing necrotic tissue from the wound, but it often not possible to carry out in view of the risk of haemorrhage.

Diathermy can be helpful in controlling bleeding points but should be used with caution given the necrosis it causes. In severe cases of bleeding topical adrenaline may also be applied; this too should be used with caution.

NURSING PRIORITIES AND MANAGEMENT: FUNGATING BREAST TUMOURS

Major considerations

Assessment

The nursing assessment of a woman with a fungating breast tumour must include far more than an assessment of the wound itself. It must consider factors such as age, marital status, concurrent disease and disabilities, drug therapies and pain. All of these factors may influence the possibility of wound healing or infection.

Assessment of the woman's psychological state, her reactions to her wound and her ability to cope with it, and of the way in which it has affected her life and her family is equally important. The nurse should bear in mind that anxiety and depression can have a significant impact on treatment outcome. Frequently it is the community nurse who has the greatest involvement with these women and their families, as hospitalisation is rarely required. Women often live for many years with a slowly progressing fungating tumour, which makes it all the more important that every effort is made to improve their quality of life.

Wound management (see also Ch. 23)

Malignant breast lesions have a pathological cause, i.e. cancer. Unless this cause is being treated wound healing is unlikely to occur. It is important that the nurse promotes realistic expectations in the patient, so that she is not hoping for complete healing of the wound if she is not receiving treatment for breast cancer.

The general aims of wound management are:

- to control the symptoms produced by the wound
- to minimise possible complications, e.g. infection
- to maximise comfort, minimise discomfort
- to promote healing where possible.

Many types of wound dressings are available. In order to choose products which are likely to be most effective for a given wound, the nurse must first identify the problems that are present. The most common problems associated with ulcerating lesions are:

- tissue necrosis
- infection
- excessive wound exudate
- odour
- haemorrhage/capillary bleeding
- pain.

These will now be considered in turn. (See also Nursing Care Plan 7.3.)

Tissue necrosis. Where tissue necrosis exists it is likely to increase the risk of infection. Debriding the wound of dead tissue will reduce this risk. Although it may be possible to remove the bulk of necrotic tissue by surgical debridement, the risk of haemorrhage sometimes prohibits this, making chemical debridement the preferred treatment even though it is a slower process. Products such as Varidase, Sorbsan, Debrisan and Granuflex may be useful as chemical debriding agents.

Infection is suspected where there is a purulent wound discharge, odour, inflammation and a raised body temperature. A wound swab should be taken by the nurse so that the right type of systemic antibiotic can be prescribed. Preparations such as metronidazole gel may be applied topically to help fight infection. The pharmacist and the infection control team will advise about the use of particular cleaning solutions when there is wound contamination by particular organisms such as Pseudomonas.

Excessive wound exudate is often due to a wound infection. Hence the first action would be to treat the infection and to debride the wound as necessary. The aim of wound dressing is to absorb the maximum volume of exudate with the minimum bulk of dressing. This requires the use of a high-absorbency primary dressing such as Sorbsan, and a high-absorbency secondary dressing such as Lyofoam C, which has the added benefit of containing charcoal to reduce odour from the wound.

It is important to remember that once there is 'strike-through' of the secondary dressing (i.e. saturation of the dressing) a pathway for bacteria to move from the outside through the dressing into the wound exists. This should be prevented with frequent changes of the outer dressing. Waterproofing is also important. Dressings such as OpSite or Tegaderm may sometimes be used as a tertiary dressing. Disposable nappies are used by some nurses effectively where great absorbency is needed.

Odour. Despite the lack of research to legitimise the use of natural live yoghurt in reducing wound odour, it is in fact widely used and appears to be effective. It is thought that the application of yoghurt creates an acid medium in which bacteria find it difficult to live, and that the lactobacilli in the yoghurt also act directly on the bacteria within the wound.

Yoghurt is usually applied thickly for around 20 min before it is removed with saline or gently showered off in the bath. A further dressing such as Sorbsan or Kaltostat can then be used on the wound. Where odour is a severe problem, yoghurt can be applied 3 or 4 times a day to try to reduce the odour as quickly as possible. A secondary dressing containing charcoal can also be used.

Metronidazole gel is also effective, but the problem of bacterial resistance to antibiotics must be considered.

External deodorisers may be helpful e.g. Ozium, Neutradol, Nilodor, but sometimes the smell of air fresheners or deodorisers are unacceptable to the patient or her family, or even cause nausea. Fresh air is probably the most effective agent for removing smells from a room, and changing clothes daily will help prevent odours from penetrating clothing.

Nursing Care Plan 7.3 Mrs S Caring for a woman with an ulcerating breast tumour (See Case History 7.4)

Nursing considerations	Action	Rationale	Expected outcome
April 6			By April 13:
1. Ulcerating left breast cancer: the wound is malodorous, necrotic, and has a profuse discharge	❐ Take wound swab for culture and sensitivity	Odour and discharge may be due to infection in wound	An improvement in wound odour
	❐ Twice a day: • Cleanse wound with saline using syringe and quill • Remove any areas of *loose* necrotic tissue with forceps and sterile scissors • Apply thick layer natural live yoghurt and leave for 15 min, covering patient with sterile towel • Remove yoghurt using saline in syringe again	Quill allows gentle but thorough cleansing (no cotton wool as fibres may be left which act as focus for infection). This will increase speed of debridement but should only be done on loose dead tissue and should not be painful. Natural *live* yoghurt very good at deodorising but need to leave 15 min to work	Reduction in necrotic tissue Amount of wound drainage will be reduced and controlled by wound dressings Mrs S will state that she finds her dressing comfortable and that the symptoms have improved.
	❐ Pack with Varidase-coated gauze or Varidase gel (Discontinued 10/4)	Varidase is very strong debriding agent but cannot be used if wound is bleeding as it affects clotting of blood.	
	❐ Cover with occlusive dressing, taking care to protect sore and friable areas with Vaseline (Discontinued 10/4)	Occlusive dressing necessary to ensure Varidase is not deactivated.	
	❐ Apply absorbent secondary dressing containing charcoal, e.g. Lyofoam	Absorbent secondary dressing used because of profuse discharge. Charcoal helps to deodorise.	
	❐ Keep in place with Netelast	Using Netelast reduces trauma to friable skin on chest wall	
	❐ Suggest change bedclothes frequently and open windows each day	These measures will help to prevent the odour lingering in the house	
	April 10		
	❐ Apply Sorbsan instead of Varidase. Occlusive dressing no longer necessary. Continue with rest of dressing.	Sorbsan has a debriding action. Though more gentle than Varidase, it is also very absorbent	

Evaluation

April 10
Varidase debriding wound well but wound bleeding close to medial edge; therefore stop Varidase and use Sorbsan. Will continue with yoghurt.

April 13
Discharge reduced and now controlled by Sorbsan dressing. Odour much less obvious but still present, therefore will continue with yoghurt, Sorbsan and charcoal dressings.

Wound swab indicates *Staph. aureas* infection. GP will visit tomorrow and prescribe a course of antibiotics.

Cont'd

Haemorrhage/capillary bleeding. Capillary bleeding is commonly seen in malignant wounds and is often difficult to stop. Dressings such as Kaltostat have a haemostatic property and are particularly useful where capillary bleeding exists.

It is extremely important that dry dressings are not applied to wounds that bleed, as removal is likely to cause further bleeding. To reduce trauma, adherent dressings should be removed only after soaking. Dressings such as Kaltostat and Sorbsan absorb exudate and turn to a gel which is then easily removed by syringing the wound with saline. Where possible, wounds which are liable to bleed should be irrigated, for even the gentle use of cotton wool may be enough to cause bleeding.

Silver nitrate and Flamazine also have haemostatic properties. The use of pressure and ice may help control bleeding, but if a major vessel is eroded bleeding may be very difficult to control and alarming to the patient.

Weak solutions of adrenaline may be advised by medical

Nursing Care Plan 7.3 *(cont'd)*

Nursing considerations	Action	Rationale	Expected outcome
April 6			
2. Embarrassment and disgust at wound causing:	❒ Dress wound to control symptoms of odour and discharge	If symptoms of odour and discharge are controlled Mrs S will be more likely to go out again and not feel so self-conscious.	
a. Difficulty in communicating with husband b. Social isolation c. Reduced self-esteem	❒ Encourage Mrs S to express her feelings about her wound and the way it is affecting her life	This may help Mrs S to 'let go' of tension, to see her situation more clearly and to allow her to accept support from the nurse. It will also help the nurse to identify specific problems/concerns	Mrs S will verbalise her feelings about her wound
	❒ Encourage her to talk about her relationship with her husband and how it has altered	This will help the nurse to understand how they used to communicate and how close their relationship was. This will help her to plan intervention which may improve communication and mutual support	She will identify how her relationship with her husband has changed
	❒ Assess her social support and what sort of activities she used to do	This will indicate what the norm was for Mrs S and how things have changed. It will allow the nurse to know what activities and relationships she might encourage Mrs S to take up again	
	April 10		
	❒ Suggest that Mr and Mrs S sit down together and discuss how they feel about the cancer, the wound and how it has altered their life	This would allow Mr and Mrs S to begin communicating again and to break down barriers so that they can support each other	Mr and Mrs S will discuss together how they both feel about Mrs S having breast cancer and an ulcerating lesion
	April 13		
	❒ Suggest Mrs S should go out to her daughter's next week for tea	Mrs S is close to her daughter. As her wound is improving, this is an appropriate first step in taking up her social life again	She will arrange to go out to visit her daughter by 20 April.
	❒ Arrange for Mrs S to visit hospital for partial prosthesis to be fitted	Mrs S has voiced concern about her appearance in clothes. A partial prosthesis will enable her to regain a balanced appearance	
	❒ Discuss the choice of loose clothing to minimise the altered shape due to the dressings		

Evaluation

April 10
Mrs S says she feels very down today. Expressed feelings of guilt that she hadn't sought help before and believes she has let her husband down. She knows that he loves her but believes he cannot possibly want to be near her because of her wound's odour. She describes her marriage as very strong previously. They used to talk about most things but both find it difficult to express their feelings to each other and have not spoken of the cancer diagnosis or what will happen now. She has spoken to her daughter, who has said they should all talk about it. She would like to but doesn't feel she can. I reinforced that I felt it would be a good idea and offered to be present if that would help. She will think about it.

April 13
Mrs S is feeling better. She is very pleased that her wound is more manageable and particularly that it is less smelly. I suggested she might consider going out. She is hesitant about this but I suggested perhaps a couple of hours with her daughter. She is still conscious of the wound and feels everyone will know something is wrong because her appearance is not balanced due to the dressings and tumour itself distorting her breast shape. I suggested partial prostheses may help this and she is very keen on this idea.

Cont'd

Nursing Care Plan 7.3 *(cont'd)*

Nursing considerations	Action	Rationale	Expected outcome
April 6			
3. Fear of breast cancer	❒ Assess Mrs S's information needs by finding out what her knowledge of breast cancer is and identifying misconceptions she may have	Providing appropriate information may help to allay anxiety and remove misconceptions	Mrs S will specify the fears she has about breast cancer
	❒ Encourage Mrs S to express and explore her feelings concerning breast cancer.	This is often therapeutic in itself but also allows the nurse to more accurately identify the fears	She will define her information needs concerning breast cancer and its treatment
	❒ Offer literature about breast cancer	Written information reinforces verbal information	
April 7			
4. Fear of dying in pain. Fear of nausea and vomiting.	❒ Reassure Mrs S that effective pain control is available. (Discuss worries about taking opiates if this is a problem for her.) Stress that nausea and vomiting can normally be controlled by medication		Mrs S will understand that pain from cancer can be effectively controlled and that nausea and vomiting, if they occur, can also be controlled by medication

Evaluation

April 7
Very upset today. Feels very guilty that she didn't go to the GP before. Feels she has let her husband down. Has always been frightened of having breast cancer, although she doesn't know anyone who has had breast cancer. She knows that it is likely that she will die from this, in spite of any treatment she may be given, and she is frightened how this will happen. She equates cancer with a painful death and cannot bear the thought of pain or feeling nauseated.

April 10
Given booklet by the Breast Cancer and Mastectomy Association. Suggested that she should let her husband read it too. Also wanted to know about possible treatments for breast cancer of this stage. Discussed chemotherapy, radiotherapy and hormone therapy.
cont'd

staff in such a situation, but should be used with caution because of the possibility of systemic absorption.

Care must also be taken when using tapes to hold dressings in place. The skin around an ulceration is often inflamed, tender and delicate. As tapes may cause trauma it is a good idea to rotate the sites to which tape is applied. It is in fact preferable for dressings to be held in place by net body bandages such as Netelast which obviates the need for tape.

Pain. Wound pain may be severe or very slight. The nurse must assess the severity and type of pain being experienced and whether it is always present or affects the patient only during dressing changes. Pain assessment should be ongoing so that the effectiveness of pain control measures can be evaluated (see Ch. 19). Where dressing changes cause discomfort analgesics should be offered to the woman at least 30 min before each dressing change. The use of Entonox during the dressing procedure may also be helpful. The use of non-adherent dressings and cleansing the wound by irrigation where possible will also reduce discomfort.

Patient education

Wound care. As much information as the woman requires concerning her wound, dressings and general condition should be given. The degree to which the patient and her family are involved in wound management will depend largely on their own wishes and sensitivities. Some women prefer to be taught how to dress their own wounds completely at home, with only minimum supervisory involvement by the community or hospital nurse. This may originate in a desire to be independent, or it may be prompted by embarrassment. Some patients feel unable to have anything to do with their wound and do not want family members to intervene either. No-one should be made to look at her wound if this is intolerable to her; to do so may destroy the only way in which she knows how to cope.

Diet. Dietary advice may be appropriate if a woman is malnourished, has an infection, is anorexic, or is considering starting a 'cancer diet'. The nurse should be able to give basic advice about a balanced diet (see Ch. 21) but may wish to refer the patient to a dietitian for further advice. The decision to go on a cancer diet rests with the patient. There are many such diets: some are reasonably well-balanced, but others are likely to cause extreme weight loss. Where this is likely to be detrimental to the individual the nurse should discuss this with her; ultimately, however, the nurse should support the patient in whatever decision she makes.

Prostheses and clothing. Practical advice about clothing may be appreciated if the disease has radically altered the contour of the chest or where a large amount of absorbent dressing is necessary to control the wound exudate. Frequently the use of partial prostheses fitted over the dressings may restore a more normal breast contour. A larger soft bra may enable the dressing to be held in place comfortably but securely whilst maintaining a normal appearance in clothing. Where a bra cannot be worn due to discomfort, loose clothing will help

Nursing Care Plan 7.3 *(cont'd)*

Nursing considerations	Action	Rationale	Expected outcome
April 6 **5. Anxiety of Mr S due to Mrs S's condition and withdrawn behaviour**	❒ Arrange a time to sit down and talk to Mr S	This will ensure the nurse has time specifically with Mr S	By April 13, Mr S will define areas of anxiety
	❒ Encourage him to express and explore his feelings and define the particular anxieties he has regarding his wife and any other areas of stress	Expression and exploration of feeling is itself therapeutic in reducing anxiety and will enable the nurse to more fully assess the home situation	Mr S will discuss his feelings concerning Mrs S's illness, behaviour and the ulcerating cancer
	❒ Assess the support systems that Mr S has and emphasise that the nurse is concerned for his welfare as well as his wife's	Many carers do not consider their own needs and consider the nurse only as a support for the patient	
	❒ Provide information about breast cancer and its treatment	Appropriate information may help to reduce anxiety by enabling Mr S to feel more involved and more in control of the situation	

Evaluation

April 6
Arranged to speak to Mr S tomorrow following visit to his wife.

April 7
Reluctant to discuss his feelings about his wife, preferring to dwell on his wife's problem and her feelings. Fought back tears when discussing the future. However, he did say he feels angry with himself and his wife that the cancer got to this stage before medical help was sought. He feels guilty he didn't know about it and frustrated with his wife's withdrawn behaviour as he believes she will just give up and die. We discussed how control of the wound problems may give her the confidence to go out again, and how she will require his support, which he appears very willing to give.

Mr S appears to have very little support, only talking to his daughter on rare occasions about his wife. He used to talk over everything with his wife but now she won't allow this.

April 6
Seen briefly. Looks more relaxed. Has talked to GP re possible treatments and appointment to see consultant oncologist has been made for next week. Also believes that his wife is brighter because her wound has improved.

to disguise any altered shape without causing any restrictions around the wound.

> **?** **7.11** Consider the following questions with reference to Case History 7.4.
> a. Identify the main problems that Mrs S has.
> b. Consider the effects a fungating lesion might have on a woman's body image.
> c. It is important that Mrs S does not feel that her nurse is disgusted by her wound. Consider how the nurse might demonstrate this verbally and non-verbally.
> d. How might the nurse endeavour to reduce Mr S's anxiety about his wife?
> e. What properties should the wound dressing have? Can you suggest any appropriate products for such a wound?

BENIGN BREAST DISORDERS

Benign breast disorders probably account for 90% of all breast problems. Of the most common, benign mammary dysplasia and breast infections, are considered here. Gynaecomastia is also mentioned because, although it is rare, it is the most common breast disorder in men.

BENIGN MAMMARY DYSPLASIA

PATHOPHYSIOLOGY

This is a common condition amongst women of all ages but particularly affects women between the ages of 30 and 55. It is often called fibrocystic disease, but this term is misleading in that it is really not a disease but a natural occurrence in women as they approach menopause. It is thought to be caused by the incomplete involution of breast tissue during each menstrual cycle, leading to cystic changes, fibrosis and nodularity.

Mammary dysplasia is usually a completely benign condition which does not predispose a woman to breast cancer. If biopsied, the cells show hyperplasia, but with no alteration in the cellular appearance. However, where atypical hyperplasia is present the risk of breast cancer developing in the breast is raised, and regular screening may be advised.

Benign mammary dysplasia may present as areas of diffuse nodularity or thickening which may contain single or multiple cysts. Commonly it is bilateral, although it may occur in only one breast. Premenstrual tenderness is often experienced coinciding with an increase in nodularity. Cysts are tender and round and are shown to be fluid-filled on ultrasound. They may increase in size or stay the same; sometimes they disperse by themselves.

MEDICAL MANAGEMENT

Investigations. Assessment of a woman who complains of a lump or lumpiness within her breasts will involve clinical examination, mammography, ultrasound and sometimes fine-needle aspiration cytology. Cystic fluid is usually sent for examination only if the fluid is blood-stained, as this may indicate cancer.

Whenever a cyst or area of nodularity is slightly suspicious in its presentation, excision biopsy will usually be recommended to exclude cancer (see p. 270). Follow-up examinations are not usually required unless histology reveals atypical hyperplasia or there is a family history of breast cancer.

Medical intervention. Benign mammary dysplasia is sometimes aggravated by oral contraceptive pills. If this appears to be the case, a change of pill may be recommended. Where severe breast pain is also experienced, drug treatments using bromocriptine (Durning & Sellwood 1982), danazol (Mansel et al 1982) and evening primrose oil (Pashby et al 1981) have all been found to be of benefit for some patients.

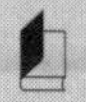

See Blamey (1986) for further information on the medical management of benign mammary dysplasia.

NURSING PRIORITIES AND MANAGEMENT: BENIGN MAMMARY DYSPLASIA

Major considerations

Assessment

Nursing assessment should include the presenting symptoms of the problem and, in particular, the presence of any discomfort and any aggravating or alleviating factors. The nurse should determine the patient's knowledge about her condition, her fears and concerns, and the ways in which the condition is affecting her normal life.

Perioperative care

General pre- and postoperative nursing practices are discussed in Chapter 27. Surgery is usually minor, involving excision of a small area of nodularity or a cyst, but the presence of a lump may give rise to great anxiety. Reassurance that this is not cancer may be needed. However, the nurse should not give false reassurance where doubt exists as to the nature of the lump. As postoperative recovery is usually rapid surgery is frequently performed as a day case or may require a one-night stay in hospital. Postoperatively, the priority of nursing will be wound management and pain control. Because the breast is very vascular there may be large amounts of bruising and wound drainage even though the surgery is minor. A wound drain is sometimes needed, but is usually removed the following morning.

The breast is likely to be very sore for several days. Paracetamol is usually sufficient for pain relief, but if bruising and oedema is very extensive stronger medication may be required. Wearing a supportive bra is usually advised for the first 2 weeks postoperatively to improve comfort and avoid strain being placed on the wound.

Patient education

The nurse can take the opportunity to promote breast health by discussing breast-screening and breast examination. It may be appropriate to discuss how breast comfort can be enhanced by a correctly fitting bra. Women who have premenstrual breast discomfort may find reducing salt or omitting caffeine from their diet helpful. Others find a course of Vitamin B_6 or evening primrose oil brings relief.

BREAST INFECTIONS

PATHOPHYSIOLOGY

Breast infections are relatively common in causing swelling, tenderness and pain, which may be associated with a breast abscess or nipple discharge. Breast abscesses are most commonly seen during or following lactation. Infection may arise from a cracked nipple but often there is no apparent cause. Staphyloccocal organisms are the most common causes.

MEDICAL MANAGEMENT

Systemic broad-spectrum antibiotics are the usual treatment. However, a persistent abscess may require surgical drainage and excision of the surrounding capsule. A persistent nipple discharge may be treated by a microductectomy, which involves removing one of the major ducts behind the nipple, or a Hadfield's procedure, which involves removing the major duct system behind the nipple. Surgery is usually through a circumareolar incision, and an overnight stay in hospital is generally required.

NURSING MANAGEMENT AND PRIORITIES: BREAST INFECTIONS

Giving psychological support

Until the presence of infection has been established fear of a more serious problem, particularly cancer, may remain. An explanation of the nature and possible cause of infection may be necessary to reassure the patient, particularly as recurrent infections are quite common and may cause frustration and distress.

Reducing discomfort

The discomfort and pain accompanying a breast infection is usually the most distressing feature of the condition. A supportive bra, applications of heat or cold and padding to protect a sore nipple may all reduce discomfort, but mild to moderate analgesic medication is usually necessary to achieve a satisfactory level of comfort.

Where surgical excision of an abscess is required, nursing management will be similar to that of a woman undergoing an excision biopsy. The nurse must be particularly vigilant for signs of infection postoperatively.

Surgical management

Where surgical excision of the abscess is required, nursing management will be similar to that for a woman undergoing an excision biopsy (see p. 270). The nurse must be particularly vigilant in observing for signs of wound infection.

GYNAECOMASTIA

This is a rare benign disorder which occurs in men and involves overdevelopment of male breast tissue as a result of oestrogen production either in puberty or at a later age. This may be due to idiopathic excess oestrogen, e.g. in choriocarcinomatous teratoma or cirrhosis, or by decreased testosterone, e.g. in Klinefelter's syndrome (see Ch. 6, p. 198), or by drugs, e.g. amphetamines, antidepressants, certain antihypertensives, digoxin, spironolactone, or oestrogen administration.

MEDICAL MANAGEMENT

Surgery is not usually recommended, unless the gynaecomastia is mistaken for a possible carcinoma; in such instances a biopsy may be advised. If the condition has arisen following the administration of a particular drug, modification of that medication can be considered. Hormone manipulation may be of benefit where gynaecomastia is due to the oversecretion of oestrogen.

NURSING PRIORITIES AND MANAGEMENT: GYNAECOMASTIA

?	**7.12** What effect might the overdevelopment of breast tissue have on a man?

Giving psychological support

Breasts are considered to be a female characteristic, and for this reason the overdevelopment of breast tissue in a man may cause an altered body image and emotional distress. Some men with gynaecomastia believe they have lost their masculinity and experience anxiety and depression as a result. When gynaecomastia occurs in adolescence such feelings may be particularly acute.

The nurse must be sensitive to such feelings and show her understanding of them. It may be difficult for a man to express these feelings to a female nurse, especially if she is relatively young, but he is more likely to do so within a professional relationship where trust exists. A clear explanation of why the breast tissue has developed and of any treatment that may be given will be essential.

REFERENCES

Atkins H, Hayward J L, Klugman D J, Wayte A B 1972 Treatment of early breast cancer: a report after ten years of a clinical trial. British Medical Journal 2: 423–429

Baum M 1988 Breast cancer: the facts. Oxford University Press, Oxford

Boore J R R 1978 Prescription for recovery. Royal College of Nursing, London

Cancer Research Campaign 1991 Factsheets 6.1 and 6.2: Breast Cancer

Clifford E 1979 The reconstructive experience: the search for restitution. In: Georgiade N G (ed) Breast reconstruction following mastectomy. Mosby, St Louis

Coleman D J, Foo I T H, Sharpe D T 1991 Textured or smooth implants for breast reconstruction? A prospective controlled trial. British Journal of Plastic Surgery 44: 444–448

Dean A, Chelty N, Forrest A P M 1983 Effects of immediate breast reconstruction on psychosocial morbidity after mastectomy. Lancet i (Feb): 459–462

Denton S, Baum M 1983 Psychosocial aspects of breast cancer. In: Margolese R (ed) Breast cancer. Churchill Livingstone, Edinburgh

DHSS 1986 Breast cancer screening: The Forrest report. HMSO, London

Durning P, Sellwood R A 1982 Bromocriptine in severe cyclical breast pain. British Journal of Surgery 69: 248–249

Early Breast Cancer Trialists' Collaborative Group 1988 Effects of adjuvant tamoxifen and of cytotoxic therapy on mortality in early breast cancer. New England Journal of Medicine 319(26): 1681–1692

Fallowfield L J, Baum M, Maguire G P 1986 Effects of breast conservation on psychological morbidity associated with diagnosis and treatment of early breast cancer. British Medical Journal 293: 1331–1335

Fisher B, Redmond C, Poisson R et al 1989 Eight year results of a randomized clinical trial comparing total mastectomy and lumpectomy with or without irradiation in the treatment of breast cancer. New England Journal of Medicine 320: 822–828

Goin M K, Goin J M 1988 Growing pains: the psychological experience of breast reconstruction with tissue expansion. Annals of Plastic Surgery 21(3)

Goldberg P, Stolzmann M, Goldberg H M 1984 Psychological considerations in breast reconstruction. Annals of Plastic Surgery 13(38)

Hayward J 1975 Information: a prescription against pain. RCN, London

King's Fund Forum 1986 Consensus development conference: treatment of primary breast cancer. British Medical Journal 293: 946–947

Maguire P, Lee E G, Bevington D J et al 1978 Psychiatric problems in the first year after mastectomy. British Medical Journal (15 April): 963–965

Maguire P, Tait A, Brooke M, Thomas C, Sellwood R 1980 Effect of counselling on the psychiatric morbidity associated with mastectomy. British Medical Journal 281: 1454–1456

Mansel R E, Wisby J R, Hughes L E 1982 Controlled trial of antigonadotrophin danazol in painful nodular benign breast disease. Lancet i: 928–931

McKinna A 1983 Clinical features of breast disease. In: Parsons C A (ed) Diagnosis of breast disease. Chapman & Hall, London

Meyer L, Aspegren K 1989 Long term psychological sequelae of mastectomy and breast conserving treatment for breast cancer. Acta Oncologica 28: 13–18

Meyer L, Ringberg A 1986 A prospective study of psychiatric and psychosocial sequelae of bilateral subcutaneous mastectomy. Scandinavian Journal of Plastic Reconstructive Surgery 20: 101–107

Morris T M, Greer H S, White P 1977 Psychological and social adjustment to mastectomy: a two-year follow-up study. Cancer 40: 2381–2387

Morris T 1979 Psychological adjustment to mastectomy. Cancer Treatment Reviews 6: 41–61

Northouse L 1989 The impact of breast cancer on patients and husbands. Cancer Nursing 12(5): 276–284

Page D L, Anderson T J 1987 Diagnostic histopathology of the breast. Churchill Livingstone, Edinburgh

Pashby N L, Mansel R E, Hughes L E et al 1981 A clinical trial of evening primrose oil in mastalgia. British Journal of Surgery 68: 801

Regnard C, Badger C, Mortimer P 1988 Lymphoedema: advice and treatment. Beaconsfield Publishers, Beaconsfield

Salter M 1988 Altered body image: the nurse's role. Wiley, Chichester

Shapiro S, Venet W, Strax P, Venet L, Roeser R 1982 Ten to fourteen year effect of breast cancer screening on mortality. Journal of the National Cancer Institute 69: 349–355

Simpson G 1985 Are you being served? Senior Nurse 2(6): 14–16

Tabar L, Gad A, Holmberg L H et al 1985 Reduction in mortality from breast cancer after mass screening with mammography: randomized trial from breast cancer screening working group of Swedish National Board of Health and Welfare. Lancet i: 829–832

Tait A, Maguire P, Faulkner A et al 1982 Improving communication skills. Nursing Times 22(9): 2181–2184

UK National Case-Control Study Group 1989 Oral contraceptive use and breast cancer in young women. Lancet (May 6): 978–982

Veronesi U, Saccozi R, Del Vecchio M et al 1981 Comparing radical mastectomy with quadrantectomy, axillary dissection and radiotherapy in patients with small cancer of the breast. New England Journal of Medicine 305(1): 6–12

Veronesi U, Banfi A, Salvadori B et al 1990 Breast conservation is the treatment of choice in small breast cancer: long term results of a randomized trial. European Journal of Cancer 26(6): 668–670

Watson M, Denton S, Baum M, Greer S 1988 Counselling breast cancer patients: a specialist nurse service. Counselling Psychology Quarterly 1(1): 25–34

Wellisch D K, Jamieson K K, Pasnan R C 1978 Psychosocial aspects of mastectomy II: the man's perspective. American Journal of Psychiatry 135: 534

FURTHER READING

Balhere 1982 Breast cancer. Clinical Oncology International Practice and Treatment 2(1)

Blamey R W 1986 Complications in the management of breast disease. Bailliere Tindall, London

Bostwick J 1987 Breast reconstruction after mastectomy. In: Harris J R et al (eds) Breast diseases. Lippincott, Philadelphia

Faulder C 1985 Whose body is it? Virago Press, London

Gateley C A, Mansel R E 1990 Management of cyclical breast pain. British Journal of Hospital Medicine 43: 330–332

Lamb M A, Woods N F 1984 Sexuality and the cancer patient. Cancer Nursing 4: 137–144

Margolese R (ed) 1983 Breast cancer. Churchill Livingstone, Edinburgh

Marks-Maran D J, Pope B M 1985 Breast cancer nursing and counselling. Blackwell Scientific, Oxford

Pfeiffer C H, Mulliken B 1984 Caring for the patient with breast cancer. Reston Publishing, Reston

Sims R, Fitzgerald V 1985 Community nursing management of the patient with ulcerating fungating malignant breast disease. Royal College of Nursing, London

Tiffany R, Borley D (ed) 1989 Oncology for nurses and health care professionals, 2nd edn. Vol. 3: Cancer nursing. Harper & Row, Beaconsfield

USEFUL ADDRESSES

BACUP (British Association of Cancer United Patients)
121–123 Charterhouse Street
London EC1M 6AA

Breast Care and Mastectomy Association of Great Britain
15–19 Britten Street
London SW3 3TZ
helpline: 071–867 1103

Publications: 'Living with Breast Surgery', *Coping with Cancer;* 'Looking Good after Breast Surgery', 'Coping with Breast Surgery' (cassette tape)

Royal Marsden Hospital
Fulham Road
London SW3 6JJ

CHAPTER 8

The urinary system

Maureen Morrison   Theyaga Shandran   Frances Smithers

Josephine N. Fawcett (Additional material and advice)

CHAPTER CONTENTS

Introduction 291

Anatomy and physiology 291

DISORDERS OF THE URINARY SYSTEM 296

Urinary tract infections 296
Nursing priorities and management: acute pyelonephritis 297
Nursing priorities and management: chronic pyelonephritis 298

Obstructive disorders of the urinary tract 298
Nursing priorities and management: acute renal colic 302
Nursing priorities and management: urethral strictures 304

Disorders of the penis and male urethra 305
Nursing priorities and management: phimosis 305

Disorders of the prostate 306
Nursing priorities and management: benign prostatic hyperplasia 307
Nursing priorities and management: carcinoma of the prostate 312

Disorders of the bladder 313
Nursing priorities and management: total cystectomy and urinary diversion 315

Renal disorders 316
Nursing priorities and management: glomerulonephritis 318
Nursing priorities and management: acute renal failure 320
Nursing priorities and management: chronic renal failure 321

References 323

Further reading 323

INTRODUCTION

The practice of urology as a specialism in its own right is now commonplace in many general hospitals. Many patients that once would have been treated by a general surgeon are now referred to consultants in urology. This has come about partly in response to advances in technology, especially in the field of endoscopic and laser surgery. It has also become an accepted view that patients with urological disorders deserve the same level of understanding and sensitivity as those with gynaecological problems.

The movement within nursing toward patient-centred care in combination with the evolution of new, less traumatic and non-invasive treatments has allowed more individuals to be treated as outpatients or day cases. The appointment of specialist stoma care nurses and continence advisors has also done much to improve standards of care.

It is important for nurses to bear in mind that patients with urological disorders often suffer from intense psychological distress. Nurses in this area of practice must develop good interpersonal skills so that they can discuss problems openly, sensitively and non-judgementally.

This chapter begins with a brief overview of the anatomy and physiology of the urinary system and of the male reproductive organs. With respect to the latter, this chapter complements the anatomy and physiology described in Chapter 7. Common disorders of the urinary tract and their treatment are then described, including infections, obstructive disorders, disorders of the bladder, and some of the more important renal disorders. With regard to the male urinary system and reproductive organs, only prostatic disorders and conditions primarily affecting the urethra are considered here. Conditions more directly affecting reproductive and sexual function, such as testicular cancer and impotence, are discussed in Chapter 7.

ANATOMY AND PHYSIOLOGY

The urinary system comprises the kidneys, the ureters, the urinary bladder and the urethra. Its function is to excrete in the form of urine the waste products of metabolism.

The kidneys

Structure

The kidneys are a pair of slightly lobulated organs which lie on the posterior abdominal wall. Because of the position of the liver, the right kidney is normally slightly lower than the left. Anteriorly, the kidneys are covered by the peritoneum and the contents of the abdominal cavity. Three layers of supportive tissue surround each kidney: an inner fibrous layer, a middle fatty layer, and an outer fascia. This fatty encasement is necessary for maintaining the kidneys in their normal position. Beneath this a dark outer cortex surrounds a paler medulla, which consists of pale conical striations called the renal pyramids (see Fig. 8.1).

At the hilus, i.e. the concave medial border of the kidney, blood vessels, lymph vessels and nerves enter and leave the organ. Medial to the hilus is the flat, funnel-shaped renal pelvis, which is continuous with the ureter leaving the hilus. Extending from the pelvis into the medulla are the cupped-shaped calyces; these receive from the renal papillae the urine that has been formed in the nephrons and has passed through the collecting tubules. From the calyces the urine passes into the renal pelvis, which acts as a reservoir.

The nephron. Each kidney is composed of about 1 million functional units called nephrons, which channel urine into collecting tubules. A nephron consists of a convoluted tubular system and a tuft of capillaries known as the glomerulus. The glomerulus is enclosed in the cup-shaped upper end of the tubule (Bowman's capsule; see Fig. 8.2).

The tubule has three sections: the proximal convoluted tubule, which is the longest segment; the loop of Henle, which forms a hairpin-shaped curve; and the distal convoluted tubule. The distal convoluted tubules merge to form straight collecting tubules; these ultimately terminate at the renal papillae. Some nephrons lie entirely within the cortex; others lie further within the organ such that the tubules extend deep into the medulla.

Blood supply. The kidney is supplied with blood by renal arteries arising directly from either side of the abdominal aorta immediately below the superior mesenteric artery. The renal arteries branch into smaller and smaller vessels, ultimately becoming afferent arterioles which lead into the nephrons. Each afferent arteriole subdivides further into a glomerulus. These capillaries then merge again to form an efferent arteriole which leaves the capsule and subdivides into a second network of peritubular capillaries which supplies the proximal and distal tubules, the loop of Henle and the collecting ducts. The capillaries merge into venules and then veins, eventually joining the renal vein, which in turn flows into the vena cava.

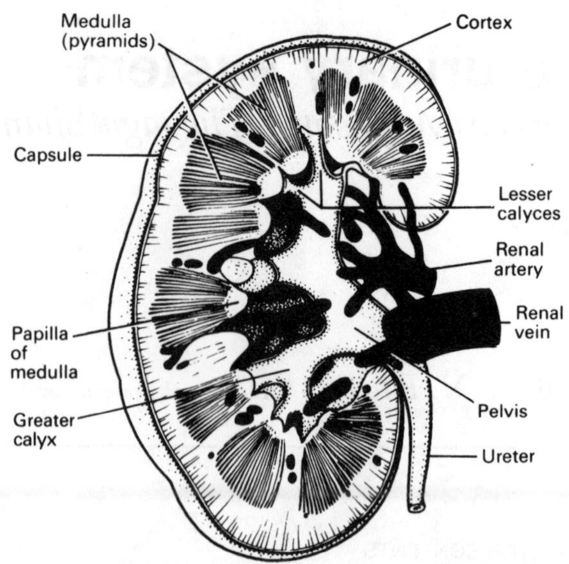

Fig. 8.1 Longitudinal section of the right kidney. (Reproduced with permission from Wilson 1990.)

Function

The kidneys process about 180 l of blood-derived fluid daily. Of this only about 1–2 l actually leaves the body as urine; the remainder is returned to the blood. The kidney's basic function of producing urine takes place in the nephron. Here, the processes of glomerular filtration, tubular reabsorption and tubular secretion result in the removal of wastes and toxins from the blood as it passes through the kidney (Marieb 1989). The characteristics of normal urine are summarised in Box 8.1.

Glomerular filtration. The initial filtration of blood takes place across a semipermeable membrane in which fluid, electrolytes and certain non-electrolytes pass into the Bowman's capsule. Filtrate formation is a passive process and follows the same principles that account for all tissue fluid formation (see Ch. 20). However, the glomerulus is

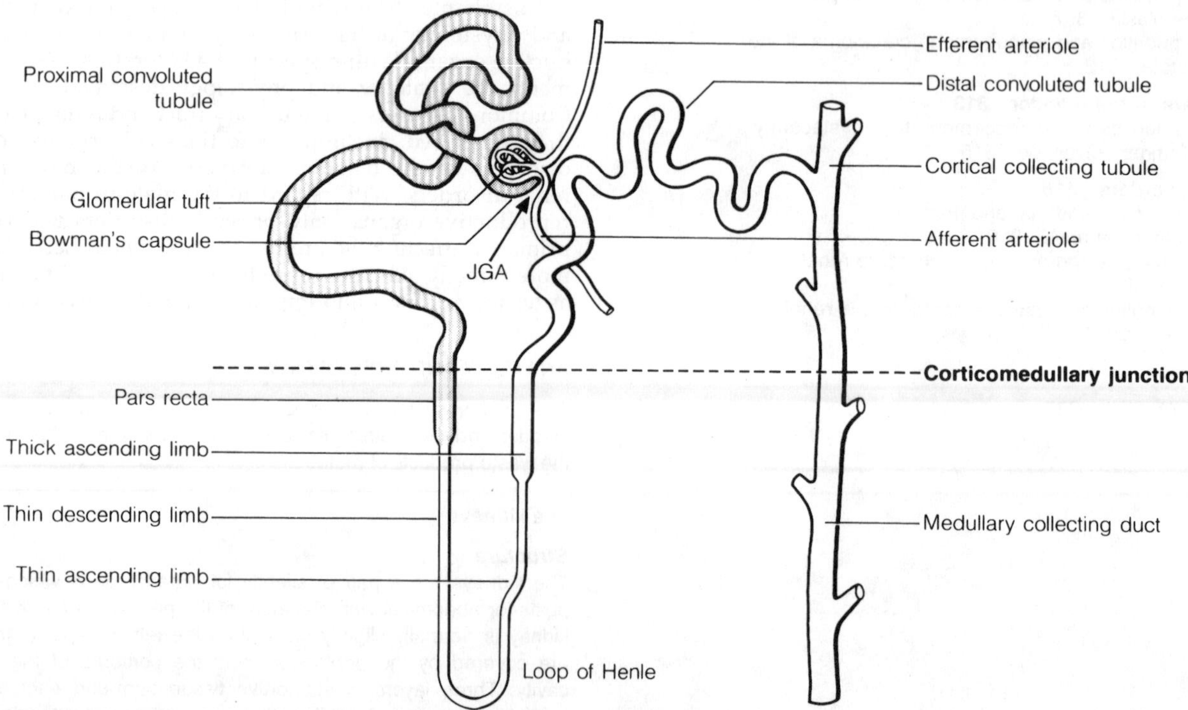

Fig. 8.2 Nephron with long loop of Henle (deep nephron). (Reproduced with permission from Edwards & Bouchier 1991.)

Box 8.1 Physical characteristics of urine (Adapted from Anthony & Thibodeau 1983.)

Volume (24 h)	1500 ml, but varies greatly according to fluid intake and insensible losses
Clarity	Transparent or clear; on standing, becomes cloudy
Colour	Amber or straw-coloured; varies according to amount voided; diet may change colour (e.g. reddish colour from eating beetroot)
Odour	'Characteristic'; on standing, develops pungent odour from formation of ammonium carbonate
Reaction	Acid, but may become alkaline if diet consists largely of vegetables. A high-protein diet increases acidity. Stale urine has alkaline reaction from decomposition of urea forming ammonium carbonate. Normal range for urine pH is 4.8–7.5, with the average about 6; it rarely becomes more acid then 4.5 or more alkaline than 8.
Specific gravity	1.015–1.020; highest in morning specimen

CHEMICAL COMPOSITION

Urine is approximately 95% water, in which is dissolved several kinds of substances. The most important of these are:

1. Nitrogenous wastes from protein metabolism such as urea (most abundant solute in urine), uric acid, ammonia, and creatinine
2. Electrolytes, mainly the following ions: sodium, potassium, ammonium, chloride, bicarbonate, phosphate, and sulphate; the amounts vary according to diet and other factors
3. Toxins. During disease, bacterial poisons leave the body in the urine; this is an important reason for 'pushing' fluids on patients suffering from infectious diseases, as a high fluid intake dilutes the toxins that might damage the kidney cells if they were eliminated in a concentrated form
4. Pigments
5. Hormones
6. Abnormal constituents such as glucose, albumin, blood, casts or calculi are sometimes found.

much more efficient because the filtration membrane is highly permeable and the glomerular pressure much higher than in other capillary beds. Hence the kidneys are able to produce 180 l of fluid daily, as compared to the 3 l daily produced by other capillary beds in the body.

The chemical composition of the glomerular filtrate is identical to that of plasma, with the following exceptions:

1. The formed elements of blood are absent, i.e. red and white blood cells and platelets
2. Plasma proteins are absent. (The presence of protein in the urine can therefore be an indication of abnormality.)

In order for glomerular filtration to take place there must be adequate blood volume in the intravascular space and sufficient glomerular hydrostatic pressure. It is the glomerular hydrostatic pressure that essentially forces the water and solutes across the filtration membrane. This pressure (55 mmHg) is opposed by the colloid osmotic pressure exerted by the glomerular plasma proteins (30 mmHg) and the capsular hydrostatic pressure (15 mmHg). Thus the net filtration pressure responsible for filtrate formation is 10 mmHg. The rate at which fluid filters from the blood to the glomerular capsule is directly proportional to the net filtration pressure. The normal filtration rate is 120–125 ml/min.

Tubular reabsorption. The greater part of reabsorption takes place in the proximal convoluted tubule. Sodium, chloride, bicarbonate and potassium are by passive or active transport returned to the blood. Glucose is actively reabsorbed. Normally, all of the glucose is reabsorbed such that none appears in the urine. However, if blood levels of glucose are too high some will be excreted in the urine.

About 99% of the water in the filtrate is reabsorbed. The continuous removal of sodium, chloride, bicarbonate, glucose and other materials from the tubule increases the osmotic forces such that water follows the dissolved materials. This is often referred to as obligatory water reabsorption.

One of the major functions of the kidney is to maintain a constant concentration of body fluids by regulating urine concentration. It is still uncertain exactly how this is achieved, but it would seem to be the result of the function of the loop of Henle, which may function as a 'counter-current multiplying system' in which the concentration of sodium and negative ions move through a gradient, being greatest at the base of the loop. This allows the urine to be more dilute leaving the loop of Henle than when it left the proximal tubule. This dilute urine remains essentially unaltered unless the need to conserve fluid results in the release of antidiuretic hormone (vasopressin) by the posterior pituitary (see p. 134).

For further information, see Marieb (1989), Ch. 26.

Tubular secretion. In the distal convoluted tubule and the collecting duct sodium is reabsorbed from the tubular fluid while hydrogen and potassium ions are secreted into the fluid. This helps to regulate acid–base balance and rid the body of excessive potassium. In addition, tubular secretion can eliminate substances such as urea and uric acid, which may have been returned to the blood by passive processes, and can also dispose of substances not already in the filtrate, for example certain drugs.

Hormonal control of the kidney

Two hormones, antidiuretic hormone (vasopressin) and aldosterone, are important regulators of renal function.

Antidiuretic hormone (ADH) (vasopressin) is produced in the hypothalamus and stored and secreted by the posterior lobe of the pituitary gland. It acts upon the distal convoluted tubule and the collecting ducts, allowing sodium, other ions, and water to be reabsorbed, making the urine more concentrated. In the absence of ADH, sodium and other ions are reabsorbed, but not water. This makes the urine more dilute.

Pain, exercise, emotion, and the use of narcotics or barbiturates can increase the secretion of ADH. Factors that decrease output are low plasma osmotic pressure, venous distension and alcohol consumption.

Aldosterone is produced in the outermost layer of the adrenal cortex. It acts on the distal tubule, where it increases the reabsorption of sodium (see Ch. 5, p. 137).

Other functions of the kidney

In addition to its role in removing waste products from the blood the kidney has the following functions:

1. It helps to regulate blood pressure through the maintenance of fluid volume
2. It produces the hormones renin, erythropoietin and 1,25-dihydroxycholecalciferol.

Renin is liberated through the juxtaglomerular cells and acts on angiotensinogen (a glycoprotein made in the liver and normally found in plasma), converting it into angiotensin I. Another enzyme in the pulmonary capillary bed acts on angiotensin I to convert it into angiotensin II. Angiotensin II has the following functions:

1. It stimulates the release of aldosterone, which helps to enable sodium reabsorption and therefore water reabsorption. This in turn helps to maintain plasma volume.
2. It has a powerful vasoconstricting effect, acting on the arterioles and precapillary sphincters to shut down the capillaries, allowing blood volume to be maintained.

Erythropoietin is produced in response to lowered O_2 in the blood. It acts on the bone marrow, stimulating the production of red blood cells (erythropoiesis; see Ch. 11, p. 407).

1,25-dihydroxycholecalciferol is synthesised in the renal tubule cells and is the active form of vitamin D which enables calcium uptake from the small intestine (see Box 5.1, p. 137).

The ureters (see Fig. 8.3)

Urine is conveyed from the pelvis of each kidney to the bladder via the ureters. The ureters are tubular structures approximately 30 cm long, ranging in diameter from 2 to 8 cm at various points along their length.

Each ureter descends behind the peritoneum from the renal hilus to the level of the bladder, and comes obliquely through the bladder wall before opening into the bladder cavity on its posterior inner surface. This arrangement is such that when the bladder fills or empties the bladder is compressed, closing the distal ends of the ureters, and no backflow into the ureters occurs.

Each ureter is composed of three layers of tissue:

- an outer fibrous layer which is continuous with the fibrous renal capsule
- a middle layer consisting of muscle fibres spiralling clockwise and anticlockwise. Contraction of the muscle layer produces peristaltic movement of urine along the ureter into the bladder
- an inner mucosa of transitional epithelium.

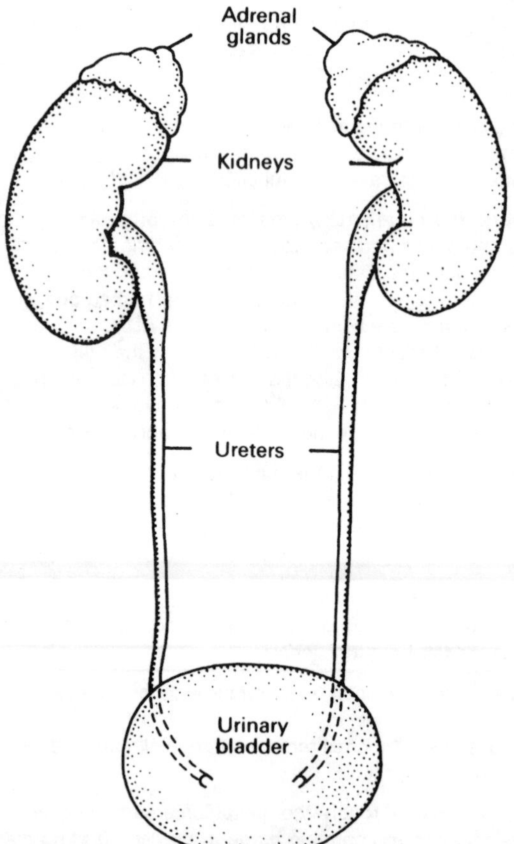

Fig. 8.3 The ureters and their relationship to the kidneys and the bladder. (Reproduced with permission from Wilson 1990.)

The urinary bladder

The bladder is a muscular sac which acts as a reservoir for urine before it is expelled from the body. It lies behind the peritoneum in the pelvic cavity, with its anterior surface located just behind the symphysis pubis. In the male the bladder lies in front of the rectum, inferiorly to the urethra and the prostate gland. In the female it lies just anterior to the ureters and the superior section of the vagina.

Structure

The bladder is composed of four layers: an outer fibrous adventitia (except where the peritoneum covers the superior surface); a muscular layer; a submucosal layer of connective tissue; and a mucosal layer of transitional epithelium. The muscle layer consists of intermingled smooth muscle arranged in inner and outer longitudinal layers and a middle circular layer and is called the detrusor muscle.

The interior of the bladder has three orifices, two for the ureters and one for the opening of the urethra. This forms a triangle called the trigone (see Fig. 8.4).

Nerve supply to the bladder is both sensory and motor. Sympathetic nerves arise from T9 to L2 and parasympathetic somatic nerves from S2 to S4. The motor innervation involves the parasympathetic supply to the detrusor muscle and the sympathetic supply to the trigone. Pudendal nerves under voluntary control supply the external sphincter and muscles of the perineum.

The urethra

The urethra is a tube 8–9 mm in diameter which extends from the neck of the bladder to the exterior. In the male it is about 21 cm long and in the female about 4 cm long. It has an outer layer of smooth muscle continuous with that of the bladder. Beneath this lies a thin, spongy layer supplied with blood vessels, lymph vessels and nerves. The innermost layer is a lining of mucous membrane continuous with that of the bladder.

The male urethra is a shared pathway by which both urine and semen reach the exterior. Originating at the urethral orifice in the bladder neck, it is surrounded by the prostate gland and ends at the tip of the glans penis. It is lined with a large number of small mucus-producing glands (Littre's glands). It has an internal sphincter composed of smooth muscle which responds to parasympathetic and sympathetic stimulation. The external urethral sphincter lies at the

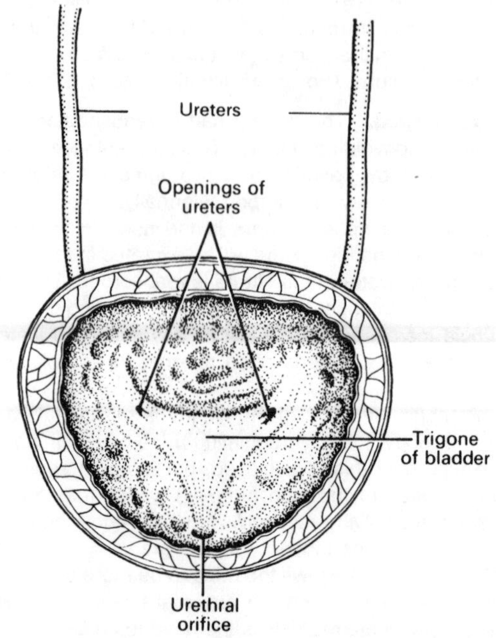

Fig. 8.4 The trigone. (Reproduced with permission from Wilson 1990.)

point where the urethra leaves the prostate; this sphincter is composed of skeletal muscle and is hence under voluntary control.

The female urethra runs behind the symphysis pubis, opening at the external urethral orifice (the meatus) just in front of the vagina. The passage of urine from the bladder through the urethra is governed by two sphincter muscles. At the opening from the bladder is an internal sphincter composed mainly of elastic tissue and smooth muscle and controlled by autonomic nerves. Near the external urethral orifice the smooth muscle is replaced by striated muscle to form an external sphincter under voluntary control.

Micturition

Micturition, the act of passing urine, is a complex physiological process governed by a number of neural controls. The bladder is very distensible, as is necessary for the storing of urine. When empty the bladder is no more than 5–8 cm long, and its walls are thick, falling into folds. As urine fills the bladder it expands to accommodate the increasing quantity of fluid. The muscle walls stretch and become thinner such that the bladder can comfortably hold 500 ml of urine. In extremis the bladder could hold more than 1 l. If this occurs it can be palpated above the symphysis pubis.

When the bladder contains 200–300 ml of urine nerve fibres in the bladder wall which are sensitive to stretch are stimulated (Wilson 1990). In the infant or young child this triggers a spinal reflex which results in contraction of the bladder muscle and relaxation of the internal urethral sphincter. When the nervous system is more mature the individual is aware of a desire to pass urine and can inhibit the reflex action for a time.

Micturition is normally a painless function that occurs 4–6 times during the day. Decreased bladder capacity and weakened sphincter and detrusor muscles can in elderly people and others necessitate voiding once or twice during the night.

The composition of urine is described in Box 8.1.

?	**8.1** Keep a fluid balance chart for yourself over a 24-h period. Record all your fluid intake and the amount and frequency of all urine output. In addition, record your activities for this period. Then compare your results with those of your colleagues. If possible, also compare your results with a patient's fluid balance chart.

The male reproductive organs

The male reproductive organs are those structures responsible for the production, the maturation, and the delivery into the female reproductive tract of spermatozoa necessary for the fertilisation of ova. The essential organs of this system are the two testes, in which spermatogenesis occurs. The accessory organs which support the reproductive process include:

- the genital ducts: the epididymis (2), vas deferens (2), ejaculatory ducts (2) and urethra, which convey sperm to the exterior
- the glands: the seminal vesicles (2), the prostate gland, and the bulbourethral (Cowper's) glands (2), which produce fluid as a vehicle for sperm
- the supporting structures: the scrotum, penis and spermatic cords.

The essential organs

The testes are oval organs 4–5 cm in length weighing 10–15 g each. They are suspended in the scrotum by the spermatic cords and are encased in three layers of tissue, as follows:

- the tunica vaginalis, or outer layer: a downgrowth of the abdominal and pelvic peritoneum
- the tunica albuginea: a layer beneath the tunica vaginalis which consists of fibroelastic connective tissue containing some smooth muscle cells
- the tunica vasculosa: an inner layer made up of delicate connective tissue and supplied by a network of capillaries.

Each testis contains 200–300 lobes, within which are tightly-coiled seminiferous tubules. It is here that the primitive sex cells (spermatagonia) present in male babies at birth become transformed into spermatozoa (spermatogenesis). This process starts at puberty and continues throughout life.

A spermatozoon provides one half of the genetic material required to create a new life. Each spermatozoon has a head, neck, body and tail, each with a specialised function. The head contains a highly compact package of genetic material encased in a specialised covering, called the acrosome, which contains digestive enzymes that can penetrate the ovum during fertilisation. The body contains mitochondria and the tail adenosine triphosphate ATP; these provide energy for sperm locomotion.

The testes also produce androgens (masculinising hormones), the most important of which is testosterone, which is produced by interstitial cells (Leydig's cells). Testosterone promotes:

- maleness and male sexual behaviour
- the development and maintenance of male secondary sex characteristics and the functions of the accessory organs
- protein anabolism
- growth of bone and skeletal muscle and closure of the bony epiphyses
- a mild stimulant effect on the kidney tubule, with reabsorption of sodium and water and excretion of potassium
- inhibition of anterior pituitary secretion of the gonadotropins follicle-stimulating hormone (FSH) and interstitial cell stimulating hormone (ICSH). FSH stimulates the seminiferous tubules of the testes to produce spermatozoa. A negative feedback mechanism operates whereby when testosterone levels are high FSH and ICSH production is inhibited.

At the upper pole of the testis the tubules combine to form the Rete testis and then penetrate the tunica vaginalis to empty into the epididymis. The epididymis leaves the scrotum as the deferent duct (vas deferens) through the spermatic cords. The testes are well supplied with blood, lymph vessels and nerves from both divisions of the autonomic nervous system.

The ductal system

The epididymis is the first part of the ductal system and forms a collection of tubules arising from the testis. The vas deferens, which is continuous with the epididymis, loops through the inguinal canal and joins the ejaculatory ducts, which pass through the prostate gland and lead into the urethra (see Fig. 8.5).

Sperm undergo a ripening process as they pass through the ductal system before ejaculation. They remain in the vas deferens for varying periods of time, depending upon the individual's degree of sexual activity. Sperm may remain in storage in the vas deferens for more than a month with no loss of fertility.

The accessory glands

The seminal vesicles are small, lobulated glands lined with secretory epithelium which lie to the posterior of the bladder at the base of the prostate. The lower end of each vesicle opens into a short duct, which joins with the deferent duct to form the ejaculatory duct.

The seminal vesicles secrete a thick, nutritive alkaline fluid that mixes with sperm on ejaculation. This fluid accounts for 30% of the volume of the seminal fluid and contains fructose and protein, which are essential to sperm motility and metabolism.

The prostate gland is a lobulated structure which lies in the pelvic cavity in front of the rectum and behind the symphysis pubis, surrounding the uppermost part of the urethra. It is palpable on rectal examination. The prostate gland secretes a thin, milky, alkaline fluid that makes up 60% of the seminal fluid; this fluid creates an environment more hospitable to sperm by giving protection from the normally acidic environment of the male urethra and female vagina. A neutral or slightly alkaline medium also increases sperm motility.

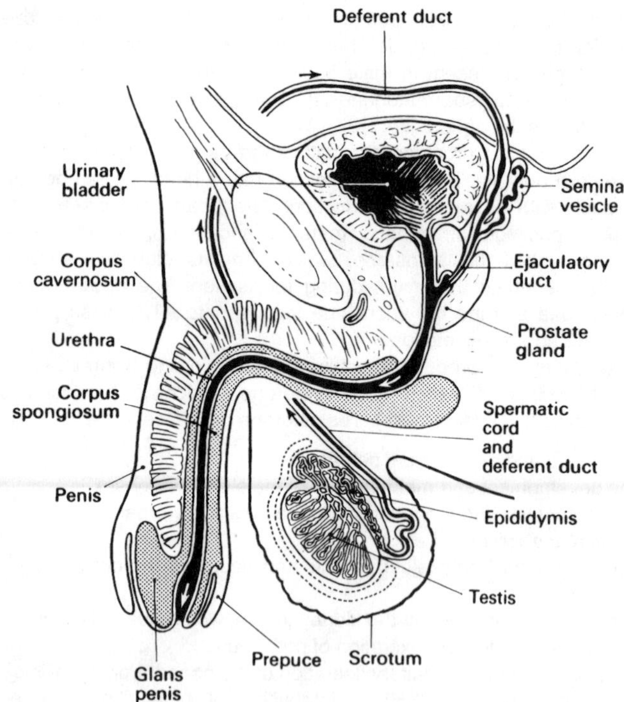

Fig. 8.5 Section of male reproductive organs. Arrows show the structures through which the spermatozoa pass. (Reproduced with permission from Wilson 1990.)

The prostate is susceptible to hyperplasia, which because of its proximity to the urethra can lead to urinary problems (see p. 306).

The bulbourethral glands are two pea-sized glands opening onto either side of the urethra. They produce a lubricating alkaline mucus that is expressed into the urethra during ejaculation, reducing its typically acidic state, and contribute less than 5% to the volume of seminal fluid.

The supporting structures

The penis is a pendulous, soft-tissue structure with a root and a body. The root lies in the perineum and is attached to the anterior and lateral walls of the pubic arch. The body, which surrounds the urethra, consists of three elongated masses of erectile tissue and involuntary muscle.

The erectile tissue is supported by fibrous tissue and covered with skin. The three elongated masses, which are longitudinal in shape, consist of an encompassing central column (the corpus spongiosum) containing the urethra and two parallel columns (the corpora cavernosa), which provide the organ's main structural support. These structures are richly supplied with blood vessels.

At the distal end of the penis the corpus spongiosum and the corpora cavernosa expand to become the glans penis, which surrounds the urethral meatus. The covering of skin folds upon itself at the glans penis to form a movable double layer called the prepuce.

Coitus and fertilisation. The penis is supplied by autonomic and somatic nerves. Tactile, visual or mental stimulation causes a parasympathetic reflex leading to engorgement of the penis with blood and consequent erection. In the next phase, emission, sperm and secretions from the accessory glands are deposited in the posterior urethra. Finally, during ejaculation, the bladder neck closes and is followed by relaxation of the distal sphincter mechanism and spasmodic contraction of the bulbourethral muscles. This forces semen out through the urethra in spurts and is accompanied by the intensely pleasurable sensation of orgasm. Once ejaculation has taken place the corpora cavernosa and the corpus spongiosum empty their excess of blood, and the penis resumes its flaccid state.

The sperm, although anatomically complete and highly motile, undergo a further maturation process referred to as capacitation after introduction into the vagina. This enables the head of the sperm to use its hydrolytic (splitting) enzymes to penetrate the encasing membrane (the zona pellucida) of the ovum.

The millions of sperm ejaculated act collectively to produce hyaluronidase to liquify the intracellular substance surrounding the ovum. This mass action is necessary for a single sperm to penetrate the ovum and bring about fertilisation.

The scrotum is a thin-walled pouch continuous with the abdominal wall. It is deeply pigmented and divided into two compartments, each of which contains one testis, one epididymis and the testicular end of the spermatic cord. The temperature of the testes is 2–3°C below body temperature; this helps to preserve sperm viability.

The spermatic cords. Leading from each testis is a spermatic cord consisting of a testicular artery, a testicular venous plexus, lymph vessels, a deferent duct (vas deferens) and nerves; these are all surrounded by a fibrous connective sheath.

DISORDERS OF THE URINARY SYSTEM

URINARY TRACT INFECTIONS

Urinary tract infections are second only to respiratory infections in incidence. If bacterial as opposed to viral infections are considered, the urinary tract is the most commonly infected organ system (Corriere 1986).

Infection can occur in both the upper and lower urinary tract. The risk of developing a urinary tract infection varies throughout life. In childhood and adulthood urinary infections are common in females; however, they are rarely seen in adolescents. In the over-60 age group urinary infections are more common in men, and are often associated with bladder outflow obstruction and with the presence of a urinary catheter (Brocklehurst 1989).

The onset of urinary infections in women is often related to the onset and frequency of sexual intercourse (Edwards & Bouchier 1991). In healthy individuals, bacteriuria of the lower urinary tract increases transiently following sexual intercourse.

PATHOPHYSIOLOGY

Normally, the anterior urethra and, in women, the entrance to the vagina contain microorganisms. The posterior urethra and the urinary tract are sterile. The urethral mucosa has antibacterial properties and is frequently washed by sterile urine which discourages the passage of bacteria up the urethra to the bladder, ureters and kidneys. The female ureter is short, wide and straight, and allows the passage of organisms into the urinary tract, more readily than in the longer male ureter.

The predisposing factors for urinary tract infections are as follows:

1. Vesico-ureteric reflux
   a. Congenital primary reflux. This occurs when there is a defect of the muscles around the vesico-ureteric junction (i.e. junction of the bladder and ureter). Abnormalities such as duplication and ectopic ureters can give rise to vesico-ureteric reflux and are one of the major causes of primary and recurrent infections in children (Forrest et al 1991).
   b. Acquired reflux. This may be seen in patients with neuropathic dysfunction, urethral valves, and (more rarely) in those with bladder outflow obstruction due to strictures. Injury to the ureteric orifice during surgery may also result in reflux. Tuberculosis and interstitial cystitis are other causes.
2. Obstruction. Stones or strictures can prevent the free flow of urine

and interfere with the ability of the kidneys to decontaminate themselves of organisms.

a. Tumours of the prostate, bladder and kidney can give rise to urinary tract infections.
b. Pregnancy. Hydroureter (distension of the ureter with urine) and hydronephrosis (distension of the kidney pelvis) can occur during pregnancy and persist for some months after childbirth. It is caused by relaxation of the muscles due to the high level of progesterone and by the obstruction of the ureters by the uterus.
c. Intubation. Nephrostomy tubes inserted into the kidney pelvis, urethral or suprapubic catheters and other drainage tubes that communicate with the urinary tract predispose the individual to infection.

3. Fistulae. Abnormal communication between the urinary tract and other structures (especially between the bladder and the colon) will allow organisms to enter the urinary tract.
4. Sexual trauma. During sexual intercourse the female urethra can be traumatised. The movement of the penis in the vagina may also milk organisms along it into the bladder and cause infection. Varied sexual practices, inadequate personal hygiene and the use of foreign bodies can all play a part.
5. Iatrogenic factors. Surgical and diagnostic procedures such as urethral and ureteric catheterisation, cystoscopy and other endoscopic instrumentations may exacerbate existing infections or send infection further up the urinary tract.

Pyelonephritis

Pyelonephritis, or inflammation of the renal pelvis, may occur in one or both kidneys. Bacteria may enter the urinary tract, especially the kidneys, via the bloodstream, or more commonly the bladder. Most organisms causing urinary tract infection are found in the bowel and the perineum. They are Escherichia coli, Klebsiella, Proteus, Pseudomonas, Streptococcus faecali and Staphylococcus albus.

Acute pyelonephritis

PATHOPHYSIOLOGY

In acute pyelonephritis the kidney is usually swollen and soft and the pelvis and calyces may contain pus. The mucosal lining of the pelvis may be congested and oedematous.

Common presenting symptoms. The patient typically experiences a sudden onset of severe pain in the loin (the area of the back immediately above the buttocks) radiating to the iliac fossa. Other common features are pyrexia, rigor, nausea and vomiting.

Where cystitis (inflammation of the bladder) coexists, dysuria, frequency of micturition and discoloured urine will be noted.

MEDICAL MANAGEMENT

Investigative procedures will include the following:

- the collection of a midstream specimen of urine (MSU) to be cultured for evidence of a causative organism and antibiotic sensitivity. The specimen must be collected in clean conditions to prevent the introduction of contaminants (Jamieson et al 1992)
- a full blood count and urea and electrolyte estimation. A raised white blood cell count and erythrocyte sedimentation rate (ESR) may be revealed in response to infection
- an intravenous urogram (IVU) to locate any obstruction in the urinary tract (see Box 8.2). An ultrasound scan may also be performed for the same purpose.

> ? **8.2** While the patient is undergoing investigations, what might the nurse do or say to reduce anxiety and help him to understand the reasons for the tests?

Medical intervention. The main aim of treatment is to eradicate the infection by means of antibiotic therapy. This may be commenced even before organism sensitivities are known. A more specific antibiotic can then be used following urine culture results. Analgesics, antiemetics and antipyretics may be prescribed. Oral fluids c. 3 l/24 h.

In addition, the doctor will endeavour to determine and resolve any predisposing cause. Urine cultures will be repeated at 7 days to ensure that the infection has been eradicated.

Box 8.2 Intravenous urogram or pyelogram (IVU or IVP)

This investigation, which involves the i.v. injection of an iodine-based contrast medium which is then excreted by the kidneys, allows a series of X-ray pictures of the kidneys, ureters and bladder to be taken.

Prior to the IVU a control X-ray of the kidneys, ureters and bladder (KUB) is taken. The patient is requested to abstain from food and fluids several hours before the start of the X-rays. This helps the contrast medium to be excreted more quickly. The patient is also given an aperient to clear the bowel and thus ensure a clear image of the contrast medium on the X-ray.

Following the investigation, the patient is allowed to eat and drink again. The contrast medium will be passed when the patient voids urine, with no after-effects or change in the colour of the urine.

The IVU X-rays may show:

- absence of kidney
- obstruction of kidney
- obstruction of the ureter
- irregularities of the bladder wall. This finding may indicate the presence of a bladder tumour, diverticulum, calculi, or foreign body.

NURSING PRIORITIES AND MANAGEMENT: ACUTE PYELONEPHRITIS

Major considerations

The patient with acute pyelonephritis of sudden onset is likely to require nursing on bedrest; he will feel lethargic and may be unable to care for himself fully.

In the acute phase nursing priorities will include the administration of prescribed antibiotics and other medications. Attention should be given to the patient's personal hygiene and comfort, as well as to maintaining an accurate fluid balance record. Increasing fluid intake to as much as 3 l/24 h is to be encouraged as this may reduce the osmotic pressure in the renal medulla and thereby decrease the proliferation of bacteria (Pitt 1989).

As the patient recovers, the nurse should focus on giving advice regarding hygiene. The importance of attendance at outpatient appointments for assessment of renal function and investigation of further urine infection should be stressed. Follow-up may be particularly problematic if the patient feels well and is symptom free.

> ? **8.3** Mrs V is 6 months pregnant and has been admitted to the antenatal ward for investigation and monitoring of a raised blood pressure. Early one evening she complains of feeling very unwell and feverish and is visibly shivering. She is known to have a history of recurrent urinary tract infection. Refer now to Chapter 22. What would be your priorities for Mrs V's immediate care?

Chronic pyelonephritis

Chronic pyelonephritis results from recurrent urinary tract infection. In children, vesico-ureteric reflux is often present.

PATHOPHYSIOLOGY

Chronic pyelonephritis is focal and irregular and may affect both kidneys. Progressive infection causes fibrosis and scarring, which gradually destroys the parenchyma. Eventually, the kidney becomes small, granular and infected.

Common presenting symptoms. This condition may be asymptomatic until the patient finally presents with features associated with renal failure. These include uraemia, lethargy, hypertension and proteinuria. Urinary frequency and dysuria may be reported.

MEDICAL MANAGEMENT

Investigative procedures. As with acute pyelonephritis, diagnosis can be made by IVU. Urine culture should be performed and urinary tract obstruction excluded.

Medical intervention. Antibiotic treatment can be administered as either a short course in response to organism sensitivities or a long-term course where chronic infection proves difficult to eradicate. Where inflammation persists renal impairment may progress to end-stage renal failure requiring treatment by dialysis (see p. 321).

NURSING PRIORITIES AND MANAGEMENT: CHRONIC PYELONEPHRITIS

Major considerations

Where the patient experiences acute episodes of inflammation, priorities may be as those for patients with acute pyelonephritis. However, some individuals with chronic pyelonephritis only experience feelings of tiredness or of being 'under the weather'. Nevertheless, recurrence of infection is common and disturbances of renal function and end-stage renal failure are possibilities that must be taken seriously. The nurse should advise the patient of the importance of attending outpatient clinics for assessment even when he has no symptoms. Where long-term antibiotic therapy is required the patient may have concerns about the necessity for such treatment and the chronic nature of his condition. The nurse should provide the opportunity for the patient to ask questions and voice his concerns.

In the event that progressive renal failure occurs, the nurse should help to prepare the patient and his family for the treatment options available and for the lifestyle adjustments that will need to be made.

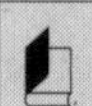
For further information, see Preshloch (1989).

Cystitis

Cystitis may be chronic or acute and is characterised by severe inflammation of the bladder walls. More commonly affecting women, cystitis may result from predisposing factors such as the presence of foreign bodies or stones, obstruction, tuberculosus, carcinoma in situ, chronic urinary infection and schistosomiasis.

PATHOPHYSIOLOGY

Common presenting features are scalding pain on micturition, often followed by bladder spasm resulting in an urge to pass urine a second time. Frequency, urgency, nocturia and incontinence may also be present. The patient may have a fever and complain of fatigue and abdominal discomfort.

MEDICAL MANAGEMENT

Investigative procedures. Urine culture will identify the causative organism, although antibiotic therapy may be commenced before sensitivities are known.

Medical intervention. Repeat urinary cultures should be examined. Persistent infection may require long-term antibiotic treatment. The patient should be encouraged to maintain a fluid intake of at least 3 l/24 h (Pitt 1989) and to void urine frequently. This may help to wash out contaminating bacteria. The measurement and recording of fluid balance, temperature and pulse are necessary until the patient's clinical symptoms are eradicated.

Many people, however, suffer from recurrent cystitis over several years and attempt to manage the associated problems, often depending on such things as lemon barley water, over-the-counter (OTC) preparations, and advice found in popular magazines. This is an example of a condition for which self-help often plays an important role.

For further information, see Kilmartin (1989).

OBSTRUCTIVE DISORDERS OF THE URINARY TRACT

Disorders that cause obstruction to the flow of urine (see Fig. 8.6) are not uncommon. Although the early stages may cause only mild symptoms which are easily ignored, the progressive damage caused by abnormal pressure, infection and stone formation can lead to renal failure. The importance of early detection and intervention cannot be over-emphasised.

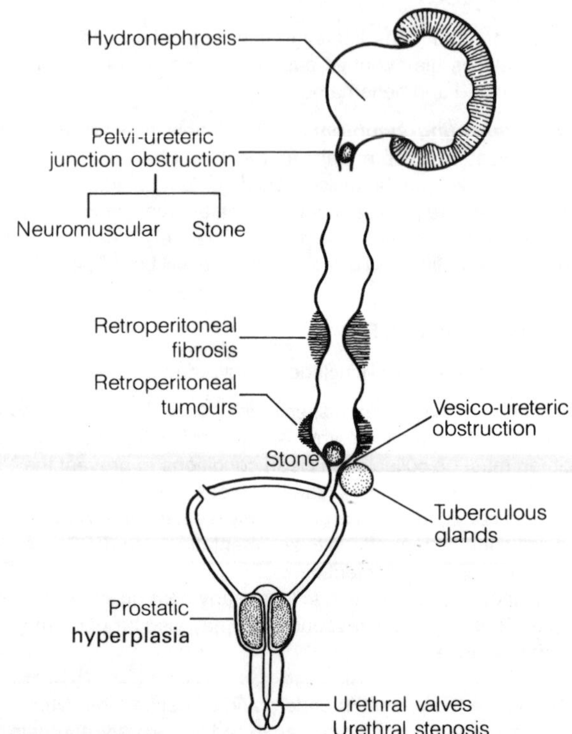

Fig. 8.6 Disorders causing obstruction to the urinary tract. (Reproduced with permission from Edwards & Bouchier 1991.)

Table 8.1 Chemical composition, clinical features and aetiology of urinary tract stones (Reproduced with permission from Burkitt et al 1990.)

Chemical composition	%	Clinical features	Aetiology
Calcium oxalate	40	3 types of stone are described: — small smooth 'hempseed' stones — small irregular 'mulberry' stones — small spiculate 'jack' stones	Most cases are idiopathic; predisposing factors include urinary stasis, infection and foreign bodies. Some are due to metabolic disorders: — hyperparathyroidism causing hypercalcaemia rather than hypercalciuria — hyperoxaluria (rare inherited disorder)
Mixed calcium oxalate and phosphate stones	15		Some are due to disorders associated with hypercalcaemia, e.g. sarcoidosis, multiple metastases, multiple myeloma, milk-alkali syndrome, overtreatment with vitamin D
Calcium and phosphate (hydroxyapatite)	15		Some patients excrete abnormally large amounts of calcium (idiopathic hypercalciuria, but without hypercalcaemia)
Magnesium ammonium phosphate	15	Typical of large 'staghorn' calculi of pelvicalyceal system and some bladder stones	Caused by chronic infection by organisms capable of producing urease. This enzyme splits urea, forming ammonia if the urine is alkaline
Uric acid	8	Stones tend to absorb yellow and brown pigments. Pure stones are radiolucent	Occur in primary gout, and hyperuricaemia following chemotherapy for leukaemias and myeloproliferative disorders. Childhood urate bladder stones occur in some underdeveloped countries when urine pH is low
Cystine or xanthine	2	Excess urinary excretion of cystine or xanthine. Pure stones are radiolucent	Autosomal recessive inherited disorders

Urinary stones (renal calculi)

The formation of stones or calculi in the urinary tract is common in Europe, North America and Japan. Worldwide, however, the incidence varies between 45 and 80 per 100 000. In the UK the incidence of stone formation is about 2–3% of the population. Stone formation is more common in men than women (M:W = 3:1) but when associated with urinary tract infection it is more frequently found in women (Hanno & Wein 1987). Children and people of Black African extraction are rarely affected.

PATHOPHYSIOLOGY

Table 8.1 summarises the features of the main types of stone that can form. In the majority of cases, however, unless there is an underlying disorder, no cause is evident. Box 8.3 identifies the predisposing factors.

Clinical features. Stone formation may occur at any point in the urinary tract. Presenting symptoms and features will depend on the stone site.

Stones that have formed in the renal calyces are often asymptomatic, but obstruction can occur at the calyx neck, resulting in infection and giving rise to pyrexia and pain. Scarring, renal atrophy and pyocalix can occur.

Stones found in the calyx can travel to the renal pelvis, causing pyrexia, nausea, vomiting and renal colic.

The main presenting symptom of upper ureteric stones is colicky pain extending across the abdomen. Haematuria (gross and microscopic) may also be noted.

The main presenting feature of midureteric and lower ureteric stones is colicky pain radiating towards the scrotum, together with urgency, frequency and abdominal distension.

The main presenting symptoms of stone formation in the bladder are pain, dysuria, frequency, and urgency.

Medical intervention. Small calculi may pass unobstructed through the urinary tract and be excreted in the urine. Intervention is indicated if there is evidence of anaemia, infection or hydronephrosis.

Conservative management. Calcium-chelating agents and avoidance of calcium-rich foods may be indicated where increased absorption of calcium is responsible for calculi formation. Acidification or alkalination of urine may prevent stones which form in these conditions. Fluid intake should be adequate but not excessive (Edwards & Bouchier 1991). The drinking of large quantities of fluid serves no useful purpose. The rationale behind this practice is to produce sufficient urine flow to flush out the stone, but in practice the presence of a continued obstruction will simply result in further distension of the collecting system and make matters worse. Normal hydration is therefore recommended.

Box 8.3 Predisposing factors in stone formation (Reproduced with permission from Burkitt et al 1990.)

- Idiopathic (most common)
- Stasis of urine, e.g. congenital abnormalities, chronic obstruction
- Chronic urinary infection (urea-splitting organisms, e.g. Proteus, cause alkaline urine and the development of magnesium-ammonium-phosphate stones, typically the 'staghorn' calculi of the renal pelvis)
- Excess urinary excretion of stone-forming substances, e.g. idiopathic hypercalciuria (calcium stones), hyperparathyroidism (calcium stones), hyperoxaluria (oxalate stones), gout (uric acid stones), cysteinuria (cysteine stones), xanthinuria (xanthine stones)
- Foreign bodies, e.g. fragments of catheter tubing, self-inserted artefacts, parasites (Schistosoma ova)
- Diseased tissue, e.g. renal papillary necrosis
- Multifactorial, e.g. prolonged immobility, children in the third world

Table 8.2 Some investigations used for patients with renal calculi (Adapted with permission from Edwards & Bouchier 1991.)

Type of investigation	Test	Purpose
Investigation of urinary tract	Examination of urine for protein, r.b.c, w.b.c.	Indicates abnormality of urinary tract
	MSU	Urinary infection
	Plain film abdomen	Shows opaque calculi, nephrocalcinosis
	IVU	Shows all calculi obstruction and abnormalities of urinary tract
Investigation of renal function	Blood urea, plasma creatinine	
	Creatinine clearance	
Investigation to determine underlying cause	Chemical analysis of calculus	Provides information as to what investigations to pursue
	Plasma calcium, phosphate	Hypercalcaemia
	Plasma parathyroid hormone	If hypercalcaemia is present to investigate possible hyperparathyroidism
	24 h urine calcium (× 2)	Hypercalciuria
	Plasma urate 24 h urine urate (× 2)	In patients with urate stones or calcium stones
	24 h urine cystine (× 2)	In patients with cystine stones
	24 h urine oxalate (× 2)	Hyperoxaluria

For further information, see Foster et al (1990).

MEDICAL MANAGEMENT OF ACUTE RENAL COLIC

Investigative procedures are listed in Table 8.2.

Symptom control. The patient with renal stones may be acutely ill, suffering from excruciating, spasmodic pain arising in the loin region and radiating to the groin. Pain is caused by small calculi being moved along the ureter by peristaltic movements, by impaction, and by obstruction of urine. Bedrest and analgesia are the first line of treatment.

Medications include i.m. pethidine (50–100 mg given 3–4 hourly), which produces prompt but short-acting relief as well as an antispasmodic effect. Diclofenic sodium (100 mg given per rectum, usually at night) is a prostaglandin synthetase inhibitor which reduces renal blood flow and urination. It has an antispasmodic and anti-inflammatory effect and is long acting. Nausea may be relieved by an antiemetic such as i.m. prochlorperazine (12.5 mg) (Trounce & Gould 1990).

Flush back of calculi and stenting. This procedure affords temporary relief when a small calculus causes obstruction and pain in the ureter. The stone is flushed back to the pelvis of the kidney. A small silicone tube, called a stent, is positioned in the ureter from the pelvi-ureteric junction to the bladder. This stent is left in position to hold the stone in place. Further treatment to remove the stone can now be planned. The stent should not be left more than 6 weeks. If the planned treatment cannot be carried out by the end of this period the stent should be changed.

Insertion of a nephrostomy tube is indicated when obstruction in the kidney of the ureter cannot be relieved by flush back and stenting (see Fig. 8.7 and Box 8.4). This is carried out under X-ray control, usually with a local anaesthetic. A small silicone tube is placed percutaneously into the collecting system of the kidney. The tube is held in place by a suture, and connected to a closed-system drainage bag.

Ureteroscopic removal of calculi. This procedure is suitable in the treatment of small calculi in the ureter. The ureteric orifice is dilated cystoscopically (see Box 8.5) and a ureteroscope to which a 'stone basket' is attached introduced into the ureter. The basket is opened out to ensnare the stone. The basket and stone are then withdrawn.

Rigid ureteroscopes are now available which can be inserted under direct vision. The surgeon is able to see the stone and can disintegrate it in situ before removing the smaller fragments in a 'basket' (see Burkitt 1990, p. 457).

Extracorporeal shock wave lithotripsy (ESWL). This procedure can be used to remove calculi in the kidney or the upper third of the ureter. Large calculi are broken up by means of this technique before percutaneous removal.

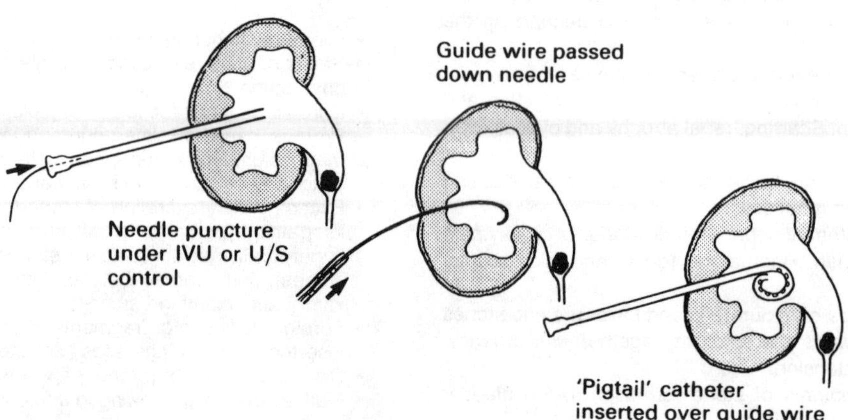

Fig. 8.7 Percutaneous nephrostomy. (Reproduced with permission from Bullock et al 1989.)

Box 8.4 Stenting

The stents used by most surgeons are called 'double-J' or 'pigtail' stents and have small holes down most of the length of their tubing. These stents are self-retaining and must be removed endoscopically.

Some surgeons use an infant feeding tube as a stent following pyeloplasty, pyelolithotomy, or ureterolithotomy. Infant feeding tubes are self-retaining to a degree, but the patient will need a urethral catheter in situ to keep the tube in place. When the catheter is removed the patient may pass the feeding tube without intervention. If this does not happen within 24 h endoscopic removal will be required.

There are several lithotripsy centres in the UK, but some patients have to travel some distance for this treatment. Second-generation lithotripsers allow most patients to be treated without anaesthetic. However, sometimes the patient's age, the degree of pain, or the size and position of the stone make general anaesthetic necessary. Some patients may require more than one treatment.

The patient lies on a special table, with the area to be treated over a special dish containing water. This dish produces shock waves from a spark generator, which are then reflected to focus the kidney stone, causing it to disintegrate. The whole procedure is performed under specialised X-ray and ultrasonic control. The disintegrated or powdered calculus is then allowed to pass down the ureter over the next few days.

Capital outlay for this procedure is currently high, but it is expected that in future 60–80% of calculi will be dealt with in this way.

Percutaneous nephrolithotomy (PCNL). This procedure is used to remove calculi lying within the kidney. Large staghorn calculi may need breaking up by ESWL first.

PCNL is performed under X-ray and ultrasound control. The patient will normally have a general anaesthetic. The kidney is punctured and the tract into the kidney is dilated to allow the nephroscope and a variety of grasping instruments to be inserted. The stone can then be removed or broken down into fine powder by ultrasonic probes (see Fig. 8.8). This powder can be aspirated through the centre of the probe.

Sometimes an electrohydraulic probe is used. This produces shock waves in the irrigating fluid to the kidney, and results in the stone splitting into several fragments.

At the end of the procedure, a large nephrostomy tube with a smaller tube running down its centre is left in position to allow drainage and to prevent haematoma formation. This also allows access

Box 8.5 Cystoscopy

This procedure allows the surgeon to visualise the interior of the bladder and to take biopsies where suspicious lesions are evident. It may be carried out either under general anaesthetic with a rigid cystoscope, or under local anaesthetic with a flexible cystoscope. The method selected will depend on the condition of the patient.

CYSTOSCOPY UNDER GENERAL ANAESTHETIC

The standard procedures for preparing a patient for general anaesthesia will apply. The lower bowel should be free of faeces so that insertion of the cystoscope is not impeded or the view restricted.

Once recovered from the anaesthetic, the patient should be encouraged to drink. He should be able to pass urine within 6 h of the procedure. The nurse should collect the first specimen passed and record its colour and amount.

Upon discharge, the patient should be advised that he may experience some frequency of desire to pass urine. He should watch for blood in the urine, and should this appear, increase his fluid intake. If the frequency doesn't settle, or if any bleeding continues, the patient should contact his GP or the hospital.

CYSTOSCOPY UNDER LOCAL ANAESTHETIC

There is no restriction on the taking of food or fluids prior to this procedure, but the lower bowels should be free of faeces. The local anaesthetic is placed directly into the urethra in the form of lignocaine gel. In a male patient, a penile clamp is applied to the penis to allow the gel to move along the urethra. A period of 10–20 minutes should normally be allowed for the local anaesthetic to take effect.

Following the procedure, the patient will normally pass urine sooner than under general anaesthetic, as there will have been no restriction applied on fluid intake prior to the operation.

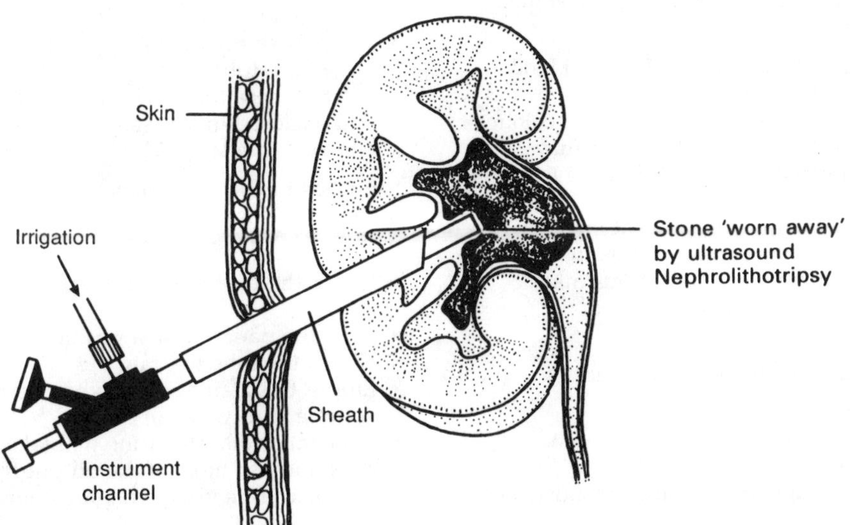

Fig. 8.8 Percutaneous nephrolithotomy. (Reproduced with permission from Bullock et al 1989.)

for a nephrogram 24–48 h postoperatively to assess effectiveness of treatment.

Nephrogram. No anaesthetic is required for this procedure. A contrast medium is injected down the smaller tube of a nephrostomy tube into the kidney. X-rays can then be taken and any fragments of calculi identified. Provided that there are no fragments left the tubes can be removed.

Ureterolithotomy. This open surgery is appropriate in the treatment of calculi occurring mid-ureter and causing obstruction that cannot be dealt with any other way. An X-ray to identify the position of the stone will determine the incision the surgeon will make. The ureter is exposed and opened and the stone removed. The ureter is repaired either by removing a small section or by suturing the opening. A stent is usually left in place, positioned along the length of the ureter. This allows the ureter to heal and prevents leakage. A wound drain will be left in position in the normal way to prevent haematoma formation. The stent will normally be removed after 7 days.

Pyelolithotomy. This open surgery can be used for calculi in the pelvis of the kidney which are causing an obstruction that cannot be removed in any other way. The procedure involves first exposing the affected kidney and then opening the pelvis of the kidney to remove the stone. Sometimes it is not possible to remove all of a staghorn calculus (see Table 8.1) in this way, in which case further incisions into the surrounding renal tissue (nephrolithotomy) is necessary. A stent will be left in place for 7 days.

NURSING PRIORITIES AND MANAGEMENT: ACUTE RENAL COLIC

Major considerations

A patient admitted with renal colic can often do little more than cope with his pain. He is often unable to answer questions or to follow advice and instructions until the pain is relieved. Once the acute attack has subsided, the patient should be allowed to rest. Only then will he feel able to attend to all the necessary explanations relating to investigations and treatment. Nursing Care Plan 8.1 outlines the priorities of nursing care for a patient admitted with acute renal colic.

Nursing care following specific interventions

Flush back and stenting

The patient should be prepared for a general anaesthetic as discussed in Chapter 27 (see p. 781). Normally only a short-acting anaesthetic is required. Priorities in postoperative nursing care are as follows:

1. To record observations, temperature, pulse and blood pressure and watch for signs of infection
2. To monitor urine output and record volume and colour of urine on the fluid chart. A decrease in volume may indicate obstruction. Haematuria may indicate trauma, but some haematuria is to be expected
3. To encourage a fluid intake of 3 l to prevent infection
4. To administer analgesics if the patient is in pain. Severe pain must be reported to medical staff, as this may indicate trauma, a misplaced stent, or return of obstruction.

Discharge advice. The patient should be advised:

1. To continue to drink 3 l daily
2. To take mild analgesics such as paracetamol or co-coproxamol if he is in pain
3. To seek help from the GP if urine output is bloodstained or 'burning'.

The patient should also be advised when follow-up treatment will take place and what this will entail. If treatment is not within 6 weeks, it must be impressed upon the patient that it is very important to have the stent changed. If it is not changed sediment and crystals will build up around it and form more calculi.

Extra-corporeal shock wave lithotripsy (ESWL)

The role of the nurse in the ESWL unit includes giving reassurance to the patient and his family, explaining what to expect, administering any prescribed medication, encouraging the patient to drink following the procedure, and giving discharge advice.

The patient may receive an oral premedication such as Diazepam, or Temazepam prior to treatment. The treatment is not normally painful. Anxiety may be experienced due to the noise from the shock waves and the requirement to lie still for 1 to 1½ h. Playing recorded music may help to alleviate anxiety and boredom.

Following treatment frusemide may be given orally to increase diuresis and help the stone fragments to pass. The patient will normally stay in the lithotripsy unit until he has passed urine. Prophylactic antibiotics and analgesics may also be given.

Most patients will be able to return home and continue with their normal daily activities. However, a small percentage will need hospital admission during the first week post-treatment, because of colicky pain, oedema and, occasionally, obstruction of the ureter. This will sometimes settle with no further treatment, but a stent may need to be inserted to allow the oedema to settle down.

Discharge advice. The patient should be advised:

1. To drink 3 l of fluid a day, to help prevent infection and to help the gravel to pass down the urinary system
2. To expect some haematuria and gravel when passing urine
3. To take prescribed analgesics, but if pain increases to see the GP or report back to the hospital
4. To attend a follow-up appointment about 6 weeks later to have further X-rays taken to assess the effect of the treatment.

Percutaneous nephrolithotomy (PCNL)

Preoperatively, the patient should be prepared for a general anaesthetic (see Ch. 27, p. 781). Postoperatively, the patient is likely to return to the ward with:

- a urethral catheter in situ
- an i.v. infusion of clear fluids
- a nephrostomy tube in the affected kidney. This will be a large-bore tube with a narrower tube running down its centre. These tubes will normally be sutured into position and enclosed in a System-2 urostomy drainage bag attached to a large 2 l drainage bag.

Priorities in the management of the nephrostomy tube are to maintain a closed drainage system to prevent infection, and to monitor drainage. The nurse responsible must:

- Check the position and the placement of the nephrostomy tube
- Help the patient into a position that is comfortable and allows the tube to drain
- Empty the drainage bag when necessary and record the volume and colour of output
- Remember that the urine will take the path of least resistance, so most of the output from the affected kidney will discharge via the nephrostomy tube.

The urethral catheter is normally removed 24 h following surgery. The i.v. infusion is discontinued at the same time, if the patient is able to drink normally. A nephrogram is carried

Nursing Care Plan 8.1 Nursing care for a patient admitted with acute renal colic

Potential problem	Action	Desired outcome
1. Pain of a potentially excruciating nature	❒ Administer prescribed analgesics ❒ Evaluate effect of analgesics: return to patient in ½ h • ask if he is pain free • observe for evidence of pain e.g. raised pulse rate, sweating and evidence of neurogenic shock (see Ch. 18, p. 604)	Pain is relieved
2. Frequency and urgency of micturition	❒ Locate urinal within reach of patient	Sensations decline as pain is relieved
3. Nausea and vomiting	❒ Administer prescribed antiemetics ❒ Evalute effect of treatment: return to patient in ½ h ❒ Locate vomit bowl within patient's reach	Patient obtains relief from feelings of nausea and from vomiting
4. Fluid and electrolyte imbalance	❒ Institute i.v. fluids if patient is unable to take adequate fluid orally	Fluid and electrolytes are maintained at satisfactory levels
5. Ureteric obstruction	❒ Check and record blood pressure ❒ Observe BP trends and report elevations ❒ Measure urine output; report reduction in volume ❒ Observe for haematuria and passage of stones	Any obstruction is recognised immediately
6. Urinary tract infection	❒ Check and record temperature; report pyrexia ❒ Check and record pulse rate; observe trends and report elevations	Infection is prevented, or immediately recognised
7. Non-passage of small calculi	❒ Encourage normal volumes of fluid intake ❒ Alleviate nausea and vomiting ❒ Check urine for presence of calculi (use plastic urinal to prevent sticking of calculi)	Passage and collection for analysis of small calculi
8. Inability to perform personal hygiene	❒ Offer wash and change of bed gown as required, particularly if sweating is profuse	Patient is clean and comfortable Self-esteem is maintained
9. Difficulty in finding a comfortable position in bed	❒ Assist patient to find a comfortable position ❒ Evaluate position regularly; ask the patient if he is comfortable	Patient is relaxed and comfortable
10. Anxiety	❒ Give patient the opportunity to voice concerns ❒ Provide information about the condition, investigations and treatment	Patient has an understanding of his condition and has reduced anxiety about outcome

out 48 h following surgery, and the nephrostomy tube removed if treatment has been successful. Following removal of the nephrostomy tube, the patient may continue to pass urine via the puncture site. This will normally cease after 12–24 h.

The patient may have colicky pain following the removal of the tube, as the urine must now redirect itself via the correct route. Analgesia can be given, and the patient should be asked to lie on the affected side. This will take the pressure off the affected kidney, and the drainage will pass via the puncture site.

Once the drainage has ceased from the puncture site, a small, dry dressing can be applied and the patient discharged home. Occasionally the nephrostomy tube may need to be left in situ for a prolonged period because further treatment may be necessary. In this case the patient may be discharged home into the care of the GP and community nurse.

Ureterolithotomy or pyelolithotomy

Preoperative preparation is as normal, including skin preparation and shaving the area to be operated upon (see Ch. 27, p. 785).

If the patient has an uneventful 2- or 3-day postoperative period, and a double-J stent or pigtail stent has been used, the patient may be discharged home into the care of the GP and community nurse, returning as a day case to the hospital for removal of the stent. The community nurse will check the wound, and take note of the patient's temperature and urine output. Sutures are removed from the wound at 7–10 days. If an infant feeding tube has been used as a stent (see Box 8.4), then the urethral catheter will remain in situ for 5–6 days. In this case the patient may need to stay in hospital until the stent and sutures have been removed.

Urethral strictures

PATHOPHYSIOLOGY

A stricture is a narrowing within a structure which may arise from inflammation, muscular spasm or neoplastic occlusion. Most urethral strictures are caused by trauma, as in pelvic fracture, self-inflicted introduction of foreign bodies, investigative instrumentation of the urethra (e.g. cystoscopy) or the presence of an indwelling urethral catheter (see Fig. 8.9). Infections such as non-specific urethritis and gonorrhoea may result in stricture formation. In women, inflammation caused by endometriosis and the trauma of pregnancy may in some cases result in strictures.

Common presenting symptoms which can prove to be both distressing and frustrating are poor urinary flow, a feeling of incomplete bladder emptying, frequency, dysuria or haematuria, and dribbling incontinence secondary to chronic urinary retention.

MEDICAL MANAGEMENT

Tests and investigations required are flow rate studies, urethrography, urethroscopy, IVP, renogram, and full blood screening.

Medical intervention. Options for treatment include the following.

Urethrotomy. The optical urethrotome allows the surgeon to divide the urethral stricture under direct vision. A silicone catheter would normally be left in place for up to 48 h postoperatively.

Self-dilatation. Often used in conjunction with urethrotomy, this technique involves using a self-lubricating urethral catheter on a regular basis to increase the urethral diameter and keep the urethral passage open.

Urethroplasty. Usually performed in two stages, this procedure aims to open the narrowed urethra by insertion of a split-skin graft. This surgery requires a longer stay in hospital and is normally performed only after other treatments have failed.

NURSING PRIORITIES AND MANAGEMENT: URETHRAL STRICTURES

> ? **8.4** As a nurse looking after Mr E (see Case History 8.1), what could you do to help him come to terms with the idea of performing self-dilatation and to feel more positive about it?

Major patient problems

Urethral strictures can cause lifelong disability (Burkitt et al 1990) and when any catheterisation or instrumentation of the urinary tract is necessary great delicacy is required. Catheterisation should be performed only when absolutely necessary, and as Burkitt et al (1990) put it, urological instruments should be 'hammered into place with a feather'.

Self-dilatation

The patient faced with the prospect of needing to perform self-dilatation on an ongoing basis will need moral support and encouragement from the health care team. A specialist nurse will explain the procedure initially and guide the patient through the procedure. She will also ensure that the patient receives continuing support as needed. It will also be helpful for the primary nurse to emphasise the following points:

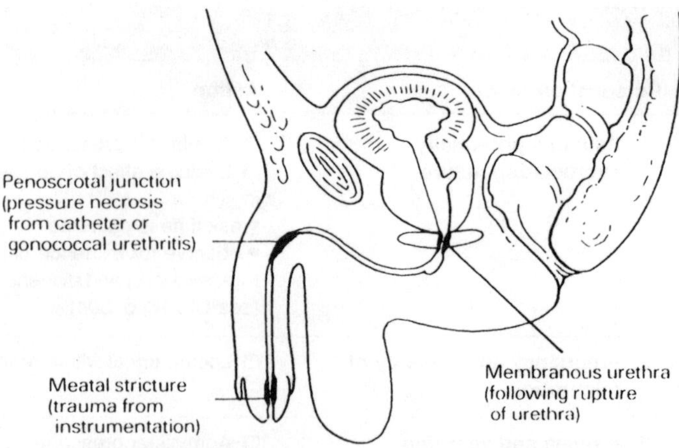

Fig. 8.9 Common sites and causes of urethral stricture. (Reproduced with permission from Forrest et al 1991.)

- No-one need know that the individual is using this technique
- Although the idea is not very appealing, this treatment will minimise the risk of further admission to hospital and time off work
- There is always a risk of infection, but this can be minimised with good hygiene, washing of hands and meatus, and adequate intake of fluids
- Dilatation will be necessary once a day at first, but as time goes on it can normally be reduced to once a week
- Irregular working schedules should not pose a problem; the patient can work out a routine that is convenient for him.

Fibrosis

PATHOPHYSIOLOGY

Fibrosis is the formation of excessive fibrous connective tissue within a structure. Fibrosis around the ureters predisposes them to obstruction; the cause of the fibrosis is often unknown. This condition, known as retroperitoneal fibrosis is not neoplastic but can result in damage to

Case History 8.1 Mr E

Mr E, a 35-year-old fireman, was having difficulty in passing urine. Two years previously, he had been involved in an accident in which he suffered crush injuries to his pelvis and urethra. At that time he had had a suprapubic catheter (i.e. a catheter inserted into the bladder via the abdominal wall) for 6 weeks.

On the more recent occasion he was referred to the urologist by his GP for two reasons. Firstly, Mr E had had repeated urinary tract infections over the last year. Secondly, he had noticed that for the last 6 months there was a difference in the time it took him to pass urine and that the stream was thinner than normal.

After a full investigation, the surgeon decided that the best course of action would be to perform an optical urethrotomy, followed by the patient being taught to perform self-dilatation. Mr E agreed to have the operation, although he did not like the idea of performing self-dilatation. When given the opportunity to discuss this, he expressed the following concerns:

- 'What if my friends and relatives find out?'
- 'I don't want to put a tube up there. How do I do it?'
- 'What about infection?'
- 'How often will I need to do this?'
- 'I work shifts. How can I do this?'

renal function. Other external causes of fibrosis are post-radiotherapy treatment, scarring arising from other surgical procedures, and aortic aneurysm. Fibrosis within structures (e.g. ureters/urethra) is usually secondary to traumatic procedures.

DISORDERS OF THE PENIS AND MALE URETHRA

Phimosis

Phimosis is a condition in which the foreskin or prepuce of the penis is too tight to be retracted over the glans penis. It may be caused by early attempts to draw back the foreskin before it has naturally separated or has developed fully in size. Retraction before separation is complete tears the still adhered surfaces. These will heal, forming scar tissue, but may later cause difficulty with retraction and hygiene.

A poorly performed circumcision operation may also contribute to a phimosis. The scar tissue will need to be separated and a recircumcision performed. Phimosis is very rarely a congenital defect.

PATHOPHYSIOLOGY

The natural separation of the two layers of skin from the glans penis normally occurs by about the age of 2. Following separation, the prepuce should be retracted to permit daily hygiene. Retained smegma (the white collection) which results from poor personal hygiene can give rise to inflammation and infection and has been implicated as a cause for carcinoma of the penis.

Common presenting symptoms. Phimosis often causes balanoposthitis, which is an inflammation of both the glans penis (balanitis) and the prepuce (posthitis). Presenting features include itching, a white discharge, pain, discomfort and bleeding at sexual intercourse, and sometimes urinary retention.

MEDICAL MANAGEMENT

Medical intervention. Initial treatment may be with antibiotics or anticandidal agents. If the individual is sexually active, he and his partner will both require treatment to prevent the infection being passed back and forth. Circumcision is the treatment of choice and may have to be performed as an emergency if urinary retention has occurred (see Box 8.6 and Case Histories 8.2 and 8.3).

NURSING PRIORITIES AND MANAGEMENT: PHIMOSIS

Prevention

Health education of the parents is important in the early years. It should be stressed that retraction of the foreskin for cleansing is unnecessary before puberty. Normal bathing or showering routines should suffice. After puberty the boy will need to pull back the foreskin to clean away smegma that accumulates around the glans penis.

Promoting wound healing after circumcision

The nurse can promote wound healing by the following means:

- teaching good personal hygiene to the newly circumcised person
- washing the wound area daily with soap and water and applying a protective, non-adhesive dressing to prevent clothing disturbing wound healing
- providing more frequent washing and dressing changes should urine leakage onto the wound or dressing occur

Box 8.6 Circumcision

Circumcision, the surgical removal of the prepuce (foreskin), may be indicated for penile carcinoma (Hanno & Wein 1987), balanitis or posthitis (which usually occur simultaneously), candidal infection, phimosis, or adherent prepuce. Circumcision may also be performed in accordance with religious beliefs.

The main complications of circumcision are infection and bleeding. Painful erections in the immediate postoperative period can usually be relieved by the application of a local anaesthetic gel. Postoperative swelling or oedema may make micturition difficult. Dribbling or urinary leakage to the wound area can delay or prevent wound healing and cause secondary infection. The insertion of a urethral catheter may be necessary to relieve this problem in order that wound healing may take place.

Case History 8.2 Mr A

Mr A, aged 20, presented to his GP with bleeding from the foreskin following sexual intercourse. He was concerned as this was the 6th occurrence.

On examination the foreskin was found to be very tight, and the GP advised circumcision. Referral was made to the local consultant urologist, and Mr A was put on the waiting list. After only a few weeks he was admitted as a day case for circumcision.

Before discharge, he was given the following advice verbally and in written form by nursing staff.

1. Take daily baths
2. Do not go straight back to work. Avoid walking around for the next few days.
3. Change underwear daily. Do not wear anything tight until the wound has healed.
4. You must be able to pass urine before leaving hospital, and you should drink at least 3 l of fluids in 24 h to prevent urinary tract infection.
5. If you have pain, take a simple analgesia such as paracetamol at 4–6 hourly intervals for the first 48 h.
6. At any sign of swelling, redness, or fever, go and see your GP.
7. Sexual intercourse should be avoided until the skin is healed and feels normal.
8. Should any other problems arise, report to your GP or if necessary return to the hospital.
9. Change the dressing if it becomes wet with urine. Use a non-stick dressing.

Case History 8.3 Mr C

Mr C, a 70-year-old widower, was referred by his GP to a urologist as an emergency, because he was in pain and having difficulty in passing urine. On examination it was found that he had a tight foreskin and it was difficult to see the meatus. On abdominal examination he appeared to be retaining urine. Ultrasound confirmed that there was approximately 500 ml in his bladder.

Mr C was admitted to the ward with instructions given that he would be operated on within the next 2 h for circumcision and urethral catheterisation. He was told that the catheter may need to stay in position for 24–48 h, depending on his general condition, and that his stay in hospital would be from 48 h to 1 week.

- counselling the sexually active patient to refrain from sexual intercourse until the wound is well healed.

> ? **8.5** How would your discharge advice to Mr A in Case History 8.2 compare with your advice to Mr C in Case History 8.3? Would you make any changes, omissions, or additions in your advice to the older man? What assumptions would prompt such changes? Are all of these assumptions fair?

Paraphimosis

Paraphimosis is a condition in which a foreskin that has been retracted over the glans penis cannot be returned to its usual position. The swollen band of foreskin obstructs the circulation to the glans, which in turn becomes swollen and painful. The condition may subside in a few hours, with general relief gained from taking a mild analgesic.

Cold compresses applied to the penis may help to relieve the swelling and pain. The doctor or nurse may be able to manipulate the glans back under the foreskin with or without anaesthesia. If this is unsuccessful a dorsal slit may be made in the foreskin. There remains a risk of recurrence of the paraphimosis and a circumcision may be advisable at a later date.

Congenital disorders of the urethra and penis

At birth an infant is examined to confirm its sex and to make sure that expected bodily structures are present. In boys the urethral meatus is normally seen at the anterior tip of the glans penis. Occasionally a malformation of the urethra is identified as a congenital defect.

Hypospadias

In the condition of hypospadias the meatus of the urethra is found in a position on the undersurface of the glans penis. The condition is usually treated quite effectively by enlargement of the meatus by plastic surgery. In some cases the urethral orifice is positioned further back on the lower surface of the penis, and this will complicate treatment. To allow a series of operations to take place, a temporary perineal urethrostomy may be formed, so creating a urinary diversion. Time is gained for the promotion of wound healing as a new urethral meatus is created.

Epispadias

The condition of epispadias is one in which the urethra opens on to the upper surface, or dorsum, of the penis. The meatus of the urethra may be positioned anywhere along the length of the penile surface. The epispadias may coexist with other serious congenital abnormality involving a poorly developed anterior section of the urinary bladder and abdominal wall. Surgical reconstruction is likely to be complex and may involve transplantation of ureters.

DISORDERS OF THE PROSTATE

Benign prostatic hyperplasia

The prostate gland increases in size with age, reaching about 20–25 g by the time the individual is 20 years old. In individuals over the age of 45 the smooth muscle segments atrophy and are replaced by collagen fibres. As ageing progresses, connective tissue accumulates, resulting in benign prostatic hyperplasia. The latter condition is the most common neoplastic growth in men, occurring with particular frequency in those aged 60 years or more. The cause of benign prostatic hyperplasia is unknown, but it is thought that it may be associated with reduced androgen secretions.

Bladder outflow obstruction can occur for a number of reasons (see Box 8.7), but the most common cause is benign prostate hyperplasia.

PATHOPHYSIOLOGY

Stasis of the urine in the bladder and a build-up of pressure in the bladder and ureters predispose the individual to infection, the formation of stones and possible renal failure. The bladder becomes enlarged, forming bundles called trabeculae. Diverticula may also be noted. If left untreated obstructive effects will develop (see Fig. 8.10).

Common presenting symptoms. The enlargement of the gland may be asymptomatic, perhaps noted only on a routine rectal examination. However, as the hyperplasia increasingly distorts and compresses the

Box 8.7 Bladder outflow obstruction

CAUSES

- Benign prostatic hyperplasia
- Bladder calculi
- Bladder tumour
- Diuretics
- Neurological disturbances
- Phimosis
- Prostatic carcinoma
- Urethral strictures, stenosis, trauma

COMMON SYMPTOMS

- Double voiding
- Dribbling post voiding
- Dysuria
- Force of urine flow/stream
- Frequency
- Hesitancy
- Haematuria (occasional)
- Nocturia
- Incontinence
- Interrupted stream
- Urgency
- Urinary retention

Inadequate emptying of the bladder can result in a build-up of residual urine, increasing the risk of urinary tract infection and the incidence of bladder stone formation.

DIAGNOSIS

Diagnosis of bladder flow obstruction may be assisted by:

- Blood screen of urea, electrolytes and creatinine
- Endoscopy: urethroscopy and cystoscopy
- History of symptoms
- Physical examination
- Ultrasound scan: residual urine volume and upper urinary tract
- Urinalysis
- Urine culture
- Urodynamic evaluation
- Voiding cystometrogram

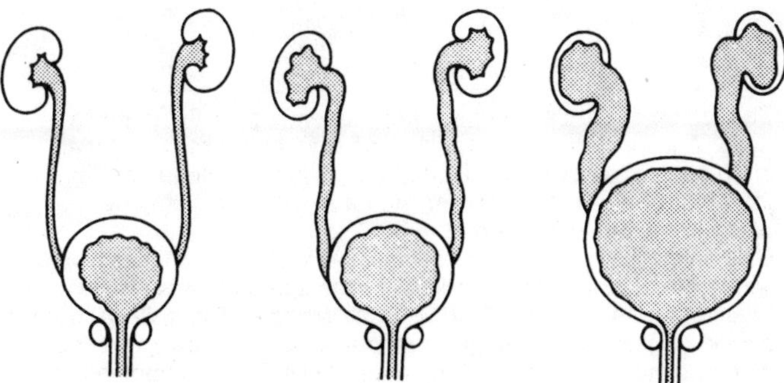

Fig. 8.10 The progressive effects of obstruction from an enlarged prostate. The bladder, ureters and kidneys all become affected. (Reproduced with permission from Charlton 1984.)

urethra and even the bladder, an inability to void normally will become obvious. Many men tolerate symptoms indefinitely, seeing them as just 'old men's problems' that have to be accepted.

Presenting symptoms include:

- difficulty in starting micturition
- difficulty in stopping micturition
- frequency and urgency
- poor flow and force in the urine passed
- dribbling and incontinence
- a feeling that the bladder is never completely emptied.

In addition, a history of recurrent urinary tract infections may be given. Increasing pressure due to obstruction can eventually result in renal impairment.

Acute urinary retention may be the single presenting feature, particularly if the prostate gland suddenly increases in size or if infection occurs. Some patients present with chronic urinary retention, sometimes associated with haematuria and urethral bleeding. Abnormal voiding patterns and disruption of daytime activities or sleep patterns can affect the individual's ability to work and interact normally with colleagues, partners and family. Bedwetting or urinary incontinence may cause embarrassment and distress. Embarrassment about such symptoms may also result in failure to seek professional help until the condition becomes unbearable.

MEDICAL MANAGEMENT

Investigative procedures. Diagnosis can be made by rectal examination; the prostate gland will feel large, elastic and uniform (Edward & Bouchier 1991). Investigations will include:

- IVU (see Box 8.2)
- urinary flow rates
- renal function tests
- full blood count
- serum acid phosphatase or serum prostatic specific antigen (PSA) to eliminate diagnosis of carcinoma
- MSU
- chest X-ray
- ECG
- cystoscopy (see Box 8.5) and biopsy, usually performed at surgery.

Medical intervention. Treatment by prostatectomy is indicated if there is significant outflow obstruction. Transurethral resection of the prostate gland (TURP) is the operation of choice. Where the gland is too large to resect transurethrally, an open procedure is used, most commonly taking the retropubic or transvesical approach. The use of a microwave heat treatment applied to the prostate gland via the rectum is being considered. This may reduce the size of the gland and perhaps obviate the need for surgery (Bolesha et al 1993).

For further information, see Willis (1992), Wozniak-Petrofsky (1991) and Khoury (1992).

Surgical intervention: TURP. Prior to commencing the resection a cystoscope is passed to view the bladder. A resectoscope is then passed and small sections are chipped away from the prostatic lobes, removing the material that had been intruding into the urethra and bladder neck. Irrigation fluid of a non-electrolyte solution, glycine, constantly flushes out the bladder during the procedure. (An electrolyte solution is contra-indicated in the presence of diathermy.) Most commonly, irrigation continues postoperatively, as the operative bed can give rise to considerable bleeding and clots could lead to obstruction.

Complications. Potential postoperative complications of TURP are:

- haemorrhage: (evident as haematuria)
- clot retention
- extravasion: escape of urine into surrounding tissue due to bladder or urethral drainage
- infection: urinary tract, epididymis or testis
- deep vein thrombosis and pulmonary embolism.

Possible late complications are:

- urethral stricture
- incontinence
- impotence
- retrograde ejaculation
- bladder neck stenosis.

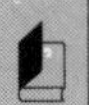

For further information, see Hanno & Wein (1987).

NURSING PRIORITIES AND MANAGEMENT: BENIGN PROSTATE HYPERPLASIA

General considerations

Patients with acute retention

Those men who present with acute urinary retention as a result of prostatism will normally be catheterised and referred to hospital care for prostatectomy. There is no urgency to perform surgery once the obstruction is relieved; therefore treatment of any associated medical conditions should be undertaken first and, when appropriate, the patient can be placed on the operating list. Should social conditions or hospital resources not permit this, the individual may be discharged to community care with catheter-in-situ until a mutually convenient date can be set for surgery. Normal procedure would, however, be for the patient to have his operation on the next available list.

Patients with chronic retention

Chronic urinary retention is usually the result of a crescendo of symptoms of prostatism. These men do not always complain of symptoms of bladder outflow obstruction, but mainly of urge incontinence, dribbling urine or wet beds at night. They usually have no pain and although they have a large residual urine, their bladder distension is not always obvious to the eye or palpable on physical examination.

Because of the large residual urine, these patients are at risk of developing upper urinary tract dilatation and impaired renal function. However, if there is no renal impairment it is not essential that these individuals are catheterised. It *is* urgent to make a diagnosis and proceed to prostatectomy once rehydration and renal function have returned to normal.

Catheterisation will permit bladder drainage and allow renal function recovery (see Boxes 8.8 and 8.9). Once catheterised,

Box 8.8 The use of catheters

INDICATIONS FOR CATHETERISATION

- Acute or chronic retention of urine
- Diagnostic investigations of the bladder function
- Pre- and postoperative needs
- Following trauma, burns, road traffic accidents or any trauma to the lower urinary tract
- Therapeutic instillations of medication specifically prescribed
- Intractable incontinence where all other methods have failed
- Protracted loss of consciousness

CHOICE OF CATHETER

Points to consider when choosing a catheter are:

- The purpose of the catheterisation
- The length of time the catheter must remain in situ
- Whether a self-retaining catheter is necessary
- The sex of the patient

FEATURES OF THE CATHETER

- The *smallest* catheter which will adequately drain the bladder should be used: size 12–16 Fg. for adults with clear urine; size 18–22 Fg. for adults with haematuria
- The lumen of the catheter will vary depending on the material used. A latex catheter is made up of several layers of material, often coated inside with silicone, and its lumen will be smaller than that of a silicone catheter, which is extruded from one piece of material (Pullman et al 1982)
- Balloon size: the larger the balloon, the higher the drainage eye lies in the bladder. This can impair drainage and cause more irritation to the sensitive trigone of the bladder. The balloon should be just large enough to stop the catheter falling out or being pushed out if the patient bears down. The recommended balloon size for routine use is 5–10 ml. A 30 ml balloon should be used only following surgery on the prostate gland.
  Note that underinflation of a large-capacity balloon causes distortion of the tip of the catheter and occlusion of the drainage eye. Therefore a large balloon should be filled with at least 20 ml of water. A smaller-ballooned catheter, because the water must reach the balloon, should be filled with at least 10 ml
- Short-term catheters are made of a latex material that can cause irritation of the urethra and buildup of crystals in the bladder. Therefore it is not recommended to use this type of catheter for longer than 2 or 3 weeks
- Long-term catheters are made of 100% silicone material; they are less irritating, softer, and cause less buildup of crystals

the patient may have a huge diuresis. His thirst mechanism will not allow adequate fluid replacement, making parenteral fluid replacement necessary. Large fluid replacement volumes put the patient at risk of heart failure and it should be borne in mind that renal function may have precipitated anaemia.

Once the patient has been catheterised, and his renal function has been restored and any anaemia corrected, there is no urgency to proceed to surgery. The individual may in fact benefit from a period of recuperation and bladder rest with the catheter in place. Depending upon the general well-being of the individual and upon community resources, care may be given in hospital or in the patient's home.

A trial without the catheter should not be made, as this would again lead to chronic retention followed by renal failure.

Whilst receiving community care pending hospital referral or surgery, some patients will develop acute or acute on chronic urinary retention. Hospital admission must be expedited to permit urgent or emergency hospital treatment.

For those with milder symptoms, it is matter of discussion between the patient and his doctor whether symptoms are interfering with the individual's lifestyle sufficiently to warrant an operation and whether he stands a good chance of improvement from surgery. In rare cases where there is poor life expectancy or the patient is too unfit for surgery, prostatectomy may not be offered and a permanent indwelling catheter may be considered the best management.

Specific considerations for the patient undergoing TURP

Informed consent

The patient must be given a clear explanation of the after-effects of TURP, so that he can give his informed consent prior to the procedure. Since almost all men have retrograde ejaculation after prostatectomy it is essential that they are counselled adequately beforehand. Retrograde ejaculation does *not* cause impotence, but a patient who has not been given adequate reassurance on this point could suffer psychological upset resulting in impotence. Retrograde ejaculation will *not* render the patient sterile, but neither will it necessarily permit him to father children easily. It should not be presumed that all elderly men are not sexually active, and all patients are entitled to preoperative information (see Case History 8.4, Box 8.10 and Research Abstract 8.1).

?	**8.6** Identify and consider all the information that will be necessary to give Mr M in Case History 8.4. How could this information best be given to ensure he can really understand and remember the details?

Major patient problems

Patients who have undergone TURP may have the following problems and concerns postoperatively:

- anxiety
  — about the success of the surgery and the outlook for recovery
  — about bleeding from the prostatic bed
  — feelings of embarrassment about having a catheter.
- pain
  — from the raw area in the bladder
  — from clots forming in the prostatic bed, blocking the catheter
  — from the catheter itself
  — from bladder extravasation.
- immobility
  — due to inability to get out of bed because of the surgery
  — because of irrigation
  — due to fear of moving
  — due to i.v. infusion.
- difficulty eating and drinking
  — due to nausea
  — due to immobility.
- disturbed sleep
  — due to irrigation changes, checks on temperature, pulse, blood pressure
  — due to pain
  — due to noise in the ward.

Box 8.9 Principles of catheter management

PERFORMING CATHETERISATION

The nurse performing catheterisation must introduce the catheter into the bladder using aseptic technique, without causing trauma and with minimum discomfort to the patient. The following considerations are essential:

- Adequate cleaning of the genital area
- Working under good light, especially when catheterising females
- Positioning the patient correctly
- Ensuring the patient's privacy
- Providing adequate anaesthetisation of the urethra; this is especially important in male catheterisation. An anaesthetic-containing antiseptic should be instilled and left to take effect for a minimum of 5 min

MANAGEMENT OF THE INDWELLING CATHETER

The main priorities of catheter care are to prevent infection and to safeguard the dignity of the patient.

To minimise the risk of infection the nurse should:

- Establish and maintain a closed system of drainage
- Promote good personal hygiene
- Provide catheter toilets 4 hourly and after each bowel movement, with soap and water
- Encourage a fluid intake of 2–4 l daily, according to the individual's needs
- Encourage maximum mobility
- Change the catheter only when necessary, rather than routinely
- Avoid causing trauma to the urethra and bladder neck
- Give bladder washouts only when absolutely necessary, i.e. when the catheter is blocked or when washouts have been prescribed as a treatment. Bladder washouts should not be employed as a prophylactic treatment for urine infections (Roe 1990)

MAINTAINING THE DIGNITY OF THE PATIENT

The following measures will help to preserve the patient's dignity and self-esteem:

- Providing education and promoting self-care where possible in catheter toilet, the use of a bidet, emptying and changing bags
- Using a female length catheter for a female patient to allow her to wear skirts
- Encouraging the use of leg bags so the catheter is not in view
- Encouraging maximum mobility to promote confidence and give better drainage.

PROBLEMS AND POSSIBLE INTERVENTIONS

The nurse should be prepared for the following potential problems

1. Bypassing:
   - Check to see if the catheter or drainage tube is blocked or kinked
   - Consider reducing the water in the balloon or changing to a smaller catheter. It is a misconception that if the catheter bypasses then a larger catheter is required (Foster et al 1990)
   - Check whether or not drugs which can cause spasm have been prescribed
   - Exclude constipation: relieve constipation immediately and emphasise the importance of a high-fibre diet
   - Check with the doctor about the possibility of prescribing anticholinergic drugs if the bypassing still persists
2. Balloon not deflating:
   - Attach syringe to the valve in position without aspiration. It may self-deflate
   - The balloon may be burst by injecting 2–5 ml of dilute ether via the balloon inflating channel
   - A fine sterile wire may be passed up the inflating channel and the balloon burst
   - Never cut off the end of the inflation channel of the catheter
3. Blockage:
   - This may be caused by drugs, e.g. aperients causing phosphatic debris in the urine; change or stop the drug, encourage the patient to take a high-fibre diet and encourage him to exercise more
   - Infection will need to be treated with the correct antibiotic. Check the amount of fluid intake and where possible try to increase this. Check the standard of personal hygiene.
   - If clots occur perform a bladder washout with normal saline
4. Urethral discharge:
   - Normal secretion of the urethral mucosa is increased with the presence of a foreign body, i.e. the catheter. To prevent this becoming troublesome to the patient adequate meatal toilet should be instituted from the first day of catheterisation

Case History 8.4 Mr M

Mr M was admitted for a TURP. He was 73 and had been suffering from the miserable symptoms of an enlarged prostate gland for some time. He was glad to be in hospital but did not feel well. His joints and bones ached from long-standing osteoarthritis. His chest was not good and his feet and hands were always cold. He knew smoking did not help and he had been cutting down.

The surgeon and anaesthetist visited him and explained the surgery and that he would have an epidural anaesthetic. The physiotherapist visited him and discussed breathing techniques and encouraged him with giving up smoking. Nursing staff were always at hand. They explained all the tests and procedures involved in preparation for surgery as well as how he could expect to feel after the procedure.

Major nursing considerations

Risk of haemorrhage

Since bleeding or haemorrhage is a major risk after prostatectomy, preoperative care should involve determining baseline haematological values. Careful consideration must be given to those individuals receiving oral anticoagulants for other disease, since the risk of haemorrhage is so great. It may be necessary to discontinue oral therapy preoperatively and to use i.v. heparin postoperatively until the oral regimen can be recommenced and stabilised. This may take some weeks to achieve and will require the patient to make additional visits to the hospital or GP surgery.

Anaemia

Preoperative anaemia should be corrected, and blood transfusion given postoperatively to replace blood loss. It would be normal to cross-match two units of blood for each patient

Box 8.10 Information for patients undergoing prostatectomy (Reproduced with kind permission of Department of Urology, The Freeman Hospital, Newcastle upon Tyne)

Your Doctor has already explained to you that you require an operation on your prostate gland. The prostate is situated at the base of the bladder and it is quite common in older men for the prostate to enlarge, causing the symptoms which you have been experiencing. In order to relieve these symptoms it is necessary to remove that part of the prostate gland which is causing a blockage to the flow of the urine from the bladder.

THE ANAESTHETIC

The operation may be performed under a general anaesthetic, when you will be completely asleep, or a spinal anaesthetic, which involves an injection in your back and makes the lower half of your body completely numb. This decision is usually made by the Anaesthetist. If you wish, you may have something else to make you relaxed or sleepy. The power and feeling of your legs recovers within a few hours and by the morning after the spinal anaesthetic you will be completely normal.

THE OPERATION

There are 2 ways of removing the prostate gland. Generally it is possible to do the operation through a telescopic instrument which is passed up through the penis. This operation is known as a transurethral resection or TUR. The prostate tissue is cut away in small pieces which are washed out of the bladder and any bleeding is stopped using a special electrocautery probe.

Alternatively, it is sometimes necessary to remove the prostate by an open operation through an incision in the lower part of the abdomen. The same amount of tissue is removed by both operations and the end result is the same. Your Surgeon will naturally try to remove your prostate with the tele-endoscopic instrument but it may be necessary to perform the 'cutting' operation, especially if the prostate is unusually large.

After the operation you will have a tube (catheter) draining the urine from your bladder into a bag which will be emptied regularly by the Nursing Staff. Immediately after the operation the catheter will contain blood so the bladder, prostate and catheter are washed continuously with fluid that runs through an extra tube attached to the catheter. This is disconnected when the urine is clear, usually the morning after the operation. After the operation you will also have an infusion into a vein for about 24 hours to provide extra fluid or blood if necessary.

AFTER THE OPERATION

As soon as possible we like you to start drinking large quantities of tea, squash, fruit juice or water after the operation but fizzy drinks are not recommended. An occasional can of beer is permissible. This will speed up your recovery by producing more urine to wash away the blood in the catheter and prevent infection. The catheter will be removed between 2 and 5 days after the operation. This is not painful. After it has been removed you should continue to drink as much as possible and pass urine every 2–3 hours. This may be uncomfortable to start with and you may have to hurry or experience some dribbling but these minor symptoms improve rapidly. Once you are satisfied that you are passing urine well and your Surgeon is satisfied with your progress you may return home, usually 1–2 days after removal of the catheter.

AT HOME

When you get home you should continue to drink well and avoid constipation, strenuous exercise and heavy lifting. You should not drive a car for 1 week nor play golf or go jogging for at least 3 weeks. Sometimes you may see some blood in your urine 7–10 days after the operation. This is rarely serious and if you drink plenty of fluids and rest it should disappear. If bleeding persists you should contact your Family Doctor. Infection and other problems are unusual. The bladder may be 'irritable' for several weeks after a prostate operation with frequency and urgency but any remaining symptoms should disappear within 12 weeks.

You will be seen again in the Urology Outpatient Clinic in about 2 months after your operation. You can return to light work at that time or even sooner, if you feel able to do so.

SEXUAL ACTIVITY AFTER PROSTATECTOMY

This operation will alter your sex life but it is unlikely that there will be any change in the quality of the erections or climax. Sexual intercourse can take place 5–6 weeks after the operation. During sexual climax, however, you will not emit any semen from your penis. The ejaculation (semen) may flow into the bladder instead of down the penis and the first time you pass urine after intercourse it will be cloudy. This is not harmful. You are unlikely to produce any children following this operation but this should not be relied on as safe contraception.

so that should transfusion be required postoperatively the blood will be available on demand. Future trends may change this protocol, since protein and plasma products are now more readily available.

Research Abstract 8.1 Preoperative information-giving

However commonplace certain surgical procedures might become to medical and nursing staff, they will never be so for the actual patient, who will wish to know about the operation. Understanding illness and surgery can help in the recovery process and reduce stress (Argyle 1981). However, the giving of information and support is not always as effective as the doctor or nurse may believe. A small research study in Edinburgh assessed the quality of the perioperative information given to patients undergoing a TURP. In a two-phase study the researchers were able to show that the use of a booklet both complemented and enhanced verbal communication (Brewster 1992).

Brewster J 1992 Operations explained. Nursing Times 88(39): 50–52

Fluid and electrolyte balance

Preoperative determination of urea and electrolyte levels will provide baseline measurements and permit correction before surgery if required. This may involve urethral catheterisation to permit adequate bladder drainage, the use of i.v. fluid to achieve hydration and, if necessary, the provision of saline (see below).

During TURP the bladder is irrigated with fluid (see below) to provide a clear view for the surgeon. Some of this fluid is usually absorbed, and if there is an interruption in the venous system during the resection the fluid absorbed can be excessive. The fluid used in irrigation is usually isotonic glycine, excessive absorption of which can cause the patient to become hyponatraemic. This can cause confusion, a restless mental state and, in some cases, unconsciousness. This imbalance can be corrected by restricting fluid intake and encouraging the patient to increase the amount of salt in his diet.

Water is not used for irrigation because it can be readily absorbed and cause haemolysis. Saline interferes with the use of diathermy, and so is also unsuitable for irrigation during surgery. It is, however, the solution of choice for postoperative bladder washouts.

Urinary infection
Men who have an indwelling urethral catheter preoperatively are at a high risk of developing infective complications. The effectiveness of prophylactic antibiotics is uncertain, but it would seem that those who do not receive systemic therapy at the time of operation followed by a postoperative course will be likely to develop bacteraemia and become unwell.

Urinary infection is common after prostatectomy, even in those who had sterile urine preoperatively. About one third of men who have bacteria in their urine postoperatively are asymptomatic but should receive the appropriate oral therapy. This reduces the incidence of secondary haemorrhage caused by infection.

Management of irrigation

An irrigation set with a Y-connection will be used to allow two 3 l bags of normal saline to be erected at any one time, with one bag running at a time. The irrigation runs into the bladder via the irrigating channel of the catheter, and then out through the outlet channel from a classic system drainage bag, thus preventing the introduction of infection.

The irrigation is regulated via a clamp to run at a speed sufficient to keep the bladder clear of blood clots. The bags are numbered and the amount of irrigation fluid recorded on a fluid chart. The patient's total output, i.e. urine and irrigation fluid, should be measured and recorded. The amount of irrigation fluid used should be subtracted from the measured output to give the urine output volume.

Specific assessment points are as follows:

1. Observe and feel the size of the patient's lower abdomen. Abdominal distension may indicate clot retention or extravasation. Clot retention is a common complication in the first 12–24 h. Bladder washout or deflation and reinflation of the catheter balloon may be required.
2. Note the colour of the irrigation fluid. A bright red colour may indicate fresh bleeding. A dark red colour would suggest old blood.
3. In an uncircumcised male patient, check that the foreskin is over the glans penis to prevent paraphimosis.

The morning following surgery, the irrigation will be discontinued provided that the patient is able to drink large quantities of fluid to help flush the prostatic bed of any further bleeding or clots.

Pain relief should be adequate to allow the patient to rest and feel comfortable. Opiate analgesics such as morphine or oral co-proxamol may be prescribed.

Catheter care (see also Boxes 8.8 and 8.9)
A common problem while the catheter is in situ is the bypassing of urine around the catheter. This is sometimes difficult to resolve, and the nurse should take the following preventive measures:

1. Check that the catheter is not blocked by clots or debris and that it is in the bladder
2. Check the amount of water in the balloon. If it is 30 ml, then reduce it to 20 ml or so, but not less than 15 ml
3. Give anticholinergic medication as prescribed
4. Encourage the patient to continue to drink large quantities of fluid.

The catheter will stay in position for 2–3 days following surgery or until the output is clear. Before removing the catheter, the nurse should ensure that the patient's bowels have moved, as straining following catheter removal can lead to further urethral bleeding.

Following catheter removal, the patient may experience urgency and frequency as before. He should be reassured that this is normal and that it may take up to 8 weeks for a normal voiding pattern to be established. The patient should be educated to tighten the sphincter muscle, and to hold on as long as possible before passing urine.

Patients who had chronic retention before surgery often fail to void following surgery. A long-term catheter will normally then be inserted in such cases, and the patient allowed home for several weeks (usually 6). This time allows the bladder to rest and regain its elasticity.

Patient involvement
The patient's dependence on nursing care will gradually decrease as blood loss and hence the need for irrigation lessens. Involvement of the patient in aspects of his own care is to be encouraged and may include:

1. Making entries in his own fluid chart; drinking at least 3 l in 24 h; emptying own drainage bag; recording amount and colour (most patients will be happy to do this but may need guidance on colour and amount).
2. Attending to own personal hygiene; this would include cleaning the urethral catheter at regular intervals (4 times daily is recommended). It is a good idea to suggest this is done either before or after mealtimes.
3. Taking regular if somewhat gentle exercise. (It should be remembered, however, that some patients feel embarrassed about carrying around a urinary drainage bag.)

Discharge

Once the urine is clear, the catheter can normally be removed. This is usually done in the morning to allow the patient to establish a normal voiding pattern before retiring to bed. Provided the patient is able to pass urine without difficulty, he may be discharged from hospital the following day.

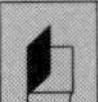
For further information, see Glenister (1990), Roe (1991) and Barnett (1991).

Many patients feel after the operation that they have gained no relief from their problems. It must be understood that it will take about 6 weeks for healing of the prostatic bed to occur such that full urinary control is possible. During the early postoperative weeks the patient should refrain from vigorous exercise. He should drink plenty of fluids and avoid becoming constipated. The community nurse will give advice and support should urinary problems occur.

It should be noted that at about 14 days postoperatively, when dessicated tissue has sloughed off the prostatic bed, haemorrhage can occur (secondary haemorrhage; see Ch. 27, p. 792).

Occasionally, urethral stricture occurs as the urethral mucosa in the prostatic region heals (see p. 307).

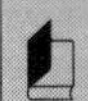
For further information, see Reynolds (1993) and Sueppel (1992).

Cancer of the prostate

Cancer of the prostate gland is rapidly becoming the most common malignancy among the Western male population (Debruyne 1991). The incidence of prostatic cancer increases with age and postmortem studies have shown that about 30% of asymptomatic men over the age of 50 and 90% over the age of 90 have microscopic foci, evident only on histological examination. About 10% of men thought to have benign prostates on examination are later found by histological examination to have prostatic cancer. This is the fourth most common malignancy in British men (over 5000 deaths annually).

PATHOPHYSIOLOGY

The cause of prostatic cancer is not clear, but there is some evidence to show that hormonal activity plays a part in the transformation of certain normal cells into cancerous ones. Benign hyperplasia and carcinoma arise in different parts of the gland. Carcinoma occurs in the peripheral gland. Metastases often move to bone, where they are associated with severe pain. In cases of extreme bony destruction, pathological fractures may occur. It has been known for spinal destruction to cause paraplegia.

Common presenting symptoms. Diagnosis of this disease is difficult because the patient is often asymptomatic. The GP is likely to see patients who present with advanced disease which is already beyond cure. Patients with locally advanced disease are likely to complain of bladder outflow obstruction, a sudden onset of urgency to void urine, and possibly haematuria.

Chronic urinary retention secondary to bladder outflow obstruction may cause renal damage by dilating the upper renal tracts. The patient may present with a palpable bladder or with renal failure; he is likely to be generally unwell and losing weight. Renal failure may also be caused by ureteric infiltration of tumour or by para-aortic lymph node obstruction causing ureteric obstruction. Those who feel unwell and are anaemic are likely to have suffered bone marrow infiltration and/or renal failure. A complaint of persistent backache may suggest bone metastases.

An irregular, enlarged, hard prostate gland does not prove diagnosis, although most advanced carcinomas will be felt as such on rectal examination. However, prostatitis or prostatic stone disease may feel similar on rectal examination. Moreover, if there is a tumour within the anterior part of the gland rectal examination will reveal no abnormality.

MEDICAL MANAGEMENT

Tests and investigations. The only certain means of making a diagnosis is by histological examination. Fine-needle transrectal prostatic biopsy can be done without anaesthetic for this purpose. Specimens (prostatic chips) resected at the time of transurethral or open prostatectomy should be sent for histological examination. However, this may yield a false negative if the sample is not taken from the peripheral part of the gland. Prostatic cancer is graded histologically to assess malignant potential (see Ch. 32, p. 883).

Additional investigations to provide evidence of local and metastatic spread include IVU, CT scanning, magnetic resonance imaging (MRI), ultrasound scanning, skeletal X-rays and lymphangiography.

Medical intervention. The nature of the treatment offered and whether it is given on an outpatient or an inpatient basis will depend upon the extent of the disease and on how the patient presents symptomatically and clinically. Transurethral resection of the prostate gland (TURP) is normally carried out to relieve urinary symptoms and retention. This does not, however, afford a cure.

In a small number of cases, radical prostatectomy and clearance of any pelvic lymphatic involvement is performed in the hope of achieving a cure. The patient should be counselled preoperatively about his disease and the almost certain complication of urinary incontinence.

Radical radiotherapy. If the patient is generally fit and quite well, he will probably attend for daily treatment as an outpatient. Should the patient or medical team prefer, inpatient treatment may be given.

The side-effects of treatment will vary from person to person. Liaison with the patient's relatives and with the community health care team will help to ensure that the patient is given optimum support in dealing with the side-effects of treatment (see Ch. 32, p. 888). In some cases the side-effects will necessitate hospitalisation, as when nausea, vomiting and diarrhoea cause dehydration, or when urinary frequency or incontinence cause severe physical and psychological distress.

Treating advanced disease. The aims of treatment in advanced disease are to provide symptomatic relief and to preserve an acceptable quality of life for the individual. The outlook for improvement will depend upon various factors; those with renal failure, anaemia or urinary retention and metastases have a poor prognosis.

Those who have metastatic disease and are symptomatic are normally offered hormonal treatment. Hormonal manipulation can be achieved by bilateral orchidectomy (excision of the testes) or by the administration of oestrogens or of LHRH (luteinising hormone releasing hormone) agonists. Of patients given hormonal treatment, 70% will experience symptomatic relief for a period but will have recurrent symptoms in the long term.

The treatment of those with metastatic disease who are not symptomatic will usually be deferred until symptoms develop. Once hormonal treatment has been given and relapse occurs the outlook is very poor.

It would appear that chemotherapy is ineffective in treating advanced prostatic carcinoma. However, radiotherapy is sometimes beneficial in the relief of bony pain caused by metastases. Vertebral collapse caused by metastatic disease of the spinal cord requires emergency radiotherapy or laminectomy and hormonal manipulation. If effective, these measures may prevent neurological symptoms and/or paraplegia from developing.

Pain control by means of opiate analgesics may cause secondary constipation; this in turn can cause urinary retention. It may be more appropriate to administer non-steroidal anti-inflammatory medication to avoid this side-effect. Should analgesics be required, they should be given in doses which prevent pain occurring (see Ch. 19, p. 624). Sustained or slow-release drugs are often very useful.

NURSING PRIORITIES AND MANAGEMENT: CARCINOMA OF THE PROSTATE

General considerations

The nursing management of prostatic cancer is very much influenced by the particular presentation of the disease in each individual. The nurse should take a problem-solving approach to care and promote independence and self-care for as long as possible. The nurse should bear in mind that constipation and urinary retention or urinary incontinence are commonly encountered and can be very distressing both for the individual and for his family. Ongoing liaison between hospital and community teams will help to ensure that care is effective and genuinely responsive to the individual's unique situation (see Ch. 34).

A range of medical interventions may be necessary at different stages in the disease process. Nursing involvement will then include assisting with procedures such as:

- correction of anaemia by blood transfusion
- TURP to relieve retention
- bilateral subcapsular orchidectomy to reduce the hormone level, help prevent the spread of metastases, and reduce pain.

In many cases, medical intervention can offer only temporary improvement, and the emphasis of care will turn to palliation. Treatment of advanced disease is usually shared between hospital and home, and the patient and his family will need a great deal of moral support in both settings. It is important to convey a sense of optimism so that life can continue to be enjoyed to the fullest degree possible. In the last stages of the illness, however, it should not be seen as a defeat or failure to help the patient to let go of life and face death with dignity (see Ch. 34, p. 935).

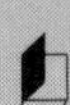

Marsh (1992) examines early detection and treatment and discusses the management of local and advanced disease, highlighting the importance of patient education and family support.
Deans (1988) and Brown & Lunt (1992) are also recommended.

DISORDERS OF THE BLADDER

Cancer of the bladder

Tumours of the bladder (usually transitional cell carcinoma) occur more commonly in men than in women (M:W = 4:1). About 9000 new cases of bladder cancer are registered each year. Bladder tumours are histologically similar to tumours of the renal pelvis and ureter. About 95% are malignant, and benign tumours often recur after apparently successful treatment.

Worldwide, the main cause of bladder cancer is urinary schistosomiasis, a parasite which invades body tissue. This disease in endemic in the tropics (Edwards & Bouchier 1991). Industrial exposure to dyes and printing agents containing aniline may be an important factor. Other possible causative agents or factors include:

- rubber
- cigarette smoking
- calculi
- diverticula
- chronic inflammation due to indwelling catheterisation.

Screening of those in high-risk groups may help to reduce incidence. Controls do exist to monitor factors associated with bladder cancer, but as many years may elapse between exposure to a carcinogen and the development of cancer, direct connections are difficult to establish.

8.7 What part can the occupational health nurse play in prevention?

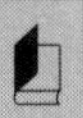

Refer to RCN 1991.

PATHOPHYSIOLOGY

Tumour growth usually commences in the epithelial lining of the bladder, often as a papillary growth. (Papilla are minute nipple-shaped projections.) Benign growth will without treatment usually progress to malignancy and then by stages from superficial to deep muscle tissue involvement, eventually spreading locally into surrounding tissue or organs. Metastatic spread to other parts of the urinary tract will also occur.

Common presenting symptoms (see Table 8.3). About 80% of people with bladder cancer will notice haematuria. This may be the only presenting feature of the disease. Dysuria, frequency, symptoms of obstruction and infection may also be noticed, but embarrassment may prevent the individual from visiting the GP's surgery. Symptoms may not persist following initial presentation, e.g. if associated infection is resolved by a course of antibiotics. Investigations should, however, be undertaken if the cause of haematuria is unclear.

? **8.8** A 35-year-old man notices blood in his urine each morning. He has no discomfort and is otherwise well. Unless the haematuria persists this man may decide not to visit his GP. How might you encourage him to report the haematuria? What anxieties might he have about reporting to his GP?

Table 8.3 Presenting features of bladder cancer

Sign/symptom	Reason
Haematuria, urine retention	Tumour growth Tumour spread
Dysuria, urgency, hesitancy, frequency. Urinary incontinence	Stimulation of reflex micturition arc Secondary infection Irritability of bladder
Chills and cystitis	Obstruction/infection
Back ache, pain	Ureteric obstruction Dependent upon the stage: infiltration Symptoms of cystitis or burning
Lower limb oedema	Venous obstruction Lymphatic obstruction
Infection	Obstruction Tumour necrosis
Malaise, anaemia	Frequency causing lack of rest or sleep Bleeding
Suprapubic mass, abnormal mass on rectal examination	Tumour size Tumour spread

MEDICAL MANAGEMENT

Investigative procedures. Diagnosis may be aided by physical examination, a full blood count, urea and electrolyte estimation and other biochemical assays. Examination of an MSU specimen will exclude evidence of infection. Table 8.4 lists the principal diagnostic investigations; in many respects these will be similar to those used in diagnosing prostatic disorders.

Staging. The staging of bladder tumours is illustrated in Figure 8.11 (see also Ch. 32, p. 883). In addition to staging according to the actual tumour, the pathologist will grade transitional cell tumours according to invasion differentiation of the lesion (Burkitt 1990).

Medical intervention. The choice of treatment will depend on the type of tumour and degree of invasion of local tissue, as determined by cystoscopy (see Table 8.5). Superficial lesions without muscle invasion can be treated by excision of the tumour through the urethra: transurethral resection of tumour (TURT). Irrigation of the bladder may be used to keep the bladder clear of blood clots following transurethral resection (see p. 311). The 5-year survival rate for well-differentiated superficial tumours is about 90% (Edwards & Bouchier 1991).

Table 8.4 Principal diagnostic investigations for tumours of the bladder

Investigation	Reason
Intravenous urogram (IVU)	If presenting feature is haematuria, IVU may exclude renal pelvic carcinoma
Cystoscopy and biopsy	Suspicious lesions can be examined for abnormal cells
CT scan	If local spread of tumour is suspected
Chest X-ray Bone scan Liver function tests	If metastatic spread is suspected

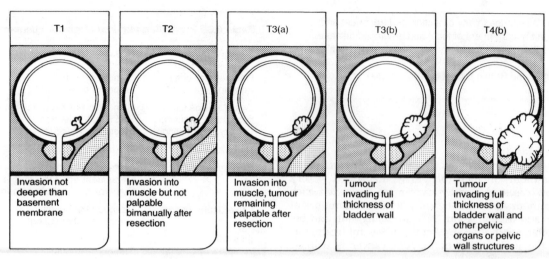

Fig. 8.11 System for staging bladder tumours. Note: stage T3(b) indicates tumour invasion of prostate gland. (Reproduced with permission from Burkitt et al 1990.)

A significant number of people with locally invasive bladder tumours have metastatic spread when they first present. The 5-year survival rate for poorly differentiated tumours is about 30% (Edwards & Bouchier 1991).

For invasive bladder tumours a combination of surgery (i.e. total cystectomy), radiotherapy and chemotherapy may be used.

Total cystectomy involves removing the lower ureters, bladder, prostate, urethra and lymphatics in men, and also the gynaecological organs in women. Urinary diversion is required and is most commonly ileal conduit and stoma formation (see Fig. 8.12). With this type of diversion, the ureters are anastomosed to an isolated section of the bowel (ileum with blood supply) and the loop brought to the abdominal surface as a stoma. This is a major procedure which will fundamentally affect the lifestyle of the patient and his family.

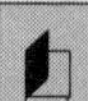

For further information, see Blandy (1986).

Table 8.5 Treatment choices in tumours of the bladder

Tumour	Treatment	Comment
Localised, well-differentiated tumour	Diathermy	Annual cystoscopy to check for recurrence
Histologically malignant tumours i) extensive superficial ii) locally invasive	Chemotherapy: intravenal Radiotherapy TURT	Annual cystoscopy to assess effect and check for recurrence
Failure to control tumour spread/severe symptoms	Cystectomy and ureter transplant to ileal conduit (urinary diversion)	Radiotherapy may be used to reduce size of tumour prior to surgery
Inoperable tumour	Analgesia Palliative radiotherapy	
Metastatic spread	Systemic chemotherapy	An option although success is limited

Radiotherapy is normally given as an external treatment for bladder carcinoma over a 6-week period. It may be used as a palliative measure or in conjunction with surgery and/or chemotherapy, pre- or post-treatment. The age and general condition of the patient will determine whether treatment is given on an outpatient or inpatient basis. Sometimes the severity of the symptoms encountered leads to conversion from outpatient to inpatient care and a rest in the treatment plan to allow the patient to recuperate before progressing to the next treatment.

Chemotherapy. Treatment of invasive bladder cancer with systemic chemotherapy is under investigation. Regimes of treatment vary. Some patients receive care on a day care basis, receiving i.v. injections, while others attend for inpatient hospital care involving 2–3 days in hospital for each cycle of treatment. (For further details on systemic chemotherapy the reader should refer to Chapter 32.)

Intravesical chemotherapy may be offered in some cases. The recurrence of superficial bladder tumours resected endoscopically is about 65%. Recurrent tumours are usually of the same type and stage as those previously resected. Further endoscopic resection may be the treatment of choice, but sometimes intravesical chemotherapy is also given. This involves the introduction of a variety of drugs via a urethral catheter. Treatment may be weekly, monthly, or bimonthly, depending upon the type of tumour and the drug used. A urethral catheter is inserted and the chosen drug instilled via the catheter. The catheter can then be removed. The patient is requested to avoid passing urine for an hour and is asked to turn from back to front to sides every 15 min, in order to wash the drug around the bladder.

The nurse administering the treatment should bear in mind that this patient may have difficulty in postponing the passing of urine for up to 1 h because of symptoms of frequency, irritability, and so on. The patient should be reassured he has not 'failed' if he is unable to comply with this request.

The side-effects of the drugs used in this treatment vary, but chemical cystitis leading to inflammation and bladder irritability, urgency and frequency is common. Sensitivity rashes are seen less commonly, as are more severe effects such as systemic toxicity and bone marrow suppression.

Since the drugs used are toxic agents, precautions such as wearing protective goggles, gloves and gowns should be taken when preparing and administering treatments and when discarding used equipment.

After the treatment is completed, the patient should be advised that the urine he passes will contain chemical substances that will irritate the skin. Leakages or dribbles to the skin should be washed off immediately.

Treatment with intravesical chemotherapy seems to reduce the

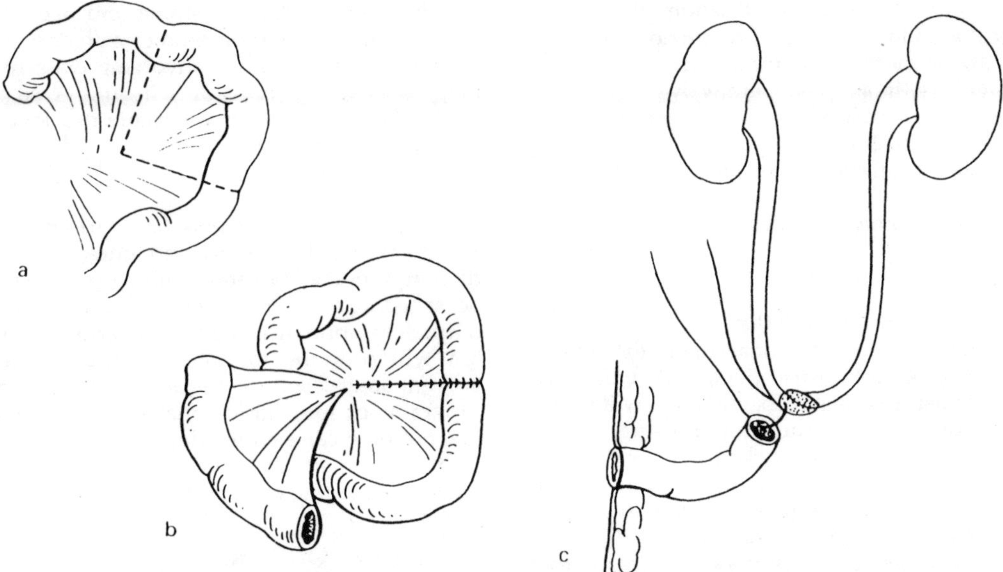

Fig. 8.12 Ileal conduit urinary diversion. (a–b) Isolation of segment of ileum. (c) Ureteroileal anastomosis. (Reproduced with permission from Forrest et al 1991.)

incidence of tumour recurrence, but it does seem to be less effective in the treatment of invasive bladder tumours.

NURSING PRIORITIES AND MANAGEMENT: TOTAL CYSTECTOMY AND URINARY DIVERSION

Preoperative care

Psychological preparation (see Case History 8.5)
The patient admitted for cystectomy and urinary diversion may already know the nursing and medical staff on the ward from a previous admission. Staff should try to build upon this rapport and provide information both verbally and in written form to prepare the patient for the physical effects of the operation, particularly the formation of a stoma. Considerable psychological adjustment may be required on the part of the patient to come to terms with the lifestyle changes that will be necessary and with the alteration in body image that may occur.

The patient is likely to have concerns relating to: any pain that will be experienced; whether the operation will effect a 'cure'; how his family will cope in his absence and after his return home; and how he will appear to other people. The contribution of the primary nurse and the stoma therapist in answering questions and allaying fears in the preoperative period is invaluable. It may be helpful to arrange for the patient and his family to meet with someone who has a stoma (Dyer 1988a, 1988b).

Case History 8.5 Mr L

Mr L, a 58-year-old married man employed as a bus driver was diagnosed 5 years ago with cancer of the bladder. He was treated with regular cystoscopies and transurethral resections of tumour. Six months ago the tumour was found to be stage T2, and a course of chemotherapy was prescribed. Recent cystoscopy showed that this treatment has not been successful. Total cystectomy is now being considered for this patient.

It should be noted that patients rarely ask about the effect surgery may have on sexual function. However, one of the side-effects for male patients of this life-saving procedure is impotence. This important matter must be discussed with the patient and his partner prior to the surgery (see Chapman 1990).

The patient may gain confidence from the knowledge that his community nurse and GP as well as a stoma nurse are available to support him. He should be given a contact telephone number to use in the event of difficulty. He should be reassured that any problems and concerns, however small, can be discussed as he makes the challenging adjustment from hospital to home.

?	**8.9**	How can the nurse help Mr L in Case History 8.5 to come to terms with this disappointing news and the prospect of total cystectomy?
?	**8.10**	Mr L is provided with an indwelling catheter which will remain in situ until he can be admitted to hospital. What advice and support could you offer Mr L and his wife to ensure that no catheter-related problems develop? What part can the community nurse play? Review Boxes 8.8 and 8.9.

Physical preparation
The stoma will be sited on the abdomen below the waist, normally on the right-hand side. Considerations in choosing the exact site include:

- the patient's build
- access for the surgeon
- previous surgery
- access for the patient following surgery
- type of clothing to be worn after the surgery.

The following procedures are carried out in preparation for surgery:

1. the patient is kept on a fluid-only or low-residue diet at commencement of bowel preparation
2. the bowel is cleared of faeces. This may be by means of an enema or a high colonic wash-out and is carried out 2

days prior to the operation. Bowel sterilisation with systemic and local antibiotics may be prescribed
3. prophylactic antibiotic therapy is commenced preoperatively (and continued postoperatively)
4. the skin is shaved from nipple to knee, or according to the surgeon's wishes (see Ch. 27)
5. the patient is assisted to take a shower on the day of the operation
6. the chosen site for the stoma is marked.

Postoperative care

Return from theatre (see Nursing Care Plan 8.2)
Following surgery and recovery from anaesthetic the patient will return to the ward. A nasogastric (NG) tube will be in place for aspiration of gastric contents. Examination will reveal a midline incision, covered by a surgical dressing, and a wound drain. The stoma, in the pre-marked position, should have a moist, red appearance and be covered by a collection bag fitted with a drainage tap and autoreflux valve to prevent backflow of urine when the patient is lying flat.

Infant feeding tubes which form temporary splints across the ureteroileal anastomosis may be seen protruding from the stoma. The splints, one for each ureter and inserted at surgery, pass through the ileal loop and along the ureters across the junction of the anastomosis. The support provided by the splints reduces the risk of urine leakage from the anastomosis before healing has taken place.

The recovery period
The NG tube will be in place for 24–48 h, or until bowel sounds have returned. Drains may be removed when discharge is less than 50 ml/24 h; this is usually at 4–5 days postoperatively. Removal of splints from the stoma can usually be done at 10–14 days, and removal of sutures at 10 days. Assessment by the dietitian and provision of a diet plan may aid wound healing and recovery.

During this time, the stoma nurse will visit. Working with the primary nurse, she will teach the patient how to clean the stoma and change the bag and flange on a daily basis. The patient should be shown how to cut the flange to shape and fit it in position with the bag.

Patients differ in the time it takes them to come to terms with management of their stoma. Some show no interest at first in looking after the stoma and need a lot of encouragement. Planning a programme with the patient, identifying goals to be attained and involving close relatives/carers will help to ensure successful self-care. A second visit with an individual who has already made the adjustment to life with a stoma may also help.

Discharge
Provided no complications have arisen, by 10–14 days after the operation the patient and nurse should be planning for discharge home. The first follow-up appointment will usually be scheduled for 6–8 weeks after the operation. Thereafter, outpatient appointments will be arranged at longer intervals, but will continue for life. To ensure optimal function and prevent long-term complications (see Box 8.11), periodic i.v. urograms or loopograms may be performed. A loopogram is the radiological examination of the bowel segment used to form the urinary diversion; this investigation may reveal any disorder of filling or capacity (Hanno & Wein 1987).

RENAL DISORDERS

Glomerulonephritis

The term 'glomerulonephritis' refers to a group of disorders characterised by the presence of a lesion in the glomerulus of the kidney. The disease may be primary to the glomerulus or secondary to a systemic disorder. Box 8.12 lists primary and secondary causes.

Proteinaemia, haematuria, hypertension and renal impairment characterise this disease but the severity of these effects will vary between individuals. Presentation is usually described in terms of a range of clinical syndromes, but accurate diagnosis requires histological investigation.

PATHOPHYSIOLOGY

Histological examination of renal tissue will demonstrate inflammation in the majority of cases, but it is also possible to find minimal change and no evidence of an inflammatory process. The disease process results from a defect in the immune response, such as a hypersensitivity to an exogenous antigen. The antigen–antibody reaction results in the formation of insoluble immune complexes that circulate in the blood and, instead of being ingested by macrophages, reach the kidney, where they become 'trapped' and set up a damaging

Box 8.11 Complications following total cystectomy

SPECIFIC COMPLICATIONS POST-CYSTECTOMY

- Breakdown of anastomosis
- Breakdown of blood supply to stoma (necrosis)
- Pelvic abscess
- Poor wound healing post-radiotherapy
- Prolapse of stoma
- Renal failure
- Retraction of stoma
- Urinary infection

LATER COMPLICATION

- Depression
- Prolapse of stoma
- Recurrence of tumour
- Retraction of stoma
- Stenosis of stoma
- Stone formation
- Urinary infection
- Urinary reflux

Box 8.12 Causes of glomerulonephritis

PRIMARY CAUSES

- Minimal change glomerular disease
- Proliferative glomerulonephritis:
  — mesangial
  — diffuse capillary
  — focal
  — IgA nephropathy
  — mesangiocapillary
  — crescentic (Goodpasture's syndrome)
  — membranous glomerulonephritis
  — focal segmental glomerulonephritis

COMMON SECONDARY CAUSES

- Systemic lupus erythematosus
- Polyarteritis
- Diabetes mellitus
- Amyloidosis
- Henoch–Schönlein purpura
- Malarial nephropathy

Nursing Care Plan 8.2 Nursing care in first 24 h following total cystectomy and urinary diversion

Potential problem	Action	Desired outcome
1. Cardiovascular instability and hypovolaemic shock due to haemorrhage and pain	❒ Record vital signs and report any deviations from normal range ❒ Monitor and mark extent of blood loss evident on wound dressing ❒ Record blood loss in drains and report if in excess of 100 ml/h	Cardiovascular stability Minimal blood loss Minimal pain
2. Pain	❒ Observe patient for distress (N.B. generalised abdominal pain may indicate peritonitis caused by leakage from anastomosis) ❒ Administer prescribed analgesics ❒ Evaluate effect after 30 min by asking patient if pain has been relieved	Patient is pain free
3. Fluid and electrolyte imbalance	❒ Measure and record hourly urine output (N.B. output < 30 ml could indicate obstruction or possible leakage from ureteroileal anastomosis leading to peritonitis ❒ Balance all fluid output against all fluid input in 24 h ❒ Observe for evidence of dyspnoea, dehydration, e.g. dry skin and mouth ❒ Observe for vomiting	Fluid and electrolytes maintained at satisfactory levels
4. Paralytic ileus	❒ Allow nil by mouth ❒ Perform NG aspirations hourly/free drainage ❒ Administer antiemetics as necessary	Comfort is maintained until return of bowel sounds
5. Deep vein thrombosis (DVT) and/or pulmonary embolism (PE)	❒ Supply antiembolic stockings preoperatively ❒ Encourage movement of lower limbs ❒ Observe for evidence of DVT or PE	Circulatory integrity is maintained
6. Chest infection	❒ Encourage deep breathing and coughing ❒ Refer to physiotherapist ❒ Position patient as upright as possible	Chest is clear with no evidence of infection
7. Wound infection	❒ Observe wound for leakage, check drains hourly ❒ Record temperature and report pyrexia ❒ Leave dressings undisturbed for 48 h	Wound heals without infection
8. Development of pressure sores	❒ Change patient's position regularly and observe for reddening ❒ Use a risk assessment scale to assess patient's needs ❒ Ensure skin is clean and dry ❒ Use Spenco mattress if necessary	Skin integrity is maintained
9. Inability to perform personal hygiene tasks	❒ Provide bedbath and mouth care	Patient is clean and comfortable
10. Anxiety	❒ Discuss patient's concerns with him. Provide information, but take post-anaesthetic drowsiness into account ❒ Evaluate patient's understanding of information given. Return next day and ask if there are further questions or concerns	Patient understands what is happening and feels secure in the care provided

inflammatory reaction in the delicate filtration structure. As a result of this:

- protein and red blood cells pass through the filtration fenestration
- the osmotic pressure of the blood plasma falls, leading to oedema
- sodium and water is retained, as are waste products and potentially toxic substances.

It would seem that most cases of acute glomerulonephritis occur 1–3 weeks after an 'innocent' streptococcal infection such as tonsillitis or otitis media (Guyton 1991); this most commonly occurs in children or adolescents. The disease can range from a mild, transitory, asymptomatic condition to a very severe form that precipitates acute renal failure, cardiac failure and convulsions.

Common presenting symptoms are exemplified in Case History 8.6.

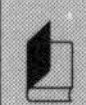

For further information, see Edwards & Bouchier (1991) Ch. 12.

MEDICAL MANAGEMENT

Tests and investigations. A patient such as T (see Case History 8.6) would probably be admitted to hospital, where investigations would confirm the diagnosis. This would especially be the case if there were symptoms of breathlessness or a risk of convulsions, which would indicate cardiac or cerebral complications. Investigations would include:

- urinalysis
- MSU
- full blood count and urea and electrolyte estimation
- throat swab
- chest X-ray
- ECG
- intravenous pyelogram (IVP).

Medical intervention. There is no cure as such for glomerulonephritis. The aim of treatment is to reduce renal workload, restore and maintain fluid and electrolyte status and prevent uraemia. Thus management aims to prevent serious complications from occurring (see Box 8.13).

Box 8.13 Life-threatening complications of glomerulonephritis

1. Acute hypertensive encephalitis leading to convulsions (see Ch. 9)

Management:

- maintain airway
- monitor level of consciousness (e.g. with Glasgow Coma Scale)
- give anticonvulsant therapy, e.g. i.v. diazepam
- give hypotensive agents, e.g. hydralazine

2. Pulmonary oedema/cardiac failure (see Chs 2 and 3)

Management:

- give oxygen therapy
- monitor cardiovascular status
- give diuretic therapy, e.g. i.v. frusemide
- give opiate analgesics, e.g. i.v. morphine combined with an antiemetic

3. Acute renal failure

Management:

- dialysis

NURSING PRIORITIES AND MANAGEMENT: GLOMERULONEPHRITIS

Major nursing considerations

Promoting rest

Bedrest is a necessity, especially in the early period, to reduce the workload of both the kidneys and the heart. This can pose quite a challenge in the care of younger patients. Time needs to be spent with the patient explaining why rest is so important.

Maintaining fluid and electrolyte balance

While renal function is impaired and fluid overload poses a very real problem, fluid and sodium intake must be restricted. Potassium levels in the blood must be closely monitored and if necessary dietary modification made or ion exchange resins given (see p. 320). If hypertension is marked, hypotensive medication may be required.

Case History 8.6 T

T was an active 15-year-old schoolgirl. In September she developed a sore throat which completely robbed her of her voice for several days. It didn't last long and she was used to such minor ailments. In early October she began to notice a feeling of weariness that was quite uncharacteristic. She found herself longing for her bed as the day progressed and declined evening invitations for the usual lively events. On waking one morning, she noticed that her face appeared rather puffy and on close inspection found she had puffy ankles. Her parents became concerned and T made an appointment to see her doctor. T now began to consider other problems. She had lost her appetite, often felt rather sick and had noticed her urine had been rather smoky and darker in hue.

T's GP identified significant proteinuria and haematuria, an elevated blood pressure and marked oedema. A diagnosis of acute glomerulonephritis was made.

Preventing uraemia

While the kidney is impaired the waste products of metabolism will build up in the blood. To prevent this a low-protein diet will be necessary. Calorie intake can be maintained with carbohydrates, and vitamin supplements can be given. This diet must also be low in salt and many patients find meals most unpalatable. The dietitian can contribute tremendously to the patient's well-being by ensuring that the restricted diet includes at least some favourite foods.

Preventing infection

If a streptococcal link is confirmed, penicillin may be prescribed. All patients with renal impairment are prone to infection (see p. 320). All procedures necessary for the prevention of cross-infection must be adhered to (see Ch. 16, p. 548).

Promoting convalescence and the maintenance of health

Most patients make a full recovery, but convalescence may take as long as 2 years. The acute condition can resolve fairly rapidly. Such patients often feel better quite quickly and it can be hard to persuade them that restrictions are still needed. Proteinuria can persist and regular monitoring will be necessary. After discharge, support for the patient and family will ensure that necessary lifestyle adjustments are made for the initial months. Exercise should be gentle and energetic sports activities avoided. *Any* infection should be treated seriously and medical advice sought.

Incomplete resolution and permanent glomerular damage can result in chronic glomerulonephritis and all the associated symptoms of renal impairment. Failure of function may be such that dialysis is required (see p. 322).

Nephrotic syndrome (see Case History 8.7)

Nephrotic syndrome can be a manifestation of certain forms of glomerulonephritis but may also result as a complication of diabetes mellitus or amyloid disease whereby insoluble

Case History 8.7 Mrs Y

Mrs Y, aged 29, presented to her GP with a 3-week history of anorexia and tiredness. Examination revealed no muscle wasting but did show a moderate degree of ankle and sacral oedema. Mrs Y said that her complexion was naturally pale but that her face seemed to have become puffy in the last week or so. Urine testing showed heavy proteinuria. Blood samples were taken for biochemical analysis.

A clinical diagnosis of nephrotic syndrome was made and 80 mg of frusemide daily and a no-added-salt diet were prescribed. Mrs Y was advised that a renal biopsy may be necessary. She resisted immediate admission to hospital and the GP and district nurse arranged to attend Mrs Y's home on alternate days.

Mrs Y wished to stay at home as she had a 3-year-old son and a 6-month-old daughter to care for. On weekday mornings Mrs Y took her son to a nursery half a mile away and collected him at midday. The family were dependent financially on Mr Y, who worked 200 miles away and was able to return home only at weekends.

One of the major difficulties Mrs Y will face is dealing with the increased diuresis that results from diuretic therapy. A heavy diuresis will occur for about 4 h following each dose. This may make it virtually impossible for Mrs Y to leave the house. Taking her son to the nursery and shopping for household necessities may become difficult. Confined to the house with two small children and a husband 200 miles away Mrs Y may become socially isolated. The 'no-added-salt diet' may also pose a problem for Mrs Y, particularly if she enjoys salty foods.

The symptoms that Mrs X has experienced are uncomfortable and frightening. It has been suggested to her that she might need a renal biopsy to determine the cause of her symptoms. It is likely that she will be worried and may need time to voice her concerns and perhaps obtain information and reassurance about her physical condition. It is possible that she may feel unable to carry out all the care for her children and require assistance at some times during the day.

starch-like deposits occur in kidney tissue. Often no cause can be found.

PATHOPHYSIOLOGY

In the normal kidney, protein molecules passing across the glomerulomembrane are reabsorbed in the kidney tubules. However, where increased glomerular permeability occurs, increased numbers of protein molecules enter the tubules. When the capacity of the tubule to reabsorb protein is exceeded, protein is lost in the urine. Further protein is lost following catabolism of protein reabsorbed in the tubule, resulting in hypoproteinaemia. Muscle wasting can result from the catabolism of muscle protein as the body tries to maintain normal plasma protein levels. A low plasma protein reduces plasma osmotic pressure and fluid leaks into the extracellular areas. The resultant oedema occurs in dependent areas and may give rise to ascites in severe cases. Intravascular volume is maintained in many cases. How this occurs is not fully understood, but activation of the renin–angiotensin–aldosterone mechanism is thought likely.

Clinical features. This syndrome is characterised by heavy proteinuria and hypoproteinaemia and by oedema. These patients generally have a low urine output and low urine sodium. Derangement of lipoproteins is evident and loss of fibrinogen in the urine can occur. Infection and thrombosis are common complications.

MEDICAL MANAGEMENT

Medical intervention. The main aim of treatment is to reduce oedema. Diuretic therapy can be adjusted according to the severity of the oedema and small maintenance doses can be administered when the oedema is under control. Severe oedema may also be treated by the administration of salt-poor albumen to temporarily increase plasma osmotic pressure. Patients are advised to adhere to a diet free from added salt.

Identification of the underlying disease process, possibly by renal biopsy and histological examination, will dictate the nature of ongoing treatment. In many patients, chronic renal failure will eventually develop.

8.11 Since Mrs Y in Case History 8.7 has young children, the health visitor will already know this family well. The effectiveness of intervention will depend on the quality of communication between members of the primary health care team. What are the essential features of teamwork that will contribute to the well-being of Mrs Y and her family? Draw from the following references as you consider these issues in a discussion group.

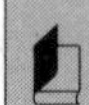

For further information, see de Guzman & Joyce (1991), Johnson (1989), Gregson et al (1991), Pearson (1992) and Waine (1992).

Acute renal failure (ARF)

Acute renal failure, the sudden and severe reduction in previously normal renal function, may result from primary renal disease but is more frequently associated with other organ failure. In the UK the incidence of failure is reported to be as high as 80 million cases per year (Allen 1990). Failure is often reversible, but should the kidneys fail to recover permanent treatment will be required.

A mortality rate of 40–70% is associated with acute renal failure, the actual risk depending on the type of patient, the cause of failure and other organ involvement (Allen 1990). Where death occurs renal failure is often not the primary cause.

PATHOPHYSIOLOGY

Causes. The causes of acute renal failure may be classified by the point of their effect on the kidneys.

Pre-renal causes are those in which a loss or decrease in renal perfusion results in renal ischaemia. They include:

- extracellular depletion, e.g. large GI loss such as vomiting, diarrhoea or NG aspiration; urinary loss due to polyuria or diuresis; loss from the skin, e.g. sweating or burns
- circulating volume loss, as in haemorrhage or hypoalbuminaemia
- reduced cardiac output, as in cardiac arrest, valvular disease, cardiac tamponade
- vascular disease, e.g. renal artery thrombosis or embolism.

Renal causes include conditions that impair renal function by damaging the structure of the kidney (tubules, interstitium, glomeruli or capillaries). If tubular damage occurs this is termed acute tubular necrosis (ATN) although microscopically the tubules usually show dilatation rather than necrosis (Thomson & Woodhouse 1987). ATN is said to account for 75% of all acute renal failure (Holloway 1988).

Pre-renal causes can cause destruction of the renal parenchyma. Nephrotoxic substances can also result in acute failure. These include:

- drugs, e.g. the antibiotics kanamycin and gentamicin
- exogenous chemicals, e.g. heavy metals, phenols, carbon tetrachloride, chlorates, ethyl glycol
- bacterial toxins, particularly those released in Gram-negative septicaemia (see Ch. 18, p. 601).

Post-renal causes are mainly attributed to obstruction. The most common of these is bladder output obstruction. In males, this is usually due to prostatic hypertrophy and in females to carcinoma of the cervix (Chatto & Power 1988).

Other causes include calculi, blood clots and tumours.

Clinical features. Acute renal failure proceeds through three phases: the oliguric stage, the diuretic stage and the recovery stage. If oliguria persists for more than 48 h, major metabolic problems can arise.

Oliguria and abnormal plasma levels of creatinine, urea and electrolytes are the principal features of presentation. The effects of acute fluid overload and hyperkalaemia ($K^+ > 6$ mmol/l) can result in sudden death.

The patient may complain of anorexia, nausea and vomiting. Increased respiration due to pulmonary oedema and acidosis can occur. Drowsiness, confusion and coma may follow.

MEDICAL MANAGEMENT

Tests and investigations will depend on the suspected cause and on the immediacy of the presentation but may include:

- full blood count and urea and electrolyte estimation
- urinalysis, MSU, 24 h collections of urine for creatinine clearance
- X-ray of kidneys, ureters and bladder
- IVU
- CT scan
- ultrasound
- renal biopsy.

Medical intervention. The goal of treatment is to restore biochemical balance and prevent ARF progressing. The onset of renal failure must be identified early to minimise damage and, if possible, prevent the necessity for dialysis. The priorities of treatment are as follows:

1. Treating the cause, e.g. correcting hypovolaemia and increasing renal perfusion; managing sepsis; relieving any urinary obstruction
2. Reversing, restoring and maintaining fluid and electrolyte status:
   - *Hyperkalaemia*: Immediate measures may be required to correct hyperkalaemia, which could cause lethal dysrhythmias. Cardiac monitoring is essential and particular attention must be paid to the T-wave (Hampton 1992). Hyperkalaemia can be corrected in the short term by i.v. insulin–glucose infusion or sodium bicarbonate, either of which will shift potassium into the cells. Other measures include the administration of ion exchange resins such as calcium, which administered orally or rectally removes potassium ions
   - *Hyponatraemia and hypernatraemia*: In the oliguric state there is a real danger of hyponatraemia, due to the very real risk of fluid overload and to the failure of the damaged tubules to reabsorb sodium. However, hypernatraemia can also be a problem in pre-renal ARF, as mechanisms instituted retain sodium in order to restore blood volume. Fluid intake must be restricted to the equivalent of insensible loss plus the previous day's urinary output. Sodium intake must be monitored closely
   - *Uraemia*: The inability to excrete the waste products of metabolism is managed by reducing protein intake and maintaining a high calorie intake in the form of carbohydrates. Total parenteral nutrition (TPN) may be necessary and potassium intake will be restricted (see Ch. 21, p. 672)
   - *Metabolic acidosis*: The loss of the kidneys' buffering function, the electrolyte imbalance and the increased anaerobic respiration by damaged renal cells all result in acidosis. In the short term this is managed by i.v. sodium bicarbonate.

If acute renal failure is very severe, persists or worsens, dialysis will be necessary.

NURSING PRIORITIES AND MANAGEMENT: ACUTE RENAL FAILURE

Major nursing considerations

The care of patients with ARF may involve a large multidisciplinary team and be carried out in an intensive care setting. However, many may be nursed in a general ward and require close monitoring and support by the nursing staff. Priorities of nursing intervention will be as follows:

- to reduce the patient's very real anxieties and recognise the risk of altered consciousness due to uraemia and electrolyte imbalance
- to control fluid and electrolyte balance by:
  — monitoring cardiac status for signs of dysrhythmias
  — monitoring pulse, respiration and blood pressure for signs of overload and hypertension
  — restricting fluid intake and measuring and recording urine output and other losses. Daily weighing may be required
  — administering prescribed medication and carrying out urinary assays as required
- to maintain nutritional status within the necessary limitations by the oral or parenteral route and to monitor the nutritional status of the patient
- to prevent infection due to uraemia by strict asepsis with regard to infusion sites and catheter management and by close monitoring of temperature and patient's reported symptoms
- to manage anaemia by the safe administration of blood transfusions, if required
- to promote comfort at all times.

?	**8.12** Reconsider the care of T, who had acute glomerulonephritis (see Case History 8.6). Severe forms can result in acute tubular necrosis and acute renal failure. Draw up a care plan that would have met T's needs should ARF have developed.

The diuretic and recovery stages

So far we have considered the oliguric stage of renal failure. This may last 1–3 weeks and is followed by the diuretic stage, which indicates that renal function is returning. This is often a time of relief, but because the kidneys will have not yet regained their capacity for selective reabsorption, urine output can be as much as 4 l a day. This in itself could potentiate dehydration and electrolyte imbalances. Close monitoring must therefore continue. The recovery phase that follows can last several months and will require close medical follow-up of renal function. Convalescence in the form of rest, restricted activity, the avoidance of infections and alertness to any symptoms that might indicate renal problems may be a source of considerable stress to the patient, who may also be concerned about fulfilling family and work responsibilities.

?	**8.13** What community support services might help alleviate such stress?

Chronic renal failure

Chronic renal failure is the gradual and progressive reduction in renal function. Failure may occur over weeks, months or even years. Each year, approximately 55 new patients per million of the population require renal replacement therapy to maintain life. The available treatments are dialysis or transplantation.

Box 8.14 Aetiology of chronic renal failure (Reproduced with permission from Edwards & Bouchier 1991.)

CONGENITAL AND INHERITED DISEASES

- Polycystic kidney disease (infantile or adult)
- Alport's syndrome
- Fabry's disease

VASCULAR DISEASE

- Arteriosclerosis
- Vasculitis (polyarteritis nodosa PAN, systemic lupus erythematosus SLE, scleroderma)

GLOMERULAR DISEASE

- Proliferative GN
- Crescentic GN
- Membranous GN
- Mesangiocapillary GN
- Glomerulosclerosis
- Secondary GN (PAN, SLE, amyloidosis, diabetic glomerulosclerosis)

INTERSTITIAL DISEASE

- Chronic infective interstitial nephritis (chronic pyelonephritis)
- Vesicoureteric reflux
- Tuberculosis
- Analgesic nephropathy
- Nephrocalcinosis
- Schistosomiasis
- Unknown origin

OBSTRUCTIVE UROPATHY

- Calculus
- Retroperitoneal fibrosis
- Prostatic hypertrophy
- Pelvic tumours
- Other causes

PATHOPHYSIOLOGY

Any disorder which damages kidney function can result in renal failure (see Box 8.14).

Clinical features. In the initial stages of failure the patient may be asymptomatic. Proteinuria, hypertension, anaemia, or an elevated blood urea are, however, common presenting features.

As renal failure progresses the patient may complain of fatigue, lethargy, pruritus, nausea, vomiting and indigestion. Breathlessness on exertion, headaches, visual disturbances, pallor and loss of libido may also be noted. A reduced immune response occurs, making the patient prone to infection, particularly of the urinary tract (see Ch. 16).

Metabolic bone disease, generalised myopathy, neuropathy and metabolic acidosis can be seen in advanced stages of renal impairment. Atherosclerosis due to altered lipid and carbohydrate metabolism and hypertension may also occur. Vascular calcification and pericarditis may also be identified.

MEDICAL MANAGEMENT

Medical intervention aims to identify the cause, extent and complications of the renal failure and to preserve useful renal function for as long as possible.

Where hypertension is evident, antihypertensive drugs may be used to gradually reduce and control blood pressure.

Fluid restriction may be required if the glomerulofiltration rate is less than 5 ml/min. Poor concentration can, however, result in a urine output of more than 2.5 l/24 h, in which case an intake of about 3 l is required.

Dietary restrictions are likely to include protein restriction to about 40 g daily if the serum creatinine is greater than 300 μmol/l. Sodium restriction is not indicated unless there is evidence of oedema, hypertension or cardiac failure. In the case of salt-losing conditions sodium supplements may be required. A no-added-salt diet may be appropriate in some cases.

Regular monitoring of biochemistry and assessment of symptoms allow treatment to be readjusted and progression of the disease to be assessed.

Dialysis in the form of haemodialysis or continuous ambulatory peritoneal dialysis are the treatments available to replace the excretory functions of the kidneys (see Box 8.15). At present, transplantation is restricted by a lack of available cadaver donor kidneys. In some cases it may be possible to consider a close family member as a live donor.

NURSING PRIORITIES AND MANAGEMENT: CHRONIC RENAL FAILURE

General considerations

Nursing management requires a strategy to help the patient and his family come to terms with an illness for which there is no cure and in which sudden death can occur. Nursing intervention should aim to help the patient develop a way to cope with the constraints of the available treatments and the possibility of other disorders associated with the renal failure occurring, for example, bone disease.

Compliance

Patient beliefs about the value and benefit of a treatment may differ markedly when compared with the priority given to the same treatment by the nurse. Non-compliance with diet and fluid restrictions is a common area of potential conflict between nurse and patient (Roper 1988). On occasion, drug therapy may not be taken — particularly if the drugs taste unpleasant or have unpleasant side-effects. An understanding of the patient's social and cultural background can give insight into his behaviour with regard to a particular treatment.

Major patient problems

Fatigue and lethargy characteristic of chronic renal failure can reduce both ability and performance at work. Absence from work due to sickness or attendance at hospital may result in unemployment or reduction of income. Feelings of helplessness, hopelessness and depression are often expressed by patients with a chronic illness (Devines et al 1981, 1983). Loss of control over many aspects of life and low self-esteem are likely to influence family relationships. Transplantation may be seen as a cure or an escape from dialysis, and indeed a more normal lifestyle and a feeling of physical well-being can follow transplant. The patient may be poorly prepared to deal with graft failure and the need to return to dialysis, or with inadequate graft function and the need for continued restrictions. The need to return regularly to hospital for check-ups, and continued problems associated with complications of renal failure or a second disease process such as diabetes can contribute to disappointment in transplantation as a treatment. On the other hand, some patients who undergo a successful transplant have difficulty abandoning the sick role. (see Ch. 33).

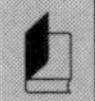

For further information, see Beckman et al (1992), Holechek et al (1991) and Locking-Cusolito (1990).

Living with CAPD

Continuous ambulatory peritoneal dialysis offers patients a

Box 8.15 Dialysis (Based on Ames & Kneisl 1988)

PRINCIPLES

Dialysis combines three principles — diffusion, osmosis and filtration — in order to permit the removal of metabolic wastes, excess electrolytes and fluids, from patients with renal failure.

Diffusion
Diffusion involves the movement of substances (solutes) across a semipermeable membrane that separates two fluid compartments containing substances of different concentrations. This process continues until the concentrations in each compartment are the same.

Osmosis
Osmosis is the movement of a fluid or solvent from a lower concentration to a higher one.

Filtration
Filtration is the movement of both solvent and solute across a semipermeable membrane under pressure.

Dialysis affects only fluid, electrolytes and acid–base imbalance, during the time it is performed. It cannot be a complete substitute for renal function.

TYPES

Haemodialysis
Haemodialysis requires a means of vascular access. In ARF this will usually be via a subclavian or femoral cannula with a Y-connection. In CRF access is normally via an arteriovenous (AV) fistula in the forearm.

The AV fistula is created by anastomosing an artery and a vein. After about 6–12 weeks increased pressure on the vein walls will cause it to become thickened and more muscular ('arterialised'), making the repeated insertion of needles for dialysis possible. The fistula becomes prominent and can be seen as well as felt.

The blood is pumped from the patient to an artificial kidney (the dialyser) and back to the patient, having now been cleansed by the dialysate. The artificial kidney is normally a disposable hollow fibre or flat plate dialyser.

Peritoneal dialysis
Here the peritoneal membrane serves as the semipermeable membrane for dialysis. A temporary or permanent Tenckhoff catheter is placed into the abdomen. The dialysate is instilled into the abdomen (usually 2 l each session). A set time elapses and the dialysate is drained out.

Continuing ambulatory peritoneal dialysis (CAPD)
The patient instils 2 l of dialysate and leaves this in place for several hours, usually exchanging the fluid 4 times a day.

Once the patient has been instructed in this method, he can be independent, visiting the hospital only for clinic appointments or when any problems arise.

The main potential problems are peritonitis, dehydration and constipation.

degree of control over their treatment. While the number of fluid exchanges per day will be prescribed by the doctor, the timing of each exchange can be decided by the patient to fit in with family life or work commitments. In addition, freedom to be away from home for visits or holidays is possible. For holidays abroad, the dialysate manufacturer may be able to deliver fluid requirements to the holiday destination.

The need for regular fluid exchanges and aseptic technique can be limiting for some patients. Performing the exchange in a designated area at home can give confidence and reassure patients that they have done all they can to reduce the risk of peritonitis. Reluctance may be expressed to perform exchanges in the homes of friends and relatives, particularly if the patient's illness is poorly understood and a source of embarrassment.

? **8.14** How might you help a patient to gain confidence dealing with his treatment so that he can take advantage of the relative freedom that CAPD offers?

The insertion of a tube and presence of fluid in the abdomen can alter body image and discourage those who are conscious of their appearance. A further disadvantage of CAPD is that it presents a constant reminder to the patient of his illness.

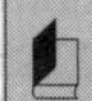
For further information, see Galpin (1992) and Simmons et al (1984).

Living with intermittent haemodialysis
For some patients, haemodialysis requiring treatment on an outpatient basis 2–3 times a week may be the preferred option. This form of treatment does have a number of drawbacks, which include the following:

- the need for transport to and from hospital
- the need to be away from home and dependants 2 or 3 times a week
- the difficulty of fitting in dialysis sessions with work and family commitments
- the increased fluid load prior to dialysis
- the need to restrict the diet
- the financial implications of lost work time
- the side-effects of dialysis and the continuing feeling of not being fully fit
- living with the uncertain hope of a kidney transplant
- the stress and strain on the family of dealing with the lifestyle constraints imposed by treatment.

? **8.15** Consider the problems listed above and, for each, suggest ways in which the health care team can help. **A**

Nursing support during dialysis. Assessments to be performed before haemodialysis are:

- patient's weight: compare with weight after last dialysis
- temperature, pulse and blood pressure. Compare these with recordings after last dialysis. Any temperature increase could indicate an infected dialysis site. Raised blood pressure may indicate fluid overloading
- inquire of the patient if he has been encountering any problems
- assess any known specific medical problem, e.g. blood sugar level in diabetics
- take blood for urea and electrolytes' level check. A full blood count for haemoglobin, white blood cells and platelets should be taken on a weekly basis.

During dialysis, the nurse should record pulse and blood pressure. A drop in blood pressure may mean that the patient needs extra fluid. If necessary, she should check the patient's weight half-way through the session. Some patients may be nursed on weigh beds during haemodialysis.

At the end of dialysis, the patient's temperature, pulse and blood pressure should be measured to assess the effectiveness of the treatment. A blood sample should be taken for urea and electrolyte estimating. Any prescribed medications should be administered, and the patient should be given the opportunity to raise any further concerns he might have.

REFERENCES

Allen M J 1990 Renal replacement therapy in the intensive care unit. Hospital Update (Oct): 828–837
Ames S W, Kneisl C R 1988 Essentials of adult health nursing. Addison Wesley, Menlo Park, CA
Anthony & Thibodeau 1983 Textbook of anatomy and physiology, 11th edn. Mosby, St Louis, MO
Argyle M 1981 Social skills and health. Methuen, London
Bolesha A S et al 1993 Transurethral microwave treatment for benign prostatic hypertrophy: a randomised controlled trial. British Journal of Medicine 306: 1293–1295
Brewster J 1992 Operations explained. Nursing Times 88(39): 50–52
Brocklehurst J 1989 Urinary investigations in old age. Nursing the Elderly 12(2): 17–18
Bullock N, Sibley G, Whitaker R 1989 Essential urology. Churchill Livingstone, Edinburgh
Burkitt H G, Quick C R G, Gatt D 1990 Essential surgery: problems, diagnosis and management. Churchill Livingstone, Edinburgh
Chapman E 1990 Facing the impossible. Nursing Times Community Outlook (April)
Charlton C A C 1984 The urological system. Churchill Livingstone, Edinburgh
Chatto G R D, Power D A 1988 Nephrology in clinical practice. Edward Arnold, London
Corriere J N 1986 Essentials of urology. Churchill Livingstone, Edinburgh
Devines G M et al 1981 Helplessness and depression in end stage renal disease. Journal of Abnormal Psychology 90(6): 531–545
Devines G M et al 1983 The emotional impact of end stage renal disease. Importance of patients' perception of intrusiveness and control. International Journal of Psychiatry in Medicine 13(4): 327–343
Dyer S 1988a The development of stoma care. Professional Nurse 3(7): 226–230
Dyer S 1988b Stoma care: choosing the right appliance. Professional Nurse 3(8): 278–283
Edwards C R W, Bouchier I A D (eds) 1991 Davidson's principles and practice of medicine, 16th edn. Churchill Livingstone, Edinburgh
Forrest A P M, Carter D C, Macleod I B (eds) 1991 Principles and practice of surgery, 2nd edn. Churchill Livingstone, Edinburgh
Foster M C, Upsdell S M, O'Reilly P H 1990 Urological myths. British Journal of Urology 64: 1421–1422
Guyton A C 1977 Basic human physiology, 2nd edn. W B Saunders, Philadelphia
Hampton J R 1992 The ECG made easy. Churchill Livingstone, Edinburgh
Hanno P M, Wein A J 1987 A clinical manual of urology. Prentice-Hall, London
Jamieson E M, McCall J M, Blythe R 1992 Guidelines for clinical nursing practice, 2nd edn. Churchill Livingstone, Edinburgh
Pitt M 1989 Fluid balance and urinary tract infection. Nursing Times (Jan 4)
Pullman B R, Phillip J I, Hickey D S 1982 Urethral lumen cross-section shape: its radiological determination and relationship to function. British Journal of Urology 54: 399–407
RCN Society of Occupational Health Nursing 1991 A guide to an occupational nursing service: a handbook for employers and nurses. Scutari Press, Harrow
Roe B 1990 The basis for sound practice. Nursing Standard 14(51): 22–25
Roper N 1988 Principles of nursing in a process context, 4th edn. Churchill Livingstone, Edinburgh
Trounce J & Gould D 1990 Clinical pharmacology for nurses. Churchill Livingstone, Edinburgh
Wilson K J W 1990 Ross & Wilson anatomy and physiology in health and illness, 7th edn. Churchill Livingstone, Edinburgh

FURTHER READING

Barnett J 1991 Catheters: preventative procedures. Nursing Times 87(10): 66–68
Beckman N J et al 1992 Kidney transplantation: a therapy option. Clinical Issues in Critical Care Nursing 3(3): 570–584
Blandy J 1986 Operative urology, 2nd edn. Blackwell Scientific, Oxford
Brown I, Lunt F 1992 Health promotion: evaluating a 'well man clinic'. Health Visitor 65(1): 12–14
Deans W 1988 Well man clinics. Nursing 26: 975–978
de Guzman L, Joyce K 1991 Case study of a patient with severe nephrotic syndrome. Journal 18(5): 502–503
Edwards C R W, Bouchier I A D (eds) 1991 Davidson's principles and practice of medicine, 16th edn. Churchill Livingstone, Edinburgh
Foster M C, Upsdell S M, O'Reilly P H 1990 Urological myths. British Journal of Urology 64: 1421–1422
Galpin C 1992 Body image in end stage renal failure. British Journal of Nursing (April/May): 21–23
Glenister H 1990 Caring for the catheterised patient. In: Worsley M A (ed) Infection control: guidelines for nursing care. Infection Control Nurses' Association, London
Gregson B A, Cartlidge A, Bond J 1991 Interprofessional collaboration in primary health care organisations. Occasional paper 52. Royal College of General Practitioners, London
Holecheck M J, Burrell-Diggs D, Navarro N O 1991 Renal transplantation: an option for end stage renal disease patients. Critical Care Nursing Quarterly 13(4): 62–77
Johnson D L 1989 Nephrotic syndrome: a nursing care plan based on current pathophysiologic concepts. Heart & Lung 18(1): 85–93
Kilmartin A 1989 Understanding cystitis: the complete self-help guide. Arrow Books, London
Khoury S 1992 Future directions in the management of hyperplasia. British Journal of Urology 70 (Supplement): 27–32
Locking-Cusolito H 1990 Renal transplant and uncertainty. Canadian Nurse 86(7): 27–28
Marieb E N 1989 Human anatomy and physiology. Benjamin/Cummings Publishing, California
Marsh M 1992 Malignant disease of the prostate gland. Nursing Standard 6(36): 28–31
Pearson P 1992 Defining the primary health care team. Health Visitor 65(10): 358–361
Preshloch K 1989 Detecting the hidden urinary tract infection. Registered Nurse 52(1): 65–69
Reynolds R 1993 Coping successfully with prostate problems. Sheldon Press, London
Roe B H 1991 Catheters: looking at the evidence. Nursing Times 87(33): 72–74
Royal College of Nursing 1991 A guide to an occupational health nursing service: a handbook for employers and nurses. Scutari Press, London
Simmons R G et al 1984 Comparison of quality of life of patients on continuous ambulatory peritoneal dialysis, haemodialysis and after transplantation. American Journal of Kidney Diseases 4(3): 253–255
Sueppel C 1992 Prostate poundage perks. Urologic Nursing 12(4): 147
Waine 1992 The primary care team. (Editorial) The British Journal of General Practice 42(365): 498–499
Willis D 1992 Taming the overgrown prostate. American Journal of Nursing 92(2): 39–40
Wozniak-Petrofsky J 1991 Treating older men's most common problem. American Journal of Nursing 54(7): 32–8

CHAPTER 9

The nervous system

Douglas Allan Elizabeth Craig

CHAPTER CONTENTS

Introduction 325

Anatomy and physiology 325

Head injury 336
Nursing priorities and management 341

Cerebrovascular disease 344
Nursing priorities and management: stroke 346

Intracranial tumours 349
Nursing priorities and management 352

Epilepsy 353
Nursing priorities and management 353

Multiple sclerosis 356
Nursing priorities and management 356

Parkinson's disease 360
Nursing priorities and management 360

Infections 363
Nursing priorities and management 364

Glossary 365

References 365

Further reading 366

Useful addresses 367

INTRODUCTION

Many nurses will have only brief contact with patients suffering from neurological disorders, either while they are waiting to be transferred to a specialist neurological unit or following their return from such a unit. Community staff are increasingly involved with patients recovering at home from acute neurosurgical interventions and long-term neurological disorders requiring supportive therapies, where the disorder cannot be cured.

This chapter covers the more common neurological and neurosurgical disorders and, where appropriate, makes reference to the more uncommon disorders. The specialised neuroscience textbooks listed at the end of the chapter provide more detailed information. It is hoped that the information contained here will help to alleviate any apprehension that the student may have regarding this specialised field of nursing, and that it stimulates further discussion as to how best to meet the needs of the neurologically impaired patient and his family.

ANATOMY AND PHYSIOLOGY

The nervous system is a complex, inter-related body system responsible for many functions including communication, coordination, behaviour and intelligence. It constantly receives data from the external and internal environment, interprets this and then makes adjustments to cope with this.

The nervous system can be considered in two distinct parts. The central nervous system (CNS), comprising the brain and spinal cord and the peripheral nervous system (PNS), consisting of the cranial and spinal nerves. The peripheral nervous system has two functional parts:

- the sensory division
- the motor division, which is further divided into
  - the somatic nervous system, which conducts impulses from the central nervous system to skeletal muscles
  - the autonomic nervous system, which conducts impulses from the central nervous system to smooth muscle, cardiac muscle and glands.

The autonomic nervous system is usually classified as part of the peripheral nervous system but it also exerts an influence on the central nervous system.

Basic tissue structure

Nervous tissue consists of neuroglia (or 'glial cells') and neurones (or 'nerve cells'). The neuroglia markedly outnumber the neurones and form a supportive and protective network for the nervous system, for example, by attaching neurones to their blood vessels and protecting the nervous system through phagocytic action, as the white cells do elsewhere in the body. In the peripheral nervous system, supporting cells, called 'Schwann cells', form the myelin sheath as well as having a phagocytic role.

Myelin protects and electrically insulates nerve fibres from one another, and speeds up nerve impulse transmission. Myelinated nerve impulses are transmitted by saltatory conduction whereby the impulse jumps from one node of Ranvier to the next. Impulses in myelinated nerves therefore are transmitted very much faster than in unmyelinated nerves and require very much less energy. The importance of myelin in nerve impulse transmission is painfully clear to those suffering from demyelinating diseases such as multiple sclerosis. In multiple sclerosis, the myelin sheath disappears, impulse conduction ceases and the affected individual loses the ability to control voluntary muscle movement (see p. 356).

Neurones

Although fewer in number, neurones form the basis of the structural and functional unit of the nervous system. They are capable of conducting impulses throughout the nervous system and to other excitable tissues, including the muscles and glands. The structure of the neurone is shown in Figure 9.1.

Most of the peripheral nerve fibres and nerve fibres in the spinal cord, and some of the myelinated nerve fibres in the brain, are arranged in bundles or tracts in the central nervous system (see Fig. 9.2).

Classification of neurones. Neurones are classified according to their function and structure. The functional classification is determined by the direction in which the impulse travels.

Sensory or afferent neurones transmit impulses from receptors in the skin, sense organs and viscera *to* the brain and spinal cord.

Motor or efferent neurones transmit impulses in the opposite direction, *from* the brain and spinal cord to muscles and glands in the body (the effectors).

A third function is to convey impulses *within* the central nervous system. The structural classification is based on shape and in particular the number of poles on the cell body, as follows:

- unipolar — cells with processes projecting from one pole
- bipolar — cells with processes projecting from two poles at opposite ends of the cell
- multipolar — cells with processes projecting from many points all over the cell body.

The nerve impulse

A nerve impulse can be initiated by a stimulus such as a change in temperature, pressure or the chemical environment, or impulses can be generated spontaneously by pacemaker cells. The impulse is described as a self-propagating wave of electrical charge along the membrane of the neurone, effecting changes crucial to the conduction of the impulse.

At rest, the nerve cell has an unequal distribution of ions on either side of the plasma membrane. This chemical difference also produces an electrical difference: the inside of the cell is negatively charged in relation to the outside. This has been measured at –70 mV and this is termed the resting membrane potential. The cell is maintained in this condition by a system whereby ions are exchanged between the intracellular and extracellular fluids. A property of all nerve cells is their ability to respond to stimuli by producing an impulse when the stimulus is sufficient to initiate certain electrical and chemical changes within the cell membrane. These positive–negative changes occur in rapid succession, spreading to the end of the axon.

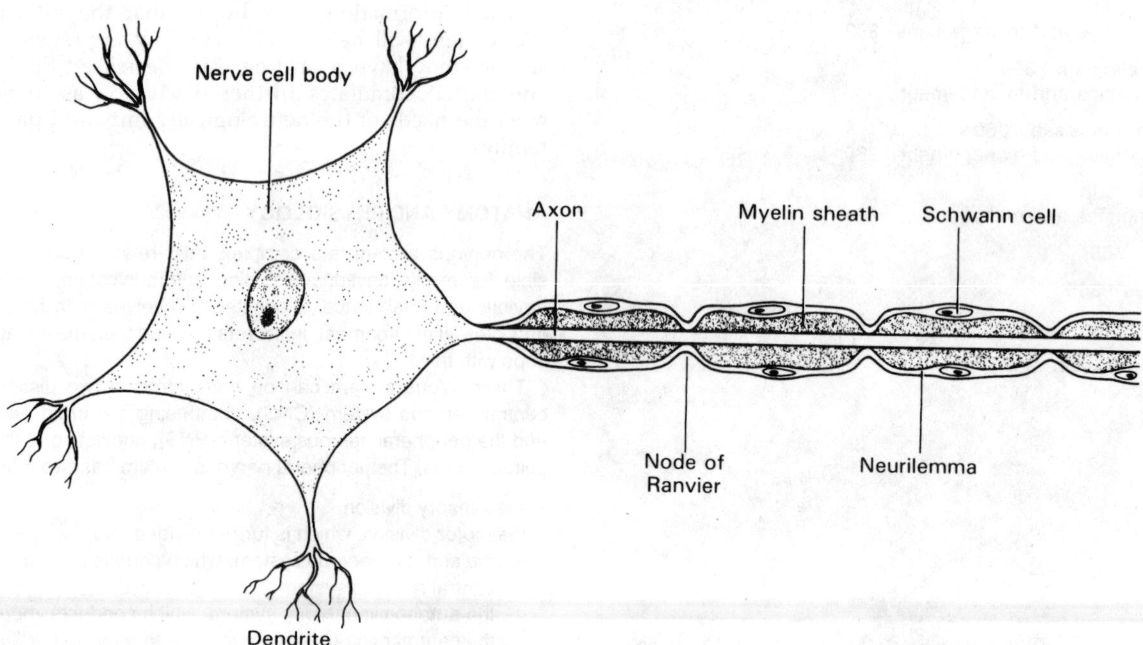

Fig. 9.1 Structure of a multipolar neurone. A neurone consists of three parts.
(1) The nerve cell body, which is grey in colour. Each cell body is enclosed in a selectively permeable membrane, which also extends along the cell process. The cell body contains a nucleus surrounded by cytoplasm which also contains other structures called organelles.
(2) The nerve processes or dendrites are thread-like extensions of the cell body, one of which is more elongated, forming the axon.
(3) The axon is a single long process that conducts impulses away from the cell body. In many large peripheral axons, the axolemma is surrounded by another covering called the myelin sheath. This is a multiple-layered covering of fatty material which is white in colour. Its function is to insulate the neurone electrically and thus speed up the conduction of the nerve impulse, by segmentation. Each interruption of the sheath is known as a Node of Ranvier and the speed of the impulse is increased by its 'jumping' from node to node. The axon and its collaterals branch into axon terminals, the ends of which form a bulb-like structure. These help transmit an impulse from one neurone to another across the gap (synapse) between them or at the junctions with effector cells.

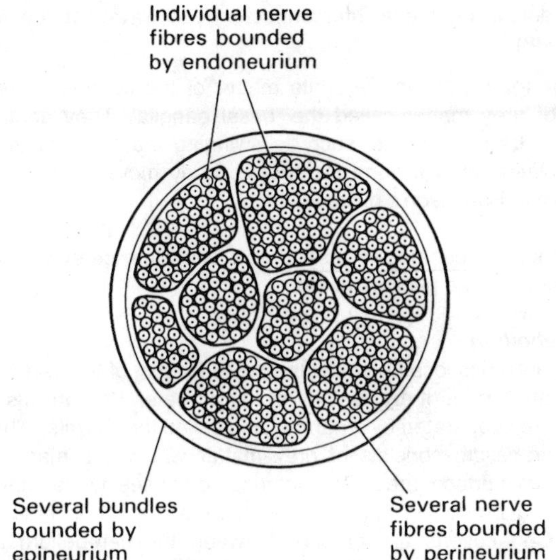

Fig. 9.2 The nerve fibres are surrounded by a fine connective tissue covering called the endoneurium. Several nerve fibres are bound together by another connective tissue covering called the perineurium and a number of these bundles may be surrounded by another covering called the epineurium.

Other more subtle and complex changes also occur.

Generally, the larger the diameter of the axon the quicker the nerve impulse travels but the alternative device of saltatory conduction is found in myelinated neurones, as shown in Figure 9.3 (see also p. 365).

The junctions between one neurone and another, and between neurones and muscles or glands, are known as synapses.

Neurotransmitters

Nerve impulses are transmitted across the gap between the adjacent tissues by chemical transmitters (neurotransmitters). The chemical is stored in vesicles in the expanded end of the axon and is released when the nerve impulse reaches this point. Several chemical transmitters have been identified, the most common ones being acetylcholine and noradrenaline. Many of these neurotransmitters are excitatory, resulting in the nerve impulse being transmitted to the adjacent tissue, but some have an inhibiting effect and prevent the transmission of impulses from neurones situated nearby.

The receiving membrane is specially constructed to receive the neurotransmitter thus effecting changes in the tissue, e.g. the contraction of a muscle.

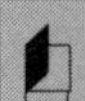 Detailed information appears in: Hubbard & Mechan (1987).

Neurotransmitters are destroyed by enzymes or reabsorbed into the axon after use. For example, acetylcholine is destroyed by cholinesterase.

The central nervous system

The central nervous system consists of the brain and spinal cord.

The brain

The cerebrum, the largest constituent of the nervous system, forms the bulk of the brain. The outer surface, the cortex, is of grey matter and consists of nerve cell bodies. The surface area of the cerebral cortex is increased by a series of grooves, (sulci), and ridges (gyri). The deeper grooves are termed fissures and some form landmarks, for example, the longitudinal fissure, which almost splits the brain into two hemispheres (see Fig. 9.4).

Each hemisphere is subdivided into four lobes:

- frontal
- temporal
- parietal
- occipital

each named according to the skull bones they underlie.

The cerebral cortex is responsible for three main functions:

1. Receiving and interpreting a mass of sensory information from various sources in the internal and external environment.
2. Initiating and controlling voluntary movement in response to the sensory information received.
3. Integrating crucial functions such as memory and consciousness.

Certain areas of the cerebral cortex have been identified as those responsible for these functions and these form a map, illustrated in Figure 9.5.

Relative size. The lips, thumbs and face use more receptors than the trunk and legs. Similarly, the thumbs, fingers, lips, tongue and vocal cords are more sensitive than the trunk due to the greater number of receptors found in them. The size of the represented area is determined by its functional importance and the need for sensitivity.

Concept of dominance. The functions of speech and motor control are usually more highly developed in one cerebral hemisphere than in the other. This is referred to as dominance. Approximately 95% of the population are dominant in the left hemisphere and, as most of the spinal pathways cross over, they are right handed. However, if the dominant hemisphere is damaged the opposite hemisphere can take over and assume a dominant role.

Association areas. Some areas remain unmapped (see Fig. 9.5). These are called 'association areas' and are thought to be responsible for complex functions such as integration of the senses, memory, learning, thought processes, behaviour and emotion.

Connecting pathways. Below the outer cortical layer can be found areas of white matter (myelinated nerve fibres) that form connections between the cerebral cortex and other areas of grey matter in the CNS. Three connecting pathways (Fig. 9.6) have been identified:

1. Association fibres, which connect between gyri in the same hemisphere.
2. Commisural fibres, which connect between gyri in different hemispheres. One important group of commisural fibres is the corpus callosum.
3. Projection fibres, which provide connections between the brain and spinal cord in ascending and descending pathways; one example is the internal capsule.

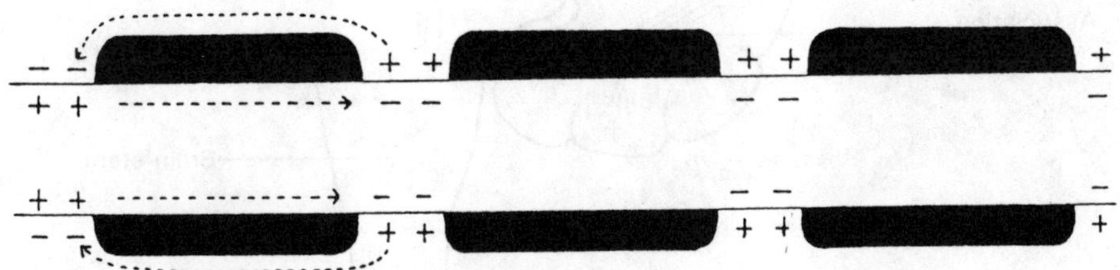

Fig. 9.3 Saltatory conduction in a myelinated nerve.

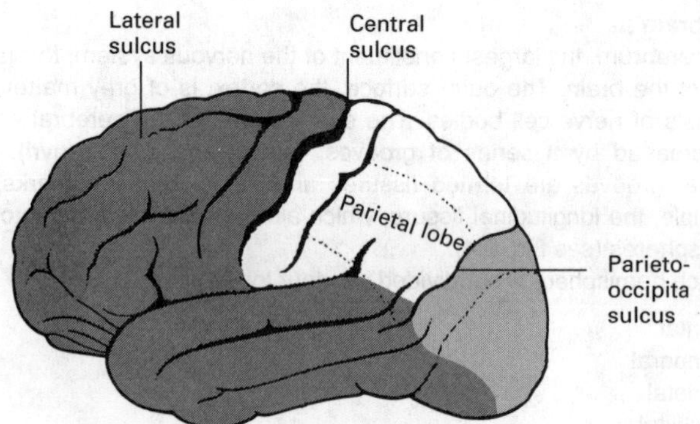

Fig. 9.4 The lobes and sulci of the cerebrum. Each of the lobes is bounded by 'landmark' fissures: the frontal lobe is separated from the parietal lobe by the central sulcus; the temporal lobe is separated from the frontal and parietal lobes by the lateral sulcus; and the occipital lobe is separated from the temporal and parietal lobes by the occipital–parietal sulcus.

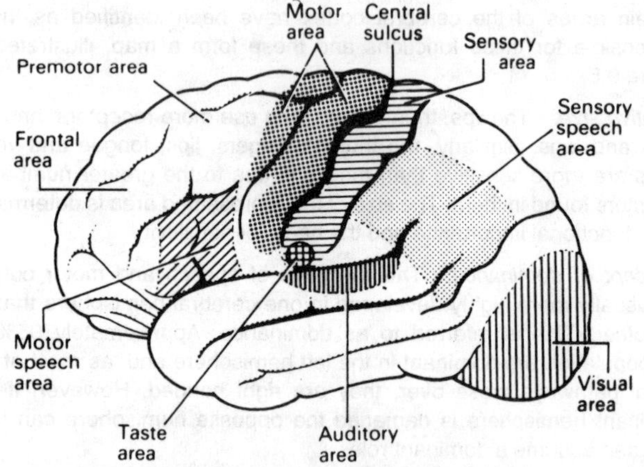

Fig. 9.5 The cerebrum showing the functional areas.

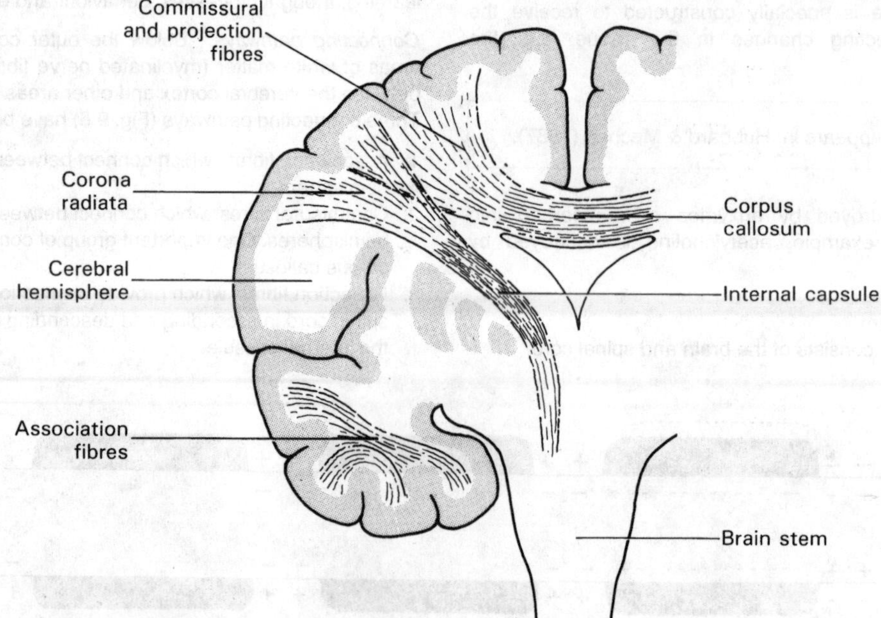

Fig. 9.6 White matter of the cerebrum.

Further details on these interconnecting pathways can be found in Allan (1988).

Basal ganglia. Within the white matter of the cerebrum are paired islands of grey matter called the 'basal ganglia'. They control large subconscious movements, such as swinging the arms while walking and regulating muscle tone for specific body movements, a function that is lost in Parkinson's disease.

Other structures closely associated with the cerebrum are the cerebellum and the pituitary gland.

The cerebellum

The cerebellum is located below the posterior part of the cerebrum and is separated from it by a fold of dura mater. It consists of two hemispheres separated by a narrow strip called the 'vermis'. The cortex of the cerebellum consists of grey matter which has many folds to increase its surface area. The interior comprises white matter presented in a branching configuration termed the arbor vitae or 'tree of life'. Connections are present between the cerebellum and the brain and spinal cord. These allow the cerebellum to receive sensory information and thereby to modify voluntary movement by making it smooth and coordinated, and maintain equilibrium. Voluntary movements cannot be initiated by the cerebellum.

There are three connections, called the 'cerebellar peduncles'.

Further detail can be found in Hubbard & Mechan (1987).

Pituitary gland

The pituitary gland is situated at the base of the brain in a depression in the sphenoid bone called the 'sella turcica'. It is attached to the brain via a stalk which is continuous with the hypothalamus and communication is by means of nerve fibres and blood vessels. It has three lobes, an anterior, middle and posterior lobe which secrete hormones that exert an influence on other parts of the body. See Chapter 5 for details of the actions of pituitary hormones.

Diencephalon

Three bilaterally symmetrical structures comprise the diencephalon:

- the thalamus
- the hypothalamus
- the epithalamus.

Collectively, these three structures enclose and form the boundaries of the third ventricle.

Thalamus. The thalamus consists of two oval-shaped masses (thalami), mainly consisting of grey matter with some white matter, and is situated within the cerebral hemispheres just below the corpus callosum. Sensory impulses associated with pain, temperature, pressure and touch are conveyed to the thalamus, which acts as a 'filter'. Chaos would reign if all the sensory information flooding into the nervous system were allowed to reach the sensory cortex.

Hypothalamus. The hypothalamus is situated below the thalamus and forms the walls of the third ventricle. It controls the output of the hormones from the pituitary gland and is located directly above it. Other functions include controlling hunger, thirst and body temperature. (See Ch. 22.) The latter function is significant for patients with a hypothalamic disturbance following head injury.

The complex control of body temperature is explained in more detail in Hubbard & Mechan (1987).

Epithalamus. The epithalamus is the most dorsal part of the diencephalon and forms the roof of the third ventricle. Extending from its posterior border is the pineal gland, thought to be concerned with body rhythms, acting as some sort of biological clock and concerned with melatonin synthesis, although the function is as yet obscure for both melatonin and the pineal body.

The brain stem

The brain stem is the collective name given to three structures, the medulla, the pons and the midbrain. Inferiorly, the medulla is continuous with the upper spinal cord and connects with the pons above. The pons is continuous with the midbrain, which connects with the lower portion of the diencephalon.

Three major structures of the brain stem have been identified.

The medulla. All the spinal pathways pass through the medulla, constituting its white matter. Some of these cross to the opposite side in triangular-shaped structures called the 'pyramids', a process known as 'decussation'. (The purpose of this has never been established.)

- It contains the reticular formation, a diffuse area of grey and white matter that has connections with other parts of the reticular formation in the rest of the brain stem and cerebral cortex. It is responsible for consciousness and arousal.
- It accommodates three reflex centres, which control vital functions. These include:
  - the cardiac centre, which regulates heartbeat and force of contraction
  - the medullary rhythmicity area, which adjusts the basic rhythm of breathing
  - the vasomotor centre, which regulates the diameter of blood vesels (important in control of blood pressure).

Other non-vital centres include those responsible for coordinating swallowing, vomiting, coughing, sneezing and hiccuping.

- It also contains the nuclei of cranial nerves VIII to XII (see Table 9.1).

The pons. The pons acts as a bridge between the medulla and the midbrain. It comprises fibres and nuclei; the fibres run in two directions. The transverse fibres connect with the cerebellum and the longitudinal fibres maintain the vital link between the spinal cord and the brain. The nuclei are the origins of cranial nerves V to VIII inclusive (see Table 9.1). Other important nuclei also exert an influence on respiration.

The midbrain. The third component of the brain stem is the midbrain, which contains the central centres for visual, auditory and postural reflexes. It is located above the pons and is the origin of the nuclei of cranial nerves III and IV (see Table 9.1). Cranial nerves I and II originate in the cerebrum.

The meninges

The brain and spinal cord are surrounded and protected by three meninges:

- the outer layer, the dura mater
- the middle layer, the arachnoid mater
- the innermost layer, the pia mater.

Dura mater. The dura mater is a double layer of dense fibrous tissue. The outer, periosteal layer adheres closely to the underside of the cranial bones whilst the inner, meningeal layer is much thinner. The spinal dura mater has only one layer, which corresponds to the meningeal layer of the cranium. The two layers of the dura mater separate at several locations and these spaces contain the venous sinuses, for example, the falx cerebri and the tentorium cerebelli. The former forms an incomplete division dipping down between the two cerebral hemispheres and is attached to the ethmoid bone at the front and the occipital protuberance at the back (see Fig. 9.7).

The tentorium cerebelli forms a division between the occipital lobes of the cerebrum and the cerebellum. It is attached along the midline to the falx cerebri, which draws it upwards to produce a tent-like appearance.

Arachnoid mater. The arachnoid mater consists of collagenous and elastic fibres, covered by squamous epithelium. Fine strands of connective tissue connect the arachnoid with the pia below. The arachnoid water projects into the sinuses as arachnoid villi, which are the structures responsible for the absorption of cerebrospinal fluid, and at certain points it joins the linings of the ventricles to form the choroid plexus, where cerebrospinal fluid is produced.

Pia mater. The pia mater is of the same structure as the arachnoid, except that it has its own blood supply. The pia closely follows and adheres to the contours of the brain and spinal cord.

The ventricular system

The ventricular system consists of four fluid-filled irregular cavities (ventricles) interconnected by narrow pathways (see Fig. 9.8) and is connected with the central canal of the spinal cord and the cranial subarachnoid space. There are two lateral ventricles, one in each cerebral hemisphere, and one ventricle (the third) located in the diencephalic region and another located in the medulla, called the fourth ventricle.

The cerebrospinal fluid. Cerebrospinal fluid (CSF) circulates within the closed ventricular system. Healthy cerebrospinal fluid is crystal clear and colourless and its normal features are as outlined in Box 9.1.

The cerebrospinal fluid production–absorption cycle is continuous and a fairly constant volume of 120–150 ml is maintained. When this process is interrupted and the volume is increased beyond normal limits, hydrocephalus occurs (see p. 347).

The main source of production is the choroid plexus, a collection of specialised capillaries located within the internal lining of the ventricles, the largest amount being produced in the lateral ventricles. From here the cerebrospinal fluid passes through two interventricular foramina (foramen of Monro) to the third ventricle; then via the single cerebral aqueduct (aqueduct of Sylvius) to the fourth ventricle; and via two lateral foramina upwards in the subarachnoid space around the brain and midline, through one foramen around the subarachnoid space in the spinal cord and into the central canal of the spinal cord. Reabsorption occurs into the arachnoid villi.

Cerebrospinal fluid. The functions of cerebrospinal fluid are:

- protection and cushioning of the brain and spinal cord
- provision of nourishment

Table 9.1 Cranial nerves (Allan 1988)

Nerve		Origin	Termination	Functions
I	Olfactory	Olfactory mucosa	Olfactory cortex	Sensory: Smell
II	Optic	Retina	Visual cortex (synapses in lateral geniculate body)	Sensory: Vision
III	Oculomotor	Midbrain	Upper eyelid muscle	Motor: Eyelid movement
			Extrinsic eye muscles (superior, medial and inferior recti, inferior oblique)	Eyeball movement
			Ciliary muscles	Accommodation of lens
			Sphincter muscle of iris	Pupillary constriction
		Proprioceptors in extrinsic eye muscles	Midbrain	Sensory: Proprioception
IV	Trochlear	Midbrain	Extrinsic eye muscle (superior oblique)	Motor: Eyeball movement
		Proprioceptors in extrinsic eye muscle (superior oblique)	Midbrain	Sensory: Proprioception
V	Trigeminal	Pons	Muscles of mastication	Motor: Chewing
		Ophthalmic branch takes sensory fibres from skin of upper eyelid, eyeball, lacrimal glands, nasal cavity, side of nose, forehead and anterior half of scalp	Midbrain, pons and medulla	Sensory: Touch, pain, temperature, proprioception
		Maxillary branch takes sensory fibres from mucosa of nose, palate, parts of pharynx, upper teeth, upper lip, cheek and lower eyelid		
		Mandibular branch takes sensory fibres from anterior two thirds of tongue, lower teeth, skin over mandible and side of head in front of ear		
VI	Abducens	Pons	Extrinsic eye muscle (lateral rectus)	Motor: Eyeball movement
		Proprioceptors in lateral rectus	Pons	Sensory: Proprioception
VII	Facial	Pons	Facial, scalp and neck muscles.	Motor: Facial expression
			Lacrimal and salivary glands (sublingual and submandibular)	Salivation Lacrimation
		Taste buds on anterior two-thirds of tongue	Gustatory cortex (synapses in pons and thalamus)	Sensory: Taste
		Proprioceptors in muscles of face and scalp		Proprioception
VIII	Vestibulo-cochlear	Cochlear and vestibular portions of the ear	Cochlear nuclei in pons	Sensory: Hearing
			Vestibular nuclei in medulla	Equilibrium
IX	Glossopharyngeal	Medulla	Swallowing muscles in pharynx	Motor: Swallowing
			Parotid gland	Salivation
		Taste buds on posterior one-third of tongue	Gustatory cortex (synapses in medulla and thalamus)	Sensory: Taste
		Carotid sinus		Regulation of blood pressure.
		Proprioceptors in swallowing muscles		Proprioception
X	Vagus	Medulla	Visceral muscles (muscles of pharynx, larynx, respiratory tract, oesophagus, heart, stomach, small intestine, proximal half of large intestine, gall bladder, liver, pancreas)	Motor: Swallowing, digestive movements and secretions
		Receptors in the same structures that the motor portions innervate	Medulla and pons	Sensory: Range of sensory inputs from organs supplied and proprioception from muscle
XI	Accessory	Bulbar portion: medulla	Muscles of pharynx, larynx, soft palate	Motor: Swallowing
		Spinal portion: cervical spinal cord	Sternocleidomastoid and trapezius muscles	Head movements
		Proprioceptors in muscles supplied by motor fibres	Medulla	Sensory: Proprioception
XII	Hypoglossal	Medulla	Muscles of tongue	Motor: Tongue movements
		Proprioceptors in tongue	Medulla	Sensory: Proprioception

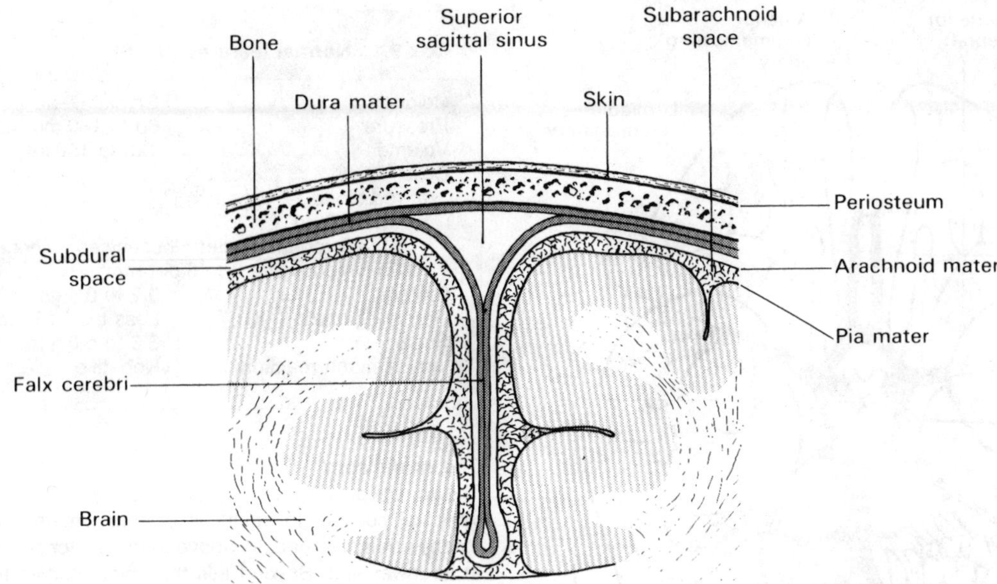

Fig. 9.7 Meninges of the brain.

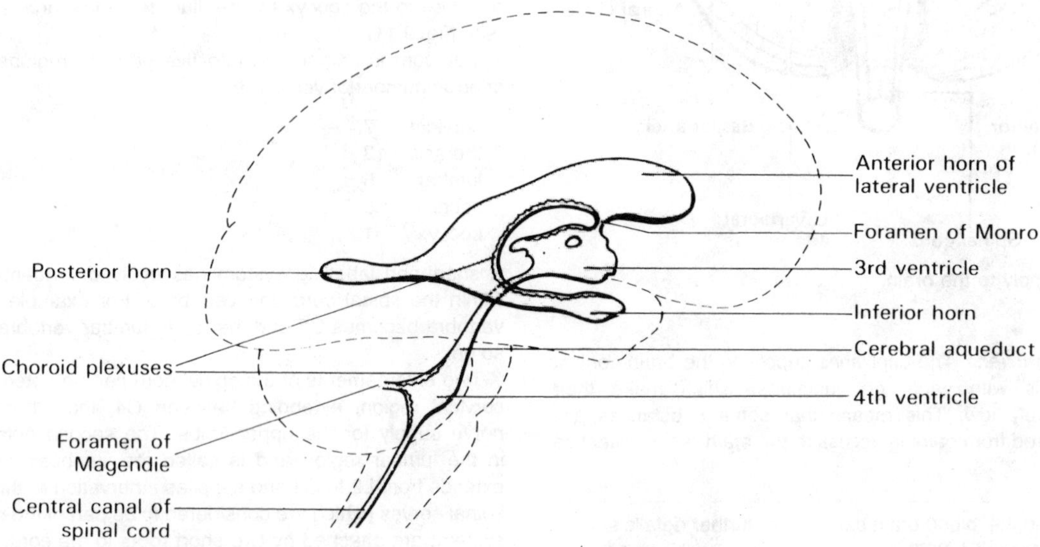

Fig. 9.8 Ventricular system.

- maintenance of a uniform intracranial pressure
- removal of waste products.

Blood supply and drainage

The supply of blood to the head arises from the left and right common carotid arteries, which subdivide to form the internal and external carotid arteries. These supply blood to the anterior part of the brain and the vertebral arteries supply the posterior part.

The greater part of the brain is supplied with blood by the Circle of Willis, an unusual configuration of anastomosed blood vessels located in the base of the brain. See Figure 9.9.

 More detailed information on the areas of the brain supplied by the cerebral circulation can be found in Allan (1988).

Venous drainage is by small veins in the brain stem and cerebellum, and external and internal veins draining the cerebrum. Some of the external and internal veins empty into one large vein called the vein of Galen (great cerebral vein). Unlike other parts of the body, these veins do not correspond with their arterial supply. All these veins empty directly into a system of venous sinuses, which are shown in Figure 9.10.

The principal sinuses are the superior and inferior sagittal, the straight, transverse, sigmoid and cavernous sinuses.

The limbic system

The limbic system comprises an interconnected complex of structures, including the hypothalamus. These are thought to be responsible for special types of behaviour associated with emotions, subconscious motor and sensory drives and the intrinsic feelings of pain and pleasure.

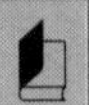 Further information is given in Tortora & Grabowski (1993).

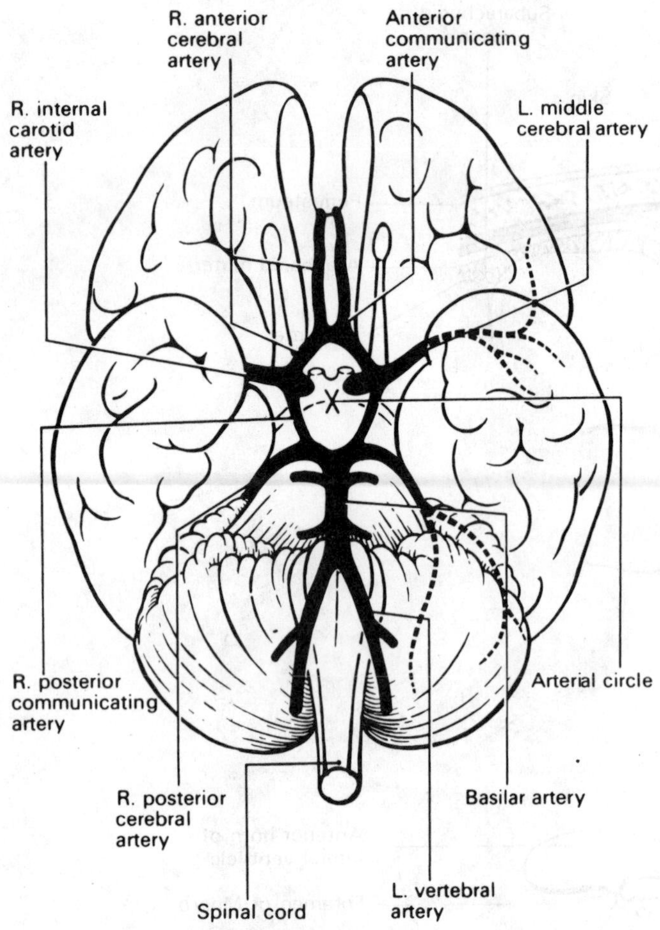

Fig. 9.9 Blood supply to the brain.

The blood brain barrier. The capillaries supplying the brain consist of endothelial cells with very tight junctions, which make their permeability relatively low. This means that some substances are prevented or hindered from gaining access to the brain, as a protective mechanism.

This is termed the 'blood brain barrier'. For further details see Hubbard & Mechan (1987).

Box 9.1 Normal features of CSF

Colour	Crystal clear
Pressure	80 to 160 mm water
Volume	120 to 150 ml
Cells	
a. red blood — none	
b. white blood	
(i) polymorphonuclear leucocytes — none	
(ii) lymphocytes 0 to 5 per mm^3	
Protein	0.2 to 0.4 g/l
Gamma globulin (IgG)	Less than 13% of total protein
Sugar	3.6 to 5.0 mmol
Wassermann reaction	Negative

The spinal cord

The spinal cord is an oval cylinder that lies within the spinal cavity of the vertebral column. In adults, it is approximately 45 cm in length and extends from the medulla above to the first or second lumbar vertebrae at its lower end. Beyond this the spinal nerves from the lumbar and sacral segments of the cord form the cauda equina, or 'horse's tail'. The cord is surrounded by the three meninges and cerebrospinal fluid circulates in the subarachnoid space. The lower part of the cord is attached to the coccyx by the filum terminale and is tapered in shape (see Fig. 9.11).

The cord is segmented into five parts or regions and each has a specific number of vertebrae:

cervical	7
thoracic	12
lumbar	5
sacral	5
coccyx	1

A shorthand labelling system has evolved to identify different levels within the spinal cord and vertebrae. For example, the third cervical vertebra becomes C3 and the fourth lumbar vertebra becomes L4 and so on.

Two enlargements of the spinal cord can be noted. The first is in the cervical region, extending between C4 and T1 and containing the nerve supply for the upper limbs. The second enlargement is lower in the lumbar region and is called the 'lumbosacral enlargement'. It extends from L2 to S3 and supplies innervation to the lower limbs. The spinal nerves (which are considered to be part of the peripheral nervous system) are attached by two short roots to the cord. There is a pair of spinal nerves equivalent to each of the vertebrae outlined above and

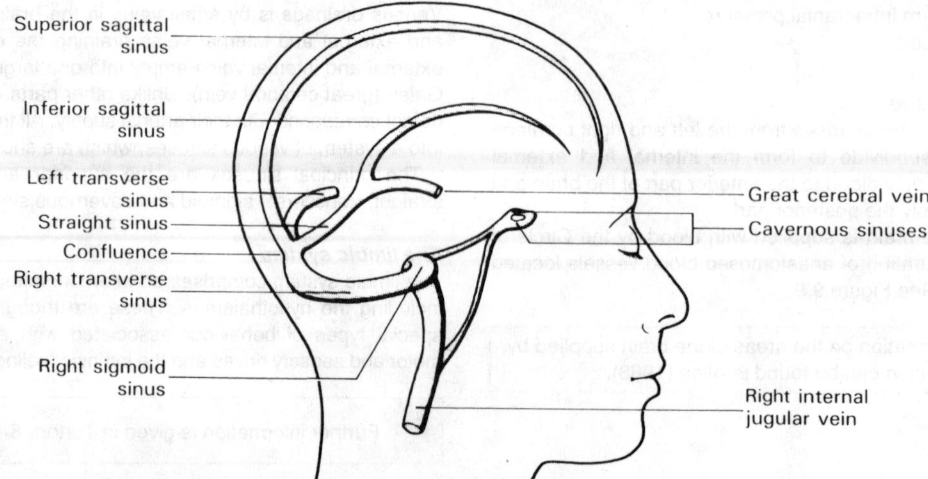

Fig. 9.10 Venous drainage of the brain.

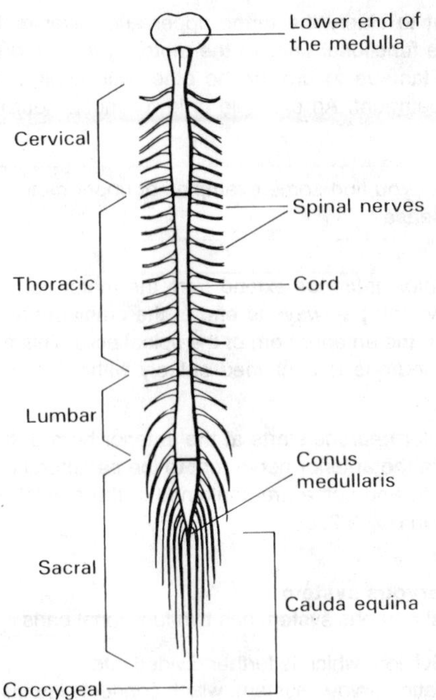

Fig. 9.11 Spinal cord.

these are labelled and numbered in a similar way. More detail on the spinal nerves can be found in the section on the peripheral nervous system, p. 334.

The structure of the spinal cord is illustrated in cross section in Figure 9.12.

The spinal pathways are described as:

- sensory, which *ascend* from the periphery of the body, for example, cutaneous receptors in the hand, and are conveyed to the sensory cortex for interpretation
- motor, which *descend* from the brain down to the periphery of the body, for example, to skeletal muscles, where they initiate a motor response.

Each pathway has a name, derived from the white column in which it travels, the origin of the cell bodies, and the termination of the axon. For example, the anterior spinothalamic tract is located in the anterior white column, originates in the spinal cord and terminates in the thalamus.

The sensory pathways consist of:

- the posterior column pathway
- the spinothalamic pathway
- the cerebellar pathway.

The posterior column pathway. Each pathway consists of a chain of three neurones, which transmit information such as discriminative touch and vibration sense from the appropriate receptors to the sensory cortex (see Fig. 9.13).

The spinothalamic pathways are:

- the lateral spinothalamic tract
- the anterior spinothalamic tract.

The first order neurone in both pathways connects the receptor with the spinal cord where it synapses with the second order neurone in the posterior grey horn. The pathway crosses over to the opposite side of the cord and ascends in either the lateral or anterior spinothalamic tract to the thalamus. The second order neurone synapses with the third order neurone which then continues, terminating in the sensory cortex. The lateral tract is responsible for conveying information about pain and temperature and the anterior tract conveys light touch and pressure. Further information on pain can be found in Chapter 19.

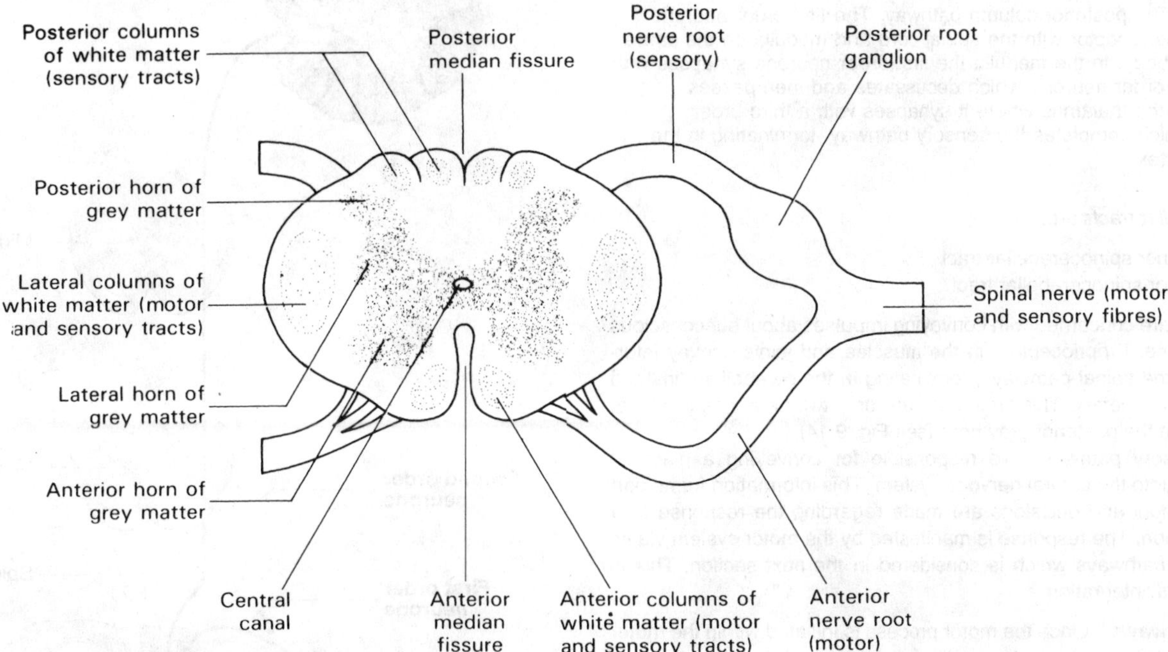

Fig. 9.12 Cross section of spinal cord. It can be seen that the cord is incompletely divided into right and left halves by the posterior and anterior median fissures. In the centre is the central canal which contains cerebrospinal fluid originating from the fourth ventricle. Extending the entire length of the cord, this is located within an H-shaped area of grey matter with posterior and anterior, and at some levels, lateral horns. The remainder of the cord is made up of white matter organised in columns in the posterior, lateral and anterior segments.

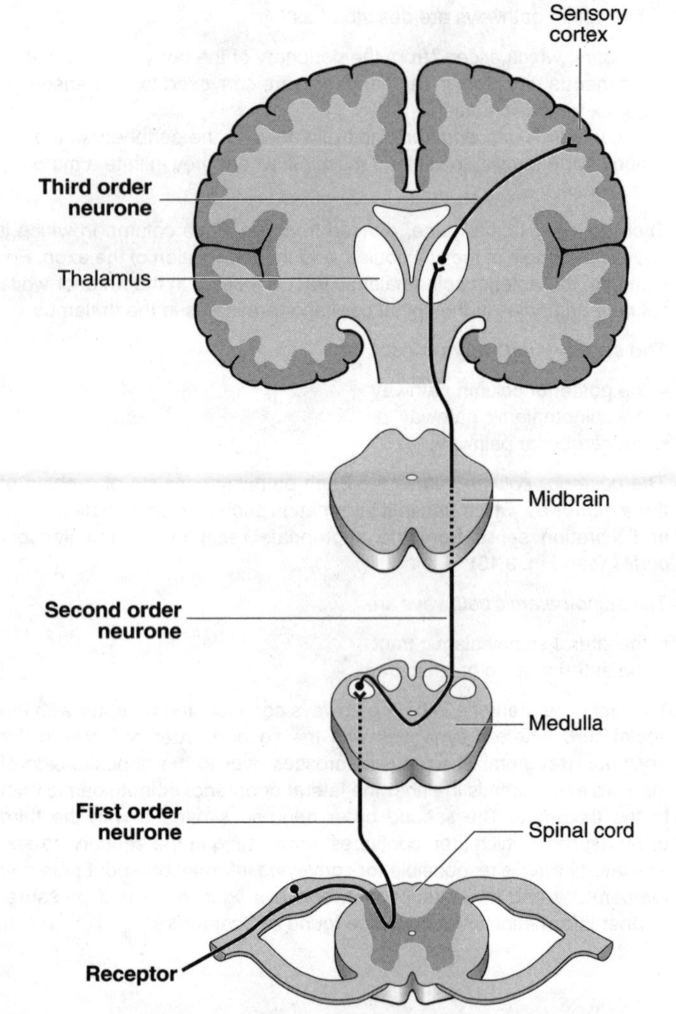

Fig. 9.13 The posterior column pathway. The first order neurone connects the receptor with the spinal cord and medulla on the same side of the body. In the medulla the first order neurone synapses with the second order neurone which decussates and then passes upwards to the thalamus where it synapses with a third order neurone which completes the sensory pathway, terminating in the sensory cortex.

The cerebellar tracts are:

- the posterior spinocerebellar tract
- the anterior spinocerebellar tract.

Both tracts are concerned with conveying impulses about subconscious muscle sense. Proprioceptors in the muscles and joints convey information via the spinal pathways, terminating in the cerebellum, instead of the cerebral cortex. This time there are only two neurones involved, synapsing in the posterior grey horn (see Fig. 9.14).

The sensory pathways are responsible for conveying a mass of information into the central nervous system. This information forms part of a large pool and decisions are made regarding the response to a given situation. The response is manifested by the motor system via its own set of pathways which is considered in the next section. This is described as 'integration'.

Motor pathways. Once the motor process is initiated within the motor area of the cortex, the impulses descend via two main motor pathways. The motor pathways are classified as:

- pyramidal, which indicates that the pathway passes through the pyramids in the medulla
- extrapyramidal.

It is important to clarify the terms upper and lower motor neurones. These are the functional units of the motor system and convey motor impulses as damage to one or the other will result in very different functional impairment. An example of lower motor neurone disease is poliomyelitis.

?	**9.1** Can you find some examples of upper motor neurone disease?

The upper motor neurones extend from the motor cortex of the brain and pass down the pathways to end at the cranial nerve nuclei in the brain stem and the anterior horn of the spinal cord. This means that the upper motor neurone is contained entirely within the central nervous system.

The lower motor neurone starts at the anterior horn of the spinal cord and passes via the anterior nerve root to the peripheral nerves and the motor end plate and some are contained in the cranial nerves. These are described in Box 9.2.

Peripheral nervous system

The peripheral nervous system has two functional parts:

- the motor division, which is further divided into
  - the somatic nervous system, which conducts impulses from the central nervous system to skeletal muscles
  - the autonomic nervous system, which conducts impulses from the central nervous system to smooth muscle, cardiac muscle and glands
- the sensory division.

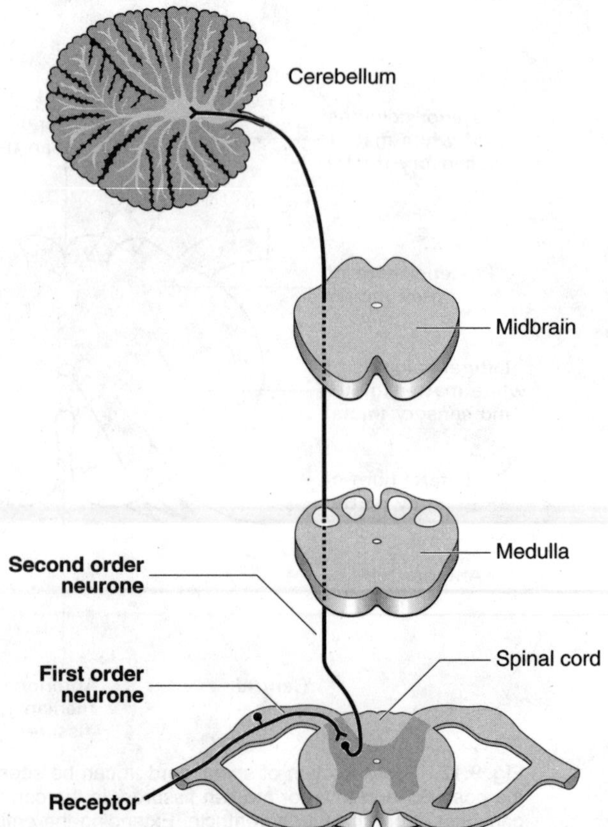

Fig. 9.14 The spinocerebellar tracts.

Box 9.2 The motor pathways

PYRAMIDAL TRACTS

The pyramidal pathway comprises three main tracts:

- lateral corticospinal
- anterior corticospinal
- corticobulbar.

The lateral corticospinal tract
This is the actual pyramidal tract. It originates in the motor cortex and descends to the medulla where 85% of the fibres decussate. They continue downwards in the lateral white column of the corticospinal tract. Most synapse in the anterior grey horn with the lower motor neurone, which then exits the spinal cord via the spinal nerves to terminate on the appropriate skeletal muscle.

The anterior corticospinal pathway
These fibres follow a similar pathway to the lateral, except that they travel in the anterior white column and most of the fibres do not decussate.

The corticobulbar tracts
These are important in that they terminate in the nuclei of the cranial nerves in the medulla. They follow the same pathway as the corticospinal pathway.

EXTRAPYRAMIDAL TRACTS

These consist of all the descending motor pathways that do *not* pass through the pyramids. They are concerned with functions of tone and posture such as control of head movement and maintaining balance.

There are three of these pathways:

1. The rubrospinal tract, which originates in the midbrain, decussates and descends in the lateral white column. It is concerned with tone and posture.
2. The tectospinal tract also originates in the midbrain, decussates and descends in the anterior white column and enters the anterior grey horns of the cervical cord.
3. The vestibulospinal tract originates in the vestibular nucleus of the medulla and descends on the same side in the anterior white column and terminates in the anterior grey horn at the cervical and lumbosacral levels of the cord. It is concerned with regulating muscle tone in response to movements of the head and therefore has an important part to play in maintaining equilibrium.

The cranial nerves
The cranial nerves pass from their origin, principally from the brain stem, out via small openings in the skull to innervate the appropriate structures. Each pair of nerves is named according to its distribution or function and is also numbered I–XII (see Table 9.1). Cranial nerves were formerly described as either motor, sensory, or a mixture of both but more recently, most motor nerves are considered to be mixed, but with a dominance of motor fibres.

Spinal nerves
There are 31 pairs of spinal nerves, named and grouped according to the vertebrae with which they are associated:

Cervical	8
Thoracic	12
Lumbar	5
Sacral	5
Coccygeal	1

Note that there is one more cervical spinal nerve than there are vertebrae. This is because the first pair leave the vertebral canal between the occipital bone and the atlas and the eighth pair leave below the last cervical vertebra. Thereafter, the spinal nerves are named and numbered according to the vertebra immediately above.

As can be seen from Figure 9.12, each spinal nerve has an anterior and posterior root. The anterior root consists of motor nerve fibres whilst the posterior roots are sensory. The posterior root can be distinguished by its root ganglion, a cluster of nerve cell bodies.

Shortly after leaving the intervertebral foramina, both roots join together to form a mixed nerve. From here the spinal nerves continue to form a complex network all over the body, carrying motor signals to effectors such as the skeletal muscles and conveying sensory information such as touch to the CNS for interpretation.

Further details of this complex network can be found in Wilson (1990).

Autonomic nervous system
The autonomic nervous system is the most complex and perhaps least understood part of the nervous system. Its involvement in, and effect upon, everyday activities is vague until its delicate mechanisms are upset. The effects are then readily felt by the individual.

The autonomic nervous system consists only of the nerves carrying motor impulses to the internal organs; thus it is exclusively peripheral and motor. The nervous mechanisms involved include sensory information from the internal organs, the effects of numerous peptides and hormones, and pathways that control the peripheral ganglia and nerves. It is described as having two divisions, the sympathetic and parasympathetic, each imposing different effects (see Figs 9.15 and 9.16).

For more detailed information see Guyton (1991).

HEAD INJURY (INCORPORATING RAISED INTRACRANIAL PRESSURE)

Head injury is difficult to quantify and estimates suggest that 1 million people in the UK each year are affected, of which 5000 will die. It predominates in the 16–35-year age group and has a distinct male bias of 3:1. Head injury accounts for a quarter of trauma deaths and almost half of those are caused by road traffic accidents. The financial cost is inestimable and this is of major significance, particularly as it is preventable. This is an area in which nurses could exercise their health education skills, for example, by emphasising the dangers associated with head injury and its detrimental effects to those patients and their families who have suffered a minor head injury and made a good recovery. Depending on the original cause, this may include consideration of driver behaviour or unsafe work practices. The Health and Safety at Work Act (1974) has done much to reduce this hazard. The use of seat belts for all car passengers has led to a reduction in head injuries as has the use of protective headgear for motorcyclists and horse riders (Pownall 1985). A common contributing factor in head injury is over-indulgence in alcohol and, where appropriate, the patient can be encouraged to consider his personal lifestyle and the consumption of alcohol.

PATHOPHYSIOLOGY

The adult skull can be considered as a rigid box divided into two major compartments, containing non-compressible components. A uniform

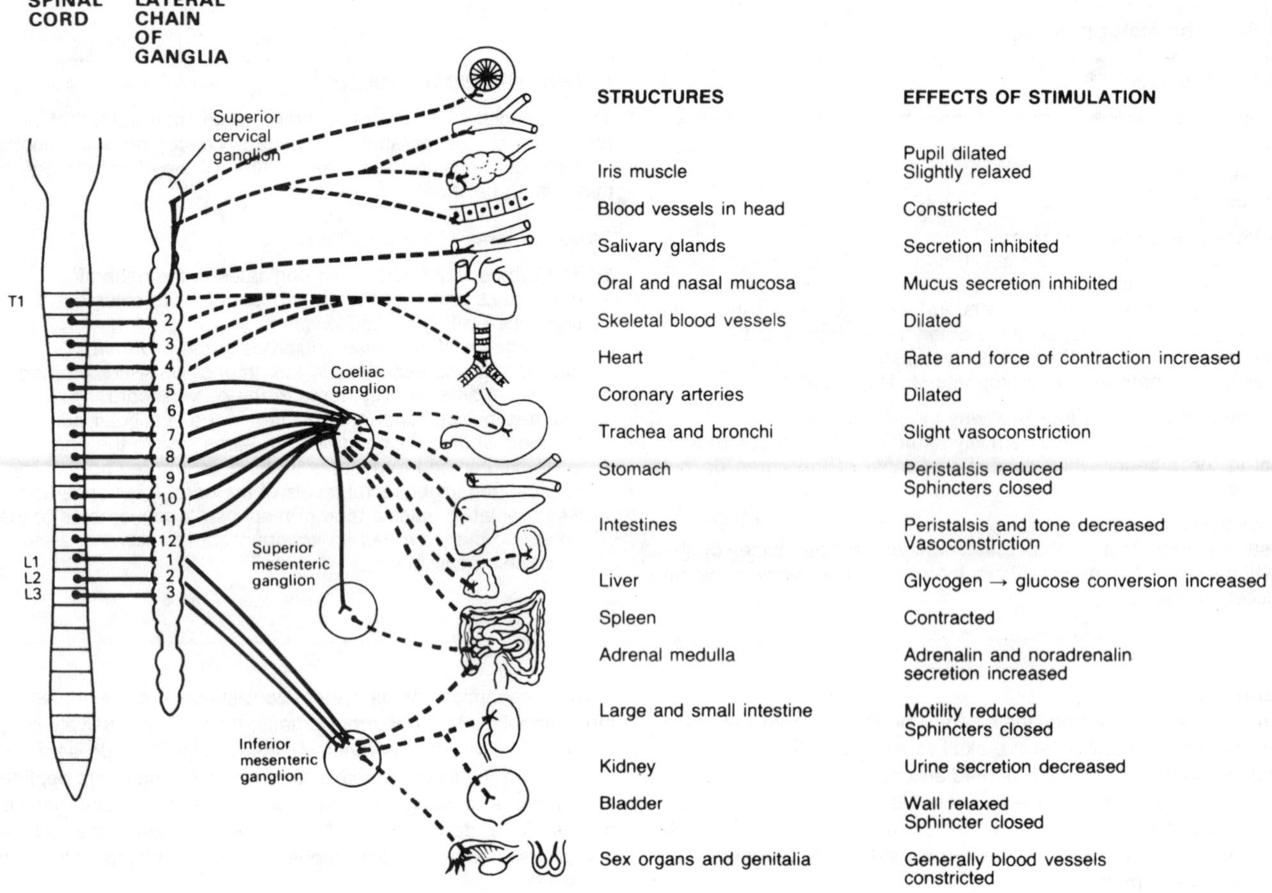

Fig. 9.15 The sympathetic outflow, the main structures supplied and the effects of stimulation. Solid lines — preganglionic fibres; broken lines — postganglionic fibres. (Reproduced with kind permission from Wilson (1990).)

pressure, called 'intracranial' pressure (ICP), is maintained. It is defined as the pressure exerted within the cerebral ventricular system. When an individual sustains a head injury or there is some abnormal pathology, for example, a tumour, it can alter this delicate balance. When an increase in ICP occurs, the pressure in one compartment is higher than in its counterpart and abnormal movement of tissue from an area of high pressure to one of low occurs, a process known as '**herniation**' or '**coning**'.

Three intracranial components are involved in the process of maintaining ICP:

- the brain
- the cerebrospinal fluid
- blood.

The brain is the largest of these, occupying 80% of the content. The remaining 20% is taken up in equal proportion by the cerebrospinal fluid and the blood. Under normal circumstances, ICP is maintained within normal limits but when there is an alteration to the volume of one of these components within the confined space of the skull, the other two are compressed, resulting in a rise in ICP. The normal range of ICP is 0–15 mmHg and anything over 15 mmHg is considered abnormal. Transient rises in pressure occur with activities such as coughing or sneezing and this is a normal physiological response.

Changes to the brain and its associated structures, following trauma, may cause intracranial pressure (ICP) to rise to a dangerous level, resulting in coma leading to permanent brain damage.

The causes and presenting symptoms of raised ICP

Causes of raised ICP can be classified according to the intracranial components involved.

Brain. Brain tissue volume can be increased due to the presence of an expanding intracranial lesion, such as a brain tumour or a haematoma following head injury.

CSF. Increased production, decreased absorption or blockage of a CSF pathway will result in hydrocephalus.

Blood. Cerebral blood flow can be increased, principally as a result of an abnormally high level of carbon dioxide in the blood (hypercapnia) and to a lesser extent lack of oxygen in the tissues (hypoxia). These lead to congestion within the cerebral circulation, culminating in a raised ICP. Such a situation can be precipitated by neglect of the patient's airway during the post-operative period following neurosurgery or following head injury.

A rise in ICP can develop over a variable period of time. It can occur over a number of years in a slow-growing brain tumour, with the patient hardly noticing any symptomatology, or it can occur in a matter of minutes following severe head injury, when the patient becomes profoundly unconscious. The underlying principle remains the same and is centred on the volume–pressure relationship curve (Fig. 9.17).

A correlation exists between ICP and conscious level. As ICP rises, conscious level deteriorates.

During the initial rise in ICP, compensatory mechanisms come into play, principally, the ability of the cerebral ventricular system to reduce the volume of CSF by displacing it into a distensible spinal dural sac. A reduction in cerebral blood volume also occurs as a result of autoregulation, the ability of blood vessels to alter their diameter according to local conditions. This is represented by the flattened part of the curve. However, this is only a temporary measure and as the volume of the expanding lesion increases, compensation is overcome

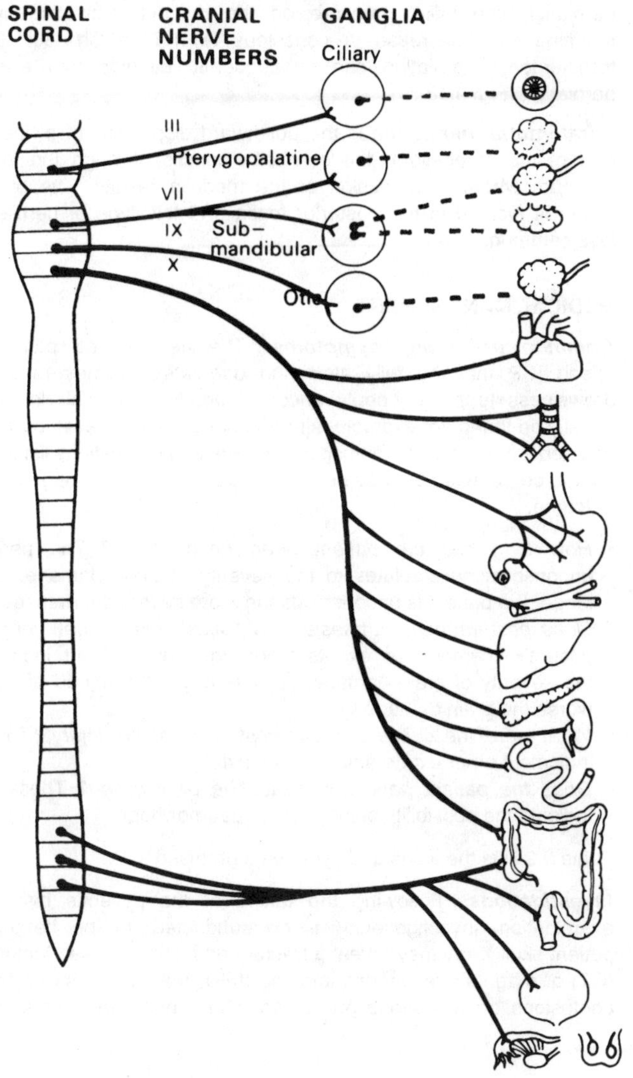

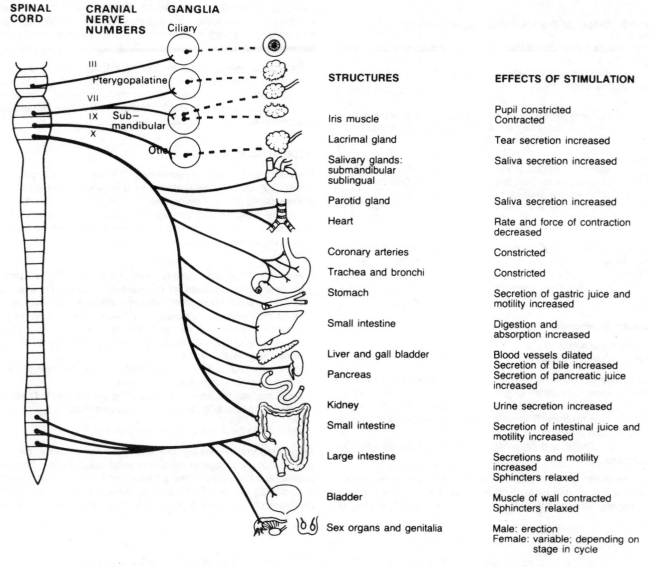

SPINAL CORD

CRANIAL NERVE NUMBERS

III

VII

IX

X

GANGLIA

Ciliary

Pterygopalatine

Sub-mandibular

Otic

STRUCTURES	EFFECTS OF STIMULATION
Iris muscle	Pupil constricted Contracted
Lacrimal gland	Tear secretion increased
Salivary glands: submandibular sublingual	Saliva secretion increased
Parotid gland	Saliva secretion increased
Heart	Rate and force of contraction decreased
Coronary arteries	Constricted
Trachea and bronchi	Constricted
Stomach	Secretion of gastric juice and motility increased
Small intestine	Digestion and absorption increased
Liver and gall bladder	Blood vessels dilated Secretion of bile increased
Pancreas	Secretion of pancreatic juice increased
Kidney	Urine secretion increased
Small intestine	Secretion of intestinal juice and motility increased
Large intestine	Secretions and motility increased Sphincters relaxed
Bladder	Muscle of wall contracted Sphincters relaxed
Sex organs and genitalia	Male: erection Female: variable; depending on stage in cycle

Fig. 9.16 The parasympathetic outflow, the main structures supplied and the effects of stimulation. Solid lines — preganglionic fibres; broken lines — postganglionlic fibres. Where there are no broken lines, the 2nd neurone is in the wall of the structure. (Reproduced with kind permission from Wilson (1990).)

and the steep part of the curve is entered. The addition of the same volume to that which was added previously and produced very little change in ICP, now results in dramatic increases in ICP. This process has four identifiable stages as illustrated in Box 9.3.

Other factors which have an influence on this complex process include cerebral blood flow and cerebral oedema.

Further information on influencing factors can be found in Allan (1988).

Herniation

Herniation is the process by which tissue in a high-pressure compartment is compressed and forced through an available opening into an adjoining low-pressure compartment. Such a situation can exist in the patient with raised ICP. The skull has two compartments; the supratentorial, that is, the region above the tentorium and infratentorial, that is, below the tentorium. The opening that permits supratentorial herniation is the tentorial notch and that which permits infratentorial herniation, the foramen magnum.

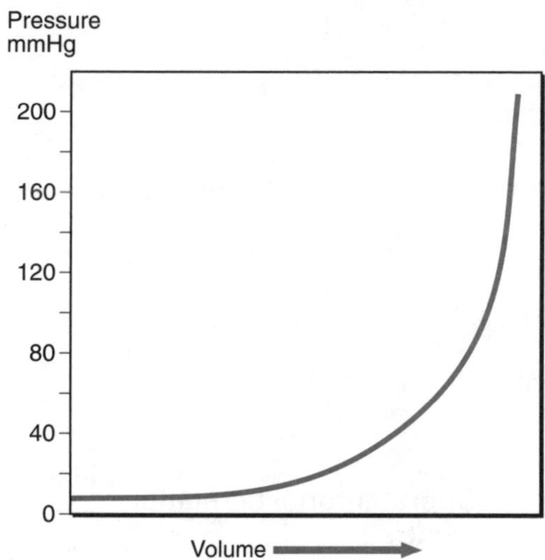

Fig. 9.17 Volume pressure curve.

Box 9.3 Stages of the volume–pressure relationship in raised ICP

Stage 1
The compensation phase: there is no rise in ICP, and conscious level remains unaltered.

Stage 2
The early phase of reversible decompensation: a slight increase in brain mass will produce an elevated ICP. Early signs of deterioration in conscious level noted.

Stage 3
The late phase of reversible decompensation: ICP now very high and conscious level now deteriorating rapidly. Detrimental changes occur in the respiratory rate and pattern. ICP will soon equal mean arterial pressure with, ultimately, cessation of cerebral blood flow.

Stage 4
The irreversible decompensation phase: in which further deterioration leading to death will occur if intervention is not initiated.

Supratentorial herniation is either:

- central tentorial herniation, or
- lateral transtentorial herniation.

Central tentorial herniation is when symmetrical herniation is produced by a midline expanding lesion or generalised swelling of brain tissue. It involves the downward displacement of the cerebral hemispheres, diencephalon and midbrain. The nerves and posterior cerebral arteries are stretched and compression of the oculomotor nerve (third cranial nerve) occurs. These and other structures are displaced into the posterior fossa.

Lateral transtentorial herniation occurs in the presence of an expanding lesion located close to the temporal lobe. The medial part of the temporal lobe (the uncus) is forced downwards. This type of herniation can inflict pressure on the reticular activating system, resulting in a decrease in conscious level (see Ch. 30). Lateral transtentorial herniation can subsequently develop into a central herniation (Fig. 9.18).

Infratentorial herniation is the downward displacement of the lower part of the cerebellum (the cerebellar tonsils) through the foramen magnum where compression of the medulla results. The offending lesion is located in the posterior fossa and this type of herniation is less common.

MEDICAL MANAGEMENT

Common presenting symptoms. The head-injured patient with raised ICP may be fully alert and orientated or may range from drowsiness to being deeply unconscious. Neurological deficits can usually be found, for example, alteration of conscious level, occurrence of a seizure or onset of confusion. Answers to the questions listed below should be obtained as they bear an influence on the management and outcome.

- *How long has the patient been unconscious?* The period of unconsciousness relates to the severity of brain damage, i.e. the longer the patient is unconscious the more severe the damage.
- *Does post-traumatic amnesia (PTA) exist and for how long?* The patient's memory for events following injury are an indicator of the severity of brain damage, i.e. the longer the period of PTA the worse the brain damage.
- *What were the cause and circumstances of the injury?* This may indicate if other extracranial injuries exist.
- *Does the patient have any headache or vomiting?* These would indicate the possibility of intracranial haemorrhage.

Table 9.2 lists the signs and symptoms of raised ICP.

Investigations. Following the taking of the patient's history and examination, investigations will be conducted. In the head-injured patient skull X-ray may reveal a fracture and computerised tomography (CT) or magnetic resonance imaging (MRI) may demonstrate cerebral contusions or lacerations and/or an intracranial haematoma (Hickey

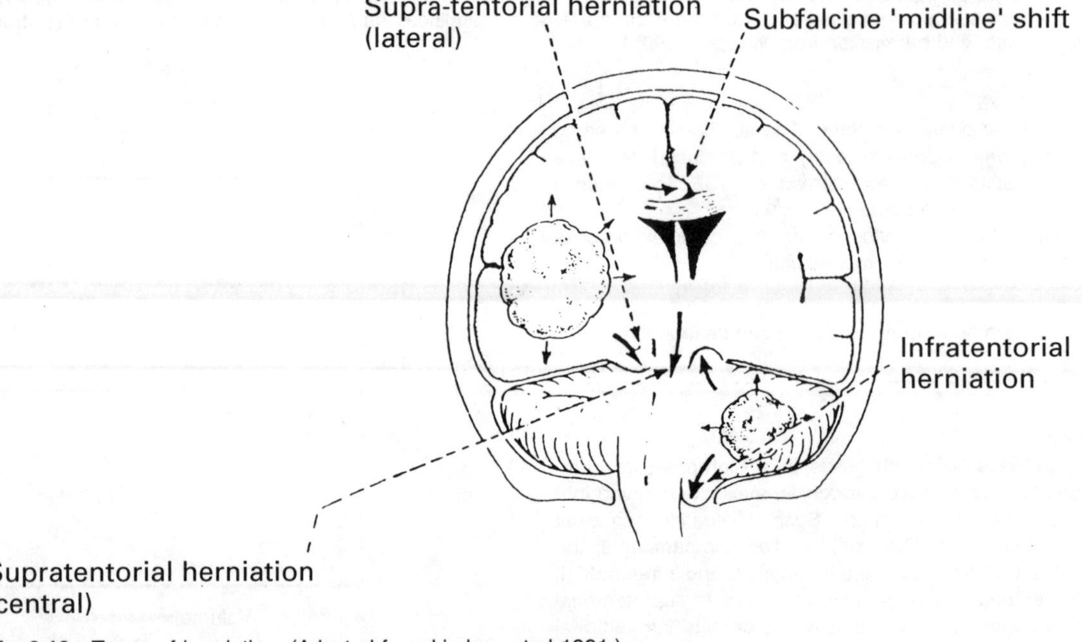

Fig. 9.18 Types of herniation. (Adapted from Lindsay et al 1991.)

Table 9.2 Signs and symptoms of raised intracranial pressure. (Adapted from Allan 1988.)

Clinical parameter	Signs/symptoms	Reasons
Conscious level	Deterioration in conscious level	Raised intracranial pressure will reduce the amount of oxygen received by the oxygen sensitive cells of the cerebral cortex.
Respiration	Deterioration in respiratory pattern	A particular respiratory pattern will be seen in relation to the non-functioning area in the medulla and pons. *Breathing pattern* — *Non-functioning area* Cheyne-Stokes — affects various areas Apneustic — Pons varolii Ataxic — Medulla Central neurogenic — Lower mid-brain Hyperventilation — Upper pons Cluster breathing — Medulla
Pupils	a. Alteration in pupil size b. Reaction to light c. Blurring of vision/diplopia d. Ocular muscle paresis/paralysis	All the pupillary and eye movement responses to raised intracranial pressure are as a result of compression of the 3rd cranial nerve (oculomotor). The ipsilateral pupil is usually affected first followed by the other one.
Blood pressure	a. An increase in systolic blood pressure followed by b. a fall	The increase in blood pressure occurs as a result of ischaemia, due to raised intracranial pressure, of the vasomotor centre. Implicated in this is a widening pulse pressure. If this is not corrected, the intracranial pressure continues to rise, and the blood pressure then begins to fall dramatically until it is unrecordable.
Pulse	Initially bradycardia (< 60 bpm) develops with a full and bounding pulse. In the later stages the pulse becomes weak and thready.	This is brought about as a result of increased workload on the heart which is attempting to overcome cerebral blood vessel resistance by pushing more blood into the cerebral circulation.
Motor function	Contralateral hemiparesis/hemiplegia	The raised intracranial pressure affects pyramidal tract function and continued deterioration will ensue until the limbs are unresponsive to deep painful stimuli.
	Headache usually in the early morning	Headache due to raised intracranial pressure is thought to be the result of displacement of the cerebrospinal fluid cushion producing dilation of cerebral blood vessels, stretching of arteries at the base of the brain and traction of bridging veins. Intracranial pressure will be adversely affected following REM sleep and by the retention of carbon dioxide during sleep resulting in exacerbation of intracranial pressure in early morning.
'Cushing's triad'	Headache, becoming more severe or persistent	This indicates that the ICP is rising and the intracranial contents are being compressed; 'herniation' may occur.
	Vomiting: may occur with early morning headache.	The mechanism involved is not well understood.
	Projectile vomiting and problems with swallowing	These indicate that there is increasing pressure on the brain stem, where the control centres for these functions are located.
	Papilloedema	Occurs as a result of raised intracranial pressure being transmitted down the optic nerve to produce a swollen nerve head. This may be seen on direct fundoscopy. An unreliable sign, which is not constantly seen in all patients with raised intracranial pressure.
	Problems with speech or comprehension	These may indicate that ICP is rising and that there is pressure on the cerebral cortex.

No order is implied within the above set of signs and symptoms. Any combination in varying degrees can occur in each patient. Individually, each of the signs and symptoms can be caused by other pathology, including extracranially.

1992). Box 9.4 gives a description of the types of injury the brain may suffer.

Intracranial pressure monitoring

One of the most important diagnostic measures is the monitoring of intracranial pressure. This is an invasive technique involving direct measurement of ICP. The Camino system comprises a fibre-optic transducer-tipped catheter, which can be placed in either the lateral ventricle, sub-dural space or extra-dural space. The level of ICP is then transmitted to a digital data display or as a wave form. A pulsatile waveform will be demonstrated along with a pressure level indicating if the patient's ICP is within normal limits (less than 15 mmHg). See Figure 9.19.

Treatment. The treatment of head injury focuses primarily on the interventions required to reduce ICP and treat other injuries. These can be considered under non-surgical or surgical interventions and some patients may undergo a combination of therapies.

Medications and other non-surgical interventions. If no operative lesion is present the patient is treated symptomatically and will

Box 9.4 Description of injury to the brain

Contusions
Described as a bruising of the cerebral tissue. Most commonly affects the frontal, occipital and undersurface of the temporal lobes. There are two types:

- coup, indicating haemorrhage and oedema immediately under the injury site
- contrecoup, where damage occurs directly opposite the injury site. This is caused by the rapid acceleration or deceleration movement of the brain within the skull, following severe trauma. Contused brain tissue affects the blood supply to that area resulting in swelling of the brain which will raise ICP.

Lacerations
Brain tissue is lacerated as a result of, for example, a skull fracture, resulting in disruption to cellular activity which will produce focal neurological deficits such as hemiparesis. Contusions and cerebral oedema may also occur.

Haematoma
A localised collection of blood. These are named according to their location:

- extradural — situated or occurring outside the dura mater
- subdural — between the dura mater and the arachnoid
- intracerebral — within the brain substance.

Diffuse brain injury
Here there is no specific focal pathology. Shearing of the white matter occurs, causing disruption and tearing of the axons.

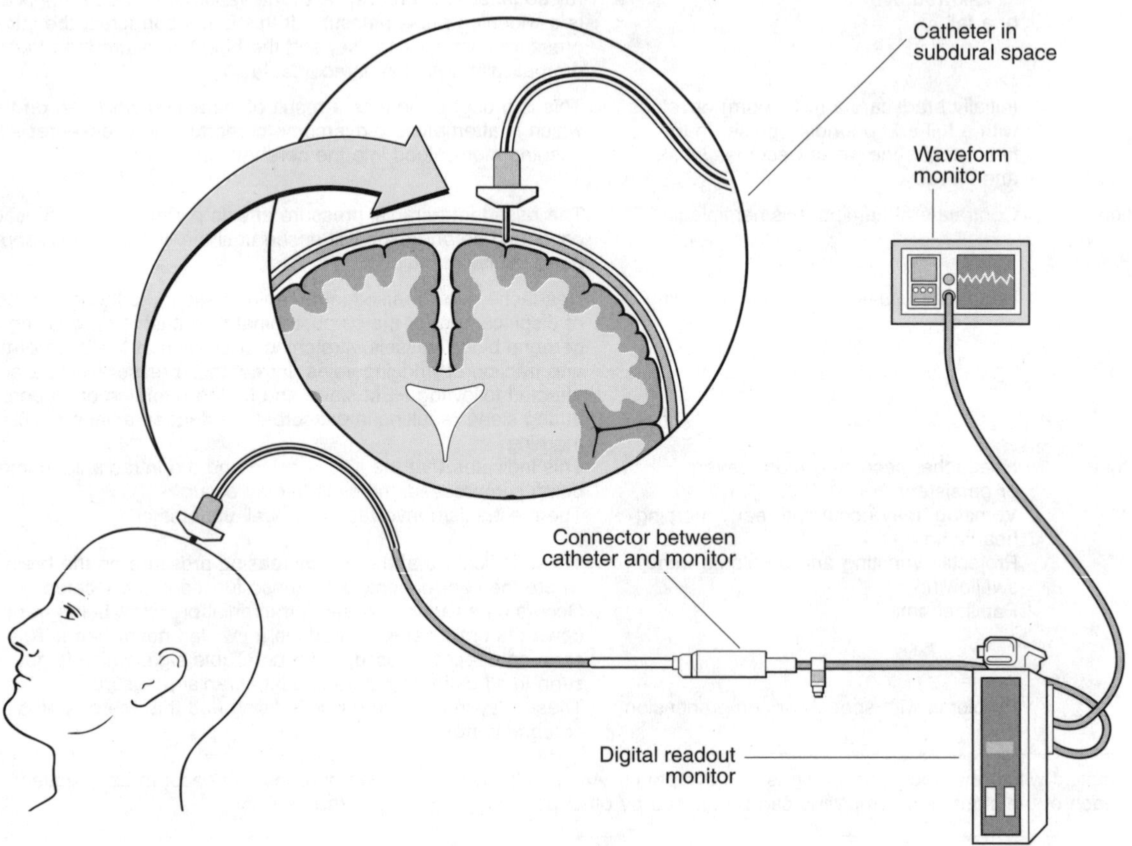

Fig. 9.19 The fibre-optic transducer-tipped catheter system for monitoring intracranial pressure (Camino System). (Adapted from Hickey 1992.)

continue to have his neurological status closely monitored. Examples of conservative treatment are as follows.

Hyperosmolar agents. An intravenous infusion of 100 ml of 20% mannitol over 15 minutes will reduce ICP by establishing an osmotic gradient between the plasma and brain tissue, thus removing water from the oedematous brain tissue to the blood. This will 'buy' time to allow the patient to be prepared for transfer to a specialist unit or for the preparation for surgery. However, if repeated boluses are administered its effect is neutralised, leading to a rebound increase in ICP.

Hyperventilation. To achieve this, the patient requires to be paralysed, intubated and mechanically ventilated. The objective is to reduce the P_aCO_2 to encourage vasoconstriction, thus reducing cerebral blood volume and ICP. However, it is thought that the patient eventually adapts to the new P_aCO_2 level and that ICP then returns to its previous high level.

Fluid restriction. Some advocate the use of fluid restriction in order to induce slight dehydration. By controlling intake, the extracellular fluid, including that of the brain, is decreased thus reducing ICP. The intake may be set at 1–2.5 litres per 24 hours.

Surgical intervention. Surgery may be performed to remove a focal

Box 9.5 Neurosurgical approaches

Burr hole
A burr hole is a hole drilled through the cranium to allow access to the brain, usually to obtain a biopsy of tumour tissue.

Craniotomy
Access is gained to the brain via the formation of a bone flap, which is fashioned by several burr holes in a circular formation. The bone between the burr holes is cut with a wire saw and usually replaced at the close of surgery.

Craniectomy
This is a hole made in the skull by chipping away the bone which means that it cannot be replaced. Usually used in the posterior fossa approach where the bone is particularly thick.

Transphenoidal approach
This approach gains access to the pituitary gland and the incision is upper submucosa. This allows easier access to the pituitary gland. (Allan 1988)

An additional surgical technique only recently developed, is the trans-oral route. To gain access to the base of the brain and upper cervical spinal cord an approach via the patient's mouth has been successfully used. This particular approach is not usually indicated for tumour removal.

Box 9.6 Respiratory care priorities in a patient with raised ICP

1. Assess the rate, depth and pattern of respirations to indicate the patency of the airway. Report if the rate is less than 14 and more than 24, and any irregularities in rate or rhythm, as these would indicate a rise in ICP.
2. Assess the skin for cyanosis, which would indicate inadequate respiration.
3. Apply oro-pharyngeal and tracheal suctioning only as required to remove secretions. Suction for no more than 15 sec. and consider pre-oxygenation prior to suctioning with 100% oxygen to prevent a build-up of carbon dioxide in the blood, resulting in further elevation of ICP.
4. Institute measures to achieve optimal respiratory status including insertion of a Guedal airway, positioning the patient on his side with a 30° head-up tilt and administer oxygen as prescribed.
5. Assist with monitoring arterial blood gases and mechanical ventilation as required.

mass lesion such as an expanding haematoma and this may be combined with decompression. Withdrawal of small aliquots of CSF via a ventricular catheter results in a reduction of ICP but this only provides temporary relief. To be effective, drainage would require to be continuous but this is often impractical. Examples of neurosurgical approaches are given in Box 9.5.

NURSING PRIORITIES AND MANAGEMENT OF HEAD INJURY

Head injured patients with raised ICP can present in different ways on admission to hospital. The person may appear to have sustained no injury initially but can become drowsy or confused, or develop speech problems or limb deficits. Epileptic fits may occur.

Immediate priorities

The immediate nursing aim is to prevent further damaging rises in ICP and the first priority is to identify any alteration in respiratory function due to an obstructed airway or an absent cough or gag reflex. The appropriate interventions are described in Box 9.6.

The nurse should be aware of the presence of other injuries, for example, multiple injuries if the patient has been in a road traffic accident. Elaboration of the assessment and appropriate interventions for this can be found in Ch. 28 and Ch. 18.

Assessment of neurological status
This is performed in order to:

- make an initial assessment of the patient, which may influence any immediate action that needs to be taken
- have a baseline with which to compare the patient's condition, to facilitate observation of changes in his condition.

Any deterioration in neurological status may be an early indication that ICP is rising further, thus increasing the likelihood of herniation. Neurological assessment is important as this may be the only indication that the patient's condition is deteriorating and a standardised method of monitoring neurological status will enhance this process. One commonly used method is the Glasgow Coma Scale (Rowley & Fielding 1991). This is described in Ch. 30.

A study of head-injured patients shows that a group treated in a neurological intensive care unit made better recoveries than a group treated in a non-specialist ward before the unit was set up (Warme, Bergstrom & Perrson 1991).

The frequency of observations is determined by the patient's condition, ranging from intervals of 15 minutes to 4 hours. Medical staff should be promptly informed of any changes in the patient's neurological status.

The nurse is normally the health care professional who spends most time with the patient and she should learn to observe changes in the patient's behaviour which may herald an impending change in neurological status. These may include the patient who does not answer questions so readily or who is becoming more agitated and restless.

The expert neurosurgical nurse (Benner 1984) will be alert to the early warning signs which it is so important to recognise, so that either surgical or conservative treatment can be carried out as soon as possible (see pp. 331–339). Quite subtle changes in the patient's condition may be the only initial indication that ICP is rising.

? **9.2** Explore, as a group, your experience of caring for patients with raised intracranial pressure. What range of signs and symptoms have you and your fellow students noted?

Cardiovascular assessment
The final life-threatening concern in a patient with a rising ICP is the effect of alterations to systemic and cerebral circulation due to shock and cardiovascular instability. The nurse should report if:

- systolic pressure is less than 90 or more than 170 mmHg
- diastolic pressure less than 50 or more than 100 mmHg
- the pulse rate is less than 50 or more than 100 beats per minute

unless requested to do otherwise by medical staff.

Readings which exceed these parameters will render the patient more susceptible to brain damage as a result of raised ICP and a lowered cerebral perfusion pressure.

Table 9.3 Complications of neurosurgery

Complication	Cause	Interventions
Altered conscious level.	Increased ICP due to cerebral haemorrhage/oedema.	Frequent assessment of neurological status.
Onset of seizures.	Cerebral irritation.	Observation of seizures. Appropriate intervention if they occur (see p. 353).
Limb weaknesses.	Increased ICP due to cerebral haemorrhage/oedema.	Frequent assessment of limb movements.
Speech problems.	Increased ICP due to cerebral haemorrhage/oedema.	Frequent assessment of verbal responses.
Respiratory problems.	Increased ICP due to cerebral haemorrhage/oedema.	Frequent assessment of respiratory status.
Loss of swallow reflex.	Increased ICP due to cerebral haemorrhage/oedema.	Frequent assessment of swallowing reflex.
Loss of corneal reflex.	Increased ICP due to cerebral haemorrhage/oedema.	Frequent assessment of corneal reflex.
Peri-orbital oedema.	Direct result of surgery.	Observe for swollen/bruised peri-orbital tissues.

Surgery

Pre-operative. Urgent surgery may be indicated shortly after admission or in response to subsequent deterioration. The nurse will need to prepare the patient in a very short time, and also to provide adequate explanation and reassurance. (See Ch. 27.)

The approaches used in surgery are as outlined in Box 9.5.

Post-operative: The overall goals of care for patients following neurosurgery are:

- continuous assessment of the patient's neurological status (see p. 341)
- instituting measures to avoid secondary brain damage
- administration of appropriate therapies.

The main complications of neurosurgery are outlined in Table 9.3.

As the patient progresses, his needs will require to be reassessed and the nursing interventions adjusted accordingly. Each patient will progress at a different rate, so continuing assessment and meeting the identified needs on an individual basis are important. The aim of care is to ensure that optimum function is obtained and early detection of complications.

Subsequent considerations

All of the nursing interventions identified in Ch. 30 will apply. Only those interventions specific to the patient who is unconscious due to raised ICP are included here. The main aim of care remains that of preventing further rises in ICP.

The patient care outlined in the following sections uses the Roper, Logan and Tierney (1990) framework of the Activities of Daily Living (ADL).

Communicating

Unpleasant stimuli are known to cause a rise in ICP, so the nurse should take a calm, reassuring approach. Relatives should be encouraged to talk to the patient and, although they may feel a bit foolish at first, they will be encouraged if they see the nurse talking to him. They should be warned to avoid discussing upsetting topics, however. Everyone should be made aware that the unconscious patient may still be able to hear (Allan 1988), and should be careful what they discuss in the patient's presence.

Non-verbal communication, particularly touch, has been shown to decrease ICP so relatives should be encouraged to touch the patient, for example by holding hands or gently stroking the patient's arm, despite the extensive equipment which may surround him.

Any investigations that are to be performed should be explained to the patient and his family, who will be anxious and distressed at this time, particularly as there may be uncertainty about the likely outcome for the patient. See Research Abstract 9.1.

Breathing

Respiratory assessment and appropriate intervention, as outlined in the previous section, will continue as long as the ICP remains elevated. In adition, the patient's position should be changed every 2 hours and physiotherapy should be instituted as this helps prevent pooling of secretions in the lungs and the development of atelectasis. The patient, if able, should be encouraged to undertake deep-breathing exercises.

Maintaining a safe environment

The patient should be positioned in the ward where he can easily be observed. If the patient is restless or agitated, the nurse should attempt to find out why. Adequate pain relief can cure a headache, which will minimise the risk of raising ICP. Non-narcotic analgesics, such as codeine phosphate and dihydrocodeine, are the first choice as they do not mask conscious level. If the patient is confused he may attempt to climb out of bed, despite explanations as to why he shouldn't. He may not appreciate that he has a limb deficit and attempt to walk, thus endangering himself. If appropriate, relatives can help persuade him to stay in bed and, as a last resort, sedation may be used. The use of side rails should be considered, but the correct precautions must be used. If the patient proves very difficult to manage, it may be necessary to place a mattress on the floor and to nurse the patient on it, however this should be fully explained to relatives beforehand. Some patients may respond to sitting up in a chair with a table secured in front.

The nurse should always be aware of the possibility of a

Research Abstract 9.1

Bruya's study set out to demonstrate the need for planned rest periods in patients with raised intracranial pressure (ICP), but this was not satisfactorily proven due to the short rest period time identified.

A chance finding was that for the majority of patients who had loved ones visit them in the morning, it was almost always noted that the patient's ICP dropped when the families approached the bedside or touched the patient's arm. The visitor did not necessarily have to speak to the patient to achieve this reduction in ICP. Touch on its own was often sufficient.

Bruya M A 1981 Planned periods of rest in the ICU: nursing care activities and ICP. Journal of Neuroscientific Nursing, 13(4): 184.

seizure. The appropriate first aid action as outlined in the section on epilepsy (see p. 355) should be adopted.

Controlling body temperature

Each 1°C rise in body temperature increases the metabolic demand of the brain by 10% (Allan 1988). This increases blood pressure and encourages vasodilation, which will increase ICP. Body temperature should be recorded at least 4-hourly. Pyrexia may indicate hypothalamic damage or the presence of infection. Any source of potential infection, such as cerebrospinal fluid (CSF) rhinorrhea should be identified and reported. Leakage of CSF from the patient's ears (ottorhea) or nose (rhinorrhea) may occur from a base-of-skull or anterior-fossa fracture. Confirmation is obtained by testing the fluid for the presence of glucose using a reagent dipstick. A positive result indicates the presence of CSF, although it is not absolutely conclusive. The identification of a fracture on the skull X-ray will confirm the evidence. If CSF leakage is left undetected the patient will be at risk of developing meningitis.

Measures to reduce the patient's temperature should be adopted. These might include tepid sponging, cool fanning or medication such as paracetamol suppositories.

Mobilising

The patient will require frequent positional changes to avoid pressure sores. Semi-prone and lateral positions are both suitable. Moving the patient also encourages expansion of the lungs and prevents pooling of secretions. A slight head-up tilt of 30° will not only reduce ICP but will aid respiration, thus helping to prevent chest infection. The patient's body should be maintained in neutral alignment, avoiding neck flexion and rotation. The hips should be carefully positioned avoiding flexion over 90°. These positions aid venous drainage as they minimise intra-abdominal and intra-thoracic pressure which will help to decrease ICP.

Passive movement exercises should be performed to prevent muscle wasting and limb contractures as these will hinder rehabilitation. Isometric exercising should be avoided as this raises ICP. Anti-embolism stockings should be used to minimise the risk of deep venous thrombosis.

As the patient's condition improves he should be encouraged to move around more. The physiotherapist will provide specialised exercises if there is a limb deficit (Hickey 1992). Sitting in a chair will help reduce respiratory complications and encourage limb movements. It may also act as an important psychological boost for the patient and his family as they will view this as progress.

Eating and drinking

As soon as the patient is able, an oral fluid intake and diet should be encouraged. Intravenous fluids may be required, however, and any fluid restrictions should be carefully observed and the intake recorded to avoid inadvertent increases in ICP due to worsening cerebral oedema. Some patients will require nasogastric or intragastric feeding and this should be facilitated by the nurse observing all the usual precautions, as detailed in Ch. 4. The patient with a basal skull fracture must not have the tube passed nasally as there is a danger of further damage and infection.

Eliminating

Observation of output should be monitored, in line with any restricted intake. Some patients require urinary catheterisation. The precautions and associated nursing care for this can be found in Ch. 8. As the patient regains consciousness, he may attempt to remove the catheter, an indication that normal functioning is returning.

Constipation should be avoided to minimise rises in ICP caused by straining at stool.

> **?** **9.3** Choose an alternative nursing model and, using the information you now have, create a nursing care plan for a patient with a head injury, using that model.
> Which model do you now feel is more appropriate to the care of the unconscious patient?

Rehabilitation

This forms a crucial part of the recovery process and the principles outlined in Ch. 35 apply. The aim is to maintain and promote function, improve or prevent further deterioration and also to prevent further complications occurring.

The neurological deficits which can impede progress during the rehabilitation process are described in Box 9.7.

The patient with a head injury may experience neurological deficits including limb weaknesses, speech problems and visual problems. He may also experience changes in personality, memory and intellect and a combination of all these factors can prove very difficult to rehabilitate.

The ward team, with the help of the patient's family and friends, should aim to assess the patient's needs and provide the optimal care and support to achieve these. Realistic goals are set and the rehabilitative process may take months or years to achieve, or the patient may remain in a persistent vegetative state requiring constant nursing care in an institution.

Often, the patient's role within the family changes. He may previously have been the provider within a family, and now have to revert to being dependent on others. Employment prospects may alter and for some a return to work is impossible. This can affect the family's long-term plans and will also have financial implications. An alteration to the patient's personality may affect relationships within a family, resulting in much stress and disagreement. Some families will report that the person has completely changed and is now different from the person they knew before, as described by a nurse who wrote of her recovery from a severe head injury (Faulkner 1989).

Very often, repeated explanations of the patient's change in behaviour toward his family are required, as they find this change distressing. The reaction of the family can range from apparent calm acceptance to rudeness and verbal aggression towards nursing staff. This should be accepted and seen as the family's method of coping.

Box 9.7 Neurological deficits that can impede rehabilitation

- motor impairment, for example, spasticity or ataxia
- sensory impairment, for example, loss of sense of pain or touch
- communication disability, for example, dysphasia
- psychologic disability
  - cognitive intelligence, for example, memory loss
  - perceptual, for example, eye–hand coordination
  - emotional, for example, irritability
  - behaviour or personality, for example, poor self image
- social disability, for example, social withdrawal
- educational or vocational disability.

All the above have an effect on the patient's ability to resume educational or vocational activities.

The multi-disciplinary approach
Early and close liaison between the many health-care professionals involved in hospital and community work is essential. The resources of the voluntary sector and self-help groups should be brought in, as well as the patient's family and friends.

Preparation for discharge
Many patients and their families will be particularly anxious as the time for discharge approaches. Much of this anxiety can be allayed if adequate preparation and reassurance is provided, along with an effective plan for discharge. The residual problems that may persist vary widely, ranging from headache to major behavioural changes, with or without neurological deficits. The degree of residual difficulty will determine what action is required in the discharge plan. Other influences may include whether the patient requires further surgery or other therapies, necessitating attendance at a hospital or rehabilitation centre. A home assessment can be performed by the occupational therapist and district nurse. Brief pre-discharge visits home may be considered and will help to identify potential problems. If there is a community liaison nurse, a referral should be made for assessment and support within the community and, if not, referral should be made to the primary health care team.

Despite these preparations, it is not usually until the patient is at home that the family fully appreciate the difficulties before them. Much of the home routine requires to be adjusted and whilst this may be easy in the early stages, it becomes more difficult to accept in the long term. Other members of the family will often view the disruption to their personal lives negatively and eventually much of the early support gradually disappears. If the patient is still at a stage in which he requires support, this withdrawal can be catastrophic. Very often the patient's partner can be left to shoulder the burden alone, and in this situation, a support group such as Headway (see p. 366) may help. This organisation seeks to provide help and assistance to the patient and his family. Regular meetings and other special outings are arranged along with helpful literature (Allan 1988). Relatives can be provided with a forum for discussion of the problems that they face and many appreciate sharing their problems with others who are similarly placed. Some families have to acknowledge a sense of failure should the patient require to be admitted for institutional care in either the short- or long-term. They may feel that they have let the patient down and do not like to admit that they are unable to cope.

> ? **9.4** Using the information on care of the head-injured patient, select a nursing model other than Roper, Logan & Tierney (1990) and write a nursing care plan for the first post-operative day following craniotomy. (See also Ch. 30.)

CEREBROVASCULAR DISEASE

'Cerebrovascular disease' can be defined as brain disease occurring secondarily to a pathological disorder of the blood vessels or of the blood supply. This section considers:

- cerebrovascular accident, the most common cerebrovascular disorder
- subarachnoid haemorrhage, an uncommon but major life-threatening situation that demands acute neurosurgical intervention.

Cerebrovascular accident

The term 'cerebrovascular accident' (CVA) is often used interchangeably with 'stroke' although, clinically, stroke refers to the sudden dramatic development of focal neurological deficits.

CVA can occur at any time during adult life but is uncommon in children. Thrombotic CVA is seen in the 60–90 year age group and embolic and haemorrhagic CVA in the 25–60 year age group.

CVA is the third commonest cause of death in developed countries: 200 per 100 000 will have a CVA each year. Age increases the risk. Most CVAs occur in the 65–75 age group and are more common in men (Allan 1988). In the UK 100 000–120 000 CVAs occur per annum, of which 70 000 result in death. The mortality rate rises in proportion to the length of time the patient is unconscious. Of patients unconscious for 48 hours or more, 98% will die, compared with 12% where there is no loss of consciousness.

Subarachnoid haemorrhage

Subarachnoid haemorrhage is often wrongly referred to as 'cerebral' or 'brain haemorrhage'. A subarachnoid haemorrhage is experienced by 10–15 000 people, with 15% dying before they reach hospital. It has a male bias in the under-40s, but this reverts in the over-40s Lindsay et al (1991).

PATHOPHYSIOLOGY

Causes of cerebrovascular accidents
There are three main causes of CVA:

- cerebral thrombosis
- cerebral embolus
- cerebral haemorrhage.

Cerebral thrombosis
This is the most common cause of CVA, in which atherosclerosis causes narrowing of the lumen of the affected blood vessels (Lindsay et al 1991). See also Ch. 2. It occurs either during sleep or shortly after wakening and is thought to be due to the older person's poorer reflex response to changes in position (postural hypotension). As the atheroma builds up it only partially occludes the blood vessel initially, until the blood supply is suddenly disrupted. During the 24–48 hours following this, neurological deficits frequently worsen.

Cerebral embolus
An embolus may lodge in the narrowed lumen of a bifurcation in the cerebral circulation. The usual origin of the embolus is a cardiac thrombus, in the presence of cardiac disease such as myocardial infarction. Air or fat can also act as an embolus. Embolic stroke can occur at any time.

Cerebral haemorrhage
Haemorrhage can occur into:

- the cerebral tissues — intracerebral haemorrhage
- the subarachnoid space — subarachnoid haemorrhage.

The most common cause of subarachnoid haemorrhage is a weakness in the wall of a cerebral blood vessel, an 'aneurysm'. Other causes include arteriovenous malformations (AVM) but in some patients no cause is identified. Hypertension, although seen in some patients, is not always present but damage caused by arteriosclerotic changes is common. Cerebral aneurysms may be described as 'berry' or 'saccular'. Most aneurysms form on the anterior part of the Circle of Willis. (See Ch. 2.) Some patients have multiple aneurysms.

The exact cause of aneurysm formation remains unknown and some remain silent, causing no symptoms. Some bleeding can occur through the very thin aneurysmal wall and produce mild signs and symptoms of subarachnoid haemorrhage without rupture occurring.

Box 9.8 Classification of CVA

Transient ischaemic attacks
Onset and disappearance of a neurological deficit within 24 hours due to temporary disturbance of blood supply to the brain.
No residual neurological deficit.
Symptoms commonly last from several minutes to 2–3 hours but may last up to 24 hours.

Reversible ischaemic neurological deficit
Neurological deficit persists longer than 12–24 hours.
Symptoms may last days or weeks.
Minimal, partial or no residual neurological deficit.

Stroke in evolution
Symptoms persist beyond 24 hours with an associated progressive deterioration of neurological status.
Residual neurological deficits.
Probably due to a failure of collateral circulation.

Completed stroke
Condition stabilises and neurological deficit remains.

Risk factors

Certain predisposing contributory factors increase the likelihood of cerebrovascular disease (see p. 347 and Ch. 2, p. 14).

The effects of a CVA

The occurrence of a CVA, for whatever reason, will result in an interruption of the cerebral blood supply, diminishing the essential oxygen and glucose levels of the brain. Within hours, oedema occurs at the site of the main lesion. This gradually worsens, peaking between the 5th and 7th day and then gradually resolving.

A classification system of CVA is given in Box 9.8.

The damage caused by a stroke can be thought of as moving out from a central area, with progressively less damage:

- at the centre, where the cerebrovascular accident occurs, the brain cells are totally destroyed and will not recover. The affected area of the brain loses its ability to carry out its function, for example:
  - control movement in a specific part of the body
  - control mental or emotional processes, speech or language
  - experience sight, sound, taste or touch
- surrounding this is an area where the cells stop functioning after the stroke but may start to function again in the course of time
- beyond that area, swelling causes fluid to press on the brain cells but does not damage them permanently. As the swelling goes down, cells in the outer area start to function again, causing rapid progress to be made in the first 2–3 weeks.

After this period, recovery is slower and is due partly to other cells taking over the functions of the permanently damaged cells. At this stage the patient also learns ways of handling his disability and regains his self-confidence and interest in general affairs.

Generally speaking, if a patient shows marked improvement within the first week, then minimal deficit will result and, conversely, if little or no improvement is made during this time, the outcome is likely to be poorer. The most common types of disability are listed in Box 9.9.

MEDICAL MANAGEMENT

Common presenting symptoms. The true onset of cerebrovascular disease can be difficult to pinpoint. In thrombotic and embolic stroke the patient usually seeks medical intervention after a major episode. Earlier symptoms will not have been noticed by the patient. Early symptoms, for example, tingling and weakness of a limb, are the result of mild transient interruptions of neurological function. Major episodes requiring medical intervention include loss of consciousness, speech difficulties and hemiplegia, which may be accompanied by loss of vision on the affected side.

Subarachnoid haemorrhage typically causes sudden, severe headache, often accompanied by vomiting. The patient may be alert and orientated, and may feel intense fear at what he is experiencing. Alternatively, there may be loss of consciousness, seizures and evidence of neurological deficits such as third-nerve palsy, hemiplegia or hemiparesis. Many of these symptoms are related to the effects of raised ICP (see p. 336).

The patient may still have a residual headache and neck stiffness which may be confirmed by passive neck flexion. This indicates meningism, caused by the presence of blood in the subarachnoid space irritating the sensitive tissue of the meninges. Kernig's sign, extending the knee to stretch the nerve roots, thus causing the patient some pain, is another indicator of meningism. Conscious level may be depressed and there may be evidence of epilepsy. Other findings may include hypertension and pyrexia. Signs and symptoms will depend on a variety of factors and can occur according to the area of the brain affected. (See Fig. 9.5.)

Box 9.9 Common types of disability caused by stroke

Motor deficits
- speech difficulties, such as
  - loss of movement in the limbs on one side of the body, called hemiplegia
  - weakness in the arms and legs (hemiparesis)
  - dysarthria, where the patient has distorted and indistinct speech but is able to understand what is said to him and can still read and write
  - dysphasia, that is, loss of the ability to talk, read and write
- facial paralysis on the affected side, causing drooling, indistinct speech and difficulty in chewing and swallowing

Sensory deficits
- visual deficits
  - partial loss of the visual field
  - double vision
  - poorer vision than previously
- poor response to superficial sensation, for example, heat and cold
- perceptual deficits, such as correct perception of the environment, or loss of sense of smell
- lack of awareness of the disabled part of the body

Loss of consciousness
- from mild impairment to coma
- loss of memory or shortened attention span

Emotional deficits
- emotional disturbances, for example, change of personality, from quiet and pleasant to surly and aggressive, or vice versa
- loss of self control or inhibitions
- confusion
- depression

Bladder dysfunction
- loss of bowel control (incontinence)
- frequency
- urgency.

?	**9.5** Think of two patients you have cared for, who have had a stroke. For each patient, write a short word picture of how you recall them, then compare your notes with the common presenting symptoms you have just read about. How similar were they?

Investigations will be as follows.

CT scan. A CT scan may be performed to determine the location and type of CVA and to ensure that there is no other, potentially treatable, lesion to account for the stroke. If a subarachnoid haemorrhage is diagnosed and the patient is alert and obeying commands and has no focal neurological deficits, lumbar puncture is indicated (Allan 1989a, Jamieson et al 1992, pp. 66–71). Confirmation of the subarachnoid haemorrhage will result when examination of the cerebrospinal fluid reveals uniform blood staining or if 6 hours have elapsed since the original bleed, straw-coloured cerebrospinal fluid, called 'xanthachromia'. This is due to the breakdown of haemoglobin.

If the patient is displaying any signs of raised ICP, for example, is in coma or has a neurological deficit, lumbar puncture is contra-indicated because of the risk of coning. The safe alternative of computerised tomography is used which may reveal the presence of blood in a variety of locations such as the surface of the cerebral hemispheres or in the ventricular system.

Angiography. If blood is detected either by lumbar puncture or computerised tomography, angiography is indicated (see Appendix 1). The presence and location of aneurysms and other blood vessel anomalies such as stenosis will be demonstrated. Angiography is not without risk and its performance may be delayed if the patient is in a poor clinical condition. Four-vessel angiography is most commonly performed. A new technique, digital subtraction angiography, produces a clearer image as surrounding anatomical structures do not show up.

Electroencephalography (see Appendix 1) may assist in differentiating between a haemorrhagic stroke, which has high-voltage slow waves, and thrombotic stroke, which has low-voltage slow waves.

In addition electrocardiography may be performed to exclude or confirm cardiac disease.

Treatment approaches in stroke vary widely because of the huge variety of presentations.

They will depend on:

- the site of the occlusion or aneurysmal rupture
- the degree and extent of the ischaemia or haemorrhage
- the effectiveness of medical and nursing intervention
- the patient's response.

The aims are to prevent further brain damage, reduce the risk factors, provide supportive care and regain functional independence.

Treatment can be conservative or surgical.

Conservative management will be as follows.

Anticoagulant therapy has been used in an attempt to halt further deterioration and to improve the patient's recovery, however some doubt has now been cast on its usefulness as a risk of further haemorrhage into the infarcted brain has been identified. To minimise this, anticoagulant therapy should be initiated gradually over several days. One example of an anticoagulant is warfarin.

Anti-fibrinolytic agents have been used in patients following subarachnoid haemorrhage. Their use is thought to prevent rebleeding by delaying dissolution of the clot around the aneurysm but their effect on the overall outcome is questionable.

Anti-platelet agents. The use of aspirin as an anti-platelet agent has received attention in recent years and research into its use continues. The patient suffering from transient ischaemic attacks may benefit from its use.

Other factors. Pre-existing contributory disorders may be treated with drug therapy, for example, anti-hypertensive agents and diuretics may be used in the patient with raised blood pressure.

Surgical management uses two techniques:

- carotid endarterectomy, which involves the removal of stenosing or ulcerating atheromatous lesions at the bifurcation of the common carotid arteries
- a superficial temporal to middle-cerebral artery anastomosis (ST–MCA bypass), which provides an artificial collateral blood supply to the affected part of the brain.

Aims of treatment in subarachnoid haemorrhage. The main aim of treatment is to avoid potentially fatal recurrence of bleeding. In untreated patients, 30% will bleed again within 28 days, and 70% of these will die.

Preventing rebleeding. An effective way to prevent rebleeding is to place a metal clip across the neck of the aneurysm. This entails a craniotomy, a major neurosurgical procedure. This procedure is not suitable for all patients, either due to their general condition or to the location of the aneurysm. Alternative surgical procedures include wrapping, which involves the application of muslin gauze around the fundus of the aneurysm. Wrapping may be combined with clipping in some patients. A third technique, known as 'trapping', may be indicated. This involves clipping the feeding vessels supplying a large aneurysm.

The timing of surgery is crucial and opinions vary with regard to this. When surgery is carried out as soon as possible to avoid the risk of rebleeding, there are higher morbidity and mortality rates during the operation. Delayed surgery decreases the operative risks but increases the risk of rebleeding. Antifibrinolytic therapy may be used in an attempt to prevent this.

There are now well-established grading systems to identify the patient most at risk from deterioration after subarachnoid haemorrhage.

Complications of subarachnoid haemorrhage that may influence treatment are as follows.

Rebleed. This is a risk which peaks between days 7 and 10 following the original bleed. This is due to the process of fibrinolysis, which dissolves the clot that formed over the ruptured vessel.

Cerebral ischaemia. Reduction of the blood supply to any part of the brain can have serious consequences for the patient. The extent of its effects will depend on the site and extent of the ischaemia (see p. 345). About half the patients who develop ischaemia will be left with a permanent deficit. Arterial narrowing (vasospasm) is common following subarachnoid haemorrhage and can have similar results.

Hydrocephalus. The normal drainage of cerebrospinal fluid may be impaired by the presence of a haematoma or by-products of blood in the cerebrospinal fluid. About one-fifth of patients are affected, although only one-third require treatment (see Box 9.10).

Intracerebral haematoma. Bleeding during a subarachnoid haemorrhage may result in a localised collection or haematoma. This will contribute to a rise in intracranial pressure and may demand treatment.

Epilepsy. Seizures may occur, necessitating treatment with anticonvulsants (see p. 353).

NURSING PRIORITIES AND MANAGEMENT: STROKE

Prevention

One of the most important aspects of stroke management is prevention, by identifying at-risk individuals and dealing with early predisposing factors such as hypertension.

Transitory ischaemic attack

If the sufferer or a relative notices the symptoms of a mild

Box 9.10 Hydrocephalus

This is a condition in which there is a progressive dilatation of the cerebral ventricular system due to a production of CSF which exceeds the absorption rate. This may be brought about by an obstruction of one of the pathways by, for example, a tumour. Other causes include congenital stenosis and infection.

It can occur at all ages; it may be congenital in the newborn or be secondary to some other intracranial pathology in the older child and adult.

Treatment is by insertion of a ventriculo-peritoneal shunt. This is a long narrow plastic tubing, valve and reservoir device. One end is inserted into the lateral ventricle and the other end is sutured into the child's peritoneum via a subcutaneous route. The excess cerebrospinal fluid is now 'shunted' from the ventricles into the peritoneum, from where it then returns to the bloodstream.

transitory ischaemic attack (TIA), they should contact a doctor immediately, as TIAs can be treated. A TIA is caused by insufficient blood reaching the brain, for a brief period. It is similar to a stroke but the symptoms last for only a few minutes (The Stroke Association 1992). These are:

- weakness of one side of the body
- tingling and twisting of the mouth
- loss of speech
- disturbance of vision.

Reducing the risk of stroke

The following factors put people at greater risk of having a stroke, but action can be taken to reduce the likelihood of stroke occurring.

High blood pressure. Using drugs to reduce high blood pressure does reduce the risk of a stroke. Blood pressure should be checked periodically, for example, every 4 years until the age of 40, and every 2 years after that. Drinking alcohol raises blood pressure. A daily maximum of 1.5 pints of beer for men and 1 pint for women, or the equivalent is recommended by the Stroke Association (Hopkins 1992). The daily equivalent in wine would be approximately 3 units for men and 2 units for women.

Cigarette smoking. In people who smoke 20 cigarettes a day, the risk of having a stroke is three times greater than that for people who do not smoke (Hopkins 1992). Smokers should therefore be encouraged to stop smoking, and young people discouraged from starting to smoke.

High blood cholesterol may lead to coronary heart disease. Patients with high blood cholesterol can reduce the amount of cholesterol-rich foods they take, by the following measures:

- using soft margarine instead of butter, and using vegetable oil for cooking
- using skimmed milk, not full-cream or milk
- avoiding cream and cheese, and cutting down on the number of eggs eaten
- choosing lean cuts of meat, or removing the fat.

Being overweight may increase the likelihood of high blood pressure, so at-risk patients should watch their weight.

Diabetic patients are more likely to have a stroke, so the level of sugar in the blood and urine should be checked regularly.

The contraceptive pill increases the risk of stroke in younger women, particularly if there is a family history of arterial disease. Other forms of contraception are therefore more suitable.

Nursing care following a stroke

Often the immediate priorities and follow-up care overlap and are separated here for the purposes of explanation only. A successful outcome is more likely when the optimum techniques and resources are utilised, encompassing every member of the multidisciplinary team. The outcome can also be influenced by other factors such as recognising the need to start the rehabilitative process as soon as possible.

Life-threatening concerns

Airway

Techniques for maintaining a patent airway and adequate ventilation, outlined in Box 9.6, are a priority. See Ch. 30.

Safety and comfort

Hemiplegia is often caused by stroke, so the care of paralysed limbs and the hazards of immobility are important.

Similarly, the patient with a decreased level of consciousness will require to have his safety needs met and this is dealt with in Ch. 30. This includes an accurate assessment of conscious level. Raised intracranial pressure will pose a number of dangers for the patient. See interventions outlined on p. 341 for care of a patient with a head injury.

The patient who has experienced a haemorrhage will be assessed for headache and an analgesic administered if required. The drugs of choice are codeine phosphate and dihydrocodeine, which do not mask conscious level. Patients often have a sore neck which can be alleviated by cold packs and a position in bed which avoids extreme flexion and sudden movement of the neck. A quiet darkened room will also relieve discomfort particularly if the patient is photophobic. An anti-emetic may also be prescribed for nausea and vomiting.

Patient safety and comfort is greatly enhanced when consideration is given to the patient's ability to communicate, and for their emotional wellbeing, as well as that of their family.

Communicating

Speech impairment or loss can be a frightening experience for the patient and his family. Early referral to a speech therapist is important in order that an expert assessment can be performed and a strategy identified. It is crucial to ascertain the type and nature of the speech deficit, for example, whether the patient's difficulties are related to expression or comprehension. The nurse should encourage the patient to perform the prescribed exercises, with her help, between sessions with the speech therapist (Johnstone 1987).

Powerful emotions are often displayed by the patient following stroke. Many of these patients display anger at or frustration with the frightening situation in which they find themselves. This can be vented onto the nurse and can manifest itself as lack of cooperation or physical abuse. Patients who are unable to communicate their feelings verbally may feel trapped inside a body that refuses to do as they want (Clark 1983). Some patients are convinced that their words are properly formed and fail to realise that what the nurse or family is hearing is indistinct or jumbled. The patient needs to be repeatedly reminded of what has happened to him and why he feels the way he does, in order to try to reassure him. Patients can become very distressed when family and friends come to visit and this needs to be handled with sensitivity. See also Ch. 26.

Mobilising

Patients with walking difficulties require a clutter-free environment and this may necessitate re-arrangement of furniture. The nurse should ensure that any obstacles likely to pose a danger are removed and that the patient is wearing appropriate clothing and footwear, for example, outdoor shoes rather than loose-fitting slippers.

Visual impairment may also be dangerous for the patient. See Box 9.9. Simple interventions that may help include providing an eye patch to eliminate double vision and approaching the patient from the side with the intact field of vision. The patient's family should also be advised about basic safety precautions at home, following discharge, for example, removal of loose rugs and any necessary rearrangement of furniture.

Differences of opinion exist with regard to mobility following subarachnoid haemorrhage. One approach advocates that patients should have strict bedrest and that their visitors should be restricted, however, this approach can heighten the patient's anxiety particularly when he feels well. An alternative approach is to allow the patient up to the toilet provided he is symptom-free. The patient with a neurological deficit or alteration to his conscious level should be kept in an easily observable bed with cot sides if required. Seizure precautions should also be adopted as outlined on page 353.

Eating and drinking

Initially the patient's fluid intake is likely to be via an intravenous infusion and the nurse will be responsible for maintaining this at the correct rate. A patient who has had a subarachnoid haemorrhage may be prescribed a fluid regime of 2.5–3 litres per day. This helps to maintain arterial blood pressure, which encourages adequate cerebral perfusion and, in turn, prevents cerebral ischaemia and infarction. An accurate record of fluid balance should be maintained. As the patient progresses, an oral diet may gradually be introduced, providing that swallowing and cough reflexes are intact. The patient may need help with feeding, or can be given adapted eating utensils which allow him to feed himself. Being spoon-fed can be embarrassing and sensitivity is required on the nurse's part to preserve the patient's dignity and self-esteem. The nurse should determine what the patient is capable of, for example, hemiplegia may prevent the patient from cutting up his own food but does not stop him from feeding himself. The patient with a facial paralysis should be instructed to chew food on the unaffected side only.

Dysphagia will hinder this progress. If the patient experiences swallowing difficulties these should be assessed to determine the extent of the difficulty before attempting oral feeding. A combined asessment may be performed by the dietitian and speech therapist. Recommendations may include the use of a nasogastric feeding tube and a prescribed proprietary liquid diet, and the use of specialised exercises and techniques. Increased oral hygiene is important in both instances. The patient with dysphagia receiving nasogastric feeding will be more prone to a dry mouth and the patient on an oral diet may leave food debris in the mouth, particularly on the affected side. (See Ch. 15.)

Eliminating

Interruption of the patient's usual elimination pattern is due to loss of consciousness and enforced immobility. Urinary incontinence is best dealt with by retraining the patient to use bedpans or urinals at specified intervals, rather than resort to catheterisation. Condom-type urinary appliances may be suitable for male patients but no successful female equivalent is yet available.

Rehabilitation

The overall aim of rehabilitation, as outlined in Ch. 35, is the active promotion and restoration of independence, and this applies equally to the patient following a stroke, whether at home, in hospital or in a rehabilitation centre. See Case History 9.1. Thomas (1988) describes the common complications following a stroke and provides advice on how to deal with these.

Case History 9.1 Mrs F

Mrs F had her stroke on May 21. She was completely paralysed on the right side and had lost all power of speech. A CT scan on May 25 showed a large area of brain loss on the left side. By June 1 her speech was normal, yet she still could not walk at all, or use her right arm. She took her first steps on June 21, and one month later was walking alone using a tripod. Her arm also developed a little movement six weeks after her stroke. She returned home on July 16, and by early November she was walking to the local shops, talking normally and was able to use her right hand and arm for holding cans. (Hewer & Wade 1986)

Mrs F's story is not unusual, and illustrates several points.

1. There was a rapid recovery over the first month, when her speech returned and leg movements started.
2. Her recovery continued, although slowly, for about 6 months.
3. This happened despite the scan showing that Mrs F had lost a lot of brain tissue.

Dead brain cannot regenerate, yet people known to have brain loss can recover quite well. How is this?

Processes of recovery

1. Learning new ways of coping
2. Use of other parts of the brain
3. Possible growth of nerve axons
4. Reduction of brain swelling around the stroke area
5. Adaptation by others to the person who has had a stroke.

Behind this success story must be close collaboration between community nurses and other members of the health care professions.

? **9.6** Can you seek out an example of such a multidisciplinary approach in support of a patient and his family from your own placement experience of nursing in the community?

Johnstone (1987) makes clear the need for the nurse to know and understand any rehabilitative exercises and positioning instructions. The work of the physiotherapist in initiating these can be destroyed if nurses in hospital and in the community do not continue these exercises and assist carers to learn the necessary skills. Johnstone emphasises that the patient needs to live in the recovery pattern, otherwise rehabilitation is doomed to failure.

Therapy

Different types of therapy can aid rehabilitation. These are not necessary immediately, as many people recover spontaneously, but can be of help once it is apparent that specific problems remain.

Physiotherapists can assist people to walk again and suggest suitable aids such as canes, Zimmer frames or foot splints. They can also help the patient regain movement in paralysed arms.

Occupational therapists can train patients to dress and cook for themselves, and can suggest suitable home aids.

Speech therapists help patients to overcome problems with speech, often involving the patient in attending speech-therapy sessions at the hospital.

Hewer & Wade (1986) state that therapists will:

- assess the main problems
- show the family how to handle the patient properly, to avoid complications
- supervise the first attempts to move paralysed limbs
- teach patients how to manage their disability
- teach helpers how to be most useful
- give exercises and advice that encourages recovery
- advise on the most useful aids
- give emotional support.

The nursing interventions identified during the acute period will often be continued during the rehabilitative phase, for example, care of the paralysed limbs must be maintained. Other areas of nursing will include attention to speech difficulties and sensory deficits and preparing the patient for discharge home with adequate support and advice. Involvement of the patient's family in the recovery phase is crucial as their cooperation can result in the increased likelihood of success (see Box 9.11). The use of self-help leaflets and pamphlets from the Chest, Heart and Stroke Association should be considered along with help and support from appropriate community groups.

The patient will have been referred to the local primary health-care team for assessment and support. Once home the patient's ability to live independently can be enhanced by aids such as handrails in the bathroom and adapted cutlery. Advice on re-arranging the patient's furniture at home may facilitate easier mobility and reduce the likelihood of an accident (Johnstone 1987). (See Research Abstract 9.2.)

?	**9.7** How many people in the UK suffer from stroke every year? Have you looked after a stroke patient with severe physical and behavioural problems? If not ask a fellow student to help you with this question. How many different members of the hospital and primary care teams do you think were involved in the patient's care? Consider each team member's role, then try to draw a circle with the patient and his wife in the middle, surrounded by each team member. What might be their feelings about having to meet so many people?

INTRACRANIAL TUMOURS

Brain tumour is the best-known disorder affecting the nervous system and primary brain tumour occurs in only 6 per 100 000. These constitute about 15% of all malignant tumours. The incidence of secondary brain tumour from a primary lesion sited elsewhere in the body is 11 per 100 000. Of patients with a primary malignancy in the breast or bronchus, 25% will develop a secondary brain tumour (Thomas 1983).

Astrocytoma, a malignant tumour, occurs twice as often in males than females and is most common in the 40–60 year age group (Allan 1988). Up to 50% of brain tumours are multiple. Approximately 2250 people die from a brain tumour every year. Causes such as toxoplasma infection, head injury and exposure in the rubber and petrochemical industries have been speculated but no definite cause other than therapeutic irradiation has been established (Thomas 1983).

There are two age peaks for intracranial tumours: the first decade of life and the 50s and 60s. There is a slight male preponderance, except for meningiomas and neurilemmomas (Allan 1988).

Box 9.11 Some do's and don'ts for home carers (adapted from Mulley 1990)

- Do not overprotect him.
- Do encourage him to exercise.
- Do not accuse him of 'not trying'.
- Do not pull his weak arm.
- Do encourage his friends to visit him.
- Do not become gloomy and pessimistic.
- Do think twice before selling the double bed.
- Do continue a normal sex life.

Research Abstract 9.2 Service needs of stroke survivors and their informal carers

In a small pilot study, McLean et al (1991) interviewed 20 stroke survivors and their informal carers to identify their main areas of perceived need for services. The areas identified included: physical care, affective needs, physical health, respite needs, health education and hospital aftercare.

Several areas of unmet need were found, mostly in the areas of personal or emotional advice. Over half of the sample had significant psychological problems.

Some of the carers' needs resulted from their inability to provide adequately for the stroke survivor's basic care. Since informal carers are responsible for much of the care given to the stroke survivor at home, the researchers suggest that it is important that carers receive preparation which will equip them mentally and with the appropriate skills to meet these needs.

The services most appreciated by the carers were those of the community nurse and the home help. Day hospital care and respite care were also greatly valued. Once discharged from hospital, it was the community nurse who organised social service support. However, help was mainly provided by family members since access to services was patchy and respondents often reported feeling 'abandoned' once away from the hospital.

McLean J, Roper-Hall A, Mayer P, Main A 1991 Service needs of stroke survivors and their informal carers: a pilot study. Journal of Advanced Nursing 16(5): 559–564

PATHOPHYSIOLOGY

Intracranial tumours can be classified according to their pathology as outlined in Table 9.4 but the presence of a benign tumour in a crucial location such as a confined space, can prove fatal. Intracranial tumours can grow in one of two ways; they may encapsulate or spread and infiltrate surrounding tissue. Their rate of growth can be very slow or extremely rapid.

The pathological phenomena of tumours are:

- cerebral oedema
- raised ICP
- focal neurological deficits
- seizures
- altered pituitary function
- hydrocephalus.

Common presenting symptoms are extremely variable. Presentation will be determined by the location, type, size and speed of growth of the tumour and its effect on surrounding structures. Symptoms are therefore extremely variable.

McKeran and Thomas (1980) state that neurological symptoms of brain tumours may occur alone or in combination. There may be

Table 9.4 Classification of tumours (Allan 1988)

Tumour	Description	Usual sites	Incidence % of total	Remarks
Tumours of neuro-epithelial tissue				
Astrocytoma Grade 1	Well differentiated, insidiously invasive, relatively benign	Cerebral hemispheres of adults; most commonly the frontal lobes followed by the temporal and parietal sites (Occipital lobe astrocytoma is rare.)	10%	A cystic type of astrocytoma is sometimes located in the cerebellum. A childhood tumour of the first decade of life
Intermediate astrocytoma Grades II & III	Will possess some of the characteristics of Grade 1 astrocytomas but cell differentiation less well defined			
Glioblastoma multiforme (anaplastic astrocytoma) Grade IV	Rapidly growing, undifferentiated cells, extremely malignant, and highly vascular. Infiltrates brain tissue extensively. Peak age is 48–52 years with a male bias. Can produce extensive brain swelling while still relatively small in size	Grade IV shown to spread into the white matter of both hemispheres via the anterior corpus callosum	18%	
Oligodendroglioma	Rare, slow growing tumour, age of onset = 40 years. Relatively benign — minor signs and symptoms can be present for a number of years before diagnosis is confirmed. Shows a marked tendency to calcify. (May be seen on skull X-ray.)	Demonstrates a predilection to grow in close proximity to the ventricular wall and commisural midline structures in the frontal region of the cerebral hemispheres. Can also be found in the temporal lobes	4%	Can 'mimic' a meningioma upon presentation. Unlike many tumours, raised ICP is a late sign in the patient with an oligodendroglioma. Sudden deterioration can occur, thought to be due to spontaneous haemorrhage and cystic degeneration within the tumour body.
Ependymoma	Rare undifferentiated slow growing glioma. Often seen in childhood and young adult	Arises from the ependymal layer of the ventricular system, therefore may be found in any of four lobes	5%	Due to involvement of the CSF pathways hydrocephalus and raised ICP are early common features
Optic nerve glioma	Occurs mainly before the age of 20 years. Follows a relatively benign course, remaining localised to the optic nerve and chiasma	Optic nerve and chiasma	4%	Approximately 60% of patients have an associated neurofibromatosis called a spongioblastoma
Medulloblastoma	Rapidly growing, malignant tumour of childhood. Composed of round, undifferentiated cells. Commonest intracranial neoplasm of childhood. Usually occurs before the age of 10 years	Cerebellar vermis or 4th ventricle roof	3%	Can 'seed' throughout the subarachnoid space. Slight male bias. Hydrocephalus is common
Tumours of nerve sheath cells				
Neurilemma/ Schwannoma	Slow growing, benign tumour. Well encapsulated. Usually unilateral, predilection for females, occurs in the middle years of life	The Schwann cell sheath of cranial nerves VIII, V & VII located within the confined cerebello-pontine angle		A tumour of the sheath of the eighth nerve. Referred to as an acoustic neuroma. Other tumour types may be seen in this location, e.g. meningioma, but a differential diagnosis may not be made till surgery
Neuroma (Neurofibroma)	A complex familial disorder characterised by widespread benign tumours throughout the nervous system. Inherited as an autosomal dominant trait. Known as Recklinghausen's disease. Manifests itself in young adulthood	The neurilemma of nerves, therefore tumours may appear intracranially, i.e. VIIth nerve, acoustic neuroma or extra-cranially, i.e. spinal roots and peripheral nerves	10%	Patient will present with cutaneous pigmentation of the skin termed 'café au lait' spots. Some of these patients will also have a meningioma or glioma as well

(cont'd)

Table 9.4 *(cont'd)*

Tumour	Description	Usual sites	Incidence % of total	Remarks
Tumours of meningeal and related tissues				
Meningioma	Benign, slow growing tumour arising from the arachnoid cells of the arachnoid villi. An irregular single mass usually well encapsulated.	Intracranial venous sinuses — most common, superior sagittal sinus known as a parasagittal meningioma. Other sites include sphenoid ridge convexity of hemispheres and suprasellar region and olfactory groove	15%	Can become very large before signs and symptoms appear. Predilection for females in 40–60 year age group. Do not show any malignant change
Tumours of blood vessel origin				
Haemangio-blastoma	Slow growing, vascular tumour of developmental origin. Single or multiple lesions occur. Manifests in children and young adults, male bias. May be familial	Cerebellar hemisphere	2%	May be associated angiomatosis of the retina or abnormal organs. von Hippel-Lindau disease
Germ cell tumours				
Teratoma	Rare tumour of childhood and young adulthood	Pineal parenchymal cells therefore located around the pineal gland		Terms pinealoma and teratoma are often interchanged
Local extensions from regional tumours				
Chordoma	Soft tumour with a jelly like consistency	Arise extra-durally at the base of the skull		
Metastatic tumours				
Metastatic tumour	Well defined, usually multiple secondary deposits of a primary growth elsewhere in the body. Common primary sites are bronchus and breast	As lesions are often multiple, can occur anywhere in the cerebrum or cerebellum	12%	The symptoms and signs of a secondary intracranial growth may precede those of the original growth
Other malformative tumours				
Craniopharyn-gioma	A tumour of developmental origin, may be cystic or solid. Does not usually present until adolescence. May calcify	Arises from embryological remnants of the cranio-pharyngeal duct (Rathke's pouch) into the suprasellar region and the posterior fossa.	3%	Sometimes referred to as a cholesteatoma
Epidermoid cyst	Congenital fluid-filled cyst of the ectodermal layer. May contain keratin and cholesterol. Occurs in childhood	Posterior fossa		
Dermoid cyst	Similar to epidermoid cyst; arises from the ectodermal layer but contains more solid material such as hair, sebaceous glands or even teeth	Posterior fossa		Difficult to differentiate from other posterior fossa tumours until direct visualisation at surgery
Colloid cyst of the third ventricle	Rounded cystic tumour of childhood	Choroid plexus within the third ventricle		Often presents with an acute, sometimes intermittent hydrocephalus
Vascular malformations				
Angioma	Arterial and/or venous congenital abnormality comprising enlarged and tortuous vessels. Usually have a 'feeder' artery and a 'draining' vein	Anywhere in the cerebral cortex, most commonly in the region of the middle cerebral artery		A unilateral capillary-venous malformation and the presence of a facial naevus is termed the Sturge-Weber syndrome. Hamartomas are small vascular malformations
Angioblastoma	Cystic tumour comprised of angioblasts	Cerebellum		The patient may also exhibit an angioblastoma of the retina

(cont'd)

Table 9.4 *(cont'd)*

Tumour	Description	Usual sites	Incidence % of total	Remarks
Tumour of the anterior pituitary				
Pituitary adenoma	Benign, slow growing, well encapsulated tumour. Classified by the clinical syndrome, i.e. the hormone produced. Three types of hypersecreting adenomas: prolactin secreting (prolactinoma); excess growth hormone (acromegaly); ACTH secreting (Cushing's disease). Hyposecreting tumours are very rare	Anterior lobe of the pituitary gland.	8%	Hyposecreting tumours will produce panhypopituitarism and chiasmal compression

general symptoms, for example, epilepsy, focal symptoms such as hemiparesis or cranial nerve deficits and signs of raised intracranial pressure such as headache (see pp. 331 and p. 339).

MEDICAL MANAGEMENT

Investigation. In non-specialist centres, skull X-ray, EEG and isotope scanning may be performed. These investigations may suggest a lesion but be unable to identify the pathology.

In specialist centres, CT scanning is likely to be the investigation of first choice. Others may include MRI scanning and cerebral angiography. Additional investigations include measuring the ESR and taking a chest X-ray to establish the presence of a primary lesion. If a pituitary tumour is suspected, endocrine studies and visual field testing will be performed. If acoustic neuroma is suspected, audiometric studies will be performed.

Identification of tumour with imaging. Burr hole biopsy, in which a small piece of tissue is removed for pathological examination, may confirm the diagnosis. This technique relies upon the ability of the operator to remove a specimen of tumour tissue which reflects the true extent and pathology of the growth.

Treatment. The usual option is surgery, with or without radiotherapy.

Surgery. The tumour is removed (if possible) using one of four different approaches as outlined in Box 9.5.

Radiotherapy may be indicated for malignant tumours and pituitary tumours, in combination with surgery.

NURSING PRIORITIES AND MANAGEMENT: INTRACRANIAL TUMOURS

Assessment should be made of the patient and his family's understanding of the reason for admission. The doctor may suspect a brain tumour but may wish to perform the investigations to confirm this before telling the patient and his family.

Someone with an intracranial tumour can usually carry out his normal daily activities unless there is a rise in intracranial pressure caused by swelling or by the tumour becoming larger. The onset of symptoms can be slow and progressive or almost immediate, in which case the person's condition deteriorates rapidly.

Immediate priorities

The patient should be assessed for increasing intracranial pressure (see section on Head Injuries), and the nurse should observe for any deterioration in the patient's condition. If this patient has experienced seizures before admission, this should be carefully noted and the nurse should be prepared if a seizure occurs (see p. 353).

If the patient has speech problems, for example, dysphasia, time should be taken to give careful explanations.

Subsequent considerations

After neurological and physical assessment the speech therapist, physiotherapist and occupational therapist should be involved in assessing the patient and offering advice and assistance.

Support during investigations

The patient will be anxious to know the results of investigations but will also be worried about the diagnosis. The investigations can confirm the diagnosis or identify the type of tumour and the patient should be encouraged to discuss his fears and anxieties (Amato 1991). He may be aware of the possibility of neurological deficits or even death. The nurse should be aware of the grieving process and accept the patient's reactions. Some of the fears and anxieties may be unfounded and the nurse may be able to alleviate some of these.

Non-surgical interventions

Medication. Steroids are prescribed once a tumour is diagnosed. The drug of choice is dexamethesone, which helps to reduce swelling around the tumour, decreasing the overall mass of the brain and therefore ICP. The patient can feel better after one day of steroids, finding relief from headache, nausea, vomiting and from the improvement of neurological deficits. However, there are side-effects from steroid medication:

- irritation of the lining of the stomach; antacids are routinely prescribed to counteract this
- glycosuria; urine is routinely tested for glucose and ketones
- adrenal insufficiency, which will occur if medication is withdrawn suddenly.

Radiotherapy. The radiotherapist can assess the patient in the ward or the patient can attend as an out-patient. If the patient requires urgent radiotherapy, this will be discussed by the radiotherapist but the nurse should be available if the patient wants to discuss his feelings about the treatment. See Ch. 32.

Inoperable tumours

A tumour may be inoperable due to inaccessibility or to the type and size. Surgery could involve great risk of neurological deficits post-operatively. This situation offers a great challenge to the nurse: to be able to communicate effectively and offer adequate support (see Chs 32 and 34).

Ongoing care

Major deficits

The patient's condition may be very poor and the doctor may advise the family that his condition will not improve. The nurse should ensure that the relatives are made welcome in the ward at any time of the day or night and reassure them that they are not 'in the way'.

It is important to tell the relatives that the patient is as comfortable as possible and that adequate pain relief is being administered.

Preparation for discharge

The patient may have no neurological deficits or only slight deficits such as limb weakness and may decide to go home and try to continue a normal life.

If the patient has a severe neurological deficit and requires a lot of assistance with the activities of daily living, the situation should be discussed with both patient and family.

If the family is anxious to have the patient at home their wishes should be discussed with the ward team, community nurses and the patient's GP in order to ensure adequate support is available and in place prior to the patient's discharge.

Hospice care should be discussed prior to discharge and if the patient and family wish, further information on this can be obtained by the nurse.

A home visit by the occupational therapist or physiotherapist may be advisable to assess the patient's requirements when he is at home.

EPILEPSY

Epilepsy can be a symptom, for example, of head injury, or a disorder with no identifiable cause. 5% of the population will have a seizure in their lifetime, but with recurrence in only 0.5% (Lindsay et al 1991). Box 9.12 shows causes at different stages of life.

Epileptic seizures can occur at any age, although the age of onset can provide a clue as to the cause, e.g. in childhood it can be due to pyrexia whereas in the middle years of life, a brain tumour is more likely (Hickey 1992). The occurrence of an isolated seizure does not mean that that person is 'epileptic'.

PATHOPHYSIOLOGY

An intermittent, uncontrolled discharge of neurones within the central nervous system results in a seizure. It can range from a major motor convulsion to a brief period of lack of awareness and can occur in any individual at any time, even in an apparently healthy nervous system. Each individual is susceptible to seizure if a threshold level, which is different for everyone, is breached. In some instances the cause is obvious, for example, a seizure can be secondary to structural damage to the brain; in others no apparent cause can be detected and it is described as an 'idiopathic' or 'primary' seizure.

Common presenting symptoms depend on when the person is examined. During certain types of seizure the patient may be unconscious, apnoeic and incontinent of urine whilst in others, changes are barely noticeable. Between seizures the patient may show no neurological impairment or deficit. Seizures are classified as outlined in Box 9.13.

MEDICAL MANAGEMENT

Investigations. Electroencephalography (EEG) will be carried out. Other investigations such as CT scanning and magnetic resonance imaging may also be considered to identify possible causes.

The most reliable diagnostic tool is a reliable eye-witness account of the seizure.

Treatment. The mainstay of therapy is medication, which is effective in keeping many people free from seizures. Anti-epileptic drugs such as phenytoin sodium and sodium valproate are given.

A small number of patients who have an identifiable focus which is amenable to surgery may be offered this option. The most commonly employed technique is temporal or other cortical area resection. Over half of the patients treated become free from seizure or acquire easier control.

NURSING PRIORITIES AND MANAGEMENT: EPILEPTIC SEIZURES

Many individuals with seizures are managed at home with regular monitoring by their GP or at an epilepsy outpatients' clinic. However, occasionally treatment is no longer effective and the patient requires to be admitted to hospital for re-assessment.

Immediate priorities

Once notification is received at the ward that a patient is to

Box 9.12 Causes of epilepsy at different stages of life

Newborn
Hypocalcaemia
Hypoglycaemia
Asphyxia
Hyperbilirubinaemia
Water intoxication
Inborn errors of metabolism
Trauma
Intracranial haemorrhage
(Vit. K deficiency, thrombocytopaenia, etc.)

Infancy
Febrile convulsions
Inborn errors of metabolism
Congenital defects
CNS infection

Childhood
Trauma
Congenital defects
Arterio-venous malformation
CNS infection

Adolescence and adulthood
Trauma
Neoplasm
Withdrawal from drugs or alcohol
Arterio-venous malformation
CNS infection

Late adult
Trauma
Neoplasm
Drug/alcohol withdrawal
Vascular disease
Degenerative disease
CNS infection

be admitted due to a worsening of his seizures, the following essential equipment should be assembled and be readily available.

- oxygen and suction in good working order
- a selection of various sizes of artificial airways
- charts for recording neurological status, vital signs and seizures
- bedside rails should be in place (may be padded for additional safety)
- supplies of anticonvulsant medication, particularly in the intravenous or intramuscular form.

If the patient is having a seizure the following actions must always be carried out:

- use suction if necessary to prevent aspiration of secretions
- ensure privacy is provided for the patient
- ensure bedside rails are in place, using pillows as padding if required
- if the patient is on the floor, ensure safety by removing any objects or furniture likely to cause harm
- loosen any restrictive clothing
- insert an airway only when teeth have unclenched (after the tonic stage); any attempts to insert objects into the patient's mouth prior to this serve no purpose and may endanger the nurse (bitten fingers) or the patient (broken teeth)
- record pupillary activity: pupils will begin to react as the patient recovers.

Immediately following a seizure the nurse should:

- turn the patient on his side to facilitate the drainage of secretions
- allow the patient to sleep
- allow time for the patient to waken and provide reassurance and assistance to encourage reorientation
- record a description of what happened on the seizure observation chart.

The nurse's record should include a note of:

- the time at which the seizure occurred
- what the patient was doing at the time
- any aura or crying out prior to the seizure
- any loss of consciousness
- which parts of the body were affected
- any stiffening or jerky movements and the length of each phase
- any urinary or bowel incontinence
- the length of the recovery period
- the patient's behaviour after the seizure
- any weakness in part of the limbs.

The doctor should be informed about the seizure and any prescribed anticonvulsant medication should be administered.

Further considerations

The patient should be allowed to express his feelings and fears and he and his family should be given adequate explanations and support. Explanation about the medication prescribed will encourage compliance by the patient. Side-effects should be discussed. Blood-level monitoring of drug serum levels will be carried out and it should be explained to the patient that this test will show if there is an adequate or inadequate dosage of the drug. It will also indicate if the blood levels are too high. If too high, the patient may be experiencing side-effects of the drugs and if too low, it will indicate that seizures will occur again. Common side-effects of anticonvulsant drugs are:

- drowsiness
- dizziness
- gastric upset
- diplopia
- ataxia.

The patient should be allowed time to come to terms with the diagnosis of epilepsy. He may experience feelings of anger and grief.

> ? **9.8** What information does your local library have about self-help groups for people with epilepsy?

The nurse should discuss with both the patient and his family the social implications of epilepsy and encourage a positive outlook.

The patient should be told that he may experience an aura (see Box 9.13) prior to a seizure and that it may be advisable to use the time available to ensure his personal safety.

It is important for the patient to recognise certain 'triggers' that may induce a seizure, such as:

- lack of food and sleep
- excessive heat
- constipation
- menstruation
- alcohol
- anxiety or stress.

Medical opinion varies as to whether someone with epilepsy should drink alcohol, as it can interfere with anti-epileptic drugs, preventing them from reaching the levels that control seizures. Large amounts of any liquid can trigger a seizure; heavy drinking is often associated with late night, irregular eating habits and forgotten tablets (Epilepsy Association of Scotland, (undated)). This is an individual decision, bearing in mind medical advice on the particular case.

It may be suggested to the patient that he consider carrying a card or wearing a Medic-alert to inform strangers about his condition, if a seizure occurs.

Advice should be given prior to discharge about safety in the home (see Box 9.14) and the patient should be made aware that an occupational therapist can be invited to become involved, especially if the patient is elderly or lives alone.

Employment

The patient's employment situation should be discussed, especially if it entails driving or operating machinery. The patient must be told that he is required to inform the DVLC of his liability to have seizures and should be advised to stop driving, meantime (Scambler 1989). This may present major problems to the patient, as he may have to look for alternative employment, and will not help the patient's self-esteem or his outlook for the future.

> ? **9.9** Discuss with your fellow students what may be some of the social implications of epilepsy. (See Box 9.15, p. 357.) Try to find out whether someone with epilepsy is permitted to drive a car.

The patient must realise that some employers may not be prepared to employ someone with epilepsy and that his current position may have to be reviewed. Epilepsy is common in adolescents and it may be necessary to warn them that they may experience a change in outlook for the future or that they may have to consider a change to their career structure.

Physical activity

The patient should be encouraged to continue normal physical

Box 9.13 Classification of seizures

PARTIAL SEIZURES

Focal seizure
Localised twitching, usually of the face and hands. Consciousness is maintained and the duration is brief.

Jacksonian seizure
As for focal seizure, except that the seizure activity spreads to affect other parts of the body, for example, twitching of the finger may spread to involve the hand, arm and side of face.

Psychomotor seizure
The origin is usually the temporal lobe and these seizures are characterised by subjective symptoms, for example, the patient may experience hallucinations prior to its onset. The patient will exhibit altered behaviour for which he is amnesic, followed by a period of automatism. Consciousness may be lost and the seizure may last 1–4 minutes.

GENERALISED SEIZURES

Absence seizure
Affects children. There is a brief lapse of consciousness lasting 5–10 seconds following which the child will continue what he was doing prior to the attack. Can easily go undetected. During the attack the child will appear blank and the eyes become vacant. Can occur repeatedly in one day.

Tonic–clonic seizure
Has several stages which are characteristic of this type of seizure.
Aura. A warning of the impending seizure. May be a smell or other feeling which the patient can learn to recognise. Not all patients experience an aura.
Tonic phase. Loss of consciousness occurs, with stiffening of the body's limbs. If the patient is standing he will fall to the ground and may bite his tongue. The muscular contraction will expel air via the vocal cords thus a shrill cry may be heard. Both bladder and bowels may empty. The patient will become apnoeic and cyanosed for a period of 15–30 seconds. During this period the patient is unresponsive.
Clonic seizure. The phase of stiffness passes to give way to clonus in which there is a violent rhythmical jerking of the limbs, accompanied by hyperventilation and the production of excess saliva. The pulse is rapid and the patient is sweating profusely. This phase can last for several minutes.
Coma. Once the clonic phase subsides the patient will lapse into coma, and be difficult to rouse. This can last for 1 hour or longer. If the patient wakens at this stage he may complain of headache and tiredness and will appear confused.

Tonic seizure
This is the tonic phase as described in the tonic–clonic seizure above. Usually occurs in children.

Clonic seizure
This is the clonic phase as described in the tonic–clonic seizure above.

Myoclonic seizure
Characterised by sudden jerky movements, usually of the limbs, accompanied by a brief lapse of consciousness. Usually occur in clusters and following these the patient can become confused.

Atonic seizure
Characterised by sudden loss of postural tone with alterations of consciousness.

Akinetic seizure
Characterised by sudden loss of postural muscle tone sometimes called 'drop attacks'.

Box 9.14 Safety measures at home

- Fireguards are essential, and should be securely fixed to the wall.
- Smokers should consider the dangers of smoking in an armchair or in bed.
- Cordless kettles and irons are safer than trailing flexes.
- Pot handles should point to the back of the cooker. Hot food or liquid should not be carried.
- Sharp corners can be covered by rounded plastic pieces, available from supermarkets, children's departments and ironmongers.
- Glass doors should either use safety glass or be covered in safety film, available from children's departments, etc.
- If seizures are frequent and unpredictable, the patient should let someone know when he is taking a bath or shower. The water should not be very hot and the depth should only be a few inches. The patient should turn the taps off before getting in. A shower is more suitable, particularly if the patient can sit, unless it has a high lip where water can gather.
- If the toilet door can be hung to open outwards, the person won't block it if he falls. Locks should not be used, except for special safety locks that can be opened in an emergency. An 'engaged' sign can be used, instead.
- Soft pillows can be dangerous. It is best to avoid pillows or to obtain special safety pillows.
- In a small proportion of people with epilepsy, a seizure may be triggered by flickering light. These people should place the television set at eye level, at least 3 metres away, with a small, lit lamp on top.
- An epileptic parent should ensure that garden gates have locks to prevent children from wandering off during a seizure.

activities, with some emphasis being placed on the need to take adequate precautions, for example, when swimming. It should be suggested that the patient lets someone know or takes a friend who can deal with a seizure when he is considering some physical activity. Some activities, such as hill-walking, should be avoided, as these can easily endanger the patient.

Involving the patient's family

The patient's family should be given time and the opportunity to express their fears and worries and the nurse should be prepared to provide advice and explanations when necessary. The nurse should explain about the type of seizure the patient is experiencing, for example, a generalised seizure. They should be told what to expect if a seizure occurs, for example, that the patient will have sudden uncontrolled movements and will appear to be holding his breath. They should know exactly what to do and why they are doing it. The Epilepsy Association issues helpful Fact Sheets, for example, helping lay people, including those with epilepsy, to understand more about the condition (see Useful Addresses). Advice should include the following:

- Ensuring the safety of the patient, which can involve removing harmful objects and ensuring that all restrictive clothing is loosened.
- After the seizure the patient should be placed on his side

and allowed to sleep. He should be given adequate time to waken up and re-orientate himself.

- The family should know that they should seek medical advice if a seizure lasts longer than usual or if seizures continue without time for the patient to recover.
- The family should be aware that the patient may have feelings of shock, anger, lack of self-esteem and should allow time for him to come to terms with these feelings.

The Royal College of Midwives, in conjunction with the Epilepsy Association of Scotland, have published *Guidelines for Women with Epilepsy* (see Useful Addresses) to help women and their husbands or partners to understand the precautions to be taken when pregnant or when looking after their children.

The ward team should work together to give the patient and his family encouragement and advice about being at home. As one person in every 200 has epilepsy, so they can recognise that they are not alone. Involvement in groups for people with epilepsy provides advice and support.

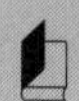
For further information, see Chadwick & Usiskin (1987).

Box 9.15 A teenager's viewpoint

I am 18 years old and in my last year at school. My friends are all making plans to go to college in the autumn and for most it will mean leaving home for the first time. I have had epilepsy since the age of 7 and my parents have always accompanied me everywhere. Even now, I am not allowed to go to the shops on my own in case something happens.

Since having my treatment reviewed 2 years ago, my attacks are under much better control and I cannot understand why I am not allowed more freedom. They do not seem to have noticed the improvement or my age.

My friends ask me what I plan to do when I finish school and I have told them that I want to go away to college. I know that I will have to discuss this with my parents, who will be upset and angry when they find out. They will think of all sorts of reasons why I cannot go and I know they worry about me but feel they don't think about what I want for myself. How can I convince them to let me go?

MULTIPLE SCLEROSIS (DISSEMINATED SCLEROSIS)

The occurrence of multiple sclerosis is not consistent in different parts of the world. Its incidence in the Orkney and Shetland islands of Britain is 128 per 100 000 whereas in South Australia, it is 7 per 100 000. It is therefore described as a disorder of temperate climates. Those who move from an area of high risk to low do not lessen the chance of the disease occurring. Multiple sclerosis is not hereditary but the risk of a child developing multiple sclerosis where the parent is afflicted is approximately 15 times greater than in the unaffected population (Lindsay et al 1991).

The age of onset is 20–50 years, and it is slightly more common in females. The cause is unknown and the disorder typically follows a pattern of relapses and remissions (Lindsay et al 1991). (See Research Abstract 9.3.)

Definitive diagnosis is usually very difficult because demyelination develops over a varying period of time. To be conclusive, there must be dissemination over a period of time and in several locations within the nervous system. In Stubbs (1992) a nurse suffering from multiple sclerosis describes her vague, but often frightening symptoms and their almost random occurrence, and how it took 11 years for her own suspicions that she had the disease to be confirmed by a neurologist.

Research Abstract 9.3

French researchers have detected autoantibodies to an endogenous protein in CSF, which may be a useful criterion for the diagnosis of multiple sclerosis. Out of 51 patients with multiple sclerosis, 47 of them tested positively for autoantibodies in their CSF compared with only 30 out of 188 patients with other neurological disorders. The researchers concluded that with a specificity of 85% and a sensitivity of 93.5% this test was as accurate as magnetic resonance imaging.

Zanetta J P et al 1990 Antibodies to cerebellar soluble lecithin (CSL) in multiple sclerosis. Lancet 335(8704): 1482

PATHOPHYSIOLOGY

Sporadic demyelination (destruction of the myelin sheath) occurs and 'plaques' may be seen on the myelin at one or more locations.

Common presenting symptoms. Clinical features vary considerably, depending on which nerves are affected, but may include:

- blurring of vision or double vision
- weakness and dragging of limbs and extreme fatigue
- slurred speech
- nystagmus
- loss of sensation in a specific area of the body, for example, part of the arm
- difficulty in determining the position of limbs in space
- 'stiff limbs'
- intention tremor
- clumsiness/difficulty with movement
- incontinence/retention of urine.

MEDICAL MANAGEMENT

Investigations

Lumbar puncture. Examination of the CSF may reveal:

- a mild rise in cell count
- an elevated total protein and gamma globulin fraction (in 60% of cases)
- oligoclonal bands in the gamma globulin in 80% of cases.

Visual evoked responses. A delay in conduction is noted in the pathways.

Magnetic resonance imaging identifies areas of demyelination.

Computed tomographic scan to exclude other disorders. (See 'Tests and Investigations'.)

Treatment. There is no specific treatment. Steroid therapy may be helpful in acute exacerbations and physiotherapy is helpful to the rehabilitation of numb limbs. Many complementary therapies exist with varying degrees of success, for example, special diets and hyperbaric oxygen (Engel 1989).

Essentially, care consists of supporting the patient and his family and alleviating the symptoms.

NURSING PRIORITIES AND MANAGEMENT: MULTIPLE SCLEROSIS

The extensive tests involved in obtaining a diagnosis may necessitate admission to hospital.

Box 9.16 A carer's view

"It's the 'not knowing' what I'll be like tomorrow that I find so difficult to cope with," was the heartfelt cry of one MS sufferer. Caught up in the turmoil of wanting desperately to make plans for the following day, she was weary of the continual conflict between her desire to be independent, and her body's limitations. The uncertainty and unpredictability of MS makes it particularly wearing, and difficult to come to terms with. As both a nurse and the relative of an MS sufferer, it would appear to me that coping with frustration becomes a major part of everyday life:

- frustration at having to rely heavily on family and friends
- frustration at loss of bodily function
- frustration at some members of society who don't seem to understand
- frustration at feeling a burden.

Coming to terms with limitations is only one aspect of living with MS; making the most of life within the confines of such restrictions is another. When caring for someone with MS, whether in hospital or in the community, the most important part we can play is in helping the patient to maintain his or her integrity and adapt to changes imposed by further degeneration.

Many patients with multiple sclerosis lead a normal lifestyle at home, requiring admission to hospital only if they are experiencing a deterioration in their condition. Many have made adjustments to their home and lifestyle in order to lead as independent a life as possible.

For the patient who is experiencing difficulties, hospitalisation will not only provide an opportunity for nursing and other health care staff to help the patient and his family to deal with problems that are disrupting the patient's daily life but often enable the nurse to learn more from the patient about the experience of living with multiple sclerosis. (See Box 9.16.)

Immediate priorities

Communicating

The patient admitted for investigations is likely to be fearful and will require adequate explanation about the tests and examinations to be carried out. Frequently, the nurse is asked about these tests and she should be prepared to answer questions or, if unable to do so, should try to find the answer for the patient. It is important that she is aware of the patient's knowledge regarding his condition, as the patient will either fear the worst, often with only a partial understanding of what the diagnosis may be, or may not be aware of the possibility of having multiple sclerosis until the diagnosis is confirmed.

It is advisable for the nurse to be present when the doctor is speaking to the patient as this allows the nurse to know what information the patient has received. Often the patient wishes to discuss certain points and will find it re-assuring to speak to the nurse when the doctor has left.

The patient will require time to consider his condition and what effects it will have on his outlook for the future. Patients often experience the range of feelings and emotions related to the loss of self-esteem and body image and may worry about how the condition will eventually affect them. Expressed feelings may include shock, denial, depression and anger (Purchese & Allan 1984). The nurse requires to accept these feelings and provide adequate support to facilitate coping mechanisms.

The patient's family must also be included and will require explanations about their relative's condition. They should be provided with opportunities to discuss their feelings and fears.

A deterioration in the patient's physical condition can cause major psychological and social problems. Carers may experience difficulties in coping and may require help and advice.

Admission to hospital can cause considerable stress, especially for the patient who has a set routine at home that allows him to maintain his independence. The nurse should encourage the patient to maintain his independence and to follow his daily routine as far as possible when in hospital. People often have well-developed coping mechanisms and if nurses think they know best it can cause the patient frustration and anger. They can then seem difficult to look after and a vicious circle develops, where the patient dreads even more having to come into hospital.

Subsequent considerations

Problems with communication

Communication impairments in the patient with multiple sclerosis can include difficulties in pronouncing words, slow, slurred speech and poor concentration. This can create major problems with everyday communication for the patient. People do not understand that, although the person has speech problems, his intellectual capabilities are not affected and their reactions towards the patient may cause him to lose confidence in his ability to communicate.

The speech therapist should be involved in the patient's care as she can give advice on how to improve the patient's ability to express himself. Useful techniques to help the patient communicate are to:

- ensure that an erect posture is maintained as this aids breathing and assists with speech
- reduce background noise as much as possible
- encourage the patient to express the most important points at the beginning of a sentence, when energy and concentration are greatest
- use communication aids such as picture boards or computer boards.

Maintaining a safe environment

The patient with multiple sclerosis can experience difficulties with:

- movement, for example, ataxia, unintentional tremors or paralysis
- vision, for example, diplopia
- sensory disturbance, for example, detection of pain and temperature.

Account needs to be taken of the patient's immediate environment both at home and in hospital in order to avoid accidents.

The patient may already be aware of the potential dangers at home and may take care to avoid them, or may be experiencing a deterioration in his condition and realise that adaptations are required in order to maintain safety.

Some patients may be unable to accept that their condition is deteriorating and that they are not able to perform certain tasks safely. When in hospital, an accurate assessment of the patient's condition, his level of understanding and, if necessary, of his home conditions should be made. This will involve assessments by the community nurse, occupational therapist and physiotherapist.

In hospital, the nurse should involve the patient in making any necessary changes to his new surroundings, as he will know best what suits him, for example, the location and height of the bed, depending on his ability to mobilise. Ensure adequate space to manoeuvre a wheelchair properly. The nurse-call system should be within easy reach and the patient should be instructed on its use. The patient with clumsiness of movement or tremor may require assistance with some activities, for example, at meal times, when there is a risk of spilling liquid and food, possibly risking a burn.

Mobility

Maintaining independence and mobility plays a large part in being independent. A problem for the patient with multiple sclerosis is the uncertainty of the rate at which deterioration in mobility will occur. The patient's family should be aware of any limitations that are necessary and also encourage the proper use of any mobility aids required when at home.

The attitude of the ward team is very important; the members should work together to encourage a positive outlook for the patient while making time to understand his and the family's feelings and fears.

If the patient uses mobility aids at home, they should also be used when he is admitted to hospital. This enables the patient to maintain independence and also allows the physiotherapist to assess the effectiveness of any aids. For example, if the patient's mobility is deteriorating, is a walking stick sufficient to maintain safety? Common problems may include ataxia, limb weakness and lack of co-ordination. Techniques which may be useful to help these problems are:

- maintain a good posture
- when walking, make contact with the ground with the heel of the foot first
- take care to place feet firmly in the direction of travel
- look straight ahead rather than down at the ground
- relax and try not to feel self-conscious.

The physiotherapist may suggest exercises to maintain the function of a limb and to prevent muscle wastage. The nurse and the patient's family can give encouragement for the exercises to be practised.

Skin care

The patient and his family should be taught the importance of regular skin inspection, for example to observe the sacrum and heels closely and to look for redness or blanching of the skin. If this occurs the patient should be aware of the importane of relieving the pressure from the problem area, for example, by lying on his side in bed.

Using a wheelchair. The physiotherapist and occupational therapist may advise that the patient requires a wheelchair in order to maintain mobility. It can be very distressing for the patient to realise that he has reached such a stage. It must be emphasised that this does not mean that the patient becomes totally reliant on the wheelchair and is unable to maintain his independence. He may require to use the wheelchair outside the house only if required to walk a long distance, or around the house only when he is feeling tired.

The patient may have become unable to stand and be able to weight-bear for short periods only. In this instance, the patient is dependent on the wheelchair for mobilising but he should be encouraged to continue to perform tasks involving his hands, for example, shaving and washing, in order to maintain a degree of independence.

If the patient requires physiotherapy when at home, advice and support can be obtained from the community physiotherapist. Some local multiple sclerosis societies also offer a physiotherapy service.

Advice should be given to the patient about when to use the wheelchair, what in particular, to look for, and why:

- the wheelchair should be used only when necessary, so that the patient utilises any residual walking ability thus helping to prevent muscle weakness
- the importance of relieving pressure, especially on the sacral area, should be discussed, as the immobile patient may lie or sit in the same position for a period of time
- careful positioning of limbs should be ensured, taking into account any weakness or paraesthesia
- the footrest on the wheelchair should always be used; care should also be taken that no part of the foot or ankle is rubbing against the footrest or wheel
- the legs should be placed in proper alignment and the patient should check regularly that the limbs are safely in position on the footrest.

Balance of rest and exercise. The patient should be advised about the importance of rest periods to avoid becoming overtired or overstressed, which will exacerbate the condition. Relaxation techniques and a specific rest/exercise programme may be beneficial for the patient and should be discussed with him and his family.

Fatigue is a symptom of multiple sclerosis and can enforce changes to the patient's existing lifestyle. The patient may have to learn to ask for help when feeling very tired and this can be difficult for someone who normally leads an active, independent life.

Although rest is very important for the patient with multiple sclerosis, exercise is also vital to maintain muscle strength and help reduce spasticity. It will also improve circulation and prevent pressure sores and joint stiffness. These will contribute to maintaining the patient's independence.

Employment. If the patient's current employment involves a lot of physical exertion then this may prove problematical with regard to returning to work. He may have to consider how his disorder will affect current employment and think about finding alternative work, although in many cases this may prove impossible. Stubbs (1992) gives a sensitive account of her sheer determination to stay at work and fulfil normal duties, driving herself to overwork and severe exacerbation, with resulting numbness and inability to walk.

Eliminating

The patient may experience incontinence, urinary frequency or urine retention, and problems with constipation. The urinary problems are due to the reflex action of the bladder having been disturbed due to damage to the nerve pathways in the lower spine.

The social implications of incontinence can be enormous and some patients will avoid going out for fear of embarrassment (see Ch. 24). The patient should be encouraged to take his time when passing urine and to ensure that the bladder is completely empty. Journeys can be planned to take account of the availability of toilets and this will reassure the patient. If a urine infection is suspected a specimen should be sent to bacteriology for culture and sensitivity.

The patient may find it necessary and useful to use aids such as protective pants and pads (see Ch. 24).

Urinary catheterisation may be required if the patient experiences persistent urinary retention. Some patients will prefer self-catheterisation at set intervals and many become very competent at performing this procedure. Adequate instruction on hygienic technique can facilitate this (see Ch. 8). Advice from a continence advisor may also be useful.

Some patients will require an indwelling catheter, and support should be provided to enable the patient to come to terms with this alteration to her body image. The community nurse can provide support at home.

The importance of an adequate fluid intake of 2–2.5 litres

per day should be stressed. Many patients mistakenly think that if they stop drinking they will no longer be incontinent.

The immobile patient will be especially prone to constipation, which will aggravate co-existing urinary problems. The patient and his family should be taught how constipation can be avoided by means of an appropriate diet, an adequate fluid intake and by maintaining mobility. Regular aperients may be required and the occasional use of enemas and suppositories may be indicated.

Expressing sexuality

The patient may experience a change in body image, and the nurse should try to encourage a positive attitude in order to improve the patient's self esteem.

Sexual counselling may be beneficial for both partners. Men may experience impotence due to neurological damage and female sufferers may experience diminished libido. The patient may be too embarrassed or worried to discuss such difficulties with a nurse or doctor and external counselling services such as SPOD (Sexual Problems of the Disabled) and Marriage Guidance services may be a good alternative.

?	**9.10** Find out where the Marriage Guidance and SPOD counselling services are in your area.

Advice on contraception may be required, especially by women, as some oral contraceptives may interfere with existing medication. Pregnancy should be avoided during active stages of the disease as this may exacerbate the symptoms, although successful pregnancy is not completely ruled out.

Eating and drinking

There has been considerable research into the link between diet and multiple sclerosis and a number of specialised diets have been identified for example, Swank & Dugan (1990). It has been shown that people with multiple sclerosis have higher levels of saturated fats and lower levels of polyunsaturated fats in the myelin sheath and the dietary advice outlined below may be useful to patients. They should

- decrease the intake of saturated fats and increase unsaturated fats
- try to include more chicken and white fish in the diet
- when cooking red meat, ensure that visible fat is trimmed off prior to cooking
- note that liver contains vitamin B12 and arachidonic acid, an essential fatty acid (see Ch. 21)
- use semi-skimmed or skimmed milk
- ensure a high-fibre content, that is wholemeal and wheaten bread, pulses and cereals and should eat plenty of fruit and fresh vegetables.

The speech therapist and dietitian may be able to offer assistance and advice if the patient has swallowing difficulties. The nurse can assist by encouraging the patient to

- sit up straight with the head supported, if necessary
- eat in a quiet, relaxed atmosphere and not to speak when eating
- to avoid choking, encourage the patient to take his time when eating
- eat certain types of food that are easier to swallow, for example, semi-solid or liquidised foods.

Personal cleansing and dressing

In hospital and at home the patient should be encouraged to maintain his independence with regard to washing and dressing himself. It may seem to the patient and at times to the nurse or to the patient's family that it would be quicker and easier for the nurse to do these activities for the patient. The patient may feel under stress to hurry in order to release the nurse to go and attend to other patients. The nurse should explain that there is no hurry to have everything finished for a set time.

?	**9.11** Many people with multiple sclerosis develop particular patterns of behaviour over the years. Have you, or any of your fellow students observed this in such patients, either at home or in hospital? If so, can you describe them? How did you adapt your work to fit in with these routines?

The carer should be encouraged to allow the patient to perform these activities at home to allow the patient to have some degree of independence. The occupational therapist can assess the patient when in hospital and give advice regarding washing and dressing. She can offer a range of dressing aids and suggest specially adapted clothing, for example, with Velcro instead of buttons and zips. The patient can be referred to the community occupational therapist if further difficulties are expected to arise in the future due to the possible deterioration in the patient's condition.

Patient education

The patient and his family should be as well informed as possible about the diagnosis of multiple sclerosis. They should be aware of the most successful methods of maintaining independence. They should know their primary care team and know that they can increasingly call on the community services, for example, the community nurse, physiotherapist or general practitioner, as the patient's condition worsens.

The patient and his family should be aware of the possibility of the occurrence of behaviour and mood changes, to help them cope with these problems and understand the patient's behaviour. Euphoria, depression, apathy and emotional lability are common. See Research Abstract 9.4.

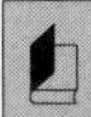

For a study of the impact of multiple sclerosis on caregivers, see Dewis & Niskala (1992).

Preparation for discharge

Episodic hospitalisation may become necessary as the multiple sclerosis condition becomes more widespread, and the patient and his family should be given the opportunity to voice any worries or fears to allow adequate preparation for discharge. A comprehensive assessment of the patient's home situation should be performed if possible, well before there is any mobility problem and should involve all members of the multidisciplinary team in order to gauge the suitability and likely success of discharge.

In cases where there is decreasing ability to perform the Activities of Daily Living, a home visit for the patient involving the nurse, occupational therapist and physiotherapist may be indicated. Assessment of the patient's home situation, layout and the patient's ability to adapt maintaining safety and independence can be carried out. Some adjustments may be required in the house, for example, bath aids, re-arrangement of furniture. If the patient depends on a wheelchair for mobility, the doorways may have to be widened, cupboards may have to be lowered, and a shower may be required instead of a bath.

The patient may have to be rehoused to be at ground floor level in order to accommodate access to and from the house

Research Abstract 9.4

Twenty multiple sclerosis patients admitted to hospital for treatment of exacerbation of their disease were asked to identify stressors and the coping mechanisms they employed to deal with stressors. They completed the MS Stressor Scale (a 20-item Likert-type scale) and the Jalowiec Coping Scale (60-item Likert-type scale). Disability level was measured using the Barthel Index. Results showed an overall mean stress score of 1.49 on a scale of 1 to 3.

The most stressful items identified were:

- feeling tired
- inability to walk
- uncertainty about the future.

The most prevalent coping theme used was self-reliance and the most prevalent individual coping responses were a sense of humour and trying to learn more. A positive correlation was found between uncertainty about the future and fatalistic coping, and a negative correlation between depression and optimistic coping. No relationship was found between degree of disability and stressors.

Buelow J M 1991 A correlation study of disabilities, stressors and coping methods in victims of multiple sclerosis. Journal of Neuroscientific Nursing 23(4): 247–252

in a wheelchair. This involves major changes not only for the patient but also the family.

Advice regarding income and benefits available, for example, mobility and attendance allowance, can be given by the social worker. Outpatient appointments can be arranged for physiotherapy, occupational or speech therapy, if necessary.

Some doctors advocate discussing the possibility of relapse so that the patient is better prepared when it occurs. On the other hand, some patients may not have a period of relapse for up to 20 years and may worry unnecessarily.

Some patients may benefit from being informed of the availability of support groups. It may even be possible for the patient to be seen by a member of the support group prior to discharge. They offer a range of services, including general advice, physiotherapy, counselling.

PARKINSON'S DISEASE (PARALYSIS AGITANS)

Chronic neurological disorders typically run an unremitting course often resulting in premature death. Parkinson's disease is not usually seen prior to the age of 50 years, affects both sexes and afflicts one individual in every 1000. It is a chronic degenerative disorder of the basal ganglia, with a slow onset that progresses gradually (Lindsay et al 1991). A disorder indistinguishable from Parkinson's disease is now emerging in some drug abusers. Some 'designer' drugs contain a substance called MPTP (1-methyl-4-phenyl-1,2,3,6, tetrahydrapyridine) which, when injected into animals, has resulted in typical Parkinsonian features. It is thought that this breakthrough may lead to further developments in the treatment of this disorder (Lindsay et al 1991).

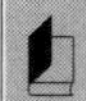

For further information on the causes of Parkinson's disease, see Cole (1988).

PATHOPHYSIOLOGY

The Parkinsonian patient is known to have a decreased level of dopamine in the basal ganglia. This is a neurotransmitter essential for the control of movement, coordination and posture. Several causes have been identified, including drug-induced Parkinsonism with, for example, the use of phenothiazines. Another unusual cause was an outbreak of encephalitis lethargica in 1916–28 and those afflicted, now 75–90 years old, developed Parkinson's disease. No new such outbreaks have occurred (Allan 1988).

Common presenting symptoms. The clinical features may include:

- a triad of symptoms; tremor, rigidity and dyskinesia
- muscle rigidity
- tremor
- a mask-like face
- disturbance in free-flowing movement
- loss of postural reflexes
- autonomic manifestations, for example, excessive perspiration
- general weakness and increased fatigue.

MEDICAL MANAGEMENT

Investigations. Investigations such as CT scanning may be considered to eliminate other disorders. There is no specific diagnostic test for Parkinson's disease. Diagnosis is usually based on clinical presentation.

Treatment. Treatment is limited. Apart from dealing with the problems symptomatically as they arise, dopaminergic preparations such as levodopa are administered to replace the depleted dopamine. Alternatively, dopamine agonist, for example, bromocriptine, are given to stimulate the surviving dopamine receptors in the basal ganglia. Anticholinergic agents such as benzhexol may be considered to treat the cramps, tremor and rigidity associated with parkinsonism. All of these medications need to be carefully titrated to gain maximum benefit for the patient. They can also have major side effects, usually necessitating admission to hospital. Another curious aspect is an 'on-off' phenomenon, whereby, at certain times of the day the patient loses the benefit of the dopamine and becomes rigid and immobile for a period of time. It is important to recognise this as alteration to the drug regimen can reduce the likelihood of this happening.

NURSING PRIORITIES AND MANAGEMENT: PARKINSON'S DISEASE

Parkinson's disease has an insidious onset. Some of its effects may be attributed by the patient and his family to old age. The progressive nature of the disease combined with the potential embarrassment of many of its symptoms can result in a patient who is aware of what is happening but at a loss as to how to obtain help (see Box 9.17).

The importance of the role taken by the patient's family cannot be overstressed. Their ability to cope with the mobility and other problems associated with Parkinson's disease can make the difference between a level of independence, with the patient living in his own home, and enforced, frequent hospitalisation or long-term care with total dependence on others for everything. Mobility aids may be of limited use.

Immediate priorities

Typically, many of the early symptoms of Parkinson's disease may be treated by the family doctor with the patient and his family making necessary adjustments to their home, for example, removal of rugs and other obstacles over which the patient may trip.

As the patient's condition worsens, admission to hospital becomes necessary in order to confirm the diagnosis and establish the patient's medication regimen where appropriate. Hospitalisation will also provide an opportunity for nursing and other health-care staff such as the physiotherapist, speech therapist and occupational therapist, to advise the patient

Box 9.17

We are 7 years into living with Father's Parkinson's disease. There have been so many challenges for him and for us over the years, and the challenges keep changing as the disease progresses. Here are just three of them.

- *'They didn't know him as he was.'* With each new admission to care, we are having to work harder to make sure that staff understand that the painfully slow speech from an expressionless face still conveys humour, awareness of world events, kindness and insight.
- *'Food goes everywhere, from face to shoelaces.'* It is hard to accept that it is probably now right to use that large bib at mealtimes. It lets him enjoy his meals independently and keeps his clothes clean, which matters a lot to him . . . but I still don't like it.
- *'He's changing.'* We knew it would happen, but it's been a shock to watch the first signs of mental change. It is painful to listen patiently to his attempts to sort out delusion from reality.

and his family on how to deal with the problems which are interfering with the patient's daily life.

Once stabilised, and if the home circumstances permit, the patient is discharged. Re-admission to hospital will only become necessary should further problems arise, such as worsening of symptoms. The stabilised patient is nursed in his own home until this is no longer possible; therefore, much of the care and advice which the patient receives during hospitalisation is directed towards maintaining the patient's independence, dignity and self esteem in what is a profoundly distressing disorder.

Mobility

Problems for the patient can include initiating walking, shuffling, tottering, being unable to stop walking, 'freezing' and stiffness.

Many of the techniques employed to assist the patient can be used by the relatives in the patient's home. The patient's strength and range of motion needs to be improved in conjunction with the drug therapy programme. Warm, relaxing baths, and passive and active range of movement exercises are a good starting point. Relatives should be advised to continue this activity at home. Effort should also be directed towards improving the patient's gait, with the assistance of the physiotherapist. Useful tips to consider can be found in Box 9.18.

If the patient experiences difficulty in rolling over in bed or getting in and out of bed, he can be advised to use a low bed with a firm mattress, or place a board under his existing mattress. Additional techniques are given in Box 9.18 (Franklin et al 1982).

Exercise

Some patients may benefit from an exercise programme to assist mobility and improve posture. It is important that this programme is performed under supervision initially, until the patient and his helper are conversant with the techniques. Again, the importance of continuing these at home should be stressed to both the patient and his family.

Box 9.18 Useful tips to encourage mobility

General tips

- Gently rocking the patient to and fro encourages initiation of walking when he 'freezes'.
- Instruct the patient to consciously lift each foot as he is walking and to place his heel on the ground first. To encourage this, tell the patient to think that he has a series of imaginary steps to climb. These techniques help to counteract the usual propulsive movement.
- Remind the patient to swing his arms when walking.
- Teach the patient to broaden his stance to provide a more stable base.
- Remind the patient to think about his posture and to stand erect.
- If the patient starts to shuffle, tell him to stop and start again.
- Tell the patient to adopt the habit of taking small steps when he is turning and to turn only in a forward direction.

Rolling over in bed

- The patient is advised to bend his knees so that his feet are flat on the mattress and then swing the knees in the direction that they wish to turn.
- The next move involves gripping the hands and lifting them straight up, straightening the elbows as they do so, then turning the head and swinging the arms in the same direction as the legs.
- The patient then grips the edge of the mattress and adjusts his position until comfortable.

To turn in the opposite direction, the process is reversed.

Some patients find a 'monkey pole' helpful. Whilst this is easy to attach to a hospital bed it is not usually possible in the home; however, an alternative the patient may consider is tying a stout rope to the bottom of the bed, and ensuring that the free end of the rope is within the patient's reach. This may allow the patient to alter his position in bed without help.

Getting in and out bed independently

- To get into bed the patient sits on the edge of the bed near the pillow so that when he lies down his head is in the correct position on the pillow.
- Once this manoeuvre has been mastered, the patient only has to lift his legs onto the bed and then adjust himself into a comfortable position.

Finding the correct spot to sit on the mattress may take some practice but once mastered the patient will find this a convenient way to get into bed.

Getting out of bed is more complicated and several techniques can be suggested. One example is as follows.

- The patient lies on his back with his arms at his side.
- He then lifts his head, tucking his chin into his chest, and sits up supported by the elbows.
- The patient then sits up, pushing the trunk so that he is leaning forward, bent at the hips.
- Support is now achieved by using his outstreched arms behind him.
- He should now move his legs towards the edge of the bed until he is sitting up and ready to stand up.

Rising from a chair

The patient should avoid low chairs, choosing instead firm, high-backed chairs. In the home the height of a low chair can be increased with blocks under the legs and it will help to raise the back of the chair slightly higher than the front. Cushions or a spring-ejector seat will also help. Placing a sturdy armchair in a frequently used location within the home is ideal. The patient can use the arms of the chair to assist him to rise from it.

Eating and drinking

The patient with Parkinson's disease may have difficulty with eating and drinking due to abnormal posture, tremor, poor swallowing and excessive saliva. The patient will be embarrassed by his untidiness when eating and the length of time it takes him to eat often results in food going cold. People will often choose to eat alone rather than endure the social embarrassment of seeing others watching them eat.

The speech therapist may be asked to assess the patient's swallowing ability and to draw up a programme of swallowing management. This could include facial exercises and techniques to encourage swallowing, for example, taking a sip of iced water to stimulate the swallowing reflex.

The dietitian's advice should also be sought. It is usual to establish what kind of foods the patient likes best. A review of his current dietary intake will alert the nurse to any deficiencies or inappropriate foods; for example, it is easier to swallow semi-solid food rather than lumpy food. If tremor is a problem, the patient can be taught to hold his arm close in to his body, using his elbow as a pivot. Bendable straws could be used and cups containing hot liquids should only be filled halfway to avoid spillage or scalding.

It is important for the patient's self esteem to resist the temptation to feed him before this is absolutely necessary. Many patients may still be able to feed themselves if their food is cut up for them. Feeding the patient for the convenience of speed is to be condemned.

Some of the swallowing difficulties which the patient may experience (Franklin et al 1982) are as follows:

- coughing within a few seconds following the act of swallowing
- food sticking in the throat
- nasal regurgitation
- fear of swallowing
- drooling
- food which remains in the mouth once the meal is completed.

The Parkinsonian patient who wears dentures should have these checked frequently to ensure that they fit properly. The importance of good oral hygiene should be emphasised. Patients should check their body weight weekly, and keep a record of this, so that they notice any changes. Some hospitalised patients need to have suctioning equipment readily available while they are eating, in case they choke.

Communication

The communication impairments seen in the Parkinsonian patient include a mask-like facial appearance, which often leads to the assumption that the patient is stupid, and loss of eye contact and normal body language due to the abnormal stooping posture.

The speech therapist should be involved in the care of the patient at a very early stage, if communication problems arise. A programme of exercises and therapy should be instituted as quickly as possible. Facial exercises encourage the patient to pronounce sounds more clearly, for example, by mouthing words slowly and clearly. Imagining that someone else is trying to lip read his words can help the patient. There are also exercises for breathing, strengthening the voice and controlling the speed of speech. Many can be continued in the patient's home. Other simple measures include reading out loud or singing in the bath. Alternatively, the patient could stand in front of a mirror, watching his lips as he talks.

Eventually the voice may become so weak that meaningful communication is impossible and an alternative means of communication becomes necessary. Communication aids must be appropriate to the patient's needs and advice regarding their use should be taken from the speech therapist. Aids can range from a simple picture board through to sophisticated computer devices.

More simply, it may be possible for the patient to write down messages using pen and paper. However, the ability to write also deteriorates progressively; and the writing becomes smaller and smaller as muscle stiffness increases. An alternative device which may be useful for some patients is a portable amplifier which will make a weak voice sound louder but this will not improve slurred speech (Franklin et al 1982). Reading books and newspapers also becomes difficult when muscle rigidity interferes with the ability to hold them and to turn pages.

?	**9.12** Work out how many day-to-day abilities need to be considered in helping a person with advanced Parkinson's disease to continue to enjoy watching television.

Elimination

The impairment of mobility in conjunction with urinary frequency or hesitancy can lead to embarrassing episodes of incontinence. This can be difficult to deal with and initially the patient is encouraged to visit the toilet regularly. The use of continence aids may be indicated (see Ch. 24). The advice of a continence advisor should be sought.

Eventually catheterisation of the bladder may be unavoidable. Many patients and their families reach a stage where they would prefer to have a catheter inserted rather than suffer the continual embarrassment of incontinence and odour. For some, the increasing expense associated with laundering clothes and bed-sheets may become overwhelming. It is important that patients are encouraged to maintain a fluid intake of 2.5–3 litres per day.

Constipation is a common accompaniment to Parkinson's disease, so the patient and his family should be taught preventative action. A high-fibre diet and plenty of fluids will encourage regular bowel motions. Failing this, it will be necessary to administer faecal softeners or bulking agents regularly. Some patients may require an enema from time to time.

Personal cleansing and dressing

The oily skin and excessive perspiration seen in patients with Parkinson's disease demand more frequent washing and bathing. If tremor is present, men will find an electric or battery-operated shaver easier to use.

Slowness in performing voluntary movement (bradykinesia) can make dressing difficult for the patient. For example, buttoning clothes and tying shoe laces may become impossible. Adaptations to clothing and the use of appropriate aids will allow the patient to continue to dress himself for as long as possible, thus maintaining his independence. Fastenings can be replaced by Velcro and cardigans are sometimes easier to take off and on than pullovers. A change of style may be indicated, for example, pull-on tracksuit trousers and front opening skirts with an elasticated waistband. Slip-on shoes or elastic shoelaces are also easier to manage.

Discharge

Every opportunity should be taken to teach the patient and his family the best way to manage the disorder at home. Each of the areas already outlined should be included in the discharge plan.

Additional points to consider if the patient has been hospitalised are as follows:

- The names and times of the medicines to be taken should be written down. The importance of maintaining the correct dosage is emphasised and some indication of the possible side effects should be given.

- A daily exercise programme should be devised for the patient, along with instructions about how much the patient should do.
- Contact should be established with the appropriate community services such as nursing, social services, physiotherapy, occupational therapy and speech therapy who may be providing the patient and his family with support at home.
- Advice on dietary aspects along with sample menus should be provided.
- Advice on safety should be provided. The removal of loose rugs and identification of other similar dangers in the home should be highlighted.

The patient should be encouraged to remain as active as possible for as long as possible but should also be warned to pace himself. Each individual patient will approach this situation in his own unique way and this has to be taken into account when proffering advice. The attitude and approach of the patient's family (where appropriate) can be crucial to the patient's progress toward maintaining his independence for as long as possible.

INFECTIONS

There are many infections of the central nervous system of which the following are considered, bacterial meningitis (infection of the meninges), viral encephalitis (infection of the brain) and brain abscess.

A serious outbreak of bacterial meningitis occurred in Stroud, Gloucestershire in 1985 (Cartwright et al 1986) and since then sporadic outbreaks have occurred in other parts of the UK. Many of the victims are young children and teenagers. It is estimated that there are about 5000 cases per year in England and Wales, with 500 deaths and approximately 1000 patients being left permanently disabled. Approximately 10 000 people contract viral meningitis annually. As a result of this, the National Meningitis Trust was set up with the following aims:

- to raise funds for research into all aspects of meningitis
- to provide help and support for the victims and families
- to educate the public about the disease and its symptoms in the hope that awareness and early diagnosis will save lives.

PATHOPHYSIOLOGY

In bacterial meningitis, purulent exudate is found in the subarachnoid space. The most likely route of entry is via the bloodstream which can carry micro-organisms from, for example, an infected middle ear. Other routes of entry include direct extension from a skull or facial fracture, via the cerebrospinal fluid, and extensions along cranial and spinal nerves. The circulating cerebrospinal fluid acts as an effective means of spreading the micro-organisms. Causative organisms in adults include streptococcus pneumoniae and neisseria meningitidis.

Viral encephalitis may accompany viral infections elsewhere in the body, for example, the respiratory tract. The commonest virus in the UK is the herpes simplex virus. Some viruses, such as in Jakob-Creutzfeldt disease, appear to be latent for many years and are called 'slow viruses' (Lindsay et al 1991).

Cerebral abscess most commonly occurs following middle ear and mastoid infections. Pus accumulates in the brain, its location depending on the source and method of spread of infection. Other related conditions are extradural abscesses (pus accumulates in the extradural space) and subdural empyema (pus accumulates in the subdural space). The offending organisms include the streptococcus and staphylococcus aureus. Once formed, the abscess comprises a mature capsule containing necrotic tissue, inflammatory cells and necrotic debris. The presence of an intracranial abscess can result in raised ICP.

Common presenting symptoms. A patient with meningitis may have had some pre-disposing infection and be receiving treatment for it, for example, antibiotics and ear-drops for an ear infection, or may have experienced a head injury and have a compound skull fracture, a fractured base of skull or a facial fracture. (See section on 'Head Injuries').

The patient may not have realised the extent of his injury, initially deferring medical attention after the accident but may begin to feel unwell over a period of time. His GP may suspect a serious problem as the patient's condition deteriorates. Admission to hospital will be necessary and, if the patient's condition is serious, referral to a neurosurgeon will be made, as the condition can rapidly become fatal, especially in children.

Infections of the central nervous system affect all age groups. Common symptoms include headache, fever, loss of consciousness, meningism, seizures, raised ICP and cranial nerve deficits. See Box 9.19.

Box 9.19 Features of presentation in CNS infections

Bacterial meningitis (abrupt onset)

- severe fronto-occipital headache
- fever (38–39°C)
- level of consciousness affected gradually. Patient may be lethargic, non-responsive and drowsy. Becomes disorientated
- neck stiffness and positive Kernig's sign present
- photophobic
- focal or generalised seizures are common
- ICP may be raised due to hydrocephalus caused by purulent exudate and cerebral oedema
- 15% of patients will have cranial nerve deficits, for example, ocular palsy, and 10% will have focal neurological signs such as hemiparesis.

Viral encephalitis (insidious onset)

- headache and fever are both present
- consciousness level deteriorates gradually. Confusion common
- moderate neck stiffness
- seizures can occur
- ICP may be elevated as a result of cerebral oedema
- cranial nerve deficits and focal neurological signs may be present.

Cerebral abscess (insidious onset, 2–3 weeks or more)

- headache is recurrent and fever usually present
- patient becomes confused and drowsy
- neck stiffness indicative of circulating CSF infection
- partial or generalised seizures occur in 30% of patients
- ICP is elevated as abscess expands
- cranial nerve deficits occur and focal neurological signs include speech disorders, motor and sensory deficits and ataxia.

MEDICAL MANAGEMENT

Examination. Typically, the patient, often a child, is pyrexial, compaining of headache and may be disoriented and drowsy. This is highly distressing for the mother. The patient's reaction to interference is often aggressive and they find all external environmental stimuli, such as strong light (photophobia), painful. See Box 9.19.

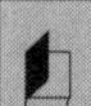

For information relating particularly to children, see Robinson (1990).

Investigations. The patient in coma or with any focal neurological signs should have a CT scan performed to exclude an intracranial mass, such as an abscess. A lumbar puncture may be performed to identify the offending organism. A moderate increase in lumbar cerebrospinal fluid pressure may be noted. The changes seen in the cerebrospinal fluid are outlined in Table 9.5.

Other investigations include blood cultures and X-rays to detect the source of infection. In the patient with a cerebral abscess, there may be a rise in the ESR. This may be confirmed by the identification of the organism on cerebrospinal fluid analysis or a lesion, such as an abscess, on CT scanning. Brain biopsy guided by CT scan may be helpful. When an abscess is suspected, the CT scan should be enhanced with contrast medium to highlight small lesions which may otherwise be missed.

Treatment. The patient with bacterial meningitis or a cerebral abscess requires to commence antibiotics as soon as possible. Penicillin is the antibiotic of choice and is usually given intravenously in high doses, such as penicillin 24 million units over 24 hours, but it should be remembered that a significant proportion of the population is allergic to this drug, and so other antibiotics may be used. Surgery will be performed on a cerebral abscess and adequate explanations should be given to the patient and his family of what is involved in this course of treatment. (See Game et al 1989 for complications.) This may involve burrhole aspiration (repeated, if necessary), primary excision of the whole abscess or evacuation of the abscess contents leaving the capsule intact (this avoids damaging the surrounding brain).

When there are signs of high intracranial pressure, the patient may be taken to theatre immediately to drain the abscess. This will relieve the intracranial pressure and will prevent coning and herniation of cerebral contents (see section on 'Head Injuries').

The patient may be in a coma or have a focal neurological deficit. (See Ch. 34 and Ch. 30.)

Table 9.5 Changes in cerebrospinal fluid which is infected

CSF	Acute bacterial meningitis	Viral encephalitis
Appearance	Yellow	Clear
Cells	Polymorphs 1000–2000 per cubic mm or more	Mononuclear 50–1500 per cubic mm
Protein	Increased 1.0–5.0 g/l	Mildly elevated
Chloride	110–115 mmol/l	Normal
Glucose	Much reduced or absent	Normal
Organisms	Present on culture	Absent on culture. Require specialist virological testing to identify.
Pressure	Increased	Increased.

NURSING PRIORITIES AND MANAGEMENT: INFECTIONS

Pre- and post-operative care

For those patients who require surgery, the general pre- and post-operative care is as given in Ch. 27. The nurse should observe the patient for signs of the abscess re-collecting: this will present as raised intracranial pressure.

Care of the dying patient

The patient's condition may deteriorate rapidly after admission if medication and surgery have not treated the cause of infection successfully. In these circumstances all of the patient's needs should be attended to. Adequate pain relief should be given and the patient should be comforted. (See Ch. 30.)

The patient's family will also require explanations, support and comfort. (See Ch. 34.)

Immediate priorities

Neurological status and vital signs

Because the patient with an intracranial infection may have a decreased conscious level and because this may deteriorate rapidly, observations should be recorded, reporting any change in condition immediately. Vital signs are very important as the patient may be pyrexial and as the infection continues, the patient's temperature can increase further. Pulse, blood pressure and respirations may be high when recorded due to infection: any changes in these observations should be reported. There may be signs of raised intracranial pressure (see p. 339).

Breathing

The patient's respiratory pattern should be observed for rate, depth and frequency, as a change may indicate a rising ICP. Any respiratory distress should be reported immediately. Oxygen may already have been prescribed and the nurse should encourage the patient to tolerate it, giving explanations when necessary. Nursing the patient in a bed with a head-up tilt of 30° will not only help to decrease ICP, but will also encourage lung expansion. The nurse should be aware of the risk of a chest infection developing.

Controlling body temperature

In order to reduce pyrexia, the patient's temperature should be recorded frequently and any further rise reported immediately, as this may indicate that the antibiotics are not controlling the infection and that the patient's condition could deteriorate. Each 1°C increase in temperature increases the body's demand for oxygen by 10% which encourages vasodilation and increases ICP.

Nursing measures to reduce pyrexia include tepid sponging, use of a fan and the administration of paracetamol, either per rectum or orally. The effects of these measures should be assessed.

Seizure activity

If seizures are observed, they should be recorded, noting the type of seizure, its duration and exactly what happened (see section on 'Seizures'). An airway, oxygen and suction should be at hand.

Communication

Communication can be difficult, as the patient may be experiencing severe headache, nausea and vomiting, have photophobia, and be disorientated and drowsy. A calm darkened environment will comfort the patient, who will be distressed about his condition and what is happening to him.

Explanations should be given to the patient about what is happening and why and the patient should be given time to ask questions and express his feelings.

His family will also require reassurance and explanations but they should be advised not to over-stimulate the patient, although touch could be suggested as this can be comforting to the patient.

Maintaining a safe environment
Bed rails should be placed in position to prevent the patient falling out of bed due to restlessness or confusion.

Medication
In order to give the patient adequate relief from pain, analgesics should be administered.

The nurse should ensure that prescribed antibiotics are taken at the correct time by the patient, to ensure maintenance of the drug at a therapeutic level in the bloodstream. An accurate fluid-balance chart should be maintained as the patient can become dehydrated due to pyrexia, nausea and vomiting. Signs of dehydration include dry skin or mouth or a diminishing urinary output and these should be reported. Intravenous fluids will be prescribed until the patient is able to tolerate adequate oral fluids.

Personal cleansing and dressing
Once an assessment of the patient's needs has been carried out, he should be assisted with personal cleansing and dressing. If the patient has a decreased conscious level, care should be exercised in meeting his needs and, as his condition improves, independence should be encouraged.

Mobilising
The patient should be mobilised as far as his condition allows. Initially, bed rest may be necessary and all care should be taken to ensure that the patient's position is changed 2-hourly. Examination of the skin should be carried out at frequent intervals in order to detect signs of pressure, such as redness.

Preparation for discharge home

If the source of the infection has been identified, it will be treated or, if necessary, further investigations carried out. If it has been treated successfully, for example, in sinusitis or an ear infection, the patient should be informed that he should contact his GP if there is a recurrence of the infection. The need to continue medication on discharge should be fully explained, with emphasis on the importance of completion of the course of antibiotics.

Further investigations may be required to ensure proper healing, if the reason for the introduction of the infection was an injury, such as a skull or facial fracture.

The patient will have been assessed by the ward team while rehabilitating in the ward. Maintenance of optimum function of the patient is a priority, both physically and mentally and out-patient appointments may be required, for example, for physiotherapy. The patient's family should be involved in the patient's rehabilitation programme and planned discharge home, with advice and encouragement for this should be given by the ward team. Advice should also be given on employment, driving and other activities, especially if the patient has experienced seizures (see p. 354). Any limitations on the patient's activities should also be explained and advice given on when to return to work.

GLOSSARY

Hydrocephalus — an excess of cerebrospinal fluid inside the skull due to an obstruction to normal cerebrospinal fluid absorption.

Isometric exercises — exercise carried out without movement, intended to maintain muscle tone.

Photophobia — inability to expose the eyes to light.

Saltatory conduction — a means of increasing the speed of nerve conduction, whereby the impulse 'jumps' from one node of Ranvier to the next.

REFERENCES

Aldenkamp A P et al 1990 Emotional and social reactions of children to epilepsy in a parent. Family Practice 7(2): 110–115

Allan D 1984 Glasgow coma scale. Nursing Mirror 158(23): 32

Allan D 1986a Management of the head injured patient. Nursing Times 82(25): 36

Allan D 1986b Raised ICP. Professional Nurse 2(3): 78

Allan D 1988 Nursing and the neurosciences. Churchill Livingstone, Edinburgh

Allan D 1989 Making sense of lumbar puncture. Nursing Times 55(49): 39–42

Amato C A 1991 Malignant glioma: coping with a devastating illness. Journal of Neuroscience Nursing 23(1): 20–23

Benner P 1984 From novice to expert: excellence and power in nursing practice. Addison Wesley, London

Bruya M A 1981 Planned periods of rest in the ICU: nursing care activities and ICP. Journal of Neuroscientific Nursing 13(4): 184

Buelow J M 1991 A correlation study of disabilities, stressors and coping methods in victims of multiple sclerosis. Journal of Neuroscientific Nursing 23(4): 247–252

Cartwright K A V, Stuart S M, Noah N D 1986 An outbreak of meningococcal diseases in Gloucestershire. Lancet 2: 558–561

Cobell R 1989 Facing up to my epilepsy. Nursing Times 85(2): 26

Collings J A 1990 Epilepsy and well-being. Social Science and Medicine 31(2): 165–170

Engel J 1989 Seizures and epilepsy. F A Davis, Philadelphia

Epilepsy Association of Scotland Undated Factsheet 5. Epilepsy Association of Scotland, Glasgow

Faulkner A 1989 Back from the edge. Nursing Times 85(4): 29

Franklin S, Perry A, Beattie A 1982 Living with Parkinson's disease. Parkinson's Disease Society, London

Game C, Anderson R E, Kidd J R 1989 Medical-surgical nursing: a cpre text. Churchill Livingstone, Melbourne

Guyton A C 1991 Textbook of medical physiology, 8th edn. W B Saunders, New York

Health and Safety at Work Act 1974 HMSO, London

Hewer R L & Wade D T 1986 Stroke: a practical guide towards recovery. Positive Health Guide. Martin Dunitz, London

Hickey J V 1992 The clinical practice of neurological and neurosurgical nursing (3rd edn). Lippincott, Philadelphia

Hopkins A 1992 Reducing the risk of a stroke. Copyright Stroke Series Leaflet S3. The Stroke Association, London

Jamieson E M, McCall J M, Blythe R 1992 Guidelines for clinical nursing practice, 2nd edn. Churchill Livingstone, Edinburgh

Johnstone M 1987 The stroke patient, 3rd edn. Churchill Livingstone, Edinburgh

Lindsay K, Bone I, Callander R 1991 Neurology and neurosurgery illustrated (2nd edn). Churchill Livingstone, Edinburgh

McKeran R O, Thomas D G T 1980 In: Thomas D G T, Graham D I (eds) 1980 Brain tumours: scientific basis, clinical investigation and current therapy. Butterworth, London
McLean J, Roper-Hall A, Mayer P, Hain A 1991 Service needs of stroke survivors and their informal carers. Journal of Advanced Nursing 16(5): 559–564
Mulley G 1990 Stroke: a handbook for the patient's family. CHSA stroke series, booklet S7. The Chest, Heart and Stroke Association, London
Pownall M 1985 Clunk click. Nursing Times 81(48): 14
Purchese G, Allan D 1984 Neuromedical and neurosurgical nursing (2nd edn). Bailliere Tindall, London
Rowley G, Fielding K 1991 Reliability and accuracy of the Glasgow Coma Scale with experienced and inexperienced users. Lancet 337(8740): 535–38
Scambler G 1989 Epilepsy. Tavistock/Routledge, London
The Stroke Association 1992 Stroke: questions and the answers. Copyright Stroke Series Leaflet S1. Stroke Association, London
Stubbs C 1992 Facing up to MS. Nursing Times 88(8): 34–36
Swank R L, Dugan B B 1990 Effect of low saturated fat diet in early and late cases of multiple sclerosis. Lancet 336(8706): 37–9
Thomas D J 1988 Strokes and their prevention. British Medical Association, London
Thomas D G T 1983 Brain tumours. British Journal of Hospital Medicine 29(2): 148
Totora G J, Grabowski S R 1993 Principles of anatomy and physiology, 7th edn. Harper Collins, London
Warme P E, Bergstrom R, Persson L 1991 Neurosurgical intensive care improves outcome after severe head injury. ACTA Neurochir Vienna 110(1–2): 57–64
Zanetta J P et al 1990 Antibodies to cerebellar soluble lecithin (CSL) in multiple sclerosis. Lancet 335(8704): 1482

FURTHER READING

Allan D 1984 Glasgow coma scale. Nursing Mirror 158(23): 32
Allan D 1986a Management of the head-injured patient. Nursing Times 82(25): 36
Allan D 1986b Raised ICP. Professional Nurse 2(3): 78
Allan D 1989 Assessment of the head injured patient. Nursing Review 7(3): 19
Anderson M S 1984 My head hurts. Nursing 84 14(9): 34–39
Barron M 1992 Life after stroke. Nursing Times 88(10): 32–34
Becker D 1989 Textbook of head injury. W B Saunders, Philadelphia
Benz C 1988 Coping with multiple sclerosis. Optima, London
Chadwick D, Usiskin S 1987 Living with epilepsy. Macdonald Optima, London
Cheney D L 1981 Coping with neurologic problems proficiently. Intermed Communications, Horsham
Clark M 1983 Diary of a stroke victim. Nursing Times. 79(34): 27
Cole K 1988 Is Parkinson's disease preventable? Professional Nurse 4: 1–15
Dawson P 1983 Rehabilitation after cerebrovascular accident. Nursing Times. 79(6): 23
Dennis M S, Warlow C P 1987 Stroke: incidence, risk factors and outcome. British Journal of Hospital Medicine 37(3): 174
Dewis M E, Niskala H 1992 Nurturing a valuable resource: family caregivers in multiple sclerosis. Axon 13(3): 87–94
Gehrke M 1980 Identifying brain tumours. Journal of Neurosurgical Nursing 12(2): 90
Gibbon B 1991 Measuring stroke recovery. Nursing Times 87(44): 32–34
Holloway N 1988 Medical surgical care plans. Springhouse Corporation, Pennsylvania
Holmes P 1988 A world turned upside down (Bobath technique). Nursing Times 84(6): 42
Hubbard J L, Mechan D 1987 Physiology for health care. Churchill Livingstone, Edinburgh
Isaacs B 1992 Understanding stroke illness. Copyright Booklet S5. The Stroke Association, London
Jacoby A 1992 Epilepsy and the quality of everyday life: findings from a study of people with well-controlled epilepsy. Social Science and Medicine 34(6): 657–666
Johnstone M 1987 Home care for the stroke patient. Churchill Livingstone, Edinburgh
Konikow N S 1982 Head injury. University of Washington, Seattle
Laidlaw M V, Laidlaw J 1984 People with epilepsy. Churchill Livingstone, Edinburgh
Larson E 1980 Epidemiology of brain tumours. Journal of Neurosurgical Nursing 12(3): 121
MacLellan M 1989 Nursing care of a patient with multiple sclerosis. Nursing 3(33): 28
McCarthy N 1990 Epilepsy: the facts. Nursery World. May 1990 10: 15–18
McManus J C, Hausman K A 1982 Cerebrospinal fluid analysis. Nursing 12(8): 43
Mitchell M 1989 Neuroscience nursing — a nursing diagnosis approach. Williams and Wilkie, New York
Martyn C N 1989 Neurology student notes. Churchill Livingstone, Edinburgh
Phillips A 1987 Speech problems following a stroke. Geriatric Nursing and Home Care 7(6): 12
Pinel C 1989 Cerebrovascular accident. Nursing 3(33): 24
Quigley J et al 1989 Neurological investigations. Nursing 3(33): 12
Readman S 1990 The challenge of epilepsy: patient education. Practice Nurse 3(4): 219–222
Richardson E 1989 Surgery for epilepsy. Nursing 3(33): 20
Robinson M J (ed) 1990 Practical paediatrics, 2nd edn. Churchill Livingstone, Edinburgh
Roper N, Logan W, Tierney A J 1990 The elements of nursing: a model of nursing, based on a model of living, 3rd edn. Churchill Livingstone, Edinburgh
Ross D 1988 Dealing with epilepsy. Occupational Health 40(12): 741–743
Tallis R 1990 Epilepsy in old age. Lancet 4 August: 295–296
Totora G J, Grabowski S R 1993 Principles of anatomy and physiology, 7th edn. Harper Collins, London
Whitney Jess L 1987 Assessing your patient for increased ICP. Nursing 87 17(6): 34–41

USEFUL ADDRESSES

Headway
7 King Edward Court
King Edward Street
Nottingham
NG1 1EW

0602 240800

British Epilepsy Association
Anstey House
40 Hanover Square
Leeds
LS3 1BE

0532 439393

Chest, Heart and Stroke Association
CHSA House
123/127 Whitecross Street
London
EC1Y 8JJ

071 490 7999

The Multiple Sclerosis Society of Great Britain
25 Effie Road
Fulham
London
SW6 1EE

071 736 6267

Royal College of Midwives
15 Mansfield Street
London W1M OBE

The Meningitis Trust
Fern House
Bath Road
Stroud
GL5 3TJ

0453 751738

Parkinson's Disease Society
22 Upper Woburn Place
London
WC1H 0RA

Association to Aid the Sexual and Personal Relationships of Disabled People
286 Camden Road
London
N7 0BJ

Relate — National Marriage Guidance Council
Herbert Gray College
Little Church Street
Rugby
Warwickshire
CV21 3AP

0788 73241

CHAPTER 10

The musculoskeletal system

Liz Jamieson   Catherine McFarlane

CHAPTER CONTENTS

Introduction 369
Anatomy and physiology of the musculoskeletal system 370
General principles of nursing management of musculoskeletal disorders 373
SKELETAL DISORDERS 373
Fractures 373
Fractures of specific sites 379
Nursing priorities and management: fracture of the femoral shaft 379
Nursing priorities and management: fracture of neck of femur 380
Nursing priorities and management: fracture of the tibia and fibula 381
Nursing priorities and management: fracture of neck of humerus 382
Nursing priorities and management: Colles' fracture 383
Nursing priorities and management: fracture of clavicle 383
Nursing priorities and management: spinal injuries 384
Nursing priorities and management: bone tumours 388
Nursing priorities and management: amputation of a limb 389
Bone infections 391
Nursing priorities and management: osteomyelitis 391
Nursing priorities and management: tuberculosis 391
DISORDERS OF JOINTS 391
Disorders of the knee 391
Nursing priorities and management: meniscus lesions 392
Disorders of the lumbar spine — back pain 392
Nursing priorities and management: acute back strain 392
Nursing priorities and management: prolapsed intervertebral disc 393
Nursing priorities and management: dislocated shoulder 394
Joint infection 394
Nursing priorities and management: septic arthritis 394
Inflammatory and degenerative joint disorders 394
Nursing priorities and management: rheumatoid arthritis 394
Nursing priorities and management: joint replacement 399
SOFT TISSUE INJURIES 401
Nursing priorities and management: ligament injuries 401
Nursing priorities and management: muscle and tendon injuries 402
Nursing priorities and management: peripheral nerve injuries 402
Conclusion 403
References 403
Further reading 403
Useful addresses 404

INTRODUCTION

A fully functioning musculoskeletal system is fundamental to optimal health in the normal active human being. Injury or disease involving this system can have a profound effect on an individual's ability to perform the activities of daily living and can result in either temporary or permanent disability, one of the main problems usually being in the degree of decreased mobility. The overall aim of nursing care is to prevent further injury, promote healing, maximise independence within individual constraints of the existing condition and promote optimal rehabilitation.

This chapter will describe some of the more common disorders of the musculoskeletal system that are caused either by trauma or disease and will outline relevant principles of nursing management.

Epidemiology

The main causes of musculoskeletal trauma or disease in the UK mirror cultural influences, changing patterns of social activity and the prevailing climatic conditions. They include road traffic accidents (RTAs), industrial and other work-related accidents, sporting accidents and damage due to underlying disease.

Road traffic accidents

In 1989 5000 people died and 317 000 were injured in road traffic accidents in Great Britain (Central Statistical Office 1990). These figures represent a substantial decrease in RTA injuries in recent years in spite of the increasing number of motor vehicles on the roads (Harvey & Durbin 1986). This could be due in part to the introduction of legislation to make wearing seat belts compulsory for front seat passengers in 1981 and similar legislation covering back seat passengers in 1991 will probably accentuate this trend.

RTAs account for a significant proportion of the workload in accident and emergency (A & E) departments throughout the country, and it should be emphasised that it is often the immediate treatment of injury or suspected fracture that determines the ultimate outcome; this applies particularly to fractures of the spinal column and major long bones.

Work-related injuries

The number of these injuries is increasing, with the construction industry, agriculture and forestry having the highest proportion (Health and Safety Council 1989). This is occurring in spite of government legislation such as the Health and Safety at Work Act 1974, 1933 and the Control of Substances Hazardous to Health Act 1989.

Back pain is commonly work related and has a high incidence in the UK, resulting in millions of work days lost.

Occupational health nurses have an increasingly important role to play in the education of workers and employers regarding accident prevention. Most nursing roles, in fact, offer the opportunity to raise public awareness of risks and preventive measures available.

Sporting injuries
With increased leisure time and facilities and the many health campaigns promoting the benefits of exercise, more time is being spent in sporting activities with a resultant increase in sporting injuries. In many cases these are minor but they can also be serious and result in permanent disability: diving into shallow water can cause serious injury to the cervical spine; knee and lower limb injuries are common in football and skiing; and shoulder and upper limb injuries often result from horse riding accidents.

There is increasing emphasis in sport's medicine on the importance of initial correct treatment and thorough rehabilitation. This often involves major physiotherapy input and can significantly affect the degree of residual musculoskeletal damage (Dirix et al 1988).

Damage due to underlying disease
Relatively minor trauma may also serve to highlight a previously undiagnosed underlying disease process. For example, osteoporosis in a postmenopausal woman may only be diagnosed when she presents with a fractured wrist or femur. Osteoporosis is loss of bone mass leading to increased porosity and brittleness and is due to an imbalance between calcium reabsorption and bone formation. Its presence may also indicate dietary deficiencies or endocrine disturbances.

Rheumatoid arthritis is a chronic or sub-acute disease of the musculoskeletal joints and is one of the most common rheumatic diseases in the UK. It usually affects more than one joint (polyarthritic) and can be extremely disabling. It is estimated that 1.5% of the population will develop rheumatoid arthritis, with the sex ratio being 3 females to 1 male (Currey 1988).

Osteoarthritis (degenerative arthritis) is mainly due to wear and tear on the articular cartilage of the larger weight-bearing joints and to the degenerative changes associated with the ageing process. When it is associated with old injury or strenuous sport or work it can affect any age group and both sexes but has a higher incidence in women over 55 years old. Prevalence increases with age until the condition is almost universal, in varying degrees, in people aged over 75 years (Royle & Walsh 1992).

The contribution of the science of bioengineering
Musculoskeletal conditions involve, or are caused by, disruption of the mechanics of the human body. Through research, bioengineers are making vital contributions to understanding these mechanics and, with the availability of more biologically compatible materials, are able to design a wider and more refined range of replacement joints and limbs. Joint replacement surgery is now a common procedure and has revolutionised the quality of life for thousands of injured or elderly people.

ANATOMY AND PHYSIOLOGY OF THE MUSCULOSKELETAL SYSTEM

This section will give a brief overview of the anatomy and physiology of the musculoskeletal system. For detailed information refer to anatomy and physiology textbooks and become familiar with the model skeleton in your classroom.

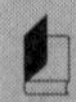
For further information, see Marieb (1992).

For ease of reference, the skeletal system and the muscular system will be outlined seperately.

The skeletal system
The skeleton is a supportive framework of bones bound together by ligaments. It can be divided into an axial part (the bones of the head and trunk) and an appendicular part (the bones of the limbs). Its main functions are to provide the basis for the mechanics of movement and to protect the internal organs and vital structures.

Bones store the body's supply of calcium and release it to maintain the constant level in body fluids that is necessary for normal muscular activity, heart action and blood clotting. Red bone marrow also plays an essential role in the manufacture of blood cells.

Structurally, the skeletal system consists of two types of connective tissue — bone and cartilage.

Bone

? **10.1** Look up the factors involved in the development and growth of healthy bone. Describe them.

Unlike other connective tissue, bone contains large amounts of mineral salts (mainly tricalcium phosphate and calcium carbonate) which when deposited on the collagen fibres results in hardening. There are two types of bone tissue — compact and cancellous.

The hard outer layer of a bone is compact bone tissue (cortical bone) while cancellous tissue fills the inside. Cancellous tissue is more spongy in appearance and the larger spaces contain the highly vascular red bone marrow and the fatty yellow bone marrow. The thickness of each type of tissue varies, depending on the type and function of the particular bone. In long bones such as the femur, the shaft (diaphysis) is enclosed by a thick layer of cortical tissue which gives strength for weight bearing; while at each end (epiphyses) the cortical tissue is thinner and encloses a greater mass of cancellous tissue.

Flat bones, such as the sternum and the pelvis, have a thinner layer of cortical tissue and a relatively greater amount of cancellous tissue. This is the reason they are chosen for bone marrow biopsy.

Tissue renewal. Like the skin, bone tissue is constantly being replaced but at variable rates in different parts of the body. The upper end of the femur is replaced about every 4 months in an adult in contrast to the shaft of the femur which will never be completely replaced during a lifetime. This process of growth and repair is dependent on balanced activity between the three types of bone cell: osteoblasts, osteocytes and osteoclasts (see Fig. 10.1).

? **10.2** Referring to an anatomy and physiology text, define the function of each type of bone cell.

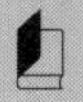
For further information on bone, see Wilson (1990) pp. 352–373.

Cartilage
This is a form of connective tissue which is tough, flexible, avascular and devoid of nerve fibres. It forms part of the support mechanism of the body.

There are three types of cartilage:

- hyaline cartilage — which is firm yet pliable and forms the articular cartilage that covers the articulating surfaces of synovial joints
- fibrocartilage — which is strong, compressible and tension resistant and is found in areas such as the intervertebral discs
- elastic cartilage — which contains more elastin fibres than the others and therefore has a greater ability to stretch whilst retaining its strength; it is found in the external ear and the epiglottis.

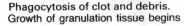

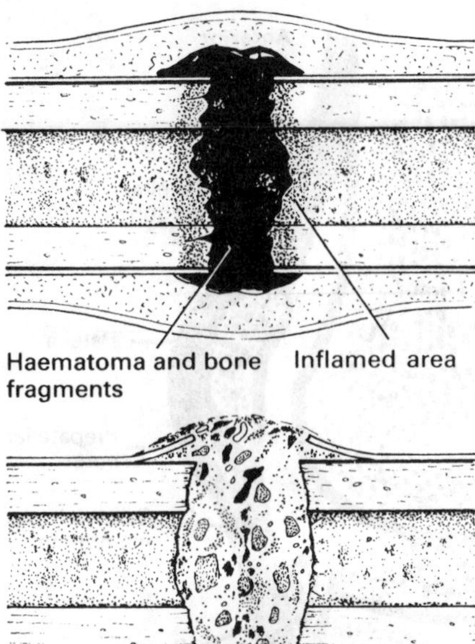

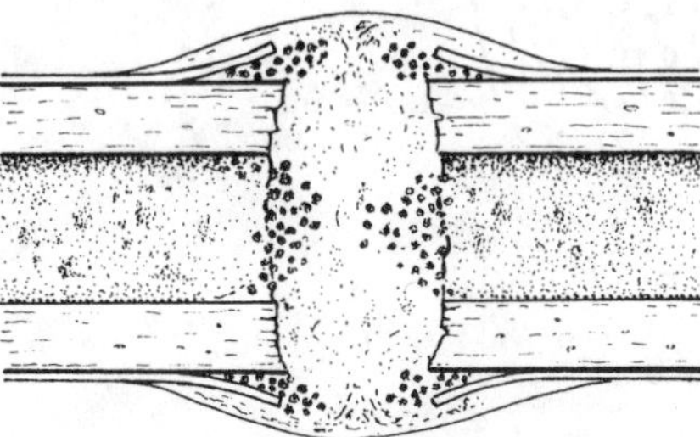

Phagocytosis of clot and debris.
Growth of granulation tissue begins

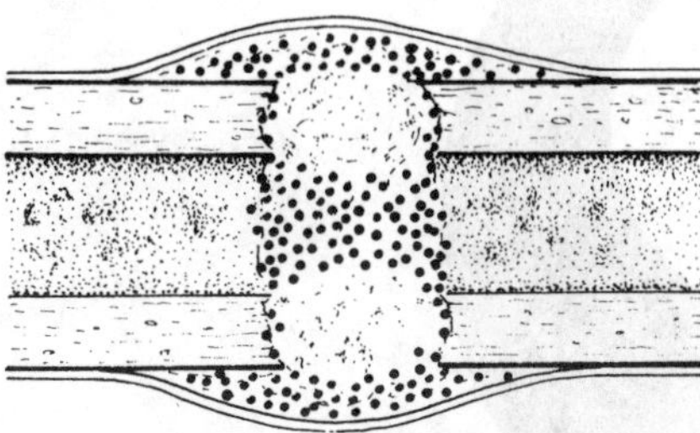

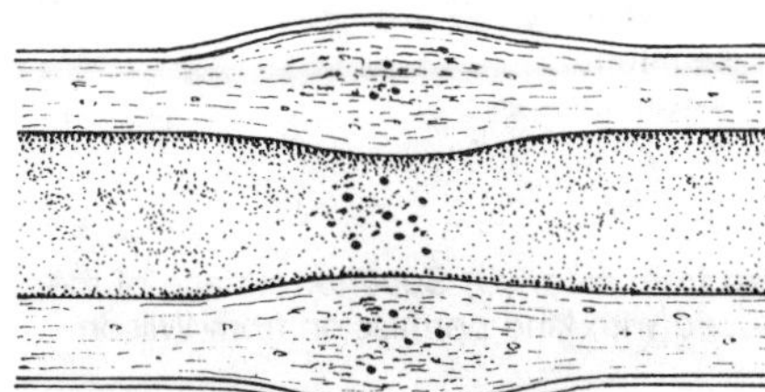

Gradual spread of new bone to bridge gap
Bone healed. Osteoblasts reshape and canalise new bone

Fig. 10.1 Stages in bone healing. (Reproduced with kind permission from Wilson 1990.)

The axial skeletal system

The vertebral column forms the central axis of the skeletal system. It is a strong, flexible column of 33 bones, 24 of which are 'true' vertebrae — the cervical, thoracic and lumbar — the remainder being fused to form the sacrum and coccyx (see Fig. 10.2). Between each of the vertebrae from C2 to S1 is a strong joint created by the fibrocartilaginous intervertebral discs which allow flexibility and act as shock absorbers when the spine is exposed to vertical forces.

The spinal column functions to protect the spinal cord, support the skull and act as a point of attachment for the ribs and muscles of the back.

The appendicular skeletal system

The upper and lower limbs are the main parts of the appendicular skeletal system and are characterised by the presence of synovial joints which connect the articular surfaces of adjoining bones. (See Fig. 10.3.) The bones that make up the joint are held within a fibrous capsule, which consists of two layers.

The outer layer is dense connective tissue which allows movement but resists dislocation. In some joints the fibres of this connective tissue are arranged parallel to each other and in bundles and are known as ligaments. The inner layer of the fibrous capsule is lined with synovial membrane which secretes synovial fluid. This provides nourishment and lubrication. The articular surfaces of the bones involved are covered in hyaline cartilage — articular cartilage. Many synovial joints

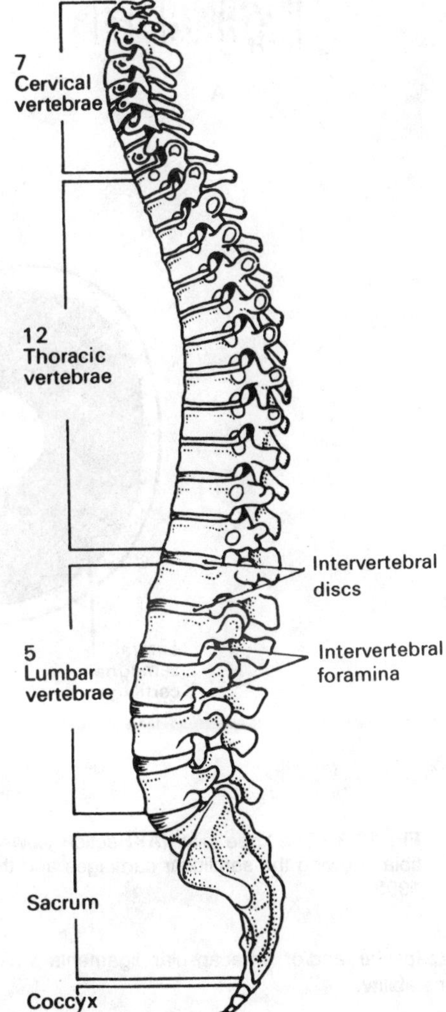

Fig. 10.2 The vertebral column — lateral view. (Reproduced with kind permission from Wilson 1990.)

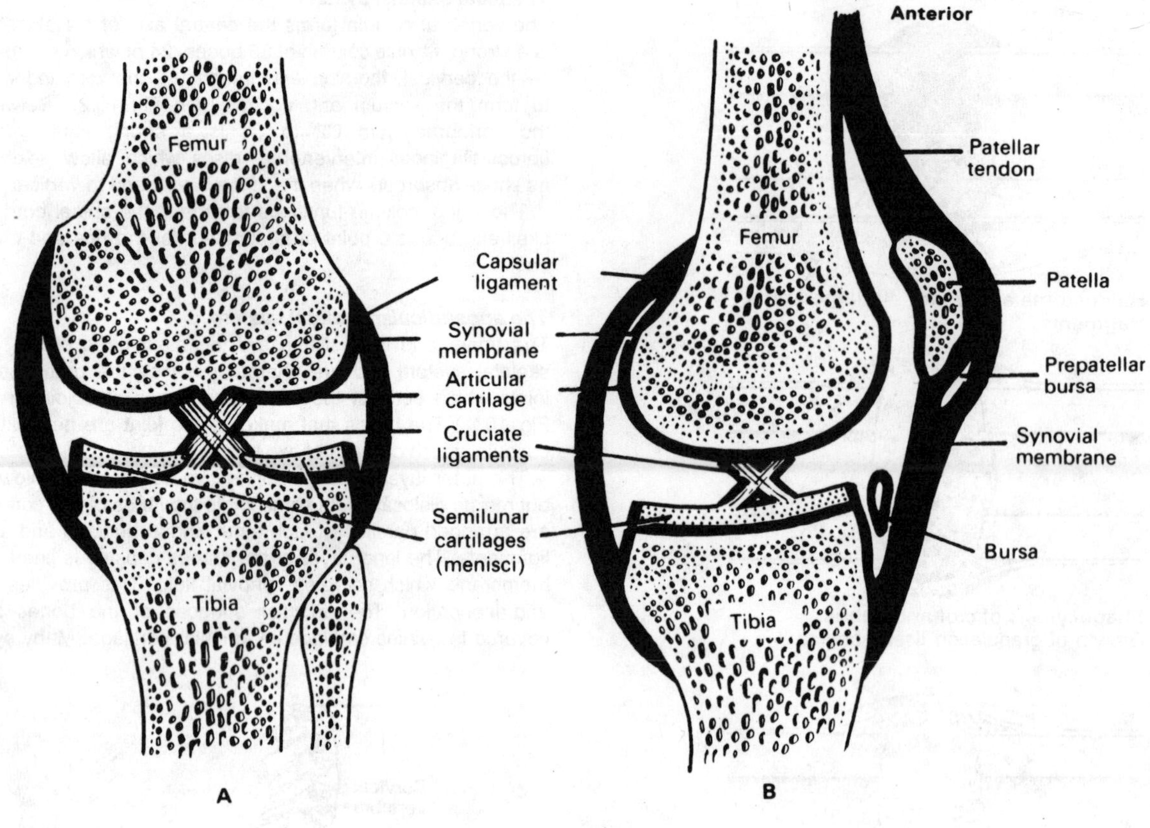

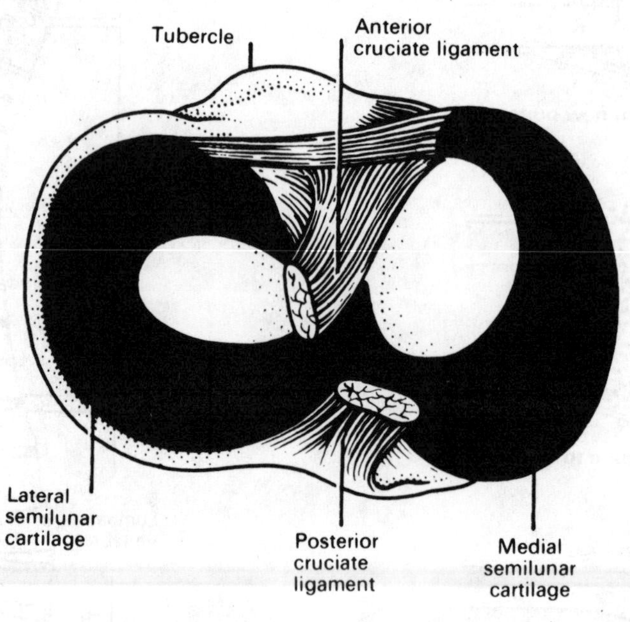

Fig. 10.3 The knee joint. (A) Section viewed from front. (B) Section viewed from side. (C) Superior surface of the tibia showing the semilunar cartilages and the cruciate ligaments. (Reproduced with kind permission from Wilson 1990.)

contain extracapsular and/or intracapsular ligaments which help to increase their stability.

The muscular system

Skeletal muscle tissue is composed of multinucleated muscle cells which are long and cylindrical in appearance. Each muscle is made up of muscle fibres and connective tissue and is attached to periosteum or other muscles by tendons. A good blood and nerve supply is essential for muscle function and the mechanics of movement.

?	**10.3** Find a chart or model of the muscular system. Identify and name the main muscle groups.

 Information on the muscular system can be found in Wilson (1990) Ch 18.

Components of the musculoskeletal system

There are various components involved in musculoskeletal injuries and disease, i.e. skeletal, joint, muscle, skin, neurovascular, and the patient's perception of cause and abnormal sensation and pain. These interacting components, although often present at the same time in varying degrees, will be addressed under the following headings: skeletal disorders, joint disorders and soft tissue disorders.

Assessment

Assessment of the condition and function of the musculoskeletal system is by:

- patient history
- visual inspection
- palpation
- measurement
- radiological and imaging studies (see Box 10.1).

GENERAL PRINCIPLES OF NURSING MANAGEMENT OF MUSCULOSKELETAL DISORDERS

Nursing assessment

This will involve general observation and nursing history. The selected philosophy and model of nursing will influence the focus of care planning. Orem's model (1990) is often suggested as being particularly useful because of the emphasis on self-care, independence and the progression towards the supportive educative role of the nurse.

Observations are made on:

- life-threatening priorities
- abnormal position or appearance of limbs or affected part with loss of function (compare with contralateral side)
- presence of shock
- report or signs of pain
- abnormal posture or gait
- use of walking aids or prostheses.

The nursing history includes:

- comprehensive cover of universal health care requisites, concurrent health problems, allergies and medications
- patient's perception of cause of primary problem and impact on Activities of Daily Living (ADLs) (Roper, Logan & Tierney (1990)) especially relating to impaired mobility
- patient's description of pain and other symptoms
- patient and his family's expectations, coping strategies, alteration to normal roles and educability.

Problems and strengths (actual and potential) are identified in the following categories:

- life-threatening priorities
- pain
- shock
- impaired mobility
- potential for further injury — physical safety and neurovascular complications
- psychosocial consequences
- rehabilitation
- patient and family strengths — these should be defined and used constructively.

Nursing intervention

- Treat life-threatening priorities — CPR.
- Relieve pain.
- Monitor and treat shock.
- Maintain an appropriate degree of therapeutic splintage and mobility.
- Constantly monitor and prevent neurovascular complications.
- Maintain a safe environment.
- Coordinate multidisciplinary intervention for psychosocial problems.
- Prevent the boredom of greatly reduced mobility.
- Facilitate rehabilitation.
- Promote patient and family strengths to support adaptation and rehabilitation.

Box 10.1 Investigations for musculoskeletal abnormalities

Radiological and imaging studies

- X-ray — to detect abnormal position, fractures, bone density and presence of fluid or abnormalities in joint capsules.
- Tomogram — X-ray technique for detail of specific plane (slice) of bone.
- Computer assisted tomogram (CAT scan) — makes use of the fact that different tissues have varying radiodensities. A series of radiographs are made at different angles and planes and the computer integrates the information to produce pictorial slices (sometimes 3D) which can be used to detect soft tissue injuries or tumours and inflammatory or metastatic skeletal disease or fracture.
- Magnetic resonance imaging (MRI) — magnetic fields used to show the difference in hydrogen density of various muscle and soft tissues indicating the presence of abnormalities.
- Arthrogram — injection of a radiopaque substance or air into a joint followed by X-ray to identify abnormalities of joint structures.
- Myelogram — a contrast medium injected into the subarachnoid space of the lumbar spine in order to visualise disc herniation or tumours.
- Discogram — injection of contrast medium into lumbar disc to show up abnormalities.

Joint examination

- Arthroscopy — endoscopic visualisation of structures inside a joint. May also involve withdrawal of synovial fluid for analysis.

Muscle and nerve studies

- Electromyography (EMG) — measures electrical potential of muscle during rest and activity.
- Nerve conduction velocities (NCVs) — measures speed of nerve impulse conduction.

Other tests

- These include bone biopsy, densimetry, total body calcium and various haematological studies for hormone and mineral levels.

SKELETAL DISORDERS

This section will focus firstly on fractures and their management and then more briefly on tumours and infections of the bone.

FRACTURES

PATHOPHYSIOLOGY

A fracture is loss of normal bone continuity, and can be caused by direct or indirect violence, weakening of the bone due to underlying disease (pathological fracture) or repeated bending stresses on a bone (stress fracture).

Box 10.2 Types of fracture

Transverse: straight across the bone
Oblique: at an angle across the bone
Spiral: twists around the shaft of the bone
Comminuted: bone splintered into several fragments
Depressed: fragment(s) indriven (seen in fractures of the skull and facial bones)
Compression: bone collapses in on itself (see in vertebral fractures)
Avulsion: fragment of bone pulled off by ligament or tendon attachment
Impacted: fragment of bone wedged into other bone fragment.

Classification of fractures. When direct contact between the fracture and the external environment occurs it is known as a compound or open fracture. A simple or closed fracture is where there is no communication between the external environment and the fracture site.

A fracture may be described as stable when the bone ends are lying in a position from which they are unlikely to move or as unstable when the bone ends are displaced or have the potential to be displaced.

Common fracture patterns are shown in Box 10.2.

MEDICAL MANAGEMENT

Priorities of treatment. A fracture is often associated with some degree of general trauma and first aid is very important as mishandling can add to the severity of the injury. Priorities are established: the ABC of resuscitation is attended and accompanying shock, which may be severe due to pain and blood loss, is treated. (See Ch. 28 and Ch. 18.)

The jagged edges of broken bones can cause further major injury if they penetrate or sever internal organs, nerves or blood vessels. Immediate immobilisation and maintenance of alignment is imperative until the full extent of the fracture has been established. This is especially important when spinal injury is suspected as irreparable damage may be done to the spinal cord.

Once the patient's physical condition has been stabilised specific treatment of the injuries will continue.

Reduction of fractures. Fractures are said to be reduced when displaced bone fragments are pulled into their normal anatomical position. In many cases a general anaesthetic will be necessary to overcome the protective muscle spasm and severe pain.

There are four objectives of reduction:

- good apposition — ensuring nothing lies between bone ends
- good alignment
- maintaining full length of limb
- normal rotation.

Splintage or reduced mobility. It is important following reduction that the fracture is held in the correct anatomical position until bony union occurs. Various methods are used depending on the site of the fracture. These include skin or skeletal traction, external splintage using plaster of Paris (POP) or synthetic casts, or an external fixator frame. Open operative reduction with internal fixation by metal pins, plates and screws may also be used to hold the bony fragments in position. When the supply of nutrients is grossly affected it may be necessary to implant prostheses to replace the affected bone, for example, in some cases of fractured neck of femur.

Maintenance and restoration of function. When one part of a limb is immobilised there is a tendency for related joints and muscles to become stiff and weak; for example, during splintage of a wrist fracture, the finger and shoulder joints can be affected. Appropriate physiotherapy is essential.

Rehabilitation. Patients require varying degrees of rehabilitation which involves a multidisciplinary team approach (see Ch. 35).

Traction

Traction is force applied in a specific direction by various systems of ropes, pulleys and weights attached to skeletal pins or skin appliances in order to maintain anatomical alignment and overcome the natural pull of muscles. It is used in the following circumstances:

- to reduce and immobilise fractures and maintain normal alignment of all injured tissues
- to prevent deformity
- to reduce muscle spasm
- to relieve pain
- to immobilise an injured or inflamed joint.

Types of traction

Balanced or sliding traction. This uses weights and pulleys as mobile counterbalancing forces and skeletal pins and external slings as suspensory devices. For example, in order to achieve the degree of traction needed to maintain reduction of a fractured femur, a Steinmann or Denham pin or a Kirchner wire is inserted through the upper end of the tibia to provide a firm point of attachment for the stirrup, ropes and pulley and the required weight (see Fig. 10.4). The extremity may be suspended within the apparatus and a fairly constant line

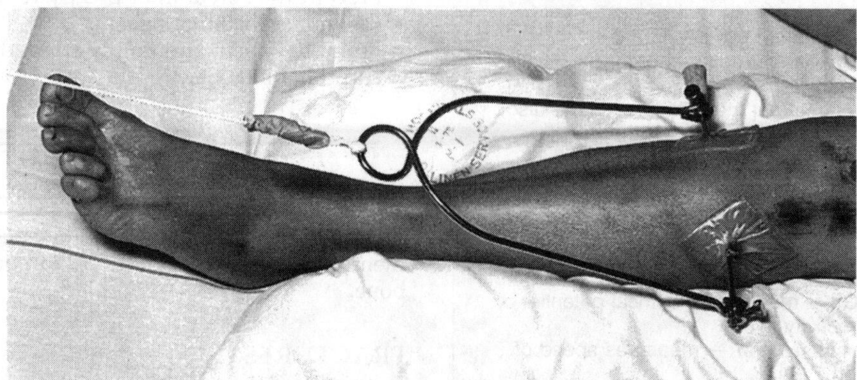

Fig. 10.4 Skeletal traction at the upper tibial site. A Böhler stirrup clamped on to a Steinmann or Denham pin carries the traction cord to the weight. Note the cork on the sharp end of the pin and the occlusive dressings at the pin insertion sites. (Reproduced with kind permission from Taylor 1990.)

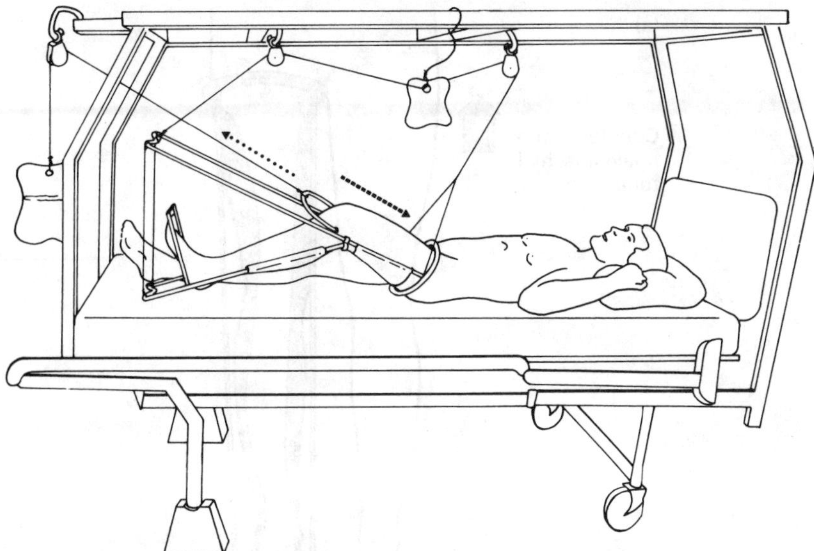

Fig. 10.5 Skeletal traction in balanced suspension in Thomas' splint. Countertraction is achieved by elevating the foot of the bed. (Reproduced with kind permission from Taylor 1990.)

of pull maintained even when the patient changes position. Together with an overhead trapeze this allows greater freedom of movement. The patient in balanced or sliding traction may lift himself up and move up and down the bed (see Fig. 10.5).

Fixed traction. This is traction between two points with the pull exerted in one plane. Skin or skeletal traction may be used (Fig. 10.6A & B). Methods used to establish skin traction are outlined in Box 10.3.

For further information, see Taylor (1987).

PRINCIPLES OF NURSING MANAGEMENT: TRACTION

In addition to the general principles outlined earlier for management of musculoskeletal injuries the following are specific to a patient in traction:

Traction equipment and purpose

The nurse should have a thorough working understanding of the type and purpose of the particular traction in use and explain these simply and clearly to the patient in order to get his active participation in overall treatment, rehabilitation and prevention of complications. He is taught how to lift himself up using the overhead lifting aid and which movements are safe. All parts of frames, pulleys, ropes and slings should be inspected at regular intervals every day to ensure that they are correctly positioned and in good working order.

Observation of neurovascular status and prevention of complications

Keen and constant observation of colour, sensation and movement of the injured limb must be carried out throughout the patient's stay in hospital. His involvement in this is essential and he should be helped and encouraged to describe changes in sensation and levels of pain. Any complaint of discomfort, pain or paraesthesia must be thoroughly investigated (Davies 1989).

External pressure can come from any part of the traction or be caused by restricted movement. Internal pressure may be the result of tissue damage and swelling.

Be alert for:

- increased risk of pressure sores
- drop foot caused by excessive pressure on the common peroneal nerve located around the head of the fibula
- compartment syndrome — increased tissue pressure resulting in inadequate tissue perfusion and anoxia which can lead to permanent loss of function within 6–8 hours.

It is vital to be aware that compartment syndrome is a hazard of the complex nature of musculoskeletal trauma that can occur even when a pulse is present and there is capillary refill (see Box 10.4).

Prevention of infection at skeletal pin sites

- The pin should be immobile in the bone and the insertion sites kept clean and free from infection. They may be dressed initially with sterile dressings around the pin and left open when dry.
- The pin ends are cleaned regularly with sterile applicators and a prescribed agent, and kept dry. Corks or adhesive covers are used to cover the sharp ends.
- The site is inspected regularly for signs of infection such as heat, redness, or oozing. Crusts and exudates are cleared from the tract to facilitate drainage and dressings applied as necessary. Be alert for pyrexia.

Maintaining normal body system functions

Traction with its accompanying degree of restriction on movement and positioning can create special problems and the following interventions are important:

- Work with the physiotherapist to coordinate and encourage breathing exercises and active and passive exercises to maintain joint mobility and prevent muscle wasting and deep vein thrombosis. In particular encourage regular dorsiflexion to counteract foot drop.
- Ensure adequate fluid intake (aim at over 2000 ml daily) and a balanced diet with plenty of fibre.
- Pay early attention to signs of constipation.

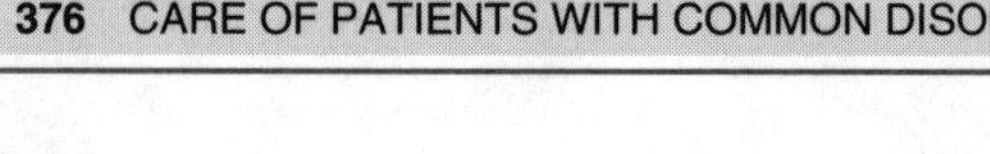

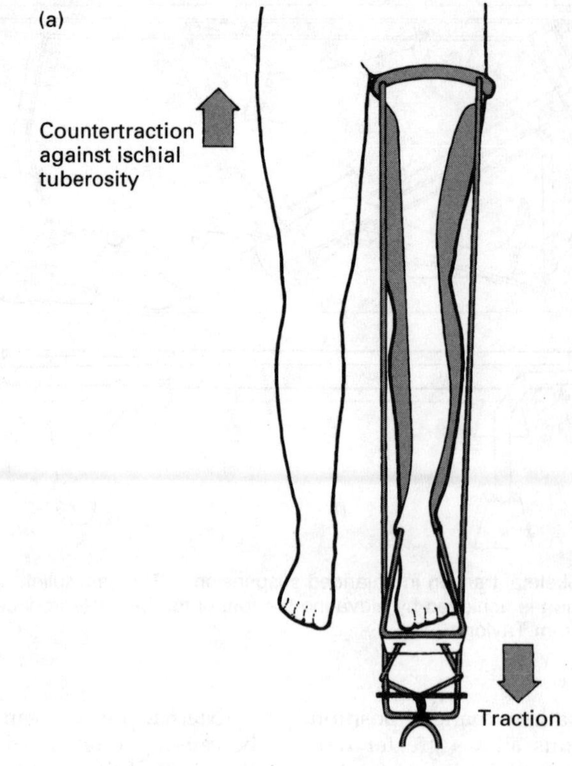

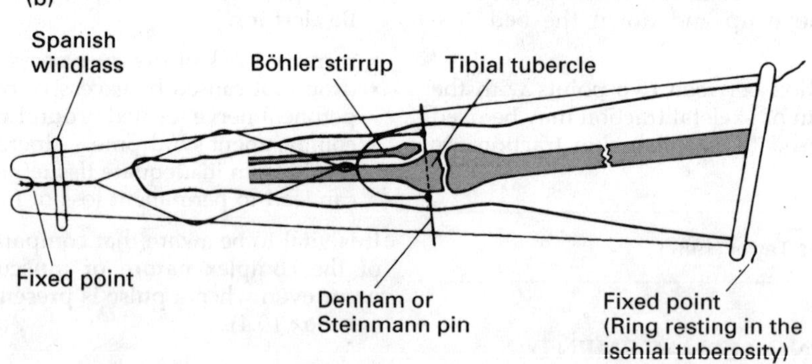

Fig. 10.6 (A) Fixed traction using skin traction and Thomas' splint. (B) Fixed traction using skeletal pin and Thomas' splint. (Reproduced with kind permission from Royle & Walsh 1992.)

- Awkwardness in using bed pans and urinals and fear of soiling the bed are dealt with sympathetically. Initially, adequate protective covering for the bed and appliances such as the leather ring of the Thomas splint will help to allay this anxiety.
- Normal sleep position and pattern will be disturbed and every attempt should be made to make the patient comfortable and relaxed before resorting to regular sedation.
- Often patients are in traction for a long time and will feel the need for close physical contact with their partners. Ensure undisturbed privacy for them.
- Boredom is a hazard of lengthy hospitalisation, particularly when movement is restricted.
- An issue that occurs more frequently on orthopaedic wards than others, because the patients are often young men and women, is that strong attraction develops between a patient and a nurse. If this becomes serious, it must be dealt with according to the Code of Professional Conduct (UKCC 1992). If the nurse is transferred to another ward, the relationship can continue normally.

?	**10.4** Discuss ways in which you can help relieve the boredom of a patient who is in traction. Which other health professionals could you call upon to help in this respect?
?	**10.5** Ask the physiotherapist in your clinical area to show you how to measure a patient for crutches and how to use them. Try this for yourself.
?	**10.6** How many different kinds of walking aids can you identify in your clinical area? Discuss each with the physiotherapist.

Casts

A cast is a splinting device consisting of layers of bandages impregnated with plaster of Paris (POP), fibreglass or resin, which are applied wet and solidify as they dry out. Their main uses are to immobilise and hold bone fragments in reduction and to support and stabilise weak joints.

Box 10.3 Application of skin traction

Skin traction can be applied using a ready prepared skin traction kit made of either elastoplast or of Ventfoam.

Elastoplast kit

First ensure that the patient is not allergic to tincture of benzoin compound by doing a patch test. Then prepare the skin carefully by shaving, drying gently and spraying with tincture of benzoin compound. This protects the skin and gives added adhesion. The elastoplast strips are then applied directly to the skin on either side of the injured limb with the spreader parallel to, and a few inches away from, the sole of the foot. The elastoplast is bandaged over with crepe bandages to give added strength. Pulleys are attached to the foot of the bed and ropes and weights attached; 15 kg is the maximum that can be applied without causing damage to the skin. The foot of the bed is elevated to provide traction counterbalance.

Ventfoam kit

Made of non-adhesive, soft foam padding this can be applied directly to the skin and held in position with a crepe bandage. It will take approximately 2–3 kg of weight and is often used as a method of pain relief for patients with fractured neck of femur or in paediatric fractures. It must be reapplied twice a day because of loss of bandage pressure.

There are different methods of application, and the manufacturer's instructions should be followed. The advantages and disadvantages of the main categories of casting types are summarised below.

Plaster of Paris. POP takes 48 hours to become completely dry; therefore no weight can be placed on the cast during this period. It requires several layers to ensure adequate strength; therefore it can become very heavy. POP is most commonly used for patients who have just received their injuries as it is relatively easy to mould into the shape of the limb and will, if well padded, allow for a certain amount of swelling before interfering with circulation and sensation. It is relatively inexpensive.

Synthetic casts. These casts are completely dry within 20 minutes and allow early weight bearing. They are stronger than POP due to the fibreglass content; thus, fewer layers are required and they are lighter. They do not allow for swelling and therefore should not be used immediately following trauma. Ideal use is in the older patient, allowing early mobilisation. A disadvantage is that they are more expensive than POP.

Cast bracing

All fractures of a long bone of the upper or lower limb can be immobilised in a cast brace to permit early mobilisation. Fractures of the shaft of femur may take 16 weeks or more to heal enough to permit weight bearing. However, in many cases once there is adequate callus visible on X-ray, a functional brace can be fitted and the length of time spent in traction can be reduced to about 6 weeks.

The top cast is applied snuggly to the femur and moulded carefully to the shape of the limb. Minimal padding is used — usually stockinette and a cast sock. The ischium will take the weight load. A cast is also applied to the lower part of the leg and may include the foot. The casts are joined by a set of hinges which can be left free or locked at the knee in various degrees of flexion (Dandy 1989, p. 126). The patient is encouraged to be mobile and fully weight bearing, initially with the help of a walking aid.

Advantages of using a cast brace include early mobilisation and discharge home, and immobilisation of the fracture site with free movement of the joints above and below.

Box 10.4 Impending compartment syndrome

Dialogue between student (S) and mentor (M):

S You've explained what compartment syndrome is but how do I know that it is actually happening, especially when I can still feel a pulse and the capillary refill appears to be normal?

M Well, the first thing to keep in mind is that there is always a possibility of it happening where there is fairly extensive musculoskeletal trauma and constricting devices or traction are in use. Also don't depend solely on observation of capillary refill and pulse — they can give a false sense of security. Obviously, degree of swelling, colour, pulse and capillary refill are very important and you may be able to feel a tight and tense muscle mass on palpation — but what the patient *feels* and can describe to you will be the deciding factor.

S I've noticed that you spend a lot of time talking to the patients about how things feel and really pursuing their answers — but what are the critical clues that you're looking for?

M I get red alerts when they describe deep throbbing pain and a persistent sensation of pressure or pain on stretch, or if they complain of abnormal sensations such as numbness, tingling, loss of sensation, increased sensitivity or weakness.

S How can we prevent compartment syndrome?

M Attention to all the basic principles of treatment such as correct tissue alignment, splinting the affected part but encouraging normal movement of other parts, elevation, keen and constant observation of neurovascular status, assessment of major nerve function such as in the peroneal, ulnar and median nerves, prompt action to relieve constriction from bandages, slings and plaster casts, educating the patient to detect adverse signs and symptoms and possibly anticipating fasciectomy, i.e. surgically opening the skin and fascia to allow the tissues to expand and relieve pressure.

S What action should we take if we suspect impending compartment syndrome?

M Report signs and symptoms immediately to a member of the surgical team and take any necessary nursing action, such as reassuring the patient, elevating and supporting the affected part, checking and possibly reapplying the traction, relieving the constriction and continuing to monitor changes. It is possible to measure tissue pressure with a direct needle measurement device — and anything above 30 mmHg needs action.

PRINCIPLES OF NURSING MANAGEMENT: CASTS

In addition to the general principles of nursing management for musculoskeletal injury (p. 373) the following will also apply.

Potential for neurovascular problems

Although padding such as Velband will allow for some swelling within the restricting cast, tissue pressure may build up and result in pain, tingling and discoloration. Pain is a valuable indicator that something is wrong and must never be masked by narcotics until it has been investigated and the cause ascertained. If not attended to immediately, pressure could lead to tissue necrosis and nerve palsy, signs and symptoms of which include severe pain, odour and discoloration on the cast.

Always be alert for signs of thromboembolic complications in patients with trauma and reduced mobility.

Prevention of neurovascular complications

- Elevate the limb above the level of the heart on cloth-covered pillows.
- Avoid denting a moist cast by handling it only with the palms of the hands and not allowing it to rest on a flat, hard or sharp surface. Use a bed board under the mattress to prevent sagging.
- Ensure that physiotherapy is carried out regularly.
- If signs and symptoms of neurovascular compromise do occur have plaster cutting equipment ready and bivalve the cast — that is split it down both sides into two halves. Spread it enough to relieve pressure and remember to cut the padding, which may have shrunk due to drying blood and exudates.
- An inspection and treatment window can be cut if pressure sore symptoms occur. The window must be replaced so that swelling does not rise into the space and cause more problems.

Care of the cast

Avoid getting the cast wet. Do not cover a leg plaster with plastic or rubber boots because of condensation. Teach the patient how to protect the cast when washing and when using bedpans and urinals. Casts can be cleaned by wiping with a damp cloth.

Many patients will go home wearing casts, so be sure to give them clear verbal and written instructions specific to their cast (for an example, see Box 10.5). Ensure that they can read English or provide a translation.

Removal of a cast

Application of a cast takes several experienced nurses or other health professionals, but all nurses need to be aware of the procedure for removal of a cast, to be familiar with the equipment used and to know where it is located.

Casts may need to be removed and renewed if they become too loose or are damaged in any way; and where serious signs and symptoms of neurovascular compromise have developed, bivalving may become an orthopaedic emergency. Guidelines for removal of a cast are given in Box 10.6.

Box 10.5 Advice to patient with hand to elbow plaster

The plaster holds all the broken bones firmly in place to allow them to heal in the correct position. To prevent your fingers swelling, support your arm in the sling provided during the day and on pillows at night. It is important that you exercise the finger, elbow and shoulder joints of your injured arm at regular intervals otherwise they will become stiff and painful to move.

The following exercises should be carried out at least four times each day:

- make a firm fist then stretch the fingers as wide as possible
- try to touch each fingertip with the thumb of that hand
- bend and stretch the elbow joint
- lift your arm high above your head — use the other arm to help
- move your arm behind your back as if you wanted to scratch between your shoulder blades.

Do not wet, heat or otherwise interfere with the plaster and do not insert sharp objects between the plaster and the skin to scratch — this could cause skin damage and infection.

Report to the doctor or the Accident and Emergency Department AT ONCE:

- if the plaster cracks, becomes loose, or uncomfortable
- if there is pain
- if the fingers become numb or difficult to move
- if the fingers become more swollen, blue or very pale
- if there is discharge
- if you have any other problems.

External fixation

With this kind of fixation the bone fragments are held in position by skeletal pins inserted into the bone on either side of the fracture and held in alignment by external rods (Dandy 1989, p. 126).

Box 10.6 Guidelines for removal of a cast

Equipment

- Plaster cutter — a small electric saw with a circular oscillating blade
- Plaster spreader
- Large flat-bladed bandage scissors
- Plaster shears
- Plaster knife.

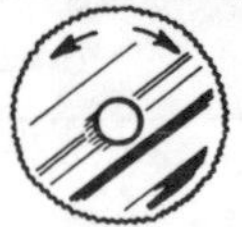

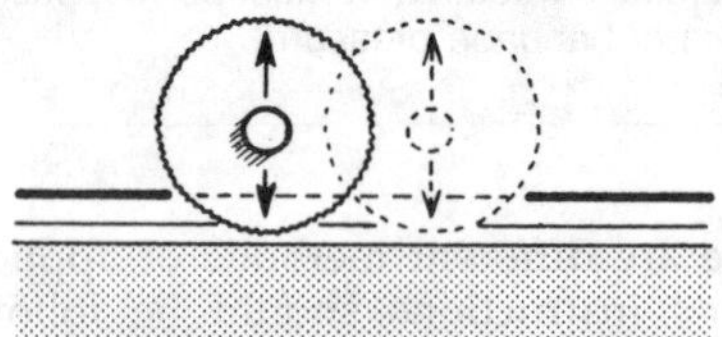

Procedure

- Explain to the patient what the procedure entails and if the cast is padded demonstrate the plaster cutter by turning it on and explaining its action (the electric cutter is not used on plasters that are not padded). Shears will be used on unpadded casts. Instruct the patient to shield his eyes as the saw could throw off fragments of plaster. Give reassurance that the saw will not cut the skin because of its oscillating action and the depth of padding.
- Mark where the cutting line will be with a felt pen and dampen it to reduce plaster dust. This line should avoid bony prominences; it is usually in front of the lateral malleolus and behind the medial malleolus in the lower limb and along the ulnar or flexor surface in the upper limb.
- Grasp the electric cutter.
- Rest the thumb on the cast to serve as a depth gauge and act as a guard.
- Turn on the cutter and push the blade firmly and gently through the cast, at the same time allowing the thumb to contact the cast as the blade oscillates. When you feel a 'give' or lack of resistance you know you are through.
- Lift the cutter blade up a degree but not out of the groove and repeat until the line of cut is complete. The movement is one of alternating pressure on the oscillating blade and lifting slightly, at right-angles to the plaster within the groove of cut. It is wise to get the 'feel' of this by practical experience with discarded plasters and then in actual practice under the guidance of an expert.
- Cut the cast down both sides.
- Insert the blades of the plaster spreader at several sites along the line of cut then separate the cast with the hands.
- Cut the padding with the bandage scissors.
- Lift the limb carefully out of the posterior portion of the cast maintaining the same position.
- After removal of the cast wash the skin gently with pure soap and water, pat dry and apply skin cream. Expect a scaly appearance, some muscle atrophy, pain and stiffness. Reassure the patient that prescribed exercise will help to regain normal feeling, appearance and function.

PRINCIPLES OF NURSING MANAGEMENT: EXTERNAL FIXATION

In addition to the general principles related to altered neurovascular status, positioning and potential for pin site infection that have already been stated, the following is specific to external fixation.

Appearance

The appearance of the appliance may cause the patient some concern. Full explanation and support in managing it will often help him to gain confidence. Early assisted weight bearing and mobilisation together with information about the beneficial effect this has in reducing the potential for complications will also reinforce a positive attitude.

Internal fixation

Fractures may also be stabilised by open surgical intervention where various nails, wires, screws and rods hold the bone fragments in place (Fig. 10.7). Again this permits earlier mobilisation and reduces the potential for complications. All perioperative principles of nursing management apply in this instance. See Ch. 27.

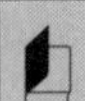

For further information, see Dandy (1989).

FRACTURES OF SPECIFIC SITES

Fracture of the femoral shaft

Femoral shaft fractures are most commonly seen in young men following motorcycle or car accidents.

MEDICAL MANAGEMENT

Following X-ray to confirm the diagnosis:

- The fracture may be reduced under general anaesthetic and skeletal traction applied. Any accompanying wounds are debrided or sutured at the same time. If there is adequate callus formation within 2–6 weeks a cast brace may be applied.
- Operative treatment may consist of either external or internal fixation as described earlier.
- Blood samples will be taken for cross-matching and repeated at regular intervals throughout hospitalisation for blood gas analysis.

NURSING PRIORITIES AND MANAGEMENT: FRACTURE OF THE FEMORAL SHAFT

In addition to the principles of management relating to fracture, traction and operative intervention the following are specific to fracture of the shaft of femur.

Haemorrhage. An early complication may be damage to the femoral artery from bone fragments, in addition to bleeding from other damaged tissues and bone marrow. As much as a litre of blood can be contained within the thigh, and this hidden haemorrhage can result in hypovolaemic shock (see Fig. 10.8 and Ch. 18).

Be alert for signs of haemorrhage and shock and ensure that intravenous replacement therapy is ready and that blood is sent for cross-matching.

Fat emboli. Fat emboli are a particular hazard following fracture of the shaft of the femur but can occur following fracture of any long bone. There are two theories relating to the cause. One is that fat cells from damaged tissue migrate into ruptured veins. The second is that catecholamines released through the stress of trauma mobilise lipids from fatty tissue. In the lung these droplets are converted into free fatty acids which are toxic to lung tissue and disrupt alveolar function. Additionally, the droplets may become enmeshed in the capillary network of the alveoli and disrupt gas exchange. This can lead to cerebral hypoxia and, if large vessels in the pulmonary system

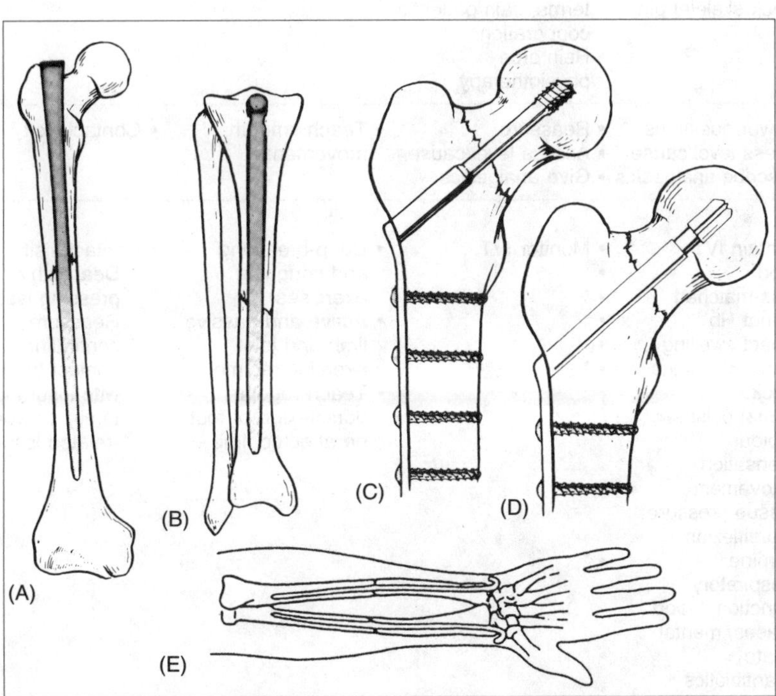

Fig. 10.7 Types of internal fixation. (A) and (B) Intramedullary nails. (C) Compression nail for fixation of femoral neck. (D) Sliding nail fixation of the femoral neck. (E) Rush nails to radius and ulna. (Reproduced with kind permission from Dandy 1989.)

are involved, respiratory failure and death. Early signs of fatty emboli are increased respiratory rate, anxiety, transient petechial haemorrhage and confusion. The latter two are the classic and most important clinical signs.

Be alert for early signs of altered mental status — anxiety, irritability and especially confusion. Report this immediately and be prepared to deal with respiratory failure and arrest and to transfer the patient to intensive care. Have equipment ready for blood gas analysis.

Collaborative care

The contributions of different health professionals to the care of a patient with fracture of the femoral shaft are summarised in Table 10.1 The nurse has an important role in coordinating the care provided.

?	**10.7** Complete Table 10.1, giving the rationale for your interventions. Say how you would evaluate them. You may refer to the text.

Fracture of neck of femur

Fracture of the neck of the femur is a fairly common injury especially in elderly women with osteoporosis. It may be associated with a fall or may be purely pathological.

MEDICAL MANAGEMENT

History and examination. The patient may have been found on the floor following a fall and, if living alone, could have been there for some time and be suffering from hypothermia and dehydration. She will complain of severe pain in the hip or knee with visible shortening and external rotation. Diagnosis will be confirmed by X-ray.

Treatment. Depending on the site of the fracture, and the age and condition of the patient, the treatment will be either internal fixation with a plate and screws or replacement of the head of femur with a metal prosthesis. Intracapsular fractures high in the neck of the femur have a serious effect on the blood supply to the femur head (Fig. 10.8) and would certainly need operative replacement. The general condition of some patients will dictate that they be treated conservatively with 10–12 weeks in traction.

NURSING PRIORITIES AND MANAGEMENT: FRACTURE OF NECK OF FEMUR

In addition to the general principles relating to musculoskeletal injury and fractures, the following priorities need to be addressed.

Complications. As a result of age and general physical condition when found, the patient will probably be confused and fearful and need a great deal of comfort and reassurance.

Table 10.1 Collaborative care of 18-year-old man with closed, comminuted fracture of femoral shaft that has been reduced under general anaesthetic

Problem focus	Surgical	Nursing	Physiotherapy	Social work	Occupational therapy
Maintain reduction and alignment of fractured left femoral shaft Balanced, sliding skeletal traction Steinmann tibial pin 6 kg weight	• X-ray Check reduction alignment • Check traction equipment — adjust weight p. r. n. • Check skeletal pin	• Assist radiographer • Reassure patient • Monitor and maintain traction • Explain principles and aims in lay terms, gain patient's cooperation • Reinforce physiotherapy	• Explain and demonstrate safe movements within limits of traction apparatus		
Pain/anxiety	• Answer questions • Assess level/cause • Prescribe analgesics	• Reassure • Assess level/cause • Give analgesics	• Teach smooth movements	• Contact visit	
Prevent complications • Shock • Further haemorrhage into thigh • Neurovascular compromise (compartment syndrome) • Cardiopulmonary complications (Pulmonary embolus, fat embolus) • Infection	 • Maintain IVT • Blood cross-matched • Repeat Hb • Inspect swelling • Check vital signs • Check: distal pulses colour sensation movement tissue pressure dorsiflexion • Examine: respiratory function, blood gases, mental state • I.v. antibiotics	 • Monitor IVT • * • * • * • * • * • * • *	 • Deep-breathing and coughing exercises • Active and passive limb and joint exercise regime • Teach regular dorsiflexion of foot on affected limb	 • Contact visit Deal with pressing issues Reassure continuing contact to deal with insurance, family or work -related issues	 Admission noted — to visit when acute symptoms resolve

*See Question 10.7.

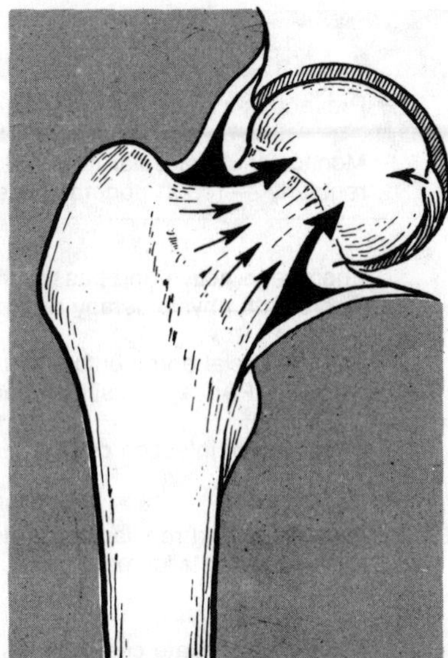

Fig. 10.8 Blood supply of the femoral head via the capsule, intramedullary vessels and ligamentum teres. (Reproduced with kind permission from Dandy 1989.)

Measures will be taken to reverse hypothermia and dehydration. Vital signs will be monitored at 4-hourly intervals to detect early signs of complications.

Pain. There is often extensive bruising which adds to the severe pain. When the cause has been established, this may be treated by re-positioning and supporting the body and limbs, and administering prescribed analgesics.

Increased risk of multisystem complications. For an elderly patient in long-term traction there is a high risk of complications developing in all body systems, especially the cardiopulmonary system, and all nursing measures should be taken to prevent these. The patient's risk rating for pressure sores is also very high.

Fracture of the tibia and fibula

Fracture of the tibia and fibula is one of the most common injuries dealt with by orthopaedic surgeons. This fracture usually results from direct violence to the limb and extensive skin and soft tissue damage may be present. Road traffic accidents and sports injuries are a common cause.

MEDICAL MANAGEMENT

Treatment. There are three choices of treatment.

Cast immobilisation. This is the treatment of choice for closed stable injuries. If the fracture requires manipulation, the patient will receive a general anaesthetic which will necessitate a stay in hospital, otherwise they may be discharged home from the A & E department. Following reduction of the fracture, a long leg plaster cast will be applied and plain radiographs taken to confirm the position of the fracture. Repeat X-rays will be taken at 1 week, 2 weeks and then at monthly intervals following reduction. The patient will not be allowed to bear weight on the injured leg for at least 1 month following injury. At this point in time a Sarmiento-type plaster (patellar tendon bearing) will be applied and the patient allowed to take weight through the injured limb. The average length of stay in plaster for this type of injury is 12–16 weeks.

Internal fixation. Fractures which are closed but unstable will benefit from internal fixation using a plate and screws. The patient will be placed in a plaster cast for 6–8 weeks following surgery. Routine postoperative care as discussed in Chapter 27, and cast care (see p. 377) will be required. The patient will be mobilised on crutches once fully recovered from the effects of surgery.

External fixation. If there is skin loss or an infected wound at the fracture site, the choice of treatment is commonly an external fixator. This enables frequent observation of the wound and easy access for wound dressing changes. An external fixator is applied under a general anaesthetic in an operating theatre.

This type of fixator is not as rigid as internal fixation but the patient can be mobilised without bearing weight on the injured limb, and discharged home to allow the community nurse and general practitioner to attend to the wound. The patient would be reviewed at regular intervals at the outpatient clinic (see Case History 10.1).

NURSING PRIORITIES AND MANAGEMENT: FRACTURE OF THE TIBIA AND FIBULA

The principles of nursing management for each type of treatment are given on pp. 377, 378 and 379.

Case History 10.1 Mr K

Mr K is a 40-year-old man who lives alone. He sustained a compound fracture to his left tibia and fibula while skiing with friends in the Highlands of Scotland. One friend stayed with him on the mountain side while the other alerted the emergency services, who arrived within an hour. The paramedical team applied a clean dressing over the open wound and splinted his leg.

On arrival at the hospital, Mr K was in obvious pain although he had been using the analgesic gas Entonox, so the doctor administered intravenous analgesia.

In the A & E department, his named nurse, Bill, noted his temperature, pulse, blood pressure and respirations, all of which were within normal limits. A clean sterile dressing was applied to the wound following inspection by the doctor.

Confirmation of the diagnosis was made by radiography and it was decided to take Mr K to the operating theatre for application of an external fixator to his left leg. This was explained to him and a picture of an external fixator in position was shown to him and the two friends who had accompanied him. His first reaction was revulsion at all the metal, pins and scaffolding, but as his friends joked about his 'bionic parts' his anxiety subsided.

After an uneventful postoperative period, Mr K was allowed to sit in an armchair on day 1 with his leg elevated on a stool to reduce the swelling. The wound had been dressed in theatre and a moisture-retaining dressing applied. The pin sites were dressed with non-adherent dressings. The physiotherapist gradually mobilised Ken to walk with the help of crutches without bearing weight on his left leg, and showed him how to manage the awkward appliance to avoid injuring himself. He was helped to widen two pairs of trousers below the knee so that he could cover the external fixator.

As Mr K lived on his own, the social worker made arrangements for a home help to be provided on discharge. His two friends agreed to visit him and provide him with food and other provisions at the weekends.

The nurse contacted the community nurse attached to Mr K's GP practice with information on the treatment he had received and the proposed date for discharge. Written confirmation of these details was given to Mr K to pass on to the community nurse. He was discharged home 6 days after his accident with a return appointment for 2 weeks later.

Table 10.2 Prevention of complications of fractures

Complication	Cause	Prevention
Damage to soft tissue — neurovascular compromise	Trauma Sharp fragments/edge of bone	Monitor neurovascular function regularly — report abnormalities
Complications associated with immobility		
Diminished function of all body systems	Decreased physical stimulation	Encourage active and passive exercise
Muscle atrophy — decreased range of movement — contractures	Lack of normal exercise	Coordinate physiotherapy programme
Altered psychological processes	Decreased social stimulation	Provide social and mental stimulation
Pressure sores	Casts — prolonged pressure	Regulate PAC and position change
Infection	Open wound postoperatively Skeletal pin sites	Principles of infection control
Mal-union	Mal-apposition of bony fragments Inadequate mobilisation (e.g. swelling subsides — cast becomes loose)	Meticulous and regular monitoring of cast fit and traction alignment
Delayed union	Unstable fracture Poor blood supply	Maintain adequate circulation and splintage
Non-union	Infection Soft tissue intrusion	Infection control
Fat embolus — emergency	Fat globules released into circulation from bone marrow at fracture site — usually associated with fractured femur or multiple fractures	Early reduction and splintage Report confusion, chest pain, dyspnoea immediately. See p. 379
Osteoarthritis	Extension of fracture into joint surface	Early physiotherapy

? **10.8** Jot down the complications associated with fractures. Discuss with colleagues the causes of each complication and say how you can prevent it. Then check your findings with Table 10.2.

Fracture of neck of humerus

Fracture of the neck of the humerus commonly occurs in adults after a fall on an outstretched hand. Often it is not displaced or badly impacted and normally heals well depending on its stability.

MEDICAL MANAGEMENT

Treatment. This injury can usually be treated at home following the initial visit to the A & E department providing there is no gross displacement or neurovascular complications. The arm is supported in a broad arm sling or collar'n'cuff for approximately 2 weeks. Movement is gradually introduced followed by outpatient physiotherapy in order to avoid the major complication which is development of a stiff shoulder joint.

NURSING PRIORITIES AND MANAGEMENT: FRACTURE OF NECK OF HUMERUS

Assessment of ability to carry out normal activities of daily living. This is made before the patient is disharged home from the A & E department. Home nursing and home help are arranged accordingly.

Skin care of injured arm. It is wise to have the community nurse attend to washing the injured arm two or three times a week taking particular care of the axilla. The sling is reapplied and neurovascular status and degree of mobility monitored. Case History 10.2 outlines the continuing care of an elderly lady with fractured neck of humerus.

Case History 10.2 Mrs L

Mrs L is a 70-year-old lady, living alone in sheltered housing. She was admitted to hospital overnight following treatment for fractured neck of humerus. As the evening progressed she became more steady when walking, obviously recovering from the initial shock of her fall. Oral analgesia was given for pain relief. When in bed, she found the most comfortable position was sitting up, well supported with pillows. The following day she was discharged with arrangements having been made for a community nurse to call to see her. The social worker had arranged for twice-weekly home help and meals on wheels three times a week.

When the community nurse called, she washed and dried the skin around Mrs L's injured shoulder, inspecting it for any signs of friction or pressure. Extensive bruising was noted all over the shoulder region. The broad arm sling was reapplied. The nurse checked that Mrs L was moving her joints as instructed and that no joint stiffness was present. On identifying where Mrs L had slipped, the nurse found a bath mat lying over a shiny floor covering in the toilet. She advised Mrs L to remove the mat in order to reduce the chance of further accidents, and suggested a non-slip mat for the base of the bath. She checked whether Mrs L needed a further prescription for the analgesic and arranged to call on alternate days.

Mrs L was to attend the hospital outpatient department 10 days later when she would be seen by an orthopaedic specialist. Her GP would then be contacted to arrange physiotherapy at her local health centre.

?	**10.9** After initial instruction from your tutor or mentor and using a fellow student, practise applying a broad arm sling, a high sling and a collar'n'cuff.

Colles' fracture

This is one of the most common fractures seen at the A & E department and is often found in elderly women after a fall on an outstretched hand. It usually involves the lower end of the radius within 2.5 cm of the wrist joint and may have an associated fracture of the ulnar styloid. The obvious feature of a Colles' fracture is the classic 'dinner fork' deformity (Fig. 10.9).

MEDICAL MANAGEMENT

Examination. Diagnosis will be confirmed by the appearance of the patient's wrist and by plain X-rays.

Treatment. A regional anaesthetic is advisable in order to reduce the fracture. A Bier's block is usually performed and as this involves a degree of risk of reactive cardiac arrest it must only be performed where resuscitation facilities are available. The patient is fasted in case the nerve block is unsuccessful and a general anaesthetic is needed.

Prevention. This fracture is more often seen in the winter months, and elderly people should be advised to avoid slippery surfaces.

NURSING PRIORITIES AND MANAGEMENT: COLLES' FRACTURE

In addition to the management principles already discussed which relate to musculoskeletal trauma, fractures and plaster casts, the following priorities should be noted.

Removal of rings. Marked swelling of the fingers is likely to occur and it is important to remove all rings and bracelets from the injured hand as soon as possible. If swelling has already made this impossible it will be necessary to get the patient's permission to cut the rings off using the special ring cutter found in all A & E departments.

The arm should be kept elevated to reduce swelling.

Splinting. Following successful reduction, a POP back (dorsal) slab is applied and will be completed when the swelling has subsided — usually in about a week's time.

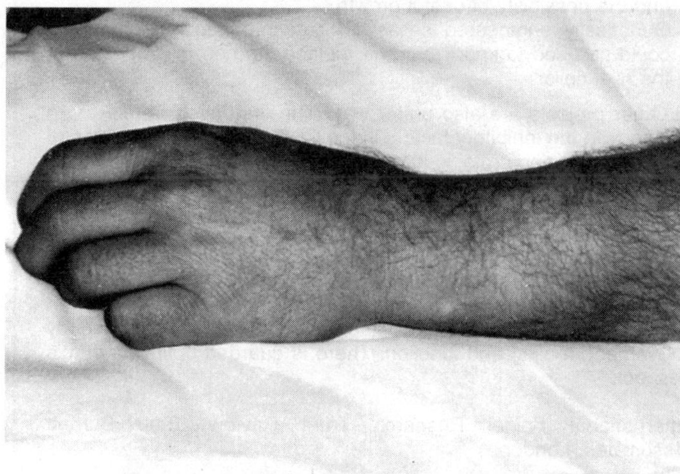

Fig. 10.9 The 'dinner fork' deformity of Colles' fracture. (Reproduced with kind permission from Dandy 1989.)

Advice. Ensure that the patient is given written and verbal advice as for 'Advice to patient with hand to elbow plaster' (see Box 10.5).

Fracture of the clavicle

This fracture is given brief mention because it is a common sporting injury (see Fig. 10.10).

NURSING PRIORITIES AND MANAGEMENT: FRACTURE OF THE CLAVICLE

Treatment is usually managed at home and the GP practice and community nurse will be called upon to assist with hygiene to the axilla and regular reapplication of the figure-of-eight bandage (Fig. 10.11) or special shoulder brace and arm support. The aim is to maintain comfortable alignment and supervise exercise of distal joints.

SPINAL INJURIES

PATHOPHYSIOLOGY

Fracture, dislocation, whiplash or any other injury to the spine is potentially serious because of the danger of injury to the spinal cord.

The main causes of spinal injury are motor vehicle, motorcycle and sporting accidents. However, inflammatory and degenerative disease, pathological conditions such as metastatic disease, and also poor surgery can result in spinal trauma. The resultant damage can involve compression, contusion, laceration or interference with blood supply to the spinal cord, accompanied by varying degrees of paralysis and sensory deficit below the level of the lesion. In some cases the paraplegia or quadriplegia that results is permanent because of the inability of the adult spinal cord to regenerate, although recent research indicates that there is room for guarded optimism in this respect (see Research Abstract 10.1).

Injury to the spine and surrounding structures need not always involve spinal cord damage; in many instances damage can be prevented by correct handling. The basic principles are to suspect spinal injury until proven otherwise, and to maintain anatomical alignment and immobilise the spine immediately.

MEDICAL MANAGEMENT

Management of spinal injury is critical throughout, with immediate immobilisation, early reduction and stabilisation, full assessment of the extent of the injury and its consequences, and ongoing specialist treatment and rehabilitation. For this reason, following initial treatment in the receiving A & E department, it is vital to get the patient to a spinal injuries or neurology unit as soon as possible.

Refer to Chapter 28 for reception and handling of the patient in the A & E department.

Investigations. History, loss of function and sensation, X-rays and CAT scans will confirm the diagnosis and indicate the extent of the injury. (See Fig.10.12.)

Treatment. Treatment depends on the type and level of injury and whether or not there is spinal cord involvement. (See Fig.10.13.)

Some types of fractures are amenable to reduction and stabilisation by either traction or open surgical reduction and fixation and others by positioning and rest.

Cervical spine fractures or dislocations are often treated with skeletal traction attached to the skull by Crutchfield or Gardner–Wells tongs or a halo device or halter (see Fig. 10.14).

The damage that can be done following injury in which the spinal ligaments are torn or stretched should never be underestimated as this can leave a potentially dangerous unstable spine. Cervical whiplash injury is a prime example of this (see Fig. 10.15).

Some fractures, especially lower thoracic and lumbar fractures, can be treated by bed rest on a firm base.

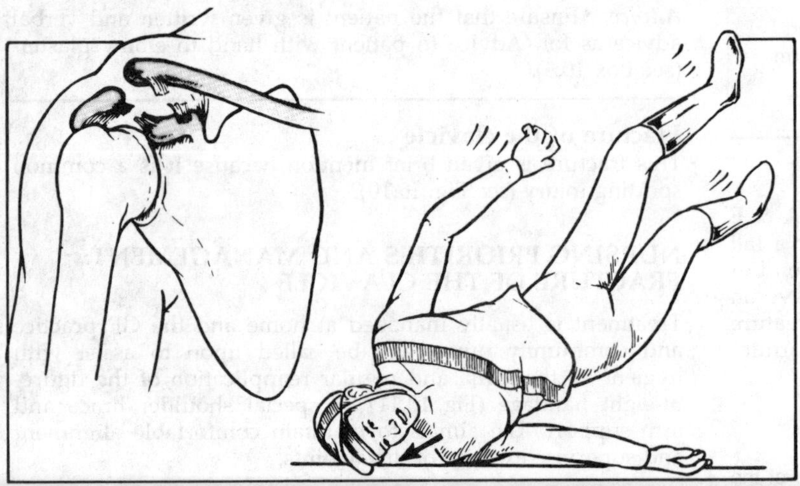

Fig. 10.10 Fracture of the acromioclavicular joint. (Reproduced with kind permission from Dandy 1989.)

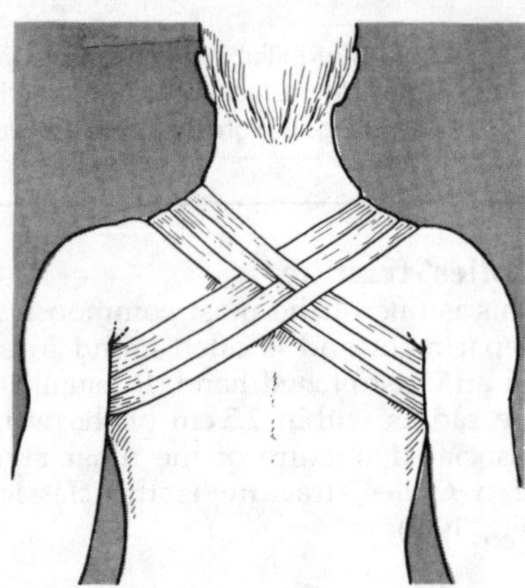

Fig. 10.11 Figure-of-eight bandage for fractured clavicle. (Reproduced with kind permission from Dandy 1989.)

NURSING PRIORITIES AND MANAGEMENT: SPINAL INJURIES

In addition to principles of nursing management for musculoskeletal disorders, traction and perioperative care, the following specific points are of importance here.

First aid. Knowledge and application of the basic principles of first aid for spinal injuries is essential in many areas of nursing practice.

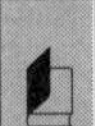

First aid manual: the authorised manual of St John's Ambulance, St Andrew's Ambulance Association, the British Red Cross Society 1992 Dorling Kindersley, London

Additionally, nurses in the community have the opportunity to teach the general public these same principles of management in order to prevent the potentially serious consequences of spinal cord injury (see Box 10.7).

? **10.10** What do you suspect are the main reasons for such a different outcome for the accident victims described in Box 10.7?

Basic principles of positioning and moving patients with spinal injury. As indicated earlier it is vital to maintain anatomical alignment and fracture reduction. Manoeuvres such as log rolling the patient, using special frames such as

Research Abstract 10.1 International spinal research

Until recently it was thought that damaged spinal cord nerves, unlike peripheral nerves, could not regenerate. A report from the International Spinal Research Trust (ISRT), however, gives new hope that it may eventually be possible to overcome the hostile conditions preventing regrowth and provide conditions that encourage it (ISRT 1993).

It is known that the mechanism that gives foetal CNS cells the ability to grow long connecting fibres is weakened in adult CNS cells and although injured adult nerves sprout new fibres they lack the ability to continue this growth over a distance long enough to repair the lesion.

Researchers have isolated two kinds of glial cells that act to block the regenerative process:

- oligodendrocytes, which form the insulating sheath
- astrocytes, which form almost impenetrable scarring at the site of the injury.

By introducing CNS nerve fibres into a culture medium that contains a high density of astrocytes and that behaves in a similar way to glial scarring, several factors involved in blocking regrowth have been defined and are influencing the direction of research:

- Whereas adult nerve cells sprouted but soon lost impetus, embryonic nerve cells continued to grow strongly through the glial tissue. This suggested that an alternative to disarming astrocytes may be to implant embryonic nerve cells to help the repair process.
- Growing nerve fibres produce enzymes to break down proteins and make a pathway through the hostile CNS tissue. The balance of enzyme and inhibitory proteins can be altered by using nerve-growth factors, thus increasing the permeability of the glial tissue and the possibility of useful growth.
- Genetically engineered cells with growth-enhancing properties could be used to knock out and replace the hostile properties of the glial cells.

Other projects are also under way. The first involves use of an antibody to the inhibitory factors in the CNS, and another the use of growth-enhancing proteins identified within the body and able to be reproduced in the laboratory. By combining these two approaches in the laboratory it is possible to get some adult CNS nerve fibres to grow over a long distance.

Eventually a combination of several of these research findings should bring success in the actual repair process of the adult spinal cord. The task will then be to find out whether these fibres can successfully reactivate appropriate target areas to restore body movement, feeling and function. There is guarded optimism in this respect.

International Spinal Research Trust Review 1993 Burnett Associates, London

THE SPINEX CARD

SPINAL CORD INJURY CARD

THE LEVEL AT WHICH SENSATION IS ALTERED OR ABSENT IS THE LEVEL OF INJURY

IT IS VITAL TO CARRY OUT MOTOR AS WELL AS SENSORY EXAMS AS THE PATIENT MAY HAVE MOTOR DAMAGE WITHOUT SENSORY DAMAGE AND VICE VERSA

SENSORY EXAMINATION

1 EXAMINE BY:
A. Light touch.
B. Response to pain.

2 USE:
The forehead as your guide to what is normal sensation.

3 EXAMINE:
A. Upper limbs and hands.
B. Lower limbs and feet.

4 EXAMINE;
Both sides.

5 T.4 EXAMINATION:
Must be carried out in the MID-AXILLARY lines, NOT the MID-CLAVICULAR line, as C2, C3 and C4 all supply sensation to the nipple line.

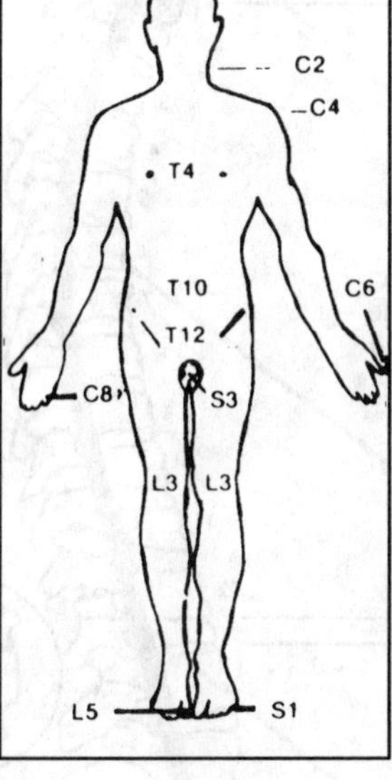

IT IS IMPORTANT TO CARRY OUT ALL OF THE ABOVE AS A VARIETY OF SENSORY CHANGES MAY OCCUR

Sponsored by: COBURG LIONS & A.S.M.
Supplied by: BROADMEADOWS BRANCH A.S.M.
Thanks to: Dr J. TOSCANO

MOTOR EXAMINATION

THE LEVEL AT WHICH WEAKNESS OR ABSENT MOVEMENT IS NOTED IS THE LEVEL OF INJURY

MOTOR EXAMINATION: EXAMINE BOTH SIDES

UPPER LIMB MOTOR EXAM	LOWER LIMB MOTOR EXAM
ASK PATIENT TO:	ASK PATIENT TO:
A Shrug Shoulders =C4	A Flex Hip =L1 & L2
B Bend the Elbow =C5	B Extend Knee =L3
C Push Wrist back =C6	C Pull Foot up =L4
D Open/Close Hands=C8	D Push Foot down =L5 & S1

THORACIC AND ABDOMINAL MOTOR EXAMINATION
LOOK FOR ACTIVITY OF INTERCOSTAL AND ABDOMINAL MUSCLES

DIAGNOSIS OF SPINAL CORD INJURY IN THE UNCONSCIOUS PATIENT

A Look for paradoxical respiration (a Quad has lost intercostal muscles so he relies on the diaphragm to breathe).

B Flaccid limbs.

C Loss of response to painful stimuli below the level of the lesion.

D Loss of reflexes below level of lesion.

E Erection in the unconscious male.

F Low B.P. (systolic Less than 100) associated with a normal pulse or bradycardia indicates Pt. may be QUADRIPLEGIC.

IF YOU DON'T THINK ABOUT A SPINAL CORD INJURY YOU WILL MISS IT!!!

TREATMENT:

1 A.B.C.
2 Immobilise injured part.
3 Lift Pt. in one piece in position found.
4 Don't move patient too many times.

Fig. 10.12 The Spinex card. (Reproduced with kind permission from Toscano 1988.)

the Stryker and electric turning beds are best initially practised under expert guidance.

Spinal shock. Be aware of the phenomenon of spinal shock, which is a response to sudden loss of continuity between the spinal cord and higher centres of the brain caused by trauma to the spine. This involves a complete loss of all motor, sensory, reflex, and autonomic activity below the level of the lesion whatever the actual damage consists of. Main features involve falling blood pressure, paralysis below the level of the injury and of bladder and bowel function. It can therefore be life threatening especially in cervical spine injury where respiratory function is compromised. It is temporary but may last for weeks. Refer to Chapter 18 for further details and management of shock.

Autonomic dysreflexia. This is a potentially dangerous syndrome in paralysed patients (both recent and long-term) where there is a sudden and exaggerated autonomic response to stimuli such as a distended bladder or bowel, catheter manipulation or unexpected skin stimulation. Arterial blood pressure can be instantly elevated to a critical level. It is characterised by a severe headache, profuse sweating, bradycardia, severe hypertension and flushing of the skin above the level of injury.

Management. This is an emergency. Alert the medical team

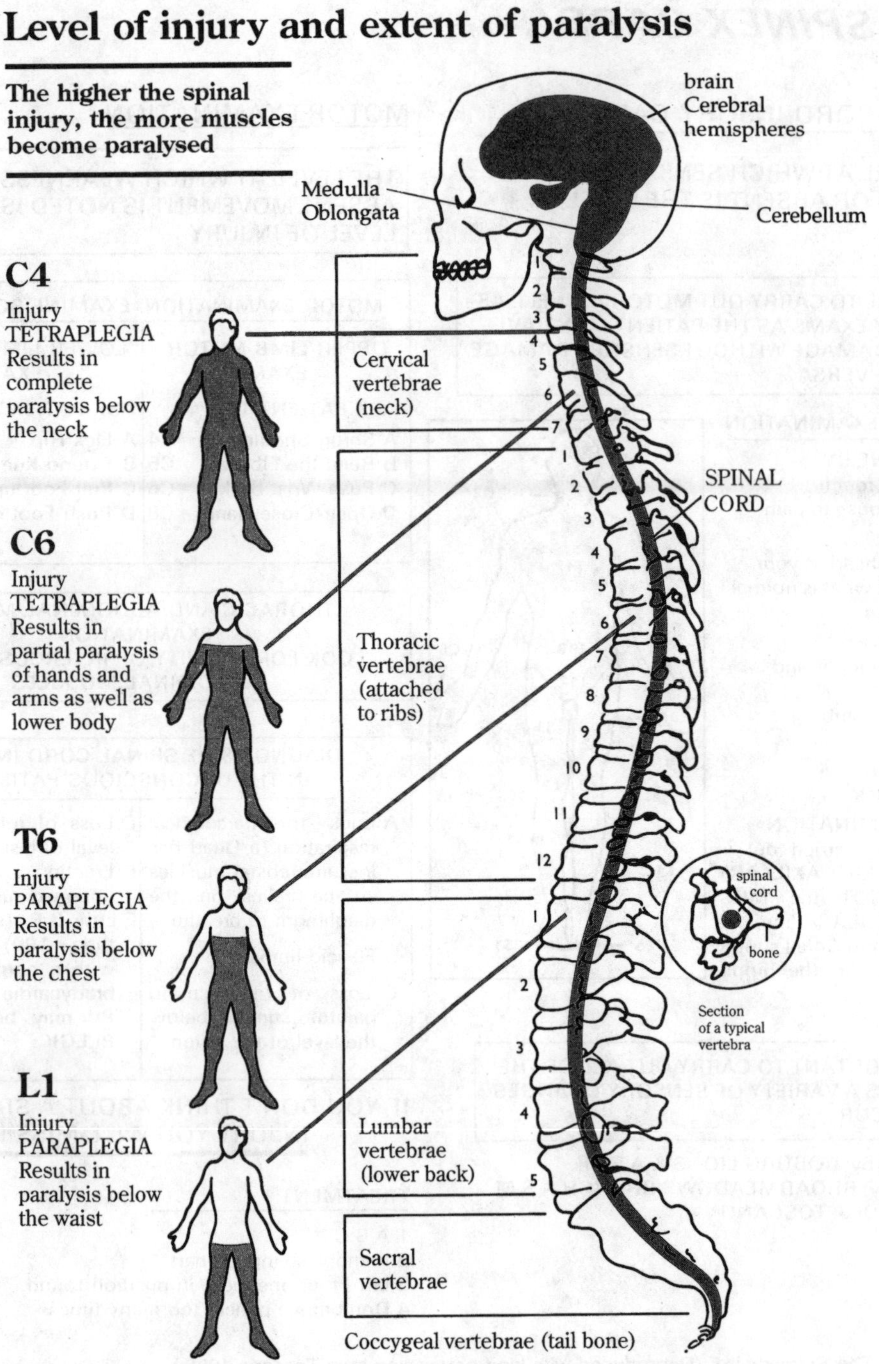

Level of injury and extent of paralysis

The higher the spinal injury, the more muscles become paralysed

C4 Injury TETRAPLEGIA Results in complete paralysis below the neck

C6 Injury TETRAPLEGIA Results in partial paralysis of hands and arms as well as lower body

T6 Injury PARAPLEGIA Results in paralysis below the chest

L1 Injury PARAPLEGIA Results in paralysis below the waist

Cervical vertebrae (neck)

Thoracic vertebrae (attached to ribs)

Lumbar vertebrae (lower back)

Sacral vertebrae

Coccygeal vertebrae (tail bone)

brain Cerebral hemispheres

Medulla Oblongata

Cerebellum

SPINAL CORD

spinal cord

bone

Section of a typical vertebra

Fig. 10.13 Level of injury and extent of paralysis. (Reproduced with kind permission from the Spinal Injuries Association 1993.)

immediately. Elevate the head of the bed to 45° unless contraindicated (the aim is to reduce blood flow to the head). Remove the triggering stimulus if known. Monitor vital signs and note the trigger to try to avoid repetition of the episode. Intravenous hypotensive drugs may be administered.

Adaptation to paraplegia or quadriplegia. This adaptation is particularly long and painful for most people especially if they are young. The International Spinal Research Trust publishes reports and newsletters which often include in-depth perspectives of how different people learn to cope.

> ? **10.11** You are a community nurse responsible for health education classes. Outline the key points you would cover in a teaching session relating to first aid in spinal injury.

BONE TUMOURS

A satisfactory classification of primary bone tumours is difficult to achieve. A bone tumour can consist of many different

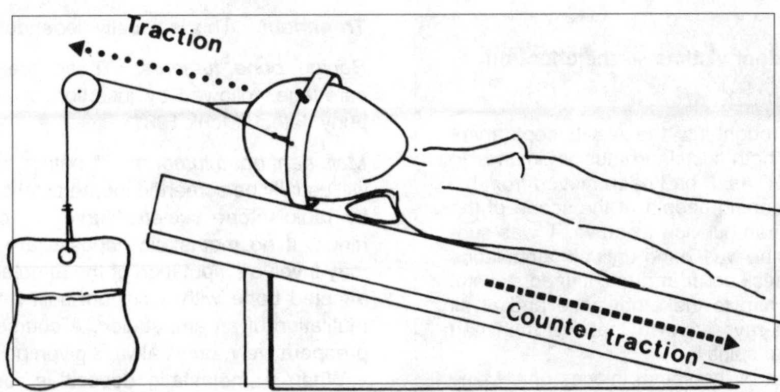

Fig. 10.14 Balanced skeletal traction. Traction is exerted on the cervical spine by means of a halo and pin fixation to the outer table of the skull. Countertraction is achieved by the patient's body weight and gravity when the end of the bed is raised. (Reproduced with kind permission from Taylor 1990.)

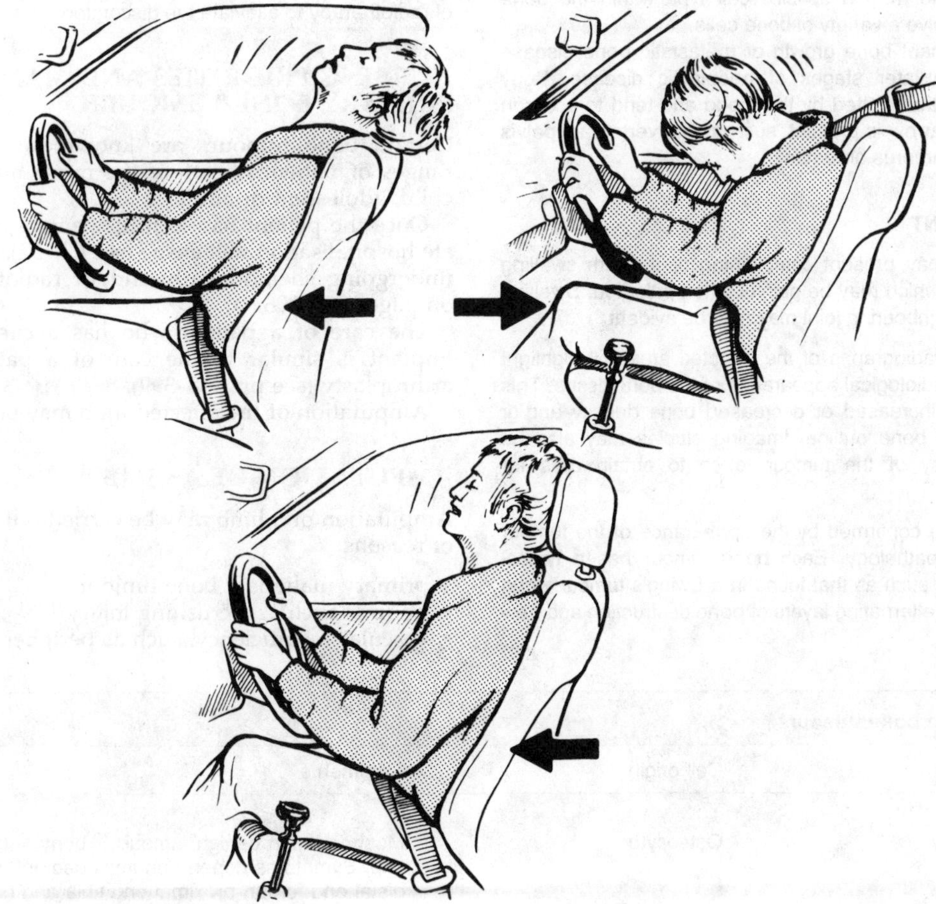

Fig. 10.15 Combined flexion/extension (whiplash) injury of the cervical spine. Movement of the head is limited by a head restraint. (Reproduced with kind permission from Dandy 1989.)

cells; therefore classification by the original cell type may not be accurate. However, separating the tumours into benign and malignant categories can be helpful, providing one is aware that benign tumours can undergo a cell change and become malignant (see Table 10.3).

Metastatic bone disease is malignant bone disease due to secondary deposits in bone tissue from a primary neoplastic site elsewhere. (See Ch. 32.)

PATHOPHYSIOLOGY

Primary bone tumours are known to occur in specific age groups and certain sites of bone tissue. Osteosarcoma, for example, is rarely seen after the age of 20 years and usually occurs in the metaphyseal region of the lower end of the femur, upper end of the tibia and upper end of the humerus.

As the bone tumour grows, eruption into the surrounding tissue can

Box 10.7 First-aid for accident victims — the effect on outcome

Two 18-year-old men were brought into the A & E department on the same night. They had both sustained multiple injuries to the head and body in similar RTAs. P had been moved from his overturned vehicle by well-meaning people at the scene of the accident whilst waiting for the ambulance to arrive. T was supported in the position in which he was found until the ambulance men arrived. They applied a neck collar and maintained skeletal alignment whilst transferring him to the ambulance and at all times subsequently. Spinal X-rays showed that the men had identical injuries to the cervical spine.

2 months later T walked out of the spinal injuries unit. Many months later P was wheeled out of the same unit as a quadriplegic.

occur, which may be noted as a warm swelling of the affected area. The tumour will originate from a specific cell type within the bone tissue, but may then involve a variety of bone cells.

The secondary malignant bone growth of metastatic bone disease normally occurs in the later stages of neoplastic disease. Bony metastases are usually transmitted by the blood and tend to occur in sites where red bone marrow is present, such as the vertebrae, pelvis and upper ends of the humerus or femur.

MEDICAL MANAGEMENT

History. The patient may present complaining of a warm swelling over the affected bone, which may be painful when palpated. Swelling and restriction of the neighbouring joint may also be evident.

Investigations. Plain radiographs of the affected area will highlight changes in the normal radiological appearance of the bone tissue. This may be in the form of increased or decreased bone density and/or distortion of the normal bone outline. Imaging studies may also be performed and a biopsy of the tumour taken to obtain cells for examination.

Diagnosis. This will be confirmed by the appearance of the tumour on X-ray and positive pathology. Each bone tumour has a typical radiological appearance, such as that found in a Ewing's tumour when the radiograph will show alternating layers of bone destruction and new bone growth.

Treatment. This is usually dependent on the type of bone tumour.

Benign bone tumours. These are usually treated by excision or curettage, followed by insertion of a bone graft into the subsequent bony defect (Monk 1981).

Malignant bone tumours. A patient with a confirmed malignant tumour will usually be screened for metastatic deposits. This may be performed by radioisotope skeletal survey or other radiological scanning technique. If no metastatic deposits are found, the method of treatment may involve amputation of the affected limb or total replacement of the affected bone with a custom-built artificial implant, thus avoiding the mutilation of an amputation. A course of chemotherapy may be given preoperatively, but is always given postoperatively.

When a metastatic deposit is found, the patient may be given a course of chemotherapy and/or radiation, but seldom would an amputation be carried out as the prognosis is very poor.

Metastatic bone disease. The treatment of a patient with metastatic bone disease tends to be symptomatic. The major problem for the patient is pain which can be very severe and debilitating. Adequate analgesics should be prescribed, often with the addition of a course of radiotherapy to alleviate the discomfort.

NURSING PRIORITIES AND MANAGEMENT: PRIMARY BONE TUMOURS

Certain bone tumours are known to affect particular age ranges of patient, therefore the nurse may care for a young child, adolescent or adult.

Once the patient has seen his general practitioner, immediate hospitalisation will ensue (see Ch. 32). The care of a patient undergoing chemotherapy and/or radiotherapy is described on pages 885–896.

The care of a patient who has a custom-built prosthetic implant is similar to the care of a patient following joint arthroplasty (see pp. 398–399).

Amputation of the affected limb may be a necessity.

AMPUTATION OF A LIMB

Amputation of a limb may be carried out for any of a number of reasons:

- primary malignant bone tumour
- trauma, such as a crushing injury
- vascular insufficiency, such as peripheral vascular disease

Table 10.3 Common bone tumours

Tumour type	Cell origin	Comments
Benign tumours		
Osteochondroma	Osteocyte	Most common benign tumour — bony outgrowth with cartilage cap. Symptoms depend on impingement. Common sites: distal end femur, proximal end tibia and humerus
Osteoclastoma	Osteocyte	Rarefaction of bone occurs. Femur, tibia and humerus. Young adults. Treat: curettage, resection and bone graft. May become malignant. Treat with chemotherapy and amputation
Malignant tumours (primary)		
Chondrosarcoma	Chondrocyte	Age group 30–40 years. Sites: femur, scapula, pelvis, humerus. Treat: excision, amputation or chemotherapy and endoprosthetic replacement
Osteosarcoma	Osteocyte	Destroys medullary and cortical bone tissue. Sites: end of long bones — 50% knee joint. Severe pain, swelling, tenderness. Treat: amputation and chemotherapy or chemotherapy and endoprosthetic replacement

- congenital anomaly
- severe infection, such as chronic osteomyelitis with systemic manifestations.

It has been estimated that a large number of the patients who undergo amputation of a limb, or part of a limb, in the Western world do so due to the effects of peripheral vascular disease (see p. 48), while trauma remains the commonest reason in the developing countries.

Sites for amputation

The aim of surgery is to provide a useful, functional, healthy, well-moulded stump which will permit the application of a prosthesis. Factors taken into account when deciding on the site are:

- total excision of all diseased tissue
- maintenance of an adequate blood supply to the tissue around the stump
- provision of a stump which is of an appropriate length to allow fitting of a prosthesis with optimum function.

As the stump will be exposed to some friction and, if a lower limb, to weight bearing the surgeon must ensure adequate cover and padding of the bone end with the surrounding tissues, otherwise breakdown of the skin tissue could occur.

NURSING PRIORITIES AND MANAGEMENT: AMPUTATION OF A LIMB

Counselling and support when surgery is planned

The patient who has been diagnosed as suffering from a malignant bone tumour will be devastated by the information on two counts: firstly that he has cancer of the bone; secondly that treatment may involve amputation of the affected limb, which appears to him to be totally healthy.

Coping with loss. Loss of a limb through amputation is like any other major loss. If the surgery is performed as an elective procedure, the patient and relatives will need support and understanding from the health care team to help them accept and adjust to the mutilation of the patient's body. The impending loss may cause the patient to display some of the initial characteristics of the bereavement process as described by Kubler Ross (1973) (see Ch. 34).

As the majority of amputations are carried out as elective procedures, the patient will usually have some time to try to adjust and to acknowledge the impending surgery.

Occasionally a patient may undergo an amputation as an emergency procedure following a severe crushing injury. In this case, the psychological preparation of the patient and family can be only very limited. They may require extra support and understanding during the postoperative period.

A visit to the local limb-fitting centre should be arranged and/or an introduction to a previous amputee who is of similar age and sex. This will help the patient to be aware of the level of mobility and lifestyle that can still be achieved after such a mutilation, and to accept his altered body image. If time permits, these visits should be arranged before the patient is admitted to hospital.

The details of specific pre- and postoperative care that follow are as for a patient undergoing a mid-thigh amputation.

Preoperative care

Standard preoperative care as outlined in Chapter 27 should be delivered.

Specific care

Mobilising. Information regarding the initial change in mobility level should be given. The physiotherapist will usually teach the patient to use crutches or other form of walking aid. Attention will be paid to maintaining the muscle power of the other limbs when a lower limb amputation is planned, as the arms and remaining lower limb will be used to support the patient during the early days of postoperative mobilisation. The patient should experience lying prone as this position will need to be adopted at least twice a day postoperatively. A patient with respiratory problems may not be able to tolerate lying prone.

The surgeon will usually mark the limb for amputation with a waterproof marker pen the day before the patient's operation, thus reducing the risk of amputating the wrong limb.

Postoperative care

A standard postoperative care plan may be utilised (see Ch. 27) with additional specific care on an individualised basis.

Specific care

Comfort measures. A bedcage should be utilised to relieve pressure on the stump during the immediate postoperative period. The stump should be maintained in the neutral position, lying parallel to the other limb in a non-flexed and non-abducted orientation.

Wound dressing. Most commonly, this is in the form of a soft dressing and stump bandage. The bandage will need to be re-applied at regular intervals, usually after the first postoperative day. After the initial postoperative period, a special stump bandage, such as an 'Elset' or a 'Juso sock' which have better elastic properties and are lighter than a crepe bandage, is used to maintain compression on the wound, thereby reducing oedema and promoting wound healing (Fig. 10.16). One or two vacuum wound drains will usually be in position and are removed within 48 hours unless the drainage is excessive.

Alternatively, the patient's stump may be encased in a plaster cast dressing, which helps healing by maintaining the stump in a neutral position and reducing swelling and oedema. The main disadvantage of this type of dressing is that regular assessment of the wound for signs of infection cannot be undertaken; therefore any rise in temperature, offensive odour and/or any complaint of pain must be reported as this may indicate wound infection or tissue breakdown.

Phantom pain. This is the name given to the painful sensation experienced by some patients that the amputated limb is still attached to the patient's body. The causal mechanism of this sensation is still not fully understood by either doctors or psychologists (Mouratoglou 1986). The sensation can be very distressing for the patient and may continue for many months after surgery. Regular, effective analgesics in the immediate postoperative period are thought to reduce the incidence of phantom pain. If it becomes a chronic problem, treatment in the form of transcutaneous nerve stimulation, ultrasound, local nerve blocks, relaxation therapy or medication such as carbamazepine (Tegratol) has been shown to be effective. Some patients may find benefit from the use of one of the many alternative complementary therapies that are available.

Preventing flexion contracture. Where possible, the patient should lie prone at regular intervals from the first postoperative day to prevent the development of a flexion contracture of the stump. The patient who normally sleeps lying prone can return to this position.

Mobilisation. The patient will normally sit out of bed within 48 hours of surgery and may use a wheelchair initially to assist with mobilisation. Practice in standing, transferring from bed to chair and from wheelchair to toilet will be given. This increases the patient's independence and morale. The physiotherapist will supervise walking. The patient may find his

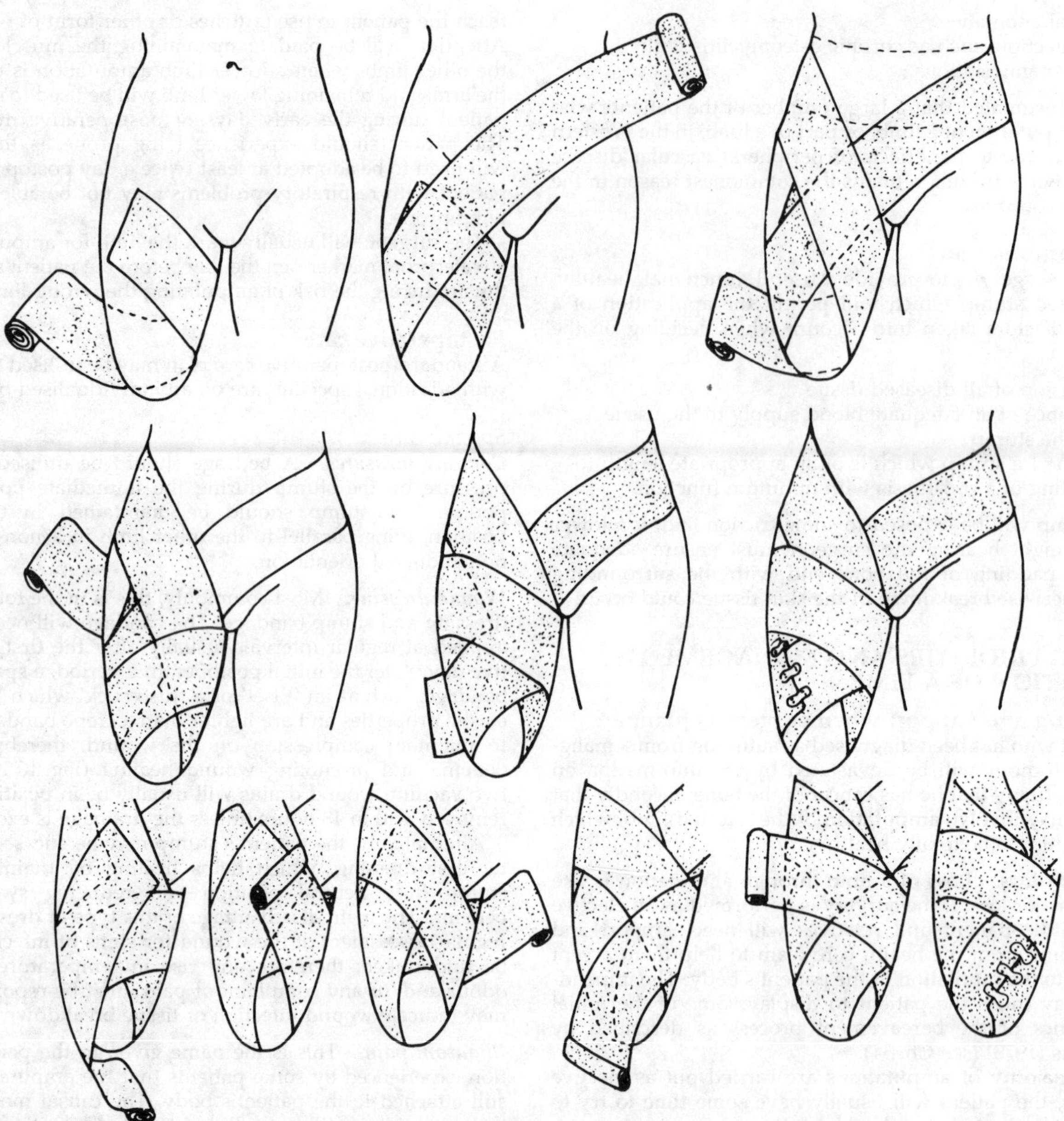

Fig. 10.16 Stump bandage. (Reproduced with kind permission from Smith Suddarth 1991.)

sense of balance has been temporarily altered, but with advice and support this problem will be overcome.

Pneumatic post-amputation mobility aid. Some centres use a prosthesis known as a pneumatic post-amputation mobility (PPAM) aid to help the patient regain balance and encourage early walking. The aid consists of an inflatable plastic tube which is placed around the patient's stump. The tube is encased in a metal frame with a rocker foot. The use of the PPAM aid can help the patient adjust to the change in body image as the time without an artificial limb is reduced.

Clothing. The patient's clothing may need to be adapted temporarily until the prosthesis is supplied. The tucking of an empty arm of a jacket or the leg of a pair of trousers into the body of the garment is an apparent detail but failure to do this can often be the last straw for a patient who, until then, has been coping well.

Promoting independence. The patient should be taught how to care for the stump once the sutures are removed, by maintaining skin hygiene, moisturising the skin surface if required and, twice daily, inspecting the whole stump for potential pressure points. This care will be reinforced during visits to the prosthetic department where further information about care of the prosthesis will be given.

The patient or a relative should be taught to apply the stump bandage so that necessary compression is maintained to help mould and firm the tissue in preparation for fitting a prosthesis. Should the patient for any reason be unable to wear his prosthesis at a later date, he must be advised to apply the stump bandage instead in order to maintain the shape of the stump.

Social adaptation. The amputation of a limb can markedly affect a person's ability to continue his previous pattern of work and play. The nurse should encourage the patient to voice anxieties that relate to this and, if necessary, refer him to a social worker.

Discharge. Prior to discharge, the patient's home will be assessed by the occupational therapist to define any need for aids to assist with activities of living. Referral to the local occupational retraining officer may be needed if the amputation makes it impossible for the patient to continue in his former occupation. The patient will attend the limb-fitting centre at regular intervals following discharge until he has achieved a safe, correct walking pattern. Some patients may be supplied with more than one definitive limb, depending on their age and the level of use/abuse to the prosthesis. Thereafter, the patient may attend annually or as the need arises should any problem with the prosthesis develop. Outpatient attendance for review by the surgeon will continue during the period of rehabilitation.

BONE INFECTIONS

In order to raise awareness of infective bone conditions and the problems associated with them a brief outline of osteomyelitis and tuberculosis will be given below.

Osteomyelitis

PATHOPHYSIOLOGY

This disease is more common in children and adolescents. It often follows minor trauma which probably causes a small haematoma at the epiphyseal plate in which blood-borne bacteria proliferate and infection develops. It is the marrow that is primarily involved. As the infection spreads, the patient develops pyrexia and severe pain and the affected part is hot and swollen. If untreated, the infection spreads through the marrow, erodes the cortex and the periosteum and an abscess forms, which will eventually discharge through the skin. By this stage it has become chronic osteomyelitis. If the infection is within a joint, it will discharge into that joint causing septic arthritis.

MEDICAL MANAGEMENT

Investigations. The patient is hospitalised, the limb elevated and blood is sent for culture and to estimate the erythrocyte sedimentation rate (ESR), white cell count and haemoglobin level. Radiography will show destructive bone changes.

Treatment. After the blood has been sent to the laboratory, antibiotic therapy is commenced. At first this will be the 'best guess' then, when the culture sensitivity is known, it will be specific to the causative agent.

If there is no response to the antibiotic treatment within 2 days, the infected area can be opened surgically and the pus drained.

NURSING PRIORITIES AND MANAGEMENT: OSTEOMYELITIS

This condition is very distressing for the patient and the parents.

Early detection. Community nurses need to be alert to the condition so that early referral and treatment can be instituted to prevent progression.

Elevation of the affected part. Pillows or bed elevation can be used.

Pain and comfort. Rest, gentle handling, use of bed cradles to relieve pressure of bedclothes, prompt administration of analgesics, reassurance and distracting activity will all help to relieve pain to some extent.

Antibiotic therapy. Antibiotics will be given regularly either intravenously or by injection and it would be wise to learn the special techniques for administering injections to children and young adults from an experienced paediatric nurse.

Tuberculosis

Tuberculosis, previously rare in developed countries is now on the increase and is rampant in undeveloped countries. It affects all age groups. The course of the disease is similar to osteomyelitis although the pace is much slower. Treatment is by antitubercular drugs and addressing the symptoms.

NURSING PRIORITIES AND MANAGEMENT: TUBERCULOSIS

Management involves implementation of principles of infection control, health education and comfort measures to alleviate symptoms.

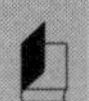

The *Tubercle and Lung Disease Journal* is a useful source of additional information.

DISORDERS OF JOINTS

Review the anatomy and physiology of joints.

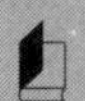

For further information, see Wilson (1990) pp. 378–390.

This section gives examples of the management of disorders of the knee and the lumbar spine, shoulder dislocation, and rheumatoid arthritis and osteoarthritis.

DISORDERS OF THE KNEE

There are many disorders of the knee. Only the more common are outlined below.

Meniscus lesions

PATHOPHYSIOLOGY

The menisci are part of the load-bearing mechanism in the knee joint and absorb much of the weight of the femoral condyles. They can be torn or injured in relatively minor sporting accidents and when not intact cause mechanical problems as loose gristly fragments move around within the joint.

MEDICAL MANAGEMENT

Diagnosis is confirmed by arthroscopy or arthrography.

Treatment. Loose fragments are excised arthroscopically — arthroscopic meniscectomy (removal of the menisci). This is a minimally invasive technique which permits visualisation of the fragments and preservation of as much healthy tissue as possible. This is important because meniscectomy exposes the articular cartilage to the full downward thrust of body weight. This may eventually lead to degenerative osteoarthritis in about 75% of patients 10 years after total meniscectomy (Dandy 1989).

NURSING PRIORITIES AND MANAGEMENT: MENISCUS LESIONS

These follow the principles for all musculoskeletal injuries and orthopaedic surgery. Additionally, community and practice nurses should be aware of the background procedures and processes because they will advise the patient and follow up his treatment.

DISORDERS OF THE LUMBAR SPINE — BACK PAIN

Disorders of the lumbar spine and 'back pain' are responsible for more human suffering and time lost from work in any one year than any other medical condition (Dandy 1989).

PATHOPHYSIOLOGY

Back pain in itself need not be an orthopaedic problem; rather it is a symptom and once the cause has been determined it is best managed by the appropriate speciality. For example, it may be related to rheumatoid, gynaecological or urological conditions; to poor posture, obesity, lack of exercise; to metastatic or infectious bone disease; or to degenerative disc disease. However, often it is classified as musculoskeletal and brought within the orthopaedic remit. This section will focus on management of acute back strain, recurrent back strain and management of prolapsed intervertebral disc.

Acute back strain

This is associated with a sudden sharp movement or an attempt to lift a heavy object from an extended position, or it may occur when people with sedentary occupations indulge in bursts of excessive exercise. It is manifest by sudden severe pain radiating from the lumbar region to the back of the knee. There are no other neurological symptoms and it is usually due to an acute muscle or ligament strain in the lumbar spine.

MEDICAL MANAGEMENT

The history indicates the cause, and differential diagnosis excludes two similar but serious conditions:

- lumbar disc protrusion — which would be accompanied by pain extending below the knee in the presence of other neurological symptoms.
- metastatic spinal tumours — which can be excluded by imaging studies.

Treatment:

- Rest in the most comfortable position.
- Analgesics.
- Gradual mobilisation.
- Advice on application of heat.

NURSING PRIORITIES AND MANAGEMENT: ACUTE BACK STRAIN

Prevention through health education. Nurses have many opportunites in the work place, community and hospital to teach people how to organise their environment and activities in order to avoid acute back strain. Much research has gone into the ergonomics of correct lifting techniques (see Box 10.8) and many teaching aids such as videos and leaflets are available.

Prevention of back injury in the workplace has been given greater emphasis with the Health and Safety at Work Regulations (1993) on Manual Handling of Loads. It is important that both workers and employers are kept aware of their responsibilities in this respect.

Nurses in particular are a high risk group for back injury and a Code of Practice has been published by the RCN Advisory Panel for Back Pain in Nurses (1992). Both employer and employee responsibilities are set out and there are specific guidelines for assessment and planning of patient care (see Box 10.9).

Box 10.8 Correct lifting technique (Dandy 1989)

1. Do not lift with the spine flexed: in this position, the weight is hanging on taut ligaments and stretched muscles which makes them vulnerable to additional load. Instead, lift with the lumbar spine extended.
2. Keep the weight to be lifted as near to the body as possible. The further the weight is from the body, the more effort has to be expended in lifting it.

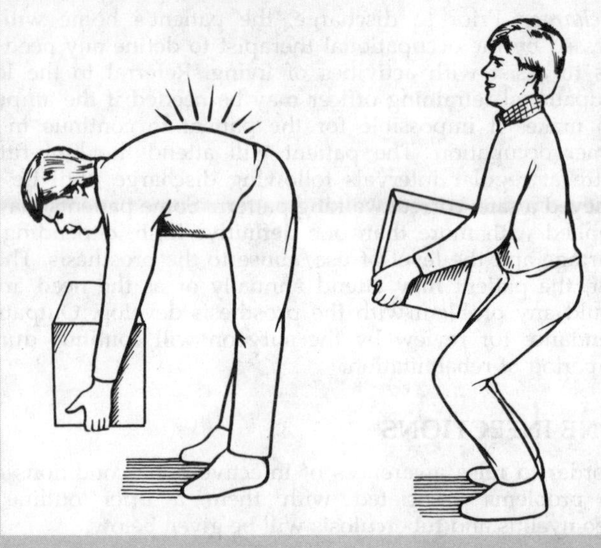

3. Lift with the knees, not the back.
4. Make the job as easy as possible. Ensure that there is good access to the load, if possible split it into lighter loads and if it cannot be split, share the job with two or more people.

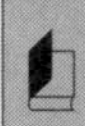

For information about lifting practices, see Jamieson, McCall & Blythe (1992) pp. 292–297 and National Back Pain Association and the Royal College of Nursing (1992)

? **10.12** Find out what lifting aids are available in the clinical area you are currently attached to. How often are they used? What different techniques for lifting and handling patients have you personally used?

Recurrent back strain

A patient who suffers recurrent back strain should be referred to a rheumatologist or rehabilitation specialist.

Prolapsed intervertebral disc

PATHOPHYSIOLOGY

The intervertebral discs consist of a firm nucleus pulposus surrounded

Box 10.9 The management of patients/clients (RCN 1992)

Assessment and planning

1. Particularly heavy patients, or helpless patients with no ability to assist nurses, need to be individually assessed by a competent patient handling team. Nurses in training and support workers should not be expected to undertake these assessments without competent supervision.
2. The care plan or profile should include the following information:
   - The current weight of the patient
   - The extent of the patient's ability to assist, weight bear and any other relevant information
   - The technique to be employed to handle that particular patient which should be consistent with the activity undertaken. This should be based upon:
     — the task
     — the patient
     — the environment
     — the equipment
     — the lifters.
3. Where the patient weighs 50 kilos (8 stones) or more, or the conditions are less than ideal, mechanical handling devices must be used.
4. Mechanical handling devices or equipment should be used for moving totally dependent patients from bed to chair, trolley, toilet, etc. Sliding equipment should be used for moving totally dependent patients in bed.

by a ring of fibrocartilage and fibrous tissue which links two vertebrae together. They tend to flatten slightly during the day and re-expand at night. Repeated exposure to excessive pressure from heavy lifting can result in flattening and weakening of the disc and supporting structures. Disturbance of fluid physiology within the disc can exacerbate this process. The disc will protrude and cause lower back pain. Eventually it may rupture and the soft contents will prolapse causing compression and stretching of nerve roots or fibres. 90% of lumbar disc protrusions involve L4–5 or L5–S1 (Fig. 10.17).

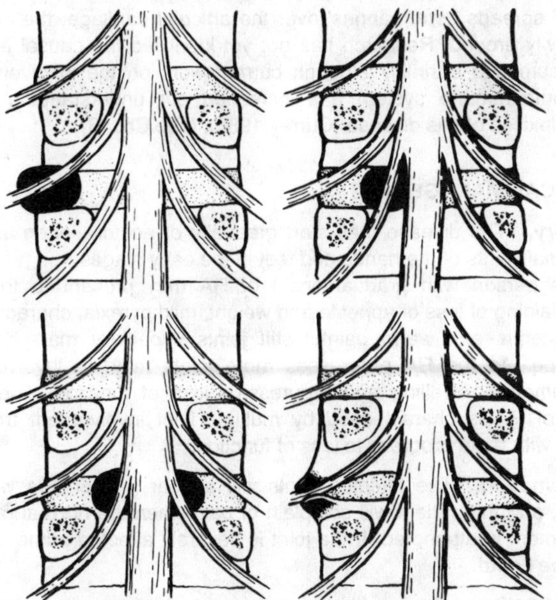

Fig. 10.17 Disc prolapse and root compression in the lumbar spine. A laterally placed prolapse may compress the L4 root, a more central prolapse will compress L5 and a central prolapse, the cauda equina. Osteophytes in the lateral canal will also produce root compression. (Reproduced with kind permission from Dandy 1989.)

MEDICAL MANAGEMENT

History. The patient will present with acute lumbar pain radiating down the thigh and lower leg — the precise position being dependent on the spinal nerve root affected. He may also be 'locked' in the classic bent position. There may be a history of dull lower back pain.

Examination. Muscle spasm and an intense focal area of pain may be identified. The straight leg raising test will indicate restriction of movement well below 90° of hip flexion and there may be sensations of numbness or tingling. If necessary, a CAT scan or myelogram will confirm the diagnosis.

Treatment. Current orthopaedic opinion suggests that conservative treatment should always be tried before surgical intervention. This would consist of rest, analgesics, muscle relaxants and traction. Manipulation of a spine with acute disc prolapse is said to be dangerous (Dandy 1989).

The indication for disc excision is when there is proven disc protrusion with accompanying neurological signs and no improvement after 6 weeks of conservative treatment, or if any neurological deficit worsens. Intervention will comprise either disc excision or chemonucleolysis:

- Disc excision involves excision of the ligamentum flavum and inferior portion of the lamina (laminectomy) overlying the affected nerve root. The herniated portion of the disc and all disc material is excised relieving the pressure on the nerve root. Symptoms are relieved in about 75% of cases.
- Chemonucleolysis is injection of an enzyme (chemopapaine) into the prolapsed disc which breaks down the disc material, thus relieving pressure on the nerve root. This procedure is done under image intensifier control and can be accompanied by severe pain. There is a small possibility of anaphylactic shock. Symptoms are relieved in about 70% of cases.

Both procedures effectively remove the disc and therefore its shock absorbing function, and unnatural stresses trigger degenerative reactions with the result that between 30–60% of patients will suffer degrees of stiffness and back pain permanently (Dandy 1989).

NURSING PRIORITIES AND MANAGEMENT: PROLAPSED INTERVERTEBRAL DISC

Myelography. For care of a patient undergoing myelography, see Box 10.10.

Conservative treatment

As most of the conservative treatment can be carried out at home, it is the community nurse who will have responsibility for advising and supporting the patient and his family in all comfort measures. The care that might be given by the community nurse is described in Nursing Care Plan 10.1; Box 10.11 provides background information about the patient.

Traction. If traction is necessary, the patient will be admitted to hospital and care will follow the principles already discussed under management of care for a patient in traction.

Operative treatment

In addition to the general principles for perioperative care, the following points are specific to postoperative management of patients having a laminectomy and chemonucleolysis.

Pain. This can be expected to be severe following chemonucleolysis but it may be complicated by developing neurological deficit — therefore neurological status should be monitored carefully and prescribed pain relief administered promptly where indicated.

Positioning and mobilising. Frequent position changes should be encouraged, always maintaining spinal alignment.

Box 10.10 Care of a patient undergoing myelography

This investigation is used to provide clear radiological detail of the spinal cord, nerve roots and nerve root sheaths.

The patient will usually be admitted to hospital for 24–48 hours when myelography is carried out. As it is an invasive procedure performed under local anaesthetic, preoperative preparation should be implemented. The patient may have a light snack before the investigation. The radiopaque contrast medium is injected into the subarachnoid space through a lumbar puncture. An adverse reaction to the contrast medium may occur during the procedure, such as anaphylactic shock, convulsions, hypotension or cardiac arrest. All emergency equipment should be present in the radiological department and the staff should be skilled in emergency patient care.

Care following the procedure depends on the type of contrast medium used. This should be clearly defined in the patient's notes, along with specific instructions for positioning. For example, if a water-based solution is used (Amipaque) the patient will need to sit up for at least 6 hours until the remaining contrast medium has been absorbed. If he lies flat the medium will move towards the brain and act as an irritant, which may cause chemical meningitis or convulsing.

20% of patients are said to suffer from headache and some experience nausea for 24 hours after a myelogram (Powell 1986). A mild analgesic and antiemetic may be prescribed to alleviate these symptoms. Pulse, blood pressure and respiration rate are monitored at regular intervals until the patient is fully ambulant. If the headache persists for longer than 48–72 hours after discharge from hospital, the patient should be advised to contact his GP.

The patient should be turned carefully, with a pillow between the legs (log role). Slight flexion of the knees using the knee rest or a pillow for support while in the prone position will allow spinal muscles to relax. A pillow between the knees will provide comfortable alignment when in the lateral position.

Early mobilisation is usually prescribed. The bed should be lowered and the patient taught to roll himself to the edge of the bed, swing his legs to the floor and stand up in one smooth movement.

DISLOCATED SHOULDER

Shoulder dislocation is addressed here because it is a fairly common sporting injury and can occasionally be treated quite simply if a health professional is present at the time of injury or very shortly afterwards. It is a very painful condition and if not attended to immediately muscle spasm will make it impossible to reduce the dislocation without intravenous diazepam or pethidine, or even a general anaesthetic.

NURSING PRIORITIES AND MANAGEMENT: DISLOCATED SHOULDER

The immediate treatment is to support the arm and assist the patient very gently and carefully to roll face down on to a raised surface as shown in Figure 10.18. If this is done before the muscles go into spasm there is a good chance that the shoulder will slip back into position because of gravitational pull and the slight outward movement. If this manoeuvre is not successful then the arm should be supported in a sling until it can be manipulated following analgesic and muscle relaxant drugs.

Often the first person to see the patient is a nurse who can carry out this first-aid manoeuvre and make the patient comfortable.

JOINT INFECTION

Septic arthritis

PATHOPHYSIOLOGY

Septic arthritis can be caused by osteomyelitis, infection from a penetrating wound or bacteraemia. It should be suspected in systemic conditions — especially diabetes — which present with swollen and painful joints. In bacteraemia it is part of a potentially fatal condition. In every case, if untreated, it destroys articular cartilage and eventually the joint becomes ankylosed (fused together).

MEDICAL MANAGEMENT

Treatment consists of arthroscopic joint lavage and division of adhesions with aggressive antibiotic therapy.

NURSING PRIORITIES AND MANAGEMENT: SEPTIC ARTHRITIS

Emphasis is on early detection, promotion of comfort, support, rehabilitation and specific management of arthroscopic procedures.

INFLAMMATORY AND DEGENERATIVE JOINT DISORDERS

This section focuses on two common inflammatory joint diseases: rheumatoid arthritis and osteoarthritis.

Rheumatoid arthritis

PATHOPHYSIOLOGY

Rheumatoid arthritis (RA) is a systemic disease of connective tissue, characterised by a chronic/subacute non-bacterial inflammation of synovial joints and the surrounding tendons and their sheaths. The disease also has extra-articular features.

The joints are acutely inflamed due to inflammatory changes in the synovial membrane. The synovium becomes thicker, very vascular and the site of increased cell infiltration which may cause an effusion within the joint that manifests as a swollen joint. As the proliferative tissue spreads as a 'pannus' over the articular cartilage, the cartilage is slowly eroded. Research has not yet identified the causal agent(s) of rheumatoid arthritis, although current work on the involvement of the auto-immune system has increased our understanding of the complexities of this disease (Currey 1988), (see Ch. 16).

MEDICAL MANAGEMENT

History. The disease may start gradually or acutely, often affecting the small joints of the hands and feet in the early stages.

The person with gradual onset of RA may present to their GP complaining of loss of appetite and weight, mild pyrexia, characteristics of anaemia and warm painful stiff joints especially marked in the morning. As the RA progresses more joints may be involved with inflammation, swelling and progressive loss of function. The acute form of RA is characterised by multiple joint involvement from the onset with rapid progress to loss of function.

Examination. The affected joints will appear swollen, be warm to touch, and the patient will complain of pain when the normal range of movement is attempted. If the joint is severely affected some crepitus may be heard.

Investigation. X-rays of both hands and feet will usually be sufficient to confirm the diagnosis. A blood specimen will be taken for assessment of the level of haemoglobin, number of white blood cells, erythrocyte sedimentation rate and the presence of rheumatoid factor.

Diagnosis. The diagnosis will be confirmed by the patient's history

Nursing Care Plan 10.1 Community nursing care of patient with prolapsed intervertebral disc

Problem (A) actual (P) potential	Goal	Nursing intervention	Evaluation
Communication **Pain (A) related to disc prolapse**	Improvement and control	Advise on: ❐ Self-administering medication ❐ Self-assessment on pain chart	Significant improvement in level of experienced pain
Anxiety (A) related to chidren's welfare and reduced mother role	Reduce anxiety by addressing causes	❐ Define problems — discuss with Mrs S and husband ❐ Neighbour willing to help Mon./Wed./Fri., husband at weekend ❐ Arrange nursery care for Emma Tues. and Thur. (social worker)	Mrs S will report satisfaction with arrangements Enquire daily Children and husband adapting and appear happy
Reduced mobility (A) related to bed rest	Maintain Mrs S at bed rest — ensure comfort	❐ Advise to lie supine on firm mattress ❐ Up to toilet ❐ Assist with shower ❐ Bed cradle over legs ❐ Ensure radio, TV, telephone, magazines available	Mrs S states she is happy to stay in bed and is more comfortable Adequate diversional therapy observed
Maintaining a safe environment (P)	Prevent accidental ingestion of Mrs S's medication by children Prevent other accidents	❐ Discuss problem with Mrs S, husband and neighbour ❐ Locate safe place ❐ Ensure child-proof medication cap ❐ Discuss potential home accidents — give RoSPA leaflet	There are no preventable incidents or accidents Family and friends demonstrate raised awareness of safety — discuss leaflet
Nutrition (P)	Maintain balanced diet	❐ Arrange friend to assist ❐ Advise flexi-straws ❐ Home help Tues. and Thur. ❐ Mrs S to ease on to side to eat	Mrs S describes balanced diet

of pain and morning stiffness, radiological changes showing bone erosion, a raised erythrocyte sedimentation rate and possibly a positive test for rheumatoid factor. Rheumatoid factor will be detected in 80% of patients who suffer RA (Currey 1988).

Treatment. There is no known cure for RA; therefore intervention is directed towards treatment of the disease characteristics. This will be the primary responsibility of a consultant rheumatologist in conjunction with an orthopaedic surgeon. The patient may receive non-operative and operative treatment.

The objectives of the rheumatologist's care are to:

- reduce the patient's pain with the use of analgesics and non-steroidal anti-inflammatory drugs (NSAIDs)
- reduce joint destruction by curtailing the inflammatory process within the joint with the use of NSAIDs
- prevent or minimise deformity of a joint by splinting damaged or painful joints
- assist the patient to adapt his lifestyle.

The orthopaedic surgeon will manage any surgical procedures which may be required during the course of the disease, such as:

- synovectomy — removal of excess synovial membrane from within the joint capsule of the affected joint
- osteotomy — division of a bone which may be done to alter the weight distribution within a joint

Box 10.11 Mrs S

Mrs S is 30 years old and married to a builder. The couple have two children, 7-year-old Tim and 4-year-old Emma. Mrs S is being treated at home for a prolapsed intervertebral disc, her prescribed treatment being bed rest, pain control and neurovascular assessment. The community nurse plans to visit Mrs S daily until her condition begins to improve. She has already ascertained that Mrs S's next-door neighbour is also a friend.

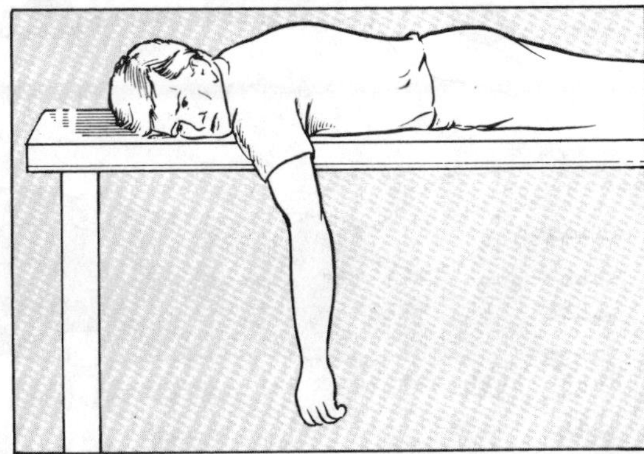

Fig. 10.18 Hanging-arm technique for reducing dislocated shoulder. (Reproduced with kind permission from Dandy 1989.)

- arthroplasty — remodelling an affected joint using synthetic materials and/or metal
- arthrodesis — surgical fusion of a joint which will reduce/eliminate the joint pain but create a stiff immovable joint.

NURSING PRIORITIES AND MANAGEMENT: RHEUMATOID ARTHRITIS

The aim of care is to maintain independence as long as possible and provide comfort and support. A multidisciplinary approach is essential but coordination of care and implementation of major comfort measures are mainly nursing responsibilities which span both hospital and home. For this reason, these are given in detail below.

Controlling pain

Pain is the overriding and chronic problem. The use of analgesics and non-steroidal anti-inflammatory drugs (NSAIDs) will help to control it. Corticosteroids are used as a last resort if the pain is severe and other pain-relieving methods have failed, but these do have serious side effects which can be life threatening (Currey 1988). Nurses need to be alert to these and to ensure that patients are also aware of these. Narcotics are avoided because of their addictive nature.

In an acute exacerbation of RA, the patient's affected joint(s) will be rested until the pain and inflammation process subside. This may require the use of a lightweight splint to hold the joint in the optimal position (Fig. 10.19). The splint will be removed for gentle physiotherapy, which will be increased as the inflammation subsides.

The patient should avoid cold environments, as low temperature has an adverse effect on joint stiffness. Where possible, the patient with RA should be helped into a warm immersion bath in the morning to ease pain and stiffness. At home, he may require bathing aids, such as a non-slip bath mat and a bath stool, which can be supplied by the occupational therapist. Cold packs placed over warm swollen joints and wax baths for the hand joints can give effective pain relief.

Maintaining independence and fostering well-being

Exercise and mobility. The patient will be involved in a daily programme of isometric and resistive exercises under the supervision of a physiotherapist. This will enable full joint movement to be maintained. If possible, the programme should include a routine of lying prone at least twice a day to prevent formation of joint contractures which can further reduce mobility. Alternately sitting and standing that is, regularly changing position will also reduce development of joint contractures.

When handling an inflamed joint, the nurse should avoid

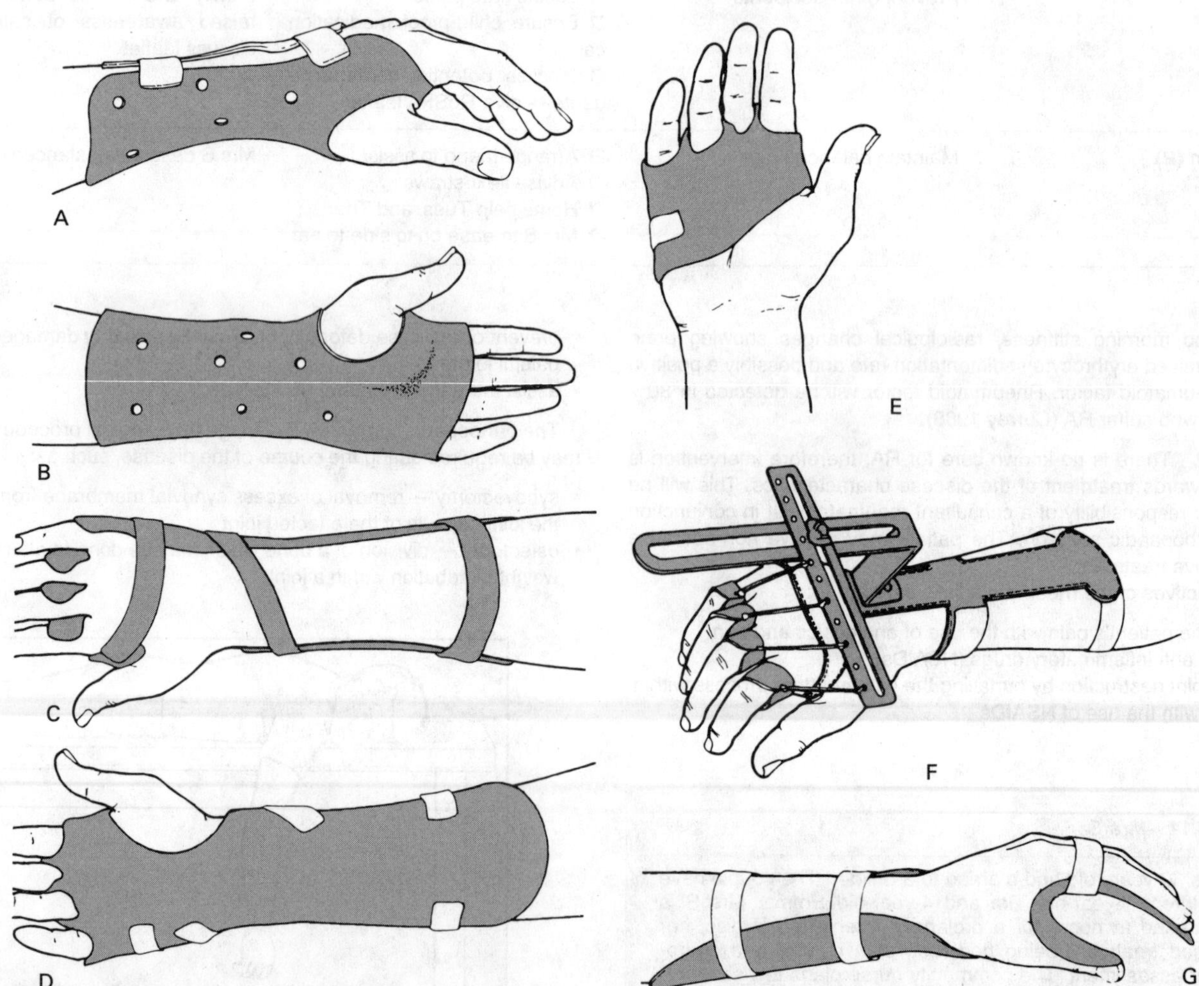

Fig. 10.19 Different types of splint. (A)–(E) Resting splints. (F) Functional splint used to stabilise a joint during activity. (G) Corrective splint to immobilise a joint, realign soft tissue or correct contractures or deformities. (Reproduced with kind permission from Royle & Walsh 1992.)

grasping movements. The limb should be supported above and below the joint using an open-handed technique.

The muscle power of the patient with RA is reduced; therefore the use of aids such as a variable-height bed, raised chair and an ejector chair may be of assistance.

Walking aids, such as a stick or elbow crutches, may help to retain the patient's level of mobility by reducing the weight load placed on specific joints. The hand pieces of the aids may need to be adapted to accommodate the finger and wrist deformities that are common features of the disease.

The patient should be reminded not to carry heavy objects as this will increase the load on the affected joints. Stress and strain on small joints such as the fingers should also be avoided.

Safety. The nurse should assist the patient to identify potential hazards in the home and workplace, such as the storage of medications and the suitability of floor coverings. The hospital environment should be hazard free.

Diet. A patient with RA is likely to develop anaemia due to the chronic inflammatory process of the disease. Iron supplements may be prescribed. Advice about dietary iron supplements should be given.

A number of NSAIDs have the common side effect of causing constipation. This should be explained to the patient and an increased dietary intake of fibre advised. The patient with RA may require assistance in maintaining his nutritional status due to anorexia and/or difficulty in using eating and drinking utensils. Frequent, light, appetising meals should be served. The occupational therapist can supply a variety of utensils, such as large-handled cutlery and a tilting kettle stand, which will help the patient to retain independence.

Clothing. The fastenings of clothing may need to be adapted; the use of Velcro is of great benefit to patients with RA.

The patient may suffer from a prolonged, mild pyrexia resulting in the need for frequent attention to personal hygiene and changes of clothing.

Skin care. The patient's skin can be extremely fragile due to the disease and/or the side effects of some of the medications. Ongoing risk assessment of skin breakdown caused by restriction of movement and the effects of equipment is necessary. Preventive measures should be taken, such as regular position changes and the use of pressure-relieving aids.

Eliminating. The use of a raised toilet seat will be beneficial, as the necessity to flex the hips and knees to 90° is reduced. A grab rail on the wall next to the toilet will also help when attempting to sit or stand.

Sleep. The physical and psychological recuperative benefits of sleep are such that the patient should be advised and encouraged to maintain as regular a sleep pattern as the painful nature of the disease will allow (see Ch. 25). In order to facilitate beneficial rest it may be necessary to control the patient's pain and discomfort by the administration of analgesics. With more severe cases, it may be necessary to fit night-resting splints, which will restrict painful movements due to muscle spasm. The patient may require assistance to position, secure and remove these splints.

Patient education. The patient should be alerted to possible side effects of the drugs he is taking and told what action to take should they occur. Information about the disease and the various treatment regimes should be freely available because this tends to help reduce anxiety. There are numerous information booklets that can be used by patients; some will have been written by local staff, others are supplied by national charity organisations such as the Arthritis and Rheumatism Council (ARC). (See p. 404.)

Counselling and support

It may be necessary for patients with RA to modify or change their jobs due to limitations of mobility. Long periods of illness and absence from the work place may cause employment to be problematic. The disablement resettlement officer's assistance in finding appropriate employment may be of benefit. Some patients will reach a stage where full-time employment is impossible. When this happens, the patient will become a registered disabled person who is eligible for various benefits and allowances, available from the Department of Social Security (Robertson 1993).

Modification of the structure and content of the home may also take place when the patient's disability increases. This may involve minor additions, such as extra handrails to external and internal stairs. A major change may be the creation of toilet facilities at ground level. Frequently a patient may need to move to more suitable housing.

Self-image. As rheumatoid arthritis progresses, the joints may become so distorted that the patient may develop a negative body image. Helping the patient to maintain individuality and self-esteem will help to create a more positive body image. The nurse can help by suggesting alterations to the style of clothing, such as wearing a longer skirt over swollen knees in order to camouflage them.

Due to the nature of the disease and the effects RA has on a person's quality of life, the patient may suffer from periods of depression which may necessitate the use of antidepressive medication.

Sexual activity. Counselling regarding sexual activity may be required. The Arthritis and Rheumatism Council and the Association to aid the Sexual and Personal Relationships of People with a Disability (SPOD) have both produced booklets containing useful information for RA patients and their partners. See p. 404.

Social contact. It is important that every effort is made to maintain social contact, even when the patient may be housebound. Family, friends and rheumatoid arthritis self-help groups will assist in this sphere.

Rheumatoid arthritis inevitably affects the lives of the patient's family; they too have need for counselling and support (see Research Abstract 10.2).

Osteoarthritis

PATHOPHYSIOLOGY

Osteoarthritis is a non-inflammatory degenerative condition affecting the hyaline cartilage of synovial joints. This is the most common condition causing disability in Great Britain with the large weight-bearing joints of the lower limb such as the hips and knees the most commonly affected.

People with osteoarthritis are not normally systemically ill and the disease can be primary or secondary in its origin. As primary osteoarthritis is a progressive condition of unknown origin, it is more common in the older person, and females are more frequently affected. Secondary osteoarthritis can affect any age or sex.

MEDICAL MANAGEMENT

History. The first indication the patient may have that something is wrong is usually a dull nagging pain most commonly felt when bearing weight on or moving an affected joint, but which can also manifest itself during periods of rest or sleep. The patient may suffer from referred pain in the knee or thigh and may visit her GP erroneously complaining of a knee problem when a hip joint is affected. Loss of function and movement of a joint may occur if the pain is severe. The

Research Abstract 10.2 Rheumatoid arthritis: effects on the family

Prior to this study there has been little research into the impact of rheumatoid arthritis (RA) on the families of people with this crippling and painful disease.

A qualitative study was undertaken on 22 patients with RA, their well partners and their 40 children.

The findings suggest that the disease had wide-ranging effects on work patterns and family roles depending on personality types, pre-existing relationships and ability to adapt to increasing restrictions. The frustration of not being able to go out and do 'useful' work was more evident in men than women. Lack of social support networks and professional awareness of the total impact of the disease on both the patient's and the partner's work patterns, along with the impact of altered financial status on the family, was perceived to be problematic.

Sexual relationships were affected by physical symptoms and changed body image but this was seldom discussed between the partners and for the majority did not result in a real threat to the marriage although it added to the stresses of coping.

For most children the effects of living with a parent with a chronic and disabling disease were not detrimental although a minority did suffer physical and verbal abuse as a result; many expressed fear of getting the disease but most said they themselves would like to have children. Very few took on extra duties within the home, because the partner usually compensated for the patient's role. Stresses were evident but in some instances family bonds were strengthened by the increased awareness of relationships and everyday values.

Recommendations coming from the families were that they should have ready access to more information about the disease and earlier involvement in caring for the patient's changing needs. This information is actually available, as are support groups, but does not appear to reach many families. There was an obvious need for counselling and support at two critical points; firstly with initial diagnosis and secondly when work patterns for both partners become radically changed. The role of the community nurse and the specialist rheumatology nurse is obvious here.

Le Gallez P 1993 Rheumatoid arthritis: effects on the family. Nursing Standard 7(39): 30–34

patient may not be aware of a shortening of the limb which will cause a limp.

These characteristics may develop over a short span of time or take years to become manifest (Powell 1986).

Examination. The normal range of movement of a joint will be reduced. A fixed flexion deformity and wasting of the hip muscles may be present.

Investigations. Plain radiographs (X-ray) of the affected joint will be taken.

Diagnosis. This is confirmed by the appearance of the joint on the X-ray showing narrowing of the joint space and possible osteophyte formation.

Treatment. This can be classified into non-operative and surgical (Box 10.12).

The decision regarding which treatment is suitable for the individual is made by the orthopaedic surgeon in consultation with the patient and his or her family. There are many facts to be considered before deciding which mode of treatment would be the most beneficial, such as the age of the person, general medical status, home and family circumstances, level of disability and most importantly the level of pain the person is experiencing and how disruptive it is of normal life.

Examples:

- An overweight 50-year-old male patient who has a physically demanding occupation which causes stress and strain to his joints would benefit initially from conservative treatment. He may require surgical intervention at a later date
- An elderly lady who places less stress and strain on her joints would benefit greatly from an arthroplasty. The incidence of complications arising following an arthroplasty is increased when the patient is under 60 years of age, obese or physically highly active (Dandy 1989).

Box 10.12 Treatment of the patient with osteoarthritis

Non-operative
- Explanation
- Analgesic and non-steroidal anti-inflammatory drugs
- Physiotherapy
- Walking aids
- Occupational therapy
- Shoe raise
- Modification of life

Surgical (Fig. 10.20)
- Osteotomy — removing parts of a bone to correct line of weight bearing
- Arthrodesis — fusion of a joint
- Arthroplasty — creation of a joint

Operative treatment

There are many variations on surgical procedures for osteoarthritis which usually involve either partial or total joint replacement (see Fig. 10.20).

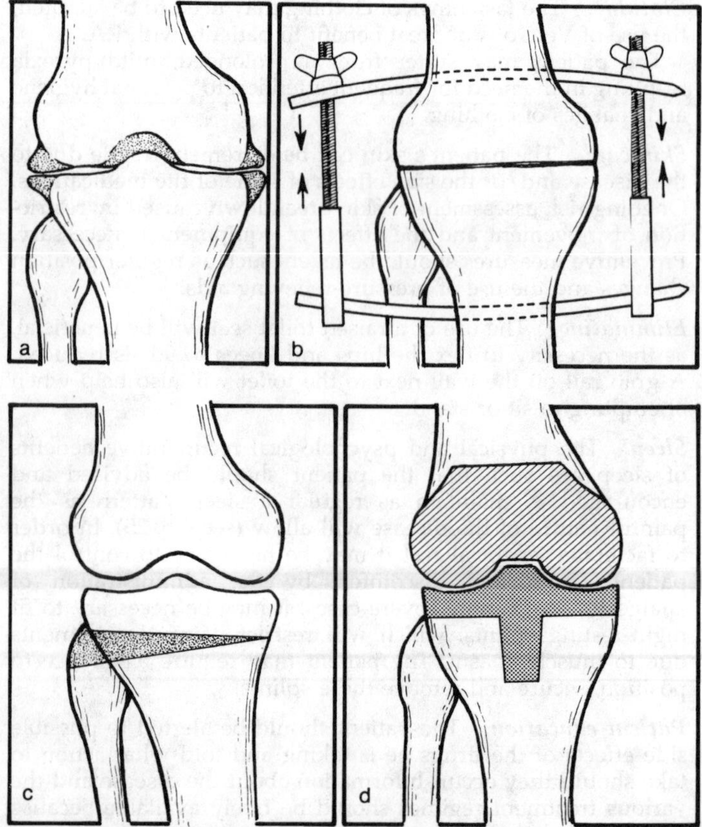

Fig. 10.20 Operations for osteoarthritis: (A) debridement and removal of osteophytes; (B) arthrodesis; (C) osteotomy to correct alignment; (D) total joint replacement. (Reproduced with kind permission from Dandy 1989.)

Joint replacement has revolutionised the lifestyle of thousands of patients who have suffered severe chronic pain and the disabling effects of this degenerative condition.

Hip replacements are now a common procedure although there are still problems associated with loosening of prostheses and failure due to infection in 0.5–1% of cases in every year (Dandy 1989). Research continues into technical and material improvements. See Figure 10.21 for types of prostheses used in hip replacement. (See Case History 10.3.)

Postoperative complications

Dislocation of the femoral component. 2% of patients who receive a total hip joint replacement will develop the complication of dislocation of the femoral component from the acetabular component (Smith 1987). To help prevent this, some orthopaedic surgeons request that the patient is nursed sitting at no more than a 45° of flexion at the hip joint. A Charnley wedge, or foam troughs in which the patient's lower legs rest, may also be used to reduce excessive adduction which can increase the incidence of dislocation of the hip joint replacement. These two measures are thought to decrease the physical strain placed on the operation site and thus prevent the development of laxity of the hip joint by stabilising tissues following the trauma of surgery.

The patient will usually have one or more wound drains of the closed vacuum type in position postoperatively. The femoral bone tissue has an excellent blood supply; therefore blood drainage can be excessive compared to other forms of surgery. Accurate recording of the volume is essential and if excessive the patient may need a blood transfusion. When emptying the wound drain(s) the nurse must ensure that contamination of the drainage system does not occur.

NURSING PRIORITIES AND MANAGEMENT: JOINT REPLACEMENT

Perioperative care

Perioperative care will follow the basic principles outlined in Chapter 27 with the following additions.

Prevention of infection. Bacterial infection of the bone around the prosthesis can have a severe debilitating effect and the prosthesis may have to be removed leaving a grossly unstable joint. Vigorous prophylaxis is therefore essential. In addition to basic attention to infection control, especially when undertaking invasive procedures, and attention to clearing up any septic foci, intravenous antibiotic therapy is commenced preoperatively and continued until healing has taken place.

Communication and information. If the patient is to have a spinal anaesthetic, the procedure is discussed and questions answered. The rationale behind vigorous infection control and antibiotic therapy is explained in order to obtain full co-operation. A full explanation of the hip replacement procedure is given and the prosthesis is demonstrated if requested. Opportunity is taken to explain the reason for limitations on the degree of hip flexion and the patient is encouraged to practise safe positions for sitting and for transferring out of bed (see below).

Deep vein thrombosis (DVT). Measures are taken to prevent the development of DVT. Antiembolic stockings will be fitted preoperatively and kept in situ postoperatively. They should be removed and replaced twice daily for skin inspection and hygiene. An exercise programme will be supervised by the physiotherapist.

Urinary retention. This is a potential problem. If all purely nursing measures fail then intermittent catheterisation may be advised. The insertion of a self-retaining catheter should be avoided because of the risk of creating a septic focus and of infecting the wound.

Mobility and rehabilitation

The patient may begin to mobilise on the second or third post-operative day depending on the type of artificial joint and the surgical approach used. This will be supervised by the physiotherapist and the nurse. A hydraulic bed is essential for correct manoeuvring as care must be taken not to flex the hip more than 45° when helping the patient out of bed. This 45° angle must not be exceeded when sitting out of bed and a special armchair with angled cushion is used.

A walking frame may be used at first and the physiotherapist will re-educate the patient to use a normal walking gait. Depending on progress, crutches may be used before discharge.

Aids to living. The occupational therapist will provide aids for dressing such as tights or a stocking applicator, elastic shoe laces and an 'extended hand', and any other aids found to be necessary after an assessment of the home environment and the patient's capabilities.

Discharge planning

The patient will be given a letter for the GP and one for the

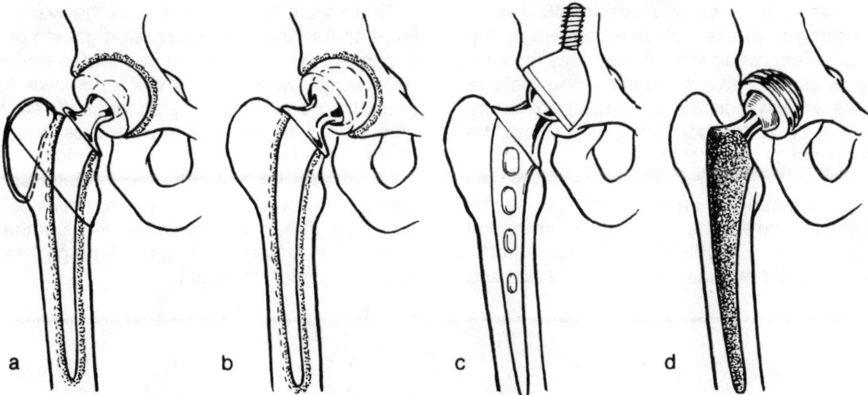

Fig. 10.21 Total hip replacement: (A) Charnley hip replacement with greater trochanter reattachment; (B) Müller-type replacement with larger femoral head; (C) Ring-type replacement using a long, threaded acetabular component without cement; (D) uncemented prosthesis with sintered surfaces and screw-in acetabular prosthesis. (Reproduced with kind permission from Dandy 1989.)

Case History 10.3 The patient's perception of experiences surrounding a total hip replacement

Two months after an operation for hip replacement I am trying to record my experiences, but one thought predominates to such an extent that everything else fades into insignificance. I can think of nothing other than the fact that I have no pain: no pain walking, no pain sitting, no pain lying in bed, no pain at all. Two ideas arise from this: one, that it does not seem at all healthy to be so conscious of the absence of pain. The hope must be that sooner or later being pain free will become the normal unobserved fact of life. The other is a retrospective awareness of the debilitating effect of continuous chronic pain, the insidious way in which everything developed. People now keep exclaiming that I look so well, that my colour has improved so much. They never in the past told me that I looked old and grey. This must have been as unremarkable to others as the experience of continuous pain was to me.

There were many different kinds of pain. The worst in intensity was probably the pain on weight bearing, but somehow it did not bother me so very much, I felt I could anticipate it, control it by leaning on a stick or furniture, or by refraining from walking altogether. There were sudden and very acute bouts of pain, sharp like toothache, on sudden movements or jolts, but these passed and did not matter much. There was the impossibility of ever sitting or lying in comfort, much less severe pain, but the most difficult to bear. It was when that particular pain suddenly got much worse that I first told the general practitioner how I felt. When in spite of anti-inflammatory painkillers even the weight of the sheet became intolerable and lack of sleep became difficult to cope with, an appointment was made with the Orthopaedic Specialist Services. The nature of the worst of the continuous pain, however, was none of these, it was almost not experienced as pain at all. It was a deep nagging, dragging, twisting sensation which was nauseating and depressing, not responding to analgesics at all, analgesics which I took in maximal dosage and which added to the feeling of nausea, depression and apathy. Neither the general practitioner nor I myself was keen on the thought of surgery, the GP no doubt because he was conscious of obesity being a contraindication for surgical intervention, I myself because I knew of many cases when no great improvement followed hip replacement. As soon as my friends had heard that I had been put on the waiting list, example after example was related to me of how wonderful Mr or Mrs X, Y, Z were as a result of this operation — 'a new lease of life', 'years younger' 'never looked back'. But my own attention focused, not on their reassurance, but on those people I had met who had developed infections, whose prosthesis had broken down, who had to have a second operation. It was no help to see a television programme and read a newspaper article about the inferior quality of the prostheses which were coming on the market at present.

Now after the operation I have joined the ranks of those who extol the virtue of the operation, but even the most enthusiastic supporters had not prepared me for the speed with which it would be possible to lead a normal life: walking within 48 hours, discharged from hospital within two weeks, fully independent by the time of the follow-up outpatient appointment six weeks after operation. Here in summary are the events which I now believe made the whole experience entirely positive: on first appointment at the Orthopaedic Outpatient clinic the thorough examination, the fact that the surgeon appeared to understand how much pain I had – perhaps even better than I did – and did not belittle what I was saying. The fact that he arranged immediately, before the operation, to start physiotherapy and that he promised an operation as soon as possible. I was on the waiting list for only four months. A week before the operation there was a day of tests and examinations in the ward to which I was to be admitted giving a good opportunity to allay anxiety. I was glad that I had explanations of the operation, the anaesthetic and the possible risks. I appreciated the time taken to answer my questions and the sensitivity of the staff though I do not think I could have entered into any decision making in spite of the explanations. My anxiety about the post-operative phase, about living alone, upstairs, in a relatively large flat was well understood and arrangements were made by the occupational therapist, at that early stage, for various pieces of helpful equipment to be delivered to the house. I was assured that I would be fully rehabilitated by the time of discharge which was anticipated to be after about two weeks, but I found this difficult to believe.

On admission I was immediately aware of the cordiality and friendliness of the nursing staff and of the community spirit of the patients who made me feel welcome and who augmented the very adequate information given to me by the staff, both in print and in discussion.

Pre-operative relief of anxiety and post-operative pain control were superb; after the initial intravenous analgesic cover, painkillers were offered every four hours, but not really needed except before physiotherapy after the first few days. It was interesting to observe that all patients who had hip operations went through the same progression of skill acquisition and setbacks, learning how to get in and out of bed, how to turn in bed, how to walk, first with a Zimmer frame, then with two and later one stick, how to pick things off the floor, to put on stockings and shoes, to shower independently, to dress and undress, to climb stairs and to get in and out of a car. It was evident that all the nurses knew exactly what each patient was capable of doing. All were willing to help but clearly expected and encouraged independence. Primary nursing was not practical, it would have made no sense to deploy the skills of the most highly trained and most experienced nurse on a patient approaching discharge, when newly operated patients needed them so much more. But their awareness of patients' progress and the supervision of the activities of less highly qualified staff were always in evidence. It was reassuring to notice that there was vigilance in case deep vein thrombosis arose and to see the speed with which one patient was advised to go to bed, the foot of which was raised, and how speedily support stockings were offered. With the emphasis throughout on what one can do by oneself and encouragement to get moving, it was a boost to self confidence to know that nurses were vigilant for complications and setbacks. I found it helpful to have been shown the X-ray of the new hip as it makes it possible to visualise what the joint is doing during various activities, and to understand why one is advised never to cross the legs, to get on all fours or to pick things up off the floor from the sitting position. A pillow between the legs during sleep helps not to cross the legs accidentally.

There were twelve women in the ward, most of them for hip or knee operations. The impression gained on admission of a friendly, supportive group spirit was reinforced throughout. What a wealth of experience, what a reservoir of knowledge, what abundance of empathy, goodwill and helpfulness. There was also a tremendous amount of fun and humour, perhaps enhanced by the experience all had of being painfree all of a sudden.

I learned a lot, not only about health and illness, but also about emotional, social and economic stress, and about coping strategies. The importance of the patient community and its therapeutic potential is seldom recognised in general nursing but it should never be underestimated.

community nurse should that be necessary. The continuing medication regime will be clarified. Written instructions on adapting to the artificial hip will be given to the patient and discussed in detail. These will include restrictions to normal mobility such as avoiding rotational movements, extreme abduction and hip flexion, leg crossing and any activity that puts stress on the new joint. Counselling regarding sexual activity should be included in the pre-discharge discussions. It is a subject often avoided by doctors and nurses but must be addressed because of the possibility of hip dislocation if the correct advice is not given, i.e. that sexual activity should be avoided for 6–8 weeks and that, once resumed, any position involving extreme hip flexion and abduction must be avoided.

Physiotherapy may be continued and a gradual return to a fairly active lifestyle pursued.

(Read Case History 10.3 again.)

> ? **10.13** From information provided above write a concise discharge plan for a patient who has undergone an uncomplicated total hip replacement.

SOFT TISSUE INJURIES

LIGAMENT INJURIES

PATHOPHYSIOLOGY

Excessive extension, flexion and/or rotation of a joint may result in a partial or complete rupture of a ligament. Whiplash injury is the term used to describe a ligamentous injury to the cervical spine area often occurring after a road traffic accident (see Fig. 10.15). This injury is due to excessive flexion and extension movements to the neck. A sportsman's knee joint can often be subjected to extreme rotational force which results in a severe ligamentous injury with often permanent disability.

MEDICAL MANAGEMENT

History. People who suffer these injuries are often young and will complain of severe pain around the injured area after feeling or hearing something snap or tear. Pain may be increased when the person's body weight is exerted through the injured limb. Frequently if other serious injuries have been sustained this injury may be overlooked until the patient complains of pain from the ligamentous injury at a later time.

Examination. Limitation of normal joint movement may be found with swelling of the injured part. Joint instability may be noted during the physical examination.

Investigation. Plain radiographs are taken to rule out a bony injury to the area. An arthroscopy may be performed or the patient may need to have the joint examined under general anaesthesia.

Treatment. Non-operative management is the usual mode of treatment. If bleeding into the injured joint (haemoarthrosis) has occurred this may be aspirated under anaesthesia. The injured area will be splinted, for example using a cervical collar (Fig. 10.22) for a whiplash injury or a Plaster of Paris cylinder for a knee injury. Surgical intervention is usually only needed when the injury affects the knee joint or where there is damage to more than one ligament and/or gross instability of the joint.

NURSING PRIORITIES AND MANAGEMENT: LIGAMENT INJURIES

The patient may arrive at the accident and emergency department within a few hours of injury (see Ch. 28). In other cases, the patient may present as much as 12–24 hours after injury when the pain and swelling have greatly increased. If no other injury has been sustained the patient may be treated and discharged to attend as an outpatient.

Pain. This will be the major patient problem on presentation at hospital. An effective analgesic such as dihydrocodeine (DF 118) may be prescribed, to be administered orally or by the intramuscular route. As ligamentous injuries are sustained following severe trauma to the body, the surrounding soft tissues will also be traumatised. This will cause further bleeding which will increase the swelling and irritate the surrounding tissues thus increasing the patient's pain.

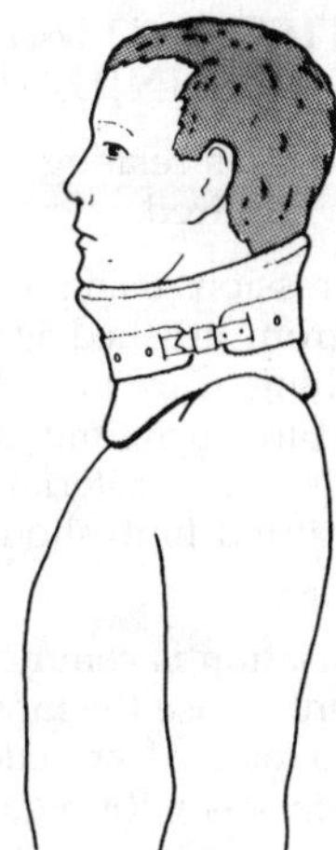

Fig. 10.22 Cervical collar. (Reproduced with kind permission from Allan 1989.)

Muscle spasm. This is a common sign of soft tissue irritation and if severe the patient may need a mild antispasmodic such as Diazepam as well as an analgesic.

Splinting. Refer to priorities and management of patients in casts. In addition, when a cervical collar is worn, it can usually be removed to allow daily skin care. Men should be advised to shave regularly, in order to keep the skin under the mandibular and neck regions stubble free to prevent irritation.

MUSCLE AND TENDON INJURIES

PATHOPHYSIOLOGY

These injuries are most often caused by either direct trauma at the site of the injury or by a sudden sharp movement of the joint associated with sports such as tennis and squash.

The large tendons and muscles of the lower limb are the most common sites of injury.

MEDICAL MANAGEMENT

History. The patient will experience a distressing tearing sensation or a kick at the site of the injury and possibly an inability to put the foot down. Swelling and tenderness will develop within a few hours following the injury. Bruising will appear later and may be extensive and alarming for the patient.

On examination a gap between the ends of the muscle or tendon may be felt.

Treatment. Initial treatment is by cold compression and elevation to reduce the extent of the swelling. Contraction of the muscle should be avoided during the first few days following the injury as this will increase the extent of the swelling. Rest in the most comfortable position is advisable initially. A padded crepe bandage may be applied to help reduce the swelling. The physiotherapist may use ultrasound to help disperse the haematoma. The injury may take 6 weeks or more before it is healed.

Surgical intervention is seldom indicated in muscle injuries. Complete muscle tears and tendon injuries will require total immobilisation in a cast or splint until healed. A ruptured tendon may require surgical repair.

NURSING PRIORITIES AND MANAGEMENT: MUSCLE AND TENDON INJURIES

Comfort. General principles relating to comfort and support will be implemented as required.

Swelling. Cold compression using commercial cold packs or an ice pack made from crushed ice in a plastic bag will help to reduce the swelling. Care must be taken to protect the patient's skin from a cold burn, and the cold pack must be wrapped in a towel or similar material before it is applied to the skin surface. The injured limb should be kept elevated as much as possible.

Mobility. Once mobilisation is commenced, the physiotherapist will teach the patient to use the most appropriate walking aid, which is usually a pair of crutches. Assessment of the patient's home circumstances with regard to his mobility will be required. It is unlikely that any active physiotherapy will be given over the first 6 weeks following injury; thereafter the patient will attend as an outpatient. An ambulance may be required to transport the patient to and from hospital for these appointments.

Should the patient have a cast applied, advice and information about cast care will be given (see p. 377).

PERIPHERAL NERVE INJURIES

Nerves can be damaged due to underlying disease or following trauma. In this section the focus will be on injuries following trauma.

PATHOPHYSIOLOGY

A single nerve or group of nerves may be damaged depending on the site of injury. Nerve injuries can be due to either direct or indirect force.

MEDICAL MANAGEMENT

History and examination. Following an accident, a patient may become aware of tingling (paraesthesia), numbness and/or loss of movement of the affected part. A common cause of a severed nerve is a cut from a sharp knife, piece of glass or bone fragment. Road traffic accidents are frequently the cause of a crushing or stretching nerve injury.

Examination of the distribution of the loss of sensation and movement will assist the medical practitioner to a diagnosis.

Investigation. Plain radiographs are useful to assess bony injury and the presence of any foreign material, such as glass fragments, which may have caused the injury.

Diagnosis. This is confirmed by the absence or alteration of neurological function and sensation of the affected part. The specific nerve(s) can often be identified due to the distribution of the change in movement and/or feeling.

Treatment. Primary surgical repair is indicated only when a nerve has been cleanly divided. Secondary repair may include suturing and grafting of nerve tissue from a less important nerve within the patient's body. Non-operative management involves immobilisation of the affected part in the anatomical position, using a lightweight cast or splint. Peripheral nerves are capable of regenerating at the rate of 1 mm a day (Dandy 1989). It is possible to calculate roughly the length of time of recovery although there is no guarantee that each nerve cell will heal.

NURSING PRIORITIES AND MANAGEMENT: PERIPHERAL NERVE INJURIES

A patient who suffers a nerve injury may come to hospital immediately after being injured or there may be a time delay before the full extent of the injury is realised.

As the patient will have been involved in some form of trauma, nursing care as outlined in Chapter 28 will apply.

Should the patient require surgery, general peri-operative care will be as described in Chapter 27.

Preventing further injury

The major problem will be loss of function and sensation of the body area supplied by the injured nerve. As the patient will have partial or complete loss of the protective mechanisms of touch and pain, care must be taken to prevent further injury to the affected part. Movement of the injured limb must be through the normal range of passive joint movements otherwise joints, muscles, tendons, ligaments and other nerves could be damaged further. To prevent the development of joint contracture and deformity the patient will be fitted with a lightweight splint which holds the joints in their anatomical position. This may be needed for a long period. Exposure to extremes of temperature should be avoided, thus preventing the development of a skin burn. Loss of function and/or sensation of any part of the body is extremely frightening. The members of the health care team need to give easily understood explanations to the patient and his relatives during the period of treatment and rehabilitation to help reduce anxiety.

Subsequent considerations

Pain. Sharp shooting pain and a constant tingling sensation can be very troublesome and the patient may need prolonged use of analgesics. Diversional therapy as organised by both the physiotherapist and the occupational therapist can be helpful should the acute pain become a chronic problem.

The nurse may also wish to suggest as an adjunct the use of one of the many alternative therapies that are widely available.

Washing and dressing. The patient will need advice and information to assist in adapting his usual mode of personal cleansing and dressing. For instance a patient with a median nerve injury due to a laceration of the wrist of his dominant hand may have difficulty in brushing his teeth or combing his hair. The occupational therapist can provide appropriate aids.

Splints. If a splint is used the patient will need information and advice about the correct method of application and removal. The patient with sensitive skin has to be taught to inspect it for signs of pressure by removing the splint at regular intervals throughout the day.

Exercise. The physiotherapist will exercise the joints of the injured limb passively to prevent stiffness and muscle wasting. The patient may be able to use his own hands to exercise his joints, or a relative can be taught the skill of passive exercises. Not only will this assist physical recovery but can also be of psychological benefit.

Support. As a peripheral nerve injury may take many weeks to recover the patient will require support and understanding from family, friends and the members of the health care team to relieve boredom and prevent the development of depression. Group sessions for patients with similar injuries receiving physiotherapy, occupational therapy and/or diversional therapy can create an excellent psychological support mechanism for all concerned. The social worker can assist with any social and/or financial problems which may develop due to the possible lengthy absence from employment.

Permanent disability. If the nerve injury prevents the patient from returning to his previous occupation it will be necessary for the local occupational resettlement officer to be contacted. For example, a butcher who sustains a severe injury to the nerves of his dominant hand, which leaves a permanent paralysis, will not be able to continue his previous employment. With retraining, he could be employed, for example, as a driver of an automatic vehicle with a slightly altered steering wheel.

In some instances, alteration to body image could have a severe psychological effect. Nurses should be aware of this and provide support and counselling as requested by the patient.

CONCLUSION

This chapter has outlined the basic principles of nursing management that relate to the more common musculoskeletal disorders and has focused on some of the critical factors that influence management and care in specific disorders. It has stressed that the focus of care is the patient and his family; and that the challenge to nursing increases with changing trends in health orientation, care in the community, early discharge home and an ageing population whose lifestyle has been revolutionised by joint replacement surgery and multidisciplinary care and support.

Trauma is a constant in human societies and musculoskeletal injuries will always be a fact of life. However, continuing research and more attention to health screening and health promotion has shown that many accidents and conditions are preventable and many diseases amenable to treatment.

A wide knowledge of musculoskeletal disorders is essential for both hospital- and community-based nurses to enable them to respond to the needs of patients and their families, to work actively to prevent accidents and complications, and to give appropriate information and advice.

REFERENCES

Allan D 1989 Nursing and the neurosciences. Churchill Livingstone, Edinburgh

Central Statistical Office 1990 Annual abstract of statistics. HMSO, London

Currey H 1988 Essentials of rheumatology, 2nd edn. Churchill Livingstone, Edinburgh

Dandy D 1989 Essential orthopaedics and trauma. Churchill Livingstone, Edinburgh

Dirix A, Knuttgen H G, Tittel K (eds) 1988 The Olympic book of sports medicine. Blackwell Scientific Publications, Oxford, vol 1

Harvey A, Durbin J 1986 The effects of seat belt legislation on British road casualties: a case study of structural time series modelling. Journal of the Royal Statistical Society 149(3): 187–209

Health and Safety Council/Health Executive 1989 Annual report. HMSO, London

Kubler Ross E 1973 On death and dying. Tavistock Publications, London

Le Gallez P 1993 Rheumatoid arthritis: effects on the family. Nursing Standard 7 (39): 30–34

Monk C 1981 Orthopaedics for undergraduates. Oxford University Press, Oxford

Mouratoglou V 1986 Amputees and phantom limb pain: a literature review. Physiotherapy Practice 2: 177–185

National Back Pain Association and Royal College of Nurses 1992. The guide to the handling of patients. NBPA/RCN, London

Orem D 1990 Nursing: concepts of practice, 4th edn. Mosby, New York

Powell M 1986 Orthopaedic nursing and rehabilitation. Churchill Livingstone, Edinburgh

Royal College of Nursing Advisory Panel for Back Pain in Nurses 1992 Code of practice for the handling of patients. RCN, London

Robertson S 1993 Disability rights handbook April 1993–1994. Educational and Research Association, London

Roper N, Logan W W & Tierney A J 1990 The elements of nursing, 3rd edn. Churchill Livingstone, Edinburgh

Royle J A, Walsh M (eds) 1992 Watson's medical–surgical nursing and related physiology, 4th edn. Baillière Tindall, London

Smith C 1987 Orthopaedic nursing. Heinemann, London

Smith Suddarth D (ed) 1991 The Lippincott manual of nursing practice, 5th edn. J B Lippincott, Philadelphia

Taylor I 1987 Ward manual of orthopaedic traction. Churchill Livingstone, Melbourne

Taylor I 1990 Ward manual of orthopaedic traction, 2nd edn. Churchill Livingstone, Edinburgh

Toscano J 1988 Prevention of neurological deterioration before admission to a spinal cord injury unit. Paraplegia 26(3): 148

Trounce J 1988 Clinical pharmacology for nurses. Churchill Livingstone, Edinburgh

Wilson K J W 1990 Ross & Wilson anatomy and physiology in health and illness, 7th edn. Churchill Livingstone, Edinburgh

UKCC 1992 Code of professional conduct for the nurse, midwife and health visitor. UKCC, London

FURTHER READING

Boore J 1978 Prescription for recovery. RCN, London

First aid manual: the authorised manual of St John's Ambulance, St Andrew's Ambulance Association, the British Red Cross Society 1992 Dorling Kindersley, London

Footner A 1987 Orthopaedic nursing. Baillière Tindall, London

Hayward J 1975 Information — a prescription against pain. RCN, London

Jamieson E, McCall J, Blythe R 1992 Guidelines for clinical nursing practice, 2nd edn. Churchill Livingstone, Edinburgh

Jayson M 1987 Back pain — the facts, 2nd edn. Oxford University Press, Oxford

Lowthian P 1989 Pressure sore prevention. Nursing 3(34): 17–23

Marchette L, Marchette B 1985 Back injury: a preventable occupational hazard. Orthopaedic Nursing 4(6): 25–29

Marieb E 1992 Human anatomy and physiology, 2nd edn. Benjamin Cummings, California

Royal College of Nursing 1979 Avoiding low back pain injury among nurses. RCN, London

Tubercle and Lung Disease Journal

USEFUL ADDRESSES

Arthritis Care,
18 Stephenson Way,
London NW1 2HD

The Arthritis and Rheumatism Council,
Copeman House, St Mary's Gate,
Chesterfield,
Derbyshire SH 7TD

The Association to Aid the Sexual and Personal Relationships of People with a Disability (SPOD),
286 Camden Road, London N7 OBJ

Disabled Living Foundation,
380–384 Harrow Road,
London
W9 2HU

RCN Orthopaedic Forum,
20 Cavendish Square,
London
W1M 0AB

CHAPTER 11

Blood disorders

Fiona M. Duke

CHAPTER CONTENTS

Introduction 405
Anatomy and physiology 406
DISORDERS OF RED BLOOD CELLS: ANAEMIAS 411
Nursing priorities and management 413
Iron deficiency anaemia 414
Nursing priorities and management 415
Megaloblastic anaemias 416
Nursing priorities and management 419
Aplastic anaemia 420
Nursing priorities and management 421
Haemolytic anaemias 421
Sickle cell anaemia 423
Nursing priorities and management 423
Anaemia resulting from blood loss 424
Nursing priorities and management 424
DISORDERS CAUSED BY OVERPRODUCTION OF RED BLOOD CELLS 425
Polycythaemia vera 425
Nursing priorities and management 425
DISORDERS OF WHITE BLOOD CELLS AND LYMPHOID TISSUE 426
Leukaemia 426
Acute leukaemia 426
Nursing priorities and management 428
Chronic leukaemia 434
Nursing priorities and management 434
Lymphoma 434
Nursing priorities and management 436
Multiple myeloma 436
Nursing priorities and management 437
Agranulocytosis 438
Nursing priorities and management 439
DISORDERS OF PLATELETS AND COAGULATION 439
Nursing priorities and management 440
References 440
Further reading 441
Useful addresses 441
Glossary 441

INTRODUCTION

Blood is a vital body fluid which, via the cardiovascular system, reaches all body tissue and cells. Its three primary functions are:

- to transport oxygen, nutrients and other substances
- to protect the body against microorganisms and antigens
- to regulate homeostatic systems.

Disorders of the blood are diverse and may be acute or chronic. All age groups may be affected, although some disorders are more common in certain age bands than in others. Some disorders, such as haemophilia, are sex-linked. Others, such as sickle cell disease and thalassaemia, are more prevalent among certain ethnic groups; still others, such as nutritional anaemia, occur worldwide.

Causes of blood disorders

Contributing factors in the development of blood disorders can be divided into eight types:

1. Developmental. Infants and elderly people can be predisposed to anaemia, the former group because of increased nutritional requirements for growth and development, and the latter because of poor eating habits resulting from such factors as depression and reduced mobility.
2. Genetic. Inherited disorders include certain abnormalities of the red blood cells (e.g. spherocytosis), haemoglobin abnormalities (e.g. thalassaemia and sickle cell anaemia) and the lack of a clotting factor (haemophilia and von Willebrand's disease).
3. Dietary. Nutritional deficiencies can be related to poverty, lack of knowledge about nutrition and healthy cooking methods, and to overriding political and economic circumstances.
4. Sociocultural. Dietary habits leading to nutritional deficiency may be related to values and beliefs. Strict vegetarians, for example, may develop vitamin B12 deficiency anaemia. Lifestyle factors, such as a reliance on fast foods or a habit of skipping meals, can also lead to nutritional anaemias. Other social factors such as homelessness and unemployment can contribute to poor nutrition leading to the development of blood disorders.
5. Environmental. Exposure to industrial chemicals (e.g. benzene, lead, sodium chlorate) and to ionising radiation has been linked to the development of blood disorders such as aplastic anaemia, agranulocytosis and leukaemia.
6. Pharmacological. Over-the-counter and prescription drugs have been known to cause several blood disorders (Firkin 1987). Agranulocytosis can be caused by dapsone (an antileprotic) and by some antithyroid drugs (e.g. carbimazole).

Quinine, quinidine and heparin can cause thrombocytopenia by damaging the platelets. Prolonged use of aspirin and non-steroidal anti-inflammatory drugs (NSAIDs) can lead to iron-deficiency anaemia. Most cancer chemotherapy agents cause myelosuppression and thus anaemia, neutropenia and thrombocytopenia.

7. Iatrogenic. Medical interventions that cause blood disorders include the use of prosthetic heart valves that can damage red blood cells and after a gastrectomy resulting in a lack of intrinsic factor, leading to Vitamin B12 anaemia.

8. Pathological. Diseases which can cause blood disorders, particularly anaemia, include inflammatory diseases, malabsorption syndromes, cancers and infections.

9. Idiopathic. In some cases of anaemia, especially aplastic anaemia, no cause can be discovered.

The nurse's role in the treatment of blood disorders

The nurse's role in caring for patients with blood disorders in a community, hospital or occupational setting will include the following functions:

- promoting health, e.g. by encouraging good dietary habits
- detecting early signs of illness such as fatigue, pallor, frequent absence from work
- assisting with medical investigations, e.g. bone marrow aspiration, dietary histories
- explaining tests, diagnoses, treatments and prognoses to patients
- educating patients about lifestyle, diet and medication
- providing emotional support to patients and their families
- referring patients to other professionals such as genetic counsellors.

Depending upon their work setting and specialism, nurses will play a variety of roles in the care of patients with blood disorders. Primary health care nurses, e.g. district nurses, health visitors, and practice nurses may be involved in health screening and may be the individual's first point of contact with the health care team. Hospital nurses may come across anaemic patients in all types of wards and units. Specialist nurses may work as sickle cell disease counsellors or in haemophiliac centres. Macmillan nurses may provide care for patients with leukaemia in their homes.

The particular needs of patients with blood disorders will vary in accordance with the nature of their illness. Some patients may present with one very acute episode of illness, e.g. massive haemorrhage, and then return to full health after treatment. More commonly, patients are diagnosed with blood disorders after a prolonged period of malaise.

ANATOMY AND PHYSIOLOGY

Blood is red viscous fluid which is pumped from the heart via the arteries to the capillaries in the tissues and returns via the veins to the heart. Its central role is to help maintain an optimal environment for the functioning of the body cells. It fulfils this role by performing the following functions:

- transporting oxygen, essential nutrients and other important substances (e.g. hormones, enzymes, chemicals) to all cells
- removing carbon dioxide and other waste products from the cell
- maintaining haemostasis
- protecting the body from microorganisms and antigens
- regulating water, electrolytes and acid–base balance
- regulating body temperature.

The total volume of blood circulating in an average adult is 5 l. Blood consists of cellular and fluid components, the main constituents of which are:

- water
- plasma proteins
- electrolytes
- nutrients
- hormones
- enzymes
- waste products.

Cellular components of blood

There are three different cellular components of blood, namely:

- red cells
- white cells
- platelets.

These cellular components are developed in the active bone marrow found in the medullary cavity of certain bones of the adult. The sites of the active bone marrow are:

- ends of the long bones (e.g. humerus)
- ribs
- sternum
- ilia of the pelvis
- vertebrae.

These sites can be extended when there is an increased demand for blood cells. There is evidence that each blood cell is derived from a pluripotent cell or stem cell (Allan 1991).

Red blood cells (erythrocytes)

Red blood cells are biconcave discs. Haemoglobin (the molecule involved in the transport of oxygen within the red cell) makes up 95% of the cell and gives blood its characteristic red colour. The thin membrane cell allows gaseous exchange between the cell and surrounding tissues. The cell is also soft and pliable, allowing it to pass along the capillary lumen easily. During maturation the red blood cell extrudes its nucleus. The mature cell therefore has no capacity to reproduce, repair, grow or make haemoglobin.

Function. Oxygen is carried in the form of oxyhaemoglobin by the red blood cells from the lungs to the tissues. Carbon dioxide, as carboxyhaemoglobin, is transported from the tissues to the lungs.

Maturation. (See Fig. 11.1.) The total number of circulating red blood cells remains fairly constant at 4.5–5.4 $\times$ 10^{12} cells/l to ensure that the optimum amount of oxygen is available to the tissues. To ensure this number the body has to maintain a balance between the number of cells produced and the number broken down.

The reticulocyte numbers are increased when there is a greater demand for red blood cells. Therefore, a reticulocyte count can be used as a measure of response to treatment for anaemia (a deficiency of haemoglobin in the blood due to a lack of red blood cells and/or haemoglobin content). Treatment should stimulate production of more reticulocytes.

The essential factors required for red cell production are:

- iron: part of haemoglobin molecule (see below)
- amino acids
- vitamin B12: for synthesis of DNA
- intrinsic factor: for absorption of Vitamin B12 from gut
- folic acid: for DNA synthesis
- vitamin C
- thyroxine } Promote erythropoietin formation
- androgens }
- adrenocortical steroids }
- human growth hormone.

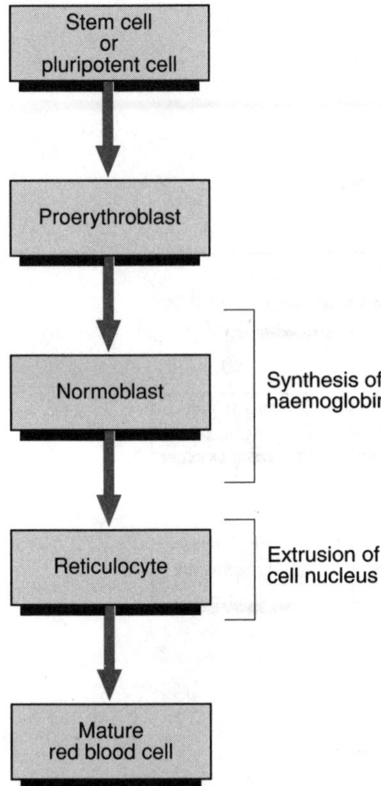

Fig. 11.1 Maturation of red blood cell.

Haemoglobin is a complex molecule of haem and globin. The haem fraction is the combination of porphyrin and iron. The globin complex is composed of polypeptide chains.

Destruction. The average lifespan of a red blood cell is 120 days. At the end of its lifespan the cell is broken down in the spleen and liver by macrophages. The haemoglobin molecule is split into its major components: haem and globin. The globin is further split into amino acids which then are stored in the body's amino acid pool. The haem is split into iron, which is stored in the liver and reused by the marrow, and porphyrin, which is converted to bilirubin. The bilirubin (insoluble in water at this stage) is transported to the liver, converted into soluble bilirubin and excreted into the small intestine as a constituent of bile. From there some is reabsorbed and excreted by kidneys as urobilinogen. The majority of the bilirubin is excreted in the faeces as stercobilirubin.

White blood cells (leucocytes)

There are three types of white blood cells:

- granulocytes
- lymphocytes
- monocytes.

Granulocytes are characterised by the presence of granules in the cytoplasm and are divided into three subtypes: neutrophils, eosinophils and basophils. Lymphocytes are subdivided into T-lymphocytes and B-lymphocytes. Of the lymphocytes circulating in the blood, 75% are T-lymphocytes and 25% are B-lymphocytes. Monocytes are of one type only.

Normal numbers and percentages of each type and subtype are given in Table 11.1.

Function. The white blood cells are involved in the defence of the body against microbes and antigens. (For further details of their functions see Ch. 16.)

Maturation. All white blood cells develop from a pluripotent or stem cell in the bone marrow and mature through several stages as illustrated in Figure 11.2. Granulocyte formation is regulated by humoral factors, some of which may be produced locally in bone marrow.

Lymphocytes mature in either bone marrow (B-lymphocytes) or in the thymus (T-lymphocytes); (see Ch. 16).

Lifespan. The different types of white blood cells have variable lifespans. Neutrophils, once they enter the blood, circulate for about 7 hours and then migrate into the tissues, where they die after a few days. Lymphocytes have a variable lifespan ranging from 100 days to several years. Monocytes, which mature into macrophages (scavenger cells) in the tissues, can survive for many years.

Platelets (thrombocytes)

Platelets are small, granular, non-nucleated blood cells that play a vital role in haemostasis (arrest of bleeding).

Function. Platelets are involved in the first three phases of haemostasis:

- phase 1: vasoconstriction of injured vessel
- phase 2: formation of platelet plug
- phase 3: formation of fibrin clot

The fourth and final stage, fibrinolysis (dissolution of the fibrin clot), does not involve platelets.

During phase 1 of haemostasis narrowing of the damaged blood vessel occurs in response to the release of powerful vasoconstrictors, serotonin and thromboxane A, by the platelets. This reduces blood flow and thus decreases the likelihood of the platelet plug being sloughed off. In phase 2 platelets adhere to the site of the damage and release adenosine diphosphate (ADP), which causes the platelets to

Table 11.1 Normal number of different subtypes of white blood cells

Type	Subtype	Normal value (cells/C)	% total	
Granulocytes		$2.5–8.0 \times 10^9$	40–75%	
	Neutrophils	$2.0–7.5 \times 10^9$	40–70%	% of total white blood cell count
	Eosinophils	Up to 0.4×10^9	1–6%	
	Basophils	$< 0.1 \times 10^9$	<1%	
Lymphocytes		$1.5–4.0 \times 10^9$	20–50%	
	B-lymphocytes		15–30%	% of total lymphocytes
	T-lymphocytes		40–80%	
Monocytes		$0.2–0.8 \times 10^9$	2–10%	

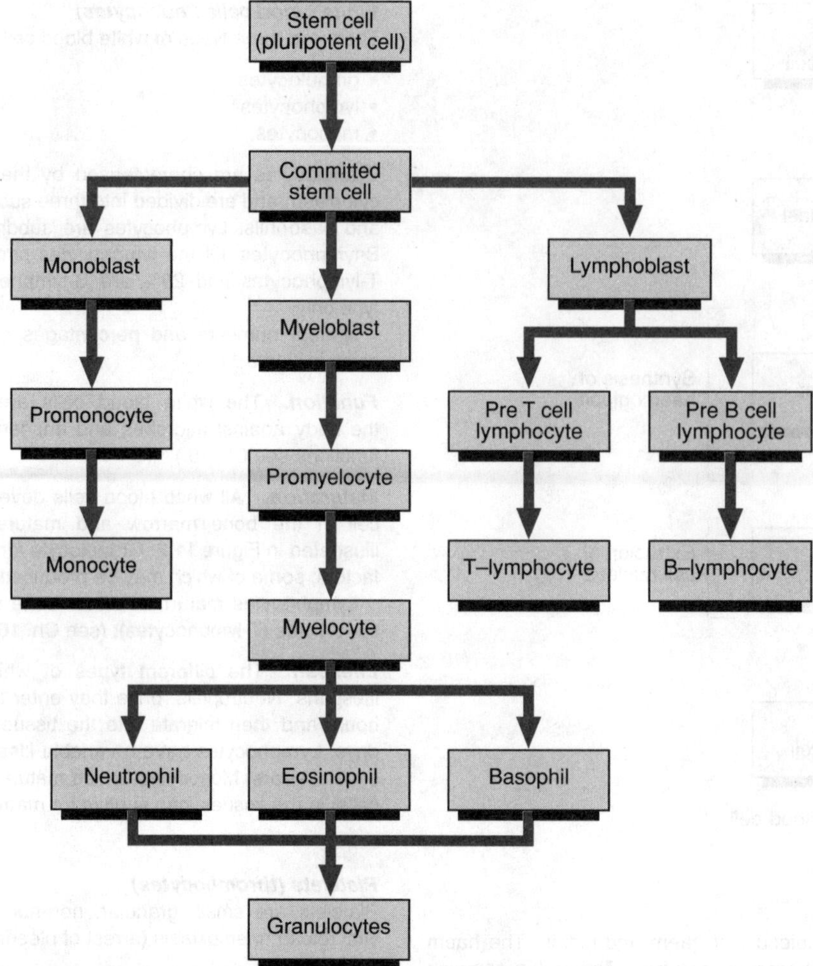

Fig. 11.2 Development of different types of leucocytes.

adopt a spherical shape conducive to aggregation. In phase 3 a fibrin clot is formed. This involves the conversion of prothrombin to thrombin, which then acts on fibrinogen (a plasma protein) to form fibrin. This fibrin clot is soluble at first but becomes insoluble in the presence of calcium and clotting Factor XIII (fibrin-stabilising factor).

The formation of fibrin in stage 3 is made possible by two cascades of events known as the extrinsic pathway (events outside the damaged blood vessel) and the intrinsic pathway (events inside the vessel). See Fig. 11.3. The extrinsic pathway is activated by the tissue damage. The intrinsic pathway is activated by exposed collagen. Each stage in the intrinsic pathway is regulated by a particular clotting factor. Together, the two cascades act on clotting Factor X, which then activates the prothrombin.

Vitamin K, a fat-soluble vitamin, is required for the synthesis in the liver of the following clotting factors (Hinchliff & Montague 1988):

- Factor II (prothrombin)
- Factor VII
- Factor IX (Christmas factor)
- Factor X (Stuart factor).

?	**11.1** What foods contain vitamin K?	A
?	**11.2** Where is vitamin K synthesised in the body?	A
?	**11.3** Which patients are likely to have a prolonged clotting time because of vitamin K deficiency?	A

Plasma

Plasma is the straw-coloured fluid part of the blood which is left after the cellular components are removed. It contains none of the blood clotting factors. Serum is the term for the fluid which separates from blood when it coagulates. It contains some of the blood clotting factors. The main constituents of plasma are shown in Figure 11.4.

Further details on the anatomy and physiology of blood can be found in Wilson (1990) and Tortora & Anagnostakos (1990).

Blood groups

ABO blood groups

In Great Britain 53% of the population have a specific antigen, called an agglutinogen, on the red cell membrane. These agglutinogens are referred to in terms of the ABO blood group system. A person can have either the A or B agglutinogen on the red blood membrane, or neither, or both. Agglutinogens are inherited and are present from birth.

The importance of these agglutinogens is apparent when a person is given blood from another person. A person with the agglutinogen A (blood group A) has anti-B antibodies in his serum. (Antibodies are substances that cause clumping to occur when attached to particular antigens.) A person with agglutinogen B (blood group B) has the anti-A agglutinin (or antibody). A person with both agglutinogens A and B, (blood group AB) has no agglutinins, whilst a person with neither A nor

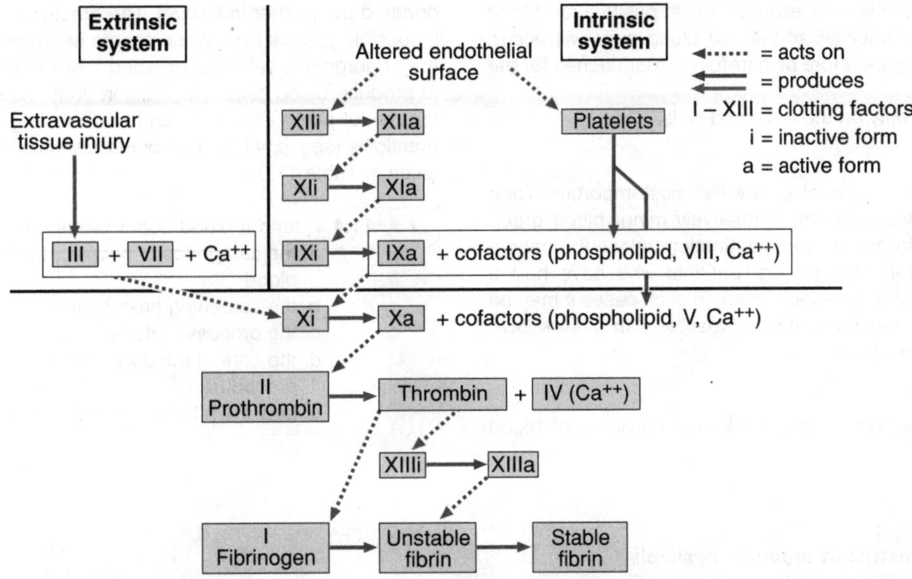

Fig. 11.3 Blood coagulation.

B agglutinogens (blood group O) has both anti-A and anti-B agglutinins (see Table 11.2). Therefore, if a person is given a transfusion of blood of a different group from his own, the red cells will clump together and haemolyse (break down). In a blood transfusion it is the reaction between the donor's red cells and the recipient's serum (i.e. between the introduced agglutinogen and the agglutinin already present) that causes an adverse reaction which can be fatal. Thus, if the recipient's serum has anti-B agglutinin present then the donor's cells must be either blood group A or O.

Table 11.2 Antigens and antibodies present in different blood groups

Blood group	Agglutinogen present on red cell membrane	Agglutinin present in serum
A	A	Anti-B
B	B	Anti-A
AB	AB	None
O	O	Anti-A and anti-B

Not only the red cells but also the white blood cells and platelets have ABO agglutinogens. Therefore, if a patient is to receive a transfusion of other cellular components, the correct blood group should be used.

The Rhesus factor

In Great Britain, 85% of the population have a second important antigen present on their red cells: the Rhesus (Rh) factor. A person is either Rh positive or Rh negative. The antibody, anti-D, does not occur naturally in the plasma of Rh negative blood, but stimulation to produce it can occur if a person receives a Rh positive blood transfusion or if, during childbirth, red blood cells from a Rh positive baby cross the placental barrier into the circulation of a Rh negative mother. In either

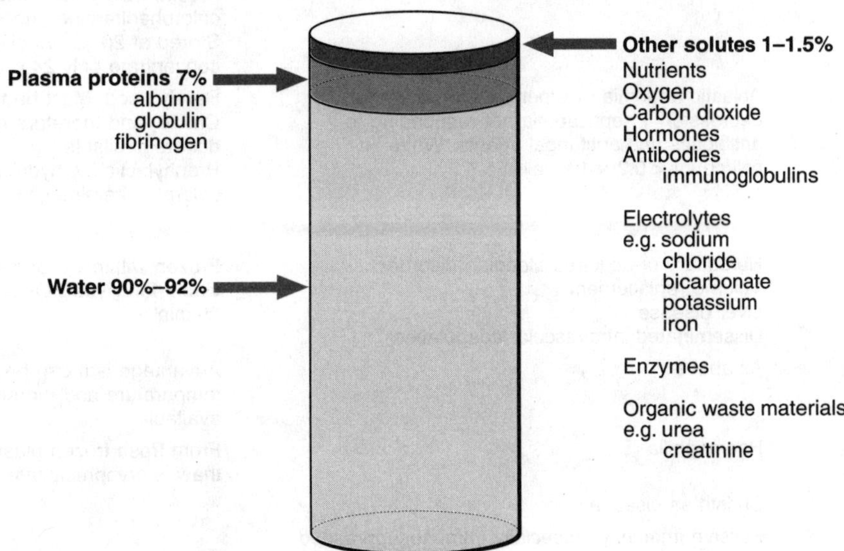

Fig. 11.4 The main constituents of plasma.

of these cases, if the person is later exposed to Rh positive red blood cells, agglutination and haemolysis of the red blood cells will occur. Blood to be transfused must therefore be carefully crossmatched for the Rh factor.

The Rh factor is carried only on the red blood cells.

Other blood groups

The ABO and Rh factor blood groupings are the most important blood classifications but there are many other relatively minor blood group systems which normally do not cause agglutination unless the patient requires multiple blood transfusions, e.g. patients who have had a massive haemorrhage or who have leukaemia; in such cases it may be necessary to ensure the donor's blood is compatible with other known antibodies in the recipient's serum.

Blood transfusion

A blood transfusion is the administration to one individual of blood donated by another individual. The practice of blood transfusion makes it possible to save lives when severe haemorrhage has occurred, when major surgery is required or when there is failure of the bone marrow to produce blood cells. Transfusion does, however, expose patients to the risk of potentially fatal complications, e.g. infection and haemolytic reactions (see p. 417). The blood transfusion products available are given in Table 11.3.

?	**11.4** Attend a blood donor session to find out about: a. the categories of people who are allowed to donate blood b. the screening process for blood donations c. the process of donating a unit of blood d. the care of the donor before, during and after the procedure e. how the blood is stored after donation.	A

Table 11.3 Blood transfusion products available

Product	Indications for use	Special points
Whole Blood	Acute, severe bleeding requiring replacement of red blood cells and plasma and clotting factors	Stored at 4 °C Remains viable for 35 days Platelets and clotting factors have much reduced viability
Fresh whole blood	As above	Blood <24 hours old, therefore more likely to contain viable clotting factors
Red cell concentrate	Replacement of red blood cells only. Therefore used when haemoglobin level is low	Up to 200 ml plasma removed per 500 ml blood
Leucocyte-poor red cells	Indicated for patients who have had febrile reactions during previous transfusions: • patients undergoing transplant • prevention of cytomegalovirus transmission	White blood cells and platelets removed to minimise the risk of an incompatible reaction Cytomegalovirus (CMV) could be transmitted to a person who has no CMV antibodies. This could be fatal in a patient who is immunocompromised (see Ch. 16)
Washed red cells	As for red cell concentrate. Specially prepared to remove antigens	Prevents anaphylactic transfusion reactions
Frozen red cells	As for red cell concentrate	Storage lifespan lengthened, therefore useful for rare blood groups
Platelet concentrate	Patients with platelet count $< 20 \times 10^9$ cell/l but not actively bleeding	Platelet units from blood banks contain platelets from many units of blood, therefore there are frequent reactions. Patient may require i.v. hydrocortisone + i.v. chlorpheniramine prior to transfusion. Stored at 20 °C. Viability of platelet concentrate only 24 h
White cells	Aplastic anaemia or other severe bone marrow depression + septicaemia not responding to antibiotics and antifungal agents. White cell count $< 0.2 \times 10^9$ cells/l	Rarely used. Must be tissue-typed (see Ch. 16) and therefore few compatible donors available. Prophylactic i.v. hydrocortisone and chlorpheniramine given
Other blood components		
Fresh frozen plasma	Hereditary or acquired bleeding disorder Volume replacement Liver disease Disseminated intravascular coagulation	Frozen within 6 h of cell separation and viable for 1 year. Once thawed, use within 30 min
Dried plasma	As above	Advantage is it can be stored at room temperature and therefore is readily available
Cryoprecipitate (factor VIII, fibrinogen)	Haemophilia	From fresh frozen plasma. Last part to thaw is cryoprecipitate
Factor IX	Christmas disease	
Human immunoglobulin	Passive immunity, especially immunosuppressed patients	

Crossmatching

Before a unit of blood or blood component is transfused into another person the blood from the donated unit must be crossmatched with that of the recipient's serum i.e. the blood from the donated unit is mixed in the laboratory with a sample of the recipient's serum. The donor's blood should be of the same ABO blood group to prevent a potentially fatal agglutination reaction. A Rh negative recipient should receive Rh negative blood. Details of the results of the crossmatching are recorded along with the blood unit number on the documentation sent with the unit of blood when the blood transfusion is given. This documentation is retained after the unit of blood has been used in case of the occurrence of any transfusion reactions. (See p. 417 for the nursing care of patients receiving transfusions.)

For further details on blood groups consult Tortora & Anagnostakos (1990).

DISORDERS OF RED BLOOD CELLS: ANAEMIAS

These disorders can be divided into:

- disorders in which there is a deficiency of haemoglobin in the blood due to lack of red cells and/or their haemoglobin content
- disorders due to blood loss
- disorders due to excessive production of the red blood cells.

Anaemias are those disorders in which the blood has a reduced oxygen-carrying capacity. The red blood cells are reduced either in total number or in size because of:

- decreased production
- blood loss
- rapid destruction.

There are three main types of anaemia (see Fig. 11.5):

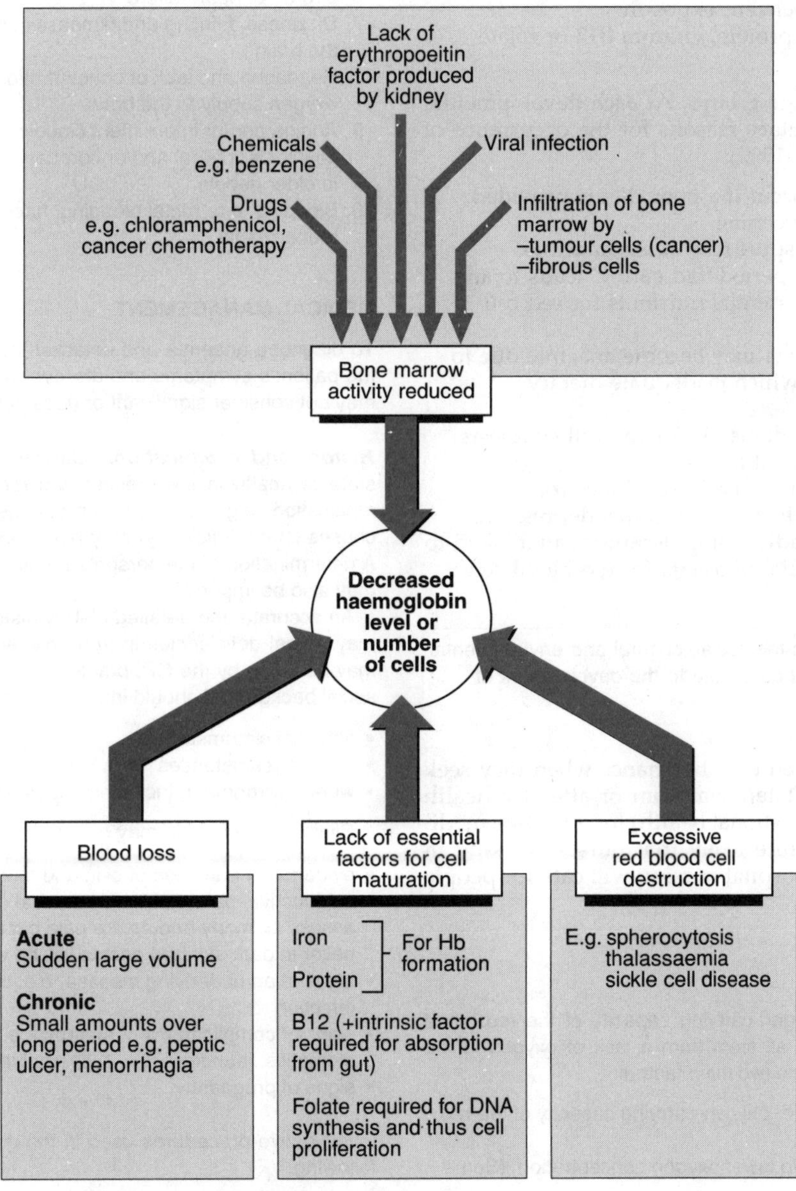

Fig. 11.5 Main types of anaemia.

1. anaemia due to decreased red cell production resulting from:
   - reduced bone marrow function
   - lack of essential factors for cell maturation
2. anaemia due to blood loss
3. haemolytic anaemia: due to excessive destruction of the red cells.

Anaemia is extremely common worldwide: the overall incidence of iron deficiency is 20% of the world population (Barnard et al 1989). The World Health Organization (WHO) defines anaemia as a haemoglobin level of less than 13 g/100 ml blood for men and less than 12 g/100 ml for women.

The anaemias are a complex group of red blood cell disorders which may be:

- primary, i.e. the presenting illness
- secondary to another disease, e.g. infection, cancer, gastrointestinal malabsorption syndrome, chronic renal failure, or an inherited disorder of haemoglobin synthesis or formation
- acquired:
  — iatrogenic, e.g. drug-induced
  — environmental, e.g. benzene exposure
  — nutritional, e.g. iron, protein, vitamin B12 or folate deficiency.

Anaemia is found in all age groups. At each developmental stage there are potential dietary reasons for the occurrence of anaemia, as follows (Davies 1990):

- In infancy, anaemia can occur if a poor diet is provided, especially at the time of weaning
- In adolescence, a growth spurt may cause anaemia particularly if during this period 'fad eating' leads to an inadequate intake of the essential nutrients for red cell formation
- Women of child bearing age may become anaemic due to menstrual blood loss for which inadequate dietary compensation is made
- In pregnant women extra demands for red cell synthesis may lead to the development of anaemia
- In elderly people poor eating habits resulting from difficulty in shopping, reduction in income, depression, poor dental hygiene or badly fitting dentures can all lead to a reduced intake of essential nutrients for red blood cell formation.

?	**11.5** In a group, discuss the social, cultural and environmental factors which might contribute to the development of anaemia.

Many people are diagnosed only by chance when they seek medical advice for an unrelated symptom or attend a health clinic (e.g. antenatal or occupational health) for a routine medical examination. It is therefore likely that nurses working in any area of community or hospital nursing will care for people with anaemia.

PATHOPHYSIOLOGY

Anaemia occurs when the oxygen-carrying capacity of the red blood cells is reduced. Its symptoms all stem from a lack of oxygen in the tissues; their severity depends on two main factors:

- haemoglobin concentration, i.e. oxygen-carrying capacity of the red blood cell
- ability of the person to adapt to lower oxygen concentration. (Some patients with chronic anaemia live very active lives with a haemoglobin level that in other people would cause severe symptoms.)

Common presenting symptoms. The clinical features of anaemia are diverse. Each type of anaemia has specific clinical features but there are common presenting symptoms, as follows:

1. Tiredness and lethargy: a very subjective symptom for which the person is unlikely to consult his general practitioner (GP). Some people have a variety of explanations for tiredness, e.g. the season, social life, stress, and workload
2. Breathlessness: a compensatory mechanism to overcome low oxygen concentration, which may be present only on exertion. The person may dismiss this symptom, thinking he is just 'not fit'
3. Palpitations: due to heart increasing its rate to increase blood flow to tissues
4. Loss of appetite: often an unexplained feature (Fitzsimmons & Jacobs 1983) but may be due to dysphagia and sore mouth
5. Dysphagia (difficulty in swallowing) and sore mouth due to epithelial lining fragility
6. Oedema of ankles, especially at the end of the day: due to a degree of heart failure
7. Dizziness, fainting and dimness of vision due to lack of oxygen to the brain
8. Headache and lack of concentration: resulting from insufficient oxygen supply to the brain
9. Angina and/or intermittent claudication because of impaired blood flow to peripheral and/or coronary arteries; this is especially likely in older people
10. Bleeding, e.g. rectal bleeding, haematuria, haemoptysis or menorrhagia.

MEDICAL MANAGEMENT

To diagnose anaemia and establish its cause it is necessary to clarify the patient's symptoms and discover if he has any other symptoms he may not consider significant or does not wish to volunteer.

History and examination. Careful questioning about the patient's state of health in the present and recent past and about his use of medication (e.g. aspirin, which causes bleeding, or phenytoin, which causes folate deficiency) may help uncover the cause of the anaemia. A determination of the person's social circumstances and dietary intake may also be important.

An accurate and detailed dietary history is often difficult to obtain but may reveal deficiencies in iron, folic acid or vitamin B12. This history may be taken by the GP, practice nurse or dietitian. Questioning about social background should include consideration of:

- financial circumstances
- home circumstances
- work environment, including exposure to harmful substances.

Clinical examination may reveal:

- evidence of paleness of skin and mucous membranes (e.g. conjunctiva, palms of hands, buccal cavity). This may be difficult to assess as many people are pale but not anaemic; assessment of pallor in dark-skinned people will be especially difficult
- signs of an underlying disease, e.g. cancer, hypothyroidism or infection
- signs of complications of anaemia, e.g. cardiac failure, glossitis, stomatitis, jaundice (due to haemolytic breakdown); see p. 114
- signs of pregnancy.

Investigative procedures used in the diagnosis of anaemia include the following:

1. Blood tests (not all of the following will be relevant for all patients):
   - full blood count: to establish total number of red cells, white cells and platelets. The result is compared with normal values (See Appendix 2)
   - blood film: examination of blood cells under the microscope to detect any abnormality in size or shape
   - haemoglobin concentration: a level 10% below normal is usually considered a sign of anaemia
   - haematocrit or packed cell volume (PCV): proportion of total blood volume which consists of red cells. Dehydrated patients have a high PCV as the plasma volume is reduced
   - reticulocyte count: a small percentage of reticulocytes are normally present in blood. A larger percentage may indicate increased bone marrow activity if the red blood cell count is low (see p. 407 on maturation of red cells)
   - mean corpuscular volume (MCV): measures the average red cell volume
   - mean corpuscular haemoglobin concentration (MCHC): measures the average concentration of haemoglobin in each red cell. A low MCHC may be found when haemoglobin is low
   - erythrocyte sedimentation rate (ESR): measures the speed at which red cells settle in uncoagulated blood left standing for 1 h. The height of the plasma column above the sedimented blood cells is measured (in mm) and compared with normal height. ESR may be raised because of an underlying problem causing the anaemia, e.g. infection.
2. Bone marrow aspiration: the removal with a special needle of a small quantity of bone marrow which can then be mounted on slides and stained for examination under a microscope. This is not done routinely but is indicated if the anaemia is severe or has no apparent cause, or if there is evidence of another blood disorder such as aplastic anaemia or leukaemia (see Box 11.1).

Medical intervention. The type of treatment given for anaemia will depend on the cause and severity of the condition. A few patients will need to be hospitalised but most can be treated in the community by their GP. The treatment may involve medication and health education. Blood transfusions may be needed either initially or repeatedly over a period of time. Intervention will also include treatment of the underlying cause of the anaemia.

Treatment may be short term (a few weeks), long term (months or years) or, as in the case of pernicious anaemia, lifelong. Follow-up care for all anaemic patients is important to encourage compliance with medication and to prevent recurrence and long-term effects. This care may be provided by the GP or at an outpatients clinic.

NURSING PRIORITIES AND MANAGEMENT OF ANAEMIAS

As the anaemias are such a diverse group of disorders, nursing intervention can take a variety of forms. It is vital that the patient is considered as an individual and that psychological, social and environmental concerns are taken into account along with the medical considerations pertinent to his specific form of anaemia.

Certain nursing interventions will be common, of course, to all cases. The first task to be carried out is an assessment of the patient's background, illness, needs and goals. Following assessment, a treatment plan will have to be agreed between the patient and the health care team.

Life-threatening complications

The patient may present with any of the following potentially life-threatening problems:

- cardiac failure

Box 11.1 Bone marrow aspiration

PURPOSES

1. Diagnosis: to examine cell populations and thus determine type of anaemia, leukaemia or lymphoma
2. Monitoring: to assess progress of disease and response to treatment.

SITES

Red bone marrow is found in the cavities of the flat bones of the adult, e.g. skull, clavicle, scapula, iliac crest. The sites which are usually chosen (for ease of access to minimise trauma to nearby structures) are:

1. Iliac crest: left and right, anterior and posterior
2. Sternum: care is required to avoid cardiac tamponade (pressure on heart caused by pericardial haemorrhage).

THE NURSE'S ROLE

The patient may be anxious about this investigation, especially if he knows that the results may show that he has a malignant condition. This anxiety may be heightened if the patient has been talking with others who have undergone the procedure.

Providing the patient with information on all aspects of the test — the use of premedication and local anaesthetic, the site to be used, the degree of discomfort to be expected, the time that it will take, and when the results will be reported — will help to reduce his anxiety (Wilson Barnett 1978).

It is the policy of some doctors, especially where repeated aspiration will be required, to give a sedative such as lorazepam or a light general anaesthetic.

The individual may undergo the procedure as an outpatient, inpatient, or in a day ward. Whatever the setting, the nurse's role will include:

1. Assessing the patient's understanding of the test and providing more information if necessary
2. Preparing the equipment
3. Ensuring that the patient is comfortable and is positioned correctly
4. Observing the patient throughout the procedure and drawing attention to any change in his condition
5. Assisting the doctor
6. Applying a pressure dressing and making the patient comfortable after the procedure
7. Inspecting the aspiration site frequently for haemorrhage or haematoma formation
8. Documenting the patient's response to the procedure
9. Preparing the patient for discharge by explaining care of puncture site, what discomfort may be expected, whom to contact if ill effects arise, when results will be available and timing of next appointment.

POSSIBLE COMPLICATIONS

1. Haemorrhage: patient's platelet count should be checked before aspiration
2. Infection
3. Cardiac tamponade if sternum site used: needle should be fitted with a guard to prevent overpenetration.

- breathlessness
- shock.

These complications may arise if there has been severe blood loss over a short period of time or if a chronic condition suddenly enters an acute phase. This is more likely to occur in individuals who have other conditions such as hypertension, chronic obstructive airways disease (COAD) and/or pre-existing chronic blood loss (see Ch. 2, Ch. 3, Ch. 18).

Major problems of nursing anaemic patients

Tiredness

Anaemic patients will tire easily because of poor oxygenation of cells and tissues. Patients with severe anaemia will be exhausted on even the slightest exertion. It is important that their daily routine in hospital or at home ensures periods of rest. If cardiac failure is evident, they will need to be nursed in bed or a chair. The nurse should be aware of the potential problems of immobility, paying particular attention to pressure areas. Such patients may require assistance with personal hygiene and dressing. They should be reassured that their tiredness is not imaginary but is part of the anaemia and that it will lessen as treatment progresses.

Breathlessness (See Ch. 3)

This problem will not be present unless the anaemia is severe (haemoglobin level below 8 g/100 ml of blood). The breathlessness may be mild, arising only on exertion, or it may be a major problem causing great distress.

The most important aspects of nursing the breathless patient are to ensure good perfusion of oxygen to the tissues and to reduce the patient's distress. This can be achieved by nursing the patient in an upright position (to allow maximum lung expansion and use of accessory respiratory muscles), administering oxygen as prescribed, explaining to the patient the reason for his breathlessness, and reassuring him that it will lessen as the anaemia improves.

Breathlessness, if incapacitating, will require the nurse to assist the patient with personal hygiene, changing position in bed and mobilisation.

Nutrition

The anaemic patient will require a high-protein diet which includes all the nutrients necessary for red cell production (see p. 406). Breathlessness, a lack of energy to shop and prepare food, a sore mouth and dysphagia may all contribute to anorexia. A sore mouth can be especially distressing and the nurse will need to carry out an initial evaluation using an assessment tool such as that described in Eilers et al 1988 (see p. 433). Care should include not only care that will improve and heal the mouth but also relevant health education about oral hygiene and care of dentures (Crosby 1989).

It will be necessary for anaemic patients who have a low income and/or a poor understanding of nutrition to receive instruction in budgeting and the components of a balanced diet as well as advice about social security allowances. The multidisciplinary team may therefore include a dietitian and a social worker.

Other important considerations include dietary restrictions deriving from the patient's cultural background and/or spiritual beliefs. Dietary restrictions may also be imposed by a pre-existing medical disorder such as diabetes mellitus. Elderly patients may have ill-fitting dentures which lead them to rely on a poorly balanced 'soft' diet. In such cases referral to a dentist may be appropriate.

Safety

Giddiness, faintness, lightheadedness and reduced sensitivity to cold may make the anaemic patient prone to injury. Since the body responds to poor oxygenation by preserving the blood supply to the essential organs, anaemic patients will have poor peripheral circulation and, consequently, fragile skin. The reduced attention span typical of anaemic patients will also make them vulnerable to falls, minor injuries, and hypothermia. Anaemic patients should be warned against changing position suddenly (especially from lying to standing) and be given instruction on first aid for minor injuries and on the prevention of hypothermia (see Ch. 22).

Skin integrity (See Ch. 12, Ch. 23)

The anaemic patient's reduced oxygen and nutrient supply to the skin will make him susceptible to pressure sores. Hypoxic skin will not necessarily break down quickly but if damaged will take longer than usual to heal. When the patient's mobility has been impaired, either as a result of the anaemia or because of a concurrent condition (e.g. arthritis), the nurse must be alert to the importance of maintaining skin integrity.

An initial assessment of all pressure points should be made using such tools as the Norton Scale or Waterlow Scale (see pp. 713–714). Once the patient's level of risk from pressure sores has been determined an appropriate intervention should be planned. Prevention of pressure sores is likely to include ensuring that the patient changes position two-hourly, the use of appropriate medical aids (e.g. silicone-filled mattresses and cushions, sheepskin pads, alternating pressure beds) and instructing the patient about the importance of regularly changing position.

Communication

Anxiety and fear may present a barrier to communication by preventing the patient from asking for information about diagnosis, prognosis and treatment. The patient's physical condition (e.g. breathlessness, sore mouth) may also impede communication. The nurse caring for anaemic patients must be aware of these potential difficulties and of the effect that they can have upon patient–staff relationships.

The nurse should assess actual and potential communication difficulties and help the patient and the health care team to overcome obstacles as they arise. The patient should be allowed the opportunity to voice his fears and should be given the appropriate reassurance and information. Here, the nurse should try to involve other relevant members of the team. The nurse should be receptive to the patient's non-verbal as well as verbal messages and, in doing so, anticipate those times when he will need support and reassurance.

Anxiety

Prior to diagnosis the anaemic patient may fear that he has a life-threatening illness, particularly if he has been experiencing symptoms such as breathlessness, palpitations and chronic headaches.

The disorientation, confusion and general slowing of intellectual responses arising from cerebral hypoxia can be especially distressing. Explanation of the causes of these symptoms and reassurance that they should improve as the anaemia responds to treatment will help to reduce the anxiety suffered by the patient and his family.

IRON DEFICIENCY ANAEMIA

Iron deficiency anaemia is the most common anaemia worldwide. It affects an estimated 500 million people (Chanarin & Pippard 1991) and is recognised as one of the most prevalent diseases of nutritional origin (Davies 1990). The onset of this form of anaemia is usually insidious, taking place over a period of months. This may be explained by the fact that iron stored in the body is usually reused after the breakdown of red blood cells and only a very small proportion is lost (less than 1 mg/day), mainly from cells shed from the skin and gut (Roberts 1990).

PATHOPHYSIOLOGY

Iron is part of the haem component of the haemoglobin molecule: each haemoglobin molecule is composed of four molecules of haem with one ferrous ion, which is the oxygen carrier that transports oxygen from the lungs to the tissues (Tortora & Anagnostakos 1990).

A typical Western diet contains 16–25 mg of iron/day, whereas only 1.0–2.0 mg is required (Chanarin & Pippard 1991). Most iron ingested is not absorbed. The ferrous form is more soluble than the ferric form; a low pH in the duodenum maintains iron in ferrous form — the form in which it can be absorbed from the gut.

Iron deficiency anaemia may be caused by:

- inadequate intake, i.e. poor diet
- increased iron requirement, e.g. in pregnancy
- lack of gastric acid, e.g. following total gastrectomy or gastric atrophy
- duodenal or jejunal malabsorption.

Common presenting symptoms. As the onset of iron deficiency anaemia is usually very gradual, the patient may not consult his doctor until some time after symptoms have begun to appear. The most common presenting symptoms are tiredness and pallor, but any of the other general symptoms of anaemia (see p. 412), may be apparent. Symptoms specific to iron deficiency anaemia include:

- painless glossitis (40% of cases; Fitzsimmons & Jacobs 1983)
- smooth tongue (Fitzsimmons & Jacobs 1983)
- angular stomatitis (14% of cases; Fitzsimmons & Jacobs 1983)
- koilonychia: brittle spoon-shaped nails (Bloom & Bloom 1986)
- dysphagia and glossitis; with the formation of a pharyngeal web (5–15% of cases), also called Plummer-Vinson syndrome (Fitzsimmons & Jacobs 1983)
- atrophic gastritis and achlorhydria (40% of cases; Fitzsimmons & Jacobs 1983).

MEDICAL MANAGEMENT

History and examination. The patient may give a history suggesting chronic blood loss (e.g. menorrhagia). Examination may reveal general signs of anaemia; koilonychia may be noted.

Investigative procedures. Blood samples will be taken for a number of tests, such as full blood count, haemoglobin level, blood film, MCV, MCHC and total iron binding capacity (TIBC); see Appendix 1. Estimates will also be made of plasma iron levels and plasma TIBC; this can be done in a GP's surgery. Other investigations, e.g. faecal occult blood and endoscopy, may be made to establish the cause of the deficiency. Such tests will be selected according to the patient's symptoms and medical history.

Bone marrow aspiration may not be required; if it is performed it will show a bone marrow with no iron stores (see p. 413) if iron deficiency anaemia is present.

Medical intervention. If dietary adjustment is insufficient to correct the anaemia, medication is given and, in very severe cases, blood transfusion is carried out.

Medication. Iron supplements will be prescribed, usually in the following forms:

1. Oral iron supplements: usually ferrous sulphate 200 mg 3 times a day after food (to prevent gastric irritation). Ideally, medication should be continued for 6 months after the haemoglobin level is normal to build up iron stores (Allan 1991). Side-effects, which include constipation, nausea, abdominal pain and diarrhoea, often lead to poor compliance. Alternative iron preparations which may be better tolerated, but are more expensive, include ferrous gluconate and ferrous fumarate.
2. Intramuscular iron injections. These are given only where there is proven malabsorption syndrome or poor compliance.

Administration of i.m. iron via the 'Z track' technique to minimise skin discolouration is recommended. 'Z track' prevents or minimises back tracking of iron and skin discolouration. *Blood transfusion.* If the anaemia is very severe (less than 7 gms/dl), a slow infusion of red cell concentrate will be administered. However, there is a danger, particularly in elderly or very young patients, of blood volume overload leading to cardiac failure.

?	**11.6** What accounts for this risk of cardiac overload?	A

NURSING PRIORITIES AND MANAGEMENT OF IRON DEFICIENCY ANAEMIA

Many of the general nursing considerations for the care of anaemic patients (see pp. 413–414) are relevant to the treatment of iron deficiency anaemia. Patients with this condition will most likely be cared for by a community nurse.

Nursing considerations

Blood transfusions

A few patients with iron deficiency anaemia will require a blood transfusion (see Case History 11.1). This measure may be interpreted by the patient and his family as a sign that the condition is very grave; therefore, it is important that the nurse clarifies the reason for the transfusion, explains what is involved, and gives reassurance that the procedure is safe. Many people fear being infected with a transmittable disease, especially AIDS, and it may be necessary to explain screening

Case History 11.1 MRS B

Mrs B, a frail lady aged 82 years, has been admitted to hospital as an emergency after collapsing at home. She used to enjoy an active social life until her husband died a year ago. Since then her family and friends have noticed that she has become withdrawn and depressed and rarely goes out except to shop.

Mrs B has always enjoyed good health until recently. On admission to hospital she admitted that over the past few months she has become increasingly tired and breathless when she climbs stairs or walks uphill. She has noticed that her ankles tend to swell, especially in the evening. She also finds that she has become forgetful; her neighbours have noticed that she appears confused at times.

A blood test has revealed that Mrs B has a haemoglobin level of 7 g/100 ml blood and other blood test results have proved that she has an iron deficiency anaemia. Mrs B has been prescribed three units of red cell concentrate to be given prior to any further investigations of the iron deficiency anaemia.

See Nursing Care Plan 11.1.

Box 11.2 Jehovah's Witnesses and blood transfusions

Devout Jehovah's Witnesses believe that it is against God's law to receive transfusions of blood or blood products. This belief is based on three biblical references: Gen. 9:4, Lev. 17:14, and Acts 15:28–29. Members of the faith consider that those who disregard God's law will be deprived of eternal salvation (Clark 1982).

If a Jehovah's Witness requires a blood transfusion as an urgent or essential part of treatment he or his next of kin will need to be approached by the medical practitioners and informed of the gravity of the situation. If the treatment is refused this must be documented.

procedures for blood donations. Practising Jehovah's Witnesses will refuse blood transfusions (see Box 11.2). Some Muslims may be reluctant to accept a blood transfusion and may wish to consult their families or a religious leader before agreeing to the procedure.

The nurse must be familiar with local policies for prescribing and checking blood products prior to transfusion to minimise the risk of administering incompatible blood. Any doubt about the unit of blood to be given should be referred to the haematology laboratory medical staff.

The unit of blood must be administered at the correct rate and temperature unless there are indications of a transfusion reaction (e.g. slight pyrexia). If any symptoms occur advice must be sought from the doctor. A reaction to incompatible blood usually occurs within an hour after transfusion begins; therefore, the nurse must observe the patient very carefully for the first hour, assessing his condition quarter-hourly and reporting any symptoms to the doctor immediately (see Nursing Care Plan 11.1).

Patient education

By helping the patient to understand the nature of his disorder and to come to terms with the fact that although the anaemia is not a life-threatening illness it may become very severe if left untreated, the nurse will encourage the patient to comply with treatment.

The patient will need to be informed about which foods are rich in iron and may need advice on budgeting for a well-balanced diet. The nurse will need to assess the patient's perception of the problem, his level of knowledge and his sociocultural background in order to ensure that the advice she offers is relevant and comprehensible. Referral to a social worker (e.g. for advice about social security benefits) may be appropriate.

Careful and clear instruction should be given to reinforce the doctor's and pharmacist's directions regarding medication. Important points to emphasise are:

- how frequently the medication should be taken.
- that it is to be taken with food.
- possible side-effects and how to overcome them. (The side-effects of constipation and indigestion are frequently the cause of poor compliance. To avoid undue alarm, the patient should be warned that oral iron supplements will turn his stools black.)
- safe storage
- the importance of the continuation of medication and the importance of follow-up.

If iron injections are required they will be given daily for about 5–7 days. This treatment can cause an unpleasant taste and induce palpitations. They are also painful and so the patient may need to be encouraged to comply.

Discharge planning

If the person has been hospitalised for treatment the following considerations should be discussed before discharge:

- socioeconomic conditions at home
- social services available (e.g. home helps, lunch clubs) if family members are unable to help
- the importance of a follow-up appointment with the consultant or GP.

In elderly individuals, there is often a link between recent bereavement (i.e. in the last 6–12 months) and the onset of iron deficiency anaemia, as grief and depression may lead to self-neglect. This problem may be accentuated if the bereaved person is physically unable to look after himself. Care needs to be taken that such patients are not returned to their former social circumstances without the necessary follow-up and support by the GP, health visitor, social worker or grief counsellor.

?	**11.7** A 72-year-old widower is admitted to hospital with general tiredness, breathlessness and mild congestive heart failure. He is diagnosed as having iron deficiency anaemia. His wife died 6 months ago and his only daughter, who is married and has two young children, lives a considerable distance away. With regard to the patient's discharge: a. identify potential problems b. discuss how these might be resolved c. identify what community services might be required.	A

MEGALOBLASTIC ANAEMIAS

These anaemias stem from a lack of one or more of the essential factors for the synthesis of DNA, resulting in a reduction in red blood cell proliferation. There are two types of megaloblastic anaemia (see Table 11.4):

- folate deficiency
- vitamin B12 deficiency.

In Britain, 60% of megaloblastic anaemias are due to folate deficiency (Allan 1991), and one in 100 people over the age of 60 have pernicious anaemia.

PATHOPHYSIOLOGY

Red blood cells proliferate continually and have a lifespan of approximately 120 days (see p. 407). Folate and vitamin B12 are essential factors for the synthesis of DNA required by each cell (see Figs 11.6 and 11.7). If DNA synthesis is reduced (because of lack of folate or vitamin B12), the time between each cell division will be prolonged. This results in the normoblasts (see p. 407) becoming larger than normal (macrocytic). While macrocytes may contain a greater amount of haemoglobin than normoblasts the total amount of haemoglobin will be reduced as the total number of red blood cells is reduced. There may also be large, primitive nucleated red cells (megaloblasts) in the peripheral blood.

Common presenting symptoms. Vitamin B12 is required by rapidly dividing cells. Lack of Vitamin B12 affects the gastrointestinal epithelium, giving rise to glossitis, anorexia, diarrhoea and malabsorption. It also causes spinal cord and peripheral nerve damage which can give rise to the following symptoms:

- paraesthesia (pins and needles or tingling)

Nursing Care Plan 11.1 Care of Mrs B during blood transfusion (See Case history 11.1.)

Nursing considerations	Action	Rationale	Evaluation
1. **Anxiety** a. About cause of anaemia	❒ Reduce anxiety and stress of receiving blood transfusion by explaining and clarifying information given	Information given about procedures and care reduces anxiety and discomfort (Wilson Barnett 1978)	Appear calm, not anxious
b. About safety of blood transfusion	❒ Reassure Mrs B by explaining screening and crossmatching of blood	Mrs B may fear receiving infection from donor, especially HIV, AIDS or hepatitis B virus. Fear of receiving wrong blood group	Accept blood transfusion
c. About possibility of complications	❒ Reassure Mrs B she will be observed and monitored frequently for any signs of complications. Tell her she must inform nurses of any new symptoms		
2. **Correct blood given to correct patient**	❒ Check blood unit details against blood transfusion crossmatching form, prescription and patient's details with a registered nurse as per local policy. Document blood unit transfused	Prevention of wrong blood being given to wrong patient, with possible incompatible reaction	Correct blood given to correct patient as detailed on prescription sheet
3. **Condition of blood to be transfused is optimal**	❒ Ensure blood stored at correct temperature prior to commencing transfusion. Blood is commenced within 30 min of removal from special refrigerator. Blood is not artificially warmed (unless directed by doctor because of special antibodies)	Blood not stored at correct temperature may undergo haemolysis (red cell breakdown) Risk of microorganisms contamination increased	Blood is given at correct temperature
4. **Early detection of blood transfusion incompatibility**	❒ Record Mrs B's temperature and pulse quarter-hourly during first hour of each unit of blood and then hourly until completion of each unit ❒ Observe Mrs B for any restlessness ❒ Record and report any nausea or vomiting	Signs and symptoms of blood transfusion incompatibility usually occur very soon after the unit of blood is commenced	Any symptoms or signs of incompatibility are detected immediately
	❒ Observe and record any complaints of: • burning sensation in arm above cannula • chest tightness or pain • dyspnoea • loin pain • lumbar pain ❒ Report any signs or symptoms to doctor	Symptoms of pain in arm, chest lumbar region and loin and dyspnoea are due to agglutination of red blood cells in blood vessels, causing obstruction to blood flow	
	❒ Summon doctor immediately if Mrs B develops circulatory collapse ❒ Stop blood transfusion if any signs or symptoms of incompatibility occur	Incompatible blood transfusion rarely causes sudden collapse	
	❒ Keep unit of blood and infusion-giving set if incompatibility occurs Return both to haematology laboratory	Blood will be further tested for cause of incompatibility. Mrs B's unit of blood may have been wrongly crossmatched or labelled or her red blood cells may have other rare antibodies which require special crossmatching	

Nursing Care Plan 11.1 *Cont'd*

Nursing considerations	Action	Rationale	Evaluation
5. Circulatory overload	❐ Monitor Mrs B's pulse, respiratory rate and blood pressure. Report any abnormal measurements ❐ Observe and report to medical staff any dyspnoea or wheezing ❐ Ensure transfusion is regulated at prescribed rate ❐ Measure urinary output	Mrs B has developed some cardiac failure due to her anaemia and the transfusion could increase her blood volume to a level at which the cardiac failure deteriorates. It is important that signs of cardiac failure and pulmonary oedema are detected early	Any signs of cardiac overload are detected immediately
	❐ Give frusemide as prescribed and monitor urinary output	Frusemide, as a diuretic, will increase fluid output and thus reduce circulatory volume	
6. Pyrexia	❐ Monitor temperature and pulse as in 4 ❐ Report any abnormal temperature and pulse recordings to doctor	Fever can occur for unknown cause at start of each unit. Temperature falls if transfusion slowed. High fever with rigors may be due to white cell antibodies. May occur 1.0–1.5 hours after transfusion. Subnormal temperature which rises later may be a sign of infection	All episodes of abnormal temperature are recorded and reported. Any further action requested by doctor is implemented immediately
	❐ Report any chest pain or sign of infections		
	❐ Ensure blood used has been out of special blood fridge for maximum 30 min	To prevent blood temperature rise with the increased risk of growth of organisms	Blood unit always commenced within 30 minutes of removal from special blood fridge
	❐ Do not continue transfusion of a unit of blood after 8 hours	Greater risk of contamination by microorganisms	
	❐ Report if transfusion rate becomes slow ❐ Administer any drugs as prescribed, e.g. antipyretics, antibiotics		
7. Allergic reactions	❐ Observations of temperature and pulse as in 4 ❐ Observe for any skin rashes ❐ Observe for any oedema around eyes ❐ Observe for any signs of laryngeal oedema (see Ch. 3) ❐ Observe for shortness of breath ❐ Record and report any of above signs to doctor immediately. If symptoms are mild slow transfusion. If severe stop transfusion, treat patient for shock (see Ch. 18)	Allergic response to protein in the plasma	Any signs of an allergic reaction are detected immediately and the appropriate action implemented

- coldness or numbness in limbs
- ataxia (lack of coordination of movement; staggering)
- paralysis.

MEDICAL MANAGEMENT

History and examination. Medical investigation will follow much the same outline as that for iron deficiency anaemia. However, in suspected megaloblastic anaemia the doctor will be alert to the following specific features:

1. Folate deficiency:
   - underlying causes such as pregnancy, malabsorption, malignancy
2. Vitamin B12/intrinsic factor deficiency
   - slow, insidious onset (especially in older person)

Table 11.4 Causes of the megaloblastic anaemias

Type	Causes
Folate deficiency	Inadequate dietary intake Disease of upper small bowel (malabsorption or extensive surgical resection of small bowel) Increasing body demands because of: • very active cell proliferation e.g. in haemolytic anaemia or leukaemia (see p. 421 and p. 426) • pregnancy Interference with folate metabolism by drugs (e.g. methotrexate; see Ch. 32) Unexplained mechanisms, e.g. ingestion of alcohol and anti-epileptic drugs (e.g. phenytoin and primidone)
Vitamin B12: pernicious anaemia	Inadequate Vitamin B12 in diet (especially vegans) Gastric surgery, gastric atrophy or intrinsic factor deficiency Disease of terminal ileum (where Vitamin B12 is absorbed e.g. Crohn's disease; see Ch. 4)

- glossitis; smooth, raw tongue
- lemon-yellow skin pallor with possible skin irritation (megaloblastic red blood cells are fragile and may be misshapen, resulting in haemolysis; see p. 441)
- paraesthesia (pins and needles) in fingers and toes
- symptoms of subacute combined degeneration of the spinal cord resulting in muscular weakness, loss of muscular coordination and paralysis. These symptoms, which may arise before any others, occur in approximately 10% of all cases of pernicious anaemia
- weight loss
- excess urobilinogen in urine (because of haemolysis).

Investigative procedures. The following diagnostic blood tests are performed in cases of suspected megaloblastic anaemia: full blood count, haemoglobin level, blood film, MCV, serum B12 levels and red cell folate level. Other investigations include:

- assessment of gastric parietal cell antibodies
- Schilling test (see Appendix 1)
- bone marrow aspiration (see p. 413)
- neurological examination (see Ch. 9)
- past medical history for gastric or intestinal surgery, alcohol abuse or epilepsy.

Medical intervention. Treatment for megaloblastic anaemia is as follows:

1. Folate deficiency:
   - 5 mg folic acid daily until anaemia is corrected, followed by 5 mg maintenance dose weekly
2. Vitamin B12 and intrinsic factor deficiency:
   - injection of hydroxocobalamin 1000 μg i.m. twice during first week, then weekly until blood count is normal
   - maintenance dose of hydroxocobalamin 1000 μg i.m. every 3 months for life.

?	**11.8** What might the implications be for the patient of the lifelong necessity for 3-monthly injections?	A

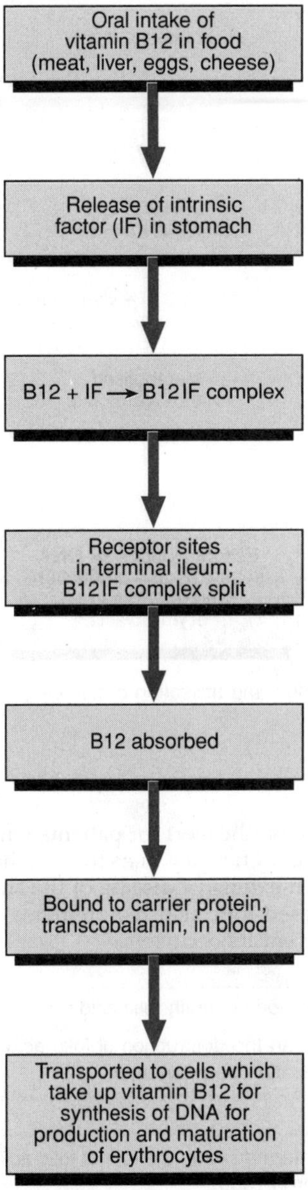

Oral intake of vitamin B12 in food (meat, liver, eggs, cheese)
↓
Release of intrinsic factor (IF) in stomach
↓
B12 + IF → B12IF complex
↓
Receptor sites in terminal ileum; B12IF complex split
↓
B12 absorbed
↓
Bound to carrier protein, transcobalamin, in blood
↓
Transported to cells which take up vitamin B12 for synthesis of DNA for production and maturation of erythrocytes

Fig. 11.6 Vitamin B12 absorption and transport.

NURSING PRIORITIES AND MANAGEMENT OF MEGALOBLASTIC ANAEMIAS

Folate deficiency

Individuals with folate deficiency are usually diagnosed and treated by a GP or at an antenatal clinic and are referred to a haematology outpatient department only if further tests are necessary (e.g. bone marrow aspiration). The setting for nursing intervention will therefore be a community health centre or the patient's home. Patient education with regard to diet and acceptance of medication will be the most important aspect of nursing care.

A patient with folate anaemia will need to know which foods contain folic acid, how to budget for these if his income is low, and how to avoid destroying folic acid in food preparation. He will also need to understand how to take folic acid supplements correctly. The nurse should also emphasise the importance of follow-up check-ups with the consultant or GP.

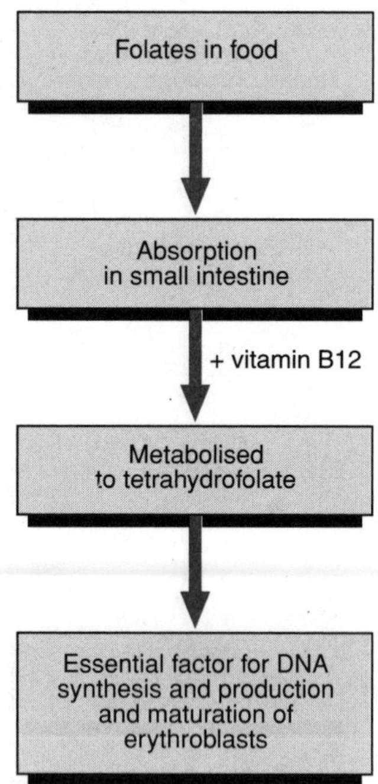

Fig. 11.7 Absorption and utilisation of folates.

Nurses must be on the alert for patients who may be susceptible to folic acid deficiency (i.e. those whose diet is inadequate, those with extensive disease of the small intestine, and those with increased folic acid requirements) and advise them as to how to prevent its occurrence.

?	11.9	What foods contain folic acid?	A
?	11.10	How can the destruction of folic acid in food preparation be prevented?	A

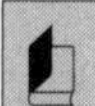
For further information on the role of folic acid in health see Fox & Cameron 1989.

Vitamin B12 and intrinsic factor deficiency

Many patients will need to be admitted to hospital for diagnosis and treatment in the initial stages. Others will have been diagnosed by their GP. If the anaemia is not yet acute, treatment can be commenced immediately by a community or practice nurse, who will administer vitamin B12 injections according to the doctor's directions. The nurse should bear in mind that the patient may be very dyspnoeic at first and will need some degree of assistance with personal care tasks (see p. 414).

He will need support in adjusting to the illness and to a regime of regular injections. The patient and his family should be encouraged to participate in the management of the anaemia, possibly by learning how to administer the hydroxocobalamin injections themselves.

Patients in the advanced stages of pernicious anaemia are rarely seen today. If cardiac failure and severe neurological problems do develop, major nursing interventions will be required (see Ch. 2 and Ch. 9).

APLASTIC ANAEMIA

This form of anaemia results from the failure of bone marrow stem cells to mature and proliferate. In 20–50% of all cases of this very rare disease, onset can be connected with exposure to one of the following:

- chemical compounds, i.e. industrial chemicals, especially benzene
- drugs, e.g. choramphenicol, therapeutic cytotoxins, phenothiazines, antiepileptics
- ionising radiation, whether therapeutic or industrial
- viral infection, notably hepatitis
- bone marrow infiltration by disease, e.g. multiple myeloma, metastases from primary tumours.

The remaining 50–70% of cases are idiopathic, having no detectable cause.

PATHOPHYSIOLOGY

Bone marrow failure causes:

- lack of red blood cells: anaemia
- lack of white cells: leucopenia
- lack of platelets: thrombocytopenia.

These three conditions together are referred to as pancytopenia. In aplastic anaemia the degree of anaemia, leucopenia and thrombocytopenia (and therefore the severity of the disorder) is variable.

Common presenting symptoms. The onset of aplastic anaemia is often insidious. One or two months may elapse between the individual's exposure to the causal agent and the development of symptoms. The presenting symptoms are the result of pancytopenia and include:

- bleeding, e.g. in the skin and mucous membranes, especially the gums
- epistaxis
- infections of the throat, upper respiratory tract, etc.
- general symptoms of anaemia.

MEDICAL MANAGEMENT

History and examination. Medical investigation may uncover no abnormality other than the presenting symptoms; for example, careful examination will reveal no enlarged liver or spleen. However, questioning might bring to light the patient's exposure to chemicals or the use of a self-prescribed medicine. It may require very careful and extensive questioning to uncover the causative factor, which may have seemed trivial to the patient at the time. The recollections of family and friends may be of help.

Investigative procedures will include:

- blood film and blood count to reveal pancytopenia
- bone marrow aspiration to reveal the degree of stem cell failure. This procedure gives a definitive diagnosis.

Medical intervention. If the patient was not admitted to hospital on presentation, he will be hospitalised immediately if a diagnosis of aplastic anaemia is made.

In mild to moderately severe cases, supportive therapy with blood and platelet transfusion will be given. Antibiotic therapy will be essential to treat any infections. Steroids to stimulate bone marrow cell synthesis (e.g. oxymetholone orally or high-dose methylprednisolone) may be tried (see Ch. 5). Such treatment must be applied with caution, given the possible side-effects of inflammatory response suppression, fluid retention, and development of diabetes mellitus.

If the aplastic anaemia is severe or the above treatment is unsuccessful, allogeneic bone marrow transplantation will be considered as an urgent treatment (see p. 427).

NURSING PRIORITIES AND MANAGEMENT OF APLASTIC ANAEMIAS

Life-threatening complications

The nurse must be on the alert for the development of grave complications of aplastic anaemia. The nurse's role will therefore include:

- prevention of infections
- early detection of infections
- immediate implementation of nursing care of septicaemic patients on detection of infection
- prevention and early treatment of bleeding.

Nursing considerations

Psychological state

The patient or his family and friends may experience feelings of guilt if and when the causative agent of the anaemia is identified; they may believe that they were to blame for the patient's contact with the toxin. The nurse must be sensitive to the patient's concerns as he assimilates information about his diagnosis and prognosis (some patients will not survive a year) and copes with the sudden transfer to hospital and, possibly, with being nursed in protective isolation.

Patient education

It is vital to inform the patient how to prevent, and detect the signs of, injury, bleeding and infection. He should be warned to avoid overexertion. The aims of instruction will depend on the severity of the disorder and the patient's response to treatment. The teaching programme should include not only the patient but also his family, friends and carers.

The patient will need to know the purpose of his medication and what to do if any medication is missed. The patient should be told how to proceed with medication after the initial supply is finished. A patient prescribed steroids (e.g. prednisolone) should be warned that it is important to continue taking them even when he feels ill. He should also be advised to inform any doctor or dentist treating him that he is taking steroids and always to carry a card giving details of his medication.

The nurse will also need to instruct the patient, his family and any members of staff unfamiliar with caring for pancytopenic patients about reducing the risk of infection and haemorrhage.

Test coordination

The nurse will act as coordinator in the programme of diagnostic tests and will prepare the patient for bone marrow graft if this is performed. Further details on caring for profoundly pancytopenic patients are given in the section on nursing management of acute leukaemia (p. 428). For details on nursing care in allogeneic bone marrow transplantation see pp. 426–427.

Rehabilitation

Rehabilitation commences even before the patient's discharge from hospital and must be planned in response to his potential for recovery, motivation and needs. The multidisciplinary team involved may include a physiotherapist, occupational therapist, dietitian, social worker, district nurse, health visitor, counsellor and psychologist.

Realistic goals must be set in discussion with the patient. Consideration must be given to avoiding the causative agent of the anaemia in the future. It may be necessary for the patient to change his job. This may require liaison between medical staff, the patient's employer, and a social worker.

Discharge planning

Before discharge it will be important to discuss with the patient any fears or apprehensions he may have and to clarify details of whom to contact if he has any further episodes of illness. Written information about the disorder, any precautions to be taken, and medication is particularly helpful.

HAEMOLYTIC ANAEMIAS

These anaemias result from the premature destruction of red blood cells, in response to either an inherited or an acquired defect. Many of the haemolytic anaemias are rare or very rare. The most common inherited anaemias are sickle cell disease and thalassaemia. The most common acquired forms result from direct cell injury following infection or medical treatment. Causes of haemolytic anaemias are listed in Box 11.3.

PATHOPHYSIOLOGY

In this type of anaemia the lifespan of the red blood cells is reduced because of a condition called red blood cell fragility, leading to excessive breakdown of these cells. This results in a reduced oxygen-carrying capacity in the blood and thus hypoxia in the tissues. This causes stimulation of the production of erythropoietin, which stimulates the bone marrow to increase erythropoiesis (see p. 406). A healthy person with mild haemolytic anaemia will not experience symptoms. However, if the red cell lifespan is greatly reduced (<15 days) the bone marrow will not be able to compensate adequately and the person will experience symptoms of haemolytic anaemia. This will occur more quickly if for any reason the bone marrow is not healthy. The resulting haemolytic anaemia gives rise to increased bilirubin and urobilinogen (see Fig. 11.8).

Medical and nursing management

The medical and nursing care provided will vary according to the specific type of haemolytic anaemia in question. This chapter will discuss only the management of sickle cell anaemia.

Box 11.3 Causes of haemolytic anaemias

INHERITED

- Red cell membrane fragility, e.g. spherocytosis
- Haemoglobin defects:
  — structure: sickle cell
  — synthesis: thalassaemia
- Red cell metabolism defect, e.g. glucose-6-phosphatic dehydrogenase deficiency

ACQUIRED

- Antibody attack, e.g. mismatched blood transfusion
- Direct cell injury:
  — traumatic e.g. prosthetic heart valve
  — chemical or drug induced, e.g. sodium chlorate, vitamin K analogues, Salazopyrin, nitrates
- Paroxysmal nocturnal haemoglobinurea.

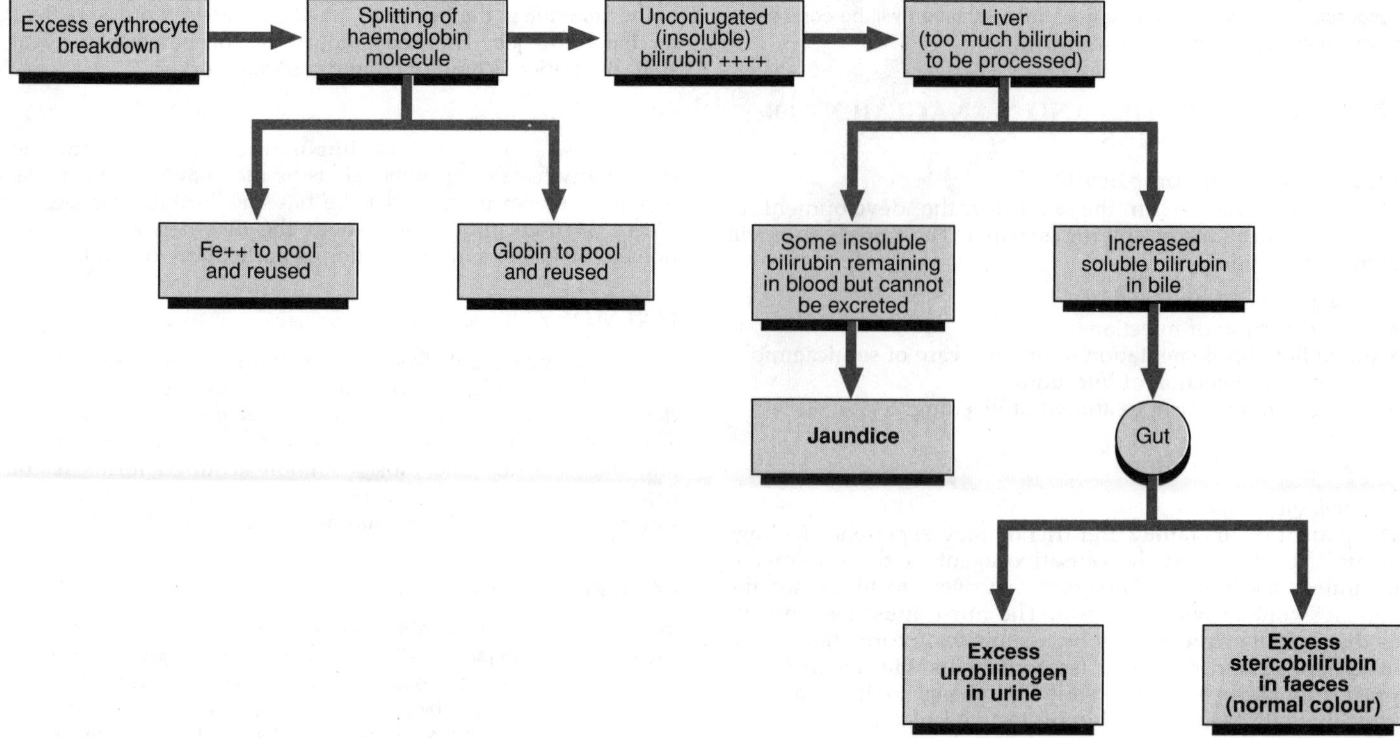

Fig. 11.8 Development of symptoms of haemolytic anaemia.

Sickle cell anaemia

The sickle cell anaemias are a group of haemolytic anaemias in which there is an inherited structural abnormality in the haemoglobin molecule (HbS). This abnormality is the result of the substitution of one amino acid in the haemoglobin molecule for another. The abnormal haemoglobin causes a characteristic sickle-like shaping of the red blood cell when it is in the deoxygenated state. It is a recessively inherited blood disorder of which there is a homozygous and a heterozygous variant (see Ch. 6 'Genetic Disorders'). In the heterozygous variant the person inherits the abnormal haemoglobin gene (HbS) from one parent and the normal (HbA) gene from the other parent. This person has the sickle cell trait (HbSA) and will usually be unaware of the abnormality unless he is tested for the trait or develops symptoms when exposed to severe hypoxic conditions (e.g. high altitude flying in an unpressurised cabin). The trait will be passed on to any children. In the homozygous variant the abnormal gene is inherited from both parents and the person will suffer from sickle cell anaemia.

This inherited sickle cell trait or sickle cell anaemia occurs among people of African, Caribbean, East Mediterranean, Middle Eastern, Indian and Pakistani origin. It is thought that this geographical distribution might be explained by the fact that sickle cell trait (not sickle cell anaemia) offers some protection against malaria.

Of people with sickle cell anaemia, 80% lead normal lives; 20% will have severe complications and die early.

PATHOPHYSIOLOGY

The normal pattern of the amino acids in the beta chains of the globin part of haemoglobin (see p. 407) is altered in the sickle cell haemoglobin by the substitution of a different amino acid for the normal one (HbS). HbS has certain properties which distinguish it from normal HbA haemoglobin. It is less soluble, especially when in a deoxygenated state and when the blood pH is below normal. Under these conditions crystals are formed within the red blood cell, making it more rigid and distorting it into a sickle shape. The effects of this abnormal cell are shown in Figure 11.9.

Common presenting symptoms. Sickle cell anaemia normally presents in childhood but might not become apparent until adulthood. Often the presenting symptoms are those of haemolytic anaemia (see p. 412 and Fig. 11.8) or of a painful 'sickle cell crisis' in response to a triggering factor (see Box 11.4). The clinical features of a crisis are:

- pain caused by the obstruction of small blood vessels in the tissues. Characteristics of the pain are the acuteness of the onset and its unresponsiveness to mild analgesia. The location of the pain depends on the location of the obstruction
- anaemia: although these patients are usually anaemic, the body often compensates so that the symptoms of anaemia occur only as the result of a very severe crisis
- infection: there is an increased incidence of minor infections, septicaemia, pneumococcal meningitis and osteomyelitis.

MEDICAL MANAGEMENT

Investigative procedures. A blood film will demonstrate the presence of the sickle-shaped red blood cells. The presence of HbS can be demonstrated when the red blood cells are mixed with a special solution of sodium metabisulphite and left for 20 min.

The screening test for sickle cell anaemia and sickle cell trait uses electrophoretic analysis to measure the rates of movement of the different haemoglobins in an electrical field.

Medical intervention. There is no cure for sickle cell disease. Management is based on alleviation of symptoms and promotion of a lifestyle that minimises crisis events and includes the following elements:

- early treatment of any infections, even minor ones
- avoiding situations in which the person could become chilled
- avoiding dehydration

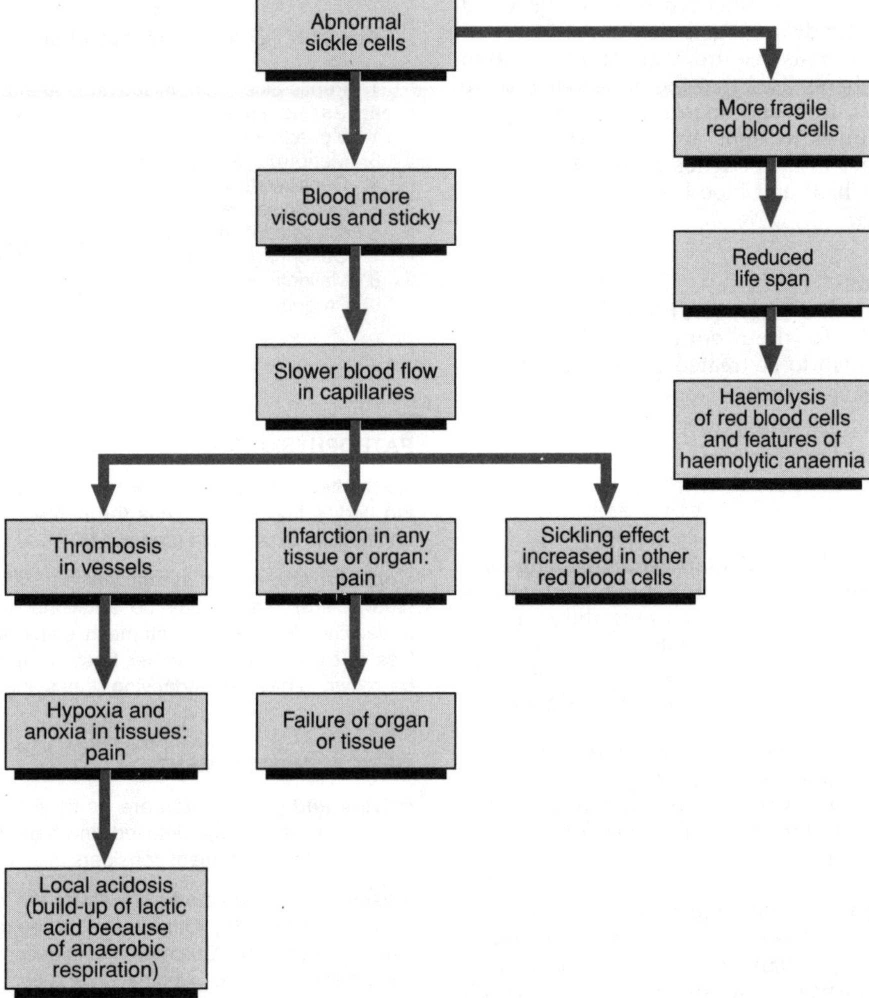

Fig. 11.9 Pathophysiology of sickle cell anaemia.

- managing crisis situations with prescribed analgesics (opiates are often required during crises)
- taking folic acid supplements
- alerting other practitioners, e.g. surgeons and anaesthetists, to the condition
- obtaining support from sickle cell centres and social work departments in improving home conditions
- learning to recognise complications of sickle cell disease, including bone and joint pains, leg ulcers, priapism in males, gallstones, blurred vision, kidney disease (in patients over 50 years old), peptic ulcers
- frequent follow-up in special clinics
- blood tests for haemoglobin and reticulocyte counts to monitor disease
- blood transfusions where necessary
- genetic counselling
- good antenatal care
- education on general health and nutrition.

Box 11.4 Trigger factors in sickle cell anaemia

1. Reduced oxygen, e.g. during strenuous exercise
2. Anaesthetics
3. Dehydration
4. Infection
5. Fever
6. Pregnancy
7. Sudden change in temperature
8. Alcohol: possibly because of dehydration
9. Emotional stress.

NURSING PRIORITIES AND MANAGEMENT OF SICKLE CELL ANAEMIA

Life-threatening concerns

Patients in sickle cell crisis admitted as emergencies to hospital may be very frightened. The nurse needs to appreciate the severity of the pain and the need for the administration of opiates. These should not be withheld and addiction problems rarely occur. The severe pain of a crisis does not respond to mild analgesics. Some hospitals within areas with a population in which sickle cell anaemia is relatively common have set up protocols for the management of patients admitted with sickle cell anaemia crisis to minimise the trauma of admission and to ensure the appropriate management of care.

Of equal importance to the alleviation of pain in sickle cell crisis is the management of the underlying cause of the crisis. An i.v. infusion will be commenced to maintain good hydration and to administer drugs (e.g. antibiotics).

Patients admitted in a crisis require vigilant observation and monitoring. It must be realised that the underlying cause may not be apparent at first and therefore monitoring of the patient may alert nurses to signs and symptoms of the cause as well as to changes in the patient's condition.

Oxygen therapy (see Ch. 3) and blood transfusion may be necessary.

Nursing considerations

Because these patients are often frightened, the nurse should listen carefully to their concerns. They often know the best way for them to be treated when in a crisis as they may have had several previous episodes.

> ? **11.11** It may not always be appropriate to ask a family member to act as interpreter. Why?

Men may be admitted with a particularly embarrassing condition, priapism (prolonged penile erection due to thrombosis in the corpus cavernosa). This requires not only the administration of analgesia but also i.v. hydration and possibly exchange blood transfusion (to reduce the percentage of sickle cells). Chronic priapism can occur and the patient's sexual function may be impaired.

Before the patient is discharged from hospital, he should be made aware of the importance of recognising and avoiding situations that may cause a sickle cell crisis and of the need to seek medical advice at the onset of a painful episode, especially if it is accompanied by symptoms of another illness (including minor ailments).

A newly diagnosed patient will require a comprehensive education programme about the disorder, the ways to minimise complications, and any adaptations to be made to lifestyle. Arrangements should be made for the screening of all members of the family if this has not been done previously. Genetic counselling should be offered. Some areas with a high incidence of sickle cell disease employ special nurse counsellors to carry out screening and to advise patients and their families about the disorder and its consequences.

The emphasis in caring for a person with sickle cell anaemia is on promoting health and minimising ill-health.

ANAEMIA RESULTING FROM BLOOD LOSS

The blood loss responsible for these anaemias may be either acute or chronic:

- acute: loss of large volume of blood over a short period of time, as in haemorrhage. (For pathophysiology, medical management, and nursing priorities and management, see Ch. 18, Ch. 20 and Ch. 29.)
- chronic: loss of a small, even microscopic, amount over a long period of time. Chronic blood loss is very common and is the form that will be considered here.

There are a number of disorders in which there is a constant or intermittent loss of small amounts of blood. Thus, this type of anaemia is secondary to another disorder, although it may be the presenting illness. Frequently, it is only when a diagnosis of anaemia has been established that the causative illness is suspected. The most common causes of chronic blood loss are listed in Box 11.5. Some patients realise that they have been bleeding but are too afraid to seek advice and discover what underlying condition the bleeding signifies.

Box 11.5 Common causes of chronic blood loss

1. Peptic ulceration, including side-effects of steroid therapy
2. Gastric irritation: side-effect of alcohol and some drugs, e.g. aspirin
3. Menorrhagia: excessive regular menstrual flow
4. Genitourinary bleeding, e.g. with bladder carcinoma
5. Liver disease
6. Chronic inflammatory disease
7. Oesophageal varices (blood loss may be acute)
8. Malignancy
9. Pregnancy.

PATHOPHYSIOLOGY

No ill effects will be felt until the blood loss has caused depletion of the body's iron stores. Thus the pathophysiology is similar to that of iron deficiency anaemia (see p. 415).

Common presenting symptoms are as for iron deficiency anaemia (see p. 415). There may be additional symptoms according to the underlying disorder, e.g. stomach pains, heavy menstruation, weight loss or blood in stools (either fresh or as melaena). The patient may be known to have an underlying illness, e.g. peptic ulceration.

MEDICAL MANAGEMENT

History and examination are as for the diagnosis of iron deficiency anaemia (see p. 415). Detailed and careful questioning may uncover symptoms that the patient considers insignificant or is afraid to report.

Investigative procedures are as for the diagnosis of iron deficiency anaemia (see p. 415). Other tests may be required according to clinical features presented. Common investigations include barium meal and barium enema, rectal examination and endoscopy.

Medical intervention will depend on the specific cause of the blood loss. Possibilities for treatment include oral iron therapy (see p. 415) and blood transfusion (see p. 410).

NURSING PRIORITIES AND MANAGEMENT OF ANAEMIAS RESULTING FROM BLOOD LOSS

Life-threatening concerns

If anaemia is very severe the nursing care will be implemented according to the complications that arise (see Ch. 2, Ch. 3 and Ch. 18). If immediate transfusion is required nursing care will be as on page 417. The nurse will need to monitor the patient very closely for possible cardiac failure and pulmonary oedema.

Nursing considerations

In her initial interactions with a patient who presents with unexplained bleeding, the nurse should bear in mind that he is likely to be feeling apprehensive about receiving a diagnosis. He may also be feeling guilty about not seeking medical advice earlier. Giving the patient clear information about the tests and investigations to be done will help to allay anxiety. If the patient is to undergo tests at an outpatient's department he will need to know about any necessary preinvestigative preparation, how long the tests will take and what they will involve, and whether he will be fit to return home unaccompanied afterwards.

Thorough nursing assessment can be invaluable in establishing the cause of bleeding and will include questioning, observation, monitoring of vital signs and discussion with the patient's family and friends.

The patient will need to be informed about the implications of the diagnosis and the proposed treatment. In planning care, the nurse must attempt to prioritise the patient's needs and problems; in so doing, she must be sensitive to individual values and perceptions. Counselling may help the patient, especially if the diagnosis is cancer or any other chronic disorder that will affect the patient's lifestyle. Counselling may also be appropriate if the patient has a self-inflicted disorder, e.g. alcohol-induced gastritis.

The patient with anaemia caused by blood loss may be treated in hospital, in an outpatient's clinic or health centre, or at home. Good liaison among all staff involved in the various stages of treatment is vital in ensuring continuity of care. Whether the patient's care is long or short term, follow-up must be emphasised to ensure that the disorder has been cured or is being adequately monitored.

DISORDERS CAUSE BY OVERPRODUCTION OF RED BLOOD CELLS

A raised haemoglobin level usually indicates an absolute increase in the number of circulating red blood cells. This may be a false finding if the plasma volume is reduced, as in dehydration.

There are three situations in which the number of red blood cells is increased:

1. Physiological response due to hypoxia, e.g. at high altitudes or with pulmonary disease
2. Inappropriate production of erythropoietin (or similar substance) in certain pathological conditions, e.g. malignant tumours
3. Pathological proliferation of red blood cells with no erythropoietin stimulus. This is called polycythaemia vera.

POLYCYTHAEMIA VERA

This disease occurs most commonly in men over the age of 40. The prognosis may be up to 20 years. There is usually an increased white cell and platelet count as well as a high red cell count.

PATHOPHYSIOLOGY

The raised red cell and platelet count and haemoglobin level have a number of consequences, including hyperviscosity of the blood, thrombosis, and hypertension, both of which could precipitate cardiac failure. Thrombosis alone may precipitate peripheral vascular disease.

Common presenting symptoms. Patients may present with one or more of the following symptoms:

- peripheral vascular disease
- headaches
- dizziness
- blackouts
- lack of concentration
- angina
- hypertension
- dyspnoea
- epistaxis
- pruritus (especially on exposure to heat or cold)
- gout
- indigestion (peptic ulceration).

MEDICAL MANAGEMENT

History and examination. The patient may not present to the doctor with any symptoms but attend for a health check-up and be found to have hypertension. He may have a ruddy complexion and the palms of the hands and the oral mucosal membrane may be a deep red colour. An enlarged spleen is found in 75% of patients.

Investigative procedures. Blood analysis will include full blood count, haemoglobin level, PCV and blood viscosity. Estimation of the red blood cell mass will be made using radioactive chromium-51. Bone marrow aspiration will be performed and usually demonstrates a hypercellular state and an increased number of megakaryocytes (large nucleated cells of the marrow that produce platelets).

Medical intervention. Venesection (the removal of whole blood) is the simplest form of treatment. It is repeated until the PCV is reduced below 0.50 and leads to a dramatic alleviation of symptoms.

If the diagnosis is certain, radioactive phosphorus – ^{32}P may be given by intravenous injection. This treatment is given in an outpatient's department, as the radioactive level within the body will not be high enough to present a risk to other people within the community provided the patient complies with certain guidelines. This treatment takes up to 3 months to be effective.

Myelosuppressive drugs (e.g. busulphan, melphalan) may be given orally until the disorder is controlled (see Ch. 32).

All patients will require frequent monitoring to minimise the effects of the disorder. Possible complications are thrombosis, haemorrhage, myelofibrosis (fibrosis of bone marrow tissue which interferes with all blood cell production) and acute leukaemia.

NURSING PRIORITIES AND MANAGEMENT OF POLYCYTHAEMIA VERA

The main aims of nursing care are:

- to support the patient during diagnostic tests
- to help the patient understand diagnosis, treatment and possible long-term effects
- to teach the patient how to detect the onset of complications.

Nursing considerations

The patient and his family will need to come to terms with a chronic disorder that may alter the patient's lifestyle and shorten his life. The patient will probably undergo tests as an outpatient or day patient. The nurse should provide the patient with information about all investigations. She will be required to assist the doctor perform a bone marrow aspiration (see p. 413).

The patient undergoing venesection (which will be commenced by the doctor) must be monitored for signs and symptoms of shock (see Ch. 18). One complication of venesection in patients with polycythaemia vera is difficulty in maintaining flow because of the hyperviscosity of the blood.

If the patient is to receive ^{32}P he must be given, preferably in writing, clear instructions regarding limitations of activities or contact with people (e.g. children or pregnant women) in view of being radioactive. If this care is impossible at home, arrangements will have to be made to admit the patient to a single room in a ward. If admission is required, the need for isolation to protect patients, visitors and staff must be tactfully explained to the patient (see Ch. 32).

Patient education

Once treatment has begun, it is important to teach the patient to monitor himself for any signs of thrombosis, e.g. pain. If medication has been prescribed he will need detailed instructions about taking oral cytotoxins (see Ch. 32). Emphasis should be placed on the importance of continued monitoring via blood tests and outpatient appointments.

DISORDERS OF WHITE BLOOD CELLS AND LYMPHOID TISSUE

The following sections will consider the nurse's role in the treatment of the following disorders:

1. leukaemia
2. lymphoma
3. multiple myeloma
4. agranulocytosis.

LEUKAEMIA

The leukaemias are a group of disorders in which there is an abnormal proliferation of immature white cells which is *usually* confined to one specific subtype of white cell, i.e. granulocyte, lymphocyte or monocyte.

The leukaemias are divided into two types: acute and chronic. Acute leukaemia is characterised by the malignant proliferation occurring at the 'blast' level of maturity (see p. 407). In the chronic form, the malignant proliferation occurs at a later, but still immature, stage of development.

Leukaemia occurs in all age groups, in both sexes and in all races. The total number of new cases in England and Wales of all types of leukaemia is approximately 4200 per year, i.e. 8 new cases per 100 000 of the population per year (OPCS 1985).

Within the United Kingdom, the incidence of leukaemia varies from region to region. This variance might be explained by certain of the aetiological factors listed below.

Aetiology

1. Ionising radiation
2. Viruses
3. Chemicals, especially benzene, toulene and other petroleum derivatives
4. Alkylating cytotoxic drugs
5. Down's syndrome.

There is also an association between acute myeloblastic leukaemia and multiple myeloma (see p. 436), lymphoma (see p. 434), and breast and ovarian cancer but the precise connection is not known.

PATHOPHYSIOLOGY

As leukaemic cells proliferate they gradually crowd out the bone marrow so that it produces fewer and fewer normal blood cells. In acute leukaemia, there is an abnormal and excessive proliferation of immature (and therefore ineffective) white blood cells. In chronic leukaemia, even though the abnormal proliferation occurs at a later stage in white cell development, the leukaemic cells still serve no useful function. Chronic leukaemia can develop into acute leukaemia.

The results of the leukaemic process are:

- anaemia
- leucopenia, especially neutropenia
- thrombocytopenia.

Acute leukaemia

PATHOPHYSIOLOGY

Common presenting symptoms: (see Table 11.5). The most common symptoms, which derive from the effects of the disease on bone marrow function, are:

Table 11.5 Summary of symptoms of acute leukaemia

Result of leukaemic process	Symptoms
Anaemia	Pallor Dyspnoea on exertion Palpitations
Leucopenia	Fever Malaise Joint pain Sore throat Mouth infection
Thrombocytopenia	Bleeding gums Petechiae Purpura Bruising

- acute infections (associated with fevers), e.g. upper respiratory infections, influenza, dental abscesses, oral *Candida albicans*, skin infections. More than one infection may occur at once, or there may be a succession of acute infections
- bleeding of gums, epistaxis, skin petechiae, purpura, bruising
- symptoms of anaemia (see p. 412).

?	**11.12** How can these symptoms be explained in terms of blood cell function?

Another symptom of acute leukaemia which is sometimes present is bone pain. This may occur because hyperplasia of bone marrow may cause the periosteum to stretch.

MEDICAL MANAGEMENT

History and examination. The patient usually describes an abrupt onset of symptoms — sometimes less than 72 hours' history of being unwell. He is usually pyrexial, tachycardic and often tachypnoeic with signs and symptoms of acute infection. He may be pale and often has cold sores on his lips (see Case History 11.2). On examination, evidence may be found of lymphadenopathy (enlarged lymph glands), petechiae, purpura and bruising.

Investigative procedures. Diagnosis can usually be established on examination of a blood film, which usually shows a picture of:

- high white blood cell count (mainly blast cells)
- low red blood cell count
- low haemoglobin
- low platelet count
- raised MCV.

A bone-marrow aspiration and biopsy are always required to establish the exact type of acute leukaemia (myeloblastic, lymphoblastic or some other, rarer, form). The bone marrow will show replacement of normal marrow by leukaemic cells. This examination is important as a baseline measurement; further aspirations are done during and after treatment to show response to treatment. The response to treatment will also help to indicate prognosis.

A lumbar puncture (see Ch. 9) will be performed if the patient has acute lymphoblastic leukaemia, as there is a high risk of central nervous system involvement, especially in the cerebrospinal fluid.

Careful examination of the testes will also be carried out in male patients with acute lymphoblastic leukaemia as this is another region where leukaemia often spreads.

Case history 11.2 Mrs D

Mrs D aged 40 years, is a housewife. She and her husband have two sons, aged 12 and 14. Mrs D's husband often works overtime so she is kept busy looking after the household. She enjoys gardening, keep-fit classes and reading.

Over the past two or three months she has been excessively tired. Although she sleeps well at night, she does not feel rested in the morning. She has had mouth ulcers, cold sores and a persistent sore throat. At first, she attributed these symptoms to being run down. Finally, she sought her GP's opinion about the sore throat. He prescribed antibiotics but because of her other symptoms took a blood sample for a full blood count in case she was anaemic. He advised her to contact the surgery in a few days for the blood test results and to return to see him if the sore throat continued.

Mrs D was very shocked when the next day the GP telephoned to tell her she was very anaemic and that he had arranged an emergency appointment for the next day at the local hospital for her to see the haematology consultant. At that appointment Mrs D was advised that she needed urgent investigation into her abnormal blood count; arrangements were made for her immediate admission to hospital.

Further investigation confirmed a diagnosis of acute myeloid (myeloblastic) leukaemia. After further discussion with the consultant and her husband Mrs D has consented to chemotherapy.

A central infusion long line (Hickman catheter) has been inserted to provide long-term access for repeated drug administration, blood specimen collection, blood product transfusion and possible parenteral nutrition. Mrs D has received a blood transfusion so that her haemoglobin level immediately prior to the first course of treatment is 11 g/100 ml. She is neutropenic and thrombocytopenic.

Her nursing care for day 2 of her first course of chemotherapy is given in Nursing Care Plan 11.2. The chemotherapy drugs she is receiving are i.v. Adriamycin, cytoscine arabinoside and oral 6-thioguanine.

Medical intervention. Treatment is directed towards controlling the disease process by means of powerful chemotherapeutic agents and, by so doing, bringing the leukaemia into remission. Remission is indicated by a reduction of blast cells to < 5% of the total white cell count in the bone marrow. Remission is then consolidated with the aim of eliminating all leukaemic cells. If remission continues, treatment will be in the form of maintenance therapy for up to 3 years.

Chemotherapy

The aim of chemotherapy is to suppress the abnormal cell production and prevent the major complications of infection and bleeding. Nursing care during treatment aims to support the patient both physiologically and psychologically during the rigours of the chemotherapeutic programme.

The major drawback of this form of treatment is that as well as destroying abnormal cells the chemotherapeutic agents used can be highly toxic to normal cells as well, especially those that, like the neoplastic cells, divide rapidly, e.g. those in the skin and the gastrointestinal tract.

Although chemotherapy is discussed in detail in Chapter 32 for the purposes of the present chapter it is important to understand how the various drugs used are classified and how they act on both leukaemic and healthy cells.

The stages of chemotherapy may be briefly described as follows:

1. Induction chemotherapy. A combination of chemotherapeutic agents is given until remission is achieved. An additional two cycles are then normally given. The common chemotherapy agents used are
   - acute lymphoblastic leukaemia:
     — vincristine
     — Adriamycin (doxorubicin)
     — L-asparaginase
     — prednisolone
   - acute myeloblastic leukaemia:
     — Adriamycin (doxorubicin)
     — 6 thioguanine
     — cytoscine arabinoside
2. Consolidation chemotherapy. At this stage some change in chemotherapeutic agents may be made, or a single drug at a high dose (e.g. cytoscine arabinoside) may be given. Radiotherapy to the cranium may be given during consolidation therapy as part of central nervous system prophylaxis.
3. Maintenance therapy: oral drugs may be given but intravenous or intrathecal chemotherapy drugs may also be administered as part of central nervous system prophylaxis. Patients with acute myeloblastic leukaemia who are under the age of 50 and whose leukaemia goes into complete remission usually have a bone marrow transplant at that stage. Patients of a similar age group with acute lymphoblastic leukaemia whose leukaemia goes into complete remission may not have a bone marrow transplant at this stage, but if the acute lymphoblastic leukaemia recurs and further chemotherapy achieves a second remission, they are usually given a bone marrow transplant at that time. This difference in timing is based on the finding that there is a higher rate of maintaining complete remission in acute lymphoblastic leukaemia than in the acute myeloblastic form.

The transplanted bone marrow may be allogeneic, i.e. from a donor — usually with matched human leucocyte antigen (HLA) — or autologous, i.e. from the patient himself, collected and stored while he is in complete remission (see Ch. 16).

Preventing infection and promoting healing

The failure of white blood cells and platelets in the leukaemic patient may require the following medical interventions:

Transfusions. Blood transfusions to minimise the effects of anaemia may be needed (see p. 417). Platelet transfusion will be required if the platelet count is $< 10 \times 10^9$ cells/l; it may also be required with a higher count if the patient is having bleeding problems. Platelet transfusions should be crossmatched for ABO blood group.

Platelet transfusions may be required daily and can cause allergic reactions to foreign antibodies. Consequently, i.v. hydrocortisone and i.v. chlorpheniramine are given to minimise this risk.

Antibiotic therapy. If pyrexia occurs as a consequence of septicaemia, i.v. antibiotics will be prescribed. In such cases blood cultures will be taken and an agreed protocol of antibiotic therapy commenced while the results of the culture are awaited. Therapy is then adjusted in accordance with the blood results.

Oral antibiotics that will not be absorbed through the gut wall will be prescribed to reduce the incidence of endogenous infection (i.e. arising from a bacterial source already present in the body, such as commensal organisms in the gut).

Antifungal and antiviral agents will be administered to minimise the incidence of infection (e.g. *Candida albicans* and herpes). These agents will also be used as part of a mouth hygiene regime.

Protective isolation may be necessary to reduce the incidence of septicaemia.

Monitoring. A central intravenous infusion line (e.g. Hickman line) will be inserted prior to treatment. This long line i.v. catheter, the tip of which lies in the right atrium of the heart, can be left in situ for many weeks, allowing easy access to obtain the many blood samples that will be required to monitor the patient's haematological profile and electrolyte balance and to administer i.v. drugs.

Prevention of tumour lysis syndrome. Allopurinal (a drug used in the treatment of gout) will be prescribed from the commencement of treatment to prevent the development of tumour lysis syndrome, i.e. metabolic upset caused by the rapid breakdown of tumour cells during the induction phase of treatment. This syndrome can also lead to renal failure.

If, despite prophylaxis, tumour lysis syndrome does occur, i.v. normal saline should be given to improve diuresis; the urine should be kept alkaline by the administration of sodium bicarbonate and chemotherapy should be discontinued.

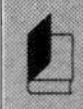

For further details on the medical care of patients with malignant blood disorders see Souhami & Tobias (1986).

NURSING PRIORITIES AND MANAGEMENT OF ACUTE LEUKAEMIA (See Nursing Care Plan 11.2.)

The aims of nursing care for the patient undergoing chemotherapy are:

- to help the patient cope with the diagnosis
- to support the patient as complications of the disease arise
- to support the patient during the therapy and while he experiences side-effects.

During the diagnostic process the nurse's role will be to keep the patient and his family informed about the tests to be performed and any necessary preparations, and to discuss the implications of the results once they are known. Particular reassurance should be given prior to and during bone marrow aspiration, as this procedure will need to be repeated frequently in the course of treatment.

Psychological support is vital for patients who are faced with a serious diagnosis that demands immediate and prolonged treatment and which is likely to give rise to life-threatening complications. The nurse must exercise good communication skills and show a sympathetic understanding of the patient's emotional state.

Nursing considerations

Preventing infection

The overwhelming concern of nursing care for patients undergoing chemotherapy will be to minimise the incidence and effects of septicaemia (see Ch. 16, Ch. 18). The nurse must be aware of potential infective agents (e.g. *Pseudomonas aeruginosa, Escherichia coli, Candida albicans*) and of their source, routes of transmission and portals of entry.

Of key importance in the prevention of crossinfection are good handwashing technique and the use of protective isolation. Also of crucial importance is the strict aseptic management of central intravenous infusion.

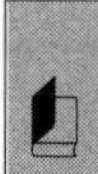

For research findings and advice on handwashing techniques see Campbell (1988), David (1988), Gidley (1987), Phillips (1989) and Taylor (1978). For details on aseptic i.v. management see Milne (1988).

Vigilant and accurate monitoring of vital signs, fluid balance and consciousness level may give the first indication of septicaemia. The nurse must bear in mind that in immunosuppression there are few symptoms of infection; close monitoring is therefore crucial. Moreover, it is only by virtue of early detection that potentially fatal septicaemic shock can be avoided.

It is essential to realise that an infected mouth can be the cause of septicaemia and that frequent mouth inspection is consequently extremely important. An objective oral assessment tool such as that described by Eilers et al (1988) may be found useful (See Table 11.6).

The patient should be given instruction in maintaining a high standard of oral hygiene. He should be advised to use a very soft toothbrush and a bactericidal mouth-wash (e.g. chlorhexidine); he may also need to use a topical antifungal agent (e.g. nystatin) along with an antiviral ointment (e.g. acyclovir). If the mouth is very sore the patient may find a local anaesthetic solution (e.g. Difflam) or lozenges (e.g. Merocaine) helpful (Crosby 1989).

Chest infection should it occur, may cause considerable distress arising from breathlessness and (due to weakness) difficulty expectorating sputum. The patient should be taught breathing exercises to ensure good lung expansion. If an infection occurs he may need oxygen therapy, administration of bronchodilators and chest physiotherapy. If haemoptysis occurs he may be particularly frightened.

Preventing haemorrhage

Careful observation and monitoring must be practised to detect any bleeding. This should include:

- hourly pulse and blood pressure readings. The nurse should be aware of the risk of bruising from the sphygmomanometer cuff in thrombocytopenic patients; the frequency of blood pressure readings may have to be reduced
- daily urinalysis for visible and occult blood
- testing of all stools for visible or occult blood
- observation of changes in consciousness level or development of headaches (signs of cerebral haemorrhage)
- observation of sputum and vomit for blood
- daily inspection of skin for petechiae, purpura and bruising
- observation for pain, especially in the abdomen, as this may be an indication of haemorrhage.

All signs and symptoms of bleeding must be reported immediately to the doctor. At no time should intramuscular or subcutaneous injections be given.

Platelet transfusion will also be given to minimise the risk of haemorrhage. The transfusion units must be stored at 20 °C and therefore must never be kept in a refrigerator. Each unit must be checked for the same details as for a blood transfusion. Particular note should be made of the expiry date, as platelet transfusions have a short lifespan. The transfusion will normally be administered over 30 min. The patient must be closely observed for allergic reactions (see p. 418).

Minimising the side-effects of therapy

The side-effects of chemotherapy may include nausea and vomiting, which in turn may cause dehydration and electrolyte imbalance. Stomatitis may also develop. Each cytotoxic chemotherapeutic agent will have characteristic side-effects; the nurse should be well-informed about these (see Ch. 32).

During the induction and consolidation phases of chemotherapy the patient may feel very lethargic and ill; it will be important for the nurse to assist him with personal hygiene in order to help minimise infection. Special skin cleansing

Nursing Care Plan 11.2 Care of Mrs D during chemotherapy for myeloid leukaemia (See Case history 11.2.)

Nursing considerations	Action	Rationale	Evaluation
1. Risk of infection (because of neutropenia and chemotherapy)	❒ Wash hands using antiseptic solution before giving any nursing care, with scrupulous attention to wrists and between fingers and careful drying	To remove commensal bacterial skin flora that may cause infection in patient; single most important preventive action against cross-infection	All symptoms and signs of infection are noted and reported immediately and thus treatment for any infection commences early
	❒ Instruct and assist with personal hygiene using antiseptic solution	To reduce skin bacterial flora and risk of endogenous septicaemia	
	❒ Inspect skin daily for infection, especially folds of buttocks, axilla, perineum, breasts, puncture sites, skin breakdown, skin lesions and rashes	To detect any skin infection early	
	❒ Explain mouth care regime: • use of chlorhexidene 0.4% solution after meals and at bedtime • use of antifungal agent in mouthcare as prescribed by doctor (after all meals and at bedtime)	To prevent bacterial and fungal infections of mouth and reduce risk of septicaemia by early detection of any infection	
	• gentle brushing of teeth using a soft toothbrush	To reduce risk of bacterial infection	
	• application of antiviral cream to lips as prescribed	To reduce risk of viral infection	
	Inspect mouth daily for signs of infection using Oral Assessment Guide (see p. 433). Take swabs from any new lesions	Early detection of mouth infection	
	Record of axillary temperature, pulse and BP 4-hourly (unless patient is receiving blood products)	Early detection of infection. Axillary route used because of sore mouth and risk of infection	
	Report any elevation of temperature to doctor immediately	To ensure any infection is treated appropriately and immediately	
	❒ Take nasal, throat and skin swabs from axilla, groin, umbilicus	To detect any microorganisms that might cause skin infections and septicaemia	
	❒ Inform patient and visitors of the restrictions re plants and flowers	Earth is a source of *Serratia murcesens*, stagnant water a medium for *pseudomonas aeruginosa*	
	❒ Advise Mrs D about dietary restrictions: no raw unpeeled fruit or raw vegetables	Raw, unpeeled fruit and raw vegetables may be contaminated with *Pseudomonas aeruginosa*, klebsiella species and *Escherichia coli* and cause septicaemia	
	❒ Administer no drugs or evacuant enemas or suppositories	Can cause rectal abscesses and septicaemia in immunosuppressed patient	
	❒ Report any symptoms e.g. dysuria, to doctor immediately.	To commence appropriate antibacterial/antifungal or antiviral treatment immediately	
	Report any change in patient's condition, especially increased drowsiness, headache, irritability or restlessness	Changes in central nervous system may be first indication of septicaemia	
2. Inadequate oxygenation of tissues due to anaemia ***(cont'd)***	❒ Assist with all activities of living as appropriate	To conserve energy and reduce oxygen requirements	Patient is not unduly tired
	❒ Observe pressure areas twice daily	To detect any skin breakdown due to hypoxia of skin	Any pressure sore is detected at first sign, if not prevented

Nursing Care Plan 11.2 *Cont'd*

Nursing considerations	Action	Rationale	Evaluation
2. Inadequate oxygenation of tissues due to anaemia (cont'd)	❐ Organise nursing care or assistance to allow periods of rest	To conserve energy	
	❐ Use Spenco mattress on bed	To reduce risk of pressure sores	
3. Easy bleeding due to thrombocytopenia	❐ Inspect skin daily for signs of new bruises, petechiae, purpura ❐ Inspect mouth daily for bleeding ❐ Test urine daily for protein and blood ❐ Test and inspect all stools for blood ❐ Observe any vomit for blood ❐ Observe any headache and/or change in conscious level ❐ Observe any other overt episodes of bleeding, e.g. epistaxis	To detect any bleeding immediately	Bleeding is detected early and prompt treatment is given
	❐ Report to doctor immediately any signs or symptoms of bleeding	To ensure treatment is given as soon as possible	
	❐ Record pulse and BP 4-hourly	To detect any hidden bleeding apparent because of tachycardia and hypotension	
	❐ Administer platelets as prescribed, ensuring compatibility of donor blood, observing and monitoring for any allergic or other reaction by recording quarter-hourly pulse and BP and asking patient about any complaints ❐ Ensure i.v. chlorpheniramine and hydrocortisone are given prior to platelet transfusion	To ensure platelets are given safely	
4. Side-effects of chemotherapy			
a. Bone marrow suppression	See 1, 2, 3		All side-effects of chemotherapy agents are observed and prompt relevant nursing care is implemented so that Mrs D experiences as few effects as possible
b. Extravasation of chemotherapeutic agents especially Adriamycin	❐ Observe cannula site vigilantly for signs of extravasation Report any soreness at cannula site to doctor		
c. Nausea and vomiting	❐ Reassure patient that nausea will stop when chemotherapy course has been completed	Patient already aware of possibility but symptoms can be very depressing	
	❐ Record all episodes of, and measure all vomit	To assess possibility of dehydration and possible electrolyte in balance	
	❐ Administer antiemetics according to prescription	To prevent or minimise nausea and vomiting	
	❐ Report to doctor nausea and vomiting not controlled by antiemetics	So that antiemetic regime can be reviewed	
(cont'd)	❐ Encourage patient to try alternative measures of controlling nausea and vomiting, e.g. relaxation tapes	Prevent or minimise episodes of nausea and vomiting	

Nursing Care Plan 11.2 *Cont'd*

Nursing considerations	Action	Rationale	Evaluation
4. Side-effects of Chemotherapy (cont'd)			
d. Stomatitis	❒ As for mouth regime in 1		
e. Flu-like symptoms due to cytoscine arabinoside	❒ Observe and report any symptoms to doctor immediately of shivering, headache or pyrexia. Monitor temperature 4-hourly	Early detection	
f. Conjunctivitis due to high doses of cytoscine arabinoside	❒ Administration of prednisolone eye drops as prescribed by doctor	To reduce conjunctivitis inflammation	
g. Red urine after i.v. Adriamycin	❒ Reassure patient that red urine is temporary consequence of i.v. Adriamycin		
	❒ Test all urine for blood during and immediately after bolus injection of Adriamycin	Difficult to differentiate between red colouring and bleeding due to thrombocytopenia	
h. Hyperuricaemia because of rapid breakdown of rapidly dividing tumour cells following chemotherapy	❒ Observe and measure output. Encourage oral fluid intake especially between administration of chemotherapy drugs ❒ Administer Allopurinol as prescribed	To reduce uric acid crystal formation and possible renal failure; to prevent or minimise high uric acid levels	
5. Anxiety about diagnosis, treatment, side-effects, prognosis	❒ Be prepared to listen to any anxieties		Mrs D feels able to talk with staff and feel she fully understands as much as she wishes to know about her disorder, its treatment and the consequences
	❒ Answer questions honestly and ensure, by reporting in writing, that all members of the multidisciplinary team know what information was given and what anxieties Mrs D is voicing	May require reiteration of information previously given by doctors, nurses or other members of the team, because of mental adjustment to diagnosis	
	❒ Request further discussion with doctor or registered nurse as required		
	❒ Arrange for support from other relevant personnel if appropriate, e.g. social worker, chaplain, special organisations e.g. BACUP, Cancerlink		
6. Altered body image **a. Alopecia**	❒ Reassure Mrs D that hair loss is temporary: reinforce information given about when hair loss will occur, likely duration and rate of regrowth	To try to reduce emotional trauma of alopecia. Accurate information will help her to adjust and explain to her husband and her children	Mrs D is able to feel she is still attractive to her husband and that her appearance is acceptable to her children
	❒ Advise Mrs D to reduce handling of hair but encourage her to keep hair style attractive	To reduce trauma to weak hair and minimise loss	
(cont'd)	❒ Discuss ways of enhancing her appearance once hair loss starts, e.g. wearing wigs, turbans, scarves	Help her to feel as attractive as possible when alopecia is complete	

Nursing Care Plan 11.2 *Cont'd*

Nursing considerations	Action	Rationale	Evaluation
6. Altered body image (cont'd)			
b. Herpes	❐ Give written information to read	To help her understand information given and a basis to ask further questions	Mrs D will feel staff understand the disfigurement of the herpes and she is helping herself
	❐ Educate and assist Mrs D to carry out mouthcare regime as in 1		
c. Sexuality	❐ Be sensitive to possible worries about sexuality ❐ Listen to worries; give truthful answers to any questions about sexual functioning ❐ Offer written information for her to read	To help her explore feelings about changes in sexual functioning and help her discuss this with husband when she feels able	Mrs D will feel she received relevant information and feels able to discuss this topic
7. Inadequate nutrition and hydration			
a. Anorexia	❐ Ensure oral hygiene regime continued as in 1	To maintain infection free mouth and because absence of blood improves taste	Weigh weekly: Mrs D should maintain admission weight
b. Nausea and vomiting	❐ Administer antiemetics as prescribed by doctor	To prevent or minimise nausea and vomiting	
c. Hypermetabolic state	❐ Help her choose a high protein/high carbohydrate diet from menu	To reduce or minimise effects of malnutrition, minimise weight loss and maintain protein intake	
	❐ Arrange for dietition to talk to her daily to help meet dietary needs ❐ Discuss with Mrs D and her husband possibility of him bringing certain foods she particularly wishes within restrictions (see 1) ❐ Encourage high protein/high energy drinks between meals ❐ Ensure meals are attractively served and small portions if appropriate	To improve or minimise effects of malnutrition and immunosuppression	
	❐ Ensure 2–3 l fluid intake	To prevent hyperuricaemia (see 4)	Fluid balance assessed daily: Mrs D does not develop negative fluid balance

solutions (e.g. povidone iodine) may be advised. If the patient is very weak, preventive measures should be taken against the complications of immobility. Of particular importance is the observation of pressure areas. A rating scale (e.g. Norton, Waterlow, Douglas) should be used as a basis for estimating pressure sore risk and planning appropriate intervention. The Waterlow scale (Waterlow 1988) and Douglas scale (Pritchard 1986) both consider risk factors additional to those addressed by the earlier Norton scale (Norton et al 1975); these include medication (e.g. steroid and cytotoxic therapy), nutritional states and skin condition. Any pressure sore that does develop must be carefully assessed; intervention must be carried out without delay as the sore can become infected and cause septicaemia.

The patient may lose his appetite, especially if he has a sore mouth (from infection or stomatitis) or suffers from nausea and vomiting (from cytoxic and other medication). A high-protein, high-carbohydrate diet is recommended. The dietitian will be able to suggest supplementary high-protein drinks. It may be possible to involve the family as well in providing food that the patient might find tempting. Nonetheless, it may be necessary to give total parenteral nutrition for a time. If this is the case the patient will require special monitoring to ensure that his optimum weight is maintained (see Ch. 21).

Altered body image may pose major difficulties for the patient. Weight loss, alopecia (as a result of cytotoxic chemotherapy), herpes lesions on lips and bleeding gums may all contribute to him feeling unhappy about his appearance. Central i.v. infusions can accentuate the problem, especially if total parenteral nutrition is required. Loss of libido, fears of sterility and anxiety about losing the affection of a partner may result in low self-esteem and depression. The topic of

Table 11.6 Oral assessment guide (reproduced with kind permission from Eilers et al 1988). This assessment tool, based on clinical experience and research, requires the nurse to score on a scale of 1–3 eight different indicators of mouth hygiene and health, thus obtaining a total score of between 8 and 24. If a score of 8–10 is obtained, assessment should be repeated morning and evening. For scores of > 10, assessment should be carried out 8-hourly.

Category	Tools for assessment	Methods of measurement	Numerical and descriptive ratings 1	2	3
Voice	Auditory	Converse with patient	Normal	Deeper or raspy	Difficulty talking or painful
Swallow	Observation	Ask patient to swallow	Normal swallowing	Some pain on swallowing	Unable to swallow
Lips	Visual/palpatory	Observe and feel tissue	Smooth, pink and moist	Dry or cracked	Ulcerated or bleeding
Tongue	Visual/palpatory	Feel and observe appearance of tissue	Pink and moist; papillae present	Coated or loss of papillae with a shiny appearance with or without redness	Blistered or cracked
Saliva	Tongue blade	Insert blade into mouth, touching the centre of the tongue and the floor of the mouth	Watery	Thick or ropy	Absent
Mucous membranes	Visual	Observe appearance of tissue	Pink and moist	Reddened or coated (increased whiteness) without ulcerations	Ulceration with or without bleeding
Gingiva	Tongue blade and visual	Gently press tissue with tip of blade	Pink, stippled and firm	Oedematous with or without redness	Spontaneous bleeding or bleeding with pressure
Teeth or dentures (or denture-bearing area)	Visual	Observe appearance of teeth or denture-bearing area	Clean and no debris	Plaque or debris in localised areas between teeth if (present)	Plaque or debris generalised along gumline or denture-bearing area

sexuality will need to be explored sensitively and the help of a psychologist or special counsellor might be required.

Communication may be difficult for the patient because of his mood, sore mouth and debilitated state. It is important for staff to listen to his anxieties, fears and wishes. He should be given as much autonomy in lifestyle choices as possible, especially if he feels he has lost control of his life. He should also be encouraged to be responsible for as much of his own care as is feasible. If he is being nursed in an isolation unit the staff should ensure they do spend time interacting with him so that he does not feel cut off.

Patient education

Teaching the patient about his illness and its management right from the start of treatment will help him to feel in control even when he is very ill. This information will also equip him to cope during periods at home. The active involvement of the family should be encouraged as the patient is given instruction in the following areas:

- monitoring body temperature
- recognising the symptoms of infection
- maintaining a high standard of oral hygiene
- managing the Hickman line and administering i.v. drugs and/or parenteral nutrition
- responding to symptoms of infection or bleeding
- taking oral medication: which drugs; how much; how often.

Discharge planning

Before the patient's discharge, arrangements must be made with his GP and district nurse regarding continuing care and a plan of action should complications arise. It may be necessary to prearrange special emergency care (e.g. platelet transfusion) with a local hospital. Other professionals who will be involved in discharge planning include:

- the social worker: for help with housing, financial problems, home help arrangements, social security benefit claims
- the occupational therapist: to assess the patient's ability to cope with everyday activities and to determine what adaptations might be needed to the home environment
- the physiotherapist: to assess the patient's mobility and help him to achieve and maintain optimal fitness
- the dietitian: to advise on nutrition, supplementary foods and, if necessary, parenteral nutrition.

Sadly, many patients will require frequent readmission after their initial discharge, and their condition may deteriorate despite the therapeutic team's best efforts. These patients and their families will need support from team members in hospital and in the community as they come to terms with their situation. Well-coordinated support can help families to care competently for their loved ones and to have confidence in the professional team (see Ch. 34 'The Terminally Ill Patient').

?	11.13 A 21-year-old woman who is engaged to be married in 6 months is diagnosed as having acute leukaemia. She has undergone chemotherapy and is in remission (i.e. there is no evidence of the leukaemia in the peripheral blood film or in the bone marrow). She has been in hospital for 3 months and is now about to be discharged. She has experienced a degree of alopecia, has lost a great deal of weight and is sensitive about her appearance. Discuss the following:	
	a. What do you think her main fears and anxieties might be?	A
	b. How could you help her to enhance her appearance?	A
	c. What support services are available in the community for the patient, her fiancé, and her family?	A
	d. What practical advice should she be given prior to discharge?	A

Chronic leukaemia

PATHOPHYSIOLOGY

Unlike that of acute leukaemia, the onset of chronic leukaemia is insidious, and the disease may be present for some time before the nature of the patient's symptoms prompt him to seek medical advice. Indeed, a proportion of patients are diagnosed as the result of blood tests done for some other medical reason.

Common presenting symptoms. These may be similar to those of acute leukaemia, and include:

- tiredness, lethargy
- anorexia, weight loss
- abdominal discomfort (caused by grossly enlarged spleen)
- visual defects and priapism (due to increased blood viscosity and slower blood flow).

MEDICAL MANAGEMENT

History and examination. In addition to the above symptoms, the patient may have a history of persistent low-grade infections. On examination, he is often pale and has an enlarged spleen and liver. Petechiae, purpura and bruising may be found. In patients with chronic lymphocytic leukaemia, enlarged, rubbery lymph glands may be palpable.

Investigative procedures. Diagnosis is based on blood count and blood film results (see Appendix 1). Results indicating the presence of leukaemia include:

- low haemoglobin
- abnormal white cell count: may be extremely high (100×10^9 cells/l) or very low
- low platelet count.

Bone marrow aspiration is performed to determine what specific type of chronic leukaemia the patient has.

Medical intervention. Patients with chronic leukaemia are rarely admitted to hospital unless their symptoms make it impossible for them to cope at home. The aim of treatment is to control the disease, usually by means of oral chemotherapy. The treatment regime employed will depend on whether the leukaemia is of the chronic lymphocytic or chronic myeloid type.

Chronic lymphocytic leukaemia is a malignant disorder of the B lymphocyte (or, occasionally, T lymphocyte) white blood cells. Chronic myeloid leukaemia is a malignant transformation of the myeloid white blood cells (notably neutrophils and monocytes; see p. 407). Treatment for these two conditions is as follows:

1. Chronic lymphocytic leukaemia: oral chlorambucil or cyclophosphamide is administered until control is achieved
2. Chronic myeloid leukaemia: if the patient has overt symptoms, oral busulphan is given to control the disease. Chronic myeloid leukaemia can transform into acute leukaemia; treatment would then be as for acute leukaemia.

Patients with chronic leukaemia may require blood transfusions to maintain a satisfactory haemoglobin level. Platelet transfusions, however, are rarely required and infections are not as common as with acute leukaemia.

NURSING PRIORITIES AND MANAGEMENT OF CHRONIC LEUKAEMIA

These patients may well be nursed at home. Some require little nursing care but others may need considerable support. In either case it is likely therefore that community nurses rather than hospital nurses will be involved. However, hospital nurses may be involved in assisting with diagnostic procedures and/or the administration of blood transfusions.

The nursing care required will include:

- giving information about tests, diagnosis and treatment
- providing psychological support to help the patient come to terms with a chronic and potentially life-threatening disease
- educating the patient about medication, including the importance of continuing with intermittent courses of chemotherapy, perhaps over several years
- supporting the patient as he experiences concurrent symptoms, e.g. tiredness and abdominal discomfort
- giving advice about the level of work and activity that can realistically be attempted
- stressing the importance of follow-up in outpatient clinics.

In the terminal stages of the disease, the patient and his family will require sensitive care (see Ch. 34).

LYMPHOMA

The lymphomas are a group of malignant disorders of the lymphoid tissue. They are divided into two types:

- Hodgkin's lymphoma (Hodgkin's disease)
- non-Hodgkin's lymphoma.

Hodgkin's lymphoma is the more common form. Its incidence in Great Britain is 3–4 new cases per year per 100 000 of the population (OPCS 1985). It is most common among people aged 15–35 or over 50 years of age. It is more common among men than among women by a ratio of 1.5:1 (Colvin & Newland 1988). Non-Hodgkin's lymphoma is most prevalent among people aged 50–70 and has an overall incidence in Great Britain of 2–3 new cases per year per 100 000 of the population (OPCS 1985).

PATHOPHYSIOLOGY

Cells in the affected lymph tissue (usually lymph nodes) show a disruption of their normal structure or architecture. In Hodgkin's lymphoma, abnormal, giant, multinucleate cells known as Reed-Sternberg cells are usually present.

In non-Hodgkin's lymphoma, these structural abnormalities are very varied. There may be a close resemblance to the normal architecture: this is referred to as follicular or nodular non-Hodgkin's lymphoma. In other cases there can be a complete loss of architecture: this type is referred to as diffuse non-Hodgkin's lymphoma. Another way of subdividing non-Hodgkin's lymphoma is into high, intermediate or low grades according to complex criteria. Each type has a different prognosis and response to treatment. Low-grade lymphoma carries the best prognosis and high-grade lymphoma the worst. However, high-grade lymphoma may respond better to treatment and achieve long-term remission.

For further details on the pathophysiology of lymphomas, see Whitehouse (1987).

Common presenting symptoms. Patients with Hodgkin's lymphoma often feel well but have accidently found a painless, enlarged lymph gland that they may describe as 'rubbery'. Such glands are often found in the cervical, axillary or inguinal regions.

Patients with non-Hodgkin's lymphoma may present with a wide variety of symptoms, including:

- dyspnoea, as a result of enlarged mediastinal lymph nodes or obstruction of the superior vena cava, affecting respiratory function
- oedema, especially of limbs, due to lymph node obstruction
- backache, due to retroperitoneal lymph node enlargement
- acute or subacute bowel obstruction, due to small bowel lymphoma
- nausea, anorexia and upper abdominal discomfort, due to lymphoma of stomach
- bone pain, due to bone involvement
- symptoms of anaemia, due to bone marrow involvement
- weakness or paralysis of one or more limbs (often involving both legs), due to compression of spinal nerve roots.

Some patients, more commonly those with Hodgkin's lymphoma, also present with some or all of the following constitutional symptoms:

- low-grade fever (this may sometimes be a swinging fever)
- drenching night sweats (requiring patient to change bed linen and night clothes)
- weight loss (more than 10% of body weight).

The above symptoms are referred to as B symptoms and are significant in staging the lymphoma (see 'Staging', below). Other possible symptoms include pruritus and pain on consuming alcohol.

The reason for the above symptoms is not altogether clear. They may be due to the secretion of a cytokine by malignant cells.

MEDICAL MANAGEMENT

History and examination. Patients with Hodgkin's lymphoma often give no history of feeling unwell and seek medical advice only because a painless lump has failed to disappear or is increasing in size. They may give a history of any of the B symptoms over several weeks.

Patients with non-Hodgkin's lymphoma may also feel well on presentation but often give a longstanding history of tiredness, lethargy, weight loss and other symptoms according to the lymphoid tissue involved.

As it is very difficult to feel certain lymph nodes clinical examination must be very thorough. Careful examination will also detect any other signs of the disease, e.g. oedema, muscle weakness, splenomegaly and hepatomegaly.

Investigative procedures. Diagnosis is by means of lymph node biopsy. The patient typically undergoes this procedure as a day-inpatient under local anaesthesia. Blood tests include:

- full blood count and differential count
- serum biochemical estimations
- tests to exclude infections that also cause enlarged lymph nodes, e.g. glandular fever, tuberculosis, toxoplasmosis.

Other tests include:

- bone marrow aspiration
- chest X-ray
- computed axial tomography (CAT scan).

Staging. After all the results of the investigations are known, the lymphoma is staged, i.e. the extent of the disease is classified according to the number and location of involved lymph nodes or extralymphatic sites (see Box 11.6). B symptoms are also taken into account. The staging of the disease provides a basis for making a prognosis and planning care.

Medical intervention: Hodgkin's lymphoma

Stages I and II. As the disease is localised to one or the other side of the diaphragm, it is treated with radiotherapy (see Ch. 32). Disease localised in lymph nodes above the diaphragm is usually treated using a mantle-shaped field. If involve-ment is confined to below the diaphragm, an inverted-Y technique of radiotherapy is usually used. Chemotherapy may be given in stage II.

If the lymphoma appears to be in either advanced stage I or advanced stage II, this may be confirmed by a staging laparotomy whereby biopsies are taken from the spleen, the liver and from lymph nodes. In such cases a splenectomy would also be performed (Allan 1991).

Stages III and IV. As the disease is present both above and below the diaphragm, combination chemotherapy (see Ch. 32) with or without radiotherapy is usually the treatment of choice.

Since it is delivered via the blood, chemotherapy will treat a greater volume of disease than will radiotherapy. Radiotherapy is either directed at specific affected nodes or applied more extensively in a 'mantle' or 'inverted Y' field.

Drugs employed in the treatment of stage III and IV lymphoma include combinations of at least three of the following:

- chlorambucil tablets
- prednisolone tablets
- procarbazine capsules
- i.v. vincristine
- i.v. vinblastine
- i.v. etoposide
- i.v. cyclophosphamide.

The drugs are often given in 2-week 'pulses' every 4 weeks for 6–12 pulses, depending on how the disease responds. If there is no response or if relapse occurs during the course of chemotherapy, the combination of drugs will be changed (see Ch. 32).

Box 11.6 Staging of lymphomas

STAGE I
One lymph node involved or one extralymphatic site (e.g. stomach, Peyer's patches, thyroid)

STAGE II
Two or more lymph nodes involved but on the same side of the diaphragm or an extralymphatic site plus lymph nodes on the same side

STAGE III
Lymph node involvement on both sides of the diaphragm with or without extralymphatic sites

STAGE IV
Diffuse involvement of extralymphatic sites, e.g. bone marrow, liver.

Most of these treatments can be given in a day ward. The patient need never be admitted to hospital unless side-effects of therapy occur, or unless he lives too far away to attend hospital as a day patient.

Prognosis. In localised Hodgkin's lymphoma, 80% of patients will be alive and well 5 years after treatment. Many of these can be considered cured. In advanced Hodgkin's lymphoma, 40–50% will be alive and well 5 years after treatment.

Patients who are ineligible for radiotherapy and/or chemotherapy because their disease is too extensive on first assessment or because they are too frail will receive palliative single-agent chemotherapy (see Ch. 32).

Medical intervention: non-Hodgkin's lymphoma. The type of treatment chosen will depend upon the type of lymphoma as well as on the stage of the disease. Specific chemotherapy regimes are prescribed according to the type of lymphoma in question and are constantly being refined as clinical understanding of these lymphomas improves.

The general outlines of treatment for non-Hodgkin's lymphoma are as follows:

Low-grade lymphoma. A low-grade lymphoma is one which follows an indolent course. The median survival is in excess of 8 years. In most patients, the lymphoma will regress partly or completely as the result of treatment with chlorambucil or cyclophosphamide. Autologous bone marrow transplantation may be considered in young patients, in whom low-grade lymphoma can be fatal.

High-grade lymphoma is an aggressive disease for which the prognosis varies widely. It tends to be associated with high mortality, but there is a 70% response rate to treatment. A small number of patients will be cured (Whitehouse 1987).

In the early stages of the disease, a combination of chemotherapy and radiotherapy is used. If complete remission is achieved, further high-dose chemotherapy is given with autologous bone marrow transplantation. Bone marrow transplantation may also be considered if relapse occurs and complete remission is obtained again.

In a more advanced stage of the disease, combination chemotherapy is used.

NURSING PRIORITIES AND MANAGEMENT OF LYMPHOMA

Many patients with lymphoma do not need to be admitted to hospital, even for original diagnosis and staging, unless they have to have a staging laparotomy.

Patients who are to receive radiotherapy using one of the extended fields (mantle or inverted Y) may need to be admitted as they may experience considerable tiredness, nausea, vomiting, dysphagia and diarrhoea.

The effects of treatment are in fact very variable. Some individuals are able to attend as out-patients and manage to carry on with their jobs with minimal side-effects. The distance that the patient must travel for treatment may be a consideration, as daily travel for up to 6 weeks can prove to be exhausting. The patient's age is also likely to have a bearing on arrangement for hospitalisation, as older people generally do not cope as well with treatment as younger patients.

Nursing considerations

During diagnosis, staging and planning, the nurse should explain all tests and investigations to the patient and his family. Testing should be coordinated to minimise delay. Some tests, such as bone marrow aspiration, will require the direct involvement of the nurse (see p. 413).

The patient may have previously considered himself fit and well and may be shocked to find himself faced with the possibility of serious illness. He will need to be prepared for an unfavourable diagnosis and for a course of treatment that may last for up to 9 months. The nurse should be prepared to cope with a range of emotional responses and should be sensitive to the patient's changes of mood, allowing him time to absorb the implications of his situation, to voice his feelings and concerns, and to seek clarification as needed.

The specific nursing care required will depend upon whether radiotherapy or chemotherapy is the prescribed treatment. For a detailed description of patient care during either of these therapies, see Chapter 32.

After the initial course of treatment, the patient and his family should be given detailed, individualised advice on post-radiotherapy or post-chemotherapy care. The patient should be given the name of someone to contact when he is in need of advice, see Ch. 32. Preparation for coping after therapy should address the following areas:

- medication: how to take it and for how long; how to obtain prescription refills
- diet
- level of activity; return to work
- self-monitoring for signs of infection or bleeding; whom to contact should either of these occur
- the importance of attending follow-up clinics for check-ups and assessment
- appropriate self-help groups
- sexual counselling as appropriate (see Ch. 32)
- referral to district nurse, social worker, and GP.

As the lymphomas are such a diverse group of blood disorders, and their treatment is so varied, nursing care cannot be definitively prescribed. Some patients will remain independent of any nursing assistance whilst others will be hospitalised throughout the course of the disease. After the course of treatment, nursing care may be required continually or intermittently. For some patients, terminal care will be required from an early stage. The key to providing high-quality nursing care lies in recognising the needs, values and concerns that are unique to each individual.

MULTIPLE MYELOMA

Multiple myeloma, or myeloma, is a rare haematological disorder in which there is a malignant proliferation of the plasma cells which develop from the B-lymphocytes.

The incidence of multiple myeloma is 3.5 new cases per 100 000 of the population per year in Europe. About 50% of cases are under 65 years but the average age on diagnosis is 60 years. There are only 0.1 new cases per 100 000 of the population per year aged 23–34 years, but 21 per 100 000 of the population per year aged 75 and over (Selby 1987).

There is no known cause or factor associated with the occurrence of myeloma.

PATHOPHYSIOLOGY

Normal plasma cells develop from B-lymphocytes following antigen stimulation. Each plasma cell releases a specific immunoglobulin with a special immune function. In myeloma there is a malignant proliferation of plasma cells, which then release an immunoglobulin, or paraprotein as it is called, which is incapable of normal function.

The paraprotein has a number of effects on the body which can be summarised as:

- bone marrow infiltration
- skeletal destruction

- production of the abnormal protein, with subsequent effects in the blood, kidneys and other tissues
- depression of production of normal immunoglobulins.

Each of these effects has pathophysiological consequences. The bone marrow infiltration will lead to pancytopenia. The skeletal destruction can lead to characteristic lesions in the bone, bone pain, hypercalcaemia and pathological fractures. The abnormal protein may cause renal failure (due to its deposition in the renal tubules). Depending on its specific properties, the paraprotein may cause hyperviscosity of the blood, bleeding disorders and the presence of cryoglobulins (abnormal proteins which are insoluble at low temperatures and therefore cause obstruction in small blood vessels). If the abnormal protein is deposited in the tissues, the formation of amyloid tissue (an abnormal complete material which accumulates and is deposited in an organ, e.g. kidney or liver, causing failure) can result. Reduction in immunoglobulin levels will lead to the patient becoming immunocompromised.

Common presenting features. The most common presenting symptoms are:

- pain in the lumbar or thoracic spine due to the myeloma deposits, pathological fractures, demineralisation, muscle spasm or periosteal pressure (87% patients on first presentation)
- tiredness, lethargy, cardiac failure and other symptoms of anaemia (74%).

Other presenting features are:

- weight loss
- bone tenderness and pathological fractures
- infections
- spinal cord compression.

MEDICAL MANAGEMENT

History and examination. The patient may have had symptoms for a number of months but not considered them significant enough to report to a doctor. Back pain, for example, is often not reported until it becomes incapacitating. Alternatively, the patient may have been receiving treatment by a GP and/or physiotherapist for a condition which did not improve or even became worse.

Some patients have a history of sudden-onset bone pain caused by pathological fracture. Others present with pneumonia due to neutropenia and lowered immunoglobulin levels. Some patients may have noticed lumps on their forehead, or extreme bone tenderness throughout the body.

Abdominal examination may reveal splenomegaly and hepatomegaly. There may be abnormal neurological symptoms such as reduced sensation and muscle power.

Investigative procedures. Test and investigations are aimed at establishing the diagnosis, staging the disease and assessing the effects of the disease on the body.

To confirm a diagnosis of myeloma and determine its stage, evidence of two of the following three features is required:

- presence of paraprotein
- bone lesion
- bone marrow infiltration.

Evidence of the paraprotein is established by means of electrophoresis examination of serum and urine. Serum electrophoresis reveals the unique patterning of the different immunoglobulins. It is then determined whether this patterning is normal and, if it is not, which paraprotein is involved. Urine electrophoresis will show whether paraprotein is present. The paraprotein present in urine is called Bence-Jones protein.

A skeletal survey and isotope bone scan will demonstrate the presence and extent of any bone lesions. On X-ray these appear as circular lesions resembling punched-out holes. They are often seen in the skull, long bones and vertebrae (Armstrong 1977).

Bone marrow aspiration and trephine biopsy are performed to establish any bone marrow infiltration.

To establish the systemic effect of multiple myeloma on the body, the following tests are performed:

- full blood, differential white blood cell count and ESR
- serum urea and electrolytes
- serum calcium and alkaline phosphatase levels
- uric acid levels
- plasma viscosity.

Medical intervention. If the patient presents with severe complications of the disease, these must be treated first.

Specific treatment of the myeloma will include chemotherapy with or without radiotherapy. Radiotherapy will target specific bony lesions to reduce bone deposits, prevent fractures and reduce pain.

The chemotherapeutic agents commonly used are cyclophosphamide, vincristine, adriamycin, melphalan and prednisolone. These are used usually in a combination regime intermittently over several months (see Ch. 32 'The Patient with Cancer'). Certain patients under 50 years of age may be considered for high-dose chemotherapy and autologous bone marrow transplantation.

Plasmapheresis (the removal of blood from the patient followed by removal of the plasma fraction and the return of the blood cells with donated plasma) may be used to reduce a high blood viscosity, as the removal of the patient's plasma will also reduce the paraprotein level. This is done only as a temporary measure whilst other treatment is given.

NURSING PRIORITIES AND MANAGEMENT OF MULTIPLE MYELOMA

Myeloma is a serious disorder with multisystemic effects, some of which are potentially life-threatening. The most serious of these are:

- renal failure (due to myeloma paraproteins causing degeneration, blood hyperviscosity, hyperuricaemia, hypercalcaemia, dehydration and anaemia)
- spinal cord compression (due to vertebral collapse)
- hypercalcaemia (due to bone destruction)
- severe cardiac failure (due to anaemia and hyperviscosity)
- immunosuppression (due to reduced normal immunoglobulin formation).

For the patient, the most distressing symptom may be bone pain. As the disorder is insidious in onset, bone pain may have existed for some time but may have been ignored or rationalised until it became too much to bear. Assessment must take this into account as the patient may well be exhausted and depressed by chronic pain (see Ch. 19 'Pain'). The patient's distress will be compounded if spontaneous fractures occur, severely curtailing activity, (which may already be impaired). Frequent and debilitating infections may also be experienced, along with fatigue, anaemia and bleeding tendencies, such that every daily activity becomes an effort. Many patients are in their middle years and have considerable family and financial responsibilities. For them, the stress of ill-health and of coming to terms with the diagnosis of a malignant disease will be keenly felt.

Close monitoring by health professionals in the community will be required to ensure that activity is maximised and pain kept to a minimum. Hospital admission may not be necessary until the more serious effects of the disease become apparent. Of these, renal failure can cause the most concern. Optimal hydration is crucial in preventing renal failure and hypercalcaemia, the requirement often being as much as 4–5 l/day. Sensitive and creative nursing strategies will help the patient to maintain a good fluid intake; even then, the renal impairment may still progress and perhaps necessitate haemodialysis.

Nursing considerations

Communication

As always, good communication skills will be vital to effective nursing intervention. On admission, the patient may or may not know his diagnosis and may be trying to cope with debilitating symptoms, e.g. paralysis, severe pain and immobility. The nurse should be sensitive to the patient's anxieties and should bear in mind that individuals with myeloma often have a reduced attention span as a result of fatigue, weakness and pain. The patient will need clear explanations of the reasons for investigations, the implications of diagnosis, and the options for treatment. He and his family should be given honest and accurate answers to their questions and requests for clarification. Written information which the patient can read at his own pace and discuss with the nurse later is often helpful.

Back pain often prompts patients to enquire about complementary forms of treatment such as osteopathy or homeopathy. The nurse should be able to provide enough background information to enable the patient to make up his own mind about these and other therapies.

Mobility

The nurse will work alongside the physiotherapist and occupational therapist in helping the patient to attain an optimal level of mobility. In setting goals for rehabilitation a balance must be struck between the need to reduce the risk of hypercalcaemia (which is increased with immobility) and the danger of fracturing weak bones. As pain will be a restricting factor the assessment and constant evaluation of pain levels will form an integral part of the therapeutic process.

For a patient on bed rest, mobilisation may need to commence with passive movement of joints and limbs, progressing to gentle muscle-strengthening exercises. The next step will be for the patient to practise mobilising out of bed with the appropriate aids and assistance. Before the patient is discharged, it will be necessary for his home to be assessed for any adaptations needed to facilitate access and accommodate the use of aids.

Patient education

Acquiring knowledge about his disease and its management will help the patient to feel that he is in control of his life. In preparation for discharge, he should be fully briefed on the following:

- self-monitoring for side-effects of chemotherapy (see Ch. 32)
- the importance of continued follow-up with the GP for medication and blood tests, as well as attendance at outpatients clinics
- safe techniques for lifting and carrying
- preventing or minimising complications, e.g. taking extra fluids
- reducing muscle weakness.

Discharge planning

The nature of arrangements for discharge will depend on the patient's physical and psychological state, the type of treatment he is receiving, and the availability of carers at home or in the community. Important aspects to consider in planning are:

- How dependent is the patient and how willing is he to participate in his own care?
- Who are his family carers and what type and degree of support will they need? (e.g. Macmillan nurses, Marie Curie nurses)
- What skills will carers need to learn? (e.g. lifting or turning the patient)

Prognosis

Myeloma is a progressive, debilitating condition for which palliative care will eventually be the only treatment option. However, 90% of patients show a response to treatment of up to a 75% reduction in tumour mass. Many patients will be able to enjoy an acceptable quality of life for some time; some who enter hospital immobile and in considerable pain return home able to walk and independent in all activities of daily living.

AGRANULOCYTOSIS

This rare disease is caused by the partial or complete absence of neutrophils, resulting in susceptibility to infection, septicaemia and death. The causal factor may be unknown (idiopathic agranulocytosis). Known factors include drugs (e.g. antithyroid drugs, rarer chemotherapy drugs, allopurinol, gold salts, phenothiazines, tricyclic antidepressants) and excess exposure to ionising radiation. Agranulocytosis may also be part of pancytopenia following bone marrow failure.

PATHOPHYSIOLOGY

Common presenting symptoms. Onset may be acute or chronic. The common presenting features of the acute-onset form include a history of sore throat, often progressing rapidly to necrotic throat ulceration with no pus formation (because of an absence of phagocytes) and septicaemia. The patient is very ill, hyperpyrexial, and often has rigors.

Onset of chronic agranulocytosis is insidious. The patient complains of vague general symptoms of malaise and weakness; sore throat follows but the progression of the disease is much less dramatic.

Agranulocytosis differs from other bone marrow failure in that it is only the granulocytes that are involved, in contrast to aplastic anaemia (in which there is pancytopenia), thrombocytopenia (in which only the platelets are involved) and the pancytopenia caused by myelofibrosis, leukaemia and bone marrow infiltration. Therefore, the patient with agranulocytosis will have a problem with infection but not the additional problems of anaemia and thrombocytopenia. However, anaemia and thrombocytopenia may both occur as the result of septicaemia.

MEDICAL MANAGEMENT

Investigative procedures. Diagnosis is based on the results of full blood count, white blood cell differential, blood film and bone marrow aspiration. These tests will confirm a very low neutrophil count, or a complete absence of neutrophils. They may also point to an underlying cause, e.g. leukaemia or cancer metastases. A careful and detailed clinical history may reveal exposure to a possible cause of the agranulocytosis, e.g. medication.

Medical intervention is aimed at removing the cause of the illness (if this is known) and establishing control over the disease process by means of antibiotic therapy. If the bone marrow has not been badly impaired the prognosis is good and neutrophil production will resume.

NURSING PRIORITIES AND MANAGEMENT OF AGRANULOCYTOSIS

The nursing management is that required for any patient with severe infection and risk of septicaemia. It must be remembered, of course, that because of the absence of neutrophils the patient's response to infection will be atypical and, as with patients with acute leukaemia, endogenous infection may well occur. Progression to a state of septicaemia may be rapid and vigilance is required to prevent and detect early signs of potentially serious infection (see Nursing Care Plan 11.2).

The disease is indeed life-threatening and, as has been said, may arise suddenly. Newly-diagnosed patients are often frightened and disbelieving, and need to be given time and support as they adjust to the diagnosis and learn to cope with treatment. Information and counselling is of a multidisciplinary nature and should involve other family members and possibly friends. If the patient survives the acute phase, rehabilitation will take time and patience. Lifestyle issues will have to be addressed in order to ensure that any identified cause is avoided in the future and that the patient understands how to avoid infections and when to seek medical advice. Such constraints can be unwelcome and advice should always be framed positively. This is especially important if fundamental changes are required, e.g. a change in occupation to avoid a causative agent. The support and advice of the community nursing team can do much to make necessary adjustments acceptable to the patient and to ensure his future health.

DISORDERS OF PLATELETS AND COAGULATION

Disorders of coagulation can be subdivided into three types:

- disorders due to lack of clotting factors
- platelet disorders
- disorders due to another cause.

These disorders may be inherited or acquired. All age groups are affected, but some coagulation disorders are sex-linked; for example, haemophilia occurs only in males but is genetically carried by females.

CLOTTING FACTOR DISORDERS

These disorders all involve a deficiency in one or more of the blood factors required for haemostasis. Inherited clotting disorders result from the lack of specific clotting factors whereas the acquired disorders involve the failure of certain clotting factors to be activated. Usual causes are Vitamin K deficiency and liver disease.

Haemophilia

The haemophilias are a group of inherited disorders in which there is a lifelong deficiency of one of the substances necessary to blood clotting. These deficiencies include:

- haemophilia A (lack of Factor VIII)
- haemophilia B or Christmas disease (lack of factor IX)
- von Willebrand's disease (lack of von Willebrand factor, which is necessary for normal platelet adhesion and for Factor VII production; not sex-linked).

A full discussion of haemophilia A is given in Ch. 6.

PLATELET DISORDERS

Thrombocytopenia purpura

Any disturbance in the number or function of circulating platelets will affect the normal coagulation process (see p. 409). The condition thrombocytopenia (TCP) implies a reduction in the number of platelets and may be either inherited or acquired.

PATHOPHYSIOLOGY

Inherited TCP is fortunately rare. Acquired TCP may occur as a result of factors which either decrease normal platelet production or increase platelet destruction (see Box 11.7). Decreased production is usually caused by drugs or some other agent whereby the bone marrow is suppressed. The most common form of TCP due to increased platelet destruction is idiopathic thrombocytopenia purpura (ITCP). This commonly affects individuals in their teens or early 20s and is thought to be autoimmune in origin. Whatever the cause, TCP will result in a prolonged bleeding time, which may give rise to bruising, purpura or petechiae. Less obviously, visceral bleeding can also occur.

Common presenting symptoms include a history of bleeding episodes, e.g. bleeding gums, epistaxis, melaena and haematuria. In contrast to haemophilia, if pressure is applied to the bleeding point, bleeding will stop and not recur unless further trauma occurs. As with leukaemia, symptoms of anaemia may be presenting features in chronic thrombocytopenia.

MEDICAL MANAGEMENT

History and examination. A careful clinical history is required, especially to pinpoint any recent minor illness or drug therapy (including medicines bought at a pharmacy). Thorough clinical examination is made for any signs of bruising, petechiae, purpura or any underlying disorder.

Box 11.7 Causes of acquired thrombocytopenia

- Decrease in platelet production
- Aplastic anaemia
- Vitamin B12/folic acid deficiency
- Bone marrow infiltration:
  — leukaemia and lymphoma
  — carcinoma
  — myelofibrosis: formation of fibrous tissue within the bone marrow cavity
- Other disorders:
  — viral infection
  — bacterial infection
- platelet destruction
- idiopathic autoimmune disorder
- idiopathic thrombocytopenia purpura (ITCP)
- large volume blood transfusion: due to the short lifespan of platelets, there may be no viable platelets in the blood transfusion units and the patient will, if requiring a large volume of blood, have insufficient platelets
- disseminated intravascular coagulation (DIC) — see Ch. 29.

Investigative procedures. These will include:

- full blood count to demonstrate low platelet count, identify anaemia and exclude any other blood disorder
- coagulation screen to exclude other coagulation disorders
- Paul-Bunnell test to exclude glandular fever
- bone marrow aspiration to exclude aplastic anaemia or some other cause of bone marrow infiltration.

Medical intervention. Many cases of thrombocytopenia (acute or chronic) resolve spontaneously, possibly because the formation of antibodies against the person's own platelet membrane antigens is transient. In cases where an exacerbating factor such as a drug or chemical is withdrawn, spontaneous remission may also occur.

Steroid therapy may be given until resolution occurs, as steroids improve platelet survival. Response to steroid therapy is usually seen within days or weeks; however, thrombocytopenia may recur when the steroids are withdrawn.

Immunoglobulin G i.v. may be given for 3–5 days (see Ch. 16). Splenectomy may be required, as the spleen is a major site of platelet destruction.

NURSING PRIORITIES AND MANAGEMENT

Nursing considerations

In hospital

Nursing priorities during the patient's stay in hospital will include:

1. Controlling superficial bleeding by application of external pressure. The bleeding tendency is not generally life-threatening
2. Observing patient for evidence of bleeding and determining severity of bleeding by means of:
   - regular monitoring of patient's pulse during diagnostic stage and initial treatment. Blood pressure is not usually measured using an inflatable cuff as this may cause bruising and petechiae
   - daily inspection of the skin for petechiae, purpura and bruises and of the mouth for bleeding and infection. Precautions must be taken to minimise the occurrence of infection in soft tissue which has been damaged
   - regular testing of urine, stools and vomit for less obvious sources of blood loss.
3. Being alert to complaints of headaches and drowsiness, as these may indicate cerebral bleeding
4. Ensuring that the patient is protected from injuring himself by advising him on environmental hazards and making him aware that feelings of faintness may indicate anaemia or low blood pressure
5. Giving explanations and support during tests and treatment, looking and listening for indications of anxiety.

Discharge planning

The aim of discharge planning is to enable the patient to make the transition from depending upon the nurse to monitor his condition to becoming competent and confident in monitoring himself. The importance of monitoring all bleeding episodes must be stressed, along with the need for regular follow-up to monitor platelet levels.

?	**11.14** What adjustments might be required to enable the individual to lead a fulfilling life without risk to health?

Precautions which the patient should be advised to take include:

- taking medicines as prescribed
- avoiding aspirin preparations
- avoiding i.m. injections
- carrying a Medicalert card
- minimising potential for soft tissue injury
- avoiding contact sports.

The family should be included in the patient's education programme to ensure that all members of the household understand the necessity of certain restrictions upon lifestyle. However, it should also be stressed that it is important for the patient to maintain a balance between being overcautious on the one hand and taking unnecessary risks on the other.

The aim of rehabilitation is to allow the patient to achieve an optimal level of function until his spontaneous recovery or throughout the remainder of his life.

REFERENCES

Allan N C 1991 Diseases of the blood. In: Edwards C, Bouchier I (eds) Davidson's principles and practice of medicine, 16th edn. Churchill Livingstone, Edinburgh, p 699

Armstrong P 1977 X-rays in focus: bone tumours. Nursing Times (Supplement) 73(7): 7

Barnard D L, McVerry B A, Norfolk D R 1989 Clinical haematology. Heinemann Medical, Oxford, p 12

Bloom A, Bloom S R 1986 Toohey's medicine for nurses, 14th edn. Churchill Livingstone, Edinburgh, p 227

Chanarin I, Pippard M J 1991 Nutritional anaemias. Medicine International 96: 3995–4002

Clark J M F 1982 Surgery in Jehovah's Witnesses. British Hospital Journal of Medicine 27(5): 497

Colvin B T, Newland A C 1988 Haematology. Blackwell Scientific Publications, Oxford, p 188, 232

Crosby C 1989 Methods in mouthcare. Nursing Times 85(35): 38–41

Davies J 1990 Anaemias of nutritional origin. Nutrition and Food Science (300): 5–7

Eilers J, Berger A M, Peterson M C 1988 Development, testing and application of the oral assessment guide. Oncology Nursing Forum 15(3): 325–330

Firkin F C 1987 Haematological side-effects of drugs. Medicine International 29(42): 1758–1761

Fitzsimmons E, Jacobs A 1983 Iron deficiency anaemia. Medical International 1(25): 1150–1155

Hinchliff S M, Montague S E 1988 Physiology for nursing practice. Baillière Tindall, London

Norton D, McLaren R, Exton-Smith A N 1975 An investigation of geriatric nursing problems in hospital. Churchill Livingstone, Edinburgh

Office of Populations Censuses and Surveys 1985 Registrations of newly diagnosed cases of cancer: sex, site and age. HMSO, London

Pritchard A P 1989 The Royal Marsden Hospital manual of clinical nursing procedures, 3rd edn. Harper & Row, London

Pritchard V 1986 Calculating the risk. Nursing Times 82(8): 59–61

Roberts A 1990 Systems of life no. 182 — senior systems — 47. Disorders of the blood in later life — 1. Nursing Times 86(15): 55–58

Selby P G 1987 Multiple myeloma. Medicine International 2(40): 1664–1667

Smith P G 1991 Case-control studies of leukaemia clusters. British Journal of Medicine 302(6778): 672–673

Souhami R, Tobias J 1986 Cancer and its management. Blackwell Scientific, London
Tortora G J, Anagnostakis N P 1990 Principles of anatomy and physiology, 6th edn. Harper & Row, London
Waterford S 1989 Blood investigations. Nursing 3(40): 24–25
Waterlow J 1988 The Waterlow card for the prevention and management of pressure sores: towards a pocket policy. Care: science and practice 6(1): 8–11
Whitehouse M 1987 The non-Hodgkin's lymphomas. Medicine International 2(40): 1671–1674
Wilson Barnett J 1978 Patient's emotional response to barium X-rays. Journal of Advanced Nursing 3(1): 37–46
Wilson K J W 1990 Ross and Wilson anatomy and physiology in health and illness, 7th edn. Churchill Livingstone, Edinburgh

FURTHER READING

Alkire K, Collingwood J 1990 Physiology of blood and bone marrow. Seminars in Oncology Nursing 6(2): 99–108
Borley D (ed) Cancer nursing, 2nd edn. Vol 3 of Tiffany R (series ed) Oncology for nurses and health care professionals. Harper & Row, London
Campbell C 1988 Could do better. Nursing Times 84(22): 66–71
Cluroe S 1989 Blood transfusions. Nursing 3(40): 8–11
David J 1988 Care of the hands. Nursing 3(30): 24–26
Fox B A, Cameron A G 1989 Food science, nutrition and health, 5th edn. Edward Arnold, London
Freedman S, Halsford M E, McGuire D B et al 1990 Nursing considerations in the administration of blood component therapy. Seminars in Oncology Nursing 6(2): 155–162
Gidley C 1987 Now, wash your hands. Nursing Times 83(29): 40–42
Levenson J A, Lesko L M 1990 Psychiatric aspects of adult leukaemia. Seminars in Oncology Nursing 6(1): 76–83
Milne C 1988 Hickman catheters. Nursing Standard 3(8): 34–35
Oniboni A C 1990 Infection in the neutropenic patient. Seminars in Oncology Nursing 6(1): 50–60
Phillips C 1989 Hand hygiene. Nursing Times 85(37): 76–79
Sneum M 1986 General aspects of handwashing procedures in preventing nosocomial infection. In: Tierney A 1986 Recent Advances in Nursing 14; Clinical Nursing Practice. Churchill Livingstone, Edinburgh, pp 165–169
Taylor L J 1978 On evaluation of handwashing techniques. Nursing Times 74(2): 54–55
Webb P (ed) 1988 Care and support. Vol 2 of Tiffany R (series ed) Oncology for nurses and health care professionals. Harper & Row, London
Wujcik 1990 Options for post-remission therapy in acute leukaemia. Seminars in Oncology Nursing 6(1): 25–30

USEFUL ADDRESSES

BACUP
3 Bath Place
Rivington Street
London EC2A 3JR
Tel. 071 613 2121
Freephone (outside London) 0800–181199

CLIC (Cancer & Leukaemia in Childhood Trust)
12 Freemantle Square
Cotham
Bristol B56 5TL

Haemophilia Society
123 Westminster Bridge Road
London SE1 7HR
Tel. 071 928 2020

Leukaemia Research Fund
43 Great Ormond Street
London WC1N 3JJ
Tel. 071 405 0101

Leukaemia Care Society
14 Kingfisher Court
Vinny Brage
Pinhoe
Devon EX4 8JN
Tel. 0392 464848

OSCAR (Organisation for Sickle Cell Anaemia Research)
4th Floor
Cambridge House
109 Mayes Road
Wood Green
London N22 6U
Tel. 081 961 7795

Sickle Cell Society
54 Station Road
London NW10 4UA
Tel. 081 961 4006

GLOSSARY

Cell Architecture is the distinct cell pattern or structure that means the pathologist can identify the pathological disorder, in this case Hodgkins lymphoma or any of the non-Hodgkin lymphomas.
Haemolysis The breakdown of red blood cells with the liberation of haemoglobin.
Haemostasis The homeostatic process which prevents the loss of blood from the vascular system and ensures the patency of the blood vessels.
Neutropenia Reduction in number of neutrophils, usually less than 1000×10^9 cells/l, resulting in the neutropenic patient being highly susceptible to infection.
Pancytopenia Reduction in the number of red blood cells, neutrophils and platelets, i.e. there is an anaemia, neutropenia, and thrombocytopenia.
Petechiae Small haemorrhagic spots in the skin or mucous membranes.
Pluripotent or stem cell A blood stem cell is the original blood cell from which all other blood cells are derived.
Purpura Extravasation of blood from the capillaries into the skin or onto or into the mucous membranes. Appears as small red dots (petechiae) or large bruises.
Stomatitis Inflammation of the oral mucosa.
Thrombocytopenia Reduced number of platelets, usually less than 100×10^9/l cells which can result in the occurrence of purpura and spontaneous bleeding.

CHAPTER 12

Skin disorders

Christine Docherty   Carmen Rose

CHAPTER CONTENTS

Introduction 443
Anatomy and physiology of the skin 445
Principles of therapy in skin disorders 446
DISORDERS OF THE SKIN 447
Psoriasis 447
Epidemiology 447
Classification 447
Nursing priorities and management: psoriasis 449
General nursing considerations 449
Nursing considerations in outpatient treatment 449
Nursing considerations in inpatient treatment 450
Eczema 451
Endogenous eczema 451
Exogenous eczema 452
Nursing priorities and management: eczema 453
General nursing considerations 453
Nursing considerations in topical therapy 453
Other considerations 454
The contribution of the nurse 454
Skin infections and infestations 454
Fungal infections 454
Nursing priorities and management: athlete's foot 455
Nursing priorities and management: ringworm 455
Nursing priorities and management: thrush 455
Infestations 455
Nursing priorities and management: scabies 455
Nursing priorities and management: head lice 456
Nursing priorities and management: body lice 456
Nursing priorities and management: impetigo 456
Nursing priorities and management: folliculitis 456
Nursing priorities and management: cellulitis 457
Nursing priorities and management: shingles 458
Bullous disorders 458
Nursing priorities and management: bullous disorders 459
Disorders of sebaceous and apocrine glands 460
Nursing priorities and management: acne 461
Nursing priorities and management: rosacea 461
Photodermatoses 461
Nursing priorities and management: photodermatoses 462
AIDS and dermatology 463
Skin tumours 463
Conclusion 463
Glossary 464
References 464
Further reading 464
Useful addresses 465

INTRODUCTION

Although the skin is the largest organ in the body its crucial importance for our health and well-being is often taken for granted. The skin is essential to a range of complex functions fundamental to our survival; these include protection and insulation of the internal organs, sensation, temperature regulation, and the synthesis of vitamin D. Disorders of the skin range from minor if irritating conditions which can be quickly resolved with over-the-counter preparations to those which are genuinely life-threatening and require intensive treatment in hospital. Other conditions can be of a chronic nature, requiring long-term management and making a significant impact upon the lifestyle of the individual and his family.

Approximately 10% of consultations with general practitioners in the United Kingdom are related to skin problems (Hunter et al 1989). As many diagnoses do not necessitate referral to a dermatologist, the importance of the role of the practice or community nurse in promoting good skin care and the maintenance of treatment regimes is clear. Indeed, nurses in virtually every specialism will encounter individuals with skin disorders, and may have many opportunities to detect early disease, to give knowledgeable advice on treatment, and to provide emotional support to patients and family members coping with chronic conditions. Nurses in many areas of practice can do much to help dispel the myths about the contagious nature of many disorders, thus helping to reduce the social discomfort and isolation suffered unnecessarily by many people with skin disease.

Social attitudes

The social and emotional implications of skin disease should not be dismissed lightly. Images of the soft-skinned baby, the blemish-free teenager and the smooth-skinned, sophisticated adult are familiar to all of us from advertising and entertainment media. The cosmetic industry is sustained by the 'selling' of such images, and millions of pounds are spent every year by women and men hoping to attain some kind of cosmetic perfection. Consider, then, the potential impact of a disfiguring skin disorder on the psyche of a patient living within a society in which success, power and achievement are so dependent upon appearance and 'image'.

Many patients will put up with a skin disorder if it can be hidden by clothing, and a visible eruption, e.g. on the face or hands, is often the factor that prompts an individual to seek help. The status of social outcast — the 'leper' image of skin disease — is often anticipated by the patient. Most dermatology patients who are asked to describe how their skin problem restricts normal socialisation will quickly give such examples as their fear of communal changing rooms, being asked to leave swimming pools, or even having people refuse to eat meals prepared by them. Many patients restrict all activities, social and professional. Relationships break down because of a drop in self-esteem and the trauma of an altered body image, and many patients hide from view, considering themselves to be socially unacceptable.

How can the nurse help

The nurse's role in educating patients, the public and her own colleagues about skin disorders and their treatment is vital. Patients who have limited information about their disorder and who are ill-informed about the benefits of topical therapy may refuse to comply with treatment. The skills of dermatology nursing embody the very essence of the nurse – patient relationship: creating comfort, facilitating rest and healing, and educating and motivating the patient to acquire the skills essential to controlling his condition. 'Cure' is not a word widely used in dermatology, as unfortunately many conditions go into remission only to recur later.

The hospital nurse

Most dermatology units achieve a 'cocoon' effect whereby the patient feels safe in an environment where staff and fellow patients understand his condition and his consequent rejection by society. The dermatology ward is an area where perhaps for the first time the patient meets others with similar skin disorders; indeed, peer group support will be a beneficial adjunct to therapy. On the ward the patient has access to trained professionals who can dispel myths about skin disease and who have the time to teach the correct implementation of treatment programmes. The patient will acquire a better understanding of his condition and will be encouraged to maintain therapy after discharge.

The community nurse

Given the fact that most patients with a skin disorder are treated by their GP, the supportive role played by community nursing staff is essential. Many topical treatments can now be bought over the counter from trained pharmacists and the community nurse is in an ideal position to provide additional advice. School nurses can provide teachers with information that will ensure that children with skin disorders are given maximum support to cope at school without disrupting their class. For example, a child suffering from eczema may appear to be uncooperative, when the simple measure of allowing him to leave the classroom for a few minutes to apply a moisturiser to reduce itch would allow him to be more attentive.

Dermatology liaison is a new nursing role which is enabling a useful link between hospital and community to be forged. In addition, nursing and medical staff can work in conjunction with a range of support groups to share knowledge and experience and thereby enhance the resources available to the patient in clinical and non-clinical settings (see Useful Addresses, p. 465).

> ? **12.1** Before reading further, try this simple exercise. Imagine that you are in a communal changing room in a busy clothes shop when you realise the person trying on clothes next to you has a generalised rash. It appears to be very itchy, and as the person scratches, numerous flakes of skin are shed. Stop now and write down your immediate reaction to this scenario. Ask your colleagues to join you in this exercise.
>
> Repeat this exercise when you have read through this chapter. Evaluate any changes in your answer.

Epidemiology

The pattern of skin disease in a population is determined by many factors. It is projected that at any given time approximately 22% of the adult population of the UK will have a skin disorder meriting medical attention (Hunter et al 1989). Growing industrialism has contributed to a rise in the prevalence of industry-related dermatoses, with associated problems of lost working time and an increase in compensation claims for work-induced disorders (Hunter et al 1989).

Age is also an important factor in the distribution of skin disorders within a population. For example, acne generally arises in the teenage years and wanes by the late 20s. As the proportion of elderly people in our society increases the incidence of skin tumours, both benign and malignant, rises. Approximately 27% of our elderly population will present with some form of skin tumour. However, some skin disorders such as psoriasis and eczema occur in all age groups (MacKie 1991).

Research has confirmed an increase in skin malignancies in the UK. In the decade between 1979 and 1989 the incidence of skin tumours increased by 82% in Scotland and 50% in England (Fenton 1992). This has been attributed to changes in the ozone layer along with the increasing popularity of holidays in sunny locations. In Australia where 1 in 3 of the population will potentially develop skin cancer, a shift in public attitudes about skin protection was achieved by the 'slip, slop, slap' campaign in which an animated seagull mascot persuaded sun-lovers to slip on a T-shirt, slop on some sunscreen and slap on a hat (Apelgren 1992). This campaign helped people to realise that a suntan is, rather than a desirable attribute, merely a sign of damaged skin. If statistics continue to bear out an increase in skin cancers in the UK, this type of campaign may become relevant here.

Social factors such as unemployment and poverty are viewed as associated factors in some skin disorders. Many sufferers identify external stressors such as exams, divorce, bereavement and trauma as contributing to the development of skin problems. Genetic or hereditary factors may also be implicated. The range of internal and external factors that may come into play in the development of skin disease is summarised in Figure 12.1.

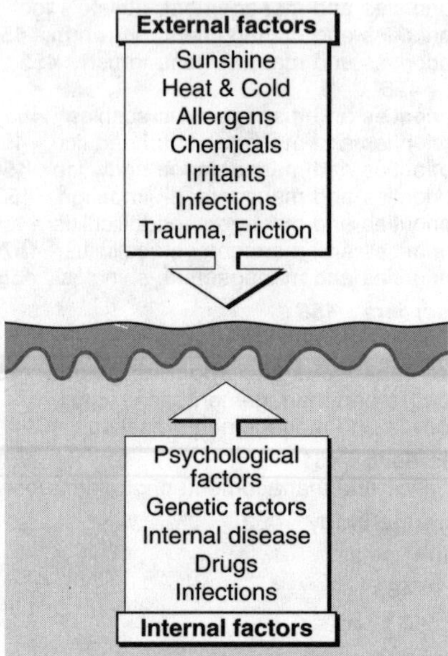

Fig. 12.1 Internal and external factors causing skin disease. (Adapted with kind permission from Hunter et al 1989 Blackwell Scientific Publications.)

ANATOMY AND PHYSIOLOGY OF THE SKIN

The structure of the skin

Originally formed from the embryonic ectoderm and mesoderm, the skin is composed of two layers: the epidermis and the dermis. Beneath these two layers lies a bed of subcutaneous fat which protects and insulates the underlying organs. In an adult, the surface area of the skin measures 1.5–2.0 m^2 and weighs approximately 9 kg (Hinchliff & Montague 1988).

The epidermis

The epidermis is composed of stratified epithelium and varies in thickness in different areas of the body. The skin on the palms of the hands and soles of the feet is much thicker than the skin on the face or back. There are no blood vessels or nerve endings in the epidermis and the cells are nourished by interstitial fluid from the dermis. Structures which track through the epidermis include hair follicles and sweat and sebaceous glands (see Fig. 12.2A). The epidermis is composed of several layers; its health depends on three factors involving these layers (Wilson 1990):

1. Regular division and migration of epidermal cells to the surface of the skin
2. Gradual keratinisation of these cells
3. Desquamation or rubbing away of these cells.

The layers of the epidermis may be described as follows (see also Fig. 12.2B).

Basal layer (stratum basale). The cells which lie nearest the dermis form the germinative layer where cell division occurs. Cells migrate upwards from this layer, becoming keratinised over a period of 21–28 days before being shed.

Prickle cell layer (stratum spinosum). In the light microscope these cells appear to be connected by fine processes or prickles. These are intercellular connections which act as protection against shearing forces or trauma to the skin.

Granular layer (stratum granulosum). Within this layer fine granules form in the cells. This granular substance, known as Keratohyalin, is a precursor of keratin, which begins to gradually replace the cytoplasm of the cells.

Clear cell layer (stratum lucidum). This layer is present only where the skin is thickened, as in the soles of the feet. The cells exhibit nuclear degeneration and contain large amounts of keratin. Injury or friction to the skin causes an increase in the production of these cells, resulting in a callus or corn.

Horny layer (stratum corneum). This layer is composed of thin, flat, non-nucleated cells, the cytoplasm of which has been lysed and is totally replaced by keratin. Normally, up to 1 g of skin cells are shed every day. Shed skin cells form the main constituent of household dust.

The junction of the epidermis and dermis is convoluted into dips and ridges. These projections into the dermis are called *rete pegs* and help prevent damage to the skin caused by shearing forces. The configuration of these ridges is visible at the surface of the epidermis as corresponding characteristic patterns, most notably on the fingertips (Hinchliff & Montague 1988).

The dermis

The dermis is composed of fibrous connective tissue and provides a supportive meshwork for the structures and organelles within it. The papillary layer has many capillaries and lies next to the basal layer of the epidermis. The reticular layer has fewer blood vessels and is less reactive. It lies above the subcutaneous fat layer. Some of the structures contained within the dermis are described below.

The ground substance of the dermis is a jelly-like material which acts as a support and as a transport medium and fills spaces. It functions as a water reservoir which may be utilised by the body in an emergency (e.g. haemorrhage).

Tissue mast cells. These are often found near hair follicles and blood vessels. They produce heparin and histamine when damaged.

Tissue macrophages. These cells have the protective function of engulfing foreign particles within the dermis.

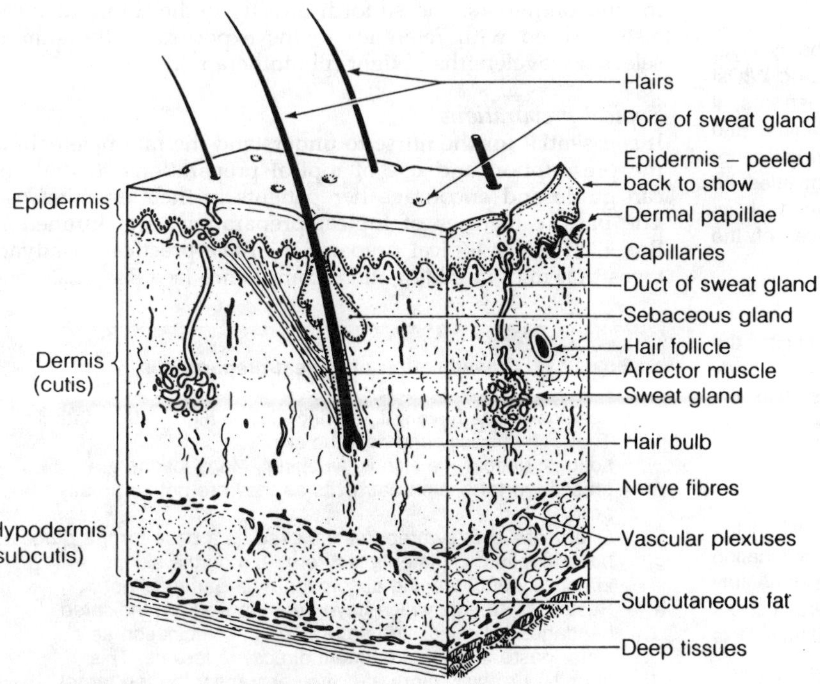

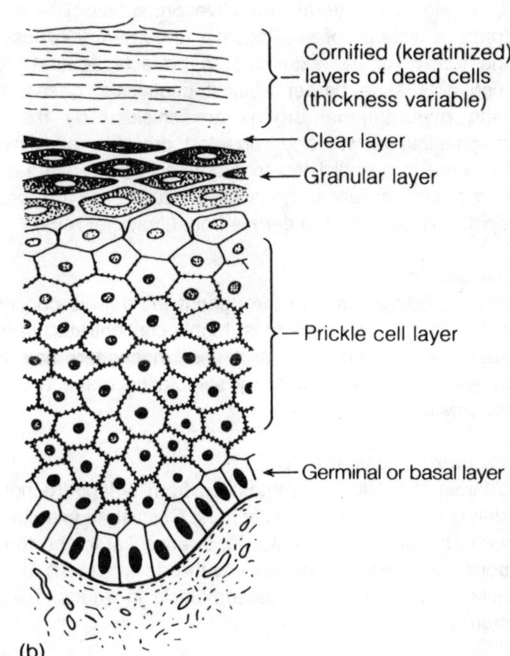

Fig. 12.2 (A) The structure of the skin. (B) The layers of the epidermis. (Reproduced with kind permission from Hinchliff & Montague 1988 Bailliere Tindall.)

Collagen fibres. Ascorbic acid is required by fibroblasts to generate these extremely strong fibres. Collagen fibres have the property of binding with water molecules to give the skin its tight, 'plump' appearance; 40–80% of the total body water is thought to be accommodated within the dermis. Wrinkling is thought to occur when collagen fibres lose their water-binding properties. Collagen fibres may rupture during growth spurts, pregnancy or obesity, leaving fine white scar-like striae.

Elastin fibres. These yellow fibres, also formed by fibroblasts, are bound loosely around bundles of collagen. In combination with the ground substance and collagen, they help the dermis maintain its characteristic properties.

Lymph vessels have a major role in draining excess tissue fluid and plasma proteins from the dermis, thereby maintaining correct volume and composition of tissue fluids.

Nerve endings. Specialised sensory receptors present in the dermis detect mechanical and thermal changes (see Ch. 22).

Glands

Sweat glands. These coiled tubes of epithelial tissue open as pores onto the surface of the skin. Sweat glands have individual nerve and blood supplies and secrete a slightly acid fluid which contains excess excretory products (water and salts). Sweat also helps keep the keratin supple. Sweat glands are of two types. Eccrine glands are under the control of the sympathetic nervous system and produce secretions in response to temperature elevation or fear. Release of latent heat in the evaporation of sweat helps lower body temperature. Apocrine glands in the pubic and axillary areas are not functional until puberty. They are thought to secrete pheromones, chemical signals released into the external environment.

The sebaceous glands. These glands are lined with epidermal tissue. They secrete sebum, a greasy, slightly acid substance which helps to form a waterproof covering over the skin and to keep the keratin supple. The acidity of sebum has anti-bacterial and antifungal properties. Most sebaceous glands open onto hair follicles. Sebum production is influenced by hormone levels.

Functions of the skin

Protection

The skin has several protective properties. The greasy horny layer forms a waterproof seal against undue entry or loss of water. Whilst the acidity of the skin surface protects against microorganisms, it also acts as a barrier against chemicals, gases, and gamma and beta rays. Internal organs are shielded by the skin from minor mechanical blows, and repeated pressure or friction stimulates an increase in cell division to produce thickened areas of skin such as corns and calluses. Melanin produced in the basal layer of the epidermis screens the dermis from ultraviolet rays.

Sensation

Nerve endings present throughout the dermis continually monitor the environment. They are most highly concentrated in areas of the body such as the fingertips and lips. Innervated hair follicles help the individual to avoid injury by stimulating reflex action in response to touch stimuli.

Formation of vitamin D

Vitamin D is slowly synthesised from 7-dehydrocholesterol when the skin is exposed to ultraviolet rays. Circulatory vitamin D, in combination with phosphorus and calcium, is essential to the formation of healthy bone. Deficiencies can lead to the development of disorders such as rickets in children and osteomalacia in adults. Excess vitamin D is stored in the liver.

Temperature regulation (see Ch. 22)

Core body temperature is usually static at around 37°C. Heat is produced in the body by the metabolic processes of the liver, muscles and digestive system. Temperature is controlled by the heat-regulating centre in the hypothalamus of the brain. The hypothalamus responds to changes in the temperature of the circulating blood and influences cardiovascular centres in the medulla oblongata. These centres control the size of the lumen of the arteries and arterioles and thereby control the rate of blood flow through the capillary beds of the dermis.

In cold conditions heat is retained by vasoconstriction and generated by the involuntary muscular action of shivering. During overheating, such as in fever, sweating is induced and vasodilation occurs. As sweat evaporates from the skin, latent heat is lost from the skin surface, causing it to cool. Vasodilation allows large quantities of blood to circulate in the uppermost layers of the dermis. Heat is then lost through convection, radiation and conduction. Blood flow is controlled by the precapillary sphincters, which direct the blood either to the capillary bed closer to the skin surface, resulting in maximum heat loss, or to the deeper tissues of the skin in order to minimise heat loss.

Other functions

During starvation, subcutaneous fat is converted into an energy source and used as a water reserve. Water can also be mobilised from the dermis during haemorrhage or shock. In addition, the skin has some excretory function in that urea and salts are excreted in small amounts through sweat production.

PRINCIPLES OF THERAPY IN SKIN DISORDERS

Before we consider specific disorders of the skin, it will be helpful to look briefly at the types of therapy available within dermatology and the basic principles of their application.

Topical therapy

The skin as the target organ of treatment is easily accessible, and the pathology of many skin disorders requires topical therapy to be used as the first line of management. Topical therapy refers to treatments which are applied directly to the skin, as opposed to medications administered orally or by an intravenous route to deliver the drug internally. The term 'topical therapy' thus usually refers to the application of lotions, ointments, and so forth directly to the skin, but it can also be used with reference to the exposure of the skin to selected wavelengths of light (phototherapy).

Topical preparations

It is essential for the nurse to understand the rationale behind the prescription and use of topical preparations so that she can guide and encourage her patients in their effective use. The basic categories of topical preparations are outlined in Box 12.1. Many topical preparations have practical disadvantages that may impede patient compliance (see Box 12.2), and

Box 12.1 Classification of topical preparations

- Creams: these have a light effect due to high water content. They rub in easily and cool the skin
- Lotions: used if the skin is 'weeping'. Many lotions are prescribed for scalp treatments as they are not so greasy to apply
- Ointments: greasy preparations used as a base for the drug being applied. Ointments last for 6–8 h on the skin, effectively encouraging absorption by a barrier effect
- Pastes: ointments which have been applied to medicated bandages for occlusive use or used in combination as a stiffer paste to apply treatment directly to lesions. This permits a slower, more effective, absorption on the target sites.

Box 12.2 Advantages and disadvantages of topical therapy

ADVANTAGES	DISADVANTAGES
• Drug delivered directly to the target area	• Time consuming
• Reduces systemic absorption	• Messy
• Patient can view improvement	• Treatment preparations may smell or stain the skin
• Side-effects easily identified	• Patient can view deterioration or lack of improvement

thus it is important for the nurse to be able to emphasise the need for perseverance in order to ensure the satisfactory outcome of a treatment programme. The specific choices made in planning a treatment regime must, however, be sensitive to the patient's needs in relation to his lifestyle and personal priorities. Treatment programmes may also need to be altered in view of the unique therapeutic response of each individual.

Phototherapy

Patients with certain skin disorders can be treated with ultraviolet light B (UVB, found in natural sunlight) in carefully measured doses. This treatment requires outpatient attendance 2–3 times weekly over a period of weeks. A test dose is administered to the patient's back to determine his normal reaction to sunlight. This dose is gradually increased over the treatment period. Treatment is given in a light cabinet. UVB is commonly used to treat eczema (see p. 451) by inducing a tan to toughen the skin and reduce itch. In certain photodermatoses, e.g. polymorphic light eruption (see p. 461), a course of UVB is administered early in the year to desensitise the patient and thus provide protection for the rest of the year.

Photochemotherapy (PUVA)

In this type of light therapy the patient takes an oral light-sensitising drug, psoralen, which makes the skin more receptive to ultraviolet light A. Psoralen is a natural plant extract in tablet form taken 2 h before exposure to UVA in a light cabinet. This delay before exposure allows the drug to be absorbed. Bath PUVA is a treatment option in which a measured amount of psoralen is added to a measured volume of bath water. The patient dries after bathing and is then exposed to UVA in the light cabinet. PUVA therapy in psoriasis (see p. 449) reduces the rapid skin cell production characteristic of this condition.

All patients undergoing light therapy must wear protective eye goggles during UVB/PUVA exposure. A patient taking oral psoralen will be instructed to wear dark glasses for a few hours after taking the drug to protect the lens of the eye. UVB/PUVA is administered only in specialist units to ensure accurate recording of the amount of light therapy given to the patient. Most units have a maximum permissible treatment level to prevent the possibility of skin malignancy.

DISORDERS OF THE SKIN

PSORIASIS

Psoriasis is a chronic, non-infectious inflammatory disease of the skin, characterised by well-defined plaques with adherent silvery scales. It manifests in a variety of types and degrees of severity.

Epidemiology

Psoriasis is prevalent in 1–2% of the population of the UK but displays great ethnic variation. The sexes are equally affected and onset can occur at any age. The causes of psoriasis are as yet unproven. but associated factors include family history, infection, drugs, hormone changes and stress (Erdash 1983).

Classification

Guttate psoriasis (see Fig. 12.3)

The term guttate, from the ancient Greek word for 'drop', refers to the salmon-pink lesions over the trunk and limbs that occur in this type of psoriasis. This eruption is usually of sudden onset, often following a streptococcal throat infection (tonsillitis) and therefore commonly presents in children and adolescents. This type of psoriasis responds well to therapy.

Plaque psoriasis (see Fig. 12.4)

This is the most common type of chronic psoriasis and is identified by well-demarcated plaques with dry, silvery-white scales. Many people have these plaques constantly on the elbows and knees without seeking treatment. In an exacerbation of the condition the plaques extend to cover all areas of the trunk and scalp.

Flexural psoriasis

This type of psoriasis presents in skin folds, i.e. in the submammary, axillary and anogenital regions. It is not a scaly condition but plaques are clearly defined and the skin appearance is of a glistening erythema.

Pustular psoriasis

This type of psoriasis presents in two forms. On the hands and feet, it is a chronic condition in which small pustules and brown macules arise on an erythematous base. The feet and

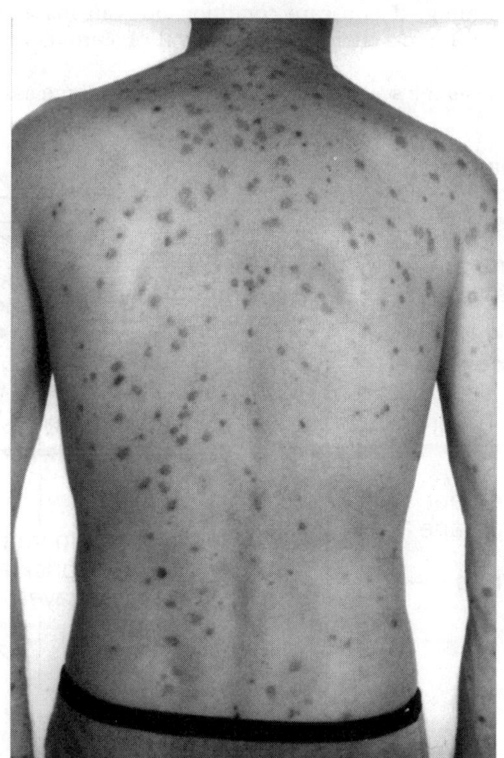

Fig. 12.3 Guttate psoriasis.

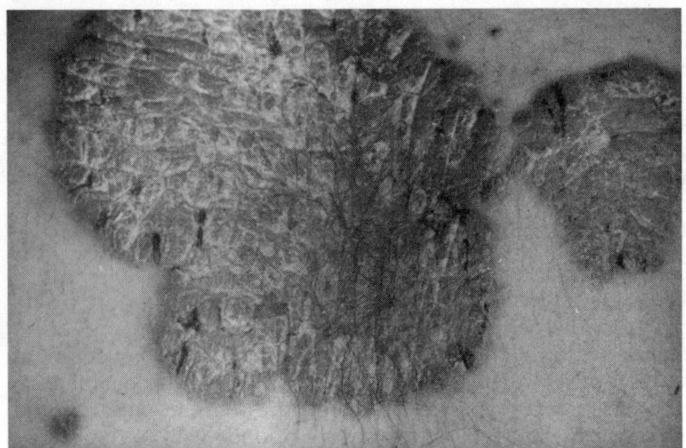

Fig. 12.4 Plaque psoriasis.

hands become fissured and painful as the psoriasis extends. Generalised pustular psoriasis is a rare but serious condition unlike any other form of psoriasis. It occurs as a result of withdrawal of systemic steroids. Sheets of sterile pustules develop and merge; these later peel off, leaving raw, painful areas generally over the whole body.

Psoriatic arthropathy

Among people with psoriasis, 5–7% have associated arthritis (Althoft 1983). The severity of the skin condition and of the arthritis can vary separately. The hands and feet are generally involved, with eventual changes in the spine and sacroiliac joints.

Erythrodermic psoriasis

In this type of psoriasis the skin becomes uniformly red with variable scaling. It is a rare condition but can manifest after irritation by topical therapy, withdrawal of steroids or a drug eruption.

In psoriasis the scalp is often involved, with some associated hair loss. The thickened plaques can be felt and often merge down onto the forehead and behind the ears. Involvement of fingernails and toenails is common and difficult to treat. The nail starts to separate from the nail bed due to psoriatic activity (oncholysis) and the nail itself becomes pitted.

PATHOPHYSIOLOGY

The pathophysiology of the various forms of psoriasis is characterised by the following general processes (see also Fig. 12.5). The epidermis thickens and becomes raised to accommodate the skin changes. There is an increase in the epidermal cell proliferation rate. In normal skin the transit time of epidermal cells maturing in transit through the skin is about 27 days. In psoriasis the transit time is 4 days. This suggests that psoriasis results from an increase in activity of dividing cells associated with an increase in their rate of reproduction, with the trigger factors as yet unidentified (MacKie 1991).

Common presenting symptoms may be summarised as follows:

1. Pain due to fissures which form, particularly on hands and feet, because of loss of flexibility in the thickened epidermis
2. Erythema. Within the dermis the blood vessels dilate and increase blood flow to the skin, creating a generalised redness. Heat loss due to erythema is a major consideration in management
3. Scaling. The horny layer of the epidermis sheds easily in normal skin but in psoriasis the cells become 'sticky' and build up to create the silver-scale appearance diagnostic of psoriasis
4. Pustules. In inflammatory conditions an infiltration of white blood cells is normal. Increased infiltration in pustular psoriasis accumulates as micro-abscesses in the outer layer of the skin
5. Itch. Many textbooks describe psoriasis as non-itchy, but patients often find itch to be troublesome even though it may be difficult to define why. Localised nerve endings can be stimulated by the itch/scratch/itch cycle.

MEDICAL MANAGEMENT

Where possible psoriasis is managed on an outpatient basis, but the severity of activity in erythrodermic/pustular psoriasis may warrant hospital admission to prevent possible life-threatening complications of an unstable psoriatic state.

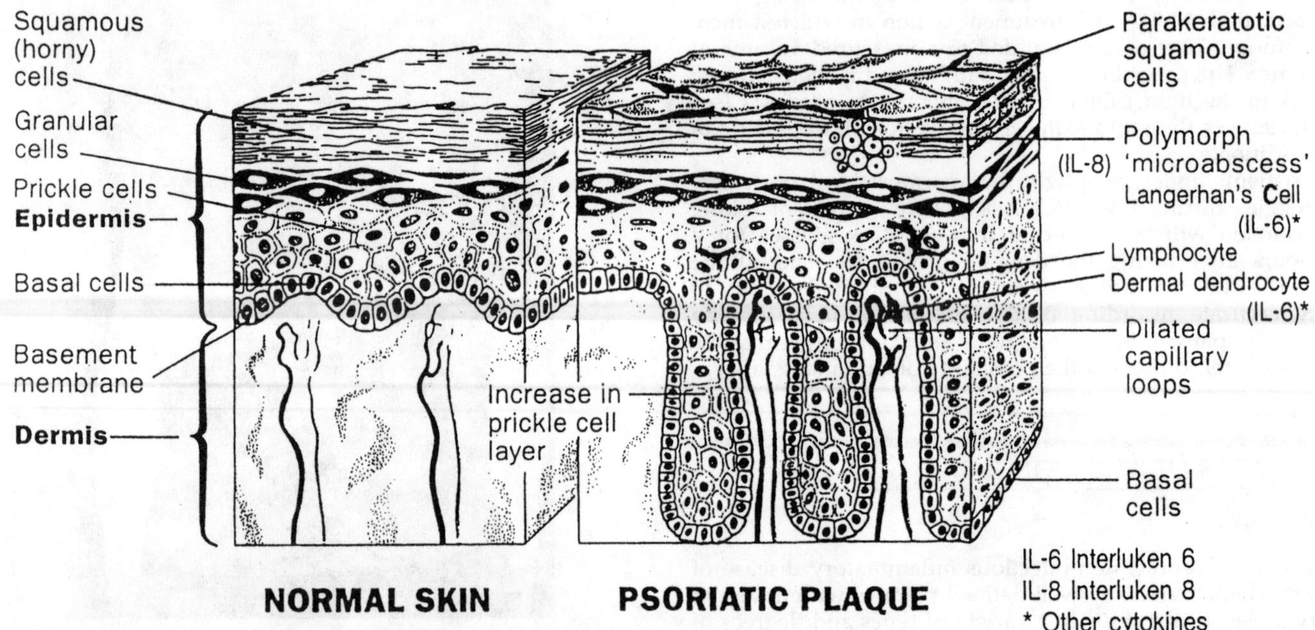

Fig. 12.5 Epidermal changes in psoriasis. (Reproduced with kind permission from the Psoriasis Association 1992.)

Investigative procedures. Diagnosis of psoriasis can be made from the clinical picture and relevant history. Diagnosis and subsequent management may require all or a combination of the following examinations and tests:

1. Skin biopsy. When diagnosis is in doubt due to the appearance of the skin, a biopsy will determine diagnosis by histological criteria
2. Throat swab. This may be taken to determine if streptococcal throat infection has been a trigger factor
3. Skin swab. This is particularly relevant in flexural psoriasis to discount the differential diagnosis of candidal infection in flexures
4. Auspitz sign. If gentle removal of the silvery scale from a plaque reveals pin-point bleeding from the dilated superficial capillaries, the diagnosis of psoriasis is confirmed
5. Routine blood tests. This will include viral check and full blood count.

Medical intervention may involve topical and systemic drug therapy as well as phototherapy. PUVA/UVB have proven to be very effective therapies for psoriasis which may be delivered on an outpatient basis. The exact combination of therapies that is chosen will depend upon the specific diagnosis and the severity of the disorder. Topical prescribed therapies remain, however, the mainstay of psoriasis treatment.

Drug therapy. A combination of systemic and topical medication will be useful in the management of psoriasis. Categories of drugs used include:

- antihistamines to alleviate itch and produce a sedative effect promoting sleep and rest
- analgesics to reduce the discomfort of inflamed skin
- antibiotics to treat secondary infection or resistant viral infections such as tonsillitis.

Drug therapy in the treatment of psoriasis must be carefully monitored. The majority of psoriatic patients respond to topical therapies but the more extensive forms of psoriasis may require a systemic approach (Hunter et al 1989). Two drugs which are particularly important in this regard are methotrexate and etretinate. Their applications and potential side-effects are described on page 451.

Box 12.3 The impact of psoriasis on socialisation as reported by psoriatic patients (Adapted from Stankler 1981)

ACTIVITY RESTRICTIONS

Avoidance of:

- swimming
- sunbathing
- going to the hairdresser
- buying clothes
- socialising
- communal baths
- dancing

CLOTHING RESTRICTIONS

Avoidance of:

- short sleeves
- dark clothing
- summer clothing

CAUSES OF EMOTIONAL UPSET

- Condition regarded as infectious
- Real or imagined stares from non-sufferers
- Questioning by non-sufferers
- Feeling that body is unclean ('leper status')
- Shedding of scales in bedroom

Case History 12.1 Miss J

Miss J, aged 22, had developed psoriasis after recurrent throat infections. At each outbreak of the psoriasis she was becoming more depressed, and she resented the constant demands of treatment. Her main physical problem was a scalp psoriasis which distressed her and restricted her social life. Miss J was independent in basic skin care but required practical help with her scalp psoriasis. She was also in need of support.

Miss J was given help in the application of overnight oil soaks to her scalp and in shampooing carefully afterwards. This helped to remove scaling and reduce discomfort, and aided the absorption of prescribed treatments.

Following counselling, she was referred to a local support network for help in achieving maximum independence, re-establishing social contacts and building confidence.

Miss J soon felt secure enough to 'open up' to nursing staff and confide her fears of social isolation. Her family became aware of her feelings and were keen to help. Joining the support group allowed her to take more control over her situation and greatly improved her self-esteem.

NURSING PRIORITIES AND MANAGEMENT: PSORIASIS

General nursing considerations

Setting priorities

The goals of nursing management will vary considerably according to the particular needs of each patient and the severity of his condition. Potentially life-threatening conditions merit skilled bedside nursing, while the patient with minimal psoriasis will require support and education in order to cope with outpatient treatment. Whatever the extent of the disease, the psychological impact of this visually disturbing condition should never be underestimated. Care planning should involve the patient and his family in setting goals for physical, emotional and social rehabilitation.

Giving psychological support

Many people with chronic psoriasis impose social restrictions upon themselves to avoid embarrassment and to prevent friends and colleagues from realising the extent of the problem (Stankler 1981; see Box 12.3). An open, informative approach will benefit the patient and help to reduce his feelings of social unacceptability (see Case History 12.1). In addition, the nurse in community or occupational health should take every opportunity to correct popular misconceptions about the nature of psoriasis and other non-contagious skin disorders.

Introducing the patient to a local support group will help him to obtain more information about his condition and to combat feelings of alienation. The Psoriasis Association (see Useful Addresses, p. 465) is a major self-help group which was founded in 1968. It has a nationwide network and is highly active in raising public awareness, giving support to psoriasis sufferers and their families, and raising funds for research.

Nursing considerations in outpatient treatment

Management of topical therapy

A range of topical therapies are used in the outpatient management of psoriasis; these include pharmaceutical prepara-

Box 12.4 Examples of topical therapies used in psoriasis management

Emollients	Emulsifying ointment, aqueous cream, 50/50 white soft paraffin/liquid paraffin
Bath oils	Oilatum, Hydromol
Soap substitute	Emulsifying ointment
Coal tar ointments	Coal tar solution and crude coal tar mixtures, e.g. Carbo-Dome, Alphosyl
Dithranol	Psoradrate, Dithrocream, dithranol — Lassar's paste
Dovonex	Vitamin D analogue
Olive oil	Relevant in scalp psoriasis
Cocois ointment	Used for scalp psoriasis
Phototherapy	UVB
Photochemotherapy	Psoralen + UVA (PUVA)

tions as well as phototherapy (see Box 12.4). The nurse should encourage patients to attend regularly for treatment and should emphasise the importance of meticulous adherence to prescribed treatment regimes. The nurse should explain why the different preparations are used, and give advice on their correct application. She should reassure the patient that any staining of the skin will fade once the topical therapy is discontinued, but advise him to discontinue applications if the skin becomes irritated or burned. Most of the prescribed topical therapies are not appropriate for use on the face. Psoriasis extending from the scalp to the forehead and ears can be treated by a mild steroid to lessen obvious redness.

By providing clear information and ongoing psychological support, the nurse can do much to ensure the patient's compliance with treatment. Specific considerations in the use of certain topical preparations are as follows.

Emollients. The application of emollients is fundamental in the management of psoriasis. Bland emollients moisturise and lubricate the skin, helping to ease scaling and thereby promoting patient comfort. Regular applications help to seal the stratum corneum, thus reducing transdermal heat and fluid loss; this is, of course, particularly relevant in erythrodermic psoriasis.

Patients with an unstable psoriasis are often treated with emollients initially, to allow the fiery skin to 'settle' before the next line of treatment is introduced.

Coal tar ointments are distilled from coal in the production of gas. They are usually blended with white soft paraffin and have an anti-pruritic and keratoplastic effect. Initially, treatment starts with a low concentration which is gradually increased according to the tolerance of the patient's skin. As tar applications are messy, smelly and stain, they tend to be used in hospital. Proprietary blends of tar creams such as Alphosyl and Carbo-Dome are available for outpatient therapy.

Tar is never applied to the face or to flexures. Patients must be advised that if the ointment appears to irritate or burn their skin they should remove it immediately in an oily bath and seek advice.

Dithranol is a potent plant extract which suppresses cell proliferation. It is available in many forms, but as it stains skin, clothing, floors and furnishings it tends not to be a popular choice among patients.

In hospital units dithranol is applied by spatula to the affected areas, dusted with maize starch to let it set, and then dressed with stockinette gauze to prevent the ointment spreading to burn or irritate surrounding skin. This procedure is time consuming and messy, but effective. For outpatient therapy, short-contact treatment is an option. Here, the patient applies the cream to the plaque area after protecting the surrounding skin with Vaseline and then removes it 30 minutes later.

Dovonex is a vitamin D analogue applied in cream form to the affected lesions. It is thought to act on the keratinocytes (MacKie 1991). It is well tolerated and is not messy but due to possible systemic absorption it is still prescribed in restricted quantities. Patients are advised to apply it to lesions but avoid the face and flexural areas.

PUVA/UVB (see p. 447). Both therapies are available to patients on an inpatient and outpatient basis. The treatment programme will vary for each individual after identification of their skin type and tolerance of sunlight. Phototherapy is a pleasant treatment option and acquiring a gentle tan will boost the morale of many patients.

Goeckerman regime. This is a long-established and effective combination treatment in which the patient takes tar baths prior to exposure to ultraviolet light (Williams 1985).

Ingram regime. This combination therapy involves tar baths, ultraviolet exposure and dithranol applications.

Cocois ointment. This is a blend of tar, emulsifying ointment and salicylic acid used in the treatment of scalp psoriasis. It can be gently massaged into the scalp, left on overnight, and then removed with a tar-based shampoo that the patient tolerates, e.g. Polytar, or Capasal.

Olive oil can be used in maintenance therapy to reduce further buildup of scale on the scalp. Patients should be advised to warm the oil before applying it to the scalp for maximum benefit.

Nursing considerations in inpatient care

Generalised pustular psoriasis and erythrodermic psoriasis can be life-threatening conditions. Patients with these conditions must be considered as urgent cases and will require skilled nursing management.

Monitoring vital signs

Body temperature. The patient will have difficulty in adapting to changes in environmental temperature and can quickly become pyrexial or hypothermic. Body temperature must be monitored regularly, as skin temperature will fluctuate and can mask a subnormal core temperature (see Ch. 22, p. 680).

Blood pressure must also be checked regularly. Hypotension can develop as a result of the shunt of blood to the peripheral circulation, leading to reduced cardiac output and possible cardiac and renal failure.

Maintaining fluid balance

Given the insensible loss of fluid from the skin in these conditions, rehydration will be important. The majority of patients will be able to maintain a balance if they are encouraged to supplement their oral intake. The liberal use of topical emollients will help to reduce fluid loss from the skin.

Other fundamentals of care

Basic hygiene. Soothing oily baths are ideal in psoriatic conditions to lubricate the skin and prevent further heat and fluid loss. In severe cases, however, it may be necessary to omit bathing given the disruption in the patient's thermoregulatory control caused by a high blood volume flushing the skin. In this situation, the regular and liberal use of emollients will suffice until the patient's condition is stable enough to permit bathing.

Rest is of paramount importance to the patient's recovery. Although isolation is not essential, nursing the patient in a sideroom will help him to rest (Champion 1992).

Diet. Protein loss through the skin may occur, and so an adequate, nutritious diet is advisable. The dietitian can advise the patient and nurse on making appropriate choices from a menu. Supplementary protein drinks can enhance a basic diet. Vitamin supplements may be indicated if dietary intake is insufficient due to the patient's diminished appetite.

Physiotherapy. Referral to the physiotherapist will be beneficial to minimise any side-effects of bedrest. For patients with psoriatic arthropathy the physiotherapist can work in cooperation with the occupational therapist to initiate joint preservation exercises to maintain mobility and flexibility and thus promote independence. A home assessment visit can help to identify problems in the patient's residence associated with limited mobility and function.

Systemic drug therapy

The severe nature of pustular and erythrodermic psoriasis usually merits systemic drug therapy. The nurse must understand the rationale behind the use of these drugs and should prepare the patient for any likely side-effects. The main systemic drugs used are methotrexate and etretinate.

Methotrexate. This cytotoxic drug is a folic acid antagonist which inhibits mitosis. It is given in a weekly dose with careful monitoring of the patient's liver and renal function. Many patients report generalised tiredness 24–48 h after taking their weekly dose, so the informed nurse can advise the patient that rest and avoidance of strenuous activity might be appropriate on treatment days. Antiemetics should be made available if nausea is reported.

Etretinate (Tigason). This is a vitamin A derivative taken in a capsule form on a daily basis in a dosage related to the patient's body weight. The drug influences the activity of the epidermis, normalising the plaques by thinning down the hyperkeratotic lesions. Some of the side-effects reported affect patients until the dose is reduced as the psoriasis improves. Dryness of the mouth, lips and nose are common and unpleasant. The nurse can advise the patient to use basic emollients and lip salves to ease discomfort. Reassurance that side-effects will abate once treatment is reduced or discontinued may help the patient to persevere with treatment.

Female patients taking etretinate require counselling by nurses or family planning services to take adequate contraceptive measures during the treatment programme. This can be a difficult request for a young female patient; and adequate counselling is vital, as this drug can be harmful to a developing fetus.

Alternative therapies

Many 'cures' have been offered in psoriasis. These include treatment programmes involving holidays at the Dead Sea in which therapy takes the form of exfoliation with Dead Sea salt and natural exposure to sunlight. Acupuncture and hypnotherapy are tried by some people. Others take fish oil capsules as an adjunct to therapy on the principle that the low susceptibility of Invit (Eskimos) to psoriasis in comparison to Western races is related to the high fish oil content of their diet (MacKie 1991). Research findings on the effectiveness of fish oil capsules remain inconclusive, however.

ECZEMA

The word eczema comes from the ancient Greek for 'to boil out of' and is the term applied to a range of inflammatory skin disorders. Most classifications of eczematous skin disorders use the term 'eczema' synonymously with 'dermatitis', as both terms apply to the inflammatory skin changes provoked by either internal (endogenous) or external (exogenous) factors. Eczema may occur as a result of one or both type of factors.

Priorities of medical and nursing management are similar for all classifications of eczema, and are therefore discussed following a brief description of the different conditions referred to as eczema.

Endogenous eczema

Atopic eczema (see Fig. 12.6)

This may be described as a clinical hypersensitivity in the presence of a genetic predisposition to develop an allergy.

It presents as a chronic itchy cutaneous disorder and occurs in approximately 1–3% of infants in the UK. In older children and adults the incidence is lower. The word 'atopic' points to the genetic disposition of the disease process. A family history usually reveals the triad of eczema, asthma and hay fever. In a proportion of children with infantile eczema the disease may resolve spontaneously. Some children, however, progress from an acute phase to the chronic pattern of episodic exacerbations of the condition.

In young children the eczema is often generalised. In older children the sites of chronic involvement tend to be the face and wrists, with flexural involvement of the elbows and knees.

Pompholyx eczema

This is a blistering eczema localised to the palms of the hands and soles of the feet. It develops rapidly and causes acute discomfort. The hands and feet may also develop secondary infections. The cause of this form of eczema is unknown. Outbreaks do not appear to be related to any external factors.

Asteatotic eczema

This condition is seen mainly in the elderly population and appears to be associated with excessive dryness of the skin, although the use of central heating, diuretic therapy and over-frequent washing can be implicated as possible causes. The stratum corneum develops a 'crazy paving' appearance due to a network of fine red superficial fissures. The individual will find the affected area itchy. Asteatotic eczema is readily treatable at the early stages with liberal use of emollients and

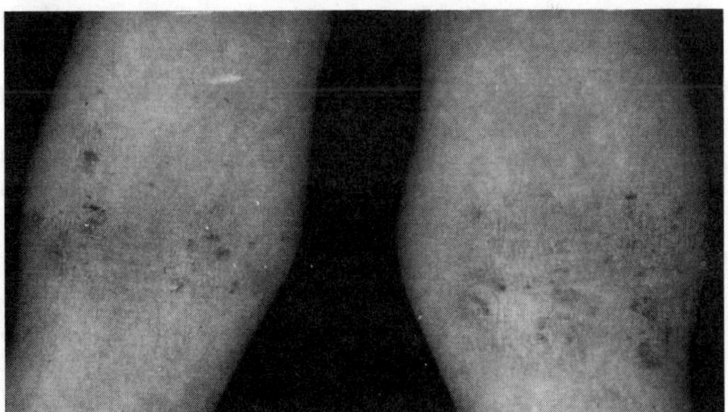

Fig. 12.6 Atopic eczema.

bath oils. If the itch is persistent, scratching will create a more resistant eczema which may merit topical steroid therapy.

Varicose eczema

This usually presents as a chronic patchy eczema of the legs with or without the presence of a varicose ulcer (see Ch. 23, p. 715). The eczema arises due to associated chronic venous stasis and the area involved can become itchy. Scratching will lead to ulceration. The eczema is often accompanied by the presence of varicose veins, oedema and pigmentation of the skin. Patients often develop a secondary response to this initial area of eczema and may produce associated eczematous areas of skin on other parts of the body.

Exogenous eczema

Irritant eczema is very common, especially in industrial settings. The eczema usually erupts at the maximum point of contact and so commonly presents on the hands. Presentation will vary according to the nature of the irritant contact. For example, the epidermis may be damaged by abrasion, and the effect of the irritant (coal dust, cement, etc.) exacerbated by being rubbed by clothing. Epidermal necrosis may occur within hours following contact with strong chemicals, while eczema triggered by milder substances (e.g. detergents) may take longer to evolve.

Many patients who have had atopic eczema appear to be prone to irritant eczema and therefore should be warned not to take up work where exposure to irritants could be problematic (Gawkrodger 1993).

Allergic contact dermatitis

Allergic contact dermatitis is a condition in which the skin develops a specific immunological hypersensitivity. The most common allergic response of this type, particularly amongst women, is to nickel as found in inexpensive jewellery. Continued exposure to the allergen will result in an eczematous response, which may be severe or quite mild. Allergic contact dermatitis may be triggered by rubber, certain plants, cosmetics, and many other substances. In many cases a change of job or avoidance of the allergen will help. The most difficult cases to treat are those in which allergic contact dermatitis is suspected but no definitive triggering factor can be proven.

PATHOPHYSIOLOGY OF ECZEMA

Acute eczema presents with redness and swelling caused by increased vasodilation and generalised oedema of the skin. The erythema may be generalised all over the body. Vesicles erupt and can in some conditions lead to blistering. Generally, however, acute eczema exacerbated by scratching will extend to an exudative, scaling and crusting phase.

In chronic eczema involving recurrent exacerbations, the skin is scaly, excoriated, thickened and pigmented. The eczematous areas will be localised to more defined parts of the body and a condition described as lichenification will be apparent. Lichenification is a skin response to repeated scratching in which the affected areas become thickened and toughened and show a marked exaggeration of normal skin markings. Chronic scratching and thickened skin also combine to allow the development of deep, painful fissures as the skin loses its normal elasticity.

Common presenting symptoms may be described as follows:

Itch (pruritus). Most eczematous conditions present with an itch which can cause the patient considerable annoyance and distress. The itch–scratch–itch cycle quickly becomes established. The skin is well supplied with sensory nerves which respond quickly to the mechanical stimulation of scratching (or any external stimulation). Itch has two components because of the manner in which sensory impulses are transported (see Ch. 19, p. 616). Thus a quick, localised prickly sensation will be followed by a slow and diffuse burning itch.

Redness. Blood supply to the skin is prolific and in normal circumstances is only required to function at low volume. Any inflammatory skin disease adjusts this balance by causing dilatation of the blood vessels feeding the skin, leading to a generalised total body redness (erythroderma). In atopic eczema white dermographism can be evoked due to the abnormal response of the skin's vascular change. Firm strokes of the skin should normally produce a 'weal-and-flare response', but in atopic patients a simple white line arises leaving the pressure site with no erythema.

Fissures/lichenification. As already described, the chronic stages of eczema create a thickening of the skin over the flexures or any area traumatised by scratching. Open fissures will be painful and slow to heal. In the chronic stages there is also a generalised thickening of the prickle cell and horny layers of the skin.

Summary. Most eczematous conditions present in varying degrees of severity. An acute phase of eczema may present as a weeping, inflamed response, while a chronic condition will give rise to fissures and clearly defined excoriated areas. All conditions are pruritic. All patients will describe itch, pain and tenderness. Loss of the normal barrier of intact skin will have associated fluid and heat loss. Excoriations may lead to secondary infections which contribute to keeping the eczema active. Patients with atopic eczema tend to be more susceptible to viral infections such as warts, herpes simplex virus and eczema herpeticum (see p. 457).

MEDICAL MANAGEMENT

An initial diagnosis will be made from the clinical picture of the disease process and history taken from the patient. Many of the exogenous conditions will be managed wholly at an outpatient clinic or treatment centre. Severe exacerbations, however, warrant hospital admission to initiate management.

Investigative procedures. Precise diagnosis may require all or a combination of the following tests and investigations.

Laboratory investigations. These will include:

1. Skin swabs. Excoriated lesions contribute to secondary infection. As many atopic patients are thought to be *Staphylococcus aureus* carriers, a full range of swabs may be taken from nasal, perineal and axillary areas prior to commencing a course of oral antibiotics. The secondary infection will be treated topically and orally, depending on laboratory results
2. Skin scrapings to identify bacterial, fungal or viral involvement
3. Skin biopsy. A small section of skin may be taken for immunohistological examinations. This is not generally done in eczematous conditions except where the diagnosis is in doubt.

Patch testing may be carried out to confirm a diagnosis of allergic dermatitis. A range of patch tests are available in which suspected allergens (e.g. hairdressing products, plant material, rubber, etc.) are made up in a concentration which would normally produce no reaction unless the patient has developed a sensitivity. The allergens are applied to the patient's back and left in situ for 48 h and then removed. The site of the test is 'read' at 96 h. Positive results may vary from mild erythema to small blisters. Patch tests should not be carried out while the patient is in the acute phase of eczema or using topical steroids, to avoid the possibility of exacerbating the condition or obtaining misleading results.

Blood tests may indicate the presence of specific antibodies which can confirm an eczematous response to an external factor, e.g. dust mite, cat and dog hair, certain foods. In acute erythematous reactions careful observation of urea and electrolytes will be essential in primary treatment due to the fluid and heat loss caused by the condition.

Drug therapy. Antihistamines, antibiotics and analgesics may be prescribed as appropriate.

Antihistamines are prescribed to reduce itch. Many antihistamines block histamine receptors and are best used prophylactically. Most antihistamines have the side-effect of causing drowsiness and may in fact be prescribed as a sedative to aid sleeping and resting.

Antibiotics. If bacterial infection is present due to excoriation a course of oral antibiotics will often be necessary. A broad-spectrum antibiotic would be appropriate.

Analgesia. The short-term use of simple analgesics in the form of an anti-inflammatory such as paracetamol may also ease heat, tenderness and localised pain.

Topical therapy. The topical therapies commonly used in eczematous conditions include the prescribed preparations listed in Box 12.5 as well as UVB treatment. Eczema also improves in some patients on exposure to natural sunlight.

NURSING PRIORITIES AND MANAGEMENT: ECZEMA

General nursing considerations

Setting priorities

Nursing management is of central importance in the treatment of eczematous conditions. The goals of any nursing care plan must be discussed with the patient and his family, whose involvement in all stages of decision-making will be crucial to the successful management of the condition.

The short-term priority of management will be to alleviate the patient's discomfort. A tired, hot, itchy patient is not in an ideal state to absorb information and learn self-care techniques.

Ongoing support and reassurance will be fundamental to the achievement of long-term goals. Informing the patient about his eczema will create a greater understanding of the disease process and its outlook. Treatment sessions present the ideal opportunity to familiarise the patient with different topical therapies and explain their effects and the rationale behind their use.

Giving psychological support

The patient must be viewed holistically. Background information that is confided to the nurse may bear upon the outcome of treatment. For example, a brash teenager who appears to be unconcerned by his condition and appearance may be putting up a front in response to feelings of social rejection. The nurse who recognises the existence of such defence mechanisms may be in a better position to help the patient to acknowledge his feelings and to improve his situation by complying with treatment regimes. The patient may also benefit by being put in contact with a support group such as a local branch of the National Eczema Society (see Useful Addresses, p. 465).

Box 12.5 Examples of topical therapies used in the management of eczematous conditions

Emollients	50/50 white soft paraffin/liquid paraffin, emulsifying ointment, aqueous cream, E45 cream, Unguentum Merck, Diprobase cream, Lipobase
Bath oils	Oilatum, Balneum
Soap substitute	Emulsifying ointment
Steroids	Dermovate, Betnovate, Eumovate
Steroids/antibiotics	Dermovate-NN, Betnovate-C
Bandages	Icthopaste, Quinaband, Coltapaste

Nursing considerations in topical therapy

Emollients

These are moisturisers used to make dry and scaly skin smoother. They can take the form of bath oils, creams and ointments and are the mainstay of treatment. Itchiness, heat and dryness all respond promptly to adequate lubrication. Many emollients create a barrier for the inflamed skin, thus preventing further fluid and heat loss. Eczema is a condition in which the skin is chronically dry, so the nurse must promote the long-term use of emollients to maintain good skin tone. Patients should be asked to avoid perfumed products and to use prescribed bath oils and soap substitutes. The nurse should advise patients with eczema to bath daily, using adequate bath oil. Continued use of emollients throughout the day is essential and a major adjunct to the treatment programme.

In hospital the patient will be asked to use very greasy moisturisers and emollients, but these products may be totally unsuitable for use at home or in the workplace. For community use most manufacturers produce bland emollients which are effective, non-messy, non-staining. Many of these emollients are available in pump dispensers and are attractively packaged to encourage compliance.

Steroids

The application of steroid creams and ointments constitutes the next line of management in inflammatory skin disorders. These preparations are absorbed into the skin to dampen down the inflammatory response mechanism. Because steroid therapy will have a major impact on the eczematous skin it is vital for the nurse to inform the patient of correct methods of application. Absorption of topical steroid and the volume of cream necessary will be greater if the skin is dry and excoriated. If is therefore essential to ensure that skin is being regularly moisturised with the prescribed emollient as an adjunct to steroid therapy. The nurse can advise the patient to apply a treatment cream after bathing when the skin is soft, well-lubricated and warm. Using the 'fingertip unit' method (see Finlay et al 1989) small amounts of cream can be gently massaged into the affected areas for maximum effect.

In some eczematous conditions potent steroids are essential to switch off the inflammatory process. A treatment programme would involve starting with a medium to strong steroid applied twice daily and then gradually reducing the strength of the creams used as the condition improves. Many patients are aware of the side-effects of topical steroids and are therefore reluctant to use them effectively. The nurse must emphasise that it is the prolonged use of strong topical steroids with the inadequate use of emollients that produces chronic side-effects, i.e. striae and loss of subcutaneous fat. In eczema, secondary bacterial infection may be present and treatment may include a combined steroid antibiotic cream (see Box 12.5).

Bandaging

A variety of occlusive, medicated bandages are available for dermatological therapy. Applied overnight they provide a cooling effect and their occlusive action creates a moist environment which aids the absorption of emollients and steroid applications. They also provide a mechanical barrier to prevent damage being inflicted to the skin if the patient scratches in his sleep. Bandaging is appropriate for infants with atopic eczema who may disrupt normal family living by waking in the night. The skilled community nurse who can teach bandaging techniques to parents may help to restore harmony to the whole family unit.

Other considerations

Rest

Rest is imperative for recovery in eczematous conditions. In hospital, the child or adult is afforded the opportunity to suspend activities of socialisation and take time out to repair. In the home setting, disruptive, manipulative behaviour is often described in the child with atopic eczema, who may merely be distraught by itch and inadequate sleep. The nurse must give clear information and reassurance on the safe use of antihistamine drugs for children. Many parents are not keen to give their child drugs, but the judicious use of antihistamines will provide rest and relief for the eczema sufferer and his family.

Diet

Diet is implicated in some forms of infantile eczema where the child is allergic to milk or milk products. The best advice to give to eczema sufferers is to maintain a well-balanced diet while avoiding any foods that they are aware create any irritation. An exclusion diet to identify a food allergy is very difficult and should be attempted only with maximum supervision from a dietitian. The theory that breastfeeding babies reduces the incidence of infantile eczema remains a matter of debate amongst dermatologists; a mother should be advised to choose the feeding method that is most appropriate to her particular circumstances and her family's needs.

Alternative therapies

Patients will often question nurses about the value of alternative therapies in the treatment of eczema.

Any alternative remedy which offers relief from the distressing symptoms suffered by eczema patients must be considered a treatment option without scepticism from traditional practitioners. Some of the alternative (or complementary) therapies available are indicated below.

Evening primrose oil. Gamma linolenic acid (GLA); in this plant extract is an essential fatty acid, deficiencies of which have been associated with the symptoms of atopic eczema. It may be prescribed to relieve the symptoms of eczema but must not be considered a cure. It is available in capsule and chewable tablet form.

Homeopathic medicine. Many dermatologists refer patients to homeopaths in the hope that a combination of therapies will improve the condition. Homeopathy may have much to offer this client group.

Chinese herbalism. Over the past few years a new source of treatment for eczema has become available in the form of herbal drinks. This form of treatment is becoming increasingly popular among people with resistant eczema but has had varying degrees of success.

The contribution of the nurse

The specific role of the nurse in supporting the patient with an eczematous condition will vary considerably, depending on the severity of the patient's condition and the setting in which he is being treated. In hospital, the nurse often meets the patient during an acute phase of the disease. Care planning must include teaching the patient about the management of his condition both in acute phases and during periods of remission. Practical tips on treatment application and bandaging may improve the quality of daily living for the sufferer and his family.

In the community, nurses will fulfil a variety of roles. For example, the community nurse visiting an elderly patient with diabetes in order to give an insulin injection may detect an area of varicose eczema requiring treatment. The health visitor will adopt an educative and supportive role for the parents of children with atopic eczema. The occupational health nurse is trained to identify problems at work and can suggest changes in working practice that will reduce the incidence of industrial dermatoses. The school nurse is ideally placed to help a child with atopic eczema to maintain topical therapy regimes; she can also inform teachers about the nature of the disease and the discomfort the affected child is likely to be experiencing.

In every professional setting, the skilled nursing practitioner will take full advantage of all available resources and refer patients as appropriate to the relevant professionals, agencies and support groups. This will help to ensure that the difficulties posed by chronic skin disease for the patient and his family in all areas of daily life are addressed.

> **?** **12.2** Ms H is the single parent of three children aged 5 years, 3 years and 1 year. She is unemployed and lives in rented one-bedroom accommodation while on a council house waiting list. Her 3-year-old son has severe eczema. He is kept awake at night by severe itch and disrupts the household.
>
> Discuss with a health visitor how this mother might be helped to cope with this situation.

SKIN INFECTIONS AND INFESTATIONS

This section describes infections and infestations more commonly encountered in the community than in hospital settings. An awareness of these disorders is thus particularly relevant for the community practitioner (district nurse, health visitor, school nurse, occupational health nurse). Many of these conditions create great consternation among those affected because of their real or perceived social implications. Sound common sense, the ability to dispel myths, and practical skill in identifying, assessing and treating the conditions described are essential to the nurse's role.

Fungal infections

This group of skin disorders tend to be superficial infections caused by fungi that thrive in non-viable keratinised tissue of the skin, i.e. nails, hair and the stratum corneum. The word 'tinea' is used as the generic description for these infections (Fitzpatrick et al 1992).

Athlete's foot (tinea pedis)

This condition presents as maceration and scaling of the skin between the toes causing pain and itch. It tends to be a chronic problem with exacerbations precipitated by occlusive footwear or hot weather.

MEDICAL MANAGEMENT

Skin scrapings from the affected area can be examined under a microscope to confirm diagnosis. Treatment includes:

- dusting shoes with antifungal powder
- applications of antifungal creams or lotions, e.g. clotrimazole, Nizoral, ketoconazole
- prescription of oral antifungal drugs, e.g. griseofulvin.

A combination of oral and topical therapy may be required on a long-term basis.

NURSING PRIORITIES AND MANAGEMENT: ATHLETE'S FOOT

Many patients, if given the appropriate advice, will cope independently with treatment. The nurse should give advice on the following aspects of maximising skin care:

- gently daily bathing of the feet
- careful drying between the toes
- use of cotton socks
- avoidance of occlusive footwear, e.g. synthetic sports shoes
- use of own towels, etc. to prevent spread of infection.

Ringworm (tinea corporis)

This infection is acquired from an active lesion on an animal or by direct human contact. It presents as scaling, red, annular lesions anywhere on the face, trunk or limbs. It is particularly common amongst children and in adults working with animals.

MEDICAL MANAGEMENT

Skin scrapings can be taken for examination under the microscope to confirm diagnosis. Topical antifungal cream (e.g. clotrimazole) applied twice daily is usually effective in resolving the condition.

NURSING PRIORITIES AND MANAGEMENT: RINGWORM

The nurse should give the patient the relevant information to support a treatment programme. Investigating the cause and isolating the source will be helpful. Basic hygiene at home (e.g. not sharing towels and face cloths) will prevent further spread to other family members.

Thrush (candidiasis)

Thrush is a fungal infection occurring on moist skin sites and mucosal surfaces. It affects all age groups, but is an opportunistic infection affecting in particular those patients whose resistance may be reduced by antibiotic therapy, diabetes, infection or pregnancy. It can have a major impact on immunosuppressed patients or HIV infected individuals. Thrush takes a number of forms, which may be classified as follows.

1. Oral thrush. This presents as milky spots on the tongue and cheeks and affects mainly babies and elderly people
2. Vaginal thrush. This presents as vulval/vaginal itch with a creamy white discharge. The mucosa becomes red and inflamed and infection will spread to the perineum and groin
3. Nappy rash. If caused by thrush infection the genitalia and buttocks will be reddened, raw and excoriated with the lesions extending to the thighs and buttocks
4. Paronychia. This is a candidal infection of the nail plate occurring in people whose occupation involves repeatedly immersing the hands in water (e.g. hairdressers and bartenders). The nails become distorted and the nail base is painful, red and swollen.
5. Intertrigo. This is the term given to a candidal infection of skin folds (submammary, groin, natal cleft). Increased heat and humidity in the skin folds associated with obesity exacerbate the problem. The skin displays erythematous, well-demarcated erosive lesions and is tender, moist and painful.

MEDICAL MANAGEMENT

Swabs, skin scrapings or nail clippings may be taken to confirm the diagnosis. Treatment is specific to the area infected. Antifungals in the form of creams, ointments and pessaries are effective, but oral antifungal drugs may be indicated, particularly in paronychial infection where it is difficult to effectively treat the nail bed topically.

NURSING PRIORITIES AND MANAGEMENT: THRUSH

By giving advice and information on basic skin hygiene and maintenance therapy, the nurse can help to resolve the condition. An awareness of the predisposing factors for this infection will help nurses to identify clients who may be at risk from this opportunistic infection. In her role as counsellor, the nurse will be able to advise female patients with vaginal thrush on the dual role of pessaries and cream for the condition. Sexual partners of the patient should be treated concurrently to prevent further transmission; the nurse should stress the importance of this without breaking confidentiality.

Infestations

Scabies

Scabies is a condition in which the skin is infested by the mite *Sarcoptes scabiei*. The mite burrows into the skin; the primary target site tends to be the hand webs. The infestation creates an intense, generalised pruritus which is particularly uncomfortable at night. Vesicles, nodules and secondary bacterial infections will develop if the condition persists untreated. These lesions may be generalised over the whole body.

Transmission is generally by skin-to-skin contact, although the scabies mite can remain in bedding and clothing for 48 h and so can be acquired without direct interpersonal contact. Scabies tends to be associated with overcrowding, promiscuity and poverty. Outbreaks also tend to occur, however, in hospitals, day nurseries and in day care centres for elderly people.

MEDICAL MANAGEMENT

The scabies burrow extends approximately 1 cm into the skin. The mite can often be extracted by needle from the minute vesicle at the end of a burrow and examined under the microscope to confirm the diagnosis.

Topical treatment with the appropriate scabicide (e.g. Quellada, Derbac-M) will follow. Once the infestation is treated, further therapy with a topical steroid/antibiotic cream is often required to reduce the itch and clear any secondary infection from excoriated lesions. Antihistamine tablets can be useful if intense itch is distressing the patient.

NURSING PRIORITIES AND MANAGEMENT: SCABIES

The nurse must provide clear and specific advice on following treatment regimes. Family members and visitors will also need advice.

Department of Health (DOH) guidelines change the prescribed therapy on a rotational basis to reduce the probability of producing a 'super mite' resistant to all conventional preparations. General advice for patients on carrying out treatment is given in Box 12.6.

> ? **12.3** A family of five (two adults, and three children aged 15, 6 and 3 years) have to treat themselves for a scabies infestation. Their GP suggests that a leaflet could be given to them to ensure they follow the correct advice.
>
> Devise a printed sheet with treatment advice for this family.

Box 12.6 Patient advice sheet for the self-treatment of scabies

1. Bathe or shower.
2. Apply the prescribed treatment from the neck down (avoiding the face) to the feet. Pay particular attention to the webs of the fingers and toes. The lotion will be left on the skin for 12–24 hours, depending on the prescription instructions.
3. Change clothing and bed linen. Normal laundering is adequate.
4. Take a bath or shower at the end of the 12–24 hour period.
5. All personal contacts and family members will need to be treated during the same period.

POINTS TO NOTE

- If the hands are washed during the 12–24 hour period, re-apply the treatment lotion to the hands.
- Weaker strengths of treatment creams will be available and prescribed for infants and pregnant women.
- The treatment can be repeated in 7 days in a particularly resistant infection.

Head lice (pediculosis capitis)
Infestation of the scalp by the head louse is commonly epidemic among schoolchildren and creates great consternation among parents. The louse feeds on the scalp and deposits its eggs (the 'nits') on the hair. Transmission is by close proximity of heads and sharing combs and brushes.

NURSING PRIORITIES AND MANAGEMENT: HEAD LICE

In schools, once the problem is identified, parents will require notification and help in treating and preventing further transmission to the family. Clear, reassuring advice will reduce anxiety and distress. The child's hair will be treated with the appropriate lotion (e.g. malathion, Prioderm) and left on the scalp for a specified number of hours. It can then be shampooed. Repeat treatments can be carried out as advised if necessary. Gentle combing with a fine-toothed comb will aid the removal of the nits. Nits look like dandruff but are totally immobile, being cemented to the hair shaft, so combing is desirable over a number of days.

Secondary infection from scratching lesions can create an impetigo which will require oral or topical antibiotic therapy. The nurse's role is to offer guidance in the prevention and detection of head lice. Parents will thus be supported in preventive action, which will help to reduce the incidence of transmission and to isolate the source. As in scabies, the prescribed treatment lotions are changed regularly to prevent a treatment-resistant strain of head lice from arising.

Body lice (pediculosis corporis)
Infestation with body lice tends to be associated with poverty and poor social hygiene. Patients are often unkempt and the skin is excoriated, itchy and smelly. In some countries body lice are associated with typhus and relapsing fever. Lice and their eggs are found in seams of clothing.

NURSING PRIORITIES AND MANAGEMENT: BODY LICE

This will be a difficult problem to manage, as without basic changes to the social environment reinfestation will occur. However, bathing and replacement of clothing will resolve the problem initially.

Oral antihistamines and topical calamine lotion will soothe itching. Secondary infection due to scratching will require antibiotic therapy. If appropriate and practicable, the nurse can refer the patient to the social work department and voluntary agencies to assist in a change of environment. Social workers can assess the individual patient and offer relevant funding to improve social conditions.

Fleas and mites
Fleas from animals can create irritating urticarial lesions on humans. General cleansing of carpets and furniture and a trip to the veterinarian for treatment of the family pet will help to remove the problem. Topical therapy with a mild antipruritic such as Eurax or calamine lotion will reduce itching.

Mites tend to be found in bulk foodstuffs such as cheese, flour and grain. Topical treatment is similar to that used for flea bites. However, if the sufferer feels he has been infested in the workplace referral to the environmental health department is appropriate to instigate an assessment of storage practices.

Bacterial infections

Impetigo
This is a superficial epidermal infection of the skin caused by staphylococcal, streptococcal or a combination of infections. It presents as transient thin-roofed vesicles which burst and develop into characteristic golden-yellow crusted lesions. The lesions spread rapidly and the infection is particularly common amongst preschool children, predominantly affecting the face. Impetiginisation also occurs in the lesions of eczema and scabies (Fitzpatrick et al 1992). Very rarely, an impetigo affected by certain streptococcal organisms leads to glomerulonephritis (Fitzpatrick et al 1992).

NURSING PRIORITIES AND MANAGEMENT: IMPETIGO

Clear advice to parents about the transmission and infectious nature of the disorder will help in source isolation. Basic hygiene and avoidance of communal use of towels and face-cloths will reduce the incidence of transmission. Treatment advice will involve demonstrating how to soak the lesions in mild antiseptic solutions before gentle removal of the crust. Topical antibiotics can then be applied directly to the affected areas.

Folliculitis
This term is given to a superficial bacterial infection of the hair follicles. The skin may be slightly tender, showing discrete pustules around the hair follicle. Factors contributing to a folliculitis include:

- bacterial infection
- topical contact with tar, adhesive plaster or occlusive dressings
- physical damage, e.g. caused by shaving legs or beard
- background of seborrhoeic eczema.

NURSING PRIORITIES AND MANAGEMENT: FOLLICULITIS

Isolating and removing the factor contributing to the folliculitis may resolve the problem. Hirsute patients using tar lotions, etc. should be advised to apply these preparations in the direction of the hair growth to reduce the effect of physical irritation. Any active eczema should be treated promptly (see p. 451).

Topical therapy will include applications of ointments effective against staphylococcal infections, e.g. mupirocin. Systemic therapy may be required if the folliculitis is resistant to topical applications.

Cellulitis

This term is given to an acute, spreading and potentially serious infection of dermal and subcutaneous tissue, characterised by a red, tender area of skin often at the site of bacterial entry. Organisms isolated in cellulitis include *Staphylococcus aureus* and *Streptococcus pyogenes*. Infection enters the skin in a variety of ways, including through surgical lesions, stasis eczema or leg ulcers, nasal fissures, and i.v. drug injection sites.

In adults the most common presentation is a cellulitis of the lower limbs, with the point of entry of infection usually a fissure between the toes. The site affected will be oedematous, red, hot and painful. An associated general malaise with rigors and fever develops. Enlarged lymph nodes are evident due to the severity of the infection.

MEDICAL MANAGEMENT

Medical intervention concentrates on diagnosis, isolation of the offending organism by blood cultures, and relevant antibiotic therapy. Analgesia will be prescribed to reduce the pain of inflammation.

NURSING PRIORITIES AND MANAGEMENT: CELLULITIS

The basics of bedrest, close monitoring of temperature and appropriate action if rigors occur are the first line of nursing management. Pain assessment and regular analgesia will ease the patient's discomfort.

Cellulitis of the lower limbs requires bedrest and elevation of the affected limb in bed to reduce oedema. Encouragement in passive exercising will reduce the complications of prolonged bedrest. Once the condition resolves, general advice on basic skin care and on avoidance of predisposing factors may be helpful to the patient.

Viral infections

Warts (see Fig. 12.7)

Infection by the human papilloma virus affects the DNA in epidermal cells, creating warts. Different clinical manifestations are specific to different viruses (Fitzpatrick et al 1992).

Warts are benign, highly contagious and usually cosmetically unacceptable. Group transmission is the mode of contact, as for example in gyms, swimming baths or schools. The classification of warts is briefly outlined in Box 12.7.

MEDICAL MANAGEMENT

Diagnosis is by history and clinical appearance. A histological examination of curetted lesions will confirm diagnosis. Treatment may involve topical application of ointments or premedicated plasters containing salicylic acid to soften and remove the wart, curettage under local anaesthetic, or cryotherapy.

The nurse should provide a full explanation of the virus transmission and encourage the meticulous continuation of treatment. Many patients become disheartened by the slow resolution of the problem and discontinue treatment. A visit for regular assessment to the practice nurse may encourage treatment compliance.

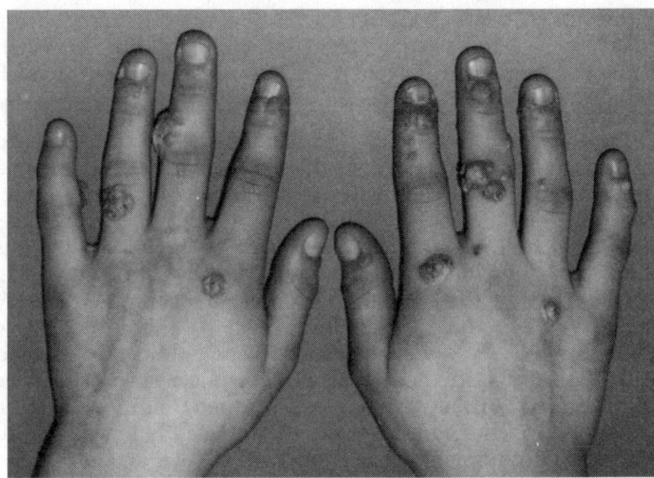

Fig. 12.7 Hand warts.

Molluscum contagiosum

This is a pox virus which causes solid, skin-coloured or pearly-white papules to appear on the skin. It affects both adults and children, arising over a period of 2–3 months. The lesions may be single or multiple and occur on the neck and trunk. In adults this condition is often considered to be a sexually transmitted disease; it frequently presents on the faces of HIV infected patients (Fitzpatrick et al 1992).

MEDICAL MANAGEMENT

Diagnosis is by history and clinical appearance. Removal and microscopic examination of the centre of the molluscum will confirm the diagnosis. If the condition does not resolve spontaneously freezing with local applications of liquid nitrogen may be carried out. When the condition occurs in children, parents will require careful explanation and reassurance that the condition tends to be self-limiting. Normal basic hygiene rules in the home will prevent further spread.

Herpes simplex virus (HSV)

The herpes simplex virus may be transmitted by direct contact or droplet infection. Two types of the virus are known: Type (I) produces smaller vesicles affecting the nose, lips and mouth. Type (II) produces larger vesicles affecting the genitalia.

Diagnosis is usually made through tissue fluid culture. After an incubation period of 4–5 days, infectious red blisters which are itchy and sore appear on the lips or skin. These heal after 7–10 days. The vesicles are treated using acyclovir creams or ointments (see herpes zoster, below). Reactivation of the latent virus is often preceded by tingling sensations

Box 12.7 Classification of warts

- **Common warts:** hyperkeratotic nodules occurring on the hands and feet of children. These often resolve spontaneously
- **Plane warts:** smooth flat-topped warts appearing on the face and hands
- **Plantar warts:** commonly known as veruccae where the papilloma virus is pressured into the dermis, creating a callus. The commonest sites are the feet
- **Genital warts:** a mass of warts with a cauliflower-like appearance present on the perianal and genital areas.

in the affected areas. Sufferers must avoid kissing, sharing food utensils and sexual contact (if genitalia are involved) while the herpes virus is active. Care must be taken to wash the hands after touching vesicles.

Eczema herpeticum. This is a cutaneous infection caused by the herpes simplex virus. Patients with atopic eczema commonly develop this condition as a primary or recurrent infection. The vesicles of herpes simplex erupt on the face, neck and trunk and are initially confined to the eczematous skin. The skin will be tender and painful with developing purulent lesions due to staphylococcal infection. A primary episode of eczema herpeticum runs a self-limiting course resolving in 2–6 weeks. Mild localised forms are treated with topical acyclovir. In a severe episode acyclovir will be administered intravenously. Any impetiginisation of the lesions will be treated by oral antibiotics. Nursing advice to patients with atopic eczema should be to seek active therapy if they develop cold sores or are in contact with people who have cold sores. Topical or oral acyclovir should be held in reserve at home to treat any developing lesions promptly.

Herpes zoster (shingles)

Herpes zoster is an acute localised infection caused by the varicella zoster virus. During childhood it manifests as chickenpox, after which the virus remains dormant in the sensory root ganglion of the spinal cord. The chickenpox infection is transmitted by direct contact and is also thought to be airborne. Herpes zoster is caused by a reactivation of the virus and is prevalent in elderly people and in immunosuppressed patients.

PATHOPHYSIOLOGY

Once reactivated the virus multiplies by invading host cells and utilising the replicatory mechanisms of the host cell to produce new DNA . The cell is lysed and virus particles are released to invade another cell. The virus particles migrate along the nerve fibres (dermatome) towards the skin surface, causing nerve damage and consequent pain. 'Balloon degeneration of the prickle cell layer of the epidermis results in the formation of vesicles ' (Gawkrodger 1993).

Common presenting symptoms are pain, fever and general malaise. These symptoms precede the eruption of vesicles along a thoracic or cranial dermatome in a characteristic unilateral band-like distribution. Fluid from the vesicles is infected with virus particles. Once the vesicles crust over they become less infectious and separate from the skin within 2 to 3 weeks.

MEDICAL MANAGEMENT

Diagnosis is confirmed by viral cultures and clinical history. Treatment is by acyclovir, which inhibits replication of the virus. Oral or i.v. acyclovir will be used depending on the severity of the disease process.

Possible complications of herpes zoster are

- disseminated herpes zoster
- post-herpetic neuralgia
- herpes zoster ophthalmicus
- Ramsay Hunt's syndrome — facial paralysis with otalgia and eruptions in the skin of the external ear and auricle.

NURSING PRIORITIES AND MANAGEMENT: SHINGLES

Major considerations

In an acute attack of shingles hospitalisation with source isolation of the patient is desirable. Assessment of the patient will highlight the priorities in care. Nursing staff should pay particular attention to hospital disinfection policies until the infectious period resolves.

Pain relief is a priority as the pain of shingles is excruciating and unrelenting. Increasing pain and itch can precede recrudescence of the disease. Rest and quiet within the ward will aid recovery; visitors, while encouraged, should be advised to make short visits. The patient should ideally be nursed by seropositive staff in order to contain nosocomial infection (Krasinski et al 1986). Topical therapy in the form of acyclovir cream will be applied regularly to affected skin.

Certain groups of people are particularly susceptible to the transmission of herpes zoster, and the clinical nurse should be aware of those at risk. These are patients having radiotherapy and / or chemotherapy, immunocompromised patients on oral or topical steroids, and people under any form of stress.

Community nursing staff need to be aware of the long-term problems associated with shingles. A small proportion of patients report persistent pain (post-herpetic neuralgia) continuing for many years. Chronic pain will have a major impact on daily living and requires full assessment. Treatment options available for post-herpetic neuralgia include transcutaneous electrical nerve stimulation (TENS), ultrasound, and antidepressants and / or anticonvulsant therapy (Galer & Portenoy 1991). Referral to a pain control clinic is advisable for the patient with intractable pain (see Ch. 19).

BULLOUS DISORDERS

The term 'bullous disorders' covers those skin conditions in which large watery blisters (bullae) arising within or immediately under the epidermis are a presenting feature (Hunter et al 1989). There are many causes of bullae (see Fig. 12.8). Histological location of the bullae will influence the classification of the disorder.

Early detection and treatment are essential, as many of the bullous conditions are severe and potentially life-threatening. The toxic effect of therapy in itself may prove fatal.

This section will highlight the bullous conditions most commonly encountered.

Pemphigus (intraepidermal bullae)

PATHOPHYSIOLOGY

This is an autoimmune disease occurring in adults. It is characterised

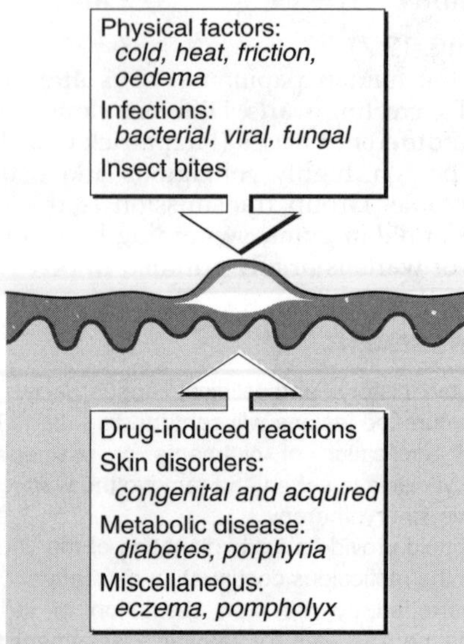

Fig. 12.8 Causes of blisters (bullae).

by the development of auto-antibodies against epidermal cell surface molecules creating superficial erosions and blisters on epidermal and mucosal surfaces (MacKie 1991).

Common presenting symptoms. The main presenting feature is the presence of superficial fluid-filled blisters within the epidermis. The patient often presents with oral lesions, with involvement of the skin developing later. These blisters are flaccid, thin-roofed and offer little resistance; consequently they shear, leaving raw, denuded skin. Pain from the exposed sites is a major factor in management.

Clinical diagnosis is confirmed by a positive Nikolsky's sign, in which when lateral pressure is applied on the skin surface with a thumb, the epidermis shears and appears to slide over the dermis (MacKie 1991).

Pemphigoid (sub-epidermal bullae)

PATHOPHYSIOLOGY

This is a common condition among elderly people; 80% of patients presenting are usually aged 60 and over (Graham, Brown & Burns 1990). Like pemphigus, pemphigoid is an autoimmune disease. Antibodies bind to the junction between the dermis and epidermis, and blisters are formed in response to enzymes released from inflammatory cells.

Common presenting symptoms. The patient reports generalised intense itch, followed by erythematous plaques on the skin (pre-pemphigoid stage), followed by the development of tense blisters affecting any area of the body. Nikolsky's sign is negative.

Toxic epidermal necrolysis (sub-epidermal)

PATHOPHYSIOLOGY

This condition presents as a dermatological emergency and is often precipitated by a drug hypersensitivity. The skin split is sub-epidermal and the entire dermis shears off in layers, leaving raw, denuded areas. A review of the patient's drug therapy and removal of the causative factor is essential to management.

Common presenting symptoms. The skin is erythrodermic and painful, with the skin shearing off in sheets. Nikolsky's sign is positive. The patient will be distressed by pain, and may have erosions in the mouth, oesophagus and bronchus.

MEDICAL MANAGEMENT OF BULLOUS DISORDERS

Early diagnosis is imperative due to the life-threatening potential of bullous disorders. Hospitalisation is a major aspect of treatment and management.

Investigative procedures will include the following:

1. Skin biopsy: to identify the type of skin split and exclude differential diagnoses
2. Blood tests: to monitor urea and electrolytes in view of the associated fluid loss from the eroded skin. In pemphigus the serum contains antibodies binding to the intracellular areas of the epidermis; titration of these antibodies is relevant to building a picture of the disease activity
3. Skin swab: to define the bacteriological status of exposed skin to secondary infection.

Drug therapy will involve treatment with the following systemic drugs:

1. Antibiotics. These are necessary for controlling secondary infection as indicated by the results of skin swab examination
2. Steroids. In pemphigus and pemphigoid, high-dose oral steroids (prednisolone 60–100 mg daily) will be the first line of management and will be maintained until the blistering stops. A gradual reduction in dosage will then be commenced, aiming for low-dose maintenance therapy
3. Analgesics. These will be a priority to alleviate pain from eroded skin lesions and may range from paracetamol to opiates, depending on the patient's needs and on disease activity
4. Antihistamines such as trimeprazine and terfenadine will be prescribed to reduce itch
5. Immunosuppressants such as cyclophosphamide and azathioprine are used in combination with oral steroids to control the disease process of pemphigus and pemphigoid.

Other interventions include plasmapheresis, which is considered only in severe cases, and allows monitoring of circulating pemphigus antibodies. Topical therapy is non-specific, aiming for patient comfort. It is discussed along with nursing management, below.

NURSING PRIORITIES AND MANAGEMENT: BULLOUS DISORDERS

This section focuses on general nursing care of the three disorders described above. Although rare conditions, they are commonly seen in dermatology units. It may assist the reader in understanding the rationale behind nursing priorities to bear in mind that these patients have needs which are similar to those of patients with severe burn injuries (see Ch. 31). The nurse's role in giving reassurance, careful explanation and psychological support to the patient and his family will be essential in promoting a partnership in care.

Major nursing considerations

Analgesia

The nurse can make an important contribution to care by ensuring that analgesia is effective and consistent. Pemphigus and toxic epidermal necrolysis are distressing, painful conditions when shearing of the skin is active. Pain assessment tools (see Ch. 19) will permit the nurse and patient together to determine pain control needs, ensure accurate delivery of analgesics, and evaluate their efficacy. This is particularly relevant prior to dressing changes.

Many hospitals have pain clinics which make expert help available to assist in prescribing appropriate analgesia by the most effective route for this type of pain.

Bedrest

Patients must rest to avoid further trauma to the skin. Special beds which are helpful in nursing patients with these conditions are described on page 460.

Hygiene

The maintenance of good personal hygiene and the prevention of crossinfection are extremely important. Gentle washing or the application of soaks, i.e. potassium permanganate, for their mild antiseptic/antipruritic effect can be soothing and will help to minimise further trauma.

Isolation nursing may be necessary due to skin loss. The patient will be susceptible to infection, and the use of immunosuppressants will increase this susceptibility. In severe cases barrier nursing may be required.

Diet

Approximately 20% of an adult's dietary protein is used for skin repair and growth in normal health (Hinchliff & Montague 1988). Therefore, an increased intake of dietary protein is advisable in bullous conditions. Referral to a hospital dietitian will ensure the prescription of any necessary supplements. Constipation induced by fluid loss, or as a side-effect of analgesia, is an associated problem. A mild laxative may be indicated to prevent added discomfort.

Monitoring vital signs

Temperature. Body temperature may vary as a result of loss of fluid and heat from the skin, and so regular observations must be maintained. Variations in environmental temperature can be reduced by nursing the patient in a sideroom.

Blood-pressure should be checked regularly due to associated fluid loss, rehydration by i.v. fluids and steroid-induced hypertension.

Monitoring electrolyte and fluid balance

This is imperative in any condition associated with skin loss. Rehydration may initially be achievable by increasing the patient's oral intake and monitoring output. An i.v. infusion will be appropriate in severe cases. If skin loss presents problems in siting a peripheral infusion, a central line can be inserted. In such a case, monitoring of central venous pressure will be wholly accurate as an assessment of fluid requirements.

Urinalysis. After the initial admission check, urinalysis should be continued to monitor for a potential diabetic state induced by oral steroid therapy.

Dressings and topical therapy

A dressing procedure provides the best opportunity for the nurse to complete a skin assessment and evaluate disease activity. In pemphigus and toxic epidermal necrolysis, raw areas are recorded and dressed. The tense bullae of pemphigoid are identified and must be left intact to permit reabsorption of blister fluid, thereby minimising further trauma.

Blisters restricting movement are uncomfortable for the patient and can be aspirated using a sterile alcohol swab, syringe and needle, leaving the blister roof intact (Stone et al 1989). The administration of analgesics prior to the application of topical therapy is important to reduce the patient's apprehensions about dressing changes. The individual patient's needs and disease severity will determine dressing requirements, but the main aims of management must be:

- to keep dressing changes to a minimum
- to maximise patient comfort
- to ensure dressings are easily removable.

By following these guidelines, the nurse will reduce further trauma and promote healing of the skin. Simple applications of a soothing emollient or a paraffin gauze dressing (Jelonet) secured by a gauze stockinette (Tubifast) will possibly be all that is tolerated. Heavier pads and bandaging will create constriction and pain. The skilled practitioner will be guided by the patient's comments and adjust dressings appropriately.

Special beds

Creating rest and comfort is a primary aim in care, and the use of special beds has revolutionised dermatological nursing practice. Low-pressure, air-fluidised beds (i.e. Clinitron) remove the need for positional changes which contribute to shearing forces on the skin. The temperature regulator in these beds maintains an appropriately warm environment, helping the patient to maintain body temperature. Dressings can be kept to a minimum and remain moist with the use of these beds, and so tend to be easily removed.

Care in the community

Although these conditions are rare, as our elderly population increases, their occurrence will become more common. The community nurse has a dual role. Firstly, she is able to identify these disorders and to coordinate the referral of the patient for specialist help. After the patient's discharge from hospital, the community nurse plays a supportive role in ensuring that the patient understands the rationale behind long-term maintenance drug therapy, thereby encouraging compliance; she will also monitor for side-effects of systemic therapies.

DISORDERS OF SEBACEOUS AND APOCRINE GLANDS

The two disorders of this type most commonly encountered are acne and rosacea.

Acne (see Fig. 12.9)

Acne is a disorder of the pilosebaceous glands. Many factors combine to cause this condition.

PATHOPHYSIOLOGY

During puberty increased levels of male hormone stimulate excess sebum production causing the pilosebaceous glands to produce increased amounts of abnormal keratin. This creates a plug, forming either 'blackhead' or 'whitehead' spots. Colonisation of the blocked glands by *Propionibacterium acnes* (a normal skin commensal) of the duct precipitates an inflammatory reaction. Diet plays no major role in the development of acne.

Common presenting symptoms include the presence of blackheads (comedones), whiteheads, papules, pustules, cysts and residual scarring of lesions.

MEDICAL MANAGEMENT

The medical management of acne varies according to the severity of the condition.

Mild acne. Antiseptic washes.

Moderate acne. Benzoyl peroxide gels and lotions are used as an antimicrobial. Topical antibiotics and Tretinoin a vitamin A derivative, create a combination therapy.

Severe acne. A prolonged course of low-dose systemic antibiotics, e.g. erythromycin can be beneficial. Women with hormonal imbalance can be treated with systemic hormones, e.g. cyproterone acetate with ethinyloestrodiol.

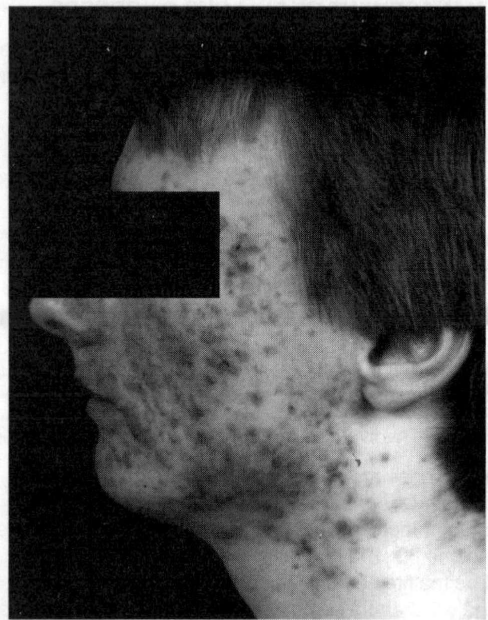

Fig. 12.9 Acne.

Severe cystic or nodular acne can respond to a potent systemic drug, e.g. isotretinoin (Roaccutane).

NURSING PRIORITIES AND MANAGEMENT: ACNE

The nurse should endeavour to identify the social and psychological problems experienced by the acne sufferer. She should give practical advice on basic skin hygiene and advise the individual to avoid heavy applications of cosmetics to disguise the problem. She should emphasise that any prescribed lotion will require regular, meticulous application over a number of weeks before improvement will be apparent, and that causing mechanical irritation by squeezing or scratching should be avoided to reduce residual scarring.

Female patients of childbearing age prescribed isotretinoin (Roaccutane) for severe acne must be advised to use an effective contraceptive for 1 month before treatment, during treatment and for 3 months afterwards in view of the teratogenic effect of the drug.

> ? **12.4** You are asked to provide a series of health talks for a group of high-school students. Acne is one of the topics requested. Devise a plan for your talk with relevant aims for this age group. Consider answers to some of the questions you may be asked on diet, cosmetics, infection and social impact.

Rosacea

Rosacea is a chronic acneform inflammation of the pilosebaceous glands in combination with an increased reactivity of the capillaries to heat, creating a 'flushing' effect. The term 'rosacea' derives from the Latin, 'like roses'.

The condition affects both sexes in the 30–50-year age group but tends to be predominant among women. It is thought to be less frequent in pigmented races (Fitzpatrick et al 1992).

PATHOPHYSIOLOGY

The dermal capillary dilatation gives a shiny, erythematous appearance to the facial skin. Sebum production is normal despite a sebaceous gland hyperplasia.

Common presenting symptoms. The patient complains of frequent flushing which eventually becomes a chronic erythema. In severe cases, evidence of telangiectases, pustules and papules helps to confirm the diagnosis. The nose can become bulbous and swollen; a condition known as rhinophyma.

MEDICAL MANAGEMENT

Microscopic examination will reveal inflammatory cells and lymphoedema (Gawkrodger 1993). The absence of comedones and whiteheads will distinguish the condition from acne. Topical therapies will include metronidazole in combination with oral antibiotics such as tetracycline and erythromycin.

NURSING PRIORITIES AND MANAGEMENT: ROSACEA

Once a diagnosis is confirmed, nursing management will involve supporting the patient in self-treatment. As facial flushing will worsen as a skin response to heat stimuli in the mouth, the patient can be advised to avoid hot drinks or spicy food. It is also a good idea to avoid alcohol, as its vasodilating effect will exacerbate flushing. Although rosacea is not a photosensitivity, the patient should be advised to avoid direct sunlight by the use of sunscreens, hats, and so forth until the condition resolves. Social distress caused by rhinophyma can be successfully treated by surgery (Fitzpatrick et al 1992). As the course of the disease may be prolonged, ongoing support is essential, particularly during recurrences. In some patients the disease resolves spontaneously after a number of years.

PHOTODERMATOSES

This term applies to a group of skin disorders which are induced or aggravated by sunlight. Most of these conditions are uncommon, but when they do occur they can impose severe limitations on daily life.

This section will highlight specific conditions and briefly describe diagnostic techniques and the treatment options which are available. The discussion of nursing management will focus on assisting the patient to maintain independent living within the limitations imposed by a photosensitivity.

Sunlight

Sunlight is composed of ultraviolet A + B and visible light. Ultraviolet light B (UVB) is responsible for sunburn. Ultraviolet light A (UVA) produces erythema in larger doses, passes through window glass, and is less variable in intensity. Visible light has longer wavelengths and easily penetrates the epidermis with minimal significance. Some conditions, however, demonstrate a sensitivity to visible light.

Certain factors affect the intensity of sunlight, i.e.:

- time of day
- geography
- season
- reflective effect of snow, water, sand.

It should be noted that clouds do not protect against sunburn, as UVB penetrates through cloud cover.

Types of photodermatosis

PATHOPHYSIOLOGY

Polymorphic light eruption. This common photodermatosis presents as itch or burning on exposure to sunlight immediately or within a few hours. The erythema and rash can be mild or severe.

Solar urticaria. This uncommon condition presents as urticaria and erythema after sunlight exposure. The symptoms fade 3–4 hours after initial exposure.

Photo-aggravated dermatoses. Some pre-existing skin conditions are described as photo-aggravated when exacerbations are triggered in patients on exposure to sunlight, e.g. atopic eczema, psoriasis, herpes simplex.

Photo-contact dermatitis. This term refers to disorders in which direct contact of the skin with a substance (e.g. tars, sunscreens) followed by exposure to ultraviolet light initiates a dermatitis. Certain genetic disorders e.g. xeroderma pigmentosum also produce a photosensitive reaction.

Photosensitive dermatitis/actinic reticuloid syndrome (see Case History 12.2). This syndrome describes patients who have contact dermatitis, photo-contact dermatitis and photosensitivity. It is the commonest form of cutaneous photosensitivity, affecting predominantly men (20:1) in the late age group (Frain-Bell 1986). Symptoms arise as a major pruritus, with erythema affecting exposed sites, predominantly the face, neck and hands a few hours after exposure to sunlight.

Case History 12.2 Mr L

Mr L is a 70-year-old gentleman admitted to hospital with a facial and hand dermatitis. This started as a minor reaction but has become gradually worse over the past few years. His hobbies include gardening and walking. He is very aware that sunlight appears to aggravate the condition.

Phototesting is carried out and confirms that he has a marked sensitivity to sunlight. Patch testing produces an allergic response to numerous plants that he comes into contact with in his garden, e.g. chrysanthemums and dahlias. In combination with the clinical picture this provides a diagnosis of photosensitive dermatitis/actinic reticuloid syndrome.

The treatment programme planned after assessment includes:

- use of a bland emollient to cleanse the skin
- careful explanation of the meticulous use of a prescribed sunscreen for all exposed sites, i.e. face, neck and hands
- education on how to use a topical steroid when the dermatitis is active, that is starting with a strong/medium cream and reducing the strength gradually over a few days as the skin improves
- advice on avoiding sun at its peak.

Avoidance of the material causing his allergic response is discussed with Mr L. He is not keen to give up gardening but will be cautious and protect his skin where possible. He does agree, however, to remove plants from his house to avoid potential problems. The social worker visits him to discuss the possibility of grants to pay to have his house (windows and garden shed) screened with yellow sunscreens.

Mr L is discharged once his investigations are completed. An outcome assessment confirms that he understands his diagnosis and feels confident about self-treatment. Phototesting will be repeated yearly to review Mr L's light sensitivity, and any appropriate changes to his therapy will be made at these times.

MEDICAL MANAGEMENT

Medical management will begin with a full medical history and an assessment of the factors and presenting symptoms relevant to diagnosis (see Box 12.8).

Investigative procedures. Diagnosis is specified by phototesting and patch testing.

Phototesting provides an objective assessment of photosensitive disorders and is available only in specialist photobiology/dermatology units. The patient's back is used as a test site and small areas are exposed to varying doses of light, after which the erythemic reaction is assessed. This reaction is compared to the known response of a control group, and helps to determine the degree of photosensitivity and the wavelengths of light to which the patient is sensitive.

Patch testing. In combination with phototesting, patch testing is carried out to determine specific contact allergies. Many patients demonstrate multiple allergy responses which are relevant to diagnosis and subsequent management.

Box 12.8 Influencing factors and common presenting symptoms of photosensitive conditions

INFLUENCING FACTORS

- Drug history
- Family history
- Hobbies
- Known allergies
- Occupation
- Sites involved
- Skin type

COMMON PRESENTING SYMPTOMS

- Eczema
- Erythema
- Heat
- Itch
- Oedema
- Pain
- Urticaria

Medical intervention involves systemic and topical therapy as well as UVB/PUVA therapy. Drug therapy can include antihistamines, immunosuppressants and both oral and topical steroids. Sunscreen creams offer a sun protection factor (SPF) either by chemically absorbing and filtering ultraviolet light or by physically reflecting and scattering ultraviolet rays to protect the skin. A combination sunscreen cream creates an effective block.

Some light-sensitive conditions (e.g. polymorphic light eruption) respond to a programme of desensitisation, in which the patient is given a short controlled course of light therapy (UVB/PUVA) to thicken and pigment the skin. This does not effect a cure, however, and must be repeated yearly.

NURSING PRIORITIES AND MANAGEMENT: PHOTODERMATOSES

Giving practical support

Patients with diagnosed photosensitive disorders require practical and supportive help from nursing practitioners. Many patients are relieved that investigation has produced a concrete diagnosis rather than a dismissal of symptoms as merely 'a bit of sunburn'. Factual information from nursing staff is vital if the patient is to cope with the changes in lifestyle imposed by a photodermatosis.

General advice to the patient should cover the following topics:

- meticulous, regular applications of prescribed sunscreen to exposed areas
- treatment with a reducing steroid cream regime if the condition flares
- avoidance of sun at its peak (10 a.m. to 4 p.m.)
- careful choice of clothing to provide further effective barrier to sunlight. (In severe cases: hat, scarf, gloves — even in summer.)

Giving psychological support

Social isolation is a major problem for individuals with severe photosensitive disorders. Many patients, distressed by their diagnosis and the restrictions it entails, reject management regimes, finding the maintenance of topical therapies to be time consuming, messy and cosmetically unacceptable. Others stoically accept the limitations and persevere with the use of sunscreens to permit them freedom to continue a restricted form of daily living.

The nurse must display a sympathetic understanding of the psychological trauma associated with the restrictions imposed by the diagnosis of a photosensitive disorder. The overall aim of nursing support should be for the patient to control management in an informed and motivated manner, with instant access to professional help as needed.

AIDS AND DERMATOLOGY (See Ch. 38)

Patients with acquired immunodeficiency caused by the human immunodeficiency virus (HIV) will often require dermatological help. Treatment of recurrent infections such as thrush, warts, etc. and prophylactic therapy to prevent recurrences of herpes infections can alleviate distressing problems for the patient.

The clinical nurse should be aware of patients in her care who may fall into the 'at risk' category. Persistent susceptibility to skin infections in an 'at risk' patient might alert the practitioner to consider the possibility of HIV/AIDS. If indicated, the nurse can initiate counselling and eventual testing for the patient.

Kaposi's sarcoma

Kaposi's sarcoma is a malignant tumour of the capillary endothelium and manifests as multiple bruising on the skin. The sarcoma presents in patients with and without AIDS, and does respond to chemotherapy and radiotherapy. The role of the nurse in identifying susceptible patients and then supporting them through counselling and testing is as important as the practical skills of skin care.

SKIN TUMOURS

A wide variety of tumours, both benign and malignant, can arise in the epidermis and dermis (MacKie 1991). These include squamous cell carcinoma, basal cell carcinoma and malignant melanoma (see Box 12.9).

These disorders are treated with a variety of therapies specific to the location of the tumour. The nurse's primary role is to alert patients to attend for diagnosis if a skin lesion develops or changes in any way. If a lesion changes shape, size or colour and becomes elevated, itchy or bleeds, referral to the GP for assessment is desirable. Skin biopsy or excision of the lesion will aid in defining the histology of the lesion and in planning specific therapy.

The skilled nursing practitioner will also be alert to the skin manifestations of systemic disorders, i.e. cutaneous lymphomas/mycosis fungoides. Early detection will be important to the outcome of treatment, and nurses carrying out basic hygiene with patients must consider themselves at the forefront of skin assessment and detection of abnormalities.

See also Beck Prigel (1987), Apelgren (1992) and Fenton (1992), as well as Chapter 32 of the present text.

CONCLUSION

This chapter has focused on the more common skin conditions encountered in community and hospital settings. Reference to a specialist dermatology textbook will be of further interest and reveal the full scope of dermatology as a major speciality.

In this area of care, the bond created between patient and nurse may develop over a number of years, due to the variable remissions and exacerbations of dermatological disorders. The importance of the nurse's counselling and teaching role has been emphasised; the value of practical advice in coping strategies must not be underestimated, for it is this background support which often motivates a patient to comply with treatment (Noble 1991).

Advice leaflets that reinforce verbal instruction given at clinic or treatment sessions can be very helpful. Many patients leave a clinic or GP appointment totally bewildered by the array of ointments that has been prescribed. Advice pamphlets pertinent to the patient's needs to be read quietly at home will reinforce treatment instructions and help to ensure compliance in treatment.

In skin disorders, maintenance therapy is a fundamental component of care requiring a meticulous, time-consuming, restrictive pattern of life. Skin care programmes should be practical and flexible, to fit around the individual's needs. Realistic goals should be set to generate a positive outlook and raise the patient's self-esteem. In planning care the unique and complex needs of the individual and his family must be sensitively assessed to ensure the best possible prognosis for each individual.

Box 12.9 Sunlight and malignant melanoma

Sunbathing is a 20th-century phenomenon of Western society; one which would have baffled our forefathers and is nonsensical to our contemporaries in hotter countries. In bygone days a suntan was associated with poverty and undesirable outdoor work. The peoples of India, Africa and the hotter parts of Asia have long recognised that excessive sunlight is damaging to the body. It is interesting to note that sunbathing is effectively illegal in the British Army, where to be incapacitated by sunburn is an offence against military discipline.

Underlying the problem of sunbathing is the ultraviolet light content of sunlight, which damages genetic material and can cause skin cancer. Under the influence of ultraviolet light a genetic mutation can take place in the melanocytes, the cells containing melanin pigment, which leads to excessive growth and division and formation of a tumour (or 'melanoma'). The incidence of melanoma worldwide has been increasing at a significant rate despite a decrease in the incidence of other skin cancers. This is probably due to the year-round promotion of 'healthy tans' in travel brochures, consumer magazines and by tanning studios.

The susceptibility to melanoma shows racial variation, with the darker-skinned races being less susceptible and, within races, fairer-skinned people more susceptible. That sunlight is responsible for the incidence of melanoma can be deduced from the fact that there is an association between this form of cancer and geographical latitude, which in turn is directly related to the intensity of sunlight. It is also apparent that the longer a person resides in a sunny climate, the more susceptible he will be to melanoma. A complicating factor is that city dwellers show a higher incidence of melanoma than people in rural areas.

Any sudden change in pigmented areas of the body such as growth and darkening of moles can be indicative of melanoma and should be investigated. The best way to avoid melanoma is to avoid the sun. Sun-hats, 'modest' clothing, and creams which absorb ultraviolet light can all provide an effective barrier. Ultimately, however, a change in our perception of what is healthy-looking and attractive skin will have the greatest influence.

GLOSSARY

Atopy. A clinical hypersensitivity state.
Comedone. 'Blackhead': a sebum plug which occupies the hair follicle.
Emollients. Agents that soften and soothe skin.
Erythroderma. Abnormal redness of skin over widespread areas of body.
Excoriation. Abrasions.
Exfoliation. Shedding of tissue in layers.
Infestation. The presence of animal parasites in or on the human body.
Macules. Non-palpable localised area of change in skin colour.
Nodules. A small node or swelling.
Papules. Small circumscribed elevation of the skin.
Plaque. Patch or flat area.
Pruritus. Itching.
Pustules. Small inflammatory swellings containing pus.
Recrudescence. Return of symptoms.
Telangiectasis. Dilatation of capillaries on a body surface.
Vesicles. Skin blisters.
Weal. Localised area of oedema, accompanied by itching.
Xeroderma pigmentosum. A familial dermatosis caused by photosensitisation.

REFERENCES

Althoft D C 1983 Psoriatic arthritis. Orthopaedic Nursing 2(5): 50

Apelgren J 1992 Pale is beautiful: skin cancer. Nursing Times 88(25): 24–26

Champion R H 1992 Textbook of dermatology. Blackwell Scientific, Oxford

Erdash M T 1983 A matter of skin. Psoriasis Nursing 2(9): 257–262

Fenton D 1992 Safe in the sun. Nursing Times 88(25): 27–28

Finlay A Y, Edwards P H, Harding K G 1989 'Fingertip unit' in dermatology. Lancet 2: 155

Fitzpatrick T, Johnson R, Polano M, Suurmond D, Wolff K 1992 Colour atlas and synopsis of clinical dermatology, 2nd edn. McGraw-Hill, New York

Frain-Bell W 1986 The photodermatoses. In: Vickers C F H (ed) Modern management of common skin diseases. Churchill Livingstone, Edinburgh

Galer G, Portenoy R 1991 Acute herpetic and post herpetic neuralgia: clinical features and management. The Mount Sinai Journal of Medicine 58(3): 257–265

Gawkrodger D J 1993 Dermatology: an illustrated colour text. Churchill Livingstone, Edinburgh

Graham-Brown R, Burns T 1990 Lecture notes on dermatology, 6th edn. Blackwell Scientific, Oxford

Hinchliff S, Montague S 1988 Physiology for nursing practice. Baillière Tindall, London

Hunter J A A, Savin J A, Dahl M V 1989 Clinical dermatology. Blackwell Scientific, Oxford

Krasinski K, Holzman R S, La Couvre R N, Forman M D 1986 Hospital experience with varicella zoster virus. Infection Control 7(6): 312–316

MacKie R M 1991 Clinical dermatology: an illustrated textbook, 3rd edn. Oxford Medical, Oxford

Noble C 1991 Are nurses good patient educators? Journal of Advanced Nursing (16): 1185–1189

Psoriasis Association 1992 Patient Journal 2 Psoriasis Association, Northampton

Stankler L 1981 The effect of psoriasis on the sufferer. Clinical and Experimental Dermatology (6): 303–306

Stone L A, Lindfield E M, Robertson S J 1989 A colour atlas of nursing procedures in skin disorders. Wolfe, London

Williams R 1985 PUVA therapy vs. Goekerman therapy in the treatment of psoriasis. Physiotherapy Canada 37(6): 361–366

Wilson K J W (ed) 1990 Ross & Wilson anatomy and physiology in health and illness, 7th edn. Churchill Livingstone, Edinburgh

FURTHER READING

Alderman C 1990 Whose skin is it anyway? Nursing Standard 11(4): 26–27

Beck Prigel C L 1987 How to spot melanoma. Nursing 17(6): 60–62

Cameron I H, McGuire C 1990 Are you dying to get a sun-tan: the pre and post campaign survey results. Health Education Journal 49(4): 166–170

Clarke A 1991 Nurses as role models and health educators. Journal of Advanced Nursing (16): 1178–1184

Cunliffe W, Patel F 1988 Learning to live with acne: a handbook for patients. Mediscript, London

Dolezal R, Cohen M, Schultz C 1985 Use of Clinitron therapy in immediate post operative care of pressure ulcers. Annals of Plastic Surgery 14(1): 33–36

Fenton D 1992 Safe in the sun. Nursing Times 88(25): 27–28

Graham-Brown R, Burns T 1990 Benign and malignant skin tumours. Lecture notes on dermatology, 6th edn. Blackwell, Oxford Ch. 9, pp. 109–130

Harper J 1991 Coping with eczema: an information booklet for parents. Oakleaf Press, London

Libbus K 1982 Psoriasis and body image. Nursing Practitioner 7(4): 15–18

Lowe J G 1993 The stigma of acne. British Journal of Hospital Medicine 49(11): 809–812

Marrz D 1991 Motivation: the key to control. Professional Nurse 7(2): 103–108

Patel F, Burns D 1989 Learning to live with psoriasis: a handbook for patients and family. Mediscript, London

Patchett T 1991 Achieving a competitive edge: an assessment of the cost effectiveness of Clinitron therapy. Professional Nurse reprint. Wolfe, London

Updike J 1990 Self consciousness memoirs. Penguin Books Harmondsworth

USEFUL ADDRESSES

Acne Support Group
16 Dufour Place
Broadwick Street
London W1V 1FE

British Dermatology Nursing Group
3 St Andrew's Place
Regents Park
London NW1 4LB

National Eczema Society
4 Tavistock House East
Tavistock Square
London WC1H 9SR

The Psoriasis Association
Milton House
7 Milton Street
Northampton NN2 7JG

The Dystrophic Epidermolysis Bullosa Research Association (DEBRA)
1 King's Road
Crowthorne
Berkshire RG11 7BG

CHAPTER 13

Disorders of the eye

Ruth Gardner Margaret A. Studley

CHAPTER CONTENTS

Introduction 467
Anatomy and physiology 468
Assessing the eye and visual function 470
Preservation of vision 473
The visually impaired person 473
DISORDERS OF THE EYE 474
Nursing priorities and management: general ophthalmic procedures 474
Nursing priorities and management: conditions requiring surgical intervention 475
PAINLESS LOSS OF VISION 477
Nursing priorities and management: cataract 478
Nursing priorities and management: POAG 480
Nursing priorities and management: retinal detachment 481
Nursing priorities and management: corneal grafting (keratoplasty) 482
Nursing priorities and management: temporal arteritis 483
RED EYE 483
Nursing priorities and management: PCAG 484
Nursing priorities and management: uveitis 484
Nursing priorities and management: keratitis 485
Herpes Zoster 485
Stye 486
DIPLOPIA (DOUBLE VISION) 486
EYE INJURIES 486
Nursing priorities and management: hyphaema 487
Nursing priorities and management: penetrating injury 488
Nursing priorities and management: chemical burns 488
Nursing priorities and management: radiation injuries 489
Minor eye injuries 489
SURGICAL REMOVAL OF AN EYE 490
AGE-RELATED CONDITIONS 492
Senile macular degeneration 492
Entropian 492
Ectropian 492
SYSTEMIC DISEASE 492
Nursing priorities and management: diabetic retinopathy 494
Nursing priorities and management: CVA 494
Hypertension 494
Nursing priorities and management: AIDS 495
Conclusion 495
References 495
Further reading 495
Useful addresses 496

INTRODUCTION

The aim of this chapter is to equip general and community nurses with a sound understanding of the causes and treatment of common eye disorders. It is also intended to raise awareness of the importance of vision to all activities of daily living and of the disabling effects, both physical and psychological, of visual impairment. In outlining the principles of ophthalmic nursing practice it also acknowledges the need for individualised care and encourages a patient-centred approach.

Although most serious ophthalmic disorders are treated in specialist hospitals, many conditions are encountered and treated in other contexts. The trend towards early discharge home and outpatient department treatment has resulted in the increasing involvement of community nurses in supporting, educating and caring for the perioperative patient and the patient with chronic or age-related eye conditions. In taking on this expanded role it is important for nurses in the community to be able to recognise adverse signs and symptoms and to provide early referral for specialised care.

Nurses in the community are also responsible for first aid and for health promotion and screening, and should bear in mind that the eye is a sensitive indicator of health and health breakdown. Many eye conditions are diagnostic of systemic disease and intercurrent with other conditions treated in medical, surgical, care of the elderly or ITU wards. A good ophthalmic knowledge base is therefore an essential component in preparation for practice.

Incidence of blindness

Although it is difficult to quantify the incidence of blindness in the world with any degree of accuracy it is estimated that it affects 27–35 million people. World Health Organization (WHO) statistics for 1969–80 indicate that 80% of blind people live in the developing countries and that there are approximately 20 million blind people in Asia and roughly 6 million in Africa. The risk of blindness in developing countries is 10–14 times higher than in developed countries, although it is estimated that about 80% of cases of blindness in poorer countries would be preventable given appropriate resources and improved environmental conditions (Riordan-Eva 1992).

The main causes of blindness worldwide include:

- cataract (opacity of the lens): the leading cause; responsible for about 50% of all blindness
- trachoma: corneal opacity caused by repeated infection of the cornea and conjunctiva by *Chlamydia trachomatis*
- glaucoma: raised intraocular pressure causing retinal and optic nerve damage

- xerophthalmia: dryness and ulceration of the cornea associated with vitamin A deficiency
- onchocerciasis: a microfilarial infestation transmitted by a fly; it can invade and eventually destroy all the structures of the eye, causing 'river blindness' (Perry & Tullo 1990).

In developed countries such as the UK, where the necessary resources are available, cataract extraction and lens implantation is a common surgical procedure which prevents all but a few people with cataracts from progressing to blindness (see p. 477). In these countries the main causes of blindness are senile macular degeneration and glaucoma, which so far are not preventable and are difficult to treat (Perry & Tullo 1990).

?	**13.1** Using library resources such as CD-ROM, investigate the present epidemiological trends in relation to blindness and its causes.

ANATOMY AND PHYSIOLOGY

The components of the sensory mechanisms responsible for sight are the eyes, the optic nerves and tracts, and the visual cortex and association areas of the brain.

Accessory structures play a vital role in enabling the eyes to scan and focus on objects in the environment and in protecting and maintaining the optical properties of the eyes.

The eye

The eyeball (see Fig. 13.1)

With minor individual variations the eyeball is spherical in shape, with the cornea on the anterior aspect being slightly more steeply curved. The adult eye is about 24 mm in diameter.

The eyeball or globe is a hollow structure composed of three main layers of tissue.

The outer layer of the globe consists of the fibrous white sclera posteriorly, and the transparent cornea anteriorly. The junction of the two is called the limbus. The cornea is transparent due to its avascularity and the regular arrangement of its fibres. It is well supplied with nerve endings.

The middle vascular layer, known as the uveal tract, consists of the choroid, the ciliary body and the iris. The choroid lines the sclera in the posterior compartment of the eye and continues into the muscular ciliary body, into which are inserted the suspensory ligaments. These ligaments extend to the lens and hold it in position. This diaphragm-like ligamentous structure is known as the zonule. The contraction and relaxation of the ciliary body changes the shape of the lens and controls its refractive and focusing power. The iris is the pigmented anterior portion of the uveal tract. It contains both circular and radial muscle fibres which control the size of the pupil.

The inner layer of the eyeball is the retina. It contains several million photoreceptive cells which are responsible for converting light into electrical impulses. The retina arises just behind the equator of the eyeball in an area known as the ora serrata. This leaves a small anterior section of the choroid, called the pars plana, exposed. This is important because it allows surgical access without retinal damage.

The retina consists of two layers: the pigmented outer layer, which lines the choroid; and the innermost neural layer, which is in contact with the vitreous humor. Rod cells predominate in the periphery and function best in dim light. Cone cells predominate near the centre of the retina and are adapted for bright light and colour vision. The greatest concentration of cone cells is at the macula, a small area in the centre of the retina which has as its midpoint the fovea centralis, the most vital part of the retina for high-definition vision. These photoreceptor cells are linked through a series of synapses to ganglion cells whose axons run together to form the optic nerve.

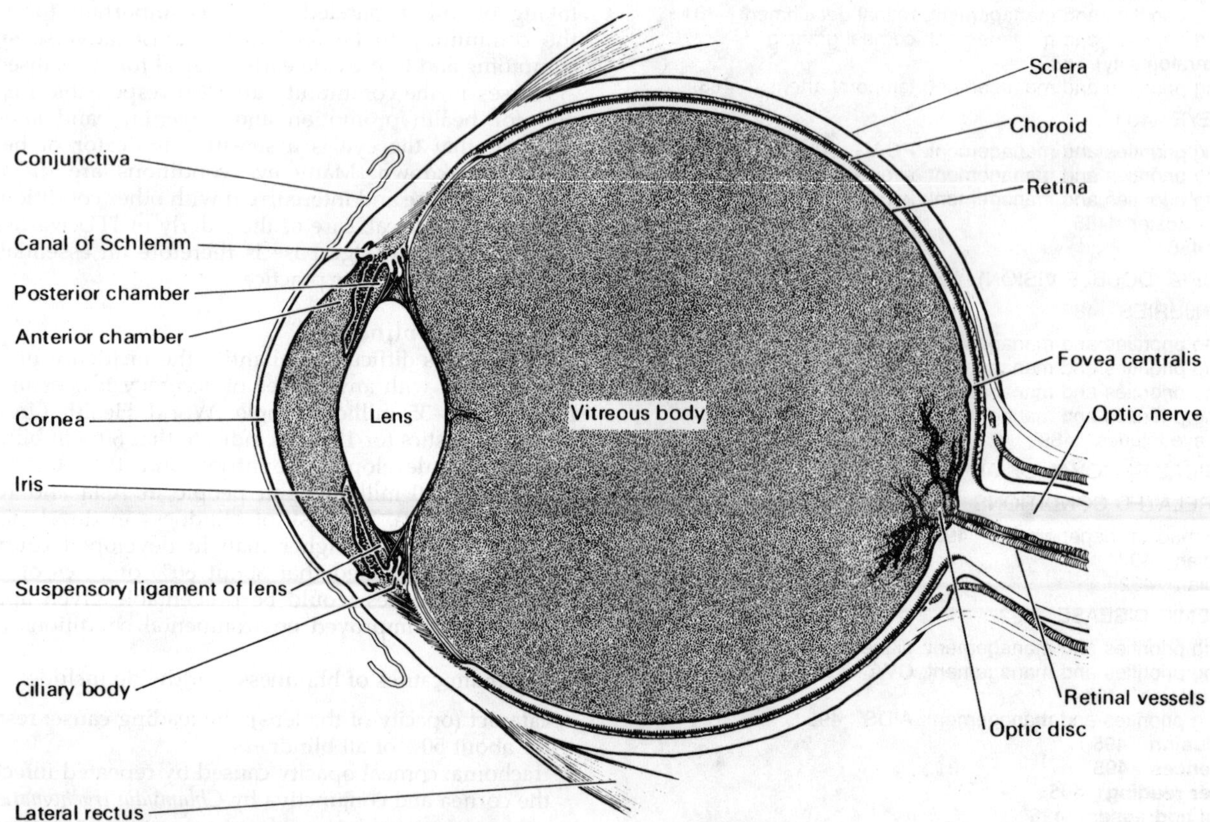

Fig. 13.1 Section through eyeball. (Reproduced with kind permission from Chilman & Thomas 1987.)

The two compartments and three chambers of the eye
Inside the globe the lens, suspended by the zonule, divides the eye into two main compartments. The anterior compartment is itself divided into two chambers: the anterior chamber in front of the iris and the posterior chamber behind the iris. The compartment behind the lens is sometimes referred to as the third chamber of the eye or the vitreous chamber, as it contains the clear jelly-like substance called the vitreous humor. The boundaries of each chamber are defined by the three tissue layers described above.

Internal environment and intraocular pressure (IOP). The anterior compartment is bathed in a clear fluid called the aqueous humor or, simply, aqueous, which is produced by the ciliary body and provides nutrients to the lens and cornea. Aqueous flows from the posterior chamber through the pupil to the anterior chamber and drains away through the sieve-like fibrous trabecular meshwork located in the angle between the iris and cornea around the circumference of the eye (see Fig. 13.2). This in turn drains into the vascular canal of Schlemm and thereby into the systemic venous circulation. The production and drainage of aqueous must be constant in order to maintain a normal IOP, which is variable over a 24 h period within the range of 12–20 mmHg (Perry & Tullo 1990).

The shape of the eye can, by determining the depth of the anterior chamber and the angle between the cornea and iris, affect the functioning of the drainage system. The larger, elongated eye of the myope has a naturally occurring deep anterior chamber with an open angle, whilst the small eye of the hypermetrope has a shallow anterior chamber with a closed angle. Any interference with normal production or drainage of the aqueous humor raises the IOP, leading to the decreased blood supply, pain and impaired vision associated with conditions such as glaucoma and postoperative or traumatic complications. IOP can be measured by tonometry (see Appendix 1).

The visual pathways and interpretative centres
The optic nerve runs from the posterior aspect of the globe and enters the cranial cavity via the optic foramen. The medial nerve fibres cross over to the opposite side at the optic chiasma (see Fig. 13.3) to join with the lateral fibres and form the optic tract before synapsing in the lateral geniculate body of the thalamus. From the lateral geniculate body the fibres run in the optic radiations to the occipital cerebral cortex of the brain.

The main blood supply to the eye is via the ophthalmic artery, a branch of the internal carotid artery which runs along the optic tract.

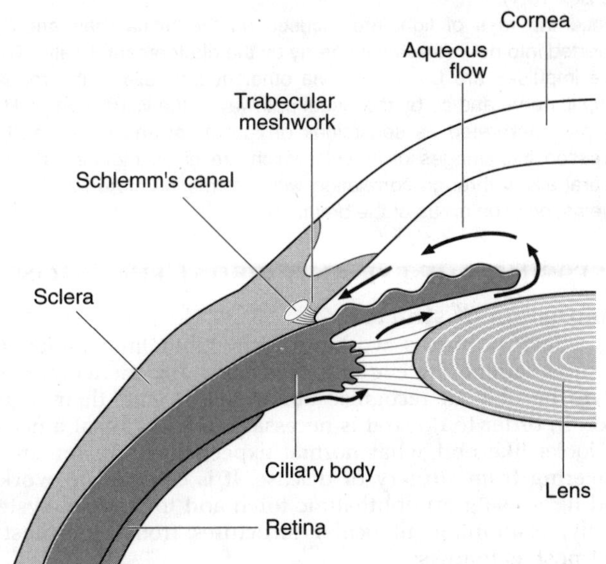

Fig. 13.2 Flow of aqueous humor from the posterior to anterior chamber of the eye.

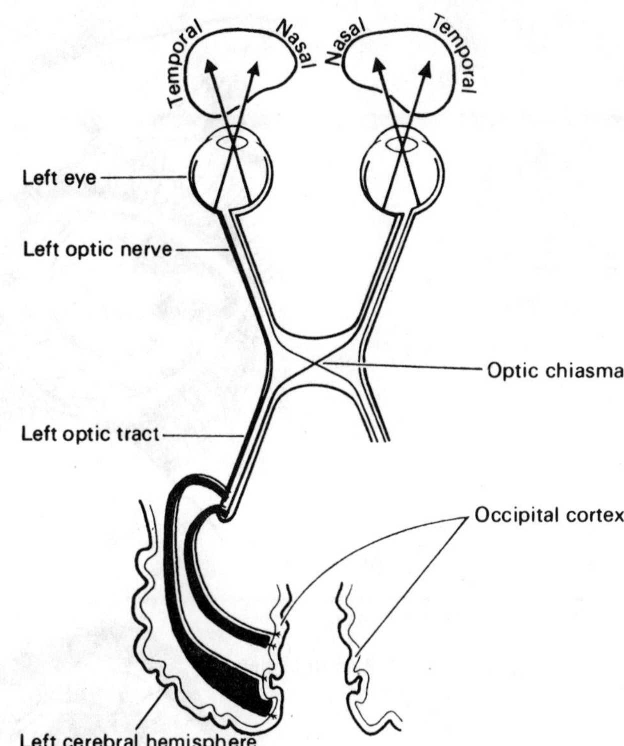

Fig. 13.3 The visual pathways from the eye. (Reproduced with kind permission from Chilman & Thomas 1987.)

Accessory structures
The exposed anterior aspect of the eyeball is protected by the eyebrow, eyelids and eyelashes. To facilitate free movement over the globe, the lids are lined with the conjunctiva, a mucous membrane which is reflected back on itself to cover the exposed sclera. This fold forms the conjunctival sac or fornix and is an ideal site for the instillation of topical drugs.

The exposed surface of the eye is also covered by a three-layered film of tear fluid. Mucous secretion from conjunctival goblet cells forms the first layer of the tear film and ensures an even spread of tears over the cornea. The second, middle layer of the tear film is the watery fluid secreted by the lacrimal glands (situated under the outer aspect of the upper orbital rim) and by the accessory glands in the conjunctiva. The third, outer, oily layer of tear film is secreted by the meibomian glands of the lids. This is thought to reduce the evaporation rate of tears and to prevent the lids sticking together during sleep. The main functions of tear fluid are: to lubricate the eye; to facilitate O_2 and CO_2 exchange; to provide an optically smooth corneal surface; and to wash the eye with a bacteriostatic enzyme, lysozyme.

Excess tears are drained from the eye via the lacrimal apparatus at the inner canthus (nasal end of the lid margins) into the lacrimal sac and thence into the nose through the nasolacrimal duct (see Figs 13.4(A) and (B)).

Posteriorly and laterally the globe is protected by the bony orbit, the extraocular recti and oblique muscles (responsible for tracking movements) and by orbital fat.

The physiology of vision
Light rays are bent (refracted) as they pass through the varying densities of the clear media of the eye to focus on the retina. The cornea is responsible for about two thirds of the refractive power of the eye and is constant. However, by virtue of its elasticity, the lens has the ability to change shape and thereby vary the amount of refraction for clarity of focus. This is known as accommodation and is necessary in order for objects at different distances to be visualised with equal clarity.

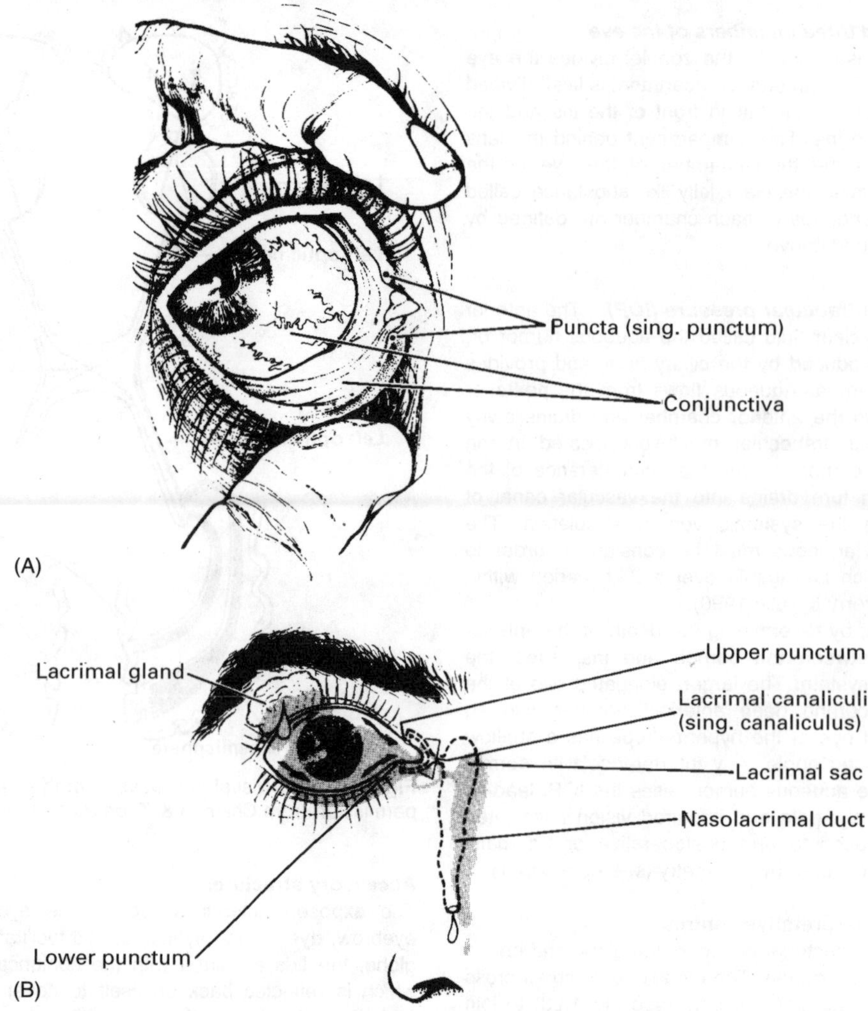

Fig. 13.4 (A) The eyelids and conjunctiva. (B) The lacrimal apparatus. (Reproduced with kind permission from Chilman & Thomas 1987.)

The normal eye in its relaxed state brings rays of light from distant objects into sharp focus. However, for clear focusing on near objects, an autonomic reflex known as the synkinetic near reflex comes into play. This reflex involves accommodation, miosis and convergence, as follows.

- Accommodation: the ciliary body contracts and changes shape, thus releasing tension on the zonular fibres and allowing the lens to thicken and increase its refractive power
- Miosis, or constriction of the pupil, accompanies accommodation and ensures that light rays are concentrated to pass through the centre of the lens and focus on the macula
- Convergence, or inturning of the eyes, seeks out the object to be focused on.

Failure to focus may be described as ametropia, or refractive error (see Box 13.1).

Once the rays of light are focused on the retina their energy is converted into neuroelectrical energy by the photoreceptor cells. These nerve impulses are transmitted via other neural cells in the retina to the optic nerve and so by the visual pathway to the visual cortex. Here, they are interpreted as sensations of light, form and colour and are processed into images of objects which are given meaning by other cerebral areas through correlation with information stored as memory in the association areas of the brain.

Box 13.1 Terms associated with visual acuity and refractive errors

- Emmetropia: normal sight; light rays focus on the retina
- Ametropia: defective sight due to refractive error
- Myopia: shortsightedness; light rays focus in front of the retina
- Hypermetropia: longsightedness; light rays focus behind the retina
- Presbyopia: loss of focused reading/near-vision capacity, resulting from loss of lens elasticity due to ageing
- Astigmatism: irregular curvature of the cornea which prevents light rays from focusing at a single point

ASSESSING THE EYE AND VISUAL FUNCTION

Examination of structure

It is vital for nurses working with ophthalmic patients to learn to examine the eye in a systematic and meticulous way and to be able to recognise abnormalities and their significance. In order to do so it is necessary to know what a normal eye looks like and what normal expectations are for an eye recovering from surgery or disease. It is essential to work in good light using an ophthalmic torch and to proceed systematically, examining all ocular structures from outermost to innermost as follows:

- lids: observe position, closure, bruising, discharge
- conjunctiva: observe degree of injection (visible blood

vessels), chemosis (thickening due to oedema), discharge, wounds
- cornea: observe clarity, type and extent of any opacity, shape, suture lines, wounds
- anterior chamber (AC): observe depth, clarity, presence of hyphaema (blood in AC) hypopyon (pus in AC)
- iris: observe colour, position, appearance
- pupil: observe size, shape, position, colour of reflection from lens
- intraocular lens (IOL): if appropriate, observe position
- retina: examine through dilated pupil using ophthalmoscope.

The possible implications of clinical features that may be found in the course of an eye examination are listed in Table 13.1.

Table 13.1 Significance of clinical features found on eye examination

Structure	Clinical features	Possible significance
Lids	Bruising (ecchymosis) Swelling Drooping Increased lacrimation Discharge	Surgical handling Trauma Infection
Conjunctiva	Redness (injection) Swelling (chemosis) Allergy Infection	Surgical handling Trauma
Cornea	Cloudy Crinkled Fluorescein staining Suture line not intact Penetrating injury	Increased IOP Infection Loss of AC Ulceration
Anterior chamber (AC)	Hyphaema (blood in AC) Hypopyon (pus in AC) Shallow AC	Hyphaema due to surgery should gradually resolve Increasing IO = bleeding Hypopyon = infection Shallow = ? aqueous loss
Iris	Muddy	Inflammation
Pupil	Irregular shape	Iris prolapse Adhesions Trauma

Testing visual function

Visual acuity (VA)

VA assessment is frequently carried out by nurses and is the mathematical estimation of visual function for different distances.

Distance vision. This is tested using test-type charts. These charts display letters or pictures arranged in rows of diminishing size (see Fig. 13.5). A person with normal visual acuity would be able to see the top letter (i.e. the 60 m line) at a distance of 60 m and successive lines at progressively shorter distances. In normal testing the individual is asked to stand 6 m away from the chart and to read each line aloud until he can no longer make out the letters. The result is recorded as a fraction of the distance from the chart in metres over the normal reading distance of the last complete line read, plus the number of extra letters read from the line below,

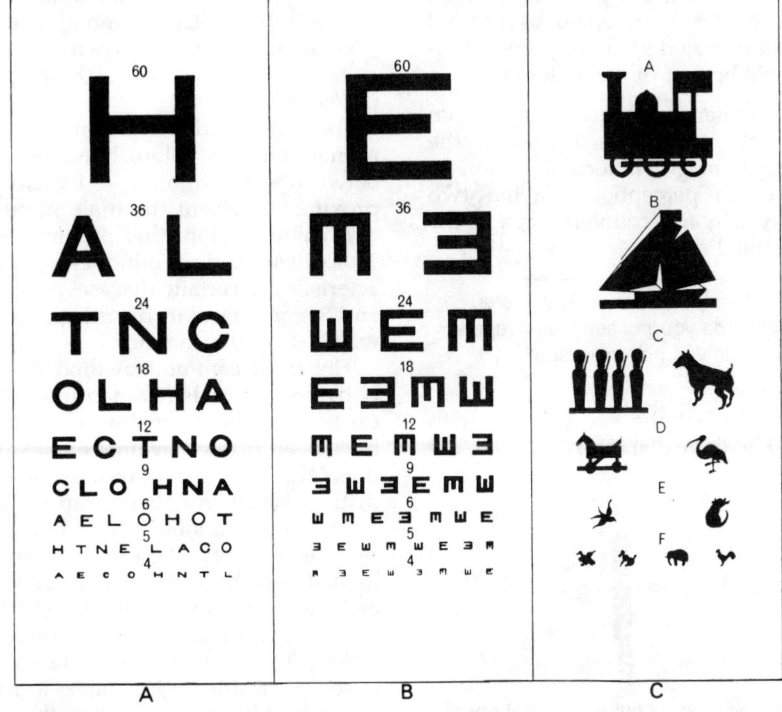

Fig. 13.5 Eye testing charts. (A) Snellen test-type chart. (B) 'E' chart for children, non-English speakers, etc. The person is given a wooden E which he moves to indicate the positions he 'reads' on the chart. (C) Object recognition chart. (Reproduced with kind permission from Chilman & Thomas 1987.)

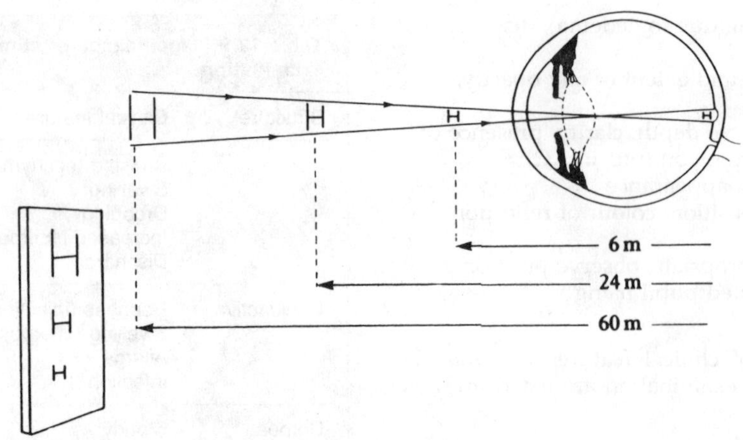

Fig. 13.6 Normal vision. 'The 6 m letter at 6 m and the 60 m letter at 60 m appear the same to the eye. The nearer the larger one approaches the eye the bigger it will appear, because it throws an angle of increasing size at the macula.' (Reproduced with kind permission from Chawla 1988.)

minus the number of letters read incorrectly, e.g. 6/9 – 2 or 6/12 + 1. If glasses or contact lenses are worn this is recorded as i/c gl. and i/c CL respectively.

Normal vision is recorded as 6/6 (see Fig. 13.6). The client may be asked to read the chart again, looking through a pinhole disc. A pure refractive error should improve by 2 lines with this simple method of sharpening focus. The improved score would be recorded as 6/9 i/c PH (see Fig. 13.7).

If the patient cannot read the test letters even when he stands closer to the chart, his ability to count fingers (CF), detect hand movements (HM) or perceive light (PL) is tested. Awareness of direction of a light source may also be noted (projection).

Near vision is tested in similar fashion by asking the patient to read charts in various sizes of standard print, all graded and prefixed with the letter N. N5 is accepted as normal reading acuity. Each eye should be tested separately, because if both eyes are used the score will be that of the better eye.

Binocular vision involves simultaneous perception of an image by both eyes and fusion of the two images in the visual cortex to form a single image. Binocular vision is thought to play a role in depth perception. Having two eyes also widens the field of vision and counters gaps in the visual field caused by natural blind spots.

?	**13.2** Look carefully straight ahead and note what you see. Now close one eye. What do you *not* see? Now repeat with the other eye. What do you no longer see?

The visual field. The range of what the eye can see with respect to angle of view (rather than distance) is called the visual field. Normally this is about 60° nasally, 90° temporally, 50° superiorly and 70° inferiorly. Assessment of the integrity of the visual field is an important aid to diagnosis of retinal detachment and neurological disease and is essential in the management of open-angle glaucoma. Visual field testing can be carried out in the following ways:

- simple confrontation test: the examiner compares the subject's field of vision with his own. Facing the subject, he moves a finger from various points on his own periphery of vision and asks the subject to indicate when it appears in his field of vision. The examiner's own visual field must be normal in order for this to be meaningful
- the Bjerrum screen: used for greater refinement in testing the central 30° of field
- Field analyser systems (some computerised), for example, Friedmann or Goldmann give accurate measurements of visual field defects known as scotomata.

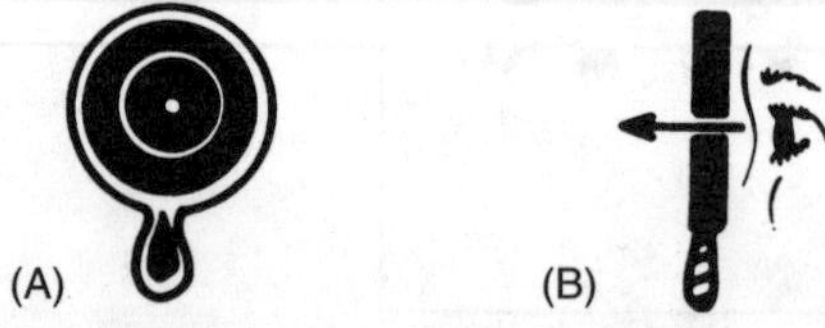

Fig. 13.7 The pinhole disk. (A) By omitting all but the central ray of light reaching the macula this simple apparatus demonstrates whether poor central vision is due to refractive error or not. (B) How the apparatus works. (Reproduced with kind permission from McKenzie, Chawla & Gordon 1986.)

Colour-blindness

Colour vision depends on the normal functioning of the retinal cones. A colour-blind person is unable to distinguish between some colours — usually red and green. While approximately 7% of the male population are born with defective colour vision, this problem is rare in females (Perry & Tullo 1990). Colour-blindness can also be acquired; it is characteristic of certain disease processes such as optic neuritis and some macular disorders, and may develop in people with a drug dependency.

The most common method of testing for colour blindness is by means of Ishihara colour plates. These are a series of cards on which numbers composed of red and green dots have been printed against a background of different coloured dots. A person with defective colour vision would be unable to distinguish the numbers from the surrounding background.

Some occupations require normal colour vision, usually for reasons of safety. For example, an electrician needs to be able to distinguish between coloured wires and an airline pilot between the coloured lights on his instrument panel. Applicants for positions such as these will be tested for colour vision. There are no restrictions on driving cars, lorries or buses as traffic lights have a fixed sequence and can be recognised by position rather than colour.

?	**13.3** What other occupations can you think of that require normal colour vision?

Eye changes with ageing

By age 70 most people will need some form of visual aid, since with advancing years the ability of the lens to accommodate decreases as it becomes less elastic. Focusing is affected as the cornea flattens, causing astigmatism (see Box 13.1). A decrease in pupil size reduces the amount of light entering the eye, and retinal cells become less efficient due to deposits laid down by ageing pigment epithelial cells. Tear film is reduced in volume and altered in structure, with the result that tears evaporate more quickly. This results in dryness and irritation of the eye. The corneal periphery often develops a marked grey ring at its junction with the sclera; this is known as the arcus senilis.

For further information, see Caird & Williamson (1985).

PRESERVATION OF VISION

Nurses can do a great deal through health education and active intervention to help people to preserve their vision. The following list suggests how nurses working in a range of specialisms can make an important contribution to this aspect of health promotion.

- Nurses in every area of practice should take all appropriate opportunities to promote general health and a well-balanced diet.
- The community nurse's observation of behavioural changes in her patients can often bring ophthalmic problems to light and result in early diagnosis and treatment. Prompt referral to the appropriate community health team professional is essential.

> ? **13.4** What behaviours would lead you to suspect that a person's sight is deteriorating?

- Regular eye examination and sight testing should be encouraged — especially in children, people over 40 years of age and those belonging to high-risk groups (e.g. diabetics). The NHS provides free sight testing to certain high-risk and socially deprived groups.

> ? **13.5** On your next community placement talk to the social worker about free sight testing and benefits for visually impaired people.

- Nurses can give advice regarding the use and cleanliness of spectacles and contact lenses. In particular, contact lenses should be cared for properly and used strictly in accordance with the optician's instructions. There is a danger of corneal ulceration if such instructions are not followed.
- Care in monitoring oxygen therapy in babies can prevent retinal damage.
- Prompt treatment of eye infections can often prevent residual damage.
- Work- and leisure-related eye injuries can be prevented by appropriate eye protection (see Box 13.2). Statutory health and safety regulations and better supervision by occupational health nurses has helped to reduce the number of industrial eye injuries. Non-compliance is, however, still a problem.
- Individuals should be urged in the workplace and at home to heed the labels on chemical products indicating whether they are harmful to the eyes; careful note should also be taken of first aid instructions in case of accidental splashing.
- The increasing use of visual display units (VDUs) carries potential for eye damage. The Health and Safety Executive recommends short, frequent rest periods to prevent eye fatigue (Health & Safety Executive 1993).

Box 13.2 Preventing eye injury

Protective eyewear should always be worn during any prolonged exposure to strong sunlight or to snow, as well as for the following activities:

- Chipping masonry
- Chopping wood
- Drilling
- Laying insulation
- Playing squash
- Pruning trees or shrubbery
- Stripping paint
- Sun-bed bathing
- Welding
- Working under the chassis of a car

THE VISUALLY IMPAIRED PERSON

> ? **13.6** Sometimes it is difficult for sighted persons to fully appreciate the importance of vision to carrying out the activities of daily living. Working through the following activity may help you to gain some understanding of the daily experience of blind people. Ask a colleague to blindfold you by padding and bandaging both eyes (good practice too!) and then to assist you through as many of the activities of daily living as possible. Try to include basic hygiene, eating a meal, going into a busy room and travelling on public transport. Swap roles. Then, using a structured framework such as Roper, Logan and Tierney's ADLs (1990), discuss how being 'blind' affected each activity. Additionally, ask yourself how it affected the essential 'you'. Did you feel any less intelligent? How great was the potential loss? Did it change the way others reacted to you? How did it feel to be the helper? Share your experiences and insights with the other members of your student group.

Registration of blindness and partial sight

There are few totally blind people, as most visually impaired people have some residual sight or perception of light. A consultant ophthalmologist will certify the degree of blindness and arrange for follow-up care.

Registration, which is completely voluntary, entitles the individual to many local and national benefits. These will be explained by the social worker, who visits eligible individuals in their homes and helps to arrange for additional support. Some areas also have the benefit of a mobility officer who is specially trained to help newly registered individuals to relearn daily living skills and to mobilise safely in their own environment. This may involve the use of special canes or guide dogs. Mobility officers also teach communication skills and Braille and advise on retraining for employment. Their overall aim is to enable the visually impaired person to function as independently as possible.

People with impaired vision may be referred to a low-visual clinic and provided with aids which can help them to make the most of residual sight and with information and advice on adaptation or retraining for employment. Employers can also be advised by the Manpower Services Commission (MSC) or the Royal National Institute for the Blind (RNIB) on the sophisticated electronic equipment now available for blind employees.

Considering the needs of the visually impaired person

All nursing care should be thought out using a structured approach to assessment and a care plan informed by a particular nursing philosophy. This will help to ensure that nothing is overlooked and that members of the nursing team have a common purpose and a shared language with which to communicate with one another. It also provides a mechanism for accountability.

One useful approach has been suggested by Rowell (1990). This is an adaptation of Orem's model (Orem 1990), which takes account of universal needs but focuses on specific areas of self-care deficit, builds on the individual's strengths and promotes personal responsibility for health maintenance. Education and counselling are also essential components of this model.

Some general principles of care for the visually impaired person are outlined below:

- Orientation to place. If the person is at home he will know his own environment and it is therefore important to keep things in their usual place. Every assistance should be given to help him to move around the community and workplace until he is confident to do so on his own. Appropriate visual aids should be used. If he is admitted to hospital it is the nurse's responsibility to orientate him adequately. Old people in particular can become very confused and are likely to need constant guidance.
- Maintaining a safe environment. In organising the environment it is essential to remove objects that the individual might fall over or bump into. Doors should be fully open or closed properly. Fires should have guards. Individuals who smoke should be warned about the high inflammability of eye pads.

> ? **13.7** Look at a ward in your hospital and identify problems that a patient with impaired vision might have. How could you make it safer?

- Communication. A visually impaired person will develop heightened perception in his other senses — especially hearing and touch — and it is important to provide additional sensory input to facilitate this. Make sure the person has access to radios, talking books and other more sophisticated means of communication if he wants them. Identify yourself when you approach the person and address him by name. Describe what you are doing so that he feels involved. It is equally important to inform the person of your intention to leave so that he is not embarrassed by being left talking to himself.
- Eating and drinking. In hospital, food should be placed directly in front of the patient and the position of what is on the plate described using a clock-face analogy. Plate guards, non-slip mats and other aids may be offered. Many safety devices are available for use in the home to help with cooking. After proper training a good degree of independence can be achieved.
- Personal hygiene and grooming. After initial orientation and help the individual should be encouraged to carry out personal self-care tasks for himself.
- Mobility. When other factors permit, early mobilisation should be encouraged in hospital and every assistance given. The preferred method of guiding a person with visual impairment is illustrated in Figure 13.8.

> The RNIB leaflet 'How to Guide a Blind Person' (1987) gives valuable advice.

With good mobility training and family support the visually impaired person should be able to get around in his environment safely and effectively. It will take courage, time and patience to achieve this level of competence, however, and the individual will require understanding and unflagging moral support.

DISORDERS OF THE EYE

The more common eye disorders and their management will be described in the sections which follow. The coverage is by no means exhaustive and the reader is urged to consult specialist ophthalmic texts as the need arises.

> For further information, see Perry & Tullo (1990) and Kanski (1992).

The present survey of common eye disorders and their management will begin, however, by setting out the basic principles that must be followed when carrying out ophthalmic nursing procedures.

NURSING PRIORITIES AND MANAGEMENT: GENERAL OPHTHALMIC PROCEDURES

The eye is a delicate organ which can be easily damaged — even in the course of treatment. The nurse must be scrupulous in observing the following principles in any situation in which she provides ophthalmic care.

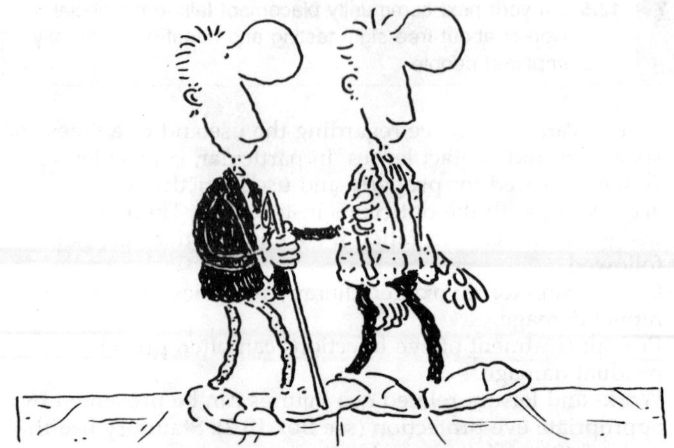

Fig. 13.8 Guiding a blind person. The blind person grasps the helper's arm firmly just above the elbow. The helper then walks beside and half a pace in front of him. In this way the blind person can sense any manoeuvre or turning of the helper's body and can walk more confidently. (Reproduced with kind permission from RNIB 1987.)

Strict asepsis must be observed by the nurse and taught to patients and relatives. Each eye should be treated separately. Drops and ointments should only be used in the eye for which they are prescribed. In hospital, topical medication should be dated upon opening and discarded after one week (after four weeks in the community). These precautions will reduce the risk of eye infection, which can quickly destroy vision.

Gentle handling is essential. *Pressure on the eyeball must be avoided at all times.* This applies particularly to cleansing of the eyelids, which should be drawn open and clear of the eyeball using the orbital margins as traction points. A sterile, moist swab is then used to wipe from inner to outer canthus outside the eyelash line and is discarded after single use. Patients should be cautioned against rubbing their eyes. The eye is a delicate organ which is easily damaged. The cornea is especially sensitive. Pressure can damage corneal suture lines and displace intraocular lenses.

Irrigation. When irrigating the eye the warmed solution should be directed onto the nasal side of the sclera. This will wash harmful foreign material away from the lacrimal duct to the side of the cheek, where it can be caught in a kidney dish.

Examination. Both eyes should be examined systematically (see p. 470) before and after any treatment using a good ophthalmic torch. Any abnormality must be reported immediately to the ophthalmologist. Visual acuity should be assessed and any significant change reported at once. The patient should be asked how each eye feels. Severe pain must be reported immediately. Systematic examination will ensure that no detail is overlooked. As eye complications can develop rapidly it is vital to refer patients immediately to avoid permanent damage. Both eyes should be examined because there is a tendency for the unaffected eye to react in sympathy with the affected one. Photophobia is to be expected postoperatively and with trauma.

Instilling eye drops and ointments. Eye drops are inserted into the outer third of the lower conjunctival sac. To facilitate this the patient is asked to tilt his head back and look up while the lower lid is gently pulled down (see Fig. 13.9). Dropping the solution onto the sensitive cornea will cause discomfort and trigger a reflexive squeezing shut of the eye. If the drop is placed in the inner canthus it will run straight down the lacrimal duct into the nasopharynx and will not be absorbed by the conjunctiva.

Eye ointment is instilled into the lower conjunctival sac with the patient's head tilted back as described above. Contact of the tube with the eye should be carefully avoided.

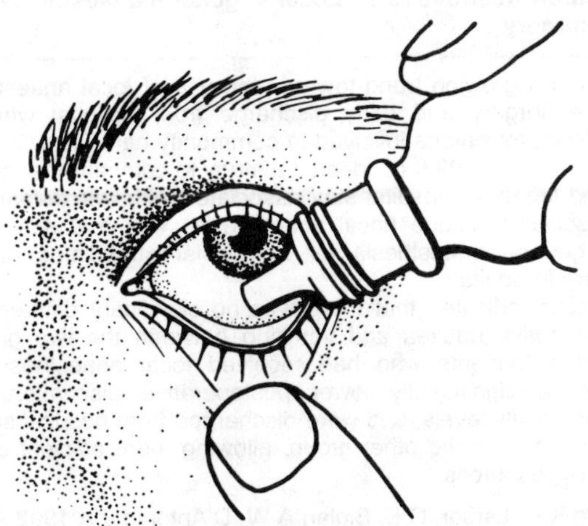

Fig. 13.9 Instilling eye drops. (Reproduced with kind permission from McKenzie, Chawla & Gordon 1986.)

Topical drugs used in ophthalmology are listed in Table 13.2.

Padding the eye. Eyepads are applied to promote healing or to apply pressure to the eye and occasionally for comfort, when photophobia or lacrimation is excessive. It is important to appreciate that the term 'double padding' does not mean that both eyes are covered but the application of two pads to the treated eye.

Eyepads are applied after eyes have been cleansed (if required), examined and treatment instilled. Ensure that the eye is closed underneath the pad at all times to prevent corneal damage.

The eyepad is held in position and non-allergenic tape applied by first attaching an end lightly to the forehead, diagonally across the eyepad towards the lateral aspect of the cheek, before the end is secured with light pressure. The downward movement maintains lid closure. The diagonal position of the tape facilitates comfort, permitting facial muscle movement. To facilitate removal, the tape is cut below the eyebrow, the pad is folded down and the skin of the cheek supported to ensure no pressure on the eyeball. The skin of the forehead is supported in a similar method for the removal of the remaining tape. Pads must be inspected for signs of infection or haemorrhage before discarding.

When the eye cannot be closed voluntarily, for example in the unconscious patient, care should be taken to avoid corneal abrasion from bedclothes or other articles when turning or attending to the patient. The cornea must be kept moist with artificial tears.

NURSING PRIORITIES AND MANAGEMENT: CONDITIONS REQUIRING SURGICAL INTERVENTION

The term 'intraocular surgery' describes procedures that are carried out inside the globe of the eye and which may involve structures in the anterior, posterior or vitreous chambers. Although there are many ophthalmic conditions requiring operative intervention, the present discussion will focus on some of the more common of these, including cataract, retinal detachment, glaucoma and perforating injuries. These conditions will have in common certain general priorities for ophthalmic and perioperative nursing management along with specific priorities relating to each condition. The general principles of perioperative ophthalmic nursing care are outlined below, followed by a discussion of nursing care specific to particular conditions. The reader is also referred to Chapter 27 for the principles of pre- and postoperative nursing management.

General nursing considerations

Assessing visual status

The patient's visual acuity and functional status is determined following his admission to the ward through formal testing and interview. It is important to establish the patient's normal visual status so that he can retain his self respect and independence and is not demeaned by inappropriate restrictions. It is equally important to determine any deficits to ensure that a safe environment is maintained for him.

The patient should be orientated to the ward area with a view to maintaining his normal degree of independence as far as possible. His dependency level will fluctuate during the peri-operative period due, for example, to anaesthesia, treatment, padding. The potential difficulties should be discussed fully.

Table 13.2 Some topical drugs used in ophthalmology (Vail & Cox 1978)

Drug	Strength	Remarks
Mydriatics		
Cyclopentolate (G.)*	0.5% and 1%	Short-acting. Used for refraction, ophthalmoscopy, fundal photography, treatment of anterior uveitis
Tropicamide (G.)	0.5% and 1%	Short-acting. Used for refraction, ophthalmoscopy
Homatropine (G.)	1% and 2%	Moderate-acting. Used for refraction, treatment of anterior uveitis
Atropine (G.)	1%	Long-acting. Used for refraction in children, treatment of anterior uveitis
Phenylephrine (G.)	2.5% and 10%	Short-acting. Used for ophthalmoscopy, fundal photography
Miotics		
Pilocarpine (G.)	0.5% – 4%	Short-acting. Treatment of glaucoma by constricting the ciliary muscle and helping to open the trabecular meshwork
Beta blockers		
Timoptol (G.)	0.25% and 0.5%	Used for treatment of chronic open-angle glaucoma and secondary glaucoma by reducing aqueous humor production
Betoptic (G.)	0.5%	As above
Steroids		
Betnesol (G.)	0.1%	Used to treat ocular inflammation. Can be combined with neomycin, an antibiotic
Chloramphenicol (G.)	0.5%	Broad spectrum. Can also be given as an ointment
Fucithalmic (G.)**	1%	Broad spectrum. Viscous eye drops
Anti-viral		
Zovirax (Oc.)	3%	Used for treatment of herpes simplex virus
Anaesthetics		
Benoxinate (G.)	0.4%	Short-acting. Used for tonometry, removal of corneal and conjunctival foreign bodies, gonioscopy
Amethocaine (G.)	0.5% and 1%	Short-acting. Used for tonometry, removal of corneal and conjunctival foreign bodies, gonioscopy
Staining agents		
Fluorescein (G.)	1% and 2%	Stains damaged living tissue. Detects corneal abrasions and demonstrates leaking corneal wound
Rose Bengal (G.)	1%	Stains dead, devitalised tissue. Detects corneal and conjunctival involvement in keratoconjunctivitis sicca (xerophthalmia)
Lubricants		
Hypromellose (G.)	0.3%	Most commonly used
Liquifilm (G.)	1.4%	More viscous by added polyvinyl alcohol
Lacri-Lube (Oc.)		White soft paraffin based. Useful overnight

* guttae — drops
** Oc. — Oculentum ointment

Alleviating stress

Anxiety levels are normally high for patients admitted to hospital and this may be exacerbated in ophthalmic patients by fear of blindness and loss of independence. The patient should be given the opportunity to discuss particular fears and should be provided with clear and realistic information. Care should be taken not to raise false expectations about operative results and the patient should be referred for counselling if the need is identified. Realistic expectations will provide a more functional base for adaptation to any remaining disability. The patient may have practical concerns about managing the activities of daily living following the operation; these should be addressed and the individual should be reassured that he will be able to receive continuing guidance and support from the health care team and from community organisations.

Giving information

Most patients are anxious to know the time of their surgery and how long it will take. If a local anaesthetic is to be used they may be concerned about their level of awareness during the procedure and about whether they will be able to cooperate. (See Research Abstract 13.1.) Depending on the patient's visual acuity it is often helpful to discuss the operation using a model of the eye. It is important to anticipate and dispel any misconceptions that the patient may have about eye surgery. However, not everyone will want to know the details of the surgery and the individual's wishes in this regard should be respected.

Procedures for preoperative eye preparation should be explained. If the patient is able to carry out self-medication, instruction in the instillation of drops can provide a good opportunity to begin a teaching programme for postoperative self-care.

Managing positioning and activity

As a general rule, any position or activity that increases venous pressure in the head should be avoided in ophthalmic patients. It is usually recommended that they are nursed with the head slightly raised, with the patient either semirecumbent or lying on the unoperated side. Exceptions to this are:

- in cases of retinal detachment — the surgeon will prescribe both pre- and postoperative positions, depending on the site of the detachment
- following vitrectomy — the surgeon may prescribe the position.

Research Abstract 13.1 Local v. general anaesthesia in eye surgery

There is a growing trend towards the use of local anaesthesia in eye surgery and early discharge from hospital which is significant for nurses involved in community care (see Ch. 1).

Cheng et al (1992) conducted a study to compare the morbidity and length of hospital stay associated with retrobulbar neuromuscular blockade (local anaesthesia) with that associated with general anaesthesia for monocular strabismus (squint) surgery in adults.

Results indicated that there was no significant difference in postoperative nausea and vomiting between the two groups. However, patients who had received local anaesthesia experienced significantly lower postoperative discomfort, had higher activity levels, and were discharged from hospital sooner than patients in the other group, allowing more efficient use of hospital resources.

Cheng K P, Larson C E, Biglan A W, D'Antonio J A 1992 A prospective, ransomized, controlled experiment of retrobulbar and general anaesthesia for strabismus su surgery. Ophthalmic Surgery 23(9): 585–590

It is vital that such instructions for positioning are followed precisely.

Postoperative vomiting should be prevented by ensuring that an antiemetic is ordered and that it is given promptly if the patient complains of nausea. The patient should also avoid bending down, lifting, and straining during bowel movements. Increased blood flow caused by a head-down position or straining will raise IOP and can result in damage to optical structures or suture lines. Many patients go home shortly after surgery and restrictions on activity and positioning should be adhered to for at least 2 weeks postoperatively, or longer if the patient's occupation involves strenuous activity. The reason for these activity and positioning regimes should be carefully explained to the patient to encourage compliance. The duration of restrictions should also be clearly defined.

Examining the eye

The eye should be examined systematically using an ophthalmic torch. Preoperatively, it is checked for signs of infection, and postoperatively for signs of abnormal healing and other problems. Early recognition of abnormalities is critical, as irreversible damage resulting in loss of sight can result if action is not taken immediately (see p. 471).

The surgeon or an ophthalmic trained or skilled nurse undertakes the procedure of first dressing. Haemorrhage is abnormal, although there may be some slight operative bleeding into the anterior chamber (hyphaema). If a hyphaema is present it will be recorded and a diagram indicating size relative to the anterior chamber entered in the medical and nursing notes. Normal postoperative expectations may include some degree of lid bruising and swelling, especially following local anaesthetic. Conjunctival injection and oedema (chemosis) should be confined to the wound site. The cornea and anterior chamber should be clear. A fine suture line may be evident. The depth of the anterior chamber should be noted, as this may relate to the disease process, the surgery, or a leaking wound.

A systematic approach to eye examination will help to ensure that no detail is missed.

Managing dressings

The eye is protected by a plastic cartella shield for the first 24 h postoperatively. Pads and dressings are removed on the surgeon's instructions according to the type of surgery that has been performed. Dark glasses may be worn to reduce the discomfort of glare. The patient should be taught to put the glasses on over his forehead to avoid accidentally poking the ear-pieces into his eye. The cartella shield is worn at night to protect the eye.

PAINLESS LOSS OF VISION

CATARACT

Any opacity of the lens can be defined as a cataract. Cataracts can develop as part of the ageing process.

They can also be congenital or may develop following trauma, as sequelae to inflammatory and degenerative disease, or as a result of the prolonged use of some drugs, for example, corticosteroids.

PATHOPHYSIOLOGY

The lens of the eye is normally transparent due to the regular arrangement of its crystalline fibres and the nature of the proteins inside them. These fibres, which originate in the epithelium of the lens capsule, continue to be laid down throughout life. This results in thickening and a loss of elasticity; opacity may eventually develop with ageing.

Clinical features. The main feature of a mature cataract is that it reflects as a grey or milky white lens behind the pupil, which normally appears black.

Common presenting symptoms. The nature of the symptoms experienced by the patient will depend upon the cause of the cataract, as follows:

1. Age-related cataract:
   - gradually decreasing acuity affecting distance vision more than near vision
   - general dimming of vision because of the reduced amount of light reaching the retina
   - more frequent refractive errors because of reduced elasticity of the lens
   - increased dazzle and glare in bright light and haloes around lights at night
   - monocular diplopia (double vision in one eye)
   - alteration in colour and depth perception
2. Cataract related to inflammation or trauma:
   - pain due to an acute inflammatory response in which the lens swells, causing acute closed-angle glaucoma
   - opacity following trauma.

Whatever the combination of early presenting symptoms, the patient will eventually experience greatly reduced visual acuity and may describe this as being 'like looking through ground glass'.

?	**13.8** Wrap several layers of clear adhesive tape around both lenses of a pair of glasses. Alternatively, smear both lenses with petroleum jelly. Wear them for a while to experience something of what it feels like to have bilateral cataracts. Then try it with vision totally occluded in one lens and the other lens wrapped in just a few layers of tape or smeared with a thin film of jelly. How would this affect your daily activities? Discuss the experience with your colleagues.

MEDICAL MANAGEMENT

During the developmental stages of cataract spectacles and the controlled use of mydriatic drops may provide a degree of improvement in visual acuity. It is impossible, however, to reverse the opacification process. Surgical removal of the mature lens will ultimately be the only effective treatment. Cataract removal is one of the surgical procedures which may now be done as day surgery, provided the ophthalmic surgeon, general practitioner and patient agree there are no contra-indications to this (Audit Commission 1990).

Tests and investigations. Preoperative investigations must ensure that retinal function is adequate, as it would be pointless to remove a cataract if the retina were non-functional.

Surgical procedures. Cataract removal is usually delayed until vision in the better eye is reduced to 6/18, as the brain is required to make considerable visual adjustments following surgery.

There are several methods of cataract extraction in common use, many of which are performed with only local anaesthesia. Before the operation the pupil is dilated to facilitate lens delivery and to reduce the risk of damage to the iris. An incision is then made into the globe, and the lens, or the contents of the lens capsule, are removed. Methods of lens removal include:

- intracapsular extraction: total removal of the lens
- extracapsular extraction: removal of the nucleus and cortex, leaving the posterior capsule intact
- lensectomy: guillotine cutting instruments are used with or without ultrasonic fragmentation to break up nuclei and aspirate soft lens material.

Intraocular lens implantation. Although corrective spectacles and contact lenses can be used following extraction, the best correction is achieved by the insertion of an intraocular lens (IOL) at the time of cataract removal. This is possible in approximately 95% of cases. Pre-existing eye disease or unforeseen surgical complications are the main contraindications (Bartholomew 1986).

There are two main kinds of IOLs: those which are positioned in the anterior chamber in front of the iris; and those which are positioned in the posterior chamber behind the iris. It is important to know which kind of lens is in situ in order to ensure appropriate postoperative care.

Postoperative medication. The inflammatory response which accompanies all healing is controlled postoperatively by a combination of topical steroids and antibiotics and, mydriatics if prescribed. It is vital that the patient understands the reasons for compliance with regular instillation of drops.

NURSING PRIORITIES AND MANAGEMENT: CATARACT EXTRACTION AND IMPLANTATION OF INTRAOCULAR LENS

Using an agreed nursing model, an individual care plan is drawn up for each patient by the nursing team, taking into account the basic perioperative management principles covered in Chapter 27 and those relating to intraocular surgery on p. 475. Additionally, the following points specific to cataract extraction and IOL implantation should be noted.

Major nursing considerations

IOL management

It is important to find out which method has been used for extraction and whether or not an IOL has been implanted. If an IOL is in situ its position must be checked at each eye dressing.

The most common problems which arise following IOL implantation are displacement, corneal endothelial damage, and the 'UGH syndrome' i.e. uveitis + glaucoma + hyphaema. Should any of these be present instant action is required in order to circumvent permanent eye damage. Severe pain is an important symptom of raised IOP.

For this reason, while mild analgesia can be given to reduce discomfort, narcotics must *not* be given as they will mask the severity of pain and thus remove a valuable indicator of serious problems.

Aphakic management

An aphakic eye is an eye without a lens. If the patient does not have an IOL implanted, his aphakic vision will have to be corrected (focused) by either the use of aphakic glasses or contact lenses.

In order to avoid disappointment at the immediate operative results it should be explained to the patient that there will be a period of adaptation as the brain adjusts to changes in visual perception. During this time the patient can expect a certain amount of visual distortion resulting in central field magnification and peripheral blurring and rounding. This will affect distance and depth perception and the individual should be cautioned to take care on steps and stairs and to turn his head more to scan the whole visual field.

> **?** **13.9** One of your patients has undergone a cataract extraction and IOL implantation. At the third dressing, as you systematically examine the eye, you note the following clinical signs:
>
> - eye pad: slightly damp
> - eye lids: slightly bruised and swollen but less than previously
> - conjunctiva: pink
> - cornea: cloudy, suture line intact
> - anterior chamber: formed, hyphaema noted and more extensive than at previous dressing
> - iris: muddy
> - pupil: dilated and round
> - posterior chamber IOL: in situ and reflecting.
>
> Which of these clinical signs are within normal expectations and which would alert you to a problem that demands immediate attention? What could this problem be? What action will you take?

Nursing Care Plan 13.1 outlines some considerations that might arise in the care of a patient undergoing cataract extraction and IOL implantation.

GLAUCOMA

Glaucoma can be defined as raised intraocular pressure (IOP) which, if untreated, will lead to pathological changes in the eye. The condition may be acquired or genetic in origin. Acquired glaucoma can be further classified as primary open-angle glaucoma (POAG), primary closed-angle glaucoma (both acute and chronic), and glaucoma secondary to pathological processes (secondary glaucoma).

> **?** **13.10** Revise your knowledge of aqueous dynamics within the eye.

Primary open-angle glaucoma (POAG)

This type of glaucoma (also known as chronic simple glaucoma) causes progressive and irreversible loss of the peripheral visual field, with the central 10% being spared until a later stage. It is initially symptomless.

PATHOPHYSIOLOGY

Raised IOP develops when there is interference with aqueous drainage as a result of degenerative changes in the angle structures. The normal range of intraocular pressure is 12–20 mmHg; this varies throughout a 24 h period, being lower during the day than at night when the individual is lying down. In POAG the pressure is persistently elevated and the diurnal variation is greater.

Raised IOP decreases the blood flow in the optic disc capillaries with resultant excavation and atrophy of the optic nerve head and subsequent loss of nerve fibres passing through it (cupping). A progressive loss of the visual field results from damage to nerve fibre bundles as they enter the optic disc.

Clinical features. The outward appearance of the eye is normal but on examination three features present which are diagnostic of glaucoma. These are: raised IOP; cupping of the optic disc; and visual field loss.

Common presenting symptoms. There is usually a gradual and painless loss of vision. The patient rarely notices this deterioration until considerable damage has been done. The glaucoma is often discovered by an optician during a routine eye examination.

MEDICAL INTERVENTION

The main aim of treatment is to reduce IOP to allow better capillary perfusion at the optic nerve head. This involves improving the aqueous drainage system, or decreasing the production of aqueous, or a combination of both. Medical treatment is the mainstay in the majority of cases, although there is a growing trend towards early surgical or laser intervention.

Tests and investigations. Diagnosis and medical assessment of the nature and severity of the condition will rely on the following:

Nursing Care Plan 13.1 A patient undergoing intraocular surgery

Nursing consideration	Action	Rationale	Evaluation
Preoperative preparation			
1. Anxiety relating to local anaesthetic; being awake during the procedure; draping procedure in theatre; communication with staff during procedure	❒ Explain that local anaesthetic (LA) ensures painless procedure, reduces postoperative discomfort of GA, and enables earlier discharge (see Research Abstract 13.1) ❒ Explain that draping and skin cleansing are carried out to reduce the risk of infection ❒ Explain that the unoperated eye needs to be closed to protect the cornea from accidental damage and reduce eye movement	Information given about procedures reduces patient anxiety and discomfort (Wilson-Barnett 1978)	Patient is able to recall details of preparation and appears more relaxed
	❒ Explain that whilst the eye is anaesthetised it is possible to overcome muscle activity and position the eye in the orbit so as to permit easy access to most surgical sites	Patients fairly commonly express a fear that the eye will be placed on the cheek to facilitate surgery. Placing the eye on the cheek is impossible without total destruction of the optic nerve, which, together with the extra-ocular muscles and cheek ligaments, tether the eye securely within the orbital cavity	
	❒ Explain that throughout the patient's time in theatre one nurse will hold his hand and that they will agree on a signalling system so that if he has any discomfort or pain he can communicate this; remedial measures will be taken immediately	An agreed communication system reduces anxiety and increases well-being	He communicates appropriately during the procedure and tolerates the operation well
Discharge considerations			
1. Anxiety about visual function following surgery	❒ Explain that visual recovery is not complete until the eye is fully healed. This may not be for several months	Improved knowledge reduces anxiety (Wilson-Barnett 1978)	Patient is able to recall information given
	❒ Visual function is to be assessed regularly and must be no worse than discharge level. (NB the 'unaffected' eye must be closed during assessment process) ❒ If vision decreased then urgent review in OPD is advised		Patient can demonstrate procedure used
	❒ Explain that 'floaters', which occur following discharge, and the experiencing of flashing lights may precede the development of complications and urgent review in OPD should be sought		Patient states arrangements he would make to obtain urgent OPD review
2. The patient has a Parkinsonian tremor and is unable to instil his own eyedrops	❒ Contact community nurse and discuss plan to approach neighbour and teach her how to assist the patient	Rehabilitation and discharge planning should begin on admission. Early liaison with the community nurse will help to ensure that treatment continues and that the nurse is fully informed of individual aspects of the case. It will also reassure the patient that a supportive health care team exists	

- tonometry: measurement of IOP by specialised instruments
- phasing: measurement of IOP by tonometry at different times of the day
- visual field studies
- gonioscopy: examination of the state and depth of the angle of the eye
- ophthalmoscopy to examine the optic nerve head and estimate the degree of cupping.

Medical management. Whether the medical regime is implemented alone or in combination with a surgical procedure it is important to maintain monitoring of the efficiency of treatment indefinitely. The regime may include the administration of some combination of the following medications:

- topical miotic drops to constrict the pupil and stretch open the trabecular meshwork, thus facilitating aqueous drainage
- topical beta blockers to inhibit the production of aqueous or systemic carbonic anhydrase inhibitors to reduce its production (see Table 13.2). Topical regimes may be prescribed for long-term continuous use; systemic drugs are generally prescribed for short-term or intermittent use.

Surgical treatment for POAG is usually employed when conservative management has failed (progression of visual field loss and persistent elevation of IOP) or when drug compliance is unsatisfactory.

The principle of surgery is to create a fistula between the anterior chamber and the subconjunctival space in order to bypass the existing drainage system and increase the outflow of aqueous. The most commonly used procedure is trabeculectomy.

Postoperatively a small bleb under the conjunctival flap will be visible as well as a small V-shaped hole in the iris (peripheral iridectomy).

The success of surgery is measured by whether the IOP remains within normal limits, but there can be no actual improvement in visual acuity. However, there may be a subjective improvement in vision. If a trabeculectomy drains well there may be no need to continue miotic drops and the pupil will revert to normal size. Consequently the world will seem brighter, colours will be truer and night vision will be improved.

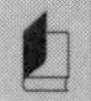
For further information, see Perry & Tullo (1990) pp. 260–262.

Laser treatment. This involves applying short bursts of a laser beam through a lens resembling a gonioscopy lens, targeting selected areas of the trabecular meshwork. Application of argon laser burns to the trabecular meshwork (argon laser trabeculoplasty) has been found to be effective in selected cases in reducing IOP. The scarring caused by the laser burns appears to stretch the tissues between the burns, thus opening up spaces in the trabecular meshwork and facilitating drainage of aqueous.

NURSING PRIORITIES AND MANAGEMENT: POAG

Major nursing considerations

Screening

Measurement of IOP and visual field testing may be carried out by a nurse working in a general practice or community department setting if she has been taught to use the required instrumentation (applanation tonometer and field analyser). The screening service is most usually undertaken by the optometry service.

Patient compliance

This is a major concern, especially in the outpatient department and the community setting where most cases of glaucoma will be seen. It is a nursing responsibility to assess the patient's understanding of his condition and the rationale for treatment and his ability to instil his own drops and comply with other aspects of treatment.

Self-administration of drops is difficult and demands flexibility of the hand, arm and neck and dexterity and judgement in managing the drop dispenser bottle. Various appliances are available to help with the procedure but it still requires skilful instruction and demonstration to ensure success. Where deficits occur additional follow-up and nursing support must be organised. In some cases relatives or carers must be taught to carry out the treatment regimes.

? **13.11** Miotic drops such as pilocarpine constrict the pupil. How can you monitor compliance in a patient who is prescribed regular miotics? What visual effects does the patient experience when his pupil is constricted?

Postoperative observation and monitoring

Depth of anterior chamber (AC). Postoperatively, the depth of the AC in the operated eye should be equal to that of the unoperated eye. Variations must be reported. It is possible for over-drainage to result in a shallow AC or for under-drainage to result in a deeper AC.

Signs of raised IOP. Severe postoperative pain accompanied by a cloudy cornea and flat AC is abnormal and must be investigated. Raised IOP must be suspected in the presence of these symptoms.

Administering laser treatment

During application of laser treatment it is vital for the nurse to understand the potential hazards to the patient and to staff and to gain the patient's cooperation in keeping still and maintaining a steady direction of gaze. If the patient moves, the laser beam may inflict accidental burns. A full explanation of what is involved and reassurance that he will be supported throughout the procedure and carefully monitored afterwards will help to ensure compliance (see Nursing Care Plan 13.2). Protective goggles are mandatory for all staff in attendance.

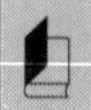
For further information, see Frost (1993).

RETINAL DETACHMENT

Retinal detachment describes a separation between the neural and pigmented layers of the retina.

PATHOPHYSIOLOGY

Retinal detachments most commonly occur secondary to a tear or hole in the retina caused by degenerative disease or by traumatic or postoperative vitreous loss and traction. The light-sensitive cells in the neural layer are detached from the essential pigments in the pigment layer as fluid effusion between the layers gradually causes more separation. Sometimes there is no obvious cause for the detachment, but predisposing factors include myopia, aphakia, trauma, or retinal/choroidal tumour. If one eye is affected the other is also at risk (see p. 487).

Common presenting symptoms. The patient may present at various stages with painless visual disturbances or loss of vision. The external appearance of the eye is unchanged unless recent traumatic injury or surgical intervention has taken place. During the early stages the rods and cones are falsely activated, causing sensations of flashing light. As flakes of pigment are shed into the vitreous, the patient may see showers of floating shapes and strands in the vitreous field. Later,

Nursing Care Plan 13.2 Ensuring patient cooperation in laser treatment

Nursing consideration	Action	Rationale	Evaluation
Anxiety due to: • **Lack of understanding of laser treatment** • **Fear of pain and discomfort during procedure**	❒ Explain to the patient that he will be asked to sit as for gonioscopy and that a similar lens will be applied to his eye Describe the anatomy of the eye, how the laser beam is targeted on the problem areas and what the expected outcome will be Explain the importance of maintaining a steady position and gaze	The patient will have experienced gonioscopy as part of his earlier examination and will therefore be familiar with the procedure Expectations of a positive outcome will reduce anxiety The patient's cooperation is necessary in order to ensure that only targeted areas are exposed to the laser	The patient can demonstrate awareness of what the procedure entails and has confidence in the medical and nursing team. He is cooperative during the treatment, keeps a steady direction of gaze and does not appear unduly anxious. Accidental burns are avoided
	❒ Reassure the patient that the treatment may be uncomfortable but should not be painful. He will experience bright flashes of light and there may be a slight headache afterwards Reassure him that the procedure is well controlled and that there will be careful follow-up	Information given about procedures reduces patient anxiety and discomfort (Wilson-Barnett 1978)	

he may describe an impression of a curtain coming down or drifting smoke passing across his line of vision.

MEDICAL MANAGEMENT

The exact nature and extent of the retinal detachment and the presence of retinal fluid will dictate the specific procedure for repair that is used.

Surgical procedures. The aim of surgery is to produce a controlled inflammatory response to seal the detachment, release the subretinal fluid and bring the retinal layers into normal apposition. Differentiation between emergency and non-urgent cases depends on the state of the macula. If the macula has been detached for just 24 h or is at risk of becoming detached an emergency situation exists.

Cryosurgery is used to produce the inflammatory response, the cryoprobe being applied to the sclera behind the detachment. This is often explained to patients as 'spot welding'. Release of subretinal fluid aids repositioning of the layers, which may be supported by internal tamponade created by intravitreal air or by volume-expanding gases. A silicone explant may be temporarily sutured into position on the outside of the eye, encircling it like a belt. Once it is seen to be in the correct position and of the correct size it is permanently tied with non-absorbable sutures. Complex cases may require more extensive intraocular surgery such as vitrectomy (removal of the vitreous humor from the vitreous chamber).

Outpatient treatment with argon laser and volume-expanding gases may be satisfactory in cases of dry retinal detachments. Here, the inflammatory response is controlled by mydriatic and steroid eye drops.

For further information, see Schutz (1984).

NURSING PRIORITIES AND MANAGEMENT: RETINAL DETACHMENT

Major nursing considerations

Patient positioning

Correct posturing is a vital adjunct to the management of retinal detachment. Individualised regimes determined by medical staff and prescribed in the case notes must be strictly observed. The positioning that is prescribed will depend on the site of the retinal hole and on the nature of the surgical repair procedure. The patient must be fully informed of the reasons for posturing, for his compliance is very important to the success of the treatment. Normal functional positions are usually allowed at mealtimes and for toilet purposes. Posturing is seldom necessary longer than 24 h postoperatively, following which mobilisation follows the same pattern as for cataract surgery (see Nursing Care Plan 13.1).

The overall aim is to help the detached area to fall back into position preoperatively and to maintain normal apposition postoperatively. Generally, if the patient has a superior detachment he will be nursed lying flat with one pillow, and if the detachment is inferior he will be nursed sitting up in bed or in a chair. In the case of a temporal or nasal detachment, the patient will be nursed on the opposite side to the affected area. These positions are reversed post-operatively if surgery has included the internal tamponade, i.e. pressure. Nursing actions that can help to encourage patient compliance with positioning regimes are described in Nursing Care Plan 13.3.

Postoperative pain

Postoperative pain can be expected to be fairly severe, depending on the complexity and the duration of the surgery. (Retinal repair procedures may take 1–4 h.) Narcotic analgesia may be necessary for effective pain control but if severe pain persists it must be reported and investigated immediately. An acute rise in IOP can be precipitated by retinal surgery and persistent severe pain reported by the patient should alert the nurse to this possibility. To avoid permanent damage action must be taken immediately to reduce raised IOP. If severe pain persists after the fifth day and the IOP is within normal limits some problem with the explant must be suspected.

Postoperative appearance of the eye

In retinal surgery the conjunctival incision is encircling, there is extensive handling of the globe and, if vitrectomy instruments have been used, there may be considerable trauma to the conjunctiva. The nurse can therefore expect to observe marked chemosis with bruising and swelling of the eyelids. Pressure dressings or regular cold compresses may be applied postoperatively. The eye must be monitored closely to ensure that the conjunctival incision heals cleanly and that there is

Nursing Care Plan 13.3 Positioning of a patient with retinal detachment

Nursing consideration	Action	Rationale	Evaluation
The patient has knowledge deficit re enforced positional bedrest to prevent further detachment of retina and help postoperative recovery	❒ Establish knowledge base by preparing and presenting a teaching session using a model of an eye. Include a family member if patient has significant visual loss. Include: • description of normal retina and its function • possible cause of detachment • description of surgical procedure • positioning before and after surgery to help retina fall back into place. Explain that this will be prescribed by the specialist and that every attempt must be made to observe it	Misconceptions about eye surgery are often lurid and frightening. Understanding what really happens will reduce fear and make compliance with instructions more likely. The informed patient experiences a significant reduction in anxiety levels and is more likely to comply	The patient is able to describe what happens in retinal detachment, how it can be repaired and asks questions which indicate an acceptable level of knowledge He appears more relaxed about the need for positioning and is very co-operative
	❒ Encourage questions	Given time and encouragement patients may express a variety of questions and individual concerns	
	❒ Reinforce explanations frequently	Due to blocking effect of anxiety patients do not always absorb information and it may be necessary to repeat or rephrase it	

no evidence of rejection or extrusion of the silicone explant. Careful observation and meticulous reporting are essential in order to measure progress and circumvent complications.

CORNEAL GRAFTING (KERATOPLASTY)

Indications for corneal grafting include destruction of the cornea by injury or disease, some cases of advanced keratoconus (conical cornea), and corneal opacity. Grafts may be full thickness or partial thickness. In full-thickness grafting the central part of the affected cornea is removed and replaced with corneal tissue taken from a donor, and which must be harvested within 10 h of death. The tissue should be accompanied by blood samples which are tested for HIV and tissue-matched. However, because of the avascularity of the cornea it is not absolutely essential to use a tissue-matched graft.

The donor eye is screened to ensure that it is disease-free. If stored in a refrigerator at 4°C, the tissue must be used within 48 h. This entails an emergency-type situation for the recipient. A National Eye Bank in Bristol accepts donor material for storage under freezing programmes. This material is then supplied for elective surgery.

The perioperative period is managed as for other intraocular surgery. In addition, both the surgeon and the nurse must ensure that the patient and his family are fully informed and have realistic expectations of what is involved and of the outcome.

NURSING PRIORITIES AND MANAGEMENT: CORNEAL GRAFTING

Special considerations

The use of donated tissue

Recipients rarely ask questions regarding the source of a donated cornea but nurses must be prepared to give a carefully worded answer to those who do; they must also be ready to give reassurance and support, as the use of donor grafts can be an emotive issue. Sometimes the donor's relatives ask if the tissue has been used. Confirmation is usually given by medical staff but nurses may also be involved. Care should be taken not to violate confidentiality whilst still providing adequate information. Ideally, the entire team caring for the patient should invest time in preparing and delivering relevant, individualised information.

Postoperative examination

Following surgery the degree of conjunctival injection (redness) may be considerable. This should lessen progressively. If the conjunctiva does not soon return to the 'white eye' state the cause may be: (1) raised IOP; (2) failure of the graft; (3) graft rejection. These three possibilities must also be considered when inspection of the cornea reveals a loss of clarity, a finding which must be reported immediately. The wound should be examined to ensure the suture line remains intact and the corneal disc (graft) has stayed in position, as disruption of either may affect the optical power of the graft.

Patient involvement and cooperation

The patient and his family should be made aware that corneal grafting requires a lengthy follow-up period. The cornea is an avascular structure, therefore healing will be slow. The corneal suture will remain in situ for several months or, if a good optical result has been obtained it may be decided to leave the sutures in indefinitely rather than risk disturbing the graft.

It must also be emphasised that it is vital to continue topical medication prescribed to avoid rejection of the graft and to prevent infection. The patient should be warned that optimum visual recovery cannot be expected until some months after surgery. Some may be disappointed by the initial outcome when vision may seem to be poorer than before grafting; these patients should be reminded of realistic expectations.

Prior to discharge, patient and carer teaching should ensure that the importance of early recognition of symptoms of graft rejection is understood. These symptoms could include:

- increased redness of the conjunctiva
- cloudiness of the cornea
- reduction of visual function and/or
- discomfort.

TEMPORAL ARTERITIS (GIANT CELL ARTERITIS, CRANIAL ARTERITIS)

This is a disease process affecting the over-60 age group, in which the middle layer of medium-sized arteries becomes inflamed. When the external carotid system is involved, ocular damage results with sudden loss of vision, which may be preceded by, or accompany, polymyalgia rheumatica (stiff aching muscles, especially around the shoulders).

PATHOPHYSIOLOGY

There is degeneration of the retina, which results from thrombosis or occlusion of the ophthalmic artery, secondary to necrotic inflammatory changes in the middle layer of the temporal and cranial arteries. The cells in the destroyed middle layer are replaced by collagen. During the active phase of this process there is a raised erthrocyte sedimentation rate (ESR).

Clinical features. Patients often complain of general malaise, loss of weight and lethargy, or a 'flu-like illness which may last for a few days or weeks and which precedes a sustained visual disturbance. This is in contrast to the prodromal phase, in which fleeting episodes of blurred vision may occur, accompanied by unilateral temporal or occipital headache. The loss of vision is sudden in onset, usually affecting one eye before the other. The length of time between both eyes being affected is extremely variable, ranging from several hours to several days.

MEDICAL MANAGEMENT

Diagnosis is made following ophthalmoscopy and a raised ESR. It has to be remembered that the ESR may not be high in the early stages of the disease and repeat tests may be necessary. The diagnosis may be confirmed by carrying out a temporal artery biopsy.

Treatment. Systemic corticosteroid therapy reduces the ESR to within normal limits. The starting dosage may be given intramuscularly to achieve the effective therapeutic level. The starting high-dosage rate, that is, 80–120 mg daily, is reduced to a maintenance dose, which will be administered for at least 2 years. Topical treatment is not usually prescribed unless a secondary condition, for example, iritis, develops.

NURSING PRIORITIES AND MANAGEMENT: TEMPORAL ARTERITIS

Nursing effort is directed towards the care of a patient undergoing corticosteroid therapy. In particular, monitoring and recording regimes for example, of BP urinalysis and body weight, will be required to give warning of any complication arising from the therapy. If vision deficit is severe, help and support will be necessary and blind or partially sighted registration will become inevitable. This entails a multi-disciplinary approach to rehabilitation care, in which the nursing staff participate fully.

RED EYE

Primary closed-angle glaucoma

Closed-angle glaucoma usually presents as an acute episode affecting one eye, although it may be sub-acute or chronic. *It is an ophthalmic emergency* and needs specialist attention within 24 h to prevent permanent visual damage. It is also necessary to initiate early prophylactic treatment in the other, 'quiet' eye.

PATHOPHYSIOLOGY

Raised IOP develops as a result of disruption of the circulation of aqueous humor in a narrow anterior chamber, which is often associated with hypermetropia. Pupil dilation is accompanied by forward displacement of the iris which occludes the trabecular meshwork, blocking the flow of aqueous to the canal of Schlemm. The pupillary margin of the iris also comes into contact with the lens, causing the pupil to become semi-dilated and fixed, further impeding the flow of aqueous and increasing forward displacement of the iris. Aqueous buildup results in corneal oedema and disturbance of sensory nerve fibres.

Common presenting symptoms are as follows:

- Onset is usually sudden, with severe pain in one eye accompanied by frontotemporal headache on the affected side
- The patient often complains of nausea and may vomit
- Vision is reduced
- The individual is photophobic and experiences increased lacrimation
- The eye is red, particularly around the limbus (due to marked ciliary injection)
- The cornea is hazy due to oedema
- The pupil is semi-dilated and does not react to light
- Iris details are poorly defined (muddy in appearance)
- On palpation over a closed lid the eye feels hard because of raised IOP.

MEDICAL MANAGEMENT

Tests and investigations. These include medical history, systematic structural examination, slit lamp and gonioscopy examination of the angle of the eye (see Appendix 1), and measurement of IOP. (A slit lamp illuminates the eye with a narrow band of light which allows particular structures (e.g. cornea, lens, anterior chamber) to be examined through a binocular microscope.)

Medical treatment. Acute signs and symptoms will be controlled by the following means:

- pain relief by analgesics, including i.m. opiates
- control of nausea and vomiting with i.m. antiemetics
- increase in outflow of aqueous humor by freeing the iris angle. To achieve this a regime of intensive topical miotic therapy is commenced to constrict the pupil rapidly and draw the iris away from the angle. Prophylactic therapy is also prescribed for the 'quiet' eye
- reduction in production of aqueous humor by administration of carbonic anhydrase inhibitors such as acetazolamide (Diamox). If the response to this is unsatisfactory, osmotic diuretics such as oral glycerol or i.v. mannitol can be used.

Surgical intervention. Once the acute signs and symptoms have been controlled, surgical intervention may be decided upon. The method depends on the appearance of the angle and may be any of the following:

- laser iridotomies (small holes in the iris) to both eyes
- surgical iridectomy to the acute eye and laser iridotomy to the 'quiet' eye
- surgical drainage, for example, trabeculectomy to the acute eye and prophylactic treatment to the 'quiet' eye.

Following laser iridotomies, steroid treatment may be given to reduce tissue irritability and ensure normal IOP. The eye is inspected at frequent intervals.

For surgical procedures such as peripheral iridectomies or

trabeculectomies the preparation and perioperative care is as for glaucoma (see p. 480).

NURSING PRIORITIES AND MANAGEMENT: PRIMARY CLOSED-ANGLE GLAUCOMA

Screening

The nurse working in a general practice, community or emergency department setting frequently has to assume a screening role and prioritise patients' needs for specialist attention in ophthalmic conditions. She should be aware of the significance of various signs and symptoms such as severe pain in one or both eyes, a hazy cornea and a significant deterioration in vision. Failure to do so may result in the patient suffering unnecessary loss of vision.

In primary closed-angle glaucoma priority is given to the immediate control of acute signs and symptoms and to the delivery of prescribed intensive therapy regimes. Otherwise, nursing priorities and management are as for primary open-angle glaucoma (see p. 480). The initial pain and distress experienced by patients with primary closed-angle glaucoma will be severe. A satisfactory pupillary miosis with resolution of corneal oedema generally occurs about 4 h after commencement of treatment and can be maintained thereafter by medical management or surgical intervention or a combination of both. Some aspects of the nursing support that can be given to patients undergoing laser treatment are described in Nursing Care Plan 13.2.

UVEITIS

PATHOPHYSIOLOGY

Uveitis is inflammation of the uveal tract. Anterior uveitis (or iritis) can involve the iris, the ciliary body, or both. Posterior uveitis involves the choroid (choroiditis). It is an acute condition the precise cause of which is unknown, although it is often associated with rheumatoid conditions, ankylosing spondylitis and sarcoidosis. Recurrent episodes are relatively common; they usually respond to immediate treatment and carry a fairly good prognosis. Secondary iritis may accompany other eye infections or trauma.

Clinical features:

- pain, probably due to pupillary spasm; pain may mark the onset of iritis and may be severe
- redness due to vascular congestion in the conjunctival vessels at the limbus of the cornea and sometimes on the iris
- photophobia
- cloudy aqueous due to the increase in aqueous protein content and presence of white blood cells (the debris floating in the aqueous is known as 'flare and cell')
- reduced vision, proportional to the severity of the attack
- cellular exudate (keratic precipitates (KP)) may be present on the posterior surface of the cornea
- loss of iris details (muddy iris)
- swelling of the iris may cause it to adhere to the anterior surface of the lens (synechia formation); this will interfere with aqueous flow
- IOP may be raised and, if untreated, may progress to secondary glaucoma.

MEDICAL MANAGEMENT

Patients with acute iritis are treated on an outpatient basis whenever possible. Inflammatory episodes are controlled using a combination of topical and systemic drugs. Steroids and mydriatics are administered as eye drops or as sub-conjunctival injection. Steroids may be prescribed systemically when the response to topical medication is poor. In some complicated cases, immunosuppressive drugs may be necessary. In addition, when the intraocular pressure is raised, acetazolamide or topical beta-blockers will be prescribed. Pain-relieving drugs are given as required. Dark glasses are supplied to relieve the discomfort of photophobia.

NURSING PRIORITIES AND MANAGEMENT: UVEITIS

Major nursing considerations

Setting priorities

Screening for potential health problems and prioritising patients' needs are two interrelated aspects of the nurse's role in the community. It is vital that community nurses are able to recognise ophthalmic conditions which need urgent medical attention. Uveitis is one such condition, as raised IOP and/or severe infection will quickly cause irreparable damage if treatment is delayed.

?	**13.12** State the ophthalmic conditions that must receive the most urgent attention.

Providing instruction

Once the diagnosis is confirmed and treatment has been commenced the nurse's role will include providing support and instruction for the patient and his family and ensuring compliance with the treatment regime. If a pattern of recurrence emerges it is advantageous to instruct the patient on early initiation of self-medication. This will reduce the severity of the attack and the risk of complications.

Ensuring a safe environment

Dilated pupils allow an increased amount of light to enter the eye, causing photophobia. Patients experience dazzle when in bright sunlight or when facing car headlights from oncoming traffic at night. Appropriate adjustments to lifestyle may be required for the duration of the treatment.

KERATITIS

The term keratitis refers to inflammatory conditions of the cornea. These may be caused by certain bacteria, viruses or fungi and result in corneal ulceration. If the epithelium only is affected, there is minimal damage with little visual loss. If the stroma is involved, loss of transparency and altered corneal curvature may lead to significant loss of vision. Severe inflammation may result in inflammatory debris being shed into the anterior chamber, producing hypopyon.

PATHOPHYSIOLOGY

Bacterial keratitis

Causative agents of bacterial keratitis include pneumococcus, streptococcus and pseudomonas, which invade the cornea and cause an inflammatory reaction. The condition tends to be recurrent. Severe, deep ulceration erodes the corneal stroma to the level of Descemet's membrane, which herniates to form a descemetocele due to the pressure of the aqueous humour. Corneal perforation will occur if the descemetocele ruptures.

Clinical features. The lesion appears as a grey circular area on the surface of the cornea, with oedema of the surrounding epithelium which dulls the corneal reflex. Other features include:

- a painful red eye
- photophobia with spasm of the eyelid
- excessive lacrimation in most cases, although there are some instances of dry eye presentation.

Viral keratitis

The most common form of viral keratitis is dendritic ulcer, which is caused by the herpes simplex virus. Its distinguishing feature is the

Research Abstract 13.2 Contact lenses and keratitis risk (Matthews et al 1992)

Disposable soft contact lenses have been marketed as a safer alternative to conventional soft lenses. A study of patients in the casualty department at Moorfields Eye Hospital by Matthews et al (1992) set out to investigate the validity of this claim and to establish patterns of use (n = 242).

The results did not support the claim but indicated that keratitis, microbial and sterile, was the most common complication found in disposable lens users, and that disposable lenses were associated with a significantly higher risk and incidence of keratitis than any other lens type. Matthews et al concluded that lens type, poor hygiene and failure to follow instructions for cleansing and use could account for these statistically significant trends.

Matthews T D, Frazer D G, Minassian D C, Radford C F, Dart J K G 1992 Risks of keratitis and patterns of use with disposable contact lenses. Archives of Ophthalmol Ophthalmology 110(11): 1559–1562

branching, tree-like pattern it forms on the cornea, which is visible only on corneal staining with fluorescein.

Fungal keratitis

Fungal infections of the eye are an increasing problem in eye departments. The damage they cause is severe and specific antifungal treatment agents are few. Complications can develop rapidly. The distinguishing feature of this kind of ulceration is that it appears as fluffy, feathery extensions over the cornea. Often it can be associated with minor trauma from vegetation or with contact lenses. (See also Research Abstract 13.2.)

MEDICAL MANAGEMENT

Diagnosis can be confirmed by conjunctival and corneal swabs and fluorescein staining. The fluorescein fixes to damaged corneal tissue and turns the affected area a bright fluorescent green, indicating the extent of the damage. Topical antibiotic, antiviral or antifungal therapy is usually commenced immediately to avoid rapid development of complications. Any accompanying iritis or rise in IOP is treated as necessary. It is important to note that steroids are generally contraindicated for keratitis. Some exceptions to this rule do occur, but can be determined only by an ophthalmic specialist.

NURSING PRIORITIES AND MANAGEMENT: KERATITIS

Management may be on an inpatient or outpatient basis and follows the principles outlined earlier for uveitis, with the following additions:

- The patient should be taught not to touch or rub his eye as this may extend the ulceration.
- Careful hygiene is essential to prevent cross-infection. Tears should be wiped from the cheek only. A clean disposable tissue should be used on each occasion. Principles of isolation and infection control will be observed in the hospital situation (see Ch. 16, p. 548).
- With regard to dendritic ulcer it is important to note that anyone who has an outbreak of herpes simplex — commonly known as 'cold sores' — should be advised to guard against touching the sores and then rubbing their eyes. Nursing staff with active sores should not be on duty on wards where there are ophthalmic patients.

CONJUNCTIVITIS

Conjunctivitis, i.e. inflammation of the conjunctiva, is a common condition, which may be acute, sub-acute or chronic. It can be unilateral or bilateral in presentation, the latter form often due to cross-infection. Causative agents are bacteria, viruses, fungi, parasites, toxins, chemicals, foreign bodies and allergies.

PATHOPHYSIOLOGY

The activating agent causes vascular dilation (injection) of the palpebral and bulbar conjunctiva, cellular infiltration leading to formation of papillae and follicles, and serous exudation. In severe cases oedema of the conjunctiva (chemosis) may occur.

Clinical features include:

- brick-red appearance
- gritty feeling and varying degrees of pain
- in bacterial conjunctivitis: often mucopurulent discharge; the eyelids may stick together at night.

The eye is not usually photophobic, nor is vision affected. Eversion of the lids will reveal follicle formation, which is the cause of the gritty sensation.

Medical and nursing management entails treating the cause, educating the patient in eye hygiene and self-medication, and monitoring for complications. Conjunctivitis is highly infectious and family members, peers and other patients should be guarded against it by active education to alert them to the danger. Scrupulous hand-washing and the use of individual towels should be emphasised.

Herpes zoster ophthalmicus (ophthalmic shingles)

This is an acute unilateral infection of the trigeminal ganglion which extends from the scalp to the nose and includes the eye. It is caused by the chickenpox virus and is fairly common in people over 50 years of age (see Ch. 16, p. 570).

PATHOPHYSIOLOGY

Common presenting symptoms are as follows:

- the eruption is usually preceded by pain, regional adenopathy and general malaise
- the eyelids swell on the affected side
- the skin of the forehead above the eye becomes red
- characteristic vesicular eruptions occur over the course of the nerve
- there may be serious inflammatory complications, including uveitis, keratitis, conjunctivitis and visual impairment.

Medical and nursing management. Treatment with systemic antiviral agents should begin immediately. Ocular involvement should be treated symptomatically and with equal vigour. Prevention of cross-infection is a priority.

Allergy to topical medication

Allergic reaction to topical eye medication manifests as inflammation of the eyelids extending to the cheeks. The lids become red and oedematous and may be moist in the acute stage, drying to form light crusts later. There is intense itching, which may result in excoriation. Common causative agents are atropine and neomycin eye drops.

Management consists of reviewing medication, suspending all medication for 24 h if possible, and substituting an alternative agent. Cortisone lotion may be prescribed for the affected skin area to relieve itching and oedema.

Stye (hordeolum)

A stye is a staphylococcal infection of the eyelash follicle or its associated sebaceous gland. It may be treated by hot spoon bathing and application of an antibiotic ointment. Principles of prevention of crossinfection should be observed. (See Box 13.3.)

Box 13.3 Hot spoon bathing

This is a method of applying moist heat locally, to the eye or abscess site, in order to relieve pain, improve the effectiveness of local treatment and to assist in the 'pointing' of abscesses.

Requirements. A wooden spoon, cotton wool to pad the bowl of the spoon, a gauze swab to cover the cotton wool and a rubber band or muslin bandage to secure the padding. A jug containing nearly boiling water standing in a tray or a basin large enough to contain the volume of water if accidentally spilt. A plastic cape or towel to protect the patient's clothing.

Method. The procedure is explained to the patient and he is positioned comfortably with his legs beneath a table. The bowl or tray containing the filled jug, is placed within easy reach on the table, which should be checked for stability. The cape or towel is draped over the shoulders. He is instructed to soak the spoon in the hot water, to remove excess water by pressing it against the rim of the jug, which must be held firmly during this part of the procedure. The steaming spoon is then held close to the affected area to provide comfortable heat *without* skin contact in order to avoid any possibility of a scald. As the spoon cools it is re-dipped to maintain an effective temperature. The process is continued for 10–15 minutes and is usually carried out four times daily. All patients require supervision during the procedure. The frail, the handicapped and children must always have assistance in order to prevent accidents.

DIPLOPIA (DOUBLE VISION)

Diplopia refers to a person's experience of seeing the same object in two different areas of his visual field. If this occurs with one eye closed it usually means that the light entering the eye is broken up, as in the presence of a cataract. If it occurs with both eyes open it is caused by an imbalance in the extraocular muscles (a squint). In adults this is usually acquired and is associated with systemic disorders or trauma. These include meningitis, multiple sclerosis, cerebral aneurysm, myasthenia gravis, neoplasm, hypertension, thyrotoxicosis, diabetes and head injury. Different factors are involved in childhood squints and for further information reference should be made to paediatric texts.

NURSING PRIORITIES AND MANAGEMENT: DIPLOPIA

Symptomatic treatment in the community. Diplopia caused by a squint can be alleviated by occluding one eye with an eye patch. This can be initiated by the nurse until the patient is seen by a specialist or, in the case of paralytic squint, during treatment of the underlying disease. If one eye is occluded there is no conflict of images in the visual cortex. This reduces the dizziness and nausea often associated with the sense of imbalance caused by diplopia.

MEDICAL MANAGEMENT

The treatment of the underlying cause is given in the appropriate chapter.

Treatment can be given for double vision:

- occlusion of one eye
- prism spectacles
- surgical squint correction – This would not be contemplated for at least six months after stabilisation of the squint as spontaneous improvement is possible
- injection of Botulinum A Neurotoxin to the overacting muscle which gives temporary flaccid paralysis (approx. three months) during which the opposing muscle undergoes contraction reducing the angle of deviation. The Botulinum blocks the transmission of the nerve impulses at the neuromuscular junction by interfering with the release of acetylcholene (see Ch. 9).

EYE INJURIES

The eye is susceptible to many types of injury, most of which are frightening and painful. A careful history (Table 13.3), which must include a record of visual acuity and a systematic eye examination (Table 13.1), is taken to establish a diagnosis and for medico–legal reasons. Chemical burns are the only exception to this; the main priority is first aid treatment. A triage system for ophthalmic injuries is outlined in Box 13.4 (see also Ch. 28, p. 810).

Careful history-taking is especially important if it is suspected that a particle may have entered the eye at a high velocity. In such a case there could well be no external evidence of injury and no pain and if the particle were left in situ it could result in blindness many years later. Some of the more commonly occurring types of eye injury are described below.

Box 13.4 Ophthalmic triage

Ophthalmic patients attending an A & E department are placed in one of three categories depending on the severity of their disorder (York 1990).

CATEGORY 1

True emergencies requiring immediate specialist attention:

- Chemical burns (initiate first aid immediately)
- Penetrating injuries
- Intraocular foreign body
- Acute glaucoma
- Extensive retinal detachment
- Sudden loss of vision in one eye (initiate first aid immediately)

CATEGORY 2

Specialist attention required as soon as possible:

- Hyphaema
- Corneal foreign body, abrasion or ulcer
- Radiation and welding burns
- All acute infections or allergies
- Recent inpatient who suspects complications

CATEGORY 3

Minor irritations and longstanding visual disturbances

HYPHAEMA

The term 'hyphaema' refers to a haemorrhage into the anterior chamber of the eye.

PATHOPHYSIOLOGY

A primary hyphaema is usually caused by a direct blow to the eye for example, a clenched fist, golf ball or champagne cork causing rupture of the small iris blood vessels. It may be microscopic with

Table 13.3 Systematic approach to history taking

Assessment	Question	Rationale
History of injury	How did accident occur? When did accident occur? Where did accident occur? Which eye is affected? Is injury unilateral/bilateral? Were safety goggles worn?	To aid diagnosis For medico–legal reasons
Ophthalmic history	Are glasses worn? Has similar accident occurred before? Has patient attended eye hospital before?	 To ascertain if preventive lessons are learnt
Medical history	Does patient have a general health problem? Has patient had previous surgery?	Some systemic disorders may affect eye, e.g. diabetes Patient may require surgery and may have had a reaction to an anaesthetic previously
Medications	Is patient taking medication at present?	Some drugs may affect the eye, e.g. aspirin and the contraceptive pill Patient may have an allergy to a drug
Allergies	Is patient allergic to any substance e.g. drugs, Sellotape, Elastoplast?	Patient may be given inadvertently a substance to which he is allergic

diffuse red cells visible only with the aid of a slit lamp, or severe with a level of blood seen. Rarely, the blood can completely fill the AC.

The degree of pain and reduction in vision depends upon the severity of the bleeding.

A secondary hyphaema may occur after intraocular surgery or a penetrating eye injury.

MEDICAL MANAGEMENT

A systematic approach of history taking is carried out as outlined in Table 13.3.

A patient with a microscopic hyphaema or moderate hyphaema will not be admitted but advised to rest at home for several days. These hyphaemas rarely rebleed.

A patient with a severe hyphaema may be admitted for observation as there could be an associated rise in IOP. Quiet activity will be allowed. If a rebleed occurs it usually happens between the 3rd and 5th day.

NURSING PRIORITIES AND MANAGEMENT: HYPHAEMA

Observation of the level of hyphaema is made 2–4 times daily. Any increase in pain or discomfort may be caused by raised IOP or a rebleed.

The patient is advised to bend at the knees to reach things from below waist height, and not to lift or strain.

Diversional therapy may be required to occupy the time of these, usually young, men.

Topical antibiotic and/or steroid eyedrops may be prescribed. On discharge, the patient will be advised to avoid active or contact sports until the first follow-up appointment. He will be told to assess visual function in the injured eye, daily, to detect possible complications, for example, retinal detachment (see page 480 and Nursing Care Plan 13.1). Protective eyewear may be necessary in the future, for example, whilst playing squash, to prevent a similar injury again (see Box 13.2).

PENETRATING INJURIES

Whatever the apparent extent of a penetrating injury it must always be treated as an emergency and thoroughly investigated. Depending on the results of history-taking and examination, X-rays and ultrasound scanning may be necessary to confirm the presence, location and type of a foreign body.

MEDICAL MANAGEMENT

Treatment will depend on the cause of the injury and on the extent of involvement of ocular structures. It will usually include the administration of mydriatic, steroid and antibiotic eye drops, and possibly of systemic antibiotics to reduce the risk of complications from inflammation and infection. In addition, the measures described below will be taken.

Perforating injuries. The patient will be admitted to hospital for surgical repair of the wound and possible excision of iris prolapse. If the lens is damaged it may be removed at same time. If facial or other injuries are present these will be repaired by the appropriate specialists (see Ch. 15).

Small puncture wounds. These may seal themselves, but the patient is admitted to ensure that the wound stays closed and that intraocular infection does not develop. If the wound is not completely sealed acrylic glue may be instilled onto the cornea to seal the wound, or a contact lens may be applied.

Intraocular foreign bodies. Admission is essential for surgical removal of the foreign body, which could be embedded in the iris, vitreous humor or lens. If the foreign body is metallic, it may be removed with the aid of a magnet. If it is found in the lens, a lens extraction is carried out. Vitrectomy may be necessary if there has been vitreous haemorrhage (see p. 494).

Complications following penetrating injury. Many complications can occur after a penetrating injury — some immediately, others months later (see Table 13.4). Severe infections can occur in any injury, making intensive treatment with antibiotic eye drops and systemic antibiotics necessary.

It is always very important to examine the uninjured eye regularly for signs of a rare complication known as 'sympathetic ophthalmitis', which presents as a low-grade iritis. The cause of the sympathetic inflammatory process is thought to involve an immune response to damaged uveal tissue. The use of topical steroids has reduced the occurrence of this potentially sight-threatening condition, which was formerly managed by enucleating the injured eye.

Table 13.4 Possible complications following penetrating eye injury

Structure	Complication	Cause	Onset	Treatment
Cornea	Astigmatism	Sutures and scarring	After surgery	Remove sutures
	Scarring	Wound	After surgery	Contact lens in future Corneal graft in future
Anterior chamber	Hypopyon: sterile	Iritis	1–3 days	Intensive steroids
	Hypopyon: infected	Infection	1–7 days	Intensive antibiotics
	Hyphaema	Bleeding iris vessels	1–7 days	Treat as secondary hyphaema
	Raised IOP	Damage to drainage angle	1–7 days	Beta blocker eyedrops and acetazolamide
Iris	Prolapse through wound	Original injury or loose suture	1–7 days	Excision of prolapse and resuturing
Lens	Cataract	Original trauma	Immediate/weeks later	Intra/extracapsular lens extraction
	Dislocation	Original trauma to suspensory ligaments	Immediate	Lens extraction or no treatment
Vitreous chamber	Haemorrhage	Bleeding into vitreous humor	Immediate	Vitrectomy
	Fibrous bands		Weeks later	Vitrectomy
Retina	Retinal tears	Original trauma	Immediate/weeks later	Cryotherapy
	Detachment	Original injury	Immediate/weeks later	Surgical repair
		Fluid vitreous	Immediate/weeks later	Surgical repair

A severely damaged eye with no prospect of useful vision may become very painful and unresponsive to analgesics. It may be necessary to remove the eye to give relief to the patient.

Following repair of large penetrating injuries (or severe infections) the eye may collapse entirely and become a shrunken mass in the orbit. This wasting of the globe (phthisis bulbii) can be unsightly and the patient may wish the eye to be removed.

NURSING PRIORITIES AND MANAGEMENT: PENETRATING INJURIES

Major patient problems

Anxiety

Many injuries are severe and mutilating and pose a grave danger to sight. Fear of becoming blind will heighten the patient's anxiety. Comforting the distressed patient and his relatives is a nursing priority. Enabling the patient and his carers to express their feelings and fears is an important part of the comforting process. All questions must be answered honestly, with a uniformity of approach, so that no false or unrealistic expectations are raised.

Post-operatively, the patient's main concern will be to know how severely affected the vision will be and the duration of the visual loss.

Fears about body image, work and lifestyle will be paramount. The patient and his relatives may approach different members of staff for answers to their questions. This may reflect their high level of anxiety or it may indicate that explanations have been inadequate. Discussion and good communication among staff is vital to prevent misunderstanding. Where the prognosis is poor, clear and consistent information will dispel false expectations and help the patient and his family to adapt to the reality of the situation. The loss of sight is like any other significant human loss and will be accompanied by a process akin to grieving.

Return to the community

If the eye is damaged to the extent that there is no useful vision left, the patient will need continuing support in the community. This should be arranged before his discharge. Patients in this situation are particularly susceptible to depression when they return home and begin to grapple with the full implications of their disability. They will need practical and psychological support through the grieving and adaptation period.

CHEMICAL BURNS

Treatment should begin immediately after a chemical has entered the eye. The sooner the eye is irrigated with copious amounts of water the less damage will be caused. Speed is essential and it may be necessary to plunge the whole head into a basin of water and force the eyelids open or to hold the head under a running tap. Many chemical substances have antidotes but no time should be wasted in finding one. Immediate irrigation is paramount (see Box 13.5).

PATHOPHYSIOLOGY

The burn may be caused by an acid or by an alkali. In general, acids cause only superficial burns because coagulation of the tissues prevents further penetration. The structures involved are usually the palpebral (i.e. lining the eyelids) and bulbar (covering the eyeball) conjunctivae and the cornea. Alkalis penetrate the eye structures more deeply and, as well as severely damaging the eyelids, conjunctivae, cornea and sclera, readily penetrate the internal structures.

Many of the substances which cause burns are contained in aerosol cans, but car battery acid and cement are frequent culprits. Superglue can be particularly dangerous. The patient is often a manual worker or a DIY enthusiast who has not taken necessary precautions (see Box 13.2).

The patient will complain of severe, burning pain due to the exposure of the pain receptors of the trigeminal nerve. Absence of pain does not mean the burn is mild: the burn may be so severe that it has destroyed the nerve endings. There will be extreme watering of the eyes due to reflex action. The lids will be very swollen and red. Burns to the surrounding skin may be evident.

MEDICAL MANAGEMENT

On arrival in the Accident and Emergency (A & E) department the patient is taken for immediate irrigation of the eye. This is one time when visual acuity is not assessed before treatment. Anaesthetic eye

Box 13.5 Occupational health nurse

Many industries employ an occupational health nurse, who educates staff in the first aid treatment of a chemical entering an eye, which is immediate irrigation of the eye.

This has made a significant reduction in the number, and the extent, of these injuries.

drops are instilled to reduce the pain and ensure the patient's cooperation with irrigation. The irrigating fluid will be either sodium chloride 0.6% or a neutralising fluid for alkaline burns, e.g. Limclair. (See Box 13.6.)

Once the nurse is sure that all traces of the chemical have been removed a full history can be taken and visual acuity assessed.

After irrigation the doctor will examine the eyes using a slit lamp (see p. 483) to assess the extent of the injury. Many chemical injuries are successfully treated before any lasting damage can occur. Occasionally, however, the burn can cause extensive damage to the cornea and conjunctiva.

Treatment for minor burns. The patient is allowed to return home. He is prescribed an antibiotic ointment. An eye pad is applied, to remain in place for at least 6 hours. If both eyes require padding, the better eye is left exposed until the patient arrives at home, where he is instructed to pad the other eye. The antibiotic ointment is prescribed for several days and the patient is given a follow-up appointment.

Box 13.6 Irrigation of an eye

The irrigation can be carried out with an i.v. giving set, or a syringe (in an emergency), and should continue for at least 10–15 min to each eye. The patient should be lying down or seated with his head supported. He should be asked to look up, down, and from side to side, to ensure that as far as possible the fluid washes over all parts of the eyeball. The upper eyelids should be everted to ensure that any particles (e.g. of lime or cement) have been washed out. If not, they can be removed with a moistened cotton bud or fine forceps.

The irrigation is discontinued once litmus paper shows that the chemical has been neutralised.

In some cases the patient may require a general anaesthetic while all traces of the chemical are removed.

Treatment for severe burns. The patient is admitted to the ward for intensive treatment and observation. Depending on the severity of the pain, i.m. analgesia is given for at least the first 24 h. An antibiotic ointment is applied at least 4 times daily to lubricate the fornices and mydriatic eye drops are instilled to relieve accompanying iris spasm and iritis. To prevent the development of conjunctival adhesions (symblepharon) rodding of the fornices may be required (see Box 13.7).

NURSING PRIORITIES AND MANAGEMENT: CHEMICAL BURNS

Major patient problems

Anxiety

It will be important for the nurse to provide reassurance and emotional support for patients who have suffered chemical burns to the eye, as their anxiety level is likely to be high. The patient may have bilateral eye pads in situ, and may find this very stressful. Once the eyepads are removed, dark glasses may be necessary to reduce the photophobia caused by iris spasm and pupil dilation.

Box 13.7 Rodding of fornices

This procedure is carried out by a nurse. Local anaesthetic eyedrops are instilled. A glass rod is lubricated with antibiotic ointment and inserted under the upper eyelid. The patient is asked to look down and the rod is passed gently, but firmly, from side to side several times whilst outward pressure is exerted. This breaks down any adhesions already formed and leaves a film of ointment in the fornix to prevent any occurrence.

The process is repeated under the lower eyelid with the patient looking up.

Return to the community

The patient will be advised to maintain prescribed treatment for several weeks and to attend follow-up outpatient appointments.

If there is permanent damage to one or both corneas a keratoplasty may be carried out (see p. 481).

It may be necessary, in cases of significant sight loss, to ensure that the patient and his carers are fully supported and are offered appropriate advice by special community services for the blind and partially sighted person.

RADIATION INJURIES

Irradiation from ultraviolet, infrared or laser light can cause eye damage.

PATHOPHYSIOLOGY

Ultraviolet radiation causes corneal epithelial damage (arc eye, welders' flash) and most commonly occurs when approved eye goggles with protective sides are not worn during welding or when the individual is using a sun bed or sun lamp (see Box 13.2). Usually the signs and symptoms do not appear until several hours after exposure, when the patient presents with photophobia, pain and excessive lacrimation. The reason that there is this latent period is not fully understood. Fluorescein drops show dot-like staining of the cornea. Treatment is symptomatic and includes pain relief and the use of eye pads or dark glasses. The cornea should heal in 3–5 days and there should be no long-term effects.

Infrared radiation penetrates the eye through the cornea and can cause cataracts.

Laser radiation can cause irreversible damage to the retina.

NURSING PRIORITIES AND MANAGEMENT: RADIATION INJURIES

Prevention

Health education and accident prevention is a major part of the nurse's role. The need for protective eyewear wherever there is danger of radiation must be actively stressed. Nurses working in occupational health, general practice, in the community, in A & E departments and in outpatients departments with laser equipment could implement a programme of health education which focuses on this topic. It is also important to stress that other people working in the immediate environment of the radiation source may sustain injuries.

?	**13.13** Can you think of reasons why people might fail to use appropriate eye protection? Is there any legislation governing the provision of protective eyewear? Discuss this issue with your tutor and reflect on how it applies to your own workplace.

MINOR EYE INJURIES

Corneal foreign body

The patient can usually give an accurate history of something entering the eye. The eye will be extremely painful, especially on blinking. On examination a foreign body will be visible on the anterior surface of the cornea. Anaesthetic eyedrops are instilled and the foreign body is removed with a moistened cotton bud or a 10 G needle. This can be carried out by the doctor or a trained ophthalmic nurse (see Box 13.8.)

Subtarsal foreign body

The nurse should suspect the presence of a subtarsal foreign body when despite the patient's complaint of something entering his eye nothing can be seen on normal inspection. There will be discomfort, especially on blinking. The upper lid should under this circumstance be everted and the foreign body, if present, removed with a moistened cotton bud. (See Box 13.9.)

Corneal abrasion
This can be caused by a fingernail, a twig or other sharp object. It is an extremely painful condition with profuse lacrimation. Fluorescein eyedrops should be instilled in order to determine the extent of the abrasion.

An eye pad need not be applied after treatment for abrasion or removal of a foreign body but if the patient feels more comfortable with one it may be worn for about 6 h. Antibiotic ointment may be prescribed to prevent infection. A follow-up appointment may be given depending on the severity of the abrasion or the depth at which the foreign body was embedded. (See Box 13.10.)

Box 13.8 Rust ring

If a metallic foreign body is left in contact with the cornea for more than 4 hours, a rust ring may develop round its perimeter.

It can usually be very easily removed after 1 or 2 days of the application antibiotic ointment. This is done with a 10 G needle or a small battery-powered instrument called a burr.

Box 13.9 Eversion of an eyelid

This procedure is carried out if the presence of a foreign body is suspected under the upper eyelid. With the patient's eyes open and looking down, the upper lashes are grasped at the same time as depressing the edge of the tarsal plate (at the crease of the eyelid), allowing the eyelid to turn over.

Box 13.10 Contact Lenses

The wearing of contact lenses is the single largest factor for the development of microbial keratitis. The absolute risk is low but there is significant variation between different lens types.

The lowest risk is associated with the use of daily wear rigid gas permeable lenses. The danger is increased with the use of soft lenses (including disposable lenses) and the greatest risk is with contact lenses that are worn overnight.

In certain cases, infection may be related to poor compliance by patients, but this is not always the case. (Royal College of Ophthalmologists 1993)

Inflammatory conditions of the eye

? **13.14** Review the anatomy and physiology of the uveal tract, the cornea and the conjunctiva.

SURGICAL REMOVAL OF AN EYE

There are three methods of removing an eye:

1. Enucleation. This is surgical removal of the globe. The extraocular muscles are cut at their insertion and the optic nerve severed. Usually a plastic implant is inserted and the muscles are sutured around it to give support and movement to an artificial eye which is made to fit over the implant.
2. Evisceration. This is the removal of the contents of the globe, leaving the scleral shell.
3. Exenteration. This is a more extensive operation which involves removing the eye and surrounding tissues.

Special considerations

The choice of operation performed is dependent upon the diagnosis necessitating the removal of an eye. A badly injured eye may be enucleated (see Nursing Care Plan 13.4) whilst an infected eye would require to be eviscerated. Exenteration would be required when a malignant tumour extended beyond the globe.

Maintenance of good cosmetic appearance post-surgery has led to the development of a range of socket and orbital implants, which may reduce the psychological trauma experienced (Carraway et al 1990).

Management is as for extensive penetrating injuries. The nurse may find that if a patient has suffered severe pain and blindness in an eye the relief from pain after it has been removed is often so great that this helps him to cope with the loss. Contact with others who have had an eye removed may help to reassure the patient that it is possible to adapt and to live a full life following this distressing experience.

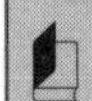
For further information, see Dutton (1992) pp. 306–325.

Artificial eye fitting

The Artificial Eye Service, Blackpool provides training to enable personnel to make and fit artificial eyes. Patient education, support and follow-up services are also provided by technicians in local ocular prosthetic departments.

An artificial eye is individually designed to fit the socket and implant exactly and is painted by an ocular artist to match the patient's other eye. The prosthesis is shell-like in shape and form and not, as anticipated, ball-shaped. In most cases, the artificial eye will move in unison with the natural eye because the extraocular muscles have been preserved and attached to the orbital implant.

Unfortunately, lack of information about artificial eyes can cause a great deal of anxiety and often a degree of revulsion. This is usually dispelled by explaining that the appearance of the socket is similar to the inside of the mouth. Anxiety is further reduced by contact with people who have adapted successfully to living with an artificial eye and by an opportunity to see and handle an artificial eye before surgery and thereby gain reassurance that they look quite natural. (See Nursing Care Plan 13.4.)

Principles of artificial eye care
Nurses should be prepared to assist or advise on the care of an artificial eye. Principles of daily management are as follows.

Removal of an artificial eye. A special extractor is provided by the ocular prosthesis department. The eyelids are opened with the thumb and forefinger and the lower edge of the eye is gently levered out with the aid of the extractor. If an extractor is not available, then a finger will suffice (see Fig. 13.10(A)).

Insertion of an artificial eye. The eyelids are opened with the thumb and forefinger. The eye is inserted under the upper lid with the curve of the eye towards the nose. The lower lid is depressed slightly. The eye can then be slipped into position (see Fig. 13.10(B)).

Care of the artificial eye. An artificial eye should be cleaned at least once a day with ordinary soap in cold or lukewarm water. It should be thoroughly rinsed afterwards under running water. Chemical cleansers or disinfectants must not be used.

Nursing Care Plan 13.4 A patient undergoing enucleation: post operative

Nursing considerations	Action	Rationale	Evaluation
Anxiety/distress			
• **due to having eye removed**	❒ Reassure and spend time with the patient. Encourage him to express his feelings and talk about his fears. Reassure him that it is normal to grieve over the loss of an eye	Giving information reduces anxiety and aids recovery	The patient will come to terms with the necessity of having his eye removed
• **due to altered body image**	❒ Discuss what the wound and socket will look like after surgery, likening it to the inside lower lip of the mouth. Discuss after-care of socket and show him an artificial eye, allowing him and his family to handle it, if he wishes. Arrange for someone who has had similar surgery to come and talk with the patient. Suggest dark glasses can be worn until he is fitted with artificial eye.	Reduces fear about the after effects of the operation	The patient will be adjusted to altered body image and will accept the situation of wearing an artificial eye
• **due to fear of having wrong eye removed**	❒ Eye to be removed is identified and checked with patient, doctor and case notes. (Some units mark the forehead with an arrow to identify correct eye.)	Relieves anxiety and reassures the patient	Correct eye will be removed. Patient will be reassured of this
	❒ Reassure patient that many checks are made prior to the operation to ensure correct eye is removed		

The patient is encouraged to wear the eye both day and night. If he prefers not to, the eye should be placed in cold water or a saline solution in a clean, labelled receptacle.

When not in regular use, the eye should be stored in cotton wool or tissue to prevent scratching. Through normal wear the eye may lose its high polish. It can be sent to the nearest ocular prosthetic department for repolishing, free of charge. Replacements can be obtained cost-free (NHS patients) from the same department.

The community nurse may need to prompt elderly patients in particular to take advantage of this service, and may need to approach their GP for initial referral to a consultant.

Care of the socket. The socket should remain clean if the artificial eye is kept clean in the recommended way. Occasionally, infection or irritation may result from scratches on the eye and lead to ulceration.

The socket can be irrigated with normal saline and treated with an antibiotic ointment for a short term. The artificial eye

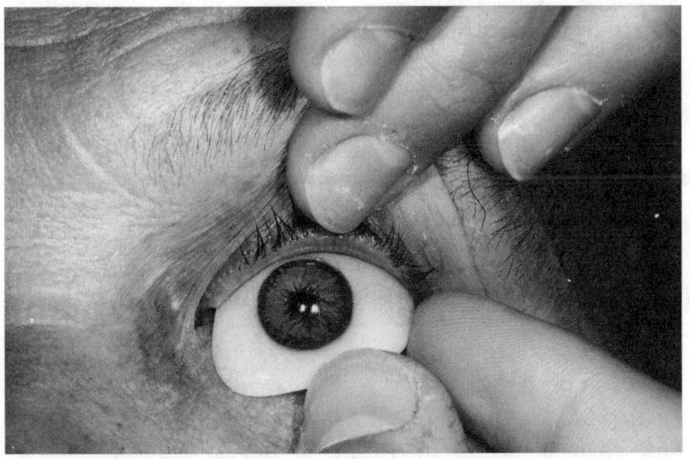

A

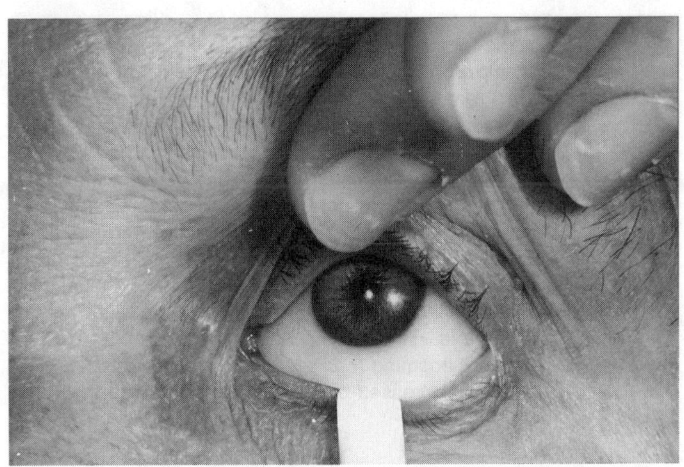

B

Fig. 13.10 (A) Removing an artificial eye. (B) Inserting an artificial eye. (Reproduced with kind permission of Blackpool, Wyre and Fylde Health Authority Artificial Eye Service.)

should not be inserted until the infection or irritation has cleared up.

It is not advisable to leave the eye out for long periods as shrinkage of the socket can occur, causing difficulty and discomfort on reinsertion of the eye.

AGE-RELATED CONDITIONS

Senile macular degeneration

Macular degeneration is the major cause of blindness in the elderly in developed countries.

Sufferers are described as being 'walking sighted – reading blind' as the peripheral retinal function is retained.

PATHOPHYSIOLOGY

Retinal pigment epithelial cells (RPE) wear out with age and are never replaced. As they degenerate they deposit material on the underlying membrane which accumulates to form yellowish white spots on the retina. Initially this process does not affect vision but eventually the cell loss will result in atrophy of the RPE layer, which may then disperse pigment into the macula. This condition is called macular degeneration. It affects form and colour vision first and the patient notices difficulty with activities such as reading and sewing and problems in identifying faces and coins.

In some cases a new blood vessel membrane may develop and cause lifting of the central retina. This results in distorted and blurred central vision.

Macular degeneration can occur in the presence of other eye conditions such as cataract and glaucoma and each will complicate the diagnosis and treatment of the other.

MEDICAL MANAGEMENT

There is no treatment for RPE degenerative changes but any underlying disease should be diagnosed and treated. If there are early symptoms of new blood vessel membrane formation krypton or argon laser treatment could be of some benefit. In some cases a degree of vision can be regained following this, although if there is foveal damage there will be a persistent central scotoma (blind spot). Those affected severely will need encouragement to make adjustments to daily living skills to maintain their independence. Advice on the use of low vision aids, contact with the Macular Degeneration Society and social work services may be advised, in addition to blind or partially sighted registration (see p. 473).

? **13.15** Mr and Mrs S are both 70 years old and live in a bungalow on the outskirts of a large town. Over the past 2 months, Mrs S has noticed a marked reduction in her near vision. Increasingly Mrs S noticed that she required help to identify her shopping items correctly and to clean her house. The pleasure obtained from completing the crosswords and reading had been lost. After a visit to her optician, she was referred to her GP and then to the eye hospital. At her appointment, the Consultant told her she had macular degeneration and that, although she will not go blind, her sight will not improve. He recommended that she should consider becoming registered as partially sighted. Mrs S is quite distressed by this and goes home to think about it.

You are a community nurse who visits Mr S daily to give him his insulin injection. Mrs S breaks down whilst you are there. What advice would you offer her and where would you advise her to go for assistance?

Entropion

This is a malposition of the eyelid in which the lid margin is turned towards the globe. It most commonly affects the lower lid and is caused by reduced elasticity of the connective tissue, which may be the result of trauma, a badly applied eye pad or the ageing process. The eyelashes irritate the cornea and can cause discomfort and ulceration.

Nursing and medical management. Discomfort can be relieved by the application of tape to the affected lid margin in such a way that downward traction of the tape when applied to the cheek restores the normal position of the lid. If the entropion persists the lid can be repositioned by a simple surgical procedure.

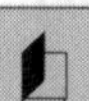

For further information, see Kanski (1992).

Ectropion

This is a malposition of the eyelid in which the lid margin is turned away from the globe. It mainly affects the lower lid and is associated with atonic tissue around the eyes. Because the punctum of the lacrimal duct is not in position to drain them, tears overflow and run down the cheeks. The sufferer constantly wipes his eyes, drawing the lid even further down and exacerbating the condition.

Nursing and medical management. Minor surgery can reposition the lid if necessary. Cautery to the inner eyelid contracts the tarsal conjunctiva and inverts the lid. Plastic surgery may be required to reposition the eyelid.

Both entropion and ectropion are fairly common conditions in the elderly, who often do not complain because they do not realise that the remedy is so simple or because they feel that they are too old to bother. Both conditions cause great discomfort and it is often the community nurse who is in a position to detect them and to advise on treatment.

SYSTEMIC DISEASE AND DISORDERS OF THE EYE

The eye is a sensitive indicator of systemic disease. Visual disturbance or abnormal appearance of the retina or optic disc may be the first manifestation of health breakdown. In this section ophthalmic conditions associated with some of the more common systemic diseases will be described to alert the nurse to the possibility of their coexistence within a disease process and to assist her in her screening role. Other conditions are described in Table 13.5.

Nursing priorities and management should be based on the general principles of ophthalmic management as well as the specific principles that pertain to the disease process in question. The reader should refer to relevant chapters in the present text as well as to more specialised ophthalmic texts.

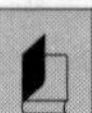

For further information, see Kanski & Thomas (1990).

DIABETES MELLITUS

Diabetes is a fairly common disorder in developed countries and its incidence is increasing in developing countries as diets include more processed foods and refined sugars. Poorly controlled diabetes can lead to retinopathy, early cataract development, vascularisation of the iris (rubeosis) and a high incidence of minor eye conditions.

Table 13.5 Further eye problems secondary to systemic diseases

Disorder	Main ophthalmic clinical features	Cause	Treatment
Thyroid function imbalance (Graves' disease)	Upper lid retraction	Sympathetic nerve innervation	Lubricating drops during day and antibiotic ointment nightly
	Exposure keratitis	Exposure of eyeball	As above
	Swelling of lids and conjunctiva Exophthalmos Compression of optic nerve	Infiltration of lymphocytes in orbital tissue and associated oedema	Partial tarsorrhaphy Systemic steroids Surgical decompression
	Diplopia	Infiltration of lymphocytes in muscle tissue leading to fibrosis	Prism spectacles Botulinum A neurotoxin injection Strabismus surgery
Migraine	Headache with visual disturbances Characteristic aura: multicoloured, jagged shape, firework-like	Idiopathic; possibly chemical changes in the brain caused by various triggers, e.g. stress or dietary, e.g. eating oranges or chocolate	Feverfew herbal remedy Ergotamine Rest
Multiple sclerosis	Uniocular	Localised demyelinating lesion to the cranial nerves	Symptoms may recover spontaneously but will always reoccur
	Small unequal pupils: do not react to light but do with accommodation, unable to dilate with atropine	– III IV VI	
	Optic neuritis		
	Rapid reduction of central vision		
	Sudden onset of pain especially when looking upwards		Systemic painkillers
	Central scotoma		
	Diplopia		• Prism spectacles • Botulinum A neurotoxin injection • Strabismus surgery
Intracranial aneurysm	Uniocular/binocular Diplopia Blurred vision Ptosis Visual field defects	Pressure on visual pathway Pressure on cranial nerves III IV VI	• Detection and clipping of aneurysm • Botulinum A neurotoxin injection • Strabismus surgery
Nephritis	a) Blurred vision b) Papilloedema c) Retinal haemorrhage d) Retinal detachment	Hypertension	• Reduce hypertension • Laser treatment • Vitrectomy • Surgical repair of detachment

Diabetic retinopathy

PATHOPHYSIOLOGY

Retinopathy involves breakdown of the microcirculation of the retina and the formation of fatty and haemorrhagic lesions. The patient will usually complain of gradual and painless loss of vision — unless there is bleeding into the vitreous humor, in which case loss of vision may be sudden and very frightening. The diagnosis and progression of the disease can be confirmed by fluorescein angiography. Diabetic retinopathy is the major cause of blindness in the 20–65 year age group in Western countries. There are two forms of the condition: background and proliferative.

Background retinopathy is more commonly associated with maturity-onset diabetes. The small retinal vessels become fragile, aneurysms form, and leakage occurs, causing localised oedema and haemorrhage. Background retinopathy can cause loss of central vision if macular oedema occurs and the hard exudates encroach on the fovea. Peripheral vision will be retained.

Proliferative retinopathy is more common in insulin-dependent diabetes. In this condition there is further deterioration as new blood vessels and fibrous bands form in response to breakdown and occlusion of the normal circulation. The main complications that can arise from this are bleeding into the vitreous humor and traction retinal detachment. Eventually, proliferative vascularisation can affect the angle of the eye, blocking the trabecular meshwork and causing glaucoma.

MEDICAL MANAGEMENT

Early diagnosis is critical, as is good control of blood sugar levels and regular monitoring of ophthalmic status. Complications are treated as they arise. Laser treatment may be used to delay the progress of proliferative retinopathy. This involves bombarding the peripheral retina with laser burns (panretinal ablation) so that the oxygen requirement of retinal tissue is reduced. This in turn reduces the stimulus for new vessel formation. Focal burns may also be used to seal off leaking blood vessels.

Severe vitreous haemorrhage or tractional retinal detachment may be treated by removing the vitreous humor (vitrectomy) and replacing it with clear infusional fluid, gas or silicone oil.

NURSING PRIORITIES AND MANAGEMENT: DIABETIC RETINOPATHY

Patient education. Ongoing education and encouragement to comply with diabetic regimes are important in the attempt to delay the onset or progression of complications and to encourage early awareness of visual changes. The community nurse often has a key role to play here. Explanation and support during laser treatment will be particularly important to encourage the patient's co-operation to prevent accidental burns (see page 480).

Vitrectomy management. Perioperative care for patients undergoing vitrectomy procedures is as for other intraocular surgery, with a particular emphasis on ensuring that the prescribed postoperative position is maintained. Where vitreous has been removed from the posterior compartment of the eye and the cavity has been filled by fluid, gas or silicone oil, strict positioning is vital. The objective is to ensure continued apposition of the retina and to minimise contact of the gas or silicone oil with the posterior surface of the lens or cornea, as this could lead to opacification of either structure.

CEREBROVASCULAR ACCIDENT (CVA)

A CVA involves an interruption of the blood supply to a part of the brain and may be caused by blockage or rupture of a blood vessel. CVA results in ischaemia of the affected part and development of neurological defects. If the visual pathways are involved, vision will be affected and the damage may be permanent. When a patient suffers a transient ischaemic attack (TIA), vision may be temporarily affected but will usually be restored when the attack subsides. (See Ch. 9, p. 345.)

NURSING PRIORITIES AND MANAGEMENT: CVA

The extent of the visual deficit must be assessed to facilitate rehabilitation and maintain patient safety. This may be difficult if the patient's ability to communicate has been affected. The accuracy of the assessment is dependent upon the nurse's observational skills.

> ? **13.16** You have a patient who has recently suffered a right-sided CVA. He is aphasic (unable to speak) and has left hemiplegia (paralysis down the left side). Discuss how you might go about detecting visual field loss just by observing his activity. Having done this, describe how your findings would affect your care plan.

CENTRAL RETINAL ARTERY OCCLUSION

This condition is an ophthalmic emergency. Treatment must begin within minutes if any degree of visual recovery is to be achieved. The compelling reason for seeking medical help is sudden, complete and painless loss of vision in one eye. Obstruction of the central retinal artery is associated with arteriosclerotic emboli, hypertension and cranial arteritis in the elderly. In younger people it may be a result of a clot being released into the circulation in valvular heart disease. The retinal artery and some of its branches may be obliterated; the damage to retinal cells is irreparable.

MEDICAL AND NURSING PRIORITIES AND MANAGEMENT

Emergency intervention. This must be attempted within minutes of the episode. The aim is to flush the clot along from the main artery to a peripheral branch. IOP can be reduced by massage of the globe and administration of drugs to draw fluid from the eye by osmosis. Paracentesis of the anterior chamber will further reduce the IOP. This should allow the retinal artery to dilate and the clot may be flushed along.

Continuing management. Once the emergency stage has passed the patient is given a full examination. The underlying medical condition is diagnosed and treated appropriately. Residual blindness is assessed and the patient given all necessary support.

HYPERTENSION

The condition of the retina and optic disc are used to aid the diagnosis of hypertension; fundal examination of the eye is in fact part of the screening process for hypertension (see Ch. 2, p. 44).

Hypertensive retinopathy in a young adult appears as widespread narrowing of the arteries caused by spasm of the arterial walls. In an older person with arteriosclerosis the arteries are narrow and rigid. As hypertension increases in severity haemorrhages and exudates are visible. The haemorrhages are flame-like in appearance and are found close to the disc. The exudates are due to lipids and occur around the macula. Oedema of the retina occurs in malignant hypertension and may also be present in some cases of mild hypertension. The optic disc is swollen and hyperaemic. The patient will complain of varying degrees of visual disturbance. The condition is painless. The outward appearance of the eye remains normal.

The eye condition improves as hypertension is brought under control by appropriate treatment (see Ch. 2).

ACQUIRED IMMUNE DEFICIENCY SYNDROME (AIDS)

Ophthalmic complications develop in about 75% of patients with AIDS. They are caused by HIV infection, opportunistic infections, and AIDS-related neoplasms and may affect any part of the eye (Kreiger & Holland 1988).

HIV retinopathy

Clinical signs are yellowish-grey cotton-wool spots, dot-like haemorrhages and microaneurysms over the retina. Vision remains normal unless the macula is involved. Some patients respond to antiviral agents.

HIV encephalopathy nystagmus

In central nervous system involvement nystagmus, gaze palsies and visual field defects may occur. No treatment is available at present.

Opportunistic infections

AIDS patients are prone to all types of eye infections. The most common infections include severe herpes zoster ophthalmicus, herpes simplex, candida retinitis, *Toxoplasma* choroidoretinitis and cytomegalovirus (CMV) retinitis. Some of these may respond to prolonged administration of systemic antiviral agents.

CMV retinitis, which develops in the late stages of AIDS, deserves special mention. Fear of blindness is often more distressing for the patient than fear of dying. CMV retinitis, with intraretinal haemorrhages and retinal necrosis, leads to retinal detachments and progressive loss of vision. Palliative treatment by i.v. or intravitreous antiviral agents such as ganciclovir may be offered in an attempt to prevent blindness in the last few months of life.

AIDS-related neoplasms

Kaposi's sarcoma may involve any of the ocular structures. Treatment may include cryotherapy, radiotherapy or the administration of cytotoxic drugs.

NURSING PRIORITIES AND MANAGEMENT: AIDS

The general principles of nursing a patient with AIDS (see Ch. 38), together with the principles of nursing a patient with eye infections, apply in all the above conditions. Full care and support facilities should be mobilised for both the patient and his family.

CONCLUSION

Eye disorders may be encountered in a wide range of contexts and nurses should be prepared to recognise these conditions and provide appropriate treatment or prompt referral for specialist help. Even where treatment is being carried out in ophthalmic units it is necessary for general and community nurses to have a working knowledge of what is involved so that they can prepare the patient and his family for the necessary procedures and monitor progress and after-care when the patient has returned home.

The impact of visual impairment on everyday life must never be underestimated. This chapter has stressed the importance of recognising the significance of adverse signs and symptoms and the fact that delay can result in irreparable damage and permanent loss of sight. It has emphasised the nurse's responsibility in helping to preserve sight and in supporting the patient and his family as they meet the practical and emotional challenges of visual impairment.

REFERENCES

Allen M, Knight C, Falk C & Strang V 1992 Effectiveness of a pre-operative teaching programme for cataract patients. Journal of Advanced Nursing 17: 303–309

Audit Commission for Local Authorities and the NHS in England and Wales 1990 A short cut to better services: day surgery in England and Wales. HMSO, London

Bartholomew R S 1986 A practical guide to cataract and lens implant surgery. Churchill Livingstone, Edinburgh

Blackpool, Wyre and Fylde Health Authority, Artificial Eye Service The use and care of artificial eyes. AES, Blackpool

Carraway J H, Mellor C G, Nustarde J C 1990 Use of cartilage graft for an orbital socket implant. Annals of Plastic Surgery 24(2): 139–148

Chawla H B 1988 Ophthalmology: student notes. Churchill Livingstone, Edinburgh

Cheng K P, Larson C E, Biglan A W, D'Antonio J A 1992 A prospective, randomized, controlled comparison of retrobulbar and general anaesthesia for strabismus surgery. Ophthalmic Surgery 23(9): 585–590

Chilman A M, Thomas M 1987 Understanding nursing care, 3rd edn. Churchill Livingstone, Edinburgh

Donnelly D 1987 Instilling eyedrops: difficulties experienced by patients following cataract surgery. Journal of Advanced Nursing 12: 235–243

Ewles L, Simnett L 1992 Promoting health: a practical guide. Scutari, London

Health and Safety Executive 1993 Working with VDUs. HMSO, London

Kreiger A E, Holland G N 1988 Ocular involvement in AIDS. Eye 2: 496–505

Matthews T D, Frazer D G, Minassian D C, Radford C F, Dart J K G 1992 Risks of keratitis and patterns of use with disposable contact lenses. Archives of Ophthalmology 110(11): 1559–1562

McKenzie G J, Chawla H B, Gordon D 1986 The special senses, 2nd edn. Churchill Livingstone, Edinburgh

Middlebrook P N 1974 Social psychology and modern life. Knopf, New York

Orem D 1990 Nursing: concepts of practice, 4th edn. Mosby, New York

Perry J P, Tullo A (eds) 1990 Care of the ophthalmic patient. Chapman & Hall, London

Riordan-Eva P 1992 In: Vaughan D G, Asbury T, Riordan-Eva P (eds) General ophthalmology, 13th edn. Appleton-Lange, USA

Roper N, Logan W W, Tierney A J 1990 The elements of nursing: a model for nursing based on a model of living, 3rd edn. Churchill Livingstone, Edinburgh

Royal National Institute for the Blind 1991 Eye safety campaign. RNIB, London

Rowell M 1990 Models for ophthalmic nursing practice. In: Perry J P, Tullo A (eds) Care of the ophthalmic patient. Chapman Hall, London

Vail J, Cox B 1978 Drugs and the eye. Butterworth, London

Wilson-Barnett J 1978 Patients' emotional response to barium X-rays. Journal of Advanced Nursing 3(1): 37–46

Wilson-Barnett J 1988 Patient teaching or patient counselling? Journal of Advanced Nursing 13: 215–222

Wilson-Barnett J 1985 Principles of patient teaching. Nursing Times 81: 28–29

York S 1990 Ophthalmic triage. Nursing Times 86(8): 40–42

FURTHER READING

Caird F I, Williamson J (eds) 1986 The eye and its disorders in the elderly. Wright, Bristol

Dutton J J 1992 Atlas of ophthalmic surgery, vol 2. Oculoplastic, lacrimal and orbital surgery. Mosby, St Louis, MO

Frost J 1993 Clinical application of lasers. Professional Nurse (Feb): 298–303

Hull J 1990 Touch the rock. SPK Publishers, London

Journal of ophthalmic nursing and technology. Slack, New Jersey

Kanski J J, Thomas D J 1990 The eye in systemic diseases, 2nd edn. Butterworth-Heinemann, London

Kanski J J 1992 Colour guide to ophthalmology. Churchill Livingstone, Edinburgh

Mehta V 1987 Sound shadows of the new world. Picador, London

Mehta V 1989 The stolen light. Collins, London

Mudie S 1992 Evaluating day care. Nursing 5(7): 22–23

Pavan-Langston D (ed) 1991 Manual of ocular diagnosis and therapy, 3rd edn. Little Brown, Boston

Piff C 1985 Let's face it. Gollancz, London

Perry J P, Tullo A (eds) 1990 Care of the ophthalmic patient. Chapman & Hall, London

Royal National Institute for the Blind 1987 How to guide a blind person. RNIB, London

Schutz J S 1984 Retinal detachment surgery. Chapman & Hall, London

USEFUL ADDRESSES

Royal National Institute for the Blind
224 Great Portland Street
London W1A 6AA
Tel: 071 388 1226

Partially Sighted Society
Queens Road
Doncaster DN1 2NX
Tel: 0303 68998

International Glaucoma Association
Kings College Hospital
Denmark Hill
London SE5 9RS
Tel: 071 274 6222

Talking Newspaper Association of the UK (TNAUK)
90 High Street
Heathfield
East Sussex TN21 8JD
Tel: 0962 65570

In Touch
BBC Broadcasting House
London W1A 1AA

Guide Dogs for the Blind Association
Hillfields
Burghfield Common
Reading R97 3YG
Tel: 0753 855711

CHAPTER 14

Disorders of the ear, nose and throat

Janice M. McCall   Anne Shackleton

Anne Shackleton managed a very busy Ear, Nose and Throat ward. Despite having major health problems she contributed to this chapter as she had a great enthusiasm for this specialty and a serious commitment to helping students to learn.
Unfortunately she died before the chapter was completed but her ideas and material have been incorporated into it and enable her commitment to students to continue.

CHAPTER CONTENTS

Introduction 497
ANATOMY AND PHYSIOLOGY OF THE EAR 497
Disorders of the external ear 498
Nursing priorities and management of external otitis 498
Nursing priorities and management of cerumen excess 499
Deafness and hearing loss 499
Nursing priorities and management of deafness and hearing loss 500
Disorders of the middle ear 501
Nursing priorities and management of secretory otitis media (glue ear) 502
Nursing priorities and management of acute suppurative otitis media (ASOM) 503
Nursing priorities and management of tympanoplasty 503
Nursing priorities and management of acute mastoiditis 504
Disorders of the inner ear 504
Nursing priorities and management of tinnitus 505
Nursing priorities and management of vertigo 505
Nursing priorities and management of Méniere's disease 506
ANATOMY AND PHYSIOLOGY OF THE NOSE 506
Disorders of the nose 506
Nursing priorities and management of epistaxis 507
Nursing priorities and management of anterior nosebleeds 507
Disorders of the paranasal sinuses 509
Nursing priorities and management of acute sinusitis 509
Nursing priorities and management of chronic sinusitis 509
Nursing priorities and management of nasal injury 509
Deviation of the nasal septum 510
Nursing priorities and management of deviation of the nasal septum 510
Nasal obstruction 510
Nursing priorities and management of foreign bodies in the nose 510
Nursing priorities and management of nasal polyps 511
ANATOMY AND PHYSIOLOGY OF THE THROAT 511
Disorders of the throat 511
Nursing priorities and management of total laryngectomy 512
Nursing priorities and management of tracheostomy 516
Nursing priorities and management of tonsillectomy 518
Nursing priorities and management of peritonsillar abscess 518
Conclusion 519
Glossary 519
References 519
Further reading 519
Useful addresses 520

INTRODUCTION

Some problems of the ear, nose and throat are very common. Most people at some time in their lives suffer from nosebleeds, sore throats or earaches. Many of these problems will be dealt with successfully by the patient at home, often with the advice of a pharmacist or general practitioner (GP). Some ENT problems, however, can be life-threatening, requiring a sudden visit to an accident and emergency (A & E) department, surgery, and in some cases, a period of nursing care at home following discharge.

To nurse ENT patients effectively in a home or hospital setting, a basic knowledge of the anatomy and physiology of the relevant structures along with a thorough understanding of the clinical features of common disorders is essential. The health visitor, district nurse, school nurse or occupational health nurse is often in a position to detect problems before the medical practitioner or even the patient himself is aware of them.

This chapter will describe in turn the basic structure and functioning of the ear, nose and throat, describing the most commonly encountered disorders of each, and outlining appropriate medical and nursing interventions. As in every area of nursing care, one of the most important contributions of the nurse will be in the area of communication and education as she provides support and reassurance to the patient and his family and conveys information about the causes of the patient's condition, its treatment, and measures to prevent its recurrence.

ANATOMY AND PHYSIOLOGY OF THE EAR

The ear can be divided into three sections: the external ear, the middle ear and the inner ear. The external and middle ears are primarily involved with the transmission of sound. The inner ear contains the organ of hearing as well as structures concerned with body balance (see Fig. 14.1).

The external ear comprises the cartilaginous pinna and the external auditory canal (or external meatus), the inner two thirds of which is composed of bone rather than cartilage. The purpose of the pinna and canal is to capture sound waves and funnel them to the tympanic membrane, which is located at the end of the external canal and divides the external from the middle ear. The healthy membrane has a pearly sheen and reflects light.

The middle ear is ventilated by the eustachian tube, which communicates with the nasopharynx. Three small bones called the auditory ossicles, or ossicular chain, pass on sound vibrations received by the tympanic membrane to the inner ear. The first of these, the malleus (i.e. 'hammer'), is attached to the tympanic membrane and joins with the incus ('anvil') or middle ossicle. The incus in turn is

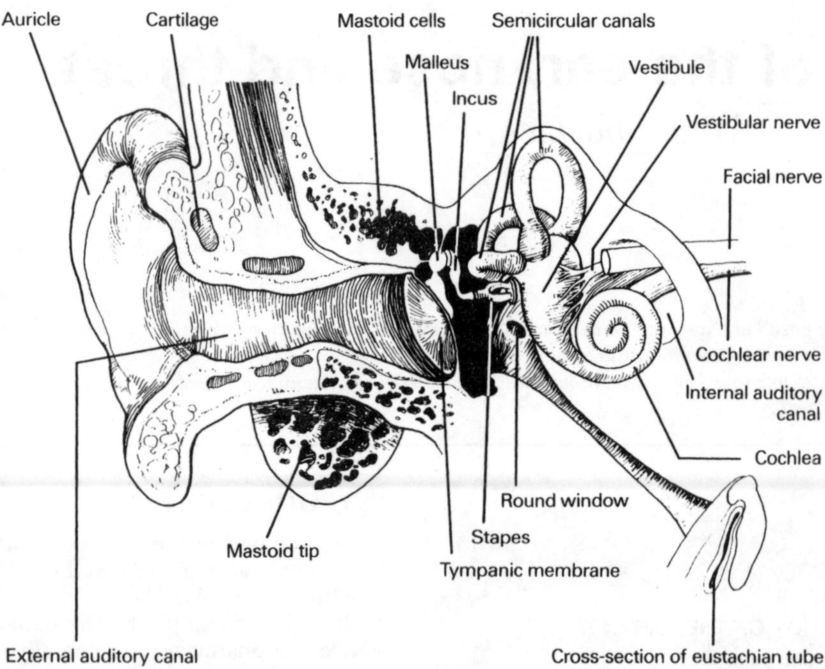

Fig. 14.1 Sagittal section of the ear. (Reproduced with kind permission from McKenzie et al 1986.)

attached to the stapes ('stirrup'), the 'footplate' of which lies against the membranous oval window or fenestra of the inner ear.

The inner ear houses the cochlea, which is shaped like a snail shell and is the organ of hearing. The cochlea contains the organ of Corti, which consists of cells with hair-like projections on a membranous layer and connects with the terminal ends of the auditory nerve. The canals of the cochlea and the organ of Corti are bathed in endolymph. Perilymph is the fluid contained within the bony (osseous) cavities of the inner ear, whereas endolymph is the fluid within membranous cavities. As sound waves are transmitted by the ossicles they travel along this fluid and disturb the hair cells. This disturbance changes to impulses which travel along the auditory nerve to the brain stem and cortex, where they are interpreted as meaningful sound.

The posterior part of the inner ear is formed by three semicircular canals and by the vestibular apparatus. These assist in the perception of body position against gravity and in the maintenance of balance. The vestibular apparatus consists of the utricle and saccule and is sensitive to linear acceleration. The semicircular canals are sensitive to rotatory acceleration. Balance is maintained by the adjustment of muscles, joints, tendons and ligaments in response to information gathered by the vestibular apparatus and the canals as well as that received by the eyes.

DISORDERS OF THE EXTERNAL EAR

External otitis

PATHOPHYSIOLOGY

The most common causes of otitis externa, or inflammation of the external ear, are infection and allergy. Infection may be caused by scratching the ear with contaminated fingernails or other sharp objects. Instruments such as auriscopes or hearing aid earpieces placed in the meatus may cause minor injuries, giving rise to infection if they have been inadequately disinfected (see Ch. 16, p. 550). Itching is an early symptom of allergy and may be caused by cosmetics or antibiotic preparations. In otitis externa multiple bacteriological flora are usually present. The condition most commonly occurs in hot, humid climates where it tends to be recurrent and may be severe.

Common presenting symptoms. The patient usually presents with a history of pain localised to the ear and a burning sensation followed by discharge, which may be watery to begin with and then become thicker. Itching may also be a symptom. If there is gross oedema of the meatus and a large amount of debris is present the patient may suffer from conductive deafness (see p. 499).

MEDICAL MANAGEMENT

If a discharge is present in otitis externa a swab is usually obtained for culture and sensitivity. Cleansing of the external meatus should be performed so that inspection can be carried out and to ensure good skin contact for any prescribed topical treatments.

NURSING PRIORITIES AND MANAGEMENT OF EXTERNAL OTITIS

The first priority of the nursing staff when caring for these patients is usually to clean the external meatus so that an examination can be carried out and any prescribed treatment can be effectively administered. Tap water and cotton wool can be used. Care should be taken not to damage skin in the folds of the ear. Gentle pulling of the auricle will allow easier access to some of the folds.

It may be necessary to administer mild oral analgesics before the external auditory canal can be properly examined as these patients often find any movement of the pinna painful.

Since the vast majority of patients are seen in the community or outpatients' department the nurse's involvement will include demonstrating how to effectively administer topical preparations. This can be quite difficult for the patient to master and will require time and careful attention. The nurse should also teach the patient safe techniques for cleansing the external ear and stress the importance of frequent, thorough cleansing of any appliances that are put in the ear.

Cerumen excess

PATHOPHYSIOLOGY

Cerumen is the normal waxy secretion of special glands in the external auditory canal. Along with shed skin scales and hair the cerumen normally migrates to the external meatus but can be hindered by coarse hair or if the individual impacts the material by attempting to clean the ears with cotton-wool buds or other instruments.

Common presenting symptoms. The patient usually presents with dulled hearing. Tinnitus may develop, causing the patient distress (see p. 504), and disturbance of balance may result from pressure of the hard material on the tympanic membrane.

MEDICAL MANAGEMENT

Ideally, the doctor, district nurse or practice nurse will be able to remove the material by syringing the external canal. Often, however, the wax is too hard and compacted for this to be carried out effectively. A course of drops containing sodium bicarbonate in glycerol, or warmed olive or almond oil may have to be prescribed first to soften the wax.

NURSING PRIORITIES AND MANAGEMENT OF CERUMEN EXCESS

Individuals with cerumen excess are usually seen in the doctor's surgery or, more rarely, in the outpatients' department and require removal of the impacted wax.

The nurse may have to teach the patient how to insert the ear drops at home over the required period before the syringing is carried out. The doctor or nurse who performs the syringing should first, if possible, determine that the tympanic membrane is intact to eliminate the danger of the solution being introduced into the middle ear and causing infection. During the procedure the patient sits upright with his clothing protected with a waterproof covering. It is helpful if he can co-operate by holding a container under his ear to receive the returning fluid. There are various types of ear syringes available. Non-disposable varieties must be sterilised after each use. Unless a special solution has been prescribed, tap water or an isotonic solution such as normal saline may be used to irrigate the canal. It is important that the solution is at 37 °C, i.e. body temperature, as any other temperature may cause the patient to experience vertigo (see p. 505).

After the syringe has been filled and any air expelled the pinna is pulled gently upwards and backwards to straighten the canal while the solution is introduced from the syringe in an upwards direction so that the wax will be washed out with the return flow (see Fig. 14.2). It is important that the flow of water is not aimed directly at the tympanic membrane as this could damage it. When the canal is clean the procedure is discontinued and the canal gently dried. To avoid vertigo the patient should be encouraged to sit for a few minutes to recover. He should also be advised that following effective ear syringing he may be hypersensitive to even quite normal sounds for a short time.

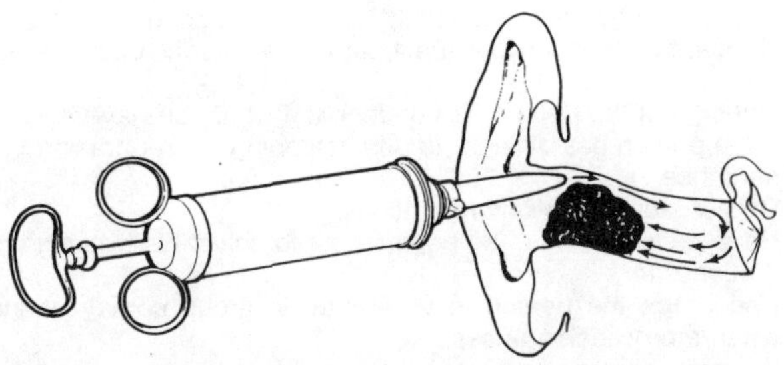

Fig. 14.2 Ear syringing. The pinna of the ear is pulled up and back and the fluid is aimed gently upwards. (Reproduced with kind permission from Jamieson et al 1986.)

Foreign bodies in the ear

Small objects may become lodged in the ear by some mishap or, as frequently occurs among children, by accident during play (Denyer 1990). Such objects may lie undetected for years unless they have damaged the tympanic membrane. Sometimes gentle syringing will wash out the foreign body but if it has become impacted it may be necessary for the patient to be admitted to hospital and for the object to be removed under general anaesthetic.

DEAFNESS AND HEARING LOSS

Although total deafness is comparatively rare, many people suffer hearing loss to varying degrees. Deafness can affect adults or children. Many children who are deaf continue to be so for all their lives but some can be helped to maximise auditory function. The present chapter will concentrate on hearing problems among adults. (See Ch. 26.) Research studies using audiometry demonstrate that 34% of people aged between 61 and 70 years have a hearing impairment and this rises to 74% in the 71+ age group (Haggard et al 1981).

PATHOPHYSIOLOGY AND MEDICAL MANAGEMENT

Deafness is usually classified into conductive and sensorineural disorders, as follows.

Diagnosis of the type of hearing loss from which an individual is suffering will be by examination and audiometry (see Box 14.1). Conductive deafness can often be helped by removing any obstruction (cerumen or a foreign body) or by amplifying sounds by means of a hearing aid. Because the external and middle ear are fairly accessible surgical intervention may also be an option. By contrast, in sensorineural deafness, where the damage is to the organ of Corti or the cochlear portion of the eighth cranial nerve, surgery does not usually have much effect (see p. 500).

Conductive deafness results from a reduced ability of the sound waves to reach the fluid in the cochlea. The sound is quieter but not distorted. This can be due to:

- otitis externa
- foreign bodies
- wax in the external canal
- damage to the tympanic membrane
- secretory otitis media (glue ear)
- damage to the incus, malleus or stapes
- tumours.

Box 14.1 Hearing tests

These have been designed to measure hearing threshold and to help ascertain whether deafness is conductive or sensorineural.

A reliable way of detecting conductive deafness is to hold a vibrating tuning fork in line with but not touching the external meatus of the ear to determine air conduction of sound, and then to place it with its base against the skull to determine conduction of sound through the bone.

Audiometric tests measure hearing acuity. Tones of variable frequency and intensity are delivered to the ear via earphones. Words can also be presented to the patient via earphones. The results are charted on graphs.

Other, more sophisticated tests are being developed which can help to pinpoint exactly which part of the ear is causing the problem.

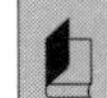

An excellent detailed description of these tests can be found in Turner (1988).

Sensorineural deafness is caused by a defect of the cochlea or its connecting nerves. The sound is quieter and also distorted. This is a result of the loss of the high frequencies which register consonant sounds. In severe cases the patient may not be able to hear the sound of his own voice. This can be due to:

- ageing
- medication
- damage to the organ of Corti by noise
- head injury or trauma
- infection
- Ménière's disease
- congenital malformation
- damage due to ischaemia.

Presbycusis, the most common type of sensorineural deafness, develops as a consequence of ageing and is becoming increasingly prevalent in western society. Audiometry initially shows loss of ability to hear high tones but there is gradual deterioration of lower tone hearing as well. Degeneration of the nervous tissue leads to loss of intelligibility in the sounds that are heard. Hearing loss in this disorder is symmetrical (i.e. affects both ears). A hearing aid may be of slight advantage but distortion and poor discrimination may cancel out any benefit from amplification. The important thing when communicating with these patients is to speak slowly and distinctly and to try to eliminate any background noise. Because the high tones are affected first the individual may have trouble hearing consonants, as these are usually of higher tone than vowels.

Medication. It has been recognised for some time that salicylates and quinine can cause deafness, but this can be reversed by discontinuing these medications. Other drugs, such as antibiotics of the aminoglycoside group, some diuretics such as intravenously administered frusemide, and cytotoxic agents of the nitrogen mustard group can cause irreparable damage.

Noise-induced hearing loss is well documented and has become recognised as an industrial disease. A single exposure to a loud noise such as an explosion can cause permanent deafness but more commonly the injury is temporary. Tinnitus usually goes along with this injury and often takes longer to improve than any deafness (see p. 504). Exposure to loud noise over a period of time leads to destruction of the hair cells in the organ of Corti. Strict standards of noise control and protection have now been laid down for employers, who are liable to be prosecuted if they do not comply. Unfortunately many people, particularly the young, willingly subject themselves to high levels of noise, for example at rock concerts, discothèques and dances, where the music is usually amplified. With audiometry early changes in hearing caused by exposure to noise are seen on the printout as a dip which gradually deepens and involves adjacent frequencies.

Head injuries or trauma resulting in deafness usually involve fractures or penetrating injuries of the temporal bone. Occasionally, concussion (see Ch. 9) can cause deafness due to haemorrhage into the middle ear or cochlea. These injuries are often accompanied by severe vertigo, nausea and vomiting.

Infection leading to deafness is usually viral in origin. The causative viruses are those associated with mumps, measles, chickenpox, rubella, poliomyelitis and influenza type A and B.

Ménière's disease. See page 505.

Congenital malformation

For information on deafness resulting from congenital malformation see Serra et al 1986, pp. 102–103.

For further information on deafness and hearing loss see Chilman & Thomas 1987.

NURSING PRIORITIES AND MANAGEMENT OF DEAFNESS AND HEARING LOSS

In the case of conductive deafness the nurse's role may be to prepare the patient for surgery and facilitate his postoperative recovery. Some of the surgical procedures that may benefit patients are myringoplasty, ossiculoplasty and stapedectomy. A patient for whom surgery is not feasible may be fitted with a hearing aid; in this case the nurse should explain to him how to obtain the most benefit from the aid.

Communicating effectively with a hearing-impaired patient is a very important nursing priority. In her assessment the nurse should obtain and record information about the patient's preferred method of conversing, e.g. lip-reading, finger spelling or sign language (see Ch. 26). For a less profoundly deaf patient it may be that speaking face-to-face with a slow distinct voice and eliminating background noise is adequate (see Box 14.2).

It is now recognised that deafness can have a profound psychological impact and that hearing-impaired individuals require support in order to cope. Nurses can make a valuable contribution by recognising the problems faced by patients with hearing loss and helping them to obtain the appropriate help. A commission of inquiry (National Deaf Children's Society 1992) into human aids in communication found that a number of deaf people were unhappy about the quality of their care in hospital and in outpatients' departments. The commission recommended that nurses should make a greater effort to ascertain what services are available to deaf people in their care.

? **14.1** How might a person with a severe hearing deficit know that his telephone or doorbell is ringing?

Community nurses can provide tremendous help and support for patients and their relatives when sensorineural deafness is a problem. They should be able to assist their patients to obtain many of the aids available which can help to overcome communication difficulties in everyday life. There are many associations, both voluntary and professional, which can provide support and help. The nurse working in the community should be a resource person for her patients and guide

Box 14.2 Talking with someone who has a hearing deficit

- Do not speak until you have the person's attention and he can see your full face. Never turn your back on the person when you are speaking.
- Ask the person if he can lip-read.
- Do not exaggerate your lip movement.
- Direct your voice to one ear if it has better hearing than the other.
- Speak slowly, enunciate clearly, and do not shout.
- Remember that vowels are heard more easily than consonants.
- Check that the person has understood what you have said.
- If the person has difficulty in understanding, try rephrasing the sentence.
- Do not laugh at misinterpretations.
- Have patience. Give the person time to adjust his hearing aid if necessary.
- Encourage the person to participate in group conversations when the occasion arises.
- If verbal communication is impossible, explore alternative means, e.g. sign language.

them to the support that is available (see Useful Addresses, p. 520).

> ? **14.2** Try to find out whether there are any professional or voluntary support groups for deaf people in your area. See if you can find out what services they offer and compile a resource list.

Hearing aids

All electronic hearing aids consist of three parts: the microphone, which picks up the sound; the amplifier, which is powered by batteries and which makes the sound louder; and the earpiece, which delivers the amplified sound to the ear via an ear mould. As there are many models on the market it is important that the most appropriate one is chosen for each person's needs and lifestyle. While most hearing aids enclose all the components in a neat package on or near the ear, they differ in such aspects as frequency response, output and ability to reduce the effects of sudden, loud noise. Hearing aids conduct sound either through air or via the bone behind the ear. Old-fashioned speaking tubes or ear trumpets can still be of surprising benefit to some people.

After the most appropriate model of hearing aid has been identified the patient will require some training in order to be able to receive maximum benefit from it. The fact that the aid makes all sounds, including background noise, louder for the patient means that he will have to develop the skill of picking out sounds essential to communication. Social interaction may be difficult until this skill is mastered and if the individual is not given enough information and support he may abandon his aid as useless.

> ? **14.3** Find out how many patients in your ward or on your community caseload have a hearing aid. How many use them? How useful do they find their hearing aids to be? What would you do if you were visiting an elderly person in his own home, and he responded to your questions by showing you a drawer containing several hearing aids and saying, 'None of these are any use.'?

All hearing aid models are battery powered and have an on/off switch which is sometimes combined with the volume control. Many models also have a switch marked 'T' which is for use with telephone and other systems fitted with an induction loop. This loop eliminates some background noise and clarifies incoming speech.

> ? **14.4** Where in your area are induction loops fitted? How can you tell?

The ear moulds are individually made to fit each user's ear. They can be disconnected from the aid for cleaning; this should be done frequently. The tube which connects the earpiece to the main aid can also be detached and washed and any blockage removed with a pipecleaner. If a hearing aid is not working make sure that:

- the switch is in the 'on' position
- the battery is still good and is of the right type
- the mould is clean and fits properly
- the connecting tube is patent.

If all of the above is in order and the aid is not working it should be returned to the hearing aid clinic for maintenance. All hearing aids supplied by the National Health Service (NHS) are maintained and replaced free of charge.

DISORDERS OF THE MIDDLE EAR

Secretory otitis media (glue ear)

Glue ear is the most common cause of deafness in children. It is thought that more than 20% of children suffer from this condition at some time (Serra et al 1986).

PATHOPHYSIOLOGY

This disorder is known as glue ear because it is characterised by a thick, tenacious fluid which collects in the middle ear. Normally, the mucosal secretions in the middle ear drain down the eustachian tube into the nasopharynx. It is not certain whether the abnormal accumulation of this fluid is caused by the viscosity of the fluid, congestion of the eustachian tubes, or by enlarged adenoids.

Common presenting symptoms. Pain is not usually associated with this condition. The adult patient usually comes to the medical practitioner complaining of hearing loss. A child might never complain, and his condition might be discovered only upon investigation into poor performance at school.

MEDICAL MANAGEMENT

Examination of the tympanic membrane by auriscope usually confirms diagnosis, as in this disorder the membrane has a characteristic dull grey or orange appearance. It will also lose its normal translucence and become retracted. Conservative treatment is to prescribe a vasoconstricting nasal spray or drops. Antihistamines may also be prescribed to reduce oedema of the nasal mucosa. This is often sufficient to allow the secretions to escape through the eustachian tube. Another treatment is to try to liquefy the mucus to help it escape, by prescribing mucolytic medicines (Turner 1988).

Surgical intervention involves the perforation of the tympanic membrane. The insertion of a grommet (see Fig. 14.3) is sometimes considered appropriate, although some specialists think this can lead to scar formation in later years which will impair hearing. Perforation allows the fluid to escape and air to circulate around the middle ear. If a grommet is inserted it usually slides out of the membrane gradually; patients sometimes find it on their pillow when they waken one morning. This can take up to a year to happen. There is usually a marked

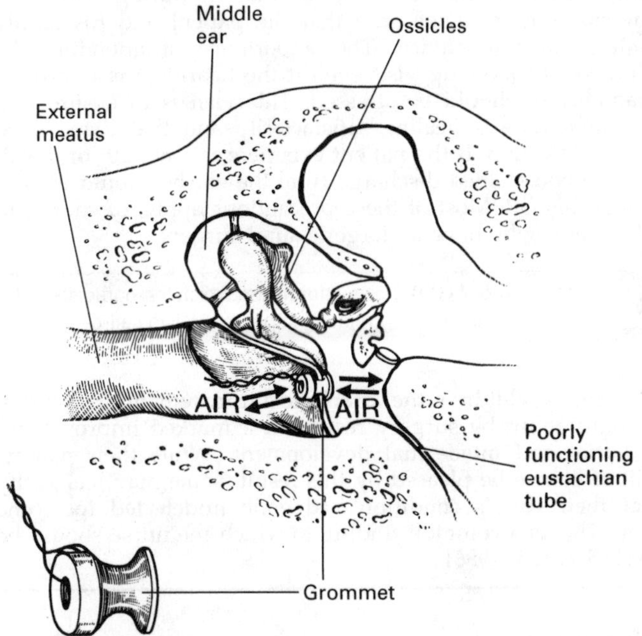

Fig. 14.3 Grommet and grommet in situ. (Reproduced with kind permission from McKenzie et al 1992.)

improvement in hearing after this procedure; this improvement is maintained in about 75% of patients.

NURSING PRIORITIES AND MANAGEMENT OF SECRETORY OTITIS MEDIA (GLUE EAR)

Throughout this chapter, the reader is referred to Ch. 27 for details of perioperative care. Only care specific to ENT patients will be outlined here.

Preoperative care

The nurse must ensure that the patient and his family are adequately informed about what any surgical procedure will entail. This may involve the use of diagrams and it may be helpful to show a grommet to them if one is to be inserted. As grommet insertion is usually performed on children and young people, it is vital that the appropriate emotional and psychological support is given.

When communicating with the patient preoperatively the nurse should make allowances for hearing loss (see Box 14.2).

Postoperative care

It is important to remember that once any packing has been removed from the patient's ear there should be a marked improvement in hearing. The anaesthetic for this operation is very light, for example, ketamine hydrochloride, and so the patient is usually discharged the day after surgery. Indeed, many patients who have undergone aural surgery are discharged within a day or two following the procedure. Ames & Kneisl (1988) suggest measures to prevent the spread of infection (e.g. washing the hands before and after touching the affected ear), how to change and dispose of cotton wool plugs in the external auditory canal, the importance of taking the full course of antibiotics which have been prescribed, and specific instructions about whether and when it is safe to allow water to enter the ear. Some surgeons allow swimming when a grommet is in place, as long as the patient does not dive or swim underwater. Others prefer their patients not to swim until the grommet has been expelled. Usually, a cotton wool plug moistened with petroleum jelly is inserted in the external canal when the hair is being washed or during a shower. The nurse must make sure that the patient and his family understand this advice. The importance of attending the clinic for a follow-up visit even if the hearing has improved dramatically should be stressed. This visit is to ensure that the membrane is healing satisfactorily and that there is no sign of infection. If the patient experiences any pain or develops a blood-stained discharge from the ear he should be told to visit his GP. Most of these precautions apply, of course, to all patients who have undergone aural surgery.

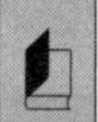

Ames & Kneisl (1988) give information which the nurse should explain to the patient in relation to postoperative self-care at home.

In many children the dramatic improvement in hearing brought about by surgery results in a marked improvement in social and intellectual development. While their parents will of course be pleased by this result, some may feel guilty that their child's condition had gone undetected for some time. This is a common finding to which the nurse should be alert (Sacharin 1986).

Otosclerosis

Otosclerosis is a condition in which the ossicles in the middle ear along with the temporal bone begin to soften. This spongy bone gradually becomes a dense sclerotic mass; the ossicles may become fixed and less effective in passing on auditory vibrations. The individual with this condition will complain of increasing hearing loss. While this loss is conductive in origin, if the damage extends to the cochlea, sensorineural loss of hearing will also occur. Mild tinnitus (see p. 505) may also be experienced, in which case some people find that they can actually hear better in a noisy environment where their tinnitus is masked.

This disorder commonly begins in adolescence and appears to affect women twice as often as men. Its cause is as yet unknown. Heredity, vitamin deficiency and otitis media have all been cited as significant factors.

Medical management and nursing priorities

Although no cure for otosclerosis is known, surgery can often dramatically improve hearing. The surgery of choice, stapedectomy, involves freeing the stapes and replacing it with a prosthesis. This restores the vibration necessary to permit the transmission of sound waves. The procedure is a very delicate one requiring the use of an operating microscope, as the stapes is one of the smallest bones in the body. Surgery may be performed under local anaesthetic and hospital admission may be no more than a few days.

Great care must be taken in the early postoperative period, as the patient may take a little while to regain his sense of balance. This short-term vertigo, if discussed and explained in the preoperative period, should cause minimal distress to the patient. Prior to discharge, advice should be given on the prevention of aural infection, the importance of preventing the entry of water into the ear and the need to guard against blowing the nose until the operative site is completely healed. Follow-up appointments in the outpatients' department and appropriate community support by the GP will ensure optimal progress and recovery.

For those for whom the symptoms of otosclerosis are not too severe or for whom surgery is inappropriate, a hearing aid may restore and maintain satisfactory hearing. For others, neither surgery nor a hearing aid will have long-term effectiveness and varying degrees of deafness will result.

Acute suppurative otitis media (ASOM)

PATHOPHYSIOLOGY

This is an acute bacterial infection of the middle ear which is especially common in childhood. The most common causative organisms are *Streptococcus pneumoniae, Haemophilus influenzae, Strep. pyogenes,* and *Staphylococcus aureus.* Onset usually follows acute tonsillitis, the common cold or influenza when infection travels up the eustachian tube to the middle ear. The whole middle ear may be affected, including the mastoid air cells, small air spaces in the posterior portion of the temporal bone, behind the middle ear (see Fig. 14.1).

Common presenting symptoms. The patient usually presents with acute ear pain. There may be deafness, general malaise and pyrexia. On examination the eardrum is red and bulging due to the collection of pus in the middle ear. The tympanic membrane may rupture releasing the discharge and dramatically and instantaneously relieving the pain.

MEDICAL MANAGEMENT

The patient with ASOM is usually seen and treated by a GP. The exact treatment given will depend on the stage of the infection, as follows.

Early stage. At this stage the tympanic membrane will still look normal. A broad-spectrum antibiotic effective against the most common organisms is usually prescribed. The initial dose may be given intramuscularly (and the rest of the course orally) in order to reduce the time it will take for the antibiotic to become effective. Antipyretic analgesics such as paracetamol will be necessary to relieve pain and reduce fever. Vasoconstricting nasal sprays may also be helpful in keeping the eustachian tubes patent and thereby allowing escape of fluid from the middle ear.

Bulging eardrum. If the infection has reached this stage a myringotomy is usually performed. This involves making an incision in the tympanic membrane to allow the fluid to escape. General anaesthesia will be required. If a myringotomy is performed in preference to allowing the eardrum to rupture the membrane will heal with less scarring and hearing should not be impaired. During this procedure a swab of the discharge may be obtained and sent to the laboratory for culture and testing for sensitivity so that an effective antibiotic can be prescribed.

Discharging ear. By this stage the tympanic membrane will already have ruptured. A swab of the discharge will be taken and the ear carefully mopped, then dressed with a small plug of cottonwool. Broad-spectrum antibiotics will be prescribed in the first instance while results of bacteriology are awaited.

The patient will have to visit his GP regularly so that healing of the membrane can be monitored. If necessary, a myringoplasty (reconstruction of the eardrum) will be performed.

NURSING PRIORITIES AND MANAGEMENT OF ACUTE SUPPURATIVE OTITIS MEDIA (ASOM)

Early stage

If at this stage a nurse (possibly a practice nurse) is involved her role will be to ensure that the prescribed course of antibiotics is completed in order to eradicate all the organisms. It may be necessary to teach the patient or a relative how to administer a nasal spray.

Bulging eardrum

At this stage the nurse will help to administer the prescribed antibiotic course and will perform mopping out of the external meatus.

Discharging ear

If the disease has reached this stage the nurse's tasks will include mopping out the external ear as often as required and helping the patient complete his course of antibiotics.

If appropriate treatment is given early enough, ASOM should resolve and hearing return to normal. Occasionally, complications do occur, namely chronic suppurative otitis media and acute mastoiditis; these are described below.

Chronic suppurative otitis media (CSOM)

PATHOPHYSIOLOGY

Common presenting symptoms. This condition follows unresolved ASOM. The patient will present with a perforated tympanic membrane, a discharging ear and some degree of conductive deafness. Pain is not usually a complaint. The discharge is mucoid, becoming purulent in the presence of secondary infection.

MEDICAL MANAGEMENT

The recommended treatment would be to keep the ear dry and if possible to correct the hearing loss by performing a tympanoplasty.

Tympanoplasty

Following removal of diseased tissue an attempt may be made to reconstruct the sound transmission mechanism in the middle ear by reconstructing the tympanic membrane (myringoplasty) using a connective tissue graft and reconstructing the ossicular chain (ossiculoplasty). This combined reconstruction is known as a tympanoplasty.

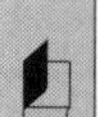

For further information on ossiculoplasty see McKenzie G et al 1986 The special senses, 2nd edn. Churchill Livingstone, Edinburgh.

NURSING PRIORITIES AND MANAGEMENT OF TYMPANOPLASTY

Preoperative care

The patient is usually admitted on the day prior to surgery. He will have a substantial hearing deficit so the establishment of a good communication system is very important. To help avoid complications the ear must be dry and free from infection. Hearing tests will be carried out to determine the degree of hearing loss and to pinpoint the problem area. If the patient has been taking aspirin regularly the dosage should be reduced to minimise the risk of bleeding. Some of the patient's hair may have to be removed and depending on local policy, skin preparation of some sort may be necessary.

To help alleviate anxiety, the nurse should give the patient information about the procedure and warn him about the sensations that he may experience afterwards, such as dizziness and tinnitus (see p. 505). It is also helpful to describe the very bulky bandage that will be present around the head and affected ear so that this does not alarm the patient and his relatives.

For patients who are having surgery on the ear in which they normally wear a hearing aid a temporary aid may be fitted to their other ear if appropriate.

Postoperative care

General postoperative care is as described in Chapter 27. The majority of patients undergoing ear surgery are given a hypotensive anaesthetic in order to reduce bleeding and thereby allow the surgeon a clearer view of the tiny operative field. This involves the intravenous administration of a hypotensive agent such as Trimetaphan or Pentolinium. Frequent blood pressure readings are therefore required until the preoperative baseline levels are regained.

Following the operation the patient should be encouraged to lie with the affected area uppermost. He should be observed for nausea, vomiting and vertigo, all of which might be present due to interference with the semicircular canals during surgery. The pressure dressing and bandage will help to prevent haematoma formation and bleeding, but the nurse should always observe the patient's bandages and pillows for bloodstains.

It is useful to ask the patient to smile, wrinkle his nose and tightly shut his eyes. The ability to perform these movements indicates that there has been no damage to the facial nerve (Turner 1988). Because of its location the facial nerve is at risk of damage in all surgery on the middle or inner ear. If infection erodes the bony canal of the facial nerve, it becomes vulnerable and, if affected, facial paralysis can result.

Most patients are out of bed on the day following surgery and return home when there is no longer any concern with regard to bleeding. The patient should be advised that he may experience dizziness during the following 2 or 3 weeks and that he should avoid movements such as quickly turning the head. The patient should return in 5–7 days to have the sutures removed. Packing is usually present in the external meatus; this will need to be changed by the patient 2–3 times daily. This packing is removed sometime between 1 and 3 weeks following surgery, when all discharge has ceased.

Patients will naturally be very anxious to know if the graft has taken and if the infection has been completely removed. Offering accurate information and giving specific answers to questions will help to alleviate these anxieties.

CSOM with choleastoma

PATHOPHYSIOLOGY

This condition is sometimes called attico-antral disease. On examination it may be possible to see the choleastoma, which is an ingrowth of keratinising squamous epithelium from the external ear into the middle ear, usually from the site of a previous perforation. The squamous epithelium growing within the middle ear produces keratin, which has the ability to erode the bony ossicles and may even spread into the inner ear.

Common presenting symptoms. The patient will complain of a foul-smelling discharge from the ear and of deafness.

MEDICAL MANAGEMENT

The treatment of choice is mastoidectomy (see below).

Acute mastoiditis

This condition arises from acute otitis media and is caused by the infection spreading to the bony walls of the cells of the mastoid process. The conservative medical management of this is by administration of antibiotics.

MEDICAL MANAGEMENT

Mastoidectomy. A cortical mastoidectomy involves incision, drainage and removal of unhealthy mucosa and bone cells from the mastoid process of the temporal bone, leaving the middle ear structures intact. A modified mastoidectomy may be performed if the disease is confined to the attic and the patient has good hearing. This is currently the most common surgical procedure for middle ear infection. It involves removal of most of the air cell system within the mastoid cavity, especially in the attic or upper area and preservation of the remnants of the tympanic membrane and the ossicles, although these are not usually functioning. Every effort is made to preserve the ossicular chain and tympanic membrane in order to retain hearing. The procedure involves extenerating (clearing out) the mastoid cells and removing the outer attic and posterior wall, thus leaving a large cavity to allow air from the meatus to circulate and dry up secretions.

NURSING PRIORITIES AND MANAGEMENT OF ACUTE MASTOIDITIS

Nursing care is as for patients undergoing tympanoplasty (see p. 503).

Other complications of middle ear infection

Less common complications of middle ear infection are facial nerve paralysis, meningitis, extra or subdural abscess, labyrinthitis, lateral sinus thrombosis, and brain abscess.

DISORDERS OF THE INNER EAR

Tinnitus

Tinnitus is a little-understood but most distressing feature of some ear diseases and disorders. It may also occur spontaneously or as a postoperative complication. Possibly because it is so puzzling, has no known cause, and is not a visible symptom, sufferers often feel that they receive very little sympathy and doubt their ability to cope.

PATHOPHYSIOLOGY

Tinnitus is a subjective sensation of sound in the ear. Its cause cannot always be determined, but it is a relatively common complaint which may arise in association with a wide range of conditions, including inner and middle ear disease, overuse of drugs such as aspirin and quinine, abnormalities of the auditory nerve, renal problems, cardiac problems and anaemia. It is often accompanied by vertigo and/or deafness. In approximately 1 million people it is severe enough to interfere with quality of life (Turner 1988).

Common presenting symptoms. Tinnitus varies in severity from a mild ringing sensation in the ear to an incessant noise loud enough to make life unbearable. The sound which is perceived varies in character from one individual to another and might be described as a 'buzzing', 'popping', 'humming' and so on. Some patients are aware of the sound only during their waking hours, while others are aware of it mainly at night or when they are somewhere very quiet.

In the worst cases individuals with tinnitus may suffer total deafness because the noise in their ear eliminates all other sounds. Understandably this symptom can cause people to become severely depressed (see Box 14.3).

MEDICAL MANAGEMENT

To aid diagnosis a careful history which includes all other symptoms and medications must be taken. A hearing test and careful examina-

Box 14.3 An experience of tinnitus

I shall never forget the first time I experienced tinnitus. It was in the dead of night when I heard a high-pitched whine in my left ear. I was so taken aback that I got up out of bed and went in search of the source of the noise. Before long, however, I realised that the noise was being carried with me.

The tinnitus had been preceded about a month beforehand by nausea and severe vertigo which I had accepted as transitory. To find that I was left with this noise made me feel very anxious indeed. I had difficulty in coming to terms with the fact that it might always be present. My reaction was 'It *can't* be! There must be *something* to combat it and make the noise go away!'

When it became clear to me that I was now a 'tinnitus sufferer' I experienced a phase of reactive depression and felt that life was not worthwhile. Naturally, I searched for a cure and eventually joined the local branch of the Tinnitus Association. This was a move which I made by myself; I was not alerted to the existence of this group by the professionals. But the Association proved to be an invaluable source of emotional and practical support.

I had no idea early on that things could get worse. With hindsight, I realise that it was just as well, as I do not think I would have had the emotional strength to carry on. Things did get worse and one New Year's night the noise changed to an intermittent, low-pitched, buzzing sound. To say I nearly went insane is putting it mildly. I recall at one point I was banging my head (none too gently) against the wall to try to dislodge the sound. I felt suicidal and realised that if this latest occurrence persisted the only way I would get peace would be to be dead.

I have been most fortunate because that phase lasted only two days and eventually the tinnitus burned itself out. My friends at the Association have not been so lucky and the suicide rate for the group has been fairly high.

tion of the ear (including radiography) may help determine the cause. Unfortunately, in many instances no treatable cause will be found. In certain patients a hearing aid can give some relief. A 'masker' which helps to cancel out the undesirable sound has become available recently and is being tried out in Britain. For patients who have become severely depressed because of the tinnitus antidepressant medication and psychological counselling may help.

NURSING PRIORITIES AND MANAGEMENT OF TINNITUS

Very few tinnitus sufferers will be patients in hospital unless their condition has arisen as an early postoperative complication. The majority will attend their GP's surgery or the outpatients' department of their local hospital. Wherever nursing staff encounter these patients high priority should be given to recognising and relieving patient anxiety and depression. Once all the necessary tests have been carried out by the medical practitioner to determine a diagnosis any prescribed treatment will be administered by nursing staff. Where there is no treatment a planned programme of explanation and information-giving will be necessary to relieve the patient's worries. Tinnitus support groups exist in many areas and can be of great help to sufferers by providing ongoing emotional support.

? **14.5** Find out if there is a tinnitus support group in your area. If there is, try to arrange to attend one of their meetings.

Vertigo

PATHOPHYSIOLOGY

Vertigo is a disturbance of equilibrium in the absence of an external cause which creates a sensation of (usually) rotating motion of one's self or one's surroundings. It is usually caused by irritation of the vestibular apparatus and is most frequently associated with disorders of the bony labyrinth and with Ménière's disease. Cardiac, neurological and psychiatric problems can also cause vertigo.

Common presenting symptoms. Vertigo is a disabling and often frightening sensation which may be transient or recurring. It is not the same as dizziness, and may be relatively mild or quite severe. The motion perceived is often described as a whirling, but rocking and swaying sensations are sometimes reported. Severe attacks of vertigo may be sudden and dramatic, accompanied by pallor, nausea and vomiting.

MEDICAL MANAGEMENT

A careful history is required from the patient and must include any precipitating factors such as neck movements. Any other symptoms such as tinnitus or deafness should be ascertained. It is also helpful to know how long the periods of vertigo last. Details of medication and any recent trauma can also aid diagnosis. A neurological and cardiovascular examination and perhaps radiography, hearing tests and blood tests may be advisable.

Occasionally, surgery will be required to treat the particular disorder of which vertigo is a symptom, but treatment is more often pharmacological (see Box 14.4).

NURSING PRIORITIES AND MANAGEMENT OF VERTIGO

As is the case with tinnitus sufferers, the majority of individuals who experience vertigo will be distressed and incapacitated by their condition. They will usually be seen in their homes, as they are likely to feel unsafe venturing out. The first nursing priority for these patients is safety. The attacks of vertigo may be unpredictable, or may be associated with particular head movements. These will be different for different individuals. For example, for one individual a precipitating circumstance might be standing on a stepladder with his head back and to one side in order to change a light bulb; for another, it may be simply a quick movement to bend down and pick up a baby from his cot. The nurse should discuss with the patient and his family how to avoid attacks.

Ménière's disease

PATHOPHYSIOLOGY

In Ménière's disease the membranous labyrinth is distended by an increase in the endolymph at the expense of the perilymph and the organ of Corti degenerates. The most widely-held theory of its cause is that it arises as a result of local ischaemia, although it has been suggested that it may be due to viral infection, biochemical disturbance, vitamin deficiency or local physiological faults.

Common presenting symptoms. Ménière's disease is characterised by four disabling features:

- vertigo
- tinnitus
- deafness
- nausea and vomiting.

It may arise at any age but is most common among individuals aged 30–50. As it runs its course over a period of many years, deafness will increase. Although this hearing loss may initially affect only one ear it will eventually affect the other as well.

During an attack the patient will be completely disoriented and unable to stand. He will want to lie down and remain as still as possible in order to relieve the vertigo. Nystagmus (see p. 519) may be present and, as a consequence of vagal stimulation, sweating, bradycardia and diarrhoea may occur.

MEDICAL MANAGEMENT

It may be difficult to arrive at a conclusive diagnosis of Ménière's disease, as many other disorders (e.g. labyrinthitis, intracranial disease and acoustic neuroma) display similar symptoms. Given that between attacks clinical examination may prove negative, diagnosis will rely heavily on careful history-taking.

The most common treatment for the symptoms of Ménière's disease is the prescription of medication (see Box 14.4). This will entail the use of diuretics and adherence to a low-salt diet to reduce the volume of endolymph. Vasodilators may be prescribed to alleviate local ischaemia, antihistamine labyrinthine sedatives to suppress the attacks of vertigo and (in very anxious patients) tranquillisers. The

Box 14.4 Examples of medications used in Ménière's disease

Antihistamine labyrinthine sedatives
Prochlorperazine maleate
Cinnarizine

Tranquillisers
Beta histine
Hydrochloride

Vasodilators
Nicotinic acid
Thymoxamine

majority of patients respond well to drug therapy and may have long periods of respite from severe symptoms.

Surgery may occasionally help to relieve symptoms. This may take the form of decompression of the endolymphatic sac, the creation of a fistula between the endolymph and perilymph reservoirs, or a vestibular neurectomy.

NURSING PRIORITIES AND MANAGEMENT OF MÉNIÈRE'S DISEASE

The main nursing priority in case of an attack of Ménière's disease is to ensure the patient's safety. Attacks are often so severe that the patient will fall to the ground: he will need to lie as still as possible, and, if in hospital, may gain a sense of security if the side rails on his bed are raised. Vomiting and diarrhoea may also be present, and can be so severe as to cause dehydration. If the patient cannot take fluids orally, intravenous fluids and antiemetic drugs will be necessary until oral medication and feeding can be tolerated.

Patients suffering from Ménière's disease often have to make lifestyle changes in order to cope with some of the symptoms of the disorder. The nurse should be prepared to offer advice on lifestyle adaptations. As an individual faced with the problems associated with Ménière's disease is likely to feel anxiety, it is vital that he be given clear information and explanations, particularly with regard to prognosis.

The involvement of the primary health care team and of the occupational health nurse will be especially important, as it is often not until the patient is back at home following diagnosis that he will begin to consider many questions with regard to participation in sport, driving, safety at home and in the workplace, and so forth.

ANATOMY AND PHYSIOLOGY OF THE NOSE

The principal function of the nose is to provide a passageway for air entering and leaving the respiratory tract. In so doing it acts as an 'air conditioner', ensuring that inspired air is humidified, sufficiently warm and free from particulate matter.

The terminal fibres of the olfactory nerve are located in the nasal cavity (see Fig. 14.4). The lower two thirds of the nose are supported by cartilage and the upper third is enclosed by bone. The cavity is divided in half by the septum which consists of cartilage anteriorly and bone posteriorly. The entrance is lined with squamous epithelium and coarse hairs and the passages with a mucous membrane of ciliated columnar epithelium. These passages are highly vascularised. A branch of the maxillary artery supplies the lower posterior section of the cavity and the anterior and posterior ethmoidal arteries supply the mucous membrane. All these vessels join at Little's area on each side of the septum (see Fig. 14.5).

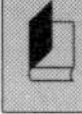

For further information, see Turner (1988).

DISORDERS OF THE NOSE

Epistaxis

PATHOPHYSIOLOGY

Epistaxis is a bleeding from the nose. It is not a disease itself but a symptom of some other disorder, which may be of a local or general nature. Local causative disorders are ideopathic; they include trauma caused by nose picking, foreign bodies, a blow to the nose, or surgery. More generalised disorders that sometimes give rise to nosebleeds can be vascular, e.g. hypertension and cardiac failure; congenital, e.g. haemophilia and hereditary haemorrhagic telangiectasia; neoplastic, e.g. leukaemia; drug-induced, e.g. a side-effect of anticoagulant therapy or of drug abuse; related to infections such as influenza, rhinitis and sinusitis.

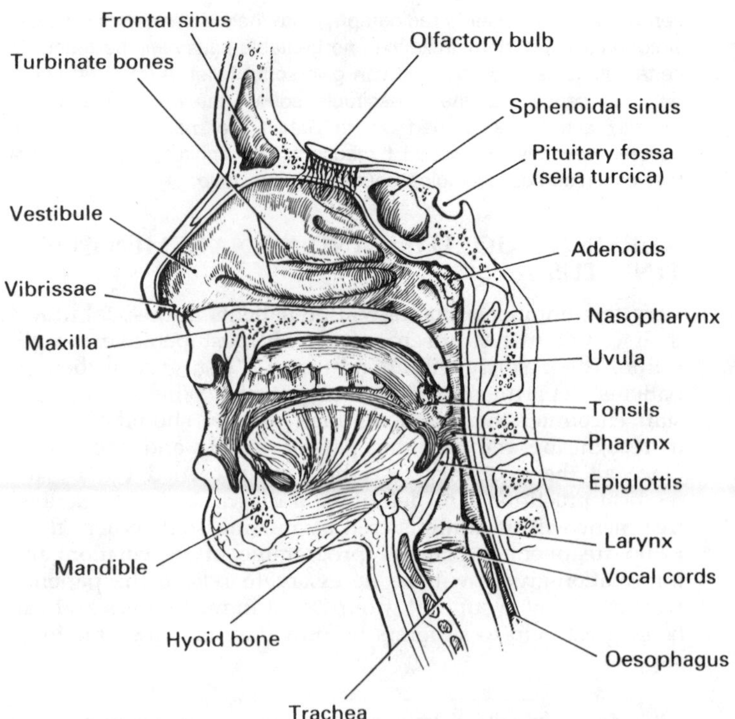

Fig. 14.4 Sagittal section showing lateral walls of nose and pharynx. (Reproduced with kind permission from McKenzie et al 1986.)

Common presenting symptoms. Epistaxis can affect males and females and can occur at any age but is most common in childhood and early adolescence, when it usually occurs in Little's area (see Fig. 14.5) and is often the result of trauma or infection. In middle-aged or elderly individuals the bleeding can also occur in the posterior part of the nose and is often associated with hypertension. This form of epistaxis may be very frightening and can be life-threatening if it proves to be difficult to control.

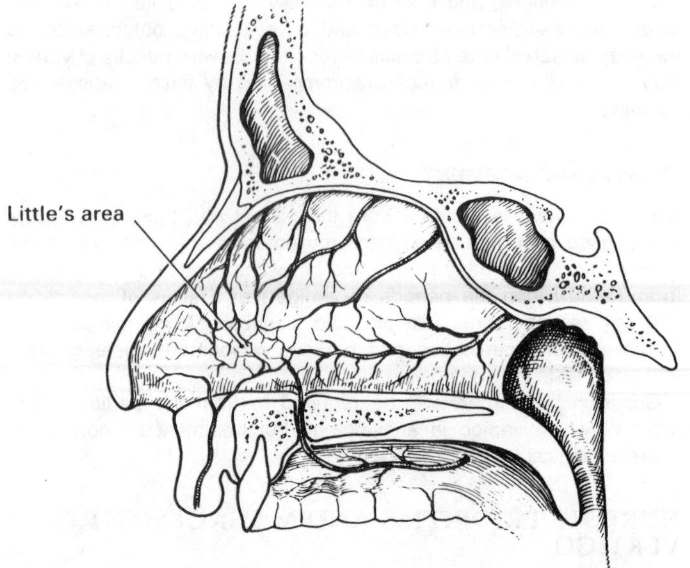

Fig. 14.5 Blood supply to nose (sagittal section). (Reproduced with kind permission from McKenzie et al 1986.)

Patients may refer themselves to the local Accident & Emergency (A&E) department when they have an active epistaxis. They may then either be given an appointment for the outpatients' clinic and sent home with an anterior pack in situ or be admitted to the appropriate hospital ward. One patient's experience of severe epistaxis is recounted in Box 14.5.

Patients often present at clinics with a history of recurrent epistaxis but rarely is a bleed in progress at the clinic visit. On examination dilated blood vessels should be apparent. The best treatment to prevent the bleeding recurring is cautery. This may be by the use of a chemical such as silver nitrate or by electric cauterisation.

MEDICAL MANAGEMENT

A patient with severe epistaxis is usually admitted to hospital as an emergency with an active nosebleed. Vital signs are recorded in case the patient is in shock. Bleeding may be severe enough to necessitate blood transfusion. Treatment is by insertion of a nasal pack. This may take the form of an inflated Foley catheter in the postnasal space and an anterior pack firmly against it, or a nasal catheter, in which case gauze packing will not be needed (Jamieson, McCall & Blythe 1992). Nasal packs are usually left in place for 48–72 hours. Antibiotics are always given to prevent any risk of infection developing and spreading to the middle ear. Occasionally, when these measures fail to control the bleeding, arterial ligation is necessary. If the bleed is the result of some underlying medical condition this will be treated at the same time.

NURSING PRIORITIES AND MANAGEMENT OF EPISTAXIS

Nursing intervention will vary, depending on the site, severity and cause of the epistaxis, as well as on the patient's age.

Anterior nosebleeds

Most patients with anterior nosebleeds will be children or adolescents and will be seen in the doctor's surgery or hospital outpatients' department and will not require hospital admission.

NURSING PRIORITIES AND MANAGEMENT OF ANTERIOR NOSEBLEEDS

The first priority of nursing intervention will be to stop the bleeding. The patient should be helped to sit upright with his head slightly forward. This prevents the blood running into the nasopharynx and causing the patient to retch. Digital pressure with the thumb and forefinger should be applied to the cartilaginous part of the nose (Little's area; see Fig. 14.5). This area has many surface arterioles which may have weakened walls. Ten minutes of this pressure is usually sufficient to control an anterior nosebleed. If these first aid measures fail or if there are recurrent nosebleeds the patient will probably be admitted to hospital for insertion of a nasal pack or cautery of the area.

Once the bleeding is under control the nurse should explain to the patient and, where appropriate, his parents how to prevent nosebleeds from recurring. Advice should be given about blowing the nose gently, avoiding picking the nose and trying to keep the nasal mucosa slightly moist by the use of soft petroleum jelly. An explanation of how to cope with and control a nosebleed should also be given.

Hospital treatment

This will be necessary for severe epistaxis which cannot be controlled by the above measures. By providing clear and concise information the nurse can help alleviate the patient's

Box 14.5 An experience of severe epistaxis

Fortunately, I was leaning forward at my desk when it started: a week earlier a nosebleed had doused my waistcoat. The next several hours were spent trying to staunch the flow. A lab technician put a small plug of cotton wool into the offending nostril, which helped for a while, and two students took my blood pressure, which as it happened was normal. When the bleeding worsened towards the end of the afternoon, I resolved to go home via my GP. With a 25-mile drive ahead of me, I donned an old lab coat back to front to protect my clothes and made for my car, leaving a trail of blood behind me. The drive, needless to say, was a strain.

The doctor's surgery was very busy and, after registering, I went over to the pharmacist's window for more cotton wool. My bloodied face evidently shocked the pharmacist; in her panic she could find neither tissues, cotton wool, nor any suitable material. At this point my GP emerged from an adjacent consulting room, took one look at me and said, 'We'd better get you laid down somewhere.' In a spare room he examined me between consultations. I made a terrible mess of his sink when he encouraged me to blow my nose in order to gain a better view of the point of bleeding. He could not find the origin and plugged the nostril with yards of ribbon-like bandage thrust high up into the nasal cavity: an excruciatingly painful procedure, leaving my nostril twice its normal size. As I rose to clean up, the other nostril began bleeding and was also packed; this was equally excruciating.

I arrived home feeling somewhat groggy and bunged up, couldn't eat much and knew I would not sleep much. Breathing constantly through my mouth made it, and my throat, uncomfortably dry. Knowing I wouldn't be able to go to work the following day, I started making the necessary phone calls, during which the bleeding started again, this time going down my throat. After some time my wife felt this couldn't continue overnight and phoned the night service GP at about 11.00 pm. He advised keeping very still, was alarmed to hear I had drunk part of a can of beer, and horrified to learn that I was swallowing the blood rather than spitting it out. He said if the bleeding had not abated in 30 minutes we were to call back. In fact it did let up during that time and, having fixed me a bed downstairs, my wife went to bed around midnight. I passed a miserable few hours of dozing and bleeding, and by 5.00 am. I had to wake my wife. She phoned the same GP who advised us to go to the casualty department of our local hospital. Leaving a note for our sleeping teenagers we drove on icy roads to the hospital, where a young houseman was roused to repack my nose. Although less painful than the first time, this was still quite horrible and left me feeling faint. I was admitted to the ENT ward and given a single room within view of the nurses' desk.

Then followed six days of hopes raised and dashed as the doctors required 24 hours clear of bleeding before I could be discharged. I needed another two repacks in that time as I had a problem with repeated sneezing, bleeding through the packs and, on two occasions, the fairly revolting experience of the pack unravelling down my throat. Each time the packs were disturbed this stimulated further bleeding and I did become anaemic. The nurses were very attentive and explained that they were relatively helpless if the bleeding continued once the packs were in place. Ice packs were their main remaining option. (One poor chap, discharged during my stay, was readmitted two days later with further bleeding.)

On being discharged I was put on a course of iron tablets and told to take a further week off work: advice I was happy to take since in the ensuing week I felt surprisingly weak. Two months later I am well and about to attend a follow-up appointment at the hospital.

anxiety and aid his recovery. The nurse will assist the medical practitioner to insert a nasal pack and will record the patient's vital signs. When a nasal pack is in place the patient will be able to breathe only through his mouth and may be afraid of suffocation. Frequent oral hygiene and plenty of oral fluids should be offered to prevent the oral mucosa becoming dry. These drinks should not be hot as this can cause local dilatation of blood vessels and exacerbate the problem. Eye care may be necessary as the packing can cause the eyes to become inflamed and weepy by obstructing the nasolacrimal duct.

Affected areas that have been cauterised may become crusted and should have soft petroleum jelly applied to them twice a day for a few weeks until the mucosa has healed.

Some patients admitted as emergencies with uncontrollable nosebleeds will be in hypovolaemic shock (see Ch. 18, p. 600).

> ? **14.6** Revise the signs and symptoms of shock so that you can visualise the likely appearance of a patient admitted with severe, uncontrollable epistaxis.

Nursing priorities in cases of severe epistaxis are to assist in stabilising the patient's condition, to arrest the bleeding by assisting with the insertion of a nasal pack or catheter and to help relieve the patient's anxiety. Temperature, pulse, respiration and blood pressure observations are commenced and if the patient has lost a lot of blood intravenous infusions of isotonic solutions or plasma are commenced. It may be necessary to give a blood transfusion.

As well as answering questions and giving information, nurses often have to administer sedatives prescribed by the medical practitioner to help relieve very anxious patients. These patients are usually nursed propped up in bed so that it is easier for them to spit out any leaking blood. Icepacks may be applied to the nose to help constrict the vessels and control bleeding. The nurse should explain to the patient how to breathe through the mouth and a sick bowl or sputum carton should be to hand into which blood can be spat. Again, it is important to offer frequent oral hygiene, plenty of cool drinks and eye care as necessary. As these patients often have dysphagia because of the pressure of the nasal pack on the soft palate a nutritious soft or even liquid diet may be appropriate. If high blood pressure or other disorders have caused the nosebleed, prescribed medication will be administered by the nurse. Bedrest is usually advised, although patients should perhaps be allowed to use the commode at the side of the bed to ease the strain of trying to use a bedpan.

Packing is usually removed in 2 or 3 days. If the bleeding has not been controlled the patient will have the nasal arteries ligated in theatre. If a deviated nasal septum (see p. 510) has been a contributory cause, corrective surgery may be performed.

If the cause of the epistaxis is hypertension (see Ch. 2, p. 44) the nurse might obtain appropriate patient education booklets or information sheets from colleagues specialising in this area. Advice may also be given about the dangers of smoking and its connection with high blood pressure and diseased arteries. Advice can also be given about diet and the dietitian may be called in as part of the health care team to give practical ideas and advice. If stress has been established as a factor in the patient's lifestyle contributing to high blood pressure, advice should be given on coping mechanisms such as relaxation exercises. Practical help from the physiotherapist may also be beneficial.

Community care

To successfully prevent the recurrence of epistaxis support should continue after the patient has returned home and resumed his normal activities. If there is an occupational health nurse at his place of work then with the patient's permission she could be alerted so that she can help to monitor the patient's progress. If the patient is at home the health visitor or district nurse should be informed of his condition so that she can encourage the patient to implement the advice he received in hospital.

> ? **14.7** Using a nursing model familiar to you, prioritise and plan the nursing interventions you think Mrs E (see Case History 14.1) will require over the next 24 hours and say how you would evaluate her care. Discuss the plan with your teacher or with a qualified member of your nursing team.

Case History 14.1 Mrs E

Mrs E is 58 years old and lives with her husband, who suffers from chronic obstructive airways disease and is unemployed. They have a son and a daughter, both of whom are married and have children. Mrs E works in a television assembly works and enjoys watching TV, going to bingo and participating in the factory social club. She smokes 20 cigarettes a day and drinks about 14 units of alcohol a week, mainly at the weekend. She often babysits for her son and daughter. She has to do all the housework, cooking and shopping as her husband's breathing problems leave him with little energy.

For the past few months Mrs E has been suffering from nosebleeds but today's was very severe and could not be controlled even with the help of the occupational health nurse at the factory. She was brought to the local hospital A & E department by ambulance. By the time she arrived her blood pressure was 90/50 and her pulse 105; she was pale and shivering. She was also very anxious and frightened.

In the A & E department an epistat catheter was inserted and an intravenous infusion commenced. Mrs E was then transferred to the ward where the staff nurse welcomed her and took her to the bed she had prepared. The staff nurse was given a report by the A & E nurse and after helping Mrs E to transfer from the trolley to bed she planned to observe her infusion closely and to monitor the bleeding and her blood pressure.

On admission Mrs E was stilll anxious and distressed. She was a very fastidious lady and the mess her nosebleed had made concerned her. She was also very worried about what her husband would do for his meal and how he would be kept informed of her condition.

In prioritising Mrs E's needs, the staff nurse took into account the details of her medical condition as well as other concerns that the patient herself felt to be important. She helped Mrs E into a hospital nightgown after washing the blood from her skin and put her blouse into cold water to soak. She checked the infusion and Mrs E's blood pressure, then brought the ward phone to the bedside and telephoned Mrs E's husband. As Mrs E had difficulty talking because of the nasal catheter the nurse assisted in a three-way conversation in which Mrs E was reassured that her husband was all right. A neighbour had made him his tea and Mrs E's daughter was on her way to the hospital, bring her mother toiletries and nightclothes. This conversation reassured Mrs E and allowed her to feel more relaxed. This in turn helped the staff nurse to concentrate on monitoring Mrs E's condition and helping to alleviate her problems.

DISORDERS OF THE PARANASAL SINUSES

The paranasal sinuses are a group of air spaces surrounding the nose which make the skull lighter and add resonance to the voice (Turner 1988). They consist of two frontal, two maxillary and two ethmoid sinuses and a single sphenoid sinus. These sinuses all drain into the nose.

Acute sinusitis

PATHOPHYSIOLOGY

Acute sinusitis is the inflammation of one or more of the paranasal sinuses. It usually develops as an infection secondary to an upper respiratory tract infection or dental disease. Because of the close anatomical connection of the sinuses with the nose, sinus infection is common. It may be acute or chronic.

Common presenting symptoms. Pain is a symptom, and may be facial, supraorbital or interocular, depending on the sinus involved. Tenderness in the area of pain may also be a feature. Nasal obstruction is also a common symptom and discharge may be present. The patient usually complains of general malaise and on examination will be found to be pyrexial.

MEDICAL MANAGEMENT

A nasal swab may be taken for culture and sensitivity. Sinus radiography may also be performed to determine which sinuses are affected. Medical treatment usually consists of the prescription of mild analgesics, antibiotics and nasal decongestant drops.

NURSING PRIORITIES AND MANAGEMENT OF ACUTE SINUSITIS

The patient with acute sinusitis is usually nursed at home. He will be advised to rest in bed, to drink plenty of fluids, to take mild analgesics such as aspirin, and to self-administer nasal drops. Oral hygiene is also important as the individual will probably be mouth breathing because of the nasal obstruction. Moist inhalations with menthol crystals can also bring some relief and help to loosen crusting in the nasal cavities. Many sufferers find inhalations very soothing first thing in the morning and last thing at night. After 2 or 3 days the individual should have improved sufficiently to be fully active again.

Chronic sinusitis

PATHOPHYSIOLOGY

By contrast to acute sinusitis, chronic sinusitis can be quite debilitating. It can develop for several reasons, including:

- inadequate treatment of an acute episode
- septal deviation or nasal polyps preventing adequate drainage of the sinuses
- pollution, e.g. cigarette smoke
- allergic nasal disease.

Common presenting symptoms. The main symptoms of chronic sinusitis are nasal discharge, postnasal discharge, a husky voice and a poor sense of smell. Pain is not always present. Complications may include throbbing of the face when the head is tilted forward, pharyngitis, recurrent tonsillitis and chronic otitis media.

MEDICAL MANAGEMENT

Treatment is usually conservative, consisting of treating any infection with antibiotics and prescribing nasal decongestant drops. It may be necessary to treat polyps or a deviated septum surgically. Antroscopy and antral lavage may also be necessary. Antral lavage, which is performed under general anaesthetic, involves the introduction through the nasal passage of a trocar and cannula into the antral sinus to wash out infected material. Occasionally more radical surgery is necessary to remove all of the diseased mucosal lining and widen the opening to the nasal passage to allow more effective drainage. This more radical surgery requires general anaesthesia.

?	**14.8** Discuss with a patient what it feels like to have a sinus wash-out.

NURSING PRIORITIES AND MANAGEMENT OF CHRONIC SINUSITIS

The nurse's priorities in caring for patients with chronic sinusitis are to administer the conservative treatment prescribed by the medical practitioner and to prepare the patient for any surgery which may be required. After any surgical procedure the patient should be observed for haemorrhage and haematoma formation; pain should be relieved with mild analgesics. Patients who smoke should be informed of the particular risks that this presents to them and should be encouraged to stop. The importance of completing any prescribed antibiotic therapy should also be explained.

Nasal injury

PATHOPHYSIOLOGY

Injuries to the nose are fairly common and usually occur in sporting activities, falls, accidents and assaults. A blow to one side of the nose may fracture and displace the bone, causing deviation on the other side. A direct blow to the front of the nose can splay out the nasal bones, resulting in a depressed bridge. An injury which is sufficiently severe to fracture the nasal bones will also cause soft tissue swelling and may cause epistaxis.

MEDICAL MANAGEMENT

Investigations will involve a radiographic examination, although this does not always reveal the fracture or may simply reveal a previously undetected fracture. An examination of the nose using a nasal speculum will allow the practitioner to see if the airways are patent and if there is any damage to the septum. Palpation of the nasal bones must be carried out very gently as they will be very tender and painful for up to 3 weeks following a fracture.

Treatment of a broken nose involves manipulating the fractured bones. Occasionally this can be done at the time of the accident but usually involves waiting for about 10 days till the oedema has subsided and manipulating the fracture while the patient is under general anaesthetic. If the corrected fracture is unstable a plaster of Paris cast is usually taped in position over the nose for about 10 days to allow the fracture to set correctly.

NURSING PRIORITIES AND MANAGEMENT OF NASAL INJURY

If nursing attention is available immediately, treatment of a fractured nose will probably involve first aid measures to stop any epistaxis and to limit the oedema. This involves compressing the end of the nostrils gently between the thumb and forefinger (unfortunately, this will be very painful to the patient) and encouraging the patient to sit with his head slightly forward so that any blood does not run down the back of his throat. If ice is available an ice pack applied to the bridge of the nose can help control bleeding and swelling. Any epistaxis which results from a blow to the nose is usually short-lived.

Common problems during nasal surgery

Bleeding. This occurs because there is such a rich blood supply to the nasal mucosa. It can be controlled by the use of ice packs, and if the surgeon suspects that the bleeding might be severe, a nasal pack may be inserted.

Oedema of the mucosa is likely to occur as a consequence of manipulation. Ice packs may help to minimise swelling.

Watery discharge. The irritation of the mucosa which results from surgery will cause an excessive amount of watery discharge to be produced. The nurse should provide an adequate supply of tissues or apply a nose bag made of gauze and cotton wool to absorb discharge. This helps to make the problem more manageable.

Pain. As there is a very good nerve supply to the nose the patient may experience quite severe pain. This should be alleviated by means of prescribed analgesics.

DEVIATION OF THE NASAL SEPTUM

The nasal septum separates the nostrils. It is usually thin and quite straight. The upper part is composed of bone and the lower part of cartilage. Deviations of the nasal septum can range from a simple bulge to a marked S-shaped deformity. It should be noted that most people have some degree of deviation; hence, when introducing a nasogastric tube the practitioner should always ask the patient which nostril would cause less discomfort.

PATHOPHYSIOLOGY

Developmental problems or trauma may result in a deviated nasal septum. Patients usually complain of nasal obstruction, infection of the sinuses or chronic otitis media due to the inability of the eustachian tubes to function properly. Any combination of these symptoms may be present. It sometimes occurs that patients with a minor deviation complain of more severe symptoms than others who, on examination, are found to have a severe deviation of the septum resulting in almost total obstruction of one nostril. Minor deviation can lead to complications such as abscesses and sinusitis.

MEDICAL MANAGEMENT

An assessment by the medical practitioner of the symptoms, correlated with the degree of the deformity should be carried out before a treatment plan is agreed. Inspection of the nose with a nasal speculum should reveal the extent of the deviation.

If surgery is the chosen treatment this is likely to be either a submucous resection or a septoplasty. There is often some confusion as to what these procedures involve. In both operations access to the bony and cartilaginous parts of the septum is gained by stripping off the nasal mucosa. In a submucous resection the affected parts of the septum are removed. During a septoplasty the septum is freed, allowing it to be repositioned along the midline of the nose. A nasal pack is usually inserted following these procedures to prevent haemorrhage.

NURSING PRIORITIES AND MANAGEMENT OF DEVIATION OF THE NASAL SEPTUM

For 24–48 hours after surgery the patient will have a nasal pack in position. Nursing care in hospital will be similar to that given for epistaxis (see p. 507). Patients are usually fit to return home 24–48 hours after the nasal packing has been removed. There will be a degree of nasal obstruction for 2 or 3 weeks after surgery, until the postsurgical swelling has subsided. Patients are usually advised to stay away from work or crowded places for 10 to 14 days after surgery to minimise the risk of infection. They are also advised to follow the surgeon's instructions with regard to steam inhalations and nasal douches or decongestant sprays.

Septal haematoma

This usually results from trauma and is a collection of blood beneath the mucoperichondrium of the septum. The patient complains of nasal obstruction; examination usually reveals a bilateral swelling in the nasal cavities. Antibiotics are given to prevent infection and it is sometimes necessary to incise and drain the haematoma.

Septal perforation

Trauma is usually the cause of a hole in the septum. Although the patient is often symptom-free, excessive crusting or minor epistaxis may occur. Occasionally the patient complains of whistling on inspiration. If symptoms are troublesome surgical closure may be attempted.

NASAL OBSTRUCTION

Obstruction of the nasal cavities can result from a number of causes but patients usually present with similar symptoms, the most common of which are obstructed breathing and increased nasal discharge. Some of the most common causes are:

- infection
- allergy
- foreign bodies
- polyps
- neoplasms.

Nasal obstruction resulting from the first two causes does not usually require hospital treatment. The others are described below.

Foreign bodies in the nose

PATHOPHYSIOLOGY

It is usually very young children, aged 2–4 years, who insert foreign bodies into the nasal cavity. These objects may be organic or inorganic. Inorganic bodies include buttons, beads, and small plastic or metal objects and may lie undetected for a long time, only to be found during a routine examination. Organic bodies such as peas, wood, paper, cotton wool or sweets cause a local inflammatory reaction which eventually will lead to the formation of granulation tissue. The resulting nasal discharge will eventually become purulent, foul-smelling and blood-stained. Characteristically, the discharge is from only one cavity.

MEDICAL MANAGEMENT

Because of the young age of the typical patient the foreign body is usually removed after he or she has been anaesthetised. This allows a thorough examination to be carried out.

NURSING PRIORITIES AND MANAGEMENT OF FOREIGN BODIES IN THE NOSE

Young children are usually accompanied by a parent. Pre- and postoperative nursing care will be adjusted according to the age of the child.

Health visitors normally spend time with parents to discuss safety in the home and the prevention of accidents. Knowledge of common types of accidents and injuries and of their relationship to a child's age and development stage can help parents of toddlers to be on the alert. For example, the most common age at which children lodge foreign bodies in the nose is around 2 years (Denyer 1990), when the toddler has developed the fine motor skill of picking up tiny objects in a pincer grasp. By increasing parents' awareness of dangers, risks can be reduced and accidents prevented.

Nasal polyps

PATHOPHYSIOLOGY

Nasal polyps are projections of oedematous mucous membrane and look like bunches of grapes. They result from prolonged infection or allergy and are usually bilateral and multiple. They occur more commonly in adult males than in women.

Common presenting symptoms. Patients usually complain of nasal obstruction and discharge. Occasionally the size of the polyps may cause broadening of the external nose. The patient may complain of headaches if there is sinus involvement and there may be loss of smell and taste.

MEDICAL MANAGEMENT

On examination a characteristic glossy, greyish swelling will be visible; if probed it will be found to be soft, insensitive and mobile. Surgical removal is the treatment of choice. This may be carried out under local or general anaesthetic. The patient will require less time in hospital for a local anaesthetic but the decongestant that it contains shrinks the polyps and makes them more difficult to identify and remove. With a general anaesthetic the polyps can be removed at a less hurried pace but bleeding may be more profuse and therefore might obscure some of the smaller polyps. Recurrences are common and an attempt should be made to treat the underlying cause.

NURSING PRIORITIES AND MANAGEMENT OF NASAL POLYPS

Nursing staff should be alert to epistaxis, which is the main postoperative complication of polyp removal. Given that polyps can be associated with allergies, many patients may also suffer from asthma and should be closely observed in this regard.

A nasal pack is sometimes inserted after the procedure; appropriate nursing care is detailed on page 508. As it is fairly common for polyps to recur, the importance of early detection and treatment should be explained to the patient.

NEOPLASMS

Nasal tumours are rare. When they occur, they usually start on one side of the nasal cavity. Malignant tumours are often infected and ulcerated, in which case they usually produce a profuse purulent discharge. Headache may also be a feature if there is sinus involvement.

Treatment may consist of surgery, radiotherapy, cytotoxic therapy or a combination of these. Patients receiving radiotherapy or cytotoxic therapy are usually treated as outpatients and may be visited by community nurses if they experience any side-effects of treatment requiring nursing intervention.

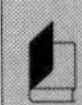

For further information on neoplasms see Turner (1988) and Serra et al (1986).

ANATOMY AND PHYSIOLOGY OF THE THROAT

The throat is usually considered to consist of the pharynx and the larynx (see Fig. 14.4). The pharynx may be divided into the nasopharynx and the oropharynx.

The nasopharynx extends from the nasal septum to the eustachian tubes and rests behind and above the soft palate. The oropharynx extends from the posterior boundary of the hard palate to the hyoid bone; it contains the uvula and the tonsils and is surrounded by lymphoid tissue.

The larynx is the organ of voice production and airway protection. It is composed mainly of cartilage and muscle and is lined with a mucosa of squamous epithelium (see Turner 1988).

DISORDERS OF THE THROAT

Benign tumours

These generally arise as a result of voice abuse or overuse and the patient usually presents with continued hoarseness. The tumours are usually attached to the vocal cords and vary greatly in size. Resolution of small nodules may be achieved by voice rest and appropriate speech therapy. Larger nodules may require surgical removal.

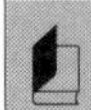

For further information on benign tumours see Turner (1988).

Carcinoma of the larynx

PATHOPHYSIOLOGY

Carcinoma of the larynx is classified according to its location and extent, i.e. glottic (confined to the vocal cords), supraglottic (above the vocal cords) or subglottic (below the vocal cords). (See Fig. 14.6.) It accounts for 1% of all malignant disease and is more common in males than in females. The majority of patients have a history of heavy smoking, although the disorder does occasionally occur in non-smokers (Turner 1988). It is also thought that high levels of alcohol consumption can be an influencing factor. The most common form of the disease is squamous cell carcinoma. About 10% of all patients with carcinoma of the larynx have a coexisting carcinoma of the bronchus.

Common presenting symptoms. Some patients with laryngeal carcinoma do not consult their medical practitioners until the disease is advanced, having ignored the symptom of hoarseness for some time. Occasionally patients are treated for laryngitis and by the time a tumour has been diagnosed it is quite advanced. Otalgia, dyspnoea, dysphagia, neck lumps and weight loss are all symptoms of advanced laryngeal carcinoma.

MEDICAL MANAGEMENT

Carcinoma of the larynx has a high rate of cure if detected early (Turner 1988) but, sadly, many people dismiss the classic symptom of hoarseness as trivial. The form of treatment offered will depend on the site of the tumour and on how early it has been detected. If the tumour is confined to the vocal cords it is usually diagnosed as a result of the patient consulting his medical practitioner with a history of hoarseness. Patients who have suffered from hoarseness for more than 4 weeks should have a mirror examination of their larynx (indirect laryngoscopy) to investigate the possibility of carcinoma. Diagnosis is confirmed by an examination of the patient's larynx under general anaesthesia (direct laryngoscopy) and a histological examination of a biopsy of the tumour.

For glottic tumours the treatment of choice is a course of radiotherapy. If the tumour has developed into the supraglottic or subglottic area, or if the vocal cords have become immobile, radiotherapy would not be the most effective treatment. The recommended treatment

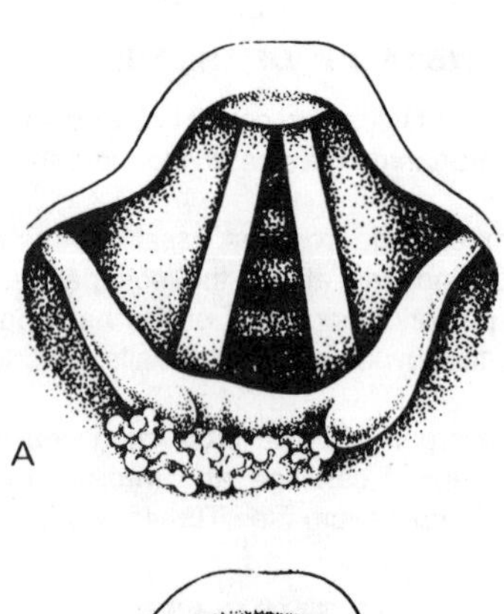

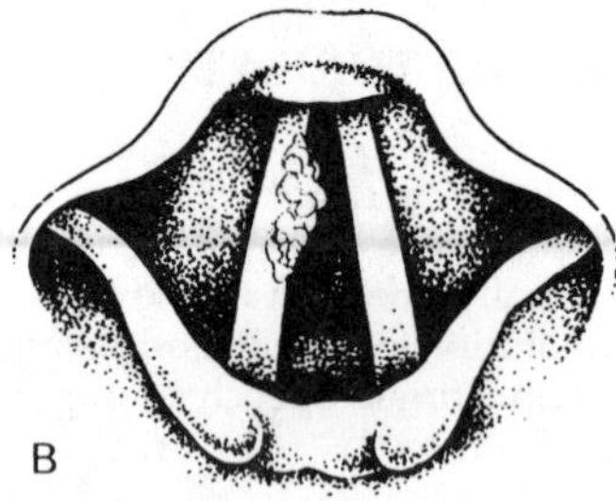

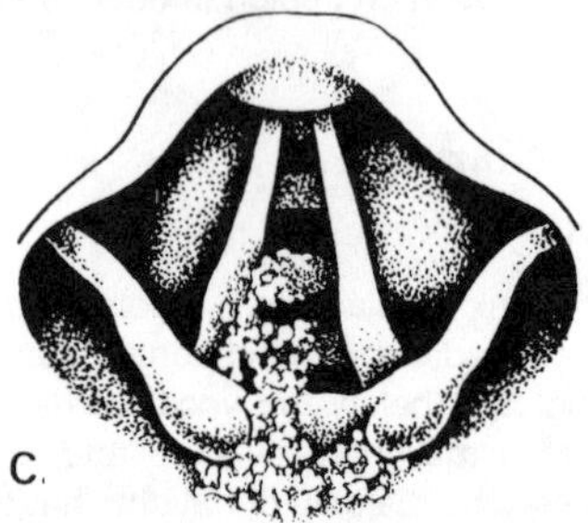

Fig. 14.6 Tumours of the larynx. (A) Supraglottic tumour. (B) Glottic tumour. (C) Subglottic tumour — extensive spread to supraglottic area. (Reproduced with kind permission from McKenzie et al 1986.)

would be total laryngectomy, which involves removal of the larynx, the creation of a permanent tracheostomy (see pp. 515–517) and the closure of the pharyngeal defect. This surgery may also have to be performed on patients who have a residual or recurrent tumour following radiotherapy. Nursing interventions appropriate to this procedure are outlined in the next section.

Very advanced tumours of the larynx may be considered inoperable, in which case the patient may be given palliative radiotherapy to relieve some of the more distressing symptoms of the disease (see Ch. 32, p. 887). In addition, a tracheostomy is sometimes performed to relieve any dyspnoea.

Total laryngectomy

Preoperative preparation

The surgeon will spend some time with the patient and his family prior to surgery to explain the operation and its after-effects. The whole health care team is usually involved at this time. This team will consist of nursing staff, speech therapists, physiotherapists, medical social workers, dietitians and, often, former patients who have had a laryngectomy.

Physical preparation. Diagnostic radiography of the neck and chest is usually performed and computerised tomography (CT scan) or magnetic imaging is sometimes carried out. A full blood analysis is made. Patients who are undergoing total laryngectomy may also require a partial thyroidectomy, in which case thyroid function must be checked pre- and postoperatively (see Ch. 5, p. 145).

An electrocardiograph (ECG) is usually ordered to check heart function (see Ch. 2, p. 12). The patient will also be given a dental check-up and receive any necessary dental treatment to help circumvent the risk of pathogenic organisms in the oral cavity. Nasal and throat swabs, a mid-stream specimen of urine and a specimen of sputum are usually collected for bacteriological examination so that any pathogenic organisms can be eliminated before surgery.

The bowel preparation of the patient will depend on the preference of the surgeon concerned but may consist of the administration of evacuant suppositories or an enema the day prior to surgery. It is important, in the period leading up to surgery, that any malnourishment of the patient is corrected by enteral or parenteral supplements.

NURSING PRIORITIES AND MANAGEMENT OF TOTAL LARYNGECTOMY

Preoperative priorities

The nurse's tasks at this stage will centre on providing support and information for the patient and his family and on preparing them physically and/or psychologically for the operation.

The patient is usually admitted several days prior to surgery to allow ample time for preparation and psychological adjustment. It is important for the patient to get to know the team members at this stage, and in some units it is possible for him to meet the community nurse who will be helping him after he returns home.

The patient and his family will need support in adjusting to the diagnosis and in facing the prospect of surgery that will disfigure the patient and alter his lifestyle (see Case History 14.2). The patient will need to be prepared for the fact that he will have a permanent 'hole' in his neck through which he will breathe. He will be unable to laugh, sing or talk normally. He will be able to swim only after receiving advice and guidance on the use of special stoma devices.

Case History 14.2 Mr G

Mr G is a 64-year-old retired labourer. A widower with no family, he lives alone but has helpful neighbours. He is a keen bowler and enjoys the social side of the bowling club. He also reads a lot and listens to music. He smokes 20 cigarettes a day and consumes about 30 units of alcohol per week. He has been diagnosed as having a subglottic tumour with extensive spread and a total laryngectomy has been recommended.

Mr E arrives at the ward with his friend Mr J and is welcomed by the staff nurse, who takes Mr G to a bed in a four-bedded room and explains that he will be there until his operation and then in a single room for a few days while he recovers from the surgery. The nurse leaves Mr G and his friend to unpack his things and then returns with a cup of tea for them both. She asks about his activities of living with a view to planning his nursing care. Since Mr G's only relative is his wife's sister in a town 200 miles away he gives her name and that of his friend as next of kin. His friend tells the staff nurse that he and his wife will visit and do Mr G's washing for him.

? **14.9** What information would you consider important to receive on this initial chat with Mr G to help you plan his nursing care?
Discuss this with your colleagues and check your ideas with your teacher or a qualified member of the nursing team.

The patient may lose his sense of smell because he may tend to gulp in air through the mouth and stoma rather than the nose. In view of these after-effects, some patients will refuse therapy altogether, a decision which may be very difficult for the patient's family and members of the health care team to accept.

To help prevent infection the patient is usually nursed in a single room. He is usually admitted into this room so that he can familiarise himself with his surroundings, although some units prefer the patient to be admitted initially to a multiple-occupancy room where he can talk with other patients and thereby relieve stress.

Prior to surgery the patient should be familiarised with the equipment and procedures that he will encounter postoperatively. For example, tracheal suction could be very alarming for the patient if he is not told about it beforehand. The nasogastric tube which will be present postoperatively for feeding, as well as intravenous infusions, oxygen supply and wound drains need to be demonstrated and explained preoperatively to help reduce anxiety and thereby aid recovery (Hayward 1975).

An appropriate means of communication which works for the patient, his family and the multidisciplinary team should be arranged before surgery. For example, a pad and pencil would usually be kept close to hand, but if the patient is illiterate or has problems with his sight other means of communication must be sought (see Ch. 26). The establishment of a good communication scheme preoperatively will help the patient to regain his confidence postoperatively and avoid frustration.

The speech therapist will visit the patient preoperatively to explain her role and offer the possibility of oesophageal speech postoperatively. She is usually the person who suggests a visit to the patient from someone who has had a laryngectomy. This visitor should be someone who presents himself well, has developed good oesophageal speech, is an effective communicator and is well integrated back into the community. During this visit it is usually suggested that the patient may like to look at the visitor's stoma but this issue is not forced. These visits can be very beneficial to the patient.

The physiotherapist will also assess the patient prior to surgery. She will explain her role in his postoperative care and teach him deep breathing and leg exercises.

It is important in the period leading up to surgery that any malnourishment is corrected by enteral or parenteral supplements. The dietitian will assess the patient's nutritional state preoperatively. She will also explain to the patient how he will be fed postoperatively and the length of time for which this may be necessary.

Box 14.6 Resuscitation of a 'neck breathing' patient

The principles of resuscitation of a 'neck breathing' patient are the same as those for any other patient, although a few alterations of technique apply. The ABCs of first aid — airway, breathing and circulation — are given top priority.

Initially, the stoma would be covered by the resuscitator's mouth, but as soon as possible a cuffed tracheal tube should be inserted, and inflated to prevent any leakage of the air which is being introduced by the rescuscitator. The tube should then be connected to an Ambu bag and resuscitation continued as normal.

Postoperative priorities

Immediately following surgery the main nursing priorities will be maintenance of a clear airway (see Box 14.6), observation of the tracheostome, establishment of good communication with the patient, and reassurance and support of the patient and his family.

The patient will be brought into his single room following recovery from the anaesthetic. He will be nursed in the semi-recumbent position initially and then gradually encouraged to sit more upright to aid respiration and neck drainage. It is important that the patient's head is always flexed slightly forward to ease tension on the suture lines. When he is being lifted a nurse should always support his head.

On return to the ward the patient's vital signs should be recorded at half-hourly intervals; as these become stable within the normal range, recordings can be reduced to 4 hourly.

In the immediate postoperative period the stomach contents should be aspirated through the nasogastric tube that will be present. This should be done at 1 or 2 hourly intervals, depending on the amount aspirated, to prevent regurgitation and the formation of a fistula (see Box 14.7).

Once bowel sounds have been detected (usually between 24 and 48 hours postoperatively) the patient can commence feeding. Water is given first, progressing to half-strength feeds and finally full-strength feeds. This gradual progression is necessary to avoid the problem of diarrhoea which may develop if full-strength feeds are administered from the beginning. Before administering each feed the nurse must check that the nasogastric tube is in the correct position.

? **14.10** What are the methods for confirming that the nasogastric tube is correctly positioned in the stomach? (see Ch. 21, p. 670)

Box 14.7 Potential complications of laryngectomy

Blockage of trachea
This potentially life-threatening complication can occur if the trachea has not been sufficiently humidified. The potential for tracheal blockage should be stressed during the teaching programme, as it tends to occur when patients have returned to the community and have not cared for their stoma as taught in hospital.

Stenosis of the tracheostome
Like tracheal blockage, this complication is potentially life-threatening and may occur when the patient has returned to the community. It arises as a result of neglect which has allowed crusting to build up. Careful toilet of the stoma should prevent its occurrence, and wearing a tube for part or all of the day can be a useful preventive measure.

Fistula formation
If the pharyngeal repair breaks down a fistula may form which allows saliva and food to leak from the incision, causing excoriation of the skin and possibly leading to infection. This is usually treated by inserting a nasogastric tube for feeding and not allowing anything to be consumed orally. Healing may take several weeks and antibiotics may be prescribed if infection is present. If the fistula does not heal by itself, surgical closure may be necessary.

Wound breakdown
This may occur in patients who are undergoing a course of radiotherapy following surgery. Careful wound care can help to prevent its occurrence.

Nasal toilet will be required while the nasogastric tube is in position, as the wide bore of the tube which is necessary for aspirating the stomach contents and preventing vomit from damaging the suture line of the pharyngeal repair will irritate the mucous lining of the nose.

Once nasogastric feeding has been established successfully the intravenous infusion with which the patient will have returned from theatre will be discontinued.

Humidified oxygen is usually administered to the patient during this time to help keep the lining of the trachea moist. On his return to the ward he may have a cuffed tracheostomy tube in position (see Fig. 14.7). The cuff pressure should be released every 8 hours to prevent damage to the tracheal lining. The tube is usually removed 24–48 hours after surgery. Some patients return from theatre without a tube in position; here, careful observation of the stoma for swelling or obstruction will be necessary. Normally, excessive secretions are moved into the trachea by ciliary action and expelled by coughing; for the new laryngectomy patient, however, this can be difficult. Frequent tracheal suction is usually necessary as in the immediate postoperative period these secretions can be profuse.

Two suction drains are usually present, one on each side of the wound. These should be observed for signs of saliva, which would indicate the formation of a fistula. The wound itself is usually closed with fine sutures or clips and may be covered by a clear plastic dressing so that it can be easily observed. Stoma care is necessary 2–4 hourly postoperatively to prevent encrustation around the opening and to keep the suture lines clear.

Good pressure area care is necessary in the first 24 hours but it can be difficult to move the patient because of the vulnerable wound in his neck. A 2-hourly change of position should be tried and full use made of aids such as special mattresses and sacral and heel protectors.

The immediate postoperative period can be very difficult for the patient and his family as they realise the full implication of the surgery. Often the patient is very agitated the first time he is awake enough to ask for something and discovers that he has no voice. The communication skills of the ear, nose and throat nurse are very important at this time. She should remind the patient of the prearranged communication plan and display patience and understanding. The patient should never be left on his own without any means of communication such as a buzzer or bell. This is very important for the patient's confidence as he may have the very natural fear of requiring tracheal suction and not being able to attract attention.

Mouth care is very important while the nasogastric tube is in position and should be offered at least 4 hourly, as well as around the time feeds are due in order to stimulate digestive juices. The specific mouth care given to each patient will be determined by individual assessment.

On the first or second postoperative day the patient is usually encouraged to sit out of bed while it is being made. Over the following days he should be encouraged to increase his activity until he is fully ambulant.

Nasogastric feeding is continued until the patient's pharyngeal repair is fully healed. This is usually tested by giving the patient a drink of dye and observing the wound for any signs of leakage as he swallows. If the wound appears to have healed the nasogastric tube is removed and the patient is allowed to commence eating a soft diet. Foods should be of gradually increasing consistency till a normal diet can be tolerated. The patient's weight should be monitored during the postoperative period to ensure that food intake is adequate. Some laryngectomy patients suffer from constipation in the postoperative period, partly due to their inability to increase their intrathoracic and abdominal pressure. This can be alleviated by including soluble fibre in the nasogastric feed and increasing fibre in the patient's diet when he is able to eat by mouth. An explanation of the causes of constipation and encouragement to drink larger amounts of fluids may also help. Sometimes it may be necessary to prescribe an aperient.

Around the 4th postoperative day the suction drains are removed from the wound. The neck sutures may be removed on about the 7th day, although they may stay in position a few days longer if the patient has had radiotherapy treatment. The stoma sutures are usually removed after 10 days.

Tracheal suction is given when necessary but the need for this should gradually diminish as the patient's cough reflexes become stronger. Stoma toilet is continued roughly every 4 hours; the nurse should encourage the patient to participate in this. Humidification may still be required at certain times and can be administered via a mechanical humidifier. Alternatively, a moistened Buchanan laryngectomy bib/protector may be worn or the patient may be given a Roger's crystal spray filled with normal saline to spray into the tracheostome. The patient should be taught how to remove any crusting which may form around the stoma. Most patients wear small soft rubber stoma buttons and find them reasonably comfortable.

Rehabilitation of the patient should start as soon as possible; ideally, this will involve the supportive participation of the patient's family and of the community nurse. The patient will first need to become accustomed to his altered appearance. If appropriate, he could be given a hand mirror on perhaps the second postoperative day after he has been told about what to expect. The presence of family members at this time might be helpful. Progress in wound healing and a decrease in face and neck puffiness over a period of days can be

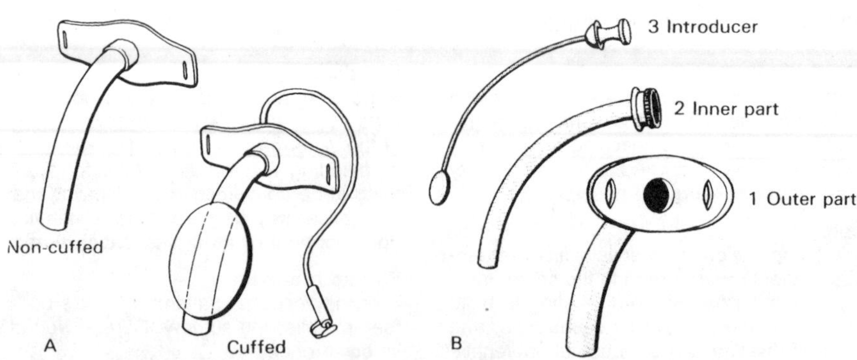

Fig. 14.7 Tracheostomy tubes in common use. (A) Disposable. (B) Non-disposable. (Reproduced with kind permission from Jamieson et al 1992.)

encouraging for the patient. Once he has become accustomed to looking in a mirror he may be encouraged to wipe away secretions from his stoma, gradually progressing to changing his stoma button by himself. When the patient goes home he will need the bib and spray and so should become confident in their use before leaving hospital.

Preparation for discharge

By demonstrating patience and understanding and sensitively implementing a planned rehabilitation programme the multidisciplinary team can help to build up the patient's confidence prior to discharge and ensure that he will be able to cope with any problem which may arise. The patient should feel at ease with his stoma and be confident in caring for it. He should be encouraged to socialise with other patients, perhaps by moving to a multi-bed room. This can be very difficult at first but should be seen as a first step to socialising after discharge.

Once the nasogastric tube has been removed the speech therapist can begin her work of teaching the patient to develop oesophageal speech. If the patient has mastered a few simple words such as 'yes' and 'no' prior to discharge his confidence may be increased tremendously. Motivation is an important factor in the acquisition of oesophageal speech; again, the participation of the patient's family can be of enormous benefit. Following discharge the patient will continue to attend for speech therapy. Speech aids which are available for individuals who have undergone laryngectomy are described in Box 14.8.

The community nursing services will be involved in preparations for the patient's return home. Ideally, the community nursing team will by now be known to the patient and his family. A community nurse will have assessed the patient's needs at home and may arrange for such things as suction equipment to be available for him there.

The medical social worker is often required to help patients and their families with practical difficulties following the surgery. Individuals who have undergone a laryngectomy are often unable to return to their former employment; e.g. since the patient will be unable to hold his breath and increase intrathoracic pressure he will not be able to do heavy manual labour. Negotiations between the medical social worker and the patient's employers for a job reallocation may allow the patient to continue working. If continued employment is impossible the medical social worker is well qualified to help the patient receive all the social security benefits to which he is entitled. She may also be able to help the patient's family with travelling expenses related to the treatment programme.

The patient will attend the ENT outpatients' clinic after discharge to ensure that no problems arise which he feels unable to handle. There is a national association of laryngectomees which circulates a regular newsletter and has clubs in most areas (see Useful Addresses, p. 520). The support which this association can give is invaluable to many patients, who greatly benefit from the opportunity to share experiences and talk about problems with others in a similar situation.

Box 14.8 Speech aids for laryngectomees

Electronic vibrator or artificial larynx
This produces a note which is articulated by the patient when the device is applied to the neck. The sound produced is very metallic and monotonous.

Blom Singer valve
This is a tube which can be inserted into the fistula created between the trachea and oesophagus following total laryngectomy. The patient can produce vocal sounds by occluding the valve.

Near-total neoglottic technique of laryngectomy
This is a primary procedure in which a tunnel (fistula) is created between the trachea and oesophagus, into which a special piece of tubing is inserted. This is connected to the Blom-Singer valve.This tubing is designed to allow expired air to go up, allowing for voice production, and to prevent fluid coming down. This procedure can be performed when the patient is undergoing a partial laryngectomy.

Amplifier
This increases the volume of the sounds produced.

For more detailed information, see Turner (1988), pp. 178–179.

Tracheostomy

The surgical procedure of tracheostomy is the making of an opening through the skin of the neck into the trachea. It is one of the earliest operations described; there is evidence that it was performed by the Egyptians in Biblical times (Turner 1988).

A tracheostomy may be temporary or permanent, and may be planned as elective surgery or performed as an emergency procedure.

Indications

The indications for a tracheostomy are as follows.

- Airway obstruction. This may be caused by the inhalation and impaction of a foreign body in the larynx. Severe inflammation may also cause obstruction. Laryngeal cancer which is being treated by radiotherapy may also cause obstruction.
- Bronchial toilet. After head injury, drug overdose, cerebral vascular accident, coma or certain neurological disorders the patient may require assistance with respiration and removal of bronchial secretions.
- Need to improve respiratory efficiency. When patients with impaired respiration are relying on their own efforts rather than assisted ventilation the performance of a tracheostomy cuts down dead space and improves respiratory efficiency by 30–50%.
- Artificial ventilation. If artificial ventilation is required for more than 72 hours a tracheostomy may be indicated, as it has been shown that endotracheal intubation for 72 hours or longer can cause laryngotracheal damage.
- Major head and neck surgery. A tracheostomy will help maintain the airway and protect it from haemorrhage during surgery (see also Ch. 30).

Box 14.9 lists some of the indications for temporary and permanent tracheostomies.

MEDICAL MANAGEMENT

Prior to performing a tracheostomy, the medical staff should explain to the patient what is involved and the effect the procedure will have. In an emergency situation, such as when the patient presents with stridor, the medical and nursing staff will have very little time to prepare the patient preoperatively. Consequently, a planned programme of support and explanation will be required afterwards.

Tracheostomy is usually carried out with the patient under a general anaesthetic but in emergencies a local anaesthetic may be used. It involves making an incision into the trachea through the third and fourth tracheal rings. An appropriately sized tracheostomy tube is then inserted. For the first 24–48 hours

Box 14.9 Indications for tracheostomy

Temporary tracheostomy
- Anaphylactic oedema
- Assisted ventilation
- Burns and scalds
- Foreign body lodged in trachea
- Major head and neck surgery
- Severe infection
- Trauma to larynx, face, mouth or oropharynx
- Vocal cord paralysis

Permanent tracheostomy
- Congenital deformity
- Trauma causing permanent damage
- Tumours
- Vocal cord paralysis

a cuffed tracheostomy tube (see Fig. 14.7) is essential to prevent blood from the wound being aspirated and aspiration pneumonia developing. A permanent tract has usually formed 2–3 days postoperatively, at which time it is possible to change the tube. Tracheal dilators must be to hand during the first few days in case the tube is expelled accidentally and it is necessary to keep the wound open.

There are several types of tracheostomy tube available, and the most appropriate one will be chosen for each patient. As mentioned above, a cuffed tube is always inserted during the operation; the cuff must be deflated regularly to prevent damage to the tracheal mucosa. For temporary tracheostomies, single-use disposable tubes are usually used. These may be cuffed or plain. They normally have an introducer which is removed immediately on insertion. Some have an inner tube which can be removed for cleaning without necessitating removal of the whole tube. For permanent tracheostomies silver tubes are often preferred. These are very expensive but can last for many years. They have an introducer, which is removed immediately on insertion, and two inner tubes. One is plain and is used at night when the patient is sleeping. The other has a small flange which allows the patient to speak by closing when air is expelled and forcing air through the vocal cords.

NURSING PRIORITIES AND MANAGEMENT OF TRACHEOSTOMY

Preoperative priorities

The physical and psychological preparation of the individual for a tracheostomy is a priority of preoperative nursing care as the procedure can present him with many difficulties. If the tracheostomy is temporary at least these problems will be of limited duration, but if it is to be permanent the patient and his family will require information and education in order to be able to cope. They may need help in coming to terms not only with the problems presented by the stoma but also with the diagnosis (e.g. cancer) which necessitated surgery. Patients who have been well prepared for a tracheostomy tend to recover better than those who have not. Unprepared patients may become insecure, withdrawn and depressed. The main problems in the immediate postoperative period for which the patient has to be prepared prior to surgery are as follows.

Loss of voice

Air will bypass the vocal cords following the tracheostomy, making speech impossible unless a tube with a speaking valve is inserted. A system of communication whereby the patient can make himself understood by staff and family members should be worked out beforehand (see p. 513).

Altered body image

Information and education must be offered to the patient to help him and his family adjust to the fact that he will have a tube in his neck. A visit from a patient who has adjusted well to having a tracheostomy may help.

Increased secretions

These are produced because of the irritation caused by the tube. This should be explained to the patient along with the need for suction; it is helpful to show the equipment required for this.

Ideally, a patient undergoing tracheostomy should be nursed in a single room initially and his care assigned to one nurse who can gain his confidence and that of his family.

Postoperative priorities

Maintenance of the airway

On his return to the ward the patient should be nursed in a sitting position with his neck well supported. Tapes round his neck and fixed to the flange of the tracheostomy tube help secure it in position. The times for deflating the cuff in the tube should be established, along with the amount of air that is to be used.

Suction should be carried out when the cuff is deflated and at any other time when secretions appear to be blocking the airway. To prevent infection it is necessary to perform this procedure with an aseptic technique (see Ch. 23, p. 710). A sterile catheter should be used each time, and should touch only the inside of the tracheostomy tube. The catheter diameter should be no more than half that of the tube. Suction should be applied only as the catheter is being removed. (Thumb-control catheters are ideal for this.) Since the patient is unable to breathe during suction it should be performed for no longer than 10–15 seconds; the patient should be allowed enough time to recover before it is repeated. The amount and type of secretions should be observed.

The physiotherapist will teach the patient how to cough into a tissue; as the patient becomes expert at this the need for suction will gradually be eliminated.

Continuous humidification is given postoperatively via a mechanical ventilator. When the patient begins to mobilise, a Buchanan bib or a gauze swab moistened with saline from a spray and held in place over the stoma will humidify inhaled air. This will also act as a filter and have a cosmetic effect by disguising the tracheostomy tube.

Care of the wound

The stoma into which the tube is inserted will require regular cleansing to prevent encrustation and infection. A dressing placed round the stoma will help prevent pressure sores caused by the tube as well as excoriation of the skin from secretions which are coughed up. Some sutures may be present; these will be removed according to local policy. (See p. 719.)

Complications

The nurse should be on the alert for the following potential complications following tracheostomy.

Blockage of tracheostomy tube

Tracheal dilators and a spare tracheostomy tube must always be kept to hand in case this problem arises. Sometimes the blockage can be relieved by suction or by changing the inner tube. At other times it will be necessary to change the whole tube.

Displacement of the tube
The tube can become displaced into the pretracheal tissue or right out of the stoma if the tapes holding it in place have not been secured correctly. Dilators should be used to keep the stoma open until the tube can be replaced.

Surgical emphysema
Emphysema is the abnormal presence of air in the tissues. Surgical emphysema is iatrogenic, being a result of faulty suturing, and can be corrected by releasing the sutures.

Haemorrhage
The insertion of a cuffed tracheostomy tube can help control bleeding and prevent aspiration of blood. It is possible, however, for a major blood vessel to be eroded by the tube, causing a massive haemorrhage.

Dysphagia, nausea, vomiting
If the tracheostomy tube is the wrong shape for the type of tracheostomy and the size of the patient it may exert pressure on the posterior wall of the trachea and oesophagus, resulting in nausea, dysphagia and vomiting. These effects can be relieved by the insertion of a different tube.

Damage to the tracheal mucosa
This can result from poor suctioning technique, badly chosen or improperly inserted tubes, or prolonged inflation of the tube cuff. Ulceration of the anterior wall or a tracheal–oesophageal fistula may result and can lead to tracheal stenosis.

Infection
A wound or respiratory tract infection can result from poor aseptic technique when performing stoma toilet, changing the tube or applying suction, or from inadequate maintenance of respiratory status.

Preparation for discharge

Before discharge can take place the patient and his family must be well prepared for all foreseeable difficulties and should be proficient in changing tubes. The teaching of self-care techniques can begin with the nurse demonstrating procedures while the patient watches in a mirror. It is wise to teach not only the patient but also his family how to care for the tracheostomy in case the occasion arises when the patient is unable to do this himself. However, some surgeons do prefer their patients to report to the ward or outpatients' department for a weekly tube change.

The community nurse will be actively involved in the patient's discharge and reintegration into the community. Ideally she will visit him in hospital and arrange for suction apparatus to be installed in his home if necessary. After discharge she should visit him regularly to ensure that he is coping with his stoma and altered body image (see Ch. 27, p. 803 and Serra (1986), Ch. 26).

Changing the tracheostomy tube

The first tube change should be performed by experienced nursing or medical staff, as it takes 5–7 days for a tract to form and there is a danger of the tube being displaced or inserted into the pretracheal tissues. Two people should be present for this procedure. One will remove the old tube and the other immediately insert the new one. The tapes are then securely tied.

Decannulation or removal of the tube

Occasionally the tube can be removed without any preliminaries but usually the patient is gradually reintroduced to breathing through his nose and mouth. A tube with a speaking valve allows the patient to breathe in through the tube and out through his larynx. Once the patient has become accustomed to this, the tube can be replaced by a 'blocker' so that he has to breathe in through his nose and mouth. When he is able to tolerate this for 24 hours the tracheostomy tube can be removed. Another method is to insert a smaller tube each time it is changed.

Whichever method is used, after removal of the tube an airtight dressing should be applied to ensure that the patient breathes through his nose and mouth. This can be a very anxious time for patients and support and encouragement are necessary. The stoma should shrink rapidly and close off in a short time.

Humidification

Humidification will prevent the tracheostomy patient breathing in cold dry air which could cause the secretions of the trachea to become dry and difficult to remove and eventually lead to infection and blockage of the tube.

Tonsillitis

The tonsils are composed of lymphoid tissue and lie between the faucial pillars (see Fig. 14.8). During early childhood they enlarge in response to upper respiratory tract infections and in adulthood should become reduced in size. In old age they normally atrophy. It is generally agreed that tonsils have a role to play in the body's defence system against infection.

Each year an average of 12 000 people in the UK undergo the surgical procedure of tonsillectomy. The majority of these patients are 14 years of age or younger. Among people aged 15–25 more females seem to require this surgery than males. Among the elderly population the tonsils are usually removed as a treatment for tumorous growths.

Common presenting symptoms. Patients usually present with a history of pain. This may be due to the many lesions caused by infection or to the presence of a tumour. Tonsil pain increases with swallowing and is often referred to the ear because of the involvement of the trigeminal nerve, which supplies both sites.

Recurrent bouts of infection are the most common reason for the removal of tonsils. Infection may take the form of acute tonsillitis, acute otitis media (see p. 502) or a peritonsillar abscess (see p. 518). Streptococci, staphylococci, and Haemophilus influenzae are the organisms most commonly present.

Patients with tonsillar tumours normally present with difficulty in swallowing food. These patients usually also com-

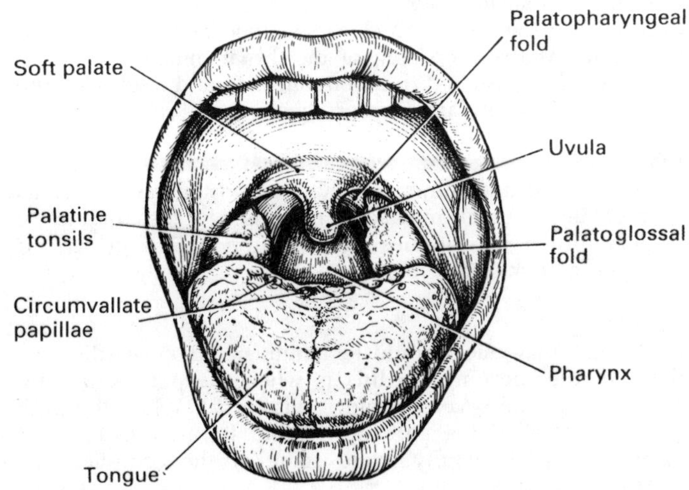

Fig. 14.8 Tonsils and surrounding area.

plain of weight loss and may have speech problems. They may also suffer from facial pain and deafness because of the involvement of cranial nerves. Tonsillar tumours are rare (Turner 1988).

Tonsillectomy

MEDICAL MANAGEMENT

There is some controversy among medical practitioners about when tonsil infections should be treated conservatively and when tonsillectomy, with or without adenoidectomy, should be performed. Each surgeon has his own criteria for the removal of a patient's tonsils. The size of the tonsils is not usually one of the main criteria, but rather the history of the effect of repeated infections on the general health of the patient. Consideration is also given to loss of appetite, speech defects, nasal catarrh or colds, hearing loss, breathing problems and abdominal pains (a sign of mesenteric adenitis which occurs because of transmission of infection through the lymphatic system; see Turner (1988)). Tonsillectomy is an elective operation and is not considered in the presence of respiratory tract infections or during the incubation period after contact with an infectious disease or if there is tonsillar inflammation.

There are two methods of carrying out the operation. The guillotine method is the more traditional but is very rarely performed nowadays as it has potential complications such as mesenteric adonitis. The current method of choice for children and adults is usually that of tonsil dissection. In this method bleeding vessels are ligated or diathermy is applied, whereas in the guillotine method the vessels are left to seal themselves by contraction.

NURSING PRIORITIES AND MANAGEMENT OF TONSILLECTOMY

Postoperative priorities

Airway

On returning from theatre, patients should be positioned in the posttonsillectomy position, that is, semi prone (McKenzie et al 1986). This allows any blood or saliva to flow out of the mouth and helps keep the airway clear.

Haemorrhage

Half-hourly recordings of pulse and blood pressure and observations of breathing and for frequent swallowing are carried out to permit early diagnosis of haemorrhage. Frequent swallowing is one of the first signs of tonsil haemorrhage and can go unnoticed unless the patient is closely observed.

Chewing and swallowing

Encouraging the patient to chew soft food and to swallow is important, as the exercising of the throat muscles seems to help keep the tonsil bed free from infection and to prevent the occurrence of secondary haemorrhage.

Infection

Pyrexia is not uncommon on the first postoperative day as part of the general metabolic response to the trauma of surgery, but if it continues antibiotics should be prescribed to avoid the risk of infection.

Analgesia

Prescribed analgesics should be administered, especially first thing in the morning, as this is when the patient usually complains of the severest pain in his throat. When the pain is well controlled the patient will find it easier to eat and drink and so hopefully avoid some of the complications which could arise.

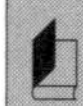

For details on the care of small children undergoing tonsillectomy see Sacharin (1986).

Preparation for discharge

Patients are discharged from hospital fairly rapidly following tonsillectomy and require a period of convalescence at home. An explanation of the expected progress of this recovery period is important. Tiredness for 7–10 days is normal. Sometimes patients experience severe ear pain on the 3rd or 4th postoperative day. Analgesics should relieve this. Slight neck pain may also be experienced. Ideally a leaflet which the patient can take home and refer to is provided. The telephone number where ENT unit or community staff can be reached should questions or worries arise should be included.

Peritonsillar abscesses (quinsy)

PATHOPHYSIOLOGY

This is a very painful condition and can be life threatening. It usually occurs as a complication of acute tonsillitis. Pus forms in the space behind the capsule of the tonsil. The abscess is usually unilateral and affects males more than females.

The patient presents with a pyrexia high enough to cause a shivering attack or rigor. There is usually a history of an episode of acute tonsillitis which has subsided only to return on one side. There is acute pain radiating to the ear on the affected side and swallowing is so difficult that saliva dribbles out of the mouth. The voice becomes muffled because of the large swelling and affected function of the palate. The neck glands on the affected side will be enlarged and tender.

MEDICAL MANAGEMENT

Antibiotic cover should be prescribed and the abscess incised and drained. Sometimes it may be necessary to administer intravenous fluids and to give the antibiotics parenterally. Analgesia will be required when the pain is severe. Occasionally the swelling will be so severe that it will obstruct the airway; it may then be necessary to perform a tracheostomy to allow the patient to breathe.

NURSING PRIORITIES AND MANAGEMENT OF PERITONSILLAR ABSCESS

Nursing care of the patient with peritonsillar abscess will include:

- physical and psychological support of the patient
- administration of analgesics
- administration of antibiotics
- administration of intravenous fluids if prescribed
- ensuring good oral hygiene
- observation and recording of patient's temperature, pulse, blood pressure, fluid intake and output
- care of the tracheostomy if the patient has required this (see p. 516).

Patients who require admission to hospital will be very anxious, agitated and in pain. They will require explanations, reassurance and swift administration of analgesics. As many will be unable to swallow, nursing staff should observe for signs of dehydration and administer intravenous fluids as prescribed by medical staff.

Good oral hygiene is important, especially once the abscess has been drained, as the patient will have had to spit out pus and will have a foul taste in his mouth. Once the pain has been relieved by analgesics and drainage of the abscess, the patient will be able to commence oral fluids and to gradually begin taking solids. As an effect of the analgesics, poor oral intake and bedrest the patient may become constipated; the nursing staff should be alert for this and offer appropriate remedies and advice.

The patient is usually discharged once he is able to eat and drink normally and has been apyrexial for 24 hours. If the abscess has been severe enough to require a tracheostomy this would be sutured and the patient would be discharged only when it had healed. Patients are often sent home before they have finished their course of antibiotics; the importance of completing the course must therefore be clearly explained to them. In 6–8 weeks most patients are admitted to have a tonsillectomy performed as peritonsillar abscesses have a habit of recurring.

CONCLUSION

The specialty of ENT care is a constantly evolving one that presents many challenges to the nurse. She will encounter patients of various ages and backgrounds who will have specific needs with respect to the intensity, duration and setting of treatment. The ENT nurse is likely to encounter a wide range of disorders, some of which will have profound implications for the patient's ability to function within his family, work, and social spheres and which will require thorough assessment and individualised care planning. As always, the nurse's ability as communicator will do much to determine the effectiveness of her interventions; in this specialty, in which many patients will suffer from disorders that will impair hearing and/or the ability to speak, the need for skill and inventiveness in communication is especially apparent.

Nurses in various fields can make an important contribution to health education and preventive care as it relates to potential ENT disorders. By helping to implement programmes for MMR vaccination, community and school nurses help to prevent the hearing impairment often seen in children whose mothers contract rubella during the early months of their pregnancy. A knowledge of how to evaluate noise levels can help occupational health nurses to protect workers from noise-induced hearing loss, and school nurses can alert young people to the fact that personal stereos are capable of producing the same volume of sound as a pneumatic drill, and thus present a serious risk of hearing impairment. For patients with a chronic condition such as Menière's disease or tinnitus, hospital and community nurses can provide ongoing psychological support, practical advice on day-to-day coping and information about local support groups. As the causes of certain ENT disorders become better understood, and as pharmacological and surgical treatments make further strides forward, ENT nursing will continue to offer challenges and rewards for nurses in a variety of care settings.

GLOSSARY

Antihistamine labrynthine sedatives. Sedatives that have an anti-inflammatory action and also reduce the levels of dizziness and nausea.

Antroscopy. Endoscopic examination of the maxillary sinuses.

Attico antral disease. Bone erosion of the middle ear, caused by chronic infection.

Auriscope. An instrument which incorporates magnification and illumination, and can be used for examining the ear.

Buchanan laryngectomy bib/protector. A covering for the stoma of a laryngectomy.

Haemorrhagic telangiectasia. A group of leaking dilated capillaries, often obvious on the surface of the skin.

Mesenteric adenitis. Inflammation of the lymph glands in the membranous support of the intestines: the mesentery. This condition must be ruled out when diagnosing appendicitis.

MMR vaccination. Measles, mumps and rubella vaccination.

Nystagmus. Rapid and involuntary movements of the eyes which may be vertical, horizontal or rotatory. The condition may be congenital and associated with poor sight or may occur due to disorders in the part of the brain responsible for movements and co-ordination. Vestibular nystagmus results when there is labyrinthine damage in the ear. Optokinetic nystagmus can occur in health when an individual tries to look at a succession of objects moving quickly across the field of vision..

Roger's crystal spray. A glass atomiser with saline to spray at the tracheostomy stoma or bib protector, in order to moisten it.

REFERENCES

Ames S W, Kneisl C R 1988 Essentials of adult health nursing. Addison-Wesley, Menlo Park, CA

Cluroe S 1989 Congenital oesophageal abnormalities. Nursing 3(35)

Denyer S 1990 Foreign bodies: where do children put them? Health Visitor 63 : 5

Haggard M, Gatehouse S, Davies A 1981 The prevalence of hearing disorders and its implications for services in the United Kingdom. British Journal of Audiology 15: 241–251

Hayward S 1975 Information: a prescription against pain. RCN, London

Jamieson E M, McCall J M, Blythe R 1992 Guidelines for clinical nursing practices. Churchill Livingstone, Edinburgh, pp 45, 50, 60, 142

McKenzie G, Chawla H, Gordon D 1986 The special senses, 2nd edn. Churchill Livingstone, Edinburgh, pp 7–8, 41–47, 52–68, 72–100

National Deaf Children's Society 1992 Communication is your responsibility. Commission of Inquiry into Human Aids in Communication. (Obtainable through C. Shaw, Panel of Four, 48 Gallows Hill Lane, Abbott's Complex, Herts, England WD5 OBY.)

Sacharin R M 1986 Principles of paediatric nursing, 2nd edn. Churchill Livingstone, Edinburgh

Serra A, Bailey C, Jackson P 1986 Ear, nose and throat nursing. Blackwell Scientific, Oxford, pp 41–47, 52–68, 72–100

Thurston-Hookway F, Seddon S 1989 Care after laryngectomy. Nursing 3(35) : 5–10

Turner A L 1988 Diseases of the nose, throat and ear, 10th edn. Birrell Wright, Bristol, pp 219–331, 409–432, 3–51, 363–372, 129–160, 381–396

Wilson K J W 1990 Ross & Wilson anatomy and physiology in health and illness, 7th edn. Churchill Livingstone, Edinburgh

FURTHER READING

Ames S W, Kneisl C R 1988 Essentials of adult health nursing. Addison-Wesley, Menlo Park, CA

Ashley J 1973 Journey into silence. Boxey Head

Chilman A, Thomas M 1987 Understanding nursing care, Churchill Livingstone, Edinburgh

Gibson I 1983 Tracheostomy management. Nursing 2(18)

Gould D 1989 Opportunities in ENT Nursing. Nursing 3(35)
Harries M 1983 Epistaxis in the elderly. Nursing 2(18)
Klein D 1983 Hearing impairment in children. Nursing 2(18)
Knowles M 1983 Infections of the ear, nose and throat. Nursing 2(18)
Levene B 1983 Hearing loss: the invisible disability. Nursing 2(18)
Ludman H 1988 ABC of ear, nose and throat. BMA, London
Lyall J 1989 Extrasensory aid. Nursing Times 85(50)
McKenzie G, Chawla H, Gordon D 1986 The special senses, 2nd edn. Churchill Livingstone, Edinburgh
Newman D 1990 Assessment of hearing loss in elderly people. Journal of Advanced Nursing 15: 400–409
Newton J 1989 Deaf, but not disabled. Nursing Times 85(47)
Rougheen M 1983 Ear syringing. Nursing 2(18)
Scott-Stevenson R, Guthrie D 1949 A history of oto-laryngology. Churchill Livingstone, Edinburgh
Serra A 1983 Lasers in ENT. Nursing 2(18)
Stokes D, Jones A 1983 Laryngectomy: nursing care and a patient's view. Nursing 2(18)
Surkitt-Parr D 1989 The removal of foreign bodies. Nursing 3(35)
Turner A L 1988 in Maran A G (ed) Diseases of the nose, throat and ear, 10th edn. J Wright, Bristol
Verney A 1989 The patient with hearing impairment. Nursing 3(35)

USEFUL ADDRESSES

British Association of the Hard of Hearing
7-11 Armstrong Road
London W3 7JL

British Deaf Association
38 Victoria Place
Carlisle

Royal National Institute for the Deaf
103 Gower Street
London WC1E 6AH

National Deaf Children's Society
31 Gloucester Place
London W1H 4EA

Scottish Association for the Deaf
158 West Regent St
Glasgow G2

National Association Laryngectomy Clubs
38–39 Eccleston Square
London SW1V 1PB

Association of Teachers of Lip-reading for Adults (ATLA)
70 Fernway
Kingswood
Watford
Herts WD2 6HQ

CHAPTER 15

Disorders of the mouth

Rosemary Kelly

CHAPTER CONTENTS

Introduction 521

Anatomy and pathophysiology 521

DISORDERS OF THE MOUTH 523

Congenital deformities of the mouth 523
Nursing priorities and management 524

Orodental disease 525
Nursing priorities and management 526

Infections and inflammatory conditions of the mouth 529
Nursing priorities and management 531

Orofacial trauma 531
Nursing priorities and management 533

Tumours of the mouth 536
Nursing priorities and management 538

References 541

Further reading 542

INTRODUCTION

The mouth is central to many activities of daily living which we often take for granted until some minor but painful problem such as toothache or an aphthous ulcer reminds us of the importance of the condition of the mouth not only to specific functions but also to our general feeling of well-being. The mouth is the source of the infant's first pleasurable activity (the sucking reflex being present at birth) and perhaps, during teething, of his first experience of *dis*-ease. For individuals approaching the end of life, or for anyone who is acutely ill, good mouth care can give much comfort and relief and help to preserve dignity.

The condition of the mouth has long been recognised as an indicator of health or illness. Because of the mouth's close relationship to other systems, structures and organs, oral symptoms may be a manifestation (sometimes the first) of generalised systemic disease, or of disease in adjacent areas.

The immediate visibility of the mouth gives any related dysfunction a particular significance for the individual. Disfigurement arising from any cause, whether congenital, traumatic or acquired, is not only a visible cosmetic defect but also a visible *functional* disability that can give rise to many difficulties affecting the person's perception of himself and his quality of life.

?	**15.1** From your own experience, how many activities of daily living (see Roper et al 1990) are affected, and in what ways, after a dental procedure (e.g. a filling or extraction requiring local anaesthesia)? Now consider how much worse it would be for a patient if any of these activities were affected in the long term or even permanently.

ANATOMY AND PATHOPHYSIOLOGY

The mouth or oral cavity is designed as a workshop, where much activity associated with chewing (mastication), drinking and speaking takes place (see Fig. 15.1).

- Entrance is between the *lips* (red, muscular and sensitive) through the *vestibule*, a small space immediately before the inner entrance which consists of *gums (gingivae)* covering *alveolar ridges* of maxillae and mandible, into which are set *teeth*.
- The opening (parotid duct) from the *parotid gland*, one of the salivary glands, is into the vestibule.
- The roof of the mouth is formed by bony *hard palate (maxilla)* and muscular *soft palate*.
- Lateral walls are formed by the muscles of the *cheeks*.
- The *floor of the mouth* is almost entirely filled by the muscular *tongue*,

1(A) Oral stage: preparatory phase
(Time taken varies.)

Lips open; saliva is stimulated
Liquid or portion of food is taken
↓
Solid material is broken down by teeth, moistened by saliva
↓
Strenous movements of jaw and cheek muscles and mobile tongue against the hard palate, teeth and alveolar ridges form food into bolus
↓
Tongue tip gathers stray food particles from between lips and teeth and from the floor of the mouth and incorporates them into bolus
↓
The lips must be closed. The soft palate is lowered and bolus or liquid is propelled backwards by strong humping movements and funnelling of the tongue

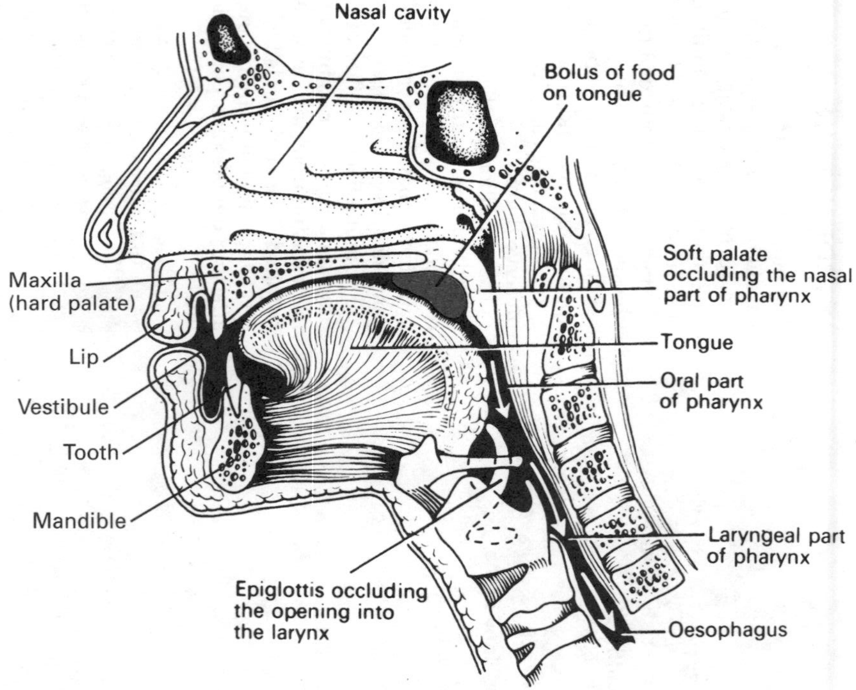

Fig. 15.1 The importance of oral competence to the process of feeding, chewing and swallowing.

1(B) Oral stage: executive phase
(Time taken should not exceed 1 second.)

The bolus of food on the tongue is propelled towards the oropharynx. The soft palate rises to close the nasopharynx and so prevent nasal regurgitation
↓
The bolus must contact pillars of fauces and the posterior oropharyngeal wall to trigger the swallow 'reflex' and initiate:
↓
2 The pharyngeal stage
(Normally lasts 0.75 seconds.)
↓
The bolus passes the laryngeal part of the pharynx, through the open cricopharyngeal sphincter, and so to:
↓
3 The oesophageal stage
(2 seconds.)

which is very mobile and sensitive. Tiny projections on it called *papillae* contain nerve endings of taste.
- There are also openings from two pairs of *salivary glands: submandibular and sublingual.*
- The rear exit to the *oropharynx* is under the border of the soft palate, through two archways, (palatoglossal and palatopharyngeal), which enclose the palatine tonsil.
- The entire oral cavity is lined with mucous membrane, much of which is *stratified epithelium* to cope with 'wear and tear'.

The mouth is situated close to many other structures, and disease or injury of the mouth may also affect, for example, eye, ear, nose, maxillary sinuses, pharynx, larynx and neck. The face and neck are richly supplied with arteries, veins, nerves, muscles, lymph vessels and nodes, and knowledge of all these is important to understanding the effects of trauma or disease arising in, or affecting the mouth.

See Wilson (1990) and, for a more detailed account, see Johnson & Moore (1989).

Functions of the mouth

The stages of normal swallowing

Only in the mouth is there normally any control over the mechanics of digestion. The first, or *oral*, stage must be accomplished (see Fig. 15.1) so that the swallowing reflex is triggered when the bolus reaches the posterior pharyngeal wall, and the second or *pharyngeal*, stage then commences. During this, and the third, or *oesophageal*, stage, swallowing is involuntary.

A deficiency in the mouth may cause difficulty in the later stages of the swallowing mechanism.

Several cranial nerves (CN) are involved in the acts of swallowing and voice production (see Table 15.1 and Wilson 1990 pp. 264–267).

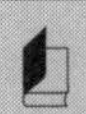
Normal swallowing is discussed in detail by Langley (1989).

A means of communication

The lips, tongue, hard and soft palate and teeth, together with throat and facial muscles, all manipulate sound to give quality and resonance to speech. The mouth also contributes to other expressions of emotion, for example, smiling, laughing, whistling and kissing. Thus any disturbance to the norm caused by trauma, cerebrovascular accident or surgery can cause diminution or failure of these very basic functions, and so reduce quality of life. Understanding some of the changes that may occur will help the nurse to assist the patient's recovery. (Refer to the sections on 'Orofacial Trauma', p. 531, and 'Tumours', p. 536, in this chapter, and to Ch. 2.)

Table 15.1 Cranial nerves involved in stages of swallowing. Damage to any of these nerves may affect the ability to eat (Adapted from Wilson 1990 and Langley 1989)

Nerve	Type	Function
CN I	Olfactory	Sense of smell
CN V	Trigeminal	Sensory to gums, cheek, lower jaw, and muscles of mastication; motor to muscles of mastication
CN VII	Facial	Taste from anterior 2/3 of the tongue; motor to muscles of face
CN IX	Glossopharyngeal	Secretion of saliva; sensory to posterior 1/3 tongue, soft palate, pillars of fauces and pharynx; taste from posterior tongue; motor to pharynx
CN X	Vagus	Sensory to larynx; motor to palate, pharynx, larynx
CN XI	Accessory	Motor to laryngeal and pharyngeal muscles, and muscles of head control
CN XII	Hypoglossal	Motor to muscles of tongue

Saliva

This is formed by a combination of secretions from the *parotid, submandibular and sublingual glands* and from mucous membrane. It keeps the mouth moist, and without it, oral functions are very difficult. *Salivary amylase* is the enzyme that assists with digestion of food.

Teeth

Teeth are important structures for biting and chewing food. Children have 20 temporary or deciduous teeth, which are gradually replaced by 32 permanent teeth between the ages of about 6 and 24 years. Time of eruption can be a measure of developmental age.

Overcrowding of teeth may necessitate extraction of third molars (wisdom teeth) during young adulthood. However, later *impaction of wisdom teeth* may result because fewer molars are now extracted.

The importance of good orodental health throughout life is discussed later in the chapter.

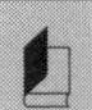
For greater detail see Wilson (1990).

Bones of the face

See Figure 15.2 and Wilson (1990), pages 355–360. Many of these bones are complex and fragile and as a result, trauma to the mouth may result in a complicated injury. Refer to the section on 'Orofacial trauma', p. 531.

DISORDERS OF THE MOUTH

Disorders of the mouth can be broadly classified into five categories:

- congenital disorders
- orodental disease
- infections and inflammatory conditions (localised or systemic)
- traumatic injury
- tumours.

Each of these categories will be considered in turn in the following sections.

CONGENITAL DEFORMITIES OF THE MOUTH

Deformities involving the mouth may require a long series of corrective procedures and may present the individual with physical, social and emotional problems in childhood, young adulthood and maturity. The most commonly occurring congenital malformations of the mouth are cleft lip and cleft palate, which together have an incidence of approximately 1 in 600 live births. Of this number roughly one third are cleft lip, one third cleft palate, and the remaining third cleft lip and palate. Other deformities of the face and mouth are comparatively rare, but can be devastating for the child and his parents. These conditions can be congenital or acquired (e.g. due to trauma or to a growth anomaly) and may be unilateral or bilateral.

Problems associated with cleft lip/palate and other deformities of the mouth may concern the following:

Fig. 15.2 The bones of the face.

- appearance
- dentition/occlusion
- eating and drinking
- speech
- hearing
- mid-face growth
- psychosocial adjustment.

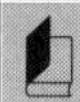

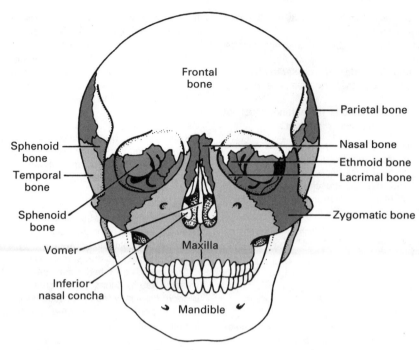

See Henderson (1985) for information on rarer deformities of the mouth and face.

PATHOPHYSIOLOGY

Cleft lip results from failure of the embryonic maxillary prominence to fuse with the intermaxillary segment and occurs 6–7 weeks after conception. Cleft lip may be unilateral or bilateral, and can vary in degree from a slight notch to a complete division of the lip and the alveolar process (gum).

Cleft palate is caused by a failure of the palatine processes to fuse with each other and with the nasal septum or with the primary palate. This occurs 7–12 weeks after conception (Roberts 1984). As a result of this failure of fusion, the soft palate is unable to meet the posterior pharyngeal wall and thus to close off the nasopharynx. Because of this, the individual's speech is affected, producing a typically 'nasal' delivery in which certain consonants, particularly C, D, K, P, S and T, cannot be properly enunciated.

MEDICAL MANAGEMENT

The medical management of cleft lip/palate requires a multidisciplinary approach extending from infancy to adulthood. Treatment protocol will depend on the extent of the deformity and on the age of the child (see Table 15.2).

Orthognathic surgery (i.e. surgery to correct major facial deformities) is an important and developing area of maxillofacial work and is carried out in only a few units in the UK. It requires a team approach involving neuro-, maxillofacial, plastic and ophthalmic surgeons, and assessment and correction takes place over many years.

NURSING PRIORITIES AND MANAGEMENT: CONGENITAL DEFORMITIES OF THE MOUTH

Nursing considerations

Referral. A parent's discovery that his or her newborn child has a facial deformity may be very traumatic, and the provision of sensitive and supportive counselling should not be delayed. Parents should be referred within a few days of their child's birth to the relevant specialist professionals (e.g. orofacial consultant, orthodontist, speech therapist, specialist nurse) and should be given information on their local branch of the Cleft Lip and Palate Association (CLAPA) (see 'Useful Addresses') or other appropriate self-help group. Professional psychological support may also be required.

Table 15.2 Treatment of cleft lip and palate

Procedure	Timing/patient's age
Lip repair	0–6 months
Palate repair	4–24 months
Bone graft to alveolus	9–11 years
Osteotomy (for correction of defect of hard palate) Rhinoplasty (for nasal defect)	Around 18 years
Pharyngoplasty (to correct the pharynx) Myringotomy revision procedures	As and when necessary
Orthodontic treatment Speech therapy	Throughout childhood and into adulthood if necessary

Oral hygiene. Good oral hygiene will be of great importance for individuals with deformities of the mouth, and the preservation of dentition will contribute greatly to the individual's well-being. Nurses should stress the importance of good dental hygiene to parents who may mistakenly feel that compared to gross abnormality the loss of a few teeth due to dental caries is inconsequential.

Pre- and postoperative nursing care of patients undergoing major corrective surgery will take into account the general considerations discussed in Chapter 27, incorporating the specialised skills and techniques demanded by each procedure.

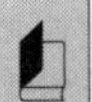

See Kemble & Lamb (1984) for the nursing care of cleft lip/palate.

ORODENTAL DISEASE

Dental and periodontal disease affects about 95% of the population of the United Kingdom in varying degrees, and accounts for the largest proportion of disorders of the mouth. Because most of this disease is preventable, this discussion of orodental disease will begin with a consideration of dental health, first with respect to recent trends, and then with regard to the promotion of orodental care.

Changing patterns of dental health

Since the early 1970s there has been a substantial improvement in dental health in the UK. More people are retaining their natural teeth into later life, and there has been a marked decrease in dental caries in children (Downer 1991).

The incidence of dental caries can be measured in terms of the number of decayed, missing and filled deciduous teeth (dmft) and/or permanent teeth (DMFT) that individuals in a population have. Another measurement is the percentage who are free from signs of caries (dmft or DMFT = 0). The World Health Organization (WHO 1988) has as its goal for the year 2000 that 50% of 5–6-year-olds will be free from caries, and that 50% of 12-year-olds will have a DMFT no greater than 3. National surveys have shown that dental caries in England and Wales fell by 50% in 5-year-olds, by 40% in 12-year-olds and by one third in 15-year-olds between 1973 and 1983. The decrease was such that the WHO goal had almost been achieved, the average DMFT for 12-year-olds being 2.9. However, there are national and regional variations. For example, in 1983 the mean DMFT for the UK as a whole was 3.1, for Scotland 4.5, and for Northern Ireland 4.8 (Downer 1991).

? **15.2** Consider why these regional variations might exist.

? **15.3** Consider also that those children who were 12 years old in 1983 are now adults. Discuss whether their approach to dental health is likely to have changed.

Promoting dental health

Nurses in all spheres of practice can help to identify orodental problems early and to minimise some of their distressing consequences (see Box 15.1). It is therefore important for nurses to undertand the factors which contribute to the maintenance of good orodental health from childhood to maturity.

Factors which affect dental health

Access to dental care. For many children the dental surgery is the first remembered clinical setting for health care. It is important for these first visits to be reasonably pleasant in order to foster a positive attitude toward regular dental checkups. Any subsequent, serious disease can then be diagnosed early and the chance of a complete cure greatly increased.

Early access to orthodontic services, particularly for those with congenital abnormalities, will also help to minimise problems in later life.

Education. Orodental disease in otherwise healthy people is caused largely by poor oral hygiene, and its incidence can be significantly reduced by the early and continued promotion of good dental hygiene and healthy eating habits. Nurses in many areas of practice can make an important contribution in providing education on the prevention of tooth decay.

Diet. The Committee on Medical Aspects of Food Policy (COMA) advocates educating the public to reduce sugar consumption as a means of preventing tooth decay (DOH 1989). Not all sugars are equally cariogenic. Sucrose appears to be the most conducive to the development of caries, followed closely by glucose, fructose and maltose. Lactose and galactose are substantially less cariogenic (DOH 1989). COMA stresses the importance of educating the consumer to be aware of 'hidden' sugars in products such as baked beans and tinned fruits, and to recognise various substances listed in food labels as sugars. Some supermarket chains produce information leaflets on interpreting food labels.

? **15.4** Examine the contents labels of the prepared foods you normally buy. Do any of these products contain more sugar than you had realised?

Oral hygiene. Parents should introduce a routine for dental hygiene as soon as their child's first teeth appear, using a soft toothbrush designed for babies. Most children will require supervision until they are 7 or 8 years old.

The teeth should be brushed last thing at night and, ideally, after every meal. The toothbrush should be held at an angle

Box 15.1 Contribution of nurses to orodental health

Health visitors
Encourage oral hygiene in childhood and visits to dentist and orthodontist. This is a primary preventive function of the health visitor

School nurses
Demonstrate dental hygiene; alert parents to need for children's visits to dentist

Occupational health nurses and practice nurses
Educate on adverse effects of smoking and excessive alcohol; raise awareness of symptoms of intraoral cancer; advise on good handwashing practices

District nurses
Identify potential problems in elderly people; advise on continued dental examination

Nurses caring for elderly people
As above; increase mouth comfort and self-esteem

Mental handicap nurses
Supervise early and continued dental care and thus minimise need for restorative dentistry

Midwives
Give dental care advice in pregnancy

All nurses
Encourage and/or assist with oral hygiene for patients' comfort and health; have dental/oral health literature available

of 45° and the teeth brushed horizontally to avoid damage to the gums. All exposed surfaces of the teeth should be cleaned and the mouth rinsed well in the course of brushing and afterwards.

Toothbrushes should be renewed regularly, but hard brushes should be avoided as they can damage tooth enamel and gums.

Toothpaste with added fluoride is recommended by many dentists. Toothpaste with sugar added to improve flavour should be avoided. Sensitivity to certain toothpaste ingredients (e.g. cinnamonaldehyde) has been noted. Oral lesions caused by sensitivity resolve spontaneously when use of the toothpaste in question is discontinued (Lamey et al 1989).

Dental floss with or without added fluoride may be used to clean between the teeth and up to the gum line. Overzealous use can damage the gums. For this reason, floss is best not used by children. Care should also be taken in the use of toothpicks to avoid damaging the gums.

Disclosing tablets can be useful in educational programmes to demonstrate how much brushing is required to remove plaque. Following cleaning of the teeth, the tablet is chewed, producing a stain on any teeth which are still covered with plaque. Correct brushing should remove the staining from the teeth (although it may remain on the tongue for some time).

Common misconceptions. Chewing gum after meals to increase saliva is of limited value in reducing decay. To be of any benefit, sugar-free gum must be chewed for 20 minutes and backed up by other forms of dental care.

Chewing an apple after a meal does not clean the teeth. Rather, it leaves an acidic deposit which predisposes the teeth to the development of plaque.

?	**15.5** How good an example do you set in the practice of oral hygiene?

Fluoride is a naturally occurring substance which is present in some areas in the water supply. It is taken up by growing teeth and makes the enamel harder and more resistant to the development of caries. Incidence of caries has been shown to be lower in areas with higher levels of fluoride (Carmichael et al 1989). Fluoride can be added to the water supply in areas where the natural level is low, although the moral and legal issues raised by this practice are still unresolved.

Fluoride supplements can be given to children from the age of 6 months. Dentists, chemists and health visitors should be able to advise on the correct amount required in view of the fluoride levels in local drinking water.

Dental and periodontal disease

PATHOPHYSIOLOGY

Plaque is a firmly adherent, non-calcified deposit of bacteria, mucus, food particles and cellular debris which accumulates on the surface of a tooth, particularly at the base. It forms rapidly in the absence of good oral hygiene and reacts with sugar to form an acid which can attack and erode tooth enamel, leading, if unchecked, to gum disease and dental caries.

Calculus is hard mineralised plaque which requires removal by a dental surgeon or dental hygienist.

Caries is a progressive and localised decay of the teeth caused by bacterial action. It is characterised by demineralisation of the inorganic portion and destruction of the organic substance of the tooth.

Gingivitis (inflammation of the gums). Normal gums are pink (e.g. in Caucasians) or brown (e.g. in Asian or African people) and are firm. In gingivitis, the gums are purple-red, soft and puffy, tender, and may bleed easily. Regular oral hygiene and dental care reduces this reversible stage of gum disease.

Untreated, gingivitis can lead to gum recession and the formation of pockets around the base of teeth, in which plaque and calculus can collect. Further infection from bacteria in plaque may lead to periodontitis.

Periodontitis is characterised by the gradual loss of the supporting membrane of the teeth, erosion of the supporting bone, and subsequent loosening of the teeth.

Acute ulcerative gingivitis is an uncommon condition caused by the abnormal growth of bacteria. Poor oral hygiene, smoking, throat infections and stress can contribute. This condition is also seen in HIV infection. The gums are sore and bleed easily and ulcers develop which may spread more deeply. A characteristic foul smell is associated with this condition. Cervical or neck lymph glands may be enlarged.

Common presenting symptoms. The patient commonly presents to his general medical practitioner (GMP) or general dental practitioner (GDP) with a combination of symptoms which may include toothache, bleeding gums and emission of pus from the gums (pyorrhoea). If oral hygiene has habitually been poor, the patient is more likely to wait until the pain is severe before presenting. Many people fear going to the dentist and delay for as long as possible.

MEDICAL MANAGEMENT

Investigations include X-rays, sialograms (see Appendix 1) and relevant blood tests.

Dental surgery or outpatient procedures. Most orodental problems are treated in dental surgeries (National Health Service or private practice). Treatments such as extractions, fillings, root treatment for dental abscess and restorative work such as fitting crowns and dentures are carried out with the patient under a local anaesthetic administered by the dentist. Some procedures necessitate general anaesthesia, which is administered by an anaesthetist. Treatment of gingivitis is with mouthwashes and metronidazole or penicillin. Scaling is carried out when swelling has subsided.

Inpatient procedures. Procedures which can be classed as minor oral surgery but generally require admission to hospital include:

- removal of impacted wisdom teeth
- removal of dental cysts
- removal of salivary glands or ducts
- apicectomy (excision of apex of tooth root)
- preprosthetic surgery
- placement of implants.

Patients may be referred to a dental hospital/school or to an oral/maxillofacial unit.

Patients with certain conditions or who are taking certain types of drugs will require hospital admission and special monitoring as follows:

- diabetes mellitus: insulin dosage must be monitored. There is a risk of delayed healing
- heart valve disease: monitoring is very important as infection can lead to bacterial endocarditis (see Ch. 2, p. 41)
- steroid drugs: must be monitored. Healing may be delayed
- anticoagulants: must be monitored. The patient has an increased risk of haemorrhage.

NURSING PRIORITIES AND MANAGEMENT: ORODENTAL DISEASE

Nursing considerations

Outpatient care. Individuals treated in dental surgeries or as hospital outpatients will require reassurance and advice on after-care at home. The nurse should make available information such as that presented in Box 15.2 and ensure that the patient understands and can carry out instructions for self-care and knows where to call for advice should problems arise.

Inpatient care. Admission is usually on the day preceding surgery and discharge on the day after. The patient's stay may be longer, however, if any of the special considerations listed above apply.

The preparation of patients for anaesthesia is described in Chapter 27. Nurses should endeavour to ascertain and relieve any anxieties the patient might have about being in hospital and facing surgery.

Postoperatively, the patient may experience considerable pain, swelling and bruising. Nursing Care Plan 15.1 gives an example of the care that would be required following a wisdom tooth extraction.

On discharge, the patient should be given clear, adequate information on self-care and a number to call should further advice be needed.

Box 15.2 INFORMATION FOR PATIENTS HAVING MINOR ORAL SURGERY

Following surgery to your mouth, you can expect some swelling and discomfort. This may last for some days. The following information will help you in the postoperative period.

ON THE DAY OF TREATMENT

1. Rest for a few hours. You do not necessarily have to lie down, however.
2. Avoid strenuous exercise for 24 hours.
3. Avoid rinsing your mouth for 24 hours, even if your mouth tastes unpleasant. Rinsing may disturb any blood clots and start up bleeding.
4. Your lips and/or tongue may be numb. Be careful not to inadvertently bite or burn them.
5. Avoid hot fluids, alcohol, hard foods and cigarettes.
6. Pain or soreness can be relieved with a mild painkiller, e.g. Co-codamol or paracetamol (no more than 8 tablets in 24 hours for an adult).
7. Should the wound begin to bleed, apply a compress (a clean cotton handkerchief rolled up is ideal). Place this on the bleeding point and *bite firmly* on it for 10 minutes, or longer if necessary.
8. If you are at all worried, or if anything untoward occurs such as prolonged bleeding, excessive pain, or swelling, please phone the oral surgery department on ________.

ON THE DAY AFTER TREATMENT

A mouthwash can now be used to cleanse the mouth. It is not necessary to purchase a proprietary mouthwash, although you can if you wish. It is the mechanical action of washing out the mouth which is of importance, rather than the substance used.

Warm salty water is very effective to cleanse and freshen the mouth. Dissolve ½ teaspoon of salt in a tumbler of warm water. Hold a mouthful of the solution in the mouth for a minute or two and then spit it out. Finish the tumbler in the same way. Repeat the procedure several times a day for 5 days.

FOLLOW-UP

You will have been given another appointment if further treatment is necessary. If you have any problems please contact the number given above for advice.

Nursing Care Plan 15.1 Care of a patient following removal of impacted wisdom teeth

Nursing considerations	Action/intervention	Expected outcome
1. Pain due to manipulation of jaw	❒ Administer adequate analgesia and monitor its effect	Patient is free of pain
2. Risk of haemorrhage	❒ Withhold mouthwashing overnight	Blood clot left undisturbed; bleeding minimised
3. Vomiting because of swallowed blood from tooth socket	❒ Give constant reassurance; stay with the patient or allow him privacy according to his wishes	Patient is comforted; dignity and self-esteem respected
4. Personal hygiene	❒ Provide frequent sponging, especially of face and hands	Comfort maintained
5. Oral hygiene	❒ Provide gentle, warm saline mouthwashes the morning after; gentle brushing, avoiding socket	Mouth is freshened; debris removed; haemorrhage avoided
6. Risk of infection	❒ Administer prescribed antibiotics ❒ Implement special precautions for patients at risk	Infection avoided; normal healing takes place
7. Discharge	❒ Evaluate outcome of treatment and post-operative care ❒ If the patient is fit for discharge: give after-care information; refer to community nurse and hygienist; arrange return appointment	Patient is confident that he can perform self-care; professional supervision is continued

Promoting dental health in special client groups

Most people are able to maintain good oral hygiene independently throughout much of their lives. Others, for reasons of physical or cognitive disability, or infirmity due to illness or advanced age, will need supervision and assistance in carrying out dental and periodontal care routines. The importance of this aspect of daily care must not be minimised, as poor orodental health can seriously compromise the individual's well-being and ability to function.

Physically and/or mentally handicapped people

Individuals with limited motor control or manual dexterity may require help with brushing teeth. Toothbrushes with adapted handles are available to aid gripping, and the nurse should be aware of how these can be obtained (often from an occupational therapist). Many people with limited movement depend on the mouth and teeth to hold or control equipment; it is thus especially important that their teeth are kept in good condition. Occasionally it is difficult to gain the cooperation of a mentally handicapped person who needs dental treatment; in such cases general anaesthesia may be required even for a simple procedure. The practice of good oral hygiene is obviously preferable to repeated general anaesthesia.

Elderly people

More elderly people now retain their natural teeth and regular dental check-ups should be encouraged and, where appropriate, arranged. Good oral hygiene should be encouraged and regular assessment of oral/dental health for elderly people in hospital should form part of any nursing care plan. Adequate dental care for elderly people can greatly enhance quality of life with regard to comfort, self-image and social interaction (Fiske et al 1990).

Elderly people often have specific problems relating to dental health, as follows:

1. Gum retraction/resorption. This occurs naturally in elderly people, causing root surfaces to be exposed. Together with the reduction in saliva which is also characteristic in old age, this increases the risk of decay.
2. Natural wear of the teeth can necessitate repair work.
3. Ill-fitting dentures. Unfortunately, it is not always possible to provide well-fitting dentures for elderly people because of the resorption of the alveoli that naturally occurs when teeth are lost. Continuous wearing of dentures can lead to the development of oral thrush (candidiasis). Dentures should therefore be removed at night, cleaned, and kept in water or a weak solution of Milton or other proprietary cleanser. Dentures left dry for any length of time can shrink.
4. Loss of appetite. Elderly people who seem to have lost interest in meals should be examined for mouth ulcers, ill-fitting dentures, pain due to thrush and early indications of intraoral cancer. Any ulcer which does not heal within 2–3 weeks should always be suspect and specialist opinion should be sought (Bramley & Smith 1990, Williams 1990).

? **15.6** Consider your nursing care of elderly patients. Do you always give the same attention to teeth as to washing face and hands and combing hair?

Acutely ill people

As far as possible, the practice of oral hygiene should follow the patient's normal routine, but there may be periods when this is not possible, e.g. if the teeth are wired together or if the mucous membrane is inflamed or ulcerated.

During the acute phase of an illness, the patient may require assistance or supervision in carrying out oral hygiene, but the objective should be to enable optimum independence as soon as possible.

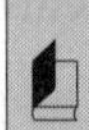

Jamieson et al (1992) describe mouth care in detail and the student is referred to that text for general procedures. Reference will be made in this section to situations in which normal procedures may need to be modified.

Gibbons (1983) summarises the objectives of mouth care as 'comfort, cleanliness, moistness and prevention of infection'. All disorders of the mouth require impeccable oral hygiene, but this must be carried out *without causing harm*, as some traditional methods of oral hygiene can further damage a mouth which is already at risk. This must be borne in mind especially with regard to patients who are immunocompromised by chemotherapy, bone marrow transplantation, radiotherapy to the head and neck region, HIV infection, and so on. Ideally, such patients should be referred to a dentist before treatment starts so that any caries can be treated. Where a dental hygienist is part of the multidisciplinary team, he or she should also be involved.

Any care given to the mouth of an immunocompromised patient must be carried out with extreme gentleness. Swabs held in forceps or wrapped round a gloved finger are best avoided as this method of removing debris can also remove a layer of regenerating epithelium. Foam sticks, cotton buds or dental rolls are more gentle. Teeth can be cleaned with a small, soft, or single-tufted brush.

If the mouth is extremely tender and painful, it should be regarded as an open wound. Mouthwashing may be all that can be tolerated, and even this may be excruciating. Taking a drink of water was once described by a patient as being 'like swallowing broken glass'.

Nurses must try to reassure the patient that frequent rinsing of the mouth will bring some relief, and may be done as often as hourly. There is, however, a lack of agreement among experts as to which cleansing agents are most effective. Advantages and disadvantages of various substances are described in the following.

Glycerine and thymol. According to Roberts (1990), 'there is no place ... in oral cavity cancer for glycerine and thymol solutions, lemon and glycerine swabs or many of the commercially available mouthwash solutions'.

Glycerine and lemon has long been used to stimulate the flow of saliva, and may have some short-term benefit. However, if used frequently, it may *inhibit* the flow of saliva. It is not appropriate for patients with a dry mouth caused by radiotherapy, chemotherapy or by surgery involving salivary glands or ducts.

Soft yellow paraffin will help to moisten lips.

Saliva substitute (if tolerated, as some people do not find it acceptable) or frequent application of *KY jelly* intraorally will help to moisten a dry mouth.

Chlorhexidine gluconate. Roberts (1990) and several others advocate the use of chlorhexidine-based solutions or gels to control bacteria that cause plaque and gum disease. These products are effective in helping prevent plaque formation for those whose teeth are wired, but may cause discoloration of the teeth and are probably of limited value to edentulous patients. Wahlin (1989) reports a study which demonstrated no significant improvement in the oral condition of acute leukaemia patients who had used chlorhexidine; rather, these patients showed an increased tendency to experience a burning sensation in the mouth and to contract certain infections.

Barkvoll & Attramadal (1989) advise that it is unwise to use nystatin and chlorhexidine together when treating candida albicans as interaction of the two may make the combination ineffective. On the other hand, Scully et al (1991) advocate the use of chlorhexidine or povidone iodine in HIV-related oral infections. Research continues to try to find the optimal treatment for oral comfort.

The British National Formulary (BNF 1993) recommends the use of all of the abovementioned preparations for oral ulceration and infection.

Benzydamine (Difflam) has been shown to reduce the discomfort of post-irradiation ulceration, but may cause stinging for some patients and may have to be diluted (BNF 1993).

Saline. It is generally agreed that it is the action of mouthwashing which is beneficial more than the specific substance used. Therefore it may be prudent to restrict mouthwashing agents to saline solution (½ tsp. salt in a glass of water at a temperature comfortable for the individual) for all patients in whom the oral mucous membrane is at risk until research demonstrates more definitively the benefit of other substances.

A simple method using easily obtained materials is more likely to be self-administered by patients after discharge than a complicated procedure with solutions which must be specially prescribed or purchased.

Other factors to be considered in minimising the discomfort of oral ulceration and other conditions are fluid intake, diet and analgesia.

INFECTIONS AND INFLAMMATORY CONDITIONS OF THE MOUTH

These conditions can give rise to considerable pain and discomfort and can set up a vicious circle whereby the individual loses interest in food, becomes debilitated by poor nutrition, and becomes even more susceptible to infection and further loss of appetite as a result. The mouth may be affected by the following types of conditions:

- local and systemic infections (see Table 15.3)
- oral manifestations of a generalised systemic disease:
  - — gastrointestinal and nutritional disorders (see Chs 4, 20, 21 and Table 15.4)
  - — blood (haemopoietic) and endocrine disorders (see Chs 11, 5 and Table 15.5)
  - — dermatological disorders (see Ch. 12).

Table 15.3 Local and systemic infections affecting the mouth (Adapted from Lamey & Lewis 1988)

Infection	Oral presentation	Cause/effect
Acute pseudomembranous candidiasis (thrush)	Soft creamy patches on mucosa	Often seen in patients on steroid therapy, particularly when also receiving broad-spectrum antibiotics
Chronic atrophic candidiasis	Erythema with demarcation from normal tissue	Poor dental hygiene and continuous wearing of dentures, especially in elderly persons
Angular cheilitis	Inflammation of corners of lips	
Chickenpox (varicella)	Occasionally vesicles develop on oral mucosa	Varicella zoster virus
Herpes labialis (cold sore)		Often follows a primary herpetic infection; stress, fever, local irritation, exposure to sunlight may reactivate the virus
Herpes zoster (shingles)	Affects one or more branches of trigeminal (CN V) nerves, usually unilaterally	As above
Herpangina	Multiple ulcers and erythema affecting palate and fauces. Mild, short lasting	Coxsackie virus group A
Kaposi's sarcoma	Skin of cheek: red/blue or purple patches	Often associated with AIDS
AIDS	May also present as hairy leukoplakia, candidiasis, oral infections	Compromise of immune system by HIV
Actinomycosis	Granulomatous tumour may develop in neck following tooth extraction, with thick oily pus discharging	*Actinomyces israeli* bacterium
Tuberculosis	Ulcers on tongue — a rare complication	*Mycobacterium tuberculosis*
Primary syphilis	Primary chancre may develop on tongue	*Treponema pallidum*
Secondary syphilis	Flat painless ulcer with grey membranous covering	*Treponema pallidum*
Tertiary syphilis	Syphilitic leukoplakia may progress to squamous cell carcinoma	*Treponema pallidum*
Bell's palsy	Lower motor neurone disorder affecting facial nerve, causing drooping of mouth, and ability to close eye or wrinkle forehead	May arise as result of viral infection

Table 15.4 Gastrointestinal and nutritional disorders affecting the mouth (Adapted from Lamey & Lewis 1988)

Disorder	Oral presentation	Cause/effect
Gastro-oesophageal reflux (bulimia)	Erosion of teeth due to exposure to gastric acid from self-induced vomiting	Tooth erosion may be first indication of disorder
Crohn's disease	Irregular swelling of lower lip, angular cheilitis, and folded thickening of oral mucosa	Mainly due to lymphoedema Sensitivity to foods, flavouring, dyes and preservatives
Coeliac disease	Recurrent oral ulceration	Caused by folic acid deficiency
Pernicious anaemia	Generalised papillary loss with mucosal atrophy	Caused by vitamin B_{12} deficiency
Iron deficiency anaemia	Atrophic glossitis	Less severe than that due to folic acid or vitamin B_{12} deficiency

Table 15.5 Haemopoietic and endocrine disorders (Adapted from Lamey & Lewis 1988)

Disorder	Oral presentation	Cause/effect
Polycythaemia vera	Bright red oral mucosa with bluish tongue	See Ch. 11
Agranulocytosis	Ulcer with minimal surrounding erythema	Oral infections are a serious complication
Thrombocytopenic purpura	Petechiae (multiple pinpoint submucosal haemorrhages)	See Ch. 11
Acute myeloid leukaemia	Haemorrhagic tendency	Chemotherapy
Acromegaly	Forward tilting of incisors	Enlargement of mandible
Diabetes mellitus	Bilateral painless parotid gland enlargement — a rare complication	See Ch. 5

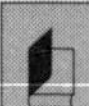

For information on dermatological conditions which may have oral manifestations see Lamey & Lewis (1988).

Thrush

PATHOPHYSIOLOGY

Thrush (candidiasis, candidosis or moniliasis) is caused by infection with *Candida (Monilia) albicans*, a yeast-like fungus normally found in the respiratory, alimentary and (in females) genital tracts of healthy people. Disease in the mouth may occur as a result of:

1. use of broad-spectrum antibiotics, steroids, immunosuppressive and cytotoxic drugs, and radiotherapy to the head and neck area. All of these cause destruction of the natural bacteria (flora) in the mouth and allow Candida to invade
2. severe debilitation, e.g. following surgery, in anaemia and other blood disorders, diabetes mellitus, Cushing's syndrome and in about 75% of terminally ill patients (Doyle & Benton 1986)
3. poor oral hygiene in elderly people or those who wear dentures at night, especially if they smoke and/or have diminished saliva
4. poor hygiene for infants (usually bottle-fed). The infection can spread rapidly to other infants
5. HIV infection (see Challacombe 1991).

Common presenting symptoms. Four different presentations of oral thrush are now recognised (Challacombe 1991):

1. pseudomembranous: soft, white or creamy yellow removable patches or plaques like milk curds; usually an acute phase
2. erythematous: red area often sharply demarcated from surrounding mucosa without removable plaques; often found in elderly people
3. hyperplastic: firm, adherent white patches or tiny nodules on an erythematous base; usually associated with HIV
4. *angular cheilitis:* deep red painful cracks or fissures at the corners of the lips.

All four types can be found at the same time, especially when associated with HIV. Anorexia is common.

Stomatitis

PATHOPHYSIOLOGY

Stomatitis, or inflammation of the mouth (stoma), is sometimes referred to as mucositis. It can be caused by:

- vitamin deficiency (B_{12}; folic acid)
- viral infection
- radiotherapy to head and neck
- chemotherapy
- bone marrow transplantation (BMT) and graft versus host disease (GVHD)
- liver failure
- renal failure.

Common presenting symptoms. In this condition, cell regeneration in the epithelium of the mucous membrane cannot keep pace with the rate of destruction which occurs as a result of any of the above. The mucosa becomes thin and there is erythema and some loss of taste. Later, oedema develops and the mucosa breaks down at the slightest trauma, giving rise to haemorrhage and ulceration.

The pain caused by stomatitis can be excruciating. A sore mouth is one of the side-effects which makes chemotherapy, or radiotherapy to the head and neck area, an unhappy experience for many people (see Ch. 32, p. 888). In health, saliva normally helps to clear the mouth of harmful pathogens, but in patients undergoing radiotherapy, chemotherapy or preparation for BMT, xerostomia (dry mouth) upsets this balance (Maximiw & Wood 1989).

MEDICAL MANAGEMENT

Medical intervention begins with the identification of the pathogen (if necessary, by culture swab). Thrush is treated with an appropriate antifungal lozenge or oral suspension (e.g. Nystan, amphotericin, fluconazole). To achieve maximum effect, these drugs should be given after oral hygiene procedures have been carried out.

If the patient is being treated for a systemic disease a review of his medication will be made with a view to adjusting his prescriptions. If the symptoms become severe, causative treatments such as radiotherapy may be withdrawn temporarily.

The administration of local or systemic analgesia will be timed so that the patient obtains maximum relief at mealtimes. Appropriate mouthwashes will also be prescribed (see p. 528).

NURSING PRIORITIES AND MANAGEMENT: INFECTIONS AND INFLAMMATORY CONDITIONS OF THE MOUTH

Oral hygiene as described on pages 525–529 and Ch. 34, pages 932–933 should be carried out, following a regime appropriate to the needs of each individual. Patients should be encouraged to master and carry out their oral hygiene routines independently as far as is reasonably possible.

Consideration should be given at all times to the importance for the patient of maintaining dignity and self-esteem. All nursing care plans for the treatment of oral conditions must take into account the patient's general condition and any therapeutic measures being implemented by other members of the multidisciplinary team.

OROFACIAL TRAUMA

Traumatic injury to the mouth or face typically gives rise to a great deal of anxiety concerning disfigurement. Moreover, because of the high vascularity of this area blood loss at the time of injury may be considerable, and the patient and his companions or relatives are likely to be very alarmed.

Soft tissue injuries to the face range from simple lacerations, knife wounds and bites to multiple injuries resulting in tissue loss. Bone injuries include fracture of the mandible, and fracture of the maxillae, malar (zygomatic) and nasal bones (middle third fracture). The signs and symptoms of different types of fracture are summarised in Table 15.6.

Causes

Violence

During the period 1974–84, recorded woundings and assaults in Britain almost doubled, rising from 62 000 to 112 000. Interpersonal violence is now the leading cause of facial fractures in many British and North American centres. In one centre in 1988, 90% of assault victims sustained fractures of facial bones (Shepherd 1989).

Injury is usually caused by a direct blow from a fist or weapon. Many injuries occur in the course of unprovoked muggings, and the victim may be in a state of shock (see Ch. 18). Many incidents are associated with excessive consumption of alcohol.

Many facial injuries are claimed to have been caused by walking into doors or 'falling down'. However, many researchers suspect that a significant percentage of assault cases go unreported. Dimitroulis & Eyre (1991) found in a study of maxillofacial injuries that 60% of men and 40% of women in a sample sustained injuries as a result of assault, while falls accounted for 36% of the injuries in women and only 12.4% in men. Domestic violence may go unreported, as many women are apprehensive of reprisals from their spouse if they take action.

Football hooliganism and attacks on public transport personnel are increasing. Shepherd (1989) argues that the reasons for the increase in violent crime in recent years include drug abuse, unemployment, inner-city deprivation and racism.

Road traffic accidents (RTAs)

Facial injuries following RTAs may involve lacerations, fractures and eye damage. Since the introduction of seat belt legislation in 1972, facial injuries from RTAs have markedly decreased. In 1978 only 3% of RTA victims had facial fractures (DHSS 1978).

Industrial injuries

Accidents in the workplace involving machinery or equipment are often followed by claims for compensation. Nurses should therefore not give any information relating to the circum-

Table 15.6 Characteristics and management of maxillofacial fractures (Note: There will be considerable variation in presentation and in the timing of manipulative procedures, in accordance with the exact site and combination of fractures)

Fracture	Signs and symptoms	Management
Fractured nasal bones	Nasal deviation or flattening; bruising	Manipulation of nasal bones and septum; nasal pack and plaster of Paris for 1–2 weeks
	Septal haematoma causing obstructed breathing	Drainage of haematoma Complicated fracture may need open reduction and fixation
Fractured malar bone	Black eye; swelling over cheek, sometimes flattening; anaesthesia of areas supplied by injured nerves (infraorbital and superior dental); inability to open mouth; diplopia	Elevation of malar bone through incision in temporal region Fixation by wiring of bone and packing of maxillary antrum is sometimes required
'Blow out' fracture of malar	Periorbital haematoma; diplopia	Insertion of implant to orbital floor to stop eye dropping
Fractured maxilla/middle third fracture	Grossly swollen face; failure of teeth to occlude properly; bilateral periorbital haematoma; fractured nasal bones; teeth may be loosened; CSF rhinorrhoea	Reduction and fixation of fractures by eyelet wires, cap splints, etc., plaster of Paris head cap, or halo frame (see Figs 15.1–15.4) Antibiotics
Fractured mandible with/without other fractured facial bones	Displaced or undisplaced; local pain and swelling; severe pain on opening mouth; sublingual haematoma	Undisplaced: usually no treatment Displaced: reduction with wires or splints depending on site of fracture

stances of any incident, either in person or by telephone, other than the standard statements agreed by hospital policy (UKCC 1992).

Sports injuries
These injuries are usually the result of a collision of players on a sports field, or of a blow from a ball, bat or other piece of equipment. The person with a maxillofacial injury in which there is minimal displacement of bone and no symptom of head injury may not present for treatment until the next day or later. Swelling and bruising may then make the injury seem more severe than was at first thought.

Burns
The treatment of burn injuries is discussed in detail in Chapter 31. It should be emphasised here, however, that contractures of the mouth can lead to great difficulty in eating, drinking and speaking and will present problems for secondary treatment (e.g. the administration of anaesthetic). To assist in the prevention of contractures of the mouth, burns patients should be encouraged to drink from a cup as early as possible and avoid the use of straws. The movement involved in sipping through a straw produces a tightening of the muscles supplying the mouth, whereas drinking from a cup encourages movement.

? **15.7** Take a few sips of a drink directly from a cup and then with a straw. What do you observe about the maxillofacial movement required for these two actions?

MEDICAL MANAGEMENT

Immediate intervention. Emergency treatment of all traumatic injuries will of course involve whatever resuscitative measures are required to maintain the patient's airway, breathing and circulation and to circumvent the development of clinical shock (see Chs 28 and 18). Priorities for intervention will have to be set if multiple injuries exist. A full physical examination will involve neurological observations and X-rays as appropriate, and will be followed by referral to the appropriate specialists, e.g. maxillofacial, orthopaedic or ophthalmic surgeons.

Treatment of maxillofacial injuries. The signs and symptoms of maxillofacial injuries, together with appropriate treatments, are summarised in Table 15.6.

Soft-tissue injuries require thorough cleansing (this may entail scrubbing of the wound under general anaesthesia) to remove glass, debris, gravel, dirt and so on. Failure to adequately clean the injury will lead to 'tattoo scarring', i.e. a permanent blue-grey scar that may later require surgical excision.

Bone injuries. Fixation of fractures may be required, and is usually carried out by a maxillofacial surgeon. Although the method of choice may vary between centres, the principle common to all methods is to immobilise the fractured bone. This is done by fixing the unstable bone and supporting it against an adjacent, stable bone by means of wires, metal bars or plates, splints or metal frames.

Methods of fixing a fractured mandible may be briefly described as follows:

- Eyelet wiring. Wires are twisted around the upper and lower teeth, leaving a loop (eyelet). The teeth are then brought into proper occlusion and wired together (see Fig. 15.3).
- Arch bar wiring. This technique is similar to eyelet wiring but is used when fewer teeth exist. A malleable bar is fitted over the gum, and wired as above.
- Interosseous plating. The fracture is exposed, reduced (i.e. repositioned) and fixed with a metal plate screwed into position. This may be left in situ permanently or removed after 3 months (see Fig. 15.4).
- Cast cap splinting. Metal alloy splints are made from dental impressions and cemented onto the teeth. The jaws are then wired together or fixed with rubber bands (see Fig. 15.5).
- Gunning splint. This is used if dentures are absent or ill-fitting. Dentures without teeth are fitted and wired to each other (see Fig. 15.6).

Undisplaced fractures of the mandible generally require no surgical treatment.

A fractured maxilla can be immobilised internally or externally,

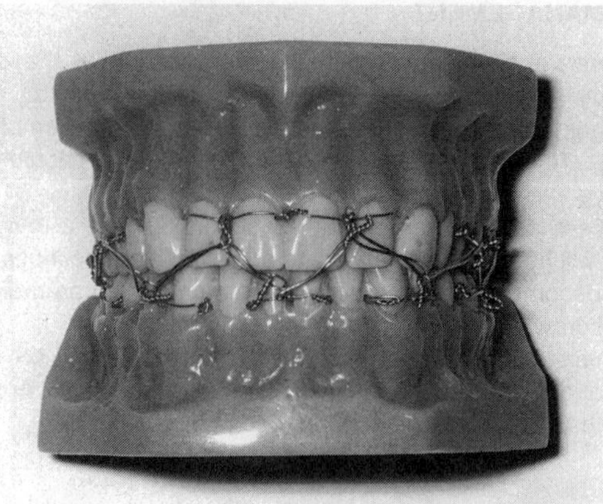

Fig. 15.3 Eyelet wiring.

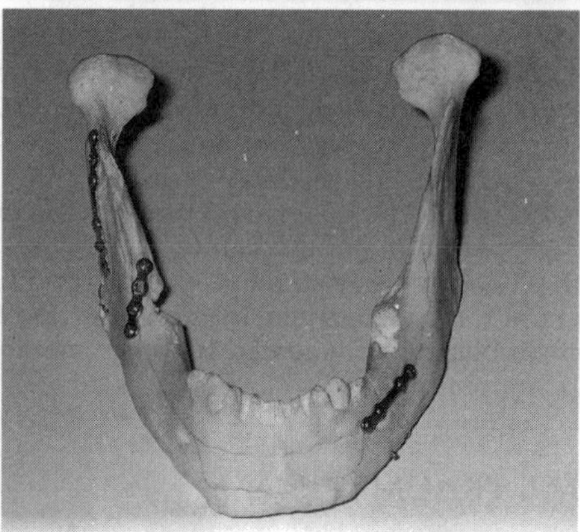

Fig. 15.4 Interosseous plating.

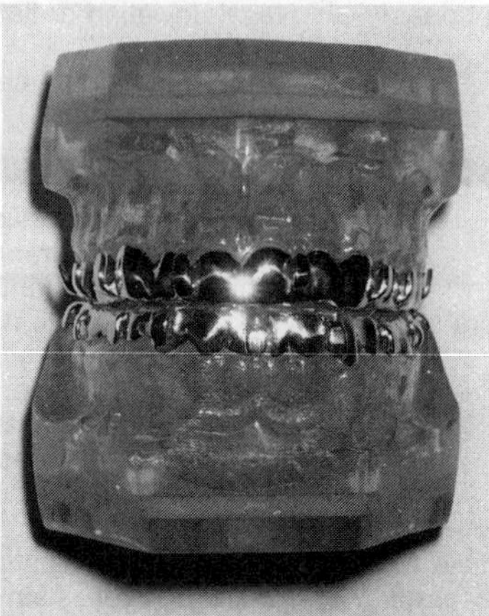

Fig. 15.5 Cast cap splinting.

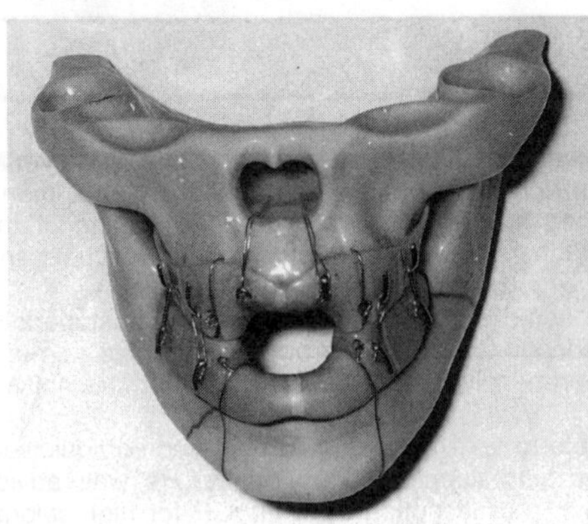

Fig. 15.6 Gunning splint.

depending on the precise nature of the injury. Internal fixation can be achieved by means of metal plates or with internal suspension wires. The latter hold the maxilla and mandible in occlusion and are fixed to the malar or frontal bone.

External fixation may be achieved by the following means:

- Le Vant or box frame. A metal frame is screwed to the skull through the supraorbital ridge. Rods are then attached to dental splints and secured to the frame. This is now the most commonly used method
- plaster of Paris head cap firmly fitted to the skull
- halo frame: a metal frame fixed to the skull.

Treatment of a fractured malar (zygoma) may take the following forms:

- elevation through incision in the temporal region
- wiring of fracture and packing of maxillary antrum to maintain stability (see Fig. 15.7)
- K-wires (rigid wires) in one or more directions. Ends are cut just clear of the skin
- an implant may be necessary to repair a shattered orbital floor (see Fig. 15.7).

Fractured nasal bones may also form part of a compound facial injury. Here, the fracture is reduced by manipulation of the nasal bones and immobilised by a plaster of Paris splint.

For further information on the treatment of maxillofacial injuries see Rowe & Williams (1985).

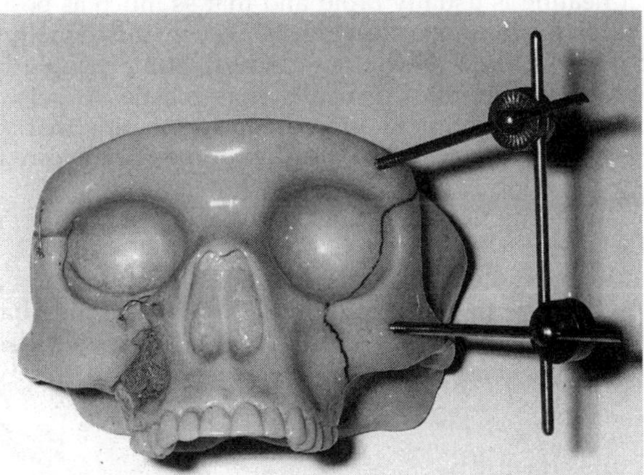

Fig. 15.7 Model showing fractures of malar or zygomatic bones and maxillae. The right bones have been wired, an implant placed in floor of orbit, and packing inserted in maxillary antrum. On the left side, fractures are stabilised by means of a form of external fixation.

NURSING PRIORITIES AND MANAGEMENT: OROFACIAL TRAUMA

Orofacial injuries vary widely both in presentation and in their impact upon the individual's lifestyle and psychological well-being. Case Histories 15.1 and 15.2 outline the experiences of two patients who are admitted to hospital after having received blows to the face. Each has different needs, priorities and concerns, and hence different requirements for nursing care. While the treatment of individuals who have suffered orofacial trauma must take into account a range of physical and emotional considerations, only that care which is specific to the mouth and face will be described here. General pre- and postoperative care is discussed in Chapter 27; reference to other chapters will be made as appropriate.

Life-threatening concerns

For patients who have suffered maxillofacial injury, the immediate priority of intervention is likely to be to maintain the airway. Respiratory difficulty and haemorrhage occur in a small number of cases and will require immediate care.

Respiratory difficulty

This problem can vary in severity and may be due to swelling of the tongue caused by oedema or haematoma, or due to the patient's inability to control the tongue because of disturbance of the muscle attachments. If the patient is conscious, he should be sat up and propped forward as soon as possible,

Case History 15.1 Ms Y

Ms Y, aged 23, was brought to the A & E department by a neighbour who heard a disturbance and found her dazed. She was found to be suffering from concussion, a fractured malar bone and facial lacerations, and was admitted to the ward. Ms Y explained that she received these injuries when she tripped and fell against a door.

Ms Y was told that she would have to have the fractured malar reduced and stabilised under anaesthetic. She was assured that the operation was not a major procedure, but that the fracture would simply be fixed by means of wires. She was also given general information on preoperative procedures and postoperative care.

As well as wiring the fractured malar bone, the surgeon inserted a gauze pack soaked in Whitehead's varnish into the maxillary antrum to support the orbital floor. A small portion was left protruding into the mouth through an incision in the upper gum. The nurse explained to Ms Y that it was important for her not to disturb this, and that she should take care not to use mouthwash too vigorously.

She was able to take a soft diet, however, and was advised to continue with soft foods for 7–10 days and to take as much protein as possible to promote healing.

After the incident, Ms Y was also suffering from diplopia (double vision) as a result of a slight displacement of one eye. This persisted, and she was later referred for orthoptic exercises.

While she was on the ward, Ms Y began to disclose some of her domestic problems, first to her primary nurse, and then with the medical social worker who, with Ms Y's agreement, had become involved. Ms Y indicated that she would consider accepting assistance from a women's support group. The social worker arranged for Ms Y's children to be cared for until she was ready for discharge.

Ms Y's discharge was planned well in advance. Through liaison with women's support agencies, she was assisted in reviewing her home circumstances and was offered alternative accommodation with her children.

Case History 15.2 Mr J

Mr J, aged 30, was assaulted while returning from an evening out with friends. He was unconsious for a short time after the incident. He was brought to the A & E department in the recovery position to prevent blood from inside his mouth trickling down the pharynx (and potentially the trachea) and causing respiratory distress. (Fortunately, he had not suffered pneumothorax, in which case he might not have been able to lie in this position.) It was difficult to restrain him as he was restless from the combined effects of blows to the head and the alcohol he had taken. He was found to be suffering from a middle third fracture, a fractured mandible, fractured ribs, and facial lacerations.

Mr J was advised that his jaws would have to be wired together and external fixation applied, but he had difficulty concentrating and absorbing information. His wife was present during the discussion. She was very anxious and mentioned that she had been concerned by the fact that her husband had been drinking more lately.

When he awoke from the anaesthetic, Mr J was quite frightened, as he did not remember much of what had been explained to him preoperatively. The nurse in the recovery ward told Mr J to breathe deeply and encouraged him to relax. She then explained again what had happened and what was preventing him from opening his mouth. She explained why it was important for him not to disturb the fixation, but also assured him that if it ever became urgent for him to release his jaw, the necessary equipment was at hand. She then stayed with Mr J until the feeling of the wires became more familiar to him, and ensured that adequate analgesics and sedation were being administered (see Ch. 19).

Mr J had some problems in the first few postoperative days when he accidently turned in bed and knocked his frame. He was somewhat apprehensive about having a visit from his active 2-year-old daughter.

He was able to take only a liquid diet, and so liquidised meals were provided with supplementary drinks. He was advised that he could obtain a prescription from his GP for high-calorie drinks during the time when the wiring was in place.

Mr J was surprised at how quickly the appearance of his injury improved. His facial wounds healed quite rapidly, and he was encouraged that within a few months the scars would fade and become less noticeable.

While he was still in hospital he was encouraged to review his alcohol intake and was given information on the effects of alcohol abuse and on local self-help groups from whom he and his family could obtain support as he addressed his dependency problem (see Ch. 37).

if other injuries allow. The airway must be kept clear. If the maxilla is fractured, it may be necessary to insert two fingers in the patient's mouth and hook behind the hard palate to re-establish the airway. In severe cases, early intubation or tracheostomy may be necessary.

Haemorrhage

There may be some bleeding initially, but it is seldom prolonged as a result of fractures, and usually stops when a free airway is provided. However, bleeding may be profuse when soft tissue injury has occurred, and immediate measures may be necessary — e.g. applying pressure on a bleeding point or pressure point — until ligation of the damaged vessel can be performed. Bleeding can also be controlled by holding the skin edges together with Steristrips until suturing can be carried out.

Shock

Nursing and medical staff must be alert to the warning signs of shock and should be prepared to take urgent action (see Ch. 18).

Major nursing considerations

Observation and monitoring

Vital signs (temperature, pulse, respiration and blood pressure) should be recorded at regular intervals.

Rhinorrhoea. The nurse should also watch for the presence of rhinorrhoea (nasal discharge) caused by leakage of cerebrospinal fluid (CSF). This can occur in fracture of the maxilla if the cribriform plate of the ethmoid bone is disturbed. CSF gives a positive reaction to Dextrostix.

Eye integrity/vision (see also Ch. 13). The nurse should check for abnormal pupil reactions, proptosis and acute pain. Vision should be checked hourly at first, especially if the patient cannot open his eyes because of oedema. Any rapid decrease in visual acuity can indicate retrobulbar haemorrhage, which can lead to blindness and requires urgent action. Double vision can indicate a fracture of the orbital floor.

Major patient problems

Pain

Pain must be assessed (see Ch. 19) but is not normally a major early problem. It is important, however, not to underestimate the patient's pain and to explain why analgesics may have to be withheld initially while investigations are carried out (see Ch. 28, p. 816).

Anxiety

Anxiety caused by fear of disfigurement and scarring may be the first concern of many patients and relatives. The high vascularity of the face may give rise to profuse bleeding even from a small laceration, and the injury may seem more serious than it is. An injury to the eye will be a source of further anxiety.

Patients and relatives should be given the opportunity to talk about their fears, particularly in the early stages when the injury may look horrific. Nurses should offer the reassurance that healing is usually rapid and that as much as possible will be done to minimise scarring. However, it is equally important not to raise expectations unduly. Some people have unrealistic ideas about the results that plastic surgery can produce, and it is unfair to allow them to imagine that what existed before can always be fully restored. Scars can fade and may be camouflaged, but it is not always possible to disguise the disfigurement caused by major tissue loss or bone displacement.

Nurses should also bear in mind that post-traumatic amnesia in which the patient has no recall of events immediately preceding the incident (see Ch. 17, p. 584) may give rise to psychological distress later should the memory of the event return.

Other considerations

Every effort should be made to clean blood and debris from the patient before his relatives see him, to avoid unnecessary distress. Dirty clothing should be removed, observing local policy for the care of patients' property.

Oral hygiene should be carried out within the limitations

of the patient's condition. For example, a blood clot should be left undisturbed as far as possible to minimise further bleeding, but broken teeth, debris, and so on should be removed if this has not already been done. Gentle irrigation with warm saline may be helpful.

Nursing care in surgical interventions

Patients who have soft tissue injury without bone damage will have suturing and/or reconstruction carried out as soon as possible.

Many patients with maxillofacial fractures will require surgical intervention to reduce and stabilise the fracture. The timing of this surgery will vary according to the patient's overall condition and the amount of localised swelling which may make assessment of the fracture difficult. In many cases, fixation is best left for a few days; if his general condition permits, the patient may be discharged home for the interim. Alternatively, direct transfer to a specialised unit may be arranged.

Postoperative management

The overall aim of postoperative management is to assist the patient as necessary with the activities of daily living and to help him to achieve independence in these activities as soon as possible.

Monitoring vital signs. In the initial postoperative period the patient's vital signs should be recorded every 15 minutes. As his condition stabilises the patient can gradually be raised to a sitting position to aid respiration, help drainage and minimise oedema. The patient should be encouraged to maintain an upright position even at night. Individuals who find it very difficult to sleep sitting up may find that resting against pillows placed in armchair fashion helps.

Respiration. The patient may have a nasal airway in situ to assist breathing, and this will need occasional suction to be kept clear. The mouth may also need gentle suction if the patient is afraid to swallow saliva for fear of choking. The patient should be encouraged to relax and to practise gentle swallowing movements.

Oral hygiene. It will be very important to help the patient maintain good oral hygiene. If the jaws have been wired, a soft tooth brush or Q-tips can be used to keep the anterior surface of the teeth and splints clean. The inside of the mouth can be cleansed with mouthwash taken through a straw (or a feeding cup with a spout) and squeezed out between the teeth. An alternative method is to irrigate the mouth through gaps between the teeth, using a rubber ball (chip) syringe, letting the fluid run out.

Preventing wound infection. The skin entry points of external fixation should be kept free of crusting by being cleaned with normal saline. An ointment such as sterile petroleum jelly should be applied to keep the area moist, and an antibiotic ointment (e.g. chloromycetin) may be used to minimise the risk of infection.

Sutures to facial lacerations can be kept clean with normal saline and removed in 3–4 days to minimise scarring. Supporting Steristrips may then be applied over the wound for a further 3–4 days. Any intraoral lacerations are usually repaired using catgut, which will be absorbed, but the mouth should be checked in case any non-absorbent sutures have been used, e.g. inside the lip.

Maintenance of fixation. The guiding principle of the treatment of maxillofacial fractures is, as for any other type of fracture, to obtain healing in the optimal position (e.g. that which maintains proper occlusion). In order for callus to form and thus for healing to take place the bone must remain immobile. Secure fixation is therefore extremely important, but appropriate instruments for releasing the fixation (i.e. wire cutters, or scissors for elastic bands) must always be available at the patient's bedside for immediate use should any danger of airway obstruction arise.

Instruments for tightening screws should also be at hand, and the fixation checked at regular intervals. Most patients will be aware if it becomes loose, but elderly people, or those with head injury may not. To avoid confusion, only those instruments appropriate for loosening or tightening the individual's particular type of fixation should be available at the bedside.

Nutrition (see also Ch. 21). A nasogastric tube may be inserted to allow for postoperative aspiration and/or drainage of old blood. Oral feeding should be encouraged as soon as possible, but this presents particular problems if the jaws must be kept wired for several weeks. A liquid diet must be taken, which may make it difficult for the patient to consume sufficient calories to maintain body weight. All food must be liquidised and supplemented with 'sip feeds', of which a wide variety is now available. Frequent, small meals should be taken throughout the day.

The dietitian should be consulted, ideally before the surgery takes place, to assess the patient's dietary requirements. Elderly patients with a low body weight will require special monitoring and encouragement. This is especially important if food is served by non-nursing personnel who may not appreciate the significance of unfinished meals.

> ? **15.8** How can a caloric intake adequate to promote healing be provided within the constraints of a hospital setting for Ms Y (Case History 15.1), who has no interest in food and Mr J (Case History 15.2), whose injuries prevent him from eating solid food?

Allaying fears. Nursing staff should bear in mind that the patient is likely to be very alarmed when he recovers from anaesthesia to find that interdental or external fixation is in place, even if he had been informed that this would be necessary. Moreover, it is not always possible for nurses to give a full explanation beforehand, either because of the patient's condition or because the precise intervention required is not known in advance of surgery. It is important that the patient is given some means of expressing his feelings and concerns and is briefed fully on how he will be able to manage basic functions such as eating and how he will be able to avoid choking should he need to cough up phlegm or to vomit.

Communication will be frustrating for the patient initially if his jaws have been fixed, but most difficulties will be overcome by otherwise healthy people, given sufficient encouragement and reassurance in the early stages. Writing pads, 'magic' slates, picture cards and other aids may be used to facilitate communication.

Mobility. When and how well the patient will be able to mobilise will depend on the nature of any other injuries incurred. Patients with facial injuries can be up on the day following surgery, but there are obvious restrictions if a maxillocranial frame is in place.

> ? **15.9** Stop and reflect on how your own activities would be affected if you had metal rods protruding from your head.

Body image. Disfigurement caused by facial injuries is of great concern to most patients. While a few individuals may be happy to display their scars, for the majority scarring will be a source of continuing anxiety.

Many people will be reluctant to look at themselves in a mirror following their surgery, and should not be forced to do so. It might help for the nurse to ask the patient if he would like her to describe how his face looks to her; if her account is matter-of-fact and accepting, he may be more willing to look for himself. Unfortunately, for many people disfigurement will give rise to deep feelings of grief and loss which may never be completely resolved.

Discharge planning
Patients who are fit and who can maintain adequate self-care can be discharged when postoperative swelling has subsided. They should be provided with written instructions on diet and oral hygiene, and given a telephone number to call in case of emergency. Referral to the community nurse should be made for care of wounds, checking of fixation, and assessment of diet. A follow-up appointment should be made for the patient to return after 4–6 weeks to have the fixation removed.

Elderly patients who are frail may never recover fully from maxillofacial injury and surgery. Some who are fit to go home may well be too afraid or self-conscious to go out again. The community nurse is in an ideal position to encourage such individuals to venture into the outside world again. Some may require long-term care, whether within the family, in sheltered housing or in an appropriate home.

See also Kemble & Lamb (1984) on the nursing care of patients recovering from maxillofacial surgery.

TUMOURS OF THE MOUTH

Oral cancer is more common than is often realised, being ranked eighth in developed countries and third in developing countries (Cancer Research Campaign 1993). Much may be preventable, and nurses by health education can make a significant contribution to its reduction.

Treatment of intraoral tumours is frequently carried out in specialised units. However, as the use of advanced reconstructive techniques becomes more widespread and patients are discharged into the community at an earlier stage, often to continue treatment as outpatients, nurses in more general areas of practice are likely to encounter patients with intraoral cancer. To help to ensure continuity of care from hospital to community, it is important for general nurses to have an understanding of the problems faced by these patients (Espie et al 1989, Freedlander et al 1989, Kelly 1990).

Treatment plans will vary considerably from centre to centre, and there are different schools of thought within the medical profession as to which treatment schedule best promotes the patient's survival and a good quality of life (McAndrew 1990). Whatever plan is chosen, it is likely that many patients will suffer some disruption of several basic functions. For example, intraoral surgery (with or without neck dissection) may cause disturbance or damage to the muscles and nerves which control the mechanisms of eating. Patients may be left with short-term, long-term or permanent malfunction. The degree of disability will vary greatly from patient to patient and is dependent on many factors. Table 15.7 indicates some of the malfunctions that may occur following this type of surgery, and as a consequence of radiotherapy.

Rehabilitation may take many months or years; it is therefore important that nurses liaise with one another and with their colleagues in other disciplines to ensure continuity and the best possible quality of care.

It must also be stressed that each patient is very much an individual whose needs and priorities will differ significantly from those of another patient with a seemingly similar problem. There can therefore be no set plan of care, and nurses must be ready and equipped to modify their ideas (working in conjunction with the other members of the multidisciplinary team and with the patient) to meet the individual's needs.

The pathophysiology and common presenting symptoms of tumours of the mouth will now be described under the following headings:

- tumours of the lips
- tumours of the floor of the mouth and tongue
- tumours of the palate
- tumours of the salivary glands.

However, because the separate functions of the mouth, e.g.

Table 15.7 The effects of intraoral disease and treatment on the mechanisms of eating

Normal mechanism	Disruption caused by intervention	Effects
Teeth bite and chew food, powered by muscles of jaw and supplied by trigeminal (5th cranial) nerve	Teeth may be extracted due to caries or to give access to tumour	Soft food only can be taken until fitting of dentures is possible
Saliva secreted by parotid (9th cranial) nerve, submandibular and sublingual glands mixes with food	Glands may be excised or damaged by radiotherapy	Dry mouth Stomatitis Thrush
Tongue and teeth powered by muscles of jaw break down food and form it into bolus	Muscles damaged or weakened by surgery and trauma	Re-education of eating skills will be needed
Mouth kept closed by superficial facial muscles (supplied by CN V and CN VII) Buccinator prevents food gathering in cheek pouches	As above	Drooling Food gathers in mouth
Tongue helps propel food to back of mouth and into contact with oral part of pharynx	Excision of part or whole tongue Tongue becomes fixed or insensate	Patient needs to push food to oropharynx
Simultaneously with above, muscles of soft palate elevate and tighten, straightening out to close off nasal cavity and preventing food from entering it	Damage to palate and nerves allows food to enter nasal space	Food, liquids come down nose unless obturator (see Box 15.3) can be fitted
Larynx rises under shelter of epiglottis to close off airway, preventing entry of food	CN IX damage causes paralysis of pharyngeal muscles	Aspiration of fluid to lungs necessitates permanent tracheostomy

speaking, chewing, swallowing, are frequently interdependent, medical and nursing management will be discussed with reference to the whole mouth.

Tumours of the lips

PATHOPHYSIOLOGY

Benign tumours include granulomata.

Malignant disease may take the form of basal cell carcinoma (BCC, often called 'rodent ulcer' because of its pattern of 'eating' or 'gnawing into' tissue) or squamous cell carcinoma (SCC). Malignant melanomas may also occur on the lips, but these are rare (see Ch. 12, p. 463).

Predisposing factors include prolonged exposure to sunlight (e.g. among outdoor workers), fair skin and pipe smoking. The lower incidence of lip cancers among women may possibly be due to the barrier effect of cosmetics.

Common presenting symptoms. Basal cell carcinoma may appear as a nodule, or as a small, unstable ulcerating area with persistent crusting. It may also be diffuse and invasive. The patient often reports, 'I thought it had healed up, but I kept knocking the top off it.' The ulcer may have 'pearlised' rolled edges. These tumours are generally slow-growing and do not metastasise, although occasionally a tendency to multiple BCCs is seen.

Squamous cell carcinoma is more aggressive, and if untreated may assume the 'cauliflower' look of a malignant ulcer and will eventually fungate and cause severe pain.

Tumours of the floor of the mouth and tongue

PATHOPHYSIOLOGY

Tumours of the tongue account for about one-third of all intra-oral tumours in the UK. Others included in the category of the floor of the mouth are found on the lower alveolus, tonsillar fossae and retromolar trigones, and about 90% are of the SCC type (Smith 1989). The incidence is twice as common in men as in women and although there had been a dramatic fall from the start of this century until the 1970s, both incidence and mortality rates now appear to be rising, especially in younger men in almost all EC countries. In Britain, a north–south divide is noted, with higher incidence in Scotland and Northern England (CRC 1993).

Spread usually involves the local lymph nodes (e.g. cervical, submandibular, submental). Distant metastases are rare, but occasionally occur in the lungs.

Predisposing factors. Heavy smoking combined with excessive alcohol consumption is associated with these cancers. In countries where tobacco-chewing is common (e.g. India) the incidence of oral cancer is relatively high (Smith 1989). Chewing tobacco teabags or nicotine chewing gum is also thought to contribute. However, tumours do occur in patients who have never smoked and who seldom or never take alcohol. There is thought to be a relationship between tumours of the floor of the mouth and chronic oral infections, e.g. syphilis, herpes simplex virus, human papilloma virus and HIV (Smith 1989). Poor oral hygiene and nutritional deficiencies are often present and may be causative factors (CRC 1993).

Common presenting symptoms. These cancers may become apparent in a variety of ways. In the early stages, intraoral SCC is easily mistaken for infection, irritation from dentures or a simple aphthous ulcer. Leukoplakia (white, thickened patches on the mucosa) may appear and may be classified as carcinoma-in-situ. This may become malignant (Williams 1990). More advanced tumours are usually unmistakable, but many patients present late for various reasons, including fear, misdiagnosis, and self-neglect.

Tumours of the hard and soft palate

PATHOPHYSIOLOGY

These tumours may arise from the epithelium of the mucous membrane (SCC), in the maxillary sinuses, in the maxilla, or in the minor salivary glands in the palate. They are less common than tumours of the floor of the mouth, but are potentially more disfiguring.

Spread usually occurs locally to the floor of the orbit or to the eye.

Common presenting symptoms. Onset may be insidious. The patient may notice a dull ache for some time and may complain of 'sinusitis'. The pain will eventually increase and swelling may develop over the cheek. There may be some displacement of the eye in advanced cases. Rarely, a malignant melanoma appears as a pigmented lesion of the palate and goes unnoticed until the individual presents with a secondary tumour of the cheek or neck.

Tumours of the salivary glands

PATHOPHYSIOLOGY

The most common cause of swelling of the parotid gland is mumps (acute parotitis), an infectious, inflammatory condition that usually resolves without treatment. Mumps may, however, be relatively severe in adults and lead to pancreatitis or orchitis.

Benign or malignant tumours may develop in the parotid, submandibular, sublingual and other minor salivary glands. Salivary gland ducts may become blocked by small accretions (see 'Orodental disease' p. 526).

Common presenting symptoms. The patient presents with a swelling, which is often asymptomatic and therefore sometimes long-standing, in the area of the affected gland. If left untreated, a parotid gland tumour may involve the facial nerve (CNV), resulting in facial palsy, a severe disfigurement.

MEDICAL MANAGEMENT

Tests and investigations. A treatment plan for malignant tumours will be devised on the basis of careful staging of the cancer (see Table 15.8 and Ch. 32, p. 883). Investigation may include the following:

- history
- physical examination: visual and by palpation
- blood tests
- diagnostic X-rays: face and jaw; chest and spine as appropriate
- orthopantomogram (OPT; see Appendix 1)
- sialogram (see Appendix 1)
- bone scan
- CT scan
- MRI (magnetic resonance imaging; see Ch. 32)
- EUA (examination under anaesthetic)
- videofluoroscopy (see Appendix 1)
- biopsy: results will be essential to staging.

Table 15.8 TNM classification for lip and oral cavity (Adapted from Hermanck & Sobin 1987)

T: Primary tumour	
T1	Tumour < 2 cm
T2	Tumour > 2–4 cm
T3	Tumour > 4 cm
T4	Tumour invading adjacent structures
N: lymph nodes (neck)	
N1	Ipsilateral single node < 3 cm
N2	Ipsilateral single node > 3–6 cm
	Ipsilateral, multiple nodes < 6 cm
	Bilateral, contralateral nodes < 6 cm
N3	Node > 6 cm
M: distant metastases	
M0	No distant metastases
M1	Distant metastases

The patient's age, general physical condition and mental outlook will also be taken into consideration.

Medical intervention. Treatment may be radical, i.e. intended to effect a cure, or conservative, i.e. intended to alleviate symptoms. Radical treatment may involve extremely difficult adjustments for the patient and a significant reduction in the quality of life (Espie et al 1989, Freedlander et al 1989).

The treatment options for oral tumours are chemotherapy, radiotherapy and surgery. These treatment modes may be used singly or in combination; their sequence and timing will vary from one centre to another.

Chemotherapy is usually given concurrently with other treatment. It may be used to reduce the bulk of some tumours prior to surgery or in cases of recurrent tumours (see also Ch. 32).

Radiotherapy can be given as the sole treatment or pre- or post-operatively. It may take either of the following forms (see also Ch. 32):

- teletherapy (external radiation) by means of megavoltage machines or supervoltage machines
- brachytherapy, in which a radioactive source is placed in or near the tumour, e.g. interstitial needles to tumours of the lip or oral cavity (Holmes 1988, McAndrew 1990).

Many tumours, (e.g. SCC) are highly curable by radiotherapy. Sarcoma and malignant melanoma, on the other hand, have a low cure rate by this method.

Surgical excision. Treatment by this method ranges from small local excisions with direct closure, to major operations with full reconstruction. Benign tumours are usually excised.

Some centres carry out excision of tumours initially with secondary reconstruction later; others carry out immediate reconstruction. Table 15.9 summarises current surgical procedures.

Both radiotherapy and surgery treat squamous cell carcinoma successfully, either independently or in combination, but there is lack of agreement among medical practitioners as to the best timing of each.

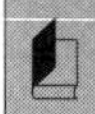
See McGregor & McGregor (1986) for detailed information on surgical and other therapies for cancers of the mouth.

Nurses should be aware of the effect of radiation on the epithelium (see Ch. 32, p. 888 and Holmes 1988). Following radical radiotherapy, healing after surgery may be delayed; occasionally, orocutaneous (between mouth and skin) fistulae may develop. Bone necrosis (osteoradionecrosis) is sometimes experienced as a late effect.

Follow-up and after-care will require outpatient appointments at regular intervals (gradually lengthening from monthly to yearly) for 5 years. Dental and/or prosthetic provision may include dentures, obturators (see Box 15.3), and other prostheses provided by members of the multidisciplinary team, as and when necessary. Referral to other consultants (e.g. ENT, ophthalmic, thoracic and neurological specialists) will be made as appropriate. Speech therapy and dietary advice will be essential for many patients.

Table 15.9 Surgery for tumours of the mouth

Site	Excision	Reconstruction
Superficial lesion of lip; leukoplakia	Shaving	None
Lip; parotid gland; T1 tumour of mouth	Simple excision	None: direct (primary) closure
Lip	Wedge excision	Direct closure
Tongue	Local excision	Split skin graft
Lip; alveolus; tongue	Local excision	Local flap (many varieties: Abbe, tongue, buccal, nasolabial, etc. See McGregor & McGregor 1986)
Mouth/pharynx (all sites); cheek; neck	Local/wide excision +/– neck dissection	Free flap common in many centres (Webster & Soutar 1986)
As above (especially for recurrent tumour as palliative procedure)	As above	Pedicled flap (deltopectoral, pectoralis major)

Box 15.3 Obturators

Obturators are prostheses which are designed to fill a defect in the palate after maxillectomy. They are fitted in three stages:

1. Surgical splint: fitted during surgery to hold a skin graft in place, and/or avoid collapse of the cheek and upper lip. After about 2 weeks, it is replaced by a temporary obturator.
2. Temporary obturator: used throughout radiotherapy. This allows the patient to become accustomed to wearing and handling an obturator.
3. Definitive obturator: fitted after shrinkage of defect. It may be composed of a soft malleable 'bung' which fills the defect, and a denture which fits over the bung.

Without the obturator, the patient will be unable to speak or eat properly, and fluid will run into the nasal cavity. With a well-fitting obturator, the patient can eat and speak normally.

The obturator must be removed after meals and cleaned by brushing or by immersion in a proprietary cleaning solution. (If the obturator has been 'built up', cleanser should not be used.) The mouth must be rinsed after all food to prevent accumulation of plaque, debris, etc.

NURSING PRIORITIES AND MANAGEMENT: TUMOURS OF THE MOUTH

The presence of an oral tumour may not give rise to immediate life-threatening concerns, except where a long-neglected tumour causes respiratory distress or haemorrhage.

Patients will vary widely in the symptoms with which they present. Individuals with early tumours and few symptoms may be admitted for assessment and staging, and will require much reassurance when their diagnosis is known. They may be discharged home, and readmitted later when appropriate treatment has been arranged. Referral to community nurses and/or Macmillan or Marie Curie home care nurses will be beneficial to many patients, including those with early disease. Patients with more advanced disease in whom the symptoms are more severe are admitted without delay.

Immediate nursing priorities

Nursing intervention in the early stages of treatment will focus on controlling pain (see Ch. 19), relieving anxiety, and on providing oral hygiene and nutritional assessment (see Ch. 21). Supplementary feeding may be necessary, as weight loss due to pain experienced when eating is common among this group of patients. Existing physical conditions must of course be taken into account in any nursing plan. An additional concern may be the assessment and control of alcoholism. Excessive consumption of alcohol is a causative factor in some cases of oral cancer, and presents a real problem for a number of patients (see Ch. 37).

Preoperative preparation

Giving information

All patients will require adequate and honest information about the proposed treatment and its implications. (See Ch. 32, p. 900 and Wells 1988.) In view of the many variations in available procedures, and the diverse presentations and responses to treatment that are possible, nurses should be wary of giving information based on limited knowledge of apparently similar cases. What is feasible for one person may not be possible for another, and expectations should not be raised unduly.

The patient should be given the opportunity to voice his concerns about the disease and its implications for normal functioning (e.g. speaking and eating) and for appearance. Many patients will also have a deep fear of cancer and may have misconceptions about their prognosis and the likely course of the disease. It is important for the nurse to listen carefully to these patients so that their needs can be recognised and any unfounded anxiety relieved.

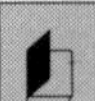

Strategies for sensitive listening are described in Porritt (1990) and in Chapter 26.

A multidisciplinary approach

A successful outcome will depend in part on the continuity of care provided by the multidisciplinary team. Along with medical staff, the team will include specialist nurses, ward nurses, community nurses and possibly Macmillan and Marie Curie nurses. In addition, the following professionals will contribute. It is important for the nurse to be aware of each team member's role and to facilitate liaison wherever possible and appropriate.

- Dietitian: assesses dietary intake and advises staff and patient on maintaining adequate nutrition when chewing and swallowing are difficult. A community dietitian may also become involved
- Speech therapist: advises patient on pre- and postoperative exercises to assist with speech and swallowing difficulties; may advise on alternative means of communicating if loss of voice is permanent (see Ch. 14, p. 515 and Ch. 26, p. 762)
- Physiotherapist: gives instruction and assistance with pre- and postoperative exercises to assist breathing, expectoration, limb and shoulder movements
- Dentist (associate specialist) or prosthodontist: assesses need for dental care (especially when radiotherapy is part of treatment) and fits obturator and/or dentures
- Dental hygienist: advises patient on care of teeth and oral hygiene, especially during radiotherapy and/or chemotherapy
- Maxillofacial technician: advises on whether provision of prosthesis is realistically possible. Designs, constructs and fits when appropriate for each individual patient
- Medical social worker: gives information and advice on availability of grants for special needs; arranges home help, day care, etc.
- Hospital chaplain or other religious counsellor: gives spiritual comfort and practical help.

? **15.10** In what ways would each member of the team be able to contribute to the care of the patient described in Case History 15.3 while in hospital and in the community?

Case History 15.3 Mrs C

Mrs C, a 45-year old housewife with two teenage children, was referred to an oncology unit from a dental hospital after she reported that she had had a lump in her mouth for some weeks. No lymphatic nodes were palpable in her neck, and Mrs C was not too concerned that she might have cancer because she had never smoked and rarely took alcohol. She and her husband were consequently very shocked when they were given the result of a biopsy which showed squamous cell carcinoma.

She was assured that the disease was treatable, and was advised to have surgical excision in the first instance, possibly followed by radiotherapy. Liaison was immediately set up with a Macmillan nurse, who visited her at home and discussed with Mrs C and her family their fears about cancer.

Mrs C felt that she did not want her husband to visit her until three or four days after the surgery. Her husband, however, felt anxious at not seeing her and came to visit of his own accord on the first postoperative day. The nurse prepared him for how his wife would look, and although he was initially shocked by her appearance, he felt that the result was not as bad as he had anticipated. He was also able to appreciate the rapid improvement which had taken place by the second day.

For herself, Mrs C was glad that he had visited. She felt more alert than she had believed possible. She also noticed the relief on her husband's face on his second visit, and was able to believe him when he said she looked much better. On the third day, having prepared them, he brought their two children.

Three years later, Mrs C is attending the outpatients' clinic for regular follow-up appointments. She has upper and lower dentures, which she wears all day, and is able to chew, swallow and speak well. She is socially very active and has adjusted well to the effects of her surgery, although she feels anxious every time she visits the clinic. Even after three years, she admits, 'I worry in case they find anything.'

Postoperative care

The postoperative nursing care of individuals who have undergone major surgery for intraoral cancer is highly specialised, and combines the skills of many specialties. There will be variations in procedures and approaches among centres, and each patient will require a highly individualised plan for care.

Many centres carry out immediate reconstruction of facial defects using free tissue transfer. Figure 15.8 outlines nursing procedures for the monitoring of free flaps.

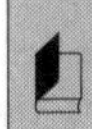

Webster & Soutar (1986) describe 20 free flaps. See also Coull & Wylie (1990) for a discussion of nursing responsibility for monitoring free flaps.

Participation of relatives

Oral tumours and the effects of treatment may have far-reaching consequences not only for the patients concerned but also for their families (Espie et al 1989, Freedlander et al 1989, Kelly 1990). Relatives must often provide care for the patient after discharge. They are likely to experience much anxiety and often have insufficient support. Nurses must help them through this very stressful time.

It is advisable to reinforce and supplement verbal advice with written information, particularly with regard to oral hygiene, diet, radiotherapy, chemotherapy, and local support groups.

Information booklets are available (e.g from the Royal Marsden Hospital and from BACUP), and written information pertaining to the centre where treatment has been carried out

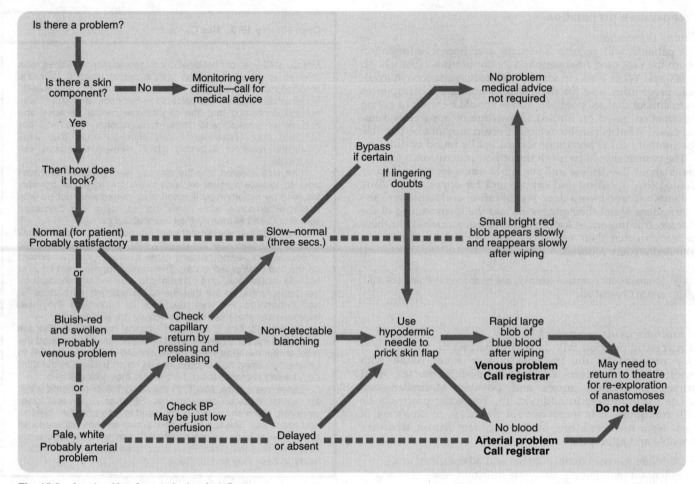

Fig. 15.8 An algorithm for monitoring free flaps.

is also helpful. Kelly (1987) found that patients and relatives who felt satisfied with the information given were half as likely to seek advice after discharge than those who were not satisfied.

Relatives will need constant reassurance, especially during the early postoperative days, and should be counselled before the first postoperative visit, which is usually very stressful (see Case History 15.3).

Altered body image

The impact of surgery to the face and mouth upon day-to-day function is visible to everyone. Basic activities such as breathing, eating and drinking may have to be performed with some loss of dignity. This, together with the disfiguring effects of the surgery will require the patient to accept an altered body image. This can be a very difficult adjustment for the individual to make, as this patient's written account of how she feels about her swollen face reveals (Kelly 1987):

> He said I was round the corner — but I don't really feel like it. He said the swelling would come down when I start moving around.
>
> I asked about my face which is freakish and he said when I start walking about gravity would reduce it. So I have now started every time I go to the toilet walking two laps of the ward — or when I am unleashed!
>
> I feel a bit shy about it. I feel a freak especially when I see in a mirror — avoid mirrors meantime!

Another patient in Kelly's study (1987), who had undergone several operations, commented: 'Each time, I feel I am a little less of the person I once was.' Remarks such as 'Of course, until I get my teeth, I can't go anywhere' are also frequently heard. Many patients, for example those who have had a tracheostomy, will be unable to speak following their surgery. It is important for nurses to bear in mind that it may be difficult for these individuals to convey their emotions in writing, and that it may be necessary to 'read between the lines' in order to fully appreciate the extent of their emotional pain.

?	**15.11** Consider how Mrs C in Case History 15.3 is likely to feel about her condition and the consequences of treatment. How is her body image likely to be affected?
?	**15.12** How can the nurse assist Mrs C to convey her feelings about her altered appearance non-verbally?

Discharge planning

Prior to the patient's discharge liaison should be established with the GP and community nurse and appropriate appointments and home visits arranged. In many cases a Macmillan nurse will have visited the patient in the ward and will continue to give support at home. Each of these professionals will coordinate subsequent visits through the local health centre according to his or her assessment of the patient's needs.

Hospital nursing staff should verify that transport arrangements are adequate for the patient's safe journey home and that all necessary preparations have been made for his return. It may be necessary for the medical social worker to assist in such matters as arranging for a home help, obtaining grants for adaptations to the patient's home, or applying for rehousing in more suitable accommodation.

Rehabilitation

Following discharge after major oral surgery and radiotherapy the process of rehabilitation may not be complete for a period of some months or even years. Patients will need ongoing support as they learn to cope with changes in lifestyle and in the activities of daily living (see Ch. 35). Planning for rehabilitation should start from the day of admission and must take into account the following considerations.

- Living arrangements. The patient may need to live with relatives temporarily or permanently, or may need rehousing if he is to live alone. Long-term nursing support (e.g. from Macmillan and Marie Curie nurses) and community-based services (e.g. Meals-on-Wheels) may need to be arranged.
- Breathing. Patients with a tracheal stoma will need to be instructed in its management and will need support in adjusting to their altered appearance.
- Oral hygiene; eating and drinking. The patient or his carer will need to be proficient in maintaining oral hygiene and using special equipment for delivering enteral feeds, if necessary.
- Communication. Training in alternative forms of communication will be needed to compensate for a loss in speech.
- Psychological support. The patient should receive pre-discharge counselling to help him adjust to an altered body image. Ongoing professional support may be needed for some time after discharge as the patient readjusts to life in the community.
- Work. The patient will need help in adjusting to new employment circumstances, whether he changes his job, stops working, or returns to his previous job and learns to cope with his changed appearance and function and with the reactions of colleagues.
- Education. The patient may need information on such matters as nutrition, giving up smoking and reducing alcohol intake. He and his family should be informed about local self-help groups where they can obtain practical and psychological support.

Collyer (1984) provides many examples of how disfigured people have been rehabilitated and of the difficulties they overcame in that process.

?	**15.13** Consider how you might go about planning the long-term rehabilitation of Mrs C in Case History 15.3.

Nursing and stress

Caring for patients with intraoral tumours can give rise to considerable stress. Nurses may find this area of care quite harrowing: unfortunately, ward nurses frequently see patients return with a recurrence of the cancer, and some may question whether radical treatment has in fact been justified.

Liaison with outpatient clinics will make it apparent, however, that many patients do in fact survive to lead fulfilling lives for many years after treatment.

Counselling and staff support in cancer nursing is discussed by Tschudin (1988). The reader is also referred to Chapters 17 and 32 of the present text.

REFERENCES

Barkvoll P, Attramadal A 1989 Effect of nystatin and chlorhexidine digluconate on candida albicans. Oral Surgery 67: 279–281

Bramley P A, Smith C J 1990 Oral cancer and precancer: establishing a diagnosis. British Dental Journal 168: 103–107

British National Formulary 1993 British Medical Association/ Pharmaceutical Society of Great Britain, London

Cancer Research Campaign 1993 Oral cancer: factsheet 14.1–5 CRC, London

Carmichael C L, Rugg-Gunn A J, Ferrell R S 1989 The relationship between fluoridation, social class and caries experience in 5-year-old children in Newcastle and Northumberland in 1987. British Dental Journal 167: 57–61

Challacombe S 1991 Revised classification of HIV-associated oral lesions. British Dental Journal 170: 305–6

Collyer H 1984 Facial disfigurement: successful rehabilitation. Macmillan, London

Department of Health (Committee on Medical Aspects of Food Policy) 1989 Report on health and social subjects No 37. Dietary sugars and human disease. Report of the panel on dietary sugars. HMSO, London

Department of Health and Social Security 1978 Road accident statistics. HMSO, London

Dimitroulis G, Eyre J 1991 A 7-year review of maxillofacial trauma in a central London hospital. British Dental Journal 170: 300–302

Downer M C 1991 The improving dental health of United Kingdom adults and prospects for the future. British Dental Journal 170: 154–158

Doyle D, Benton T F 1986 Pain and symptom control in terminal care. St Columba's Hospice, Edinburgh

Espie C A, Freedlander E, Campsie L M, Soutar D S, Robertson A G 1989 Psychological distress at follow-up after major surgery for intraoral cancer. Journal of Psychosomatic Research 33(4): 441–448

Fiske J, Gelbier S, Watson R M 1990 The benefit of dental care to an elderly population assessed using a sociodental measure of oral handicap. British Dental Journal 168: 153–156

Freedlander E, Espie C A, Campsie L M, Soutar D S, Robertson A G 1989 Functional implications of major surgery for intraoral cancer. British Journal of Plastic Surgery 42: 266–269

Gibbons D E 1983 Mouthcare procedures. Nursing Times 79(7): 30

Hermanck P, Sobin L H 1987 (eds) UICC TNM classification of malignant tumours, 4th edn. Springer Verlag, Berlin

Holmes S 1988 Radiotherapy. Lisa Sainsbury Foundation Series. Austin Cornish, London

Johnson N W, Warnakulasuriya K A A S 1991 Oral cancer: is it more common than cervical? British Dental Journal 170: 170–171

Kelly R 1987 A study of patients who have undergone surgery for cancer in the head and neck region. Unpublished paper

Kelly R 1990 Head and neck cancer. Nursing Times Community Outlook Supplement (November): 19–22

Lamey P-J, Rees T D, Forsyth A 1990 Sensitivity reaction to the cinnamonaldehyde component of toothpaste. British Dental Journal 168: 115–118

McAndrew P G 1990 Oral cancer and precancer: treatment. British Dental Journal 168: 191–198

Maximiw W G, Wood R E 1989 The role of dentistry in patients undergoing bone marrow transplantation. British Dental Journal 167: 229–234

Scully C, Porter S R, Luker J 1991 An ABC of oral health care in patients with HIV infection. British Dental Journal 170: 149–150

Shepherd J P 1989 Surgical, socio-economic and forensic aspects of assault: a review. British Journal of Oral and Maxillofacial Surgery 27: 89–98

Smith C J 1989 Oral cancer and precancer: background, epidemiology and aetiology. British Dental Journal 167: 377–383

Roberts A 1984 Systems of life No 112. Setting up the systems — 12. Development of the face. Nursing Times 80: 16

Roberts H 1990 Mouthcare in oral cavity cancer. Nursing Standard 4(19): 26–29

Roper N, Logan W W, Tierney A J 1990 The elements of nursing: a model for nursing based on a model of living, 3rd edn. Churchill Livingstone, Edinburgh

Tschudin V 1988 Counselling; staff support. In: Tschudin V (ed) Nursing the patient with cancer. Prentice-Hall, London, Chs 27, 28

United Kingdom Central Council for Nursing, Midwifery and Health Visiting 1992 Code of professional conduct for the nurse, midwife and health visitor. UKCC, London

Wahlin Y B 1989 Effects of chlorhexidine mouthrinse on oral health in patients with acute leukaemia. Oral Surgery 68: 279–287

Williams J Ll 1990 Oral cancer: clinical features. British Dental Journal 168: 13–16

World Health Organization 1988 Oral health global indicator for 2000. WHO, Geneva

FURTHER READING

Coull A, Wylie K 1990 Regular monitoring: the way to ensure flap healing. Nursing priorities following flap repair and reconstruction surgery. The Professional Nurse 6(1): 18–21

Coull A 1992 Making sense of surgical flaps. Nursing Times 88(1): 32–34

Davies S 1988 Head and neck cancer. In: Tschudin V (ed) Nursing the patient with cancer. Prentice-Hall, London, Ch. 12

Henderson D 1985 A colour atlas and text book of orthognathic surgery. The surgery of facial skeletal deformity. Wolfe Publishing, London

Jamieson E M, McCall J M, Blythe R, Logan W W 1992 Guidelines for clinical nursing practices, 2nd edn. Churchill Livingstone, Edinburgh

Johnson D R, Moore W J 1989 Anatomy for dental students, 2nd edn. Oxford University Press, Oxford

Kemble J V H, Lamb B E 1984 Plastic surgical and burns nursing. Baillière Tindall, London

Lamey P-J, Lewis M A O 1988 Oral medicine. Pocket picture guides series. Lippincott, Philadelphia, PA

Langley J 1989 Working with swallowing disorders. Winslow Press, Bicester

McGregor I A, McGregor F M 1986 Cancer of the face and mouth. Churchill Livingstone, Edinburgh

McGregor I A 1989 Fundamental techniques of plastic surgery and their surgical applications, 8th edn. Churchill Livingstone, Edinburgh

Oliver G 1988 Radiotherapy. In: Tschudin V (ed) Nursing the patient with cancer. Prentice-Hall, London, Ch. 5

Porritt L 1990 Interaction strategies, 2nd edn. Churchill Livingstone, Edinburgh

Rowe N L, Williams J Ll 1985 (eds) Maxillofacial injuries. Churchill Livingstone, Edinburgh

Towner E M L (Undated) Children's dental health: a guide for those teaching and caring for children. General Dental Council and Scottish Health Education Group, Glasgow

Webster M H C, Soutar D S 1986 Practical guide to free tissue transfer. Butterworth, London

Wells R 1988 Ethics, informed consent and confidentiality. In: Tschudin V (ed) Nursing the patient with cancer. Prentice-Hall, London, Ch. 30

Wilson K J W 1990 Ross & Wilson: anatomy and physiology in health and illness, 7th edn. Churchill Livingstone, Edinburgh

CHAPTER 16

The immune system and infectious disease

Marion C. Stewart

CHAPTER CONTENTS

Introduction 543
Anatomy and physiology 544
Control of infection 548
The nursing process and infection control 556
DISORDERS OF IMMUNITY 558
Immunodeficiency 558
Hypersensitivity 559
Anaphylactic shock 559
Nursing priorities and management 560
Farmer's lung 560
Nursing priorities and management 560
Sarcoidosis 560
Nursing priorities and management 561
Autoimmune diseases 561
Goodpasture's syndrome 561
Nursing priorities and management 561
Myasthenia gravis 561
Nursing priorities and management 562
Systemic lupus erythematosus (SLE) 562
Nursing priorities and management 562
INFECTIOUS DISEASES 563
Salmonellosis 565
Nursing priorities and management 565
Hepatitis B 565
Nursing priorities and management 567
Pulmonary tuberculosis 567
Nursing priorities and management 568
Meningococcal infection 569
Nursing priorities and management 569
Chickenpox and shingles 569
Nursing priorities and management of chickenpox 570
Nursing priorities and management of shingles 570
Conclusion 571
Acknowledgements 571
References 571
Further reading 572

INTRODUCTION

The immune system is a complex and fascinating network of cells and proteins which is programmed to respond to the many challenges presented to it by foreign particles, microorganisms (such as bacteria, viruses, fungi and protozoa) and tumour cells. Its function is to protect the body from anything that could be harmful. In order to carry out this function it has to be able to recognise 'self', which is tolerated, and 'non-self', which it attacks and attempts to eliminate or destroy.

Human beings and animals have a number of non-specific barriers to foreign substances; e.g. the intact skin protects the body from invasion and substances in some body fluids help to kill microorganisms (see Fig. 16.1). It is when these barriers fail or are compromised that the specific immune responses come into play.

Healthy individuals can fight off infection by immune mechanisms and in many cases immunity to a disease occurs after a single encounter with the infectious organism. Sometimes, the system is unable to function normally because of an immune deficiency or a functional disorder. When a large number of microorganisms enter the body, the immune system may function normally but still be too slow to prevent the person from developing the infectious disease. Immune suppression can occur as a result of other disease; it can also be iatrogenic, resulting from drug treatment or radiotherapy.

Epidemiology

Methods of reporting the diseases of the immune system vary and in some instances yield only an estimate of their occurrence. Statistics about infectious diseases, however, are more readily available because of the statutory requirement for notification of certain infections (Emond et al 1989).

So important is the immune system that few people, if any, can survive with a severe immune defect. Nonetheless, nurses are likely to encounter a range of immune disorders in their work. Hyperactive disorders such as asthma (see Ch. 3, p. 73) are thought to affect around 5% of people in Britain, while up to 10% of the population suffer from allergies to common substances such as grass pollens, animal danders, and food allergens. Genetic factors are important in these diseases, but it is thought that environmental pollution is also a contributing factor. Advances in medical treatment have meant that organs can now be transplanted with a degree of success and malignancies controlled if not eliminated. Unfortunately, organ transplantation and cancer therapy involve the destruction or suppression of vital components of the immune system, thus predisposing the patient to over-

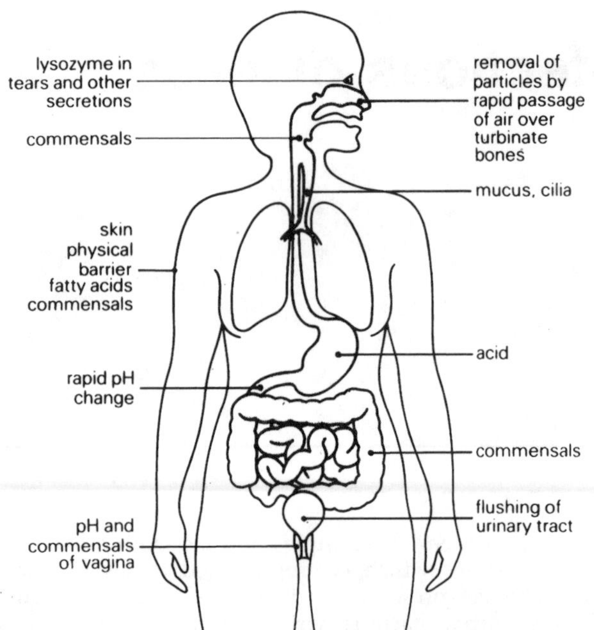

Fig. 16.1 Non-specific barriers to infection, before entry into the tissues. Invasion by potentially pathogenic organisms is limited by a variety of non-specific mechanisms.

1. The intact skin is impenetrable to most bacteria. Additionally, fatty acids produced by the skin are toxic to many organisms. The pathogenicity of some strains correlates with their ability to survive on the skin.
2. Epithelial surfaces are cleansed, for example, by ciliary action in the trachea or by flushing of the urinary tract.
3. pH changes in the stomach and vagina lead to destruction of many bacteria—both are acidic. In the case of the vagina, the epithelium secretes glycogen, which is metabolised by particular species of commensal bacteria producing lactic acid. This also limits pathogen invasion.
4. Commensals occupy particular ecological niches and so stop pathogens gaining access to these sites. Thus Candida or *Clostridium difficile* can occur when the normal flora is disturbed by antibiotics.

(Reproduced with kind permission from Roitt, Brostoff and Male 1989).

whelming infection due to an acquired immune deficiency. The autoimmune diseases, in which the body attacks its own cells, are comparatively rare, and their cause is not completely understood at present.

Infectious diseases have been around for centuries, but many factors have influenced the pattern of their occurrence in recent years. Smallpox has virtually been eradicated from the world by the widespread use of vaccination (Reid et al 1986), and vaccination has had a significant effect in reducing the incidence of many other diseases such as polio, whooping cough, measles and rubella. The decline in tuberculosis has probably been due more to improved sanitation, hygiene, nutrition, and housing than to vaccination, although anti-tubercular drugs have had a significant effect. Tuberculosis, however, is on the rise again, and is seen in some patients with human immunodeficiency virus (HIV) infection and the acquired immune deficiency syndrome (AIDS) (see Ch. 38, p. 1006).

Some infections have been recognised only in the last 15–20 years, e.g. legionnaire's disease in 1976, and AIDS in the 1980s. Others, such as campylobacter and toxoplasmosis, are recognised more frequently than in the past.

Some hazards arise from behaviour and lifestyle. The number of people suffering from sexually transmitted diseases has increased over the last 20 years (OPCS 1988). Intravenous drug misuse leads to the risk of blood-borne disease such as hepatitis B or HIV infection through the sharing of contaminated injection equipment. (These diseases are also transmitted sexually.)

Changes in cooking and eating habits (e.g. a reliance on microwave ovens and fast foods) have emphasised the necessity for thorough and adequate cooking of all foods which are known to be frequently contaminated with organisms such as the Salmonella species. Processed foods can also be a problem; for example, soft cheeses, pâté and yoghurt have on occasion been found to be contaminated with *Listeria monocytogenes*.

Increased foreign travel has meant that diseases can cross borders as easily as their hosts or victims. Malaria, for example, is often contracted abroad, but becomes apparent only after the traveller returns home.

Food poisoning is one of the most common notifiable infectious diseases in the UK. Measles is still extremely common in spite of the reduction in cases by large-scale vaccination programmes. It is likely that the increase in HIV infection and AIDS throughout the world will influence the future incidence of other infectious diseases.

The nurse's role

The nurse is in an ideal position to educate people about the avoidance and management of infectious diseases. A home visit to any patient is an ideal opportunity to assess and give advice on food safety and on the prevention of infection through good hygiene. A patient recovering from salmonellosis or hepatitis B may be anxious about transmitting the infection to others and require practical advice; such advice should emphasise what *can* as well as what *can not* be done.

For infectious patients who are unable or unwilling to act upon such advice special arrangements may have to be made to ensure that others are not put at unnecessary risk. The assessment of the patient as an individual is particularly important in these circumstances.

ANATOMY AND PHYSIOLOGY

The lymphoid system

The lymphoid (or lymphatic) system consists of organs and tissues made up of cells which are involved in the immune response (see Fig. 16.2). These structures may be described as being either primary or secondary, as follows.

Primary lymphoid organs

The thymus gland and the bone marrow are known as primary lymphoid organs. Lymphocytes develop in the bone marrow (see Ch. 11, p. 408). T lymphocytes differentiate in the thymus gland, and B lymphocytes differentiate in the bone marrow. It is in the organ where they differentiate that lymphocytes acquire the surface receptors which enable them to recognise antigens.

Secondary lymphoid organs

The spleen and lymph nodes are known as secondary lymphoid organs, as are other areas of lymphoid tissue which are associated with mucosal surfaces in the body, such as in the respiratory, gastrointestinal, and genitourinary systems. The spleen contains white blood cells or leukocytes (see Ch. 11, p. 408) and is involved in the breakdown of erythrocytes, leukocytes and platelets. The lymph nodes

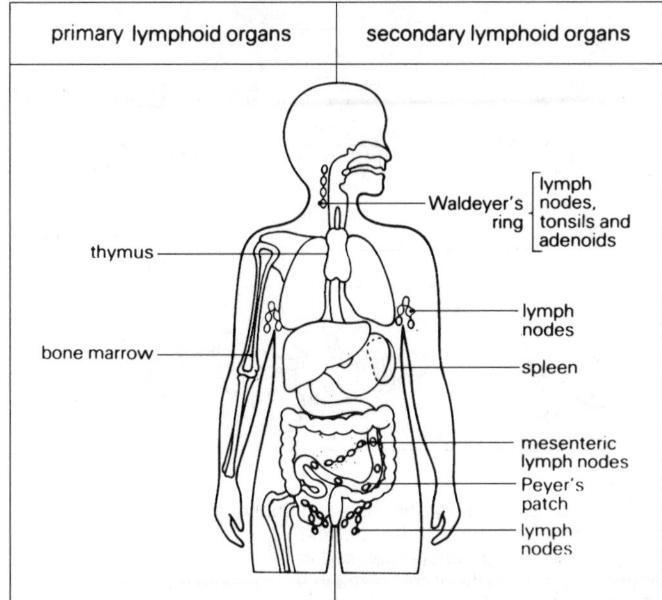

Fig. 16.2 Major lymphoid organs and tissues. The thymus produces T cells and the bone marrow, B cells. The secondary lymphoid organs and tissues contain mature T and B cells and accessory cells. In the mammalian foetus the B cells are initially generated in the liver. In man the adult bone marrow is also a secondary lymphoid organ. Lymph nodes are present throughout the body (only a few are depicted here) and are usually found at the junctions of lymphatic vessels. Lymph nodes drain the tissue spaces and the lymphocytes at these sites generally respond to lymph-borne antigens whilst lymphoid cells in the spleen respond to blood-borne antigens. Peyer's patches are unencapsulated masses of lymphoid tissue in the small intestine.
(Reproduced with kind permission from Roitt, Brostoff and Male 1989.)

are small collections of lymphoid tissue (1–25 mm in diameter) which are found all over the body, often where lymphatic vessels branch. Lymph nodes act as filters, trapping any foreign materials or antigens so that they can be attacked and destroyed by specialised white blood cells which accumulate there in large numbers.

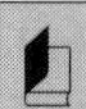
Further information: Wilson 1990.

Types of immune response

Two types of immune response are involved in recognising and eliminating any 'foreign' material which enters the body. These are:

1. *Non-specific or innate immunity*, by which any foreign cell or particle is identified as such and attacked. Even tumour cells which arise in the body's own tissues can be recognised as foreign and may be destroyed. This response is non-specific in that it is the same whether the foreign particle or antigen is a bacterium, a particle of asbestos, or anything else. The response occurs as soon as the antigen is encountered. No 'memory' is involved, and a second contact with the same antigen will produce the same response at the same rate.

2. *Specific or adaptive immunity*, in which special cells (B and T lymphocytes) are programmed to respond to recognised antigens. This response is highly specific: each lymphocyte is equipped to recognise only one antigen. Once contact has been made with that antigen and it has been destroyed, some 'memory' cells (see p. 546) remain in the body. If the same antigen is encountered again, these cells are stimulated to reproduce, and the response is both faster and greater (see p. 548).

Table 16.1 Cells and chemicals involved in immunity

Cells	Chemical molecules
Phagocytes: • neutrophils • monocytes • macrophages	Complement proteins Proteins
Accessory cells: • eosinophils • basophils • mast cells	Lymphokines Histamine Antibodies
Lymphocytes: • B lymphocytes • T lymphocytes • NK (natural killer) cells	

Cells and chemicals involved

Table 16.1 lists the cells and chemicals involved in the immune response.

Cells

The cells involved in the immune response are white blood cells (leukocytes). These may be granular (also called granulocytes or polymorphonuclear leukocytes) — the neutrophils, basophils and eosinophils — or non-granular (also called agranulocytes) — the monocytes and lymphocytes. In this section these cells will be described according to their function.

Phagocytes have the ability to recognise foreign material and to engulf and digest microorganisms by a process called phagocytosis. Three different cells are classed as phagocytes, namely neutrophils, monocytes and macrophages.

Neutrophils are small cells and live only for a few days. They originate in the bone marrow and circulate in the blood.

Monocytes are roughly the same size as neutrophils. They also originate in the bone marrow and circulate in the blood, but they may enter the tissues, where they become macrophages.

Macrophages are larger than neutrophils and monocytes. They are long-lived and are found in the tissues, principally in the liver, spleen, lymph nodes and lungs. Mainly involved in non-specific immunity, they are also activated by lymphokines, which are produced by some T cells in the cell-mediated immune response (see p. 548). Phagocytosis can take place only if the invading cell becomes adherent to the surface of the phagocyte. This occurs by a chemical attraction between the surface of the phagocyte and antigen. The process can be assisted by complement (see p. 546) and by antibodies.

Accessory cells. These cells function by releasing chemicals which are harmful to invading organisms. This group of cells comprises eosinophils, basophils and mast cells.

Eosinophils are capable of phagocytosis, but their main function is to attach themselves to larger parasites such as helminths (worms) and kill them by releasing harmful substances. They may also help to control the inflammatory response by breaking down histamine. There is an increase in the number of eosinophils in people suffering from allergic conditions or from parasitic infections.

Basophils and mast cells contain histamine and other chemicals which give rise to an inflammatory response when released. They are important in some allergies, e.g. hay fever (see p. 559). Basophils circulate in the blood stream. Mast cells, although similar in function, are located in connective tissues and mucous membranes.

Lymphocytes originate in the bone marrow as stem cells and subsequently differentiate into the following types.

B cells are the lymphocytes which produce antibodies. They differentiate in the bone marrow and then mature in the secondary lymphoid tissues. The antigen receptor on their surface is specific for one antigen only. B lymphocytes are capable of 'memory' (see p. 547) and are specialised to deal with microorganisms which do not, of their own accord, enter host cells (e.g. circulating bacteria).

T cells are the regulatory lymphocytes which control the activity of other T and B cells. They originate in the bone marrow and then mature and differentiate in the thymus gland. They are also antigen-specific. T lymphocytes are capable of 'memory' and are specialised to deal mainly with microorganisms which invade host cells (e.g. viruses).

There are four types of T cells:

- T-helper cells
- T-suppressor cells
- cytotoxic T cells.

T-helper cells assist B cells to produce antibodies by enabling the B cell to interact with the antigen to which the T cell has 'bound'. They also produce mediators called lymphokines, which activate macrophages (see below). *T-suppressor* cells regulate the activity of B cells and other T cells by, for example, inhibiting antibody production. *Cytotoxic T cells* recognise and combine with antigens on the surface of a foreign or virally-infected cell and destroy the cell by lysis.

Natural killer (NK) cells have an uncertain origin but are a type of lymphocyte. Their function is to kill some tumour cells as well as virally-infected cells before the virus has had time to reproduce within the cell. They are activated by the interferons, a class of proteins found to be effective against some viruses by rendering surrounding cells resistant to viral attack.

Chemicals

Complement is the collective name for a series of proteins which induce chemical reactions. Their three main functions are:

1. To coat microorganisms with a substance which phagocytic cells can recognise. This ensures that the microorganism adheres to the surface of the phagocytic cell.
2. To activate the destruction of the microorganism inside the phagocyte once ingestion has taken place. Complement also participates in the acute inflammatory response by inducing vasodilation and increasing the permeability of the capillary endothelium.
3. To assist in the lysis of invading cells. (See Fig. 16.3.)

Lymphokines are a series of proteins whose structure is not completely understood. They are produced mainly by T lymphocytes (after activation by an antigen) and enhance the inflammatory response at the site of infection in the following ways:

- by causing macrophages to aggregate and stimulating them to destroy foreign particles by phagocytosis
- by attracting neutrophils and monocytes.

The interferons are one example of lymphokines. Interferons are synthesised by virally infected cells as well as T lymphocytes and released into the extracellular fluid. They activate NK cells but are thought to be more significant in the recovery from viral infection than in its prevention.

Specific, sensitised T cells release lymphokines on contact with an antigen but the lymphokine itself is not specific to that antigen and may help to protect the individual from other microorganisms encountered at the same time.

Histamine is released by mast cells when they degranulate after adhering to a microorganism. It gives rise to increased vascular permeability, arteriolar dilatation, smooth muscle contraction in the respiratory and alimentary tracts, and increased secretion of respiratory mucus.

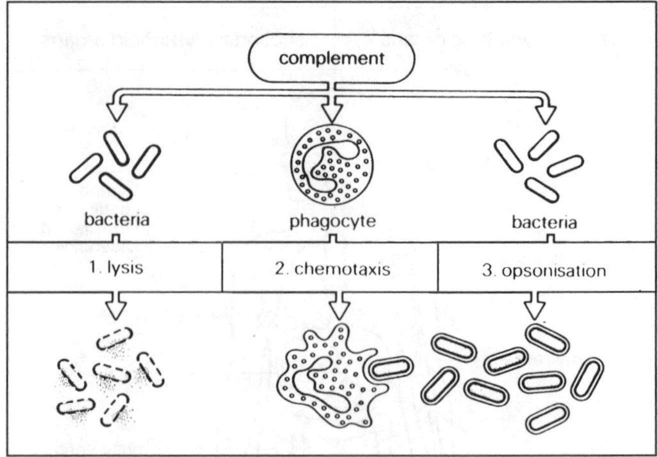

Fig. 16.3 Complement functions.
1. The complement system has an intrinsic ability to lyse the cell membranes of many bacterial species.
2. Complement products released in this reaction attract phagocytes to the site of the reaction — chemotaxis.
3. Once they arrive at the site of reaction other complement components coating the bacterial surface allow the phagocyte to recognise the bacteria and facilitate bacterial phagocytosis — opsonisation.
These are all functions of the innate immune system, although the reactions can also be triggered by the adaptive immune system.
(Reproduced with kind permission from Roitt, Brostoff and Male 1989.)

Antibodies are the principal substances involved in the adaptive or specific immune response. Collectively known as immunoglobulins, they are proteins capable of recognising and binding to their own specific antigen (usually a microorganism).

Antibodies are produced by B lymphocytes and, once formed, circulate in the plasma. They have three functions:

- to bind to antigens
- to bind to phagocytes
- to activate the complement pathway.

There are five classes of antibody: immunoglobulin G (IgG), IgA, IgM, IgD, and IgE. Each of the five classes may be produced with specificity for a single antigen. Their structure varies according to function and they are present in different amounts in the bloodstream (see Box 16.1).

The immune response

The non-specific immune response

When a foreign substance enters the body, the first line of defence is the non-specific immune response, which comprises the following components:

- mechanical barriers (e.g. cilia in the upper respiratory tract)
- phagocytes
- chemicals (complement, the interferons)
- substances found in body secretions (e.g. lysozyme, gastric acid).

These defences can be effective on their own, but help is sometimes needed from adaptive or specific immune response mechanisms.

Disadvantages of the non-specific response are as follows:

- The cells can differentiate between 'self' and 'non-self' but cannot recognise specific antigens

Box 16.1 Immunoglobulins

Immunoglobulins are proteins with known antibody activity. They form the central component of the immune system and are synthesised by lymphocytes and plasma cells. The five classes of immunoglobulins are as follows:

- IgM: the first immunoglobulin to appear in the blood stream in the primary response to infection. Since it disappears fairly quickly after the antigen disappears, it is an indicator of current or very recent infection.
- IgG: produced in large quantities in both the primary and secondary responses to infection. It is also important as a defence against infection in the first few weeks of life, being the only immunoglobulin which crosses the placenta to the fetus.
- IgA: secreted onto the luminal surface of the respiratory, alimentary and genitourinary tracts and present in saliva, tracheobronchial, and genitourinary secretions as well as in the serum. It is important in preventing the entry of microorganisms from the external orifices of the body.
- IgE: normally found on the surface membrane of basophils and mast cells. It is associated with allergic reactions such as hay fever.
- IgD: present in small quantities bound to B cells where it aids in the 'memory' function.

Immunoglobulins can be taken from a donor by plasmapheresis, and given:

- to someone who has been exposed to a pathogen and is not immune, e.g. antitetanus immunoglobulin (Humotet).
- as short-term prophylaxis, when it is known that a person will be exposed to a pathogen and vaccine is not available, e.g. hepatitis A immunoglobulin for travellers to countries where hepatitis A is common.
- to someone who is heavily immunosuppressed, following exposure to a pathogen which could cause serious infection because of an inadequate immune response.

Passive immunisation with immunoglobulins does not confer long-term protection: this requires vaccination (see p. 548).

- It does not adapt after exposure, i.e. the same level of response is produced for each exposure to an antigen
- It does not have a 'memory' and so cannot prevent the individual from developing the same infection a second time.

The specific immune response: natural immunity

The specific immune response involves the lymphocytes and comprises the humoral or antibody-mediated response (initiated by B lymphocytes) and the cell-mediated response (initiated by T lymphocytes). These responses are described separately here, but they interact with each other as well as with non-specific factors. The humoral response deals mainly with extracellular organisms and the antibodies which it produces are present in the serum. The cell-mediated response is important for dealing with intracellular organisms.

Specificity. When it is first exposed to an antigen, the circulating lymphocyte differentiates to recognise and bind to that one particular antigen. This recognition and binding is like a lock and key mechanism on a door. Many different keys may go into the same lock, but only one will fit closely enough to turn in the lock and open the door (the primary response).

On re-exposure to the antigen, perhaps many years later, the remaining progeny of that cell (memory cells) will be stimulated to replicate (the secondary response).

Antibody-mediated immune response. This response may be described in terms of its primary and secondary phases.

Primary response. The first time an antigen is encountered in the body it takes about two weeks for a corresponding antibody to be detectable in the blood. The production of this antibody is called the primary response. Although the immune system reacts immediately to antigens, the synthesis of antibodies takes some time. An antigen binds to its specific receptor on the surface of the B lymphocyte, triggering the following sequence of events:

1. The B lymphocyte is stimulated to develop into a *plasma cell* and to undergo multiple divisions so that identical plasma cells are formed.
2. The plasma cells synthesise antibodies.
3. Some B cells differentiate to become *memory cells*, which persist and replicate in the body long after the invading antigen has been dealt with (see Fig. 16.4).
4. Once sufficient quantities of an antibody have been produced to destroy all the antigen, the plasma cells die, leaving memory cells ready to respond to a future attack by that antigen.
5. Antibodies bind to the antigen, activating the complement system.
6. When several antibodies bind to one antigen, the complex thus formed is chemically attracted to the surface of phagocytic cells,

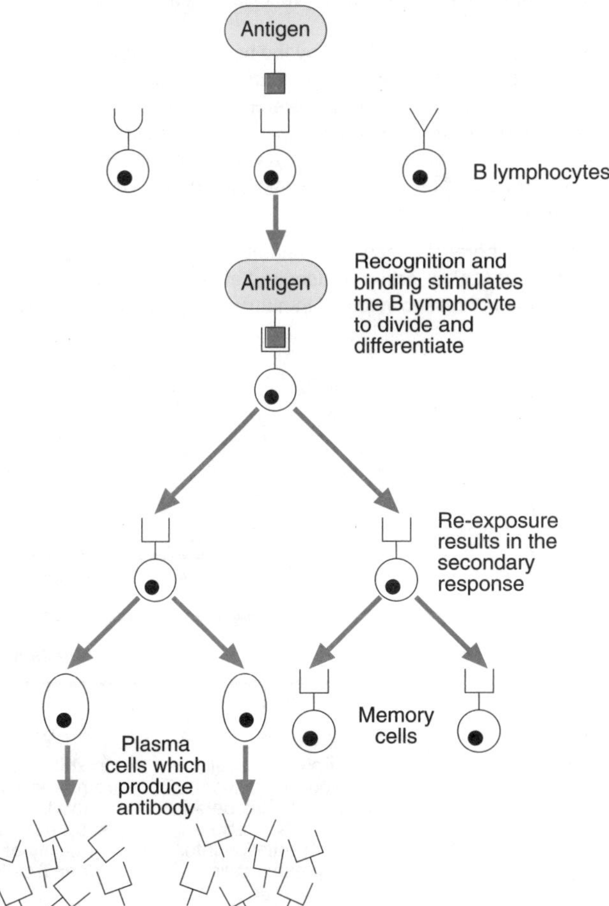

Fig. 16.4 The primary immune response.

resulting in the formation of an antigen–antibody–phagocyte complex.

7. The presence of antibodies seems to trigger the phagocyte into action, resulting in ingestion and digestion of the bacterium.

The time interval between contact with the antigen, and the production of antibodies (IgM) may allow disease to develop in the individual due to the effects of the antigen (e.g. infection from microorganisms).

Secondary response. When the body encounters an antigen for the second time (or subsequently) the memory cells respond rapidly by producing plasma cells, which then produce antibodies. This response occurs within a few days, and, together with any residual antibody from the primary response, usually prevents disease from developing. In other words, the individual is immune.

Immunisation: artificial immunity

Vaccination or immunisation is a means of artificially invoking a primary immune response to a particular microorganism (antigen) so that when the antigen is subsequently encountered the individual will be immune to it. The principle of immunisation is to introduce altered microorganisms or toxins into the body so that the individual does not develop the disease, but does mount an immune response. In other words, it mimics the natural response to infectious disease. Booster doses may be required months or years after the first dose of a vaccine in order to maintain an adequate level of memory cells. There are three types of vaccine:

1. *Live attenuated vaccines.* Laboratory culturing of virulent strains of some organisms causes them to lose their virulence. These are then capable of inducing immunity without causing disease. The BCG (tuberculosis) and rubella vaccines are of this type. It can be dangerous to administer a live vaccine to someone who is immunosuppressed.
2. *Toxoids.* The toxin produced by the bacterium is chemically modified by Formalin treatment so that its toxicity is lost but it retains its antigenicity and is therefore still capable of inducing an immune response. The tetanus toxoid is an example of this type.
3. *Killed vaccines* are preparations in which the organisms have been killed by heat or chemicals; the whooping cough vaccine is one example.

Immunity, therefore, can be natural (acquired in utero or after infectious disease) or artificial (acquired after immunisation). Fig. 16.5 illustrates the processes involved in natural and artificial immunity.

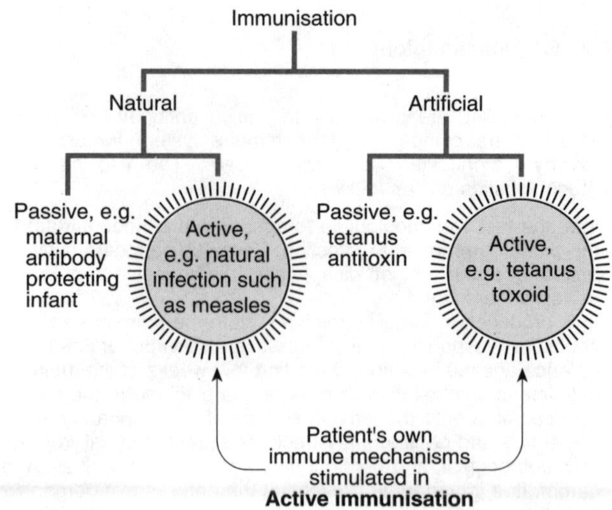

Fig. 16.5 Natural and artifical immunity. (Reproduced with kind permission from Kirkwood E, Lewis C 1989 Understanding medical immunology, 2nd edn. John Wiley & Sons Ltd, Chichester:)

Cell-mediated immune response. The first stage in this process is the binding of the antigen to the antigen receptor on the T lymphocyte, sometimes in conjunction with macrophages. This activates the T lymphocyte to divide and differentiate into T-helper cells, T-suppressor cells, and cytotoxic T cells, as illustrated in Fig. 16.6.

Once all the antigen has been dealt with, the T-suppressor cells will stop the antibody production by the B lymphocytes, and the destructive process ends — until the next time.

The involvement of other cells (e.g. mast cells) in the immune response has been discussed on page 545.

CONTROL OF INFECTION

Considering their disparity in size, the relationship between man and the microorganisms with which he shares his world is a paradoxical one. Too small to be seen except under a microscope, some of these organisms can cause severe disease and even death in their host if the conditions are favourable

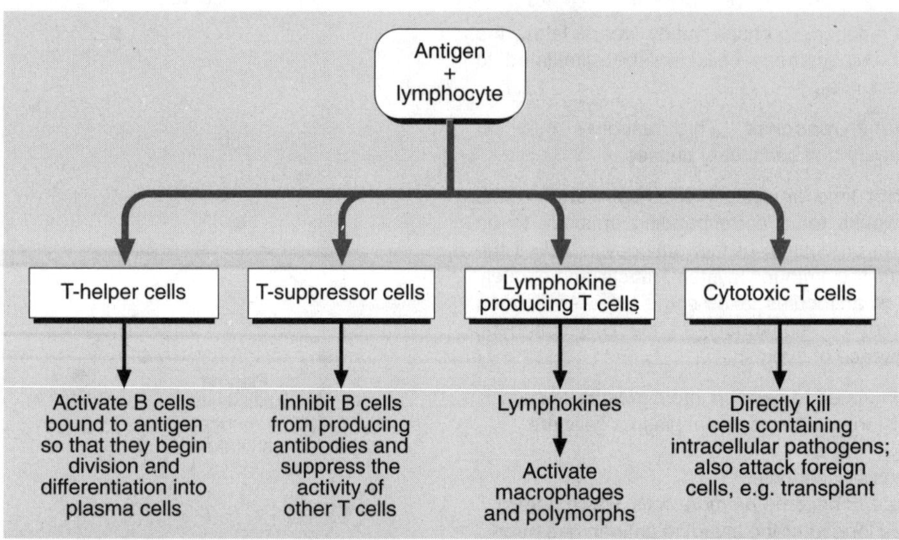

Fig. 16.6 Differentiation of T lymphocytes as a result of encounter with antigen.

for them to do so. On the other hand, some microorganisms are normal inhabitants of the human body (e.g. on the skin and in the gut), and without them we should be in grave danger of invasion by pathogenic (disease-producing) organisms. This situation can arise when people are treated unnecessarily with antibiotics which kill the useful microorganisms that normally compete with invading bacteria.

Disease-producing organisms

Why are some organisms pathogenic and others not? The extent to which an organism is capable of producing disease will depend on the nature of the organism, its location, the numbers present, and the state of the host's defences. It is not possible to classify all organisms as either pathogens or commensals (commensals are those which normally live harmlessly on or in the body), for some commensals can be pathogenic if they are transferred to a more susceptible site. For example, *Escherichia coli* is a normal commensal in the gastrointestinal tract, but it can cause urinary tract infection if it gets into the bladder.

The first microorganisms a healthy newborn baby encounters are those in the birth canal of its mother and on the hands of its attendants. The baby's skin very quickly becomes colonised, and once feeding is established the gut is also colonised. These organisms are usually those which constitute the normal flora of the body (Table 16.2), but can also include disease-producing organisms.

There are other organisms which are always considered to be pathogenic, as they inevitably produce disease if they are introduced into the body in large enough numbers; one such example is *Salmonella typhimurium*.

Control of infection in patient care

Nurses have a responsibility not only to assist individuals to return to good health, but also to prevent further illness while the healing process is taking place. Patients should also be given the information they need in order to stay healthy; for example, a patient at home with a urinary catheter should be taught how to keep the urethral meatus clean and to prevent the introduction of bowel or other organisms; or an elderly patient should be reminded that by scratching a leg ulcer infection is likely to be caused by the introduction of organisms into a site where they will happily grow and multiply. Nurses also have a responsibility to prevent the spread of infection from one person to another (crossinfection or exogenous infection), whether from patient to nurse, nurse to patient, nurse to nurse, or patient to patient. Nurses must all do what they can to ensure the safety of patients and of other health care staff.

Table 16.2 Normal commensal microorganisms

Site	Organism
Skin	*Staph. epidermidis* Diphtheroids Corynebacterium sp.
Mouth and throat	Staphylococci Streptococci Anaerobes Neisseria sp.
Nose	Staphylococci Diphtheroids
Gut	*Escherichia coli* Klebsiella sp. Proteus sp. *Strep. faecalis* *Clostridium perfringens* Yeasts (Candida)
Kidneys and bladder	Normally sterile
Vagina	Lactobacilli Streptococci Staphylococci Anaerobes

?	**16.1** How might infection spread within a hospital setting?

The patient with an infection may not know the importance of even the simplest measures (e.g. thorough handwashing) to prevent it spreading. Many people have misconceptions about how infections are acquired, and it may be helpful if the nurse asks the patient what he understands about his illness so that appropriate information can be given. At times, the nurse may have to use a great deal of subtlety to persuade the patient to change his behaviour.

The problem of infection is much greater in hospital than at home for a number of reasons, which include the following:

- Sick people are gathered together
- Each has a large number of attendants — nurses, doctors, physiotherapists, domestics and many more
- Normal skin barriers are broken by surgery and invasive procedures
- Equipment and instruments may be used for a number of patients
- Food is cooked and stored in bulk
- Stress, which is thought to lower resistance to infection, is caused by being in hospital.

Nevertheless, the principles of controlling infection should be applied in the home as well as the hospital setting; at all times, the nurse must do everything she can to prevent the spread of infection. Indeed this is part of her professional responsibility (UKCC 1992). Most health boards/authorities have a control of infection nurse who gives advice and provides information to all health care staff.

?	**16.2** How would you protect yourself from getting an infection at work?

Microorganisms can neither walk, jump, nor fly: they have to be *transferred*, usually in body fluids or on the surface of articles or hands. It follows, therefore, that any body fluid is capable of transmitting infection, and that the hands of doctors and nurses, as well as instruments and other equipment used on patients, are potential means of transfer.

Policies

Many arrangements and procedures in health care are governed by legislation or by guidelines issued from time to time by the UK Health Departments: the Department of Health (DOH) in England, formerly the Department of Health and Social Security (DHSS); the Scottish Office Home and Health Department (SOHHD) in Scotland; the Welsh Office in Wales; and the Department of Health and Social Services (DHSS) in Northern Ireland. Documents governing infection control are numerous and are updated from time to time. Health boards/authorities are expected to have up-to-date local policies based on national guidelines.

Policies that cover every eventuality are so lengthy and

cumbersome that they are unlikely to be read or used. In addition, individualised care precludes the writing of very detailed guidelines, because the assessment of the patient as an individual determines the care required. Policies that are easy to understand and apply are more likely to be followed, but in order to achieve simplicity without compromising safety it may be necessary to set general rules which are more than may be required in each individual case.

In this chapter examples are given of policy requirements as well as of additional measures that can be taken. It is important that nurses be familiar with existing control of infection policies in their place of work.

Safe working practice

Safe working practice entails making sure that one does not put oneself or others at unnecessary risk of acquiring an infection (see Box 16.2). It is not always possible to identify people who have transmissible infections; indeed, many (such as symptomless hepatitis B carriers) will be unaware of the fact themselves. By relying solely on identification the nurse may unknowingly expose herself to pathogens. Safe practice involves:

- good hand hygiene
- universal blood and body fluid precautions
- cleaning, disinfection or sterilisation of equipment, instruments and surfaces
- correct use of disinfectants
- aseptic technique
- safe disposal of waste, sharps and linen
- isolation precautions when patients have a known or suspected infection.

Each of these elements of safe practice will now be considered in turn.

Hand hygiene

Hands should ideally be washed after each patient contact. This is not always possible, however, and an alcohol wipe or handrub (if approved by the local health board/authority) may be used instead.

Liquid antibacterial soaps (e.g. those containing chlorhexidine or povidone iodine) have been shown to kill a higher percentage of microorganisms than soap and water (Lowbury & Lilly 1973). Some authorities advocate the use of an antibacterial cleanser *after* the hands have been contaminated with a body fluid (including contact with contaminated equipment) and *before* an aseptic procedure is carried out (e.g. wound dressing or emptying a urinary catheter drainage bag). Others believe that a soap and water wash is adequate, as it has not been proved that the reduction in number of microorganisms achieved by using an antibacterial soap actually reduces the incidence of infection in patients (Ayliffe et al 1988), although this has been demonstrated in intensive care units (Larson 1988).

It is important that all surfaces of both hands are washed thoroughly, taking particular care with the areas likely to be missed (Taylor 1978a–b), i.e. the fingertips, finger webs and the back of the thumbs. The hands should first of all be wetted, the soap applied and used to wash the hands, and the hands rinsed and thoroughly dried, preferably with paper towels. The taps should be turned off with the elbow or wrist.

?	**16.3** Why should you not turn the taps off with your hands?

If elbow or wrist-action taps are not available, a paper towel should be used to turn off the tap. Handwashing is essentially simple, easily forgotten, but nonetheless crucial to safe patient care: just think of all the things one does with one's hands! (See Box 16.3.)

Universal blood and body fluid precautions

The UK Health Departments (1990) consider that blood, body fluids likely to contain blood, and certain other body fluids such as cerebrospinal fluid are capable of transmitting infection, and recommend that precautions are taken in the handling of these body fluids. Some authorities believe that all body fluids should be treated as if they were infectious, given the difficulty in identifying people who have transmissible infections — for example, salmonella excretors or hepatitis B carriers. If the nurse assumes that all body fluids *might* be infectious, then she will avoid unnecessary risk.

In this chapter, the term 'universal precautions' refers to measures taken to protect health workers when they have contact with blood or other body fluids from *anyone*, regardless of whether that individual is known to have an infection or not. All patients are thus treated in the same way, except when *additional* isolation precautions are required (see p. 555; Box 16.4; Research Abstract 16.1).

Cleaning, disinfecting and sterilising equipment, instruments and surfaces

Instruments, equipment and surfaces used in patient care may be 'sterile', 'disinfected', or 'clean', depending upon the standard of cleanliness demanded by the patient's condition and by the nature of the procedure being carried out.

There are different ways of determining whether instruments need to be sterile, disinfected, or clean. Rutala (1990) makes this determination in terms of three categories of instrument use, i.e:

Box 16.2 Safe practice: preventing infection

- Wash hands thoroughly and frequently.
- Cover all cuts and broken skin with a waterproof plaster.
- Wear the appropriate protective clothing for contact with all body fluids and substances.
- Keep immunisations up to date.
- Be familiar with procedures for needlestick injury and accidental contamination with body fluid.

Box 16.3 Hand hygiene

Hands should be washed:

After
- examining or caring for a patient
- going to the toilet
- they have been contaminated with body fluids
- handling a patient in standard isolation or leaving a strict isolation room.

Before
- leaving a patient or work area
- eating or serving food
- carrying out an aseptic procedure
- entering a protective isolation room.

Box 16.4 Universal blood and body fluid precautions

- Cover cuts and broken skin with a waterproof plaster.
- Wear disposable gloves if you are going to be handling blood or body fluids.
- Wear a disposable apron (and perhaps a gown) if your uniform or clothing is likely to be contaminated.
- Wear a facemask and protective visor or spectacles if you think your eyes or mouth might be splashed.

Research abstract 16.1

A study by Kelen et al (1989) was carried out to assess the impact of the HIV epidemic on the emergency department of an American inner-city hospital, where the known prevalence of HIV infection was around 5%. Staff adherence to universal precautions was observed. The study took place after health care workers had received instruction, within the previous year, on the risks to them of acquiring HIV infection. Instructional posters were visible throughout the department, and protective clothing was available.

The results of the study showed an overall HIV seroprevalence rate of 6% (152 out of 2544 patients), of whom 3.7% (95 patients) were not known to be HIV positive.

Personnel adhered to universal precautions only 44% of the time and, in caring for patients with severe bleeding, only 19.5% of the time.

Kelen G D, DiGiovanna T, Bisson L, Kalainov D, Sivertson K T, Quinn T C 1989 Human immunodeficiency virus infection in emergency department patients. Journal of the American Medical Association 262(4): 516–522

- critical — devices which enter sterile tissue or the vascular system: these must be sterile
- semi-critical — devices which touch non-intact skin and mucous membranes: these must be disinfected
- non-critical — devices which touch intact skin: these must be clean.

The British Medical Association (1989) gives a similar classification in terms of 'high', 'medium' and 'low' risk areas of the body. These classifications are organised in terms of the *future* use of an instrument, and so do not refer to items which have *already* been contaminated by body fluids or used on patients with known infection. Such items are obviously also likely to inadvertently or indirectly transmit infection, by the oral or mucosal route, and must be disinfected.

Sterilisation. A sterile object is one which is free from all microorganisms, including spores. Sterilisation in hospitals can be reliably done only by heat, using an autoclave.

Spores are formed by some bacteria such as *Clostridium tetani* or *C. perfringens* when they encounter adverse conditions. The bacterium encases itself in a tough, resistant shell which allows it to survive for weeks or months in dust or soil. When conditions become favourable (i.e. in the presence of warmth, moisture and a food source) the spores germinate and regain all the properties of bacteria. Spores are difficult to kill, requiring a sterilisation process to ensure their destruction.

?	**16.4** When could spores germinate in a patient in hospital?

Surgery and traumatic injury present the greatest risk for infection caused by spores. This is because deep tissues or body cavities may be penetrated and inadvertently implanted with spores. Sterilisation is required for all instruments which are used subcutaneously (under the skin) or submucosally (across mucous membrane into a sterile cavity); this includes surgical instruments, injection needles, urinary catheters, and instruments being passed into the uterus. Ideally, it is carried out in a hospital sterilisation and disinfection unit (HSDU).

Once instruments have been sterilised, they must be kept sterile until they are used. This is done by packing the instrument (before autoclaving but after thorough cleaning and drying) in a special autoclave bag made of paper which is permeable to steam but impermeable when dry. The autoclave uses steam under pressure (usually at 134 °C for 3 minutes) which penetrates the bag. The packs are then dried before the cycle is complete. As long as the packaging remains undamaged and dry, the contents of the bag should be sterile. The pack should therefore be checked for damage and signs of dampness before it is used. Dentists, general practitioners and some hospital departments may use a small autoclave suitable only for naked (i.e. unpackaged) instruments. These autoclaves are useful in situations where sterile instruments are required for *immediate* use only, as sterility cannot be maintained.

Special autoclave tape, or a small coloured panel on the bag, is used to indicate if a pack has been sterilised. The appearance of dark stripes on the tape, or a colour change in the panel, indicates that the pack has been through a sterilisation process.

Instruments that have been used on patients at risk from Jakob–Creutzfeldt disease are treated differently from all other surgical instruments. Jakob–Creutzfeldt disease, which affects the central nervous system, causing senile dementia and psychosis, is caused by an organism resistant to the normal sterilisation and disinfection procedures (i.e. autoclaving at 134 °C for 3 minutes or immersion in glutaraldehyde, see p. 552).

Contaminated instruments from someone at risk of developing this disease may have to be destroyed (SOHHD, 1993a). Contaminated instruments from people with tuberculosis, HIV, or hepatitis B are sometimes autoclaved before they are handled in the HSDU. This may not be necessary if an automatic wash process at 98°C for 5 min. is performed.

Disinfection ensures freedom from harmful micro-organisms, but not spores, and is recommended for all instruments and surfaces which have been:

- in contact with body fluids, tissues, broken skin, or mucosal surfaces, pathological specimens or cultures
- used by, or on, patients with known or suspected infection
- about to be used by, or on, severely immuno-suppressed patients.

Disinfection is necessary to prevent cross-infection. It can be achieved using heat or chemicals; for small items, heat is the best method. Most micro-organisms are destroyed by a temperature of 80°C held for 1 min. but a higher temperature (98°C for 2 min.) is required to kill the hepatitis B virus (Kobayashi et al 1984). Equipment that is used in such close proximity to the patient that trauma to mucosal surfaces or contact with broken skin is likely (e.g. ENT instruments, sigmoidoscopes and breast pumps) may provide a vehicle for blood-borne viruses, such as hepatitis B, and should be cleaned and disinfected at a higher temperature such as 93°C for 10 min. in a washer disinfector.

Vaginal instruments, which may provide a vehicle for heat-resistant papillomaviruses, should be autoclaved at 134°C. Body fluid containers, for example, bedpans, urinals, suction

Research Abstract 16.2

A study by Greaves (1985) examined infection control practices relating to bed-baths and washbowls. Part of the study looked at the use and misuse of washbowls. One bowl in each of three wards was marked, and then observed twice daily for five days. In addition, 11 random bowls were sampled for microbiology by being rinsed out with normal saline and the resulting fluid sent for culture.

Articles of clothing (e.g. pants, nightdresses, scrotal supports) were found soaking in some of the bowls. Bowls were mostly communal, were frequently left wet, and were stacked upright, one on top of the other.

Questioning on other wards revealed that 9 out of 13 used some sort of disinfectant for cleaning the bowls, but most used Hibiscrub (a liquid antibacterial soap for handwashing). Of the 11 bowls randomly sampled, only 2 showed 'no growth'. Others showed the presence of microorganisms which could potentially cause infection if they reached a susceptible site.

Greaves' recommendations were as follows:

- Hospital patients should be supplied with their own bowls.
- These bowls should be washed with detergents and hot water after use, and dried and stored inverted, preferably in the patient's locker.
- Before a bowl is used for another patient it should be disinfected; stericol, a phenolic, is recommended.

Greaves A 1985 We'll just freshen you up, dear. Nursing Times Journal of Infection Control Nursing 81(10) Suppl: 3–8

jars and wash-bowls, are unlikely to be traumatic or to provide a vehicle for blood-borne transmission, and should be cleaned and disinfected at 80°C for 1 min. in a washer disinfector designed for that purpose. (See Research Abstract 16.2.)

An autoclave can be used for disinfection where a washer/disinfector is not available, in which case the items must be thoroughly cleaned and dried first. They do not need to be individually wrapped, as sterility does not need to be maintained. The disinfection process is used simply to kill any microorganisms which have been deposited on an instrument before it is used for another patient. Figure 16.7 gives an example of a policy for the disinfection of small items.

Chemical disinfectants can be used to disinfect heat-sensitive instruments (e.g. flexible endoscopes) but the process is fraught with difficulties. Some of the problems with the use of chemicals are as follows:

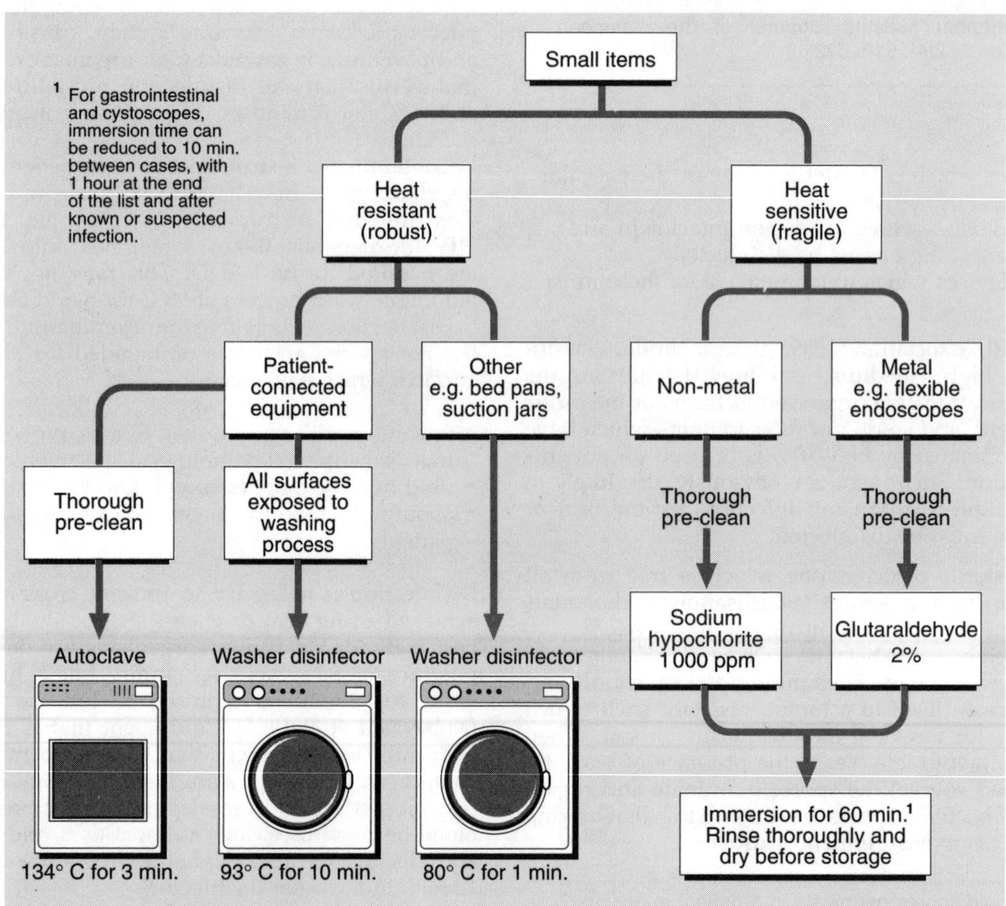

Fig. 16.7 An example of a policy for disinfection of small items. (Reproduced with kind permission from Dr A. B. White, Raigmore Hospital.)

- They are not all effective against commonly encountered microorganisms.
- They tend to be inactivated by body fluids, and so the surfaces of the item must be clean before it is immersed.
- The correct strength must be used.
- Steps must be taken to ensure that all surfaces of the instrument are in contact with the disinfectant and that all air is removed.
- Ample time is required.
- Thorough rinsing after immersion is essential, except in the case of alcohol.
- Once diluted, most disinfectants quickly deteriorate.
- It is necessary to check that the material of which the instrument is made is compatible with the disinfectant to be used. For example, soft porous rubber as well as plastic may absorb phenolics and glutaraldehyde, and hypochlorite will damage metal and some fabrics.
- Disinfectants are toxic and can cause skin reactions.

Heat-sensitive instruments may be chemically disinfected, using either sodium hypochlorite 1000 ppm (for non-metallic items) or glutaraldehyde 2% (for instruments which are incompatible with hypochlorite). A Control of Substances Hazardous to Health Regulations (COSHH) assessment is required (see below).

Recommendations for immersion time in chemical disinfectant vary, the shortest time being 4 minutes (Working Party of the British Society of Gastroenterology 1988). Most harmful microorganisms, including the hepatitis B virus, are known to be killed by immersion in glutaraldehyde for 10 min (Bond et al 1983), but 1 hour in glutaraldehyde is required to kill Mycobacterium species e.g. *M. tuberculosis*; (DHSS 1986b).

Flexible endoscopes are heat sensitive and can only be disinfected chemically. These instruments are expensive, and because of the speed with which endoscopy is performed, a large number of instruments would be required if each instrument was to be immersed for 1 hour. As a compromise, endoscopes which are considered unlikely to be contaminated with mycobacteria are generally immersed for a shorter time (see Fig. 16.7). On the basis that all bronchoscopes *could* be contaminated with mycobacteria, and that this is more likely than with gastrointestinal or cystoscopes, some authorities recommend that all bronchoscopes be immersed for 1 hour if they cannot be heat disinfected. Scopes entering a sterile cavity, such as arthroscopes and laparoscopes, should of course be sterile. This is possible chemically with a 3-hour immer-sion, but autoclavable arthroscopes and laparoscopes are now available.

COSHH (1988) require users of chemicals such as glutaraldehyde to take steps to minimise the hazards to staff in the use of such substances if there is not an acceptable alternative chemical or process. Totally closed machines to prevent the escape of vapour are being developed, and air extraction systems may also be required to keep the amount of aldehyde vapour below the mimimum acceptable level. If glutaraldehyde must be used, staff exposure to it should be minimised, and gloves, masks and visors or goggles worn. The problems of chemical disinfection and the COSHH regulations are discussed by Babb (1990).

Instruments should not be stored in disinfectants, but removed after the required immersion time, rinsed thoroughly, and stored dry. Disinfection is carried out preferably in an HSDU, but may be done on the ward: if the process is carried out correctly there should be no risk to patients or staff.

Spillage. The management of spillage must adhere to local prescribed policy. Normally, spillage of body fluid on a floor or other surface should first of all be mopped up using disposable paper, cloth, or a mop with a detachable head which is sent to the laundry after use. Gloves must of course be worn. The spillage area should then be wiped with a disinfectant, e.g. sodium hypochlorite 10 000 ppm. The disinfectant should be rinsed off and the surface dried afterwards; this is especially important if the surface will come into contact with the skin, e.g. a toilet seat. Disinfectants are also used for wiping down surfaces which have been in contact with patients with known or suspected infection. All surfaces should be left dry after cleaning or disinfection.

Strong chlorine-releasing granules (> 100 000 ppm) can be poured over fresh blood spills; these will absorb the blood and disinfect it before it is cleared up. They are, however, extremely pungent and care is necessary in their use. With other body fluid spillages, it is probably more effective and less messy to clear up the spillage first (using disposable paper) and then disinfect the area.

Hypochlorite 1000 ppm may be used where body fluid contamination is probable although the surface looks clean, and for well-sponged fabrics and thoroughly pre-cleaned metal surfaces.

Alcohol is a useful decontaminant for clean, hard surfaces such as glass, but is not suitable for disinfecting dirty surfaces, e.g. commodes, because of its poor penetration when organic material is present (Maurer 1985).

Figure 16.8 provides an example of a policy for the disinfection of surfaces. The certificate referred to in the figure is required for all medical equipment and devices sent to a third party for investigation, inspection, repair, or servicing (DHSS 1987c). It serves as a warning to the receiving department that where dismantling of the item is required a hazard may still exist and precautions will be necessary.

Cleaning. Ordinary cleaning with soap or detergent and water is adequate when there is no contamination with blood or body fluid, and no contact with patients with known or suspected infection.

Aseptic technique

An aseptic technique is carried out in a clean environment using sterile equipment. The procedure is carried out in such a way as to minimise the likelihood of infection being introduced to the site. It is used for wound dressings, urinary catheterisation, manipulation of intravenous infusions and other situations where the skin is broken. Hands should be thoroughly washed (see p. 550) and only sterile materials (gloves, instruments, etc.) should be used.

Safe disposal

Waste. Procedures in the safe disposal of clinical and household waste are as follows.

Clinical waste consists of human tissue, blood or other body fluids; excretions; drugs, swabs or dressings; and syringes, needles or other sharp instruments. It includes all waste arising from medical, nursing, dental or similar practice, investigation, treatment, care, teaching and research (HSAC 1992).

Household or domestic waste consists of all non-hazardous waste generated in the course of normal life.

Waste identification. Colour-coded bags make it easy to distinguish between clinical and household waste. Health workers should check which colours are used in their area

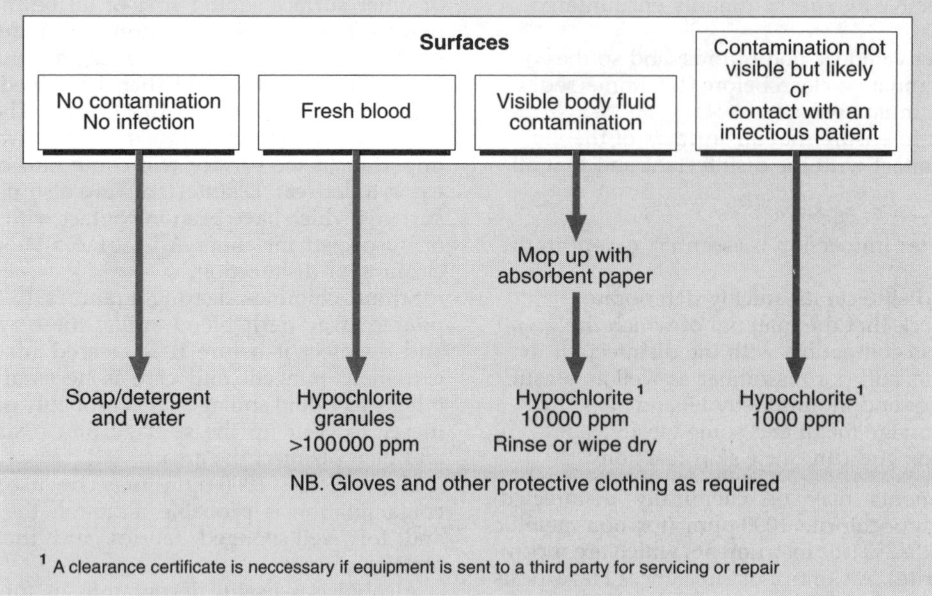

Fig. 16.8 An example of a policy for spillage: surfaces and equipment. (Reproduced with kind permission from Dr A. B. White, Raigmore Hospital.)

of work. Most health boards or authorities have adopted the national colour code (HSAC 1992) which is as follows:

- human tissue, dialysis waste, and waste from the isolation nursing of patients with infectious disease should be placed in thick yellow plastic bags
- sharps should be placed in the designated yellow sharps box immediately after use, by the person using them, and not left for someone else to clear up
- other clinical waste should be discarded in thin yellow plastic bags.

Incineration is mandatory for most clinical waste, and is the preferred option for all clinical waste. There are some exceptions to this rule. Certain items of waste can be placed in striped black-and-yellow bags, and disposed of by licensed landfill.

Clinical waste arising from home treatment must not enter the domestic waste system. Some health boards/authorities in urban areas may make special arrangements for the uplift of clinical waste through the environmental health or cleansing department, but this can be difficult in rural areas. If the colour coding of waste is done correctly, there need not be a problem of confidentiality in the community. The colour of the waste sack does not indicate a particular disease, but rather the preferred method of disposal.

Figure 16.9 gives an example of a waste disposal policy.

Linen. Procedures for the safe laundering of hospital and domestic linen are as follows.

Hospital laundry. All hospital linen is disinfected using either heat or chemicals. Heat is the method of choice, and temperatures and holding times are laid down by the DHSS (1987b) and SOHHD (1993b). Chemicals, e.g. sodium hypochlorite, may be used for fabrics which are likely to be heat labile, such as personal clothing, so that they can be washed at a lower temperature (40 °C), although if fouling is likely to be frequent it is advisable for the patient to buy clothing that will withstand the disinfection temperatures.

It is a national requirement that linen is sorted in the ward into used (soiled and fouled) linen, and infected linen. What follows in this section is an example of a local laundry policy.

Figure 16.10 outlines a laundry policy in which linen is sorted into the following categories:

- used (no longer fresh)
- fouled (contaminated with body fluid)
- infected (used for a patient with known or suspected infection)
- heat labile (unable to withstand thermal disinfection temperatures).

White outer bags identify all used linen. Red outer bags are used for potentially infected linen. Blue outer bags are used for personal clothing.

In addition, alginate stitch or soluble panel bags are used for all fouled or infected linen before it is placed in the outer laundry bags. (Totally water-soluble bags may also be used.) This prevents seepage through the outer bag during transit and protects laundry staff as the bag should be placed straight into the laundry machine without being opened. When the washing process has started, the soluble panel dissolves to allow the contents to be washed and heat disinfected. The remains of the bags must be removed before the linen is placed in the drier.

It is important that no extraneous items are inadvertently sent to the laundry, as sharp items can damage linen and cause injury to the laundry staff.

In this policy, used and fouled linen is thermally disinfected at 71 °C for 3 min. A higher temperature (93 °C for 10 min.) is recommended for all infected linen in order to inactivate the hepatitis B virus and make the linen safe to handle.

Laundry in the home. Most linen and clothing can be washed in the usual way at home. Fouled linen is washed at 60 °C, and infected linen at 90–95 °C (in an automatic washing machine). In some areas, it may be possible for contaminated linen to be collected and laundered by the hospital laundry and then returned clean.

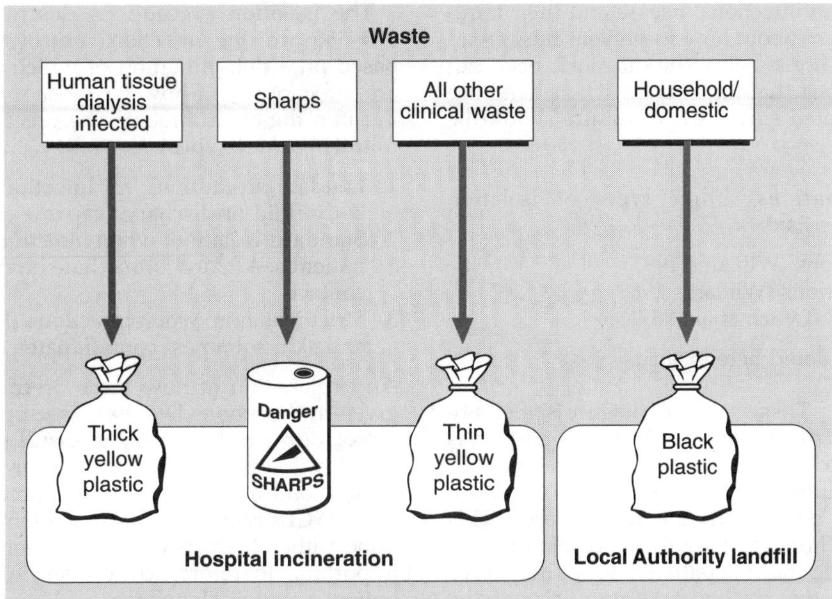

Fig. 16.9 An example of a waste disposal policy. (Reproduced with kind permission from Dr A. B. White, Raigmore Hospital.)

Isolation precautions for patients with known or suspected infection

Patients who suffer from an infectious disease are a potential source of infection to others. Isolation in this context involves keeping someone who may be an infection risk away from others who might be susceptible. This is sometimes possible in a multi-bed ward, but it is easier if the patient can be nursed in a single room.

Some people believe that if universal precautions are carried out there is no need to take further isolation precautions with patients who have a known or suspected infection. However, certain things are required when a patient is known to have a transmissible infection, namely a thick yellow waste bag (HSAC 1992), a red linen bag (DHSS 1987b, SOHHD 1993b), and an appropriate warning to other departments so that the same precautions can be taken there. In addition, we know that universal precautions are not always carried out properly (see Research Abstract 16.1) and that universal precautions do not encompass the unseen contamination which can result from patient rather than staff behaviour, for example, when a person suffering from salmonellosis has diarrhoea, does not wash his hands properly, and touches door handles and the furniture around him or even hands sweets or food to other people.

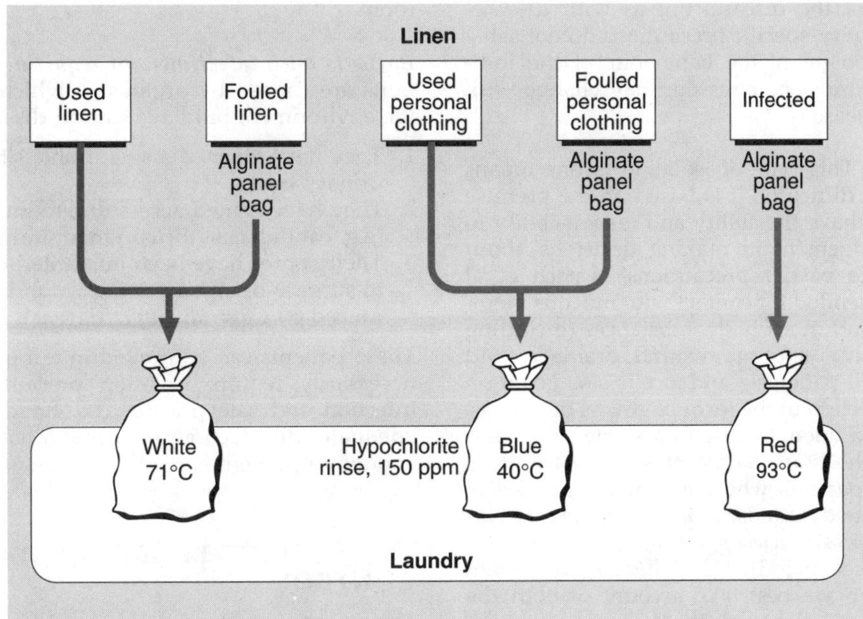

Fig. 16.10 An example of a linen laundering policy. (Reproduced with kind permission from Dr A. B. White, Raigmore Hospital.)

Patients suffering from an infectious disease and their families at home will need advice about how to prevent the spread of infection. In the case of home helps, the diagnosis need not be disclosed but precautions that are needed when handling body fluids and contaminated surfaces or furniture should be carefully explained.

Types of isolation precautions. Three types of isolation precautions have been described:

- disease-specific precautions (Williams 1983)
- category-specific precautions (Williams 1983)
- body substance isolation (Lynch et al 1987).

Each of these will be considered here in turn.

Disease-specific precautions. These rely on diagnosis and are specific for the particular disease from which the patient is suffering. Body fluids which may be infectious are identified, but this can create difficulties if the diagnosis is uncertain and universal body fluid precautions are not in force. This approach also relies on a thorough knowledge of the disease, whereas not everyone going into the patient's room may have this knowledge. Nor does this method take into account the behaviour of the patient: for example, a cooperative and continent patient with salmonellosis who is able to use the toilet may only require effective handwashing, whereas an incontinent, confused or uncooperative patient may contaminate his entire environment.

Category-specific precautions. These group together diseases for which similar precautions are recommended, based on the means of transmission of the organisms responsible. The following seven categories of precautions are used:

- strict isolation
- contact isolation
- respiratory isolation
- tuberculosis isolation
- enteric precautions
- drainage/secretion precautions
- blood/body fluid precautions.

This approach overcomes the necessity for each carer to have a thorough knowledge of the disease, but as with disease-specific precautions, category-specific precautions do not satisfactorily address the problem of the behaviour of the individual patient, which, it must be stressed, may change with the progression of the disease.

Body substance isolation. This type of isolation is one means of overcoming the above difficulty. It is based on the premise that 'health care workers have the ability and responsibility to exercise independent judgement in making decisions about when to use appropriate barrier precautions' (Lynch et al 1987). Gloves are recommended for contact with mucous membranes, non-intact skin, and moist body substances (including faeces, blood, urine, saliva, sputum, wound drainage, and other body fluids) with all patients. Guidance is also given on handwashing, extra protection in the form of gowns or aprons, safe disposal of waste and linen, the use of a single room, and the immune status of the staff. While this approach does address the problem of patients who contaminate articles in their environment with body fluids, *it does not allow for the additional arrangements necessary when a patient is known to have a transmissible infection* (see p. 563). How then, in the event of a known infection, can we best take account of both the relevant transmission categories and the behaviour of the individual patient?

The isolation precautions described below and on pages 555–556 are one infection control team's method. They are based on a determination of which body fluids or substances are infectious, and how far those infectious fluids are spreading into the environment. The precautions outlined are of the following three types:

1. Exudate precautions: for infection confined to an internal body fluid or discharge capable of occlusion
2. Standard isolation: when infectious fluid contaminates the patient's skin and immediate environment by direct contact
3. Strict isolation: when infectious fluid (including droplets and skin squames) contaminates the entire room.

An explanation of how these precautions work in practice is given in 'Infectious Diseases' (see pp. 563–565).

Isolation can be a very stressful experience (Denton 1986), but this is not in itself a reason for failing to isolate someone if his condition warrants this precaution for the safety of others. Criticism of isolation often relates to the way it is done rather than to the requirement for isolation itself. It is important, therefore, to do everything possible to lessen the patient's anxiety, loneliness and boredom.

Improving the quality of life for patients in isolation. A patient in isolation requires skilled and sensitive care, as he is in effect cut off from the outside world and from normal human contact. It is important, therefore, that the patient's needs are discussed, agreed, and recorded in the care plan. Loneliness is often a major problem: allocating one nurse on each shift to be responsible for the patient will help, as long as that nurse spends time with the patient at frequent intervals. Extra staff may be required. Encouraging relatives to visit at different times of the day can help, as can the offer of a television, telephone, radio or cassette player. Favourite leisure activities such as card games, sewing or knitting will help to pass the time.

The patient needs to have some privacy and should not feel that he is constantly being watched. Patients suffering from diarrhoea are often acutely aware of smells and may welcome the offer of a deodorising room spray, or a few drops of an essential plant oil such as lavender placed on a tissue in the room.

Patients with infections not requiring isolation. Some infections are caused by organisms which are normally found in the environment but have caused disease because:

1. They have infected a susceptible site (e.g. *Esch. coli* in the urinary tract)
2. They have gained access due to impaired host defences (e.g. candidiasis (thrush) in an immunosuppressed patient)
3. Their spores have been implanted deep in the tissues due to surgery or a penetrating wound (e.g. gas gangrene caused by *Clostridium perfringens*).

These patients can be nursed in a multi-bed ward and do not necessarily require isolation precautions. Treatment of the infection and safe practice (i.e. hand hygiene, safe disposal, adequate disinfection of contaminated articles) should be enough to prevent spread.

THE NURSING PROCESS AND INFECTION CONTROL

The assessment of a patient should always include consideration of the possible infection risks to which he might be exposed, as well as the degree to which he presents a risk to other people. This will be reflected in the care plan. All individuals are at risk of acquiring an infection while in hospital, but the very young, the very old, those who are immunosuppressed, debilitated, or undergoing surgery or invasive procedures are especially vulnerable. Urinary catheters, intravenous therapy, enteral feeding and many other procedures put the patient in danger of infection.

?	**16.5** What would be the dangers of bacterial contamination of nasogastric feeding solutions?

Enteral feeds should be prepared under clean conditions and in accordance with food hygiene regulations (DHSS 1987a). Equipment used in preparation must be adequately disinfected and correctly stored. (Feeds prepared locally are refrigerated immediately and administered as soon as possible after preparation. Commercially prepared feeds carry instructions about shelf life and storage.) Feeding solutions are an ideal breeding-ground for bacteria, particularly at room temperature. It is therefore essential to give the feed within the specified time in order to prevent bacterial multiplication and possible gastrointestinal upset (see Nursing Care Plan 16.1).

As an aid to the assessment of an individual's risk of infection, Webster & Bowell (1986) developed a guide (see Table 16.3) which is a helpful reminder.

Anticipation of potential problems is essential in patient care. For example, the passage of a urinary catheter should remind the nurse of the infection risks involved and lead her to assess how much the patient needs to be taught about subsequent selfcare. In the case of immunosuppressed patients, (see Ch. 11, p. 429) the greatest risk is endogenous infection (self-infection), caused by the patient's own microorganisms entering a susceptible site, or by reactivation of latent infection, e.g. cytomegalovirus. Although endogenous infection is more difficult to prevent than crossinfection, the nurse can still teach the patient how to minimise the risk. This not only helps the individual to stay free from infection, but also encourages a positive attitude, allowing him to feel he can contribute to his own well-being.

Health and safety

Nurses have a duty of care to others, as stated in the Health and Safety at Work etc. Act (1974). This duty can be expressed in health care situations in a number of ways, which include:

- Implementing measures in accordance with safe working practice (see p. 550) to ensure that no harm results from actions or omissions
- notifying other departments that precautions need to be taken with the body fluids of an infectious patient being transferred there
- staying home from work if one is unwell, particularly if the illness could be communicated to others, e.g. diarrhoea
- being aware of one's immune status regarding infectious diseases such as rubella, chickenpox, measles, tuberculosis, tetanus, hepatitis B, poliomyelitis, etc. Nurses can obtain advice from their general practitioner (GP) or from their employer's occupational health department. (Further information about immunisation can be found in DOH 1992.)

Confidentiality

People suffering from infection are often embarrassed and sometimes depressed because of isolation precautions and the feeling that they are in some way 'dirty'. Nurses are legally responsible for keeping confidential any information given to them by patients, and may divulge such information only when it is necessary to do so for the benefit of the patient or the safety of others (UKCC 1992). Nurses should reassure the patient that this is the case, in order to minimise any embar-

Nursing Care Plan 16.1 Preventing bacterial contamination during nasogastric feeding.
Mr W is a 46-year-old bachelor who works as a travelling salesman. He suffers from an inflammatory bowel disease which has recently become unmanageable. He has been admitted to hospital for enteral nutrition to improve his nutritional state prior to surgery.

Nursing considerations	Action	Rationale	Evaluation
1. Nasogastric tube may have caused trauma to mucosal surfaces resulting in mild immunosuppression/potential risk of infection	❒ Keep mouth clean and comfortable by giving mouthwashes every 2 h ❒ Encourage Mr W to clean his teeth regularly	The patient is not able to drink much fluid and his mouth may become dry. Salivary flow may be diminished	Patient's mouth is clean, moist, and salivary flow is adequate
2. Danger of bacterial multiplication in hospital/prepared feed unless refrigerated, and administered within given time	❒ Administer 500 ml feeds within 4 h at a consistent rate and record on fluid balance chart	If the feed is left at room temperature for longer than this, bacterial counts will rise rapidly	Feed administered to time except 12.00 h–14.00 h detached while patient at X-ray. Remaining feed discarded and fresh feed commenced at 14.00 h
	❒ Use a fresh reservoir and giving set for each 500 ml feed	Even after the feed has been given, a fine film remains on the inside of the reservoir and giving set: bacteria will have begun to replicate	Reservoir and giving set changed after each 4-hourly feed
	❒ Observe patient for nausea, vomiting, abdominal pain, diarrhoea	Any signs of gastroenteritis should be reported	No signs of gastroenteritis. Feed appears to be tolerated well

Table 16.3 The Bowell–Webster risk assessment guide for identifying patients at risk of infection (Reproduced with kind permission from Bowell 1989 Applied Microbiology, 1st edn. Scutari Press, Harrow.)

General factors	Local factors	Invasive procedures	Drugs	Disease
Age	*Oedema*	*Cannulation*	Cytotoxics	Carcinoma
Very young	Pulmonary	Peripheral		
Very old	Ascites	Central	Antibiotics	Leukaemia
	Effusion	Parenteral		
Nutrition			Steroids	Aplastic anaemia
Emaciated	*Ischaemia*	*Catheterisation*		
Thin	Thrombus	Intermittent		Diabetes mellitus
Obese	Embolus	Closed drainage		
Dehydrated	Necrosis	Irrigation		
				Liver disease
Mobility	*Skin lesions*	*Surgery*		Renal disease
Limited	Trauma	Anaesthesia		
Immobile	Burns	Wound		AIDS
Temporary	Ulceration	Wound drainage		
Permanent		Wound/colostomy		
	Foreign body	Implant		
Mental state	Accidental			
Confused	Planned	*Intubation*		
Depressed		Endobronchial suction		
Senile		Humidification		
		Ventilation		
Incontinence				
Urine				
Faeces				
Temporary				
Permanent				
General health				
Weak				
Debilitated				
General hygiene				
Dependence				
Mouth/teeth				
Skin				

rassment or unease he may feel. It is also helpful to inform the patient about infection control procedures and the reasons for them.

The notification of a department in advance of their receiving a patient of the precautions required (*not* the diagnosis) preserves confidentiality and yet alerts staff to the need for care. The labelling of patients' case notes with 'High Risk' or 'Danger of Infection' stickers is really not acceptable, as it may create fear and embarrassment in the patient and is in any case a difficult system to establish and maintain.

DISORDERS OF IMMUNITY

Four types of immunity disorder can be identified:

- immunodeficiency
- hypersensitivity
- autoimmune disease
- graft rejection after transplantation.

In this chapter only the first three are addressed.

IMMUNODEFICIENCY

Immunodeficiency can be primary or secondary in nature, as outlined in the following.

Primary immunodeficiency

Primary immunodeficiency states are very rare, but may arise under either of the following two conditions:

- There are not enough cells available
- The number of cells is adequate but they have a functional defect.

These problems will be discussed in relation to the cells and proteins involved, i.e. impairment of phagocytes, B lymphocytes or of T lymphocytes.

?	**16.6** Recall the cells and proteins that are involved in the immune response.

Impairment of phagocytes

Phagocyte impairment may occur in the following forms.

1. Neutropenia: a low number of neutrophils (see p. 429). This condition can be congenital (very rare), secondary to

drug or radiation therapy (see Ch. 32), or associated with the autoimmune diseases (see p. 561).
2. Functional defects: abnormalities in phagocyte structure or function. These can result in the inability of phagocytes to localise in an inflammatory site, or their inability to ingest and digest microorganisms.
3. Failure of complement activation. There are many steps in the complement pathway, and many components are involved or created during complement activation. Some appear to be more important than others (Roitt 1990). Absence of one of the complement components can make phagocytosis difficult, as it is easier for the granular leucocytes to ingest microorganisms if their outer surface is coated with complement.

?	**16.7** Recall the function of B lymphocytes and try to work out what will happen if they are deficient.

Impairment of B lymphocytes
Occasionally B lymphocytes fail to mature properly in the bone marrow, resulting in B cell deficiency and therefore diminished antibody production. People with B cell deficiency are particularly prone to bacterial infections, e.g. *Staphylococcus aureus* (Roitt 1990).

Impairment of T lymphocytes
T cell deficiency occasionally occurs in children in whom absence of the thymus gland means that the cells cannot differentiate to become T lymphocytes. People with T cell deficiency are particularly prone to some viral infections, e.g. varicella (Roitt 1990).

Secondary immunodeficiency

This occurs as a result of some other condition and an individual suffering from secondary immunodeficiency is sometimes called a 'compromised host'. This term simply means that the person's immune defences are in some way reduced, making him particularly susceptible to infection (Kirkwood & Lewis 1989).

HYPERSENSITIVITY

An excessive immune response (hypersensitivity) can result in damage to normal tissue. This response may be immediate or delayed. Four types of hypersensitivity reaction have been described: types I, II and III are antibody-mediated; type IV is mediated mainly by T cells and macrophages (Roitt et al 1989).

Type 1: anaphylactic or immediate hypersensitivity

In this type of immune response excessive IgE production results in IgE binding to mast cells which, when the antigen is encountered, release histamine, giving rise to an acute inflammatory reaction. This response develops within minutes of exposure to the antigen and will recur on subsequent encounters.

The reaction can be local, as in asthma, hay fever and eczema, or systemic, as in anaphylactic shock. The nature of the symptoms will depend on whether the antigen is encountered locally, systemically, or absorbed via the intestine.

Asthma (see Ch. 3, p. 73), hay fever and eczema are classical indicators of an *atopic* subject, i.e. someone who has a 'hereditary tendency to develop a hypersensitivity reaction to commonly encountered antigens' (Nurse's Clinical Library 1985).

Type II: Antibody-dependent cytotoxic hypersensitivity

In this type of response antibodies react to normal tissue cells, which then bind to complement or to phagocytes, resulting in lysis or phagocytosis of the cell. This can occur as a result of a mismatched blood transfusion (see p. 411) or can be drug induced.

Type III: Immune-complex mediated hypersensitivity

In this form of hypersensitivity immune complexes (i.e. antigens bound to antibodies; see p. 547) form in excess and are deposited in the capillary endothelium. They may activate complement and attract phagocytes, resulting in mast cell degranulation and local inflammation. The inflammation may be acute, as in serum sickness (see p. 316); chronic, as in glomerulonephritis; or both, as in farmer's lung (see p. 560). This type of hypersensitivity resembles an anaphylactic reaction, but takes longer (several hours) to develop.

Type IV: Cell-mediated or delayed hypersensitivity

In this type of immune reaction sensitised T cells, on contact with an allergen (antigen), release lymphokines (soluble chemicals) which attract phagocytes and function without the presence of antibodies. These reactions cause chronic and sometimes extensive inflammation and are apparent a few hours after exposure to the antigen.

This type of immune response is the basis of the Mantoux test (see p. 568), given to find out whether a person has tuberculosis or has developed immunity to tuberculosis. It also gives rise to contact dermatitis (see p. 452) and sarcoidosis (see p. 560), and contributes to graft rejection.

Anaphylactic shock (Type I)

Anaphylactic shock is a sudden and severe form of type I hypersensitivity reaction, where there is an inappropriate or excessive response to some foreign material such as an antibiotic or other drug, a vaccine, or a bee sting.

PATHOPHYSIOLOGY

IgE antibodies are the mediators of this reaction. The mechanism is similar to that of hay fever, except that the response is systemic rather than localised.

Common presenting symptoms. The characteristic feature of anaphylactic shock is collapse within seconds or minutes after exposure to the offending allergen. Usually this is by injection and less commonly by ingestion. Laryngeal oedema manifests as a lump in the throat, hoarseness, or stridor. Examination of the patient shows an urticarial skin rash which may be localised or widespread. The rash is itchy, and can coalesce to form giant hives. In anaphylaxis, urticaria is part of a life-threatening condition. However, urticaria can present independently as a mild type I hypersensitivity and can be alleviated by the application of antihistamine creams.

Angioedema resulting from a sudden increase in vascular permeability can lead to oedema of the skin, respiratory obstruction and vascular collapse, the result of which may be fatal (p. 604).

MEDICAL MANAGEMENT

There is not usually time for investigations in patients with anaphylactic shock. The diagnosis must be made rapidly. Treatment in mild cases is with subcutaneous adrenaline to restore haemodynamic stability. This can be repeated at 3-minute intervals. Severe cases require intensive cardiovascular and respiratory support with adrenaline given intravenously.

NURSING PRIORITIES AND MANAGEMENT OF ANAPHYLACTIC SHOCK

Life-threatening concerns

Anaphylactic shock may occur suddenly and unexpectedly and is life threatening, especially in circumstances where emergency facilities are not available. Death may ensue if prompt action is not taken. Maintenance of airway, breathing and circulation are paramount. Emergency procedures are as follows:

- Place the patient flat in the left lateral position
- Give 0.5 ml (adult dose) adrenaline 1:1000 intramuscularly (unless the patient's condition is good and there is a strong central pulse)
- Give oxygen by face mask if it is available
- Send for medical aid (GP) or ambulance (dial 999); ask a relative, if present, to stay with the patient while you do this
- Be prepared to institute cardiopulmonary resuscitation
- Check pulse and blood pressure regularly and after any drug treatment.

Major patient problems

Should the patient survive, he is likely to experience severe anxiety after the event. The question of how to prevent a similar occurrence will need to be explored and the cause of the reaction investigated.

Transfusion reaction (Type II)

This is a type II antibody-dependent cytotoxic hypersensitivity. An adverse reaction to a blood transfusion can occur when the immune system mounts an antibody response to the transfused blood. For details of this kind of reaction and the associated medical and nursing care, see Chapter 11, p. 417.

Serum sickness (Type III)

This condition is a type III immune-complex mediated hypersensitivity reaction to foreign serum i.e. that of another species. It occurs when the immune system recognises the proteins in an introduced serum as foreign and produces antibodies against them. Antigen–antibody complexes (known as immune complexes) form and may be deposited in the skin, joints, heart and kidneys, resulting in a temperature rise, urticarial skin rash, swollen lymph glands / nodes and swollen and painful joints. Serum sickness was common in the days when horse serum was used as a source of immunoglobulin. Its occurrence led to the development of blood transfusion–derived products such as Humotet (human antitetanus immunoglobulin).

Farmer's lung (Type III)

PATHOPHYSIOLOGY

Also known as extrinsic allergic alveolitis, this is a type III hypersensitivity reaction in which inhalation of fungal spores in dust from mouldy hay causes an allergic reaction in the alveoli and bronchioles. The spores act as an antigen. As the name suggests, this disease is common in farm workers.

Common presenting symptoms. Within 6 to 8 hours of exposure, the sensitised person will develop symptoms, i.e. dry cough, dyspnoea without wheeze, headache and chest tightness accompanied by fever and malaise. The symptoms usually subside when exposure to the antigen ceases. However, prolonged exposure can lead to permanent disability due to interstitial fibrosis.

MEDICAL MANAGEMENT

Diagnostic investigation includes serology (positive precipitin test; see Appendix 1) and a nasal provocation test, in which the patient inhales an aerosol containing the suspected antigen. The provocation test is considered positive if symptoms occur 3–6 hours after inhalation, pyrexia develops, and ventilatory capacity is reduced.

In severe cases, corticosteroids such as prednisolone may be given to suppress the inflammatory response. Patients with hypoxia may require high concentration oxygen therapy (see Ch. 3, p. 68).

NURSING PRIORITIES AND MANAGEMENT OF FARMER'S LUNG

Depending on the severity of symptoms, respiratory support may be required (see Ch. 3).

Prevention

Farm workers are advised to take the following precautions:

- avoid creating dust when working
- wear a suitable dust respirator if contact is unavoidable
- make sure indoor working areas are well ventilated
- use an industrial vacuum cleaner to remove dust from the inside of buildings
- wear protective clothing at work; do not take work clothing home.

Employers have a duty under the Health and Safety at Work etc. Act (1974) and the COSHH regulations (1988) to provide a safe working environment and to inform and instruct employees about health risks and the precautions to be taken. Employees have a duty to follow such advice. A leaflet entitled 'Farmer's Lungs' is produced by the Health and Safety Executive (1990) and gives helpful information to both farmers and their employees.

Sarcoidosis (Type IV)

This is a type IV hypersensitivity reaction of which the cause is as yet unknown.

PATHOPHYSIOLOGY

This disease may take a subacute or chronic form and is characterised by disturbances in cell-mediated immunity in which the balance between the different types of T lymphocyte is altered. Lesions or granulomas develop in the lungs, liver, spleen, parotid glands, skin, eyes, mediastinal and superficial lymph nodes, and phalangeal bones. In the subacute form, the lesions usually resolve spontaneously without treatment, but in chronic sarcoidosis they may lead to the production of fibrous tissue, causing permanent damage, for example: interstitial fibrosis in the lungs; myocardial damage leading to cardiac arrhythmias; skin lesions; and damage to the iris possibly leading to blindness. Although the disease may involve other organs, the severity of their involvement is variable. The disease is primarily pulmonary.

Common presenting symptoms. Most patients have pulmonary symptoms, i.e. dyspnoea on exertion and unproductive cough in addition to general malaise, weakness, loss of appetite, fever and weight loss. Lymph node enlargement may also be detected on examination.

MEDICAL MANAGEMENT

Diagnostic investigation includes Chest X-ray and lung function tests (see Ch. 3). Transbronchial lung biopsy can confirm the diagnosis.

Treatment for chronic sarcoidosis involves the administration of corticosteroids, often for several years. Oxygen is given in acute or severe cases.

NURSING PRIORITIES AND MANAGEMENT OF SARCOIDOSIS

The priorities in nursing care will depend on the level of impairment caused by the granulomatous lesions. Commonly, there is respiratory impairment and a potential for cardiac arrhythmias. Vision may be affected and liver function disturbed. Sarcoidosis may not be the prime reason for admission to hospital but must not be neglected in setting priorities for care.

AUTOIMMUNE DISEASES

These disorders occur when the body's tolerance to 'self' breaks down, and autoantibodies (antibodies against 'self' cells) are formed. There are two categories of autoimmune disorders:

- *organ specific*, for example,
  - Hashimoto's thyroiditis
  - pernicious anaemia (see Ch. 11, p. 420)
- *non–organ specific*, for example,
  - rheumatoid arthritis (see Ch. 10, p. 394)
  - Goodpasture's syndrome
  - systemic lupus erythematosus (SLE)
  - sarcoidosis
  - myasthenia gravis.

It is not properly understood why autoantibodies sometimes cause disease. Their production may be initiated by minor changes in cells or by the exposure of previously 'hidden' cells as a result of damage, infection or genetic mutation, resulting in 'new' surface antigens being presented to the immune system. Autoimmune diseases may also involve a hypersensitivity reaction, whether immediate or delayed.

Goodpasture's syndrome

(Also known as Anti-GBM Disease.)

PATHOPHYSIOLOGY

People with this non-organ specific disorder have antibodies to their own kidney glomerular basement membrane (GBM). Immune complexes are formed with the help of complement, and these are deposited in the kidney glomeruli, causing glomerulonephritis. They may also be deposited in the basement membranes of the lung alveoli. The cause of this disease is not known. It is potentially fatal, and is commoner in young men. Fortunately, it is rare.

Common presenting symptoms include:

- haematuria, mild or severe
- haemoptysis, dyspnoea, cough.

Symptoms may be severe.

MEDICAL MANAGEMENT

History and examination. The onset can be rapid, with symptoms of nephritis and pulmonary haemorrhage.

Investigative procedures. Urinalysis will confirm haematuria and a chest X-ray will determine the degree of lung involvement. The diagnosis is confirmed if serology reveals the presence of anti-GBM antibodies. Kidney or lung biopsy may be carried out. Blood chemistry shows raised serum creatinine and blood urea nitrogen. Urine collection would demonstrate reduced creatinine clearance, indicating some degree of kidney failure.

Treatment. This disease must be treated urgently, as renal and respiratory failure can occur. High-dose parenteral corticosteroids (e.g. prednisolone) in conjunction with a cytotoxic drug such as azathioprine or cyclophosphamide are given. Plasmapheresis may be carried out to remove circulating anti-GBM antibodies. If renal failure develops, dialysis will be undertaken. Kidney transplant may be required, but can be attempted only after intensive plasmapheresis to ensure that no circulating anti-GBM antibodies remain. Oxygen therapy and assisted ventilation (see Ch. 3, p. 82) may be required if respiratory failure develops.

NURSING PRIORITIES AND MANAGEMENT OF GOODPASTURE'S SYNDROME

Patients with Goodpasture's syndrome will present with both respiratory and renal failure which may require intensive nursing support.

Myasthenia gravis

This non-organ specific disease is thought to be caused by a disorder of the thymus gland whereby it produces defective T lymphocytes. It usually occurs in individuals aged between 15 and 50 years, and is more common in females than in males.

PATHOPHYSIOLOGY

The defective T cells stimulate B cells to produce antibodies to the acetylcholine receptors in the neuromuscular junction. Acetylcholine allows the normal transmission of impulses from the motor nerves to voluntary muscle (see Ch. 10, p. 327).

The antiacetylcholine antibodies react with the acetylcholine receptor, blocking the attachment of this neurotransmitter and thus preventing normal muscular activity.

Common presenting symptoms. The classic symptom of myasthenia gravis is that muscles tire quickly. Movement may be strong at first, but rapidly weakens. Localised symptoms include diplopia or ptosis (see Ch. 13) due to weakness of the extraocular muscles, as well as weakness in chewing, swallowing, talking, and moving the limbs. The muscles around the shoulder girdle are most commonly affected.

Symptoms are often worse at the end of the day or after exercising. Respiratory muscles may be affected, resulting in a weakened cough. Relapses sometimes occur after infections, or following emotional disturbance.

MEDICAL MANAGEMENT

History and examination. The patient presents with a history of muscle weakness and inability to sustain muscle power, e.g. difficulty in brushing hair. Antiacetylcholine antibodies can be detected in the serum.

Investigative procedures. Diagnosis is assisted by giving an intravenous injection of a short-acting anticholinesterase. Muscle power improves within 30 seconds of the injection and often persists for 2–3 minutes.

Treatment. Anticholinesterase drugs such as pyridostigmine or neostigmine are used. Pyridostigmine is the drug of choice; 60–120 mg orally 2–8 hourly are given, depending on the effect, which can be measured during a supervised trial of the drug. Neostigmine acts more quickly but for a shorter time: the dose would be 15–30 mg.

Thymectomy may be recommended, depending on the stage of the disease. Sometimes corticosteroids are given but they need to be carefully controlled. Plasmapheresis can be done to remove the antibodies from the blood but the effect is short-lived.

'Cholinergic crisis' may occur as a consequence of drug therapy. The patient becomes paralysed, pale and sweaty, salivates excessively and has persistently small pupils. This occurs as a result of overdosage of the longer-acting anticholinesterase drugs, which causes hyperstimulation of the acetylcholine receptor. It requires urgent medical attention.

NURSING PRIORITIES AND MANAGEMENT OF MYASTHENIA GRAVIS

Life-threatening concerns

The consequences of cholinergic (or myasthenic) crisis are life-threatening. Paralysis of the respiratory muscles can rapidly lead to severe hypoxia; consequently, the patient may require resuscitation and ventilation (see Ch. 3, p. 82).

Major patient problems

These include fatigue and muscle weakness. Patients may need help with eating, drinking, washing and dressing. Difficulty with swallowing can lead to choking, and reduced mobility may lead to pressure sores (see Ch. 23, p. 712).

Further considerations

Most people suffering from myasthenia gravis will be cared for at home. Their nursing care, when required, will depend on the severity of symptoms. The potential seriousness of their condition may not be obvious. The educational aspect of community care for family and friends will be a priority. Advice on a nutritious diet is particularly important where chewing and swallowing are impaired. Small mouthfuls of food should be chewed slowly before swallowing. Soft, moist food is usually easiest to manage. Choking is a danger, but can often be avoided by helping the patient to concentrate on chewing, and then swallowing. Eye care may be required if blinking is impaired; this may include the use of eye drops to prevent dryness of the cornea (see Ch. 13, p. 475). If breathing is made difficult by respiratory muscle fatigue, the patient may be more comfortable sitting up, or propped up in bed.

Systemic lupus erythematosus (SLE)

SLE is a multisystem disorder in which autoantibodies against a variety of cellular antigens are produced. Thus any cell or tissue can be affected. Women are more often affected than men, and onset usually occurs in young adulthood. It is commoner in people of Afro-Asian and Chinese origin.

PATHOPHYSIOLOGY

The cause of this disease is not known, although both genetic and environmental factors (e.g. the effect of sunlight, drugs, hormone levels or viral infections) have been suggested. Damage is caused by the deposition of immune complexes in the tissues (a type III hypersensitivity reaction) and by the autoantibodies reacting directly with normal tissue cells (a type II hypersensitivity reaction).

Common presenting symptoms. Joint symptoms (arthritis, polyarthralgia) and fever are the most common features. Fatigue is a common non-specific symptom, and skin rash, usually on areas which are exposed to sunlight such as the face, neck and scalp may occur; characteristically, this is a 'butterfly rash' across the nose and cheeks. Nephritis is common, along with decreased urine output.

Vasculitis, especially in the smaller blood vessels, can give rise to skin ulceration and, in the gastrointestinal tract, to diarrhoea, pain, and bleeding. There may be poor peripheral perfusion, due to inflammation and consequent occlusion of small blood vessels. There may also be cardiopulmonary symptoms, including decreased cardiac output due to pericarditis, myocarditis, endocarditis and pulmonary infarction.

Occasionally there is cerebral inflammation leading to confusion, epilepsy or psychiatric symptoms.

MEDICAL MANAGEMENT

History and examination. As the symptoms of SLE are diverse, and their severity highly variable, a thorough history will be required. There may be external signs of tissue damage (such as skin rash) which will assist the doctor in making a diagnosis. Some patients will have lymphadenopathy and an enlarged spleen. Other features will depend on the specific organs involved.

Investigative procedures. In the course of diagnostic investigation the erythrocyte sedimentation rate (ESR; see Appendix 1) will usually be found to be raised. Antinuclear antibodies will be found in the serum of most patients with this disease. Some patients will have detectable anti-DNA antibodies and circulating immune complexes. Anaemia, leucopenia and thrombocytopenia (see Ch. 11) may be present on haematological examination. Depending on the organs involved, renal, cardiac or respiratory function may be altered.

Treatment. Treatment is aimed at relieving symptoms and preventing organ damage. Non-steroidal anti-inflammatory drugs (NSAIDs) such as aspirin may help to alleviate joint pain and other symptoms. Antimalarial drugs are sometimes used, as they can reduce the frequency of exacerbations of skin and joint lesions. Corticosteroids, e.g. prednisolone, are given when major organs (heart, lung, kidney, brain) are involved.

NURSING PRIORITIES AND MANAGEMENT OF SLE

The specific care of patients with SLE depends very much on the stage of the disease and on the organs involved. In any event, the aim is to alleviate symptoms as they present.

Life-threatening concerns

Depending on the nature and severity of organ involvement, myocardial infarction, respiratory failure, and renal failure may ensue. Appropriate resuscitative measures are described in Chapters 2, 3 and 8.

Major patient problems

As fatigue is common, the patient should be encouraged to have adequate rest. For patients who have experienced alteration in bowel habit, dietary advice may help. Patients may experience confusion, depression due to CNS involvement, or fears about prognosis. Epilepsy may also occur.

Poor peripheral circulation leading to cold hands and feet may develop. Patients are also likely to become susceptible to infection due to the debilitating effects of the disease process and the immunosuppressive effects of treatment.

Further considerations

Both pregnancy and the contraceptive pill have exacerbating effects on this disease. Patients suffering from photosensitivity should be encouraged to minimise exposure to sunlight and to protect the skin when exposure is unavoidable. Emotional support will be needed as this is a chronic disease of uncertain progression.

INFECTIOUS DISEASES

'Infectious' (or 'communicable') diseases are illnesses caused by microorganisms which are not normally present in or on the body, such as salmonellosis, hepatitis B and tuberculosis. Such infections contrast markedly with those which are acquired as a result of poor asepsis in invasive techniques, or as a consequence of antibiotic therapy, immunosuppressive drugs or inadequate hand-washing. Infectious diseases can be caught by anyone, at any time, in any place, and do not usually result from a particular nursing or medical procedure. This does not mean, however, that they cannot be spread from person to person; this presents a particular danger when patients with infectious disease are nursed in hospital.

CAUSES

Infectious diseases are generally caused by:

- bacteria, e.g. salmonellosis, meningococcal meningitis
- viruses, e.g. hepatitis A and B, chickenpox
- protozoa, e.g. malaria, toxoplasmosis, amoebic dysentery.

Knowledge of the organism that is causing the disease is important in the planning of care.

TRANSMISSION

Most infectious diseases are ingested (e.g. hepatitis A), inhaled (e.g. tuberculosis), or inoculated (e.g. hepatitis B). Inoculation in this context refers to blood or body fluid entering a cut or skin abrasion or being splashed onto mucous membranes; it can also occur following needlestick injury. The organisms can be transmitted directly (i.e. straight from one person to another through direct contact with the infectious body substance) or indirectly (i.e. deposited on hands or surfaces where they can be picked up by touch).

Some infectious diseases are so common in the population that only general care is needed. Many people suffer from cold sores (herpes simplex) but the commonsense precautions of avoiding mucous membrane contact until the sores have healed, careful handwashing and washing of cutlery and cups, and not sharing toothbrushes, razors or facecloths are usually enough to prevent transmission.

Diseases like chickenpox are so common and so easily transmitted that special precautions to prevent their spread in the community are rarely necessary, although these may need to be enforced in settings such as hospitals and schools where there are particularly susceptible individuals. Other common diseases are preventable by an active immunisation programme; for example, immunisation against diphtheria, pertussis (whooping cough), tetanus; poliomyelitis; measles, mumps and rubella and Haemophilus influenzae Type B is now offered for all infants. It is still advisable, however, for pregnant women and people who are immunosuppressed to keep away from anyone known to have an infectious disease.

IMMUNITY TO INFECTIOUS DISEASES

?	16.8 Review your knowledge of how immunity comes about (see p. 546).

Immunisation against many diseases is carried out during childhood, with booster doses being required only in later life (DOH 1992). A booster dose is a smaller dose of a vaccine which boosts the level of memory cells (specific to the given antigen) circulating in the bloodstream (see Fig. 16.4).

Nurses and health visitors have an important role to play in encouraging parents to have their children vaccinated. Vaccination should be carried out by staff who are aware of the risks and the benefits. Some parents are afraid that their child might develop an adverse reaction to a vaccine; this is an uncommon occurrence, however, and few of the children so affected have developed serious complications (DOH 1992). In the late 1970s in England and Wales the percentage of infants vaccinated against whooping cough fell dramatically due to public concern about vaccine-damaged children (although such cases were very rare). There was a concurrent rise in the number of whooping cough cases reported (Reid et al 1986), a proportion of which had serious systemic complications.

MEASURES TO PREVENT SPREAD OF INFECTIOUS DISEASE

Planning the care of patients with an infectious disease requires the following preliminary steps:

- finding out the diagnosis or provisional diagnosis
- ascertaining which body fluid/substance is infectious
- assessing how far that body fluid is likely to travel from the patient into the environment
- finding out the period of communicability.

At this point the details of care planned for a patient in his own home and those for a patient in hospital will diverge. At home, the patient will have been in contact only with family and friends; in hospital he will be among other sick people who may be particularly susceptible to infection. In hospital, there is also the problem of the large number of people who will be in contact with the patient. Directly involved are nurses, doctors, physiotherapists, radiographers, domestics and porters; indirectly involved are laundry workers and staff working in sterilising and disinfecting units handling contaminated equipment.

?	16.9 Consider how measures to prevent the spread of infection would apply to a patient with urinary incontinence who is practising clean intermittent self-catheterisation at home (see Ch. 24, p. 732).

Hospital care: isolation precautions

Isolation precautions may be taken in hospital when a patient is suffering from an infectious disease which could be passed on to other patients or staff. The precautions required will vary according to which body fluid is infectious and how far that body fluid is likely to spread into the environment. Three things are required for the spread of infection:

- a source of infection
- a means of transfer
- a susceptible host.

As discussed earlier, it is advised that universal blood and body fluid precautions are adopted as safe working practice. This is important because for every person who is known to be infectious there may be many more who have not been identified. Moreover, *additional* precautions are required in the care of a patient known to be infectious, e.g. red laundry bags, thick yellow waste bags, the disinfection of surfaces that may have been contaminated, and warnings to other departments (see p. 554). There are different ways of classifying isolation precautions (see p. 555), but some arrangements for isolation precautions are standard for all types. These are as follows:

- accommodation: single room with washbasin is advisable, preferably with own toilet and shower/bath
- protective clothing: worn as appropriate
- crockery: heat disinfected or disposable
- linen: laundered as infected
- refuse: disposed of in a thick yellow plastic sack
- laboratory specimens: may need a 'danger of infection' sticker on container and request form
- body fluids: must be disposed of carefully, without splash, and any spillage dealt with using the correct strength of disinfectant
- room cleaning: should be done using the appropriate disinfectant, and cloths and mop-heads either disposed of or laundered as infected
- hands: washed and dried thoroughly before and after leaving an isolation room
- visitors: restricted if the nature of the disease and the state of the patient warrant
- repairs: external surfaces of all equipment should be disinfected before removal from the ward, and the service department should be notified in advance, in writing, if an infection hazard still exists
- transport: if it is essential that a patient is moved to another department, the nurse must inform that department of the precautions being taken in the ward, without divulging the diagnosis. Porters and ambulance staff may also need to be informed
- accidents involving blood or body fluid should be reported immediately to the nurse in charge, who will initiate the local accident procedure. Always encourage a fresh injury (e.g. needlestick injury) to bleed, and wash off any contamination
- death of a patient with an established transmissible disease: it is sometimes recommended that the body is placed in a sealed cadaver bag after the last offices have been carried out (SHHD 1988), for the protection of anyone subsequently handling the body. Undertakers must be informed that a risk of infection exists (DHSS 1988).

Three categories of isolation precautions will now be described; these are:

- exudate precautions
- standard isolation
- strict isolation.

Exudate precautions

This category is appropriate for patients with a known infection in which the infectious body fluid (exudate) is normally *contained* (i.e. not contaminating the environment). Protective clothing is required only at times when there is contact with the exudate. Examples could be changing a wound dressing for a hepatitis B carrier, or toileting a patient with salmonellosis who no longer has diarrhoea, is continent and cooperative, and practises good hand hygiene.

Standard isolation

This category is appropriate when the infectious body fluid is contaminating everything used by, or touched by, the patient, and the contamination is restricted to the patient's immediate surroundings because he is confined to bed. Staff should wear protective clothing for direct nursing care and when touching any items that may have been contaminated. Disposable crockery and cutlery are advisable. Surfaces touched by the patient must be disinfected. Examples of this are the patient with salmonellosis who has diarrhoea and is bedridden, or a hepatitis B carrier with a discharging wound where the discharge cannot reliably be contained by an occlusive dressing.

Strict isolation

In this type of isolation everything within the patient's room may be contaminated, for one of the following reasons:

- The patient has infectious diarrhoea, is ambulant and mobile, practises poor hand hygiene, and may touch anything in the room
- The patient has an infection which is spread by upper respiratory tract secretions or saliva and is highly productive of those secretions
- The disease is a skin infection and there is desquamation.

Protective clothing is required on entry to the room for any purpose. Negative ventilation (i.e. extract) should be used if available for patients with respiratory or skin infections. Disposable crockery and cutlery are advisable. All horizontal surfaces and equipment in the room must be disinfected.

It will be apparent from the above descriptions that it is not the infectious agent itself which determines what type of isolation precautions will be required, but the *mode of transmission*, the *stage of the disease* and the *state of the patient*. It is essential, therefore, that each patient is individually assessed and that care is reviewed on a daily basis. Care should be planned and discussed with the patient, where possible, and the reasons for any precautions carefully explained to him and to his relatives.

Home care

In the case of patients being nursed at home the risk of cross-infection is confined to family members and to anyone visiting the household, e.g. the community nurse, health visitor, GP, home help or friends. Isolation precautions may consist of wearing the appropriate protective clothing (gloves and apron) when contact with body fluid or contaminated surfaces is likely, and careful handwashing after removing the gloves and apron and before leaving the house. Nurses should remember that taps, towels and door handles may be contaminated if the patient's hygiene is poor; it is useful to carry some paper towels in addition to a small container of antibacterial handwash solution. The use of an alcohol hand-rub after leaving the house may also be advisable.

The patient, or his relatives, may need advice on washing clothes or dishes. Generally, hot soapy water is adequate for dishes, which are best left to drip dry, and a 'hot' wash (60 °C or 90–95 °C) is satisfactory for linen (see p. 554). A laundry service may be available through the local health board/authority. Clinical waste should be disposed of in the appropriately coloured bag designated for clinical waste in the community (see p. 554), and special collection arrangements may have to be made.

Other isolation precautions are rarely necessary at home, and many are not practicable.

Choosing a disinfectant

Most health boards/authorities have a disinfectant policy which states the disinfectants that have been tested and approved for use.

?	**16.10** Check the disinfectant policy for your health board to find out which agents are recommended.

Despite the disadvantages of chemical disinfectants, chemicals are still necessary for dealing with large surfaces after spillage or infection (see p. 554). It must be remembered that some materials are incompatible with certain disinfectants (see p. 553), and that disinfectants will not work in some situations, e.g. on carpets. Carpets are almost impossible to disinfect adequately, and it is not advisable in hospital to carpet areas where body fluid spillage is likely to occur.

SALMONELLOSIS

PATHOPHYSIOLOGY

Salmonellosis is caused by one of about 200 serotypes of the genus *Salmonella* which cause disease in humans and animals (Grist et al 1987). Only a few of these are encountered in the UK. The organism is ingested; common sources are contaminated meat and poultry products (Benenson 1990, Abbott & Robertson 1980) and untreated milk (DHSS 1987a). The incubation period is 12–72 hours.

Some salmonelli, e.g. *S. typhi* and *S. paratyphi*, can cause enteric fever.

Common presenting symptoms are highly variable, ranging from the mild or inapparent to life-threatening septicaemia. Normally, the effects of infection are acute enterocolitis with diarrhoea, abdominal pain and nausea; less frequently, they include vomiting, fever, headache and toxaemia. Rarely, arthritis, cholecystitis, endocarditis, pyelonephritis, meningitis or pneumonia occur.

MEDICAL MANAGEMENT

Investigative procedures. Diagnostic investigation includes stool bacterial culture while diarrhoea persists. If enteric fever, septicaemia or a focal infection is suspected, blood cultures during the acute stage of the illness are done. Serological tests are of little value except in the detection of a 'carrier'.

Treatment. Rehydration and electrolyte replacement may be necessary in the treatment of severe enterocolitis. Antibiotics are not generally given in uncomplicated intestinal infection as they tend to prolong the excretion of the organism. Antibiotics are given in systemic disease and in extraintestinal focal infections. Chloramphenicol is traditionally used in enteric fever; ampicillin or trimethoprim/sulphamethoxazole can be given if the organism is known to be sensitive. Ciprofloxacin is exceedingly active and can even be successful in eradicating the carrier state.

NURSING PRIORITIES AND MANAGEMENT OF SALMONELLOSIS

Many people with salmonellosis become ill at home, often after a cold buffet or an undercooked meal or after eating poultry. Eggs have also been implicated (Coyle et al 1988). Most people will wait to see if the symptoms subside before contacting their GP, but if a particular item of food is suspect they may seek help earlier.

Institutional outbreaks can and do occur (DHSS 1986a) and are usually a result of defects in food hygiene, either at kitchen or ward level. Crossinfection in the ward can occur, either directly from a patient with salmonellosis to another person, or via nurses' hands if hygiene is poor. The cause of such outbreaks is not always identified.

The nurse is unlikely to be involved in caring for a patient at home with acute salmonellosis, unless there are concurrent problems. The community nurse or health visitor may be involved in helping to obtain faecal specimens from other members of the family and in trying to trace the source of infection, in conjunction with the Environmental Health Officer and the Community Medicine Specialist (Communicable Diseases and Environmental Health; variously termed Medical Officer for Environmental Health, Consultant in Public Health Medicine, etc.). Such visits are an excellent opportunity for health education in general and food hygiene as part of a planned programme which takes into account family needs.

Life-threatening concerns

Those that may arise are septicaemia, focal sepsis, severe fluid and electrolyte imbalance, and dehydration.

Major patient problems

These include skin excoriation from severe diarrhoea, fever, abdominal pain, nausea, loss of appetite, and weakness because of constant diarrhoea. (See Nursing Care Plan 16.2.)

Further considerations

Specific ongoing nursing care

Ongoing care comprises the following aspects:

- preventing the spread of infection and teaching handwashing
- ensuring that fluid intake is adequate (see Ch. 20)
- ensuring that nutrition is adequate (see Ch. 21), while trying to accommodate the patient's wishes. (This can be difficult in hospital, where there is central catering and where meals are delivered at specific times.)
- keeping the anal region clean and dry and applying a barrier cream to prevent excoriation
- ensuring that the patient can manage to get to the toilet or has a commode at his bedside
- designating one nurse on each shift (in hospital) to look after the patient. It is important for nurses to spend time with the patient to give reassurance and counteract the loneliness of isolation
- encouraging visitors to visit at different times of day
- identifying a carer at home
- encouraging self-care and independence
- trying to ensure privacy as far as possible
- being sensitive to any odour problem; discussing this with the patient might help (see Ch. 26).

Care with faeces will be needed in the home, with particular attention to surfaces which may be contaminated. In hospital, isolation precautions will be required (see Box 16.5). The degree of isolation will depend on the state of the patient and on how far faecal matter is likely to be spread into the environment.

HEPATITIS B

Hepatitis B is a viral infection which is transmitted sexually, by blood contact (e.g. needle-sharing by intravenous drug abusers) and needlestick injury, and across the placenta from mother to child in utero. It is endemic in some parts of the world. The virus, HBV, has been found in most body secretions and excretions, but only blood, saliva, semen and vaginal secretions have been shown to be infectious (Benenson 1990). Hepatitis B was formerly seen in people who had received blood and blood products and in people who had been given

Nursing Care Plan 16.2 Managing problems of a patient with salmonellosis
Mr G is 67 years old and has been admitted to hospital from a local nursing home because he has salmonellosis. He is confined to bed and has frequent diarrhoea.

Nursing considerations	Action	Rationale	Evaluation
1. Isolation precautions required because: • **Mr G has salmonellosis** • **He is bedridden** • **He has diarrhoea and experiences difficulty in using bedpans**	❒ Standard isolation ❒ Wear disposable gloves when handling faeces or any items touched or used by Mr G ❒ Wear plastic apron and mask if there is danger of splash ❒ Wear gown if uniform is likely to be contaminated e.g. lifting	Mr G is bedridden, has diarrhoea and finds it difficult to use bedpans, and so his immediate environment (bedlinen, items touched by him) might be contaminated Protective clothing is necessary only when there is contact with faeces, or when items touched or used by the patient are being handled. The type of protective clothing worn will depend on the procedure being carried out	No spread of salmonellosis to any other patients or staff in the ward
2. Mr G will need company and distraction while in the single room	❒ Allocate one nurse to look after him on each shift.Try to ensure frequent visits and company. TV in room	Loneliness is common when patients are isolated; aim to do the same for Mr G as you would if he were in a multi-bed ward	
3. Mr G is embarrassed by constant diarrhoea and occasional accidents	❒ Try to ensure privacy		

Box 16.5 Patient education: prevention and management of salmonellosis

In discussing the management of salmonella poisoning in a home care setting with the patient and his relatives and giving instruction on how to prevent its recurrence the nurse should:

- stress the need for fluids and for nourishing and tempting meals
- teach and demonstrate good hand hygiene
- teach skin care and its importance
- explain the need to keep surfaces clean, e.g. toilets, doorhandles, taps
- offer reassurance that efforts will be made to trace the cause
- explain the importance of food hygiene, stressing the following points:
  - — Defrost frozen foods thoroughly before cooking
  - — Do not store raw foods above cooked foods in the fridge (to prevent contamination through dripping)
  - — Do not use the same utensils or surfaces for cooked and raw foods
  - — Cook food at the recommended temperature for the required time; if the food is to be stored, chill it as quickly as possible
  - — Keep foods hot or cold, not warm
- reassure the patient that recovery is the usual outcome
- ask if the patient's work involves food handling; if it does, check with the doctor about the need for clearance specimens.

In hospital, the nurse should follow the above outline but in addition:

- explain treatment and give information and reassurance about isolation procedures and why they are needed
- assure the patient that by the time he is discharged home isolation precautions should be minimal, i.e. care with faeces and exudate precautions.

Excretion of the organism may persist long after the symptoms have disappeared — sometimes for months or years. This is only significant in people whose work involves food handling.

injections with contaminated needles. These risks have largely been eliminated in the developed countries by the screening of blood donors, the testing of donor blood, and the single use of sterile syringes and needles. The risk to health care workers is that of inoculation with infected blood, either through needlestick injury with a contaminated needle, or by being splashed with infected blood on skin abrasions or mucous membranes.

PATHOPHYSIOLOGY

The virus is made up of several particles, each of which is capable of inducing an immune response. HBsAg (hepatitis B surface antigen) is the first antigen to appear in the blood after infection. The presence of anti-HBs in the blood is the best measure of immunity to the virus (Holland 1985).

Acute hepatitis B may have one of four outcomes:

- complete recovery
- fulminant hepatitis: rare but frequently fatal
- carrier state: HBsAg positive
- chronic hepatitis: may lead to cirrhosis of the liver and to hepatocellular carcinoma (See Ch. 4, p. 115).

Of all cases of hepatitis B infection in Western societies, Junge & Deinhardt (1985) have estimated that 45% result in acute disease, 5% develop chronic infection and 50% follow an asymptomatic course.

Individuals in the last group may be unaware of the infection and of their potential for transmitting the virus to others. Approximately 5–10% of these will become HBsAg carriers (Williams & Fagan 1988).

The incubation period for hepatitis B is 45–180 days (Benenson 1990). Onset is insidious.

Common presenting symptoms are highly variable, ranging from inapparent infection or malaise with abnormal liver function tests to cases of fatal acute hepatic necrosis. Normally, anorexia, nausea, vomiting, abdominal discomfort and fever occur, followed perhaps by arthralgia, urticaria or glomerulonephritis (caused by antigen–antibody complexes) progressing to jaundice.

MEDICAL MANAGEMENT

Investigative procedures are serological, e.g. radioimmunoassay, ELISA or immunodiffusion. HBsAg is indicative of infection and infectivity and occurs both before and during the acute illness. This finding must be interpreted with caution, however, as HBsAg may still be present in carriers and the chronically infected who have become jaundiced from some other cause. Another antigen, HBeAg, is a marker of replication in the liver and therefore of high infectivity. HBV DNA is a more sophisticated measure of replication, infectivity and the progression to chronic liver disease. IgM anti-HBc is an antibody to the 'c' or 'core' antigen which may be present during the diagnostically difficult 'window' when HBsAg and anti-HBs are in equivalence and neither is detectable in the serum. Serial estimation of these, other antigens/antibodies, other viruses such as hepatitis D and the liver enzymes may be necessary to establish the stage and progression of the disease.

Treatment. There is no effective treatment for the acute disease. Bedrest is not of proven value but it would seem wise to avoid strenuous exercise during the acute phase. Effective vaccines are available and are recommended for health care personnel working with patients, particularly high-risk patients, and those in contact with blood, particularly when handling instruments. Prophylaxis is also given after inoculation accidents and to sexual contacts of HBsAg positive persons as well as to infants born to HBsAg positive mothers. Chronic hepatitis B may be treated by immunosuppression with a tapering course of corticosteroids such as prednisone for 6 weeks followed by antiviral therapy with recombinant interferon or interleukin-2. Liver transplantation, however, may still be the last recourse for a patient with advancing chronic disease.

NURSING PRIORITIES AND MANAGEMENT OF HEPATITIS B

Since there is no treatment for acute hepatitis B, nursing priorities are to alleviate symptoms and to support the patient until the disease has run its course. People with acute hepatitis B may stay at home, requiring admission to hospital only when they are too ill to be looked after at home, or when they require specific medical intervention.

Life-threatening concerns

Fulminant hepatitis will lead to gross liver failure and all of the associated problems (see Ch. 4).

Major patient problems

These include lethargy, weakness, nausea, vomiting, and anxiety about transmission.

Further considerations

Specific ongoing care

This includes the following interventions:

- preventing the spread of infection
- encouraging the patient to rest; lethargy and weakness are often the first symptoms to arise and the last to go away
- ensuring that fluid intake is adequate (see Ch. 20).
- accurate recording of fluid balance
- ensuring that nutrition is adequate (see Ch. 21)
- providing skin care and change of position
- ensuring that the patient can manage to get to the toilet, or has a commode at his bedside
- designating one nurse per shift to look after the patient in hospital. Loneliness and dejection can be minimised by talking with the patient and discussing his needs. Access to a telephone, television and other diversions may be important (see p. 556)
- encouraging relatives and friends to stagger visiting times
- encourage self-care and independence (see Box 16.6)
- exercising care with blood if the nurse is caring for the patient at home.

In hospital, isolation precautions will be required during the acute illness. The patient must not share razors and toothbrushes with others.

PULMONARY TUBERCULOSIS

Pulmonary tuberculosis is now the most common form of tuberculosis infection, although other systems are sometimes affected, e.g. the genitourinary or skeletal systems. Incidence and prevalence are considerably higher among immigrants to Britain than in the native white population (Christie 1987). This disease is notifiable in the UK.

Box 16.6 Patient education: management of hepatitis B

In discussing with the patient and his relatives the management of hepatitis B infection at home, the nurse should:

- stress the need for rest and for adequate fluids and nourishment
- explain the importance of position changes and how to care for the skin
- explain about how the virus can be passed on to others
- teach hand hygiene
- discuss the possibility of hepatitis B vaccination for the patient's partner
- offer emotional support and include the family in the assessment of the patient and care planning
- provide written information if available.

In a hospital setting, the nurse should also explain about isolation precautions and why they are necessary.

Some patients may be concerned about their employment outlook because they have had hepatitis B or are carriers. In general, this is not a barrier to future employment; the patient should be encouraged to discuss the matter with his own doctor, and possibly with his employer's occupational health physician.

Depending on how the infection was contracted, the patient may need advice about the possibility of HIV infection. It could also be helpful to the patient to discuss the sharing of information about his illness with others; the patient's wishes in this regard should be documented in the care plan.

PATHOPHYSIOLOGY

Pulmonary tuberculosis is a bacterial infection caused by *Mycobacterium tuberculosis* (also known as the tubercle bacillus). The bacteria enter the body by being inhaled; once they reach the epithelial surface of the alveolus they cause swelling of the epithelial cells and local capillary dilatation. Although some organisms will be engulfed by alveolar macrophages (see p. 545), they will not be destroyed and will continue to multiply; some will escape and may enter the bloodstream, with the potential to infect any other organ in the body. Lymph nodes are often infected.

Invasion of the lung tissue gives rise to an inflammatory reaction in which the infected alveoli fill up with fluid, macrophages, and bacteria. Eventually fibrosis will be visible on a chest X-ray. The primary lesion in the lung is often asymptomatic and confined to one area. Healing of the lung tissue occurs, sometimes leaving an area of calcification.

The patient becomes Mantoux positive 4–6 weeks after primary infection; that is to say, he will develop a hypersensitivity reaction to an injection of tuberculin (see Appendix II). A chronic cough with mucopurulent sputum develops as the disease becomes more advanced.

Dormant bacilli may be reactivated by an alteration in immunity resulting from age, malnutrition or other diseases. People with AIDS (see Ch. 38) are prone to developing tuberculosis. People with pulmonary tuberculosis are considered to be infectious until they have had 2 weeks of appropriate chemotherapy (Sub-committee of the Joint Tuberculosis Committee 1990).

Common presenting symptoms. Normally the initial infection is inapparent. Pulmonary disease is characterised by cough, fever, fatigue and weight loss, and less frequently by haemoptysis, chest pain or erythema nodosum. Extrapulmonary disease is less common but can involve most organs of the body, causing, for example, meningitis, lymphadenitis, pericarditis, pleurisy, nephritis, cystitis, osteomyelitis, arthritis, laryngitis or peritonitis.

MEDICAL MANAGEMENT

Investigative procedures. Diagnostic investigation includes chest X-ray, often with tomograms. Microscopy and culture of sputum, gastric washings, urine, CSF, aspirate or biopsy material are performed as appropriate. Histology of biopsy material is done. Skin testing with tuberculin may be performed, especially in the young.

Treatment. Normally, pulmonary tuberculosis is treated with a combination of isoniazid, rifampicin, ethambutol and pyrazinamide to avoid emergence of bacterial resistance. Other antibiotics may be used when resistance is present or likely to be a problem, and particularly in patients from abroad. Ethambutol is not normally given to patients under 5 years of age or to very elderly individuals. Therapy continues for at least 6 months.

NURSING PRIORITIES AND MANAGEMENT OF PULMONARY TUBERCULOSIS

The main aims in nursing patients with pulmonary tuberculosis are to establish drug therapy and to encourage compliance. The underlying health of these patients may not be good, and their nutritional status is often poor. The prospect of having to take a large number of tablets regularly over a long period of time is daunting, and the side-effects of some drugs may make some people stop taking them. A great deal of support and encouragement will be needed (Ley 1988).

Once a person is diagnosed as having pulmonary tuberculosis, it is important that he is kept away from anyone who is immunosuppressed. Contacts may require follow-up; in the case of staff, this is done by the Occupational Health Department. Non-staff contacts such as family members can be referred to a chest physician.

A sputum specimen sent to bacteriology will be examined directly under the microscope for the presence of tubercle bacilli. If these bacilli are seen, the report will state 'AAFB (acid alcohol fast bacilli) seen on direct film', 'film positive', 'smear positive', or 'ZN (Ziehl – Nielsen) positive', and the patient will be considered to have 'open' pulmonary tuberculosis. This simply means that there are enough bacilli in the sputum for them to be easily seen in a small sample, and therefore that the sputum is infectious to others. Culture of the organism may take 3–6 weeks, and is necessary to make a firm diagnosis. (There are mycobacteria other than *M. tuberculosis*.) Infectivity also depends on whether or not the person is 'productive'; that is, a person who is highly productive of sputum and is film positive is much more likely to infect others than someone who is film positive and not coughing up any sputum at all.

Life-threatening concerns

Respiratory failure may develop if the patient is too weak to cough. Tuberculosis in people who are immunosuppressed, such as AIDS patients, can result in serious illness.

Major patient problems

These include difficulty in maintaining the drug regimen and in learning to cough in a safe way.

Further considerations

Specific ongoing care

Nursing care and physiotherapy for people with pulmonary tuberculosis is similar to that for patients with any other respiratory infection (see Ch. 3). The dietitian may be asked to advise on appropriate diet.

The risk of spreading the infection to others is greatly reduced when the person remains at home, in which case care with sputum is usually all that is necessary. There is some debate as to whether isolation precautions are required for patients with pulmonary tuberculosis in hospital. Recent advice (Sub-Committee of the Joint Tuberculosis Committee 1990) recommends that the patient who is 'smear positive' should be segregated in a single room for 2 weeks, but that other isolation precautions (gowns, masks, special crockery, etc.) are unnecessary. This document, however, also states that people who are 'smear positive' are infectious. Because of this, some isolation precautions may still be taken, for example, wearing a mask when one is within 3 feet of the patient when he is coughing.

Staff who have been in close respiratory contact with patients with open pulmonary tuberculosis may be screened by Mantoux tests and if necessary, by chest X-ray. Other staff contacts may receive TB contact cards.

Patients are sometimes found to have tuberculosis when they are being investigated in hospital for chest disease. Other patients in the same room may be notified through their GP. If these contacts are likely to have a prolonged stay in hospital, their consultant may also be notified.

There may be difficulties in explaining the importance of drug therapy, particularly if English is not the patient's native language. Tracing and follow-up of contacts of people with pulmonary tuberculosis is important. Those relatives and friends of the patient who have been in close respiratory contact are generally referred to an infectious diseases' physician for examination and follow-up. Some English inner cities are reintroducing specialist community nurses as TB visitors.

?	**16.11** Miss A is a 78-year-old lady who has lived alone since her sister's death a year ago. Recently, she lost her appetite and developed a persistent cough. A sputum specimen was taken and open pulmonary tuberculosis diagnosed. Normally a pleasant, cooperative person, Miss A was grumpy and resentful when the nurse visited her at home, and there were soiled tissues strewn all over the bed and floor. Devise a care plan to prevent the spread of infection from sputum and saliva.

MENINGOCOCCAL INFECTION

Infections caused by a gram-negative bacterium, *Neisseria meningitidis*, are commonly known as meningococcal infections.

PATHOPHYSIOLOGY

The organism is inhaled and may enter the bloodstream via the nasopharynx, giving rise to bacteraemia and, frequently, pyogenic meningitis. It is the most common cause of bacterial meningitis in the UK (MacLeod et al 1987). The disease usually starts with signs of upper respiratory infection, followed after a day or two by headache, vomiting, fever, and a petechial rash.

Common presenting symptoms are highly variable. They may be inapparent or consist of local symptoms if there is nasopharyngeal infection only. The disease may be invasive with fever, septicaemia, a petechial or macular rash and rarely, pneumonia or joint involvement. It may be meningeal, with fever, intense headache, stiff neck, nausea and vomiting. Delirium and coma may supervene. Fulminating cases may present with sudden shock, extensive purpura and disseminated intravascular coagulation (see Ch. 18, p. 613).

MEDICAL MANAGEMENT

Investigative procedures. Diagnostic investigation consists of microscopy and culture of CSF as well as CSF cellular and chemical analysis. Detection of antigens in the CSF is carried out by CCIE (countercurrent immunoelectrophoresis) or immunocoagglutination techniques. Blood and throat swab or skin lesion culture is done.

Treatment. The drug of choice in the treatment of meningococcal infections is benzyl penicillin, given in high dosage parenterally, commenced as soon as the diagnosis is suspected. If the bacteriological diagnosis cannot be established with certainty then broad spectrum treatment is often given to cover other bacterial pathogens; this consists of high-dose penicillin in combination with chloramphenicol or an injectable cephalosporin such as cefotaxime alone. Sulphonamides are not usually used in the UK as resistant strains of the bacterium are common. Close salivary contacts are given rifampicin to eradicate nasopharyngeal carriage.

NURSING PRIORITIES AND MANAGEMENT OF MENINGOCOCCAL INFECTION

Life-threatening concerns

This disease *is* life threatening. Death may occur due to fulminating septicaemic shock (see p. 601), which has a high mortality rate if not detected in its early stages.

Major patient problems

Meningeal irritation may result in neck stiffness. Vomiting and sweating may lead to dehydration and electrolyte imbalance (see Ch. 20, p. 641).

Further considerations

The patient with meningococcal meningitis is infectious, and isolation precautions, especially taking care with upper respiratory tract secretions and saliva, will be required until antibiotics have been administered.

?	**16.12** Create a care plan for a young woman admitted to hospital with all of the typical features of meningococcal meningitis.

CHICKENPOX AND SHINGLES

Chickenpox and shingles are both caused by the same virus, known as the varicella zoster virus. Primary infection causes chickenpox (varicella), and most people have chickenpox only once, since infection usually confers long immunity. The virus remains latent, however, and recurrence in a different form — shingles (herpes zoster) — can occur many years after the initial infection and on more than one occasion.

Chickenpox is highly infectious, from both respiratory droplets and from skin lesions. Although common in children, it also affects adults, sometimes causing severe disease. Shingles is usually seen in older people (50–80 years of age) and only the skin lesions are infectious. People can develop chickenpox after contact with someone suffering from shingles; but shingles cannot be contracted from a person suffering from chickenpox.

Nursing staff should be aware of their immune status (see Box 16.7). (The nurse's immune status is normally determined from her personal history. Only in the event of a unit being unable to provide sufficient immune staff would it be necessary to resort to an IgG (see Box 16.1) test for the presence of antibodies.) A nurse who is not known to be immune should not nurse someone with chickenpox or shingles. This is because people who are incubating the disease are infectious for several days before they develop symptoms, and they may inadvertently infect others before they are aware they have caught the disease themselves. It is also advisable for pregnant staff to keep away from patients with chickenpox or shingles.

Box 16.7 Staff contacts with infectious diseases of childhood

The following questions should be posed in determining which staff members should provide nursing care for patients with diseases such as measles, mumps, rubella and chickenpox:

1. Are the staff members known to be immune (e.g. rubella antibody positive, or have they been immunised)? In the case of a disease that produces lasting immunity, have they had the disease themselves?
2. Are they working with susceptible patients, e.g. neonates, young children, the seriously ill, or the immunosuppressed?

If the answer to (1) is 'Yes' it is usually all right for the staff members to work as usual.

If the answer to (1) is 'No' and to (2) is 'Yes', the staff members should be reassigned to a non-susceptible area until the incubation period is over.

In circumstances where there is any doubt, the control of infection or occupational health department should be consulted.

Chickenpox

PATHOPHYSIOLOGY

The incubation period of chickenpox is 2–3 weeks, commonly 13–17 days. The disease is communicable from 5 days before the onset of the rash until 6 days after the first crop of vesicles has appeared.

Common presenting symptoms. The first symptoms are usually a slight fever and the development of a skin rash which is maculopapular at first, becomes vesicular, and then forms a scab. The lesions do not all occur at the same time but in succession, so that on different parts of the body they may be at a different stage. Areas of the body that are normally covered by clothing often have more lesions than exposed parts.

MEDICAL MANAGEMENT

Treatment. There is no specific treatment for chickenpox, although antibiotics may be given for secondary infection of vesicles. Zoster immunoglobulin can be given to those at special risk (e.g. the immunosuppressed) who have been in contact with the disease and have not had it themselves.

NURSING PRIORITIES AND MANAGEMENT OF CHICKENPOX

Life-threatening concerns

Rarely, chickenpox can cause severe illness. The most common cause of death in adults with the disease is primary viral pneumonia. Children may develop septic complications or encephalitis. The disease can be severe in the immunosuppressed.

Major patient problems

The rash may cause irritation and discomfort, and secondary bacterial infection of lesions can occur.

Further considerations

Chickenpox is highly infectious, both from respiratory secretions and from skin discharges. Strict isolation will be required until the period of communicability is over. (Protective clothing must be worn for every entry to the room; the door must be kept closed, and negative ventilation used if available. All items in the room will be contaminated and will therefore require disinfection.)

SHINGLES

PATHOPHYSIOLOGY

Common presenting symptoms. The first symptoms the person notices are often pain and paraesthesia in the affected area; this is usually the trunk but can be the face or a limb. A rash appears, starting with a macule on which vesicles develop over several days. The vesicles, which are a grey colour, dry up and crust over, usually in a week or so. The rash is characteristically restricted to the area supplied by the sensory nerves of one or an associated group of dorsal root ganglia. Subsequent healing may take several weeks, and residual or prolonged pain occurs in about 10% of cases.

MEDICAL MANAGEMENT

Treatment involves administering analgesics, acyclovir and sometimes applying idoxuridine paint to the vesicles in the early stages.

NURSING PRIORITIES AND MANAGEMENT OF SHINGLES

Shingles can flare up spontaneously, or may follow treatment for another disease, e.g. radiotherapy.

Major patient problems

Pain and discomfort may result from the lesions, which may persist for a long time. The patient may experience anxiety and depression if the condition fails to improve; this is especially common among elderly patients. A sympathetic and optimistic attitude can do a lot to make the symptoms more bearable.

Further considerations

Care of the skin condition is similar to that for other skin disorders (see Ch. 12); it should be borne in mind that the lesions will be susceptible to secondary bacterial infection.

If the person is in hospital he should be kept apart from other vulnerable patients. Isolation precautions may be necessary until the lesions have crusted over. The type of isolation will be determined by the extent and location of the lesions and whether they can be adequately covered to prevent contamination of outer clothing or bed-linen. Only immune staff should nurse patients with shingles (see Box 16.7).

?	
?	**16.13** A 70-year-old woman is at home suffering from *Campylobacter jejuni* enteritis. She is fully mobile and has profuse diarrhoea but seems to make it to the toilet in time. Although she tells you she has understood what you told her about the disease, during your visit she went to the toilet and did not wash her hands afterwards. Her grandchildren (aged 3 years and 7 years) visit her regularly and she always has a supply of fruit and sweets for them. • Devise a nursing plan for this patient for home care. • Devise a nursing plan for hospital care. • What advice would you give to this patient and to her family about hygiene? • Think about how you might try to ensure that your advice was followed.
?	**16.14** Arrange to spend some time with the Infection Control Nurse in your health board/authority. Find out what she does and how her work relates to patient care.
?	**16.15** Ask if you can visit the microbiology laboratory in your hospital. Find out what information is required on the specimen request form and why it is important. Ask to see what happens to the various specimens and which tests are carried out.
?	**16.16** Arrange to visit your HSDU. Watch how instruments are received, unwrapped, washed, dried, packed and autoclaved, or disinfected.
?	**16.17** Discuss with a community nurse how the control of infection can be achieved in the patient's home, e.g. hand hygiene, use of protective clothing, aseptic techniques and disinfection of equipment.

CONCLUSION

This chapter has outlined the function of the immune system and explained how the components of the immune response come together to protect the body from foreign material, whether microorganisms, allergens, or tumour cells. Unfortunately, things can go wrong. Deficiencies, whether of cells or of proteins, can impair the immune system in its response.

Immune deficiency can be acquired, either through infection, e.g. HIV/AIDS (see Ch. 38) or as a result of medical treatment, e.g. immunosuppression during and after cytotoxic drug administration or radiotherapy (see Ch. 32). Hypersensitivity gives rise to a whole range of 'allergic' conditions, and the autoimmune diseases cause considerable morbidity and mortality. Infectious diseases have been with us for centuries and although some have become less common, others step in to take their place.

Nursing care, in whatever context, involves a thorough assessment of each patient as an individual. Potential problems include the risk of the spread of infection, either through people (other patients, staff) or through inanimate objects (equipment, instruments). Some of the issues surrounding hospital-acquired infection (also called nosocomial infection) will be discussed in Ch. 23. The safety of our patients is, to a large extent, in our own hands. It is up to us to do everything we can to make sure that the environment in which we care for people is, indeed, a safe one.

ACKNOWLEDGEMENTS

The author wishes to extend her thanks to Dr A. B. White, Consultant Microbiologist and Control of Infection Officer, Dr D. O. Ho-Yen, Consultant Microbiologist, and Dr M. M. Steven, Consultant Physician, all of Raigmore Hospital, NHS Trust, Inverness, for their generous assistance in the preparation of this chapter.

REFERENCES

Abbott J D, Robertson L 1980 The isolation of salmonellas from minced meat. A report from the PHLS Salmonella Sub-committee. Environmental Health 88: 123

Ayliffe G A J, Babb J R, Davies J G, Lilly H A 1988 Hand disinfection: a comparison of various agents in laboratory and ward studies. Journal of Hospital Infection 11: 226–43

Babb J R 1990 Chemical disinfection and COSHH: safe and effective work practices. Institute of Sterile Services Managers Journal July/Aug: 9–12

Benenson A S (ed) 1990 Control of communicable diseases in man, 15th edn. American Public Health Association, Washington

Bond W, Favero M S, Petersen N J, Ebert J W 1983 Inactivation of hepatitis B virus by intermediate to high level disinfectant chemicals. Journal of Clinical Microbiology 18(3): 535–538

Bowell B. In: Caddow P (ed) 1989 Applied microbiology. Scutari, Harrow, ch 8

British Medical Association 1989 A code of practice for sterilisation of instruments and control of cross-infection. British Medical Association, London

Christie A B 1987 Infectious diseases, 4th edn. Churchill Livingstone, Edinburgh, vols 1, 2

Control of substances hazardous to health regulations (COSHH) 1988 HMSO, London

Coyle E F, Palmer S R, Ribeiro C D, Jones H I, Howard A J, Ward L, Rowe B 1988 Salmonella enteritidis phage type 4 infection: association with hens' eggs. Lancet 2: 1295–1296

Denton P F 1986 Psychological and physiological effects of isolation. Nursing UK 3: 88–91

DOH 1992 Immunisation against infectious disease. HMSO, London

DHSS 1986a The report of the committee of inquiry into an outbreak of food poisoning at Stanley Royal Hospital. HMSO, London

DHSS 1986b Safety information bulletin SIB(86). Disinfection of endoscopes potentially contaminated with Mycobacterium species. DHSS, London

DHSS 1987a Health Service catering hygiene. HMSO, London

DHSS 1987b Hospital laundry arrangements for used and infected linen. HC(87) 30 DHSS, London

DHSS 1987c Decontamination of health care equipment prior to inspection, service or repair HN(87) 22 DHSS, London

DHSS 1988 Information to undertakers: infectious diseases PL/CMO (88) 7 DHSS, London

Emond B T D, Bradley J M, Galbraith N S 1989 Pocket consultant: infection, 2nd edn. Blackwell Scientific, Oxford

Greaves A 1985 We'll just freshen you up, dear ... Nursing Times Journal of Infection Control Nursing 81(10) Suppl: 3–8

Grist N R, Ho-Yen D O, Walker E, Williams G R 1987 Diseases of infection: an illustrated textbook. Oxford University Press, Oxford

Health and safety at work act 1974 HMSO, London

HSAC (Health Services Advisory Committee) 1982 The safe disposal of clinical waste. HMSO, London

Holland P V 1985 Hepatitis B surface antigen and antibody (HBsAg/Anti-HBs). In: Gerety R J (ed) Hepatitis B. Academic Press, London

Junge U, Deinhardt F 1985 The acute manifestations of hepatitis B virus infection. In: Gerety R J (ed) Hepatitis B. Academic Press, London

Kelen G D, DiGiovanna T, Bisson L, Kalainov D, Sivertson K T, Quinn T C 1989 Human immunodeficiency virus infection in emergency department patients. Journal of the American Medical Association 262(4): 516–22

Kirkwood E, Lewis C 1989 Understanding medical immunology, 2nd edn. Wiley, Chichester

Kobayashi H, Tsuzuki M, Koshimizu K et al 1984 Susceptibility of hepatitis B virus to disinfectants or heat. Journal of Clinical Microbiology 20(2): 214–6

Larson E 1988 A causal link between hand washing and risk of infection? Examination of the evidence. Infection Control Hospital Epidemiology 9(1): 28–36

Ley P 1988 Communicating with patients: improving communication, satisfaction and compliance. Croom Helm, London

Lowbury E J L, Lilly H A 1973 Use of 4% chlorhexidine detergent solution (Hibiscrub) and other methods of skin disinfection. British Medical Journal 1(5852): 510–15

Lynch P, Jackson M M, Cummings J, Stamm W E 1987 Rethinking the role of isolation practices in the prevention of nosocomial infections. Annals of Internal Medicine 107: 243–6

MacLeod J, Edwards C, Bouchier I (eds) 1987 Davidson's principles and practice of medicine, 15th edn. Churchill Livingstone, Edinburgh

Maurer I 1985 Hospital hygiene, 3rd edn, Edward Arnold, London

Nurse's Clinical Library 1985 Immune disorders. Nursing 85 Books, Springhouse, PA

Office of Population Censuses and Surveys 1988 Communicable disease statistics. HMSO, London

Reid D, Grist N R, Pinkerton I W 1986 Infections in current medical practice. Butterworth, London

Roitt I 1990 Essential immunology, 7th edn. Blackwell Scientific, Oxford

Roitt I, Brostoff J, Male D 1989 Immunology. Gower, London

Rutala W A 1990 APIC guideline for selection and use of disinfectants. American Journal of Infection Control 18(2): 99–117

SOHHD (Scottish Office Home and Health Department) 1993a Neuro and ophthalmic surgery procedures on patients with or suspected to have, or at risk of developing, Creutzfeldt–Jakob disease (CJD), or Gerstmann–Straussler syndrome (GSS). SOHHD, Edinburgh

SOHHD 1993b Hospital laundry arrangements for used and infected linen MEL (1993)7. SOHHD, Edinburgh

SHHD (Scottish Home and Health Department) 1988 The hospital infection manual. HMSO, Edinburgh

Sub-committee of the Joint Tuberculosis Committee of the British

Thoracic Society 1990 Control and prevention of tuberculosis in Britain: an updated code of practice. British Medical Journal 300(6730): 995–9

Taylor L J 1978a An evaluation of hand-washing techniques — I Nursing Times 74(2): 54–55

Taylor L J 1978b An evaluation of hand-washing techniques — II Nursing Times 74(3): 108–110

United Kingdom Central Council (UKCC) 1992 Code of Professional Conduct for the Nurse, Midwife and Health Visitor, 3rd edn. UKCC, London

UK Health Departments 1990 Guidance for clinical health care workers: protection against infection with HIV and hepatitis viruses. HMSO, London

Webster O, Bowell B 1986 Thinking prevention. Nursing Times Journal of Infection Control Nursing 82(23): 68–74

Williams W D 1983 Guidelines for infection control in hospital personnel. Centers for Disease Control, Atlanta, GA

Williams R, Fagan E 1988 Viral hepatitis in hospitals: a clinical overview. Journal of Hospital Infection II Suppl A: 142–149

Working Party of the British Society of Gastroenterology 1988 Cleaning and disinfection of equipment for gastrointestinal flexible endoscopy: interim recommendations. Gut 29: 1134–1151

FURTHER READING

Akerman V, Dunk-Richards G 1991 Microbiology: an introduction for the health sciences. Harcourt Brace Jovanovich, Sydney

Brown J, Capewell S 1986 Respiratory tuberculosis. Nursing UK 4: 132–134

Burton G R W 1992 Microbiology for the health sciences, 4th edn. Lippincott, Philadelphia

Contreras M, Mollison P L 1990 Immunological complications of transfusion. British Medical Journal 300(6718): 173–176

Davey B 1989 Immunology: a foundation text. Open University Press, Milton Keynes

Health and Safety Executive 1990 Farmer's lungs. Health and Safety Executive, London

Jenner E 1990 Aspects of isolation care. Nursing UK 4(20): 17–22

Levy J 1989 Listeria and food poisoning: a growing concern. Maternal and Child Health 14: 380–383

MacFarlane A 1989a Infection control: reducing the risk to medical patients. Professional Nurse 4(7): 344–348

MacFarlane A 1989b Using the laboratory in infection control. Professional Nurse 4(8): 393–394, 396–397

Rubin R H, Tolkoff-Rubin N E 1989 Infection: the new problems. Transplantation Proceedings 21(1): 1440–1445

Stewart M 1993 Skills for caring: hygiene for care. Churchill Livingstone, Edinburgh

Wilson K J W 1990 Ross and Wilson anatomy and physiology in health and illness, 7th edn. Churchill Livingstone, Edinburgh

Zukerman A J 1988 Hepatitis B. Hospital Update 14(4): 1389–1400

SECTION 2

Common patient problems and related nursing care

SECTION CONTENTS

17 Stress 575

18 Shock 597

19 Pain 615

20 Fluid and electrolyte balance 637

21 Nutrition 657

22 Temperature control 679

23 Wound healing 697

24 Continence 723

25 Sleep 743

26 Communication 757

The chapters in this section build on the knowledge presented in Section 1 and focus on the problems patients experience in many different disease processes and conditions.

The problems discussed are part of life and so are very much a part of nursing. They arise for any one person at different times, and in a variety of settings and circumstances.

Both patient and nurse perspectives are considered. The focus is on problem solving, based on the latest research.

CHAPTER 17

Stress

Vivian Leefarr

Prof. Margaret Cutler (Section on 'Physiological responses to stress')

CHAPTER CONTENTS

Introduction 575

Models of stress 576
The stimulus-based model 576
Response-based models of stress 576
Transactional models of stress 577
The phenomenological approach 578

Physiological responses to stress 580
The role of hormones in responses to stress 580
The chronic stress response 582

Stress and disease 582
Migraine 582
Depression 583
Anxiety attacks 584
Post-traumatic stress disorder 584
Post-viral fatigue syndrome 585

The concept of coping 585
Models of coping 585

Defence mechanisms 587

The treatment and management of stress 587
Therapy 587
Choosing therapeutic help 588
Drug therapy 588
Other means of stress reduction 589

Stress in nursing 590
Sources of stress 590
Nursing education and the expectations of patient-centred care 591
Working with dying patients 591

Conclusion 594

Glossary 594

References 594

Further reading 595

Useful addresses 596

INTRODUCTION

'Stress' is a word that frequently enters into everyday conversation as people remark on the difficulties and challenges of life. Perhaps most people would describe themselves as being 'stressed' from time to time, but what does this really mean? Is stress something that resides within the environment, in situations that are threatening, harmful or unpleasant, or is it essentially an internal state, an effect of the individual's perception of what is happening to him? Benner & Wreubel (1989, p. 59) define stress as 'the disruption of meanings, understanding and smooth functioning so that harm, loss or challenge is experienced and sorrow, interpretation, or new skill acquisition is required'.

Stress research is a highly complex field involving a number of sciences, including biology, physiology, psychology and sociology. These disciplines take different approaches to the definition, observation and measurement of stress. When biologists and physiologists talk of sources of stress they are referring to empirical phenomena. Their interest is in examining identifiable stressors and their measurable effects upon the organism or system being stressed. Anything which affects the equilibrium of the organism may be described as a stressor; this would include bacterial or viral infections, dehydration, excessive cold or heat, inadequate food, and so on.

Social scientists view stress in terms of the pressures upon the individual to conform (or not to conform) to societal norms. The inherent values expressed in a society's organisation and functioning may themselves be a source of stress to the individual. Modern industrial society, for example, provides food, safety and shelter for its members in return for a commitment to work, often at some sacrifice to personal interests, leisure, and family life.

Psychologists view stress from the perspective of the interaction of individuals and groups with the environment, describing the effects of stress on cognition, emotional well-being, and behaviour.

Nurses need to have a clear understanding of the concept of stress as they endeavour to provide the best possible care for their patients. It is essential for them to appreciate why their patients might be feeling stressed and how their anxiety might be alleviated. In relation to the nurse's own well-being, an understanding of stress and its effects is equally important. Nursing is physically and emotionally strenuous work, and it is vital for nurses to be able to recognise the signs of stress in themselves and to know how to go about managing stress in their daily work.

The present chapter begins by outlining some of the more influential models by which stress has been described. This includes definitions of stress as a type of stimulus, or as a response, or as an interaction between the individual and his environment. The second section of the chapter describes in some detail the effects of stress upon physiological systems. This provides a basis for the third section, which examines the relationship between stress and disease.

The discussion then turns to the concept of coping as various cognitive and behavioural mechanisms by which people commonly attempt to deal with stress are outlined. This is followed by a description of the therapeutic strategies that are available to assist the individual in managing stress. The chapter ends with a discussion of stress in nursing, identifying some of the most significant sources of stress in this very demanding profession and suggesting ways in which vital support can be given to nurses to enable them to meet the emotional demands of patient-centred care.

Case History 17.1

The health visitor could not understand initially why her client, J, an unsupported mother of two, appeared to be tense and unhappy when they met at the child surveillance clinic. She asked if everything was alright and J described how she had new neighbours in the flat above her who played loud music until early in the morning, preventing her and her two children from getting enough sleep. She had tried to talk with them but they had been hostile towards her and made her feel apprehensive. She didn't dare complain to them again. The lack of sleep was affecting J and her children. J had difficulty concentrating at work and felt like crying frequently during the day; the children were overtired and generally irritable, making it even more difficult for her to cope.

The health visitor asked J if she could intervene by contacting the housing department on her behalf, but J said that she was afraid that this would make matters worse.

Note: The author wishes to state that all Case Histories used in this chapter are fictional.

MODELS OF STRESS

The physicist Robert Hooke (1635–1703) used the word 'stress' in the 17th century to refer to the ratio of an external force (created by a load) to the area over which that force was exerted. The resultant strain created a deformation or distortion of the object by what became known as Hooke's Law (Cox 1989).

This use of the word stress is interestingly similar to its modern application in the realm of human emotion and behaviour; indeed, people frequently use words such as 'weight' and 'strain' when describing their feelings of anxiety and stress.

In the 20th century, the adoption of the concept of stress by the biological and behavioural sciences has resulted in the formulation of a number of models by which stress and its effects might be described. The four most influential of these are as follows:

- stimulus-based model
- response-based models
- the transactional model
- the phenomenological approach.

Each of these models and its implications for nursing practice will be described in the following sections.

The stimulus based model

In this model the person is viewed as being constantly exposed to external or environmental 'stressors' in his daily life. Examples of these might be the demands of work, family responsibilities, bereavement or disablement, or more specific stressors such as smells or poor lighting. In this model stress arises from the environment and is external to the individual. It has the potential, however, to cause distressing feelings and/or physical symptoms and to undermin : well-being.

In the stimulus-based model stress is a state that can generally be empirically observed, measured and evaluated, and which can, potentially, be removed or altered to reduce the individual's stress: it is possible, in theory, to make noisy neighbours quieter, a cold working environment warmer or poor lighting conditions more satisfactory. As an approach to iden-tifying areas that might be improved to increase productivity, this model has some appeal for industrial planners and managers (Sutherland & Cooper 1990).

Limitations of the model. In many situations, such as a bereavement or disablement, the original stressor cannot be changed or adapted to reduce distressing feelings. Even in relatively simple situations such as that illustrated in Case History 17.1, removing the stressor is not necessarily a straightforward matter. It quickly becomes apparent that the stimulus-based model has substantial shortcomings when considered in relation to the breadth of human experience (Sutherland & Cooper 1990). Whilst it has some application in limited contexts such as certain working environments it does not explain why some people experience stress in some situations whilst others in similar circumstances do not. Nor does it explain why a given situation may be stressful for a person on one occasion but not at another time. This model also offers no explanation of why a person may be stressed in response to apparently neutral stimuli such as birds, spiders or aeroplanes. Lazarus (1966) argues that it is not possible to evaluate objectively the human experience of stress; only the account or story told by the person about his own feelings and experiences can adequately convey the nature of his stress.

Response-based models of stress

In this model the word 'stress' is used to refer to the experience of the person who sees himself as being in a threatening or difficult situation. Stress is thus a person's *response* to threat and, unlike in the stimulus-based model, is not inherent in the environment or situation. By using this approach it is possible to make sense of an individual's unique stress responses and even of responses that might seem within the stimulus-based model to be irrational, such as a fear of birds, spiders or of flying.

The systems model of the human stress response

A response-based model that considers the human stress response as health related phenomena, represents 'a multifactorial, interactive, dynamic, phenomenon' is the systems model described by Everly & Sobelman (1987, p. 15). In this model the stress response is defined as consisting of the six components described below.

1. Environmental stimuli. Some environmental stimuli, or stressors, cause the activation of the stress response as a direct consequence of their physical or biochemical properties; that is, their effects are not mediated by cognitive – affective evaluation. Examples of such stressors are caffeine, nicotine and extremes of heat and cold. Many environmental stimuli are not, however, intrinsically harmful but are *perceived* as such by the individual and in this way set the stage for the activation of the stress response.

2. *Cognitive-affective domain.* Everly & Sobelman (1987, p. 30) describe this as 'the critical "causal" phase in most stress responses' in that it is the individual's interpretation of environmental stimuli that gives rise to most stress reactions. The perspective that the individual takes toward his environment will be determined by: 'biological predispositions', 'personality patterns', 'learning history' and 'available resources' (p. 17). Everly & Sobelman argue that cognitive appraisal precedes emotional response.

3. *Neurologic triggering mechanisms.* In the locus coeruleus, limbic system and hypothalamic nuclei, Everly & Sobelman (1987) locate the anatomical site for 'the integration of sensory, cognitive, affective, and visceral activity' (p. 20). In response to cognitive – affective appraisal, these structures trigger neurological and endocrine reactions. They also seem to be involved in a feedback system in which visceral and somatic efferent messages are relayed in response to emotional arousal. Everly & Sobelman suggest that 'these centers seem capable of establishing an endogenously-determined neurological tone that is potentially self-perpetuating' and which 'may, over time, serve as the basis for a host of psychiatric and psychophysiologic disorders' (p. 20).

4. *The physiological stress response axes.* The stress response itself occurs sequentially along the neurological, neuroendocrine and endocrine axes and results in neural and hormonal activity directed at target organs.

Neurological axis. Neurological activity is especially evident in reactions to sudden, acute stress and results in direct activation of the sympathetic nervous system (seen in raised heart rate and blood pressure, etc.), the parasympathetic nervous system (seen in constricted pupils, increased salivation, urinary bladder contraction, and so on) and in the transmission of messages to skeletal muscle (resulting in contraction).

Neuroendocrine axis. This is based in the adrenal medullae and plays an important role in longer-term arousal. Release of the catecholamines noradrenaline and adrenaline by the adrenal medullae results in such sympathetic responses as increased cardiac output and diminished blood flow to the skin and the gastrointestinal system (see p. 581).

Endocrine axis. This axis also plays an important role in chronic arousal. Here the hypothalamus, pituitary gland, adrenal cortex and thyroid gland are stimulated serially to release into the circulatory system the range of hormones described on page 581.

5. *Coping.* In this final phase of the stress response the individual attempts to reduce his level of arousal by manipulating the environment or making cognitive adjustments.

6. *Target-organ effects.* If coping is unsuccessful and arousal is either excessive or prolonged, the physiological processes of the stress response are likely to lead to target organ dysfunction or disease.

Limitations of the model. One of the problems in viewing stress as a response only is that this can lead to the assumption that the occurrence of stress in the life of the individual is solely his own responsibility. The descriptive term 'coping' used in a technical sense by stress researchers to describe physiological and psychological ways of adapting to stress can also be used in everyday discourse to describe an individual's lack of *mastery* in stressful circumstances. Thus someone who 'copes' with stress masters a situation in a positive way, whilst someone who does not 'cope' is lacking in this ability (see Case History 17.2). Such judgements on self or others can have a harmful emotional effect on the individual.

?	**17.1** Is shedding tears of sadness in such a circumstance a sign of one's inability to cope?

Hans Selye's General Adaptation Syndrome

Hans Selye's extensive physiological research as an endocrinologist (1936, 1946a–b, 1976) was largely based upon the response-based model of stress. His hypothesis was that all organisms placed under stress behaved in a particular way physiologically, regardless of the nature of the stress. Given the presence of a stressor such as severe heat or cold the response of the organism would be of a uniform nature. Selye concentrated mainly upon a set of physiological responses to stress, which he called the general adaptation syndrome. This syndrome is divisible into three phases: 'alarm reaction', 'resistance' and 'exhaustion'; these are described on page 581.

Limitations of the model. Whilst Selye's work was highly influential in early stress research it is now felt that his model does not take full account of the individuality of psychological and physiological responses. Nor does it consider the role of the *appraisal* of stressful situations, which is now considered to precede each response. Lazarus (1966) argues that there is a circularity about Selye's model in so far as something about the stimulus elicits a particular stress response while something about the response indicates the presence of a stressor.

?	**17.2** Physical stressors such as disease or injury may well result in death, but how might the individual respond to psychological or social stressors such as bereavement or unemployment?

Transactional models of stress

Transactional models of stress do not locate stress solely within the environment or within the responses of the individual, but rather, in the *interaction* between the individual and his environment. Within these models the individual appraises the situation in an attempt to judge how threatening it is and makes a response on the basis of that appraisal. The process of appraisal is highly individual; each person will perceive a threatening situation differently and attach to it his own meanings (Lazarus 1984, Cox 1989, Wolff 1953). Moreover, the relationship between the individual and his envi-

Case History 17.2 Nurse S

Nurse S felt very sad and upset after Mrs B died. As a charge nurse, she had looked after her in the ward for many months after she had been admitted with a fractured hip. In some ways, Mrs B had reminded her of her own mother, who had died many years before. A colleague later saw that she had been crying and remarked brusquely, 'You get too involved! You should try to keep patients at a distance. It doesn't help them or you, and if you cannot cope with the job maybe you should think of doing something else!'

Case History 17.3 Mr P

Nurse T was asked to interview Mr P on his admission to the ward for minor dental surgery the following day. Mr P, a 32-year-old engineer, was married and had two children, a girl and a boy. He lived with his family near the hospital and worked in a factory in a nearby town. During the interview, Nurse T noticed that while Mr P appeared to be in good health and to have a clear understanding of the surgery he was facing he seemed uneasy. Knowing that many patients feel apprehensive before having surgery she asked him how he was feeling. Mr P replied: 'I feel silly, stupid and embarrassed about it but I am very scared — have been since I got the appointment in the post — can't understand why! — Haven't been able to sleep for the past week and when I do I have awful dreams.'

The nurse talked further with Mr P about his feeling of fear. She asked him if he had ever been in hospital before and he recalled with some difficulty how as a small child he had been admitted as an emergency for a circumcision. As he talked he realised how frightened he had been and that when he had been readmitted for an inflamed wound his fear had become even greater.

The following day Mr P had his surgery. Before leaving the ward he said to Nurse T that he had felt better after talking with her. He had still felt afraid but the powerful feeling of terror had gone.

ronment is a dynamic one which constantly changes as the process of appraisal continues.

Nursing application. Case History 17.3 highlights how the transactional model of stress has clear advantages for the clinical nurse. Although Mr P's feeling of terror was related to the stressor of being in hospital and the prospect of surgery these circumstances *in themselves* did not fully account for his state of mind. His feeling of stress derived from his appraisal of the situation, and this appraisal reflected childhood experience. The transactional model of stress recognises that a person such as Mr P, rather than being a passive recipient of stress, interacts actively with a situation.

Cox's man–environment interaction model

Building on the work of Lazarus (1966) and Lazarus & Folkman (1984), Cox's (1989) man – environment interaction model describes the individual's conscious appraisal of a situation, his recognition of threat or harm, and the coping strategies which he then implements. According to this model the individual's interaction with a stressful situation has five stages:

1. Source of demand: a situation is perceived as threatening
2. Individual's perception of demand, and coping based upon personality and early experiences
3. Psychophysiological changes in response to the perceived threat
4. Coping responses and consequences: how the individual sets about dealing with the threat
5. Feedback: both physiological and psychological.

Cox (1989) describes the 'demand' as arising from the individual's psychological and physiological needs. The individual attempts to understand the demand and his ability to do this determines the way he sets about coping. Stress may occur at a time of hopelessness, when the person understands the nature of the threat but is unable to respond in a way that diminishes or removes the threat. At this time physiological responses also become active as methods of coping with stress. At each stage of the model the individual receives evaluative feedback.

Limitations of the model. Given the complexity of individual experiences and coping strategies, it is extremely difficult to subject transactional models of stress such as Cox's man–environment model to empirical evaluation.

? **17.3** Discuss how the terms 'stress' and 'stressor' are used differently within various models of stress.

The role of appraisal

Transactional models of stress recognise that stress is located both within the person and within the situation, and that it is the individual's conscious or unconscious *appraisal* of the situation that determines his feelings of stress or distress. These models acknowledge the complexity of the interaction between the person and his environment and recognise that the person is not the passive victim of a stressor but an active participant in stressful events.

In understanding the role of appraisal it is important to ask two questions:

1. What is it about the environment that causes the person to feel stressed?
2. What is it about the person that makes them feel stressed in this environment?

Appraisal is the interpretative process involving perception, intuition and reason by which the individual continually distinguishes between safe and threatening situations. For the purposes of discussion we may think of appraisal as taking place in the following two stages, although in reality these are concurrent, and the individual's response may be instantaneous.

Primary appraisal. The person evaluates the situation and may decide not to respond even though the situation presents the possibility of harm, loss, threat or challenge.

Secondary appraisal. This involves the longer-term management of the situation: whether the individual needs to take action, when he needs to act, and what action to take.

The phenomenological approach

Phenomenological approaches to knowledge emphasise the importance of the object as it *appears* rather than the object *in itself*. Thus a phenomenological approach to stress rests largely upon the description given by the individual of his own experience of stress. The writings of phenomenological philosophers such as Merleau-Ponty and Heidegger describe human experience as 'being-in-the-world' whereby each person is defined by his own thoughts, feelings, memories, relationships and social settings. Mind and body are not described as separate but as one integral whole (Dreyfus 1987, Benner & Wreubel 1989). The body is the physical means of knowing and sensing the world, and with disablement or disease the experience of the person will be impaired (Benner & Wreubel 1989). Whether the impairment is of the mind or the body the whole experience of the person will be affected.

This view of human experience invites the clinician to use an intuitive approach when working with people who are

Case History 17.4 L and C

L, a student nurse, notices at mealtimes that his colleague C often mentions her distressed feelings about her weight. Knowing that she frequently eats sweets and cakes, he suggests to her that all she would need to do to lose weight would be to stop eating between meals. C, however, rejects this option as being too difficult to carry through.

distressed, for it acknowledges the complexity of individual responses to stress and recognises that providing the right kind of help is, similarly, a complex and subtle task.

Nursing application. Case History 17.4 underlines the fact that solutions to a difficulty which may seem reasonable to one person may present insuperable difficulties to another. In order to understand his colleague's rejection of his suggestion, L would need to know more about why C overeats. If it were possible to ask her about her feelings she might offer one or more reasons for her behaviour. For instance:

- she may feel anxious and unhappy as a student and feel reassured when she eats sweet foods
- she may have started overeating as a child at a time of family distress
- she may have been abused as a child
- she may feel sexually unattractive and find eating a means of gaining consolation
- she may feel constantly hungry.

Nursing application. The description of human experience from a phenomenological viewpoint attributes to the person a wisdom about himself and his problems that cannot easily be gained from an 'objective' position. But does this mean that the clinical nurse is merely a passive observer when working with distressed people? If suggestions and advice cannot be offered in any but the most uncomplicated situations what help *can* be offered?

The most effective help that can be given by the clinical nurse is support in enabling the person to identify what is causing his stress and to deal with it in his own way. This does *not* entail the nurse, however subtly, suggesting what she thinks the patient should do. Rather, it involves being aware and respectful of the patient's right to choose what is appropriate for himself. This is not a passive position for the clinical nurse to take but, in fact, a highly interactive and enabling one (Rogers 1961, Kennedy 1977, Egan 1986). (See Case History 17.5.)

In Case History 17.6 the health visitor does not attempt to deal with the situation by taking action or giving suggestions, even though her concern that Miss H had not eaten or moved for some time might have prompted her to do so. Jennifer's support and concern does, however, enable Miss H to talk about how she feels and then to accept help in dealing with the body of her cat.

This example may also underline a further facet of stress, i.e. that people often experience stress when they are not themselves being threatened. Stress can arise as an empathic response through the perception of the stress experienced by another even when no personal threat is possible. When Jennifer perceives the intense distress of her client she too may experience that distress herself.

Phenomenology, appraisal and the role of stress

In a sense, all appraisal is phenomenological because it rests upon the individual's own attribution of meaning to a situation (Lazarus 1984).

Case History 17.5 Mrs K

Mrs K was admitted to the surgical ward for preliminary investigations to determine why she was experiencing stress incontinence both during the day on coughing or lifting heavy bags and during sexual intercourse.

Her nurse, Sarah, carried out a number of routine investigations. She learned that Mrs K's weight was 16 stone and that she smoked about 30 cigarettes a day. Mrs K expressed embarrassment about her weight and her high level of smoking but said to Sarah that she had never been successful at cutting down on food or cigarettes. As Mrs K's primary nurse, Sarah liaised with other members of the ward team. The general discussion focused on the need for Mrs K to reduce both her weight and her smoking before her incontinence could be helped either surgically or by pelvic exercises. Mrs K was encouraged to talk with a dietitian and to think seriously about joining a weight-reducing club where she would get help and support from others in a similar situation. She was also encouraged to stop smoking and was referred to a physiotherapist for relaxation and pelvic floor exercises.

Although Sarah could understand that it would be very difficult for Mrs K to lose weight and to stop smoking she expected that she would be anxious to work hard to overcome her incontinence. Surely Mrs K was distressed by her incontinence, particularly when it happened during sexual intercourse? Sarah felt that she herself would do anything rather than have this happen to her and felt that Mrs K would have the same resolve.

Mrs K went home from the ward determined to try to work in the way suggested to her and agreed to return in two months after having achieved the agreed aims. On Mrs K's readmission to the ward, however, it was found that her weight had not gone down. Although she had reduced her smoking by 10 cigarettes per day her consumption was still high. Mrs K became very distressed when she realised that she hadn't lost any weight. Sarah, who was now able to spend more time with Mrs K than during her previous admission, realised that she often seemed very tense and anxious. She worried about herself and her children not only while she was in hospital but in their day-to-day lives. She also worried about other patients on the ward, becoming very distressed if they did not seem contented. When Sarah questioned her about this Mrs K said that she had always felt worried, even as a small child, and could not remember a time when she had not had a feeling of apprehension. Mrs K then described the death of her twin brother when they were 5 years old. Her parents had not explained to her what had happened to him until she was much older and she had spent long periods searching for him, not understanding where he had gone. She could remember those early feelings of worry very clearly. Sarah wondered whether somehow Mrs K's feelings of worry, which were linked to childhood experience, were holding her back from working on her weight and her smoking. When Sarah suggested that this might be the case, Mrs K, after some thought, agreed.

Although Sarah did not see Mrs K again she had a greater understanding of why Mrs K could not take the necessary physical steps to improve her health.

Case History 17.6 Miss H

Jennifer had been an experienced health visitor for a number of years, working with a general practice in a rural area. She had been visiting Miss H for a year or two, and had been alerted by the home help to the possibility that Miss H was not eating as regularly as she ought. Miss H was 86 years old and had lived alone for 20 years, i.e. ever since her father had died. She had always been fiercely independent, but her home help telephoned on Thursday morning to ask if Miss H could be visited urgently.

When Jennifer visited she found Miss H sitting in her kitchen with her elderly cat on her lap. It was apparent that the cat had died. Miss H's home help thought that she had been sitting with her cat throughout the night and was worried that she had not eaten or moved. Jennifer did not know what to do and so quietly sat beside Miss H for some time. She felt it would somehow be wrong to try to separate her from her lifelong friend.

After a while Miss H and Jennifer talked quietly about her cat and how he had become ill and died during the night. Miss H said that she did not know whether she would be able to live without him. Much later, however, she agreed to put the cat out in the garden and allowed a neighbour to come and bury him. When the village heard what had occurred many people came forward to give Miss H sympathetic support and to keep her company.

In ordinary circumstances perception and appraisal of the environment are relatively unproblematic; that is, most people would interpret a given situation in much the same way. Personality can, however, play a large part in determining what features of his environment an individual attends to, and what he attends to is a feature of the meaning that a situation has for him (Lazarus 1984, Benner & Wreubel 1989). Rather than describing the individual as 'appraising' a situation, however, Benner & Wreubel (1989) prefer to speak of him 'being in' a situation. They emphasise that the attribution of meaning to a situation is unique for every individual, even though many people's interpretations appear to coincide. Taking this even further, they argue that there are no situations with an objective reality beyond the highly individual interpretations that are put upon them.

For Benner & Wreubel (1989), stress is woven into the fabric of our 'being-in-the-world' and is not 'out there' to be dealt with. From this point of view, it would be harmful to suppress painful emotions, for these assist us in our interpretations of the world. Emotions such as anger or guilt give guidance to the person as to what is happening to him in the world. To teach people to relax may give them some short respite from painful tension until they are ready to confront their problems again and may be useful for this reason, but to teach relaxation as a way of dealing with problems is surely misguided? Stress is part of the person's self, his concerns, thoughts, feelings about the past and future, memories and relationships to others and to objects.

PHYSIOLOGICAL RESPONSES TO STRESS

The role of hormones in responses to stress

In 1935, Cannon summarised the response to external threat as a 'flight, fight or fright' reaction; this has often been called the 'acute stress response'. There are, in fact, many stress-provoking events in life. Real and imagined psychosocial stressors are an essential component of living, and when present to a moderate degree have been described as 'eustress' since they optimise performance and improve learning. It is when threat is perceived to be greater, endangering either a person's reputation or even life itself, that one sees the full manifestations of the acute stress response. After events such as a car crash, bomb explosion, or unexpected physical attack, alarm occurs, activating the rapid physiological adaptations of the acute stress response. This can in some circumstances be life-saving. When, for example, smoke suddenly arises in the room and all too soon the first flames begin to spread, a person finds a sudden unexpected ability for rapid action to deal with the emergency. Along with a surge of physical strength, there is increased ability for immediate attack upon the flames and marked enhancement of ability to run rapidly out of the vicinity of danger. The adrenal medulla has been activated to release the hormones that enable these responses.

An alarm reaction of lesser magnitude is a common occurrence in the more ordinary trials of life. This occurs, for example, in such circumstances as running out of petrol on the motorway en route to an important engagement, losing one's front door keys, or being with someone who unexpectedly becomes acutely ill. The severity of the alarm reaction varies considerably between different individuals, and between different occurrences of a similar situation. Thus, on the second occasion when a person breaks down on the motorway he may feel even more distressed than on the first occasion, or perhaps more confident in his ability to deal with the event and consequently less 'stressed'.

Psychosocial stress derives not merely from external problems or dangers but from the way in which people attempt to manage these problems. Ostell (1991) describes stress as the state of affairs which exists when the way people attempt to manage problems taxes or exceeds their coping resources. When the response to a stressor is severe, normal social relationships can be affected as aspects of the 'flight, fight or fright' response impinge upon rational behaviour.

Stress-provoking events additional to psychosocial stressors include aversive physical stimuli such as excessive noise, cold or heat, and physiological imbalances such as those associated with sleep deprivation, lack of food or chronic pain. Each of these stressors not only acts to bring about hormonal changes associated with the acute stress response, but also has its own selective effects on physiological functioning.

An example of such a selective effect can be seen in the body's response to cold. In cold conditions the body seeks to maintain homeostasis by redistributing the blood supply to less exposed areas and by increasing body temperature via the mechanical act of shivering and the increased secretion of thyrotrophin-releasing hormone from the hypothalamus. Thyrotrophin-releasing hormone stimulates the pituitary gland to secrete thyroid-stimulating hormone (TSH); this causes enhanced release of the thyroid hormones thyroxine and triiodothyronine, which raise basal metabolic rate and hence increase heat production and core temperature.

Thus, in seeking to maintain constancy of the internal environment when this is threatened by a stressor, the body employs a range of physiological mechanisms. Some stressors are short-lived, in which case the body may be able to react to the situation and quickly resolve the disturbance evoked by the stressor. Other stressors may last for days, months or even years. There are many circumstances of chronic stress, as when people must live with circumstances such as chronic disease or social disharmony. Where there has been repeated exposure to a particularly stressful or aversive event, there can be a further reaction characterised by a conditioned fear response to any neutral stimulus experienced at the same time as the previous stress. This effect is responsible for many of the anxiety reactions or acts of avoidance some people show in response to specific harmless objects.

The general adaptation syndrome

The endocrinologist Hans Selye noted that diverse noxious stimuli which threatened the ability of the body to maintain homeostasis induced a common pattern of effects (Selye 1936, 1976). He had found initially that injection of extract from cattle ovaries into rats stimulated growth of the adrenal cortex, induced atrophy of lymphoid tissue in the thymus gland, lymph nodes and spleen, and produced ulceration in the stomach and duodenum. He then noted that the same effects were produced when animals had been placed in cold environments or had been forced to swim for prolonged periods or had been injected with a noxious chemical at low concentrations. He called this pattern of non-specific responses to stressors the general adaptation syndrome.

The syndrome is divisible into three phases. In the first of these, 'the alarm reaction', the adrenal glands are activated. The adrenal medulla, together with the sympathetic nervous system, prepares the body for flight or fight following cognitive appraisal of the threat. If the stress continues, the triggering of neural and endocrine responses in the alarm reaction is followed by the second phase of the stress response, 'resistance'. Stimulation of the pituitary–adrenal axis results in increased secretion of corticosteroids. In this phase, the internal responses of the body stimulate tissue defences and achieve the maximum adaptation possible. The final phase of the general adaptation syndrome is 'exhaustion', in which the body may succumb to the stressor.

The general adaptation syndrome provides a somewhat simplistic model of the actual responses of the body and fails to take full account of the individual nature of psychological and physiological responses.

The acute stress response

During the alarm reaction to stress a series of physiological responses involving limbic and brainstem structures is triggered (Fox 1990, Gray 1987). Neural pathways from the amygdaloid nuclei in the limbic system mediate responses to emotional stress, and pathways from the reticular formation in the brainstem mediate responses to traumatic stressors such as pain and injury. This activates the hypothalamopituitary–adrenal axis and results in the secretion of a range of hormones, as illustrated in Figure 17.1.

An immediate response to threat or stress involves the neural connections from the hypothalamus to the sympathetic outflow, activating both postganglionic sympathetic nerves and preganglionic sympathetic nerves passing to the adrenal medulla. This is the emergency reaction described by Cannon (1935). In the adrenal medulla, acetylcholine released at preganglionic sympathetic nerve terminals activates the chromaffin cells to secrete adrenaline and noradrenaline. In humans, adrenaline is secreted in greater amounts than noradrenaline. The release of these hormones takes place in a matter of seconds or minutes.

The hormones liberated from the adrenal medulla have many effects which facilitate emergency reactions. For example, adrenaline and noradrenaline improve cardiac and respiratory function. Heart rate and force of contraction are increased. Bronchioles are dilated and the depth and rate of respiration are increased. Blood flow is redistributed to areas of need, i.e. the heart and skeletal muscles. Blood glucose and basal metabolism are raised and blood clotting facilitated. The increase of blood glucose is due mainly to the actions of adrenaline on the liver to promote glycogen breakdown and

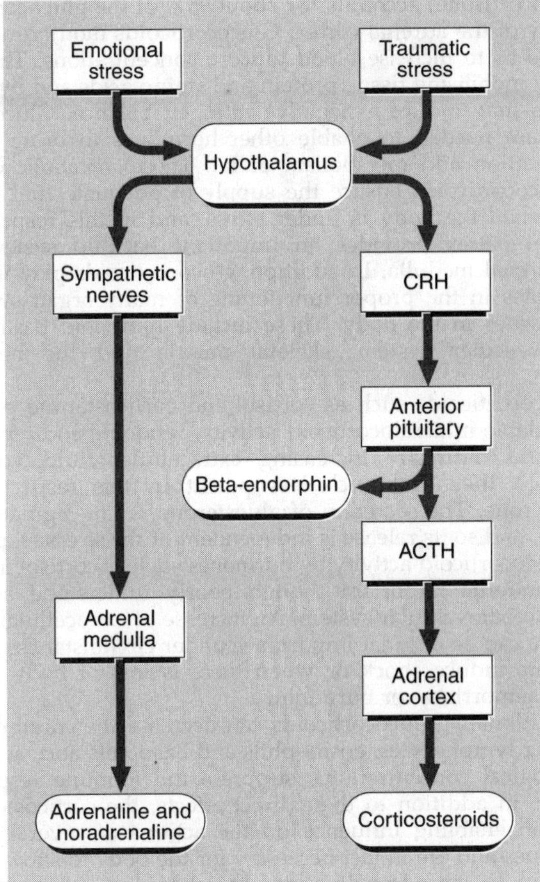

Fig. 17.1 Hormone secretion in response to stress.

enhance gluconeogenesis from lactate. Adrenaline also acts on the pancreas to inhibit insulin secretion. The piloerection and pupillary dilatation so characteristic of the behaviour of fighting cats represent yet another physiological consequence of hormone release from the adrenal medulla. Sweating by the eccrine glands is increased. In the meantime, functioning of the digestive tract is reduced and urinary sphincters are closed. The physiological effects of noradrenaline and adrenaline are explained in Chapter 5 (see p. 137). Adrenaline acts on α- and β-adrenoceptors, whereas noradrenaline acts predominantly on α-adrenoceptors.

In the more long-term responses to stress described by Selye, the centre of activity passes from the adrenal medulla to the adrenal cortex, and to the hypothalamus and pituitary, which are responsible for activating the adrenal cortex. Corticotrophin-releasing hormone (CRH) is secreted by the hypothalamus as well as by extrahypothalamic sites in the brain. CRH acts on the anterior pituitary gland, stimulating the secretion of adrenocorticotrophic hormone (ACTH) and beta-endorphin. Beta-endorphin reduces susceptibility to pain and is probably one of the means by which stress and the stimuli of conditioned fear give rise to endogenous analgesia. Other factors influence the release of ACTH. These include antidiuretic hormone (vasopressin) and hypothalamic vasoactive intestinal peptide (VIP). The ACTH liberated by the anterior pituitary acts to stimulate cells in the adrenal cortex to secrete corticosteroids.

Glucocorticoids secreted by the adrenal cortex play a key role in adaptation to stress (Bowman & Rand 1980). Cortisol (hydrocortisone) accounts for about 95% of the glucocorticoid activity of the adrenal cortex. Glucocorticoids modify metabolism so as to increase blood glucose concentrations. They do this by mobilising tissue protein and amino acids and by these actions may induce a negative nitrogen balance. Glucocorticoids are needed to enable other hormones to bring about mobilisation and metabolism of fat. These metabolic effects of glucocorticoids ensure the supply of adequate fuel to the cells when the body is under stress, and in this respect the adrenal cortex provides an important back-up system for the adrenal medulla. In addition, glucocorticoids play important roles in the proper functioning of many organ systems and tissues in the body. These include lymphoid tissue, the cardiovascular system, skeletal muscle and the nervous system.

Glucocorticoids such as cortisol and corticosterone possess appreciable mineralocorticoid activity, retaining sodium chloride and indirectly increasing extracellular fluid volume, although they are much less potent in this respect than aldosterone. The secretion of aldosterone is not regulated by ACTH, and so its release is independent of the stress response. Mineralocorticoid activity by hormones such as cortisol may in part underlie important though poorly understood actions on the cardiovascular system. An increase of extracellular fluid volume can be of great importance under circumstances when stressors induce shock or when there is loss of body fluids after haemorrhage or burn injury.

Additionally, glucocorticoids can decrease the count of circulating lymphocytes, eosinophils and basophils and, at pharmacological concentrations, suppress the immune response. Finally, in addition to their direct effects, the corticosteroids exert an enabling influence on the actions of several other hormones and are in fact necessary for the body to show a full response to the adrenaline and noradrenaline released from the adrenal medulla. As a result of its wide-ranging functions, especially in the maintenance of fluid and electrolyte balance, the adrenal cortex is essential to life.

The chronic stress response

Clearly, there are limits to the ability of the body to maintain its stage of resistance and adaptation in the face of continuing stress. Under conditions of prolonged stress enlargement of the adrenal glands and thymicolymphatic atrophy will occur (Selye 1976). When stress persists beyond a certain period of time, disturbances occur in the homeostatic balance of the body and there is an ever-increasing danger that disease processes will be precipitated.

An important part of the body's defence mechanism in the stage of resistance is the pituitary secretion of ACTH, which in turn stimulates the adrenal cortex to release corticosteroids. One of the early signs of the body's inability to meet the demands of unremitting stress is a blunting of the amounts of ACTH released by the anterior pituitary in response to that stress (Schatzberg & Nemeroff 1988). Under these circumstances, the adrenal cortex frequently shows hyperplasia, which persists despite the reduced secretion of ACTH. This blunting of the ACTH response to stress also occurs in long-standing timidity, which is possibly due to high arousal together with slow habituation to the stressors. This is coupled with an associated enlargement of the adrenal glands and hypersecretion of adrenal steroids under comparatively non-threatening circumstances. Likewise, blunting of the ACTH responses to stressors is seen in depressive illness and in many forms of anxiety. In depressed individuals there is frequently a high corticosteroid excretion associated with enlargement of the adrenal glands and an increase in the concentrations of CRH in cerebrospinal fluid.

Emotional as well as hormonal changes characterise chronic stress. These include a decreased sensitivity to rewards and a withdrawal from decision-making characteristic of fatigue. This can progress to the condition known as 'burn-out'. In burn-out the person feels physical fatigue along with a lack of involvement, sympathy or respect for colleagues and clients. At its final stage, chronic stress is followed by exhaustion and collapse. Long-lasting stress in which there is a poor coping strategy is correlated with increased occurrence of a variety of diseases (Levi 1971). These may be described as diseases of adaptation and are related to deranged secretion of adaptive hormones in the stage of resistance. These conditions include digestive disturbances, hypertension, myocardial infarction, allergies and sleep disturbances. Such chronic stress may also lead to anxiety, depression or behavioural disturbances, such as appetite disorders or increased usage of alcohol, tobacco, caffeine and drugs.

Due to the prevalence of cardiovascular disease in Western society, particular attention has been paid in recent years to the relationship of stress to hypertension, myocardial dysfunction leading to unexpected sudden death, and to coronary atherosclerosis and myocardial infarctions (Matthews et al 1986). It has been noted that vascular responses to a series of acute stresses in normotensive people living under permanent emotional stress sometimes became protracted and exaggerated. The excess of mineralocorticoid secretion in response to the stress in these persons had raised peripheral resistance, and many later developed permanent hypertension.

Unexpected sudden death arising from cardiac failure has been found frequently to follow emotional upheaval or shock. It may be caused either by adrenosympathetically-induced ventricular fibrillation or by apparent vagal stimulation and cardiac standstill. The increase in blood concentrations of glucocorticoids, mineralocorticoids and catecholamines from stress can derange the vital myocardial electrolyte equilibrium. In a series of unexpected sudden deaths, the post-mortem catecholamine concentrations in the blood were found to be excessively high, almost as high as in fatal adrenaline poisoning.

Finally, increase in the blood concentrations of adrenaline, by its enhancement of platelet aggregation, can promote thrombus formation in atherosclerotic coronary arteries and thus lead to myocardial infarction. Statistical data show a close correlation between the high incidence of ischaemic heart disease in professional persons exposed to demanding occupational stress and in the 'type A' personality, characterised by time consciousness, irritability and driving ambition (see p. 15 and p. 586).

In view of the serious consequences which can arise from excessive or prolonged stress in combination with poor coping strategies, it can be seen that improvements to the working environment and social milieu, together with 'stress education' to lessen reactivity to adverse circumstances, might have as profound an impact on the health of a community as did the improvements to diet and sanitation in the mid-19th century.

STRESS AND DISEASE

Migraine

Migraine headaches have been known about for well over 2000 years. Although it is recognised that they are not caused solely by stress it is possible that certain dietary and olfactory factors associated with migraine onset may be intensified in stressful situations. It is estimated that 10% of the population experience migraine (Blau 1987).

Predisposing factors
The most common precipitant of migraine is recognised to be stress; however, unlike other stress-related disorders migraine often occurs after the cessation of stress (Blau 1987). Various research studies have indicated that migraine sufferers handle stress 'inadequately' and may have a lowered stress threshold. Other precipitating factors include:

- hunger
- certain foods or food additives
- hormonal changes such as those associated with the contraceptive pill or with puberty
- environmental factors such as heat, noise, flashing lights, smells
- exercise
- travel
- allergies.

Possible physiological mechanism
The hypothesis has been put forward (Blau 1987) that stress causes cerebral hypoxia through increased activity in catecholamine pathways. This suggestion is supported by the observation that cerebral oxygen consumption rises when the individual is stressed. The role of the catecholamines adrenaline, noradrenaline and dopamine is to activate the cerebral metabolism. Blau says that if the nerve fibres penetrate deeply enough into the brain, the sympathetic nervous system could release noradrenaline and increase neuronal metabolism in the surrounding tissue. If this hypothesis is correct stress could increase cerebral metabolism and thereby increase the risk of migraine. The phases of a migraine attack are outlined in Box 17.1.

Treatment
The patient should identify, if possible, the precipitating factors of his migraine attacks and avoid them where this is feasible. The pain can be treated with analgesics and the nausea with metoclopramide; the latter will also improve absorption of analgesics from the intestine. Prophylactic treatment with low-dose aspirin is described by Buring et al (1990).

Depression

Frequency of occurrence
Depression appears to be a fairly common response to stress, whether that stress is being felt in the present or was experienced as a child. Paykel (1989) writes:

> The basic facts regarding rates of depression are easily summarised. About 1 per 1000 of the general population are admitted to hospital annually with depression; about 3 per 1000 are referred to psychiatrists, of whom 2 are treated as outpatients. However, about 3% are treated in this country by general practitioners and an equal number probably consult and are not recognised. The prevalence rate in the general population is about 5% although estimates vary considerably. Depression is therefore a kind of iceberg of which only the tip sticks up to reach psychiatrists.

It is difficult to formulate an exact definition of depression and its relationship to stress. The experience of depression seems to range from unpleasant but normal feelings of being 'fed up' to severe states of mental ill-health requiring psychiatric intervention. It is important to recognise that depression can be life-threatening in so far as suicide is a frequent outcome of severe depression. It is vital for health professionals to be alert to this possibility. Hawton writes: 'Among people who kill themselves, or who attempt suicide, approximately two-thirds have visited doctors, usually their general practitioners, within the month beforehand' (Hawton 1989).

Symptoms
The presence of depression is often not obvious to the clinician, as observable signs do not always indicate the unpleasantness of the feelings that the individual is experiencing. Some symptoms, however, particularly when they occur in combination, strongly indicate the presence of depression. Symptoms often associated with depressed states include early morning wakening, a feeling of grinding tiredness, loss of energy, loss of sexual interest in relationships, loss of appetite, feeling 'down' and a feeling of bad temper. Montgomery

Box 17.1 Migraine phases (Blau 1987)

Migraine attacks follow a pattern consisting of the five phases described below. The third and fourth phases are prerequisites of a diagnosis of classical migraine.

PRODROME

- Subtle symptoms; may not be noticed
- Craving to eat sweet food
- Mood variations
- Tiredness
- Mild photophobia
- Heightened visual perception

AURA

- Multicoloured visual disturbances
- Scotoma with flickering, scintillating edge
- Tingling of face, sometimes one-sided
- Numbness of face

HEADACHE

- Slowly developing throbbing pain
- Lasts 2–72 hours

RESOLUTION

- Sleep is major resolving mechanism
- Vomiting

POSTDROME

- 'Washed-out' or drained feeling
- Euphoria
- Impaired concentration
- Irritability
- Cerebral flow observations indicate that anomalies can outlast headache by 24 hours

(1989) asserts that 'the classical division into depression, anxiety states, phobic states and panic disorders is questionable'. If we dispense with this division, the list of potential symptoms of depression might be expanded to include panic or anxiety attacks.

Feelings associated with depression

The relationship between stress and depression is an extremely close one. Some people experiencing depression feel stressed by, amongst other things, their inability to continue with their day-to-day concerns. People who are burdened by overwhelming demands respond by becoming depressed. What is not understood is why some people respond to stress by becoming depressed whilst others show other emotions such as anger.

People experiencing depression often describe their circumstances in terms that denote an ongoing feeling of oppression, as of being under a cloud, or of everything looking black or grey, or of being in a tunnel without an end. Feelings of hope diminish, to be replaced by feelings of hopelessness. Depressed people often feel uncared for and alone even when this is not the case. Undertaking tasks or projects often becomes impossible as inertia takes the place of activity. Depressed individuals often blame themselves for problems in their relationships or daily lives where others who are not depressed might show anger. This leads to the hypothesis that depression is anger turned in on itself when for some reason it cannot be expressed openly.

People experiencing feelings of depression may have additional problems such as sleeplessness, anxiety and eating disorders. They may also be prey to overwhelming and terrifying urges to commit suicide as a way of freeing themselves from a seemingly hopeless situation.

Causes

Depression can occur at any time in life and may follow on from any painful event or loss, such as the death of a loved one or the loss of a job. Depression which does not have an obvious cause when it occurs in adulthood may be the result of early childhood loss or distress. Individuals who have been the victims of sexual, physical or emotional abuse as children may suffer depression as adults in a delayed response to the loss associated with abuse. Early unresolved loss has been suggested as a possible explanation for the distressing symptoms of depression following childbirth. The depression of a parent witnessed in childhood may, for some, be at the root of depression experienced in adulthood.

> ? **17.4** Identify five stressors in each of the following categories:
> a. emotional
> b. physical
> c. environmental
> d. societal.

Anxiety attacks

Anxiety or panic attacks are characterised by severe sympathetic arousal, often in the absence of any obvious or immediate stressor. Panic attacks are a common presenting problem for those visiting their general practitioner with feelings of stress. During an attack the person often experiences intense fear accompanied by physiological signs such as palpitations, sweating, trembling, rapid respiration and pallor. The fear may be associated with a fear of collapse or death or a need to escape. Sufferers often explain that they feel that their heart might burst.

By explaining the nature of these attacks the professional can sometimes bring an element of relief to the sufferer. Practical advice on the management of attacks is also helpful (see Case History 17.7).

Anxiety attacks are symptomatic of underlying distress. They can be acute and of rapid onset, occurring perhaps only once or twice or can develop into a chronic response. Attacks may occur at any time, causing intense feelings of fear where there is no obvious cause. The stressor causing the attack may only become apparent (if at all) upon later introspection or therapy.

Post-traumatic stress disorder

This condition, which has been recognised for a number of years, can affect people who have experienced any serious accident or trauma outside the range of their normal experience, such as a severe road traffic accident, rape, physical attack, plane crash, bomb blast or war. The disorder can follow one or more of such events and can occur not only in those directly involved but also in those called to assist, such as emergency workers or onlookers. The greater the scale of the accident the more likely it is for post-traumatic stress disorder to arise.

A number of somatic symptoms may present either immediately following the traumatic event or some time later.

Case History 17.7 Nursing sister D

Nursing sister D had been working very hard in her new post in the labour suite and she discussed with her colleagues her feeling of apprehension that she might make a mistake or be unable to deal with the management responsibility that her new post entailed. The suite was often understaffed, and although she realised that this was not her responsibility she felt guilty about the demands it placed upon her colleagues. On her night off she went with one or two friends to a pub and although she had not drunk a great deal she knew that she had exceeded her usual limit.

The following morning she awoke with a feeling of unease that she found difficult to describe. She experienced something like a feeling of agitation but her skin also felt as if it were 'crawling'. She had planned to go for a walk with her friends but when she reached the park where she was to meet them the feeling she had experienced throughout the morning became much more intense. She became sweaty, had great difficulty in breathing and felt very afraid. Feeling her pulse, she realised that her heart was beating very fast. Sister D later described her fear that she might collapse and die during this attack. This feeling lasted for ten minutes. Her friends took her home, and later she contacted her family doctor.

This episode was described by the doctor, following some routine investigations, as an anxiety attack. He suggested that she either attend a stress reduction workshop or talk to a counsellor, and reduce her coffee and alcohol consumption. After sister D had taken the opportunity to talk about her fears and problems with a counsellor she felt more able to deal with her new job. She noticed, however, that when she began to feel tired and worried the physical signs of sweating and palpitation would re-emerge. She used this as an indication that she needed a rest. Sister D also noticed that alcohol exacerbated the problem, as it had during her first attack.

These can be particularly difficult to recognise by the individual who has escaped serious harm; as the expectation is that he should feel relief, the occurrence of these symptoms is often unexpected and difficult to understand.

Symptoms indicative of post-traumatic stress disorder are as follows:

- heightened arousal, feelings of anxiety, exaggerated startle response
- sleep disturbances, dreams and nightmares
- flashbacks to the traumatic event, causing psychological distress
- irritability; problems, sometimes severe, with personal relationships; lack of interest in enjoyable pastimes
- poor concentration
- panic, phobias and depression
- bereavement reactions.

There may be loss of memory, although total amnesia of the event is rare. Sufferers can be psychically numbed and may report a feeling of being cut off (Mckinley & Brooks 1991).

Not everyone who experiences severe traumatic stress goes on to develop these symptoms. Where they do occur, counselling and psychotherapy can help, but the person should receive such assistance willingly. Alexander (1990) suggests that therapeutic help should be offered to the survivors of traumatic events early, as a 'first aid' to assess the extent of their distress and to establish a bond between victim and supporter that can then form the basis of a later, more long-term, counselling relationship. Alexander also emphasises that those who assist at traumatic events may require support and proposes that regular group debriefing sessions form an essential part of such support.

Post-viral fatigue syndrome (myalgic encephalomyelitis)

The symptoms of this puzzling illness, which seems to have close links with depression, include extreme muscle fatigue, poor memory and concentration and slips of the tongue (Wessley 1990). This condition can cause considerable distress and disability over a period of months and sometimes years. The individual may, with devastating consequences, be unable to continue full or even part-time work or may be forced to take frequent periods of sick leave. This and other implications of the illness can cause stress to loved ones and adversely affect the well-being of the family as a whole.

Fatigue and depression as sequelae to infection have long been recognised, particularly in relation to Epstein-Barr, coxsackie and other enteroviruses. It is important, however, that post-viral fatigue syndrome not be mistaken for psychiatric illness (Calder et al 1987). Indeed, not all general practitioners recognise the condition (Ho-Yen & Macnamara 1991).

Some commentators advise rest whilst others, recognising the adverse effects of long-term inactivity, advise exercise. Good emotional support is vital, and it is most important that depression, where present, is treated (Lynch et al 1991). Other treatments are aimed at the detection of possible allergies and/or candidiasis and at maintaining a good diet. There is an extremely active ME association which often has local branches (see Useful Addresses, p. 596).

THE CONCEPT OF COPING

Used in a neutral sense, the term 'coping' refers to the way in which the individual responds to a stressful situation or the perception of threat. It can be revealing, however, to reflect upon everyday usage of the word, as it can be a value-laden term used in intrinsically judgemental descriptions of an individual's degree of mastery over a situation or environment. Consider the degree of approval or disapproval that might be implied in the following statements:

- 'She cannot cope.'
- 'He finds it difficult to cope with exams.'
- 'He couldn't cope with the patient's relatives.'
- 'She coped well in her first managerial position.'

The association of 'coping' with mastery and of 'failure to cope' with weakness should not be automatic. It may be the case that the individual who succumbs to feelings of stress is more able to sense tension in a situation than the person who gives the appearance of coping well. The person who removes himself from a situation may in fact be 'coping' with it, by acknowledging that distancing or disengagement is the best way in the circumstances to preserve emotional health or physical safety. In some situations the determination to persevere or to achieve mastery can be a damaging choice ending in disease.

Different situations demand different strategies for coping. In some cases the individual may need to confront a difficulty or overcome an obstacle. In other circumstances the individual must learn how to carry on with his life in the face of an ongoing situation such as bereavement, disability or unemployment. What 'coping' entails will depend upon the individual's unique circumstances and needs, and various models have been put forward in an attempt to identify the factors that contribute to an individual's style of coping.

Models of coping

In many ways, models of coping are more relevant to the nurse's understanding of patients under stress than models of stress in itself. One of the most well-known approaches to the concept of coping focuses on the role of personality in the individual's response to stressful events and identifies 'type A' behaviours (see below) which characterise the individual as being particularly susceptible to the health risks associated with stress. An alternative approach (Kobasa 1979) attempts to identify those personality types which are particularly *resilient* under stress (see p. 586). Some models describe coping in terms of the palliation strategies — e.g. exercise, relaxation, prescribed medication, drug abuse, smoking and alcohol consumption — that various people use as ways of coping. Other models describe coping in terms of problem-solving, or, as in Lazarus' approach (1966), in terms of a dynamic process by which the individual engages himself with the source of stress. It is also possible to discuss coping in terms of defence mechanisms that the individual employs to preserve himself from a perceived threat. Some of the most commonly occurring of these are listed in Box 17.2.

Coping and personality

Some people appear to be relatively unaffected by traumatic events; others seem to be quite unable to withstand what might appear to the onlooker as minor upheavals. Researchers have attempted to identify personality 'types' which are more likely than others to cope effectively with stress, by isolating relatively stable and highly consistent inborn personality dispositions or traits which enable the individual to function well in difficult situations. Such traits may be related to, for example, conformity or nonconformity, conscientiousness, compulsive behaviour, or the ability to suppress, repress or sublimate feelings.

Box 17.2 Defence mechanisms

REPRESSION

Unconsciously keeping unacceptable feelings out of awareness. Not acknowledging our angry or jealous feelings towards another.

DISAVOWAL OR DENIAL

This defence blocks out a perception from memory. Someone whose father left them at birth may unconsciously think of their father as having died rather than confront feelings of loss and anger.

PROJECTION

In projection people unconsciously attribute to others their own aggressive or angry feelings. The feeling that a colleague is 'getting at' oneself may be a projection of one's own angry negative feelings towards the colleague.

INTROJECTION

The acceptance of anothers values and opinions as one's own. A young person living with a domineering parent may unconsciously accept the attitudes of the parent rather than risk confrontation.

REVERSAL

This is the process of detaching a feeling from the person or object to whom it should be directed and directing it to oneself instead. A wish to physically harm another may instead become a process of self harm.

DISPLACEMENT

Strong feelings towards another person may be directed towards someone less dangerous than the original source of the feeling. A child experiencing powerful and angry feelings towards their mother may punish their favourite doll instead.

ISOLATION

In isolation the feeling is detached from the thought to deprive the thought of emotional significance. A nurse may be able to describe how she helped at the scene of an accident without being in touch with the experience of the associated feelings.

REACTION FORMATION

Unacceptable feelings disguised by repression of the real feeling and the reinforcement of the opposite feeling. A husband caring for a disabled wife feels angry at her dependence, but instead showers her with loving attention.

RATIONALISATION

In rationalisation false reasons are found to justify unacceptable attitudes. Following the termination of an employment contract the person might claim that they were pleased to no longer be employed, not acknowledging painful feelings of worthlessness.

CONVERSION

This is the process of converting a psychological disturbance into a physical disorder. A feeling of panic or fear accompanied by physical symptoms may be seen as physical symptoms *only* by the person, to unconsciously avoid confronting the cause.

Type A behaviour. Extensive research (Friedman & Rosenman 1974) over the last 20 years into the question of whether there are certain people who experience stress more acutely than most others and who are more likely to succumb to cardiac or circulatory disease as a result has identified a 'type A' personality which is at particular risk from the effects of stress. Type A behaviour is not, strictly speaking, a *trait*; traits are by definition inborn, whereas type A behaviour appears to be learned by social modelling. Type A behaviour seems to have very positive short-term consequences; for example, in business or other organisations people who show involvement, drive and initiative are often highly valued. The long-term consequences of type A behaviour, however, are often negative.

The type A individual is typically observed engaged in polyphasic activity, e.g. driving their cars whilst dictating memos to their secretaries over their cellular phones. Characteristics associated with this personality type include time urgency, hostility, difficulty in expressing anger, impatience, desire for control and aggression. Type A behaviours are often negative and are based upon the following interrelated elements:

- a set of beliefs about oneself in relation to the world
- a set of values which merge with motivation and commitment
- a behavioural lifestyle.

Type A individuals invest a great deal of themselves in their lifestyle and expend a great deal of energy in maintaining control. When challenged their response is often highly emotional; this is likely to stimulate frequent surges of catecholamine secretion, which is likely to induce in the physically unhealthy person coronary heart disease. These people often show signs of raised serum cholesterol levels, raised serum fats, and diabetic-like traits; at the same time they are frequently smokers who do not have time for regular exercise. Understandably, type A behaviour is often highly destructive to relationships with family members, friends or colleagues.

It is important to bear in mind that people can change their learned behaviours and improve their ability to cope with certain experiences. In addition, there can be some degree of habituation to stressors such that they seem less stressful over time.

Personality and health. Kobasa (1979) examined the mediating effects of personality not in relation to stress and disease, but in relation to stress and health. Whilst much research effort had been directed towards understanding the role of mediators such as early childhood influences, physiological predisposition and social resources in relation to the onset of disease, Kobasa asked why some people can be under considerable stress but not become ill. Using the social readjustment rating scale (Holmes & Rahe 1967), she tested the following hypotheses:

1. People who have a greater sense of control over their own lives will remain healthier than those with a sense of powerlessness.
2. People who have a sense of commitment to various areas of their lives will be healthier than those who have a sense of alienation.

3. People who view change as a challenge will remain healthier than those who view change as a threat.

Kobasa postulated a state of hardiness in the personalities of those who can be stressed without becoming ill. The hardy person has certain characteristics, including:

- a clear sense of self and of personal meaning
- an understanding of values, goals and capabilities and a belief in their importance
- a vigorous involvement in and commitment to his own environment
- an internal locus of control
- active involvement in change.

The process model of coping

Lazarus (1984) described coping in terms of a *dynamic process* involving movement, force and energy within the individual and his relationship with the source of stress. An important feature of the process approach is that it reflects the fact often observed in clinical settings that an individual's response to his situation changes and evolves over time. This response is highly complex and unique to each individual and might be described as occurring in stages, although these stages are not sequential or predictable.

Worden (1983), for example, describes four tasks of mourning that the individual must complete in order to emerge from a state of grief:

- accepting the reality of the loss
- experiencing the pain of grief
- adjusting to an environment from which the deceased is missing
- withdrawing emotional energy and reinvesting it in another relationship.

For the individual, these tasks of mourning may not be sequential, but may be experienced instead as an 'ebb and flow' of feelings. For the nurse, Worden's definition of the tasks of grieving will give an indication of the direction that a person might take in his mourning. For the individual concerned, the stages passed through might be recognised only in hindsight.

The process approach emphasises that the individual copes with stress in a unique way that is governed by both childhood and adult experience. The ability to cope is shaped by the developmental processes that the individual undergoes from birth to death. The individual's perspective will change continually, and situations that may be stressful at one time may be viewed differently at another stage of life.

DEFENCE MECHANISMS

Whilst it is possible to think of defence mechanisms as both conscious and unconscious strategies of self-protection against perceived threat, these mechanisms may seriously compromise the effective functioning of the individual. Defence mechanisms operate essentially by restricting situations which are seen as threatening, narrowing down the individual's field of action to one that is manageable. They enable the individual, often against overwhelming odds, to maintain an equilibrium of feelings, thoughts and actions in daily life.

Problems arise when they feature inappropriately, as when a defence mechanism first acquired to combat severe or terrifying feelings in one domain becomes active without cause in another, perpetuating the emotional disturbance that gave rise to the mechanism in the first place. This may occur some time after the original experience, and the content of that experience may not be accessible to the person even after therapy. Whilst it is useful for the clinician to bear in mind that unresolved conflict *may* exist, the detailed and often long-term task of helping the person to understand the extent of his defences is best left to therapists and counsellors.

Defences are often like a sea wall in that the magnitude of the original intense fear and distress will determine the height, breadth and depth of the defence. These defences are not alway infallible, however; they can be breached during sleep, under the influence of alcohol and other drugs, and in conditions of stress.

A number of defence mechanisms have been identified; the most common of these are listed in Box 17.2.

THE TREATMENT AND MANAGEMENT OF STRESS

The treatment or, perhaps more to the point, *management* of stress can be approached in a number of ways. One of these is to offer the individual the opportunity to examine the sources of his stress in present or childhood experience and to consider ways of modifying his responses to that stress. This kind of therapy can be provided by a psychotherapist, clinical psychologist or qualified counsellor. The nurse should be familiar with the basic approaches available within psychological therapy; two significant models, patient-centred therapy and cognitive therapy, will be described shortly.

Some individuals suffering from acute anxiety or depression may find it impossible to confront the source of their difficulty and to make constructive changes without first being given some relief from their distressing feelings. Here, carefully monitored drug therapy can facilitate recovery and change. Again, the nurse should be familiar with the most common pharmaceutical agents used in this type of treatment; these are briefly described on pages 588–589.

The individual suffering from stress can also learn a number of techniques that will assist him to reduce or manage his stress in day-to-day life. Techniques such as relaxation, yoga, biofeedback, visualisation and meditation have all gained in credibility and popularity in recent years. When taught well and followed up with continuing support, courses in such techniques can help people to take a new approach to the problem of stress. Moreover, learning a new skill such as deep relaxation can impart to the individual a feeling of well-being which may facilitate positive change in various areas of his life. We should remind ourselves, however, that if stress lies in the interaction between the person and his environment, or in the meaning he attributes to his situation, then clearly a short workshop on relaxation (for example) cannot hope to seriously address the source of his stress. Indeed, it should be borne in mind that there is a potential for courses in stress reduction to exacerbate the problem if the individual is made to feel that any stress that is not helped by the techniques offered is intractable or somehow abnormal.

Therapy

Person-centred therapy

In person-centred therapy, first described by the psychologist Carl Rogers (1961), the therapist assumes that he and his client are *trustworthy* (Thorne 1990). It is assumed that, given the right conditions, the client is able to strive towards personal growth and understanding, and it is the therapist's task to work with the person to create the ideal conditions for the exploration and understanding of feelings. The therapist shows his trustworthiness by the unconditional acceptance, warmth and genuineness that he shows toward the client as he explores his deepest feelings in an effort to achieve personal growth. It is the therapist's open and honest acceptance of the painful and distressing feelings being expressed that enables the person to trust enough to move towards psychological health.

Thorne (1990) emphasises that the therapist's feelings and actions must be congruent; the degree of his caring cannot be feigned, for to be genuinely therapeutic it must be *felt*. This demands, Thorne writes, that the therapist first accepts *himself*:

> If I cannot trust myself to acknowledge and accept my own feelings without adverse judgement or self-recrimination it is unlikely that I shall appear sufficiently trustworthy to a client who may have much deeper cause to feel ashamed or worthless. If, too, I am in constant fear that I shall be overwhelmed by an upsurging of unacceptable data into my awareness then I am unlikely to convey to my client that I am genuinely open to the full exploration of his own doubts and fears. (Thorne 1990, p. 115.)

The person feeling despair, hurt or anger can seek help from a person-centred therapist by asking for details from the BAC Directory of Counsellors and Therapists. Therapy can take place in groups or individually and the therapist will discuss with the client the setting, duration and cost of therapy.

Cognitive therapy

In 1963–64 the psychologist A T Beck identified certain manifestations of 'thought disorder' (Dryden 1990), by which people entertain thoughts that in a number of ways harm them. According to Beck's theory, people ordinarily function effectively in their day-to-day lives as problem-solvers. For example, the nurse who considers applying for promotion may try to consider objectively whether she has the relevant experience, training and personality for the job. If, however, she is feeling depressed her thoughts might be negative or destructive, as in 'Why apply for this? I wouldn't get it anyway. I'm no good at anything'.

Cognitive therapists work closely with people to help them identify negative or dysfunctional thoughts and to replace them with positive, enabling thoughts which will help them cope with difficult situations. This approach attempts to relieve disabling psychological symptoms whilst reinforcing the person's own psychological responses. At the same time, it offers detailed analysis of interpersonal or other situations that cause problems. This type of therapy does not seek first and foremost to find the causes of distress by, for instance, reexamining childhood trauma; nor is it centred on the person's own feelings to the same degree as client-centred therapy. It is, rather, directed towards the alleviation of distressing symptoms with a view to enabling the person to have positive experiences in his day-to-day life and thus enhance his ability to deal with other new challenges.

Cognitive therapy can take place in groups or individually. It involves regular attendance, either for short-term focused therapy or for longer-term therapy, perhaps extending over several months. As in other approaches to therapy, the therapist's ability to respond to the client with warmth, genuineness and empathy will be vital to the success of the intervention.

Choosing therapeutic help

For therapy to be effective it must respond to the person within his own frame of reference and be relevant to his own life from his own unique perspective. Finding an appropriate form of therapy can be very difficult for the individual, and many people are reluctant to approach a professional agency or voluntary organisation for assistance with personal problems. Many people think and wait for long periods before plucking up the courage to seek help.

General practitioners can help individuals suffering from feelings of stress in a number of ways, e.g:

- by talking over the problem and giving counselling support themselves
- by referring the individual to another professional such as a clinical psychologist, psychiatrist or psychotherapist, as appropriate. (Some GPs have counsellors on staff within their own practice.)
- by prescribing antidepressants where indicated
- by ensuring that there is no organic cause for the person's feelings of stress, such as hyper- or hypothyroidism or anaemia
- by giving reassurance that panic attacks are not life-threatening and giving advice on how to deal with them
- by authorising official sick leave to enable the patient to rest.

The therapist-client relationship

People are highly individual in their feelings, experiences, backgrounds and personalities. A model of therapy which is helpful to one person may not suit another, and a therapist who is helpful to one person may fail to establish a good rapport with another. For this reason it is important for therapists to be clear with their clients about the way they work, what the work involves, its likely duration and, if private, its cost. It is possible for the client to change therapists if the therapy does not seem to be helpful, although there is one major proviso to this. For personal change to take place therapist and client must work closely in a relationship of trust. This will enable the therapist to reflect back and challenge the behaviour that is causing the client distress. The fact that this can be an unsettling experience for the client may not be the right reason for him to leave therapy. Nevertheless, the therapist should be willing to discuss any feeling on the client's part that the therapy is detrimental or unhelpful and if appropriate to give guidance on finding an alternative therapist.

The person wishing to become a therapist must undertake extensive training which involves the study of theory as well as supervised work with clients. Nurses working in clinical settings can undertake shortened courses which will help them to develop the necessary skills to listen in a therapeutic way to people in their daily work. An example of therapeutic listening is given in Case History 17.8.

Drug therapy

The personal experience of stress can be so severe and overwhelming that the individual finds himself unable to take any action to alleviate his feelings. Severe anxiety or depression, perhaps in combination with an overpowering feeling that a serious physical illness is lurking can have an immobilising effect on the person so that even the prospect of any action to alleviate symptoms is daunting. When people feel as severely distressed as this they may begin to entertain thoughts of suicide.

Drug therapy can help to alleviate severe distress by relieving its most acute symptoms and thus enabling emotional rest to take place. Some drugs are intended to help with sleeplessness, while others which do not have a tranquillising effect will permit those taking them to continue to work, to problem-solve, to drive, and so on. Drug therapy should always be supplemented by continuing monitoring and sup-

Case History 17.8 Mrs A

Mrs A cares for her mentally and physically handicapped son, J, at home with the help of the community nursing service and the local social work department. She is 68 years old and a widow; her son is 29. He is visually impaired and unable to communicate easily by speaking. He is always incontinent. Although he can walk, Mrs A always has to guide him. Getting him out of bed and dressed in the morning is very heavy work for her.

Mrs A has known her community nurse, Barbara, for a number of years. Barbara feels a sense of despair that Mrs A never has any freedom from J, and has rarely had any time to herself in the years she has known her. Barbara has tried repeatedly both by herself and in conjunction with social work colleagues to plan some respite care for J. This planning has taken the form of a provision for day care at a local day centre and periods of respite care at a local residential unit. But somehow when the time came for J to attend Mrs A managed to avoid sending him. The only assistance she will accept is from the local care attendant team; one helper, who has become a friend, sits with J for two hours while Mrs A does her shopping.

One day Barbara was able to sit and talk with Mrs A whilst J was asleep. By listening carefully to her Barbara realised that Mrs A felt extremely guilty about J's handicap. She felt that she had caused J's condition by not taking sufficient rest during her pregnancy, and she relieved her feelings of guilt by caring for him all the time. She was also extremely fearful of what would happen to J after she died.

Barbara listened to Mrs A carefully as she talked about her painful feelings, and was aware that she had not been able to share these feelings with anyone before. She did not try to make Mrs A feel better by taking away her feelings of guilt, nor did she try to reassure her. Instead, she simply listened carefully and attentively.

They did not talk again about this problem although Barbara was ready to listen if Mrs A wished to raise the subject again. Some time later, however, Mrs A asked Barbara if she could help her organise some day care for J, as it would help him to get used to other people. Barbara was then able to arrange respite care for J, which also enabled Barbara to get some rest.

port by the medical practitioner. The following provides a brief overview of the main types of drugs that might be used in the treatment of stress-related conditions.

For more detailed information on drug therapy the reader is referred to Lacey (1991).

Tricyclic and related antidepressants

The most common antidepressant drugs used in severe stress and depression are the tricyclic and related groups. These are used for people suffering from moderate to severe depression, although it is important to realise that they work by alleviating *symptoms*. This can be useful; for instance, the person who is debilitated by anxiety might be able to find ways of living that are more constructive once his feelings of anxiety are lifted. These drugs may not be helpful, however, when the depression is related to bereavement, an unhappy working environment, overwhelming family responsibilities or disturbing memories of abuse or neglect, for it is only when the underlying cause of depression can be understood that the person is likely to obtain any lasting benefit.

Management. The person prescribed tricyclic antidepressants must be seen frequently following prescription. These drugs can take 2–4 weeks to begin to have an effect; during this time the patient may feel isolated and helpless. Side-effects include the following:

- constipation
- sleepiness
- dry mouth
- blurred vision
- urinary retention
- sweating.

Tolerance seems to develop over time and some of the side-effects become less unpleasant.

If the individual's depression is severe he may feel like killing himself. Careful support and perhaps hospitalisation may be essential at this time. Treatment with this group of drugs should be continued for at least one month (BMA 1992). Reduction or withdrawal of the drug should be carried out *very slowly* to avoid severe symptoms such as strange, fragmented dreams, headaches, recurrence of anxiety, depression or restlessness.

Selective serotonin re-uptake inhibitors

This group of drugs block the re-uptake of 5-hydroxytryptamine (5-HT), producing an increase in the amount of neurotransmitter at central synapses.

Monoamine oxidase inhibitors (MAOIs)

This group of drugs prevents the breakdown of monoamine neurotransmitters, thereby prolonging their action. They are recommended for people with depression, anxiety and somatic complaints, for patients who do not respond to tricyclics and patients with agoraphobia.

Lithium

Lithium possibly decreases noradrenaline release and enhances its re-uptake. Lithium salts are used to treat mania and hypomania, and to prevent mania and depression.

Traxodone

This drug exhibits antiserotonin and alphareceptor antagonist properties. Its sedative properties are useful in the treatment of anxiety.

Benzodiazepine tranquillisers

The benzodiazepine group of drugs came into disrepute when people who had been taking them for long periods found that their original symptoms were often intensified and that the drugs were addictive. It is recommended that these drugs are prescribed for periods not exceeding 2 or 3 weeks and that careful supervision is provided by the general practitioner (BMA 1992).

Other means of stress reduction

Exercise

There is strong anecdotal and research evidence that regular vigorous exercise has a positive effect upon the individual's ability to deal with feelings of stress (Kraus & Raab 1961, Goodway 1987). Proponents of exercise as a means of stress reduction argue that exercise is essential for psychological, physiological and social development and that the health of

Box 17.3 Guidelines for exercise

- Any exercise is good.
- Set aside a specific time for exercise. Treat that time as sacro-sanct, but do not feel worried if it is necessary for some reason to miss a session.
- Exercise at least three times a week if possible, for at least half an hour.
- Exercise should be gentle but vigorous; build up slowly to a good exercise level.
- If in doubt, have a health check and talk over your exercise programme with your general practitioner prior to starting.

the mind is closely linked to the health of the body. Physical fitness is seen as a positive aid towards emotional stability. Guidelines for exercise as a means towards stress reduction are given in Box 17.3.

Exercise works in a paradoxical manner in reducing stress; it is itself a physical stressor causing an acute stress response (Goodway 1987) but nonetheless functions as a relaxant. The physiological effects of exercise include increased blood flow and oxygen consumption as well as changes in blood pressure, heart rate, respiration, and metabolic rate.

Physical exercise can act as a relaxant for a number of reasons:

- Most exercise involves effort and concentration and it can be difficult to sustain anxious thought whilst engaged in physical exercise.
- Meeting a physical challenge can give the individual a sense of achievement.
- During strenuous exercise the body produces norepinephrine and endorphins; these substances help to alleviate depression and bring about feelings of happiness and tranquillity (Lamb 1978).
- Exercise can be taken alongside other people and so can diminish feelings of social isolation.

Relaxation

Relaxation has long been known to help alleviate feelings of stress. Relaxation may take various forms, including relieving muscle tension (e.g. through exercise) taking time off, either on a daily or weekly basis or as a scheduled holiday, and meditation. Everly & Benson (1989) discuss the response elicited physiologically and psychologically by certain types of relaxation. They identify two components of these techniques which cause the relaxation response:

1. The repetition of a word, sound, phrase, liturgical prayer or muscular activity
2. The positive disregard of everyday thoughts when they come to mind.

There are 7 types of activity which foster this type of relaxation:

- meditation
- autogenic training
- pre-suggestion hypnosis
- prayer (repetitive or liturgical)
- yoga exercises
- T'ai chi chu'an
- Chi gong.

For many people these techniques produce a sense of well-being as well as an increase in concentration and energy. They also produce the following physiological changes (Everly & Benson 1989):

- decreased oxygen consumption and carbon dioxide elimination with no change in the respiratory quotient
- reduced heart and respiratory rates and lowered blood lactate
- reduced blood pressure (during exercise).

Everly & Benson (1989) show that during relaxation there are physiological alterations consistent with a decrease in central and peripheral adrenergic excitation, and that people who undertake regular meditative relaxation (see Box 17.4) recover faster from stressful events than those who do not relax in this way.

Paradoxically, for some people experiencing anxiety the effort of trying to relax can intensify their feelings of panic (Heide & Borkovec 1983). Feelings of not being in control intensify and the experience of relaxing, by not being achievable, becomes a negative one.

STRESS IN NURSING

Sources of stress

Nursing can be an extremely exciting and satisfying profession. The rewards of seeing patients move from ill-health to health and from disability to independence are great. To nurse a dying person in a way that enables him to die without pain and with dignity can also be very fulfilling. When nurses have the benefit of comprehensive managerial, educational and emotional support their work may not be harmfully stressful (Hawkins & Shohet 1989). When formal supports do not exist nursing is by its very nature likely to cause some degree of stress. In certain cases the nurse may find that she is unable to help the patient recover and is only able to offer support as he comes to accept permanent disablement or chronic disease. The nurse may feel that her role is a passive and unhelpful one and she may feel frustrated and distressed by her inability to help.

> Nurses are in constant contact with people who are physically ill or injured, often seriously. The recovery of patients is not certain and will not always be complete. Nursing patients who have incurable diseases is one of the nurse's most distressing tasks. Nurses are confronted by the threat and the reality of suffering and death as few lay people are. Their work involves carrying out tasks which, by ordinary standards, are distasteful, disgusting and frightening . . . . The work situation arouses very strong and mixed feelings in the nurse: pity, compassion and love; guilt and anxiety; hatred and resentment of the patients who aroused these strong feelings; envy of the care given to patients. (Menzies 1960, pp. 97–98.)

Menzies (1960) described nurses working in a task-orientated way with patients. This way of working allowed nurses only minimal contact with each patient and, Menzies hypothesised, enabled them to be emotionally defended against feelings of anxiety caused by contact with patients. Because they were always moving on to the next task, they did not have time to listen to their patients. This defence, Menzies argued, while offering protection against anxiety was a source of dissatisfaction for the nurse and impeded personal growth and maturation.

When caring for patients who are themselves experiencing high levels of stress, nurses, ideally, should be able to recognise their own feelings of stress and, where possible, to identify their cause. This is essential for three reasons:

1. Nurses cannot interact in a therapeutic manner with their patients if they cannot enter into a relationship with them.

Box 17.4 Guidelines for meditative relaxation

SETTING THE SCENE

- Find a quiet, warm, comfortable room where you are unlikely to be disturbed. (Try to exclude children, pets, ticking clocks or telephones.)
- Meditate sitting upright in a comfortable chair. Rest the feet flat on the floor and the hands loosely in your lap.
- Have a watch or clock in clear view. The session lasts 20 minutes. If you feel that it is likely that you will fall asleep set an alarm.
- Loosen any tight clothing; slip off your shoes if this makes you more comfortable.
- Meditate whilst neither too hungry nor too full.
- Try to meditate twice each day for 20 minutes. Because you may feel very relaxed it is better not to meditate close to bedtime, as this might interfere with sleep patterns.

THE PROCESS

- During the process of meditation you will remain completely conscious.
- This can be a sound, though not a word. Or it can be a prayer.
- You may prefer to meditate with your eyes closed. Take one or two deep, relaxing breaths.
- Gently begin to count, on each inhalation or exhalation, with the number one, then two, then three .... Every time a thought comes into the awareness calmly return to number one. It is unlikely, though, that in a number of years of *regular* meditating you will go beyond number one; indeed, the principle of this sort of meditation is not one of *mastery* but of the gentle pushing aside of thoughts to enable the body and the mind to achieve rest.
- You may find that you have spent the whole session thinking over a problem. If so, do not worry; before you finish the session gently return to the counting for one or two minutes.
- If you find that you have fallen asleep do not worry about this. It may be that you are very tired and your body needs sleep. Before finishing the relaxation gently return to the counting for one or two minutes. If you find that you have solved a major problem, written a poem or worked out a solution, gently return to your counting.
- At the end of the session, stretch gently, taking a slow breath in before opening your eyes.

2. Nurses are unlikely to enter into such a relationship if they are feeling the need to protect themselves by evading the emotional distress of their patients.
3. For nurses to recognise and deal with their own feelings of stress is ultimately important for their own peace of mind and mental health. Nurses often work intensely for long hours in situations that they cannot walk away from, with people who are themselves frightened, afraid, confused or perhaps dying; in order to cope effectively with this work nurses must have good support and supervision.

Nursing education and the expectations of patient-centred care

More than ever before, educational programmes for nurses are including a substantial amount of work in such areas as psychological theory, interpersonal relationships and interviewing skills. However, it is important for such education to be clinically based, to prevent nurses feeling distressed by being expected to exercise interactive skills that in reality they have practised only in the artificial setting of the classroom or workshop. Nursing education should also allow nurses the scope to appreciate and develop their own individual strengths, so that their approach to patients can be based in feelings of positive self-worth and genuine caring rather than in self-conscious attempts to listen and respond 'correctly'.

Unlike in the days described by Isobel Menzies (1960), nurses are now expected to form closer interpersonal relationships with their patients and to work cooperatively with them in devising individualised programmes of care. They are being asked to work in this way in the face of budgetary constraints and sometimes inadequate staffing levels. But, just as a building worker would not be expected to work on a building site without protective head gear and proper footwear, so too nurses should not be expected to do their difficult work without access to emotional support when they need it. After all, many nurses no longer have the benefit of the defences previously offered by task-oriented care (Menzies 1960) to protect them from the rigours of close interpersonal contact with patients. If nursing education is to give students and qualified nurses the ability to interact more closely with patients then as a concomitant to this it must also teach methods of giving and getting support.

Working with dying patients

Many studies of stress in nursing draw attention to the distressing aspects of working with people who are dying and the emotional strain of caring for them and their families through this extremely difficult time. It would be misleading, however, to say that working with terminally ill people is always distressing or stressful in predictable ways, for the experience of stress is related both to the person and to the situation.

The nurse who cares for patients who are terminally ill might herself feel intense grief, but may lack the opportunity to express her feelings (see Case History 17.9). If she feels extreme relief at the death of a patient who has suffered from a painful illness for a long period she may feel guilty about her reaction. Nurses who work in busy wards or who have heavy caseloads in the community may be obliged to set their feelings aside; as a result, unresolved grief or guilt may give rise to feelings of stress and ultimately to stress-related illnesses.

Lazarus & Folkman (1984) describe a type of coping that is not related to mastery of a situation but which is an experiential learning process. This model is particularly relevant to the situation of professionals working with dying people. For example, Jeanette in Case History 17.9 is not looking for help in problem-solving when she shares her feelings with her colleague. Rather, she is working through a process of grief and self-understanding which started at the time of her mother's death and which she finally comes to recognise through her relationship with Mrs M's family.

Grief and bereavement are generally not pathological states. They are normal, if often very painful, aspects of human experience. Coming to terms with loss is an opportunity for personal growth; if the process of mourning is suppressed, however, grief can become a source of acute or chronic stress.

Case History 17.9 Jeanette

Jeanette is a community nursing sister in a small town. She is attached to a busy general practice where other team members work together sharing patient care. They also spend some social time together and are generally able to give support to one another when it is needed.

Jeanette had been closely involved with the care of Mrs M, a 45-year-old woman suffering from multiple sclerosis. Jeanette had shared Mrs M's care with a colleague, but during the last year she had visited the family on almost a daily basis on her working days, as the nursing care required increased in complexity. Throughout the year Mrs M's condition deteriorated considerably. She died before Christmas, shortly after being admitted to the local general hospital.

Jeanette had got to know Mrs M's family well and following her death she tried on a number of occasions to visit them. This became increasingly difficult as time went on and Jeanette found herself driving longer distances than necessary to avoid passing their house. She began to feel extremely distressed by this and suffered from overwhelming feelings of guilt. She also found that she was short-tempered with her own family and began taking some sick leave just to give herself a break. She could not understand why she was feeling as she did and felt ashamed.

Later she was able to talk over her feelings with a colleague. This woman who had also been a Cruse counsellor, gently suggested that perhaps Jeanette had also 'lost' Mrs M and was also feeling grief. Jeanette soon found herself talking about the feelings she had experienced following the death of her own mother a number of years before and her strong feelings of guilt at not being with her mother when she died.

Jeanette later felt able to visit the family. She was able to talk openly and with affection of Mrs M and she was able to return to them on later occasions. Jeanette also took the opportunity offered by her colleague to informally talk over the experience of visiting Mrs M's family and of her own feelings. She felt as if a weight had been lifted from her shoulders.

* National Organization for the Widowed and their Children

The fear of death

Working with dying patients may bring to the fore feelings about death and dying that might go unrecognised in more ordinary cirucumstances. Many writers (e.g. Yalom 1968) have described death anxiety, i.e. the feeling of fear associated with the realisation that one will some day die, as having a profound effect upon the life of the individual. Yalom writes that people often go to great lengths to deny their knowledge that they will eventually die, and argues that the idea of their own death is for many people a primary underlying source of anxiety which is expressed in highly individual ways.

Diggory & Rothman (1961) have suggested that the fear of death is made up of a number of smaller fears. They asked a sample (N = 563) drawn from the general population to rank-order several consequences of death. In order of descending frequency, the following were the most common fears associated with the idea of death:

1. My death would cause grief to my relatives and friends.
2. All my plans and projects would come to an end.
3. The process of dying might be painful.
4. I could no longer have any experiences.
5. I would no longer be able to care for my dependents.
6. I am afraid of what might happen to me if there is a life after death.
7. I am afraid of what might happen to my body after death.

When in the presence of a dying patient, who is perhaps frightened or experiencing pain, the nurse may as well as feeling distressed by her patient's suffering, be acutely aware of the possibility of the same thing happening to herself or her family. It is hardly surprising that this area of care can be one that causes distressing feelings for nurses, especially in a society such as ours that does not give great recognition to the reality of death and dying.

The feeling of fear or anxiety that surrounds the experience of death may not in fact be clearly understood by the nurse or the patient as being related to death or dying. Wolff (1953) has shown how non-specific the physiological effects of stress can be; the same is true of emotional responses, which may be clearly understood or expérienced simply as freefloating, non-specific feelings of anxiety.

Support and supervision for nurses

There is a long tradition in Britain of supervision amongst counsellors and psychotherapists. This practice has become enshrined in the accreditation of counsellors currently offered by the British Association for Counselling and is a requirement of other bona fide qualifying bodies for counselling and psychotherapy. The principle is that the person who is undertaking counselling work meets regularly with a supervisor, i.e. someone who is doing similar work and has skills of giving support, to discuss her feelings about her work. Nurses who listen carefully to their patients are doing work that is intense, exacting and difficult; supervision can offer them invaluable support (Alexander 1990). Hawkins & Shohet (1989) write:

> The supervisor's work is not just to reassure the worker, but to allow the emotional disturbance to be felt within the safer setting of the supervisory relationship, where it can be survived, reflected upon and learnt from.

Supervision is essential for those who call upon their inner resources in the effort to listen empathically to others. Supervision can enable nurses to develop an awareness of the full extent of their therapeutic role with patients. Good regular supervision can also prevent the nurse from succumbing to emotional fatigue, disillusionment and apathy. (See Box 17.5.) The nurse seeking supervision, however, should be aware of the special demands that this implies:

> Before entering this relationship, however, we believe that supervision begins with self-supervision; and this begins with appraising one's motives and facing parts of ourselves we would normally keep hidden (even from our own awareness) as honestly as possible. (Hawkins & Shohet 1989.)

The search for support must be a voluntary step taken by the clinician, who recognises the value to herself of this help.

Every health worker whose job involves some aspect of counselling should be aware of the kinds of supervision that are available. Support may take the following forms:

Box 17.5 Guidelines for using supervision and support

For the patient
When support or supervision is sought by the clinical nurse in her work with a patient it is essential that the *strictest confidentiality* is maintained. The patient is *never* mentioned by name and any identifying characteristics are carefully removed from the presentation. If the patient is known to the supervisor or if in a group setting the patient is recognised by another person in the group then in the interests of the patient's privacy the person who knows the patient should withdraw from the group or the discussion should not take place.

For the nurse
The focus of supervision is upon the feelings and thoughts of the *nurse* seeking support. Although the problems she encounters in working with the patient are important, the nurse's reaction to these problems is of more importance and should be the focus of supervision. (British Association for Counselling 1990)

- individual
- group
- team supervision
- peer supervision
- ad hoc sharing
- triads.

These may be briefly described as follows.

Individual supervision. The nurse and supervisor meet regularly (for instance, one or two hours each month) to discuss areas of work and the nurse's feelings. A contract for working together is agreed at the outset.

Group supervision. Groups can be both creative and therapeutic as supervisory tools. They can be 'open', with people joining and leaving them during the life of the group, or 'closed', with not more than 8 members and a coordinator meeting regularly (Yalom 1968).

Team supervision. Many nurses work in teams, either with colleagues from the same discipline or in multi-disciplinary groups. Informal or formal sharing can take place when support is needed from a group of people who are experiencing similar stressful situations. The disadvantage of this arrangement is that the individual will have to share feelings with others who will continue to be colleagues; this may compromise the degree of openness that can be achieved.

Peer supervision. In this model the clinical nurse talks with someone who is working in the same way with patients and so understands the type of work that is being undertaken.

Ad hoc sharing. The value of sharing problems with a trusted friend, relative or colleague on an ad hoc basis should not be underestimated as a means of relieving intense feelings of stress. While this outlet for stress has the advantage of immediacy and informality, the confidante may not feel as bound to confidentiality as she might in a more formal arrangement.

? **17.5** Imagine that following a time spent nursing a particular patient you feel unhappy and troubled and that your sleep is disturbed by nightmares. You recognise that you would like to talk about your feelings with someone. Write a few lines about the advantages and the disadvantages as you see them, of talking to:
a. your line manager
b. your tutor or lecturer
c. a friend or relative
d. a colleague
e. a professional helper such as a counsellor, general practitioner or psychotherapist.

Triads. The triad model (see Box 17.6) created by the Tavistock Institute of Human Relations as a support and training model is especially suitable for people working on shifts as it requires a group of three people working together. This model is appealing in that the small number of people taking part makes it relatively easy to implement. If a working agreement is carefully formulated at the outset this model does not lose any of the formal constraints that are essential in any system of professional support.

? **17.6** Take a few moments to think about your clinical working environment. Would you like more support in the work that you do?
Write a few lines under the following headings to describe how you feel you might be better supported:
a. emotional
b. educational
c. organisational
d. managerial.

Box 17.6 The triads model of supervision

Triads provide an opportunity for three persons to 'tune into' each other on an emotional and cognitive level in a process that is unthreatening. The purpose of a triad is to create an association of the three people involved which allows them to explore issues in a positive manner with a view to facilitating insight and resolution. *Everything that takes place in a triad is confidential to its three members.*

There are three roles in the triad:

- presenter
- listener
- observer.

The presenter takes no longer than 5 minutes to talk about something that concerns him.

The listener does not interrupt the presenter, but listens until he is finished. The listener may then ask questions, make observations, obtain clarification, refresh his memory on what was said, and enable the presenter to amplify his remarks if he wishes to do so. The listener will try to be aware of whether or not a particular interpretation or conclusion was helpful.

The observer simply observes the interaction between the presenter and the listener. His role is to be alert to the feeling level of the interchange, the non-verbal messages given by both participants and the quality of the listening and responding. He then conveys his observations to the others.

The three persons in the triad then reflect on the value of the exercise. They are then encouraged to work together with parity. They will have the opportunity, in turn, to exercise each of the roles, completing the exercise within an hour.

? **17.7** Set 10–15 minutes aside for this exercise. You may find a notepad and pen useful. Think back over your last working day and of the patients with whom you worked. Try to answer in as straightforward a manner as possible the following:
Can you think of one person who has 'stayed with' you since you stopped work? Perhaps you have been thinking of this person whilst doing other activities. Ask yourself:
a. How did I feel whilst speaking with my patient?
b. What were we talking about?
c. How did we end our discussion? How did I feel about this?
d. What will happen next? How do I feel about this?

CONCLUSION

Stress is not in itself a pathological or an abnormal phenomenon. Indeed, it is hard to imagine how any individual might go through life without being faced with stressful situations. For some individuals, stress can to a significant degree be met as a challenge and as a spur to personal growth and maturation. Why it is that certain people seem better able than others to withstand stressful conditions has been the subject of a great deal of debate as researchers have attempted to identify the physiological, psychological and social factors that mediate the experience of stress.

The fact that the word 'stress' can be freely used in daily conversation without invoking the negative connotations of 'mental illness' perhaps indicates how the potentially grave effects of stress can be underestimated or obscured. As this chapter has shown, stress can be closely associated with serious physical, emotional or psychiatric illness, including heart disease, depression, and compulsions. Stress can also give rise to detrimental coping behaviours such as drug and alcohol abuse. For this reason it is vital that stress is taken seriously by health professionals, and that its mechanisms and effects are clearly understood.

From the nurse's perspective, perhaps the most important aspect of the experience of stress is its uniqueness for each individual. The experience of stress, like the experience of pain, must be assessed for each patient, and approaches to stress management must be congruent with the individual's personality, experiences and values. It is hoped that this chapter has assisted the nurse in formulating a practical understanding of stress and its effects, and will enable her to make a positive contribution to the treatment and management of stress and stress-related disorders in her patients. It is also hoped that the reader will be able to meet with greater confidence the challenge of recognising and coming to terms with the effects of stress in her professional and personal life.

GLOSSARY

Stimulus. Any factor such as heat, light, cold or drugs that will cause a response in a person or an organism. The term can also apply to any event causing emotional distress.

Response. A psychological or physiological reaction to stimulation.

Transactional. Representing an interaction between the perception of the person and the object of their stress.

Phenomenological. Offering an account of the person's own experience as a unique event or phenomenon.

Appraisal. The individual's assessment of a stressful situation and how it will affect them.

Coping. The various strategies the individual utilises to deal with the effects of stress in their lives.

Support and supervision. Regular contact with another person undertaking similar clinical work with the purpose of sharing and learning from difficult or painful situations.

REFERENCES

Alexander D A 1990 Psychological intervention for victims and helpers after disasters. British Journal of General Practice 40: 345–348

Benner P, Wreubel J 1989 The primacy of caring. Addison Wesley

Blau J N 1987 A clinico-therapeutic approach to migraine. Migraine. Chapman Hall, London pp 185–204

Blau J N (ed) 1987 Migraine: clinical, therapeutic, conceptual and research aspects. Chapman & Hall, London

Bowman W C, Rand M J 1980 Textbook of pharmacology, 3rd edn. Blackwell, Oxford, p 19.30–19.39

British Association for Counsellors 1989 Directory of Counsellors. BAC, Rugby

British Association for Counsellors 1990 Code of ethics and practice for counsellors. BAC, Rugby, sections B. 3.2, B. 3.3 & B. 3.5

Buring J E, Peto R, Hennekens C H 1990 Low dose aspirin for migraine prophylaxis. Journal of American Medical Association 264(13): 1711–1713

British Medical Association and Royal Pharmaceutical Society of Great Britain 1992 British national formulary. BMA, London

Calder B D, Warnock P J, McCartney R A, Bell E J 1987 Cocksackie B viruses and the post viral fatigue syndrome: a prospective study in general practice. The Journal of the Royal College of General Practitioners (294) 37: 11–15

Cannon W B 1935 Stresses and strains of homeostasis. American Journal of Medical Science 189: 1

Cox T 1989 Stress. Macmillan Educational, London

Diggory J, Rothman D 1961 Values destroyed by death. Journal of Abnormal and Social Psychology 63(1): 205–210

Dreyfus H L 1987 From depth psychology to breadth psychology: a phenomenological approach to psychopathology. In: Messer S B, Sass L A, Woolfolk R L (eds) Hermeneutics and psychological theory. Rutgers University Press, New Brunswick, N J

Dryden W 1990 Individual therapy. Open University Press, Milton Keynes

Egan G 1986 The skilled helper: a systematic approach to effective helping. Brooks Cole, California

Everly G S, Benson H 1989 Disorders of arousal and the relaxation response: speculations on the nature and treatment of stress related diseases. International Journal of Psychosomatics. 36(1–4): 15–21

Everly G S, Sobelman S H 1987 The assessment of the human stress response: neurological, biochemical and psychological foundations. AMS Press, New York

Fox S I 1990 Human physiology, 3rd edn. W C Brown, Dubuque, USA, pp 293–303

Friedman M, Rosenman R H 1974 Type A behaviour and your heart. Knopf, New York

Goodway J 1987 Exercise: the stressor that reduces stress? Journal of Occupational Health. (May): 164–167
Gray J A 1987 The physiology of fear and stress. Cambridge University Press, Cambridge, pp 52–66
Hawkins P, Shohet R 1989 Supervision in the helping professions. Open University Press, Milton Keynes
Hawton K Suicide and the management of attempted suicide. In: Herbst K R and Paykel E S (eds) 1989 Depression: an integrated approach. Heinmann & The Mental Health Foundation, Oxford
Hawton K & Blackstock E 1976 General practice aspects of self-poisoning and self-injury. Psychological Medicine 6: 571–5
Heide F, Borkovec T 1983 Relaxation-induced anxiety. Journal of Consulting and Clinical Psychology 51: 171–182
Hinkle L E 1987 Stress and disease: the concept after 50 years. Social Science and Medicine 25(6): 561–566
Holmes T H, Rahe R H 1967 The social readjustment rating scale. Journal of Psychosomatic Research 11: 213–218
Ho-Yen D O, Macnamara I 1991 General practitioners' experience of the chronic fatigue syndrome. The British Journal of General Practice 41: 349
Kennedy E 1977 On becoming a counsellor: a basic guide for non-professional counsellors. Gill and Macmillan, Dublin
Kobasa S C 1979 Stressful life events, personality and health: an inquiry into hardiness. Journal of Personality and Social Psychology 37(1): 1–11
Kraus H, Raab W 1961 Hypokinetic disease. Thomas, Springfield, I L
Lacey R 1991 The complete guide to psychiatric drugs. Ebury Press, London, in conjunction with MIND
Lamb D R 1978 Physiology of exercise. Macmillan, New York
Lazarus R S 1966 Psychological stress and the coping process. McGraw-Hill, New York
Lazarus R S, Folkman S 1984 Stress, appraisal, and coping. Springer, New York
Levi L (ed) 1971 Society, stress and disease, vol 1. Oxford University Press, Oxford, pp 280–366
Lynch S, Seth R, Montgomery S 1991 Antidepressant therapy in the chronic fatigue syndrome. The British Journal of General Practice 41(349)
Matthews K A et al 1986 Handbook of stress, reactivity and cardiovascular disease. Wiley, New York
Mckinley B, Brooks N 1991 Post traumatic stress disorder explained. Nursing Standard 5(19)
Menzies I E P 1960 A case study of the functioning of social systems as a defence against anxiety. Human Relations 13(2): 95–123
Montgomery S A Developments in antidepressants. In: Herbst K R and Paykel E S (eds) 1989 Depression: an integrated approach. Heinmann & The Mental Health Foundation, Oxford
Oatley K 1989 The importance of being emotional. New Scientist (Aug): 33–36
Ostell A 1991 Coping, problem solving and stress: a framework for intervention strategies. British Journal of Medical Psychology 64 (Pt 1): 11–24
Paykel E S (ed) 1989 Depression: an integrated approach. Heinemann Medical/The Mental Health Foundation, London
Rogers C R 1961 On becoming a person. Constable, London
Schatzberg A E, Nemeroff C B (eds) 1988 The hypothalmic–pituitary–adrenal axis: physiology, pathophysiology and psychiatric implications. Raven Press, New York, pp 55–66
Selye H 1936 Syndrome produced by diverse nocuous agents. Nature (London) 138: 32
Selye H 1946a The general adaptation syndrome and the diseases of adaptation. Journal of Clinical Endocrinology 6: 117
Selye H 1946b What is stress? Metabolism 5: 525
Selye H 1976 The stress of life, rev edn. McGraw-Hill, New York
Smith D L 1990 Psychodynamic therapy. In: Dryden (ed) Individual therapy. Open University Press, Milton Keynes pp 18–38
Thorne B 1990 Person-centred therapy. In: Dryden W (ed) Individual therapy psychotherapy handbooks. Open University Press, Milton Keynes
Wessley S 1990 Postviral fatigue syndrome. Update 41(12)
Wolff H G 1953 Stress and disease. Thomas, Springfield, I L
Worden J 1983 Grief counselling and grief therapy. Tavistock, London
Yalom I D 1968 Existential psychotherapy. Basic Books, New York

FURTHER READING

Asterita M 1985 The physiology of stress. Human Sciences Press, New York
Bailey R, Clarke M 1989 Stress and coping in nursing. Chapman & Hall, London
Beck A T 1976 Cognitive therapy and the emotional disorders. International Universities Press, New York
Beck A T 1989 Love is never enough. Viking Penguin, London
Bowlby J 1980 Attachment and loss. Vol 3: Loss, sadness and depression. Tavistock, London
Burnard P 1989 Existentialism as a theoretical basis for counselling in psychiatric nursing. Archives of Psychiatric Nursing 3(3): 142–147
Denton, Wisenbacker 1977 Death experience and death anxiety amongst nurses and nursing students. Nursing Research 26: 61–64
Everly G S, Smith K 1987 Occupational stress and its management. In: Humphrey J (ed) Human stress: current selected research, vol 2. AMS Press, New York, pp 235–246
Jones A Talking back to happiness. Nursing Times 85(14): 60–61
Kobasa S, Puccetti M 1983 Personality and social resources in stress resistance. Journal of Personality and Social Psychology 37: 1–11
Kubler-Ross E 1982 Living with death and dying. Souvenir Press, London
Lazarus R 1979 Positive denial: the case for not facing reality. Psychology Today (Nov.): 44–60
Liebowitz 1989 To release stress exercise. NYS Dental Journal
Mason J W 1975 A historical view of the stress field. Journal of Human Stress (March): 6–12
Parkes C M 1972 Bereavement. Tavistock, London
Parkes C M 1972 Determinants of outcome following bereavement. Omega 6: 303–23
Payne R, Firth-Cozens J 1988 Stress in health professionals. Wiley, Chichester
Price V A 1982 Type A behaviour pattern. Academic Press, London
Savage Y, West M 1987 Visitations of distress. Nursing Times 84(31):
Schatzberg A E, Nemeroff C B (eds) 1988 The hypothalmic-pituitary-adrenal axis: physiology, pathophysiology and psychiatric implications. Raven Press, New York, pp 55–66
Sedgwick A W, Paul B, Plooij D, Davies M 1989 Follow-up of stress management courses. Medical Journal of Australia. (May): 485–486, 488–489
Selley C 1991 Post-traumatic stress disorder. The Practitioner (Sept)
Stoltenberg C D, Delworth U 1988 Supervising counsellors and therapists. Jossey-Bass, San Francisco
Sutherland V J, Cooper C L 1990 Understanding stress. Chapman & Hall, London
Taylor J 1977 The rules and exercises of holy dying. Arno Press, New York. First published in 1665
Wessely S, David A, Butler S, Chalder T 1989 Management of chronic (postviral) fatigue syndrome. The Journal of the Royal College of General Practitioners 39(318): 26–30
West M, Jones A, Savage Y 1988 Stress in health visiting. Health Visitor 61(Sept)
Wilson H S, Kneisl C R 1988 Psychiatric nursing Addison-Wesley, Menlo Park, California

USEFUL ADDRESSES

British Association for Counsellors
1 Regent Place
Rugby
Warwickshire CV21 2PJ
Information Line (0788) 578328
Office (0788) 550899

British Migraine Association
178a High Road
Byfleet
Surrey KT14 7ED

CRUSE Bereavement Care
Scottish Headquarters
18 South Trinity Road
Edinburgh EH5 3PN
Tel: 031 551 1511

Depressives Anonymous
36 Chestnut Avenue
Beverly
North Humberside HU17 90U
Tel: 0482 860619

Keep Fit Association
16 Upper Woburn Place
London WC1 H OQG
Tel: 071 387 4349

Manic Depression Fellowship
51 Sheen Road
Richmond
Surrey TW9
Tel: 081 332 1087

Mental Health Foundation
24 George Square
Glasgow G2 1EG
Tel: 041 221 2092

Migraine Trust
45 Great Ormond Street
London WC1N 3HD
Tel: 071 278 2676

MIND (National Association for Mental Health)
22 Harley Street
London WIN 2ED
Tel: 071 637 0741

Myalgic Encephalomyelitis (ME) Association
P O Box 8
Stamford-le-Hope
Essex SS17 8EX
Tel: (0375) 642466

RELATE (National Marriage Guidance Council)
Herbert Gray College
Little Church Street
Rugby
Warwickshire CV21 3AP
Tel: 0788 573241

The Samaritans
17 Uxbridge Road
Slough
Berkshire SLI ISN
Tel: 0753 32713

The Scottish Institute of Human Relations
56 Albany Street
Edinburgh EH1 3QR
Tel: 031 556 0924

Tavistock Institute
Tavistock Centre
120 Belsize Lane
London NW3 5BA
Tel: 071 435 7111

Westminster Pastoral Foundation
23 Kensington Square
London W8 5HN
Tel: 071 937 6956

CHAPTER 18

Shock

Eleanor Hayes

CHAPTER CONTENTS

Introduction 597

The pathophysiology of shock 597
The stages of shock 598

Types of shock 600
Hypovolaemic shock 600
Cardiogenic shock 600
Distributive shock 601

Management and treatment of shock 604
Management and treatment of hypovolaemic shock 605
Management and treatment of cardiogenic shock 606
Management and treatment of septicaemic shock 606
Management and treatment of anaphylactic shock 607
Definitive and supportive therapy 607
First aid treatment for shock 607

Monitoring the patient in shock 608
Monitoring cardiac status 608
Monitoring respiratory status 608
Monitoring haemodynamic status 608
Monitoring level of consciousness 611
Monitoring renal function 611
Monitoring body temperature 611
Observing skin condition 613
Laboratory and diagnostic tests 613

Complications of shock 613
Renal failure 613
Adult respiratory distress syndrome (ARDS) 613
Disseminated intravascular coagulation (DIC) 613

Conclusion 614

References 614

Further reading 614

INTRODUCTION

Shock is a very complex physiological phenomenon which, when it develops suddenly, can transform a relatively well person into an acutely ill patient in a matter of minutes. Nurses may encounter patients who are in shock in any clinical area — for example, in medical, surgical and recovery wards or in specialist areas such as dermatology, orthopaedic and obstetric departments. Shock can and does occur outside the clinical setting. A business man may collapse with a bleeding peptic ulcer; disaster such as a plane or train crash may result in many cases of shock; and shock can even occur in a dentist's chair. Nurses in all areas of practice must therefore understand the processes of shock and be prepared to take part in life-saving therapy. This chapter is intended to help the student nurse to develop this competence.

In the hospital setting improvements in therapeutic and monitoring techniques have greatly improved the survival rate of patients suffering from some kinds of shock. Observant and knowledgeable nurses who are able to interpret the clinical information they help to collect are in the best possible situation to anticipate problems and initiate action. A nurse faced with a collapsed person at home or elsewhere in the community will have less clinical support, but with a sound understanding of the process of shock will be able to take appropriate action and use available resources to the best advantage.

In any environment, awareness of the predisposing factors which may lead to shock, early detection, and prompt action are vital to a good prognosis. Caring for patients who are suffering from shock requires not only an understanding of the pathophysiology of shock and the principles of its treatment and management, but also an awareness of the devastating psychological and social impact such a sudden change from health to illness can have on patients and their families.

THE PATHOPHYSIOLOGY OF SHOCK

Shock is a state in which tissue perfusion is inadequate to maintain the supply of oxygen and nutrients necessary for normal cell function. The cells may also be unable to extract and utilise normally the reduced supply of **substrates** and oxygen which is delivered. Tissue perfusion may become inadequate due to:

- decreased blood volume
- failure of the heart pump
- increased peripheral vasodilation.

Circulatory haemostasis exists when the blood volume, the heart's pumping action, and the vascular tone or resistance of blood vessels are in dynamic equilibrium. Shock syndromes have traditionally been categorised according to aetiology. By this means they may be classified into three main types:

- Hypovolaemic: due to reduction of blood volume
- Cardiogenic: due to myocardial damage and ineffective function
- Distributive: due to altered vascular resistance. This category includes septicaemic shock, neurogenic shock, spinal shock, and anaphylactic shock.

The stages of shock

Before we consider specific types of shock it is necessary to understand the basic pathophysiological processes which produce the clinical picture typically observed in shock. These processes can be divided into four stages (Quaal 1992):

1. Initial stage. There are no signs and symptoms but cellular changes begin to occur in response to a disturbance in cell perfusion and oxygenation (see Fig. 18.1). This disturbance progresses to a change from aerobic to anaerobic cellular metabolism, in which production of lactic and pyruvic acid leads to metabolic acidosis.
2. Compensatory stage. Physiological adaptations occur in an attempt to overcome the original problem, e.g. hypovolaemia
3. Progressive stage. Compensatory mechanisms begin to fail and produce adverse effects
4. Refractory stage. Pathophysiological processes set in motion cannot be arrested or reversed. Death is imminent.

Stages 2, 3, and 4 will be discussed in some detail in the following pages.

It is important to understand that the stages of shock comprise continuous and complex processes and that there is usually no sudden transition from one stage to the next. It should also be noted that in septicaemic shock the early clinical picture is altered. For example, the presence of endotoxins produces a hyperdynamic state with depressed left ventricular function. This occurs even when the endotoxin is experimentally injected into healthy people (Suffredini et al 1989).

The compensatory stage

When circulation becomes inadequate due to the reduction of circulating fluid, massive vasodilation, or pump failure, various mechanisms are activated in response to hypotension, hypoxaemia, acidosis or a combination of these. These mechanisms may be neural, hormonal or chemical, but since the body functions as a whole system they are closely interlinked (see Fig. 18.2).

Neural mechanisms. Hypotension is quickly detected by the aortic and carotid sinus baroceptors, which then decrease impulses to the vasomotor centre and thus reduce inhibition of the vasoconstrictor centre. This stimulates the sympathetic

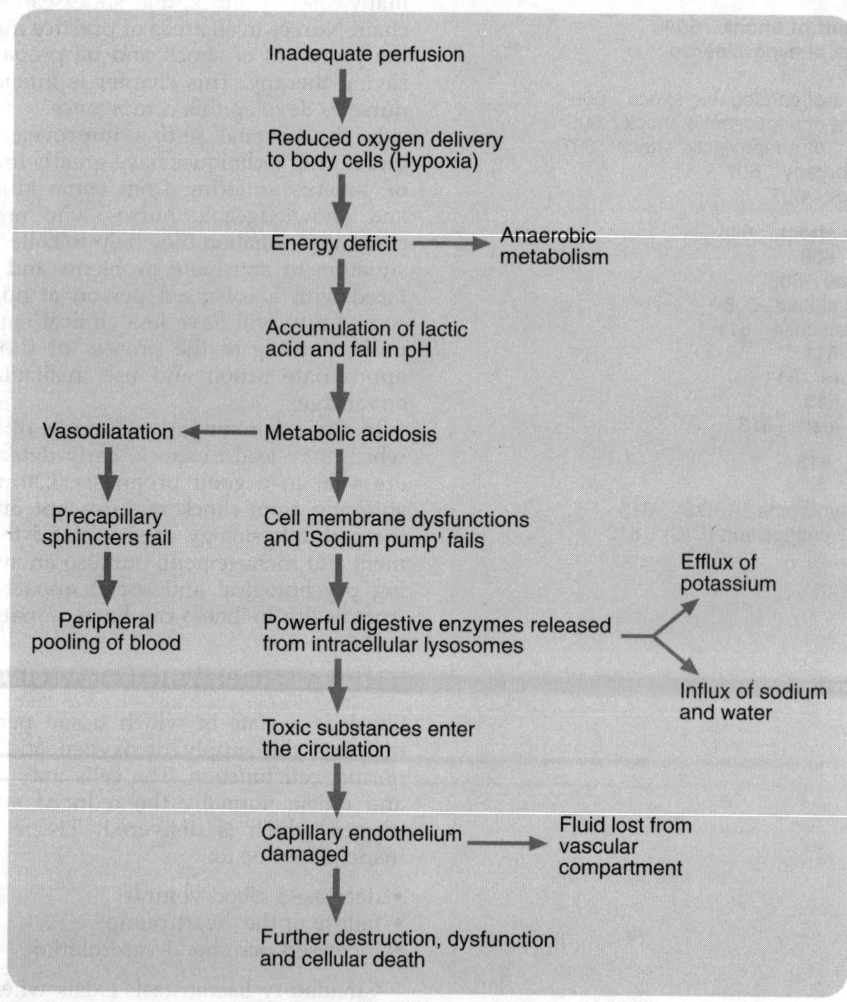

Fig. 18.1 Effects of inadequate perfusion on cell function.

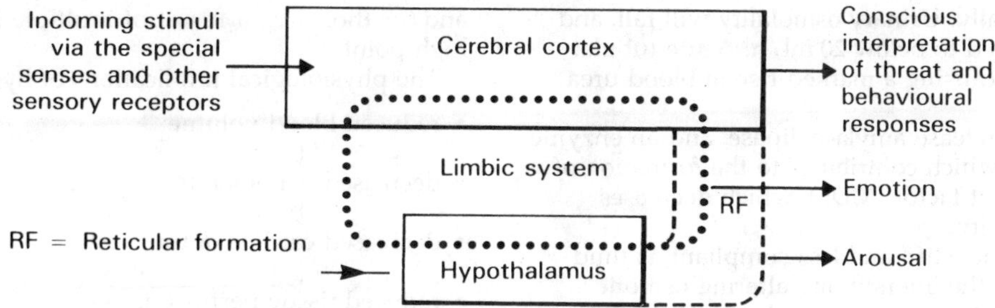

Fig. 18.2 Major control mechanisms of the stress response

nervous system so that noradrenaline is discharged from sympathetic nerve endings and the physiological stress response shown in Figure 18.3 is activated. This response includes the discharge of adrenaline and more noradrenaline by the adrenal medulla, resulting in vasoconstriction in the skin, kidneys, gastrointestinal tract and other organs while blood supply to the heart and brain is preserved. Vasoconstriction and increased heart rate may initially restore the arterial blood pressure to normal, but peripheral resistance will be raised making the myocardium work harder to maintain cardiac output. Urinary output and peristalsis will decrease, and the individual's skin will become pale and cool. Sympathetic nervous system stimulation will also result in increased respiratory rate and depth, dilated pupils, and increased sweat gland activity causing the 'clammy' skin typically found in shock (other than early septicaemic shock).

Hormonal mechanisms. Adrenaline secreted by the adrenal medulla stimulates the anterior pituitary gland to release adrenocorticotrophic hormone (ACTH), which causes the adrenal cortex to release glucocorticoids (mainly hydrocortisone) and mineralocorticoids (mainly aldosterone).

Glucocorticoids raise blood sugar by increasing glucogenesis (changing amino acids to glucose in the liver). They mobilise amino acids from the tissues (mainly muscle) and decrease protein synthesis. They also reduce glucose uptake by the cells and mobilise fatty acids from the adipose tissue into the plasma. Hydrocortisone shifts cell metabolism from glucose to fatty acids for energy, enhancing fatty acid oxidation. It also reduces tissue destruction by stabilising lysosomal membranes (Quaal 1992).

Aldosterone decreases excretion (increases reabsorption) of sodium and chloride by the kidney and increases excretion of potassium and hydrogen ions. Metabolic acidosis and hypokalaemia can occur. The high serum osmolality resulting from a high concentration of sodium chloride shrinks the hypothalamic osmoreceptors, which stimulate the posterior pituitary gland to release antidiuretic hormone (ADH).

ADH stimulates an increase in renal water reabsorption (to restore normal serum osmolality), and thus increases circulating fluid and blood pressure.

Noradrenaline secretion by the adrenal medulla causes renal artery vasoconstriction, stimulating secretion of renin by the kidney. In the circulation renin reacts with angiotensinogen, producing angiotensin I. This is converted by an enzyme in the lungs to angiotensin II, which causes venous constriction and increases aldosterone release, thus leading to increased fluid and sodium retention and increased venous return, blood pressure and renal perfusion.

Thyroxine secreted by the thyroid gland sensitises the betareceptors in the heart to noradrenaline and so increases heart rate, systolic pressure, stroke volume and cardiac output.

Chemical mechanisms. Poor lung perfusion leads to ventilation–perfusion imbalance and decreased oxygen tension in the circulating blood. This is detected by chemoreceptors in the aorta and carotid bodies, and stimulates hyperventilation in an effort to increase oxygen intake. Respiratory alkalosis and cerebral vasoconstriction then follow as carbon dioxide is removed by hyperventilation: 'blown off'. (However, the acid–base balance is further complicated by metabolic acidosis resulting from anaerobic metabolism in hypoxic cells.)

These mechanisms may initially combine to compensate for the initial problem, but unless the latter is promptly and successfully overcome more clinical signs will become evident. The typical clinical picture is of a patient with cool, pale, clammy skin, decreased urinary output, increased heart-rate, and decreased bowel sounds. Unless artificially ventilated he will be hyperventilating and will probably seem anxious. He may also be restless, agitated and confused due to the cerebral effects of hypoxia, hypocapnia and sympathetic nervous system stimulation.

It should be remembered that there are well-established pathways linking the cerebral cortex, limbic system, and hypothalamus which govern the psychophysiological stress response (see Ch. 17, p. 577). Psychological stress can intensify physiological responses and thus is undesirable for a critically ill person. Anything which can be done to reduce anxiety and psychological stress for the patient in what is often a very anxiety-provoking situation may contribute to his physical as well as psychological well-being.

The progressive stage

Although the compensatory mechanisms may at first appear to reverse the effects of shock, if the originating problem (e.g. bleeding) is not resolved they will eventually break down. With decreased perfusion supplying inadequate oxygen and nutrients, the cells will be unable to produce sufficient adenosine triphosphate (ATP). The sodium pump will fail and sodium will collect inside the cells while potassium leaks out. This can result in hyperkalaemia, which may in turn cause cardiac arrest. The anaerobic metabolism which results from an inadequate oxygen supply will create increasing metabolic acidosis, causing the arteriolar and precapillary sphincters to constrict such that blood is trapped in the capillaries. Hydrostatic pressure will rise; this, combined with increased capillary permeability due to local histamine release, will lead to the leakage of fluid and protein into the tissues. As fluid is lost, haemoconcentration and viscosity will increase. Sludging in the microcirculation may lead to disseminated intravascular coagulation (DIC, see p. 613), one of the complications of shock.

Prolonged vasoconstriction and its impact on cell function will soon compromise the functioning of the vital organs, as follows.

- The kidneys will become unable to filter, excrete and

reabsorb fluid normally. Urinary osmolality will fall, and output will be reduced to below 20 ml/h. Acute tubular necrosis may occur, causing a marked rise in blood urea and creatinine.

- Pancreatic cells will release amylase, lipase, and an enzyme, into the circulation, which contributes to the formation of myocardial depressant factor (MDF), which decreases myocardial contractility.
- The lungs will become 'stiff' and less compliant as fluid and colloid leak into the interstitium, altering osmotic pressure and leading to pulmonary oedema. This in turn may lead to adult respiratory distress syndrome (ARDS, see p. 613) with alveolar damage and collapse. Hydrostatic or cardiac pulmonary oedema may occur as the heart fails. All of these changes will increase hypoxia and acidosis.
- The heart will eventually fail as coronary perfusion and oxygen supply become inadequate to meet the demands of the myocardium, which will be working hard to maintain blood flow by pumping rapidly against high resistance (and disadvantaged by the effect of MDF).
- Ischaemic damage to the intestinal mucosa may release bacteria and toxins from the gut into the circulation.
- Alteration in cerebral function may have a number of effects, ranging from a dulling of responses to major behavioural changes.

The refractory stage

At this stage death is imminent. Continuing vasoconstriction, increasing acidosis, sludging of red cells and platelets, and decreased intravascular volume will all contribute to decreasing perfusion of tissues. Massive bleeding due to DIC may also exacerbate this effect. Inadequate ventilation of non-compliant, 'wet' lungs will lead to increasingly inadequate oxygenation. Renal failure will contribute to increasing metabolic abnormalities, and vital centres in the brain will eventually cease to function due to ischaemia and hypoxia. One abnormality may sometimes appear to be the major problem, but death will ultimately occur as a result of multiple organ failure (MOF).

TYPES OF SHOCK

Specific aspects of the pathophysiological processes of shock will be more, or less, evident according to the type of shock which is occurring. The following sections will therefore describe the distinguishing features of hypovolaemic shock, cardiogenic shock, and the different forms of distributive shock.

Hypovolaemic shock

This is the most common type of shock. Its primary cause is loss of fluid from the circulation. This fluid loss may be described as external or internal, as follows.

- external fluid loss: e.g. due to bleeding from wounds, vomiting, diarrhoea, overuse of diuretics, burns, **diabetes insipidus**
- internal fluid loss: i.e. from the circulation, internally, as in haemothorax, retroperitoneal bleeding or bleeding into tissues at fracture sites after injuries; or due to paralytic ileus, intestinal obstruction, acute dilatation of the stomach; or due to gross ascites.

While internal conditions may not be obvious as a cause of fluid loss their effect can be very serious. For example, 1 l (around 20% of the blood volume of an average man) or more of fluid may be sequestered in the gastrointestinal tract during paralytic ileus and/or acute dilatation of the stomach, and the same volume or more of blood may escape into the tissues and/or thorax as a result of multiple injuries or a fall from a high point.

The physiological implications of hypovolaemia are:

- reduced blood volume
  ↓
- decreased venous return
  ↓
- decreased cardiac output
  ↓
- reduced tissue perfusion.

In early hypovolaemic shock the compensatory mechanisms already described (see p. 598) are activated when the blood pressure starts to fall. These mechanisms allow up to 10% reduction of the circulating volume of a healthy person without the development of marked symptoms. However, if a greater volume of fluid is lost and is not replaced quickly the compensatory mechanisms may fail quite suddenly, in which case the patient's condition will deteriorate rapidly. In older people the cardiovascular system is often less able to cope with haemodynamic changes, and the heart may be less able to pump faster and harder in order to maintain cardiac output against high peripheral resistance.

Recognising hypovolaemic shock

The following signs and symptoms of hypovolaemic shock are reliable only if they are considered in relation to one another and to the patient's previous, stable condition. Nevertheless, whenever several of these indicators occur together the possibility of shock should be considered, for a successful outcome depends upon early intervention. The nurse should therefore be alert to the following:

- narrowing of the pulse pressure, i.e. a reduced difference between systolic and arterial pressure due to decreased stroke volume and increased peripheral resistance (See, for example, Daily (1992) for more information.)
- anxiety, restlessness and confusion, which may indicate decreased cerebral perfusion and oxygenation
- a rapid, weak, thready pulse, due to low blood flow despite a rapid heart rate
- cool, clammy skin due to vasoconstriction and sympathetic stimulation of sweat glands
- decreased urinary output, due to renal artery vasoconstriction and endocrine compensatory mechanisms (see p. 599)
- rapid and deep respirations in response to sympathetic nervous system stimulation, hypoxia and acidosis
- lowered body temperature, which may be related to altered metabolism, perfusion and oxygenation and, possibly, heat loss from evaporation of sweat from the skin
- thirst and a dry mouth related to fluid depletion and possibly to sympathetic nervous system stimulation
- fatigue, probably related to inadequate perfusion and oxygenation of the tissue and vital organs.

It is relatively easy to diagnose hypovolaemic shock when a patient is bleeding externally. Diagnosis is more difficult when hypovolaemia is developing as a consequence of an internal crisis. Nurses must be ready to recognise the above signs and to take prompt action and/or seek help should they occur.

Cardiogenic shock

This type of shock is caused by abnormalities in the functioning of the heart, and is particularly problematic in patients who have just suffered a myocardial infarction. Cardiogenic shock can perhaps best be understood with reference to the physiological processes that contribute to the normal circulation of blood.

Box 18.1 Key terms relating to cardiac status

CARDIAC OUTPUT

This is the product of the heart rate multiplied by the stroke volume and represents the amount of blood ejected from the heart each minute. In the adult, cardiac output is normally 5–8 l/min.

CARDIAC INDEX

This is patient's cardiac output divided by his body surface area. It indicates how many litres per minute per square metre of body surface the heart ejects. The normal range of an adult is 2.7–4.3 l/min/m^2.

STROKE VOLUME

This is the amount of blood delivered to the aorta during a left ventricular contraction (normally 80–120 ml in an adult). Three factors influence stroke volume: preload, afterload and contractility.

PRELOAD

Indicators are central venous pressure (CVP) and pulmonary capillary wedge pressure (PCWP). By means of a CVP transducer right atrial pressure can be measured. CVP reflects the pressure in the right atrium and systemic veins but does not reliably reflect left ventricular pressures. PCWP gives an indication of the compliance of the left ventricular myocardium during diastole and the left atrial filling pressure necessary to fill the left ventricle with blood prior to systole.

AFTERLOAD

This is the resistance to systolic ejection of blood from the ventricle and can be assessed by measuring pulmonary vascular resistance and systemic vascular resistance. The pulmonary vascular resistance is the ratio of the pressure drop across the pulmonary vascular system to the total flow passing through the pulmonary circulation. Systemic or peripheral vascular resistance is a measurement of the vascular resistance to blood flow.

CONTRACTILITY

This refers to the ability of the myocardium to contract effectively and act as a pump to maintain the circulation of blood.

?	**18.1** Refresh your knowledge of cardiac function by reviewing Chapter 2, pages 10–13.
?	**18.2** Review the terms listed in Box 18.1 to ensure that you understand how they would be applied in the course of treatment and monitoring for cardiogenic shock.

Haemodynamic changes leading to the development of cardiogenic shock

When myocardial ischaemia and infarction occur the contractility of the ventricles is impaired. Ischaemic muscle is deprived of adequate oxygen and substrates for effective contraction, and infarcted muscle or scar tissue is unable to contract. When there is a rapid reduction in the amount of functional myocardium (e.g. when 40–50% is damaged) cardiac output will fall to a level insufficient to maintain adequate arterial pressure and tissue perfusion. In addition, since the left ventricle is not being effectively emptied, pressure will rise in the left atrium, the pulmonary circulation and the right side of the heart. As the capillary pressure rises (reflected by a PCWP above 18 mmHg), pulmonary oedema will eventually ensue, reducing oxygenation. Thus not only will the tissues be poorly perfused, but the blood which does reach them will carry less oxygen.

Pump failure (i.e. reduced contractility of the damaged myocardium), and ensuing hypoxia and acidosis activate the compensatory mechanisms of shock. The resulting tachycardia and vasoconstriction will increase the workload of the impaired myocardial muscle. As shock progresses the release of MDF (see p. 600) will depress myocardial contractility even further. Without effective intervention the vicious circle of effects shown in Figure 18.3 will result in progressive deterioration.

The signs of cardiogenic shock include:

- systolic pressure < 80 mmHg
- tachycardia and a weak, thready pulse
- cold, clammy skin
- oliguria: urine output < 20 ml/h
- confusion
- mottling of the extremities, particularly the legs
- if measured pulmonary wedge pressure is > 18 mmHg, cardiac index is < 1.8 l/m/m^2.

Despite modern advances in haemodynamic monitoring and therapy, the mortality rate of patients with cardiogenic shock remains over 80% (Quaal 1992, Jowett & Thompson 1989).

Distributive shock

Septicaemic shock

This type of shock may arise as a consequence of any infectious disease. Although Gram-negative bacteria are most commonly associated with this phenomenon, Gram-positive organisms

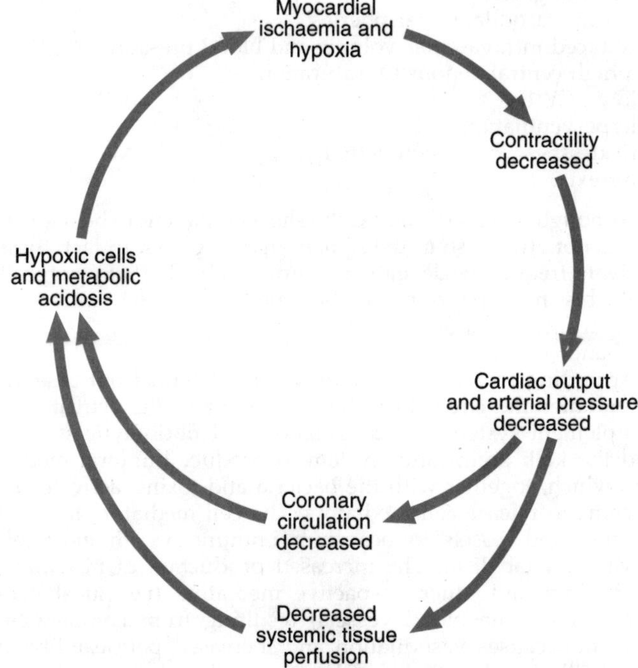

Fig. 18.3 The vicious circle of effects in cardiogenic shock.

such as streptococci, staphylococci and pneumococci can also produce the myocardial depression and haemodynamic states which characterise septicaemic shock (Natanson et al 1989), as can certain fungi. Despite the unavailability of exact figures, Hartnett (1989) suggests that the incidence of septicaemic shock has greatly increased in the last 20–30 years. Hartnett believes that this is partly due to the increased use of antibiotics, the increasing incidence of Gram-negative infections, the growing number of immuno-suppressed patients and increased use of invasive monitoring and diagnostic techniques. Indwelling catheters offer easy access to bacterial invasion and while antibiotics are commonly used in critical care, resistant Gram-negative bacteria can still prevail. According to Hartnett (1989), septicaemic shock is now a relatively common occurrence among oncology patients, who are undergoing an increasing number of aggressive and invasive forms of therapy.

Gram-negative and gram-positive organisms. Many Gram-positive organisms normally live on the skin and mucous membranes. If they attack a host, they release a protein toxin as a byproduct of their metabolism. It is this toxin which is responsible for the various signs and symptoms manifested in disease. Gram-negative bacteria normally reside in the gut, where they are harmless. However, if they migrate from their normal environment to other parts of the body they may cause infection resulting in the release of endotoxins. Gram-negative bacteria particularly favour a wet or damp environment such as that found in sinks, humidifiers and ventilators, and are therefore often a major bacteriological problem in critical care areas.

The pathophysiology of septicaemia has recently become better understood. Sibbald (1988) has suggested it is characterised initially by a hyperdynamic stage, followed by a hypodynamic phase and, finally, by multiple organ failure.

The hyperdynamic phase. The distinguishing feature of early septicaemic shock is usually a vasodilated and hyperdynamic state, with clinical evidence that intravascular volume is depleted. A focus of infection may not be immediately obvious. Rather, the diagnosis may be suspected in the presence of:

- bounding, full pulse
- warm, vasodilated peripheries
- reduced intravascular volume and blood pressure
- a high central venous O_2 saturation
- low PCWP
- hyperventilation
- restlessness, confusion, lethargy
- pyrexia.

Although it is usual to find the shocked patient to be oliguric this is not always so in the hyperdynamic phase. In fact, these patients frequently develop polyuria. Sibbald (1988) suggests that this may be due to abnormalities in the 'intrarenal compartmentalisation of blood flow leading to renal sodium loss' and consequently a form of diabetes insipidus.

According to Schuster (1990), when bacteria from a septic focus enter the circulation they and their toxins activate the complement system, the coagulation and fibrinolytic system, and the kalli krein kinin system to produce humoral mediators which, together with the bacteria and toxins, activate cell systems to release cell mediators. The cell mediators then act on the blood vessels, myocardium, immune system and intermediate metabolism. The increased production of histamine, bradykinin and other vasoactive mediators (i.e. substances which affect the blood vessels) resulting from complement activation causes vasodilation and increased permeability of the capillaries. This is helpful on a small scale in combating local infection. But when massive vasodilation and increased capillary permeability occurs throughout the body the results may be disastrous (Whitman 1988): the increased requirement for circulating volume to fill the dilated vessels and maintain blood flow to vital organs may fail to be met, resulting in inadequate circulation, perfusion and oxygenation.

At least three mechanisms are involved in the development of septicaemic shock. Schuster (1990, p. 282) describes these as follows:

- 'maldistribution of blood flow leading to a mismatch between supply and demand of oxygen within the microvasculature'
- 'cytotoxic effects damaging membranes and intracellular structures'
- 'direct inhibition of the intracellular metabolic oxidative metabolism'.

These mechanisms give rise to the following effects:

- massive vasodilation (reduced afterload)
- some loss of intravascular fluid due to increased capillary permeability together with an increase in the capacity of the circulatory system to be filled
- reduced myocardial contractility as toxins affect the myocardium
- changes in the microcirculation, which may include clotting in small vessels
- failure of oxygen delivery to meet tissue demands
- direct cytotoxic damage to the cells and inhibition of their normal utilisation of oxygen and substrates.

The hypodynamic phase. At this stage clinical findings begin to resemble more closely those typically associated with shock. Catecholamine release (adrenaline and noradrenaline) results in vasoconstriction and the patient's skin becomes cold, moist and possibly mottled at the peripheries. The pulse becomes rapid, thready and weak, and ECG changes suggest an inadequate coronary blood flow.

During this phase it is common for haematological problems to become evident. The released endotoxins damage the endothelium and cause adhesion of platelets and subsequent destruction of the microcirculation. These effects, together with the activation of the coagulation and fibrinolytic systems, may give rise to disseminated intravascular coagulation (DIC, see p. 613). Hyperventilation persists but fails to overcome hypoxia. Lactic acid builds up and there is increasing metabolic acidosis, further compromising cell function. At this point the patient is almost certain to develop multiple organ failure. See Case History 18.1 and Nursing Care Plan 18.1.

Case History 18.1 Mr R (See Nursing Care Plan 18.1)

Mr R, a 50-year-old bank manager, was admitted to the surgical unit for a hemicolectomy for diverticular disease. The surgery went according to plan and Mr R appeared to be progressing well. On the 5th postoperative day, however, the staff nurse noticed that he looked ill, and Mr R admitted that he was 'not so well today'.

Physical findings included:

- tachycardia
- tachypnoea
- warm, pink skin
- restlessness
- pyrexia
- polyuria.

The doctor concluded that Mr R was in the early stages of septicaemic shock. Nursing staff then implemented the interventions summarised in Nursing Care Plan 18.1.

Nursing Care Plan 18.1 Mr R Care of a patient with septicaemic shock (See Case History 18.1.)

Nursing considerations	Goal	Action	Rationale
1. Potential risk of fluid volume depletion due to peripheral vasodilation and capillary leakage	To restore and maintain circulating blood volume	❒ Assess vital signs, skin colour and capillary refill time	Depending on the shock phase, Mr R may present with an increased cardiac output, which causes a flushed, pink appearance. As the hypodynamic phase develops the cardinal signs of shock become evident (see p. 600)
		❒ Ensure i.v. access with a minimum of two large-bore catheters	Fluid volume loss due to redistribution requires blood, colloid and crystalloid replacement
		❒ Monitor and record vital signs and core body temperature	Alterations in vital signs determine stability, improvement or deterioration and indicate whether changes need to be made to therapy
		❒ Insert a urinary catheter	Renal function is a good indicator of overall tissue perfusion. A urine output of 0.5–1.0 ml/kg/h is desirable. In the early stages of septicaemic shock, an inappropriately large volume of urine may be passed due to renal vasodilation caused by bacterial toxins. In such circumstances urine output can be more than 100 ml/h
		❒ Assist with the insertion of a pulmonary artery catheter	Ideally the left ventricular function should be monitored by means of a PA catheter. If this is not possible then a central line will monitor the CVP and serve as a guide to fluid replacement
		❒ Administer and evaluate the effectiveness of inotropic agents: • dobutamine • dopamine • dopexamine	Inotropic agents increase cardiac output and therefore improve renal, coronary, mesenteric and cerebral blood flow
2. Potential for impaired gas exchange due to interstitial fluid overload	Restore and maintain optimal pulmonary function	❒ Assess Mr R's respiratory status, rate and rhythm: • Is he distressed? • Does he have any bronchospasm? • Monitor arterial blood gases • Monitor O_2 saturation via pulse oximetry	Escalating demands on the cardiovascular system increase oxygen consumption. In the early hyperdynamic stage the ABGs may be relatively normal and it is not until the hypodynamic stage is reached that they reflect hypoxia or metabolic acidosis
		❒ Encourage Mr R's cooperation in optimising respiratory function by means of: • breathing exercises • chest physiotherapy • incentive spirometry (see Ch. 3) • progressive O_2 therapy	Mr R may eventually need intubation and ventilation to maintain acceptable ABGs. To try to avoid this the nurse can employ these interventions
(Cont'd)		❒ Administer bronchodilators as prescribed by the physician	Bronchodilators cause airway dilatation by acting directly on β_2 receptors

Nursing Care Plan 18.1 *(Cont'd)*

Nursing considerations	Goal	Action	Rationale
3. Potential for further systemic infection	Reduce or eliminate the systemic risk of further infection	❒ Administer appropriate antibiotic therapy via i.v. route	Antibiotics are given i.v. to ensure a high level of the drug in the blood, body cavity fluids and tissues
		❒ Minimise the introduction of further infection by: • careful and frequent handwashing • maintaining aseptic techniques for all invasive procedures	Shock states alter the immune response and these patients are even more susceptible to infection. The increased use of invasive monitoring techniques offers more opportunities for invading pathogens
		❒ Perform frequent bacteriological screening	The use of antibiotic 'cocktails' to treat one organism may allow others to proliferate

> ? **18.3** Which stage of shock do the clinical findings in Case History 18.1 represent: hyperdynamic, or hypodynamic?

Neurogenic shock
This type of distributive shock is associated with the central nervous system. It can occur when a disease process, drug or traumatic injury blocks sympathetic nerve impulses from the brain's vasomotor centre and thus increases parasympathetic activity. Neurogenic shock produces a picture of vasodilation with loss of vascular tone. Venous return is reduced, cardiac output falls and hypotension rapidly follows.

Aetiology. There are a number of preconditions which may over the course of several hours or even a few weeks or months lead to the development of neurogenic shock. One of the most common causes is spinal anaesthesia, especially that which extends up the length of the spinal cord and results in a blockage of sympathetic impulses. Brain trauma, such as contusions or concussion (particularly to the brain stem or medulla oblongata) may also produce severe neurogenic shock. Another potential cause is spinal cord trauma in which all reflex activity below the level of the lesion is lost.

Spinal shock
Trauma to the head, neck, back or shoulders resulting from an accident or fall may cause injury to the vertebral column and/or spinal cord. Spinal injuries are most prevalent among young men who have been previously healthy and for whom the injury is a catastrophic event necessitating major changes in lifestyle.

The degree and type of force exerted on the spine at the time of injury will determine the nature and severity of the injury. The most frequently seen and, unfortunately, the most damaging type of spinal injury as a result of a road traffic accident (RTA) i.e. a sudden hyperflexion and rotation with fracture dislocation at C5 and C6, and T12 to L1. Within 30 to 60 minutes of the trauma, autonomic and motor reflexes below the level of the injury are suppressed. This state is known as spinal shock and it may last hours or even weeks. It is probably a result of the sudden cessation of efferent impulses from the supraspinal centres.

Anaphylactic shock
This type of shock is life-threatening if it is not dealt with immediately. It arises when the individual develops a hypersensitivity response to an antigen, drug or foreign protein in which the release of histamine causes widespread vasodilation resulting in hypotension and increased capillary permeability with loss of fluid into the interstitium.

The main causes of systemic anaphylaxis are insect bites and stings (particularly from bees and wasps) and drugs (notably penicillin). Occasionally, diagnostic contrast media may also precipitate anaphylactic reactions.

> ? **18.4** What precautions might be observed before a patient undergoes a diagnostic test involving a contrast medium?

The individual developing anaphylactic shock presents with a combination of the following symptoms:

- skin eruptions, large weals
- local oedema, particularly around the face
- a weak and rapid pulse
- laryngeal stridor, dyspnoea, cough and, occasionally, cyanosis.

Treatment will be urgently needed because of the respiratory problems caused by local tissue swelling, laryngeal oedema and/or bronchospasm in addition to circulatory insufficiency.

MANAGEMENT AND TREATMENT OF SHOCK

In its early stages, shock demands urgent intervention. Treatment must begin even before a primary diagnosis is confirmed; otherwise the pathophysiological process of the shock reaction may quickly become irreversible. Reestablishing perfusion of the vital organs is essential. Basic measures cannot be neglected, including the ABCs of resuscitation (see Ch. 28, p. 811). The patient may require immediate intubation in the A & E department or protection of his own airway by the insertion of an artificial airway. Immediate oxygen therapy will be required, possibly with assisted ventilation. In the obviously hypovolaemic patient rapid fluid replacement will be required. The nurse's role in carrying out or assisting with these measures will be crucial from the outset.

The nurse must know what actions will be necessary for the particular type of shock that has developed. She must understand the rationale behind all interventions, bearing firmly in mind the overall aims of treatment, which are:

1. To restore and maintain the circulating blood volume, ensuring that oxygenation and plasma osmotic pressure are adequate
2. To achieve and maintain effective cardiac function
3. To prevent complications.

As well as being able to recognise the warning signs of shock (see p. 600), the nurse should be able to identify those patients who are most at risk of developing shock. When obtaining a patient's initial history the nurse should take note of the risk factors listed in Box 18.2.

?	18.5 a. Read Case History 18.2. In your opinion, is Mr A suffering from shock? If so, which type? b. Why might his abdomen be rigid? c. What initial steps should medical and nursing staff take?

Management and treatment of hypovolaemic shock

Regardless of what may have triggered the patient's hypovolaemia, the restoration of circulating fluid volume is the key to management. As soon as the patient's airway has been cleared and oxygen therapy instituted, the next priority is to assess circulatory status and commence i.v. fluids via two large-bore cannulae. The nurse needs to ask:

Box 18.2 Identifying patients at risk of experiencing shock

- Has the patient experienced multiple trauma?
- Has the patient had surgery recently?
- Has the patient suffered severe burns?
- Is the patient postpartum?
- Does the patient have a history of oesophageal varices or peptic ulceration?
- Is the patient taking anticoagulant therapy?

The above factors put the patient at risk of *hypovolaemic* shock.

- Has the patient experienced chest pain recently or suffered a myocardial infarction — especially in vessels supplying the anterior wall of the left ventricle?
- Does the patient have a history of cardiac failure or cardiac dysrhythmias?

The above factors put the patient at risk of *cardiogenic* shock.

- Does the patient have impaired immunity, e.g. is he suffering from AIDS or cancer or undergoing chemotherapy?
- Does the patient have a resistant deep-seated infection?
- Is the patient seriously ill and requiring multiple invasive catheters and devices?

The above factors put the patient at risk of *septicaemic* shock.

- Does the patient suffer from any disordered state resulting in impaired nervous stimuli to vascular smooth muscle?
- Has the patient experienced recent spinal anaesthesia?
- Has the patient experienced trauma to the brain and/or the spinal cord?

The above factors put the patient at risk of experiencing *neurogenic* or *spinal shock*.

- Does the patient have significant allergies or sensitivities?
- Is the patient undergoing tests requiring contrast media?

The above factors put the patient at risk of experiencing *anaphylactic* shock.

Case History 18.2 Mr A

Mr A, aged 35, is married and has two young children. While travelling to work one morning he was involved in an RTA. Within 30 minutes he was admitted to the nearest A & E department, where initial assessment showed the following:

1. Vital signs:
   - blood pressure: systolic = 70 mmHg but diastolic difficult to hear
   - heart rate: 150/min; pulse weak, thready and rapid
   - respirations: 40/min; breathing shallow
   - temperature: 35.5°C
2. Neurological signs:
   - little response to painful stimuli
   - poor gag and cough reflex
   - right pupil unresponsive to light
   - left pupil reacting sluggishly
   - Glasgow Coma Scale score: 4
3. General examination
   - large swelling in right occiput
   - rigid abdomen; bowel sounds absent
   - obvious fracture to right femur with large gaping wound
   - possible fractured pelvis
   - skin moist and clammy; mouth dry.

1. What kind of fluid is required?
2. How much fluid does the patient need?

Clinical opinion varies with regard to resuscitative fluids. Both crystalloids and colloids are generally considered suitable, although certain disadvantages are associated with each. If the patient has haemorrhaged excessively a blood transfusion will also be necessary.

Crystalloids

Hartmann's solution (lactated Ringer injection) is probably one of the most common resuscitative fluids used in haemorrhagic shock. It mimics extracellular fluid and is therefore an ideal substitute when extracellular levels have been diminished. Essentially it is an electrolyte solution consisting of sodium chloride, potassium chloride, calcium chloride and sodium lactate in water. Since it closely resembles blood plasma it can be used as an emergency plasma expander until blood has been grouped and crossmatched. It rarely causes any adverse reactions and is inexpensive and readily available.

Normal saline solution (0.9% sodium chloride) is probably as good a resuscitative fluid as Ringer's lactate, although its large concentration of chloride ions could be disadvantageous to the patient whose renal function is already impaired. It may also cause hypernatraemia, hypokalaemia or a hyperchloraemic metabolic acidosis.

Dextrose 5% in water is not considered a suitable fluid for the patient in shock, although it may maintain water balance and supply the calories necessary for cell metabolism. Dextrose 5% may be used to establish a line, but should be replaced as soon as possible by a more suitable crystalloid.

Colloids

Normal human serum albumin or fresh frozen plasma is the volume expander of choice when non-colloidal solutions do not reverse hypovolaemia.

Dextran is a synthetic colloidal solution that simulates the effects of albumin. It is available in both high and low molecular weights. It provides rapid plasma volume expansion when compatible blood or blood products are unavailable. Advantages of dextran include its long shelf life, its reasonable cost and the fact that it presents no risk of hepatitis or AIDS transmission. It may, however, interfere with blood typing and crossmatching, as it tends to coat the cells. It has also been known to cause allergic reactions.

Other colloids include polygeline (Haemaccel), succinylated gelatin (Gelofusine) and hetastarch (Hespan).

Combined solutions

Despite their advantages, it is argued that the crystalloid group of solutions dilute the plasma proteins and reduce the plasma oncotic pressure. This leads to changes in cell wall permeability, resulting in increased fluid leakage across the capillaries into the interstitial space and hence oedema, particularly in the lungs. Ledingham & Ramsay (1986) suggest that the best results are achieved by using a combination of crystalloid and colloid solutions, citing evidence that the cell's oxygen consumption is higher with a combination of both solutions.

Blood

The rapid replacement of blood and blood products is essential in the haemorrhagically shocked patient. It is advisable to use a blood warmer to bring the blood up to body temperature in order to avoid excessive cooling of the patient. In addition serial haemoglobin and haematocrit tests should be carried out 4-hourly to gauge the patient's additional fluid needs.

Autotransfusion. This simply involves collecting the patient's lost blood and reinfusing it as packed cells after the blood has been collected and filtered and its components separated. Autotransfusion is a popular practice in large trauma centres.

MAST. Medical (originally 'military') antishock trousers are used in some parts of the world as a means of squeezing 500–1000 ml of circulating volume to the vital organs until fluid replacement has been achieved. They are not used widely in Britain.

Management and treatment of cardiogenic shock

The main goals of therapy in cardiogenic shock are:

- to reestablish circulation to the myocardium
- to minimise heart muscle damage
- to improve the effectiveness of the heart as a pump.

Damage to cardiac muscle can be minimised by improving the heart's oxygen supply and, at the same time, reducing its oxygen demand. Oxygen supply can be increased by the administration of a high percentage of O_2 via a face mask. Jowett & Thompson (1989, p. 239) state: 'high oxygen concentrations (100%) are required and toxicity rarely occurs because of arteriovenous shrinking in the lungs.' Oxygen demand can be reduced by placing the patient in a comfortable position (see Boore et al, p. 706) and keeping him at rest. Analgesics to control pain will also aid in the reduction of O_2 demand.

The effectiveness of the heart's pumping action can be enhanced by the use of inotropic agents, which increase the force of contraction and improve systolic ejection of blood (Rice 1991).

Catecholamines (see below) are commonly used to improve contractility and correct hypotension, and since the patient with myocardial ischaemia and impaired myocardial contractility will also be at risk of arrhythmias, antiarrhythmic agents may also be administered.

Drugs commonly used

Catecholamines function by stimulating the smooth muscle receptors of the myocardium. This leads to an increase in the contractility of the myocardium and thereby increases cardiac output, raises arterial pressure and improves tissue perfusion.

Dopamine is one such agent frequently used in cardiogenic shock; it does have the disadvantage, however, of producing an atrial tachycardia. Dobutamine is another catecholamine which acts directly on the beta-adrenergic receptors in the myocardium and has an inotropic and chronotropic effect. More recently, dopexamine hydrochloride has become available and is proving beneficial as an inotropic agent, as are a new generation of drugs known as inodilators (e.g. enoximone), which have inotropic and vasodilating qualities.

In some cases, drugs may be prescribed to decrease afterload. Here, the goal of therapy is to decrease vascular resistance, improve the ventricles' emptying capacity and, in so doing, to lower the filling pressure of the heart. Nitroprusside is probably the drug most frequently used for this purpose in short-term applications. For long-term therapy, oral preparations such as nifedipine are prescribed.

The intra-aortic balloon pump (IABP)

The IABP is often used in conjunction with drugs to improve afterload. It assists a weakened or damaged left ventricle by aiding left ventricle ejection and thus improving coronary artery and peripheral tissue perfusion.

There are various types of IABPs, all of which work by the same principle. The catheter is inserted via the femoral artery and the balloon is advanced into the aorta just distal to the left subclavian junction. The catheter is then attached to a pump which inflates the balloon with helium during diastole and in so doing increases intra-aortic blood pressure, thereby improving coronary artery perfusion.

Management and treatment of septicaemic shock

As in hypovolaemic shock, the restoration of adequate intravascular fluid volume is a major consideration in treatment. A balance of crystalloid and colloid solutions must be infused. Cultures should be taken from all possible sites of infection and sensitivities determined. It may in some cases be necessary to treat the septic focus surgically; e.g. by drainage of abscesses or debridement of infected or necrotic tissue.

The critically ill patient is likely to be monitored by a number of invasive devices, all of which provide an opportunity for pathogens to invade the body. In view of this risk antibiotics are usually commenced before any definitive results arrive from the bacteriology laboratory. Recent studies by Blair et al (1991) have so far shown a reduction in sepsis in critical care practice by the selective decontamination of the gut and buccal mucosa with a special 'cocktail' of antibiotics.

Blood gases

Blood gases should be monitored carefully. In many cases patients develop a sequence of hypoxia and acidosis. The hypoxia may need to be corrected with artifical ventilation, and an infusion of bicarbonate may be required to reverse the acidosis. Since severe pyrexia increases oxygen requirements, cooling measures are often instituted when the patient's temperature rises above 39°C. This is more easily accomplished when the patient is adequately sedated and mechanically ventilated and is not so aware of his cold surroundings.

Skin integrity

The patient suffering from septicaemic shock needs particular nursing attention to his skin condition. The administration of inotropic agents increases peripheral vasoconstriction and the resulting decrease in tissue perfusion puts the patient at risk of pressure sores. Moreover, the patient may not be sufficiently haemodynamically stable to allow the two-hourly turning regime used to help prevent pressure sores. When this situation arises many intensive care nurses will decide to nurse the patient on an air-fluidised system such as the Clinitron unit, which will support the patient at low pressures and thus help to prevent damage to the skin.

Management and treatment of anaphylactic shock

Anaphylactic shock results from a severe allergic reaction to a specific antigen. Intervention should aim first at identifying and removing the cause. If this is not possible the effects of the reaction must be reversed. The drug of choice is i.v. adrenaline to restore vascular tone. Aminophylline may be given to counteract bronchoconstriction and antihistamines may be administered to reverse the adverse effect of the mediator histamine involved in the reaction. As with other forms of shock, oxygen therapy and i.v. fluid replacement will usually be required.

Definitive and supportive therapy

Interventions used in the treatment and management of shock may be described as either 'definitive' or 'supportive', as follows (Rice 1991). The goal of definitive therapy is to locate and correct the cause of the shock and to restore and maintain adequate perfusion and oxygenation of the tissues. The goal of supportive therapy is to improve oxygen delivery to the tissues, to restore and maintain tissue perfusion, and to restore cellular function. See Box 18.3 for a summary of interventions used in the treatment of shock.

First aid treatment for shock

Nurses may occasionally be called upon to help people on the street or in other public places who have gone into shock as the result of an accident, heart attack or severe allergic reaction, and so should be aware of the appropriate first aid to give in the absence of clinical facilities.

The main objectives of intervention in such an emergency should be:

- to maintain an adequate supply of blood to the heart, lungs and brain
- to ascertain the cause of the shock
- to limit haemorrhaging and prevent further injury
- to arrange for transfer to hospital.

Box 18.4 lists the steps to take in the event of an emergency, especially where hypovolaemic shock is suspected or imminent.

Immediate management of severe burns or scalds

Many of the interventions listed in Box 18.2 will be appropriate to cases of severe burn injury. It would also be advisable to quickly and gently remove constricting articles such as belts and jewellery from the individual before the affected area becomes oedematous. Other specific instructions for the emergency treatment of burns is given in Chapter 31.

Immediate management for fractures

The main aim of first aid treatment for any fracture is immobilisation at the site of injury. Apart from increasing the individual's pain, movement can cause further damage to the fracture and surrounding soft tissue and muscle. However, if the person is obviously haemorrhaging from a compound wound site, then pressure will need to be applied even if this involves further damage to the fracture site.

The extent of blood loss accompanying fracture injuries should never be underestimated. To take one example, as much as one or two litres of blood may be lost by an individual who sustains a fracture to the shaft of femur. The risk of hypovolaemic shock following fracture must therefore never be discounted.

Immediate management of anaphylactic shock

Swift recognition of anaphylactic shock is vital to the individual's survival. Anyone who knows that he is allergic to bee stings should wear a Medic Alert bracelet and carry an emergency kit for self-administration of adrenaline, especially during the summer season. If an insect sting should occur a tourniquet applied proximal to the site of the sting may prevent further absorption of the antigen. If the actual sting has become embedded in the skin it should be carefully removed.

In severe cases i.v. fluids and plasma expanders may be necessary. In extreme circumstances intubation and artifical ventilation may be needed to overcome respiratory complications.

Box 18.3 Definitive and supportive therapy in clinical shock (Adapted from Rice 1991)

DEFINITIVE THERAPY

Hypovolaemic shock
- Maintain or increase intravascular volume
- Decrease any future fluid/blood loss via i.v. fluid regime
- Give supplementary O_2 therapy

Cardiogenic shock
- Reduce cardiac muscle damage by ↑ O_2 supply and ↓ cardiac demand by O_2 therapy and cardiac medication to dilate the coronary vessels and by decreasing pain and activity
- ↑ effectiveness of heart as a pump via inotropic medication

Septicaemic shock
- Restore adequate intravascular volume via i.v. fluids
- Give supplemental O_2 therapy
- Identify and control source of infection via bacterial screening
- Administer appropriate antibiotics
- Remove nidus of infection if possible

Anaphylactic shock
- Identify and remove causative antigen
- Reduce effects of mediator substances that have caused massive vasodilation, e.g. give adrenaline to restore vascular tone, antihistamines to reverse histamine effects, bronchiolators to oppose bronchial constriction
- Give O_2 therapy and i.v. fluid replacement

Supportive therapy
- Give adequate ventilation and oxygenation via optimal airway maintenance, optimal breathing technique and supplemental O_2
- Maintain or restore adequate perfusion of tissues to ensure oxygen delivery, via maintenance of cardiac pump to effectively circulate the blood and medication to improve contractility and reduce cardiac workload
- Maintain or restore metabolic equilibrium
- Reverse metabolic acidosis via hyperventilation and if severe, by i.v. sodium bicarbonate administration

Box 18.4 Emergency interventions at the scene of an accident

1. Immediately reassure and comfort the person.
2. Check his airway for patency. If his breathing is laboured or difficult lie the individual in the recovery position if it is safe to do so. This will reduce the risk of aspiration of stomach contents. The jaw may need to be lifted, without hyperextension of the neck, to aid in the maintenance of the airway. Loosen any tight clothing, especially around the neck. **NB: Do not attempt to move the person if there is any likelihood of cervical or other spinal injury.**
3. If haemorrhaging is obvious, try to control it by applying pressure.
4. Ask someone reliable to call 999. Give clear instructions, i.e. what kind of help is needed and the correct location of the accident. People tend to panic when a crisis occurs and someone needs to assume the position of leader and maintain an air of calm efficiency. Discourage onlookers from gathering as this only distresses the individual even further.
5. If relatives or friends are at the scene ask them for a quick history. This may help to ascertain the cause of the shock.
6. Someone may be able to provide a blanket or coat to cover the person. However, do not accept the offer of a hot water bottle, as the application of heat would only increase peripheral vasodilation and draw some of the blood supply away from the vital organs.
7. If the person complains of thirst, moisten his lips with water but do not allow him to drink.
8. If a cardiac or respiratory arrest develops commence artificial resuscitation immediately.
9. Transfer the person to hospital as soon as possible.
10. Try to ensure safety, considering the cause of the problem. For example, in the case of an RTA, ask someone to warn and divert traffic, taking care for his or her own safety.

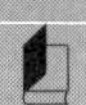
For further information on artificial ventilation see Hewett (1992).

MONITORING THE PATIENT IN SHOCK

Monitoring and observation of the patient's ever-changing condition will allow for the prompt correction of deficits. The following are the most important indicators of tissue perfusion and will be discussed in the following sections:

- cardiac status
- respiratory status
- haemodynamic status
- level of consciousness
- renal function
- body temperature
- skin condition.

Monitoring cardiac status

Electrocardiography

An electrocardiogram (ECG) is a recording of the electrical activity of the myocardium and indicates the changes which occur as a result of contraction. The contraction of any heart muscle is associated with electrical changes called depolarisation and these can be detected by electrodes attached to the surface of the body (see Ch. 2, p. 12). An ECG can be obtained quickly in an A & E department or even with a portable electrocardiograph at the site of an accident and can give useful information about the rate and rhythm of the heart. Thus if arrhythmias arise they can be detected and treated immediately. All patients who are likely to be suffering from shock should be monitored by electrocardiograph. In addition, heart sounds should be assessed, as should major arterial pulses for rate, rhythm and pressure.

?	18.6 What might cause a shocked patient to experience: a. tachycardia: heart rate 100 beats or more per minute b. bradycardia: heart rate 60 beats or fewer per minute.	A

Monitoring respiratory status

The shocked patient's respiratory status may change rapidly and therefore should be monitored at intervals of one hour or less. Constant observation will allow for the detection of potential deterioration. In the early stages, the nurse should be alert to hyperventilation resulting in respiratory alkalosis, followed by fatigue of the respiratory muscles. This may lead to shallow breathing and the risk of respiratory distress, necessitating mechanical ventilation.

Monitoring oxygen saturation

The level of O_2 saturation in the patient's blood (SaO_2) will give some indication of respiratory status. Continuous monitoring will give valuable information on the individual's response to interventions and can provide early warning of hypoxaemia. Both invasive and non-invasive techniques are available for SaO_2 measurement.

The opticath fibreoptic catheter can be used to measure the patient's venous oxygen saturation. This pulmonary artery catheter contains two optical fibres: one transmits light from the optical module to the catheter tip and the second collects reflected light at the catheter tip and transmits it back to the optical module. These signals are transmitted to a computer which calculates oxygen saturation percentage values. These values are continuously displayed in numerical form and recorded as a graph.

Pulse oximetry. Arterial O_2 saturation along with pulse rate can be monitored continuously by means of a non-invasive electronic device called a pulse oximeter. This functions by measuring the absorption of red and infrared light passed through living tissue (usually a finger, toe or earlobe). Since results correspond closely to arterial blood gas values this instrument reduces the need for blood samples. Readings are not affected by skin colour but can be distorted by high blood bilirubin levels (as in jaundice) and in cases of carbon monoxide poisoning and smoke inhalation. Results for very heavy smokers may also be difficult to interpret. Coull (1992) gives further details on the operation of the pulse oximeter.

Monitoring haemodynamic status

In the shocked patient, blood pressure may initially be kept within normal limits by the compensatory mechanisms described earlier (see p. 598). However, as shock progresses and cardiac output decreases, blood pressure will fall. In progressive decompensating shock the use of a sphygmomanometer to estimate blood pressure is inaccurate and inadequate, and more sophisticated investigation will be required.

Blood pressure should be monitored in all patients suffering from shock not only as part of ongoing physical assessment but also as a means of obtaining information about the individual's psychological response to his dilemma.

Intra-arterial pressure monitoring

An accurate assessment of blood pressure can be made by measuring the intra-arterial pressure directly. This is per-

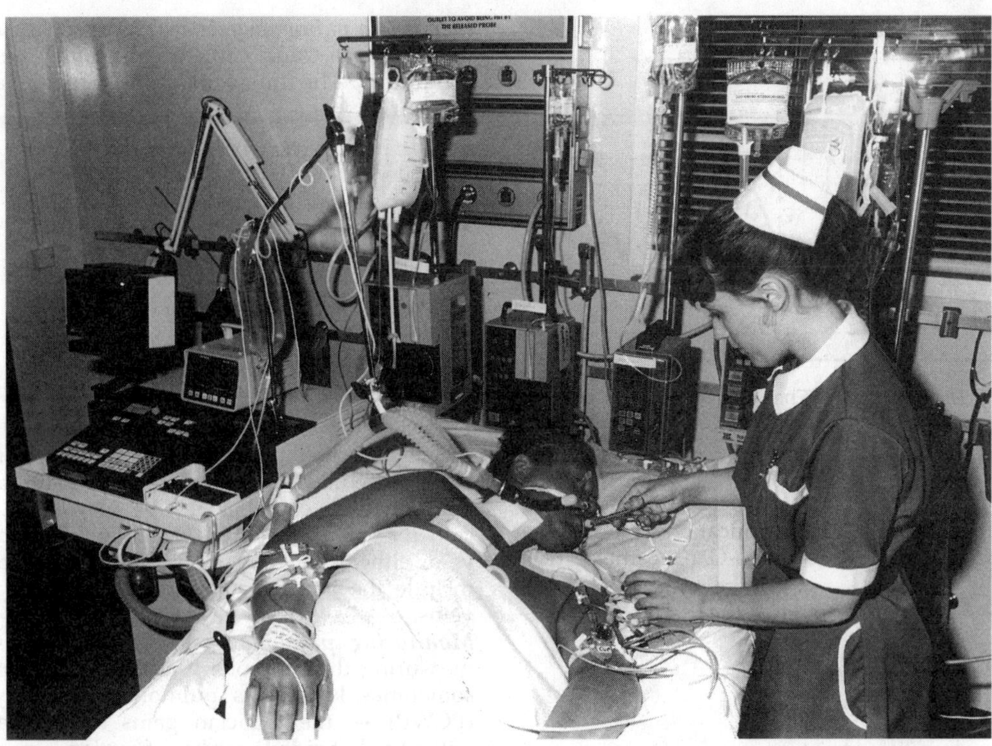

Fig. 18.4 Catheter inserted at radial artery.

formed by medical staff by the insertion of a flexible polyvinyl catheter into an easily accessible artery. The most commonly used site is the radial artery, as the line can be readily secured and observed at this point, and the hand has a good collateral circulation (see Fig. 18.4). Other frequently used sites include the brachial, femoral and dorsal arteries.

Once the catheter is inserted it is attached to a supply of pressurised and heparinised solution (see Fig. 18.5). Approximately 2–3 ml/h of the solution is delivered into the artery to maintain patency. By means of a transducer the arterial wave

Pressurised heparinised solution. Pressure maintained at 300 mmHg to prevent backflow of arterial blood

Monitor

Disposable transducer

Flushing device

Cannula in radial artery

Fig. 18.5 Arterial pressure monitoring equipment.

form is displayed on a monitor along with blood pressure readings.

It should be pointed out that as an arterial line is particularly difficult to insert in the hypovolaemic patient some fluid replacement may be necessary before the line can be established. This will have to be carried out quickly. Under these conditions the femoral artery may be chosen until the patient is more haemodynamically stable, after which a more desirable site may be found.

For further information see Allan (1989).

Once an arterial line has been inserted it is the nurse's responsibility to ensure that it is securely positioned. The arterial pressure monitoring line must be clearly labelled to eliminate any danger of its being mistaken for another line.

The normal waveform will indicate that the arterial catheter is functioning and that the digital blood pressure display is accurate. The nurse must be able to recognise its distinct pattern, which is composed of a systolic upstroke, and a dicrotic notch on the downstroke (see Fig. 18.6). The dicrotic notch occurs as a result of the aortic valve closing and a simultaneous increase in aortic pressure. If this pattern becomes dampened the nurse must be aware that it may indicate a clot in the catheter, air in the line or pressure from the tip of the catheter against the vessel wall itself.

Pulmonary artery pressure monitoring

Haemodynamic monitoring of intracardiac pressure with floating balloon catheters within the heart's chambers gives valuable information about the ventricles' capacity to receive and eject blood and helps medical staff to prescribe the most appropriate therapy. The pulmonary artery catheter is a flexible catheter made of radio-opaque polyvinyl chloride (PVC) and coated with a heparinised preparation to help prevent

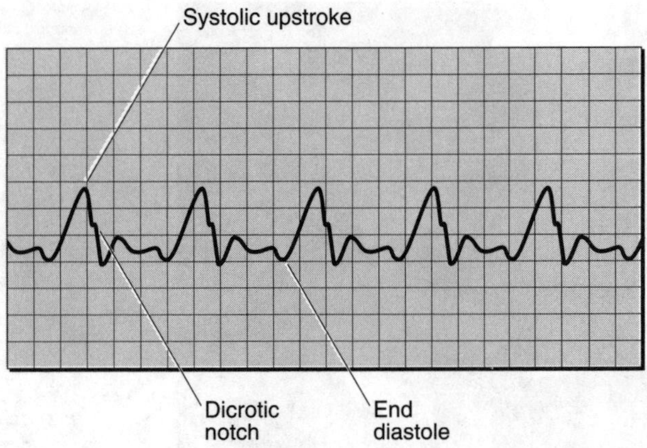

Fig. 18.6 Normal arterial waveform.

catheter-induced thromboembolitic complications. One of the most commonly used types is the Swan-Ganz catheter (see Fig. 18.7).

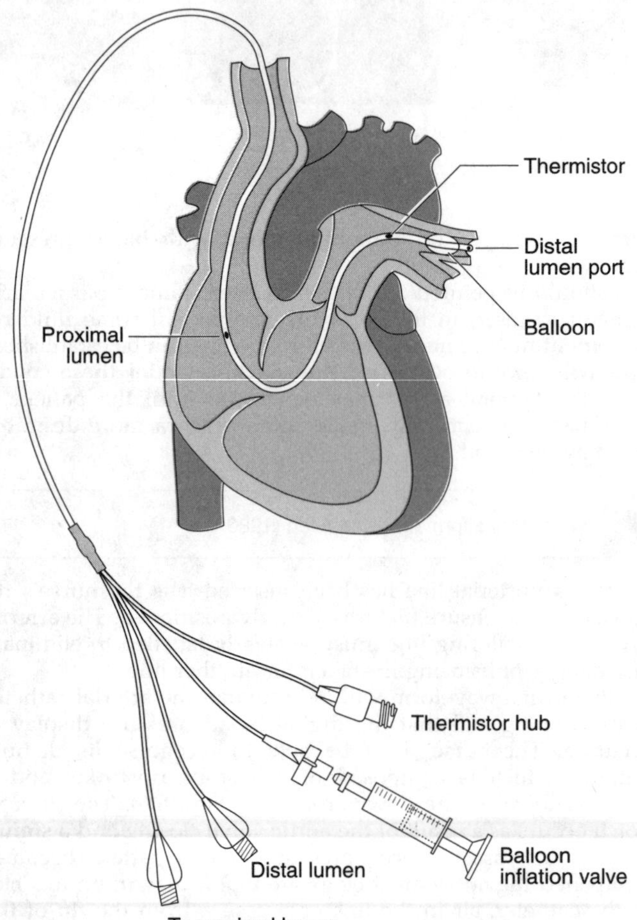

Fig. 18.7 A pulmonary artery catheter. *Distal lumen:* located at the tip of the catheter in the pulmonary artery. Pulmonary artery pressure (PAW), pulmonary artery wedge pressure (PAWP) and mixed venous gas pressures are obtained at this port. *Proximal lumen:* used for central venous pressure (CVP) monitoring or main fluid infusion lumen. It is situated in the right atrium and can also be utilised to measure the right atrial pressure. *Balloon inflation valve:* the balloon situated at the end of the catheter may be inflated to read the PAWP. *Thermistor hub:* situated 4 cm from the tip of the catheter and used to measure cardiac output by thermodilution methods (see Fig. 18.9).

Inserting a pulmonary artery catheter. Like any other central line, a Swan-Ganz catheter must be inserted under sterile conditions. The nurse needs to prepare a trolley with the following:

- large basic pack with sterile forceps
- sterile towels
- skin cleansing lotions
- scalpel blade
- suture material
- Swan-Ganz catheter
- two 5 ml syringes
- hypodermic needles
- lignocaine 1% or 2%
- 2 pressurised and heparinised 500 ml bags of normal saline.

The catheter is usually inserted at the bedside with the patient attached to an ECG monitor. An image intensifier is not required, as the characteristic pressure changes which take place in each chamber can be viewed on the monitor. The catheter can be inserted via either a peripheral or a central vein, either percutaneously or via a cutdown. Possible sites include the internal jugular, subclavian, basilic and cephalic veins.

Monitoring pulmonary wedge pressure (see Fig. 18.8). By measuring the pulmonary artery wedge pressure (PAWP) — sometimes known as pulmonary capillary wedge pressure (PCWP) — the clinician gains an accurate picture of the patient's left-sided cardiac function. In order to measure PAWP the balloon is inflated with approximately 1.0 cc of air. This will enable the catheter tip to be wedged in a smaller branch of the pulmonary artery. When the vessel has been totally occluded the catheter's distal port will detect the pressure within the occluded vessel and will display the resulting waveform and pressure reading on the monitor.

PAWP is expressed as the mean of the diastolic and systolic pressures, the normal range being 8–12 mmHg.

?	**18.7** If the patient has a PAWP of < 8 mmHg what does that indicate?	A
?	**18.8** If the PAWP is > 25 mmHg, what might be the medical diagnosis?	

The nurse's responsibilities. As soon as the PAWP reading is obtained the balloon must be deflated, as prolonged occlusion of the pulmonary artery will cause pulmonary infarction. The nurse needs to observe the catheter waveform carefully and ensure that the catheter does not migrate up into a branch of the pulmonary artery and occlude it. A flat or dampened trace will indicate that this has occurred and that the balloon needs to be checked. Sometimes if the patient is asked to cough the tip of the catheter may be freed. However, this method is not always effective and the doctor should be notified if a dampened waveform persists.

Monitoring cardiac output

By means of the pulmonary catheter with a thermistor (temperature probe) in place the patient's cardiac output (see Box 18.1) can be calculated using the thermodilution technique (see Fig. 18.9). This involves injecting a 10 ml bolus of 5% dextrose or normal saline through the proximal port into the right atrium. This fluid must be cooler than the patient's blood so that the temperature change which occurs as the blood mixes with the fluid can be detected by the thermistor bead in the pulmonary artery. The results are relayed to a cardiac output computer and displayed in l/min. This procedure is usually carried out at least 3–4 times and the mean value taken as the cardiac output.

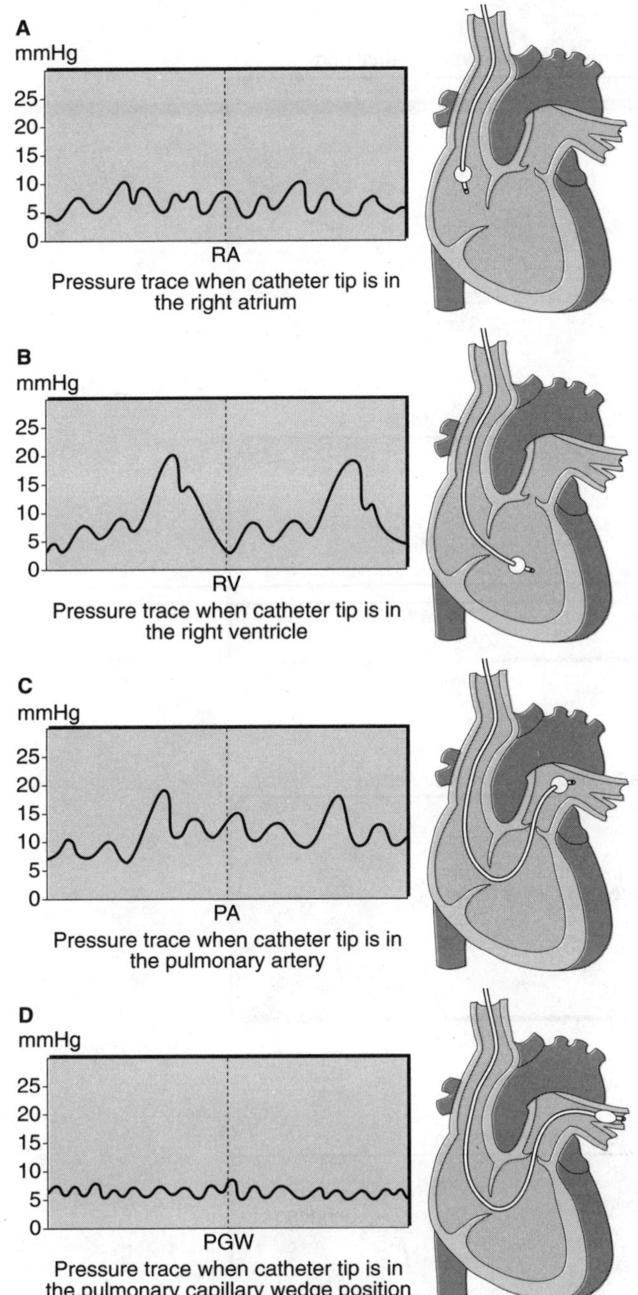

Fig. 18.8 Waveform changes during monitoring by pulmonary artery catheter. (A) The catheter is advanced by the doctor until it is in the right atrium. The balloon is then inflated. (B) The balloon carries the catheter through the tricuspid valve and into the right ventricle. (C) The pressure of blood flow carries the catheter through the pulmonary valve into the pulmonary artery. (D) When the catheter has become wedged in a branch of the pulmonary artery, the balloon is deflated and falls back into the pulmonary artery, where it can be used to monitor continously the pulmonary artery pressure.

Central venous pressure (CVP) monitoring

CVP is the blood pressure within the right atrium and vena cava. Its measurement can give information about blood volume or venous system capacity. It can also give an indication of vascular tone and pulmonary vascular resistance, as well as of the effectiveness of the right heart pump. However, it does not measure left ventricular function.

CVP monitoring reflects the rate of blood return to the right side of the heart and can be an accurate guide for fluid replacement. A CVP of about 0.5 cm water in the presence of a low arterial blood pressure usually indicates hypovolaemia, while a CVP above 14 cm in the presence of a low arterial blood pressure indicates cardiac failure (see Fig. 18.10).

Technique. A large-bore catheter should be inserted under aseptic conditions into the internal or external jugular, subclavian, or femoral veins using either the percutaneous technique via a large-bore needle or by means of a venous cut-down by a member of the medical staff. The site of the central line is checked radiologically prior to the commencement of fluid therapy.

In the intensive therapy or high dependency unit a transducer can be attached to the central line in order to obtain a waveform and digital display of the CVP reading in mmHg. Continuous monitoring will indicate the effectiveness of treatment.

Central venous lines, although extremely important for a critically ill patient, present a danger of bacterial infection. Nurses can make an important contribution to care by ensuring that aseptic techniques are adhered to when the line is inserted initially and that the insertion site is kept clean and dressed daily. Once it is no longer needed the line should be removed as quickly as possible to reduce the risk of infection.

Luer lock connections are essential in all i.v. administrative equipment to minimise accidental disconnection of lines which might allow the patient to haemorrhage.

Monitoring level of consciousness

In the early stages of shock the patient may still be quite alert and anxious. He may complain of pain and may be able to give a history which will help the clinician to establish a diagnosis. However, if his circulating fluid volume falls and cerebral hypoxia results, he will gradually become less coherent and may eventually become comatose. The nurse should observe the patient carefully at this stage and ensure that he is maintaining a safe airway. It may be advisable to place him in the lateral position. In a clinical setting medical staff may decide to intubate the patient and electively and artificially ventilate him. The Glasgow Coma Scale (see Fig 30.3) is a useful tool with which to assess the patient's cerebral function. For a detailed discussion of consciousness levels see Chapter 30, pages 844–846.

Monitoring renal function

Renal function is a very good indicator of tissue perfusion and should therefore be monitored carefully in patients suffering from shock. Since the kidneys are dependent on adequate tissue perfusion a drop in urinary output will indicate poor perfusion. Unless the patient is dehydrated urinary output should be 0.5–1.0 ml/kg/h.

Hourly urine output can be measured by means of a urinary catheter attached to a closed-system urimeter. Any drop in output should be noted and acted upon as necessary to restore renal perfusion.

Measurement of specific gravity and osmolality will reflect the concentration of the urine. In the early stages of shock, when urine volume falls, the concentration of excreted waste products rises. However, if the shock state progresses, urine volumes remain low but the ability to concentrate the urine and blood and the osmolality is fixed or low (Rice 1991).

Monitoring body temperature

The importance of obtaining accurate body temperature measurements should not be underestimated, as many clinical interventions are based on these readings. The nurse needs to be aware of those factors, such as circadian rhythm, which

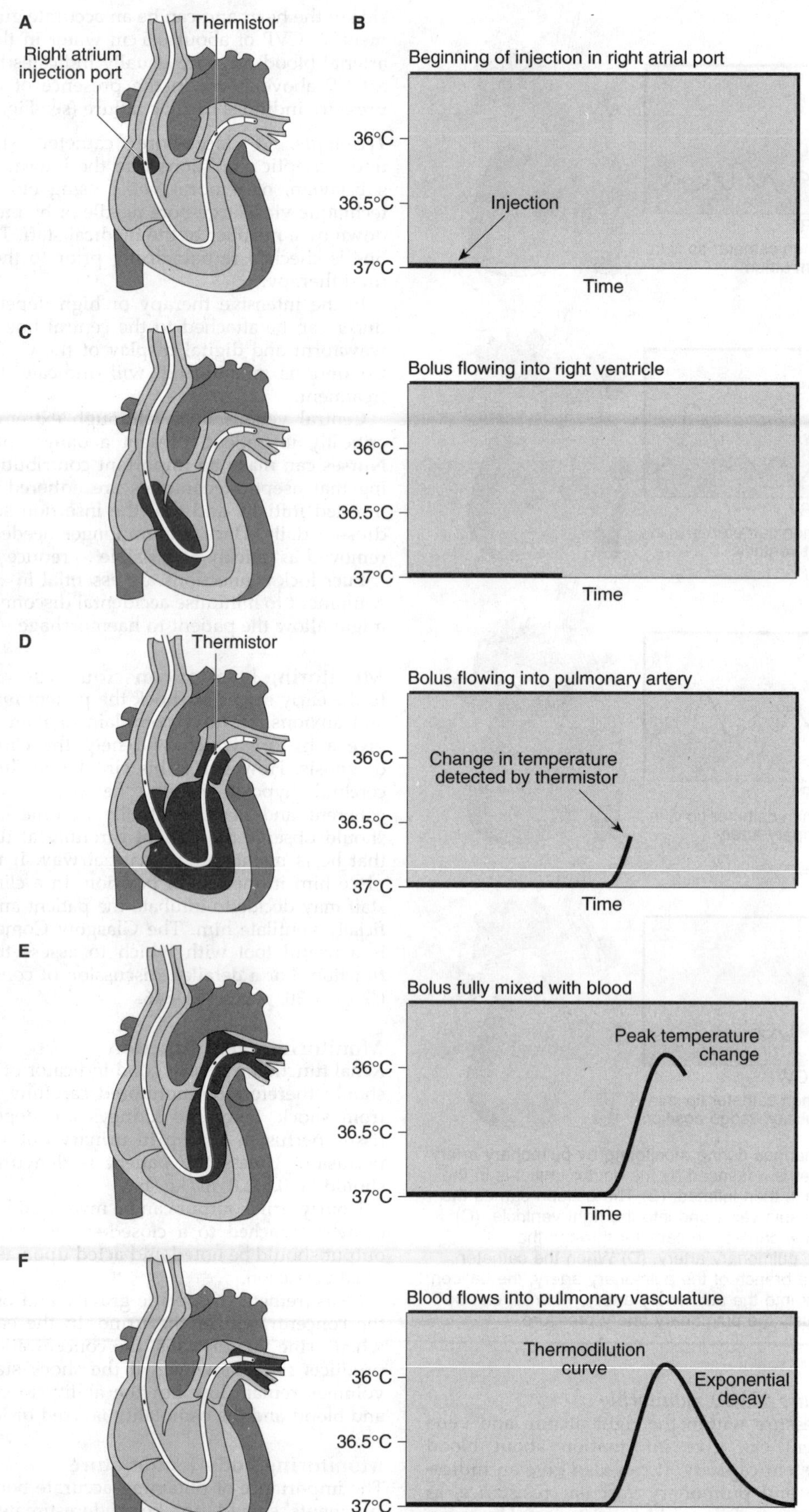

Fig. 18.9 The thermodilution technique for assessing cardiac output.

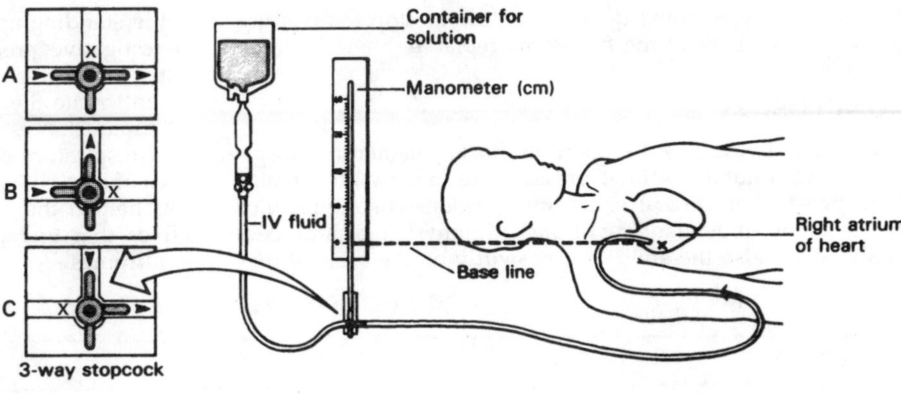

Fig. 18.10 Diagram of a CVP water manometer. (A) Before measuring central venous pressure (CVP), the infusion flow is to the patient and the three-way stopcock is closed to the manometer. (B) To measure CVP, the stopcock is turned so that it is closed to the patient. This allows the manometer to be refilled with fluid. (C) The stopcock is turned so that it is closed to the infusion fluid. This allows a free flow of fluid from the manometer to the intravenous catheter. The fluid level will fall until the level corresponds with the pressure in the right atrium or superior vena cava. (Adapted from Jamieson, McCall & Blythe 1992 Guidelines for clinical nursing practices. Churchill Livingstone, Edinburgh)

can influence body temperature. These factors, as well as procedures for obtaining accurate core temperature readings are described in detail in Chapter 22.

Observing skin condition

The state of the skin and mucous membranes will reflect the stage of shock that the patient is in. The nurse should observe skin colour, moistness and temperature. Intense activation of the sympathetic nervous system will result in pale, clammy skin and a dry mouth. Failure of capillary refill will indicate sustained and prolonged vasoconstriction. If oxygen delivery is severely impaired, the skin will become cold, mottled and cyanosed. However, it should be noted that the clinical picture in septicaemic shock is different. In the early stages of this type of shock, the skin becomes warm, dry and flushed as bacterial toxins cause vasodilation.

Laboratory and diagnostic tests

Haematological and other studies

Arterial blood gas (ABG) analysis can give some indication of circulatory efficiency. In the early stages of shock it is not uncommon to find a fall in the partial pressure of oxygen (Po_2) and a rise in the partial pressure of carbon dioxide (Pco_2). However, Pco_2 may fall due to hyperventilation. With an increase in anaerobic metabolism and in the production of lactic acid, metabolic acidosis is frequently seen in the severely shocked patient.

Other possible blood analyses include:

- serum urea and electrolytes
- blood glucose levels
- cardiac enzymes
- serum amylase levels
- full blood count
- coagulation studies
- blood cultures.

Urinary studies may include:

- urinary electrolytes
- urine osmolality
- creatinine clearance tests.

Other diagnostic tests may include:

- CAT scanning
- ultrasound scanning
- ECGs
- pulmonary function tests
- angiography.

Information on a range of diagnostic tests is given in Appendix 2.

COMPLICATIONS OF SHOCK

Renal failure

When the crisis of shock occurs, blood flow to the kidneys is reduced both by the original hypovolaemic or other circulatory problem and by the vasoconstriction which occurs as part of the body's compensatory mechanisms (see p. 598).

?	**18.9** What are the functions of noradrenaline?

In addition to the reduction of blood flow to the kidneys there is also a change in the flow *within* the kidneys. Blood flow is directed away from the renal cortex to the renal medulla to preserve the function of the juxtamedullary nephrons. This is essential if the countercurrent system of concentrating the urine is to function (see Ch. 8, p. 293). If, however, the shock persists without prompt treatment, then the countercurrent mechanism will fail and the urine will become dilute, leading to the early stages of acute renal failure.

It is important to detect and treat renal failure early. Failure of kidney function should be suspected if urinary output remains low (< 30 ml/h) when arterial pressure and circulating volume are adequate.

Adult respiratory distress syndrome (ARDS)

ARDS is a type of pulmonary insufficiency which may arise as a complication of shock. With the increase in the permeability of the patient's alveolar capillary membranes, fluid accumulates in the interstitial spaces and leaks into the alveoli, causing the lungs to become 'stiff' (non-compliant) and difficult to ventilate and oxygenate. This situation is potentially fatal. Mechanical ventilation with positive end expiratory pressure (PEEP) is the treatment of choice.

?	**18.10** What is PEEP?

Disseminated intravascular coagulation (DIC)

Some of the pathophysiological processes leading to DIC have already been described in relation to septicaemic shock (see p. 601). In DIC the patient's normal clotting mechanisms do not function correctly. Clots may be produced in capillaries where they are not required, and sites where clotting factors could be utilised are deprived of them. Fibrinolytic (clot-dissolving) factors then go into action where they are not needed, and the end result is uncontrolled haemorrhage.

Early clinical signs usually include bleeding from venepuncture sites, the mucous membranes, wounds or drain sites. Treatment is aimed at replacing the clotting factors by administering blood and blood components, platelets, fresh frozen plasma, and possibly cryoprecipitates. Sometimes it is advisable to administer some heparin to slow or stop the clotting process before the clotting factors are replaced.

CONCLUSION

Assisting individuals suffering from shock, whether in a hospital or a community setting, presents the nurse with a major challenge to her clinical skills. Intervention will require not only a sound understanding of the pathophysiological process of shock but also the ability to act swiftly on the basis of that understanding and to assist with a range of resuscitative and investigative procedures. Because the patient's survival will often depend on early intervention, the nurse must be able to anticipate the problems that might arise under a given set of circumstances and to recognise the first signs of circulatory and respiratory distress. The contribution of the nurse in this area of care will be a vital one, and it is hoped that this chapter has helped the reader to come to terms with the basic principles that underlie the recognition and treatment of shock syndromes.

REFERENCES

Blair P, Rowlands B J, Lowry K G et al 1991 Selective decontamination of the digestive tract: a stratified, randomised, prospective study in a mixed intensive care unit. Surgery 110(2): 303–309

Boore J R P, Champion R, Ferguson M C 1987 Nursing the physically ill adult. Churchill Livingstone, Edinburgh

Coull A 1992 Making sense of pulse oximetry. Nursing Times 88(32): 42–43

Hartnett S 1989 Septic shock in the oncology patient. Cancer Nursing 12(4): 191–201

Jowett N I, Thompson D R 1989 Comprehensive coronary care. Scutari, Harrow, p. 239

Ledingham I M, Ramsey G 1986 Hypovolaemic shock. British Journal of Anaesthesia 58: 169–189

Natanson C, Danner R L, Elin R J et al 1989 Role of endotoxaemia in cardiovascular dysfunction and mortality: Escherichia coli and Staphylococcus aureus challenges in a canine model of human shock. Journal of Clinical Investigation 83(Jan): 243–251

Quaal S J 1992 The person with heart failure and cardiogenic shock. In: Guzzetta C E, Dossey B M (eds) Cardiovascular nursing: holistic practice. Mosby, St Louis, M O, pp. 329–332

Rice V 1991 Shock: A clinical syndrome. Parts 1–4. Critical Care Nurse 11(4–7): 20–27, 74–82, 34–39, 28–39

Schuster H P 1990 Sepsis as a source of multiple organ failure: definition, pathophysiology, and diagnostic parameters. In: Aochi O, Amaha K, Takeshita H (eds) Intensive and critical care medicine. Elsevier, Amsterdam, pp. 281–286

Sibbald W J 1988 Synopsis of critical care, 3rd edn. Williams & Wilkins, London

Suffredini A F, Fromm R E, Parker M M et al 1989 The cardiovascular response of normal humans to the administration of endotoxin. New England Journal of Medicine 321: 280–287

Whitman G R 1988 Tissue perfusion. In: Kinney M R, Packa D R, Dunbar S B (eds) AACN's clinical reference for critical-care nursing, 2nd edn. McGraw-Hill, New York, pp. 115–159

FURTHER READING

Allan D 1989 Making sense of arterial catheterisation. Nursing Times 85(40): 45–47

Barrett J, Nyhus L M 1986 Treatment of shock: principles and practice, 2nd edn. Lea & Febiger, Beckenham

Carolan J M 1986 Shock: a nursing guide. Wright, Bristol

Caroline N L 1986 Emergency care in the streets, 3rd edn. Little, Brown, London

Colardyn F C, Vandenbogaerde J F, Vogelaers D P, Verbeke J H 1989 Use of dopexamine hydrochloride in patients with septic shock. Critical Care Medicine 17(10): 999–1003

Daily E K 1992 Haemodynamic monitoring. In: Guzzetta C E, Dossey B M (eds) Cardiovascular nursing: holistic practice. Mosby, St Louis, M O, pp. 183–184

Hayes E E 1990 Needs of family members of the critically ill patient: a Northern Ireland perspective. Care of the Critically Ill 6(1): 27–28

Hewett 1992 Beyond first aid. Churchill Livingstone, Edinburgh

Jeffries P R, Whelan S K 1988 Cardiogenic shock: current management. Critical Care Nursing 11(1): 48–56

Kram H B, Evans T, Bundage B, Shoemaker W C 1988 Use of dobutamine for treatment of shock liver syndrome. Critical Care Medicine 16(6): 644–645

Meyers K A, Hickey M K 1988 Nursing management of hypovolaemic shock. Critical Care Nursing 11(1): 57–67

Moulopoulos S, Stamatelopoulos S, Petrou P 1986 Intraaortic balloon assistance in intractable cardiogenic shock. European Heart Journal 7: 396–403

Roberts S L 1988 Cardiogenic shock: decreased coronary artery tissue perfusion. Dimensions of Critical Care Nursing 7(4): 196–208

Showronski G A 1988 The pathophysiology of shock. Medical Journal of Australia 148: 576–683

St John Ambulance 1988 First aid manual, 5th edn. Dorling Kindersley, London

Strange J M 1987 Shock trauma care plans. Springhouse Corporation, New York

Tuchschmidt J, Fried J, Swinney R, Sharma P 1989 Early haemodynamic correlates of survival in patients with septic shock. Critical Care Medicine 17(8): 719–723

CHAPTER 19

Pain

Kate Seers

CHAPTER CONTENTS

Introduction 615
Factors influencing the experience of pain 616

Anatomy and physiology of the experience of pain 616
Nociceptors 616
Peripheral nerve pathways 617
Spinal cord pathways 617
Ascending pathways 617
Brain mechanisms 618
Descending pathways 618
Endogenous control 618
Summary 618

Theories of pain 618
The specificity theory 618
The pattern theory 618
The affect theory 619
The gate control theory 619

Acute and chronic pain 619
Acute pain 619
Chronic pain 620
Pain tolerance and pain threshold 621
Referred pain 621

Issues in caring for people in pain 621
Factors affecting the quality of pain relief 621

Pain management 624
The role of the nurse 624
The role of the person in pain 624
The role of family members and carers 625
Strategies for effective pain assessment 625
Pain relief 628
Analgesics 628
Other medical interventions 629
Specialised pain services 629
Complementary methods of pain relief 630

Conclusion 632

Glossary 632

References 632

Further reading 635

Useful addresses 635

INTRODUCTION

But pain is perfet miserie, the worst
of evils, and excessive, overturnes
All patience. (Milton, *Paradise Lost*, VI: 462–464)

Although everyone experiences pain from time to time it is by no means easy to understand the experience of pain in another person. Perhaps this is because pain, as Melzack & Wall (1988) point out, is a category of complex experiences rather than a single sensation produced by a specific stimulus. Pain is not merely a sensory phenomenon, for emotional, cognitive and behavioural components come into play as well. Many factors influence the way a person feels, thinks and behaves when in pain. The experience of pain occurs against the background of the individual's personal history and is shaped by the complex interaction of physiological, psychological and sociocultural factors. Only the person experiencing the pain knows what it feels like. One can never know what being in pain is like for another person.

?	**19.1** If pain is so complex and subjective, can it be defined? How would you define pain?

The following definition of pain emphasises its complex nature:

Pain is a subjective experience that can be perceived directly only by the sufferer. It is a multidimensional phenomenon that can be described by pain location, intensity, temporal aspects, quality, impact and meaning. Pain does not occur in isolation but in a specific human being in psychosocial, economic, and cultural contexts that influence the meaning, experience and verbal and non-verbal expression of pain. (National Institutes of Health 1987, p. 36.)

Or, more succinctly:

Pain is whatever the experiencing person says it is, existing whenever he says it does. (McCaffery 1972, p. 8.)

Wall (1979) describes pain as a need state, like thirst and hunger, rather than as a sensation. Pain signals the need for recovery and recuperation to take place. The presence of pain indicates that activity should be disrupted and substituted by activity related to the prevention of further damage and to cure and recovery.

?	**19.2** If it is not only the sensation that affects how one experiences pain, what other specific factors might come into play?

Factors influencing the experience of pain

Personal factors

Past learning. Learning about pain takes place throughout life, at home as well as in hospital. For example, if a child falls over and hurts his knee, he learns that this feeling is called pain. He also learns how he is expected to react. A crying child may elicit concern, sympathy and a cuddle, or be ignored and praised only when he stops crying.

> ? **19.3** Think of a time, either in childhood or more recently, when you were in pain. How did the people around you react?

Gender. There is sometimes an expectation that males should be 'brave' whereas females may be allowed a greater freedom of expression in their responses to pain. Davitz & Davitz (1981) found that the nurses in their study tended to see female patients as suffering more physical pain and psychological distress than male patients. However, when Cohen (1980) gave nurses two sets of examples of patients in pain, differing only by gender, nurses selected less analgesia for females. The evidence on the effect of gender on pain and its expression seems to be inconclusive.

> ? **19.4** Do you think males and females react differently when in pain?

Age. There is much debate over the effect of age on pain and its expression. Many conditions common to old age are painful and older people in the community may often be in pain. Liebeskind & Melzack (1987, p. 1) report that 'Pain in the elderly is often dismissed as something to be expected and thus tolerated.' Clark & Mehl (1971) argue that it is possible that elderly people endure more pain before reporting it than do younger individuals. However, Harkins et al (1984) conclude that evidence on the effects of age on pain tolerance and pain threshold is 'conflicting'.

Personality. Different people have different ways of expressing their pain. Some may be very expressive, whereas others may prefer to keep their pain to themselves. Drawing on Eysenck's theory of the personality, Bond & Pearson (1969) conclude that introverts have more intense pain but complain less than extroverts.

Meaning of pain. Pain will have different meanings for different people. Some patients may view pain as a punishment; others may see it as having some value for self-testing or personal growth; still others may see it as something that must be cured. Pain from a recurrence of cancer is likely to have a different significance for the patient than pain following routine elective surgery. Chronic pain may also have implications for the individual's self-image by necessitating a change or loss of roles.

Body part affected. The part of the body involved may influence the expression of pain (Meinhart & McCaffery 1983). Some areas of the body such as the rectum or genitals may be difficult to refer to for some people, and thus pain in these areas may go unreported. The assessment and relief of pain in these areas therefore needs very skilled management.

Social and environmental factors

Culture. Each cultural group has its own behaviours and attitudes which it regards as normal and correct, and these expectations appear to influence responses to pain. Zborowski (1952) conducted a study of men who could be described as 'old Americans' (i.e. their grandparents or earlier forebears were born in America and they did not identify with a particular cultural group), Italian Americans, or Jewish Americans. He found that the old Americans attempted to avoid showing any pain, tended to withdraw and preferred to be alone when in severe pain. The Italian and Jewish Americans openly expressed their pain and did not want to be alone. The Italian Americans were concerned with relief of their pain whilst the Jewish Americans were concerned about the implications of their pain for the future. Moore (1990) found that whilst Anglo-American patients preferred pills and injections, Chinese patients preferred external agents such as oils, salves and massage to help them cope with pain. Differences between American and Japanese patients with low back pain were evaluated by Brena et al (1990), who found that the Americans in their study had greater dysfunction than the Japanese patients, despite similar medical findings. However, the sample size was small and such findings need to be interpreted with caution.

> ? **19.5** Discuss in a group what might happen if a patient from a culture in which pain is expressed freely was admitted to a ward where most staff and patients were used to keeping a 'stiff upper lip'?

Social conditioning/group pressure. The reactions of others may affect an individual's expression of pain. This was demonstrated in the laboratory by Craig & Weiss (1971), who studied the effect of observers on subjects experiencing apparently the same degree of pain. They found if subjects were with a passive model (neither tolerant nor intolerant of shocks) they would tolerate a shock of 6.3 milliamps (mA) before describing it as painful. With an intolerant model the shock was described as painful at 2.5 mA and with a tolerant model at 8.65 mA.

Organisational factors. Because it is common practice in hospital wards to administer medication at specific times of the day, there is a tendency to assess pain only at those times. However, asking, 'Anything for pain?' on the drug round is not the same as sitting down with the patient and discussing his pain. A degree of group pressure is likely to come into play if the patient is asked in front of others whether he needs analgesics. Edwards (1990) questions how often quality assurance programmes monitor the provision of pain relief and just what the commitment of hospital administrators and society as a whole is to the provision of pain relief. Fagerhaugh & Strauss (1977), looking at the context of pain management, point to a discrepancy between actual and possible pain relief that seems to arise due to work demands of the clinical setting, a lack of accountability surrounding pain management, and the complexity of patient–staff and staff–staff interactions.

ANATOMY AND PHYSIOLOGY OF THE EXPERIENCE OF PAIN

Nociceptors

Pain can be caused by superficial stimuli (from the skin), by deep stimuli (from skeletal muscle, tendons and joints) or by visceral stimulation (Chung & Dickenson 1981). Receptors that respond to noxious stimulation, known as nociceptors, are free sensory nerve endings that detect physical and chemical damage to the tissues and form a widespread and overlapping network in almost all tissues of the body. Nociceptors have higher thresholds than other cutaneous receptor types

(Campbell et al 1989). They respond to pressure, temperature and chemicals and show specificity of response. Some receptors respond to heat of >45 °C, some to cooling and others to intense mechanical stimulation. Polymodal receptors are responsive to thermal, mechanical and chemical stimulation; many respond to more than one type of stimulus.

Tissue damage leads to a release of chemicals into the fluid surrounding the free nerve endings. These chemicals, which include bradykinin, histamine, prostaglandins, leukotrienes, peptides and proteolytic enzymes, produce pain in themselves or sensitise the nerve endings, such that their threshold for response is lowered. The clinical significance of this is that pain can be reduced by blocking these chemical mediators. For example, the therapeutic effect of aspirin derives from its ability to inhibit prostaglandin synthesis.

Peripheral nerve pathways

Afferent (i.e. sensory) nerve fibres carry messages in the form of nerve impulses from the tissues to the central nervous system (CNS). They may also transport chemicals in their axoplasm. These pathways from nociceptors to the spinal cord are mediated by two types of afferent fibres, designated A-delta (A-δ) and C fibres. Stimulation at noxious intensities evokes activity in both systems. The A-δ fibres are small, myelinated fibres that provide a fast conducting pathway for pricking and sharp pain. C fibres are more numerous unmyelinated fibres that conduct, at a slower rate, a dull, diffuse and more persistent pain. C fibres respond to pressure, heat and chemicals. They are thus less specific than A-δ fibres and have an important role in long duration changes following injury. Chemicals such as substance P (see p. 618) and other peptides are also released from C fibres causing sensitisation, vasodilation and leaking of blood vessels. In addition, substance P induces histamine release from mast cells and serotonin from platelets. Chemicals are also released from the sympathetic fibres and contribute to pain and aspects of the inflammatory process (Melzack & Wall 1988; see also Ch. 23, p. 699).

Spinal cord pathways

The A-δ and C fibre peripheral afferents enter the spinal cord via the dorsal horn (see Fig. 19.1). This is the dorsal part of the grey, butterfly-shaped area in the spinal cord. The white matter around this is composed of axons running up and down the cord. The cells of the dorsal horn are arranged in 6 layers or laminae (the outer two of which comprise the substantia gelatinosa) and run the length of the spinal cord on both sides. The C fibres terminate mainly in these outer two layers, and the A-δ fibres mainly in laminae I, II and V. Wall (1989b) emphasises that the role of these dorsal horn cells is not simply to collect information and transmit it to its destination; like all cells in the CNS, they select and compute in combination the signals which they receive. Dorsal horn cells send impulses to cells in the same segment as well as other segments, and to the brain via ascending pathways. Many structures in the brain project to the dorsal horn and mainly inhibit the firing of dorsal horn cells.

Ascending pathways

Multiple ascending neural pathways are involved in pain transmission. Some of the fibres from the dorsal horn cross the midline and form a tract in the anterolateral (front and side) portions of the white matter of the spinal cord. Willis (1985) describes this anterolateral quadrant of the spinal cord as the most important pathway for pain in man, but Wall

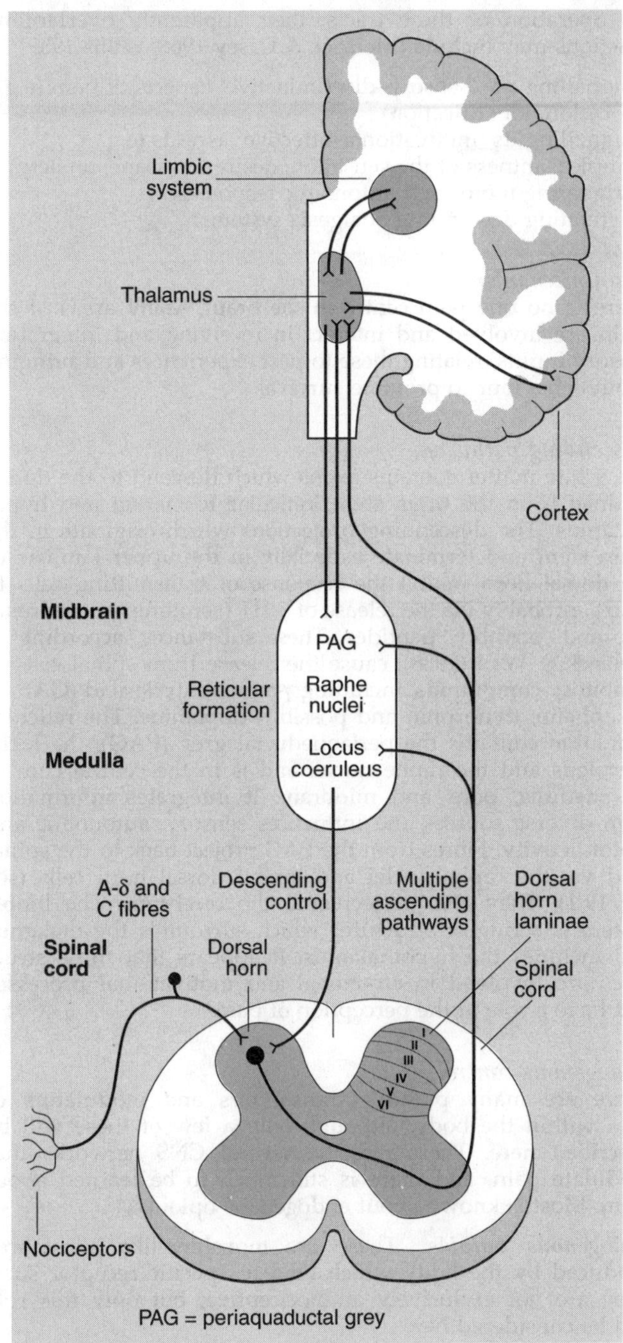

Fig. 19.1 Diagrammatic representation of some neural pathways involved in pain transmission.

(1989a) doubts if this emphasis is correct. Some fibres in the anterolateral quadrant go to the thalamus, and from there on to the cortex. Some penetrate the reticular formation, which contains systems that play a key role in the pain processes. From the reticular formation a series of pathways go on to the thalamus.

Willis (1989) describes a number of parallel ascending pathways by which nociceptive information is transmitted. These pathways include the spinothalamic, spinoreticular, spinomesencephalic, spinocervical and postsynaptic dorsal column tracts. While much remains to be discovered about the operation of these tracts, their apparently overlapping functions may include (Melzack & Casey 1968, Willis 1989):

- signalling the 'sensory–discriminative' aspects of pain (e.g. location; identification)
- signalling its 'motivational–affective' aspects (e.g. unpleasantness of the sensation; desire to escape; anxiety)
- triggering motor and autonomic responses
- activating descending analgesia systems.

Brain mechanisms
There is no one pain centre in the brain. Many areas of the brain are involved and interact in receiving and integrating sensory inputs, relating these to past experiences and bringing about behaviour to promote survival.

Descending pathways
The white matter contains axons which descend to the dorsal laminae from the brain stem, reticular formation and hypothalamus. The descending projections which originate in the brain stem and terminate especially in the upper laminae of the dorsal horn inhibit the response of transmitting cells to injury, probably via the release of 5-HT (serotonin), noradrenaline and, possibly, peptides. These substances, according to Melzack & Wall (1988), cause the release from spinal cells of inhibitory compounds, including γ-aminobutyric acid (GABA), enkephalin, dynorphin and possibly, dopamine. The reticular formation contains the periaqueductal grey (PAG), the locus coeruleus and the raphe nuclei and is in the central core of the medulla, pons and midbrain. It integrates information from diverse sources and influences sensory, autonomic and motor activity. Fibres from the PAG project back to the spinal cord via the raphe nuclei and inhibit dorsal horn cells (see Fig. 19.1). They also project onto the cerebrum. The limbic system is a ring of structures which surrounds the thalamus and includes the hypothalamus. It appears that these structures are involved in emotional and motivational processes and have a role in the perception of pain.

Endogenous control
There are many putative transmitters and modulators of pain within the body, although only a few of these will be described here. There may be several CNS networks that modulate pain, and there is still much to be learned about them. Most is known about endogenous opioids.

Endogenous opioids. These are morphine-like substances produced by the body which bind to specific receptor sites. They are not exclusively antinociceptive, but only this role will be considered here.

Endogenous opioids isolated so far include the pentapeptides leucine (leu-) and methionine (met-) enkephalin, and the peptides β endorphin, dynorphin and α neoendorphin. There is a significant concentration of endorphin-containing cells and terminals in the hypothalamic, brainstem and spinal parts of what Fields & Basbaum (1989) describe as an 'opioid-mediated analgesia system' (p. 214). This system can be activated by pain, stress and classical conditioning.

5-hydroxytryptamine (5-HT). 5-HT (also known as serotonin) appears to exert a diffuse inhibitory influence on pain sensations. The analgesic action of systemic opioids is blocked by the depletion of 5-HT, and 5-HT contributes to the antinociceptive action of opioids.

Substance P is produced when nociceptive afferents are activated and has an excitatory influence in the transmission of pain (Clement-Jones & Besser 1983).

Summary
The presence of injurious stimuli activates multiple fibre systems which converge and diverge a number of times and which are subject to modulation. Wall (1989a, p. 5) points out that 'pain is not the simple activation of a single specific, isolated signalling system but is subject to a series of controls acting in the context of a whole integrated nervous system'. All of the signals resulting from peripheral stimuli are subject to central control; the stimulation of receptors does not mark the start of the pain process, but produces neural signals that enter an active nervous system. There is no separate, specialised *pain system,* but an integrated *nervous system.* The definition of pain purely as a sensation is inadequate since:

1. Not all stimuli are known or presently detectable
2. No stimulus exists in isolation but is influenced by other, peripheral stimuli and by CNS activity
3. The way the nervous system responds to stimuli, especially after injury, is variable (Wall 1989a). The nervous system is thus mouldable and changeable, not fixed.

?	**19.6** Imagine that you have just hit your thumb. Describe how this message is transmitted from the tissues to the CNS.

THEORIES OF PAIN

Many theories of pain have been put forward, all of which contribute to our understanding of the phenomenon of pain. But as no single theory answers to all aspects of an individual's experience, four of the most influential theories of pain are briefly described in the following.

The specificity theory
This theory has been very influential and continues to dominate some people's thinking and practice today. The philosopher Descartes (1596–1650) provided a basis for the specificity theory when he proposed that there was a direct channel for pain from the periphery of the body to the brain. This concept was developed in the 19th century by thinkers who proposed the existence of a specific pain system that carried messages from pain receptors to a pain centre in the brain. Eventually the spinothalamic tract was postulated to be the pain pathway, and the pain centre was thought by some to be located in the thalamus (Melzack & Wall 1988).

Clinical evidence, however, contradicts the notion of a direct pathway for pain. For example, people who have had a limb amputated may feel pain as if the limb were still there (phantom limb pain). The causalgias and neuralgias also suggest that the relationship between stimulus and pain is not fixed or direct; Melzack & Wall (1988) describe how surgical lesions of the peripheral and central nervous systems, which one might expect to abolish pain in a direct pathway system, are unsuccessful in permanently abolishing these pains. Moreover, if a direct pathway existed, one would expect painful stimuli always to produce pain. This, however, is not the case. People who are hurt in accidents or sporting events do not always experience pain at the time of the injury.

The pattern theory
This theory describes any stimulus as capable of producing pain if it reaches sufficient intensity. The existence of specialised receptors and neurons is denied.

The affect theory

This older theory, dating back to Aristotle, describes pain as an emotion rather than as a sensation. Pain is described as the opposite of pleasure.

The gate control theory

The gate control theory of pain, developed by Melzack & Wall (1965), combines pertinent aspects of older theories with an account of what happens in clinical practice. According to this theory, the transmission of information from a potentially painful stimulus can be modified by a gating mechanism (see Fig. 19.2) situated in laminae I and II (the substantia gelatinosa) in the dorsal horn of the spinal cord. This mechanism can increase or decrease the flow of nerve impulses from the periphery to the CNS. If the gate is open, impulses pass through; if it is partially open some pass through; and if it is shut no impulses get through and pain is not experienced.

Whether the gate is open or closed is determined by:

1. Activity in small-diameter fibres (A-δ and C fibres, which transmit pain)
2. Activity in large diameter fibres (A-β fibres concerned with transmitting touch)
3. Descending influences from higher centres, including those concerned with motivational and cognitive processes.

The substantia gelatinosa is activated by large A-β fibres, which shut the gate, and is inhibited by small A-δ and C fibres, which open the gate. This influences the information sent from the spinal cord to the brain. Descending inhibitory control from the brainstem reticular formation is influenced by messages from other areas, including the cortex.

Implications of the gate control theory. The gate control theory throws doubt on the intuitive belief that the relationship between injury and pain is a direct one. It has been applied to nursing care by McCaffery & Beebe (1989), who argue that it provides 'an integrated conceptual model for appreciating the many factors that contribute to individual differences in the experience of pain.' They also use it as a theoretical base for developing various pain relief measures. For example, stimulation of the skin may, by increasing large fibre (A-β) activity, relieve pain at the spinal cord level by closing the gate. Examples would be using touch, massage and possibly transcutaneous electrical nerve stimulation (TENS; see p. 631). The advice often given to children to 'rub it better' acknowledges the usefulness of touch or massage in pain control. The gate control theory provides an explanation of *why* this kind of measure, which many people discover by experience, can be effective.

At the brainstem level the gate can sometimes be closed by ensuring sufficient sensory input, for example by using distraction and imagery (see p. 630); at the level of the cortex/thalamus it can be closed by reducing anxiety, for example, by providing accurate information about the cause, likely course and relief of pain and thereby increasing the patient's confidence and sense of control.

Developments since the gate control theory. The pain control system described by the gate control theory is one which acts rapidly, but Walls (1989a) described slower processes involved in the transmission of pain which complement gate control and may help to account for what happens in some cases of chronic pain. The research also demonstrates the existence of 'plasticity' or adaptability in the nervous system which allows for both rapidly transmitted impulses and slow-onset, long duration changes. It is thought that these slower messages are triggered by the unmyelinated C fibres, especially those originating in deep tissues, and that this prolonged mechanism results in a sustained experience of pain (Wall 1989a). Recent evidence indicates changes in central neural function may also play a significant role in the development of pathological pain (Coderre et al 1993).

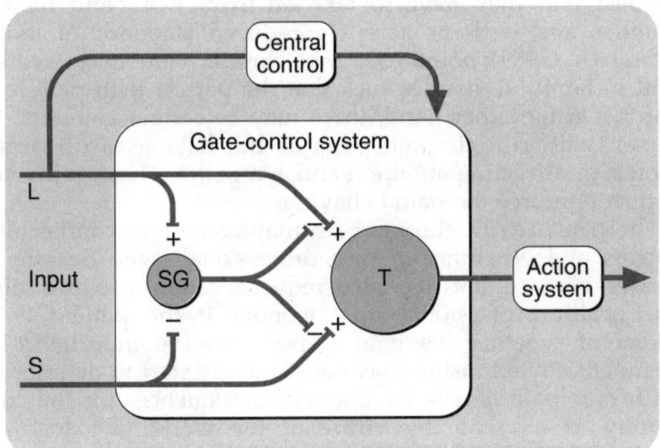

Fig. 19.2 The gate control theory of pain. + = excitation, − = inhibition, L = Large diameter fibres, S = small diameter fibres. The fibres project to the substantia gelatinosa (SG) and the first central transmission (T) cells. The inhibitory effect exerted by the SG on the afferent fibre terminals is increased by activity in the L fibres and decreased by activity in the S fibres. The central control trigger is represented by a line running from the large fibre system to the central control mechanisms; these mechanisms, in turn, project back to the gate control system. The T cells project to the action system. (Reproduced with kind permission of Penguin Books Ltd, Harmondsworth from R. Melzack & P. D. Wall, *The Challenge of Pain*, 2nd edn, 1988, copyright © Ronald Melzack and Patrick D. Wall, 1982, 1988.)

ACUTE AND CHRONIC PAIN

Acute and chronic pain are terms often used in pain management to categorise types of pain experience with a view to selecting the correct approach to management. In the following discussion it should be remembered, however, that these two types of pain are interrelated and that their management will have similarities as well as important differences. See also Ch. 34.

Acute pain

Acute pain usually warns the individual to protect himself against injury and thus prolong survival. In those rare cases of congenital insensitivity to pain, life expectancy is considerably shortened due to unrecognised trauma and subsequent infections (Sternbach 1989). The pain experienced after touching something hot acts as a disincentive to return the hand to the hot surface, thus averting additional injury. It may also result in rest, which promotes healing. Acute pain usually has a well-defined course and disappears once the injury is healed. It can, however, be intermittent. Examples of acute pain are pain after surgery and pain from a fractured bone.

Effects of acute pain on physiological mechanisms

Pain evokes the 'fight or flight' reaction, with sympathetic dominance and vagal inhibition. This results in inhibition of gastric mobility, nausea and vomiting, glycogen liberation from the liver into the blood as an energy source and an increase in oxygen consumption, blood pressure, pulse and vasoconstriction.

The implications of these responses for a patient with post-operative pain are important. For example, if he feels sick he will find it difficult to take adequate fluids. If he is in pain and cannot move around, it seems likely that his risk of stasis complications such as chest infection, deep vein thrombosis and pressure sores will be increased. However, pain causing parasympathetic stimulation may result in a decrease in pulse and blood pressure. Interpreting a pattern of responses specific to pain is difficult, especially since these responses may reflect stresses or physiological disturbances other than pain.

Psychosocial effects of acute pain

Anxiety is often linked to acute pain: increased anxiety may lead to increased pain, and increased pain may lead to increased anxiety (Peck 1986). Thus a vicious circle of pain, anxiety, and thus more pain and anxiety can be set up.

Chronic pain

Chronic pain is that which persists after healing; it usually has no clear function as a warning system. An arbitrary time element, such as a duration greater than 3 or 6 months is sometimes included in definitions of chronic pain. Sternbach (1989) argues that whilst acute pain may promote survival, chronic pain is usually destructive–physically, psychologically and socially. Types of chronic pain described in the following are chronic non-malignant pain and cancer pain.

Chronic non-malignant pain

This term can be applied to many different types and intensities of pain, which may or may not have an identifiable physical cause. Examples include chronic low back pain and phantom limb pain. Patients with non-malignant pain have often suffered with it for many years, and have typically tried various treatments without lasting success. This sort of pain is sometimes referred to as 'benign' pain, but since it can affect the patient and family in many negative ways, 'non-malignant' seems a more appropriate term.

Chronic non-malignant pain is often poorly understood and there is much controversy as to how it should be treated. Some patients whose pain has no identifiable cause are unfairly regarded as malingerers. The frustration of patient and professional alike may be compounded when intervention, e.g. surgery, only proves to make the pain worse. In many cases it must be agreed that the aim of treatment cannot be to stop the pain, but to help the patient cope with or manage it.

The most effective relief for patients with chronic non-malignant pain is often obtained through multi-disciplinary pain clinics Flor et al (1992) (see p. 630) in which the whole pain experience is considered and treatments such as graded exercise and activity, medication reduction, and cognitive and behavioural therapy are explored. Portenoy (1990) argues that long-term opioid therapy may be appropriate for a selected subgroup of patients with chronic non-malignant pain and may be pursued without the development of significant toxicity or side-effects. Whatever the approach, pain management will need to be incorporated into everyday life. McCaffery & Beebe (1989) have developed useful guidelines for the nursing case of patients with chronic pain.

Cancer pain

Stjernsward & Teoh (1990) have estimated that 3.5 million people worldwide suffer from cancer pain daily. There has been much interest in cancer pain relief since Saunders' (1976) pioneering work in the hospice movement emphasised the need to give regular analgesics and to titrate dosages in accordance with need. Not all people with cancer have pain, but cancer may produce pain by activating nociceptors in bones, soft tissues or hollow viscera, and tumours may also compress or infiltrate nerves (Scott 1989). Pain may also be associated with cancer therapy, i.e. surgery, chemotherapy and radiotherapy (see Ch. 32).

Effects of chronic pain on physiological mechanisms

The physiological responses which accompany acute pain habituate over time. However, sleep disturbance, irritability, fatigue, reduced motor activity and reduced pain tolerance are all effects of chronic pain and share many characteristics with depression (Sternbach 1989). It can be argued that these physiological responses also have behavioural components.

Psychosocial effects of chronic pain

As anxiety is often associated with acute pain, so too depression is often associated with chronic pain (Kramlinger et al 1983). However, just as patients with acute pain may also be depressed, those with chronic pain may also be anxious. Anger and frustration have also been associated with chronic pain (Wade et al 1990).

Chronic non-malignant pain presents particular challenges, and when or if it will end cannot be predicted. Chronic pain may affect the individual's work, home relationships, and social life, leading to withdrawal, depression, and lowered self-esteem. Interactions with others may centre on the pain, reinforcing the individual's 'sick role'. The pain may start to dominate the individual's thoughts and he may think of himself as chronically disabled, or believe that the pain is a warning sign of a pathological process.

If the pain affects the individual's ability to work, the family may be put under financial strain. Family members may also feel guilty that they cannot relieve the pain or resentful of the fact that they have to take on extra work and responsibilities and perhaps accept a reduced standard of living. Sternbach (1989) points out that chronic pain may create a shift in family dynamics such that the person with pain loses status. On the other hand, there may be certain gains for the person with chronic pain, such as not having to do certain chores, or attracting attention and sympathy. These gains may in turn reinforce the pain behaviour.

The person with chronic pain may come into conflict with doctors and other health care professionals who despite increased contacts and repeated requests cannot provide relief. The health professional may wonder if the patient is an addict or whether his pain is psychological in origin. The therapeutic relationship may consequently start to deteriorate.

Chronic pain also has economic consequences for the community as a whole by virtue of the work days lost and the increased use of health care facilities.

Cancer pain. In their study of the meaning of pain to cancer patients Daut & Cleeland (1982) found that patients who believed their pain symptoms meant they were getting worse reported greatest interference with activity and pleasure. Next were those who felt their pain was due to therapy and least affected were those who felt that their pain was due to unrelated causes.

Most cancer patients respond readily to established clinical treatment, whereas this is not true of many people with chronic non-malignant pain (WHO 1986). However, control of cancer pain is often inadequate; reasons for this include a lack of awareness of established methods, fear of causing addiction and lack of systematic education of health professionals (WHO 1986).

Pain tolerance and pain threshold

These are important concepts which must be carefully distinguished from one another. *Pain threshold* is 'the least experience of pain which a subject can recognise'; *pain tolerance* is 'the greatest level of pain which a subject is prepared to tolerate' (IASP 1986, pp. S220–221). Pain tolerance has also been described as 'the duration or intensity of pain that a person is willing to endure' (McCaffery & Beebe 1989, p. 15).

Referred pain

Normally, if one stubs a toe or cuts a finger, it is apparent from the pain experienced exactly where the injury has occurred. However, this localisation of pain sensations is limited to the skin. Pain from the viscera and from deep somatic tissue can be felt in apparently unrelated but predictable locations. For example, the pain of a heart attack is often referred to the left arm, and pain in the early stages of appendicitis may appear to originate from above the umbilicus. Pain is usually referred to a structure developed from the same embryonic structure or sclerotome.

Another type of referred pain is associated with trigger points. These are small hypersensitive regions in muscle or connective tissue which can be located in the area of pain or some distance from it. This referred pain does not follow any known dermatomes, but stimulation produces pain in a relatively constant and predictable location (Meinhart & McCaffery 1983).

ISSUES IN CARING FOR PEOPLE IN PAIN

> ? **19.7** Before reading this section, think about your own feelings about pain and pain relief. If you were in pain, what sorts of things would be important to you to help you cope? Would this be different if you were at home rather than in hospital? Would different things be important for different types/causes of pain?

There seems to be a gap between theory and practice in current pain management. Information on the action of analgesics, on complementary methods of pain relief and on pain assessment is readily available but there appears to be a lack of recognition and utilisation of the methods that already exist. Nurses will often note pain as a potential problem on a care plan, and aim for a 'pain-free patient', but they are not always effective in achieving this goal. Kuhn et al (1990) found that for the patients in their study pain levels were 60% of maximum during the first 24 h after surgery. Seers (1989) found that 43% of patients had 'quite a lot of pain' or more when questioned on the first postoperative day; over 86% had reported 'quite a lot' of pain or more at least once by their seventh postoperative day. The Royal College of Surgeons and College of Anaesthetists (1990) concluded that 'treatment of pain after surgery ... has been inadequate and has not advanced significantly for many years'. However, the World Health Organization (WHO 1986) has argued that the management of cancer pain has improved since the 1960s, citing numerous factors such as better cancer diagnosis and treatment, greater understanding of analgesic drug therapy, insistence of patients and their families that pain be better controlled, and consensus that adequate symptom control and good quality of life are important for patients with advanced disease. A recent report from West Germany found that for 80% of a group of cancer patients who suffered from more than moderate pain despite prior treatment the implementation of the WHO guidelines for the treatment of cancer pain (see Box 19.1) resulted in a reduction of pain to levels ranging from 'none' to 'moderate' (Schug et al 1990).

Factors affecting the quality of pain management

Professional education and training

The National Institutes of Health (1987) have expressed concern that the education and training of many health professionals does not place 'an adequate emphasis on contemporary methods of pain assessment and management'. Sofaer (1985) and the International Association for the Study of Pain (1991) have pointed out deficiencies in current education on pain and have put forward suggestions for an educational programme or curriculum on pain. Sofaer (1985) demonstrated that a ward-based educational programme for nurses can produce some significant improvements in patient outcome.

If practising nurses do not regard pain relief as a priority and are given insufficient educational input, they will perpetuate any inadequacies of existing systems for pain management when they act as role models for new staff. Well-designed educational programmes are needed, as is training in the application of this education to clinical practice. Lander (1990a) suggests that training in decision-making could help to reduce judgemental biases. Edwards (1990) argues that a lack of knowledge leads to attitudinal barriers and inappropriate behaviours in pain management.

Professional and cultural biases in inferences of pain

The inferences or assumptions that health professionals make about the amount or type of pain their patients are suffering

Box 19.1 WHO guidelines on treating cancer pain (Reproduced with kind permission from WHO 1986.)

1. Cancer pain can, and must, be treated.
2. A thorough history should first be obtained and the patient examined carefully. Acute conditions that require specific treatment should be excluded.
3. Drugs usually give good relief, provided the right drug is administered in the right dose at the right intervals.
4. For persistent pain, the drugs should be taken regularly 'by the clock' and not 'as required'.
5. For mild to moderate pain, the patient should be prescribed a non-opioid drug and the dose adjusted to the optimum level. If necessary, an adjuvant drug should also be used.
6. If or when this treatment no longer relieves pain, a weak opioid drug should be prescribed in addition to the non-opioid drug, together with an adjuvant, if appropriate.
7. If and when these no longer relieve pain, the patient should be prescribed a strong opioid, together with a non-opioid adjuvant drug, if appropriate.
8. The patient must be supervised as often as possible to ensure that treatment continues to match the pain and to minimise side-effects.

have a significant influence on the quality of care provided. It is important therefore to examine the expectations and attitudes that can colour the professional's perception of the patient's pain experience.

A study by Lenburg et al (1970) demonstrated that, in a sample of professional groups, nuns, followed by teachers and then nurses and doctors inferred the greatest levels of pain and distress among their clients, a finding that may suggest health workers regard pain as 'normal'. In a study of student health professionals, Pitts & Healy (1989) found that student nurses inferred the greatest degree of pain among patients, followed by student physiotherapists and, lastly, student doctors. Among the medical students in the sample women inferred more pain than men. Dudley & Holm (1984) found that the number of years which had elapsed since qualification did not affect nurses' inferences of pain, although Mason (1981) found that nurses with less than one year's experience inferred more pain than those with 6–10 years' experience. In burns units, Perry & Heidrich (1982) found that nurses working in a unit for fewer than 5 years rated pain as more severe than those who had been on staff for more than 5 years.

Holm et al (1989) found that nurses who had themselves experienced intense pain at some time were generally more sympathetic to the patient in pain. Davitz & Davitz (1981) found that some nurses consistently inferred a relatively high and some a relatively low degree of suffering. Most nurses reported a distinction between 'complainers' and patients who had a 'right to complain'. If a nurse felt that a patient exaggerated claims of pain, that patient was often labelled a 'complainer' and the therapeutic relationship subsequently deteriorated. Davitz & Davitz also found that patients' religious or ethnic backgrounds influenced nurses' inferences of pain and psychological distress, with Jewish and Spanish patients being thought to have most pain and Oriental and Anglo-Saxon patients as suffering least.

Taylor et al (1984) found that nurses rated pain as less intense when it was chronic and when no physical cause could be found. Halferns et al (1990) replicated Taylor et al's study with a Dutch population and confirmed that nurses rated pain as being less severe when no physical cause could be found. However, they were unable to confirm that the presence of a chronic condition influenced nurses' assessments of pain. They also found that nurses rated depressed patients as having more pain than others. It seemed to Lander (1990a) that unpopular or difficult patients were labelled as not having 'real' pain.

Assessment and evaluation

Unless the importance of assessing pain and acting on that assessment is fully appreciated there is little hope for real progress in pain control (Meinhart & McCaffery 1983). Effective assessment requires the cooperation of the entire health care team and, wherever possible, the patient's full participation. It is sometimes easy, however, for pain assessment to be given low priority in the face of more urgent or obvious patient needs. Pain is largely an invisible problem, and unless a systematic effort is made to address the issue of pain with each patient it may be inadequately treated. Without conscientious recording of pain levels and of pain relief, professional accountability for pain management will be difficult to establish.

The importance of effective communication in the assessment and subsequent management of pain must not be overlooked (see Ch. 26). The process by which a patient conveys the degree and nature of his pain and asks for help is a complex one which has the potential to break down at any of a number of stages.

Pain assessment can also fail to reflect the genuine needs of the patient because of the professional's lack of appreciation of the possible range of responses to pain and to analgesics. It cannot be assumed that a patient who does not appear to be in pain is in fact in no discomfort, or that because he has been given an analgesic he has obtained relief (Bourbonnais & MacKay 1981, Choiniere et al 1990). Nor should it be assumed that there is only one source of pain. Ten common misconceptions which may compromise effective pain assessment are listed in Box 19.2.

Expectations and attitudes surrounding pain relief

Pain may be viewed by both nurse and patient as something to be tolerated, (see Ch. 10, p. 400) and the patient may feel that an uncomplaining attitude is expected of him. As one patient explained: 'I keep quiet even if the pain is severe, I don't want to get into the nurses' bad books' (Seers 1987, p. 350). Indeed, 'good' patients who tolerate pain and do not ask for analgesics may be rewarded.

In addition, research has shown that both patients and nurses often have low expectations of analgesia, and accordingly are satisfied with pain 'relief' that allows significant levels of pain to remain (Cartwright 1985, Chapman et al 1987, Cohen 1980, Weis et al 1983). It would appear, particularly in postoperative care, that pain is generally regarded as being inevitable.

Low expectations regarding pain relief may derive from certain beliefs about the assumed risks of analgesics, as described in the following.

Fear of addiction. An unreasonable fear of causing an addiction by the administration of analgesic drugs can arise from confusion surrounding the terms 'addiction', 'tolerance' and 'dependence'.

Addiction. McCaffery & Beebe (1989, p. 68) define addiction as the behaviour of 'obtaining and using a drug for its psychic effects, not for approved medical reasons'.

Tolerance occurs when with repeated administration a given dose of a narcotic becomes less effective and larger doses are needed.

Dependence. When a narcotic has been given repeatedly, withdrawal symptoms occur if the narcotic is abruptly stopped. McCaffery & Beebe (1989) point out that symptoms of withdrawal rarely appear in a clinical setting as pain usually subsides gradually and the dosage of analgesic narcotics is accordingly reduced slowly. The overwhelming majority of patients stop taking narcotics when the pains stops.

The presence of tolerance and/or physical dependence is *not* equivalent to addiction. Nevertheless, Seers (1987) found that over 75% of the patients in her study disliked taking 'painkillers' or would take them only if the pain was severe. One said: 'Once you get used to them you've had it'; and another: 'I'd rather suffer in silence than rely on them.' Some patients do not want to take an analgesic as they feel it will not work later when they 'really need it'. McCaffery & Beebe (1989) emphasise that a patient's decision not to take an analgesic must be based on accurate information and not on unfounded fears and misconceptions; they suggest asking the patient who fears addiction, 'Would you want to take medication if you were not in pain?'

It would seem to be important for nurses to initiate dis-

Box 19.2 Ten myths and misconceptions surrounding pain assessment (After McCaffery & Beebe 1989)

Misconception 1: The health care team is the authority on the existence and nature of pain.

In fact, the professional does not necessarily see the situation as the person in pain does. He or she must accept the patient as an authority on his pain.

Misconception 2: We can rely on our personal values and intuitions to judge whether a person is lying about his pain.

This is not a professional approach. The professional response is to believe the person in pain or to give him the benefit of the doubt.

Misconception 3: Pain is largely an emotional or psychological problem, especially in a person who is anxious or depressed or whose pain is unclear.

Reacting to pain with emotion does not mean that the pain is caused by an emotional problem.

Misconception 4: Lying about pain is common.

In fact, this would seem to be rare. It is important to avoid the inaccurate labelling of patients as malingerers.

Misconception 5: A person who obtains benefits because of pain is exaggerating his pain.

Using pain to one's advantage is not the same as malingering and it is not easy to assess what constitutes using pain for advantage.

Misconception 6: If there is no obvious physical cause for pain, its existence may be doubted.

All pain is a result of physical and mental events and, whatever its cause, is real to the person in pain.

Misconception 7: Pain is accompanied by physiological and/or behavioural changes which can be used to confirm the existence and severity of pain.

Physiological signs such as an increase in blood pressure and pulse do adapt over time. Behavioural cues such as guarding, bracing, moaning and grimacing can be unreliable, and a lack of pain expression does not necessarily mean a person is not in pain. People in pain may choose to hide it, taking pride in their self-control. Fatigue can also reduce expressions of pain.

Misconception 8: Similar physical stimuli produce similar pain in different people.

There is no direct relationship between the pain stimulus and the perception of pain. Two people who have had an identical operation may experience very different levels of postoperative pain, and the duration and intensity of their pain cannot be predicted with any certainty.

Misconception 9: People with pain should have a high tolerance for pain.

Pain tolerance varies from one person to another and in the same person in different situations. What may be tolerable during the day may become intolerable at night when there are fewer distractions from the pain. If health professionals reward a high pain tolerance, this may encourage patients not to express pain. This may control pain expression, but it does not control pain.

Misconception 10: People who obtain pain relief from placebos are malingering or their pain is not real.

There is no evidence for this. Placebos may increase patients' expectations for relief, which in turn may reduce anxiety and pain. There is some evidence, moreover, that placebos activate endogenous pain relief mechanisms such as the endorphins (see p. 628).

cussions with patients and their families about fears of addiction. However, nurses must first be sure that their own understanding of the mechanisms of addiction is sound. Most of the nurses in Lander's (1990b) study believed addiction was very likely to occur with regular but short-term administration of a narcotic and considered narcotic addiction after surgery to be a far greater risk for patients than is the case. However, Porter & Jick's (1980) review of nearly 12 000 records of patients taking at least one narcotic contradicts these beliefs, finding only four cases of addiction in patients with no history of addiction, and, among these, only one which was considered major. Perry & Heidrich (1982) report that out of at least 10 000 hospitalised burn patients, among whom the prolonged use of narcotics was common, not one case of iatrogenic addiction could be documented in patients with no history of addiction.

Fear of respiratory depression. Although respiratory depression can be produced by all narcotics McCaffery & Beebe (1989) state that this should not prevent them from being used to relieve pain as this side-effect is not life-threatening or even clinically significant in most patients. However, they add that 'The only safe and effective way to administer a narcotic is to *watch the individual's response,* especially to the first dose' (p. 72). This should include monitoring respirations and level of arousal.

Other fears. The fear of losing control or of experiencing strange feelings causes some patients to avoid analgesics. As one patient in Seers' study (1987) remarked, 'It's a funny feeling — I hate it not being yourself'.

Fear of sedation may be a worry for patients; however, McCaffery & Beebe (1989) argue that the sedative effect of an analgesic usually subsides after several days.

Fear of injections may pose a problem for some patients (Seers 1987); in such cases an alternative route of administration could be considered.

Problems in the administration of analgesics

Inadequate prescribing. If analgesics are not prescribed frequently enough or in large enough doses pain relief cannot be effective. However, an 'adequate' dose may be hard to define, particularly since the effect of a standard prescription may vary, depending on the individual, from complete to negligible pain relief. Part of the nurse's role is to monitor whether prescriptions are adequate. Nursing assessment and recording of pain and of pain-relieving interventions could form the basis of discussions with the doctor should it appear that pain control is unsatisfactory. As always, teamwork and effective communication are crucial to a successful outcome.

Inadequate administration. Many analgesics are prescribed, especially after surgery, 'as needed' or pro re nata (PRN). If they *are* given 'as needed', titrated to effect, the flexibility that this mode of prescribing allows could help the patient to obtain optimum relief. The success of this approach, however, depends upon adequate assessment and on judicious timing of each dose.

McCaffery & Beebe (1989) argue strongly that analgesics should be used as soon as the pain begins, and Mather &

Mackie (1983) make the criticism that PRN is sometimes wrongly interpreted as 'as little as possible'. Similarly, a study by Closs (1990) found that only 30–35% of the maximum doses of analgesics prescribed were actually given in the immediate postoperative period.

It can also be argued that analgesics need to be given round the clock in order for adequate blood levels to be maintained (see Fig. 19.3). In the treatment of chronic cancer pain, around-the-clock administration seems particularly appropriate as it breaks the pain–anxiety cycle and decreases the patient's anticipation of pain worsening or returning. Baines & Kirkham (1989) argue that PRN administration of analgesics is inappropriate for patients with chronic cancer pain, and Keefe (1989) suggests that offering pain relief at specific times rather than PRN may also help patients with chronic non-malignant pain by dissociating their pain from the positive reinforcement of obtaining analgesia. Lutz & Lamer (1990), on the other hand, argue that in the case of postoperative care around-the-clock administration may result in patients being overmedicated.

If around-the-clock administration is used, it is important not to let the pain get out of control. This may mean that it will be necessary to wake the patient to give him an analgesic. This may not seem ideal, but pain may wake the patient later and prove to be much more difficult to control than if it were treated before becoming severe.

PAIN MANAGEMENT

The role of the nurse

> [It is] our responsibility to obtain the best pain control possible for patients, and it is part of our role to work toward this in whatever clinical setting we practise. (McCaffery & Beebe 1989, p. 42.)

The nurse works as part of a team, which most often comprises the doctor, nurse, the patient and his family, but which may include other health professionals and other people of the patient's choosing. All members have their own perspective and contribution to make. Effective communication is crucial to the effectiveness of the team, and the nurse is in an ideal position to ensure that all members have the relevant information about the patient's pain and pain relief. The nurse will often have to choose the most appropriate method of pain relief, decide when to give it, and evaluate its effectiveness. She will also have an important role to play in helping the patient to understand his pain and to explore methods of pain relief. In her role as educator, the nurse must take the time to listen to the patient's concerns; she must believe his reports of pain and value them as a valid source of information.

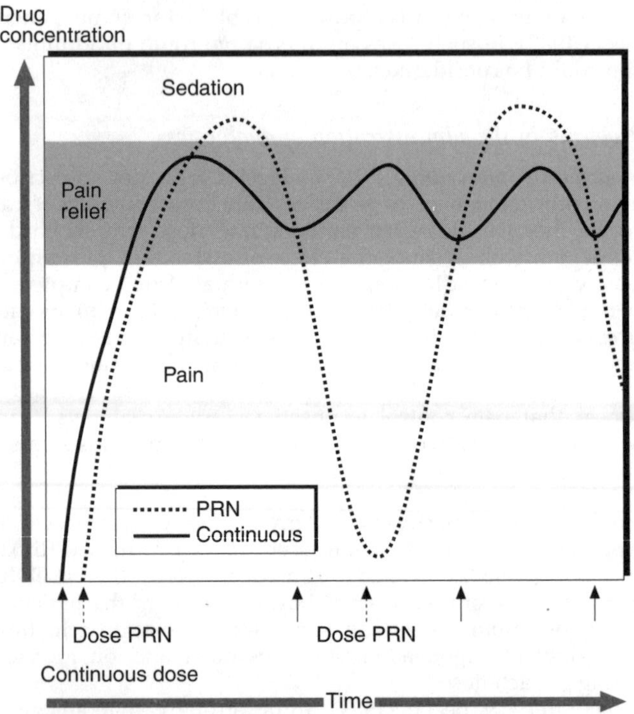

Fig. 19.3 PRN versus around-the-clock administration of analgesics.

The nurse should provide the patient with information on what can be expected in terms of pain and pain relief. In their review of this area Suls & Wan (1989) found that patients who are briefed on the procedures they are to undergo and the sensations they are likely to experience show the most consistent reductions in pain reports, negative affect and other-rated distress.

?	**19.8** If you do not know what sensations might be experienced with a particular condition or following a certain procedure, ask people who have themselves had the experience; they are a very valuable source of knowledge. You could ask what sorts of things they think would help other people who are in the same situation.

The need for patients prescribed PRN medication to be properly informed about this method of pain relief is demonstrated by one postoperative patient in Seers' (1990) study, who said:

> It would be useful if you were told you should ask for a painkiller. You drift in and out of sleep and pain. I presumed I'd had one and they would come with another. You don't realise you can ask between when they come round. One nurse on a shift mentioned it but that was way after the op. She said 'If you don't need it now you can always ask in half an hour.' If I'd known that initially it would have been helpful. (p. 109)

Owen et al (1990) found that over two-thirds of the patients in their study would wait until they were in severe pain before requesting an analgesic or would not ask at all.

The role of the person in pain

Articles and books available to a general readership such as Melzack (1990) and Melzack & Wall (1988) have helped to increase public awareness of the treatment options available to people in pain. Edwards (1990) argues that the informed consumer will be the strongest advocate for an uncompromised standard of excellence in pain management, and WHO (1986) lists consumer awareness as a contributing factor in recent improvements in the treatment of cancer pain. However, Owen et al (1990) found that postoperative patients did not have the necessary knowledge about pain relief to contribute effectively to their own pain management.

People in pain have a crucial role to play in assessing their pain and pain relief. They are, after all, the authority on their pain, and it is important to establish a partnership with them. In hospital they may be totally reliant on health professionals for pain relief; being involved in systematic assessment of pain and pain relief can help them to regain some sense of control over the situation. If part of their pain control involves the use of patient-controlled analgesia (PCA) (see p. 629), patients can take a much more active role. Similarly, people with pain who are cared for at home often take their own painkillers and thus maintain more direct control over their pain relief. All patients in pain may, given appropriate instruction and support, contribute to pain management by using complementary methods of pain relief (see p. 630) and by taking some responsibility for certain aspects of their pain relief.

The role of family members and carers

When an individual is trying to cope with pain his family members and other loved ones are likely to be affected. Taylor et al (1990) found that not only people with chronic pain but their spouses as well had elevated psychological distress when compared to a non-patient sample. It can be very frightening to see a loved one in pain, and carers may feel very helpless. Rowat & Jeans (1989) view chronic pain as a family problem and urge a collaborative approach to pain management with goals for adaptation, enhancing quality of life, improving pain control and facilitating coping. This approach avoids the pitfall of treating pain as an isolated symptom, and appears to be helpful for people with all types of pain.

Strategies for effective pain assessment

It is important to carry out a comprehensive pain assessment as part of the initial nursing assessment and at regular intervals thereafter in order to obtain a complete and evolving picture of the patient's pain. During her first meeting with the patient the nurse should discuss with him the nature of the pain that he is experiencing or is likely to experience and what can be expected of pain relief. (Of course, the patient in acute discomfort will need to be given pain relief before an extensive assessment can be made.) It is important to make sure that both patient and nurse are working toward similar, realistic goals with regard to pain management. Once defined, these goals should be continually reviewed.

Pain may be assessed by such means as observing the patient's behaviours, taking physiological measurements, interviewing the patient, and by using pain assessment tools.

Observation

?	**19.9** Discuss with your colleagues what sorts of verbal and non-verbal clues might indicate that a patient is in pain?

The patient may provide verbal and/or non-verbal clues that he is in pain. Verbal clues include direct statements as well as moaning, crying or sighing. Non-verbal indications might include grimacing, guarding, bracing and lying perfectly still. It cannot be assumed, however, that if the patient does not *appear* to be in pain he is in fact not in pain. If he is laughing at a television programme or chatting with visitors he may still be in pain, for these activities can distract the person from his pain. Caution should be exercised, therefore, in the interpretation of non-verbal signals. Keefe (1989) argues that observation techniques can be useful in the assessment of people with chronic pain, but cannot and should not replace other pain measurements. Used on its own, observation of the patient can be unreliable.

Measuring physiological responses

Pain assessment may include measurement of sympathetic responses such as increases in blood pressure and pulse. However, these responses are not specific to pain and may reflect other emotions such as anger or other physiological conditions, and they soon adapt. In addition, parasympathetic stimulation may reduce blood pressure and pulse. Therefore it is unwise for the assessor to rely purely on physiological indicators.

Asking the patient

In pain assessment the observation of behaviour and measurement of physiological responses should be subsidiary to direct consultation with the patient. Donovan et al (1987) found, however, that fewer than 50% of 353 medical and surgical inpatients could remember being asked about their pain. A tendency for nurses to discount their patients' own perceptions of pain was demonstrated by Teske et al (1983), who found a discrepancy between patients' testimony and nurses' judgement of pain; this finding was substantiated by Seers (1989).

?	**19.10** Compare your perception of a patient's pain with his own description. Do the two versions match?

It may be useful to note in the pain assessment a few of the adjectives that the patient chooses to describe his pain. Melzack & Torgerson (1971) incorporated a range of pain descriptors into their McGill Pain Questionnaire (MPQ), and the later short-form MPQ by Melzack (1987). These questionnaires are designed to help the patient draw on the sensory, affective and cognitive dimensions of pain as well as its overall intensity in describing their experience. The short-form MPQ offers the following descriptors for the patient to select from: throbbing, shooting, stabbing, sharp, cramping, gnawing, hot/burning, aching, heavy, tender, splitting, tiring/exhausting, sickening, fearful and punishing/cruel. The MPQ can be useful for some people with chronic pain, but may be too complex for use in the assessment of postoperative pain.

?	**19.11** Try to describe a recent pain, such as a headache or toothache, to your group. What was the sensation like? How did it make you feel, think and behave? Look at the differences and similarities between pain descriptions within the group.

Gaston-Johansson et al (1990) found that different cultural groups rated 'pain' as the most intense sensation, followed by 'hurt' and lastly 'ache' as the least intense. Some people may not actually use the word 'pain' when asked about their discomfort and may even deny having pain. Introducing words such as 'ache', 'hurt', 'sore' or 'discomfort' into one's line of questioning may be helpful. Pain assessment may prove to be difficult with patients who do not share a common language with the assessor; here, the observation of non-verbal signs will become especially important. Patients with cognitive disabilities can also be very difficult to assess. In such cases the family can be an invaluable source of information.

Assessment content

The general points that pain assessment must cover include:

- location of the pain
- its intensity
- patterns of the pain
- effects of the pain.

Location. The London Hospital Pain Observation Chart (see Fig. 19.4) uses an outline of the human body to help the patient to locate the site of pain. One advantage of such a chart is the opportunity it gives the patient to disclose the presence of pain in a site that is unexpected or not the present focus of concern. Such a diagram can also be useful in helping the

The London Hospital
PAIN OBSERVATION CHART

This chart records where a patient's pain is and how bad it is, by the nurse asking the patient at regular intervals. If analgesics are being given regularly, make an observation with *each* dose and another *half-way between* each dose. If analgesics are given only 'as required', observe two-hourly. When the observations are stable and the patient is comfortable, any regular time interval between observations may be chosen.

To use this chart, ask the patient to mark all his or her pains on the body diagram. Label each site of pain with a letter (i.e. A, B, C, etc).

Then at each observation time ask the patient to assess:

1. The *pain in each separate site* since the last observation. Use the scale above the body diagram, and enter the number or letter in the appropriate column.
2. The *pain overall* since the last observation. Use the same scale and enter in column marked *overall.*

Next, record what has been done to relieve pain. In particular:

3. Note any *analgesic* given since the last observation, stating name, dose, route and time given.
4. Tick any other *nursing care* or *action taken* to ease pain.

Finally note any *comment on pain* from patient or nurse (use the back of the chart as well, if necessary) and initial the record.

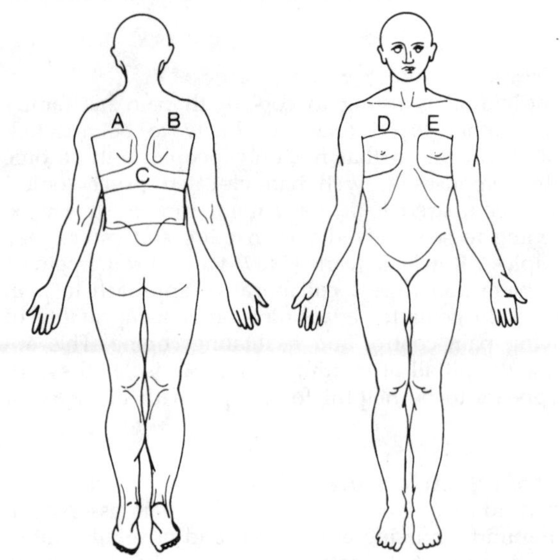

Date ______________ **Sheet number** ____________________ **Patient identification label**

Time	Pain rating: By sites A	B	C	D	E	F	G	H	Overall	Measures to relieve pain (specify where starred): Analgesic given (Name, dose, route, time)	Lifting	Turning	Massage	Distracting activities	Position change*	Additional aids*	Other*	Comments from patients and/or staff	Initials

Adapted from the London Hospital Pain Observation Chart

Fig. 19.4 The London Hospital Pain Chart. (Reproduced with kind permission from Raiman 1987.)

nurse to detect the existence of chronic pain in patients who are, for example, admitted for elective surgery.

Intensity. To determine the intensity of a person's pain it is useful to use a scale on which the patient can rate the degree of pain he is feeling. These scales can be used to note any change in pain levels following an intervention, or to indicate when the 'worst pain' or 'least pain' was felt, thus giving a profile of the pain experience over time. Scales can also be used to help the patient quantify the distress caused by the pain, or to determine at what level of intensity the patient would like to be given analgesics. It should be remembered, however, that this level is not necessarily constant, and that the patient's pain tolerance may fluctuate from day to day or within a 24-hour period.

Three pain scales in current use are described below.

Patterns. In the course of her assessment the nurse should ask the patient such questions as:

- When did the pain start?
- How long does it last?
- Is it intermittent or continuous?
- What makes it better?
- What makes it worse?
- Do you have your own methods of relieving and coping with the pain?

McCaffery & Beebe (1989) recommend that the patient be asked: 'Is there anything else that you can tell me that may help us work with you to get the best possible control of your pain?'

Effects. The nurse should also determine how the individual's pain affects daily activities such as sleeping and socialising. Patients with chronic pain, for example, may find that they are prevented from working and that they have difficulty getting adequate sleep.

Using pain assessment scales

It can be very difficult to convey the precise quality of such a complex and subjective experience as pain. The nurse may find that the use of one or more of the assessment tools described here will help the patient to communicate his needs.

Visual analogue scale (VAS). This is usually a 10 cm line with the words 'no pain at all' at one end and a phrase such as 'agonising pain' or 'worst pain possible' at the other end (see Fig. 19.5). The patient is asked to mark this line at whatever point he feels corresponds to the degree of pain he is experiencing at the moment. The assessor then measures in cm from the left-hand side of the pain scale to the mark in order to obtain the pain 'score'.

The advantages of this scale include the absence of numbers or words along the scale; the person in pain is not forced to assign a precise numerical value to his pain or to choose a word which does not exactly represent it. Some patients, however, will find this scale too abstract and will be unable to think about their pain in reference to a line. Sriwatanakul et al (1982) found that 4% of the patients in their study were unable to understand the scale; Kremer et al (1981) found that 11% of their sample were unable to complete it and that it was especially difficult for elderly people.

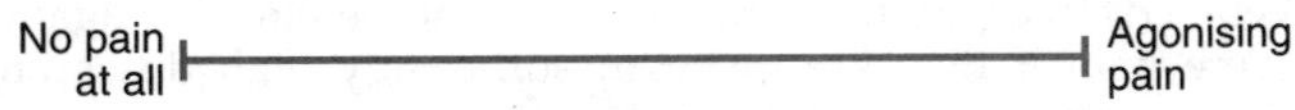

Fig. 19.5 The visual analogue scale.

Numerical rating scale (NRS). This scale is like the VAS but is calibrated with the numbers 0–10 (see Fig. 19.6). The patient is asked to make a mark at a point which indicates the intensity of his pain. Even with the added numerical guideline, not all patients find this scale easy to use. Jensen et al (1989, 1986) found that a 0–10 scale was a useful clinical index of pain intensity with postoperative patients, but that a 0–100 scale appeared to be the most effective for patients with chronic pain.

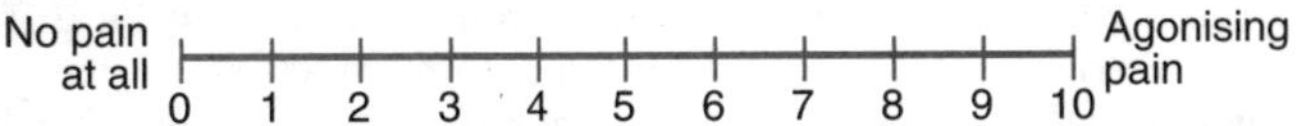

Fig. 19.6 The numerical rating scale.

Verbal rating scale (VRS). This scale provides graded categories, for example, 'no pain at all', 'slight pain', 'moderate pain', 'very bad pain' and 'agonising pain' (see Fig. 19.7). The patient marks whichever category is most like his pain and is assigned a score from 0 to 4 respectively. The advantage of this scale is that many patients find it easy to use (Kremer et al 1981). Its disadvantages include the fact that there are fewer points than on a 0–10 scale and so it is not as sensitive. For example, a patient may rate himself as being in 'moderate' pain before and after an intervention, although he has noticed some worsening, or easing, of his pain.

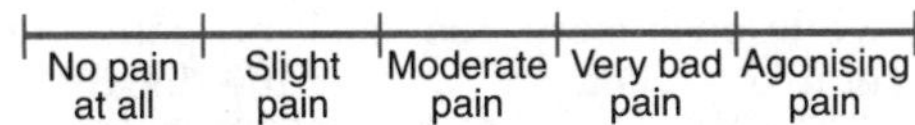

Fig. 19.7 The verbal rating scale.

The visual, numerical and verbal pain scales rate intensity, which is only one aspect of pain. They could also be used to rate how distressing the pain is, for example, from 'not at all distressing' to 'extremely distressing'. Turk (1989) points out that pain intensity may not be seen by the person in pain in a linear fashion, and that forcing a judgement onto a linear scale may constrain and distort the results. McCaffery & Beebe (1989) cite inadvertent and deliberate denial of pain as possible problems in assessment. Deliberate denial of pain may be attempted to please the doctor or nurse, to be stoic, or to avoid being forced to spend longer in hospital or off work.

> ? **19.12** How would you feel if a patient told you he had pain, but told the doctor he had no pain? How would you feel if a patient told you he had no pain, but reported pain to the doctor? Can you explain this from the patient's perspective?

Recording pain assessment

Pain levels and pain-relieving measures must be carefully documented as a basis for evaluating pain management. Recording tools such as the London Hospital Chart (see Fig. 19.4) can be useful. This chart has been adapted for use with postoperative patients by Sofaer (1984) and for use with orthopaedic patients by Davis (1988). McCaffery & Beebe's (1989) pain chart has columns for recording respirations, blood pressure, pulse and level of arousal. A 'plan and comments' column for strategies to improve or maintain pain control is also included. McCaffery & Beebe (1989) have also devised a daily diary for the patient to use at home. This includes columns for time, pain rating, medication, other pain-relieving measures and major activities (e.g. lying, sitting, walking) being done at the time of the pain rating.

The type of pain chart used should be appropriate to the care setting (e.g. hospital or home) and should be one to which the patient can respond. The frequency of recording will depend on the patient's situation and the nature of his pain, but must be adequate for continuous evaluation of interventions. Pain charts can provide an invaluable basis for discussion with other members of the health care team. Informing the doctor that a regime is not effective can be difficult for some nurses to do and for some doctors to accept. However, the systematic use of a pain chart which clearly documents results can help overcome these difficulties.

PAIN RELIEF

As a detailed review of narcotic, non-narcotic and adjuvant medications will not be undertaken here, the reader is referred to a detailed pharmacology text such as Rogers & Spector (1989). In addition, pharmacists can be a valuable source of information. It is important for the nurse to be familiar with the dosages, routes of administration, duration, mode of action and side-effects of the analgesics commonly used in her field of practice.

One important question for the nurse to consider is how much pain relief she is aiming for and whether this is the same target as that of the person in pain. Weis et al (1983) state that while in theory the goal of pain management should be complete relief, only 21% of the doctors and nurses in their study had this aim. Cohen (1980) found that during the first two postoperative days, 3.3% of nurses aimed for complete pain relief, 57% aimed to relieve as much pain as possible, 38% aimed to relieve pain just enough for the patient to function, and 1% aimed to relieve pain to a level where the patient could just tolerate it.

The nurse should ask the person in pain how much pain relief he is aiming for. In the case of patients with post-operative pain or cancer, the nurse should be able to do a lot towards relieving their pain. She may encounter problems, however, if the person with chronic non-malignant pain aims for complete relief: the best she may be able to offer in such cases is support in coping with the pain.

Analgesics

The most common pain-relieving measure is the administration of drugs to achieve analgesia, which may be defined as the 'Absence of pain in response to stimulation which would normally be painful' (IASP 1986, p. S218). Narcotic analgesics such as morphine act centrally. According to McCaffery & Beebe (1989) they are under-used, partly for fear of addiction (see p. 622); the tendency is for physicians to underprescribe them, nurses to underadminister them, and patients not to ask for them. Some pain, however, such as that caused by lesions in the peripheral nervous system or by bony metastases is unresponsive or only partially responsive to opioids.

Non-narcotic analgesics such as aspirin act more peripherally; their effectiveness is often underrated. A combination of narcotic and non-narcotic analgesics is often helpful as they relieve pain in different ways.

Adjuvant medication may be given to enhance the effects of narcotic or non-narcotic analgesics or because their own action is desirable. Drugs given in adjuvant therapy include anticonvulsants, neuroleptics, anxiolytics, antidepressants and corticosteroids (WHO 1986).

Individual responses to set dosages of narcotic and non-narcotic analgesics is not entirely predictable (Austin et al 1980, Sunshine & Olson 1989). Results must be carefully observed and documented in order to ensure that the dosage and timing are effective and that side-effects are minimised.

Placebos

The word 'placebo' comes from the Latin 'I shall please' and may be used to refer to 'any medical treatment . . . or nursing care that produces an effect in a patient because of its implicit or explicit intent and not because of its specific nature or therapeutic properties' (McCaffery & Beebe 1989, p. 16).

?	**19.13** What would your reaction be if a patient reported that an injection of saline or a sugar pill had made his pain better?

It is a common misconception that people who are helped by placebos were exaggerating their pain in the first place. One reason why placebos may relieve pain is that a high expectation of pain relief may trigger the release of the body's natural opiates, endorphins (Levine et al 1978).

The Misuse of Drugs Act 1971

The prescription, supply, administration and storage of 'controlled' drugs, i.e. medications which are habit-forming or which are liable to misuse are regulated by the Misuse of Drugs Act 1971. Many drugs used to relieve severe pain, e.g. opiates, are regulated by the Act, as well as by local health authority procedures. The nurse should familiarise herself with these guidelines as well as with any additional policies in effect at her place of work. The Department of Health (1989) has issued guidelines on the Misuse of Drugs Act and on the Misuse of Drugs Regulations 1985. A leaflet on 'Standards for the administration of medicines' produced by the UKCC (1992) also gives useful advice within a more general framework.

Routes of administration

Analgesics are administered via a number of routes — oral, intramuscular, intravenous, rectal, sublingual, buccal, transdermal, subcutaneous, by inhalation, intrapleural, respiratory, and spinal — depending on such factors as efficacy, convenience, desired onset of analgesia, acceptability to the patient, side-effects and cost. The choice of route should be made after a careful consideration of the comparative risks and benefits of the various routes possible for a given drug. The following discussion provides only a brief introduction to the routes of analgesic administration in common use. For more detailed information the reader is referred to McCaffery & Beebe (1989).

Oral. Tablets or liquids are usually easy to administer and place no restrictions on patient mobility. Sustained release preparations can be useful. Any nausea and vomiting must be controlled to ensure the patient's comfort and maximise absorption of the drug. Oral medication is susceptible to the first pass effect in the liver and intestine, by which some of the drug is metabolised and thus inactivated before it enters the circulation. The oral route is often thought to be appropriate only for mild to moderate pain, but McCaffery & Beebe (1989) argue that oral narcotics can be effective against severe pain if they are given in sufficiently high doses and a preventative approach is used.

Intramuscular (i.m.). This route is often used in the treatment of postoperative pain. Although in itself an effective route for drug delivery, it can be less satisfactory if the time required to prepare the injection and have it checked, or other factors, delays a repeat dose beyond the optimum interval.

Intravenous (i.v.). The action of analgesics administered by this route is rapid in onset but of short duration. Therefore a continuous infusion rather than bolus injection may be more effective in maintaining analgesia. Nurses currently require training and certification by their employing health authority before they can administer i.v. drugs. There are often additional regulations governing the i.v. administration of opioids.

Rectal. The patient may find this route of administration unacceptable. However, it may be useful for patients experiencing nausea and vomiting or who have difficulty swallowing. Cole & Hanning (1990) conclude that the use of sustained-release rectal opioids offers steady drug concentration with once or twice daily dosing, which could benefit terminal care patients who may be managed at home for a longer time if non-parenteral routes of drug administration are used.

Sublingual and buccal. In sublingual administration the medication is placed under the tongue; in buccal administration it is placed between the upper lip and gum or between the cheek and gum. These routes may avoid the first pass effect but the patient may inadvertently swallow the drug. Buccal administration may be difficult if the patient has upper dentures.

Transdermal. This is a relatively new method of pain relief which involves placing a drug-containing patch directly onto the skin, where absorption occurs. Gourlay et al (1990) found that when transdermal fentanyl was compared to a placebo in the treatment of postoperative pain, pain relief was similar between the two groups but significantly less supplementary pethidine was required by the fentanyl group in the first 12–48 hours after surgery.

Subcutaneous infusions may be very useful for ambulatory patients who need continuous pain control, e.g. people with chronic pain who are at home. Storey et al (1990) concluded that this method offers a simple, safe and effective alternative to i.v. or i.m. injections when oral medications cannot be used, and can be safely used in the patient's home.

Inhalation. Nitrous oxide (Entonox) administered with a mask or inhaler can help the patient to deal with bursts of pain, as in childbirth, or during dressing changes or other painful minor procedures.

Spinal. Opioids can be injected into the epidural or subarachnoid space of the spinal column. Respiratory depression is an important and potentially serious complication to which the nurse must be alert. Doses are considerably smaller than those required for i.m or i.v. use and changing a syringe requires appropriate training, expertise and certification from the employing authority. Bromage (1989) points out that these techniques are only as safe as the quality of patient surveillance. Much remains to be learned about the application of epidural and intrathecal narcotics. Local anaesthetic agents can be administered epidurally.

Changing the route of administration. McCaffery & Beebe (1989) point out that in changing from one route of analgesic administration to another care must be taken not to over- or undermedicate patients. They recommend using equianalgesic charts when determining the dosage for the new route and explaining to the patient any differences likely to occur, such as delayed or accelerated onset of action.

Patient controlled analgesia (PCA)

PCA refers to the administration of analgesics by any appropriate and safe route over which the patient has control. It usually refers to the self-administration of i.v. boluses of a narcotic analgesic via a specifically designed pump. There are pre-set 'lock-out' intervals on these machines, so that the patient cannot administer more than a certain dose in a given time. The patient has to be able and willing to use this method. Its advantages lie in the fact that the patient can have an analgesic dose whenever he needs it, which gives him more control over his pain and greater confidence that he will obtain relief. Clark et al (1989) found that a group of surgical patients receiving PCA had more morphine and went home more quickly than a group receiving i.m. injections. Thomas (1989), in a pilot study of patients using PCA, found that these patients had less pain, received less analgesic medication and were discharged earlier than patients receiving only i.m. injections.

Other medical interventions

Local anaesthesia and regional nerve blocks. These procedures, which are usually performed by anaesthetists, are reviewed in detail by Bonica (1989) and Latham (1991). Many people have had such a block at the dentist when local anaesthetic is injected into the gums. They work by injecting local anaesthetic (sometimes with a steroid) near to or in a peripheral nerve or a major nerve plexus or into the spine. There can be adverse reactions and complications. The pain-relieving effects often outlast the duration of the local anaesthetic.

Surgery. Nerves can be transected in an attempt to reduce or eliminate intractable pain. Although this measure may work initially, because there are so many pain pathways the pain often returns and may be worse. Examples of surgical methods of pain relief include sympathectomy and cordotomy. The reader is referred to Latham (1991) for details.

Radiotherapy, chemotherapy and hormone therapy may relieve pain by reducing invasive tumours. These therapies are reviewed in detail by Hoy (1989); the reader is also referred to Chapter 32 in the present volume.

Specialised pain services

Acute pain services. In response to continuing documentation of inadequate postoperative pain relief and the introduction of techniques such as PCA some centres have set up a multidisciplinary acute pain service (see e.g. Ready et al 1988, Ready 1989). These services are responsible for the day-to-day management of acute pain after surgery. They ensure that the level of pain relief and monitoring is appropriate and provide in-service training for medical and nursing staff. They may also be involved in auditing outcomes and undertaking clinical research.

Hospice/palliative care teams working in hospitals and in the community have a wealth of expertise in pain and symptom control and can be a valuable resource. A study by Bruera et al (1989) on the influence of a pain and symptom control team (PSCT) on the management of pain in patients not under the direct care of the PSCT found that higher doses of narcotics were prescribed three years after the PSCT was set up. However, two-thirds of medication was still prescribed

PRN, despite the recommendation that narcotics be administered regularly. Bruera et al concluded that while the presence of the PSCT had resulted in some changes, more instruction or discussion was needed in many areas.

Pain clinics. Chronic pain is recognised as a syndrome in its own right and pain clinics often, although not exclusively, treat patients with chronic non-malignant pain. Clinics are often multidisciplinary and may be staffed by anaesthetists, nurses, psychologists, physiotherapists, occupational therapists and pharmacists. The aim of pain clinics is to increase the person's ability to function and to lead a more active life. People with chronic non-malignant pain have been successfully treated on an inpatient basis (Gottlieb et al 1977), on an outpatient basis (Skinner et al 1990), and using 'field management' whereby behavioural assessment and treatment strategies are implemented in the patient's own home and work environments (Cott et al 1990).

Complementary methods of pain relief

'Complementary' methods of pain relief include distraction, relaxation imagery, transcutaneous electrical nerve stimulation (TENS), massage, the application of heat or cold, hypnosis, biofeedback and acupuncture. There is some overlap between certain of these techniques; for example imagery contains elements of distraction and relaxation. One advantage of these methods is that they appear to have fewer undesirable side-effects although more research needs to be done to monitor this, and to demonstrate their efficacy.

It is important that any complementary pain relief method used is appropriate to the individual. The nurse should know what the patient is capable of doing and what he *wants* to do. The patient may already be using complementary techniques without realising it. For example, he may say that his pain is better when he watches television or listens to music. It is important to build on techniques the patient already uses. Similarly, many nurses may use such techniques without valuing them as special skills. For example, the nurse may distract the patient during a dressing change by asking him about a holiday or his family.

Patients, doctors and nurses may be sceptical of complementary techniques and find it difficult to think beyond pharmacological methods of pain relief. Patients may feel that it is being implied that their pain is 'all in the mind' if they are offered these therapies; they may also think that their pain is too bad to be affected by complementary techniques.

It is important that teaching sessions for these methods are held when the patient has no pain, e.g. before surgery, or when his pain is under control, e.g. after an effective analgesic, as he will need time to become familiar with new techniques before trying to apply them.

Distraction

Distraction as a means of pain relief involves diverting the attention toward stimuli other than the pain. Distraction may be provided by conversation, watching television or listening to music, planned activities, or by focusing on everyday stimuli in the immediate environment. For example, Copp (1974) found that patients resorted to counting bricks on a wall or repeating words or phrases to cope with pain.

Distraction does not remove the pain, but can help to make it more bearable by removing it from the centre of attention. It can improve the patient's mood by allowing him to focus on pleasant things and can give him a greater sense of control over his pain (McCaffery & Beebe 1989). To help patients benefit from distraction the nurse will need to find out what sorts of things they find absorbing.

Possible disadvantages of this technique pointed out by McCaffery & Beebe (1989) include the following:

- others may begin to doubt that the individual's pain is real if he can be distracted from it
- analgesics may still be needed during and after the distracting activity
- the technique has no lasting effect following the period of distraction
- the patient may be more aware of the pain afterwards and feel fatigued and irritable.

Relaxation

People who are in pain often have tense muscles and an anxious expression. Relaxation is defined by McCaffery & Beebe (1989) as 'a state of relative freedom from both anxiety and skeletal muscle tension'. It is a skill which needs to be learned and which improves with practice. Relaxation may help to reduce the distress associated with having pain, rather than the pain itself, and it is important not to give the patient unrealistic expectations of the pain relief he will obtain by learning relaxation techniques. Teaching someone face to face has been found to be more effective than using taped instructions (Paul & Trimble 1970), although once the patient has been given personal instruction he could be given a tape to refresh his memory.

Various methods may be used to promote relaxation; some of these highlight breathing techniques, and others attempt to focus the attention sequentially on various parts of the body and then 'letting go' of the tension in those areas. Where and when a relaxation technique is used depends partly on the sort of pain in question. Someone with postoperative pain might use relaxation whilst lying in bed or sitting in a chair. Someone with chronic pain would also benefit from learning how to integrate relaxation into the activities of everyday life.

Relaxation has been found to reduce postoperative pain (Clum et al 1982), tension headache (Cox et al 1975) and chronic low back pain (Philips 1988). Sims (1987) reviewed relaxation studies involving cancer patients and concluded that the results were generally encouraging. Levin et al (1987), however, found no significant difference in the number of analgesics, number of days in hospital after surgery, pain sensation or pain distress between those who received a tape recording of a relaxation technique and those in a control group.

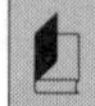
For more detailed instructions see McCaffery & Beebe (1989), Goldfried & Davison (1978) and Bernstein & Borkovec (1973).

Directed imagery

This technique involves using the imagination to help control pain. For example, the patient might imagine a favourite place or tranquil scene, invoking all of his senses to conjure it up — for example, 'seeing' the sand and waves at a beach, 'hearing' the waves and the wind, 'feeling' the sand under his feet and the warmth of the sun on his skin, 'smelling' the sea air and 'tasting' the salty sea-spray on his lips.

This technique appears to be most effective when the patient chooses his own image and is in control of whether and when he uses imagery. McCaffery & Beebe (1989) recommend that patients who are psychotic should not be encouraged to use imagery. In Swinford's (1987) study of the use of relaxation and imagery, pain was found to decrease on the first and second days after surgery. Dental patients who were given pleasant images to dwell on by Horan et al (1976) were found to have less discomfort than a control group.

Cutaneous stimulation

Transcutaneous electrical nerve stimulation (TENS). In this intervention low-voltage electrical stimulation is delivered via electrodes placed on the skin near or on the site of pain. This usually causes a sensation of vibrating or tingling and can be used in an intermittent or continuous mode. The device is powered by a battery pack and can be operated by the patient. In a review of clinical pain conditions successfully and unsuccessfully treated with TENS Woolf (1989) concluded that while TENS could be useful in a wide variety of acute and chronic conditions, reducing or eliminating mild to moderate pain, it appeared to be less effective against severe pain. McCaffery & Beebe (1989) stipulate that TENS should not be used with people who have cardiac pacemakers, over a pregnant uterus, over the carotid sinus or with people suffering from senility.

Massage. The laying on of hands is described by Haldeman (1989, p. 942) as 'unquestionably the oldest, most universally utilised and probably the most appreciated means of relieving pain and suffering'. The reader is referred to this source for a description of different massage and manipulation techniques.

The application of heat or cold may relieve pain through a 'counterirritant' effect as well as by direct effects on peripheral and free nerve endings (Lehmann & de Lateur 1989). Care should be taken with patients with impaired sensation or reduced level of consciousness who could damage their skin without realising it while using these methods.

Hypnosis

Hypnosis is an altered state of consciousness in which concentration is focused and distractions are minimised. The subject's ability to respond to suggestion appears to be important to the success of hypnosis (Orne & Dinges 1989) and this responsiveness may be inhibited by the subject if he so chooses. The nature of hypnosis and the mechanism of its effects are unclear. It seems that the type of pain being treated, the context and goals of treatment, the skill of the therapist and the expectations, motivations and responsiveness of the subject determine the way hypnosis can be used to relieve pain. This technique is not one that should be attempted without special training.

Biofeedback

This involves monitoring specific body functions, such as muscle tension, blood pressure, pulse and/or temperature, and establishing some control over these functions. The therapist usually teaches the subject to relax while feedback from the monitoring equipment tells him how he is doing. Although this technique may be useful for some people, the research suggests it is no more effective than relaxation alone for pain relief. Jessup's (1989) review of the literature on relaxation and biofeedback describes the overall finding that biofeedback and relaxation are equally effective for most pain treatment applications.

Acupuncture

Acupuncture originated in China thousands of years ago. It involves inserting needles into the skin at specific acupuncture or Hoku points which are located in a series of channels or meridians. These needles may be manipulated to maximise the effect. The mechanism of action has been the subject of much debate, and activation of endorphins has been suggested. Patel et al (1989) reviewed 14 studies which used acupuncture for chronic pain and concluded that while most results favoured acupuncture there were various potential sources of bias which precluded a conclusive finding.

In acupressure the acupuncture points are stimulated by pressing and/or rubbing rather than by the insertion of needles.

Behaviour therapy

The development of behaviour therapy programmes for pain management owes much to Fordyce (1978), who first drew attention to the rewards a person in chronic pain may receive for 'pain behaviour', such as sympathy, attention, and exemption from certain tasks. Since behavioural psychologists believe that all behaviour is governed by its consequences, they feel that by discouraging pain behaviours (such as moaning or grimacing) and encouraging 'well behaviours' the professional can help the person adopt a more normal pattern of behaviour. This has been described as operant conditioning. A cognitive–behavioural approach (e.g. Turk & Meichenbaum 1989) includes the modification of the patient's thought and feelings as well as his behaviours; it also includes a commitment to behaviour therapy procedures in promoting change, such as graded practice and homework assignments. Pain clinic programmes usually contain some element of behaviour therapy.

Chiropractic and osteopathy

Chiropractors use physical manipulation to realign the vertebrae. A recent study found that patients with chronic low back pain benefited more from consulting a chiropractor than from traditional hospital outpatient treatment and recommended that chiropractic be offered under the National Health Service (Meade et al 1990). However, this conclusion was disputed by several authors (Graham et al 1990, Greenough 1990).

Tanner (1987) describes the difference between osteopathy and chiropractic as 'subtle'. He argues that chiropractors are more likely to view the problem in terms of the *structure* of the spine whereas osteopaths emphasise abnormal *movement* of the spine. However, as Tanner points out, methods and techniques in these two disciplines overlap.

Beyond the traditional health care setting

Which approaches to pain relief may be considered outside and which inside the 'traditional' health care setting is open to debate. Some of the methods mentioned here could be considered appropriate to a conventional setting. As with all aspects of pain management, the client — therapist relationship may be crucial to the success of these treatments, since having someone take a sympathetic interest in one's problems can be therapeutic in itself. Certainly much more research needs to be done to establish the efficacy and mode of action of non-traditional approaches to pain control.

Therapeutic touch is a technique whereby the healer attempts to transmit his own healing energy to the patient. Proponents of this technique argue that energy fields alter when people are unwell. Therapeutic touch may work in a manner similar to acupressure or by virtue of a placebo effect. It may also have some effect simply by increasing the individual's sense of well-being. For further reading see Wright (1987) and Wyatt & Dimmer (1988).

Other approaches include faith healing, herbal remedies, aromatherapy and reflexology.

?	**19.14** Discuss with your colleagues whether anyone has had some experience of these therapies used in pain relief.

Support and self-help groups. People suffering from pain often seek help from relatives and friends before approaching a professional within the health care system. For example, an individual might obtain a friend's opinion as to whether he should consult his GP about a particular pain symptom. Zola (1973) argues that while people are subject to an array of bodily discomforts only a small number present to a doctor; it is therefore important to discover what 'trigger' has converted the 'person' into a 'patient'.

After the individual has sought professional help he may continue to obtain support from relatives and friends as well as from self-help organisations such as The National Back Pain Association and The British Migraine Association. The individual may also consult some of the many books now available for the general reader on pain and its relief. The nurse may help her patients in this regard by bringing their attention to such texts as Sternbach (1987), Broome & Jellicoe (1987), Gingell (1988), Hewitt (1982), Benson & Klipper (1975), Tanner (1987) and Shone (1992).

CONCLUSION

Pain and its relief are a central part of nursing in almost all care settings. Ongoing education for health professionals and an understanding of the complexities of pain and its management are crucial in forming a sound basis for practice. Lander (1990b) describes education as probably 'the single most important tool for improving pain management'. The person in pain should be believed, his pain should be systematically assessed, treated and reassessed, and he should be involved in pain management whenever possible. Pain and its relief need to be given a high priority in care and health professionals should be accountable for the pain relief of people in their care. Indeed, 'failure to treat pain is inhumane and constitutes professional negligence' (Meinhart & McCaffery 1983, p. vi). Nurses are in the fortunate position of being able to make an important contribution towards the comfort and well-being of people in pain.

GLOSSARY

Allodynia. 'Pain due to a stimulus which does not normally provoke pain' (IASP 1986, p. 5217).

Afferent nerve fibre. This is the sensory nerve fibre which runs from the tissues to the central nervous system.

Antinociceptive. This describes something that helps to reduce or stop the response to noxious stimulation.

Causalgias. 'A syndrome of sustained burning pain, allodymia and hyperpathios after a traumatic nerve lesion' (IASP 1986, p. 5218).

Dermatome. An area of skin mainly innervated by a particular spinal cord segment.

Equianalgesic. A specified drug dose or route of administration that will give about the same analgesic effect as another specified drug dose or route. The term is often applied to an equianalgesic chart. This chart is useful to help maintain the same level of analgesia when changing the type of drug and/or the route of administration. Morphine is usually used as a standard for comparison. This chart, can be used, for example, to see how much Pethidine would have the same effect as 10 mg morphine. It also shows how much of an oral dose would be needed to equate in analgesic effect to a previous i.m. or i.v. dose, or vice versa.

Hyperpathia. 'A painful syndrome, characterised by increased reaction to a stimulus, especially a repetitive stimulus, as well as an increased threshold' (IASP 1986, p. 5219).

Neuralgias. 'Pain in the distribution of a nerve or nerves' (IASP 1986, p. 5220).

Nociceptor. This is a receptor which responds to noxious stimuli or injury.

REFERENCES

Austin K L, Stapleton J V, Mather L E 1980 Multiple intramuscular injections: a major source of variability in analgesic response to meperidine. Pain 8: 47–62

Baines M, Kirkham S R 1989 Cancer pain. In: Wall P D, Melzack R (eds) Textbook of pain, 2nd edn. Churchill Livingstone, Edinburgh, ch 41, pp 590–597

Bond M R, Pearson I B 1969 Psychological aspects of pain in women with advanced cancer of the cervix. Journal of Psychosomatic Research 13: 13–19

Bonica J J 1989 Local anaesthesia and regional blocks. In: Wall P D, Melzack R (eds) Textbook of pain, 2nd edn. Churchill Livingstone, Edinburgh ch 50, pp 724–743

Bourbonnais F E, Mackay R C 1981 The influence of nursing intervention on chest pain. Nursing Papers 13(3): 38–48

Brena S F, Sanders S H, Motoyama H 1990 American and Japanese chronic low back pain patients: cross-cultural similarities and differences. Clinical Journal of Pain 6(2): 118–124

Bromage P R 1989 Epidural anaesthetics and narcotics. In: Wall P D, Melzack R (eds) Textbook of pain, 2nd edn. Churchill Livingstone, Edinburgh, ch 51, pp 744–753

Bruera E, MacMillan K, Hanson J, MacDonald R N 1989 Palliative care in a cancer centre: results in 1984 versus 1987. Journal of Pain and Symptom Management 5(1): 1–5

Campbell J N, Raja S N, Cohen R H, Manning D C, Khan A A, Meyer R A 1989 Peripheral neural mechanisms of nociception. In: Wall P D, Melzack R (eds) Textbook of pain, 2nd edn. Churchill Livingstone, Edinburgh, ch. 1, pp 22–45

Cartwright P D 1985 Pain control after surgery: a survey of current practice. Annals of the Royal College of Surgeons 67: 13–16

Chapman P J, Ganendran A, Scott R J, Basford K E 1987 Attitudes and knowledge of nursing staff in relation to management of postoperative pain. Australian and New Zealand Journal of Surgery 57(7): 447–450

Choiniere M, Melzack R, Girard N, Rondeau J, Paquin M J 1990 Comparisons between patients' and nurses' assessment of pain and medication efficacy in severe burn injuries. Pain 40(2): 143–152

Chung S H, Dickenson A 1981 The last piece in the puzzle. Nursing Mirror 152(6): 40–41

Clark E, Hodsman N, Kenny G 1989 Improved postoperative recovery with patient-controlled analgesia. Nursing Times 85(9): 54–55

Clark W C, Mehl L J 1971 Thermal pain: a sensory decision theory analysis of the effect of age and sex on d', various response criteria and 50% pain threshold. Journal of Abnormal Psychology 78: 202–212

Clement-Jones V, Besser G M 1983 Clinical perspectives in opioid peptides. British Medical Bulletin 39(1): 95–100
Closs S J 1990 An exploratory analysis of nurses' provision of postoperative analgesic drugs. Journal of Advanced Nursing 15(1): 42–49
Clum G A, Luscomb R L, Scott L 1982 Relaxation training and cognitive strategies in the treatment of acute pain. Pain 12(2): 175–183
Coderre T J, Katz J, Vaccarino A L & Melzack R 1993 Contribution of central neuroplasticity to pathological pain: review of clinical and experimental evidence. Pain 52(3): 259–285
Cohen F 1980 Postsurgical pain relief: patients' status and nurses' medication choices. Pain 9: 265–274
Cole L, Hanning C D 1990 Review of the rectal use of opioids. Journal of Pain and Symptom Management 5(2): 118–126
Copp L A 1974 The spectrum of suffering. American Journal of Nursing 74(3): 491–495
Cott A, Anchel H, Goldberg W M, Fabich M, Parkinson W 1990 Non-institutional treatment of chronic pain by field management: an outcome study with comparison group. Pain 40(2): 183–194
Cox D J, Freundlich A, Meyer R G 1975 Differential effectiveness of electromyograph feedback, verbal relaxation instructions, and medication placebo with tension headache. Journal of Consulting and Clinical Psychology 43(6): 892–898
Craig K D, Weiss S M 1971 Vicarious influences on pain threshold determinations. Journal of Personality and Social Psychology 19(1): 53–59
Daut R L, Cleeland C S 1982 The prevalence and severity of pain in cancer. Cancer 50: 1913–1918
Davis P S 1988 Changing nursing practice for more effective control of postoperative pain through a staff initiated programme. Nurse Education Today 8: 325–331
Davitz J R, Davitz L J 1981 Inferences of patients' pain and psychological distress: studies of nursing behaviors. Springer, New York
Department of Health 1989 Guide to The Misuse of Drugs Act 1971 and the Misuse of Drugs Regulations. DOH, Welsh Office, Scottish Office, London
Donovan M, Dillon P, McGuire L 1987 Incidence and characteristics of pain in a sample of medical surgical inpatients. Pain 30: 69–78
Dudley S R, Holm R 1984 Assessment of the pain experience in relation to selected nurse characteristics. Pain 18(2): 179–186
Edwards W T 1990 Optimizing opioid treatment of postoperative pain. Journal of Pain and Symptom Management 5(1 Suppl.): S24–S36
Fagerhaugh S Y, Strauss A 1977 Politics of pain management: staff–patient interactions. Addison-Wesley, California
Fields H L, Basbaum A I 1989 Endogenous pain control mechanisms. In: Wall P D, Melzack R (eds) Textbook of pain, 2nd edn. Churchill Livingstone, Edinburgh, ch 11, pp 206–217
Flor H, Fydrich T & Turk D C 1992 Efficacy of multidisciplinary pain treatment centers: a meta-analytic review. Pain 49(2): 221–230
Fordyce W E 1978 Learning processes in pain. In: Sternbach R A (ed) The psychology of pain. Raven Press, New York, pp 49–72
Gaston-Johansson F, Albert M, Fagan E, Zimmerman L 1990 Similarities in pain descriptors of four different ethnic-cultural groups. Journal of Pain and Symptom Management 5(2): 94–100
Gottlieb H, Strite L C, Koller R, Mardorsky A, Hockersmith V, Kleeman M, Wagner J 1977 Comprehensive rehabilitation of patients having chronic low back pain. Archives of Physical Rehabilitation 58: 101–108
Gourlay G K, Kowalski S R, Plummer J L et al 1990 The efficacy of transdermal fentanyl in the treatment of postoperative pain: a double-blind comparison of fentanyl and placebo systems. Pain 40(1): 21–28
Graham G P, Dent C M, Fairclough J A 1990 Low back pain: comparison of chiropractic and hospital outpatient treatment. British Medical Journal 300: 1647
Greenough C G 1990 Low back pain: comparison of chiropractic and hospital outpatient treatment. British Medical Journal 300:1648
Haldeman S 1989 Manipulation and massage for the relief of pain. In: Wall P D, Melzack R (eds) Textbook of pain, 2nd edn. Churchill Livingstone, Edinburgh, ch 69, pp 942–951
Halfens R, Evers G, Abu-Saad H 1990 Determinants of pain assessment by nurses. International Journal of Nursing Studies 27(1): 43–49
Harkins S W, Kwentus J, Price D D 1984 Pain and the elderly. In: Benedetti C, Chapman C R, Moricca G (eds) Advances in pain research and therapy, vol 7. Recent advances in the management of pain. Raven Press, New York, pp 103–121
Holm K, Cohen F, Dudas S, Medema P G, Allen B L 1989 Effect of personal pain experience on pain assessment. Image. Journal of Nursing Scholarship 21(2): 72–75
Horan J J, Layng F C, Pursell C H 1976 Preliminary study of effects of 'in vivo' emotive imagery on dental discomfort. Perceptual and Motor Skills 42: 105–106
Hoy A M 1989 Radiotherapy, chemotherapy and hormone therapy: treatment for pain. In: Wall P D, Melzack R (eds) Textbook of pain, 2nd edn. Churchill Livingstone, Edinburgh, ch 71, pp 966–978
International Association for the Study of Pain (IASP) 1986 Pain terms: a current list with definitions and notes on usage. Pain 27: S215–S221
International Association for the Study of Pain (IASP) 1991 Core curriculum for professional education in pain. IASP, Seattle
Jensen M P, Karoly P, Braver S 1986 The measurement of clinical pain intensity: a comparison of six methods. Pain 27: 117–126
Jensen M P, Karoly P O, Riordan E F, Bland F, Burns R S 1989 The subjective experience of acute pain: an assessment of the utility of 10 indices. Clinical Journal of Pain 5(2): 153–159
Jessup B A 1989 Relaxation and biofeedback. In: Wall P D, Melzack R (eds) Textbook of pain, 2nd edn. Churchill Livingstone, Edinburgh, ch 73, pp 989–1000
Keefe F J 1989 Behavioral measurement of pain. In: Chapman C R, Loeser J D (eds) Issues in pain measurement. Advances in pain research and therapy, vol 12. Raven Press, New York, ch 32, pp 405–424
Kramlinger K G, Swanson D W, Maruta T 1983 Are patients with chronic pain depressed? American Journal of Psychiatry 140(6): 747–749
Kremer E, Atkinson J H, Ignelzi R J 1981 Measurement of pain: patient preference does not confound pain measurement. Pain 10(2): 241–248
Kuhn S, Cooke K, Collins M, Jones J M, Mucklow J C 1990 Perceptions of pain relief after surgery. British Medical Journal 300: 1687–1690
Lander J 1990a Clinical judgements in pain management. Pain 42(4): 15–22
Lander J 1990b Fallacies and phobias about addiction and pain. British Journal of Addiction 85(6): 803–809
Latham J 1991 Pain control, 2nd edn. Austen Cornish/Lisa Sainsbury Foundation, London
Lehmann J F, de Lateur B J 1989 Ultrasound, shortwave, microwave, superficial heat and cold in the treatment of pain. In: Wall P D, Melzack R (eds) Textbook of pain, 2nd edn. Churchill Livingstone, Edinburgh, ch 68, pp 932–941
Lenburg C B, Glass H P, Davitz L J 1970 Inferences of pain and psychological distress II. In relation to the stage of the patient's illness and occupation of the perceiver. Nursing Research 19(5): 392–398
Levine J D, Gordon N C, Jones R T, Fields H L 1978 The mechanism of placebo analgesia. Lancet 2: 654–657
Levin R F, Malloy G B, Hyman R B 1987 Nursing management of postoperative pain: use of relaxation techniques with female cholecystectomy patients. Journal of Advanced Nursing 12: 463–472
Liebeskind J C, Melzack R 1987 The international pain foundation: meeting a need for education in pain management. Editorial. Pain 30: 1–2
Lutz L J, Lamer T J 1990 Management of postoperative pain: review of current techniques and methods. Mayo Clinic Proceedings 65(4): 584–596
McCaffery M 1972 Nursing management of the patient in pain. Lippincott, Philadelphia, P A
McCaffery M, Beebe A 1989 Pain: clinical manual for nursing practice. Mosby, St Louis, M O
Mason D J 1981 An investigation of the influence of selected factors on nurses' inferences of patients' suffering. International Journal of Nursing Studies 18(4): 251–259

Mather L, Mackie J 1983 The incidence of postoperative pain in children. Pain 15: 271–282
Meade T W, Dyer S, Browne W, Townsend J, Frank A O 1990 Low back pain of mechanical origin: randomised comparison of chiropractic and hospital outpatient treatment. British Medical Journal 300: 1431–1437
Meinhart N T, McCaffery M 1983 Pain: a nursing approach to assessment and analysis. Appleton-Century-Crofts, Norwalk
Melzack R 1987 The short-form McGill Pain Questionnaire. Pain 30: 191–197
Melzack R 1990 The tragedy of needless pain. Scientific American 262(2): 19–25
Melzack R, Casey K L 1968 Sensory, motivational, and central control determinants of pain: a new conceptual model. In: Kenshalo D R (ed) The skin senses. Thomas, Springfield, I L
Melzack R, Torgerson W S 1971 On the language of pain. Anesthesiology 34(1): 50–59
Melzack R, Wall P D 1965 Pain mechanisms: a new theory. Science 150: 971–979
Melzack R, Wall P D 1988 The challenge of pain, 2nd edn. Penguin, Harmondsworth
Melzack R, Wall P D, Ty T C 1982 Acute pain in an emergency clinic: latency of onset and descriptor patterns related to different injuries. Pain 14(1): 33–43
Misuse of drugs act 1971. HMSO, London
Moore R 1990 Ethnographic assessment of pain coping perceptions. Psychosomatic Medicine 52: 156–170
National Institutes of Health Consensus Development Conference 1987 The integrated approach to the management of pain. Journal of Pain and Symptom Management 2(1): 35–44
Orne M T, Dinges D F 1989 Hypnosis. In: Wall P D, Melzack R (eds) Textbook of pain, 2nd edn. Churchill Livingstone, Edinburgh, ch 77, pp 1021–1031
Owen H, McMillan V, Rogowski D 1990 Postoperative pain therapy: a survey of patients' expectations and their experiences. Pain 41(3): 303–307
Patel M, Gutzwiller F, Marazzi A 1989 A meta-analysis of acupuncture for chronic pain. International Journal of Epidemiology 18(4): 900–906
Paul G L, Trimble R W 1970 Recorded vs. 'live' relaxation training and hypnotic suggestion: comparative effectiveness for reducing physiological arousal and inhibiting stress response. Behavior Therapy 1: 285–302
Peck C L 1986 Psychological factors in acute pain management. In: Cousins M J, Phillips G D (eds) Acute pain management. Churchill Livingstone, Edinburgh, ch 10, pp 251–274
Perry S, Heidrich G 1982 Management of pain during debridement: a survey of US burn units. Pain 13: 267–280
Philips H C 1988 Changing chronic pain experience. Pain 32(2): 165–172
Pitts M, Healey S 1989 Factors influencing the inferences of pain made by three health professions. Physiotherapy Practice 5: 65–68
Portenoy R K 1990 Chronic opioid therapy in non-malignant pain. Journal of Pain and Symptom Management 5(suppl 1): 546–562
Porter J, Jick H 1980 Addiction rare in patients treated with narcotics. New England Journal of Medicine 302(2):123
Raiman J 1987 Pain. In: Collins S, Parker E (eds) Essentials of nursing, 2nd edn. Macmillan, London, ch 5, pp 70–90
Ready L B 1989 Acute pain services: an academic asset. Clinical Journal of Pain 5 (suppl 1): S28–33
Ready L B, Oden R, Chadwick H S, Benedetti C, Rooke G A, Caplan R, Wild L M 1988 Development of an anesthesiology-based postoperative pain management service. Anesthesiology 68(1): 100–106
Rogers R C, Spector H J 1989 Aids to clinical pharmacology, 2nd edn. Churchill Livingstone, Edinburgh
Rowat K M, Jeans M E 1989 A collaborative model of care: patient, family and health care professionals. In: Wall P D, Melzack R (eds) Textbook of pain, 2nd edn. Churchill Livingstone, Edinburgh, ch 75, pp 1010–1014
Royal College of Surgeons and College of Anaesthetists 1990 Commission on the provision of surgical services. Report of the working party on pain after surgery. Royal College of Surgeons, London
Saunders C 1976 Care of the dying, 2nd edn. Macmillan/Nursing Times, London
Schug S A, Zech D, Dorr U 1990 Cancer pain management according to WHO analgesic guidelines. Journal of Pain and Symptom Management 5(1): 27–32
Scott J F 1989 Carcinoma invading nerve. In: Wall P D, Melzack R (eds) Textbook of pain, 2nd edn. Churchill Livingstone, Edinburgh, ch 42, pp 598–609
Seers C J 1987 Pain, anxiety and recovery in patients undergoing surgery. Unpublished PhD thesis, University of London
Seers K 1989 Patients' perceptions of acute pain. In: Wilson-Barnett J, Robinson S (eds) Directions in nursing research: ten years of progress at London University. Scutari, London, ch 12, pp 107–116
Seers K 1990 Early discharge after surgery: its effects on patients, their informal carers and on the workload of health professionals. Daphne Heald Research Unit Report, Royal College of Nursing, London
Sims S E 1987 Relaxation training as a technique for helping patients cope with the experience of cancer: a selective review of the literature. Journal of Advanced Nursing 12(5): 583–591
Skinner J B, Erskine A, Pearce S, Rubenstein I, Taylor M, Foster C 1990 The evaluation of a cognitive behavioural treatment programme in outpatients with chronic pain. Journal of Psychosomatic Research 34(1): 13–19
Sofaer B 1984 Pain: a handbook for nurses. Harper & Row, London
Sofaer B 1985 Pain management through nurse education. In: Copp L A (ed) Perspectives on pain. Recent advances in nursing 11. Churchill Livingstone, Edinburgh, ch 5, pp 62–74
Sriwatanakul K, Kelvie W, Lasagna L 1982 The quantification of pain: an analysis of words used to describe pain and analgesia in clinical trials. Clinical Pharmacology and Therapeutics 32(2): 143–148
Sternbach R A 1989 Acute versus chronic pain. In: Wall P D, Melzack R (eds) Textbook of pain, 2nd edn. Churchill Livingstone, Edinburgh, ch 14, pp 242–246
Stjernsward J, Teoh N 1990 The scope of the cancer pain problem. In: Foley K M, Bonica J J, Ventafridda V (eds) Advances in pain research and therapy, vol 16. Raven Press, New York, pp 7–12
Storey P, Hill H H, St Louis R H, Tarver E E 1990 Subcutaneous infusions for control of cancer symptoms. Journal of Pain and Symptom Management 5(1): 33–41
Suls J, Wan C K 1989 Effects of sensory and procedural information on coping with stressful medical procedures and pain: a meta-analysis. Journal of Consulting and Clinical Psychology 57(3): 372–379
Sunshine A, Olson N Z 1989 Non-narcotic analgesics. In: Wall P D, Melzack R (eds) Textbook of pain, 2nd edn. Churchill Livingstone, Edinburgh, ch 47, pp 670–685
Swinford P 1987 Relaxation and positive imagery for the surgical patient: a research study. Perioperative Nursing Quarterly 3(3): 9–16
Tanner J 1987 Beating back pain: a practical self-help guide to prevention and treatment. Dorling Kindersley, London
Taylor A G, Lorentzen L J, Blank M B 1990 Psychological distress of chronic pain sufferers and their spouses. Journal of Pain and Symptom Management 5(1): 6–10
Taylor A G, Skelton J A, Butcher J 1984 Duration of pain condition and physical pathology as determinants of nurses' assessments of patients in pain. Nursing Research 33(1): 4–8
Teske K, Daut R L, Cleeland C S 1983 Relationships between nurses' observations and patients' self reports of pain. Pain 16(3): 289–296
Turk D C 1989 Assessment of pain: the elusiveness of latent constructs. In: Chapman C R, Loeser J D (eds) Issues in pain measurement. Advances in pain research and therapy, vol 12. Raven Press, New York, ch 22, pp 267–279
Turk D C, Meichenbaum D H 1989 A cognitive — behavioural approach to pain. In: Wall P D, Melzack R (eds) Textbook of pain, 2nd edn. Churchill Livingstone, Edinburgh, ch 74, pp 1001–1009
UKCC 1992 Standards for the administration of medicines. United Kingdom Central Council for Nursing, Midwifery and Health Visiting, London
Wade J B, Price D D, Hamer R M, Schwartz S M, Hart R P 1990 An emotional component analysis of chronic pain. Pain 40(3): 303–310

Wall P D 1979 On the relation of injury to pain. Pain 6(3): 253–264
Wall P D 1989a Introduction. In: Wall P D, Melzack R (eds) Textbook of pain, 2nd edn. Churchill Livingstone, Edinburgh, pp 1–18
Wall P D 1989b The dorsal horn. In: Wall P D, Melzack R (eds) Textbook of pain, 2nd edn. Churchill Livingstone, Edinburgh, ch 5, pp 102–111
Weis O F, Sriwatanakul K, Alloza J L, Weintraub M, Lasagna L 1983 Attitudes of patients, housestaff, and nurses toward postoperative analgesic care. Anaesthesia and Analgesia 62: 70–74
Willis W D 1985 The pain system: the neural basis of nociceptive transmission in the mammalian nervous system. Pain and Headache, vol 8. Karger, Basel
Willis W D 1989 The origin and destination of pathways involved in pain transmission. In: Wall P D, Melzack R (eds) Textbook of pain, 2nd edn. Churchill Livingstone, Edinburgh, ch 6, pp 112–127
Woolf C J 1989 Segmental afferent fibre-induced analgesia: transcutaneous electrical nerve stimulation (TENS) and vibration. In: Wall P D, Melzack R (eds) Textbook of pain, 2nd edn. Churchill Livingstone, Edinburgh, ch 63, pp 884–896
World Health Organization 1986 Cancer pain relief. WHO, Geneva
Zborowski M 1952 Cultural components in response to pain. Journal of Social Issues 8(4): 16–30
Zola I K 1973 Pathways to the doctor: from person to patient. Social Science and Medicine 7: 677–689

FURTHER READING

Benson H, Klipper M Z 1975 The relaxation response. Collins, London
Bernstein D A, Borkovec T D 1973 Progressive relaxation training: a manual for the helping professions. Research Press, Champaign
Broome A, Jellicoe H 1987 Living with your pain. British Psychological Society / Methuen, Leicester
Gingell J 1988 A safety net when experts fail. Action Group for the Relief of Pain and Distress, Bristol
Goldfield M R, Davison G C 1976 Clinical behaviour therapy. Holt Rinehart & Wilson, New York, Ch. 5, pp 81–111
Hewitt J 1982 The complete relaxation book. Rider, London
Melzack R, Casey K L 1968 Sensory, motivational and central control determinants of pain: a new conceptual model. In: Kenshalo D R (ed) The skin senses. Thomas, Springfield, Illinois
Shore N 1992 Coping successfully with pain. Sheldon Press, London
Sternbach R A 1987 Mastering pain. A twelve-step regimen for coping with chronic pain. Arlington, London
Tanner J 1987 Beating back pain: a practical self-help guide to prevention and treatment. Dorling Kindersley, London
Thomas V 1989 Predicting PCA. Nursing Standard 3(18): 34–35
Wright S M 1987 The use of therapeutic touch in the management of pain. Nursing Clinics of North America 22(3): 705–714
Wyatt G, Dimmer S 1988 The balancing touch. Nursing Times 84(21): 41–42

USEFUL ADDRESSES

The British Migraine Association
178a High Road
Byfleet
Weybridge
Surrey KT14 7ED

The National Back Pain Association
31–33 Park Road
Teddington
Middlesex TW11 OAB

Self-help in pain groups (SHIP)
c/o Room 27
Walton Hospital
Liverpool L9 1AE

CHAPTER 20

Fluid and electrolyte balance

Mary Gobbi Colin Torrance

CHAPTER CONTENTS

Introduction 637

Body water 638
Fluid compartments 638
Solutes and electrolytes 638
Fluid exchange 639
Oedema 639

Water and electrolyte homeostasis 640
Regulation of ECF volume, osmolality and sodium 640
Regulation of ECF volume and sodium 641

Disorders of water and sodium balance 641
Fluid volume deficit 641
Fluid volume excess 643
Fluid volume adjustments 643

The electrolytes 644
Sodium 644
Chloride 644
Potassium 645
Calcium 646

Acid-base balance 647
Acidosis and alkalosis 648
Buffers 648
Handling blood gases 649
The acidotic/alkalotic states 649

Nursing considerations in maintaining fluid and electrolyte balance 650
Assessment 650
Monitoring 651
Managing fluid and electrolyte therapy 651

Problems associated with disorders of fluid and electrolyte balance 653
Gastrointestinal disorders 653
Special needs of the patient undergoing surgery 655

References 655

Further reading 655

INTRODUCTION

Monitoring and manipulating body fluid and electrolytes is an important aspect of nursing care. For the average male, only about 18% of the body weight is protein (with 15% fat and 7% minerals); 60% is water. For health, body water and electrolytes must be maintained within a limited range of tolerances. Homeostatic mechanisms regulate parameters such as body fluid volume, pH, and electrolyte concentrations, maintaining a delicate, dynamic balance which can be destabilised during illness. In extreme cases the fluid or electrolyte deficit can lead to death, and nurses need to be able to assess fluid and electrolyte status, to recognise deterioration, and to implement corrective interventions.

Nurses need a clear understanding of fluid and electrolyte homeostasis. Nursing interventions in relation to fluid therapy may range from encouraging the patient to drink his afternoon cup of tea to managing a complicated intravenous fluid regime. Ill-defined terms such as 'restrict fluids' or 'push fluids' and instructions to record fluid intake/output or daily weight are commonly encountered, but without a knowledgeable appreciation of the physiology and pathophysiology of fluid and electrolyte balance there is a real risk that these tasks will be performed in a somewhat mechanical fashion, without sufficient thought.

This chapter will review the normal mechanisms which regulate body fluid and outline some of the basic adaptive responses to stress. The regulation of acid–base balance will also be considered, along with basic principles in the management of fluid and electrolyte disorders. Throughout the chapter typical clinical situations where fluid and electrolyte control may be embarrassed are reviewed.

Students who are unfamiliar with the physiology of fluid, electrolyte and acid–base balance are advised to read this chapter in conjunction with their physiology textbook. It is important for the reader to be familiar with units and terms such as 'moles', 'molality', 'equivalents', 'diffusion', 'osmosis', 'osmoles', 'osmolality', 'tonicity' and 'filtration'.

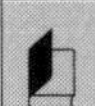

For more detailed information, see Smith & Kinsey (1991) and Timberlake (1988).

Nursing goals in the care of patients with existing or potential fluid and electrolyte problems include:

- the promotion and maintenance of a healthy pattern of fluid intake/output appropriate to the patient's lifestyle and wishes
- the detection of existing or potential fluid and electrolyte imbalances

- the re-establishment of fluid and electrolyte balance when homeostasis is disturbed
- the development of educational programmes on the maintenance of fluid and electrolyte balance.

It is hoped that this chapter will provide some of the essential background knowledge necessary to achieving these aims.

BODY WATER

Water has a range of functions within the body which are essential to sustaining life and maintaining health. These include:

- giving form to body structures and cushioning the body from shock
- acting as a transport medium for nutrients, electrolytes, blood gases, metabolic wastes, heat, and electrical currents
- providing insulation
- aiding in the hydrolysis of food
- acting as a medium and reactant in chemical processes
- acting as a lubricant.

Body tissues contain varying proportions of water, ranging from 10% for fat to 83% for blood. A young 70 kg man of average build has a total body water (TBW) of about 63% of body weight, or 45 l. The percentage of body weight represented by the TBW varies from one individual to another, depending on factors such as age, sex and build. Fat contributes little towards TBW and is the main source of this variation. A 70 kg woman of average build would have a TBW of about 52% (36 l) due to the greater proportion of adipose tissue. In both sexes the percentage of body water tends to decrease with age. Lean tissue has a fairly constant water content of 71–72 ml/100 g, and if adipose tissue is disregarded as a non-functional storage tissue, then the TBW of the lean body mass is about 73%. As water makes up nearly ¾ of the body's active tissues, homeostatic regulation of body fluids is essential to normal function and health.

Fluid compartments

Body water is distributed between two major compartments: the intracellular fluid (ICF) and the extracellular fluid (ECF). The distinction between the two compartments is maintained by the selective permeability of cell membranes. The intracellular environment is not homogeneous but varies greatly between cell types. However, all cells can tolerate only a limited variation in the volume and composition of their ICF before function is disrupted.

The large proteins that are synthesised by the cell remain trapped inside, as they are too big to pass through the membrane. However, the membrane is freely permeable to water. Selective membrane transport processes regulate the distribution of electrolytes, and hence water, across the cell membrane. The ICF has been estimated to be approximately 40% of TBW, or about 28 l in a 70 kg male.

The ECF bathes and surrounds the cells, forming a relatively constant environment. It has a smaller volume than the ICF, accounting for about 20% of TBW (or 14 l), and can be divided into four sub-compartments:

- the extravascular fluid (interstitial or tissue fluid)
- inaccessible bone water (skeletal water)
- the intravascular fluid compartment (blood plasma)
- transcellular fluids.

Interstitial fluid includes lymph and accounts for about 15% or 10.5 l of TBW. Interstitial fluid is defined by two membranes: the cell membrane separates it from the ICF, and the capillary endothelium separates it from plasma. Interstitial fluid forms the interface and exchange route between the ICF and plasma. Plasma represents about 4% of body weight, or 3 l.

Transcellular fluids are specialised fluids which are separated from the ECF by an additional epithelial cell layer. They include:

- cerebrospinal fluid (CSF)
- aqueous and vitreous humour of the eye
- glandular secretions
- synovial fluid
- pleural fluid
- peritoneal fluid
- glandular secretions
- saliva and other gastrointestinal secretions
- respiratory tract fluid
- fluid within the urinary system.

Transcellular fluid volume is highly variable, and some transcellular fluids have a very high turnover. (In the gastrointestinal tract alone it can be greater than 20 l a day.) Some water is trapped in the deeper layers of bone; this is inaccessible and, because it does not readily exchange with the rest of the ECF, is difficult to measure. The relative contribution of each compartment is summarised in Box 20.1. In infants and children, although the actual ECF volume is much smaller than in adults, the ECF:ICF ratio is larger, i.e. the ECF represents a greater percentage of the TBW and fluid loss can rapidly lead to dehydration. The consequences of ECF losses from, for example, vomiting, sweating, or diarrhoea are potentially more serious in the infant than the adult.

Solutes and electrolytes

Body fluids cannot be equated simply with water, as they also contain dissolved substances or solutes as well as larger particles in suspension (colloids). Solutes may be complete molecules (non-electrolytes) or parts of molecules (electrolytes). Measures of body fluid volume such as the litre refer to the volume of water *and* its dissolved solutes. Glucose is a good example of a non-electrolyte. It dissolves in the body water but does not dissociate into component parts. An elec-

Box 20.1 Distribution of body water in the average young adult male (After Ebelman & Liebman 1959)

FLUID COMPARTMENT	PERCENTAGE OF TBW	
Intracellular fluid	**55**	
Extracellular fluid	**45**	
Extravascular fluid		20.0
Inaccessible bone water		15.0
Intravascular fluid		7.5
Transcellular fluid		2.5
	100	

Assuming that the individual's body contained 40 l of fluid, the average distribution would be as follows:

FLUID COMPARTMENT	VOLUME IN LITRES	
Intracellular fluid	**22**	
Extracellular fluid	**18**	
Extravascular fluid		9
Inaccessible bone water		6
Intravascular fluid		3
Transcellular fluid		1
	40	

trolyte, however, will dissociate in solution into its constituent ions. Sodium chloride provides the most important example of this. In solution, a molecule of sodium chloride dissociates into a positively charged sodium ion (cation) and a negatively charged chloride ion (anion). Sodium is the dominant cation in the ECF but smaller concentrations of potassium, magnesium and calcium ions are present. Chloride and bicarbonate are the major extracellular anions.

Inside the cell, potassium is the dominant cation. Lower concentrations of magnesium, calcium and sodium are also present. Intracellular anions include phosphate, sulphate and intracellular proteins which also behave as anions. The cell regulates the movement of ions across its membrane, and maintenance of an uneven distribution of ions between the ECF and ICF is essential for cell function, particularly in excitable tissues such as nerve and muscle.

Fluid exchange

Fluid exchange between ICF and ECF

The movement of body fluids and their constituents between the different compartments involves both active and passive transport processes. The main mechanisms which enable body fluids to enter the cell membrane are:

- diffusion
- facilitated diffusion
- voltage-gated channels
- ligand-gated channels
- active transport

(Guyton 1991, Ch. 4).

Lipid-soluble substances diffuse directly through the cell membrane while water and electrolytes utilise channels formed by membrane proteins. The membrane is freely permeable to water but is only selectively permeable to electrolytes. Permeability is affected by the size and charge of the hydrated ion; for example, the membrane is 50–100 times more permeable to K^+ than to Na^+. Movement into the cell via membrane proteins may be by simple diffusion, facilitated diffusion (carrier-mediated transport) and by active transport. Glucose, for example, enters the muscle cell by facilitated diffusion under the influence of insulin. The most important example of active transport is the sodium–potassium pump. This pump is a membrane protein that couples the active transport of Na^+ out of the cell with the active transport of K^+ inwards. It requires energy derived from the hydrolysis of ATP (adenosine 5′-triphosphate) to function.

Tissue–capillary fluid exchange

Just as the cell membrane separates the ICF from the ECF, the capillary wall represents the boundary between the intravascular and interstitial compartments of the ECF. The capillary wall is selectively permeable to substances of a molecular weight less than 69 000 and to lipid-soluble molecules. The exchange of water, electrolytes, metabolites and waste products between the plasma and interstitial fluid occurs at the capillary. Fluid movement is determined by three forces: diffusion, osmosis and filtration. The capillary endothelium is freely permeable to water and solutes but the larger plasma proteins are retained. At the arterial end of the capillary, fluid is forced out of the capillary by hydrostatic pressure. As water is lost from the capillary, the plasma proteins become more concentrated and the colloid osmotic or oncotic pressure exerted by the plasma proteins increases. (Oncotic pressure means osmotic pressure caused by the presence of colloids, that is, colloid osmotic pressure.) At the venous end the hydrostatic pressure is lower and the osmotic pressure draws fluid back into the capillary.

Because the capillary endothelium is a very imperfect barrier plasma proteins may leak into the interstitial fluid, complicating the situation described above. If these proteins were not removed, the oncotic pressure of the interstitial fluid would rise, disrupting capillary fluid exchange and favouring retention of water in the interstitial spaces. The lymphatic system is central to maintaining interstitial fluid volume. Blind-ended lymphatic capillaries in the interstitium are more permeable than the capillaries and easily uptake and remove plasma proteins and fluid from the interstitial space. The fluid formed in these vessels, lymph, is carried through the lymphatic system, eventually returning to the circulation via the central lymphatic and the thoracic duct.

As approximately 20% of body fluid is found in the interstitial or tissue spaces, the maintenance of fluid volume in this compartment plays a key role in homeostasis. Normally, a dynamic equilibrium exists which maintains the extracellular fluid content of both the plasma and the tissue spaces. However, this delicate balance can easily be disturbed by the following factors.

1. Alterations in capillary pressure. Changes in pressure at either end of the capillary will alter net movement of fluid. Increased arterial pressure or venous congestion will both tend to favour the loss of fluid to the interstitial space. Examples include hypertension, hypotension, heart failure, and arterial or venous obstruction.
2. Alterations in the plasma proteins. A reduction in plasma proteins due to malnutrition, liver or renal disease, loss of circulating plasma or leakage of proteins into the tissue fluids will alter the osmotic pressure gradient and prevent fluid being reclaimed from the tissue spaces. Failure of the lymphatics to remove this fluid will increase the osmotic pressure of the interstitial fluid and favour fluid retention.
3. Changes in the integrity of the capillary membranes. Factors which alter the normal mechanisms regulating the permeability/pore size of the capillary membranes also change the osmotic or hydrostatic pressures. These effects may be local or systemic. Examples include membrane damage from burns, anoxia, pressure, septicaemia and the presence of inflammatory mediators such as bradykinin or histamine.
4. Accumulation of metabolites. An accumulation of metabolites within the tissue fluid can alter the hydrostatic and colloidal osmotic pressures with consequent changes in fluid movement. For example, in some states of shock or tissue hypoxia the accumulative effects of lactic acid and carbon dioxide when combined with vasoactive substances may result in oedema.

Oedema

Oedema is an accumulation of fluid in the interstitial spaces or other sites such as the pericardial sac, between the pleura, in the peritoneal cavity or within the joint capsule. Oedema alters the natural turgor of the tissue spaces and may be noticed by swelling or distension. If the swollen tissue is indented by slight pressure it is called pitting oedema. In the case of blocked lymphatics, protein leakage from the capillaries is not reclaimed from the tissue fluid and the oedema so caused is firm due to the presence of the proteins and does not tend to pit — a characteristic sign of lymphoedema. Oedema may be localised (as in the case of inflammation and tissue damage) or generalised (as seen in heart failure).

General features

Oedema presents several problems to the patient. Its characteristic features may be described as follows:

- It accumulates in dependent areas, especially soft tissues
- It presents as swelling and distension which sometimes 'pits' under pressure
- It hinders the diffusion of gases and transport of nutrients and waste products
- The oedematous tissues lose integrity and are easily traumatised
- Tissues adjacent to the oedema may be damaged by the pressure.

Management

It is important to ascertain the cause(s) of the oedema before initiating any nursing actions.

> ? **20.1** Consider for a moment how the management of the following situations may be vastly different.
> a. oedema caused by a deep vein thrombosis
> b. oedema caused by a soft tissue injury
> c. oedema due to arterial insufficiency and the accumulation of metabolites liberated from hypoxic cells
> d. oedema due to protein loss
> e. oedema due to cardiac failure.

Consideration of the points listed below may enable a safe, effective plan of care to be initiated which is specific to the person concerned.

1. Identify the cause of the oedema and its appropriate management by liaising with medical staff and other health professionals (for example, physiotherapists may advise in the case of sports or orthopaedic problems)
2. Consider the use and effects of gravity, which may alter fluid drainage or blood flow
3. Monitor and record the extent and nature of the oedema. Communication between day and night staff may identify oedema due to the effects of gravity/position. For example, oedematous feet in the evening may appear to be resolved by a night in bed, only to be replaced in the morning by sacral or orbital oedema (recognised by puffy eyes)
4. Assess the effects of the oedema on local tissues and take appropriate action. For example, sacral oedema increases the risk of a pressure sore, and severe oedema of the fascia may restrict blood flow and lead to tissue hypoxia
5. Implement medical therapies with appropriate interventions, e.g. administration of diuretics
6. Be aware of the implications of specific types of oedema (e.g. pulmonary or cerebral) for a deterioration in the person's condition and initiate appropriate nursing assessment
7. Be aware that oedema may restrict movement, alter a person's self-image and cause practical difficulties in daily life. Ankle oedema may be exacerbated by tight-fitting shoes, whilst ascites may cause respiratory embarrassment and affect the body image. Attention to small details may greatly enhance the comfort of a person with oedema.

> ? **20.2** Why should one try to avoid giving injections in oedematous areas?

> ? **20.3** What advice could you give to an elderly person who suffers from persistent ankle oedema and who wishes to buy a new pair of shoes?

WATER AND ELECTROLYTE HOMEOSTASIS

Constancy of the internal environment is essential for efficient cell function. In health, the volume and composition of the different fluid compartments is finely regulated, with daily fluctuations in TBW of less than 0.2%. Water and electrolytes are ingested and absorbed through the gastrointestinal (GI) tract, although a small volume of water is produced through the oxidation of hydrogen in food. Excess water, electrolytes and waste products are excreted via the kidneys and in faeces. Additional water and salt loss occurs via the skin and respiratory tract.

Since losses from the GI and respiratory tracts are not subject to fine regulation, the kidney is the main regulator of fluid and electrolyte balance. Plasma represents about 4% of the body weight or only 3 l, but the glomerular filtration rate is 125 ml/min, or about 180 l a day. This means that the 3 l of plasma contained within the body is filtered and reabsorbed about 60 times a day! With such a large turnover the kidney can exert a major influence on plasma composition and, through plasma, on the composition of interstitial and — ultimately — intracellular fluid. Basal urine production in the absence of fluid ingestion is about 300 ml/day. The maximum rate seen in some disease states is 23 l/day, and a normal volume might be around about 2–2.5 l/day. The kidney regulates not only fluid volume but electrolyte composition, osmolality and pH. Central to the renal regulation of body fluid, osmolality, and volume is the kidney's role in the handling of sodium and water.

> ? **20.4** What would be the average daily water requirement of a 70 kg adult?

Regulation of ECF volume, osmolality* and sodium

Volume and osmolality regulation involves a series of homeostatic mechanisms which regulate the constancy of the ECF. Although the plasma compartment is small, it is dynamic, with shifts in volume and pressure occurring in response to internal and external stimuli. The rapid turnover of the plasma makes it the ideal target for regulatory mechanisms. Although plasma volume and osmolality are monitored, sodium is also a major factor in the regulation of ECF. Changes will also occur in the interstitial and intracellular fluid volumes, but these are usually slower than changes in plasma volume and the body can adapt to them with less functional disruption. The kidney regulates sodium and water ingestion/excretion under the influence of two hormones, aldosterone and vasopressin also known as antidiuretic hormone or ADH with additional input from the renin–angiotensin system and other factors.

Osmolality and ADH

Within the hypothalamus are specialised cells called osmoreceptors which monitor and respond to changes in plasma osmolality. They are very sensitive and respond to changes of as little as ±3 milliosmoles (mosmoles). Plasma osmolality is normally in the range of 280–290 mosmoles/kg water. The osmoreceptors respond to variations in plasma osmolality by stimulating two mechanisms: ADH release and thirst.

ADH acts on the epithelial cells of the nephron collecting ducts to increase tubular permeability to water and therefore water reabsorption. If a large volume of water is ingested the plasma sodium is diluted, causing a fall in the plasma osmolality. This fall is registered by the osmoreceptors, with a resultant decrease in ADH release. Lowered plasma ADH then

* The concentration of a solution defined in terms of the number of osmoles per kg of solvent; this is a measure of a solution's osmotic property.

results in decreased tubular permeability; less water is reabsorbed and water is excreted in the form of a more dilute urine. Conversely, if plasma osmolality is increased, for example after fluid loss or after the ingestion of excess salt, a higher plasma ADH results with an increased permeability of the collecting ducts, and water is absorbed to dilute the hypertonic plasma.

The presence of a non-absorbable solute in the tubular lumen will increase water loss. For example, when plasma glucose levels are raised (as in diabetes mellitus) and filtered glucose exceeds the ability of the nephrons to reabsorb it, urine production is increased. The glucose exerts an osmotic force, keeping water in the tubule. Osmotic diuresis can also be induced therapeutically by the i.v. administration of a non-absorbable molecule such as mannitol.

Other factors affecting ADH regulation of osmolality. ADH release may be altered by some drugs, including nicotine and alcohol. Alcohol inhibits the release of ADH, with a resulting diuresis. Nicotine, morphine and barbiturates are drugs which increase ADH release. Adrenal insufficiency alters the renal response to water loading. Deficiency in adrenal glucocorticoids causes an increase in distal tubular permeability to water. Water reabsorption is increased and dilute urine cannot be produced. Tubular response to ADH is decreased and even in the absence of ADH permeability to water remains high.

Regulation of ECF volume and sodium

ECF volume is principally determined by sodium, and body sodium is regulated by the kidney under the influence of aldosterone and other factors. Aldosterone is a mineralocorticoid essential for sodium (with associated water) reabsorption. It has a complex effect: it stimulates Na^+ reabsorption but is not the main regulator of Na^+ reabsorption. (Excess aldosterone production does not usually lead to excess sodium retention.) When aldosterone is lacking Na^+ reabsorption does not occur; this can rapidly lead to death from sodium and water depletion. Aldosterone is also important in hydrogen/potassium ion exchange in the kidney, and to the reabsorption of sodium in the gut and from sweat and the salivary glands. Aldosterone release is stimulated by plasma potassium concentration, plasma sodium concentration, and changes in ECF volume. Increases in serum potassium levels of as little as 0.1 mmol can cause a marked increase in aldosterone release.

However, hypovolaemia, which reflects a fall in sodium content (as opposed to concentration) will increase aldosterone secretion via the renin–angiotensin system. Changes in the effective circulating volume (that is, the blood volume actually perfusing the tissues, which may be less than the total blood volume) stimulate renin release.

Renin is a proteolytic enzyme released when sodium loss causes a drop in the effective circulating volume. Renin acts on a plasma protein called angiotensinogen, causing it to release angiotensin I. Angiotensin I is in turn split by a converting enzyme into angiotensin II. Angiotensin II has several actions:

- It is a potent vasoconstrictor
- It stimulates the release of aldosterone
- It increases the reabsorption of sodium by the proximal convoluted tubule
- It acts upon the hypothalamus, which then stimulates the thirst centre and increases ADH secretion.

DISORDERS OF WATER AND SODIUM BALANCE

Water volume and sodium imbalances frequently occur in combination with other electrolyte problems, although occasionally they occur alone. Principal causes of disturbance can be related to insufficient or excessive intake or output, problems in the regulation of intake and output, or problems related to fluid shifts within the body. To begin with, we will consider the effects of water deprivation (dehydration) and excessive intake (water overload).

Fluid volume deficit (see Boxes 20.2 and 20.3)

An ECF volume deficit will arise when water loss exceeds water intake. Insufficiency of intake may be related to a number of factors. For example, a patient may be reluctant to swallow because of oral or pharyngeal pain and so may take in less fluid and food. Depressed, anorexic, nauseous, or fatigued patients may also fail to take in adequate fluid. Patients suffering from neuromuscular impairment, or who are unconscious will have an impaired ability to swallow and thus will also be prone to fluid volume deficit.

Dehydration

Strictly speaking, dehydration refers only to water losses from the body which exceed intake, leaving the person with a corresponding accumulation of sodium (hypernatraemic dehydration). However, 'free water' losses are unusual and it is more common for water to be lost in conjunction with sodium and/or in its role as the biological solvent. Dehydration may thus be isotonic, hypernatraemic or hyponatraemic with respect to the extracellular fluid. Isotonic dehydration occurs when the fluid lost is isotonic with the ECF in respect to the water and sodium content, whilst in hyponatraemic dehydration the sodium losses exceed the water losses.

Water-only depletion causes a volume deficit in the ECF. Sodium concentration is increased (hypernatraemic dehydration) with a consequent rise in osmolality and haematocrit (PCV, see Appendix 2). If the dehydration is not resolved, the cells will ultimately become dehydrated. Compensatory mechanisms initially maintain blood pressure, heart rate and haematocrit, but as the dehydration continues blood pressure falls, pulse volume weakens, and heart rate and haematocrit rise. Haemoconcentration also causes apparent rises in haemoglobin and albumin levels. Eventually the person will be unable to meet the obligatory volume necessary to excrete waste products in the urine. The sequelae of this — metabolite accumulation, acidosis, renal failure, and toxaemia — may lead to death.

Dehydration can be assessed according to the approximate percentage of body water that is lost; in the adult this may be defined as follows:

- mild: 4% (3 l)
- moderate: 5–8% (4–6 l)
- severe: 8–10% (7 l).

Management of dehydration is often complex, especially in severe states where there is gross derangement of body chemistry. In mild to moderate dehydration, fluid losses should be replaced slowly to prevent sudden shifts of water and/or electrolytes between fluid compartments which would aggravate ionic balance. However, as severe dehydration (as seen in diabetes insipidus) may lead to fatal hypovolaemia aggressive therapy is required. The effects of hyponatraemia and hypernatraemia which may accompany dehydration will be discussed later (see p. 644).

Gastrointestinal losses

Within the gastrointestinal tract there is a continuous exchange of fluids, with most of the fluid produced being absorbed. Illnesses which present with diarrhoea or vomiting, or conditions in which fistulas, drainage tubes or GI suction are involved, can result in excessive fluid volume losses (potentially up to about 8–9 l/day). Continuous GI or fistula

Box 20.2 Causes of fluid volume deficit and excess (Adapted with kind permission from Porth 1990)

FLUID DEFICIT

1. Inadequate fluid intake:
   - Unconsciousness, inability to express thirst, inability to gain access to fluids
   - Oral trauma or dysphasia
   - Impaired thirst mechanism
   - Withholding of fluids for therapeutic reasons
   - Anorexia
   - Nausea
   - Depression
2. Excessive fluid losses:
   - Gastrointestinal losses:
     — Vomiting
     — Diarrhoea
     — Laxative abuse
     — Gastrointestinal suction
     — Fistula drainage
   - Urine losses:
     — Diuretic therapy
     — Osmotic diuresis (hyperglycaemia)
     — Adrenal insufficiency
     — Salt wasting renal disease
     — Polyuria due to diabetes insipidus
   - Skin losses:
     — Fever
     — Exposure to hot environments
     — Burns and wounds that remove skin
3. Third space losses (Na^+ & H_2O):
   - Intestinal obstruction
   - Oedema
   - Ascites
   - Burns (especially in first few days)

FLUID EXCESS

1. Excessive sodium and water intake:
   - Excessive dietary intake
   - Excessive administration of sodium-containing i.v. fluids
   - Excessive ingestion of sodium-containing foods or medications
2. Inadequate renal losses:
   - Renal disease
   - Congestive heart failure
   - Cirrhosis of the liver
   - Increased corticosteroid levels:
     — Glucocorticoids (Cushing's syndrome)
     — Hyperaldosteronism

Box 20.3 Signs and symptoms of fluid volume deficit and excess (Adapted with kind permission from Porth 1990)

FLUID DEFICIT

1. Thirst
2. Acute weight loss:
   - Mild extracellular deficit: 2% loss
   - Moderate extracellular deficit: 2–5% loss
   - Severe extracellular deficit: 6% or more
3. Alteration in renal function:
   - Decreased urine output
   - Increased urine osmolality in specific gravity
4. Alteration in cardiovascular function:
   - Increased serum osmolality
   - Increased haematocrit
   - Increased BUN (blood urea nitrogen)
   - Decreased vascular volume
   - Tachycardia
   - Weak and thready pulse
   - Postural hypotension
   - Decreased vein filling and increased vein refill time
   - Hypertension and shock
5. Other:
   - Loss of intercellular fluid
   - Dry skin and mucous membrane
   - Cracked and fissured tongue
   - Decreased salivation and lacrimination
   - Neuromuscular weakness
   - Fatigue
   - Increased body temperature

FLUID EXCESS

1. Acute weight gain: in excess of 5% body weight
2. Alteration in cardiovascular function:
   - Full and bounding pulse
   - Venous distension
   - Increased ECF
   - Pitting oedema
   - Puffy eyelids
3. Alteration in respiratory function:
   - Pulmonary oedema
   - Shortness of breath
   - Râles
   - Dyspnoea
   - Cough

drainage will have the same consequences for a patient as severe diarrhoea and vomiting.

Urinary loss

Patients who have incurred head injury, who have undergone hypophysectomy (see Ch. 5, p. 139) or who have a primary diagnosis of diabetes insipidus may excrete excessive volumes of water and electrolytes. This results from a disruption to the hypothalamo-pituitary release of AVP. Diabetes insipidus occurs when there is either a deficiency in the manufacture and release of AVP, or an inability of the kidney to respond to AVP. AVP deficiency and its consequences are discussed in Chapter 5 (p. 142).

Osmotic diuresis

In osmotic diuresis, polyuria results from the presence of large quantities of solutes in the blood which enter the glomerular filtrate and are not reabsorbed. The high osmolality produced in the renal tubules inhibits the action of AVP and prevents reabsorption of water. This principle can be used to produce an osmotic diuresis therapeutically; for example, mannitol can be administered to reduce intracranial pressure.

Osmotic diuresis will occur in the following circumstances:

1. When the production of large particles exceeds the body's ability to reabsorb or excrete them. Classic examples are glucose excess in diabetes and urea excess in renal failure
2. When solutes which can be filtered by the kidney are not reabsorbed (e.g. when mannitol and polysaccharides are administered)
3. When substances are infused beyond the capacity of the nephron to reabsorb them (e.g. sodium chloride and urea).

Skin losses

The loss of sodium and water from the skin increases dramatically during excessive sweating or if large areas of the skin have been damaged. For example, in extreme hot weather as much as 1.5–2.0 l/h can be lost through sweat. In the patient with fever, water loss may be up to 3 l/24 h. Burns patients suffer excessive fluid losses; evaporation losses may be from 0.8–2.6 ml/kg for each percentage point of burn area (Porth 1989). Total loss from burns can be as much as 6–8 l/24 h.

Third space losses

The concept of the 'third space' is used to describe the presence of fluids in areas of the body where they are usually absent or present only in small quantities, for example the peritoneal cavity. Although not lost from the body, the fluid is physiologically unavailable and thus many of the effects of fluid loss may be produced. Whilst the total body weight may remain constant with no net change in body water, the distribution of fluid within the body may be altered. The difficulty in ascertaining the actual problem experienced by a patient is illustrated by the following example. Reduced urinary output is observed in a patient who has just received an opiate to relieve postoperative pain. Possible causes for this reduction are:

- administration of the opiate
- pain and related stress factors
- surgical losses and exposure in theatre
- inadequate fluid replacement therapy
- impaired renal function due to renal disease or diabetes
- a blocked urinary catheter or urine retention.

Whilst diagnosis is the physician's role, astute nursing assessment and implementation of a sound plan of care for such a patient may prevent or anticipate likely problems in relation to the patient's fluid and electrolyte balance.

?	**20.5** What might be the significance of a patient complaining of being very thirsty?

Fluid volume excess (see Boxes 20.2 and 20.3)

The retention of fluid results in a fluid volume excess. Such an imbalance can be caused by overloading with fluids or by reduced functioning of the body's homeostatic mechanisms responsible for maintaining fluid and electrolyte balance. Circulatory overload is a condition associated with an increase in the intravascular blood volume. It is most often observed during the administration of i.v. fluids or in blood transfusion, especially if the amount or rate of the administration is excessive. Isotonic fluids such as 0.9% sodium chloride (normal saline) or Ringer's lactate contain large amounts of sodium, e.g. in Ringer's lactate the sodium content is 131 mmol/l. With some patients, for example those who are elderly or who have a history of heart disease, careful attention needs to be paid to i.v. fluid therapy. Other sources of sodium gain include some proprietary drugs (e.g. Alka Seltzer) or the frequent use of hypertonic enemas.

Effects of drinking large amounts of hypotonic fluid, e.g. water. When a large volume of water is ingested it begins to be absorbed within about 15 min, in consequence of which the osmolality of the blood decreases. This causes an inhibition of the production and secretion of AVP. Absence of AVP makes the distal convoluted tubule and collecting duct impermeable to water and so more urine is excreted in the kidney, thus producing a more dilute urine and a water diuresis. Following a single large intake of oral fluid the maximum effect upon diuresis will be noticed about 40 min later. A similar effect is achieved if a bolus or fluid challenge of i.v. fluid is administered.

Water intoxication. The kidney has a maximum rate at which it can excrete fluid. If water (or hypotonic i.v. fluid) ingestion exceeds this capacity, then the extracellular fluid remains hypotonic. The hypotonic ECF results in fluid moving into the ICF, with a subsequent swelling and bursting of cells. In the brain this is most serious, causing raised intracranial pressure, convulsions and death.

Fluid volume adjustments

Chapter 2 described how the circulatory system comprises the arterial system of high pressure and low volume and the venous system which operates with a lower pressure and higher volume. Approximately 55% of the plasma volume is in the venous system, 10% in the arterial system and the remaining 35% distributed in the heart, lungs and capillaries. Thus changes in volume are usually accommodated by the venous system. The effects of gravity upon fluid in the circulatory system is marked, causing pooling of blood in the venous system with a consequent reduction in the arterial blood volume. If an individual stands for a prolonged period, particularly in a warm environment, there is a reduction in arterial flow to the cells; inadequate venous return then leads to a fall in end diastolic volume and hence cardiac output. Inadequate perfusion of the brain can then lead to fainting.

The tissue spaces can accommodate large volumes of fluid, but the process is slow and causes less disturbances to the ICF or plasma. Adults can usually tolerate changes of about 2 l in the tissue spaces before there are noticeable signs of a volume shift. This 'hidden' accumulation of fluid may, however, be noticed by changes in body weight, based on 1 kg being equivalent to 1 l of water.

THE ELECTROLYTES

Sodium

Sodium is a major cation found in the extracellular fluid, and its concentration is maintained within the range 135–145 mmol/l. Its importance for a number of body functions is related to its role in maintaining the osmolality of extracellular fluids, normal muscular functioning, acid–base balance, and a number of other chemical reactions. While hyper- or hyponatraemia usually indicates changes in body water content rather than the intake of sodium, it is not unknown for individuals to have bizarre eating habits and thus become hypernatraemic. Furthermore, as sodium is the main extracellular cation, addition of substances to the plasma may cause a dilution effect rather than an actual loss of sodium. For example, serum sodium may appear to have fallen when glucose levels suddenly rise either due to hyperalimentation or in diabetes mellitus. Sodium losses may occur from the GI tract, kidney, skin, or traumatised limbs.

Normally, the kidneys are extremely efficient in controlling sodium when the intake is reduced. Hyponatraemia, i.e. sodium depletion in the extracellular fluids, is defined as a sodium concentration in the blood of less than 135 mmol/l. The loss of sodium from the ECF is usually as a result of excessive fluid loss and not from a deficit in intake. Signs and symptoms and causes of sodium imbalance are listed in Boxes 20.4 and 20.5.

Chloride

Chloride is ingested either with sodium or as potassium chloride. Normal daily intake is about 70–120 mmol, and the minimum requirement 75 mmol. Chloride output is via sweat (15 mmol/l), gastric juice (90–150 mmol/l) and other intestinal secretions (50–100 mmol/l). Renal excretion is in conjunction with ammonia (NH_4Cl) and occurs mainly in the proximal tubule. Reabsorption occurs in the ascending limb and is passively linked with Na reabsorption. Cl^- reabsorption is

Box 20.4 Signs and symptoms of sodium imbalance (Adapted with kind permission from Porth 1990)

HYPONATRAEMIA

- Serum sodium < 137 mmol/l
- Decreased serum osmolality
- Dilution of other blood components, eg. haematocrit, BUN (blood urea nitrogen)
- Increased water content of brain and nerve cells
- Headache
- Mental depression
- Personality changes
- Confusion
- Apprehension
- Lethargy, weakness
- Stupor
- Coma
- Convulsions
- Gastrointestinal disturbances
- Anorexia, nausea and vomiting
- Abdominal cramps
- Increased ICF
- Fingerprinting over the sternum

HYPERNATRAEMIA

- Serum Na^+ > 147 mmol/l
- Increased serum osmolality
- Thirst
- Oliguria or anuria
- High specific gravity of urine
- Intracellular dehydration
- Skin dry and flushed
- Mucous membranes dry and sticky
- Tongue rough and dry
- Subcutaneous tissue firm and rubbery
- Agitation and restlessness
- Decreased reflexes
- Manical behaviour
- Convulsions and coma
- Change in body temperature
- Decreased vascular volume
- Tachycardia, decreased blood pressure
- Weak and thready pulse

Box 20.5 Causes of sodium imbalance (Adapted with kind permission from Porth 1990)

HYPONATRAEMIA

1. Excess sodium loss:
   - Sweating
   - Gastrointestinal losses
   - Diuresis
2. Sodium dilution:
   - Overinfusion of sodium-free i.v. solutions
   - Psychogenic polydipsia
   - Ingestion of tap water during periods of sodium restriction
   - Repeated use of tap water enemas
3. Hormone-induced water gains:
   - SIADH (syndrome of inappropriate ADH secretion)
   - AVP (ADH) agonists (e.g. oxytocin)

HYPERNATRAEMIA

1. Excessive sodium intake:
   - Rapid or excessive parenteral infusion of sodium chloride or sodium bicarbonate
   - Excessive oral intake
2. Decreased extracellular water:
   - Increased insensible water loss, e.g. burns, diaphoresis, hyperventilation
   - Water diarrhoea
   - Hypertonic tube feeds
3. Water deprivation
   Unconscious, debilitated patient (thirst excess)
4. Diabetes insipidus
   - Tracheobronchitis
5. Decreased water intake:
   - Unconsciousness or inability to express thirst
   - Oral trauma or inability to swallow
   - The withholding of water for therapeutic reasons

inversely linked to bicarbonate. As Cl^- is linked to Na^+ reabsorption, aldosterone is an indirect regulator.

Potassium

Potassium (K) is the major intracellular cation. The body contains 2900–3500 mmol of potassium, of which 98% is intracellular and 2% in the ECF. The intracellular potassium level is approximately 150 mmol/l, as compared with a plasma concentration of 3.5–4.8 mmol/l. Of the body's potassium, 90% is exchangeable while the remaining 10% is bound (mainly in the red blood cells). Men have about 45 mmol/kg body weight and women about 37 mmol/kg body weight of exchangeable K. The total body K declines significantly with increasing age in both sexes. Potassium continually leaks out of the cells but a high intracellular level is maintained by the sodium–potassium pump. Although extracellular K is low, both intracellular and extracellular K are essential for normal physiological function.

As the muscle cell membrane potential is largely a function of the ratio of intracellular K^+ to extracellular K^+, any alteration of this ratio can adversely effect neuromuscular function. The low ECF potassium means that large changes can occur in total body potassium without a significant effect on plasma K^+.

Potassium is acquired through the diet. Although the potassium content of food varies widely, any diet providing sufficient energy will invariably supply more than enough K, and a normal intake would be 40–200 mmol a day. Potassium is not as well conserved by the kidney as sodium and the minimum daily K loss is about 40 mmol: obligatory losses are between 15–20 mmol from the gastrointestinal tract and skin and 10–20 mmol in urine. Dietary K is usually sufficient to cover the individual's needs but additional potassium may be required during trauma and stress. Potassium excretion is regulated mainly by the kidney, and plasma K^+ levels are regulated by both renal mechanisms and by shifts between the intracellular and extracellular compartments. Although only small amounts are normally lost through the gastrointestinal tract, diarrhoea and vomiting can quickly lead to potassium imbalances.

Box 20.6 outlines some other factors influencing potassium levels. Signs and symptoms of potassium imbalance are listed in Box 20.7. Potassium cannot be conserved by the body, and so a daily intake is required. In the proximal tubule 80–90% of filtered potassium is reabsorbed; this is essentially an obligatory process little influenced by regulatory factors. Renal regulation of potassium excretion occurs in the distal tubule and collecting duct. Aldosterone is the regulatory hormone for potassium ions. A rise in plasma K^+ concentration increases aldosterone secretion, resulting in increased potassium excretion; a fall in plasma K^+ decreases aldosterone secretion.

Hyperkalaemia

Body regulation of potassium is geared mainly towards management of hyperkalaemic states, with general excretion occurring via the colon and kidney, whilst serum levels are also influenced by the catecholamines, the pancreatic hormones (insulin and glucagon) and by acid–base states. Due to the cation exchange mechanism which operates in the regulation of acid–base balance, potassium secretion is increased by the nephron in alkalotic states and decreased in acidosis. For example, in metabolic alkalosis the potassium levels rise in the ICF to compensate for hydrogen ion loss. Potassium levels are thus high in the nephron and so potassium is excreted with a resultant total body loss of potassium.

Changes in serum potassium levels tend to reflect either total body changes of potassium or movement of potassium from one fluid compartment to another. Potassium levels are interrelated with sodium and body water levels. This relationship is disturbed by illness, especially if cell membrane function is disrupted. Cell membrane function is itself very susceptible to changes in potassium concentrations; even small alterations affect membrane excitation, with potentially dire consequences for cardiac tissue. In diabetes mellitus, the administration of insulin causes potassium to enter the cells with glucose in a cotransporter system, leading to a fall in serum potassium. Thus potassium depletion decreases insulin secretion, with the cells having a lower tolerance to glucose. This action of insulin can be utilised in the management of

Box 20.6 Factors associated with potassium imbalance (Adapted with kind permission from Porth 1990)

HYPOKALAEMIA

1. Inadequate intake:
   - Inability to eat/debilitation
   - Potassium deficient diet
   - Administration of potassium-free massive parenteral solutions
   - Anorexia
   - Alcoholism
2. Excessive gastrointestinal losses:
   - Vomiting
   - Diarrhoea
   - Prolonged gastric suction
   - Fistula drainage
   - Laxative abuse
3. Excessive renal losses
   - Diuretic phase of renal failure
   - Diuretic therapy
   - Increased mineralocorticoid levels
   - Cushing's syndrome
   - Primary aldosteronism
   - Treatment with glucocorticoid hormones
4. Intercellular shift:
   - Treatment for diabetic acidosis/alkalosis, either metabolic or respiratory

HYPERKALAEMIA

1. Excessive intake or gain:
   - Excessive oral intake
   - Excessive or rapid parenteral infusion
   - Tissue trauma, burns and crushing injuries
2. Inadequate renal losses:
   - Renal failure
   - Adrenal insufficiency
   - Addison's disease
   - Potassium-sparing diuretics

Box 20.7 Signs and symptoms of potassium imbalance (Adapted with kind permission from Porth 1990)

HYPOKALAEMIA

- Serum $K^+ < 3.5$ mmol/l
- Muscle tenderness, paraesthesia, or cramps
- Weakness, muscle flabbiness
- Paralysis
- Postural hypotension
- Increased sensitivity to digoxin
- Arrhythmias
- Anorexia, vomiting, abdominal distension, paralytic ileus
- Shortness of breath, shallow breathing
- Low osmolality and specific gravity of urine
- Nocturia
- Thirst
- Confusion, depression
- Metabolic alkalosis

HYPERKALAEMIA

- Serum $K^+ > 5.5$ mmol/l
- Paraesthesia
- Weakness and dizziness
- Muscle cramps
- Nausea, diarrhoea, intestinal colic, gastrointestinal distress
- Peaked T waves
- Depressed S-T segments
- Depressed P wave & widening of QRS segment
- Cardiac arrest

patients with hyperkalaemia: insulin and glucose can be administered to reduce serum potassium.

Hyperkalaemia may also be managed by creating gastrointestinal losses through the induction of diarrhoea or by using an ion exchange (i.e. a sodium or calcium resin which exchanges with the potassium). Intravenous calcium may temporarily reverse the toxic effect of potassium upon cardiac tissue.

Hypokalaemia

Management of hypokalaemia involves the treatment of any accompanying alkalosis or potassium losses. Potassium supplements may be given orally or intravenously. However, i.v. potassium can cause peripheral vein phlebitis and overly rapid infusion may cause cardiac dysrhythmias and death. I.v. potassium should not be added to blood products, where it may cause erythrocyte lysis, nor should it be added to solutions of mannitol, amino acids or lipids, as precipitation may occur. Nursing considerations in the administration of potassium are summarised in Boxes 20.8 and 20.9.

Box 20.8 Oral potassium supplements: nursing implications (Adapted from Metheny 1992)

Common side-effects of oral potassium are nausea, vomiting, gastrointestinal discomfort and diarrhoea. These are due to gastrointestinal irritation and can be reduced by the steps listed below. Because of these side-effects patient compliance may be poor, limiting the effectiveness of the supplements. Liquid preparations are preferred to slow-release tablets. Potassium-sparing diuretics are used where possible as they do not require potassium to be supplemented, unlike other diuretics. Potassium supplements can be a cause of hyperkalaemia.

To prevent gastrointestinal irritation/ulceration:

- Always dilute potassium preparations according to the manufacturer's instructions
- Advise patients to sip the diluted solution slowly, over a 5–10 min period
- Effervescent products must be fully dissolved and should not be swallowed until they have stopped fizzing
- Advise the patient to drink a full glass of water with slow-release tablets to help them dissolve in the GI tract
- Give potassium supplements *after* meals
- Observe patients on slow-release potassium tablets for signs of GI bleeding
- Check manufacturer's information before crushing potassium tablets. Some types must not be crushed.

Calcium

Calcium is the 5th most abundant element in the body, constituting 2% of body weight. Of the total body calcium 99% is found in bone, 0.5% in teeth and the remaining 0.5% in soft tissues. Total plasma content is low (8 mmol) and over half of this is bound to albumin. Binding to plasma proteins is pH sensitive, so that acidosis can cause an increase in plasma Ca^{++} without changes in the total Ca^{++}. Spuriously high Ca^{++} levels will be obtained if a tourniquet is used to obtain blood for calcium levels. This is due to venous constriction increasing fluid loss with an apparent concentration of the Ca-binding plasma proteins. Normal plasma levels are 2.2–2.6 mmol/l and urinary excretion is 2.5–7.5 mmol per day.

Calcium is required for a range of physiological functions, including:

- calcification of bones and teeth

Box 20.9 Critical precautions to observe when administering i.v. potassium (Adapted from Metheny 1992)

- Never give a rapid bolus of potassium, as this may cause cardiac arrest
- Always dilute potassium ampoules before administration. Usual concentration is 40 mmol/l (range 40–60 mmol/l); do not exceed 80 mmol/l
- 10 mmol/h via a peripheral line and 20 mmol/h via a central line are maximum recommended infusion rates
- Maximum adult dose is 100–200 mmol/24 h
- Avoid giving higher concentrations of i.v. potassium via a peripheral vein, as this causes venous pain and sclerosis
- Use an infusion pump to control rate when giving higher concentrations intravenously. Observe closely for signs of extravasation
- Observe for signs of thrombophlebitis
- Use ready-prepared solutions when possible
- Ensure thorough mixing of the infusate when potassium is added to infusion solutions. Never add potassium to an infusion bag which is hanging in the upright position because the patient may receive a bolus of undiluted potassium due to inadequate mixing
- Avoid i.v. potassium if the patient is dehydrated or has seriously impaired renal function. Adequate urine flow is required before i.v. potassium can be administered
- Monitor the patient carefully, noting urine flow, cardiovascular parameters, infusion rate, and infusion site. Potassium is highly irritating if it leaks into subcutaneous tissues and may lead to serious tissue damage.

- regulation of cell metabolism
- excitability of nerve and muscle, synaptic neurotransmitter release, muscle contraction
- cardiac conduction
- haemostasis
- complement activation.

Calcium is an important intracellular cation, with free calcium ion levels of 10^{-7} mol/l. Within the cell, calcium may be contained within organelles or bound to proteins. A calcium/magnesium ATPase may maintain the concentration gradient of calcium across the cell membrane.

Bone calcium, found in the hydroxyapatite form, provides a large reserve of calcium. The continual formation and destruction of bone, together with soft tissue calcium and calcium in the ECF, provides a small, exchangeable pool which can compensate for decreases in plasma Ca.

Calcium is ingested through the diet. Its absorption from the gut varies according to the presence of vitamin D, parathyroid hormone, growth hormone, corticosteroids and lactose (see Ch. 5). Calcium exists in two major forms within the extracellular fluid: as plasma, namely as freely ionised calcium ions, and as a complex bound to proteins (usually albumin). It is the freely ionised calcium which is important for nerve and muscle function. In the plasma the ratio of the two forms of calcium is usually 50:50, although in the tissue fluid there is only freely ionised calcium.

The location of plasma calcium varies according to pH. The more acidic the plasma the less protein is available for binding with calcium, and thus the free calcium ion level rises. In a patient with alkalosis there may be signs of hypocalcaemia because the free ions are reduced, yet total plasma levels remain unchanged. Any sudden change in pH will change the free calcium levels and cause clinical effects. This is one reason why in the treatment of metabolic acidosis (e.g. after a cardiac arrest) any infused sodium bicarbonate should be given slowly and with caution. Where there is a low serum albumin, the free calcium ion level will be normal, although the total plasma calcium will be low. Calcium should not be added to blood, lipid, bicarbonate or amino acid preparations as precipitation may occur.

It is known that cardiac muscle contraction is dependent not only upon the concentration of calcium ions but also upon the acidity of the extracellular environment. Myocardial depression may occur when there is a rapid drop in calcium levels, as for example following massive blood transfusion when the calcium may have been chelated by the citrates and the bone reservoir cannot release calcium quickly enough to compensate.

The myocardial depression will be aggravated in states of shock where there is poor coronary perfusion. The normal ionic regulation of the cardiac cells is disturbed when there is myocardial necrosis; in this circumstance calcium ions can pour into the cells and overactivate the ATPases, which in turn aggravate and worsen the cardiac necrosis. Thus where the cell becomes overloaded with calcium ions, uncoordinated and disturbed waves of contraction spread through the muscle, inhibiting effective contraction. Unfortunately, following myocardial ischaemia, immediate reperfusion of the cells with oxygen and nutrients does not necessarily reverse the problem.

Calcium-blocking drugs such as verapamil, nifedipine and beta blockers can slow the entry of calcium into the cells, thus reducing the effects of the necrosis. Calcium antagonists may be used for their two major effects, namely, to relax muscle and cause vasodilation, and to alter cardiac rhythm.

Digoxin is known to ultimately change intracellular calcium levels through its action upon the sodium–potassium pump. It is this action which enables digoxin to improve the contractility of cardiac muscle.

The causes and symptoms of calcium deficit and excess are listed in Boxes 20.10 and 20.11.

Tetany

If there is a decrease in extracellular freely ionised calcium ions then a condition known as hypocalcaemic tetany may be observed. In the absence of sufficient calcium ions in the ECF, neurotransmission is inhibited but the deficit of calcium ions in the cell leads to an excitatory effect on nerve and muscle cells, giving rise to increased motor activity. The outcome of this neuromuscular activity is marked spasms of skeletal muscle, particularly affecting the larynx and extremities. If laryngospasm becomes severe, then the person may suffer respiratory obstruction and arrest. Signs to observe for in early hypocalcaemia are described in Box 5.4, p. 147.

ACID–BASE BALANCE

Body fluids are normally slightly alkaline, within a pH range of 7.36–7.44 (H^+ concentration ($[H^+]$) 35–45 nmol/l). Blood has a H^+ concentration of 40 nmol/l, or a pH of 7.4. Acidaemia occurs when the arterial blood pH is less than 7.36 (greater than 44 nmol/l H^+). An arterial pH greater than 7.44 (or less than 36 nmol/l H^+) is alkalaemia. The body enzymes which control most physiological processes are optimally active within the normal pH range, and variations from this range can rapidly result in severe disability or death. It is therefore essential to understand the basis of acid–base balance

Box 20.10 Causes of calcium deficit and excess (Adapted with kind permission from Porth 1990)

HYPOCALCAEMIA

- Impaired ability to mobilise calcium from bone:
  - Hypoparathyroidism
- Abnormal calcium binding:
  - Decreased serum albumin
  - Decreased pH
  - Increased free fatty acids
  - Rapid transfusion of citrated blood
- Abnormal losses:
  - Cardiovascular, inadequate vitamin D
- Impaired absorption
- Renal failure
- Liver disease

HYPERCALCAEMIA

- Excessive gains:
  - Increased intestinal absorption
  - Excessive vitamin D
  - Excessive dietary intake
  - Milk alkali syndrome
- Increased bone resorption
- Increased levels of parathyroid hormone
- Inadequate losses
- renal insufficiency

Box 20.11 Signs and symptoms of calcium deficit and excess (Adapted with kind permission from Porth 1990)

HYPOCALCAEMIA

- Serum calcium < 8.5 mg/dl
- Increased nerve excitability:
  - Paraesthesia
  - Skeletal muscle cramps
  - Abdominal spasms and cramps
  - Hyperactive reflexes
  - Carpopedal spasm
  - Laryngeal spasm
  - Positive Chvostek's sign
  - Positive Trousseau's sign
- Renal failure
- Hypotension
- Cardiac insufficiency
- Failure to respond to drugs that act via calcium-mediated mechanisms

HYPERCALCAEMIA

- Serum calcium > 10.5 mg/dl
- Altered neural and muscular activity
- Muscle weakness and atrophy
- Ataxia, loss of muscle tone, lethargy
- Stupor and coma
- Cardiovascular alterations:
  - Hypertension
  - Shortening of the QT interval
  - AV block
- Anorexia, nausea, vomiting, constipation

in health and the effects of disease on this balance. A pH outside of the range 6.9–7.7 is incompatible with life and variations outside 7.36–7.44 are serious and may be difficult to rectify. Whilst the blood pH is maintained at a slightly alkaline level, the pH of urine is frequently acidic as the body seeks to excrete surplus acids which have been produced by both metabolic and respiratory processes.

This section will outline how the body attempts to maintain its internal environment at an optimal pH and will review a few situations in which acid–base balance is disrupted. The long-term regulation of pH occurs through the lungs and kidneys, whilst buffers in the blood provide an immediate response to changes in pH. With adjustments in respiratory rate, carbon dioxide levels (and hence pH) can also change. The response involving the kidney is slower and sometimes referred to as the 'renal lag'. The kidney's ability to regenerate bicarbonate ions whilst excreting hydrogen ions enables it to aid the regulation of pH.

Acidosis and alkalosis

The terms acidosis and alkalosis refer to abnormal situations which lead to acidaemia and alkalaemia respectively if there are no secondary compensatory mechanisms to reverse the situation. Both situations can be equally disruptive.

Acidosis occurs when there is a high hydrogen ion concentration and thus a low pH (below 7.36). It can arise through:

- metabolism of proteins producing sulphuric and phosphoric acids
- anaerobic metabolism producing lactic acid
- metabolism of fats producing acetoacetic acid and ketone bodies
- excessive intake of acidic products orally or intravenously
- excessive loss of bicarbonate from the body
- hypoventilation with resulting retention of carbon dioxide.

Alkalosis occurs when there is a loss of hydrogen ions or a gain in bicarbonate ions and hence a correspondingly high pH (greater than 7.44). Alkalosis can occur through:

- excessive loss of gastric juices; vomiting, gastric aspiration, etc.
- excessive intake of alkaline products: overdose of antacids
- hyperventilation with resulting removal of carbon dioxide.

Changes in carbon dioxide tension with a respiratory origin result in respiratory acidosis or alkalosis. Changes in bicarbonate levels reflect metabolic causes: metabolic acidosis or alkalosis. Whilst the primary causes may be metabolic or respiratory, the adaptive responses involve both systems and lead to compensatory states. Occasionally both metabolic and respiratory problems occur simultaneously and a confused picture presents, as in respiratory failure in a patient with renal failure.

Buffers

?	20.6 Refer to your physiology textbook to review the Henderson–Hasselbalch equation.

Regulation of blood pH at all levels involves complex chemical reactions in which buffers play a critical role. Buffers are substances which prevent major changes in the pH of a solution by removing or releasing hydrogen ions. In humans there are three main buffer systems:

1. carbonic acid bicarbonate
2. phosphate and sulphate compounds
3. proteins and haemoglobin (main ICF system).

Buffers are found in both the ICF and the ECF and enable products to be safely transported to the site of excretion.

Carbonic acid bicarbonate

This is the main buffer in humans and will serve as an illustration of the role of buffers in the body. This mechanism operates through the following reversible reaction:

$$H_2O + CO_2 \rightleftharpoons H_2CO_3 \rightleftharpoons H^+ + HCO_3^- \text{ (bicarbonate ion)}$$

In situations where hydrogen ions are added to body fluids they combine with the bicarbonate ion:

$$H^+ + HCO_3^- \rightleftharpoons H_2CO_3$$

In situations where the hydrogen ion levels become low, or there is an excess of hydroxyl ions, carbonic acid dissociates, releasing hydrogen ions into solution:

$$H_2CO_3 \rightleftharpoons H^+ + HCO_3^-$$

In alkalotic states the level of bicarbonate ions rises (metabolic alkalosis) or the amount of carbon dioxide in solution falls (respiratory alkalosis). In acidic states the level of bicarbonate decreases (metabolic acidosis) or the amount of carbon dioxide in solution rises (respiratory acidosis). There is thus a reciprocal relationship between the levels of carbon dioxide and the bicarbonate ions. This dynamic relationship, which enables pH to be regulated, is utilised in several ways within the respiratory system and the renal tubule. The enzyme carbonic anhydrase catalyses the formation of carbonic acid from water and carbon dioxide. Acetazolamide is an example of a drug which blocks carbonic anhydrase and thus inhibits both the regeneration of bicarbonate ions and the production of hydrogen ions in the renal tubule.

Alterations in the pH of the body may be indicated by clinical signs and laboratory results. The acidity of plasma is determined using arterial blood gas samples, but changes in other body fluids may be detected by testing urine, intestinal fluids, CSF and other exudates.

Handling blood gases

Obtaining a sample for the analysis of blood gases can be effected by direct arterial puncture or the withdrawal of blood from an arterial line. The nurse responsible for the patient will need to ensure that several precautions are taken to prevent a false result. The specimen form should include details such as the following:

- temperature
- respiratory pattern
- concentration of oxygen in the inspired gases
- any relevant recent therapies (e.g. physiotherapy, administration of bicarbonate or blood)
- time the sample was taken.

The sample should be collected in a small syringe (1 or 2 ml), to which a small quantity of dilute heparin (100 units per ml) has been added to prevent coagulation. The amount of heparinised saline added should be just enough to fill the dead space of the syringe. In the case of collecting a blood sample from an arterial line, it will be necessary to first withdraw and discard the heparinised saline in the arterial line tubing (excess heparin itself reduces the measured pH). A second syringe may then be used to withdraw the arterial blood itself. As soon as the sample has been collected a bung or stopper is attached to the end to prevent air contamination. The syringe should be labelled and sent to the lab as soon as possible. If the ambient temperature is warm then the sample can be transported in ice. The arterial line will need to be flushed and reset in order to remove the blood which has been drawn back into the line. With direct puncture, firm digital pressure will be required over the puncture site for at least 5 min to prevent arterial haemorrhage or subsequent aneurysm formation. The circulation of the limb distal to the puncture should be checked later. Normal blood gas results are listed in Box 20.12.

Box 20.12 Normal blood gas results

pH	7.36–7.44
$[H^+]$	35–45 nmol/l
$Pa{CO_2}$	4.6–5.6 kPa (35–42 mmHg)
$Pa{O_2}$	11.3–14 kPa (90–105 mmHg)
HCO_3	23–31 mmol/l^{-1}
Standard HCO_3^-	22–26 mmol/l^{-1}
Base excess	–2–+2 mmol/l^{-1}
Saturation O_2	97%

(Slight variations according to local laboratory.)

The acidotic/alkalotic states

? **20.7** Disorders of acid–base balance are primarily respiratory or metabolic in origin. From the information given so far the reader should be able to draw up a chart to indicate how the respective acid/base states may influence the pH, the bicarbonate ion levels (HCO_3^-) and the partial pressure of carbon dioxide in the plasma ($P{CO_2}$) in:

a. Metabolic acidosis
b. Respiratory acidosis
c. Metabolic alkalosis
d. Respiratory alkalosis.

Recognition and management of metabolic alkalosis

Metabolic alkalosis is caused by a loss of hydrogen ions (e.g. through vomiting) or a gain of alkali, as seen in the excess intake of sodium bicarbonate (see Box 20.14). It is characterised by high pH and a high concentration of bicarbonate ions. This rise in pH decreases the ionisation of calcium, thus giving signs of hypocalcaemia. Indicators of hypokalaemia may also arise. The respiratory response seeks to compensate for the alkalosis by raising the $P{CO_2}$ through a decreased respiratory effort: thus a respiratory acidosis may accompany the metabolic alkalosis. The increasing numbers of bicarbonate ions utilise free sodium ions, thus decreasing the ratio of free sodium ions to chloride ions. There is a slight renal compensation which attempts to conserve hydrogen ions. Usually, a metabolic alkalosis is successfully treated by management of the cause with appropriate monitoring of any hypokalaemia and/or by restoration of fluid volume. Occasionally, acidification of the plasma may be required, or the administration of acetazolamide to inhibit carbonic anhydrase.

Antacid use. Antacids are bases used to neutralise the acidity of gastric juices. Injudicious use can lead to metabolic alkalosis and problems associated with other side-effects of the substances used. Most antacids comprise a combination of aluminium or magnesium hydroxides, or derivatives of carbonates. It is important that patients who take antacids are aware of the necessity to keep within the prescribed doses and to report side-effects or failure of the therapy to their physician or community pharmacist. Some of the antacids are contraindicated with peptic ulcers.

Recognition and management of metabolic acidosis

Metabolic acidosis is characterised by a low pH and low levels of bicarbonate ions. The lowered pH leads to a compensatory respiratory drive to hyperventilate, thus causing a transitory fall in the $P{CO_2}$. If this is successful the pH will return towards normal. However, if the acidosis is severe cardiac output may drop with accompanying bradycardia (because acidosis impairs cardiac contractility). Renal compensation is made through the excretion of extra hydrogen ions. Hyperkalaemia may also be present, depending upon the cause of the acidosis. The features of the underlying acidotic state (e.g. peripheral vasodilation) will also be present. Treatment may involve the administration of bicarbonates, but it is important to recall that each mmol of sodium bicarbonate given contains 1 mmol of sodium ions. The three most common causes of metabolic acidosis are renal failure, diabetic ketoacidosis and hypoxia.

Recognition and management of respiratory alkalosis

The most common cause of respiratory alkalosis is an anxiety attack which has lead to the person noticeably hyperventilating. The subsequent removal of carbon dioxide leads to a raised pH and eventually a fall in the bicarbonate level when renal compensation has occurred. The aim in managing the anxiety attack is to enable the person to breath more slowly, to calm him (with a sedative if necessary) and, if it is safe, to enable him to rebreathe his expired air, thus raising the carbon dioxide level. (This can be achieved by having the person breathe in and out of a paper bag. While this technique is effective it must be supervised to ensure that the person does not suffocate or do it to excess.) Other instances of alkalosis will require management of their specific causes.

Recognition and management of respiratory acidosis
Respiratory acidosis is caused by an excess of carbon dioxide. It is most frequently caused by primary disorders of the respiratory tract or by conditions which effect the respiratory centre (e.g. drug overdose and central nervous system problems). Faults in the management of mechanical ventilation may also lead to respiratory acidosis.

Respiratory acidosis may be detected when the underlying respiratory problem is recognised, (for example, asthma or bronchitis) and/or when the signs of acidosis become apparent. People with chronic respiratory problems may of course already have well-established compensatory mechanisms; for example, in chronic obstructive airways disease (COAD) there may be a renal compensation which retains bicarbonate ions to counter the respiratory acidosis generated by a chronic high level of $P\text{CO}_2$. In these situations biochemical results may have a different significance from those associated with acute respiratory acidosis.

NURSING CONSIDERATIONS IN MAINTAINING FLUID AND ELECTROLYTE BALANCE

Assessment

Assessing hydration
The effects of a fluid loss or gain depend to a large extent on the volume of the loss or gain and the rate at which it occurs. Effects are more acute when they develop rapidly, when the person is elderly, and when the person is debilitated. Signs and symptoms observed by the nurse will depend upon the effects of the fluid loss or gain on the serum osmolality. A major problem in the assessment of fluid and electrolyte imbalance is that significant changes occur before they can be detected by clinical measurements such as blood pressure or central venous pressure.

Changes in tissue fluid volume are noticed mainly through observation of mucous membranes and of skin elasticity. (The latter is more easily observed over bony prominences.) With an infant, the anterior fontanelle provides a good indication of hydration status. In an elderly person it is difficult to detect changes in skin turgor due to the gradual loss of skin elasticity with age. However, changes in the presence or absence of oedema may be a useful indicator. Alterations in the intracellular fluid volume are very difficult to detect — except in the brain, where changes in intracranial pressure may be manifest.

The nurse should remember, when assessing hydration status, that the mucous membranes in the mouth may become dry for a variety of reasons, e.g. the use of anticholinergic drugs, mouth breathing, oxygen administration or dehydration itself. In a patient who is mouth breathing or on oxygen therapy, hydration status may be checked by inspecting the membrane between the cheek and gum wall, which should stay moist if the patient is sufficiently hydrated. Examination of the veins in the hand can also give a useful indication of a person's state of hydration: normally, elevation or dependency of the hand causes the veins to empty or fill within 3–5 seconds.

? **20.8** What are the other indicators of a person's state of hydration? (See Box 20.3.)

Assessing fluid and electrolyte status
The nurse's frequent contact with the patient should enable her to detect any disturbances or features which may be related to fluid and electrolyte status. Unfortunately, nursing management of patients' needs for food and fluid is often neglected and notoriously full of errors and confusion (see Research Abstract 20.1). In illness certain groups of patients such as elderly people, children and pregnant women are particularly susceptible to fluid and electrolyte problems. Others are at risk by virtue of an underlying pathological problem and/or as a result of nursing or medical interventions.

? **20.9** Make a list of any reasons which may cause a person to have a problem in managing their fluid and electrolyte balance.

A number of parameters may indicate changes in fluid or electrolyte status, but minor changes are often recognised only by those familiar with the person. This emphasises the importance of communication between nursing shifts and with carers (for example, relatives may notice changes). The rapid detection of patterns and trends can be important in identifying deterioration or improvement in the patient's condition.

A structured approach to nursing assessment should facilitate the identification of actual and potential patient problems. Indeed, the initial assessment may not be completed until a 24-h observation of the patient has been undertaken. Assessment of the patient's fluid and electrolyte status frequently involves the use of a fluid balance chart.

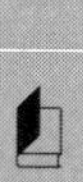

Jones (1975) published the results of a study into the nutritional care of unconscious patients being fed by a nasogastric tube. Amongst the many findings of this study were several points pertinent to the fluid status of the patient. It is suggested that the reader consult this study and its discussion of the errors commonly made in fluid measurement and administration.

? **20.10** Carry out the following exercises and consider the implications of the results for achieving accuracy in hydration assessments.

a. Measure out 100 ml quantities of liquid using a syringe or i.v. burette and inject them into the following utensils, observing the water levels:
   - urinal
   - catheter bag
   - usual measuring jugs
   - standard hospital glass, cup, cereal bowl.
b. Determine how much liquid is contained by the standard hospital glass, cup, bowl when:
   - full to the brim
   - half full
   - filled to the level usually served by the catering staff.

? **20.11** Select a suitable person on your next clinical allocation and make an assessment.

a. What is the state of the person's hydration?
b. What is his ability to regulate fluid and electrolyte intake and to excrete necessary fluids?
c. Give reasons for your conclusions.

Monitoring

The two most important components of monitoring patient's fluid balance are measurements (or estimations) of fluid intake/output and of weight. Insensible fluid losses are estimated according to standard norms, with adjustments made for factors such as the following:

- body temperature
- ambient temperature
- basal metabolic rate
- respiratory rate
- respiratory assistance: (e.g. use of oxygen, humidification)
- other pathologies
- fluid content in stools
- internal losses due to fluid movement
- losses through skin trauma.

Whilst some losses and gains have to be estimated, in appropriate circumstances others can be measured:

- content of food and fluids
- i.v. fluids
- GI gains through enteral sources
- GI losses
- losses from fistulae and drains
- urine.

Unfortunately, the fluid content of food and fluid intake is usually estimated rather than measured. Indeed, some 'fluid foods' such as soups and custards are not necessarily included in fluid recording. This is particularly important in patients who are restricted to a liquefied diet or volume control, as it is a means of getting round fluid intake restrictions!

Fluid balance charting: possible sources of error

Nurses should be aware of the many ways in which the accuracy of fluid intake/output calculations may be compromised. Examples include:

- duplication or omission of items
- use of estimations rather than measurements
- arithmetical errors
- fluids counted in theatre transferred to ward chart
- shift change errors, i.e. in carrying forward from previous shift
- mixing of colloidal and crystalloid calculations
- recording wrong i.v. bag: confusion between treatment chart and fluid chart
- failure to observe patterns in consecutive daily balances.

Measurement errors also arise when inappropriate utensils are used. To reduce the margin of error low volumes of urine should be measured in containers with graduations designed for low volumes. Large volumes measured from catheter bags may prove to be different if the bag is emptied and then measured from a rigid jug. Similarly, i.v. fluid bags may contain more than the actual amount specified. Understanding the relative acceptable margins of error is an essential but neglected aspect of fluid monitoring. In a fit, healthy person small errors may not be significant, but in a vulnerable person they can lead to inappropriate treatment regimes with consequent problems.

Managing fluid and electrolyte therapy

Aims

The aims of all fluid and electrolyte therapy are:

1. To regulate where possible the patient's fluid and electrolyte balance by controlling the content and volume of the oral/enteral route. When oral/enteral routes are inadequate venous access is used.
2. To control excessive losses and gains, for example by means of surgical intervention to prevent blood loss, or the use of diuretics to regulate fluid balance.

Both the medical and nursing management of the patient's fluid and electrolyte status will be derived from the initial assessment. The patient may require one or more of the following interventions:

- assistance with the maintenance of normal fluid and electrolyte requirements. This usually occurs for a short period of time in a previously well-nourished person, e.g. following surgery or during a brief period of coma
- correction of fluid/electrolyte imbalances
- total parenteral nutrition.

Occasionally, a person will require all three measures simultaneously: for example, someone with a major injury to the abdomen may need immediate correction of blood losses and electrolyte disturbances. There would then be a need to ensure that normal fluid and electrolyte needs are met, with consideration being given to changes in demand due to the injury. If oral/enteral feeding is unlikely to be resumed within a couple of days then immediate plans may be made to commence parenteral feeding.

In deciding on the most appropriate plan for a patient, consideration is given not only to the content of the therapy, but also to the resources available, the patient's coexisting problems (e.g. cardiac failure or diabetes) and the particular hazards associated with the respective methods of administration. The timing, rate and duration of the therapy can also determine which route is most sensible.

Determining the volume and content of the therapy

The regime prescribed for the patient will be based upon the following essential considerations:

- what needs to be replaced: measured and insensible or hidden losses from the body
- what needs to be removed: where there is excess production or excretory failure
- what needs to be adjusted: where there is translocation of fluids or electrolytes
- what needs to be halted: the cause of the problem, e.g. vomiting, haemorrhage.

The identification of these requirements will be based on nursing observation, medical assessment and laboratory analysis of specimens. However, the method of administration will influence the nature of the fluid regime. Fluids can be administered through the rectum and through ostomies, although these routes are not always efficient. When the oral route is inadequate, arteriovenous (AV) access may be used for i.v. therapy, or AV shunts for dialysis. Fluid and electrolyte regulation may also involve the use of human or artificial membranes in the case of peritoneal or haemodialysis. Subcutaneous infusions (hypodermoclysis) are infrequently used for fluid or electrolyte therapy, although they may be used in situations where facilities or personnel to administer i.v. therapy are absent. Subcutaneous infusates need to match extracellular fluid, with absorption dependent upon the vascular condition of the area concerned. Eventually the tissues will no longer be able to absorb fluid and will become swollen and hard. In complex situations a variety of routes for therapy may be employed.

Routes for fluid and electrolyte therapy

The oral route. Replacing fluids via the oral route is without doubt the safest method. In a healthy adult who has no circulatory or renal insufficiency the need for fluid is 1500–3000 ml/24 h. Replacing fluids orally will involve identifying the person's preferred drinks and making these available (where reasonable) in the desirable quantity.

In some situations the patient may be prescribed 'restricted fluids', the amount usually being stated. For example, a person with renal failure may have a restricted fluid intake of 1000 ml/24 h.

In other circumstances the nurse may be instructed to 'encourage fluids', especially when the goal is to prevent urinary stasis in the catheterised patient.

Two key points for the nurse to bear in mind when caring for persons requiring replacement of fluid and electrolytes by the oral route are as follows:

1. Always ascertain the exact meaning of any vague verbal or written orders concerning fluid replacement, e.g. 'push fluids', 'encourage fluids', 'taking sips', etc. Remember that fluid and electrolyte balance is important and that the nurse has a key role to play in preventing further problems.
2. If at all possible, know exactly how much fluid a person is required to have over a 24-h period. Medical orders can easily be written to identify appropriate daily fluid intake targets, e.g. 2000–2500 ml/24 h.

Sometimes patients on fluid replacement therapy still complain of thirst. Whilst the thirst reflex will be permanently relieved if the thirst sensors in the hypothalamus are no longer stimulated, a temporary depression of the thirst mechanism has been associated with interventions related to the oropharyngeal region (Anderson & Rundgren 1982). The patient troubled by thirst may be comforted by the following nursing actions (Woodtli 1990):

- carrying out frequent oral hygiene
- applying lubricant on lips
- giving mouth rinses
- choosing carefully the type and temperature of fluids
- offering ice chips for the patient to suck.

The parenteral route. For a number of patients, fluid and electrolyte therapy must be administered via the parenteral (i.v.) route. Parenteral fluid administration enables solutions to enter into the extracellular compartment directly, enabling a rapid and controlled method of delivery. Managing an i.v. therapy regime has become a common nursing responsibility, although in most health authorities it is clearly seen as part of an extended nursing role (Speechley & Tovey 1987).

Prior to the commencement of an i.v. therapy regime assessment should take into account the adequacy of the person's renal/cardiac function and his current fluid/electrolyte status, referring to such objective measures as laboratory studies, body surface area and intake/output.

Major complications of intravenous therapy

Whilst, thanks to advances in technology, intravenous therapy is now relatively safe, it is still possible for serious complications to arise. Unfortunately, as Speechley & Tovey (1987) remarked, these complications are sometimes regarded as routine occurrences or a mere 'nuisance'. But to overlook or underestimate the potential risks of i.v. therapy is to lose sight of the aim of therapy, which is to effectively replace fluid and electrolytes without causing the patient discomfort or further injury. (See Research Abstract 20.1.)

Phlebitis and extravasation are the two most commonly encountered problems. In their review of the literature Adams & Larson (1986) found several factors associated with an increased incidence of phlebitis:

Research Abstract 20.1

Nystrom et al (1983) published the findings of a European multicentre trial whose purpose was to survey the incidence of bacteraemia and the use of intravenous devices in surgical patients. The study sample comprised 1016 patients in 42 hospitals across 8 countries. The survey demonstrated that 62.9% of the patients received an i.v. device at some point in their hospital stay (in the UK this figure was 39.9% in those with a peripheral device and 2.5% with a central line). The incidence of thrombophlebitis was 10.3% (UK 15.1%), with the incidence of bacteraemia being as follows:

- patients without an i.v.: 1.5 in 1000, of which 0.5 per 1000 was a nosocomial infection
- patients with peripheral device only: 6.9 in 1000, of which 3.7 per 1000 were nosocomial
- patients with a central device: 59 per 1000, of which 44.8 per 1000 were nosocomial.

Nystrom B et al 1983 Bacteraemia in surgical patients with intravenous devices: a European multicentre incidence study. Journal of Hospital Infection 4: 338–349

- cannula location: insertion in the lower extremities or movable joints gave an increased risk
- duration of therapy: increasing length of time raised the incidence, especially over 24 h
- blood flow problems in the region
- inadequate sterilisation of the cannula site
- pre-existent infection within the body
- pH and osmolality of the fluid: acidic infusates in particular
- particulate matter which contaminated the delivery system.

Selecting the site

Patients who are particularly vulnerable to complications are those with existing infections or immune suppression and those whose restlessness or mental state may lead them to traumatise the cannula site. As Maki et al (1973) has pointed out, the cannula site is similar to an open surgical wound containing a foreign body and should be treated as such.

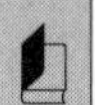
See Peters 1984 for a summary of the potential complications associated with i.v. devices.

Some practical considerations are involved in site selection, namely:

- the nature and anticipated duration of the therapy
- situational and environmental factors
- patient and safety factors
- availability of products
- staff expertise.

Insertion of the i.v. cannula is an extended role of the nurse and is usually undertaken by medical staff. However, communication between patient, nurse and doctor may enable a more effective and safe selection of site, materials and insertion technique.

In life-threatening circumstances, the selection of the i.v. site is largely dependent upon the expertise of the staff available, the products to hand and the purpose of the line. Whilst infection control measures are important, at the scene of a disaster or accident environmental contaminants may be inevitable and speed may take priority. The more invasive the procedure, the greater the importance of environmental control. Where possible, central lines (especially those involving a cut down procedure) should be inserted in an operating theatre. Local factors which may be controlled during the time of insertion include the elimination of airborne contaminants and the avoidance of debris or bacteria entering via the insertion site.

Patient factors. Patient mobility and comfort may be enhanced or hindered by site selection. It is wiser and causes less discomfort to avoid siting the i.v. cannula in movable joints, or where clothes may rub. Skin areas which are vulnerable to breakdown should also be avoided; this includes areas which are burned, oedematous, traumatised, inflamed, or affected by dermatological conditions such as eczema or psoriasis. The integrity and state of the veins themselves should influence selection.

The safety of lines in patients who are restless often poses a practical problem for nursing staff. Stability of the line may be enhanced by the method of attachment to the patient, and applying principles of counter-traction through the use of loops may prevent unnecessary trauma. Personal and environmental hygiene factors may necessitate that the insertion site be covered.

Central lines

Chapter 18 discusses the management of central lines used for the measurement of central venous pressure. Rainbow (1989) summarises the potential problems associated with the insertion, maintenance and removal of CVP lines. Similar principles apply when the central line is used for the long-term administration of infusates (e.g. patients requiring total parenteral nutrition (TPN), cytotoxic and antibiotic therapy). However, the greatly increased incidence of complications associated with the use of central lines necessitates a very cautious and competent approach to their management. Mennim (1992) provides a reminder of the danger of venous embolism associated with central line removal, although this is also a potential problem during insertion.

Types of parenteral fluids

The nature of the products to be infused determines both the number and location of the lines. Some infusates cannot be mixed, and if concurrent administration is required 2 or more lines may be needed. Infusates which increase the likelihood of microbial contamination include those used in parenteral nutrition, especially those containing high concentrations of glucose. Each infusate carries with it particular risks, and nurses should familiarise themselves with the specific potential side-effects associated with different infusates.

Broadly speaking, the infusates commonly used in intravenous therapy as opposed to TPN may be categorised as follows:

1. colloidal solutions:
   - blood and blood products
   - plasma and plasma substitutes
2. crystalloids:
   - water, electrolytes and isotonic solutions.

Infusates can also be categorised in respect to their tonicity, as described below.

Isotonic solutions have the same osmolarity (tonicity) as serum or other body fluids and expand the intravascular compartment without affecting the intracellular and interstitial compartments.

Hypotonic solutions have a lower serum osmolarity and cause body fluids to shift away from the blood vessels and into the intracellular and interstitial spaces to areas of higher osmolarity. Hypotonic solutions may be used in the case of cellular dehydration due to diabetic ketoacidosis.

Hypertonic solutions cause fluid to move from the interstitial and intracellular compartments towards the intravascular compartments. For example, hypertonic saline will increase plasma and interstitial fluid osmolality.

?	**20.12** This résumé of the numerous issues involved in the safe management of a person with an intravenous device illustrates the complexity and importance of skilful and knowledgeable nursing practice. The professional accountability of the nurse practitioner is outlined in both the UKCC Code of Professional Conduct and the October 1992 Standards for the Administration of Medicines. Whý not try and evaluate the 'customs and practices' in your own clinical areas in the light of these standards? It may also be a useful management exercise to attempt to devise some criteria/standards which could be employed to evaluate the effectiveness of local policies.
?	**20.13** How might the nurse recognise signs of a problem associated with the maintenance of i.v. therapy?
?	**20.14** What specific problems may be encountered by a person with an infusion device who is being nursed at home?

PROBLEMS ASSOCIATED WITH DISORDERS OF FLUID AND ELECTROLYTE BALANCE

This section will outline some areas in which patients commonly experience difficulties with fluid and electrolyte control. Nurses in many areas of practice will encounter patients whose fluid and electrolyte balance has been challenged with potentially dire consequences, e.g. burns patients, patients with cardiac failure, and patients with respiratory problems. The reader is referred to the relevant chapter of this book for information on fluid and electrolyte management in these more specialised contexts.

Gastrointestinal disorders

Disorders of the gastrointestinal system are very likely to lead to derangements in the normal balance of fluid and electrolytes, with subsequent problems in acid–base control. Fundamental problems can arise in circumstances such as the following:

- Fluids are lost from the body by vomiting, diarrhoea or via stomas
- The body is unable to absorb ingested fluids and foods
- The usual gastrointestinal fluids are produced either normally or in excess but the body is unable to reabsorb them; thus the gut acts as a third space, as seen in paralytic ileus
- Body fluids leak into the gut or gastrointestinal fluids leak into adjacent organs or cavities (which, again, act as a third space). Examples include gastrointestinal bleeds like oesophageal varices or gut ulcers; fistulae; peritonitis.

It is possible for several of these conditions to occur simultaneously, for example in a person with intestinal obstruction who is vomiting, has abdominal distension from the obstruction and may develop paralytic ileus. Two common problems of the gastrointestinal tract which, if untreated, can be fatal are vomiting and diarrhoea.

Vomiting

Losses of fluid through vomiting can rapidly cause dehydration and if prolonged or severe may lead to metabolic alkalosis and malnutrition. Following surgery to the thoracic and abdominal regions, vomiting can exacerbate the pain experience and delay healing due to the strain imposed upon the abdominal muscles. In the case of a person's inability to protect his airway (e.g. through coma), inhalation of vomitus may lead to inhalation pneumonia and possibly death.

Vomiting causes fluid loss through the ejection of recently ingested foods and fluids, the loss of gastric or upper intestinal juices, the loss of blood from gastrointestinal bleeds and the prevention of oral fluid and nutritional replacement. Thus prolonged or severe vomiting requires not only the prevention and/or control of the vomiting itself, but also adequate fluid replacement.

The loss of gastric juices, which contain hydrochloric acid and potassium ions, initially leads to metabolic alkalosis due to a surplus of bicarbonate ions. In severe, prolonged vomiting without adequate nutritional replacement, the body begins to metabolise fats as an energy source, producing ketone bodies and further exacerbating the metabolic acidosis.

Thus fluid and electrolyte losses caused by vomiting may be summarised as follows:

- depletion of the ECF volume
- hypochloraemia (Cl^- loss)
- alkalosis
- hypokalaemia
- possible acidosis
- anaemia due to any blood losses.

Nursing management. The actual control and the prevention of further episodes of vomiting will depend upon the triggers of the vomiting and on available resources. However, whilst the person is vomiting some practical measures can help to alleviate some of his distress. These include providing a receptacle to vomit into, ensuring privacy if possible, and providing something to wipe away the vomit and mucus. The controlled use of breathing and swallowing techniques can sometimes enable the person to regain control of the waves of contraction that accompany the vomiting episode.

The nurse's ability to enable a person to adopt such techniques often rests on her interpersonal skills and confidence. The use of touch can also help the person to relax and thus avoid unnecessary muscular contractions which may aggravate any wound pains. (In the presence of a wound, it is important for the patient or nurse to support the wound). When the immediate episode is over, a method of refreshing the mouth is essential. Judicious use of pharmacological agents may prevent vomiting episodes, especially if their timing is sequenced for maximum benefit, e.g. taken before anticipated triggers. With very severe vomiting episodes there is a risk that inhalation may occur; in such cases observation of the person's breathing pattern is essential (indeed, occasionally gastric contents may be emitted via the nose).

If a person vomits whilst a nasogastric tube is in place, the nurse should investigate the following possibilities:

- the tube is either blocked, kinked, in the wrong place or spigoted
- the tube is too fine for the aspirate
- the frequency of gastric aspiration needs to be altered
- there is a deterioration in the patient's condition, e.g. haemorrhage
- it is inappropriate for the person to have the tube in place.

The best action is to leave the tube on free drainage and consider whether aspiration is needed (this will depend upon the cause). At a suitable juncture the effectiveness of the tube should be re-evaluated.

? **20.15** What actions could be taken when the following patients seem likely to vomit?
a. A person with a spinal injury.
b. A person with a wired jaw.

? **20.16** What is the significance of the information that may be obtained through observation of vomitus and the accompanying episodes of vomiting?

Diarrhoea

Diarrhoea occurs when the body is unable to reclaim/absorb the fluids in the intestinal tract and the peristaltic contractions of the gut expel the intestinal contents. Generally, intestinal fluids are isotonic with the ECF until the colon is reached, at which point the contents gradually become hypotonic due to the colon's role in water reabsorption. Severe and prolonged diarrhoea as seen in cholera or in some forms of infant enteritis can lead to severe electrolyte imbalance, dehydration and ultimately death if treatment is unsuccessful or delayed. The fluid losses may cause:

- depletion of ECF volume
- hyponatraemia
- hypokalaemia
- metabolic acidosis due to loss of HCO_3^- in the digestive juices
- if the problem is located in the colon, water dehydration may be severe.

The causes of diarrhoea are identified and its nursing and medical management discussed in Chapter 4. Fluid and electrolyte replacement are essential components in the management of the effects of diarrhoea, with accompanying management of the causative agent. Oral rehydration therapy is frequently employed in cases of enteritis and dehydration, providing the gut is able to absorb ingested fluids (see Box 20.13).

? **20.17** Why do oral preparations to rehydrate a person suffering from diarrhoea/dehydration contain salts *and* glucose?

Box 20.13 Contents of a solution to use in oral rehydration therapy (To be reconstituted with water to make a total volume of 1 litre.) (British National Formulary 1993)

SUBSTANCE	WHO FORMULATION
Sodium chloride	3.5 g
Potassium chloride	1.5 g
Sodium citrate	2.9 g
Anhydrous glucose	20.0 g

This combination gives in mmol/l:

- sodium: 90
- potassium: 20
- chloride: 80
- citrate 10
- glucose 111.

In fact, in UK practice, where less severe forms of dehydration are found than in developing countries, the sodium content is slightly less and the glucose higher. It is important, however, to ensure that the water additive is safe.

Special needs of the person undergoing surgery

The person undergoing surgery, whether elective or emergency, is particularly vulnerable to several disturbances of fluid and electrolyte balance. Disturbances in the composition and placement of the body fluids and electrolytes accompany many procedures and include blood loss, dehydration from preoperative fasting, bowel preparation (e.g. mannitol administration to clear the gut) and surgical exposure. Problems due to the underlying pathology and the patient's general health status exacerbate the situation. Surgery/trauma causes a defensive metabolic response which conserves water and sodium and changes the plasma levels of sodium, potassium, nitrogen and albumin. The basis of the response is vasoconstriction of the renal artery and the release of AVP, whilst any changes in blood pressure which affect the juxtaglomerular apparatus will stimulate the renin/aldosterone systems. This response enables conservation of plasma volume and the retention of sodium, whilst an increase in catecholamines raises the cardiac output and heart rate.

The renal response to trauma usually takes 24–72 h to recover and during this time the patient is unable to cope normally with electrolyte control and cannot produce a hypotonic urine. The risks of fluid overload and water intoxication are thus high; yet, conversely, inadequate replacement therapy may lead to dehydration and shock. Thus, in a vulnerable person it is important not only to measure daily fluid balance but to keep record of the *consecutive* daily balances over the first 72 h. Oedema may occur due to changes in vascular permeability, with translocation of fluids into the third space. The fundamental nursing activities of patient assessment and effective implementation of treatment regimes are often critical to the patient's recovery.

By convention, it is normally assumed that intraoperative fluid losses are replaced in theatre and that fluid balance recording commences postoperatively from a state of 'zero' balance. It is important to note the losses during surgery in order to anticipate any potential problems, which should be indicated in the theatre notes and postoperative guidelines from the anaesthetist. However, the picture is occasionally confused by poor record-keeping and inadequate communication, which may cause the postoperative fluid balance data to be misleading. Insensible losses may also pass unnoticed, for example loss from sweating (as in shock or pyrexia).

? **20.18** Select a person who is to undergo surgery and whom you can follow up postoperatively. Assess your chosen patient and identify his actual and potential needs with particular reference to:

a. Comfort needs in respect to hydration and elimination
b. Potential fluid and electrolyte losses or gains
c. Other factors influencing fluid and electrolyte balance
d. The changing needs of the patient from the preoperative assessment through surgery to the postoperative phase.

Critically evaluate the planned and implemented nursing care of your selected patient in respect to the identified problems derived from items a–d.

REFERENCES

Adam S D, Killien & Larson E 1986 In line filtration and infusion phlebitis. Heart & Lung. March 15(2): 134–140

Anderson B, Rundgren M 1982 Thirst and its disorders. Annual Review of Medicine 33: 231–239

Edelman I S & Leibman J 1959 Anatomy of body water electrolytes. American Journal of Medicine 27: 256–278 (August 1959)

Guyton A 1991 Textbook of medical physiology. Saunders, Philadelphia

Jones D C 1975 Food for thought. Royal College of Nursing, London

Lamb J F et al 1980 Essentials of physiology. Blackwell Scientific

Maki D G, Goldman D, Rhame S 1973 Infection control in IV therapy. Annals of Internal Medicine 79(6): 867–887

Maki D G & Ringer M 1987 Evaluation of dressing regimens for prevention of infection with peripheral IV catheters. Journal of American Nursing 6 Nov. 258(17): 2396–2403

Mennim P et al 1992 Venous air embolism associated with the removal of CV catheter. British Medical Journal 18 July 305 (6846) 171–172

Metheny N 1992 Fluid and electrolyte balance: nursing considerations, 2nd edn. Lippincott, Philadelphia

Nystrom B et al 1983 Bacteraemia in surgical patients with intravenous devices: a European multicentre incidence study. Journal of Hospital Infection 4: 338–349

Porth C 1990 Pathophysiology: concepts of altered health state, 3rd edn. Lippincott, Philadelphia

Peters J L 1984 Peripheral venous cannulation: reducing the risks. British Journal of Parenteral Therapy March 56–68

Rainbow C 1989 Monitoring the critically ill patient. Heinemann, Oxford

Smith E K M 1991 Fluids and electrolytes: a conceptual approach, 2nd edn. Churchill Livingstone, New York

Speechley V, Toovey J 1987 Problems in IV therapy. Professional Nurse 1 May 240–242

UKCC 1992 Code of professional conduct. UKCC, London

UKCC 1992 The scope of professional practice. UKCC, London

Woodtli A O 1990 Thirst: a critical care nursing challenge: dimensions of critical care nursing 9(1): 6–15

FURTHER READING

Barta M 1987 Correcting electrolyte imbalances. Registered Nurse February 30–34

Bland J H 1963 Clinical metabolism of body water and electrolytes. Saunders, London

British National Formulary 1993 No. 26 September Pharmaceutical Press, London

Dougherty L 1992 Intravenous therapy. Surgical Nurse. April 5(2): 10–13

Fan S et al 1988 Predictive value of surveillance skin and hub cultures in central venous catheter.

Feluer L 1980 Understanding the electrolyte maze. American Journal of Nursing Sept 1980 1591–1595

Gamble J L 1954 Chemical anatomy, physiology and pathology of ECF, 6th edn. Harvard University Press, Harvard

Ganong W F 1991 Review of medical physiology, 15th edn. Prentice Hall, London

Green J H 1976 An introduction to human physiology, 4th edn. Oxford University Press, Oxford

Green J H 1978 Basic clinical physiology, 3rd edn. Oxford University Press, Oxford

Haynes S 1989 Infusion phlebitis and extravasation. Professional Nurse Dec 160–161

Haynes S 1992 CVP monitoring. Professional Nurse Sept 727–729

Hecker J, Swartz M (eds) 1982 Current topics in infectious diseases. McGraw Hill, New York
Hinchliff S & Montague S (eds) 1988 Physiology for nursing practice. Baillière Tindall, London
Lamb J F et al 1980 Essentials of physiology. Blackwell Scientific, Oxford
Maki D G 1977 Preventing infection in IV therapy. Current Research Anaesthesia and Analgesics 56(1): 141–153
Maki D G, Goldmann D, Rhame S 1993 Infection control in IV therapy. Annals of Internal Medicine 79(6): 867–887
Manley K M 1992 Flow control devices in intravenous therapy. Surgical Nurse June 5(3): 11–15
Marieb E N 1989 Human anatomy and physiology. Benjamin Cummings, California
Millam D 1988 Managing complications of IV therapy. Nursing 88, 18(3): 34–42
McVicar A, Clancy J 1992 Which infusate do I need? Professional Nurse 7 June 9: 586–591
Miller J 1988 Recording the CVP. Professional Nurse March 188–189
Miller J 1989 Intravenous therapy in fluid and electrolyte balance. Professional Nurse Feb. 237–240
Neeser M et al 1992 Thirst strike: hypernatraemia and acute prerenal failure in a prisoner who refused to drink. British Medical Journal 23 May 304: 1352
Smith E, Kinsey M 1991 Fluids and electrolytes: a conceptual approach, 2nd edn. Churchill Livingstone, Edinburgh
Smith E K M 1991 Fluids and electrolytes: a conceptual approach, 2nd edn. Churchill Livingstone, New York
Timberlake K 1988 Chemistry, 4th edn. Harper Collins, New York

CHAPTER 21

Nutrition

Colin Torrance   Mary Gobbi

CHAPTER CONTENTS

Introduction 657
Normal nutrition 657
The healthy diet 658
Food groups 659

The major nutrients 659
Carbohydrates 659
Proteins 660
Lipids 661
Vitamins 662
Minerals 662

Nutritional intervention 662
Obesity 662
Malnutrition 663

Nutritional assessment 664
The dietary and clinical history 664
Physical examination 665
Laboratory investigations 665
Encouraging the patient to eat 666
Oral intake 666
Physical factors influencing eating 666
Organising effective mealtimes 667
Assisting patients to eat 668

Enteral feeding 669
Indications for enteral feeding 669
Nasoenteral feeding 669
Selection of enteral feeds 670
Methods of administration 670
Complications of enteral feeding 671

Parenteral nutrition 672
Indications for TPN 673
Nutritional assessment and monitoring 673
Venous access 673
Administration equipment 673
Solutions for TPN 673
Complications of TPN 674
Complications of the intravenous route 674
Complications associated with the infusion fluid 675
Coexisting medical problems 676
Psychosocial effects 676

References 676

Further reading 677

INTRODUCTION

Eating and drinking are an integral part of human existence. An adequate intake of food and water is required to maintain physiological function, to allow for growth and maintenance of tissues, and to provide energy to meet the demands of daily living. Eating and drinking is identified as one of the 12 essential Activities of Living (ALs) in Roper, Logan and Tierney's (1985) model of living. Although a biological necessity, eating and drinking has a significance beyond the merely physiological, forming an important part of social and psychological well-being. In any society, food growing and preparation are central activities; even in developed countries where food is abundant, the preparation and consumption of food may take up several hours a day. Meals are used as a time for families to come together, food or drink may be offered to make a guest feel welcome, formal meals may be a feature of family, religious or national ceremonies. Illness or hospitalisation can alter eating habits with important psychological as well as nutritional effects. The AL of eating and drinking is influenced by a range of factors including physical, psychological, social, cultural, religious, environmental and economic factors. Nursing interventions need to be based on both a physiological and psychosocial assessment of the nutritional needs of the individual. Presenting a well-balanced meal is of little value if the patient is unable or unwilling to eat. Discharging a patient home with a diet sheet that includes items that are economically or culturally unacceptable is equally futile.

The importance of nutritional care within nursing has been well recognised. Henderson (1960) stated that 'There is no more important an element in the preparation for nursing than the study of nutrition', and Florence Nightingale was as influential in the development of dietetics as nursing. The nurse's role in nutritional care spans the wellness–illness continuum from involvement in health education like giving advice on a 'healthy' diet to the management of a total parenteral feeding regime. Helping an individual meet his basic need for food is as critical a component of nursing care as ensuring adequate oxygenation. In this chapter we will consider normal nutrition and the basic need for food, the role of food in health and disease, non-nutritional aspects of eating and drinking, assessment of nutritional status and the nurse's role in planning and implementing nutritional care.

Normal nutrition

To maintain healthy function an adequate supply of the essential nutrients is required. The exact composition of the diet can vary enormously, foods common in one culture may be unacceptable in another, but the constituents will belong to one of the six main nutrient groups: protein, carbohydrate, fat, vitamins, minerals and of course water. In addition, many non-nutrient components are included in the diet and have their own importance, for example fibre, whilst other non-nutrients like food colourings, flavourings and preservatives, which are useful in the cooking and commercial production of food, may be associated with disease in susceptible individuals. Food is not always 'healthy'; contaminants like microorganisms and bacterial toxins can cause disease. Improperly prepared or stored food may harbour organisms causing food poisoning; typical culprits found in under-cooked chicken are bacteria belonging to the genus Salmonella. Clostridium botulinum is an anaerobic bacterium which may multiply in inadequately preserved (often home-canned) foods and produces a powerful toxin that interferes with synaptic transmission. Box 21.1 lists some major food contaminants of possible toxicological importance.

?	**21.1** What safety precautions are taken in the hospital environment to reduce the likelihood of food poisoning? Check your local policies.

Although synthetic foods containing all the known nutrients can be formulated, no single naturally occurring food can meet all the daily nutritional demands. Many foods contain the essential six nutrients but the proportion of each varies and a range of different foods is necessary to provide the daily requirement of individual nutrients. In general, plant products are richer in carbohydrate but lower in protein and fats than animal products. Plants are the major source of fibre. Some foods are particularly rich in a single nutrient, although they may contain other nutrients, thus meat should be classed as protein rich rather than a protein as it also contains a lot of fat and other nutrients. Cereals are rich in carbohydrate, wheat flour for example is over 70% carbohydrate but it also has more than 10% protein and 1–2% fat. Very few foods, such as sugar (almost pure carbohydrate) or cooking oils (almost pure fat), fall predominantly into one nutrient group.

Nutrients have a complex role in physiological function and most nutrients are involved in several processes. Iron is required for oxygen transport within the red blood cell but is also important in several enzyme systems, for example as part of prolyl hydroxylase, an essential enzyme in collagen formation. Nutrients may form the structural material of the body, provide energy for metabolism or help in the regulation of physiological processes. A single nutrient may be necessary for one or for all these functions, for example carbohydrate, fat and protein are all sources of energy. Although carbohydrate and fat are well recognised as 'fattening' foods, protein has the same calorific value as carbohydrate and can be equally fattening when taken in excess (Box 21.2). Water, protein, fat, minerals and carbohydrate form the structural elements of the body. Minerals and vitamins are important in regulatory processes but protein and fats, as hormones and enzymes, also contribute to metabolic regulation. Non-nutrients such as fibre are important for physiological function and others such as caffeine and food additives may fulfil other lifestyle functions and possibly contribute to disease. Alcohol is calorie rich and has a complex role in many societies but is damaging if it contributes a major proportion of dietary energy.

Box 21.1 Sources of food contamination (adapted from Kilgore & Li 1980)

During food production
Animal and insect filth, whole or parts of insects.
Parasites.
Microorganisms.
Agrochemical residues (pesticides, fungicides etc.).
Drugs (antibiotic, growth hormones).
Toxic metals (especially mercury and the heavy metals).

During processing
Animal and insect filth, whole or parts of insects.
Microorganisms and microbial toxins.
Foreign bodies and processing residues.

During packing and storage
Animal and insect filth.
Labelling materials.
Microorganisms and microbial toxins.
Chemical migrants from the packaging materials.

The healthy diet

A healthy or normal diet will provide an adequate supply of all the nutrients (and important non-nutrients like fibre) that are necessary to satisfy the needs of body cells. Whilst the healthy person can tolerate short-term fluctuations in nutrient intake, a persistent deficiency of any of the nutrients will impair function (see Table 21.1). There must be enough:

- water
- protein for tissue repair, maintenance and growth
- carbohydrate and fat for energy
- vitamins and minerals for the regulation of physiological processes.

The diet must supply the essential nutrients, that is those which are necessary for survival but cannot be synthesised by the body from other sources. Some amino acids, for example, are required for health but are not dietarily essential as they can be synthesised by the body in sufficient quantities to meet metabolic needs. The diet should supply all these necessary ingredients in the correct quantities and proportions, whilst avoiding excessive intake. For optimal health, nutrient intake must balance nutrient usage, an excess intake may be nearly as damaging as a deficiency. Western society has demonstrated that the adverse effects of overeating may be as serious as chronic undernutrition. Recently, health problems have been identified due to excessive intake of a single nutrient taken in the form of vitamin supplements: a typical example being vitamin A which is toxic in high doses.

Actual requirements will vary depending on the person's size, age, gender, activity level and state of health. The recommended daily intake or amount (RDA) of some major nutrients for different groups within the British population are listed in Table 21.2 (p. 660). However, recently the Scientific Committee for Food has decided to give, not just one, but three reference values for a nutrient: the lowest threshold index (LTI), the intake below which most individuals would be unable to meet metabolic requirements; the average requirement (AR) and the population reference index (PRI) which corresponds to the RDA but avoids the use of the term 'recommended'. (See Table 21.3, p. 661.)

Box 21.2 Energy value of major nutrients

Carbohydrate	16 kJ/g (approximately 4 kcal/g)
Protein	17 kJ/g (approximately 4 kcal/g)
Fat	38 kJ/g (approximately 9 kcal/g)
Alcohol	29 kJ/g (approximately 7 kcal/g)

Table 21.1 A summary of clinical signs of nutritional significance (Miller & Torrance 1991)

Area	Signs	Deficiencies
Hair	Dull/dry Thin/sparse Easily falls out Loss of colour Alopecia	PEM Essential fatty acids
Face	Moon-face Enlarged thyroid Nasolabial seborrhoea Seborrhoeic dermatitis	PEM Iodine Riboflavin, niacin, zinc
Eyes	Dryness, softening/ inflammation of cornea Pale conjunctiva Conjunctivitis Keratomalacia Loss of vision, night blindness	Vitamin A, B complex, iron, folate
Lips	Angular stomatitis, cheilosis	Riboflavin, niacin, iron
Tongue	Glossitis, red, swollen	Folate, B complex, iron
Gums	Reddened, spongy, receding, bleeding	Vitamin C
Nails	Spoon shaped	Iron
Skin	Dryness, petechiae, ecchymoses, oedema, colour changes, texture changes Follicular hyperkeratosis Pellagrous dermatosis	Vitamins A, C, and K, niacin
Musculo-skeletal	Fat and muscle wasting Fatigue, stiffness, pain	PEM, Vitamin D
Neurological	Paraesthesia, sensory loss Irritability, confusion, depression Motor weakness, hypoflexia	B complex, thiamine, PEM

For further information on dietary requirements, see Dept of Health 1991, and Scientific Committee for Food for the European Community 1993 Editorial: Proposed Nutrient and Energy Intakes for the European Community. Nutrition Reviews 51(7): 209–212

To remain healthy the individual may need to modify his or her diet to meet changes in metabolic demand, for example during pregnancy, lactation (Box 21.3) and disease. Effective nutritional nursing depends on assessing the patient to identify current needs and helping him find ways of meeting these nutritional requirements that fit in as much as possible with his usual food habits and preferences. In addition, an RDA has not been established for all the essential nutrients, especially the trace elements. A varied diet remains the best way to ensure an adequate intake of all the essential nutrients.

? **21.2** Apart from pregnancy and lactation, when else during their lifespan may a person have sudden changes in their nutrient demand?

Food groups

For patients needing special diets, detailed assessment, food analysis and dietary planning are important, but for many patients it may be more appropriate to adopt a more general approach to nutritional education. The food group approach aims to inform and encourage the patient to eat a balanced diet, one in which major food groupings are all represented providing a sufficient variety of foods to meet all nutrient requirements. One of the most widely used divides foods into four basic groups: milk and milk products; fruit and vegetables; cereals/bread; and meat or meat alternatives. Box 21.4 demonstrates a four group plan based on an adult's daily needs. Such a plan needs modification for groups with special nutritional needs, such as children, teenagers, pregnant women and nursing mothers. A more complex food exchange system is required for those with a known metabolic condition such as diabetes mellitus. One group meriting special mention are vegetarians for whom the normal four food group plan with a reliance on meat as a protein source is obviously unacceptable. Vegetarians can be classed as lacto-ovo-vegetarians, that is those who use animal products such as milk and eggs but exclude animal flesh (meat, fish and poultry), and vegans who avoid all animal products and eat only plant foods. Box 21.5 illustrates a modified four group plan for vegetarians.

Food plans of this type provide an easily understandable guide for balanced eating but an individual following such a plan can still become deficient in some nutrients. Vitamins B_6 and E, and minerals such as iron, magnesium and zinc are often deficient. The quality of the foods consumed can also be an important factor as economic or ethnic factors may influence food choices within the groups. However, the simplicity of the approach with the division of foods into easily recognised groups can make it an effective way of providing patients with nutritional education.

THE MAJOR NUTRIENTS

The essential nutrients are water, carbohydrate, protein, lipid, vitamins and minerals. Water is the major component of the body and the diet must include sufficient to meet daily needs. Energy supply is the primary function of carbohydrate but it also has a protein-sparing action, an antiketogenic effect, a protective function and a role in the synthesis of many body materials. Proteins are required for a range of functions including structure, movement, communication and transport. They also have a role in immune function, acid–base regulation and the maintenance of osmotic pressure. Lipids (fats, oils and waxes) are necessary for a number of physiological functions, and lipid is the richest source of energy available to the body. Vitamins are required for the regulation of metabolic processes. They act as cofactors, coenzymes or as components of coenzymes and enzymes. The final group of essential nutrients is the minerals. More than 24 minerals may be required for physiological functioning and these can be divided into the major minerals, trace elements and putative trace elements.

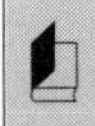

Only a brief review of the major nutrients is possible here and for further details the reader is directed to Passmore & Eastwood (1986).

Carbohydrates

Carbohydrate is the main energy source for the body, glucose is the preferred fuel for the brain. Although fat has a higher calorific value it is less efficiently used by the brain, and a high fat diet increases the risk from some diseases. Protein has no advantage over carbohydrate as an energy source and protein foods are more expensive to buy. The three major carbohydrate groups in food are sugars, starches and the complex polysaccharides, cellulose and associated materials, that make

Table 21.2 DHSS recommended daily amounts for groups within the British population (DHSS 1979)

Age range	Energy		Protein	Minerals		Vitamins				
				Calcium	Iron*	A	Thiamine	Riboflavin	Niacin	C
years	MJ	kcal	g	mg	mg	µg	mg	mg	mg	mg
Males										
Under 1	3.25	780	19	600	6	450	0.3	0.4	5	20
1	5.0	1200	30	600	7	300	0.5	0.6	7	20
2	5.75	1400	35	600	7	300	0.6	0.7	8	20
3–4	6.5	1560	39	600	8	300	0.6	0.8	9	20
5–6	7.25	1740	43	600	10	300	0.7	0.9	10	20
7–8	8.25	1980	49	600	10	400	0.8	1.0	11	20
9–11	9.5	2280	56	700	12	575	0.9	1.2	14	25
12–14	11.0	2640	66	700	12	725	1.1	1.4	16	25
15–17	12.0	2880	72	600	12	750	1.2	1.7	19	30
18–34 Sedentary	10.5	2510	62	500	10	750	1.0	1.6	18	30
Moderately active	12.0	2900	72	500	10	750	1.2	1.6	18	30
Very active	14.0	3350	84	500	10	750	1.3	1.6	18	30
35–64 Sedentary	10.0	2400	60	500	10	750	1.0	1.6	18	30
Moderately active	11.5	2750	69	500	10	750	1.1	1.6	18	30
Very active	14.0	3350	84	500	10	750	1.3	1.6	18	30
65–74	10.0	2400	60	500	10	750	1.0	1.6	18	30
75+	9.0	2150	54	500	10	750	0.9	1.6	18	30
Females										
Under 1	3.0	720	18	600	6	450	0.3	0.4	5	20
1	4.5	1100	27	600	7	300	0.4	0.6	7	20
2	5.5	1300	32	600	7	300	0.5	0.7	8	20
3–4	6.2	1500	37	600	8	300	0.6	0.8	9	20
5–6	7.0	1680	42	600	10	300	0.7	0.9	10	20
7–8	8.0	1900	48	600	10	400	0.8	1.0	11	20
9–11	8.5	2050	51	700	12	575	0.8	1.2	14	25
12–14	9.0	2150	53	700	12	725	0.9	1.4	16	25
15–17	9.0	2150	53	600	12	750	0.9	1.7	19	30
18–54 Most occupations	9.0	2150	54	500	12	750	0.9	1.3	15	30
Very active	10.5	2500	62	500	12	750	1.0	1.3	15	30
54–74	8.0	1900	47	500	10	750	0.8	1.3	15	30
75+	7.0	1680	42	500	10	750	0.7	1.3	15	30
Pregnant	10.0	2400	60	1200	13	750	1.0	1.6	18	60
Lactating	11.5	2750	69	1200	15	1200	1.1	1.8	18	60

* Iron RDA may not be sufficient to cover heavy menstrual losses.

up dietary fibre. The fruits, flowers, roots, leaves and stalks of plants provide carbohydrate, but leaves and stalks tend to have more indigestible cellulose and so provide little energy. Berries and fruits are rich in sugars while roots and seeds are usually excellent sources of starch. Carbohydrate was for many years considered 'fattening' and slimming diets used to concentrate on reducing carbohydrate intake. Now foods rich in starch and fibre are recommended as the main energy source in healthy diet. However, it is necessary to distinguish between useful carbohydrate sources, those which supply starch and fibre, and sources of questionable nutritional value which supply mainly processed sugars or 'empty calories'.

Proteins

There is no dietary requirement for protein as such but rather for the 20 or so component amino acids. Some amino acids are synthesised by the body; others, the dietarily essential amino acids, cannot be synthesised and must be obtained from food. Dietary protein is required primarily for the growth and maintenance of body tissue but proteins fulfil many roles and protein function can be summarised into three broad categories: structural maintenance, physiological regulation and energy supply. Proteins are required to build new tissue during growth or replace tissue lost through injury, for example new blood cells after haemorrhage. Less obviously, protein is required to replace tissues lost on a daily basis; hair, nail, skin cells and blood cells need constant replacement. In fact, nearly all cells need replacing on a regular basis and, in addition, cell proteins are regularly replaced and renewed. Almost all enzymes and many hormones are proteins so the regulatory role of proteins is profound. Protein is an energy source and if insufficient carbohydrates or fats are ingested than the body will use protein for energy.

Proteins are found in most foods, including meat, fish, cereals, legumes, fruit and vegetables but the amount and quality of protein varies. A high-quality protein, with a high biological value would be one that contains all the essential amino acids and is easily digested and absorbed. In general, the amino acids from animal products such as eggs, meat, milk and fish are well absorbed (over 90%), amino acids from legumes (e.g. beans, peas, lentils etc.) are about 80% absorbed, and those from grains and other plant sources are between 60–90% absorbed. Animal products represent the best sources of quality protein but tend also to increase fat intake. Legumes come close in protein quality, avoid the problem of fat and contain many additional minerals and vitamins. If plant foods are to provide the major source of protein, it usually requires a wider mix to ensure an adequate supply of all the essential amino acids. For health, it is probably better to reduce the current level of animal protein in the western diet and increase the use of legumes and cereals. However, no nutrient can be considered in isolation and animal products are good sources

Table 21.3 Multiple values proposed for adults[a] (The Scientific Committee for Food (1993))

Nutrient	Average requirement (AR)	Population reference intake (PRI)	Lowest threshold intake (LTI)
Protein (g)	0.6/kg body wt	0.75/kg body wt	0.45/kg body wt
Vitamin A (μg)	500 (400)	700 (600)	300 (250)
Thiamin (μg)	72/MJ	100/MJ	50/MJ
Riboflavin (mg)	1.3 (1.1)	1.6 (1.3)	0.6
Niacin (mg niacin equivalents)	1.3/MJ	1.6/MJ	1.0/MJ
Vitamin B_6	13/g protein	15/g protein	—
Folate (μg)	140	200	85
Vitamin B_{12}	1.0	1.4	0.6
Vitamin C (mg)	30	45	12
Vitamin E (mg α-tocopherol equivalents)		0.4/g PUFA$^+$	4 (3)/d regardless of PUFA$^+$ intakes
n-6 PUFA$^+$ (as percentage of dietary energy)	1	2	0.5
n-3 PUFA$^+$ (as percentage of dietary energy)	0.2	0.5	0.1
Calcium (mg)	550	700	400
Phosphorus (mg)	400	550	300
Potassium (mg)	—	3100	1600
Iron (mg)	7 (10,6[a])	9 (16[b],8[a])	5 (7,4[a])
Zinc (mg)	7.5 (5.5)	9.5 (7)	5.5 (4)
Copper (mg)	0.8	1.1	0.6
Selenium (μg)	40	55	20
Iodine (μg)	100	130	70

For the following, acceptable ranges of intake are given: Pantothenic acid (mg) = 3–12; Biotin (μg) = 15–100; Vitamin D (μg) = 0–10; Sodium (g) = 0.575–3.5; Magnesium (mg) = 150–500; Manganese (mg) = 1–10.
[a] Amounts per day, unless given in other terms. If that for women is different from that for men, it is given in parentheses.
[b] PUFA: Polyunsaturated fatty acids.
[c] Postmenopausal women.
[d] PRI to cover 90% of women.

Box 21.3 Calcium requirements during lactation

The calcium requirement of lactating women provides a striking example of how requirements for a nutrient can vary in health. A non-pregnant woman has a calcium RDA of 500 mg whereas the RDA during lactating is 1200 mg; therefore the woman's normal diet would need modification to meet her increased requirements for calcium during lactation.

Box 21.4 Four-food group plan for adult's daily requirements

Milk/milk products — 2 servings. Examples of serving size: 1 cup of milk; 150 g carton of yoghurt; 1–2 oz (approximately 28–56 g) cheese.

Meat/meat alternatives — servings. Examples of serving size: 3 oz (approximately 85 g) of cooked meat, fish or chicken. Additionally 2 servings of legumes or nuts, about ¾ cup per serving.

Fruit and vegetables — 4 servings (to include 1 serving of citrus fruit daily for vitamin C, 1 serving of dark-green/yellow vegetables on alternate days for vitamin A). 1 medium fruit, apple, orange, pear or banana equals one serving.

Cereals/bread — 4 servings, whole grain products are preferred. A serving equals 1 slice of bread or ½ cup of cooked cereal (e.g. rice, pasta).

In addition, 1 serving of fat or oil (for vitamin E) is recommended. This food plan has the disadvantage of having a high energy content (about 9000 kJ).

of other nutrients, for example vitamin B_{12}, vitamin D and bioavailable iron.

Lipids

Lipids (Greek *lipos* = fat) provide a concentrated energy source and are the body's main mechanism for storing energy. Fat provides an important insulating layer beneath the skin and surrounds some body organs, providing support and cushioning the organs from mechanical trauma. Fat is a structural element forming, for example, the major component of the cell membrane. It is also required for effective neural function — myelin is a form of lipid. Lipids are used in the formation of substances such as lipoproteins, cholesterol and phospholipids and the steroid hormones. Adequate dietary fat is important, the essential fatty acids and the fat-soluble vitamins are found mainly in fatty foods. Food fats provide energy and cholesterol to supplement the body's endogenous cholesterol supply.

Box 21.5 Four-food group plan for vegetarian adults' daily requirements

Milk/milk products/alternatives — 2 servings. Alternative: calcium and vitamin B_{12} fortified soya milk.

Meat alternatives — 4 servings of protein-rich plant foods (nut and legumes) should include 2 servings of legumes daily.

Fruit and vegetables — 4 servings (to include 1 serving of citrus fruit daily for vitamin C, 1 serving of dark-green/yellow vegetables for vitamin A and iron).

Cereals/bread — 4 servings, whole grain products are preferred.

In addition 1 serving of fat or oil (for vitamin E) is recommended.

Lipids are also important in foods for giving aroma and flavour and contribute to the feeling of satiety. Fat greatly increases the palatability of food and so has gained a prominent place in the western diet. In some countries 40–45% of food energy may be derived from fat. While sufficient fat is vital for health, excess intake is associated with a number of health problems including obesity, cardiovascular disease and perhaps cancer. Excess of animal fats may be the particular problem.

Vitamins

Apart from vitamin D which can be synthesised by the body and vitamin K which can be synthesised by intestinal bacteria all the vitamins must be obtained from the diet. Since they are not consumed by the reactions they regulate, only small amounts are needed and a varied diet will normally supply all the vitamins required. The two main groupings are the fat-soluble and the water-soluble vitamins. The fat-soluble vitamins are usually absorbed from the small intestine along with dietary fat. They are found in foods such as fish and plant oils. The fat-soluble vitamins can be stored in the liver and adipose tissues; therefore excessive intake (hypervitaminosis) can lead to toxic levels. Water-soluble vitamins are easily lost from foods and the body, little storage occurs and hypervitaminosis for these vitamins is rare. Vitamin deficiency often results from a more widespread nutritional disruption but some specific deficiencies and disease states are important. Vitamin deficiency usually affects the water-soluble vitamins but in severe trauma or illness the fat-soluble vitamins may also be involved.

Minerals

The major minerals (calcium, phosphorus, sodium, potassium, chlorine, magnesium and sulphur) are essential for health and required in amounts over 100 mg/day. Trace elements are required in much smaller amounts (under 100 mg/day); putative trace elements are thought to be important but an essential role in human nutrition remains to be proven. A balanced diet featuring a range of different foods is likely to meet daily requirements for the major minerals and trace elements. A mineral is established as essential when deficiency can be shown to produce an impairment which can only be reversed or prevented by supplementation with that particular element. Trace elements are important as enzyme components or as structural components. Of particular nutritional significance are iron, iodine and zinc. Iodine deficiency in the form of endemic goitre is characterised by marked enlargement of the thyroid gland. It occurs in areas where water and soil are deficient in iodine. Zinc is present in body tissues in larger amounts than all of the other trace elements except iron. It is involved in a number of enzyme reactions and is particularly important in periods of growth and during wound healing. Animal products are the main sources of zinc. Cereals and legumes are poorer sources. Marginal deficiency may occur in the elderly and the hospitalised patient with poor appetite.

The major function of iron is as a component of haemoglobin but it may also be important in many enzyme processes and in the immune response. Iron is not excreted by the body but small amounts are lost mainly through the gastrointestinal tract in blood, desquamated cells and bile. Basal losses in the female are negligible but menstruation adds an additional, variable loss and pregnancy and lactation increase requirements. Although most foods are rich in iron, iron deficiency is one of the major nutritional diseases in the world. This is due not so much to a lack of iron but to a lack of bioavailable iron. Iron in the form of haem as found in meats is 20–40% available whereas iron in most plant foods is often less than 5% available. In addition a number of dietary factors may influence iron absorption; these have recently been reviewed (Torrance 1992).

NUTRITIONAL INTERVENTION

Dietary manipulation is a useful adjunct to the treatment of many diseases, for example special diets may help in renal disease, gastrointestinal disease and cardiovascular disease, and are essential in the management of diabetes mellitus and conditions such as phenylketonuria (PKU). Diets may be used to increase or decrease intake of specific nutrients, to help control body weight or to improve nutrition in the malnourished. A detailed consideration of diet therapy is beyond our remit but before discussing the nurse's role in helping a patient meet his nutritional needs a brief discussion of obesity and its management is presented. Obesity is the major nutritional disorder of our society and provides a good example of an overall approach to diet management. Paradoxically severe malnutrition is a major problem worldwide and a degree of malnutrition may be relatively common in the hospitalised patient.

Obesity

Obesity is the condition of excessive accumulation of fat in the body, leading to an increase in weight beyond that considered desirable with regard to the individual's height, bone structure and age. It has a complex aetiology related to food habits and intake, exercise and activity patterns and individual metabolic rate. Obesity is considered a major health problem of the Western world. Fat people tend to die younger than comparable lean people and obesity is linked with many common disorders (Simopoulos 1985). The extra strain placed on the musculoskeletal system may contribute to arthritic disease, particularly of the lower spine, hips and knees. Abdominal muscle may fail resulting in abdominal hernias. Fatty leg muscle may be inefficient, reducing the effectiveness of the muscle pump and predisposing to varicose veins. Excess fat in the thoracic cavity may impair breathing (Pickwickian syndrome). Obesity is linked with cardiovascular disease including atherosclerosis and hypertension which may progress to angina pectoralis and heart failure. Other diseases associated with obesity are gall bladder disease and non-insulin-dependent diabetes mellitus. Figure 21.1 summarises some of the complications of obesity. The psychological and social effects of obesity can also be profound. Thinness is the current, perceived norm for western societies and fat people may suffer social and employment discrimination, insurance rates will be higher, and current fashions may not be available in larger sizes. Obesity may engender a negative body image and this may be reinforced by the way society views and treats fat people.

In general, obesity results from an increased food intake or a reduced level of activity, i.e. over a significant period of time energy intake exceeds energy expenditure. Overeating is the major cause but this does not mean that all fat people simply overeat. Studies on twins suggest that genetic factors may be involved in obesity. Newman et al (1937) found that fraternal twins had a greater weight difference than identical twins. However, they also showed a greater difference in weight between twins raised apart compared with twins raised together, suggesting that environmental factors (family environment) may have the greater influence. The importance of the family environment is confirmed by studies of adopted children where there is little evidence of weight differences between the adopted and biological siblings (Garn & Bailey 1976). In a later report Garn & Clark (1976) recorded a high correlation between the skinfold measurements of parents

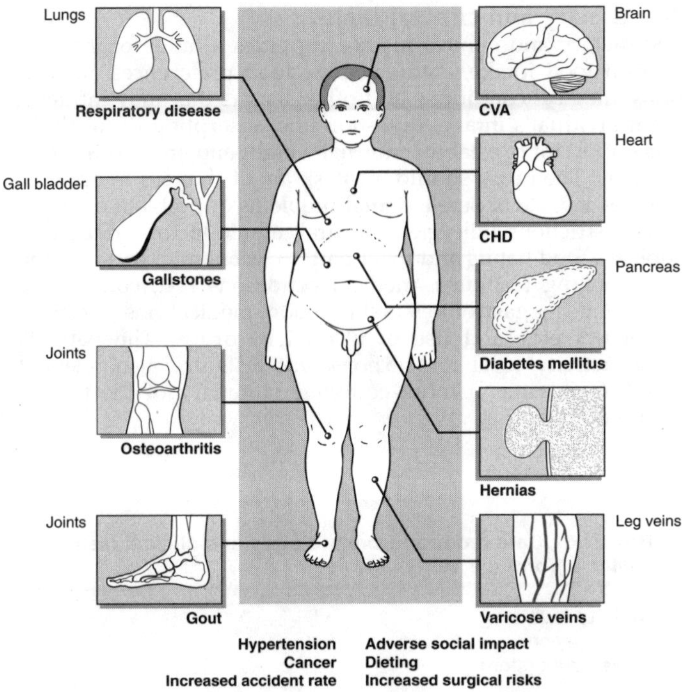

Fig. 21.1 Adverse effects of obesity.

and child. It seems likely, therefore, that the family's attitude to food and food habits are a major factor in obesity.

The importance of socioeconomic factors is clear and, although its exact nature is uncertain, the relationship between socioeconomic status and obesity is particularly strong in women. In a major American study an inverse relationship between obesity and socioeconomic status was demonstrated: 5% of upper status women; 16% of middle status women; and 30% of lower status women were obese (Goldblatt et al 1965). The situation is complicated, however, by the findings that racial, ethnic and religious factors also have an influence.

Popular opinion suggests a glandular basis for obesity but there is little evidence for an endocrine origin in most cases. Individual differences in metabolic rate and handling of nutrients has also been suggested. It is postulated that fat people are more efficient at utilising carbohydrate, i.e. they need less calories per unit of lean mass that those who are thin. This remains controversial. While individual variations in basal metabolic rate (BMR) are expected there is no clear evidence that fat people metabolise fuel foods more efficiently than lean people.

For a detailed review of obesity, see Pi-Sunyer Obesity. In: Shils & Young (eds) 1988 p. 795–816

A number of approaches are available to deal with excess weight ranging from severe diets (including wiring of jaws to decrease intake) to surgical removal of fat, from diuretics to appetite suppressors, and from fad diets to counselling and self-help groups. As the problem is in most cases due to overeating, diet therapy and counselling/support is perhaps the major approach. A balanced approach to eating and increased exercise are the mainstay of weight reduction. Reducing diets are perhaps the main area of popular interest with exponents recommending high fibre diets, low calorie diets, tropical fruit diets, banana and milk diet, and a number of specialised powder and food-bar diets. Some of these diets may restrict calories and other nutrients to such a degree that they can only be used under medical supervision. Behavioural changes, peer support and a sensible diet as typified by the Weight Watchers programme are to be recommended. Going on a diet is not enough, one must stay on a diet to lose weight and then adopt healthy eating patterns to maintain an ideal body weight. Episodic dieting where the individual swings from overeating to very low calorie intake and back to overeating may be more injurious than obesity itself.

A reducing diet should be planned after nutritional assessment and take into account the patient's lifestyle and food habits. It must supply sufficient energy for BMR and normal activity but exclude excess energy intake. Restriction of fat and an increase in the use of complex carbohydrate (including fibre) is usually recommended. Choices should still be made from the usual food groups to ensure enough vitamins and minerals. Defining the exact amount of energy required depends on the individual but most women will need at least 5 MJ (1200 kcal) a day, and bigger or more active women and men may need 6–7.5 MJ (1500–1800 kcal) daily. Diets providing less than this should probably only be undertaken on medical advice. It is important to establish a realistic level of energy intake.

Malnutrition

Malnutrition is an endemic problem; protein-energy malnutrition (PEM) affects large numbers of the world's population and contributes significantly to human mortality and morbidity. However, in developed countries, outright starvation is unlikely but levels of malnutrition exist. Certain groups including the homeless, the elderly, alcoholics, those with behavioural disturbances of eating such as anorexia nervosa, and the hospitalised patient may be at particular risk.

Illness can alter or increase the need for nutrients. Disease processes may reduce food intake or absorption of nutrients; pyrexia and infection may increase metabolic rate and nutritional demands; surgery and trauma have a profound impact on metabolism, initiating a complex neuroendocrine response which shares some of the characteristics of the body's response to starvation (Torrance 1991). Malnutrition is often associated with the chronically ill and is a risk whether they are nursed at home or in hospital but there is also evidence of significant undernutrition in medical and surgical wards. Bistrian et al (1976, 1974) found that protein-energy malnutrition (PEM) was common in both surgical and medical patients. Medical patients were more calorie depleted than surgical patients but had better protein status. In a British study of 105 surgical patients there was a significant reduction of four indices of nutritional status compared with controls (Hill et al 1977). Only 22 out of the 105 patients had any comments in their records about their nutritional status and less than one-fifth had been weighed during their period of hospitalisation. A small-scale study by Todd et al (1984) on medical, surgical and orthopaedic wards indicated that 24% of patients had a food intake below the level predicted for BMR and 16% had less than the recommended daily amount of protein.

In surgical patients, malnutrition is associated with increased postoperative morbidity and mortality and studies have demonstrated that preoperative nutritional support can reduce these rates (Mullen et al 1980, Heatley et al 1979). Postoperative infection is particularly linked to undernutrition. Infection can induce a stress-related, catabolic response similar to that seen in surgical trauma and it is also often associated with anorexia. The link between nutrition and immunodepression is complex but it is clear that a wide range of immunological functions may be affected. Nearly all dietary elements can be important in resistance to infection but adequate levels of protein, carbohydrate, types of lipid, iron and zinc may be of particular significance.

A study of nursing nutritional care is reported in Coates (1985).

? **21.3** Coates considered the issue of nutritional care in relation to the nutritional needs of patients; record keeping; and organisation of nursing care. What ward-based factors do you think influence a patient's nutritional needs and nursing management?

Hospitalisation may predispose to undernutrition due to a number of factors. The patient may find the anxiety and unfamiliarity of the environment reduces appetite. Food may not be to his taste and the presentation of meals and environment for eating less than ideal. Investigations may require periods of fasting and missed meals may not be replaced. Of particular interest is the practice of preoperative fasting, reviewed by Torrance (1991). Routine practice is to fast patients for a minimum of 4 hours before surgery to empty the stomach and avoid perioperative or postoperative vomiting and the risk of aspiration into the lungs. However, actual fasting times for elective surgery ranging from 5–22 hours have been reported and in one study only 16% of patients on an afternoon list were fasted for 6 hours or less (Thomas 1987, Smith 1972); 33% had been deprived of food for more than 13 hours. For patients on the morning list, 10 hours was the minimum length of fast. The theoretical 4–6-hour preoperative fast appears to result in practice in periods of abstinence that might be better termed preoperative starvation. Preoperative starvation could lead to a state of catabolism which may be detrimental to a patient undergoing major surgery (Short 1983).

? **21.4** Patients attending as outpatients for procedures on a day basis may have been advised to fast before or after the procedure. In respect of the patient's nutritional needs, review your hospital's practices in relation to the information given to patients attending day care.

The remainder of this chapter will explore the nurse's role in nutritional assessment and ensuring an adequate intake of food — encouraging oral intake and managing artificial feeding by enteral and parenteral routes.

NUTRITIONAL ASSESSMENT

The first stage in nutritional intervention is assessment, identifying the individual's current nutritional status, normal eating habits, risk of developing nutritional imbalances and establishing a baseline for monitoring changes in status. Important aspects of nutritional assessment are clinical and dietary history, physical examination, biochemical tests and immunological tests. Tables of normal values, expected weight for height, etc., are useful but it must be remembered that nutritional care like other aspects of nursing care must be individualised and patient centred. Obtaining the patient's confidence is as important as mastering technical procedures and measurement tools. Assessment and analysis should allow needs and goals to be set with the patient, and nursing interventions can be planned to meet these needs. As always, interventions should be recorded, and regularly evaluated and modified as the patient's condition progresses.

The dietary and clinical history

The dietary and clinical history provides a range of information on food intake, eating habits, food preferences, medications, medical conditions and other factors that may influence the individual's intake, digestion and absorption of nutrients. It is important to establish normal weight and any recent losses or gains. The nurse should also ask about changes in appetite, changes in taste or smell, dental problems or problem dentures, food restrictions (allergies, cultural/ethnic factors, individual choices), food habits and meal pattern, economic/social factors (e.g. cooking facilities), medical conditions restricting intake or influencing gastrointestinal function, medications (laxatives, antibiotics etc.) and use of alcohol or drugs. The patient's usual activity level and exercise interests are also relevant. Box 21.6 provides a more complete summary of the type of data required.

Box 21.6 Data required from a dietary and clinical history (Miller & Torrance 1991)

Activity levels
- Occupation.
- Exercise pattern.

Appetite
- Good, poor, recent changes.
- Changes and/or problems with the sense of taste or smell.
- Effects of stress.

Factors influencing food habits
- Cultural/ethnic influences.
- Religion.
- Educational level.
- Nutritional knowledge/insight.
- Eating patterns/family meal patterns.

Gastrointestinal status
- Indigestion 'heartburn'.
- Flatulence, constipation.
- Diarrhoea.

Medical conditions/special diets
- Chronic diseases (e.g. diabetes, ulcerative colitis, coeliac disease).
- Special diets (e.g. diabetic diet, low salt diet, lactose free, etc.).

Social drug use
- Alcohol consumption, amount and frequency.
- Smoking.
- Other recreational drugs.

Economic/social
- Income, spending on food.
- Social benefits/services.
- Cooking facilities and other services (e.g. meals on wheels).

Foods
- Likes/dislikes.
- Type/amounts.
- Food restrictions — allergies, intolerance.
- Fluid intake — type, amount, frequency.

Medications
- Type, dose, frequency.
- Length of treatment.
- Use of laxatives, emetics.
- Vitamins or other supplements.

Other problems
- Dental problems, dentures.
- Problems with chewing/swallowing.
- Physical or mental handicaps.

If necessary, a 24-hour recall using a questionnaire and interview is useful to determine the patient's consumption over the last 24 hours. However, it is very subjective and care must be taken to ensure that the previous 24 hours' intake was typical for the patient. If poor nutrition is suspected a daily food record might be useful and this is especially important if the patient is subjected to extensive investigations which might require fasting or risk missing mealtimes.

Physical examination

The patient's general appearance and fit of clothes should be noted as should the condition of the hair, skin, eyes, mouth, neurological and musculoskeletal system. Table 21.1 gives a brief summary of changes to look out for in the physical assessment.

Anthropometric evaluation. Anthropometric measurements provide an objective assessment of nutritional status. Height, weight, skinfold thickness and muscle mass are the commonly used anthropometric measurements. Although not routinely used by nurses, the skills could be easily taught and provide a useful addition to the physical examination. Regular checks of accuracy and if necessary recalibration are essential for all anthropometric equipment including scales.

Height and weight. Body weight is a useful indicator of nutritional status; it should be recorded on admission and monitored regularly. To ensure accuracy the patient should, if possible, be weighed on the same scales, at the same time each day and preferably in the same clothes and after emptying bladder and bowels. Single measurements of weight are of limited value, but serial measurements permit trends in weight loss to be identified; a rapid loss of 10% suggests mild malnutrition. A weight loss of 20% indicates moderate and 30% severe malnutrition. However, caution is required when interpreting rapid weight losses; factors such as dehydration or oedema can complicate the clinical picture. Height is another useful indicator of under- or overnutrition, most often combined with weight for comparison with ideal values of weight for height and sex as obtained from standard weight/height tables.

Body mass index. Another, more recent, way of classifying weight is to use the body mass index (BMI). This is simply the body weight in kilograms (kg) divided by the height in metres squared (m^2).

$$\frac{\text{Weight}}{\text{Height}^2}$$

For example, $\frac{57}{1.6^2} = 22.3$

The resulting ratio tends to vary between 20 and 30. The ideal range is 20–25; 25–30 indicates overweight and a ratio of over 30 indicates obesity.

Triceps skinfold thickness (TSF). Skinfold measurements provide a good estimate of body fat. A number of sites can be used but the triceps is the most accessible and reproducible. Skinfold callipers such as the Holtain calliper are used, the measurement being made on the posterior aspect of the upper, non-dominant arm, midway between the elbow and shoulder. A fold of skin is grasped and the callipers applied while the arm is relaxed and an average of three readings is recorded. Readings will not be accurate if oedema is present. The TSF can be compared with the value from standard tables: less than 60% of standard will indicate severe malnutrition; less than 90% moderate malnutrition. Training is required for accurate measurement using skinfold callipers and other measures such as arm circumference are recommended for routine use.

Mid-arm circumference (MAC). Estimates of muscle mass can be obtained by measuring mid-arm circumference. The non-dominant arm is bent at right angles to the body and the mid-point between the acromial process of the scapula and the olecranon process of the ulna marked. Using indelible ink will help to ensure that later measurements can be made at exactly the same place. MAC is measured at this point with the arm relaxed. The undernutrition can be recognised by comparing the measured MAC with standard tables. It is important to use a high-quality, non-stretch anthropometric tape measure.

Mid-arm muscle circumference (MAMC). MAMC is calculated by the following equation and provides an index of skeletal muscle mass alone:

$$\text{MAMC (cm)} = \text{MAC (cm)} - 0.134 \times \text{TSF}$$

MAMC is a useful indicator of PEM; less than 90% of standard indicates moderate and less than 60% severe PEM.

Laboratory investigations

Laboratory measurements are another useful source of objective data. A number of parameters, obtained from investigation of plasma, blood cells, urine and tissues (e.g. hair, liver, bone) can be measured to assess protein, fat, vitamin and mineral status.

The creatinine–height index (CHI). The CHI provides an estimate of skeletal muscle mass. Creatinine is produced in muscle by the breakdown of creatine, an energy-source compound found in muscle. It is filtered by the kidney and excreted in the urine unchanged. Urinary excretion rate is proportional to the patient's muscle mass and 24-hour urine collection provides a measure of creatinine excretion which can be compared with ideal creatinine excretion rate from a standard table:

$$\text{CHI} = \text{Urinary creatinine}/\text{Ideal creatinine} \times 100$$

The CHI provides an estimate of skeletal muscle loss: 60–80% of standard suggests moderate malnutrition; less than 60% severe malnutrition.

Nitrogen balance. Nitrogen balance studies provide an index of protein status. Nitrogen balance is determined by estimating protein intake and subtracting urinary nitrogen excretion with an allowance for nitrogen loss via hair, skin and faeces. Additionally, losses from wound drainage or gastrointestinal fistulae must be considered. A positive nitrogen balance indicates that the patient is in an anabolic state, a negative balance indicates catabolism. A loss of 5–10 g/day would be defined as a mild negative balance, 10–15 g/day as moderate and over 15 g/day as severe.

Serum proteins. Total serum protein provides an estimate of nutritional status but is a relatively insensitive measure. Measurement of individual plasma proteins is sensitive. Albumin, transferrin, prealbumin and retinol binding protein, the major plasma proteins, are synthesised in the liver. Serum albumin is the most frequently measured plasma protein; low albumin levels are a useful indicator of long-standing PEM, and hypoalbuminaemia can be predictive of complications such as anergy, sepsis and increased mortality. However, albumin has a long half-life (20 days) and there is a large reserve so serum albumin levels will only fall after sustained protein loss. Accepted standards for serum albumin vary but less than 3 g/dl suggests significant PEM. The other serum proteins have a shorter half-life and are more responsive to nutritional changes providing an earlier indication of nutritional deple-

Table 21.4 Serum proteins of nutritional significance (Miller & Torrance 1991)

Protein	Half-life	Other factors influencing levels
Albumin	20 days	Extravascular pool, stress, trauma, infection
Prealbumin	2 days	Trauma, sepsis, cancer
Transferrin	7–8 days	Iron deficiency
Retinol binding protein	12 hours	Vitamin A status

tion than albumin (Table 21.4). However, as a large number of disease conditions, including trauma and sepsis, can alter serum protein levels these parameters (like all biochemical data) need to be used with caution and in conjunction with other nutritional indicators and the clinical data.

Laboratory investigation can also assess more specific nutritional components. Fat status can be evaluated by measuring serum cholesterol, triglycerides or lipoproteins. Specific vitamins (e.g. vitamins C, D, B_1) or minerals (e.g. iron, zinc) can be assayed. Tests of immune function such as total lymphocyte count or skin testing are also useful indicators of nutritional depletion.

Accurate nutritional assessment relies on utilisation of data from a number of sources. Data from only one source can be open to misinterpretation due to the many factors such as disease processes that can influence individual parameters. A combination of dietary history, clinical examination, anthropometric measurements and laboratory studies is required to gain an accurate picture of the patient's nutritional status and to diagnose malnutrition.

Encouraging the patient to eat

Nurses are ideally placed to help patients, whether at home or in hospital, to manage their nutritional needs. However, dietitians and occupational therapists are invaluable as the members of the health care team with special expertise in dietary and functional aspects of nutritional care. Nutritional assessment identifies dietary needs but a full nursing assessment will help in identifying the patient's ability to meet those needs and the level of intervention required. Nursing interventions may include the provision of nutritional education, assisting and encouraging an oral intake or managing an artificial (either enteral or parenteral) feeding regime.

It is important to acknowledge that food has a number of non-nutritional roles, fulfilling a range of psychosocial needs. Eating will have very different expectations and associations for different people. Loss of menu choice, unfamiliar foods, food presentation, ethnic or cultural preferences, eating alone, eating in company, timing of meals, even the eating utensils can all influence the patient's motivation to eat. The patient's psychological state, for example stress due to the hospital environment or illness, may modify eating behaviour. Physical factors such as ability to manipulate cutlery, ability to chew and swallow, to taste food, even to reach food independently will also be important. Assessment of all aspects of the patient and his environment that might influence food intake and enjoyment is critical. A carefully planned, nutritionally correct diet is of no value if the patient cannot or chooses not to eat the food. In managing an artificial feeding regime, ensuring the provision of the essential nutrients is critical but an understanding of the equipment and feeds used, essential monitoring, infection risks, psychological impact, and metabolic or mechanical complications is also required.

Oral intake

A number of individual factors (physical and psychological) and environment or organisational factors will influence the patient's ability or willingness to eat an adequate diet. For an individual to successfully ingest an adequate oral diet a number of activities are required and have to be assessed:

- Is the patient able to go shopping and to choose and purchase appropriate foods?
- Is his nutritional knowledge adequate for informed choice and has he the financial resources to purchase the required foods?
- Once purchased can he easily transport food home or is a delivery service available?
- Are adequate cooking facilities available and can the patient use them safely?
- Can the patient feed himself or does he need help?

If a deficit occurs in any of these areas the nurse may need to look at alternative strategies; the occupational therapist may have a major role in assessing the home environment.

Shopping for food can be difficult for disabled people, the ill-elderly and some patients with behavioural disturbances. Mobile shops and delivery services may overcome these problems, if they are available and the individual can cope with ordering the food. However, where these services are unavailable or psychiatric or communication difficulties limit their use, the patient will require outside assistance. The family or informal carers may be involved as can social services (e.g. home helps) or voluntary agencies.

Food preparation can also be a problem. The home environment should be assessed for access to the kitchen, and access to worktops, cupboards, fridges and cookers. For example, a patient who is dependent on a wheelchair may need substantial alteration to the kitchen to enable independent food preparation. Patients with chronic illness such as multiple sclerosis or rheumatoid arthritis may have limited mobility or find food preparation tiring and need adapted equipment and lightweight cooking utensils. Perceptual problems and confusion may also interfere with independent food preparation. Again, if the patient cannot cope, or can only cope with assistance, family or community services may need to be involved.

Physical factors influencing eating

To eat and drink normally requires the ability to transfer food to the mouth, the ability to chew and the ability to swallow. Sensory function is also important; appetite is improved and eating is easier if we can see, smell and taste the food. Digestion and absorption of the nutrients is dependent on effective gastrointestinal function, and utilisation on metabolism. Box 21.7 lists physical factors that influence eating. The state of the teeth and mouth is important. Cleft lip and cleft palate are examples of congenital abnormalities that reduce a baby's ability to suck. Teeth are needed for effective chewing; edentulous patients may require food of a softer texture or cut into smaller pieces but seldom a diet of only mashed or minced foods. Edentulous patients can suffer from malnutrition. In one study of 130 healthy individuals, it was found protein intake was inversely correlated with chewing ability (Davidson et al 1962). If the oral tissues are dry, inflamed or painful the patient may be reluctant to eat. In xerostomia, artificial saliva can be used to help lubricate food. Oral health may also contribute to improving the taste/enjoyment of a meal; poor oral hygiene can mask taste and reduce appetite. The number of taste buds per papilla of the tongue decreases with age and taste changes can occur in some conditions such as cancer. Strohl (1983) has suggested the use of mouthwashes prior to food for cancer patients with taste alterations. In the elderly the sensations of sweet and salty tend to deteriorate while sour

Box 21.7 Physical factors influencing eating

Oral cavity
Congenital abnormalities, e.g. cleft lip and palate.
Dentition — natural teeth, dentures, edentulous.
Oral health — xerostomia, gingivitis, stomatitis, mouth ulcers, pain.
Sensory — temperature sensation, taste, smell.

Chewing and swallowing
Age.
Dentition.
Dysphagia.
Achalasia.

Dexterity/mobility
Perceptual problems.
Upper limb function.
Mobility.
Positioning.

Others
Dyspnoea.
Pain.

and bitter tastes are better detected. They may therefore prefer more highly seasoned food.

The odour of food is an important aspect of taste and enjoyment. Conditions such as upper respiratory tract infections can cause a temporary reduction in the sense of smell. Rare conditions causing anosmia may alter the patient's perception of food. Ageing may also be associated with alterations in the sensation of smell. Reduced oral sensitivity or confusion may cause the temperature of food to be misjudged resulting in a greater risk of scalds and burns. The visual appearance of food is also important; meals that look unappetising or are poorly presented may reduce interest in eating. The visually impaired will appreciate knowing where different foods are positioned on the plate.

The texture of food and the patient's perception of his ability to chew it are also important. Problems with mastication appear to increase with age and may often be related to poorly fitting dentures. In some conditions there may be difficulty in coordinating chewing, and the movements of the mouth may be uneven with a tendency for food to dribble out of one side.

Dysphagia is defined as difficulty in swallowing and has a number of causes. It may be due to neurological injury as in stroke, mechanical or motor obstruction of the oesophagus, oesophagitis and oesophageal cancer. Odynophagia, pain associated with swallowing, is often due to reflux of gastric acid. Achalasia is a condition in which the smooth muscle of the lower oesophagus and cardiac sphincter of the stomach fail to relax leading to dysphagia, vomiting and odynophagia. The degree of dysphagia must be assessed. It may be that only soft foods or liquids can be tolerated. If oral intake is problematic, supplementary artificial feeding can be instigated. If oral intake is not possible, parenteral or tube feeding is required.

Reduced mobility may cause problems in access to foods, choice of place for eating and attaining a comfortable eating position. Care and perhaps some dietary alterations may be required if supine or prone positions have to be adopted for eating. Any impediment of arm or hand movement or hand–eye coordination may diminish ability to eat. The patient may need assessment for eating aids such as cutlery with special grips or shapes. If the patient has to eat one-handed, stabilisation of plates and the provision of plate guards may help. Drinking may also be a problem and special cups and glasses are available. If the patient suffers from muscle weakness, special lightweight utensils can be ordered. A number of diseases may result in problems with feeding but stroke is an example of a disease which can markedly alter many aspects of feeding behaviour. The nurse can assess eating skills and an occupational therapy consultation will help in the identification of suitable eating aids.

Organising effective mealtimes

Ensuring a supply of nutritious food, at the right temperature and in an attractive and hygienic manner is the responsibility of both nursing and catering services. Although nurses remain responsible for ensuring adequate nutrition, their role in the preparation and distribution of food has tended to be reduced. Food preparation is not usually a nursing task but the nurse is responsible for ensuring that food is ordered and may have to act as a buffer between the patient and the centralised catering services. Meals are often delivered to the wards preplated in heated trolleys at times dictated by catering service needs. With the withdrawal of Crown Immunity, reheating of meals or preparation of small snacks in the ward kitchen is discouraged. However, some patients may need or prefer more frequent, smaller meals. Patients may miss meals due to investigations, treatments etc. and obtaining meals in these cases can be difficult if catering services are inflexible. In one study it was found that for some patients food had to be ordered 2 days in advance, which is not always possible in the acute areas (DHSS & Welsh Office 1976).

Mealtimes. Ideally, mealtimes should be a planned part of nutritional care; used appropriately they can be an effective therapeutic event. Meals are often the focal point of the day, providing landmarks that break up the day and lend a familiar pattern to the ward routine. For the elderly person at home the arrival of a midday meal may be an important social event; in a busy ward sharing a table may help patients break down barriers. Mealtimes must not be considered as an inconvenience, disrupting ward activities three times a day. Rather they should be orchestrated to be, where possible, a pleasurable social activity. Properly managed they can provide a useful focus for the social activities of the ward. To make the most of meals they should be planned in relation to timing, to environment, and of course to menu and nutritional value. A King's Fund study (1986) indicated that 'food should be given priority over other work when it appears on the ward'.

Ideally the timing of meals would be flexible allowing individual patients to continue with their normal pattern of mealtimes. Unfortunately the necessities of catering for large numbers preclude this. Mealtimes should not coincide with other structured ward activities such as drug rounds, shift handovers or staff breaks, since there is a risk that they will then be hurried and unsatisfactory for both nurse and patient. Some patients may like to take their time over meals and others may require assistance in eating. Hovering staff, in a hurry to clear away dishes, will not encourage appetite. Even when meals are preplated and the trays distributed by domestic staff it is essential for the nurse to be involved.

Timing of meals may have to be a compromise, reflecting the needs of the individual, the ward and the catering service. Breakfast need not be inflexible, especially if cold cereals or a continental style breakfast has been chosen. Midday is probably an appropriate time for lunch for most people but it may not be the main meal of the day for some. The evening meal is often the main meal for working people but in hospital it may occur too early at around 5 p.m. It also tends to leave a long gap before breakfast. A snack and hot drink later in the evening may be essential. In the hospital surveyed by Simon (1991) breakfast was delivered at 9.30 a.m., lunch at 11.30 a.m.

and tea at 5.30 p.m. This resulted in a gap of only 2½ hours between breakfast and lunch. Not surprisingly, the late breakfast was eaten well but lunch poorly! Kirk (1990) also found that timing of meals influenced how much was eaten. Some flexibility over mealtimes is preferable in the acute setting but it is essential that an effort is made to meet residents' needs and norms in long-term care.

Ideally the patient will have a choice of where he eats. While some may prefer to eat by their bed or in their own room, a separate dining area, distinct from the bed spaces and treatment area of the ward, is required. The nature of the open ward with inevitable sights, sounds and smells of illness are not conducive to appetite. The dining area should be decorated to provide a social atmosphere and provided with small tables to allow patients to eat in their natural groupings. Provision for those who wish to eat alone or who need assistance are also necessary. Forcing relative strangers to eat together or to have to watch a person with eating difficulties will not aid appetite. Even if the eating area has also to double as the day room it can be specifically set up at mealtimes. Tables should be bright and clean, and tablecloths, large napkins and other civilised accoutrements will help. Large numbers of visitors in the ward while patients are eating may be a disadvantage. If a patient has visitors during meals a phenomenon described by Holmes (1987) as 'feeding time at the zoo' might occur with the patient having to eat surrounded by his visitors. If possible it might be better for the patient and visitors to go to the cafeteria and eat together.

Food presentation. Although nurses do not always serve meals, it is important for them to make sure that each of their patients receives the right food in sufficient quantities. It is then easier to ensure adherence to dietary regimes and, after a meal, to estimate the patient's intake. The patient needs to be active in food selection. Helping him to fill in a menu card or offering him a choice from a bulk trolley is an important nursing function. Foods should be attractively served, with small inviting portions (usually they are too large) placed separately on the plate. Presenting a heaped plate of food to an ill person with a poor appetite will be counterproductive. For some, large portions of food can be daunting (see Box 21.8). In a study of anorexia nervosa sufferers it was found that they exaggerated the size of food portions and might find smaller portions more tempting (Yellowless et al 1988). The temperature of food is another factor that affects appetite; cold food was one problem noted in the DHSS & Welsh Office (1976) study. It is also important that food is served using a no-touch technique. Chipped or cracked crockery will not clean properly and can become a source of cross-infection.

> **Box 21.8 Improving presentation of food to the terminally ill patient**
>
> Williams & Copp (1990) carried out a study of food presentation to terminally ill cancer patients. They identified problems with ordering food 24 hours in advance. Patients often could not remember what they had ordered. 85% found portions too large and off-putting. They also felt embarrassed about leaving food. Food was often too dry; more sauces and gravy were recommended. Food was often cold, meals too early or late and food presentation was poor.
>
> The plated meals were replaced with a bulk trolley system. This allowed the primary nurses to serve their own patients. Patients made their choices from the food available and portion size, order and timing of courses could be individualised. Other changes made included the use of smaller, decorated plates and bowls (to reduce portions), serviettes and individual salt and pepper pots on each tray. These changes improved enjoyment of meals and avoided complaints about the temperature, portion size and dryness of food.

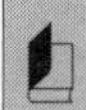

For further information, see Patients' Association (1993).

21.5 Discuss the management issues that might arise from adjusting food presentation, timing and service.

Assisting patients to eat

When someone has difficulty in eating it becomes the nurse's privilege to help him with this basic activity of living. Feeding a patient requires considerable care and sensitivity. Having to be fed is a threat to the individual's integrity and self-esteem. This should be recognised and every effort made to minimise the negative aspects. Before preparing for the meal the dependent patient should be offered a bedpan or urinal, followed by hand-washing facilities. Eating is easier and more normal sitting out of bed but the bedfast patient can be sat upright and made comfortable. An appropriate table is required so the patient can have his food set before him, allowing him to see the food and indicate preferences. The patient can be offered the opportunity to clean his teeth or use a mouthwash before (and after) the meal.

The nurse should sit level with the patient and encourage a relaxed social atmosphere. The patient's food habits must be identified and the rate and manner of feeding should be at the patient's normal pace and pattern. Plenty of time is essential to allow the patient to chew, to pause between mouthfuls, and to have a drink when desired. If protection for the clothing is required a normal serviette can be used. Plastic bibs or rolls of paper towel will damage self-esteem. Normal crockery should be used if the nurse is feeding the patient; if the patient is able to participate, then feeding aids may improve his independence. Spoons have their place but knife and fork should be used for the main course. The nurse should check that plates and food are at an appropriate temperature and ensure that any bones or fruit pips are removed.

Feeding a patient or assisting him in feeding himself is an essential nursing function. The patient should be closely observed and assessed for developing independence in eating. What he can do for himself he must be given the time and encouragement to attempt. Food and drink can be positioned on the dominant side, well within reach. If the patient cannot manage to pour a drink, a glass can be left ready filled. If he cannot manage to cut up his food, the nurse can do this but encourage him to do the rest. By giving the patient her full attention and allowing the patient to control the process of feeding as much as possible the negative effects of having to be fed can be alleviated. As with any nursing activity, assisting with eating necessitates assessment of the individual, identification of problems and the required interventions, and evaluation and reassessment as the activity proceeds or the patient progresses.

Patients with poor appetite or dysphagia may not be able to ingest enough solid food to meet nutritional needs and supplements of liquid foods between meals may be required. A number of supplementary oral or sip feeds are available. These may be powdered feeds added to milk or complete formulas. Many sip feeds can also be used as tube feeds. Although providing a range of nutrients they are particularly useful for providing a supplementary energy intake. Patients may need some persuasion to take supplementary feeds and they may reduce food intake at meals. Barnes (1989) has suggested adding supplementary calories in the form of glucose powder to foods such as porridge and soups to overcome this problem. If a patient has a poor intake or requires assistance with feeding it is useful to chart daily intakes of food and fluid and note any successful feeding strategies in the nursing records.

ENTERAL FEEDING

Enteral or tube feeding involves delivering nutrients directly to the stomach or small intestine. Its success depends on normal digestion and absorption but it provides a way of avoiding the oral route. The major enteral route is via a nasogastric tube but longer tubes can be passed directly to the small intestine (nasoduodenal and nasojejunal). Less commonly a tube can be passed via the mouth — the orogastric route. Another form of enteral feeding is via tubes surgically inserted through the body wall into the oesophagus (oesophagostomy), the stomach (gastrostomy) and jejunum (jejunostomy). Gastrostomy is the most commonly used of the enterostomies.

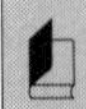

For further information, see Starkey, Jefferson & Kirby (1988).

Nasal insertion is often preferred for short-term alimentation; it is well tolerated if a small-bore, flexible tube is used. Enterostomies are more likely to be used for long-term feeding or if transnasal passage is difficult. If feeding is likely to last for longer than 6 weeks or there is a risk of aspiration, enterostomy feeding is preferable. If the expected duration is less than 6 weeks and aspiration is not a major risk then the nasoenteral route can be used (Cataldo & Smith 1980).

Tube feeding represents a more 'normal' mode of feeding than the intravenous route. It has many benefits and is based on the maxim 'if the gut works, use it', although this is not an infallible guide. With appropriate patient selection, tube feeding can be used to meet all the daily demands for nutrients and water. It has been shown to be cost effective and because digestion and absorption follow a more physiological pattern it helps to maintain normal structure and function in the small intestine (Rombeau & Jacobs 1984). In general, tube feeding can be considered as more cost effective and less hazardous than intravenous alimentation. It remains an invasive treatment with complications as well as benefits. The relative simplicity of the method may result in the nursing skills and responsibilities involved being underestimated; as reported by Jones (1975), the management of enteral feeding may often be delegated to very junior nurses. In common with many 'basic' nursing skills the management of tube feeding requires a considerable level of knowledge and expertise to ensure a satisfactory outcome for the patient.

Indications for enteral feeding

The enteral route can be considered for any patients unable to meet all their nutritional needs by oral ingestion. A voluntary oral intake of less than 80% of normal daily requirements indicates the need for supplementary feeding. Enteral feeding can be used as the sole form of nutrition or as a supplement to oral intake. The two major requirements for enteral feeding are:

- a sufficient area of functioning small intestine for absorption of nutrients
- convenient access for introduction of nutrients.

Providing access, absorption and the availability of a suitable feed can be ensured then the majority of medical and surgical patients can tolerate enteral feeding (Moghissi & Boore 1983). Indeed, relatively few conditions preclude enteral feeding, but those that do include malfunctioning of the gastrointestinal tract and major upper alimentary tract surgery. Tube feeding is contraindicated in adynamic ileus, total intestinal obstruction, some types of malabsorption and intractable vomiting, when parenteral nutrition should be considered. The unconscious patient can tolerate enteral feeding but the danger of aspiration must be recognised. If the comatose patient has serious pulmonary disease, vomiting or hiccupping and lacks a gag response then parenteral feeding is recommended; if a gag response is present and pulmonary dysfunction minimal then nasojejunal feeding can be considered (Shils 1988). High output fistulae, particularly upper alimentary fistulae which cannot be bypassed by the feeding tube, are a contraindication (Moghissi & Boore 1983, Shils 1988). Tube feeding is indicated in a wide range of clinical situations; major indications are listed in Box 21.9. As transnasal tubes represent the commonest approach to tube feeding they will be the focus of the rest of this section.

Nasoenteral feeding

Nasoenteral feeding is indicated when short-term nutritional support is required. Nasoenteric tubes include nasogastric, nasoduodenal or nasojejunal tubes. As the transnasal route does not interfere with oral function nasoenteric feeding can be used to supplement oral intake. The traditional nasoenteral tube was a wide-bore rubber or PVC tube such as the Ryle's tube. Although still used they are poorly tolerated and can cause pressure necrosis of the nares and oropharynx (Rombeau & Jacobs 1984). The wide bore may encourage cardiac sphincter incompetence and increase the risk of gastric reflux and aspiration (Cataldo & Smith 1980, Silk 1980, Janes 1982). Fine-bore feeding tubes of silicone or polyurethane are now available. These are softer, more pliable tubes that are better tolerated by the patient and less likely to cause pressure ulceration or sphincter problems. However, they are more difficult

Box 21.9 Indications for enteral feeding

Increased nutritional needs
Protein-energy malnutrition.
Persistent anorexia.
Hypercatabolic states: burns, major sepsis, severe trauma.

Compromised oral access to GI tract
Facial/oral surgery.
Head and neck surgery.
Oesophageal stricture, surgery, fistula.
Carcinoma of the mouth or upper alimentary structures.
Functional or mechanical obstructions.

Inability to eat
Unconscious.
Confused/uncooperative.

Unwillingness to eat
Odynophagia: mucositis, pharyngitis, oesophagitis.
Persistent anorexia (e.g. related to chemotherapy or radiotherapy).
Psychiatric disorders resulting in a refusal to eat (anorexia nervosa).
Cancer cachexia/anorexia.
Persistent nausea and vomiting.

Danger of aspiration
Dysphagia.
Neurological disorders with loss of cough reflex.

Gastrointestinal disorders
Fistula.
Short bowel syndrome.
Malabsorption syndromes.
Inflammatory bowel disease.

to insert (a wire introducer may be required) and due to the narrow lumen are prone to blockage. The tube can pass into the trachea without causing laryngeal spasm or respiratory distress and the position of the tube has to be checked by X-ray (the tubes usually have a weighted, radioopaque tip). A tendency to collapse on aspiration makes it difficult to check for gastric acid. Choice of tube depends on the patient and the intended feed. In general a tube with the smallest bore compatible with the viscosity of the enteral formula should be used. Ports and connections on enteral feeding tubes and equipment must not be compatible with intravenous infusion sets.

The patient should be in an upright position while the tube is being inserted to avoid the risk of intracranial insertion. The length of tube required can be estimated by measuring the distance from the bridge of the nose to the ear lobe plus the distance from the tip of the nose to the xiphisternum (Delaney 1991). In general, a 36-inch tube is used for nasogastric intubation, and a 43-inch tube for the nasoduodenal/jejunal route. If radiography is not used another method of checking placement must be adopted. Two main methods are aspiration with pH testing, and air injection. Injecting 2–5 ml of air while listening over the stomach with a stethoscope for the whoosh or gurgling of the injected air is a common practice. Research by Metheny et al (1990) indicates that this is not a reliable method. Problems associated with this method listed by Delaney (1991) include:

- small-bore tubes do not always allow the entry of sufficient air for diagnosis
- vigorous peristalsis may mimic the sound of injected air
- there is a danger of pneumothorax if the tube is in the lungs
- an inexperienced nurse may misinterpret the sounds heard.

Selection of enteral feeds

The range of enteral feeds, oral or tube, is large. Feeds may vary from liquidised meals to commercially prepared specialised products for patients with particular nutritional needs. In general, hospitals tend to use commercially prepared feeds as these are of known nutritional content, sterile and designed for ease of nasoenteral administration. Liquidised diets can be used for patients receiving enteral nutrition at home but even here the nutritional advantages, sterility, ease of use and the danger of blocking a fine-bore tube would tend to favour prepared feeds. Liquidised feeds are cheap and cause less diarrhoea than commercial feeds but usually have to be strained, diluted and require a wide-bore tube. Hospital diet kitchens may make up tube feeds from constituents such as milk, raw eggs and commercial supplements such as Complan as the protein sources, plus sugar and fat emulsions as the energy sources. Additional minerals and vitamins are included. However, the risk of infection with species of Salmonella should limit the use of raw eggs, and liquidised or hospital-prepared feeds must be stored in the refrigerator and should not hang at room temperature for more than 4 hours. Due to the risk of a break in asepsis during feed preparation and the likelihood of the patient having a degree of immunoincompetence, commercially prepared formulas are probably a safer, more cost-effective solution.

Commercial formulas vary in nutritional content, nutrient sources, digestibility, osmolality and viscosity. Energy density and the distribution of energy among protein, carbohydrate and fats are important variables. Enteral feeds may come as complete liquid preparations or as powders requiring reconstitution. An aseptic approach is required when reconstituting powdered feeds. As some tube feeds are also used for oral supplementation (sip feeding) taste or palatability is also important; if a pleasantly tasting feed is stocked it can be used for both purposes. The texture and smell of the feed should be considered. A more recent development is the addition of soluble fibre to enteral formulas. It can, however, increase viscosity and may require the use of an infusion pump. Commercial feeds may be polymeric, that is have whole protein as the nitrogen source with a mixture of carbohydrate and fats for energy. Predigested formulas have hydrolysed proteins so that the nitrogen is in the form of oligopeptides and amino acids. Fully defined or elemental feeds contain purified nutrients, that is amino acids, simple sugars and usually very little fat. Elemental formulas require very little digestion. Additional minerals and vitamins may be added to all types of feeds and many feeds are available that are lactose and gluten free.

In general, cost increases and palatability decreases as the feed is further purified. Polymeric formulas are generally the most economical choice for the majority of tube-fed patients. Predigested feeds may be required for patients with short bowel syndrome. Some fully defined feeds are designed for patients with particular nutritional needs due to organ- or system-specific disease. The use of disease-specific or modular formulas which restrict or increase availability of specific nutrients is controversial. For some conditions defined formulas may have a proven role, for others it is much less certain. There is a lack of controlled studies comparing the efficacy of defined formulas in many clinical conditions (Shils 1988).

Prescription of a tube feed depends on a complete assessment of the patient's nutritional needs. Protein content varies between 1.2 and 10 g per 100 ml, energy content from 188 J (45 kcal) to 837 J (200 kcal) per 100 ml. The osmolality of feeds ranges from 184 to over 900 mosmol/kg. As most feeds are hyperosmolar they can cause gastrointestinal disturbances when feeding is being initiated or if they are infused too rapidly.

Methods of administration

Nasoenteral feeds can be delivered by intermittent bolus or continuous feeding. Bolus feeding was the traditional approach when large-bore nasogastric tubes were used. Gravity- or pump-controlled drip infusion can be intermittent or more usually continuous. Bolus feeding can be organised to reflect more closely the normal eating pattern, it permits free movement between feeds and is particularly convenient for home enteral nutrition. Disadvantages are that it is more likely to result in feelings of nausea, vomiting, intestinal distension, cramps and diarrhoea. There is an increased risk of reflux and aspiration. Hanson et al (1975) reported that problems with tachycardia, nausea, gagging and regurgitation increased in normal subjects due to rapid feeding. To avoid overloading the stomach the bolus should be limited to a maximum of 300 ml (Janes 1982) and sufficient time, 10–15 minutes, allowed to deliver the bolus. The risk of aspiration can be reduced by feeding the patient in an upright position and maintaining this position for an hour after the feed. As discussed, the position of the tube should be checked and if the gastric residue exceeds 75–100 ml the feed should be withheld (Holmes 1987). Flushing of the tube with water after the feed will help to reduce blockage and additionally may help by reducing the osmolality of the feed. For bolus feeding it is probably better if the feed is approximately at body temperature.

Intermittent feeding by gravity or peristaltic pumps over a period of 30–40 minutes may be better tolerated than a bolus feed. However, for many patients continuous feeding is adopted. The feeding regime may extend from 16–24 hours. The advantages of continuous feeding are that it delivers a lower volume per hour resulting in a smaller residual volume, reduces the risk of aspiration and increases patient tolerance. The major disadvantages are cost and the reduction in patient mobility, although the patient can move around with the enteral feeding set supported on a wheeled drip stand. The initial delivery should be at a rate of 25–50 ml per hour and then it should be slowly increased until the desired rate is attained. It is also desirable to start with dilute feeds until the bowel has adapted (Chernoff 1983). The temperature of the feed is probably less important during continuous administration. Gormican (1970) and Kagarva-Busby et al (1980) have reported an association between cold feeds and diarrhoea but other authors have found no adverse effects from administering cold tube feeds (Holt 1962, Fason 1967, Williams & Walike 1975).

The equipment for continuous feeding consists of the nasoenteral tube, a reservoir, giving set and possibly a peristaltic pump. The reservoir may be a rigid plastic or glass bottle or a PVC bag. In addition there is a proliferation of products designed for use with particular tubes, or combining reservoir and giving set. PVC bag-type reservoirs can be difficult to fill and calibration is less reliable. Bottles require an airway but are easier to fill and allow more accurate monitoring of the volume administered. Reservoirs should not be used for more than 24 hours. A number of peristaltic pumps are available for ensuring accurate delivery of feeds and these may be required for more viscous formulas. Use of a pump is convenient but does not remove the nurse's responsibility for monitoring the delivery of the nasoenteric feed.

Complications of enteral feeding

If patient selection and monitoring has been appropriate then the complications of enteral feeding can be prevented or identified and rectified at an early stage. Complications are rarely serious enough to discontinue feeding but care is necessary to minimise their impact. Complications can be classed into three broad groups: mechanical, metabolic and gastrointestinal. Complications are summarised in Tables 21.5–21.7. Careful monitoring of the patient is essential. Monitoring is required

Table 21.5 Mechanical and infectious complications of enteral feeding

Complication	Prevention	Treatment
Tube blockage	Flush tube with water when feed stopped/interrupted Maintain continuous flow Use correct feeding tube/nutrient solutions combinations	Flush tube Replace tube
Knotted tubes	Use acid-resistant tubes Use unweighted tubes Replace regularly Remove tubes with care	Note any pain on tube withdrawal If knotted end can be seen through the mouth grip with forceps, pull out of mouth and cut; remove rest of tube as normal. If not seen further investigation required
Misplacement	Insert tube with patient in an upright position Use correct type, length of tube Check position by aspiration and pH or by X-ray Particular care needed if the patient lacks a gag reflex, is unconscious or has severe facial injuries	Withdraw and replace
Displacement	Secure firmly, explanation of need for tube to patient Check position at least daily Marking the tube at the nares will facilitate monitoring of position	Replace tube
Aspiration	Elevate head of bed during continuous feeding, 30 minutes after intermittent feeding Correct placement of tube Check position before starting feed Use nasojejunal feeding Avoid use of large-bore tubes	Discontinue tube feeding
Discomfort	Ensure hydration Encourage nose breathing Lubricate lips Provide regular oral care Secure tube firmly Use smallest appropriate bore of tube	Give water by mouth if possible
Acute otitis media	Use small-bore, soft feeding tube	Change to other nostril Antibiotic therapy
Mucosal erosion (nares, nasal septum, nasopharynx, gastrointestinal mucosa)	Secure tube firmly to avoid Keep mucosa moist (see discomfort above) Avoid Ryle's or other wide-bore tubes Inspect nares daily	
Aspiration pneumonia	Avoid aspiration as above Risk greater if patient supine, unconscious, when cardiac sphincter is incompetent or if a Ryle's tube is used	
Contamination	Avoid non-sterile feeds Take care when handling feeds or equipment Change giving sets regularly Change bags/bottles after 24 hours	

Table 21.6 Metabolic complications of enteral feeding (adapted from Forlaw & Williamson 1986)

Complication	Monitoring	Intervention
Hyperkalaemia	Routine electrolytes	Use lower potassium feed
Hyponatraemia	Routine electrolytes	Restrict water
Hypophosphataemia	Routine electrolytes	Phosphate supplements
Hyperglycaemia	Blood glucose testing	Reduce infusion rate
	Serum glucose level Urinalysis — glycosuria, ketones	Administer insulin
Uraemia	Check blood and urine urea regularly Assess hydration Assess protein intake	Deal with dehydration Correct any protein/energy imbalance
Overhydration	Accurate daily intake/ output recording Weight regularly	Reduce flow rate
Dehydration	Accurate daily intake/ output recording Weight regularly	Additional water

to prevent complications developing and to ensure that nutritional goals are being met. Daily recording of intake and output is essential including calculation of nutritional content. Nutritional monitoring using anthropometric and biochemical parameters is also required. General monitoring of the patient and equipment is necessary to identify any technical problems. Monitoring of the patient receiving tube feeding has been extensively discussed by Moghissi & Boore (1983).

The psychological effects of tube feeding should also be considered, since food has a profound influence on psychosocial well-being. For a patient with facial injuries who is unable to chew, the enteral tube may represent control and relief from his anxieties over nutrition but for others it may be yet another assault on their self-image and feelings of loss of control over their own life. Enteral feeding can lead to a marked change in a patient's attitude to food. The nurse should try to:

- understand what tube feeding means to the patient and family
- encourage the patient to express his feelings about the feeding regime
- ensure that nursing management recognises and meets the patient's needs
- discuss the duration and management of the regime with the patient.

If tube feeding is likely to be a long-term intervention or to be continued at home, then patient and family education becomes a priority. Padilla and colleagues have addressed some psychological aspects of tube feeding (Padilla et al 1979).

PARENTERAL NUTRITION

In parenteral feeding, nutrients in solution are infused directly into the venous system usually via a large, central vein into the right atrium. Parenteral nutrition may be used as a supplement to oral or nasogastric feeding or it can be the sole form of feeding — total parenteral nutrition (TPN). It is an invasive technique associated with several hazards and problems and should only be used when other methods have been excluded. The function of parenteral feeding is to provide the patient with adequate nutrients and water during a period of stress/ illness when other methods of feeding are either impractical or inadequate. The need for parenteral feeding can be identified by accurate clinical and nutritional assessment and by anticipating the patient's nutritional needs as his condition or treatment progresses. Parenteral feeding is best initiated before the patient deteriorates. Early intervention can prevent or

Table 21.7 Gastrointestinal complications of enteral feeding (adapted from Taylor 1989, and Forlaw & Williamson 1986)

Complication	Prevention	Treatment
Nausea & vomiting	Avoid high fat or hyperosmolar feeds Avoid rapid infusion rates Use low lactose or lactose-free formulas Elevate head or bed during feeds Initiate feeding with low volume or dilute feeds Increase concentration and rate slowly Use enteral pump	Reduce infusion rate Dilute feed Change to lower fat formula Change to lower lactose or lactose-free feeds
Diarrhoea	Monitor antibiotic therapy Avoid hyperosmolar feeds If patient has not been eating or has been on TPN introduce enteral feeding slowly (gut atrophy) Use isotonic formula if appropriate Use lactose-free feeds Monitor hydration	Dilute feed Change to lactose-free feed Consider i.v. antibiotics or changing to better absorbed antibiotics Oral rehydration solutions might be required Check feeds for contamination
Constipation/overflow	Use fibre-containing feed Encourage mobility Monitor frequency and consistency of stool Ensure adequate water intake	Extra fluid and bulking agents Enemas or laxatives as appropriate
Distension/cramps	Commence feeding with slow rate and dilute feeds Use lactose-free formula	Reduce infusion rate Dilute formula Change to lactose-free feed

reduce the likelihood of other complications arising. Nurses have a major role in the management of TPN and the important aspects to consider include:

- indications for TPN
- assessment of needs and selection of nutrient solutions
- infusion systems for TPN
- monitoring and management of TPN
- complications of TPN.

Indications for TPN

The risks and expense associated with TPN are significant and three general factors should be considered when deciding to use this form of feeding:

- the availability of the gastrointestinal (GI) system
- the degree of malnutrition
- the metabolic status of the patient.

TPN will be method of choice if the GI system is unavailable for use. Major abdominal surgery or injury, GI obstruction, fistula or malignancy, inflammatory disease of the bowel or malabsorption syndromes can all rule out the use of enteral feeding. Psychiatric disturbances, severe anorexia or coma may also indicate a need for TPN. As discussed earlier, undernutrition may be common in some groups of hospitalised patients. Severely malnourished patients may not be able to tolerate the oral or enteral intake required to rectify their nutrition deficits and supplementary parenteral feeding should be considered. In some cases of GI disease the patient may be severely malnourished and require preoperative TPN to prepare for the increased metabolic demands after surgery. Severe trauma, including extensive surgery, some malignancies and major sepsis can all induce a state of hypercatabolism which imposes an enormous demand on nutritional resources. If exogenous nutrients are not available the catabolic demands can result in a marked loss of body tissues.

TPN should be considered if a patient is severely malnourished before surgery or if he has not eaten for 5 days and is not expected to eat for another 7 days. TPN may also be required in patients who are likely to be starved for over 5 days and have a history of a 7–10% loss of body weight in the preceding 2 months. With these basic considerations in mind appropriate use of TPN would include:

- Nutritional preparation of severely malnourished patients prior to surgery, for example those with mechanical obstruction of the oesophagus due to stricture or cancer, swallowing difficulties, gastric obstruction, severe gastric ulceration, cancer of the stomach or congenital abnormalities.
- Trauma to the GI system which may result in an inability to ingest or absorb foods. This trauma may be due to incidents or surgery, or be secondary to other disease processes, for example fistula, perforated bowel, facial injuries, oesophageal injuries or intestinal tumours.
- Postoperative complications delaying enteral feeding, for example paralytic ileus, obstruction, short bowel syndrome, fistulas, peritoneal sepsis.
- Patients suffering from acute or chronic gastrointestinal inflammation which is not responding to treatment, for example Crohn's disease, ulcerative colitis, severe gastroenteritis.
- Insufficient oral intake or malabsorption, for example in cancer and cancer chemotherapy or radiotherapy, severe trauma, burns, sepsis and other conditions resulting in a hypermetabolic state, major hepatic disease, pancreatitis, coma, nausea and vomiting secondary to CNS disease, anorexia nervosa, severe or chronic malnutrition.

Whilst there may be 'typical' indications for parenteral nutrition each patient will have individual needs and pose a challenge to the staff. In order to successfully support and maintain a patient with parenteral nutrition, a team approach is needed involving not only the nursing and medical staff but also the nutritionist, pharmacist and community nurses if the patient is to receive therapy at home.

Nutritional assessment and monitoring

Nutritional assessment for TPN is carried out using the standard methods discussed earlier — dietary history, anthropometric measurements, laboratory and immune function data and clinical evaluation to identify requirements and deficits. Baseline measurements must be established; monitoring is critical during the stabilisation period and regular checks are still required once TPN has been established. Local protocols for monitoring the progress of TPN should be consulted.

Venous access

Parenteral nutrition can be administered through a peripheral or central vein. Peripheral cannulation is not usually suitable for parenteral feeding as the solutions infused are often hypertonic and chemical irritation will result in thrombophlebitis. If peripheral cannulation is used it should only be for 24–48 hours before resiting the cannula, and the leg veins should be avoided.

Central venous catheterisation is the route of choice. The superior vena cava is the preferred vessel as the inferior vena cava is more difficult to reach. Infusion into the vena cava promotes rapid dilution of the hyperosmolar infusates. The vena cava can be accessed by direct cannulation via the subclavian, external jugular, internal jugular or brachiocephalic veins. Catheters can be inserted by percutaneous puncture, a cut-down procedure or sometimes using a tunnelling technique. With tunnelling there is some distance between where the catheter enters the skin and the point at which it enters the vein, and so there is less danger of contamination. Central venous catheterisation can also be carried out through a peripheral vein using a long catheter that is threaded up to the vena cava. Regardless of the approach adopted an aseptic insertion technique and careful insertion site management are essential (see Ch. 20). The central venous line should ideally be inserted in the operating theatre where maximum control of the environment is possible. After insertion of the cannula, an X-ray should be performed to ensure that extravasation has not occurred.

Administration equipment

A large variety of intravenous cannulae and catheters are available for parenteral feeding. A rigid cannula is more likely to damage the internal lining of the vein and cause phlebitis. A flexible, strong catheter made from an inert material is ideal. It should also be detectable by X-ray. Silicone catheters are often used although other materials are common. Infusion sets with Luer locks should be used. Flow control is important and if infusion pumps are not available a burette can be used to limit the volume infused. In-line filters can be used to reduce phlebitis due to particulate and bacterial contamination.

Solutions for TPN

TPN must meet all of the patient's requirements for water, energy, amino acids, vitamins, major minerals and trace elements. The fluid intake should cover loss via urine, faeces (especially if diarrhoea occurs), respiration, perspiration and any abnormal losses via wounds or drains. An estimate of fluid loss for an average adult would be 2.5–3.0 l per day. Energy and protein requirements should be determined after nutritional assessment and additional demands due to the medical condition taken into account. The need for water-soluble and fat-soluble vitamins, minerals and trace elements may be increased by the disease process. To meet all these needs, a variety of intravenous solutions are required. Table 21.8 lists nutrient solutions. Energy can be obtained from carbohydrate, fat or alcohol preparations. Carbohydrate and alcohol may be provided in amino acid solutions or supplied as separate sugar (dextrose, fructose or sorbitol) solutions. Alcohol can be infused directly as ethanol but is commonly given with amino acids. A number of different amino acid solutions are available with varying proportions of essential and nonessential amino acids. They may contain additional energy sources. Fat is provided by soya bean oil emulsions with added glycerol and triglycerides. Vitamins, minerals and trace elements can be provided by a number of additive preparations (Table 21.9). Nutrients may be infused separately, but it is now common for pharmacy departments to prepare, under aseptic conditions, 3 l bags, containing all the nutrients (except possibly lipid) prescribed for the individual patient. These decrease the need to change bags and the risk of infection and are also much easier for the patient receiving home parenteral nutrition to manage.

Complications of TPN

A number of complications are associated with TPN. Some of these have been reduced by the use of the 3 l bag system which provides most of the nutrients required over 24 hours in a sterile, stable and more compatible format. When fluids had to be administered singly or in tandem the sudden changes in the nature of the fluid meant marked fluctuations in body chemistry. Lipid solutions are usually given separately but some centres practise TNA (total nutrient admixture or triple mix) with some success. Shils (1988) has listed possible problems with TNA including:

- a shorter shelf life
- support for more bacterial growth
- may need more expensive plasticiser-free bags
- may not be compatible with infusion pumps
- 0.22 μm bacterial filters cannot be used.

In addition, the 3 l system may lead to waste if the patient's nutrient needs change rapidly and bags in progress have to be abandoned.

General complications associated with TPN can be classed as:

- complications associated with the intravenous route, especially with central venous access
- complications associated with the nature of the feeding regime
- difficulties arising from coexisting medical problems
- the psychosocial impact of artificial feeding upon the patient.

Complications of the intravenous route

Chapter 20 considers the general problems of intravenous therapy. In TPN, particular risks are those related to the long-term use of a central venous catheter and the administration of large quantities of viscous and hypertonic fluid. Mechanical problems of TPN are listed in Box 21.10. Many of the complications associated with catheter insertion can be reduced by restricting insertion to experienced personnel. Bernard & Stahl (1971) report less complications when central vein catheters are inserted by medical staff with experience of 50 or more catheterisations.

Air embolism can occur during insertion when the syringe is removed; a head-down tilt will reduce the likelihood of this, because venous pressure is raised preventing air aspiration. Intravenous administration sets must have a safety valve to prevent air entry if the fluid container is allowed to run empty. Pneumothorax is a common complication, although the incidence is reduced by using experienced personnel; haemothorax, brachial plexus injury and subclavian artery damage

Table 21.8 Some examples of nutrient solutions for TPN

Product (manufacturer)	Nitrogen g/l	Energy kJ/l	K^+ mmol/l	Na^+ mmol/l	Mg^{2+} mmol/l	Cl^- mmol/l	$Acet^-$ mmol/l	Others per l
Amino acids								
Aminoplasmal L5 (Braun)	8.03	850	25	48	2.5	31	59	Acid phosphate 9 mmol Malate 7.5 mmol
Aminoplex 5 (Geistlich)	5.00	4200	28	35	4.0	43	28	Ethanol 5% Sorbitol 125 g Malic acid 1.85 g
FreAmine III 8.5% (Kendall)	13.00	1400	—	10	—	<3	72	Phosphate 10 mmol
Perfusin (Kabi)	5.00	500	30	40	5.0	9	10	Malate 22.5 mmol
Synthamin 9 (Clintec)	9.10	1000	60	70	5.0	70	100	Acid phosphate 30 mmol
Vamin 9 (Kabi)	9.40	1000	20	50	1.5	55	—	Ca^{2+} 2.5 mmol
Lipid								
Intralipid 10% (Kabi)	—	4600	—	—	—	—	—	Fractionated soya oil 100 g Glycerol 22.5 g
Lipofundin S 10% (Braun)	—	4470	—	—	—	—	—	Soya oil 100g
Carbohydrate–electrolytes								
Glucoplex 1000	—	4200	30	50	2.5	67	—	Acid phosphate 18 mmol Anhydrous glucose 240 g Zn^{2+} 0.046 mmol
Plasma-Lyte 148 (Baxter) (water)	—	80	5	140	1.5	98	27	Gluconate 23 mmol
Plasma-Lyte 148 (Baxter) (dextrose 5%)	—	880	5	140	1.5	98	27	Gluconate 23 mmol Anhydrous glucose 50 g

Table 21.9 Nutrient additives for TPN (adults)

Product (manufacturer)	Purpose	Composition	Comments
Addamel (Kabi)	Electrolytes and trace elements	Ca^{2+} 5 mmol, Mg^{2+} 1.5 mmol, Cl^{-} 13.3 mmol Traces: Fe^{3+}, Zn^{2+}, Mn^{2+}, Cu^{2+}, F^{-}, I^{-} (per 10 ml ampoule)	Addition to Vamin range (except Vamin 18)
Addiphos (Kabi)	Electrolytes	Phosphate 40 mmol, K^{+} 30 mmol, Na^{+} 30 mmol (per 20 ml ampoule)	Addition to Vamin range and glucose solutions
Additrace (Kabi)	Trace elements	Traces: Fe^{3+}, Zn^{2+}, Mn^{2+}, Cu^{2+}, Cr^{3+}, Se^{4+}, Mb^{6+}, F^{-}, I^{-} (per 10 ml ampoule)	Addition to Vamin range
Multibiona (Merck)	Vitamins	Ascorbic acid 500 mg Dexpanthenol 25 mg Nicotinamide 100 mg Pyridoxine 15 mg Riboflavin 10 mg Thiamine 50 mg Tocopheryl acetate 5 mg Vitamin A 10 000 units (per 10 ml ampoule)	Addition to infusion solutions
Solvito N (Kabi)	Vitamins	Biotin 60 μg Cyanocobalamin 5 μg Folic acid 400 μg Glycine 100 mg Nicotinamide 100 mg Pyridoxine 15 mg Riboflavin 10 mg Sodium ascorbate 113 mg Sodium pantothenate 16.5 mg Thiamine 3.1 mg	Addition to glucose infusions Intralipid (Powder for reconstitution)
Vitalipid N (Kabi)	Vitamins	Vitamin A 330 units Ergocalciferol 20 units Tocopherol 1 unit Phytomenadione 15 μg (per ml)	Addition to Intralipid (10 ml ampoule)

NB: Amino acid and lipid solutions are available in many different strengths and formulations, e.g. Intralipid 20%, Vamin 18 (18 g/l nitrogen), Synthamin 14 (14 g/l nitrogen). Paediatric and other special formulations are also available.

can also occur. Catheter displacement usually occurs during insertion and can be ascertained by radiography. Catheters may also become displaced during dressing changes especially when adhesive transparent dressing such as OpSite are used (Moghissi & Boore 1983). Displacement can result in hydropneumothorax. Displacement of a peripheral TPN cannula can result in serious extravasation and tissue necrosis. Catheters should be well secured when initially inserted. Catheter fracture and embolus is very rare with modern equipment.

Catheter blockage can be due to blood or lipid emulsions clotting within the lumen of the catheter. Lipid blocks may also form at two-way taps and connections. They are encouraged by interruption of flow. The need to change fluid bags should be foreseen and changeover accomplished with minimum delay. Slow infusion of hyperosmolar dextrose may also increase the risk of clotting at the catheter tip. Heparinisation may be useful when a catheter is not in use. Catheters should only be irrigated with caution and never if there is no blood return. As with general intravenous therapy, local and systemic infection is a serious risk. It is a particular risk for the patient with a long-term cannula who may be immunocompromised and is receiving lipid and hypertonic glucose solutions. These form an ideal growth medium if there is a breach of sterility. The sources of infection in TPN are essentially the same as those discussed in Chapter 20 for peripheral intravenous lines. Stopcocks should be avoided and giving sets and infusion bags changed every 24 hours.

Box 21.10 Mechanical complications of TPN

Air embolism
Catheter displacement/accidental withdrawal
Catheter infection and sepsis
Catheter fracture and catheter embolus
Catheter blockage

These complications can be avoided or reduced if attention is paid to the management of the line. Poor management increases the risk of infection, and Finnegan & Oldfield (1989) consider catheter infection as almost totally preventable. Scrupulous attention to the care of the insertion site, infusion lines and bag changes is essential, and hospital protocols should be observed. It is also important to reduce the number of 'breaks' in the infusion system and feeding lines should not be used for the administration of medications or the withdrawal of blood.

Complications associated with the infusion fluid

Satisfying the nutritional requirements of an individual through the intravenous route poses complex administration problems. Calorific intake, nitrogen balance and amino acids for protein synthesis, need to be regulated together with the normal and specific constituents of the diet. An understanding of the processes involved in the absorption and metabolism of the intravenous products used in parenteral nutrition enables the nurse to appreciate the potential complications that may arise during therapy. On the whole these complications are metabolic or are associated with the nature of the fluid being administered or the speed of administration, for example over-/underinfusion. The biochemical problems arise because the body's attempts to utilise different energy sources have metabolic effects, for example high carbohydrate infusions produce raised levels of carbon dioxide which in turn influence the respiratory pattern, particularly of patients with concurrent respiratory problems. Metabolic complications are identified in Table 21.10.

For further information, see Finnegan (1989) pp. 271–275.

Table 21.10 Metabolic complications associated with TPN

Nutrient	Associated complications
Carbohydrate	Hypoglycaemia Hyperglycaemia Hyperosmolar coma Respiratory distress Fatty liver
Amino acids	Raised blood urea Acid–base abnormalities Hepatic encephalopathy Raised ammonia levels, especially in the newborn
Lipids	Overinfusion Acute reactions Immunosuppression Poor utilisation of lipids, e.g. liver disease Reduced pulmonary function
Deficiencies	Fatty acids: linoleic acid Minerals: ph Vitamins both fat and water soluble Trace elements, e.g. Fe, Se, Zn, Cu
Toxicity	Vitamin A
Others	Acid–base disturbances Hepatic toxicities

In order to detect and prevent these complications, accurate and continuous monitoring of the patient's condition is necessary, for example the routine monitoring of blood glucose levels with the prescription of appropriate insulin regimes. Nursing assessment of the patient is essential to monitor the patient's progress and response to therapy. Effective management of the patient with TPN involves all members of the health care team. Body biochemistry will be monitored by both the nurse and the physician so that estimations of the patient's nutritional requirements may be made in conjunction with the nutritionist. The clinical pharmacist will then be responsible for preparing the prescribed intravenous regime and advising on any potential administration problems.

Coexisting medical problems

The complexity of managing the patient receiving parenteral nutrition is often related to underlying medical problems, for example patients with hypertension, arthritis, diabetes, renal, hepatic or respiratory diseases. Whatever the coexisting medical problems they will influence the patient's need for, or response to, nutritional support and must be considered in the patient's nursing and medical management.

Psychosocial effects

Most patients on TPN receive nothing by mouth and may rapidly lose the normal sensations and drives associated with both the physical and social aspects of eating. It is important to support the patient and family during this period, and they may require appropriate counselling related to the underlying illness. Hopefully, for those for whom parenteral feeding is not a lifetime necessity TPN will be gradually supplemented with oral or enteral feeding and the patient weaned gradually from therapy. During this adaptation period the patient may experience difficulties in ingesting food and suffer from diarrhoea, constipation, nausea, vomiting and the sensation of fullness. Loss of weight or absence of chewing may also have led some individuals to find themselves with ill-fitting dentures. Some patients find it difficult to resume normal eating habits. At this stage liaison with the family, the nutritionist and sometimes the occupational or speech therapist may prove of great value in restoring both eating habits and a pleasure in food.

REFERENCES

Barnes E 1989 Increasing energy intake in hospital food. Nursing Standard 4(5): 30–31

Bernard R W, Stahl W M 1971 Subclavian vein catheterization: a prospective study. 1 Non-infectious complications. Annals of Surgery 173: 184–190

Bistrian B R, Blackburn G L, Hallowell E et al 1974 Protein status of general surgical patients. JAMA 230: 856–860

Bistrian B R, Blackburn G L, Vitale J et al 1976 Prevalence of malnutrition in general medical patients. JAMA 235: 1567–1570

Cataldo D B, Smith L 1980 Tube feedings: Clinical application. Ross Laboratories, Columbus

Chernoff R 1983 Enteral support: introduction to nutritional support. 7th Clinical Congress of American Society for Parenteral and Enteral Nutrition, Washington, DC

Davidson C S, Livermore J, Anderson P, Kaufman S 1962 The nutrition of a group of apparently healthy aging persons. American Journal of Clinical Nutrition 10: 181–199

Delaney C J 1991 Nasogastric intubation: use and abuse. Surgical Nurse 4(3): 4–9

Department of Health and Social Security 1979 Recommended daily amounts of food energy and nutrients for groups of people in the UK. Report on health and social subjects No 15. HMSO, London

Department of Health and Social Security and Welsh Office Central Health Services Council 1976 The organisation of the in-patient's day. HMSO, London

Fason M F 1967 Controlling bacterial growth in tube feeding. American Journal of Nursing 67: 1246–1247

Finnegan S, Oldfield K 1989 When eating is impossible: TPN in maintaining nutritional status. Professional Nurse 4: 271–275

Forlaw L, Williamson I J 1986 Advances in nutritional support. In: Tierney A J (ed) Clinical nursing practice. Churchill Livingstone, Edinburgh

Garn S M, Bailey S M 1976 Fatness similarities in adopted pairs. (Letter) American Journal of Clinical Nutrition 29: 1067–1068

Garn S M, Clark D C 1976 Trends in fatness and the origins of obesity. Pediatrics 57: 443–455

Goldblatt P B, Moore M E, Stunkard A J 1965 Social factors in obesity. JAMA 192: 1039–1044

Gormican A 1970 Prepackaged tube feedings. Hospital 44: 58–60

Hanson R L et al 1975 Patient responses and problems associated with tube feeding. Washington State Journal of Nursing 47(1): 9–13

Heatley R, Williams R, Lewis N 1979 Preoperative intravenous feeding — a controlled trail. Postgraduate Medical Journal 55: 541–545

Henderson V 1960 Basic principles of nursing care. International Council of Nurses, Geneva
Hill G L, Pickford G A, Young C J et al 1977 Malnutrition in surgical patients. An unrecognised problem. Lancet 1: 689–692
Holmes S 1987 Artificial feeding. Nursing Times 83(31): 49–58
Holt E et al 1962 A study of premature infants fed cold formulas. Journal of Paediatrics 61: 556–561
Janes E M H 1982 Nursing aspects of tube feeding. Nursing 2(4): 101–104
Jones D 1975 Food for thought. Royal College of Nursing, London
Kagarva-Busby K, Heitkemper M M, Hansen B et al 1980 Effects of diet temperature on tolerance of enteral feedings. Nursing Research 29: 276–280
Kilgore W W, Li M-Y 1980 Food additives and contaminants. In: Doull J, Klassen C D, Amdur M O (eds) Toxicology. Macmillan Publishing Co., New York, pp. 593–607
King's Fund 1986 A review of hospital catering. King's Fund, London
Kirk S L 1990 Adequacy of meals served and consumed at a long-stay hospital for the elderly. Care of the Elderly 2(2): 77–80
Methaney N, McSweeney M, Wehrle M A et al 1990 Effectiveness of the auscultatory method in predicting feeding tube location. Nursing Research 39: 262–267
Miller B, Torrance C 1991 Nutritional assessment. Surgical Nurse 4(5): 21–25
Moghissi K, Boore J R P 1983 Parenteral and enteral nutrition for nurses. William Heinemann Medical Books, London
Mullen J L, Buzby G P, Matthews D C et al 1980 Reduction of operative morbidity and mortality by combined preoperative and postoperative nutritional support. Annals of Surgery 192: 604–613
Newman H H, Freeman F N, Holzinger K J 1937 Twins: a study of heredity and environment. University of Chicago Press, Chicago
Padilla G V, Grant M, Wong H et al 1979 Subjective distresses of nasogastric tube feeding. Journal of Parenteral and Enteral Nutrition 13: 53–57
Passmore R, Eastwood M A 1986 Davidson's human nutrition and dietetics, 8th edn. Churchill Livingstone, Edinburgh
Rombeau J L, Jacobs D O 1984 Nasogastric tube feeding. In: Rombeau J L, Caldwell M D (eds) Clinical nutrition volume I. Enteral and tube feedings. W B Saunders, Philadelphia, pp. 261–274
Roper N, Logan W W, Tierney A J 1985 The elements of nursing. Churchill Livingstone, Edinburgh
Scientific Committee for Food for the European Community 1993 Report on proposed nutrient and energy intakes for the European Community. Nutrition Reviews (Editorial) 51(7): 209–212
Shils M E 1988 Enteral (tube) and parenteral nutritional support. In: Shils M E, Young V R (eds) Modern nutrition in health and disease, 7th edn. Lea & Febiger, Philadelphia, pp. 1023–1066
Short E A 1983 Perioperative starvation — an often underrecognised condition. The Australian Nurses Journal 13: 47–52
Silk D B A 1980 Enteral nutrition. Hospital Update 8: 761
Simon S 1991 A survey of the nutritional adequacy of meals served and eaten by patients. Nursing Practice 4(2): 7–11
Simopoulos 1985 The health implications of overweight and obesity. Nutrition Reviews 43(2): 33–40
Smith S H 1972 Nil by mouth? Royal College of Nursing, London
Strohl R A 1983 Nursing management of the patient with cancer experiencing taste changes. Cancer Nursing 6(5): 353–359
Taylor S J 1989 Preventing complications in enteral feeding. Professional Nurse 4(5): 247–249
Thomas E A 1989 Preoperative fasting — a question of routine? Nursing Times 83: 46–47
Todd E A, Hunt P, Crowe P J et al 1984 What do patients eat in hospital? Human Nutrition: Applied Nutrition 38A: 294–297
Torrance C 1991 Preoperative nutrition, fasting and the surgical patient. Surgical Nurse 4(4): 4–9
Torrance C 1992 Absorption and function of iron. Nursing Standard 6(19): 25–28
Williams K R, Walike B C 1975 Effect of temperature of tube feeding on gastric motility of monkeys. Nursing Research 24: 4–9
Williams J, Copp G 1990 Food presentation and the terminally ill. Nursing Standard 4(5): 29–32
Yellowless P M et al 1988 Abnormal perception of food size in anorexia nervosa. British Medical Journal 296(6638): 1689–1690

FURTHER READING

Coates V 1985 Are they being served? Royal College of Nursing, London
Department of Health 1991 Report on health and social studies 41. Dietary reference values for food energy and nutrients for the United Kingdom. Report of the panel on dietary reference values of the committee on Medical aspects of food policy. HMSO, London
Finnegan S 1989 Mechanical complications of parenteral nutrition. Professional Nurse 4: 325-327
Patients' Association 1993 Catering for patients in hospital: guidelines on hospital food. Patients' Association, London
Pi-Sunyer F X 1988 Obesity. In: Shils M E, Young V R (eds) Modern nutrition in health and disease, 7th edn. Lea & Febiger, Philadelphia, pp. 795–816
Scientific Committee for Food for the European Community 1993 Report on proposed nutrient and energy intakes for the European Community. Nutrition Reviews (Editorial) 51(7): 209–212
Starkey J F, Jefferson P A, Kirby D F 1988 Taking care of percutaneous endoscopic gastrostomy. American Journal of Nursing 1(42): 42–45

CHAPTER 22

Temperature control

Charmaine Childs

CHAPTER CONTENTS

Introduction 679

Normal body temperature 679
The temperature of the tissues of the body 679
Surface temperature 679
Deep body (core) temperature 680

Regulation of body temperature 681
Mechanisms of heat conservation and heat production 681
Heat conservation 681
Heat production 682
Mechanisms of heat loss 683

Fluctuations in a healthy person's temperature 683
Normal temperature range 683
Circadian rhythm 683
Other factors which affect a healthy person's temperature 685
The source of body heat (chemical thermogenesis) 686
Metabolic rate 686

The measurement of body temperature 686
Thermometers 686
The clinical thermometer 686
Electronic thermometers 687
Infrared radiation thermometers 687
Liquid crystal thermometers 687
Taking temperatures 687

Disturbances in temperature regulation 687
Fever 688
How fever develops 689
Chills and rigors 689
Fever in myocardial infarction 689
Fever or heat illness? 690
How heat illness develops 690
Nursing care of a febrile patient 690
Hypothermia 690
Causes of accidental hypothermia 691
The importance of temperature measurements in elderly people at home 693
Rewarming the hypothermic patient 693
Local cold injuries 693
Frost bite 693
Raynaud's phenomenon 694

References 694

Further reading 695

INTRODUCTION

The aim of this chapter is to give the student nurse a basic understanding of the factors and processes which are involved in thermoregulation, i.e. the maintenance of body temperature at a near constant level. Only when the nurse has a clear understanding of these physical, physiological and biological mechanisms will she be able to provide rational treatment for patients whose thermoregulatory system is disturbed. There are a number of reasons why body temperature might rise or fall out of the 'normal' range, and it is essential that the treatment the patient receives for an alteration in body temperature does not cause the problem to worsen. Unfortunately, it often happens that a patient's condition is exacerbated by an overzealous attempt to correct a rise or fall in deep body (core) temperature. Excellence in clinical practice cannot be achieved without a proper understanding of the patterns of normal body temperature and of the pathological processes which give rise to problems.

Taking a person's temperature with a clinical thermometer is one of the most commonly used methods for detecting disturbances in health. It is therefore an extremely important clinical measurement but one which in practice is often done rather badly. The responsibility of the nurse, whether practising in the home or hospital, is to record an accurate measurement which can be used with confidence to guide decisions about treatment. Simply recording a temperature measurement without appreciating what it reflects about the person's condition is not good nursing practice. The nurse needs to understand the factors which contribute to the production of body heat, why normal body temperature is 'set' at about 37 °C, and how much this can be expected to vary in health and illness. She must also understand in what circumstances treatment should be given for alterations in body temperature.

NORMAL BODY TEMPERATURE

'Body temperature' is a general term frequently used to refer to a person's temperature without regard to the site at which that temperature was taken. However, since temperature varies so much across the skin surface and within the tissues of the body it is good practice to avoid the use of this rather vague term and to report the temperature of the site used, for example: 'Axillary temperature of Mr A on admission to hospital was 36.9 °C', or 'Oral temperature of Mrs B was 37.1 °C'.

The temperature of the tissues of the body

Surface temperature

The body is not at a uniform temperature at all sites or in

all tissues. Under most circumstances the skin surface is the coolest area. The skin is often referred to as the 'shell' and the organs, blood and deeper tissues as the 'core' of the body (Edholm 1978). Skin temperature varies very much in accordance with air temperature (see Fig. 22.1) and will be considerably lower than oral, axillary or rectal temperature.

? **22.1** After examining the temperature data given in Figure 22.1, answer the following questions.

a. What is the reason for the change in the size of the shell in A and C?
b. What is the explanation for the higher skin temperatures at the extremities in A compared with C?
c. What do you notice about the skin temperatures measured over the thigh, leg, foot and toe in A? Why is the pattern of skin temperature in A different from the pattern of skin temperature in B and C.

Deep body (core temperature)

The body core is well protected from the environment but not all of the organs contained within it are at the same temperature. The liver, kidney, brain and myocardium, for example, have a high metabolic rate and consequently a higher temperature than tissues with a lower rate of metabolic activity such as smooth muscle (Houdas & Ring 1982). One might be surprised, therefore, to learn that the highest temperature is measured in the rectum. The temperature of the liver, which is usually considered to be the warmest organ, is actually 0.1–0.2 °C lower than rectal temperature. The reason why rectal temperature is higher than that of other organs was once thought to be increased metabolic activity from bacterial fermentation in the lower bowel (Grayson & Kuehn 1979), but since sterilisation of the gut does not alter rectal temperature other explanations have been sought. It is now generally believed that rectal temperature is influenced by venous drainage from the limbs. The temperature of blood in the limbs can increase after muscular exercise and this could provide an alternative explanation for the higher rectal temperatures.

The practice of using the rectum as the site of core temperature measurement has been criticised because of the factors just mentioned. Another problem is that rectal temperature tends to react fairly slowly to thermoregulatory changes and may therefore not reflect the true central temperature at a given moment. However, providing the nurse appreciates these drawbacks, rectal temperature can provide a very useful measurement of deep body temperature, particularly in unconscious patients for whom continuous temperature measurements are needed.

It is important to be precise about the site at which temperature measurements are made. Ideally, the same site should be used each time the nurse takes a person's temperature. If this is not possible and the site must be changed, then the temperature chart should be marked to show the change of site. It is also important to be consistent in the way in which a temperature measurement is taken, for example, by leaving the thermometer in situ for the same duration each time. For these reasons the delegation of temperature-taking to

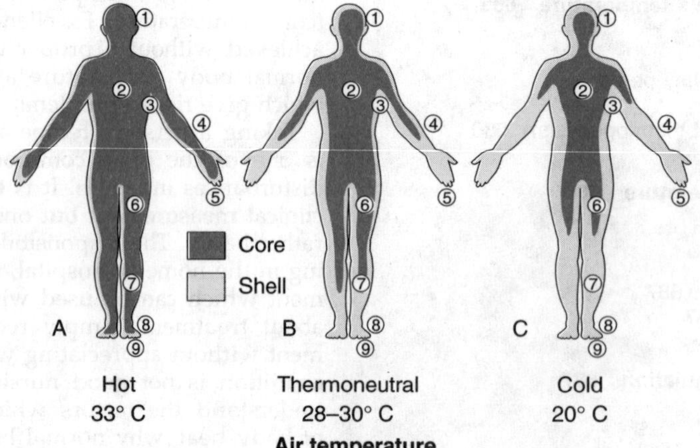

	Site	A (°C)	B (°C)	C (°C)
1	Scalp	36.0	34.8	32.8
2	Chest	35.8	34.5	31.3
3	Axilla	36.5	36.4	36.4
4	Arm	35.9	33.5	27.6
5	Finger	35.9	33.2	21.0
6	Thigh	35.2	33.4	27.8
7	Leg	35.3	30.1	25.2
8	Foot	35.5	29.7	22.7
9	Toe	36.2	29.1	21.4

Fig. 22.1 Core temperature and temperature of the skin surface at various sites in a hot, thermoneutral and cold environment. (Developed from Aschoff & Wever and Fox, cited in Edholm 1978.)

Table 22.1 Sites for body temperature measurement: advantages and disadvantages

Site	Nursing practice	Advantages	Disadvantages
Mouth (posterior sublingual pocket)	Leave mercury-in-glass thermometer in situ for 8 min.	Safe and accessible, particularly in adults and older children. Reliable indication of 'core' temperature	Inaccurate results after recent hot or cold drinks, food, or smoking. Wait 20–30 min before taking measurement in these circumstances
Axilla	Place in centre of armpit, hold arm against chest. Leave in position for 9 min.	Ideal for temperature measurement in babies and toddlers	Less accurate than oral or rectal measurements but can be a reasonable indicator of core temperature if thermometer is left in situ for the required length of time. Since it is a measurement which is not taken in a body cavity there is more chance of external influences affecting the result
Recturn	Insert rectal thermometer 4 cm into the anus (adults) or 2–3 cm in an infant. Leave in situ for 4 min.	Suitable site for babies or for unconscious patients who need continuous temperature monitoring	Unacceptable for routine monitoring in some conscious patients, although seriously ill patients with fluctuating conscious levels may require rectal temperature monitoring. Rectal temperature may be higher than at other sites. There is a lag phase between the true 'core' temperature and the rectal temperature.

untrained staff should be avoided. The advantages and disadvantages of the oral, axillary and rectal sites for temperature measurement are listed in Table 22.1.

REGULATION OF BODY TEMPERATURE

Our current understanding is that mammalian thermoregulation is controlled by the brain. Observations made in the early 19th century found that the body cooled down after severe damage to the spinal cord. This finding led people to believe that the nervous system was important in thermoregulation. Over a century later, Bazett and Penfield (Bligh 1972) showed just how important the brain was (particularly the hypothalamus) in the control of body temperature.

Even though a hypothalamic nerve cell or group of cells has still not been identified as the precise location for the control of body temperature, the pre-optic region within the anterior portion of the hypothalamus has been shown to be vital for an intact thermoregulatory system.

Information from thermoreceptors in the skin and in the deeper organs is integrated within the hypothalamus. Outgoing, or efferent signals stimulate changes in either heat gain or heat-losing processes if the temperature of the blood bathing the cells of the hypothalamus starts to change from that of the body's own thermostat or 'set-point' temperature. An intact nervous system is essential, not only to permit the transmission and reception of afferent signals but also to allow the transmission of signals to effector organs such as muscles (for shivering) and sweat glands.

If incoming information indicates that the body is above or below its normal thermostat temperature (often referred to as the temperature 'set-point'), an 'error signal' is received. The error signal is a useful concept borrowed from engineering theory to describe incoming sensory signals which differ from the brain's thermostat reference temperature. When an error signal is received the nervous system stimulates activities which protect the person from overheating or from becoming too cold. If the former situation occurs, mechanisms will be stimulated to promote heat loss; in the latter case, mechanisms to conserve or produce heat will be activated. In this way deep body temperature is prevented from fluctuating greatly from its biological set-point.

Mechanisms of heat conservation and heat production

There are many circumstances which could cause the temperature of the blood bathing the cells of the hypothalamus to rise above or fall below the set-point temperature of 37 °C. These include exposure to modest or extremely high air temperatures as well as disturbances in the rate of heat produced or lost from the skin surface. When conditions such as these alter the hypothalamic temperature, even if only very slightly, homoeostatic mechanisms are brought into operation to restore core temperature to 37 °C again.

Heat conservation (see Fig. 22.2A)

If a person becomes cold and core temperature falls slightly, signals from peripheral thermoreceptors in the skin are interpreted at the pre-optic region of the hypothalamus to stimulate the heat-promoting centre to initiate actions to retain heat and/or to increase the amount of heat produced within the body so that body temperature returns to 'normal'.

Behavioural thermoregulation. Man's ability to conserve heat by putting on more clothes or seeking shelter is often overlooked as a most important aspect of thermoregulation. But these are, in fact, the first protective thermoregulatory responses to feeling cold. Of course, very young and very old persons as well as those who are immobile due to illness or sedation are unable to protect themselves from cold and are therefore more vulnerable to changes in environmental temperature. It then becomes the responsibility of the nurse to place her patient in a warm and comfortable situation so that body temperature does not fall.

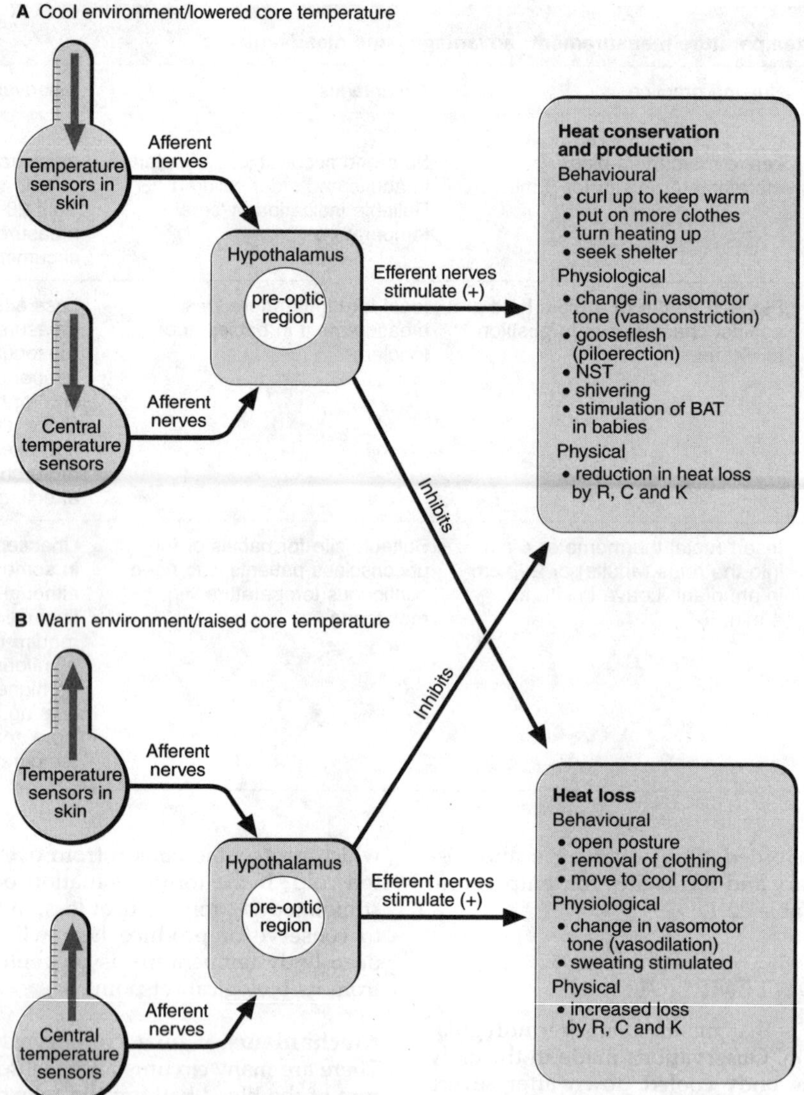

Fig. 22.2 Control of body temperature. (A) Responses to a cool environment or lowered core temperature. (B) Responses to a warm environment or raised core temperature.

Peripheral vasoconstriction. At about the same time that a person begins to recognise feelings of cold, changes in the flow of blood to peripheral tissues also occur. Nerve impulses from the area of the hypothalamus concerned with heat conservation cause blood vessels, particularly in the hands, feet, ears and nose to constrict. Sympathetic stimulation to nerves supplying the blood vessels in these regions (described as acral regions) results in peripheral vasoconstriction and a reduced flow of warm blood from internal organs to the skin. This means that heat is retained or stored in the body, where it maintains the core tissues at or close to 37 °C.

In situations where body temperature continues to fall, despite the above measures, additional mechanisms that involve heat production come into play (see NST and shivering thermogenesis) in order to restore body temperature to normal.

> **?** **22.2** What steps should a nurse take to help a patient with a low core temperature to retain body heat? What are the harmful or adverse effects of allowing a patient to shiver continuously?

Heat production

In a healthy 20-year-old adult the metabolic rate is between 35 and 39 kcal/m^2 body surface/h. In an infant the metabolic rate is 53 kcal/m^2/h. This difference can be explained by the fact that the rapid synthesis of cells in the growing body of a child contributes to an increased metabolic heat production. Metabolic rate can be increased well above the normal limit for a given age in sick or injured patients, particularly those who are febrile and/or have an infection (Barcos et al 1987). Patients suffering from serious burns (see Ch. 31) have been shown to undergo a large increase in metabolic rate (Wilmore et al 1974), but more recent studies have indicated that the increase in metabolic activity is not as great as was once thought and that the most likely explanation for this is the change in the management of burn wounds, i.e. by the early surgical removal of dead and necrotic tissue and its replacement with healthy skin grafts.

Any situation or series of events which increases the rate of chemical reactions in cells (and thus the rate of oxygen uptake by the cells) increases metabolic rate and the amount of metabolically produced heat. If deep body temperature is within the normal range the additional heat generated must be matched by an increase in the rate of heat loss from the body surface; otherwise, deep body temperature will rise.

Non-shivering thermogenesis (NST). Although peripheral vasoconstriction is very effective in helping to conserve heat, heat production itself may need to increase in order to restore body temperature to normal. Initially, this is achieved by NST. As its name implies, NST does not involve muscular contraction to produce heat, although muscle tissue is the most important source of chemically produced heat (Jansky 1979). Other important heat-producing organs are the brain and liver. NST is controlled by the sympathetic nervous system and is stimulated by the release of the hormone noradrenaline.

Shivering thermogenesis. Shivering is an easily recognisable feature of a person who feels cold or whose body temperature has fallen. The heat conservation area of the brain stimulates an increase in muscle tone (i.e. shivering) which can increase heat production by 5 times the basal rate. Shivering occurs in most skeletal muscles but is of greatest intensity in the neck and of least intensity in the legs. The repetitive contraction of muscle is not, however, a very economical process, for only 40% of the heat generated in shivering is retained by the body.

Mechanisms of heat loss (see Fig. 22.2B)
High air temperatures and strenuous exercise can raise the temperature of the blood so that heat-losing mechanisms are initiated and heat-conserving mechanisms are inhibited. The series of events which protects the brain (and core tissues) from reaching dangerously high temperatures is as follows:

1. A higher air temperature heats the skin and the resultant change in skin temperature is detected by skin thermoreceptors which signal the thermoregulatory centre.
2. The first reaction of the person is to reduce the amount of body insulation by removing some clothing.
3. At about the same time, blood vessels in acral regions dilate so that more blood is brought to the surface of the skin.
4. Providing the air temperature is lower than the skin temperature, heat will be lost by radiation and convection (see Table 22.2). If the air temperature is higher than skin temperature, the person will gain heat from the environment. This is why evaporative heat loss becomes so important when the temperature gradient between skin and air temperature is narrow.
5. Stimulation of sweat glands in hot conditions is controlled by the sympathetic nervous system. Production of a fluid consisting mostly of water (but also containing salt, urea, lactic acid and potassium ions) onto the skin causes cooling when the thermal energy needed to transfer the fluid to a gas is absorbed by the surrounding air from the skin surface. This transfer of energy from a fluid to a gaseous state is called vaporisational heat loss.

? **22.3** What is the most important route for heat loss in a warm environment?

? **22.4** What is the collective term used to describe heat loss by radiation and convection?

? **22.5** Find out which areas of the body are described as 'acral regions'. What is their specific function in thermoregulation?

? **22.6** During a hot bath, heat is transferred to the body by radiation, convection and conduction (see Table 22.2). For each route give examples of the way in which the furniture and objects in the room (the bath, walls and furniture) transfer heat to the body.

? **22.7** After a bath, patients often feel cold and uncomfortable if the nurse is slow in helping them to dry themselves. What is the cause of this feeling of discomfort when the body is wet and the room temperature low? Why would leaving the door of the bathroom open make the patient feel cold? How can the nurse improve the patient's comfort when preparing him for a bath?

FLUCTUATIONS IN A HEALTHY PERSON'S TEMPERATURE

Man is capable of surviving in a range of climates. This is because he is able to make both physiological and behavioural adjustments which prevent deep body temperature from rising above or falling below 37 °C (Stainer et al 1984). Like many mammals, man has the ability to increase the amount of heat in the body as air temperature falls or to increase heat loss when conditions become uncomfortably hot.

Normal temperature range

Although central or hypothalamic temperature is set to a relatively constant level, fluctuations do occur in healthy people, as for example following exercise. No harm is done to the cells of the body by a change in temperature, providing core temperature does not rise above or fall below certain limits. Indeed, the ability of the thermoregulatory system to stimulate changes in heat production or heat loss indicates that the system is operating efficiently.

DuBois's now classic monograph (1984) illustrates the range of 'normal' temperature in health. In the early morning or during cold weather body temperature may fall to 35–36 °C. After moderate exercise or under the influence of emotion (as in some crying babies), the temperature may rise to about 38 °C. Following hard exercise body temperature may rise as high as 40 °C. A rise of 5 °C from 37 °C indicates a serious disruption of thermoregulation and a person's life may be at risk if deep body temperature rises above 45 °C or falls below 24 °C.

? **22.8** During one shift of duty, find out how many patients are pyrexial and for each investigate the following:
a. Has the pyrexia been reported?
b. What are the possible reasons for the pyrexia?
c. Has the cause been identified and treated?
d. How frequently is the temperature being monitored?

Circadian rhythm
Body temperature fluctuates in a characteristic pattern over a 24-hour period. It is thought that this pattern derives from regular alterations in the set-point of the hypothalamic thermostat. Thus, like many other physiological functions, thermoregulation displays a circadian rhythm. This rhythm persists in health and even during short periods of night work. Eventually, however, regular night work will reverse the pattern so that lower temperatures occur during the day and higher temperatures at night.

In general, the lowest temperatures recorded over a 24-hour cycle will be approximately 0.5 °C lower than the plateau temperature. The highest temperature during the evening may be as much as 1.0 °C above the early morning temperature.

The circadian rhythm of deep body temperature does not occur in babies (Lorin 1982, Peterson et al 1991) but develops

Table 22.2 Principles of heat transfer

Route for heat loss	Principle	Relevance to clinical practice
Radiation (R)	Transfer of energy in the form of electromagnetic waves. The human body emits heat as infrared radiation. At the same time all dense objects (furniture, buildings, other people) are also radiating heat. The rate at which heat is emitted from the human body is dependent upon the temperature difference (gradient) between the skin and other objects and surfaces in the room. If the skin is hotter than the average temperature of objects in the room, heat will be lost. If the objects in the room are hotter, the body will gain heat.	A person, naked, sitting quietly in a room at 25°C loses between 50–70% of heat by R, the major route for heat loss under such conditions. As air temperature increases, the temperature gradient between skin and air falls such that less heat is lost by this route. As air temperature rises towards skin temperature (35°C) the gradient will be so small that very little heat loss can take place by this route. Evaporative heat loss then becomes an important route for heat loss.
Convection (C)	Air (or water) next to the body warms and moves slowly away because warm air is less dense and rises. As it moves away from the body, cooler air replaces it. This process can be speeded up if a strong draught (e.g. electric fan) is used to force the air away and cause a rapid replacement of warmed air with cool air.	Nurses frequently increase the rate of heat loss by convection by placing electric fans close to their patients. This can be a very efficient way to lower skin temperature but frequently the cool stimulus results in an inappropriate response; i.e. peripheral vasoconstriction. Heat retention within core tissues then causes core temperature to rise rather than fall. In febrile patients who have an elevated set-point the use of electric fans is likely to exacerbate the problem of pyrexia.
Conduction (K)	Heat loss by K involves transfer of thermal energy from atom to atom. The skin must be in contact with cooler or hotter objects for heat exchange to take place by K.	Critically ill patients are often nursed on special beds designed to reduce the incidence of pressure sores. These beds are often maintained at a constant temperature to help prevent heat loss from the body. Sometimes the thermostat can fail and patients have been known to overheat or to cool because the temperature of the bed is too high or too low. This is an example of heat loss or heat gain by conduction. Patients must be protected from body temperature disturbances of an iatrogenic nature such as this.
Evaporation (E)	Evaporation of water from the skin and respiratory passages is the most important route for heat loss in hot conditions. The evaporation of water occurs when energy transforms water and sweat droplets to a gas. The heat (or thermal energy) needed to drive this process is taken from the body. Thus the more water there is on the skin the more heat is taken from the body to turn it into a gas (vaporisation). The more heat removed from the body in the process of E the more the body cools. The function of sweat (produced under the control of the sympathetic nervous system) as an agent for vaporisational heat loss can be enhanced by spraying the body with a fine mist of warm water.	Patients with a high core temperature may not always sweat. During a rise in rectal temperature the body responds as though it were too cold and if patients are observed carefully it will be seen that their skin is dry. At this stage the hypothalamic set-point is above normal but the body continues to activate heat-conserving mechanisms to achieve the new set-point temperature. Only when the patient has reached the new central temperature set-point will heat loss by all routes (E included) be activated. Thus when nurses notice that patients with a high core temperature are sweating it is more likely to indicate that core temperature has reached the new set-point. A fall in body temperature may then follow.

during early childhood, when fluctuations may be more marked than in the adult.

An awareness of the normal changes in deep body temperature in health is necessary if nurses are to interpret temperature measurements correctly. A moderately elevated oral temperature recorded during the afternoon should be monitored closely before treatment is started. If the cyclical nature of oral temperature is not appreciated, treatment for pyrexia could be instigated for what is essentially a normal temperature.

> **?** **22.9** For this project you will need to measure the temperature of a healthy person every 2–4 hours. You will need to enlist the cooperation of a friend or family member who does not mind being woken at night for the sake of this exercise. Plot your subject's oral temperature every 2–4 hours for 24 hours onto graph paper. From the data you collect, try to identify a circadian rhythm in your subject. State the highest and lowest temperatures recorded over the 24-hour period. You should now be able to state the overall variation in body temperature of a healthy subject.

Other factors which affect a healthy person's temperature

Age. The age of a patient must be taken into account in the interpretation of body temperature.

Babies and young children. Early studies (e.g. Bayley & Stolz 1937) showed that rectal temperature begins to rise during the first 7 months of life, remaining fairly constant until the age of 2 years, after which it begins to fall. Bayley & Stolz (1937) found that average rectal temperature at one month of age was 37.1–37.2 °C, at 8 months 37.6–37.7 °C, and at 18 months 37.7 °C. By the time the children in their study approached their third birthday, rectal temperature had settled to values around 37.1 °C.

Healthy children tend to have a higher deep body temperature than adults and therefore their 'normal' range differs slightly. Higher temperatures in early childhood are thought to be a result of increased cellular and metabolic activity. The newborn baby and the young of most mammals are particularly well adapted to generating body heat. This adaptation is vital for survival; human infants have a large body surface area in proportion to their weight and are therefore vulnerable to the effects of cold. They are unable to shiver and cannot increase body insulation by adding extra layers of clothes by themselves. However, they do have an important source of body heat in the form of brown adipose tissue (BAT), a specialised fat which can be found around the kidneys, between the shoulder blades, around the great vessels and deep within the axillae (Rothwell 1989).

A large amount of heat is produced by this unique tissue, which requires a large supply of blood and oxygen in order to fulfil this function. (The dense vascular supply is responsible for the brown colour of this tissue). Brown fat becomes much less important in maintaining the temperature of the body as a baby gets older.

Adults and elderly people. The importance of BAT for heat production in an adult is not clear, but is probably minimal. Unlike small infants, who rely principally on 'switching on' heat production to maintain a stable deep body temperature, adults conserve body heat. In other words, they rely on preventing body heat from being lost, either by putting on more clothes (behavioural thermoregulation) or by vasoconstriction at the extremities (physiological thermoregulation).

Even in health, older people often have lower body temperatures than children or younger adults. There are a number of reasons for this. After the age of about 50 years, metabolic rate starts to fall. This results in a lower rate of heat production within the body; consequently, deep body temperature tends to be lower. In addition, social and economic factors contribute to the inability of some elderly people to keep warm, particularly in winter. As people grow older it is more difficult for them to detect extremes in temperature; this puts them at risk of hypothermia and hyperthermia (see Box 22.1). In warm conditions, for example, deep body temperature in the older person may rise slightly because the ability to sweat is reduced. Evaporative heat loss is therefore less efficient at a time when increased heat loss is needed to keep the temperature within the normal range (Wagner et al 1974).

Exercise. Hard exercise can raise oral and rectal temperature by several degrees. Temperatures above 40 °C have been recorded in marathon runners (Sutton 1978) and after a game of rugby rectal temperatures over 39 °C can occur (Mitchell & Laburn 1985). This rise in temperature can persist for many hours and represents an imbalance between heat production and heat loss (see pp. 682–683).

> **?** **22.10** When you have the opportunity, either at work or at home, record the temperatures of three or four people before and after they take a hot drink and before and after they smoke a cigarette. What differences do you observe?

Box 22.1 Helping the elderly to keep warm in winter

There will always be cold spells during the winter months and some will be much worse than others. Weathermen frequently refer to the more extreme conditions as a 'cold snap' and their advice, particularly to elderly television viewers, is to make sure that they keep warm. The problem is that keeping warm usually means keeping the heating on for longer than usual with a consequent rise in heating bills. Government subsidies are usually given only at times when the weather is very cold and well below the monthly average, and information about financial help sometimes arrives too late. Moreover, elderly people become cold for many reasons and at times other than during extremely cold spells.

The older housing stock in which many elderly people live becomes damp and cold if maintenance and repairs are not kept up to date. It is expensive to keep old houses warm at any time of year, but particularly in winter. If elderly people cannot be persuaded to keep their heating on during the winter it can be helpful for family, friends and neighbours to offer good advice about keeping warm.

The obvious suggestion for someone on a low pension would be to heat just one room, i.e. the room in which he spends most of his time. An alternative is to conserve body heat by wearing extra layers of clothes. These should be comfortable but effective in retaining body heat. The most important principle to remember is that there is no particular merit in one kind of material as compared to another except in its capacity to trap air. Clothes made of cotton are as good as down feathers in this respect. The problem is that feathers can be easily compressed and when this happens the insulating properties are reduced. It is worth advising people who use a down quilt to keep it 'fluffed' for maximum insulation.

Covering the parts of the body which are exposed to draughts (i.e. hands, feet and head) should be done in much the same way as for a person in a cold climate. Although the head is generally heated by a plume of warm air rising upwards from the body (Clarke & Edholm 1985) this band of warm air can be blown away if the person is in a draught. People who spend a lot of time relatively immobile in a draughty house should be advised to wear something on their head like a hat, cap or even a Balaclava. The reasons for taking so much care to keep warm are obvious: lives can be saved by these simple yet effective actions.

The menstrual cycle. It is now well recognised that 80% of healthy ovulating women have higher oral temperatures at the time of ovulation. A record of early morning oral temperature can be used to predict the time of ovulation in healthy women. On waking, oral temperature should be recorded before doing any work or exercise. These measurements should be made on a daily basis throughout the cycle. A slight drop in temperature occurs 24–36 hours after ovulation. Temperature then rises abruptly by 0.3–0.4 °C and continues at this slightly higher level for the rest of the cycle. Three days after the onset of the higher temperature is generally thought to coincide with the end of the fertile phase (Benson 1984).

The occurrence of 'hot flushes' in the menopause is discussed in Box 22.2.

Eating a meal. The process of breaking down and metabolising food produces body heat. This effect was originally described as the specific dynamic action (SDA) of food. Metabolism of protein was found to have a greater effect in generating heat than the metabolism of carbohydrate or fat (Ashworth 1969). However, the SDA of foods has recently been shown to occur with both high- and low-protein diets.

The term 'heat increment of feeding' is now used in farm animal nutrition and 'diet-induced thermogenesis' (DIT) in the study of human nutrition to refer to the heat-producing effect of a meal (Kinney 1988). DIT raises heat production by two processes: obligatory and facultative metabolism. Obligatory metabolism results from the digestion and assimilation of food. It is not clear what factors contribute to facultative metabolism but it may be a result of futile cycling, particularly of glucose metabolism. An example of a futile cycle is the conversion of glucose to its by-products and then back to glucose again. Although some authors believe that DIT can produce a slight rise in core temperature its main effect is increased heat production.

The source of body heat (chemical thermogenesis)

Heat is expressed in 'energy units' called calories (cal) or, more usually, the larger unit kilocalories (kcal; 1 kcal = 1000 cal). The SI unit for energy is the kilojoule (kJ; 1 kJ = 4.18 kcal).

> **Box 22.2 Hot flushes**
>
> The exact cause of 'hot flushes' in menopausal women is not known, but there is evidence that a defect in thermoregulatory function may be responsible for the discomfort and distress associated with the hot flush. The two physiological changes which characterise hot flushes are sweating and cutaneous vasodilation. During a hot flush central temperature falls in response to heat lost from the skin surface after peripheral vasodilation and sweating. Sufferers feel very warm and uncomfortable and want to cool themselves. Since the flushes frequently occur at night (night sweats) they can cause great distress and make it difficult to get a good night's sleep.
>
> It is thought that hot flushes are the result of a sudden fall in the central hypothalamic thermostat. This would result in the body being too hot and stimulating heat loss mechanisms such as sweating and vasodilation. Because hot flushes occur during the climacteric and are associated with cessation of ovarian function their underlying cause is thought to lie in changes in the endocrine system.
>
> Oestrogens are the principal medicines used to relieve hot flushes. The benefits of treatment with Vitamins E and K, mineral supplements and belladonna alkaloids have not been critically evaluated.

Since nurses are involved in measuring the temperature of the tissues of the body it is important for them to understand how body heat is generated. Most of our energy for growth and repair of tissues, for work and for body warmth comes from the food we eat. Different foods provide different amounts of energy. Most packaged foods have a label which gives the amount of energy (kcal or kJ) contained in an average serving when oxidised or burned by the body. Heat is a by-product of oxidation and the process by which it is produced is called chemical thermogenesis (see Ch. 21). The rate at which heat is produced is called the metabolic rate.

Metabolic rate

If a semi-nude man fasts overnight for 12 hours resting quietly (awake) in a warm (28–30 °C) room, his metabolic rate will be at a minimum or basal level. Under these conditions the only energy consumed by the body will be that needed to sustain life i.e. that used in breathing, contracting the heart, keeping ions in the correct concentration across cell membranes and in other forms of 'synthetic' work (replacement of structural protein, glandular activity, protein and red blood cell production). Under such conditions all the energy produced in metabolic processes will be transferred as heat, and so the rate of heat production will be equal to the metabolic rate. The person would be said to be under basal conditions and if his metabolic rate were measured it would represent his basal metabolic rate (BMR).

If the man fell asleep his metabolic rate would fall slightly. If after waking up he moved around, shivered or started to exercise his demand for energy and thus his metabolic rate would rise. Under these conditions some of his energy would be used to do external work (between 2% and 25%, depending on the activity) but most would be lost as heat.

A business man spending most of his day at his office and doing little exercise can expect to increase his energy requirements by 25–40% above the basal rate during the course of a day. Assuming that all his energy requirements were provided from the food he ate on that day (100%), approximately 10% would be lost as heat as a by-product of the work involved in processing his food, 50% would be lost as heat in the conversion of potential energy in food to high-energy biochemical bonds (see Ch. 21) and 20% would be lost as heat in internal work (respiration, cell pumps, glandular activity). In this example, 20% of the individual's energy intake would be used for external work in muscular contraction (Wilmore 1977) and 80% would be lost as heat.

It is clear that our utilisation of food energy is a very inefficient process. Most of our energy intake is lost as heat. However, the rate at which heat is produced does not necessarily reflect the rate at which it is lost from the body: heat can be retained and stored. One of the most important stimuli for body heat storage is a slight fall in core temperature, particularly if the person is in a cool environment.

THE MEASUREMENT OF BODY TEMPERATURE

Thermometers

The clinical thermometer

The development of a reliable thermometer was made possible only after scientists came to an agreement about the meaning of temperature and devised a scale to measure it (Keezer 1966). The scale we are most familiar with in clinical practice is the Celsius or centigrade scale determined by Anders Celsius (1701–1744). The mercury-in-glass thermometer has been the standard temperature-taking instrument for the last century. It is the simplest type of temperature-sensing device

Box 22.3 How safe are clinical thermometers?

Although the clinical thermometer (mercury-in-glass) is widely used it can be dangerous if not used properly (Campbell 1983) or if it is cracked or broken. Precautions must be taken to ensure that the patient is not put at any risk when this type of thermometer is used.

If care is not taken to clean the thermometer after each use cross-infection or reinfection can occur. Mercury-in-glass thermometers placed on bedside lockers or in holders may become contaminated with bacteria. The best way to store a thermometer is to put it inside a plastic sheath. Storage of thermometers in liquid (disinfectants, including alcohol) or even dry in a holder has been shown to cause colonisation of the thermometer with a variety of bacteria (Litsky 1976). If the thermometer is bitten down on and broken, fragments of glass can be swallowed. For this reason a clinical thermometer should not be used to take oral temperatures in young children or in the confused, unconscious or uncooperative patient.

Although the clinical thermometer is slowly being replaced by electronic thermometers in hospital wards, it is still a very popular method of taking temperatures in the community and in the home.

but is rapidly being replaced in hospitals by more sophisticated instruments which are quicker and easier to use (see Box 22.3).

Electronic thermometers

Electronic thermometers like the 'IVAC' are very accurate instruments and are often more suitable for measuring a patient's temperature than clinical thermometers because of their speed of recording. Since the early 1960s IVAC temperature monitors have gradually been introduced into hospitals in the UK. These instruments have a rapid response and enable a reading to be obtained within about 60 seconds (Erickson 1980). This is a great advantage when one considers the time needed to obtain an accurate oral or axillary temperature with a mercury-in-glass thermometer (see Table 22.1) and appreciates how difficult it can be to take a baby's or toddler's temperature if he is upset or uncooperative.

Infrared radiation thermometers

A very recent innovation in temperature monitoring is the tympanic membrane thermometer (Fraden 1991, Fraden & Lackey 1991). This thermometer determines temperature by measuring infrared radiation emitted from the tympanic membrane. For many years it was known that tympanic measurement gave the best approximation of core temperature (Benzinger 1969) because of the proximity of the tympanic membrane's blood supply to the hypothalamus. The old method of taking a tympanic temperature measurement was difficult to execute and there was always a risk of perforating the membrane. The new tympanic membrane thermometer, however, is simple to use; the probe is placed in the external auditory canal (it does not have to touch the tympanic membrane itself) and a recording is available in 10–15 seconds. The accuracy of the measurement, however, depends on directing the probe to the tympanic membrane and not to the wall of the ear canal. Instruments like the Genius (model 3000A) instant clinical thermometer can be used to measure tympanic temperature in adults and children.

Studies using a Thermoscan tympanic membrane thermometer (Talo et al 1991) compared the temperature at three different sites: the tympanic membrane with the Thermoscan thermometer and the rectum and mouth with IVAC electronic thermometers. The difference between average ear and rectal temperatures was found to be 1.1 °C (rectal temperature 37.7 °C, mean ear temperature 36.6 °C). Mean oral temperature was 36.8 °C.

There are a number of other hand-held infrared radiation thermometers on the market which can be used on the ward or in research to measure surface temperature (Childs 1992). The great benefit of these instruments is that they dispense with the need for leads or skin attachments whilst providing a measurement within seconds. In vascular surgery or after trauma the temperature of the skin surface is an indication of skin blood flow (Stoner et al 1991). In plastic surgery surface temperature measurements are a useful and often an important way to diagnose burn depth (Cole et al 1990, Cole et al 1991, Wyllie & Sutherland 1991), the deeper burn being colder than surrounding tissue (see Ch. 31, p. 866). After transplantation of skin flaps a change in temperature of a flap could, if lowered, indicate poor vascular supply or, if raised, infection.

Liquid crystal thermometers

Some liquids have rather special properties which resemble certain characteristics of crystals. When these substances are placed under a form of stress, e.g. a change in temperature, their optical properties cause them to change colour. These 'liquid crystals' can be used to indicate temperature by being mounted in a flexible plastic sheet which can then be placed directly onto the surface of the body. Obviously, this sort of thermometer cannot be used for temperature measurement in body cavities. Changes in colour at different temperatures are easily detected and provide a simple (albeit an imprecise) means of taking temperatures.

Taking temperatures

Recording accurate temperatures depends not only on having a reliable instrument but also on clinical skill. Even the most accurate of instruments will give an incorrect reading if the nurse has a poor temperature-taking technique. Table 22.1 gives some useful tips to help the nurse improve clinical practice.

?	**22.11**	Ask a qualified nurse to help you with this exercise. With a patient's cooperation measure axillary and oral temperature at intervals of 1, 3, 5 and 9 minutes. Compare the results. Are there differences in the values recorded at the two sites?
?	**22.12**	If you have some experience with a thermometer other than the clinical thermometer comment on the advantages or disadvantages of that instrument.
?	**22.13**	Ask the ward sister or charge nurse on the ward where you are working to tell you about the cost of temperature-taking and how much of the ward/unit budget is allocated to temperature measurement.

DISTURBANCES IN TEMPERATURE REGULATION

The aim of this section is to supplement the nurse's understanding of thermal physiology with examples of abnormal responses which disturb the thermoregulatory system, causing illness, discomfort or even death.

Table 22.3 gives examples of clinical conditions associated with a rise in body temperature. The causes of increased body temperature can be divided into two categories:

1. a rise due to fever and
2. an increase as a result of heat illness.

Table 22.3 Changes in body temperature

	Cause	Clinical examples	Appropriate treatment
Fever	Elevation of hypothalamic set-point by endogenous pyrogens such as cytokines, interleukin-1 (IL-1) and interleukin-6 (IL-6). Both are released from the patient's own white cells in response to bacterial or viral infection or to damage to skin and tissues	Infection: bronchitis, malaria, sepsis, meningitis Trauma: burn injury, minor and major surgery, myocardial infarction, thrombophlebitis	Antipyretic drugs like aspirin or paracetamol return altered set-point temperature to a lower level. Avoid external cooling for this may exacerbate the rising core temperature
Heat illness	Increased metabolic heat production OR Reduction in the rate of heat loss (by R, C and E) from the body surface (see Table 22.2)	Heat stroke resulting from high air temperature, overwrapping (children/elderly) and excessive clothing OR due to increased exercise or work in hot conditions where dehydration and reduced sweating are common associated factors	External cooling: 1. Increase radiant and convective heat loss by removing clothing and helping 'stir' the air around subject. Avoid cold draughts. Do not use ice packs for these can increase vasoconstriction. Increase evaporative heat loss by applying a fine mist of warm water (40°C) over the body and exposing as much of the skin surface as possible to the air.
Malignant hyperpyrexia	Largely unknown. Patients found to have an underlying inborn error of muscle metabolism (Britt 1979) usually triggered by general anaesthesia	Hyperthermia occurs shortly, or immediately, after general anaesthetic, in apparently normal patients. Once body temperature starts to go up, it does so very rapidly, and by as much as 1 °C every 5 minutes. Temperatures as high as 46 °C may be reached, with tachycardia, cyanosis and loss of consciousness (Lorin 1882).	Active cooling, maintenance of cardiac output, correction of metabolic disturbances e.g. hyperkalaemia, acidosis. Administration of dantrolene sodium

It is very important to recognise the fundamental differences between these two causes of raised body temperature and to appreciate their implications for treatment.

Fever

The high core temperature associated with fever is due to an upward movement in the central set-point temperature in the hypothalamus (see p. 681) (Bligh 1973). If the set-point is shifted from 37 °C to, say, 39 °C by pyrogens (cytokines) the thermoreceptors in the brain will detect a discrepancy between the set-point temperature and the temperature of the blood circulating through the hypothalamus. (This is the error signal described on page 681.) Since the blood temperature is lower than the new, raised set-point temperature, heat-gain mechanisms will be stimulated by the nervous system to promote an increase in the temperature of core tissues. This can be detected in a person's behaviour as he pulls on more bedclothes or turns the heating up. Patients do this even when their core temperature has started to rise. Their hands and feet will feel cold as skin blood flow is diverted away from shell tissues to the central core. The patient may also start to shiver. (Very vigorous shivering is called a rigor.) The occurrence of febrile convulsions in young children is discussed in Box 22.4.

Despite the gradual development of fever and higher core temperature the heat loss mechanisms are inhibited or 'switched off'. These thermoregulatory changes help the temperature to reach the new set-point level. At this stage the nurse should not try to lower the patient's temperature by cooling him either by tepid sponging or with electric fans, because in so doing she will counteract the heat conservation mechanisms already in operation. However, once the temperature of the blood and core tissues is at the new set-point level and sufficient heat has been stored within the body to sustain the new set-point temperature the patient will become more comfortable despite his high temperature.

The set-point will not remain at the higher level. Eventually, the pyrogenic effects will wear off and the thermoregulatory set-point abruptly returns to normal. When this happens the patient will feel uncomfortable and hot. His hands, face and feet will be red as peripheral vasodilation replaces vasoconstriction. Vasodilation allows skin blood flow to reach the most superficial layers of skin so that heat exchange from core tissues to the surface can take place. The patient should be put in the best position to allow dissipation of body heat naturally. Forcing heat loss by causing excessive draughts or allowing the temperature of the room to fall so low that the patient quickly becomes cold will make him uncomfortable and possibly induce peripheral vasoconstriction again. If this happens, heat loss by radiation and convection will be reduced. Patients often have a drenching sweat when their set-point returns to normal. It is, however, possible to encourage heat loss by evaporation by spraying the patient with a fine mist of warm water. The use of non-steroidal anti-inflammatory drugs (NSAIDs) in the treatment of fever is discussed in Box 22.5.

Box 22.4 What to do in the event of a febrile convulsion

Febrile convulsions occur in 40 out of 1000 children (Hull 1984) and it has been estimated that 30% of all convulsions in children occur during a febrile episode. About 2–5% of all children have at least one convulsion in association with fever by the time they are 5–7 years of age.

Febrile convulsions generally occur in normal children between the age of 6 months and 5 years. Simple febrile convulsions are probably not harmful. They are brief, lasting only seconds or a few minutes. They occur soon after the onset of fever and it is the height of the fever rather than the speed of the rise in temperature that is thought to be an important contributing factor. However, there are some situations in which a rapidly developing high fever (of 39–40 °C) in infants and young children is not associated with convulsions (Childs 1988) and this raises questions about the precise contribution of level of fever and rapidity of onset to the development of a convulsion.

Certain infections, particularly those of the central nervous system, have a particularly high incidence of associated seizures. Bacterial and viral meningitis have been associated with a high incidence of convulsions but these conditions may well precipitate convulsions by virtue of the nature of the underlying disease rather than because of the fever *per se*.

Nurses play an important role in the acute management of the child with a febrile convulsion. Convulsions can cause fear and misunderstanding and since they generally occur in very young children the parents may feel particularly helpless. Health visitors are often in a good position to explore these fears and misconceptions with parents and to provide them with information about what to do if their child experiences a febrile convulsion; this information will help to reduce anxiety and feelings of helplessness.

When a convulsion starts the child needs to be protected from falling on the floor or against furniture. If he is in a cot or bed, care should be taken to prevent him from falling out or hitting himself against sharp corners which may be within reach. The airway should be cleared but nothing should be inserted in the mouth. A common misconception is that the use of spoons or gags is necessary to prevent the tongue from blocking the airway. This practice is dangerous and can harm the child. As long as the nurse puts the child in the recovery position (see Ch. 27), observes the airway and takes the necessary actions to maintain a clear airway by, for example, wiping away accumulated secretions, little more can be done. However, if the convulsion does not resolve after a period of 10–20 minutes, drugs may be needed to control it. In such a case medical help will be needed.

In addition to protecting the child from injury during the fit the nurse should document the characteristics of the convulsion. Notes should be made relating to the child's temperature at the time of the convulsion or the last measurement made before it started, the type of movements made during the convulsion, where they started, how they developed and for how long they lasted. The clinical condition of the child should also be described.

How fever develops

A rapidly expanding area of biology is the study of cytokines. Cytokines are peptide molecules released from a variety of cells, including those of the immune system (see Ch. 16). They allow communication to occur between cells such that the internal environment is regulated following inflammation, injury or sepsis and during healing. To exactly what extent cytokines influence normal homoeostatic mechanisms is not clear. For many years the substances thought to be responsible for the fever associated with infection, tissue breakdown and necrosis (after traumatic injury or a myocardial infarction) was a group of peptides called endogenous pyrogens (EP). The endogenous pyrogens have recently been shown to include specific molecules and are now collectively called interleukins.

Interleukin-1 (IL-1) is generally believed to be the pyrogen which acts in the brain to raise the set-point temperature to a higher level (Stainer et al 1984). IL-1 is not easily detected in plasma (Childs et al 1990) and its role as a circulating pyrogen is unclear. Its release in the brain is probably stimulated by other interleukins produced outside the brain. Interleukin-6 (IL-6) is a cytokine produced by a number of different cells (activated macrophages, monocytes, keratinocytes, fibroblasts and endothelial cells, to name a few). It is thought that IL-6 released at the site of inflammation or injury triggers the production of IL-1 in the brain. In the brain IL-1 probably stimulates production of a group of substances called prostaglandins. These substances are thought ultimately to be responsible for elevating the thermoregulatory set-point.

Box 22.5 Non steroidal anti-inflammatory drugs (NSAIDs)

In addition to their anti-inflammatory effects NSAIDs are antipyretics. They act by inhibiting the production of prostaglandins from arachidonic acid in the cyclo-oxygenase pathway.

Since 1986 the NSAID, aspirin (acetylsalicylic acid), has been withdrawn from general use in children under the age of 12 years because of the association between this drug and a serious condition called Reye's syndrome. Paracetamol (acetaminophen) is now the most commonly used antipyretic for children. Although not an NSAID its antipyretic properties are thought to lie in its ability to prevent the synthesis of prostaglandins, which are thought to affect the temperature set-point when released into the brain (see p. 688).

Antipyretic drugs are not effective in conditions where high core temperatures are caused by heat illness; neither are they effective in lowering normal body temperature.

Chills and rigors

A sudden onset of fever with a 'chill' or 'rigor' is characteristic of some diseases. The chills associated with malaria are well known and are often portrayed in novels and films as a serious symptom of tropical disease. Repeated rigors are typical of pyrogenic infections and bacteraemia but are now also recognised as a symptom of viral as well as bacterial infections and of non-infectious as well as infectious diseases. Rigors and chills were once taken to confirm diagnosis of certain illnesses but because they are now known to be associated with a variety of diseases their diagnostic importance has been diminished.

A chill or rigor is accompanied by intense feelings of cold. The patient's skin will be white and cold and he will probably pull his bedclothes tightly around his body and curl up into a ball. His teeth may chatter and he will be very uncomfortable. Intense shivering and violent jerking movements will be uncontrollable.

Fever in myocardial infarction

Myocardial infarction is an example of a condition in which there is an acute rise in deep body temperature. Typically, body temperature rises after the first 24 hours to 37.8–39.9 °C and remains elevated for 2–3 days. Higher temperatures may be observed (Meltzer et al 1977). By day 5, however, deep body temperature returns to normal. It is thought that the pattern of elevated body temperature reflects necrosis of myocardial tissue (see Ch. 2, p. 22).

While fever is an expected clinical finding after a myocardial infarction, if it is prolonged and the temperature is above the expected range then an additional cause or supervening infection may be suspected. The possibility that pneumonia, thrombophlebitis or a systemic infection is present must be considered.

> **?** **22.14** For each of the following illnesses and conditions which may result in fever:
> - otitis media
> - meningitis
> - blood transfusion
> - acquired immune deficiency syndrome (AIDS)
>
> construct a table to give the cause of the fever and its appropriate nursing care. You will need to refer to Nursing Care Plan 22.1 as well as to other chapters in this book to complete the table. When you have done so, answer the following questions:
> a. What is the common cause of the raised deep body temperature in the above examples?
> b. Why would you expect your chosen methods of treatment to be effective in lowering deep body temperature in each case?

Fever or heat illness?

Whether the factor responsible for the development of fever is of an infectious or non-infectious nature, treatment must be planned with an understanding of the basic pathophysiology of the underlying fever mechanism. In many cases the cause of the patient's fever may not be known. If laboratory investigations are done some delay will be inevitable before the diagnosis can be confirmed. Consequently, it is possible for inappropriate treatment to be given.

It is important at this point to clear up some of the confusion which sometimes surrounds the use of the word 'fever' to describe an elevated body temperature. 'Fever' is often used as a general term to describe a rise in body temperature but in fact it has specific characteristics. To add to the confusion, the word 'hyperthermia' is often interchanged with 'fever' even though the cause of the high temperature in each case is very different. In caring for patients with an elevated deep body temperature it is important to appreciate the distinction between the mechanisms of fever on the one hand and of heat illness on the other. The nurse should ask herself when planning a treatment strategy: 'Does this patient have a high temperature because he has an altered set-point, or is he hot because he has a problem dissipating his body heat?'

How heat illness develops

Heat illness is a term which includes these three clinical conditions:

- heat cramps
- heat exhaustion
- heat stroke.

An elevated body temperature is not a diagnostic criterion for heat illness but it may occur in association with clinical symptoms secondary to environmental heat stress or to a thermoregulatory disturbance in the ability to dissipate heat.

The aetiology of heat illness is quite different from that of fever. Fever and the concept of an upward resetting of the hypothalamic set-point has already been discussed (see pp. 688–690). Heat illness can be a minor medical problem or so severe that it poses a threat to life. It is caused not by the production of endogenous pyrogens but by a variety of other factors (e.g. drugs, extremely hot and humid conditions, over-wrapping, excessive work in a hot environment) which cause an excess amount of heat to build up which cannot be dissipated quickly enough from the body surface. The mildest form of heat illness is heat cramp and the most severe heat stroke (see Case History 22.1).

> **Case History 22.1 Mr G**
>
> While making her weekly call to the home of Mr G, an 81-year-old widower, the community nurse finds her patient in the garden sitting in his wheelchair in a state of collapse. A relative arrives shortly after and explains that since it was a nice day she thought Mr G would benefit from some fresh air and sunshine whilst she did his shopping.
>
> Mr G feels hot and his hands and feet are red and sunburned. His skin is dry (he is not sweating) and his lips are slightly cracked. His axillary temperature (measured when taken indoors) is 39.2 °C.
>
> After being taken indoors, Mr G is sponged with warm water and his clothing removed or loosened. Cool drinks are given and his temperature gradually returns to normal over the next 4 hours.

Table 22.4 (p. 692) presents some of the signs which may alert the nurse that a patient is becoming overheated.

Nursing care of a febrile patient

Fever may start abruptly with a shaking chill or it can develop without the patient even being aware that his temperature has gone up. When measured, core temperature may remain high or it may fluctuate. A fluctuating temperature with peaks and troughs can occur naturally but often in hospital it is a consequence of antipyretic drugs such as aspirin or paracetamol. The nurse should be able to differentiate between fluctuating fevers brought about by repeated administration of antipyretic drugs and fevers which fluctuate independently of external factors.

The two most common occasions when patients feel uncomfortable during a fever is during a chill and when they are sweating. Nursing care should be directed not only to giving appropriate treatment (if necessary) but also to making the patient feel more comfortable.

Nursing the patient with fever is a complex practice demanding both knowledge of the mechanisms of thermoregulatory disturbance and practical ability in the provision of basic nursing care. The care that might be given to a febrile patient in the course of a few hours is described in Nursing Care Plan 22.1 (p. 691).

Hypothermia

The physiological mechanisms that lead to the development of hypothermia can be explained with reference to the hillwalker described in Case History 22.2. With nightfall a drop in air temperature would have stimulated a number of physiological reponses to limit the rate of heat loss from the surface of Mr E's body. First of all, the fall in skin temperature, detected by skin thermoreceptors, would have resulted in a reduced blood flow to the skin of the extremities. Whilst peripheral vasoconstriction is extremely effective in maintaining body temperature with a moderate fall in air temperature, the conditions on the hillside would have been much more severe and eventually peripheral vasoconstriction would have become maximal. When the vessels could not constrict any further other mechanisms had to be stimulated to prevent a fall in deep body temperature. This would have involved activation of the thermoregulatory mechanisms of heat production.

Nursing Care Plan 22.1 Care of a febrile patient

Time scale	Problem	Action	Rationale
8:00	When measured the patient's oral temperature has risen to 37.5 °C	❒ Measure patient's temperature every 10 min.	During a chill frequent measurements should be made to determine the pattern of temperature and the maximum values reached
9:00	Oral temperature continues to rise, and now does so rapidly and is accompanied by shivering. The trunk is hot but the limbs are cold	❒ Cover the patient's body with blankets and raise the air temperature slightly. Avoid exposing the patient to cold draughts	At this stage the temperature regulating system is disturbed. Mechanisms are initiated to raise body heat to meet the new, raised set-point temperature. Any attempt at this stage to cool the patient will worsen his chill and delay the time in which the new set-point temperature is reached
11:00	Oral temperature has reached a plateau of 39.5 °C	❒ Once deep body temperature has settled and is no longer rising, temperature measurements can be made every 30 min.	A person's temperature can be considered to be stable when there are at least two consecutive readings of the same value over a period of 1 h. Once the temperature is stable measurements can be made every 2–4 h but observations of the patient's general condition should continue
11:30	Pulse rate has increased to 100 beats/min. and respiratory rate to 20/min.	❒ Frequent observations of pulse and respiratory rate should be part of the overall assessment of the febrile patient	As body temperature goes up so does cellular activity; in other words, there is a rise in metabolic activity. There are direct effects upon the cardiovascular and pulmonary system as a consequence of a rise in temperature and metabolic activity. Metabolic activity increases by 13% for every 1°C rise in core temperature. Because of the increased energy demands brought about by fever, a persistent pyrexia represents a drain on energy stores. In addition, febrile patients become anorexic and are reluctant to eat and so their energy intake falls. A poor energy intake in conjunction with increased energy expenditure results in negative energy balance or weight loss.
11:45	An antipyretic has been prescribed to lower core temperature	❒ Administer aspirin/paracetamol as indicated. Note the patient's temperature at the time of giving the drug. Monitor the patient's temperature regularly (every 15 min.) and record the changes on the patient's temperature chart. This will allow the nurse to be able to describe for herself the efficacy of the treatment given	Antipyretics such as aspirin return the upwardly reset temperature to the original set-point level of approximately 37 °C. Once this happens the excess heat stored within the body represents an excessive heat load which must be dissipated. In addition to heat loss by the dry routes, radiation, convection and evaporative heat loss is switched on and patients may sweat profusely. Body temperature subsequently falls
		❒ Remove blankets and switch off any form of external heating	During the phase of heat dissipation the surface of the body needs to be exposed so that heat loss by all routes can be encouraged
13:00	The patient's mouth is dry. He is drenched in sweat and feels uncomfortable	❒ Frequent mouth care should be given if the patient cannot eat or drink but whenever possible clear fluids should be encouraged. These can be refreshing and can provide glucose for energy	Some authors claim that as much as 3 l water can be lost each day in a febrile sweating person. An inadequate fluid intake is accompanied by excretion of a small amount of concentrated urine. An inadequate urine output indicates poor hydration and this is often accompanied by the development of sordes. Drenching sweats are uncomfortable, particularly if nightwear and sheets are wet. The patient can be made more comfortable by giving him a bedbath and by sponging him with warm water. Cold water should be avoided as this causes external cooling and worsens the feeling of discomfort

Table 22.4 Clinical appearance and observations of an apyrexial patient who complains of feeling hot: evidence for behavioural and physiological thermoregulation

Observation	Response
The bedclothes have been pushed to the bottom of the bed by the patient	This is a behavioural response to the sensation of feeling too warm. Removal of bedclothes/clothing exposes a larger area of the body surface for heat exchange by radiation and convection. If bedclothes/clothing are removed then sweat can freely evaporate to the room and so facilitate evaporative heat loss.
Close inspection of the patient shows that the skin of the hands and feet are red and the veins in these areas dilated	Under control of the sympathetic nervous system, veins of the feet and hands vasodilate due to a reduction in vasomotor tone. Blood is therefore directed to the skin surface and the result is that the core tissues extend to the shell (see page 680). This is why the skin appears to be flushed. The skin is now at a higher temperature, thus creating a wider temperature gradient between the body and the environment. The greater the temperature difference between the body surface and its surroundings, the greater the heat loss by dry routes.
Small droplets of sweat appear on the forehead and trunk	Sweating is stimulated in response to either an increase in skin temperature or to a rise in core temperature. (Note the exception to this described in Table 22.2). Sweating occurs first on the forehead, followed by the upper arms, hands, thighs, feet and, finally, the abdomen. Sweating has been shown to start when the average skin temperature was 34°C; as skin temperature increased so did the sweat rate.

The first response to a modest reduction in air temperature which causes mild sensations of discomfort is an increase in non-shivering thermogenesis (NST; see p. 683). Shivering quickly follows NST as the major thermoregulatory mechanism to raise heat production as air temperature and deep body temperature fall. The main stimulus to shivering thermogenesis is a fall in skin temperature but the intensity of shivering increases when core temperature falls as well. Shivering starts first in the muscles of the jaw and progresses to all muscles. It can result in an increase in heat production of about 5 times the basal rate, but only about 48% of the heat produced is retained within the body (Glickman et al 1967). The rest is lost as wasted heat from the body surface. Although shivering is not a very economical process it is very important in increasing heat production and thus preventing an excessive fall in core tissue temperatures.

Shivering is maximal when core temperature is about 35 °C. It does not go on indefinitely in response to continued cold exposure but stops when deep body temperature falls to about 32 °C. By this time the energy stores in skeletal muscle will be exhausted (the muscular contractions of shivering rapidly utilise these stores). The cold also prevents optimum contraction of muscle tissue.

As the protective thermoregulatory mechanisms fail core temperature will fall further and body systems begin to fail. Although the hillwalker in Case History 22.2 initially took sensible steps to protect himself from the cold and exposure his loss of body heat continued. Under less severe conditions his normal thermoregulatory mechanisms would have been adequate to prevent a serious fall in deep body temperature. The duration of exposure in Mr E's case was obviously of major importance in the development of hypothermia.

> ? **22.15** What would be the main reason for Mr E to find shelter on the hillside in Case History 22.2? Would rain have made the hillwalker's problem of becoming cold worse? If so, why? (See Edholm 1978.)

Case History 22.2 Mr E

Mr E, a novice hillwalker, becomes separated from his fellow hikers and is lost for many hours in the mountains of the Lake District. As evening approaches the air temperature falls and Mr E begins to feel tired, hungry and cold. After putting on an extra woollen jumper he sets off to find shelter. He is found early the next morning huddled under an outcropping of rock. The rescue team recognise that he is suffering from hypothermia and take him to hospital.

On his admission to hospital Mr E's rectal temperature is found to be 33.8 °C. Although mortality accompanying this degree of cold exposure is approximately 50% (Houdas & Ring 1982) and Mr E is confused and unable to speak clearly when found, he does in fact recover after successful rewarming and emergency treatment.

Causes of accidental hypothermia

Although accidental hypothermia does occur in fit, young people it is more often associated with neonates shortly after birth and in the elderly living at home. These people are vulnerable to the effects of cold, particularly during the winter months. Resistance to cold in the fit and healthy person depends upon an efficient thermoregulatory system (see Fig. 22.2). Some impairment of thermoregulation may play a role in the predisposition of elderly people as a group to the adverse effects of cold. Perception of cold, for example, may be impaired and the individual may therefore not be prompted to make behavioural adaptations such as putting on more clothes. For many elderly people who are immobile it may not be possible for them to go and get extra clothes even when they do feel the cold. Those caring for elderly patients at home can help on daily visits by leaving extra clothes close at hand so that they can be used when needed. A hat may be useful to reduce heat loss from the head. Warm drinks will help warm the body but care should be taken not to

?	22.16	Why are the extremities important in thermoregulation? Why is it important to control the rate of blood flow to these regions?
?	22.17	What tissues have been identified as a source of NST?
?	22.18	Why is shivering a wasteful process? Why does it occur also in febrile patients?
?	22.19	Although shivering is a protective thermoregulatory mechanism in the cold exposed person, why should patients with a fever be protected from shivering? At what stage in a febrile response does it occur? What can the nurse do to help alleviate the symptoms of a 'chill'? Why do these measures work?
?	22.20	In what other situations would you think that a person (child or adult) coming from a deprived or affluent social environment might be at risk of exposure to extreme cold? (See Fox et al 1973.)

leave hot drinks where they can be spilled and cause scald injuries.

Although the young of most mammalian species have an additional protection from the cold in the form of brown fat (BAT) (p. 685) the elderly do not have the same resource for generating heat within the body and NST and shivering thermogenesis may not be as efficient as in the younger adult. In addition, malnutrition, paralytic disease and hypothyroidism, if present, can all reduce the ability of the body to produce heat when needed. Hypoglycaemia may also be a problem in the elderly diabetic patient for it inhibits shivering (Gale et al 1981).

Intoxication with alcohol can be an important cause of hypothermia; although alcohol was once thought to be a contributing factor to hypothermia by a vasodilator action it now seems that it predisposes to hypothermia by inhibiting gluconeogenesis (see Ch. 21) in the liver. The hypoglycaemia which follows excessive alcohol ingestion then leads to an inhibition of shivering thermogenesis in response to cold.

In Britain, accidental hypothermia in the elderly is common; 5000–10 000 cases occur every year, with a mortality rate of 40% (Stoner & Randall 1990). It is clear that accidental hypothermia is preventable and could probably be reduced significantly with adequate funding and health education directed not only to elderly people but also to the family members and health workers who are in a position to contribute to their well-being.

The importance of temperature measurements in elderly people at home

The importance of an accurate measurement of deep body temperature in an elderly person living alone is obvious. When the nurse visits her elderly patients during the winter months some assessment of their thermoregulatory system should be made. The temperature of a patient's house gives a good indication of potential problems as does the general appearance, condition and temperature of the patient's skin. Whatever site for temperature measurement is used (see Table 22.1) it is essential that the measurement is accurate. In the event of discovering an elderly person who is unconscious and cold it will be necessary to have a low-reading thermometer if deep body temperature has fallen below 35 °C.

Rewarming the hypothermic patient

Safely rewarming an individual who has developed hypothermia is a difficult task which must be undertaken with care, as late death after rescue is a common problem. In one tragic incident involving 16 people who had fallen into the water off the coast of Greenland, a rescue ship had arrived on the scene quickly and brought all 16 people on board. The survivors were given hot drinks and wrapped in warm covers. Although it appeared that they had been saved, they all died a short while later (Marcus 1979).

After a person has been rescued from cold water, his core temperature continues to fall for some time before it rises back to normal. This phenomenon has been called 'after drop', and it is thought that this provides an explanation for death after rescue operations such as the one off the Greenland coast. Death due to after drop is thought to be caused by ventricular fibrillation (Burton & Edholm 1955). As the patient is warmed, skin blood flow increases with the result that a larger volume of very cold blood flows from the extremities to the heart, leading to ventricular fibrillation and death.

The most appropriate way to rewarm a hypothermic patient after immersion in cold water also applies to the person subjected to cold exposure. The first step is to stop any further heat loss from the body. Once this is done the body will gradually warm up. This is 'passive' rewarming and can be supplemented by a number of actions such as using a metallised shock blanket. When the patient is warmed passively a rise in core temperature occurs by a gradual build-up of body heat as a natural consequence of the metabolic activity of the body. Providing most of this heat is conserved, the temperature of the body will gradually rise (Stoner & Randall 1990). If core temperature is above 32 °C, passive rewarming is the method of choice.

If core temperature is below 32 °C and the patient is a young adult who has become hypothermic through immersion in cold water or from exposure, active rewarming of the core tissues is required. The principle of active rewarming of the core can be likened to the arousal from hibernation of small mammals. After hibernation, core tissues are warmed by activation of brown fat. Since brown fat is located around central organs such as the heart and kidneys, the body warms from the inside to the outside, i.e. from the core tissues to the shell. But since the role of brown fat in adult man is probably of little thermoregulatory importance, this rewarming of tissues from the core to the shell can be done only by artificial means. There are a number of methods available (King & Hayward 1989), namely: gastric lavage with warmed saline, the introduction of warmed humidified gases via a ventilator, the administration of warmed intravenous fluids, and peritoneal lavage. Rewarming the elderly hypothermic patient by active rewarming is a safer method to use but some external heating will probably be necessary as well (Stoner & Randall 1990). If this is done the patient's cardiovascular system should be monitored carefully.

In all patients it is important to remember that if the skin surface is warmed first, blood flow to the extremities will be increased — as will the effective cardiovascular volume. For elderly people with pre-existing cardiovascular disease this could precipitate a fall in blood pressure. It should also be noted that as the circulation improves cold blood from the periphery will return to the heart and that this additional cooling can lead to a potentially fatal after drop in body temperature. With active rewarming core temperature can rise from 0.6°–1.9 °C/h (Stoner & Randall 1990). As core temperature rises, shivering may start and will become maximal at about 35 °C.

Local cold injuries

Frostbite

When tissue freezes, ice crystals form and the substances in tissue fluid become concentrated. The ice crystals can be many times the size of the cell itself. The degree of cell death after freezing depends on the concentration of the solute. Tissue damage resulting from freezing very much resembles a burn injury.

The milder form of freezing injury is called 'frost nip'. The extremities (nose, earlobe, cheek, fingertips, hands and feet) can be affected but treatment is simple rewarming of the affected area. A more serious form of cold injury is frostbite. In this condition blood vessels are damaged and blood circulation stops. The congested blood causes agglutination of cells resulting in thrombus formation. The severe conditions which result in frostbite can mean that the person is so cold that he neglects to care for the frostbitten tissues and that if rewarming does occur because of improvements in weather conditions the frostbitten areas become macerated.

Treatment for frostbitten limbs should be aimed at warming the core tissues first before treating the local damage. The affected limb can then be immersed in water at 10–15 °C. The water temperature should then be raised every 5 minutes by 5 °C to a maximum of 40 °C.

Once the core and the affected extremities have been rewarmed the patient should be put on bedrest. The limbs should be elevated and tetanus toxoid administered. Antibiotics may be necessary if there is any evidence of infection. Local treatment should consist of care of the wound with early physiotherapy.

Raynaud's phenomenon

Raynaud's phenomenon occurs most often in young women and is due to abnormal stimulation of vasoconstrictor nerves (see Ch. 2, p. 52). The cause of this abnormal vasoconstriction is thought to be emotional upset and, often, cold weather. The fingers are mainly affected; spasm of the digital arteries causes sluggish circulation in the fingers, which then become cyanosed. The intense vasoconstriction causes the arteries to empty of blood and this leads to the typical 'dead', white appearance of the fingers. When the vasoconstrictor spasm has passed the circulation starts to flow. At this stage the individual experiences intense pain, throbbing and tingling. In some patients vasoconstriction can be so severe and prolonged that the skin of the fingertips become ulcerated and necrosed, a condition known as 'Raynaud's disease'. Raynaud's phenomena generally worsens in winter.

Nursing care of individuals with Raynaud's phenomenon should be directed toward helping them to avoid the stimuli which they know cause their fingers (and toes) to go 'dead'. For some people simply wearing gloves may be sufficient precaution. Pocket handwarmers are very useful in preventing attacks but they should be used *before* the person goes out into the cold, as once the hands have become cold a pocket handwarmer is unlikely to be sufficient to prevent vasoconstriction. In severe cases vasodilator drugs or sympathectomy may be necessary.

Now try to apply the knowledge you have gained in reading this chapter to the following situations. In formulating your answers refer to the pertinent sections of this chapter as well as to relevant books and articles listed in 'References' and 'Further Reading'.

? **22.21** An elderly patient who had suffered a major stroke had been cared for at home by her husband. After his death she was cared for by relatives who made frequent visits throughout the day. The patient was very distressed by her husband's death; her appetite became poor and she lost weight. A referral from her general practitioner was made to the district nurse because she was becoming weak and debilitated. At your first visit you find the patient collapsed in the cold hallway of her home. Your initial examination reveals a cold skin and an axillary temperature of 34 °C.

a. What is the rationale for the immediate management of this patient?
b. What steps would you take to rewarm the patient at home and once admitted to hospital?
c. What method of temperature measurement might be used in both settings to record deep body temperaure?
d. What would you expect the method of rewarming to be in the accident and emergency department?
e. What advice would you give to the patient's family so that further episodes of hypothermia could be avoided?

? **22.22** In the following situations what decisions would you consider appropriate in the management of a patient with a disturbance in body temperature? (Note: you may decide that no action is necessary in some cases; if so, give your reasons.)

a. A patient admitted to hospital with abdominal pain has had a fluctuating oral temperature (between 36.5 and 37.5 °C) for 2 days. When you last took her temperature it was 39 °C and she was complaining of feeling cold. Her hands and feet were cold and looked mottled. A few minutes later the patient started to shiver.
b. A patient on his second postoperative day has had a raised axillary temperature for 6 hours. Treatment with aspirin was given 30 minutes previously. The patient is flushed and droplets of sweat are present on his forehead.

REFERENCES

Ashworth A 1969 Metabolic rates during recovery from protein–calorie malnutrition: the need for a new concept of specific dynamic action. Nature 223: 407–409

Barcos V E, Whitmore W T, Gale R 1987 The metabolic cost of fever. Canadian Journal of Physiology and Pharmacology 65: 1248–1254

Bayley N, Stolz H R 1937 Maturational changes in rectal temperature of 61 infants from 1–36 months. Child Development 8(3): 195–206

Benson R C 1984 In: Current obstetrics and gynecology diagnosis and treatment, 5th edn. Lange Medical Publications, California

Benzinger T H 1969 Heat regulation: homeostasis of central temperature in man. Physiological Reviews 49(4): 678–684

Bligh J 1972 Neuronal models of mammalian temperature regulation. In: Bligh J, Moore R E (eds) Essays on temperature regulation. North-Holland Publishing, Amsterdam

Bligh J 1973 Temperature regulation in mammals and other vertebrates. North-Holland Publishing, Amsterdam, pp. 153–147

Britt B A 1979 Etiology and pathophysiology of malignant hyperpyrexia. Federation proceedings 38: 44

Burton A C, Edholm O G 1955 Man in a cold environment. Edward Arnold, London

Campbell K 1983 Taking temperatures. Nursing Times (Aug 10): 63–65

Childs C 1988 Fever in burned children. Burns 14(1): 1–6

Childs C 1992 Cutaneous heat loss shortly after burn injury in children. Clinical Science 83: 117–126

Childs C, Ratcliffe R J, Holt I, Hopkins S J 1990 The relationship

between interleukin-1, interleukin-6 and pyrexia in burned children. In: The physiological and psychological effects of cytokines. Wiley, New York
Childs C, Stoner H B, Little R A, Davenport P J 1989 A comparison of some thermoregulatory responses in healthy children and in children with burn injury. Clinical Science 77(4): 425–429
Clarke R P, Edholm O G 1985 Man and his thermal environment. Edward Arnold, London
Cole R P, Jones S G, Shakespeare P G 1990 Thermographic assessment of hand burns. Burns 16: 60–63
Cole R P, Shakespeare P G, Chissell H G, Jones S G 1991 Thermographic assessment of burns using a non permeable wound covering. Burns 17: 117–122
DuBois E F 1948 Fever and the regulation of body temperature. Thomas, Springfield, IL
Edholm G 1978 Man: hot and cold. Edward Arnold, London
Erickson R 1980 A sourcebook for temperature taking. IVAC Corporation
Fraden J 1991 The development of the Thermoscan® instant thermometer. Clinical Paediatrics (Supplement): 11–12
Fraden J, Lackey R P 1991 Estimation of body temperature from tympanic measurements. Clinical Paediatrics (Supplement): 65–70
Gale E A M, Bennett T, Green H, Macdonald I A 1981 Hypoglycaemia, hypothermia and shivering in man. Clinical Science 61: 463–469
Glickman N, Mitchel H H, Keeton R W, Lambert E H 1967 Shivering and heat production in men exposed to intense cold. Journal of Applied Physiology 22: 1–8
Grayson J, Kuehn L A 1979 Heat transfer and heat loss. In: Lomax P, Schonbaum E (eds) Body temperature: regulation, drug effects, and therapeutics. Marcel Dekker, New York
Houdas Y, Ring E F J 1982 Human body temperature. Plenum Press, New York
Jansky L 1979 Heat production. In: Lomax P, Schonbaum E (eds) Body temperature regulation, drug effects and therapeutic implications. Marcel Dekker, New York
Keezer W S 1966 The clinical thermometer. American Journal of Nursing 66(2): 326–327
King G, Hayward J S 1989 Hypothermia and drowning. Medicine International 2964–2967
Kinney J 1988 Energy metabolism: heat, fuel and life. In: Kinney J, Jeejeebhoy K N, Hill G L, Owen O E (eds) Nutrition and metabolism in patient care. Saunders, Philadelphia
Litsky B Y 1976 A study of temperature taking systems. Supervisor Nurse 7: 48–53
Lorin M I 1982 The febrile child. Wiley, New York
Meltzer L E, Pinnto R, Kitchell J R 1977 Intensive coronary care. 'A manual for nurses', 3rd edn. The Charles Press, Maryland
Mitchell D, Laburn H P 1985 Pathophysiology of temperature regulation. The Physiologist 28(6): 507–517
Peterson S A, Anderson E S, Lodemore M, Rawson D, Wailoo M P 1991 Sleeping position and rectal temperature. Archives of Disease in Childhood 66: 976–979
Rothwell N J 1989 Brown fat: a biological furnace. Biological Sciences Review (March): 11–14
Stainer M W, Mount L E, Bligh J 1984 Energy balance and temperature regulation. Cambridge University Press, Cambridge
Stoner H B, Randall P E 1990 The metabolic aspects of hypothermia. In: Cohen R D, Lewis B, Alberti K G M M, Denman A M (eds) The metabolic and molecular basis of acquired disease. Baillière Tindall, London
Stoner H B, Barker P, Riding G S G, Hazelhurst D E, Taylor L, Marcuson R W 1991. Relationships between skin temperature and perfusion in the arm and leg. Clinical Physiology 11: 27–40
Sutton J R 1978 43°C in fun runners. Medical Journal of Australia 2: 463–464
Talo H, Macknin M L, Medendorp S V 1991 Tympanic membrane temperatures compared to rectal and oral temperatures. Clinical Pediatrics (Supplement): 30–35
Wilmore D W, Long J M, Mason A D, Skreen R W, Pruitt B A 1974 Catecholamines: mediator of the hypermetabolic response to thermal injury. Annals of Surgery 180(4): 653–66
Wilmore D W 1977 The metabolic management of the critically ill. Plenum, London
Wyllie F J, Sutherland A B 1991 Measurement of surface temperature as an aid to the diagnosis of burn depth. Burns 17: 123–128

FURTHER READING

Ashworth A 1969 Metabolic rates during recovery from protein–calorie malnutrition: the need for a new concept of specific dynamic action. Nature 223: 407–409
Central Office of Information 1991 Keep warm keep well. (HMSO, London
Cremer J E & Bligh J 1969 Body temperature and responses to drugs. British Medical Bulletin 25(3): 299–306
Edholm O G 1978 Man: hot and cold. Edward Arnold, London
Fox R H, MacGibbon R, Davies L & Woodward P M 1973 The problem of the old and the cold. British Medical Journal 1: 21–24
Graham A 1987 Cold comfort: welfare rights to heating allowances for the elderly. Nursing Times/Community Outlook (December): 21–22
Marcus P 1979 The treatment of acute accidental hypothermia: proceedings of a symposium held at the Institute of Aviation Medicine. Aviation Space Environmental Medicine 50: 834–43
Otty C, Mo R 1987 Hypothermia and the elderly: scope for prevention. British Medical Journal (15 Aug): 20–21
Taylor T G 1978 Principles of human nutrition. Edward Arnold, London
Thomas L 1989 Insulating the elderly: what measures can be taken to prevent the onset of hypothermia. Nursing the Elderly 1(5): 8–10
Tortora G J, Anagnostakos N P 1990 Principles of anatomy and physiology, 6th edn. Harper & Row, New York
Wagner J A, Robinson S, Marino R P 1974 Age and temperature regulation of humans in neutral and cold environments. Journal of Applied Physiology 37(4): 562–565
Wailoo M P, Petersen S A, Whittaker H, Goodenough P 1989 The thermal environment in which 3–4-month-old infants sleep at home. Archives Disease in Childhood 64: 600–604

CHAPTER 23

Wound healing

Sue Bale

CHAPTER CONTENTS

Introduction 697
Definition of a wound 698
Wound types and the classification of wounds 698
Epidemiology 698

The physiology of wound healing 699
Tissue repair 699
Healing by primary/first intention 700
Healing by secondary intention 701
Scar tissue 701
Why some wounds are sutured and others left open 701

Factors that adversely affect healing 702
Intrinsic factors 702
Extrinsic factors 703

Wound infection 703
Factors that predispose to wound infection 703
Sources of wound infection 704
Bacteria 704

Wound management — a holistic approach 704
Assessment of the patient 705
Assessment of the wound 705
Assessment of the physical environment 706
Creating an environment for healing 706
Dressing change techniques 708
Involving the patient in wound care 710
Nurse prescribing 711
Wound management policies 711
The transition from hospital to home 711
Provision of materials in hospitals and in the community 711
Expectations of outcome and effectiveness of treatment 711

Specific wound types 712
Pressure sores 712
Leg ulcers 715
Sutured wounds 719
Traumatic wounds 720
Malignant wounds 720
Burns 720

Psychosocial factors 720

Conclusion 720

References 721

Further reading 721

Video cassettes 721

Useful addresses 721

INTRODUCTION

For most healthy individuals the term 'wound' conjures up thoughts of a cut, a graze or even a surgical incision which heals rapidly without difficulty. For nurses, however, the management of wounds is a complex aspect of patient care, requiring much skill and expertise. A nurse may care for a patient with a wound in a variety of settings; ranging, for example, from patients with surgical incisions nursed in hospital, to patients with chronic leg ulcers nursed in their own homes, to patients with industrial injury or trauma treated in their work place.

We might be tempted to forget the impact that wounds have on an individual. Pain, fear and scarring are the most obvious, but individuals vary in their response to having a wound. For some, restriction in social activity, or the financial implications of not being able to work, should also be considered alongside the psychological effects of altered body image.

Tissue injury and the resulting wound problems have existed for as long as man (Westaby 1985). For many centuries trauma and war injury caused most wounds. A variety of readily available materials were used as wound coverings, the forefathers of today's dressing materials. Prehistoric man had a wide range of salves, which were used to achieve haemostasis, and plant extracts, herbs, cold water, snow and clay were used to ease pain. Surprisingly, throughout man's history wound management has been well documented. One of the first ever records of wounds was found in cave paintings.

Archaeologists have found skulls dating back to the New Stone Age that show evidence of healing following skull trephining. This demonstrates that not only was this procedure performed then, but also that people survived it long enough to heal. Injuries which did not result in death were likely to have been lacerations, contusions (bruises) and fractures. First-aid priorities in these situations would have been to arrest bleeding, bring the tissue edges together, hold them in place and protect the damaged tissues with a covering.

Scandinavian folklore (Forrest 1982) suggests that for thousands of years plant extracts have been applied to wounds for a variety of reasons. Of these 2500 agents some were antimicrobial, others astringent and others used to effect healing. Towards the end of the Roman era, Galen (the famous Greek physician and anatomist AD 129–200) developed his theory of laudable pus 'pus bonum et laudabile'. The basis of this principle was that, should a wound become infected, it increased the temperature of the wound and this localisation of infection should be allowed to continue. Galen wrote that, when infection localised and then discharged itself the wound would then go on to heal without problems. In the years that followed, medical practitioners became so keen on this idea that they believed not only that pus was acceptable, but also that it was essential and desirable for good wound healing. Clean, uninfected wounds were inoculated with various noxious substances in order to stimulate pus formation. These practices continued from the 7th to the 14th century. It was not until the 19th century that Pasteur and Lister managed to persuade their medical colleagues that mortality rates could be reduced by using antiseptics and aseptic principles.

Throughout time, individual species have varied in the way in which their tissues are renewed. Primitive vertebrates such as reptiles and amphibians have retained the ability to regenerate lost tissue. However, in man, only liver and epidermal tissue can regenerate. Where tissue loss in man occurs, healing is achieved by tissue repair.

The healing process depends on a number of factors, and in order for it to proceed at its optimal rate the individual concerned should be in good health. The nurse who cares for a patient with wounds has an important role in promoting health. Her skills as a health promoter and health educator will be called upon to minimise the healing time.

Definition of a wound

A wound can be defined as a defect or breach in the continuity of the skin. This is an injury to the skin or underlying tissues/organs caused by surgery, a blow, a cut, chemicals, heat/cold, friction/shear force, pressure or as a result of disease, such as in leg ulcers and carcinomas.

Box 23.1 lists the terms that are used in wound healing.

Box 23.1 Terms used in wound healing

Aseptic technique:	a precautionary method, using sterile equipment and a non-touch technique to prevent infection
Chemotaxis:	the process by which chemical attractants (kinins) stimulate polymorphs to move towards damaged cells
Collagen:	fibrous protein strands which provide the strength and structure of granulation tissue
Collagenase:	an enzyme which breaks down collagen during remodelling
Debridement:	the removal of devitalised tissues from a wound
Dehiscence:	bursting open of a wound
Elastin:	fibres in connective tissue which provide elasticity
Epithelium:	the cells which form the epidermis
Exudate:	the extracellular fluid which bathes a wound and is rich in nutrients, phagocytes and antibodies
Granulation:	the process of healing by secondary intention
Ground substance:	a gel-like material in which connective tissue cells and fibres are embedded
Necrotic tissue:	dead tissue, often black in colour
Slough:	devitalised white/yellow tissue — dead tissue that separates (and is 'sloughed' off) from healthy tissue after inflammation and infection
Tensile:	the ability to be stretched
Wound abscess:	a localised collection of pus, caused by invading microorganisms, which forms as a result of liquefaction of disintegrated tissue and an accumulation of polymorphs — the process of abscess development is in response to the defences of the body atempting to 'wall off' the damage

Wound types and the classification of wounds

The ability to deal with injury quickly and effectively has been important throughout human evolution for survival of the species.

There is no clear-cut method of classifying wounds. Some practitioners refer to wound by anatomical site, e.g. abdominal wall wounds, axillary wounds. Others classify wounds by their depth, e.g. epidermal loss, subcutaneous wounds. Another possible classification is by degree of tissue loss. In the first group there are wounds with little or no tissue loss where the skin edges can be brought together and sutured. In the second there has been substantial tissue loss and the skin edges cannot be brought together.

Epidemiology

The epidemiology of wounds is not clearly documented. Because patients with wounds can be found in almost every specialty, information relating specifically to wounds is not collected. However, although there are currently no centrally collected data on wounds, information is available for some wound types.

Leg ulcers

Venous leg ulceration has affected man over the centuries (Louden 1982) and venous ulcers account for around 85% of all leg ulcers (Wilson 1989).

The largest survey of patients with leg ulcers was carried out in the Lothian and Forth Valley Leg Ulcer Study 1985 (Callam et al 1987) (see Table 23.1).

These figures are supported by Cornwall et al (1986) who also found that leg ulcers in half of their patients remained unhealed for longer than 1 year.

The social and economic burden of managing these patients is great. Lees & Lombert (1992) estimate the costs of treatment to be up to £600M annually, and Morison (1992a) gives an estimate of between £400–800M annually for the UK. Around 100 000 patients have an open leg ulcer requiring treatment at any one time (Lees & Lombert 1992).

The cost of managing these patients in their own homes has been estimated at £1200 per patient per year, but this figure allows only one visit by a district nurse per week (Eagle 1990). Other studies had previously shown (Callam et al 1985) that district nurses spend half their time treating leg ulcer patients. Of this population, half are seen more than twice weekly with over a fifth receiving daily dressing changes.

The individual's lifestyle can be greatly affected by the presence of a leg ulcer. These are wounds which are difficult to manage, traditionally slow to heal and, even once healed, are likely to recur (Table 23.2).

Pressure sores

Pressure sores are one of the most difficult wound types to

Table 23.1 Leg ulcers — prevalence

Prevalence 10 per 1000 in adult population	
36 per 1000 in over 65s	
Age (years)	Sex ratio Male : Female
Under 65	1 : 1
65–74	1 : 2.6
75–84	1 : 4.8
85+	1 : 10.3

Table 23.2 Leg ulcers — healing time and recurrence (Dale & Gibson 1986)

Time to heal	%	Recurrence	%
< 3 months	21	1 episode	33
3 months – 1 year	29	2–5 episodes	46
1–5 years	40	Over 6 episodes	21
Over 5 years	10		

manage. Around 30 000 hospital inpatients per year develop a pressure sore related to their admission (Duthie 1990).

The incidence of pressure sores within hospital ranges from 2.7–66% (Roberts & Goldstone 1979, Verslugsen 1986). The variation in rates depends on the specialty in which the patients are being nursed; orthopaedic units and wards where patients are elderly, immobile, chronically ill and disabled having the higher rates.

In the community, rates of around 3–9% are found (Barbenel et al 1977, Hibbert 1980). The cost implications of a patient developing a pressure sore are high. Such patients need to spend longer in hospital and, even when discharged home, frequently require a district nurse to continue treatment.

This financial cost is rising. In 1973 the estimate was around £60M (Lancet Editor 1973), and in 1982 it was £150M (Scales et al 1982), increasing to £300M in 1988 (Waterlow 1988). If one takes into consideration the rising number of elderly and debilitated, the figure will be much higher today.

The personal costs to the individual of developing a pressure sore also need to be taken into account. Apart from the disappointment of having discharge postponed and return to normal function delayed, there is the pain and distress, all of which are difficult to measure.

That 95% of pressure sores can be prevented from developing (Waterlow 1988), highlights the extent of the challenge for practising nurses (p. 712).

?	**23.1** Review the structure and function of the skin (see Tortora & Grabowski 1992).

THE PHYSIOLOGY OF WOUND HEALING

A number of cell types are involved in the process of healing (Table 23.3).

Tissue repair

The wound healing process is one whereby the continuity and strength of damaged tissues are restored by the formation of connective tissue and regrowth of epithelium. The process can be divided into four phases (Fig. 23.1) but, since wound healing is a continuous biological process, there is some overlap between phases (Table 23.4).

Table 23.3 Important cells in wound healing

Cell	Function
Endothelial cells	Help to achieve haemostasis
Polymorphs	Take part in the initial inflammatory response
Macrophages	Digest debris and stimulate other cells to function
Fibroblasts	Produce collagen
Myofibroblasts	Aid wound contraction by producing mature collagen

Phase I — inflammation

As soon as wounding occurs the wound bleeds, platelets stimulate coagulation and a fibrin clot quickly forms.

An inflammatory reaction takes place at the wound site and histamine, prostaglandins and activated complement proteins are released. This causes the surrounding blood vessels to dilate and become more permeable. Inflammatory exudate, containing plasma proteins, antibodies, some erythrocytes and white blood cells (neutrophils and monocytes), flows into the damaged area.

Phase II — destructive phase

Polymorphonuclear leucocytes (polymorphs) begin the process of clearing the wound area of debris. Polymorphs ingest damaged cells and are attracted to the site of the wound by chemotaxis. During this time the numbers of monocytes (which later become macrophages) present increase. It is the macrophages which, through phagocytic activity, clear debris from the wound site. This phase can be looked on as being one of biological cleansing. It does, however, make a considerable metabolic demand on the body. Much heat and fluid can also be lost where a cavity wound exists. The shorter the duration of this phase the better, for, as it nears completion, proliferation or formation of new tissue can begin. Following the destructive phase the wound site is prepared for the repair process to begin.

Phase III — proliferation/reconstruction

During this phase tissue repair takes place. The increasing numbers of macrophages present play an important role.

Macrophages:

- have a phagocytic action on cell debris and bacteria
- are able to break down numerous complex molecules into simple sugars and amino acids which can then provide nutrition to the wounded area
- attract fibroblasts to the wounded area and also enhance their multiplication (through MDGF — monocyte-derived growth factor)
- stimulate fibroblasts to produce collagen, fibronectin and ground substance, which form the mass of connective tissue
- produce a variety of proteins (e.g. interferon and enzymes such as lysozyme) and lipids.

A comprehensive understanding of the full role of the macrophage does not as yet exist. However, its importance in coordinating tissue repair is without doubt.

The role of fibroblasts. Fibroblasts greatly increase in numbers during this phase of healing. They produce the materials which form granulation tissue. Fibroblasts will multiply rapidly in the well-nourished individual and to be most effective need adequate amounts of vitamin C, ferrous iron, oxygen and nutrients.

Fibroblasts produce:

- fibronectin which forms the framework for tissue by holding collagen and cells together whilst attaching them to the ground substance
- elastin, a protein which gives elasticity to tissue although production is limited in scar tissue
- ground substance which forms the mass of connective tissue and is made up of proteoglycans (glycoproteins formed of sub-units of polysaccharide chains with amino acids).

As the wound defect is filled with newly formed tissue, fibroblast and macrophage numbers and activity decrease.

Re-epithelialisation. Following complete filling of the wound

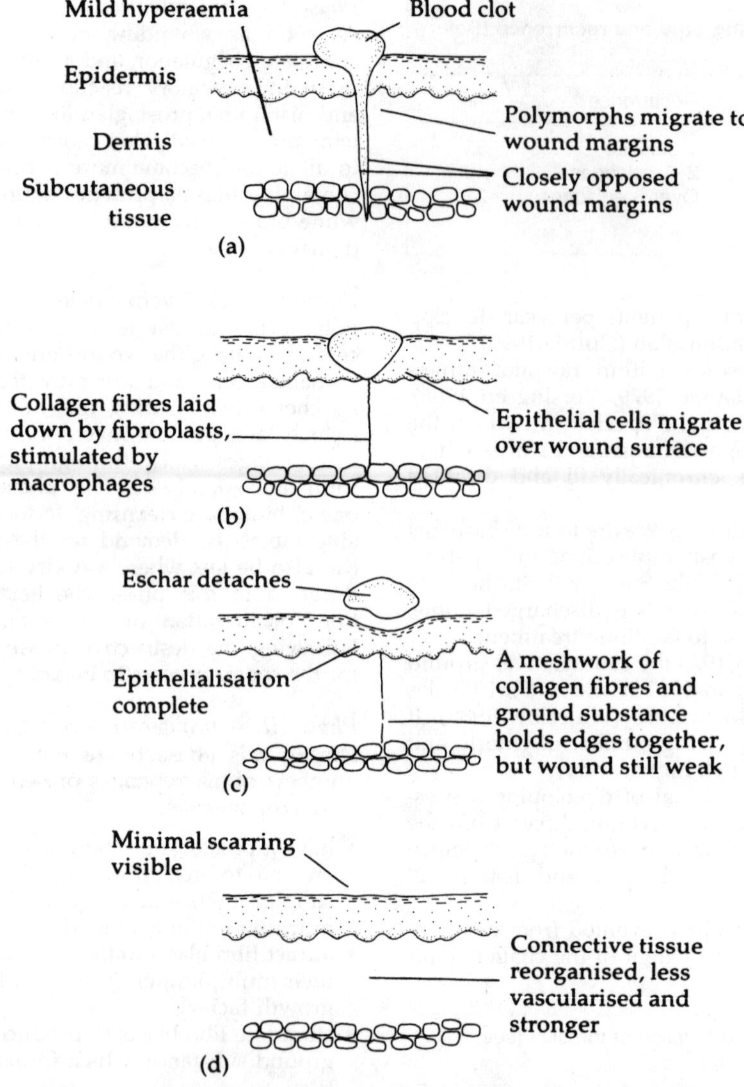

Fig. 23.1 Wound healing by primary intention. (A) Inflammation/destructive phase (B) and (C) Proliferation/reconstruction phase (D) Maturation phase. (Adapted from Morison 1992b.)

defect with granulation tissue, the open wound surface is ready to be covered by epithelium. Epithelialisation of the relatively large area is achieved by migration into it of epithelium from two sources. At the wound edges, epithelial cells divide and, gradually, epithelium migrates from the edges towards the middle of the wound. At the same time, any epithelial cells near hair follicles, which might be present deep in the dermis, divide rapidly. Islands of epithelium appear wherever a follicle is present. Cells migrate from these islands to meet each other while cells from the edges of the wound grow inwards to cover the raw surface.

Table 23.4 Phases of wound healing

Inflammation	Destructive phase	Proliferation	Maturation
0–3 days	2–5 days	4–28 days or until defect is filled	15 days–1 year

Phase IV — maturation

Vascularisation of the wounded area decreases during this phase. Although the wound appears closed or healed to the naked eye, much activity continues. The immature collagen laid down in phase II is gradually replaced by a mature collagen. The formation of new collagen and the lysis of immature collagen are balanced so that the amount of collagen present at any one time remains constant. The immature collagen is laid down in a random, haphazard fashion, its function being to fill the wound defect as quickly as possible. Mature collagen is laid down following lines of tension within the wound and, at the same time, it is cross-linked to give strength. Tensile strength at 14 days in sutured wounds is only about 10% of the original strength of the skin. Tensile strength is gained over a period of months and a year after wounding will have reached only about 70% of its original value.

Healing by primary/first intention

When injury occurs, whether through accident or as a surgical necessity, the aim of treatment is to effect complete healing as quickly as possible with minimal scarring.

To achieve this, the method of choice is healing by primary intention which occurs when wound edges are in apposition (Fig. 23.1). This is only possible where there is adequate, mobile tissue and no complicating bacterial contamination. In situations where contamination is suspected, closure of the wound is accompanied by the use of prophylactic systemic antibiotics. For healing to take place by primary intention the wound edges need to be closely approximated and held together until the wound has healed sufficiently. The skin may be closed by using adhesive tapes, clips, or continuous or interrupted sutures. The skill of the surgeon ensures that the sutures are not inserted too tightly and that the skin edges are closely apposed. The choice of suture material depends on the type of tissue being closed and on the particular function of the tissue.

Healing by secondary intention

Where there is significant tissue loss and/or bacterial contamination, wounds are usually left open to heal by secondary intention through the formation of granulation tissue and, later, wound contraction (Fig. 23.2). Due to the amount of tissue excised or lost during injury, wound healing is a longer process, taking weeks or even months to complete. The healing process itself proceeds in much the same way as for healing by primary intention. The proliferative phase is much extended, as this is when granulation tissue forms and fills the wound defect. It is generally accepted that the length of time a wound takes to heal depends on its original size, i.e. small wounds heal more quickly than larger ones, and it is therefore possible in some wound types (pilonidal sinus, abdominal and axillary wounds) to predict when wounds of a given size that are free from infection will heal (Marks et al 1983).

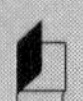

For methods of wound closure and types of suture material, see Morison (1992b), Ch. 9.

Scar tissue

A scar is the mark that may remain after a wound has healed. A scar consists of relatively avascular collagen fibres covered by a thin layer of epithelium.

Most scars fade with time (see Table 23.5) and the resultant cosmetic effect is generally acceptable, but abnormal scarring can lead to problems.

- Stretching of scar tissue — this can occur where sutures have been removed prematurely especially over areas that are under tension, e.g. the skin over the scapula and back are common sites for scars.
- Hypertrophic scar tissue — here collagen lysis and collagen production are out of synchrony and excessive tissue lies within the boundaries of the scar.
- Keloid — this is a protuberant, prominent scar which results from excessive collagen formation in the dermis during connective tissue repair.

Hypertrophic and keloidal scarring are examples of excessive scar formation. Such scarring is more common in young people, especially during pregnancy and puberty, and also in deeply pigmented skins, the peristernal area being particularly susceptible.

A number of factors influence scarring (see Table 23.6).

Why some wounds are sutured and others left open

Wound closure (enabling wounds to heal by primary intention) is considered to be the method of choice whenever possi-

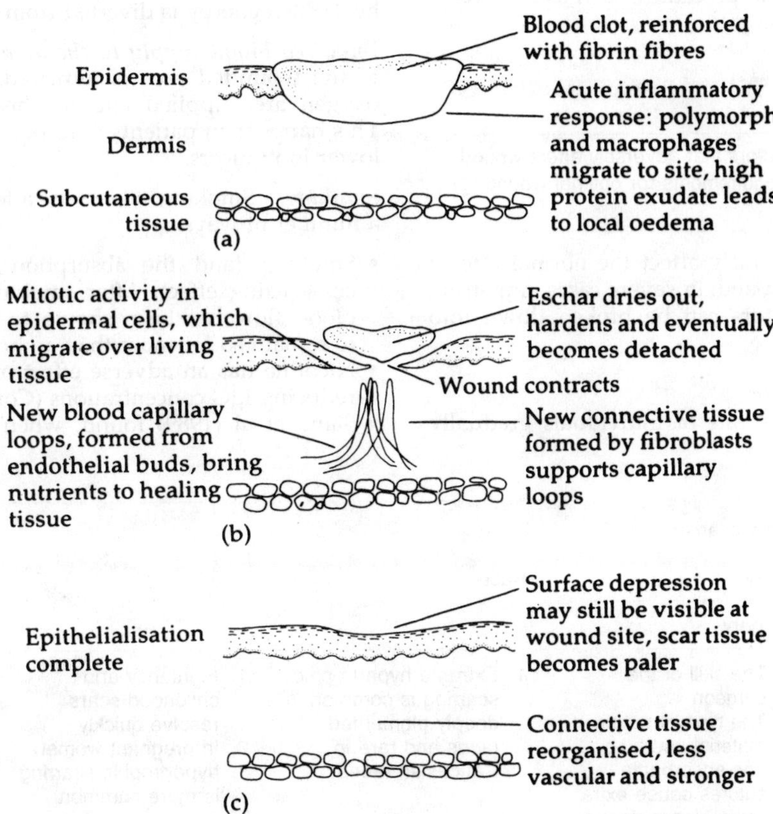

Fig. 23.2 Wound healing by secondary intention. (A) Inflammation/destructive phase (B) Proliferation/reconstruction phase (C) Maturation phase. (Adapted from Morison 1992b.)

Table 23.5 The maturation of scar tissue

0–28 days	28 days–3 months	3 months onwards
The scar is fragile and soft	The scar becomes denser, stronger and is red or purplish in colour	Over time the colour fades to white and the tissues become softer and more elastic

ble as healing by primary intention is much quicker than healing by secondary intention.

Wound closure is undertaken where:

- the procedure will result in cosmetically acceptable scars (adhesive tapes and clips can be used to avoid undesirable suture marks)
- sufficient mobile tissue exists to allow the edges of the wound to be brought together easily without tension or without causing trauma (which could lead to subsequent wound breakdown)
- the wound site is clean, e.g. when an operation is considered to be a clean procedure as in excision of lipoma (a benign tumour containing fatty tissue).

Secondary intention is chosen as the method of healing where:

- the final cosmetic effect is likely to be an improvement over either skin grafting or suturing
- there is insufficient tissue to allow the wound edges to be approximated; for example, in some chronic open wounds such as pressure sores (see p. 712) and leg ulcers (see p. 715)
- the wound area is heavily contaminated or infected, i.e. in a dirty injury or a dirty surgical procedure such as excision of an infected pilonidal sinus.

FACTORS THAT ADVERSELY AFFECT HEALING

?	**23.2** Before considering factors that adversely affect wound healing, identify the requirements for optimal wound healing.

A number of factors can adversely affect the normal rate of healing, slowing healing down and, in severe cases, impairing healing altogether. These factors can be broken down into intrinsic and extrinsic factors.

Intrinsic factors

Advanced age. The metabolic rate of individuals gradually slows down with advancing years. This is reflected in wound healing where the healing rate is relatively slow in the elderly. This is in marked contrast to the rate of healing in young children and in pregnancy when the metabolic rate is increased.

Impaired nutritional status. Well-nourished individuals have a plentiful supply of the proteins, carbohydrates, fats, vitamins and minerals that are essential for normal healing. Good nutrition should be encouraged throughout the healing period. Those patients undergoing surgery should be carefully assessed, as their nutrition may be poor in the perioperative period as a result of preoperative fasting or postoperative dietary restrictions (see Ch. 21). For some patients it is not always easy to maintain adequate nutrition, for example an elderly person living alone or a terminally ill patient who is unable to eat. The importance of diet cannot be over-stressed and wherever possible the nurse should ensure that the patient receives all the nutrients required for healing. The advice of a dietitian may be sought in an attempt to improve the nutritional status of vulnerable individuals.

Dehydration. The metabolic processes of an individual require about 2500 mls of water every 24 hours (see Ch. 20). A dehydrated individual will not be able to metabolise efficiently and this will adversely affect the healing process.

Disease processes. The generalised metabolic effects of a number of disease processes can delay healing. Diabetes, cancer, inflammatory disease and jaundice are included in this group as is any disease that impairs the body's immune response.

Fever. Febrile patients have an increased metabolic rate and use vast amounts of energy in both generating and dissipating heat. Such energy is diverted from the healing process.

Impaired blood supply to the area. Where the blood supply to the wounded area is impaired, insufficient nutrients and oxygen are supplied and the healing period is prolonged. This happens in patients with peripheral vascular disease and lower limb ulcers.

Smoking. Smoking adversely affects the healing process in a number of ways:

- Smoking (and the absorption of nicotine) has a vasoconstricting effect. After smoking one cigarette peripheral blood flow has been shown to be depressed by 50% and to remain so for more than an hour.
- Nicotine has an adverse effect on the immune response by reducing IgG concentrations (Corre et al 1971).
- Siana et al (1989) found, when looking at the healing of

Table 23.6 Factors influencing scarring

Cause of injury		Race	Age	Wound site
Burn/trauma	Surgery			
1. Over joints, contractures can occur 2. Dirty injuries caused by gravel can cause pigmentation	1. The skill of the surgeon 2. The type of suture material used, i.e. non-absorbable sutures cause extra scars alongside the wound	1. Extreme hypertrophic scarring is common in deeply pigmented races and rare in Caucasian races	1. In infancy and childhood scars resolve quickly 2. In pregnant women hypertrophic scarring is more common	1. Scars which follow the body's natural lines of skin tension do best 2. Scars which cross skin folds do less well 3. Scars on the shoulders, sternum and back produce unsightly scarring

abdominal wounds, that the overall cosmetic effect of a scar was poorer in patients who were smokers.

Extrinsic factors

Poor surgical technique. Where tissues are handled roughly during surgery they can be damaged, resulting in haematoma formation. This can lead to the development of wound infection as the haematoma is broken down. A dead space may also occur if tissues are not correctly approximated during surgery; again this encourages the development of wound infection. Where sutures are inserted too tightly the tissue becomes damaged and tissue death can occur.

Drug treatments. A whole range of drug therapies can affect the healing rate. The cytotoxic drugs given during chemotherapy can destroy healthy cells as well as malignant cells. Ideally, their use is withheld until any wound healing is complete. Steroids can also slow down, or prevent, healing taking place and their use is closely monitored in individuals with wounds.

Inappropriate wound management. The healing process may be adversely affected by the use of poor dressing technique, the wrong dressing material or antiseptics where they are not needed.

Adverse psychosocial factors. A wide variety of psychosocial factors can have an adverse effect on wound healing; for example, lack of understanding and acceptance of the treatment regime, or anxiety associated with changes in work, income, personal relationships and self-image (Morison 1992b).

Infection. Of all the factors which can delay or prevent healing, infection is the most important.

WOUND INFECTION

A wound is a breach in the skin and, until complete healing is achieved, presents a risk of infection to the individual. Infection in a healing wound delays healing and may even cause wound breakdown, herniation of the wound and complete wound dehiscence. The clinical signs and symptoms of a wound infection are summarised in Box 23.2. Despite all the technological advances that have been made in surgery and wound management, the problem of wound infection persists. This happens because the causes of wound infection are so varied and are often linked to the individual's general condition; both nutritional status and immune status are important factors in resistance to infection.

The wound environment can itself encourage bacterial growth. Some organisms (anaerobes) thrive in wounds with a poor oxygen supply. A wound bed or area which is free from haematomas and dead tissue and is clean reduces the risk of infection.

The way in which the wound is managed can also affect infection. Contamination by bacteria, through poor technique on the part of the nurse, poor hygiene, or incontinence on the part of the patient, can all increase the risk of wound infection.

The consequences of wound infection vary depending upon the environment in which the individual is being nursed.

In a hospital, a patient with a surgical wound infection poses a considerable risk to other patients with wounds on that ward. At home, that patient is less of a risk to his family and community, who are unlikely to be vulnerable.

Box 23.2 Clinical signs and symptoms of wound infection

The local effects of wound infection are:

- Pain — throbbing
- Redness
- Swelling — of the area surrounding the wound
- Discharge — haemoserous and/or purulent
- Loss of function — to protect the area
- Unhealthy appearance of the wound bed (p. 705).

Wound infection prolongs the inflammatory healing phase and delays healing by secondary intention. Systemic effects on the patient are:

- Raised temperature
- Increased metabolic rate
- General malaise
- Anorexia.

Factors that predispose to wound infection

Factors associated with the patient

There are several factors which, in addition to delaying the healing process, can predispose a patient to wound infection. These can be identified on first assessment:

- Poor nutritional status — Hill et al (1971) and Dickerson (1990) both found that as many as 30% of patients undergoing surgery were malnourished and therefore at risk, inadequate diet being a possibility both at home and in hospital.
- Immunosuppression — suppression of the immune system, (e.g. in diabetes mellitus or after steroid therapy) can lead to an increased rate of infection (Bibby & Collins 1986).
- Excessive body weight.
- Advanced age.

Factors specifically related to the hospital environment

- Adverse spatial arrangements — when too many patients are nursed in close proximity to each other, especially in an open ward, the wound infection rate increases. An increase occurs when there are more than 25 patients being nursed in an open ward (Bibby & Collins 1986).
- Length of preoperative stay — the wound infection rate is linked to the length of time a patient spends in hospital prior to operation. The longer this period the more likelihood there is of the individual being colonised by the pathogenic bacteria that are found in hospitals.
- Inappropriate preoperative care — patients who receive no shave preoperatively have the lowest clean wound infection rate at 0.9%. This increases to 2.5% when patients are shaved (Spencer & Bale 1990).
- Prolonged operative procedure — the longer the operation the greater is the risk of infection in clean wounds (Cruse & Foord 1980).
- Surgical contamination — in clean elective surgery (e.g. excision of benign breast lump), the rate of infection is between 1 and 2%. In emergency operations where the area is contaminated (e.g. for perforated bowel) the rate soars up to 40% (Westaby 1985).
- Use of drains — the presence of a drain increases the risk of wound infection. It is lowest with closed drainage systems (Redivac) and highest with open drainage systems (e.g. corrugated drains) (Cruse & Foord 1980).

As a wound infection develops, localisation of the infection leads to the formation of a wound abscess. This may drain through the suture line or into the wound in the case of cavities. Occasionally, if deep seated, the abscess will need a surgical incision to drain it properly. Where partial wound breakdown occurs extra caution is needed to ensure that the wound is surgically satisfactory (Bale 1992a).

Sources of wound infection

Endogenous. Organisms found on the patient's own skin are endogenous sources of wound infection. These organisms (usually *Staphylococcus aureus* or gut commensals) are either present under normal circumstances or are hospital pathogens that colonise the body after the patient is admitted to hospital. *Staphylococcus aureus* is found on the skin and sometimes in the upper respiratory tract. This organism does not normally affect the patient adversely, but, when a wound has been created, *Staph. aureus* can invade the wound from adjacent skin or be breathed into the wound from the nose.

Exogenous. Infections from exogenous sources are those that occur following contamination of the wound from outside of the patient. This may happen in theatre or later in the ward when pathogens are allowed to fall on to the wound and penetrate it. Bacteria such as *Pseudomonas aeruginosa* can be found in wet areas or where moisture is present, i.e. in water, fluids or ventilators. *Pseudomonas aeruginosa* is also found in flower vases, sinks and drains.

Accidental injuries are highly likely to have been contaminated by bacteria. *Clostridium tetani* and *Clostridium welchii* are present in the soil and can be hazardous to the individual. People who garden or receive minor injuries in their gardens are at risk and should be immunised.

Bacteria

Bacteria consist of a variety of single-celled organisms which have a primitive nucleus with no nuclear membrane. Bacteria do vary in size, but are larger than viruses and can be seen under a light microscope. Bacteria reproduce by simple binary fission, that is each bacterial cell divides into two, both of which can divide again. The rate of division of bacteria, and so multiplication, depends on their environment and, in suitable conditions, they divide rapidly.

There are three bacterial shapes, which give rise to three groups of bacteria.

Spherical bacteria. These are called cocci, which is a name derived from the Greek word for berry. Cocci arrange themselves in one of three patterns: staphylococci grow in clusters; streptococci grow in chains; and diplococci grow in pairs and may be encapsulated.

Cylindrical bacteria. These are called bacilli, which is derived from the Latin word for a rod or little stick.

In adverse conditions, bacilli can form spores which are resistant to such conditions. When conditions improve the organism reverts to its original form and multiplication can begin.

Spiral or helical bacteria. These are called spirilla. Their coils can be either tight or loose.

Many of the harmful effects of bacteria on man are caused by products of the bacteria, namely toxins, when these are released into the bloodstream. Endotoxins are released when a bacterial cell dies and breaks up, whereas exotoxins are continually released by thriving bacteria.

Bacteria cell walls. The cell wall of a bacterium can have a number of characteristics (Box 23.3). This ultimately influences how capable a host will be of destroying that bacteria. It is the cell wall of a bacterium that the body's immune system penetrates in order to destroy it.

Bacteria may also have a number of other features such as:

- Capsules — a polysaccharide or sometimes a protein makes up the outermost layer. The function of this is to inhibit phagocytosis, so increasing the bacteria's ability to survive the body's immune system defences (see Ch. 16).
- Flagella — the rotatory action of these hair-like projections bring about movement of the bacteria.
- Filii — much shorter projections which are thought to be connected with the passage of genetic material between bacteria.

Box 23.3 Gram-positive versus Gram-negative bacteria

The differing characteristics of the bacterial cell wall can be determined by the staining reaction first used by Professor Hans Gram in the late 19th century. Gram, who developed the procedure quite accidentally, found that due to the properties of the cell wall certain bacteria retain staining with crystal violet and resist any attempt to decolourise with ethanol. Other bacteria lose the stain, or respond to decolourisation and then respond to a pink counterstain. The former are described as Gram-positive bacteria and include such organisms as the cocci and clostridia. The latter are described as Gram-negative and include such organisms as *Escherichia coli* and *Pseudomonas aeruginosa*. This staining reaction is now considered a major classification distinction between bacteria.

? **23.3** Identify the major microorganisms that cause wound infection. Can you identify their sources?

WOUND MANAGEMENT — A HOLISTIC APPROACH

In the past many aspects of nursing care have been administered in a disjointed way using a task-oriented approach. Wound management has been no exception, all wounds being managed in much the same way, regardless of the needs of the individual or the environment in which he is being cared for.

Ideally management of a patient with a wound uses an organised approach. This begins with an initial assessment (Box 23.4) of both the patient and the wound so that the management can be planned. Following implementation, evaluation of that management is required to ensure that the needs of the patient have been met.

This approach can be adapted to suit the environment in which the patient is being cared for, whether this be in the patient's own home or in the hospital setting.

Nursing developments in wound management are under-

Box 23.4 Assessment in wound care

1. Assess the patient:
   - Identify factors that might impede healing, such as intercurrent disease processes, or certain medications (see p. 702).
   - Where disease processes are identified, attempt to ensure that they are corrected.
   - Where they cannot be corrected, build an expected delay in healing into the nursing care plan.
2. Assess the wound:
   - Consider whether the wound is healthy for the stage of healing and free from infection (see p. 705).
   - Assess the wound's physical characteristics.
   - Where appropriate, measure and record wound size.
3. Asses the environment in which the patient is being nursed.
4. Assess the appropriateness of wound agents and wound dressing materials.

going rapid change, so it is important that nurses keep pace with current research findings. Journals, study days and conferences provide access to much of the research-based data and to cost-effectiveness studies. A whole range of written material, workbooks and videos on individual products is available from pharmaceutical companies and, while these may be biased, they contain useful information on handling and application techniques, and on product range and sizes.

Assessment of the patient

When managing patients with wounds it is easy to get carried away solely by assessment of the wound. Do not forget that the whole patient needs to be cared for, not just the wound. Whether the patient is being managed in the hospital or in the home, or is young or old, assessment of the patient's general condition should be undertaken. This is done to identify any of the factors which might impair the wound-healing process and so delay or prevent healing (p. 702). For those factors discovered which are reversible, treatment should be sought. For those factors uncovered for which no treatment is possible, some degree of delay should be anticipated and allowed for in the nursing care plan.

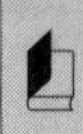

For further reading, see Bannon (1993). In this article, the author explains the importance of the holistic approach to wound care in the setting of an intensive care unit.

Assessment of the wound

Once the patient has been assessed in order to identify any factors that might affect healing, the next logical step is assessment of the wound being managed. A little time and thought taken at this stage can save much work later. When a sensible approach to wound assessment is used, treatment is quite straightforward and many pitfalls can be avoided (Bale 1992a).

Assessment of wounds that are healing by primary intention

Three questions need to be answered when assessing wounds that are healing by primary intention:

What has caused this wound? The answer may be surgical incision to perform an operation, or surgical excision of an abscess. Once the cause of the wound has been established the expected prognosis for complete healing can be estimated. For example, a surgical incision created in a fit, 20-year-old woman to remove a benign breast lump should result in a wound which will heal quickly and without complications. Compare that to an elderly lady who has had emergency bowel surgery for removal of a cancer. The expected healing potential here is not as good as in the first case (Spencer & Bale 1990).

Is the wound healthy for the stage of healing? During the first 3 days of healing by primary intention the area surrounding the wound will be swollen, indurated and often painful. This is normal during the inflammatory phase of healing. This can be illustrated by looking at a wound 2 days postoperatively. The patient experiences some difficulty in moving around and the incision area appears red, sore, swollen and inflamed. Whereas this is normal at this stage of the healing process, it would not be considered normal if the patient presented with the same symptoms 7–10 days postoperatively, and would indicate that some infection is present. Recognising what is normal throughout the healing process is essential. Only when this has been achieved can the abnormal be identified.

What needs to be done in the days before the sutures, clips etc. are removed? Nothing; if the wound remains healthy during the early days, the original dressing (if unstained and intact) can be left in place until the wound closure material is removed.

Assessment of cavity wounds

If wound management materials are to be used successfully, the appropriate product must be applied to the wound throughout the stages of healing. It is essential that the nurse is aware of what he, or she, requires from a dressing material in order to ensure that each product is used cost effectively. During the assessment the following factors should be taken into consideration (Bale 1993).

Appearance of the wound bed. In the pregranulation stage, cavity wounds often appear red, raw, and have a very uneven surface of adipose tissue. It is important to recognise that this is normal for this early stage of healing. Within 10–13 days, however, the appearance of the wound will change as granulation tissue is formed. A healthy wound should be pale pink in colour (sometimes covered with a pale yellow membrane), pain free and should not bleed easily if touched. If infection is present, the appearance of the wound will alter. The colour of the tissue may change to a dark red and the wound shows a tendency to bleed easily on light contact and become uncomfortable or painful. Superficial bridging of tissue can also be seen within the cavity. As the presence of infection can delay healing, prompt treatment is needed in these situations. For deep-seated infection, a wound swab (Box 23.5) followed by the appropriate course of antibiotics is generally indicated, but more superficial infections can sometimes be treated topically. Until the infection is cleared no dressing material will be fully effective.

Wound size. In general, the larger a wound the longer it will take to heal; therefore the size of a wound provides a useful indication of the probable healing time. The healing rate of some wound types, such as pilonidal sinus excisions, axillary wounds and abdominal wall wounds, have been carefully measured and so it is possible with these wound types to predict with some accuracy how long they will take to heal (Marks et al 1983).

The size of a wound may also influence the choice of dressing. Whilst small cavities may be dressed with one of a number of products, it may not be practical to use some products on larger wounds where multiple pieces or packs

Box 23.5 Taking a wound swab

Points to remember:

- Use an aseptic technique.
- Use a sterile, microbiological cotton wool swab.
- This swab should be moistened in a transport medium before use.
- If the wound is flat or shallow, gently rotate the swab across the middle of the wound bed. Care needs to be taken not to contaminate the swab with skin flora from the edges of the wound.
- If the wound is deep, or has a recess, insert the swab into the depths of the wound. Bacteria present in the depths of a wound are different and more likely to be pathogenic than bacteria on the surface of a wound.
- Carefully replace the swab directly into its storage tube containing culture medium.
- Deliver to the laboratory as soon as possible, but at the latest within 24 hours.
- Record antibiotic drugs being given, the site of the wound, together with any other information likely to be of help to the laboratory.

would be required. In these situations, the choice of dressing material may be limited to products which provide the bulk with just one or two packs. This is an especially important consideration in the community where the available size range of modern dressing materials is limited.

Wound measurement. In order to assess the effectiveness of a particular treatment, it is necessary to monitor changes in the size of the wound. For the majority of wound situations this should be the way a wound progresses towards complete healing. Surgically created cavities are usually of even contour and depth; the length and breadth of such a wound can generally be determined fairly easily. Weekly measurement is sufficient and steady progress should be evident (Bale 1992a).

Wound volume is more difficult to assess and does not really offer any advantages over the measurement of linear dimensions.

Chronic wounds, such as pressure sores, are often more difficult to measure as these wounds can extend under the skin edge. The simplest way of assessing the extent of these wounds is to measure by using a probe in the wound, under the edge of the cavity, and marking the boundary on the skin with an ink marker. This outline of the extent of the wound can then be traced on to paper and stored as a permanent record of wound progress.

For leg ulcers the circumference of the wound can be traced on to clean acetate or plastic sheets and, again, can be stored as a permanent record.

Remeasurement of chronic wounds may only be necessary every 2–3 weeks, as healing is generally slower in these situations. Accurate measurement and keeping of these records avoids the need to depend upon clinical impression. Ask several different nurses how they feel a wound is progressing and you are likely to get as many different answers!

> ? **23.4** How are wounds measured in the areas in which you have worked? Devise a way of recording the wound dimensions in the care plan of one of your patients.

Wound shape. When managing cavity wounds, it is necessary to recognise the importance of wound shape. Ideally, cavities created surgically should be boat or saucer shaped, with evenly sloping sides. Where pockets, tracts or sinuses occur within a cavity, drainage of exudate may be inadequate and this in turn may greatly delay healing. Poor wound shape also restricts the range of dressing materials that can be used. For example, a long narrow cavity will require a dressing material that is conformable enough to be inserted into the restricted space but can be easily removed from the depth of the wound without leaving behind fibres and particles which could then become a focus for infection.

In a wound where the shape is so poor that progress towards healing is unacceptably slow, surgical revision may be required in order to create a wound with more regular contours. This is occasionally necessary when wounds, which have undergone primary closure, subsequently break down. Pressure sores are particularly prone to develop into poorly shaped wounds and, as surgical revision here is not always possible or advisable, careful choice of an appropriate dressing material is essential (Bale 1992a).

Exudate production. Cavities vary enormously in the amount of exudate they produce. New, surgically created wounds can exude heavily, whereas some pressure sores produce very little fluid. This variation will affect management, especially the choice of dressing material. Some products are highly absorbent and able to deal with copious discharges, whereas others have a limited capacity for absorption. The inappropriate use of a dressing material can sometimes have serious consequences. If, for example, a dressing material is chosen that is unable to cope with heavy exudate production, the surrounding skin can quickly become macerated. Alternatively, a very hydrophilic dressing material applied to a lightly exuding wound may cause excessive drying of the wound surface, delaying healing and sometimes even causing pain.

Presence of slough or necrotic tissue. When slough or necrotic tissue is present on the wound surface, healing will be delayed or, in some cases, prevented altogether. This material needs to be loosened and removed to allow wound healing to progress. This is known as debridement and is a difficult task which requires intensive nursing intervention (see p. 708) (Bale 1992b).

Assessment of the physical environment

Where patients are being nursed can have an effect on their progress. Patients being nursed in a hospital are in a controlled environment. Their dietary intake and fluid balance can be monitored and their general well-being assured. For 24 hours each day nursing care is available and to a great extent the nurse 'controls' the environment in which the patient is being nursed. In the community when patients are being cared for in their own homes the nurse has far less control over what happens in the environment of the patient. As a guest, the district nurse is able to advise and recommend an adequate food and fluid intake but is unable to monitor this accurately, as she is only available for a comparatively short period once or twice a day.

Creating an environment for healing

Principles of moist wound healing

Healing proceeds at its optimal rate when the wound is enclosed in a warm, moist environment (Fig. 23.3). Under these conditions cellular activity is maximised and the benefits of such an environment have been recognised since the early 60s (Winter 1962, Turner 1985). This is true for the whole spectrum of wounds encountered, from superficial cuts and grazes to large, extensive granulating wounds. Exposure of a wound to the air precipitates drying out of the wound surface and scab formation (Thomas 1990a).

Nurses should be mindful of the importance of providing a suitable environment for wound healing when choosing a wound management material. The term dressing is a misnomer in the 1990s. The concept of a dressing 20 years ago was one of some form of absorbent cotton/gauze type material that was used to soak up excess wound secretions and protect the wound from trauma. By the 1990s a whole range of sophisticated materials have been developed to cater for the diversity of needs of individual wound situations. Many of these materials interact with the wound surface (so-called interactive materials) and are designed to optimise the local conditions for wound healing (Thomas 1990a). Box 23.6 summarises the characteristics of an ideal wound dressing material.

Principles of cleansing

Why cleanse a wound? Sutured wounds rarely need cleansing unless leakage has occurred. In this situation the suture line can be gently, aseptically cleansed with sterile normal saline. With open wounds strict asepsis is not always required. The patient can use the bath or preferably the shower to irrigate the wound using warm water (Harding 1992). All fluids used for wound cleansing should be warmed to body temperature. When using cold fluids, 'it takes wounds 40 minutes to regain original temperature and 3 hours for mitotic

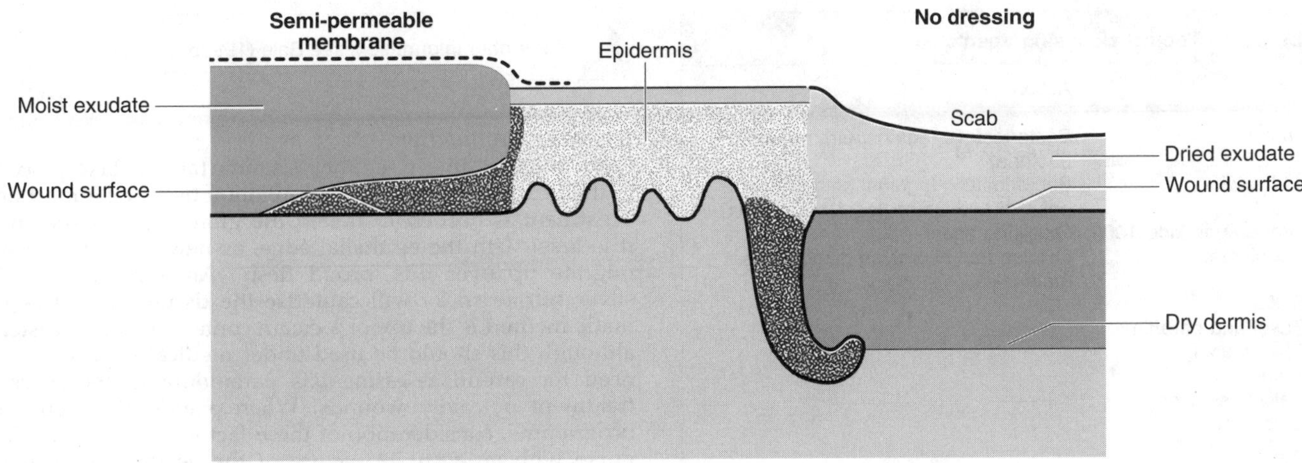

Fig. 23.3 Healing of skin wounds with and without a semi-permeable membrane dressing (Winter 1962).

activity to return to the wound' (Myers 1982). The reason for cleansing open cavity wounds is to remove any loose debris and excess wound secretions. A shower is particularly useful in achieving this. The gently flushing action of the spray will remove any particles which are loose, and flushing for 10–15 seconds is usually sufficient. In a bath the wound should be flushed by splashing water into it. Wounds of the lower limb can be bathed in a bucket or bowl, gently splashing the wound to remove loose debris. A bucket can be lined with a commercial bin liner. This protects the bucket from contamination and makes cleaning of the bucket much easier and so reduces the potential risk of cross-infection.

The role of antiseptics and topical agents. The actions of the whole range of antiseptics and cleansing agents is generally poorly understood by nurses. These lotions are widely used to mechanically cleanse wounds at dressing changes, and also as topical applications which stay in contact with the surface of the wound. In the past, nurses have been taught that all bacteria are bad for a wound and that wounds should be kept bacteria free and sterile. Along with this went teaching that antiseptics which eradicate bacteria are therefore good and should be used routinely to keep the bacterial count at the wound surface as low as possible. There are a few situations where this is the case, i.e. for the treatment of burns and some immunocompromised patients and for some wounds which have undergone primary closure. For cavity wounds the role of bacteria is somewhat different. All cavity wounds become colonised by bacteria from the surrounding skin which are particular to that individual. Their presence does not affect the healing rate in most cases and these bacteria are extremely difficult to get rid of completely (Leaper 1986).

Bacterial studies on pilonidal sinus excisions, axillary wounds and abdominal wall wounds have shown that the vast majority of bacteria present in these wound types do not cause problems to the patient or in fact delay healing (Marks et al 1983). In a similar study looking at the bacteriology of leg ulcers the presence of bacteria on the wound surface again did not delay healing (Eriksson 1984). Patients with leg ulcers appeared to keep their initial bacterial flora irrespective of the type of treatment and its eventual outcome. The organisms here included *Staphylococcus aureus, Escherichia coli* and *Pseudomonas aeruginosa.*

Nurses should use a realistic approach when cleansing wounds. Many antiseptics have a short-lived action and so bacteria will quickly recolonise the wound surface. If these organisms are not harmful then why seek to eradicate them? Since the mid-1980s there has been debate within the nursing, medical and pharmaceutical professions as to the effectiveness of antiseptics, especially chlorinated solutions. Thomas (1990b) has made recommendations on the use of hypochlorite solutions based on the available research. There are, however, many clinicians who have successfully used these solutions over a number of years and advocate their use (Langridge 1990). The problem is yet to be resolved due to the lack of in vivo studies demonstrating their effects on healthy human tissue. The general guidelines issued by Thomas (1990b) should be followed if chlorinated solutions are to be used. Their use should be restricted to infected, sloughy and necrotic wounds and then only for short periods of time (maximum 7 days). These solutions are best not used on healthy tissues due to their potentially cytotoxic effects.

Box 23.6 Characteristics of an ideal dressing (Morison 1992b)

Non-adherent
Impermeable to bacteria
Capable of maintaining a high humidity at the wound site while removing excess exudate
Thermally insulating
Non-toxic and non-allergenic
Comfortable and conformable
Capable of protecting the wound from further trauma
Requires infrequent dressing changes
Cost effective
Long shelf life
Available both in hospital and in the community

Devitalised tissue can be removed in several ways:

Chemical debridement. Before the advent of modern dressing materials a range of chemicals have been applied to sloughy and necrotic tissue in an attempt to soften and remove it (Bale 1992b), but with varying degrees of success. What often happens is that the skin surrounding the wound is affected. When hypochlorite solutions are used, bleaching of the surrounding skin is encountered and, with other agents, maceration can occur. In their use with harder necrotic tissue, which forms an eschar, these agents have difficulty in penetrating the surface and so are ineffective. About 100 ml of a solution which contains 0.25% w/v chlorine is needed to solubilise 1 g of sloughy tissue (Thomas 1990b). Further work with Eusol on necrotic tissue showed that, after immersion for 24 hours,

Table 23.7 Topical cleansing agents

Agent	Action
Cetrimide	Bacteriostatic (against Gram-negative bacteria)
Chlorhexidine	Bacteriostatic (against both Gram-positive and Gram-negative bacteria)
Hydrogen peroxide 1000	Oxidising agent
Hypochlorites	Oxidise and hydrolyse nitrogenous materials
Eusol	
Eusol and paraffin	
Chloramin T	
Milton	
Dakin's solution	
Chlorasol	
Iodine preparations	
aqueous solutions	
alcoholic lotions	Powerful antimicrobial action
Proflavin cream	Mild bacteriostatic (against Gram-positive bacteria)

the tissue remained unchanged (Thomas 1990b). Where granulation tissue is present, damage can occur due to the toxicity of the chemicals. However, it must be said that many nurses, both in the hospital and in the community, have successfully used these products for many years (Table 23.7). In these cases the chemicals are generally used in the short term, for around 5–7 days, and the surrounding skin is well protected with a barrier cream. The experience and expertise of the user is the key to their success.

Enzymatic agents. Another product designed to remove slough and necrotic tissue is an enzymatic agent (a mixure of streptokinase and streptodornase) which is thought to act on slough and necrotic tissue without affecting viable tissue. It can be applied directly to the area or injected into an eschar. The latter procedure should only be carried out by experienced practitioners (Thomas 1990a). Alternatively, an eschar can be scored with a scalpel prior to application of the enzymes. This product should be used with caution and instructions should be followed to the letter. Mixing of the two vials (one containing the enzymes, the other water) prior to application should be done gently; some inexperienced users may find the process difficult compared to using other materials. Again, the success of this agent depends upon the experience and expertise of the individual user (Bale 1992b).

Surgical debridement. It is sometimes possible for a surgeon to excise devitalised tissue with, or without, anaesthesia depending on the site and depth of the problem. The advantages of this method are that debridement is instant and a healthy cavity results. Where patients are being cared for in the community, access to the surgeon may be limited and this is not always a practical alternative for many patients.

Modern wound dressing materials. A number of these materials will effectively remove sloughy and necrotic tissue without damaging either the skin surrounding the wound or healthy tissue within the wound. Included here are the hydrogels, hydrocolloids and the polysaccharides (Table 23.8).

Hydrogels and hydrocolloids quickly rehydrate devitalised tissue which has become dehydrated. Under moist conditions the normal autolytic processes facilitate separation of viable from non-viable tissue. As the sloughy and necrotic tissue loosens it can be wiped away or carefully pared off (Thomas 1990b).

For further information, see Bale (1992b).

Excessive granulation

From time to time re-epithelialisation fails to take place due to the presence of excessive granulation tissue or 'proud flesh'. Treatment is needed to flatten the granulation tissue so that it is level with the epithelial edge, as new epithelium cannot migrate up over this 'proud flesh'. An application of 75% silver nitrate sticks will cauterise the tissue, but a less traumatic method is the use of a cream containing a corticosteroid, although this should be used under medical supervision. The need for careful assessment is paramount in the successful treatment of cavity wounds. When planning a wound-care programme, consideration of these factors should provide the nurse with an accurate picture of the needs of each wound and also provide some assistance with the dressing selection process.

Dressings of the future

Unlike traditional cotton absorbent materials some of the modern dressings available interact with the wound (e.g. hydrocolloids, hydrogels, alginates). The trend to develop interactive products continues. Outside the UK other countries are using agents to stimulate the healing process. These include the use of growth factors such as bFGF (basic fibroblasts growth factor), TGFβ (transforming growth factor, β family), the interleukin family of proteins, and PDGF (platelet-derived growth factor) (Hopkinson 1992). Research continues to determine which wounds are likely to benefit most from the application of such agents.

Dressing change techniques

Throughout the UK there are many different policies, procedures and protocols for dressing changes. However, the general principles remain the same.

A dressing needs changing when:

- there is a specific purpose, e.g. to remove sutures
- clinical signs of infection are present (see p. 703)
- wound discharge has leaked through the dressing
- cleansing of an open wound is necessary — this may be as frequently as twice a day or as infrequently as once a week (see Table 23.8 for different dressings)
- special treatments are needed, e.g. burns dressings.

Aseptic technique

In hospital. When dressing changes are being performed within a hospital, the nurse must always take into consideration the possibility of transferring bacteria from one patient to another, due to the close proximity in which patients are cared for. This is more of a risk when several patients with wounds are being nursed in the same ward and by the same nurses. Once a wound has become contaminated clinical infection can quickly develop. Aseptic technique aims to prevent pathogenic organisms from contaminating a wound (Box 23.7).

In hospital, dressings are generally changed using an aseptic technique. There may, however, be occasions when dressing changes require a technique that is socially clean without being fully aseptic.

It is an individual nurse's responsibility to understand the principles of asepsis and adapt her knowledge to the situation being managed.

In the community. In the hospital, equipment is provided which allows the nurse to manage safely all the wound man-

Table 23.8 Dressing materials

Material	Presentation	Action	Advantages	Disadvantages	Suitable for
Absorbent cotton and gauze	Variety of pads, rolls, squares and ribbon gauze	Absorbent material	Absorbent and cheap	Allows strike through Adheres to granulation tissue and can become embedded in it Need frequent dressing changes	As an outer layer for extra absorbency Should not be a primary contact material
Low-adherence dressing	Flat sheets in a variety of sizes	Absorbent for lightly exuding wounds	When used correctly has low adherence with wound surface	Allows strike through when used in moderately to heavily exuding wounds and in these situations can stick	As a primary wound contact material for lightly exuding wounds, i.e. suture lines, superficial injuries, some superficial leg ulcers and pressure sores and at the end stage of healing
Tulle	Sheets of various sizes have paraffin and other substances impregnated in them	Non-adherent when used for lightly exuding wounds	Cheap When sufficient is applied correctly will not adhere to wound surface	When used in moderately or heavily exuding wounds or when the exudate is particularly sticky can adhere to the wound surface and be difficult to remove Impregnates can be allergenic especially with leg ulcer patients	Superficial open wounds which are lightly exuding
Semipermeable film	Sheets of various sizes	Moisture-retaining adhesive film Allows gaseous exchange	Maintains moisture and fulfills a number of the criteria of a good dressing	Can peel off Can leak if wound exuding (although this can be prevented by aspiration of excess fluid)	Shallow superficial open wounds, suture lines, prophylaxis on pressure sores
Paste bandage	7.5 cm × 4 m impregnated bandages used in conjunction with a compression bandage	Depends on the substance impregnated	Cheap, low-adherent Usually only need changing weekly	Some patients develop allergies Does need skill to apply correctly, can cause damage if applied too tightly or with poor technique	Leg ulcer of venous origin, can be cut into strips for use on fungating lesions
Impregnated textile (Inadine)	Sheets of various sizes	Bacteriocidal	Low-adherence Delivers iodine to wound	Reaction if patient allergic to iodine When used inappropriately in lightly exuding wounds, can stick	Superficial leg ulcers and pressure sores and infected (especially pseudomonal) superficial open wounds
Polysaccharide (Debrisan, Iodosorb)	Beads, pads, paste, ointment	Cleansing and debriding by osmotic action at the wound surface and bacteriocidal	Will debride sloughy and necrotic matter	Beads can be difficult to hold in place Possibility of allergic reaction to iodine	Sloughy, dirty and necrotic wounds, also for leg ulcers and pressure sores
Foam (Lyofoam, Allevyn, Silastic)	Sheets of various sizes, liquid base and catalyst but also need disinfectant to clean foam stent	Absorbent foams When poured forms an exact cast of the wound	Infrequent dressing changes by the nurse, patient manageable	Not for use in irregularly shaped cavities	Superficial open wounds and cavity wounds

Table 23.8 *(cont'd)*

Material	Presentation	Action	Advantages	Disadvantages	Suitable for
Hydrocolloid	Wafers, beads, powder and paste	Dissolves into a gel on contact with wound secretions and this provides a healing environment, may stimulate formation of granulation tissue	Infrequent dressing changes Improved healing in chronic wounds	Offensive smell produced by the dressing as it degrades Not for infected wounds Occasionally, maceration of surrounding skin	Granulating wounds especially chronic wounds
Hydrogel	Sheets and sachets	Provides a healing environment	Rehydrates dry areas Soothes painful areas Quickly removes necrotic tissue and slough from a wound surface Infrequent dressing changes	Can cause maceration of the surrounding skin Can be difficult to keep in place and may leak	Painful flat areas, burns, fungating lesions, cavity wounds, leg ulcers, pressure sores, sloughy and necrotic wounds
Alginate	Sheets, ribbon gauze	Provides a healing environment when dissolved into a gel	Absorbent material Infrequent dressing changes Can be used in sinuses and irregularly shaped wounds	Can build up on the wound edge Can be difficult to keep in place	Open wounds, chronic wounds, both regularly and irregularly shaped wounds

agement situations she may encounter. Maintaining asepsis may pose different problems in the patient's own home. The district nurse may have little control over the cleanliness of the area and needs to take extra care when changing dressings. It is just as important in the community to avoid cross-infection between households and contamination of wounds. The district nurse in these situations has many opportunities for health education.

Box 23.7 Principles of aseptic technique

- Perform procedure in an area which is closed, clean and well ventilated at least 1 hour after periods of activity (bed making and ward cleaning, for example, increase the circulation of dust particles and airborne bacteria).
- Use a clean trolley (this should be thoroughly cleaned daily and wiped with an alcoholic solution before and after use).
- Wash hands (p. 550) before, after and at any point during the procedure should hands become contaminated. The use of an alcoholic hand rub can sometimes be substituted.
- Wear a clean plastic apron to protect the patient from bacteria on the nurse's uniform.
- Use sterile equipment for the procedure (be aware of how your Health Authority/Board identifies equipment which is sterile and so safe to use).
- Discard equipment which has broken or damaged packaging.
- Use sterile fluids and dressing materials.
- Prepare equipment before dressings are removed.
- Use gloves to remove any dressings and dispose of both immediately.
- Carry out the procedure using forceps or sterile gloves, discarding equipment as it becomes contaminated.
- Dispose of used equipment in the appropriate bin.

The place for a clean technique

For many dressing changes the use of a clean technique (Table 23.9) is safe and acceptable. The types of wound suitable for this method include the majority of granulating wounds.

Involving the patient in wound care

Whether the patient is being cared for at home or in hospital there are many opportunities for the nurse to involve the patient in his or her wound management. This is important in giving the patient a sense of independence and will help the individual to return to normality. Patients with sutured

Table 23.9 Clean technique

Procedure	Rationale
1. Use non-sterile gloves to remove dressing. Change gloves	Protects both nurse and patient from cross-infection
2. Shower or bathe patient's wound	Mechanically removes loose wound debris (NB ensure thorough cleansing of shower/bath whether at home or in hospital)
3. Use clean bowl/bucket with bin liner for patients with small wounds or foot/leg wounds in the home	Prevents contamination of equipment
4. Use clean paper, or a clean towel to dry area surrounding wound	Prior to application of dressing, area needs to be dry
5. Encourage patient involvement in treatment	Increases patient compliance and encourages return to normal activity

wounds can be taught to monitor themselves for clinical signs of infection, and to give good self-care in terms of nutrition, fluid intake, rest and avoidance of excessive movement of the affected area. Patients with open wounds can become much more involved. In addition to the self-care elements outlined above, they can be taught about the appearance of the wound surface and what can be expected to happen during the healing phase. In the community, patients and their relatives can be taught the basic dressing-change technique where asepsis is not necessary and the district nurse can assume a supervisory role. This obviously depends on individual circumstances and the patient's level of understanding, but certainly many patients with open wounds are able to play a major role in wound management. This is important as the patient begins to resume a more normal lifestyle and it also avoids the need for routine daily visits by the district nurse.

Patients with chronic wounds, such as leg ulcers and pressure sores, need special help but it is very important to gain their cooperation. Patients with venous leg ulcers (see p. 715) need to be taught leg elevation techniques and calf pump muscle exercises to stimulate the circulation and aid drainage of the lower limb. Patients with pressure sores (see p. 712), and their relatives, need to be taught how to correctly lift, turn and position, and handle the patient. They also need to know how the pressure-relieving aids work, so that these are used correctly all the time and not just when the district nurse is in the home.

Nurse prescribing

Nurses working in the community play an integral part in the management of patients with wounds.

The need for patients to receive a high standard of wound care in the community is of paramount importance as more and more patients are being cared for outside of hospital (Bale 1991).

For district nurses the vast majority of their wound-management workload concerns chronic wounds. Only 1% of patients with leg ulcers for example, are managed in hospital. It is the district nurse who is faced with the long-term management of such wounds. Difficulties arose in the community when, following patient assessment, district nurses had to have the necessary dressing prescribed by the general practitioner. This 'rubber stamping' was both time wasting and frustrating for the nurse. In response to a directive from the 1987 Primary Health Care White Paper 'Promoting better health', an Advisory Group was set up to investigate the professional and ethical issues surrounding nurse prescribing and make recommendations. In 1991 the Advisory Group recommended that 'suitably qualified nurses in the community should be able, in clearly defined circumstances, to prescribe from a limited list of items'.

As far as wound management is concerned this list includes an extensive range of primary wound contact materials, bandages and dressing-retention materials (Bale 1991).

Wound management policies

There has been an increasingly popular trend towards standardising wound management by Health Boards and Health Authorities throughout the UK. There are two responses on the part of the nurse to implementation of such policies. The first is that wound policies are useful. The second is that these policies take away the individual nurse's initiative when deciding on a wound treatment for an individual patient. As all wounds are different, each treatment should be tailor-made to suit the individual; it follows then that this is not possible if a strict policy is being followed. However, such policies can control the use of idiosyncratic, unproven management strategies.

Whatever an individual nurse's opinion on wound management policies, there is every possibility that she may have to work within the confines of such a policy.

The transition from hospital to home

The transition from hospital to home for patients with wounds usually happens without any problems. Liaison nurses are often available to organise the discharge home and to arrange for any visits needed by the district nurse for the newly discharged patient. In accident and emergency departments a liaison service may also be available. It is important, though, that wherever patients receive treatment they have a point of contact so that they are well supported when discharged home (Bale 1989a).

Provision of materials in hospitals and in the community

Many nurses are unaware of the vast differences which exist in the provision of wound-management materials to patients cared for in the hospital compared to those managed in the community. Although most hospitals impose some form of restriction on which materials are provided, generally all the main groups of manufactured materials are available for use in the hospital. These are supplied not only to inpatients but also to outpatients who are under the care of a hospital consultant. All materials needed for inpatient treatment are provided without direct cost to the individual patient. It is the norm then for patients treated in hospital to have access to a comprehensive range of wound-management materials for their wound care, and supplies of these continue as long as the patient remains in hospital. Patients managed in the community are in a different position. Materials needed for their treatment are generally obtained from the general practitioner, who writes a prescription for those items required. Unless the patient is exempt from paying, a charge is made for each item dispensed. Provision is made to enable patients to purchase a 'season ticket' lasting 4 months or 1 year.

Apart from direct costs, which may be incurred, the range of materials available on FP10 prescription is less comprehensive than that available within hospitals. The products that can be prescribed are listed in the Drug Tariff which is controlled by the DoH.

> ? **23.5** Ask the pharmacist what products are available on FP10 to patients in the community. Look also at the sizes of prescribable products.

The Drug Tariff shows the current list of modern products. Although at first sight it would appear that it includes materials from all groups, the range of sizes is very restricted. In turn this restricts the sizes of wounds that can be managed or increases the number of smaller packets required for each dressing change.

Expectations of outcome and effectiveness of treatment

Following individual patient and wound assessment, the nurse should have reasonable expectations regarding the prospects of achieving complete healing. In some wounds, complete healing is expected rapidly, as in primary wound closure following excision of a lipoma in a healthy young person. For others, the prognosis for healing is not so good; for example, an elderly lady with arthritis and a venous leg ulcer. The expected outcome affects the choice of treatment for individual patients. For patients with a poor prognosis for healing, treatment is often directed towards minimising symptoms and preventing further wound breakdown. This situation can arise in terminally ill patients with superficial pressure sores where the aim is to prevent deterioration of the sore into deeper tissues. Patient comfort and convenience become the priorities and provide some measure of the effectiveness of the treatment. Where healing is expected, effectiveness means complete healing achieved in the minimal number of days.

Cost effectiveness

Efficacy is also measured in terms of the cost of treatments. Hospital doctors, general practitioners and the pharmacists who supply materials for wound management can be misled into believing that, because the initial cost of a material is high then it follows that the total treatment costs will also be high. The modern wound-dressing materials are very much more expensive to buy per unit than traditional materials. However, the modern materials can often be left on the wound for several days and, in some cases, for a full week. Traditional, cheaper materials need daily or twice-daily dressing changes and the equipment needed during these frequent dressing changes increases the total treatment costs dramatically. If nursing time is also taken into consideration then the cost of using traditional, cheap materials increases again (Bale 1989b).

It is important, when comparing the costs of modern and traditional materials to look at:

- How long the product can be left on the wound
- How much nursing time is needed to change and apply dressings
- The benefits of using a material which is interactive and so stimulates tissue growth to achieve rapid healing or stimulate healing in a chronic wound.

It is in the area of materials that there has been most benefit, especially in the community where much of the chronic wound care is undertaken. Modern materials here are helping to achieve healing in these difficult wounds and enabling more efficient use of nurses' time.

Discharging such patients after many months, if not years of treatment also improves their quality of life.

SPECIFIC WOUND TYPES

Pressure sores

Definition. A pressure sore is an area of localised damage to the skin and may involve underlying structures. Tissue damage can be restricted to superficial epidermal loss or extend to involve muscle and bone (Banks 1992).

The prevention of pressure sores and management of patients with pressure sores present major problems for nurses. Patients from all walks of life and with a range of illnesses may be susceptible to develop pressure sores. The difficulties arise in trying to identify patients who might develop a pressure sore, and when they are at risk of doing so. It is a basic responsibility of nurses to:

- accurately assess the patients in their care for being 'at risk' of developing a pressure sore
- ensure that any predisposing factors are reduced
- ensure that patients are nursed on the most suitable surface, depending on their individual needs
- ensure that established pressure sores are efficiently managed
- undertake regular and ongoing reassessments of individual patients; a patient's needs vary from one day to the next, and in the very ill from one hour to the next.

Aetiology. Pressure sores result from areas of previously healthy tissue becoming devitalised, resulting in localised tissue death. Pressure sores develop in a number of ways:

- As a result of direct, unrelieved pressure of soft tissues against bone.
- Where friction occurs between the patient and the surface of a bed or chair. This can happen if the patient is moved and the skin is dragged over a sheet.
- As a result of the shear force which frequently accompanies both direct pressure and friction. Shear forces develop in tissues that are distorted and pulled, so that the blood supply is disrupted.

Classification. In order to assess the extent or degree of damage, several gradings have been developed for the classification of pressure sores (Torrence 1983, Hibbs 1988).

Hibbs (1988) describes the following:

Stage I — blanching hyperaemia. Reactive hyperaemia causes a distinct erythema after pressure is released. Light finger pressure will cause blanching of this erythema, indicating that the microcirculation is intact.

Stage II — non-blanching hyperaemia. Erythema remains after release of pressure. A degree of microcirculatory disruption and inflammation, oedema and thickening occurs. Superficial swelling, induration, blistering and epidermal ulceration will be present.

Stage III — ulceration progresses through to the subcutaneous tissue. Ulcer edges are distinct, but surrounded by erythema and induration. At this stage damage is still reversible.

Stage IV — lesion extends into the subcutaneous fat. Small vessel thrombosis and infection compound fat necrosis. There is a distinct ulcer margin, but lateral extension of necrosis continues under the skin. Deep fascia temporarily impedes downward progress.

Stage V — infective necrosis. Necrosis penetrates the deep fascia and muscle induration proceeds rapidly. Joints and body cavities can become involved. Multiple sores may communicate.

Closed pressure sores. There is deep, extensive damage to tissues, but the surface presents as a small ulcer.

Assessment of risk. As even the most unlikely individual may become 'at risk' of developing a pressure sore, all patients should be assessed on admission either to a hospital ward or unit or on to a district nurse's case load. 'The importance of assessing all patients (except perhaps some short-stay cases) cannot be over emphasised.' (Waterlow 1992). A combination of disease processes and/or drug therapies or surgery, for example, can quite suddenly put an individual into an 'at-risk' category.

The following types of patients are at risk of developing pressure sores:

- the elderly
- the immobile, e.g. paraplegic, following orthopaedic surgery
- those with sensory loss, e.g. comatose, diabetic
- those with a range of systemic diseases, e.g. anaemia, peripheral vascular disease, carcinoma
- those having a range of drug therapies, e.g. anti-inflammatories, cytotoxics, steroids
- the incontinent
- poorly nourished individuals
- the obese and those with below average body weight.

Several scales and scoring systems have been devised for assessing risk, the best-known being the Norton scale (Table 23.10) and the Waterlow score (Fig. 23.4). The Waterlow scoring system has been widely used in the UK because it takes many factors into consideration. It is comprehensive and yet

Norton risk scale (Norton et al 1962)

	B Mental condition		C Activity		D Mobility		E Incontinent	
4	Alert	4	Ambulant	4	Full	4	Not	4
3	Apathetic	3	Walk/help	3	Slightly limited	3	Occasional	3
2	Confused	2	Chairbound	2	Very limited	2	Usually/urine	2
1	Stuporous	1	Bedfast	1	Immobile	1	Double	1

Scoring sy[illegible]n: total score of 14 and below = at risk of developing a pressure sore.

easy to use (Morison 1992b). There are many other risk assessment scores available, including those of Douglas (Pritchard 1986), Lowthian (1987) (Fig. 23.5) and Bradon (Flanagan 1993).

With so many risk assessment systems available, it is inevitable that criticism has arisen. Because the Norton scale was devised using elderly patients, it has been suggested that its use is limited for younger people. It has also been criticised for not being comprehensive enough to cover other risk factors such as nutrition. Barrett (1987) reviewed the various scoring systems and came to the conclusion that more effective evaluation was needed.

The reasons for the widespread use of the Waterlow and Norton scoring systems, and for their popularity, are probably that both are easy to use and only take a matter of minutes to complete. Both reasons are important if all patients are to be regularly reassessed. Some Health Authorities and Health Boards have adapted these scoring systems to suit their own patients' needs and as part of a pressure sore prevention policy.

A risk assessment scoring system is only useful, however, if it is used regularly — on admission and again each time the patient's condition changes. The scores need to be accurately documented and then used to determine the most appropriate pressure-relieving devices on which to nurse the patient.

? **23.6** What scoring system does your ward/area use? Where is the score documented and how often are patients reassessed?

For further information, see: Goldstone & Goldstone (1982), Watson (1989) and Bridel (1993).

Prevention of pressure sores. Once patients have been identified as being 'at risk', they should be nursed on the most appropriate surface (Box 23.8). This includes not only the mattress on the bed but also any chairs in which they may sit during the day (Dealey 1992). Other areas worth considering are theatre operating tables and trolleys on which patients are transported around hospital.

For further reading, see Hibbs (1991).

Liaison with other professionals may be indicated, for example with the physiotherapist to assess the degree of mobility an individual has and where help and treatment can be given.

Attempts to reduce friction and shearing when nursing patients are essential. At home this is easier than in hospital where sheets are often starched. Where possible, nurse patients on soft sheets or use a duvet, as hard rigid surfaces increase friction.

Friction also increases with moisture. As increased skin moisture can result from incontinence and sweating, these should be avoided where possible.

Nutrition and fluid balance also need attention. It has been estimated that dehydrated patients and patients in a negative nitrogen balance are more likely to experience tissue breakdown.

Pressure sore prevention policies. These are designed to rationalise and standardise patient care so that all patients receive a reasonable level of care. They also help to ensure that the available pressure-relieving equipment is used most efficiently.

Management of patients with established pressure sores. In addition to providing a suitable surface for the patient to be nursed on, ensuring adequate nutrition, using good handling techniques when moving a patient, local care of the pressure sore needs to be considered.

Stage 1–3 sores. These superficial wounds usually need a dressing to assist tissue recovery and to protect the area. A common cause of such sores is either friction or, more usually, a combination of friction and shear force.

Elimination of the cause is needed to avoid further and more extensive damage. Several materials can be chosen as dressings which will provide a healing environment: semipermeable films, occlusion alginates, foam sheeting and hydrocolloids are all good examples (Table 23.8). Where incontinence is a problem, occlusion or semi-occlusive materials are invaluable.

Stage 4–5 sores. These deeper wounds are much more difficult to manage. They often have an irregular contour with the wound extending under the skin edge. Assessment is needed of the full extent of the wound (see p. 705). Other problems related to wound shape are sinus formation which requires careful management and packing and/or irrigation. This is a situation where surgical intervention may be needed.

The presence of necrotic tissue and slough deep within these extensive wounds requires careful consideration. This devitalised tissue must be removed if healing is to proceed, and there are several ways of achieving this (see p. 707). One important point to remember is that, until all the devitalised tissue has been removed, the full extent of the pressure sore cannot be realised. Some nurses get unduly worried when, in the process of debriding a wound, it appears to be getting bigger and so worsening. What is happening here is that the damaged tissue is still coming away and the point where only viable tissue exists has not been reached.

Other nursing considerations. The management of an established pressure sore is costly both in economic and personal terms. Prevention of pressure sores is often far cheaper than management (Hibbs 1988). Health service managers are able to cost the treatment of pressure sores more accurately and with the call for pressure sores to become a notifiable condition (Dealey 1992) more emphasis is being put on prevention.

A

WATERLOW PRESSURE SORE PREVENTION/TREATMENT POLICY
Ring scores in table, add total, several scores per category can be used

Build/weight for height	★
Average	0
Above average	1
Obese	2
Below average	3

Continence	★
Complete/ catheterised	0
Occasion. incont.	1
Cath./incontinent of faeces	2
Doubly incontinent	3

Skin type Visual risk areas	★
Healthy	0
Tissue paper	1
Dry	1
Oedematous	1
Clammy (temp.↑)	1
Discoloured	2
Broken/spot	3

Mobility	★
Fully	0
Restless/fidgety	1
Apathetic	2
Restricted	3
Inert/traction	4
Chairbound	5

Sex Age	★
Male	1
Female	2
14 – 49	1
50 – 64	2
65 – 74	3
75 – 80	4
81 +	5

Appetite	★
Average	0
Poor	1
N.G. tube/ fluids only	2
NBM/anorexic	3

Special risks	★
Tissue malnutrition	★
e.g. Terminal cachexia	8
Cardiac failure	5
Peripheral vascular disease	5
Anaemia	2
Smoking	1
Neurological deficit	★
e.g. Diabetes, M.S., CVA	
Motor/sensory paraplegia	4–6
Major surgery/trauma	★
Orthopaedic-below waist, spinal	5
On table >2 hours	5
Medication	★
Cytotoxics, High dose steroids Anti-inflammatory	4

Score	10+ at risk	15+ high risk	20+ very high risk

 Obtainable from Newtons, Curland, Taunton TA3 5SG

B

REMEMBER: TISSUE DAMAGE OFTEN STARTS PRIOR TO ADMISSION, IN CASUALTY.

ASSESSMENT : (see over) If the patient falls into any of the risk categories then preventative nursing is required. A combination of good nursing techniques and preventative aids will definitely be necessary.

PREVENTION :

Preventative aids:

Special mattress/bed: 10+ Water mattresses, e.g. Dyson, Spenco, Vaperm, Topper. 15+ Large cell ripple, e.g. Huntleigh, Water beds. 20+ Pegasus Airwave, Clinitron, Mediscus.

Chair: Correct for patient protection-side/seats, movement, e.g. Nestor, Roho, Jay.

Bed clothing: i) Cotton cellular blanket ii) Duvet iii) Vapour permeable mattress cover. iv) Pillows

Nursing care: Pain control; Turning / 30° tilt; Passive movements; Nutrition-high protein, minerals, vitamins

Mechanical aids: Real sheepskins - sacral, heel/ elbow pads, e.g. Pegasus Lamb Pads, Gel protection; Bed Cradle

Patient aids: Monkey Pole; Hand Lifts

Operating table/ Theatre trolley: e.g. 'Moulding Top'; e.g. Topper, Waffle

Skin care: General hygiene, NO rubbing. Prevent shearing force damage e.g. correct lifting & positioning. Dress with inert covering e.g. Opsite

IF TREATMENT IS REQUIRED, FIRST REMOVE PRESSURE

WOUND CLASSIFICATION :

Blanching hyperaemia	STAGE I	Is wound RED?	YES Semi-occlusive dressing Bioclusive, Tayederm. / NO
Non-blanching hyperaemia	STAGE II	Is wound RED, clean but not healed?	YES Granuflex, Lyofoam, Scherisorb, Sorbsan, Silastic Foam (deep) / NO
Ulceration progresses	STAGE III	Is wound YELLOW/ infected/inflamed?	YES Sorbsan, Scherisorb, Debrisan Granuflex / NO
Ulceration extends	STAGE IV	Infected?	YES Sorbsan packing, Isosorb, Actisorb, Flamazine (for pseudomonas), Debrisan. / NO
Infective necrosis	STAGE V	Is wound BLACK/ necrotic?	YES Debride-surgical excision Granuflex, Scherisorb, Varidase

Fig. 23.4 The Waterlow pressure sore prevention/treatment policy. (With kind permission from Waterlow 1991.)

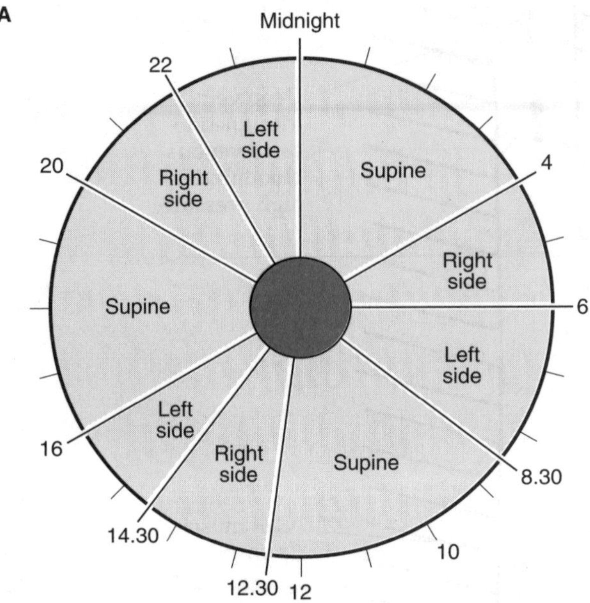

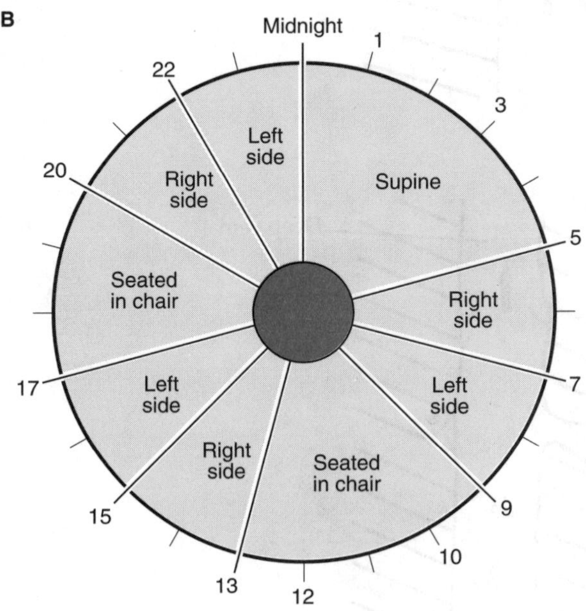

Fig. 23.5 Lowthian's 24 h turning clocks. Turning schedules for (A) bedbound patients and (B) chairfast patients. (Adapted from Lowthian 1987.)

Patient education. In the prevention and management of pressure sores, patients have an important role to play. The young, chronically disabled patients can be taught various methods of regularly relieving pressure by change of position (Thomas et al 1990). Patients who are not able to take such an active part in their own management can be taught the value of and need for the changes of position that nurses and other carers carry out for them. Compliance increases when patients understand why intervention in necessary.

Education leaflets can also be useful. An extract from a typical patient information leaflet demonstrates how the nurse and the patient share in the prevention of pressure sores (Box 23.9).

Box 23.8 The range of pressure-relieving devices (Dealey 1992)

Low-risk patients
- Sheepskins
- Hollow-core fibre pads
- Bead overlays
- Foam overlays
- Gel pads

Medium-risk patients
- Foam overlays
- Foam replacement mattresses
- Combination foam/water mattresses
- Combination foam/gel mattresses
- Alternating air pads
- Water beds
- Double-layer alternating air pads

High-risk patients
- Double-layer alternating air pads
- Air-flotation pads
- Dynamic air-flotation mattresses
- Air-wave mattresses
- Air-fluidised bed

Box 23.9 Extract from an education leaflet: preventing pressure sores (Morison 1992b)

As most pressure sores are the result of staying in one position for too long, the answer is to:

Relieve the pressure by changing position
Ideally, you should get up out of bed or your chair at least once every 2 hours during the day, and take a short walk. This activity also helps your blood circulation and stops your muscles getting lax.

If you are confined to a chair you should lift your bottom off the seat for a few moments every half hour by pushing up on the arms of the chair.

If you have to stay in bed, then your bed may be fitted with a 'monkey pole' or rope ladder — the nurse will show you how to use this to lift yourself off the bed.

If your pressure sore is extensive or deep, or your movement is very restricted, a special movement chart will be devised for you by the nursing staff to keep you off the sore as much as possible, and you may be given a special bed or mattress.

Leg ulcers

These are very difficult wounds to manage. Only about 1% of leg ulcers are managed with the patient in hospital (Callam et al 1985). The day-to-day care of patients with these wounds is undertaken in the community with the district nurse and general practitioner being responsible for their management. The major cause of leg ulceration in the UK is chronic venous insufficiency associated with venous hypertension (70–75%). Somewhere between 20–30% of patients with a leg ulcer have some degree of ischaemia. Diabetes, vasculitis and trauma are other causes of leg ulceration. It follows that one of the most important stages in the assessment of these patients is to diagnose the cause of the ulcer. The aetiology of the ulcer dictates which will be the most appropriate method of management. The use of a hand-held Doppler probe can give a guide to the aetiology of the ulcer (Moffatt 1992) (see p. 717).

Venous stasis leg ulcers

This is the most commonly encountered group of leg ulcers, occurring frequently in elderly female patients. Damage to the veins deep in the calf causes incompetence of the perforators (the veins which link the deep and superficial veins in the calf) (Fig. 23.6).

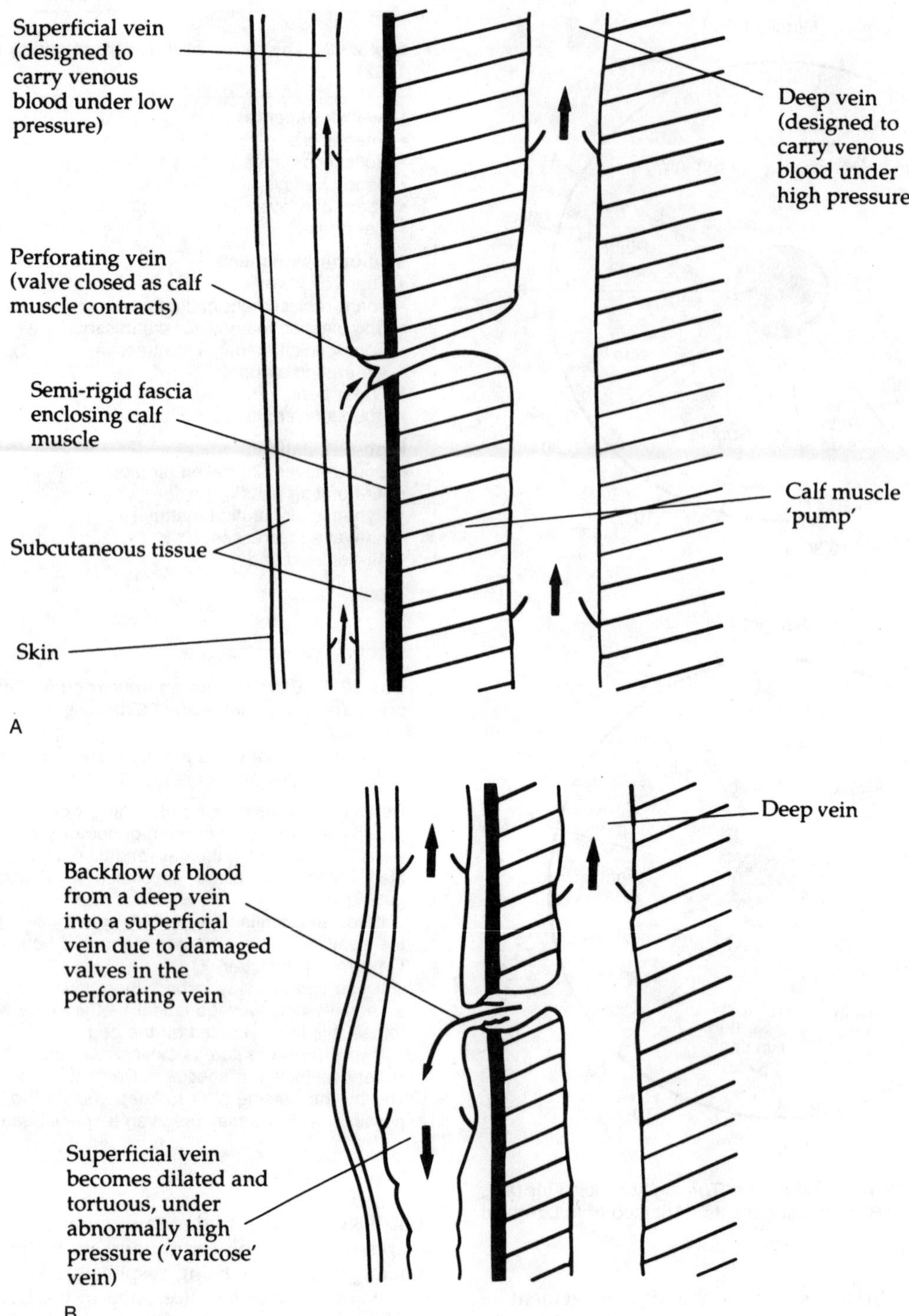

Fig. 23.6 (A) Healthy, intact valves prevent backflow of blood from the deep to the superficial veins. (B) An incompetent valve in a perforating vein allows backflow of blood from the deep to the superficial venous system (with kind permission from Morison 1992b).

Drainage of the skin in the lower leg is affected, leading to oedema, induration and pigmentation. Fibrin is laid down around the capillaries in this area which interferes with oxygen diffusion into the tissues. Following this any knock or minor injury to the lower leg leads rapidly to breakdown of the skin and ulceration. Most commonly, ulceration occurs around the medial malleolus, the ulcers being shallow and pain is not usually a factor.

A typical past history reveals previous phlebitis, deep vein thrombosis (DVT), leg fracture or severe leg injury, or varicose veins.

It can take months and even years for these wounds to heal. Because of the poor condition of the tissues, ulceration can recur and these patients need to wear compression stockings even after healing, to help maintain drainage of the affected limb.

Assessment. One of the primary aims of assessment for a patient with an ulcer is to determine the cause of that ulcer. This is frequently undertaken by both the nurse and doctor working together as part of the Primary Health Care Team. This assessment includes:

- taking a comprehensive medical history which might indicate the presence of venous disease, e.g. history of previous DVT, venous claudication, previous vein surgery or pelvic trauma
- undertaking a thorough clinical examination to support the medical history
- undertaking the appropriate investigations: a Doppler assessment will give the ankle pressure index (Box 23.10) but other investigations may include haemoglobin to exclude anaemia, ESR to indicate the presence of infection, glucose levels to exclude diabetes mellitus, wound swab where infection is suspected (see p. 705).

Management

Bandaging. The most important component in the treatment of venous stasis ulcers is the control of oedema by compression bandages or support stockings (Moffatt 1992). Compression bandages are designed to give a graduated compression that provides more support at the ankle and less at the knee to compensate for the failure of the perforators in the leg. The bandages need to be worn constantly during the day when the patient is walking and upright, to reduce oedema. It may be necessary to prescribe diuretics to assist drainage of oedema where it is particularly stubborn.

The principles of compression bandaging are to:

- bandage from toes to below knee (see Fig. 23.7)
- apply graduated compression by applying even tension to a compression bandage; more pressure is applied to the ankle and less as the circumference of the leg increases to the knee — 30–40 mmHg of pressure may be required at the ankle graduating to 15–20 mmHg below the knee (Morison 1992a)
- maintain the level of compression
- ensure that the bandage/stocking does not slip, causing constriction of the limb (Morison 1992a).

The pressure exerted by a bandaging system can be calculated using Laplace's law (Box 23.11).

Box 23.10 How to take the ankle pressure index

- Lay the patient flat and allow the patient to rest quietly for 20 minutes. This is necessary to eliminate the effects of gravity on the legs.
- Place sphygmomanometer cuff on the upper arm, apply gel over the brachial artery. Hold Doppler probe at 45° angle and measure the systolic pressure.
- Place the sphygmomanometer cuff around the malleolus (should the ulcer be sited here, place the cuff above the ulcer). Apply gel around either the dorsalis pedis or posterior tibial pulse.
- Locate the pulse, inflate cuff until Doppler sound disappears. Gradually deflate cuff and when sound returns record this as the ankle systolic pressure. The ankle pressure index is calculated by dividing the ankle pressure reading by the brachial pressure reading.

Normal ankle pressure index = 1 or >1
Abnormal ankle pressure index = <1
If ankle pressure index = <0.8 the arterial impairment is significant.

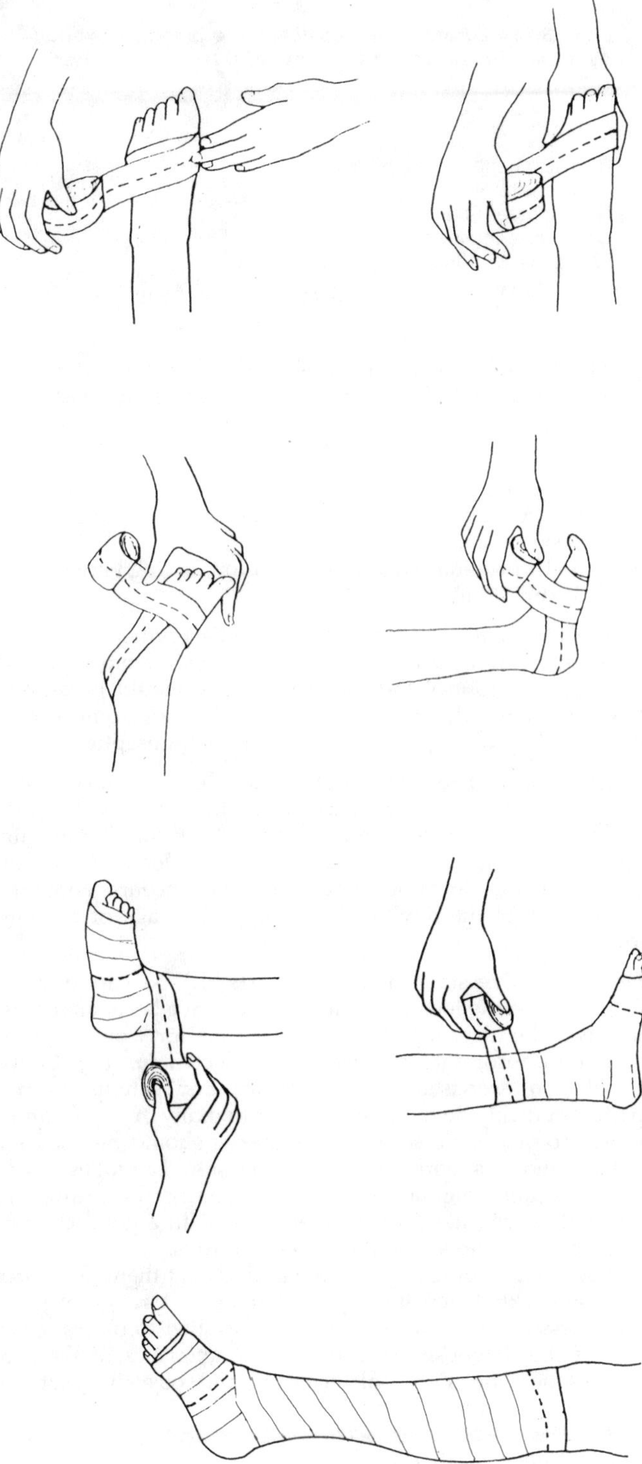

Fig. 23.7 Elastic web bandage. (1) Start bandage on the inner side of the sole of the foot, with the lower edge of bandage at the root of the toes. Turn 1½ times round the foot. (2) The thumb fixes the bandage for the start of the turn around the heel. (3) View from the outer side of the foot. Thumb and finger hold bandage in place prior to completing turn around base of toes. (4) View from the inner side of the foot. (5) View from the outer side of the foot. Continuation of the bandaging keeping lower edge of the bandage along red or blue line of the previous turn. (6) View from the outer side of the foot. Tension used is about half the full stretch of the bandage. (7) View from the outer side of the leg. Note the position of the final turn of bandage immediately below the knee. (With kind permission from Ryan 1991.)

Box 23.11 Formula for calculating the pressure exerted by a bandaging system (Moffatt 1992)

$$P = \frac{T \times N \times \text{Constant}}{C \times W}$$

P = sub-bandage pressure
T = tension
N = number of layers
C = limb circumference
W = width of bandage

Selection of a bandage depends on the amount of compression required. Three grades of compression bandage are available:

- grade I provides very light compression or support for mild oedema
- grade II provides moderate compression at the ankle of between 18–24 mmHg
- grade III provides strong compression, giving between 25–35 mmHg at the ankle.

Control of infection. Where pain, cellulitis, erythema, enlarging of the ulcer and purulent discharge occur, antibiotics may be necessary to control the infection. These should be administered systemically. Superficial infection can sometimes be controlled by the topical application of an antiseptic.

Physiotherapy. Exercises to stimulate the calf muscle pump (which assists venous return) can be taught to each patient, and these encouraged regularly throughout the day to stimulate circulation and aid drainage of the lower legs. Some period of leg elevation should also be encouraged around the middle of the day, again to allow drainage of the lower legs.

Dressings. Dressing management should be carefully considered once the factors outlined above have been successfully tackled. The ulcer should be assessed (as for wounds, p. 705) and the appropriate material then selected (p. 708). Caution should be exercised with dressings and lotions as these patients quickly develop sensitivities to many of the commonly used products. The simplest treatments should be used first. Paste bandages with elastic compression bandages, hydrocolloid wafers, alginate sheets, impregnated textile dressings and polysaccharide dressings, all used with a good compression bandage, are suitable for these wounds.

However, in practice nurses will find that there are various 'special cocktails' created by practitioners. A range of lotions and dressings have in the past been applied to ulcers regardless of the diagnosis or physical characteristics of the ulcer. Practitioners need to look critically and objectively at their management of leg ulcers.

Arterial ulcers

These are a result of ischaemia of the lower leg and so are a very different problem from ulcers arising from venous disease (see Table 23.11). Damage to the arteries supplying the leg can be caused by vascular disease and this gradually occludes and blocks them. On the other hand, infarction of smaller arteries is caused by embolus formation which causes ischaemia in the area of skin normally supplied by that artery. What follows is a very rapid breakdown of the skin. The characteristics of these ulcers are rapid onset of a deep ulcer which is often extremely painful; relief is gained by lowering the affected limb and dangling it over the edge of the bed or chair. These patients rarely go to bed to sleep, or if they do, have to get up in the night because of the pain. They tend to sleep in a chair, which allows the affected limb to hang down. These ulcers can occur anywhere on the lower leg, but present usually on the foot and lateral aspect of the lower leg. Foot pulses are often absent or very difficult to palpate. Doppler assessment reveals a pressure index of below 0.8. The patient may also have a history of hypertension, myocardial infarction, strokes or transient ischaemic attacks.

Management. Surgical intervention may be necessary to improve the circulation or to debride dead tissue within the ulcer and skin grafting may be considered. Light bandaging only is applied to keep a dressing in place; compression is to be avoided at all costs as this would further impede an already poor blood supply to the area.

Healing of these wounds is slow and the prognosis for eventual healing often poor. Treatment aims to keep the patient as comfortable as possible and to achieve debridement and cleansing where necessary. Useful dressings include alginate sheets, polysaccharide dressings and hydrogel sheets.

Mixed aetiology ulcers

Around 25% of venous ulcers also have a significant arterial blood supply deficiency (Cornwall et al 1986). This further complicates management as control of oedema is needed but without restricting the already poor blood supply.

Diagnosis

Accurate diagnosis is fundamental to successful treatment. Those giving care should be absolutely certain of exactly

Table 23.11 Characteristics of venous and arterial disease of the lower limb

Characteristic	Venous disease	Arterial disease
Site of ulcer	Around the 'gater' area, commonly above the medial malleolus	Anywhere on the lower limb including the foot but commonly affecting the toes
Depth of ulcer	Shallow and spreading	Deep, with a punched-out appearance
Presence of oedema	Common due to poor venous return	Often not detected
Onset	Gradual unless precipitated by trauma	Rapid
Pain	Often uncomfortable, nagging in character	Pain on elevation of limb relieved by lowering it (the blood flow is increased when the limb is in the dependent position) The pain of ischaemia can be unremitting
Temperature of foot	Warm and well perfused	Cool or cold and poorly perfused
Condition of the skin surrounding the ulcer	Lipodermatosclerosis present Varicose eczema	
Ankle pressure index	>0.8	<0.8

what the aetiology of the ulcer is before any type of treatment begins. Doppler assessment (p. 717) will assist diagnosis. Clearly, if arterial problems are allowed to go unrecognised and strong compression bandaging applied, treatment will not only be ineffective but could also cause the patient harm. Nurses often blame local dressings for lack of progress towards healing of leg ulcers when in fact a full and comprehensive assessment and diagnosis of the patient has not been undertaken. Information on other types of leg ulcer is summarised in Box 23.12.

Patient education
Individual education regarding wound management can have a dramatic effect on progress.

This aspect of care is particularly appropriate in patients with leg ulcers, especially venous leg ulcers — unless these patients know the cause of their ulcer they may not comply with treatment. Leg exercises, leg elevation and the need for adequate compression are the key factors to success. Without this education the patient is not fully equipped to participate in management of his or her ulcer. Patient education can be helped by providing leaflets which can be read at home (Box 23.13).

Box 23.12 Other types of leg ulcers (Browse & Burnard 1982)

Vasculitic ulcers 2.5%
These are due to connective tissue disease (e.g. rheumatoid arthritis, sclerodema), and also occur on the lower leg. They are unusual and extremely difficult to manage due to the underlying disease process and the drug therapies that these patients require.

Diabetic ulcers 5.0%
These occur most commonly on the foot. Again due to the general condition of the patient, they heal slowly. It is worth noting that diabetics may give a falsely high reading on Doppler assessment due to peripheral hypertension.

The management of rheumatoid and diabetic ulcers is generally under specialist care and treatment is prescribed by the individual consultant.

Traumatic ulcers 2%

Miscellaneous causes 1%
Neoplastic and tropical ulcers are examples of this category.

Sutured wounds

Although the vast majority of sutured wounds heal without complication, there is a need for careful observation of both the patient and the wound site (p. 705).

- Observe patient for change in vital signs, pulse, temperature, or malaise which could indicate the presence of infection, especially wound infection.
- Observe wounded area for signs of infection after the initial inflammatory response has taken place, i.e. redness, swelling, pain, discharge, heat.

When are the sutures removed? The best time for removal of suture material depends upon a number of factors:

- The site of the wound — wounds on the head and neck heal, usually, within 2 days due to the rich blood supply to the area, whereas wounds on the back may take 10–14 days to heal. The skin here is thicker and less well supplied with blood.
- Patient variation — if, during suture removal, the wound begins to gape then the nurse should stop and refer to the surgeon for advice. The skin edges can be pulled back together and held for a few more days with paper sutures.
- Cosmetic considerations — it should also be noted that leaving sutures in for too long can cause excessive scarring.

In general, the principles for managing sutured wounds are to leave the wound undisturbed and the theatre dressing intact unless either the patient or the wounded area begin to develop signs which indicate the presence of infection. Disturbing

Box 23.13 An education leaflet for patients with venous ulcers, and their carers: how to care for your legs (Morison 1992a)

How long must I keep the dressing and bandage (or stocking) in place?
Wear the support bandages or elastic support stockings as advised by the doctor and nurse. They will make arrangements for your next dressing change.

Do not be tempted to look under the bandage or disturb the dressing in the meantime as this may delay healing. It is particularly important not to scratch the skin around the ulcer as this skin is easily damaged.

Ask for help AT ONCE if:

- Your leg itches excessively, is hot, or more painful than usual.
- You feel that the bandage is too tight anywhere.
- You lose sensation in your toes, or they turn cold or blue.
- You need any other advice.

Contact person:
Contact telephone number:

Can I exercise?
Yes. Exercise is good for your circulation and your general health. If possible take a gentle walk every day. Even indoors you can bend and stretch your toes while sitting, and bend, flex, and circle your ankles to prevent them from becoming stiff. It is important not to stand still for too long. It is a good idea to do the dishes and the ironing sitting down, if you can obtain a chair of the correct height.

Should I sit with my legs up?
Yes. Sitting with your legs hanging down is almost as bad as standing in one place for too long. You should sit with your legs supported on a stool, on a cushion or pillow, that is above the level of your hips. It is also helpful to raise the foot of your bed 9 inches, as this aids return of blood from the legs to the heart overnight.

Do I need a special diet?
You do not need a special diet, but try to eat a balanced one that includes protein (meat, fish, eggs), fresh fruit, and vegetables. Being overweight does not help the circulation in your legs. Ask the doctor for advice on weight loss if this is a problem for you.

Are there any other ways I can help my legs?
Yes

- Avoid knocks to your legs, as this could lead to another ulcer.
- Keep your legs warm, but do not sit too close to the fire as this can damage the skin.
- Do not wear anything tight round the tops of your legs, such as garters or girdles, as your circulation will be hindered.
- Stop smoking.

dressings unnecessarily can lead to the entry of bacteria into the wound itself or disturb the newly forming epithelium. Local wound infection can slow down the rate of healing and also increase the amount of scar tissue produced. Ultimately a severe wound infection can spread into the tissues and also the bloodstream causing septicaemia which could be life threatening (Spencer & Bale 1990).

Traumatic wounds

Patients who present to the accident and emergency department with traumatic wounds need special consideration. These patients may be shocked or have other injuries and their wounds are often contaminated due to the nature of the trauma (see Ch. 28).

These wounds are frequently an irregular shape, with varying degrees of tissue loss. Due to contamination wound closure is often not attempted. Mechanical cleansing of the wound is undertaken to remove debris such as glass, wood or tarmac. Where wound closure is attempted antibiotic cover is given to prevent infection.

Patients with extensive injuries are admitted for inpatient treatment. However, the majority of patients with wounds are discharged home to be cared for in the community. They may be instructed to care for the wound themselves or told to return to the accident and emergency department for any dressing changes necessary, or the community nurse may be asked to take over the management.

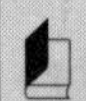

For further information, see Chapter 11, 'Traumatic wounds', in Morison (1992b).

Malignant wounds

This is one group of wounds where healing is not always the expected outcome of wound management. These wounds include fungating carcinoma of breast, fungating lesions of malignant melanoma and a variety of other non-healing, extending or fungating wounds. These patients are generally managed by a combination of hospital and home care and over a period of time become well known to both agencies.

Problems encountered with malignant wounds (see Ch. 32):

- Wound site — often these wounds are present in an area which is extremely difficult to dress in terms of keeping the dressing in place, i.e. on the chest wall, in the groin and on the lower limb.
- Exudate production — the exudate tends to be thick and sticky. Many dressings which do not adhere to other wound types will do so in the presence of this particularly viscous exudate. The hydrogel sheets and gel are very useful dressings for these wounds.
- Pain — where nerve endings are exposed, changing dressings and dressings rubbing can be problems. Keeping the wound covered reduces the irritation to the nerve endings and using gel dressings reduces pain at dressing changes.

Where healing is not the ultimate aim, wound management should maximise convenience and minimise distress.

Burns

The management of burns is a specialised area (see Ch. 31). Treatment given depends on the individual burns unit. However, all follow the same basic principles for management. Treatment will depend on the physical well-being and age of the individual, the area burnt and the depth and size of the burn.

Psychosocial factors

The presence of a wound will inevitably have some effect on well-being. There may be no difficulty when a wound is small and heals rapidly but, for many patients, some degree of anxiety is felt relating to the wound. This can disrupt sleep patterns, increase the perception of pain and even suppress the immune system. In more serious wounds, a disturbance of body image may also cause lasting distress unless anticipated and therapy begun (Lacey & Birchnell 1986).

? **23.7** How would you help these patients to overcome their fears and worries?

- An elderly lady living alone has a chronic venous ulcer requiring frequent dressing by the community nurse. She is increasingly confined to the house.
- A small girl recovering from surgery for an umbilical hernia becomes distressed when told that the sutures are due to be removed. She fears that her wound will break open when this happens.
- A young woman has been mugged on her way home from work. The knife wound to her face required suturing in the accident and emergency department. She has had no opportuniy to see the wound and is fearing the worst.

CONCLUSION

The effective management of patients with wounds requires an understanding of the healing process in conjunction with an organised approach to both assessment and management, and includes:

- assessment of the individual's overall health, taking into account factors which might impair healing
- assessment of the wound
- planning the management of the individual taking into account the social and physical environment, and using the most appropriate dressings materials available
- involving the patient, where possible, in wound care
- evaluation and reassessment of the individual until the wound heals or the needs of the patient change.

? **23.8** Which types of dressing materials are available in your hospital/community?
Cost out the treatment of dressing materials needed to manage four different patients for 1 week. Include dressing packs, surgical tapes and lotions as well as the dressing materials themselves.
How much variation is there between the four? Which patient is the most expensive to manage?

? **23.9** Go to the operating theatre and find out how pressure sores are prevented in theatre.

? **23.10** Go to the hospital pharmacy/chemist's shop to find out how dressing materials are ordered and dispensed. Who decides which products are made available in the hospital?

REFERENCES

Bale S 1989a Cost effective wound management in the community. Professional Nurse 4(12): 598–601

Bale S 1989b Research in the community. Nursing Times 84(38): 73–75

Bale S 1991 Nurse prescribing wound management in the community. Nursing Standard 5(8): 29–31

Bale S 1992a A holistic approach and the ideal dressing: cavity wound management in the 1990s. In: Horne E M & Cowan T (eds) Staff nurse's survival guide, 2nd edn. Wolfe Publishing, London, pp. 261–268

Bale S 1992b Using modern dressings to effect debridement. In: Horne E M & Cowan T (eds) Staff nurse's survival guide, 2nd edn. Wolfe Publishing, London, pp. 308–311

Bale S 1993 Wound assessment. Surgical Nurse 6(1): 641–645

Banks V 1992 Pressure sores: a community problem. Journal of Wound Care 1(2): 42–44

Bannon M 1993 Healing the whole person. Nursing Times 89(13) (Wound Care Supplement): 62–68

Barbenel J C, Jordan M M, Nichol S M, Clark M O 1977 Incidence of pressure sores in the Greater Glasgow Health Board Area. Lancet 2: 548–550

Barrett E 1987 Putting risk calculations in their place. Nursing Times 83(6): 65–70

Barton A, Barton M 1981 The management and prevention of pressure sores. Faber & Faber, London

Bibby B A, Collins B J, Ayliffe G 1986 A mathematical model for assessing the risk of post-operative wound infection. Journal of Hospital Infection 8: 31–38

Bridel J 1993 Assessing the risks of pressure sores. Nursing Standard 7(25): 32–35

Browse N L, Burnard K G 1982 The cause of venous ulceration. Lancet ii: 243–245

Callam M J, Harper D R, Dale J J, Ruckley C V 1987 Chronic ulceration of the leg: clinical history. Lothian and Forth Valley Leg Ulcer Study

Callam M J, Ruckley C, Harper D, Dale J J 1985 Chronic ulceration of the leg — extent of the problem and provision of care. British Medical Journal 290: 1855–1856

Cornwall J, Done C S, Lewis J D 1986 Leg ulcers; epidemiology and aetiology. British Journal of Surgery 73: 693–696

Corre F, Lellouch J, Schwartz D 1971 Smoking and leucocyte counts. Lancet 2: 632–634

Cruse P J E, Foord R 1980 The epidemiology of wound infection: a 10 year prospective study of 62,939 wounds. Surgical Clinics of North America 60(1): 27–40

Dale J, Gibson B (1986) The epidemiology of leg ulcers. Professional Nurse 1(8): 215–216

Dealey C 1991 The size of the pressure sore problem in a teaching hospital. Journal of Advanced Nursing 16: 663–670

Dealey C 1992 How are you supporting your patients? A review of pressure relieving equipment. In: Horne E M & Cowan T (eds) Staff nurse's survival guide, 2nd end. Wolfe Publishing, London

Dickerson J W T 1990 Hospital induced malnutrition: prevention and treatment. In: The staff nurse's survival guide. Austin Cornish, London pp. 175–178

Duthie R 1990 Foreword In: Bader D L (ed) Pressure sores: clinical practice and scientific approach. Macmillan Press, London

Eagle M 1990 Leg ulcers: the quiet epidemic below the knee. Nursing Standard 4(15): 32–36

Eriksson G 1984 Bacterial growth in venous leg ulcers — its clinical significance in the healing process. An environment for healing: the role of occlusion. The Royal Society of Medicine, London

Flanagan M 1993 Pressure sore risk assessment scales. Journal of Wound Care 2(3): 162–167

Forrest R O 1982 Early history of wound treatment. Journal of the Royal Society of Medicine 75(March): 198–205

Fountain W S 1985 The surgical incision and haemostasis. In: Westaby S (ed) Wound care. William Heinemann Medical Books, London

Goldstone L A, Goldstone J 1982 The Norton score: an early warning of pressure sores. Journal of Advanced Nursing 7: 419–426

Harding K G 1992 The wound programme. Centre for Medical Education, University of Dundee

Hibbert D L 1980 A sore point at home. Nursing Mirror 151(6): 40–41

Hibbs P J 1988 Pressure area care for the City and Hackney Health Authority. Prevention plan for patients at risk from developing pressure sores. Policy for the management of pressure sores. City and Hackney Health Authority, London

Hibbs P J 1991 The economics of pressure sore prevention. In: Bader D (ed) Pressure sores: clinical practice and scientific approach. Macmillan Press, London

Hill G L, Blackett R L, Pickford I, Barkinshaw L, Young G A, Warren J V, Schorah G J, Morgan D B 1971 Malnutrition in surgical patients: an unrecognised problem. Lancet 82(17): 33–36

Hopkinson I 1992 Growth factors and extracellular matrix biosynthesis. Journal of Wound Care 1(2): 42–50

Lacey J H, Birchnell S A 1986 Body image and its disturbance. Journal of Psychosomatic Research 30(6): 623–631

Lancet Editor 1973 Editorial: the costs of pressure on the patient. Lancet 2: 309

Langridge C J 1990 Ban on hypochlorites is stupid. Hospital Doctor 10(26)

Lawrence C 1983 Pressure sores: aetiology, treatment and prevention. Croom Helm, Beckenham

Leaper D J 1986 Antiseptics and their effect on healing tissue. Nursing Times 82(23): 45–47

Lees T A, Lombert D 1992 Prevalence of lower limb ulceration in an urban health district. British Journal of Surgery 92(Oct): 1032–1034

Louden I S L 1982 Leg ulcers in the 18th and early 19th centuries. Journal of the Royal College of General Practitioners 32: 301–309

Lowthian P 1987 The practical assessment of pressure sore risk. Care, Science and Practice 5(4): 3–7

Marks J, Hughes L E, Harding K G, Campbell H, Ribero C D 1983 Prediction of healing time as an aid to the management of open granulating wounds. World Journal of Surgery 7: 641–645

Moffatt C J 1992 Compression bandaging — the state of the art. Journal of Wound Care 1(1): 45–50

Morison M 1992a Treatment options. In: A colour guide to the assessment and management of leg ulcers. Wolfe Publishing, London

Morison M 1992b A colour guide to the nursing management of wounds. Wolfe Publishing, London

Myers J A 1982 Plastic surgical dressings. Social Services Journal 11(18 March): 336–337

Norton D, McLaren R, Exton-Smith A N 1962 Investigation of geriatric nursing problems in hospital. National Corporation for the Care of Old People, London (reissued 1975, Churchill Livingstone, Edinburgh)

Pritchard V 1986 Calculating the risk. Nursing Times 82: 59–61

Roberts B V, Goldstone L A 1979 A survey of pressure sores in the over-sixties on two orthopaedic wards. International Journal of Nursing Studies 16: 355–364

Scales J T, Lowthian P T, Poole A G et al 1982 'Vaperm' patient support system: a new general purpose hospital mattress. Lancet 2: 1150–1152

Siana J E, Rex S, Gottrup F 1989 The effect of cigarette smoking on wound healing. Scandinavian Journal of Plastic Reconstruction Surgery 24: 207–209

Siana J E, Frankild S, Gottrup F 1992 The effect of smoking on tissue function. Journal of Wound Care 1(2): 37–41

Spencer K, Bale S 1990 A logical approach: management of surgical wounds. Professional Nurse 5(6): 303–306

Thomas A, Krowskop S L, Noble G, Noble P 1990 Pressure sore management and the recumbent person. In: Bader D L (ed)

Pressure sores: clinical practice and scientific approach. Macmillan Press, London
Thomas S 1990a Wound management and dressings. The Pharmaceutical Press, London
Thomas S 1990b Eusol revisited. Dressing Times 3: 1
Torrence C 1983 Pressure sores: aetiology, treatment and prevention. Croom Helm, Beckenham
Tortora G J, Grabowski S R 1993 Principles of anatomy and physiology, 7th edn. Harper Collins, New York, Ch. 5, pp. 127–137
Turner T D 1985 Semiocclusive and occlusive dressings. In: Ryan T (ed) An environment for healing: the role of occlusion. Royal Society of Medicine Congress and Symposium Series 8
Verslugsen M 1986 How elderly patients with femoral fractures develop pressure sores in hospital. British Medical Journal 292: 1311–1313
Waterlow J 1988 Prevention is cheaper than cure. Nursing Times 84(25): 69–70
Waterlow J 1992 A policy that protects: the Waterlow pressure sore prevention/treatment policy. In: Horne E M & Cowan T (eds) Staff nurse's survival guide, 2nd edn. Wolfe Publishing, London
Watson R 1989 Sore point. Geriatric Nursing and Home Care 9(4): 26–27
Westaby S (ed) 1985 Wound care. William Heinemann Medical Books, London, p. 71
Wilson E 1989 Prevention and treatment of chronic leg ulcers. Health Trends 1989 4: 97
Winter G D 1962 Formation of the scab and rate of epithelialization of superficial wounds in the skin of the young domestic pig. Nature 193: 293–294

FURTHER READING

Bader D L (ed) 1990 Pressure sores: clinical practice and scientific approach. Macmillan Press, London
David J 1985 Wound management. Dunitz, London
Overstall P, Marchall M 1983 Mattresses to prevent pressure sores. Nursing Times 79(24): 54–57
Ryan T 1991 The management of leg ulcers. Oxford University Press, Oxford
Senter H, Pringle A 1985 How wounds heal — a practical guide for nurses. The Wellcome Foundation, London
Westaby S (ed) 1985 Wound care. William Heinemann Medical Books, London
Zederfeldt B, Jacobsson S 1980 Wounds and wound healing. Wolfe, London

VIDEO CASSETTES

Harding K G, Bale S, Banks V, Jones V 1992 Nursing chronic wounds in the community. Medical Television Productions, London
Harding K G, Bale S, Lewis B, Banks V 1992 Nutrition and wound healing. Purvis-Wickes Video Projects, London

USEFUL ADDRESSES

The Wound Care Society
PO Box 263
Northampton NN3 4UJ

The Tissue Viability Society
Wessex Rehabilitation Unit
Odstock Hospital
Salisbury

European Wound Management Association
88 White Hart Lane
Tottenham N17 8HP

CHAPTER 24

Continence

Jean Swaffield

CHAPTER CONTENTS

Introduction 723

Urinary continence 723

Promoting continence: problem-solving approach 728
Assessment 729
Planning and implementing care 731
Evaluation 734
Continence advisory services 734

Managing intractable incontinence 734
Aids and equipment 735
Long-term catheter care 736
Sexuality 738

Faecal incontinence 739

Glossary 739

References 740

Further reading 741

Video cassettes 741

Useful addresses 741

INTRODUCTION

Having control over urinary and faecal elimination is an expected norm within every society. In all but the very young, incontinence is generally not viewed with sympathy, and the real suffering it causes to the individual and his carers has not received the attention it deserves. Epidemiological research has shown that the number of people suffering from incontinence in some form or other far exceeds the number of cases reported to health professionals. An underlying theme of this chapter is the need to acknowledge the extent of the problem and to promote continence by improving screening practices and raising public and professional awareness of preventive measures against incontinence and of the range of treatments available.

Incontinence is a symptom that is often wrongly labelled as a disease. This chapter describes the underlying conditions that can prevent the acquisition of continence or provoke its loss. It is argued that a sound understanding of the causes and types of incontinence is essential for its proper investigation, treatment and management and that diagnostic assessment must recognise the individuality of each patient. Similarly, where incontinence is intractable, assessment for aids and equipment must be sensitive to the values, needs and priorities of each patient to ensure that an optimum quality of life is achieved.

Throughout the chapter the nurse is encouraged to take a positive, problem-solving approach toward this often hidden problem, to assess her own attitudes toward the subject of incontinence, and to base her nursing decisions and actions on up-to-date, research-based knowledge.

URINARY CONTINENCE

The acquisition of continence in early childhood is a much-valued developmental milestone. In the adult, the ability to control urinary and faecal elimination is largely taken for granted, and a loss of continence will have profound implications for the individual's ability to participate fully within society. While it may be deemed acceptable for a child to have an occasional 'accident', this is not generally the case for adults. The subject of incontinence is one which many people find difficult to discuss openly, and one which is badly understood. Clear definitions and sound knowledge have been lacking, and certain mistaken beliefs — such as the assumption that incontinence is untreatable — have become entrenched.

The onus is on health professionals to foster a change in social attitudes by acquiring a clear understanding of how continence is attained and how incontinence can develop. In the role as health educator, the nurse can make an important contribution to the promotion of continence among those groups who are particularly vulnerable.

Defining continence

Continence may be defined in terms of the actions and abilities necessary for the appropriate management of urinary and faecal elimination. These include:

- recognising the need to pass urine or faeces
- identifying the correct place to pass urine or faeces
- delaying elimination until the appropriate place is reached
- reaching the correct place
- passing urine or faeces appropriately once a suitable place is reached.

Acquiring continence

Urinary continence cannot be acquired until the physiological systems necessary for micturition have matured. Once the prerequisite physical development has taken place, becoming continent is a matter of imitation, skill attainment and social conditioning.

The anatomy of the bladder is detailed in Chapter 8. The bladder is a simple organ which has a dual function: it acts as a reservoir for urine and it expels urine at the volition of the individual. Urine remains in the bladder as long as the intravesical pressure does not exceed the urethral resistance.

In normal micturition, the contraction of the detrusor muscle of the bladder induces the bladder neck to open, while the pelvic floor muscles and the external sphincter relax. For a child to obtain continence, he must acquire control of the mechanisms for preventing the bladder from automatically emptying when it is full; this is usually achieved by the age of 3.

The neurological control of the bladder at birth involves a simple sacral reflex arc whereby automatic filling and emptying of the bladder is under the control of sacral segments 3 and 4 of the spinal cord. Stretch receptors in the bladder wall are activated by urine accumulation. These relay impulses with increasing frequency through the parasympathetic nerves to the spinal cord until the motor parasympathetic nerves react by causing the bladder muscles to contract and the urethra sphincter to open, where upon reflex emptying occurs.

In order to achieve continence a child needs to become aware of the sensation of the bladder becoming full and through trial and error attempt to overcome the reflex emptying mechanism by using the pelvic floor to keep the urethral sphincter closed. The sensory tracts of the spinal cord involve the cerebral cortex in the brain to overcome or inhibit the contractions; this requires practice as well as maturation of the central nervous system (see Fig. 24.1).

Continence thus involves the active inhibition of nerve impulses. When micturition is initiated, the brain ceases to send out inhibitory impulses, allowing the spinal reflex arc to be completed. Figure 24.2 illustrates the innervation of the bladder.

'Normal' patterns of micturition can vary markedly from one individual to another. Most people empty their bladders 4–6 times a day and have a bladder capacity of up to 600 ml; this may be altered, however, by age, fluid intake, perspiration, body temperature, activity and stress. People in a state of anxiety often feel the need to empty their bladders more often; in the event of acute emotional distress or sudden shock, it is possible for incontinence to occur.

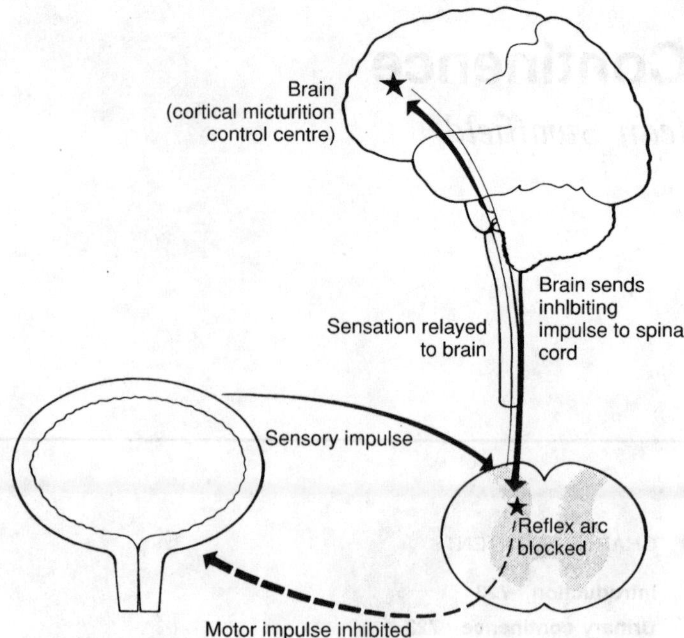

Fig. 24.1 Bladder-filling phase. The brain inhibits the spinal reflex arc. (Reproduced with kind permission from Coloplast Foundation 1987.)

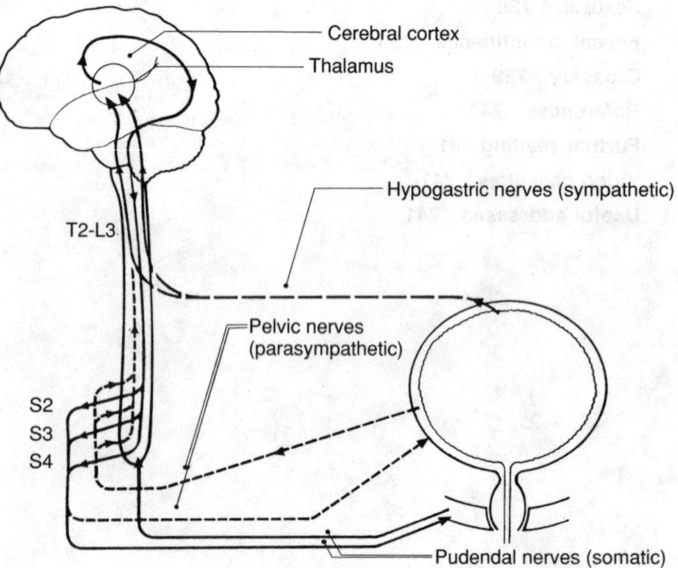

Fig. 24.2 Nerve pathways between the bladder, spine and micturition control centre. Note: nerves supplying the urethra have been omitted for clarity. (Reproduced with kind permission from Coloplast Foundation 1987.)

ATTITUDES TOWARDS INCONTINENCE

In modern British society attitudes toward many previously taboo subjects are rapidly changing. This is particularly evident in the topics that are now permissible within 'polite' conversation — for example, sex, AIDS and homosexuality.

Incontinence is also gradually becoming an acceptable subject for open discussion and is being addressed in newspaper and magazine articles (Glew 1985, Horsfield 1986, Walker 1987), radio and television programmes and medical journals. Nevertheless, certain myths still persist, such as the notion that incontinence is an inevitable consequence of old age. Such mistaken ideas must be dispelled in favour of seeking the real cause of incontinence in any given case.

For the nurse, perhaps the best starting-point in this process of re-education is an examination of her own preconceptions of incontinence, since it has been demonstrated that nurses to a large degree reflect the views of the society that they serve (Hatten 1977, Fielding 1986, Ewles & Simnett 1992). Self-appraisal of one's own attitude to the subject of incontinence may be a necessary prerequisite to the effective nursing of incontinent patients.

Types of incontinence

The International Continence Society (ICS), which has tried to regulate the terminology associated with the lower urinary tract, has defined urinary incontinence as 'a condition in which involuntary loss of urine is a social or hygienic problem and is objectively demonstrable' (ICS 1984).

Urinary incontinence may take a variety of forms; these are:

- stress incontinence
- urge incontinence
- overflow incontinence
- reflex incontinence
- enuresis
- immobility incontinence.

It is only when the specific type and cause of an individual's incontinence are known that appropriate treatment can be offered.

Stress incontinence results from a failure of the urethral sphincter to remain closed when sudden abdominal pressure on the bladder occurs, e.g. during coughing, sneezing or laughing. The weak pelvic floor allows the urethra to descend and the sphincter to open, leaking urine.

Urge incontinence results from the contraction of the detrusor muscle of the bladder as if to void, when only small amounts of urine have accumulated in the bladder. This may be caused by overactive detrusor function (motor urgency) or by hypersensitivity (sensory urgency).

Overflow incontinence occurs as a consequence of urinary retention, which may in turn result from:

- an obstruction, for example such as that caused by a tumour, faecal impaction, or an enlarged prostate gland
- an underactive detrusor muscle, producing a flaccid bladder and thus failing to generate enough pressure to open the urethra
- failure of the urethra to open.

Reflex incontinence may occur as a result of damage to the spinal cord and loss of sensation associated with the desire to micturate, leading to failure to inhibit the simple reflex arc.

Enuresis: refers to any involuntary loss of urine. Nocturnal enuresis is the term for urinary incontinence which occurs during sleep in the absence of any organic disease or infection. Nocturia refers to being woken at night by the urge to pass urine.

Immobility incontinence. The individual with this type of incontinence would in favourable circumstances be able to remain continent but is prevented by pre-existing disease or disability from gaining access to an appropriate place at an appropriate time to pass urine. Diseases which may affect mobility and dexterity, and therefore continence, are multiple sclerosis, spina bifida, arthritis and spinal cord injury. In addition, conditions associated with ageing such as slowness of movement, pain, stiffness, inability to climb stairs or difficulty in manipulating fastenings may all contribute to incontinence.

EPIDEMIOLOGY

In conducting their research into the prevalence of incontinence Thomas et al (1980) used the following definition to identify all those in two London health districts over the age of 5 who were incontinent: 'involuntary excretion or leakage of urine and/or faeces in inappropriate places or at inappropriate times and production of two or more 'accidents' a month or continuous leakage of urine'. This categorisation included individuals with 'long term catheters and urinary diversions'.

In the early stages of the study this definition was applied to known patients who were already in touch with health and social services agencies. These individuals were monitored over a one-year period, and the following information was obtained:

Age	*Percentage of incontinence in this sample*
15–64	0.2% in women
	0.1% in men
65+	2.5% in women
	1.3% in men

In an extension of the study a postal questionnaire was sent to all individuals over the age of 5 on the lists of 12 general practitioners (a total of 22 430 patients). An 89% return was obtained. The result when compared with those of the first study were illuminating, as they revealed a markedly higher incidence of incontinence, as follows:

Age	*Percentage of incontinence in this sample*
15–64	8.5% in women
	1.6% in men
65+	11.6% in women
	6.9% in men

While incontinence was the most prevalent among elderly women, its occurrence was significant across all age groups. Stress incontinence was reported less commonly by nulliparous than by parous women of all ages, and was especially prevalent among those who had borne 4 or more children. Urge incontinence also occurred more commonly among parous than nulliparous women. No significant class differences were found among men or women, but individuals of Afro-Caribbean or part Afro-Caribbean descent were more likely to have some form of incontinence than those with an Asian background.

The most important finding of the study, however, was the 1:10 ratio of known to unknown cases of incontinence. This means that for every incontinent person who is known to medical or social services professionals, there are 10 others who are unidentified and require help. As further in-depth interviews revealed, many people try to 'cope' with moderate to severe problems of incontinence without professional support. These findings identify the need for health care workers to take advantage of all appropriate opportunities in hospital or community care settings to identify those who require assessment and treatment for incontinence.

Surveys of health care institutions and social services homes have shown a high prevalence of incontinence, and suggest that this is to some extent a consequence of the quality of care given. A high failure rate in addressing the problems of incontinence is apparent; this has been attributed to insufficient knowledge (Egan 1983), a factor also noted by Townsend (1964) and confirmed by Edginton et al (1986).

The implication of these research findings is that there is a need not only to identify patients who are incontinent, but to improve public and professional understanding of incontinence, to evaluate services available for those requiring assessment and to improve methods of treatment and management.

?	**24.1** Determine how many patients in your ward or on your community list are incontinent.
?	**24.2** What percentage of your caseload does this represent?
?	**24.3** To the best of your knowledge, how many of those who are incontinent have been fully investigated?
?	**24.4** From what you have been told, try to identify the type of incontinence that each person has.
?	**24.5** Compare your findings with the work of Edginton et al (1986), Gilleard (1981) and McLaren et al (1981) or, if you are working in the community, with Thomas et al (1980).
?	**24.6** Discuss your findings with a senior member of staff in your working area.

Sociological factors in under-reporting of incontinence

The fact that incontinence remains to such a large extent a hidden problem among the general population can be attributed in part to the reluctance of many people to admit to their incontinence and seek treatment. The failure to report symptoms is of course not limited to individuals who are incontinent; indeed, it has been estimated that only 20% of people needing treatment for illness of any kind attend for medical advice (Patrick & Scambler 1986).

Sociologists have investigated the factors that may prompt an individual to seek a medical opinion; their findings suggest that such decisions are rarely made in isolation. Scambler (1986), assessing the work of Zola (1973), suggests that people present with illness not only when there is a distressing symptom such as pain, but also in response to 'triggers' that arise out of social and personal interaction. These triggers include:

- interpersonal crises
- perceived interference of the health problem with social or personal relations
- sanctioning pressures from others to consult a doctor
- perceived interference of the problem with vocational or physical activity
- reaching a personal deadline for the resolution of symptoms.

Scambler (1986) also cites cultural variations as a partial determinant of who will consult a doctor and who will try to treat himself.

The fact that it is 'comparatively rare for someone to decide in favour of or against a visit to the surgery without discussing his or her symptoms with others' (p. 49) — Freidson (1970) refers to this as 'a lay referral system' — may go some way toward explaining why incontinence is underreported. Many people prefer not to mention their incontinence to others, and so the opportunity for friends to encourage them to seek advice does not arise. Moreover, it may also be true that in the case of women the private and to some degree secretive management of menstruation gives an easily transferable model of management to follow should incontinence develop. Many women conceal the leakage of urine as they have concealed menstruation previously, and some also accidentally discover that the use of a tampon will temporarily lessen the problem of stress incontinence. The bulk of the tampon in the vagina pushes against the urethra and thus helps to keep the urethral sphincter closed.

For many people, incontinence is a source of embarrassment or shame rather than a signal to them that they should seek medical help. The dysfunction is seen mainly in terms of its social consequences rather than as a symptom of an underlying illness or disease process.

Personal and social attitudes toward incontinence are not, however, the only factors that account for the underreporting of this widespread health problem. The way that particular health services are marketed or presented can also influence an individual's decision whether to seek help or cope on his own. Armstrong (1980) suggests that there are a number of ways in which health services can be presented, all of which suggest different value systems and approaches:

- provision: it exists but we challenge you to find out about it
- offer: we will tell you of its existence
- invitation: we would like you to avail yourself
- encouragement: we will go to some trouble to convince you of the benefit
- persuasion: we will make you feel guilty if you decline
- pressure: we will reward you if you do, or exert sanctions if you do not
- compulsion: we have passed a law (Armstrong 1980, p. 26).

It is therefore important that services available through the National Health Service (NHS) reflect positive approaches to the promotion of continence and that this is demonstrated in the setting of standards by nurses and their regular monitoring via quality assurance audits.

Identifying patients

Most people who are incontinent do not regard themselves as ill. It is therefore incumbent upon nurses and other professionals working in hospitals and the community to take advantage of every opportunity to identify those who are suffering in silence. Table 24.1 outlines potential opportunities for professionals to identify patients with incontinence problems and demonstrates that it is not always medical professionals who have the greatest opportunity to help people with problems of incontinence. This supports the view that non-medical professionals and others should become better informed about this aspect of health. Chemists and home carers to choose two very different examples, are well placed to provide information and foster positive attitudes towards treatment and should be included in educational initiatives to promote continence.

Primary reasons for incontinence

Delay in achieving continence

In childhood, the acquisition of the skills needed to become continent may be delayed. Nocturnal enuresis may be a

Table 24.1 Lifespan opportunities for helping people who are incontinent

Lifespan stage	Potential problem areas	Sources of help Nurses	Others
Childhood	'Potty' training; enuresis; urinary control; mental handicap; ureteric reflux	Health visitor, clinic nurse, school nurse, practice nurse, community mental handicap nurse, nursery nurse, paediatric nurse	Doctor, consultant, **portage** staff, social worker, dietician, teachers
Teenager	Body function; sex education; cystitis	Health visitor, school nurse/ matron, family planning nurse	Teachers, health educator, product reps, youth club leader
Pregnancy, childbirth	Antenatal frequency; difficult birth: tissue/nerve injuries, postnatal stress incontinence	Health visitor, midwife, district nurse	GP, gynaecologist, obstetrician, self-help groups, chemist
Adulthood and hormone changes	Symptoms of incontinence from urological, gynaecological, neurological, psychological conditions	Well-women's nurse, practice nurse, clinic nurse, district nurse, health visitor, outpatients/ occupational health nurse, specialist ward, or urodynamics nurse	Urologist, neurologist, psychologist, physiotherapist, occupational therapist, dietitian, keep-fit teacher, GP
Old age	As above, combined with the ageing process, prostatic enlargement and disability	District nurse, health visitor, practice nurse, day/ward nurse, geriatric nurse	Home help, home carers, social workers and aides, old age club leaders, senior citizens organisers, GP, geriatrician

particular problem, especially among boys (Thomas et al 1980). Nocturnal enuresis may present as a primary or secondary feature; its cause is not known. Although it often spontaneously resolves itself, it is sometimes not resolved during childhood. In such cases it may remain a problem throughout life if it is not treated (Feneley 1987, Walker 1987, Shapiro 1989).

Sometimes mental or physical handicap will prevent a person from attaining continence. Professionals working with individuals with mental handicap, however, should base their interventions on the assumption that although the process of toilet training will be slow, continence will eventually be achieved. Some children are incapable of acquiring continence because of spinal lesions, as in spina bifida. Others are prevented by other congenital malformations. A baby who is continuously wet or leaking should always be investigated for either congenital fistula or failure to empty the bladder. Such symptoms should be taken seriously, for ureteric reflux caused by failure of the bladder to empty will put pressure on the kidney and may cause infection and life-threatening damage.

Problems in maintaining continence

Childbirth. Giving birth can cause damage to the mother's pudendal nerve, preventing the tone of the pelvic floor muscles from returning to normal. This has been shown to be particularly significant in the development of stress incontinence in women who have had 4 or more children (Thomas et al 1980). Henry et al (1982) suggest that prolonged second-stage labour, the delivery of large babies and the use of forceps put mothers at particular risk of damage to the pudendal nerve.

Chronic disorders. Cerebral, nerve or muscle damage can have varying effects on continence, as can trauma and damage resulting from injury or accident (see Fig. 24.3). Tumours or growths in the area of the bladder or cauda equina are also contributory factors, as is constipation. The process of ageing may in itself have an effect on the lower urinary tract system and its control.

Drugs. Many drugs, especially diuretics can have an effect on the bladder and its function. They may cause incontinence because of the sheer volume of output that they induce, and because of the demands they place on elderly or handicapped individuals in reaching a place to pass urine in time.

The sedative and diuretic effects of alcohol can also contribute to incontinence. Sedatives and hypnotics make people less responsive to signals from the bladder. Anticholinergic drugs and others that have some anticholinergic action, such as phenothiazines and antidepressants, can cause retention in people with previously normal bladder function. Beta blockers also generate a variety of urinary dysfunctions. Keister (1989) has shown that numerous drugs taken by the elderly have the potential to cause incontinence. For further information see Trounce (1990).

The effects of ageing. Age can also affect an individual's ability to maintain continence. It should be emphasised, however, that while incontinence is more prevalent among elderly people (especially women) than among other sectors of society, it is not an inevitable consequence of ageing. Nonetheless, research suggests that around 20% of admissions to long-term care for the elderly may be a direct result of incontinence (Shuttleworth 1970).

With age comes an increasing degeneration of the glomeruli in the kidneys; their function is reduced by up to 50% by the age of 80, thus impairing the ability of the kidney to concentrate urine. This consequence of ageing occurs alongside a decrease in the bladder's urine-storing capacity (Wysocki 1983).

The failure of the kidneys to dispose of sufficient waste products from the body means that at night they remain very active. An increased nocturnal output of urine results, leading to a change in the individual's rhythms of micturition.

Ageing may also have some effect on the cerebral control of micturition, through the diminishing of cell function. Ageing of the cerebral cortical neurones diminishes their effectiveness in inhibiting the sacral reflex arc so that involuntary emptying of the bladder occurs.

In elderly women, vaginal dryness, soreness and atrophic changes may give a number of clues as to why incontinence has developed. Glycosuria or atrophic changes in the vulva may lead to vaginitis and urethritis. (Note that the lining of the vagina is continuous with that of the urethra.) After the menopause, hormonal changes resulting in a decrease of oestrogen can cause dryness in the vagina and urethra. This may interfere with functioning of the moist seal at the urethral sphincter in the urethra, producing incompetency and thus allowing urine to leak through (Ritch 1988).

Constipation is one of the main causes of urinary incontinence. Because of the anatomical proximity of the rectum to the urethra, it is possible for the urethra to be closed off by a faecal mass (see Fig. 24.4). This can lead to failure of complete voiding and thus stasis of urine, which in turn can lead to an infection in the bladder. A full rectum, patulous anus and distended rectal walls are all signs of constipation.

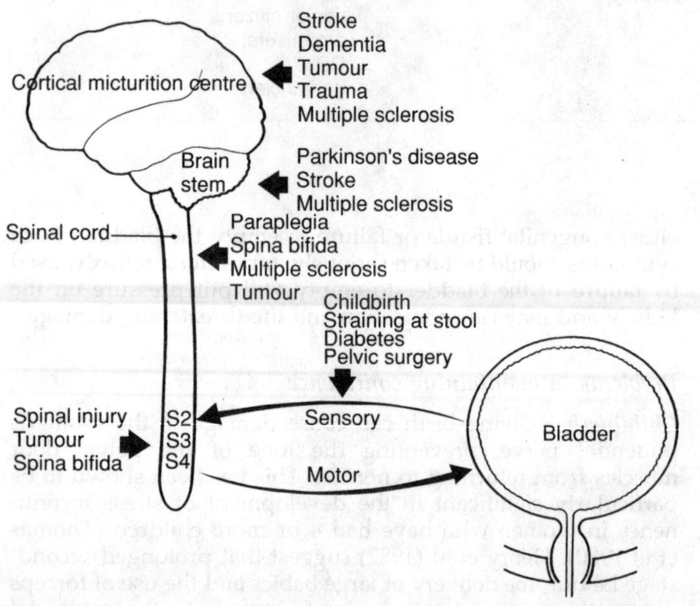

Fig. 24.3 Possible neurogenic causes of incontinence. (Reproduced with kind permission from Coloplast Foundation 1987.)

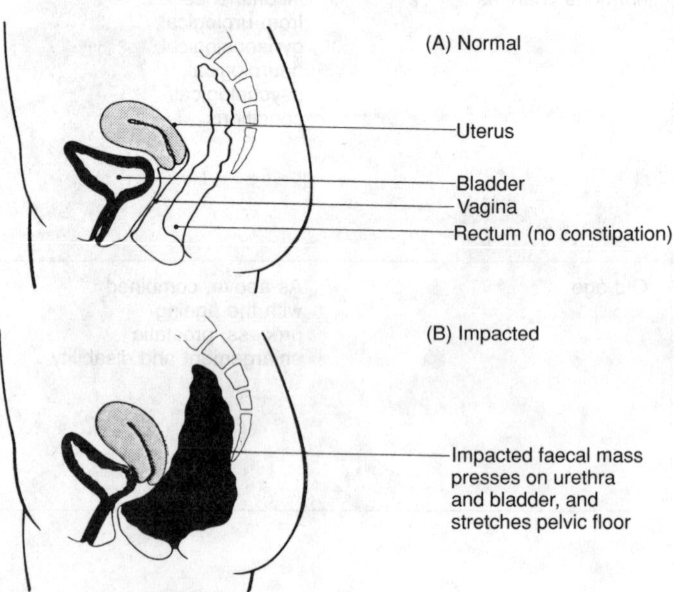

Fig. 24.4 How constipation can cause incontinence. Female, side view. (A) Normal. (B) Impacted. (Reproduced with kind permission from Coloplast Foundation 1987.)

PROMOTING CONTINENCE: A PROBLEM-SOLVING APPROACH

The problem-solving approach to nursing intervention consists of four stages:

1. Identifying the problem through assessment
2. Setting goals
3. Implementing care or treatment
4. Evaluating outcome to ascertain that the goals have been achieved.

The involvement of the patient in all aspects of the nursing process will help to improve motivation and compliance and will enhance the patient's feeling of independence and self-esteem.

Assessment

Assessment should be carried out with reference to a professionally agreed protocol and be individualised. It is vital that this assessment is conducted with a view to ascertaining the *cause* of any incontinence, for only then can the correct type of treatment be instigated. In collecting information from patients, the nurse must have a clear understanding of the rationale behind her questions and of the implications for diagnosis and treatment of the patient's responses (see Box 24.1).

A full assessment should include:

- the patient's own account of the problem
- a detailed history, using closed and open-ended questions
- recording of micturition and incontinence over a few days
- physical examination by the medical staff
- urine testing
- further investigations as required.

Assessment should take place in a private setting and allow adequate time for the patient to air his concerns and ask questions.

Questioning the patient

In order to establish a good rapport with the patient it is important to meet his own agenda when discussing the potentially embarrassing topic of incontinence. Open-ended questions such as 'Tell me about the problems with wetting that you have been having' or 'Could you describe what happens when wetting occurs' will give the patient a greater opportunity to relate his problem in detail than questions that require a simple 'yes' or 'no' response, and will allow him to set out his own agenda for the interview. However, yes/no questions are useful with patients who are acutely embarrassed and have trouble finding a comfortable vocabulary to describe their problems.

The nurse's choice of language and her sensitivity to the patient's preferred terminology will be important to the patient's comfort during the assessment interview. Patients generally use terms such as 'passing water', 'peeing' or 'making water' more often than medical terms such as 'micturition' or 'voiding' and many find words such as 'accidents', 'wetting' or 'leaking' more acceptable than the term 'incontinence'. Where the patient uses euphemism or is vague, the nurse should seek clarification if there is any danger of misunderstanding, for example by asking 'When you said "at it" did you mean "having intercourse"?' or 'What do you mean by "a little"?'

Other specific questions may be indicated when the assess-

Box 24.1 Incontinence assessment questions

Question	Rationale
How long have these symptoms been present?	The symptoms may have begun at a life crisis or on taking a new drug, or they may have been a long-standing problem, but some new development has prompted the patient to ask for help.
Are you wet every time?	It is important to establish the degree and frequency of wetting.
How many times do you pass water each day?	A baseline needs to be established in order for progress to be charted.
Are you wet at night as well as by day?	This gives an indication of the degree of the problem as well as the type of incontinence.
Are you aware of the need to go to the toilet before you are wet?	This will determine whether signals are normal or absent.
Do you have feelings of urgency to go to the toilet?	This indicates whether signals are present and their degree of urgency.
Do you lose urine if you laugh, jump or run?	A positive response often indicates genuine stress incontinence.
Do you pass small amounts of urine?	Passing small amounts of urine may be due to urge, stress or overflow incontinence. It may also be indicative of reduced fluid intake.
Do you pass a full stream?	Passing a full stream suggests the bladder capacity is normal.
Is the stream of urine poor?	The flow rate may indicate a degree of obstruction or the bladder's inability to contract.
Does passing urine sting?	Stinging urine usually indicates infection or a sore or broken area.
Does the urine have a strong smell?	Urine invaded with bacteria or concentrated often has a strong smell.
Do you have difficulty in starting to pass urine?	Hesitancy may be caused by an obstruction, e.g. prostatic enlargement.
Do you dribble urine before or after going to the toilet?	Dribbling before suggests overflow; dribbling after, a failure to completely empty the bladder or an incompetent sphincter.
Do you need to use pads or other aids, and if so how many and how often?	The answer may indicate the degree of urine loss.
Are you constipated?	Constipation is the most common cause of urinary incontinence.
Have you had any operations 'down below' (lower abdomen)?	Surgical trauma may be significant.
Have you difficulty in getting to the toilet, problems with undoing clothes or any sight problems?	If the patient has problems with mobility or dexterity, clothes may need to be adapted and toilet seats raised. Supports to steady patients and aids to help them locate the toilet may be required.
Are you taking any medication?	Many drugs can effect the functioning of the urinary tract.
Is the patient mentally aware?	Senile dementia may be the cause of incontinence due to a failure to remember the routines of the day.

ment is of a patient with a pre-existing illness, e.g. multiple sclerosis, or where bleeding, pain or discharge has occurred. Obviously, some questions (such as those concerning childbirth or prostate problems) will be gender specific. Supplementary questions can be asked by means of a written assessment form.

Box 24.1 provides a checklist of questions that can be used during the assessment interview, together with a rationale for each item of information requested. These questions should be posed only after the patient has described his symptoms and been given the opportunity to articulate his own agenda of concerns.

Charting information

The patient's history may yield enough information to determine the type and cause of his incontinence and its type. A baseline chart can confirm the accuracy of the history by supplying information indicating frequency of micturition and incontinence and where required the volume of urine passed. Charting such information at intervals of a few weeks or at the end of treatment will produce a means of evaluating the treatment implemented. Any chart provided should be straightforward and easily understood so that patients will not be discouraged from using it, for the success of any future treatment will depend upon the patient's motivation.

After careful explanation, the patient should be given the chart to fill in for a few days. Suggestions that the chart is hung with a pen on the back of the bathroom door at home, or kept available in the bedside locker in hospital, are useful in reminding the patient to fill them in. The times of voiding and times of wetting are the most important pieces of information. While amounts lost may be too subjective to be useful, unless complicated before and after testing of pads are incorporated. This is a possibility if objective testing is required (Sutherst et al 1986). Ticking or a collection of ++++ may be sufficient. A full fluid chart is rarely required, although issuing a jug and persuading the patient to measure output for a day may be useful in some cases.

The above approach is advocated for most patients, whether in the hospital or the community, and many specialists in the field of incontinence suggest that complicated investigations, and admission to hospital to discover the type of incontinence among the majority of patients seen, is not required (McGrother et al 1987).

For many patients this assessment will indicate the likely type, or cause, of the incontinence and the problem can be identified.

Physical examination

Women. In women, a physical examination can determine whether atrophic vaginal changes, vaginitis or soreness from excoriation are features, and whether prolapses or constipation is present. In the case of genuine stress incontinence, provocative testing such as asking the patient to cough while she is in a semi-recumbent position may demonstrate leakage. Assessing the ability of the pelvic floor to contract may be achieved by placing two gloved fingers in the vagina and asking the patient to tighten the pelvic floor muscles.

Men should be examined for prostate enlargement and to determine whether the bladder is palpable. If a bladder is palpable or the history suggests inability to void the bladder completely, it may be necessary to ask the patient to pass urine, after which a catheter can be introduced so that the residual volume of urine can be assessed.

Urine testing. A urine sample may be obtained and examined for signs of infection, blood or glycosuria, and a midstream sample sent for culture and sensitivity analysis. Routine testing of urine can identify problems which may contribute to incontinence; haematuria, for example, may be an indication of infection, stones in the bladder or tumours. The neuropathy that may accompany diabetes mellitus may eventually result in damage to the receptors in the bladder demonstrated by proteinuria. However, protein in urine, together with a cloudy appearance and a strong smell, is a sign of a urinary tract infection.

Further investigations

Once the *type* of incontinence in question has been diagnosed, goals can be set for the patient's achievement or recovery of continence. If the incontinence is of an intractable nature, requiring long-term management rather than cure, further assessment for aids or equipment will be required. It may also be the case that further investigation into the *cause* of the incontinence is needed and that referral is indicated.

Urodynamics. Where the information given suggests urge incontinence or mixed symptoms, patients are often referred for urodynamic testing and further investigation. Patients will want to know what this involves and it is an important part of the nurse's role as advocate to explain these procedures to them.

Urodynamic testing measures the pressure and flow relationships in the bladder and urethra. It can aid diagnosis of the type of incontinence by showing sphincter incompetence, bladder instability, overflow incontinence, urethral instability and problems with voiding due to obstruction or an underactive detrusor. The procedure is invasive, unpleasant, potentially very embarrassing, but not painful. Clear explanations and psychological support must be given to the patient throughout.

For the test, the patient usually attends with a full bladder in itself a potentially distressing requirement. Urine is passed while sitting on an adapted commode with a flow meter attached. Flow rates are recorded, as are volumes and time taken, using a transducer which relays to the urodynamic printer. On catheterisation the residual volumes can then be accurately measured.

Following the patient's emptying of the bladder, the patient lies on the couch. Two catheters are passed into the bladder, one is a filling catheter (Jacques), and the other a fine epidural cannula, and a special balloon catheter placed in the rectum. The patient is then transferred to the commode and the tubes joined up to the urodynamic equipment. Care in taping the catheter and holding them in place while transferring the patient is essential.

The bladder is then gently filled with saline via the Jacques catheter and the other catheter records the pressures. The balloon catheter in the rectum is used to record the abdominal resting pressure and the increase when coughing, talking, straining etc. This is subtracted from the bladder pressure reading to record the actual bladder pressure.

During the filling phase patients need to report their first need to pass urine and subsequently the onset of a strong desire to pass urine. During the test or at the close of the procedure, provocative testing can then be undertaken, such as coughing, standing or jumping. Any leakage is recorded by the flowmeter or by observation, possibly by listening. Urethral pressure profiles may also be recorded as the catheters are removed from the bladder.

In the case of urine flow, it is possible to time the speed and flow of urine and contrast this with normal outputs (Dove 1987).

Radiography. Radiographs can reveal signs of stones or large tumours in the bladder and may be required to assess the extent of faecal impaction in the colon and to show any narrowing or obstruction.

Videocystourethrography affords the opportunity to observe the bladder and the urethra on a video screen during filling and emptying.

Cystoscopy. A cystoscope is an instrument fitted with a fine telescope which is introduced via the urethra into the bladder. Modern types of cystoscopes are quite flexible and allow the procedure to be carried out with only a local anaesthetic. It allows the urologist the opportunity to inspect the bladder and urethra, observing for tumours, stones, strictures and the condition of the mucosa. Further information on this procedure is given in Chapter 8.

Planning and implementing care

Effective treatment can be implemented only when the type of incontinence has been correctly diagnosed. This may seem obvious, but research has shown that doctors have often prescribed the wrong treatment for incontinence because of a lack of understanding of its causes, that drugs have therefore been used wrongly and that women who have had children have been advised that incontinence is inevitable (Horsfield 1986, Walker 1987).

Treatments for incontinence include pelvic floor exercises, bladder training, anticholinergic drugs, clean intermittent self-catheterisation, advice on diet, relieving underlying medical conditions, and surgical intervention. These forms of treatment together with their application in different forms of incontinence are described in the following.

Pelvic floor exercises

These exercises are primarily intended to increase the strength of the levator ani muscles and to evoke their contraction without simultaneously increasing intra-abdominal pressure. In women, assessment of the ability to 'squeeze' the muscles around the vagina is followed by teaching the patient exercises to improve their tone, thereby counteracting any descent of the pelvic floor with their corresponding exit channels and restoring the normal anatomical relationships and sphincter function. Figure 24.5 illustrates the position of the muscles of the pelvic floor in women.

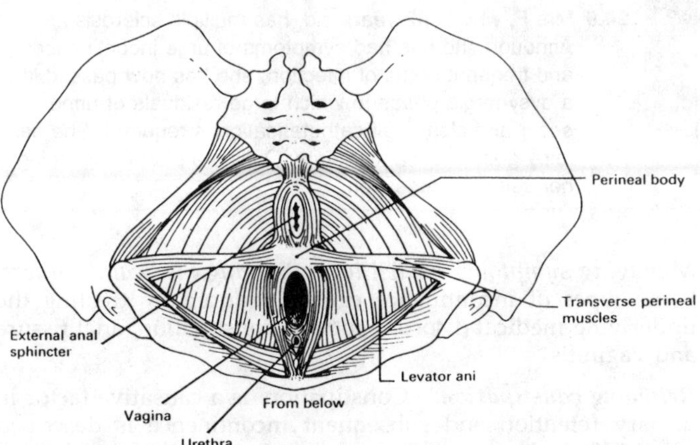

Fig. 24.5 The female pelvic floor muscles viewed from below. (Reproduced with kind permission from Farrer 1986.)

Genuine stress incontinence in men or women (see p. 725) is the main problem for which pelvic floor exercises may be used. This type of incontinence occurs when the pelvic floor is unable to absorb a sudden abdominal pressure and allows the urethral sphincter to open; that is, the intravesical pressure overcomes the intraurethral pressure.

Pelvic floor exercises can also be useful for patients with urge incontinence. Sitting down when strong 'signals' occur and carrying out pelvic floor exercises can help the patient to overcome urgency signals and encourage the bladder to fill a little more before needing to be emptied.

Pelvic floor exercises are also useful following prostatectomy to stop postmicturition dribble, and should be taught pre-operatively.

Identifying the pelvic floor muscles. Before patients can perform pelvic floor exercises they must be able to identify two specific muscles:

- the levator ani
- the pubococcygeus: the anterior portion of the levator ani (see Fig 24.5).

Patients can locate the levator ani muscle by imagining that they have diarrhoea and need to tighten their back passage muscle in order to get to the toilet without an accident.

Patients can locate the pubococcygeus when passing urine: while in full stream they should try to stop, or at least slow, the flow and then try to remember which muscle was used in order to do so.

It is essential that patients identify the correct muscles; crossing the legs and pulling in 'tummy' or buttock muscles are not correct.

Motivation and practice. In order to encourage compliance the nurse must ensure that the patient has understood the instructions on performing the exercises and is motivated to practise them over a 3-month period (Laycock 1987, Montgomery 1986). In carrying out the exercise, the patient should tighten the two muscles of the pelvic floor to the count of 5, 5 times; this should be repeated hourly through the day.

Supplementary techniques. Physiotherapists have a range of equipment and techniques that can be used to help patients to overcome stress incontinence. Electrical stimulation and **interferential** treatment are the main therapies in use (Laycock & Green 1988); not less popular is Faridism.

Recently, the use of various weight cones, which are carried in the vagina, has gained popularity and is being actively researched (Peattie et al 1988). A disposable type has been introduced which is 5 cm long and plastic coated with a string attached to the narrow end for removal. Motivation and support of patients appear to be important elements in achieving success with this treatment.

A perineometer can also be used in therapy for stress incontinence. This instrument is a probe which is placed in the vagina or rectum to measure the strength of the pelvic floor contraction. This procedure used in conjunction with biofeedback (see Ch. 17) has been shown to be a beneficial therapy for stress and urge incontinence (Taylor & Henderson 1986, Holmes 1990). In this treatment the patient watches a gauge which shows intravesical pressure in the bladder; she then experiments with relaxing muscles or holding contractions to reduce the rise in pressure or to contract the urethra in order to prevent urine escaping. With practice, the patient will then be able to apply this technique to retaining urine when necessary in everyday life.

Evaluation. Success of these conservative approaches to achieving continence may be measured objectively by recording the weight of pads for urine loss, and subjectively by the patient's reports on the number of pad changes required per day. Female patients can check their ability to tighten the pelvic floor muscles by placing two fingers in the vagina and squeezing.

> ? **24.7** While discussing the rehabilitation of her mother following a mild stroke, Mrs M confides to you that she is occasionally wet after lifting her mother. What is your role here and what advice may be given as to treatment?

Bladder retraining

For the patient with urge incontinence bladder retraining in conjunction with anticholinergic drugs is the main treatment.

The aim of this form of treatment is for the bladder to 'learn' to increase its capacity and for the urethral sphincter to maintain its ability to remain sealed as the bladder fills, thereby lengthening the intervals between voiding.

Method. The treatment begins with a baseline measurement of bladder capacity at the time of assessment. Then, in stages, the patient learns to hold on for a few minutes more between the bladder signal and going to the toilet. As each lengthened interval is achieved and maintained, new objectives are set for the next few days.

Anticholinergic drugs are a useful adjunct to bladder retraining, as they reduce the initial urge to void and thereby help to increase bladder capacity. When the patient achieves an acceptable social interval between toilet visits, the drugs are then reduced and eventually discontinued; he then tries to maintain the same regime as when he was taking the medication. If the same interval between passing urine is maintained the treatment is seen as successful.

Anticholinergic drugs are contraindicated in patients with glaucoma; see Ch. 13. The normal side-effect of a dry mouth should be explained to patients using this medication.

Evaluation. Whatever the degree of success of the treatment, toileting regimes will remain individual to each patient. In order to evaluate progress a further continence chart should be completed after a few weeks' treatment and again towards the end of treatment. Comparison of the charts, showing both voiding intervals and quantities, will allow an objective evaluation of the success of the treatment to be made.

> ? **24.8** Mrs C needs to pass urine frequently. She tells you that she has had a 'poor' bladder for about 10 years which often wakes her at night as well as 'keeping her on the run' during the day. After referral for urodynamics and further investigations, it is confirmed that she has urge incontinence. You are requested to instigate her treatment of a course of anticholinergic drugs and bladder training. What plan of action would you implement?

Clean intermittent self-catheterisation

This technique is employed by patients with voiding difficulties caused by conditions such as an atonic bladder or dysynergia (in which bladder contraction does not synchronise with opening of the urethral sphincter). It has also been used in conjunction with the passing of 'sounds' for urethral adhesion or prostate enlargement. Clean intermittent self-catheterisation has also been of particular benefit to individuals with multiple sclerosis (Sibley 1988), spina bifida (White 1990), paraplegia and prostate obstruction.

Intermittent self-catheterisation is a relatively simple treatment for incontinence which is known to have been used in ancient times. The ancient Egyptians used reeds, and the ancient Chinese onion stems. The Roman encyclopaedist, Celsus, mentions the use of catheters in his writings (circa 30 BC) and in 11th-century Europe, silver catheters are known to have been in use (Bard 1987, Seth 1987).

Assessment of the suitability of this technique for a particular patient must include identification of the specific type of incontinence in question and an evaluation of the manual dexterity, mental alertness, and motivation of the individual. Children as well as adults have been successful in learning the technique. In some cases it may be appropriate for partners or family members to be taught to carry out the catheterisation.

The procedure of self-catheterisation simulates normal voiding; the bladder is allowed to fill, the clean catheter introduced and the bladder completely emptied. This prevents the build-up of residual urine in the bladder, which otherwise may cause:

- damage to the stretch receptors
- overflow incontinence
- urine reflux into the ureters and kidneys leading to pressure which may cause renal damage and give rise to infection.

Unlike long-term catheterisation, in which aseptic technique and good management are of paramount importance, self-catheterisation may seem unhygienic. However, the clean technique is not associated with bladder infection, as the bladder is completely emptied each time a catheter is passed (Lipedes et al 1972, Murray et al 1984).

The clean intermittent self-catheterisation technique requires the patient to be able to identify the urethra. A small catheter (a Jacques catheter) is introduced several times a day. The same catheter is used repeatedly; after use it is rinsed under the tap, dried and placed in a polythene bag, ready for use again. It is replaced weekly.

Evaluation. Most patients find that inserting the catheter becomes easier with each attempt. The success of the treatment can be measured in terms of the improved quality of life it offers to patients who were continually wet or who previously had to visit hospital emergency departments to seek relief from pain caused by failure to empty.

> ? **24.9** Mrs F, who is 42 years old, has multiple sclerosis. Although she has had symptoms of urge incontinence and frequent bouts of infection, she has now passed into a dysynergia phase in which large residuals of urine occur and clean self-catheterisation is required. She has fairly good manual dexterity. Outline a plan for teaching her self-catheterisation.

Managing symptoms related to underlying medical disorders

Some types of incontinence can be reduced by treating the underlying medical disorder such as constipation, anal fissure and vaginitis.

Relieving constipation. Constipation as a causative factor in urinary retention and subsequent incontinence is described on p. 728. In the treatment of constipation the faecal mass can be cleared by such means as arachis oil retention enemas followed by a course of evacuation enemas over a period of a few days. When the main mass of faeces has been cleared, laxatives may be prescribed to clear any residual material.

An investigation of the cause of the constipation must be undertaken to establish that it is not caused by medication or by any underlying pathology. Dietary factors should also be assessed.

Preventing constipation. Patients who are prone to constipation should be encouraged to be as active as possible. Requests by elderly patients to go to the toilet should always be responded to as quickly as possible, in order to ensure that the gastrocolic reflex is never ignored. In the patient's home this may necessitate structural adaptations to make the toilet more accessible, or the installation of a chemical or macerating toilet or commode in the patient's bedroom or sitting room.

A lack of privacy, time or comfort in an institutional care setting can easily interfere with the maintenance of good bowel habits. Where patients share facilities, nurses and carers must apply standards that allow patients to retain dignity and privacy.

Constipation can be prevented by the introduction of adequate fibre or roughage into the diet, in conjunction with an intake of approximately 8 cups of fluid a day. A dental check-up may be necessary to ensure that patients will be able to manage the raw or chewy typical of a high fibre diet. Individuals who are forced by dental problems to eat only soft foods will be susceptible to constipation.

Confusional states. For patients with senile dementia or other confusional states adherence to a regular routine will help to reinforce the need to go to the toilet at particular times during the day. If a high roughage diet is encouraged and usual patterns of defaecation maintained (usually a half hour after breakfast or other meals) it may be possible to prevent constipation. Subsequent 'spurious' diarrhoea which occurs when the mass of faeces breaks down and mucus and faeces flow away — causing faecal incontinence associated with a characteristic, penetrating smell — can then be avoided. It is probably preferable for patients with senile dementia to be taken to the toilet at normal intervals than to be asked to adapt to new regimes such as using a commode in the sitting room.

Problems related to bowel evacuation. Anal fissures and haemorrhoids need to be healed and soothed in order that constipation caused through pain and avoidance can be prevented.

Analgesic medication taken over a long period, should always be accompanied by a regular laxative to prevent constipation from developing.

Vaginal dryness or vaginitis may be treated with oestrogen creams or oral supplements. Patients should be referred to a doctor if vaginal prolapse or procidentia is evident. For women who are not sexually active and prefer not to have surgery, ring pessaries may be used to correct the uterine displacement. This appliance will need to be changed at intervals of 3 to 6 months.

?	**24.10** Mr G has been drawn to your attention because of increasing agitation exacerbated by what appears as diarrhoea and incontinence of faeces. What aspects of his regime would be considered in his assessment and what therapies would you implement with his carer to promote continence?

Referring patients

It is the responsibility of the nurse to investigate the causes of a patient's incontinence by careful history-taking. The findings of the history can then be supplemented with a baseline chart which records the times that the patient passes urine and/or faeces. Patients should not be referred without this data as this would delay treatment.

In a busy surgery or hospital situation the significance of a patient's wetness may not be fully appreciated. In her role as patient advocate the nurse should make a case for further investigation, as quite often the individual feels embarrassed by his problem and is unable to convince the doctor of its impact on his social life.

For the nurse who is inexperienced in dealing with the problems of incontinence, a continence advisor or a trained nurse with a specialism in continence may be able to act as a resource person and help the nurse gain confidence in her own ability to interpret the data obtained from the patient history and the baseline incontinence chart.

Where the incontinence is not understood, or appears to be outside the scope of the treatments available to the nurse, the patient should be referred to the appropriate professional. This may be a gynaecologist, urologist, geriatrician, physiotherapist, neurologist or psychiatrist.

Surgical intervention

Surgery for stress incontinence. Although conservative measures are generally tried initially, some cases of stress incontinence in women can only be treated by means of surgical intervention. Operations for genuine stress incontinence may be carried out by the vaginal or a suprapubic route. The operation of choice for stress incontinence is suprapubic, whereby the bladder neck is hitched up or supported with sutures or with the patient's own connective tissue. The sling passes around the bladder neck and is usually attached to the ileopectineal ligaments or the rectus sheath. The most common operation is the colposuspension, in which the paravaginal fascia is sutured to the ileopectinal ligament. The care of patients during this operation is described in Chapter 8.

Intervention for prostatic enlargement. Where the prostate partially or completely obstructs the urethra, failure to empty may occur as well as overflow incontinence. Transurethral resection of the prostate (TURP) is the most common surgical intervention performed for an enlarged prostate. This operation is fully described in Chapter 8.

While patients may have experienced overflow incontinence previously, if damage occurs to the sphincter during the operation dribbling incontinence may develop postoperatively and in some cases may be permanent. Gentle pressure behind the scrotum on the perineum or bulbospongiosum can help to prevent postmicturition dribbling. Incontinence aids such as dribble pouches or Y-front marsupial pants with pads for those with a retracted penis should be available in hospitals and in the community. Also available are Y-front pants with a plastic-backed gusset to prevent leakage.

Pelvic floor exercises (see p. 731) should be learned preoperatively and practised diligently following surgery.

Incontinence within the institutional setting

The health problems generated by the institutionalisation of patients have been graphically described by Townsend (1964) and Robb (1967). In some care settings, especially long-stay wards, nurses may still find that the care they give actually causes such problems as incontinence. This is often due to a task-oriented style of nursing and a failure to individualise care, causing patients to become overdependent on the institutional regime. Studies of hospitalised patients by Miller (1984,

1985) and Donaldson (1983) showed that a number of functions of daily living tended to decline even in patients whose physical state remained steady. They concluded that increased dependency and decline in function were induced by ward routines. The loss of continence was one area in which this tendency was apparent. Miller (1984) also showed that in one ward where a systematic and individualised 'nursing process' approach was used the incidence of incontinence fell.

However, more recent research by Cheater & Hawthorn (1987) into problems of urinary incontinence among elderly patients in hospital wards still reflected some confusion in nursing approaches to incontinent patients. That study indicated that the term 'urinary incontinence' was subject to individual interpretation and that there was a low level of agreement among qualified nurses in identifying and characterising instances of incontinence.

Cheater & Hawthorn's study found that assessment was lacking in detail and that possible causes of incontinence were identified in less than 12% of cases. Incontinence charts were highly subjective; it could be inferred from the recorded periods of continence, the researchers pointed out, which nurse was on duty at a given time. The researchers suggest that if rehabilitation is to take place then 'there has to be a more consistent and systematic means of identifying, articulating and communicating the problem of incontinence'.

The King's Fund report *Action on Incontinence* (1983) revealed that in the pre-registration education and training of doctors and nurses as little as 10 minutes may be devoted specifically to incontinence, and that some textbooks fail to refer to it at all.

Clegg (1980) argued that the ward sister is the key figure in health education and that she should be re-educated in the area of incontinence therapy (cited in Syred 1981, p. 32). Copperwheat (1985) showed from her experience of caring for elderly people on a ward that it is important to start with a good basic knowledge of incontinence, to have continual communication with colleagues and work as part of a team, and to start the programme with one or two patients, building up the numbers of successful cases gradually.

Some nurses have made a start by introducing into their ward philosophy the intention 'to reduce the level of incontinence in elderly people who are resident in hospital'; Southern & Henderson (1990) reported a reduction of incontinence episodes by 40% when this standard was implemented in their units.

Evaluation

The last stage of the problem-solving approach to nursing is to evaluate the care given and assess whether the goals set have been achieved. At this point new problems may come to light, in which case the nursing process will begin again with an assessment for this new problem.

?	**24.11** Fully assess the next patient suffering from incontinence who is admitted to your ward or whom you meet in the community. Outline your strategy for care resulting from this assessment.

Continence advisory services

Health authority services

Nurses may find that within their own health area there is a well-established continence advisory service which offers support in the promotion of continence in the community and hospital setting. These services were established during the 1980s from very small but significant beginnings.

In 1977 Dame Phyllis Friend suggested that health authorities should direct attention to the problems of incontinence by taking the following measures (DHSS 1977):

- making local arrangements for the assessment and provision of aids and equipment
- holding seminars to discuss and disseminate information and research findings on matters related, in particular, to the promotion of continence
- making simple local arrangements (in nursing libraries or other suitable areas) for the exhibition of literature and examples of aids and equipment
- identifying the subject of incontinence in the workload of an appropriate nursing officer, who will then act as a resource person for nurses and health visitors in all fields of the service.

The King's Fund group made further recommendations, which included:

- the appointment of continence advisors to all Health Authorities
- the inclusion of the subject of incontinence on all nursing curricula
- activation of a major campaign of public awareness through the media, chemists' shops and public information posters, indicating where to obtain help
- the introduction of a special course for nurses and other professionals on continence promotion and incontinence management.

A recent review of Continence Services by the Department of Health, resulted in a report which recommended models of good continence services across a District (DOH 1991).

The Association for Continence Advice (ACA)

From a small group of interested people an Association of Continence Advisors was formed in 1980. The Association is multidisciplinary and now has over 700 members, including international members and representatives from appropriate manufacturers.

Continence advisors

The institution of the post of continence advisor within the Health Authorities has been of key importance in the struggle to improve care for individuals suffering from incontinence. In addition to carrying a small case load of their own, continence advisors attempt to alter public opinion through education and discussion in the media, set up services, and work to improve the knowledge base of nurses and medical professionals. Within Health Authorities networks have been set up to facilitate communication among and to give support to professionals working in the area of incontinence therapy. In order to expand the knowledge base of continence advisors and to provide peer support, the ACA organises branch meetings, and annual conferences and issues four newsletters a year. The ACA has always maintained that the role of the continence advisor is primarily that of educator or resource person (ACA 1985). The setting up of linkage schemes in some regions has helped continence advisors to disseminate information to nurses at all levels, to encourage uniformity of care across authorities and to motivate and support nurses who are trying to put improved assessment techniques into practice.

MANAGING INTRACTABLE INCONTINENCE

In some patients incontinence will unfortunately be intractable.

The key to successful assessment of these patients for aids and equipment is, as always, to determine individual needs and priorities with a view to improving quality of life. The problem-solving approach should again be applied, taking into account:

- financial considerations
- lifestyle
- home conditions
- the degree and frequency of micturition or defaecation.

Aids and equipment

Many aids and equipment are now being formally submitted to evaluation by product trials. Recent trials and reports include Fader et al (1987) and Ryan-Woolley (1987).

The type of aid that should be recommended for an individual will depend upon the specific type of incontinence from which he suffers. The assessment of a patient for aids or equipment must be informed by an understanding of the cause of his incontinence.

Aids to enhance mobility and stability, raised toilet seats, portable bidets or commodes and clothes that have been chosen or adapted for ease of access may be helpful to many individuals. Aids to personal cleansing can also be made available to help the patient maintain independence and dignity.

Urinals for women

For women confined to a wheelchair, incontinence may derive from an inability to transfer. Here a 'turtle cone' with attached tubing may be the answer, or, if the individual is confined to bed, a 'Femina bedpan' with tubing. These are fully described in the ACA *Directory of Continence and Toileting Aids* (ACA 1990).

For some women with arthritis who are taking diuretics and find that they cannot get to the toilet in time, a small slimline jug may be the solution. The patient stands and passes urine into this container and then, when able, takes it to the toilet for emptying or waits until assistance is available.

Pads and pants

For men and women who cannot achieve urinary control, a wide range of appliances, pads and pants is available. For up-to-date details on these, the reader is again directed to the ACA's *Directory of Continence and Toileting Aids* (ACA 1990) or to the nearest continence service, which will be able to provide information on the availability of particular pads in the local hospital and community.

Many pads can be obtained by mail order. Availability of aids and the process of collection or delivery vary for each area (Devlin 1985, Egan et al 1985). The type of pad and bed protection that an individual will be able to use will depend on the laundry facilities available. During assessment for aids, patients should be asked if they have a washing machine or whether they will need to use a launderette or if a laundry service is provided by their local area health authority. It should be also established whether there are local facilities for collecting large amounts of incontinence aids refuse.

The pads available fall into the following categories:

Light incontinence. To collect small amounts of urine, and in cases where frequent changes are required, adhesive sanitary towels, marsupial pants and pads, small pads with stretch net pants, disposable pants, and washable pants with protective waterproof gussets can all be used satisfactorily.

Medium and heavy incontinence. For medium and heavy incontinence larger plastic-backed pads can be used with stretch net pants. Where hygiene is a concern or where large amounts of reflux emptying occurs, all-in-one adult diapers or nappy-style pads are available. A thin liner inside the pad may be useful where faecal incontinence also occurs. The liner can easily be separated from the pad and flushed with its contents down the toilet.

Bed pads are as an extra protection for furniture and should not be sat or lain upon directly by the patient unless there are clear indications for using them in this way — for instance, where skin care of terminal patients presents a problem. Plastic mattress covers are also available to prevent soiling. Reusable bed pads can be purchased by those who have the necessary laundry facilities to cope with them, and the finances to purchase at least three. These particular aids are sometimes provided through local health services.

Products for men

Most urinary equipment designed to enable men to combat incontinence is available on prescription. New equipment is being developed and introduced quite rapidly and is frequently being tested in field trials (Pomfret 1990). Dribble pouches are available to accommodate small amounts of urine loss while sheaths (urodomes) with varying types of adhesive fixings and attachments are continually being refined.

Urethral occlusive devices are available but should be used with caution. Recently, surgical radio receiver implants have been introduced to aid continence and micturition (Schreiter 1985).

Pad and pants systems with Y-front marsupial pouches are particularly useful for men with a retracted penis and dribbling problems.

Obtaining further information

Many other aids are available in addition to those mentioned above that may prove helpful to particular patients. During assessment for aids and equipment it may be advisable to consult an occupational therapist, physiotherapist or continence advisor on the range of supplies available in a particular health area. The patient may wish to investigate aids to daily living on view in Regional Aids Centres or in shops.

Financial support and advisory service

Individuals who are incontinent or who care for an incontinent person may be eligible for a number of benefits such as Disability Living Allowance, Invalidity Benefit, Income Support, Social Fund, budgeting loans, crisis loans, Community Care Grants and support from the Independent Living Fund.

A number of voluntary agencies may also be able to offer practical support. For children the Family Fund can give help with washing machines, tumble driers and bedding. Services such as Crossroads may be available to provide respite care so that carers can have a break from their responsibilities.

For those patients needing advice concerning care in the community, a new leaflet, SSCCI, gives up-to-date information on the new policies resulting from the NHS and Community Care Act 1990.

Advisory services

Nurses should be aware of the free advice on benefits that is available to patients, e.g. through Freephone services. In some local authorities Welfare Rights Officers are also available to advise patients.

?	24.12 When you are in your local post office or library take note of any free literature or available benefits. Jot down the reference numbers of leaflets that may be relevant to your patients or build up a collection to refer to as particular questions on benefits arise.

Long-term catheter care

Long-term catheterisation is used in the management of incontinence only after all other treatment possibilities have been eliminated. It should not be undertaken without due consideration of the patient's lifestyle, preferences and likely level of compliance. The potential effect of long-term catheterisation on sexual relationships should also be considered (Webb 1985). The patient should be made aware of what catheter management will entail before the procedure is carried out (Heenan 1990). Catheter care is an important part of the nurse's role in the hospital and the community; an understanding of the principles of catheter selection and drainage system management together with skill in patient education are, of course, prerequisites for this. The anatomy and physiology of the lower urinary tract system and the selection and management of catheters are outlined in Chapter 8. The following exercise will help the reader to review her knowledge.

? 24.13 Mr A, who is 69 years old, had been sent home from hospital with a Foley catheter in place. He will need advice and information. Ascertain whether your knowledge base will be adequate to give good management care of his catheter and drainage system by considering the following questions. **A**

a. State four situations in which catheterisation would be justified.
b. Define what is meant by a Foley catheter.
c. When is a large balloon catheter (30 ml) used?
d. When is a small balloon catheter (5–10 ml) used?
e. State four other features which should be considered in the selection of a catheter.
f. What materials can be used to make catheters?
g. What is a catheter with a hole below the balloon called?
h. Can air, saline or other substances be used to fill balloons? Justify your answer.
i. How many mls of fluid are used to fill a 5 ml balloon?
j. What conditions are correct for the storage of catheters? What conditions should be avoided?

Preventing urinary tract infection

Urinary tract infection is the most common of all infections acquired in hospital, accounting for about 30% of all such infections (Meers et al 1980, Bielski 1980 and Mulhall et al 1988). However, infection in the catheterised patient is not inevitable and can be prevented when the potential entry points of infection are properly managed.

? 24.14 In Figure 24.6, can you identify the potential entry points for infection? What techniques can be used to prevent infection at each of these entry points? **A**

A great deal of research is being carried out on catheter management following the study by the Nursing Practice Research Unit at Surrey University (NPRU 1986) and other research projects such as that of Roe et al (1986). In keeping with the UKCC Professional Code of Conduct (UKCC 1992) all nurses involved in catheter care should keep abreast of new research findings in this area.

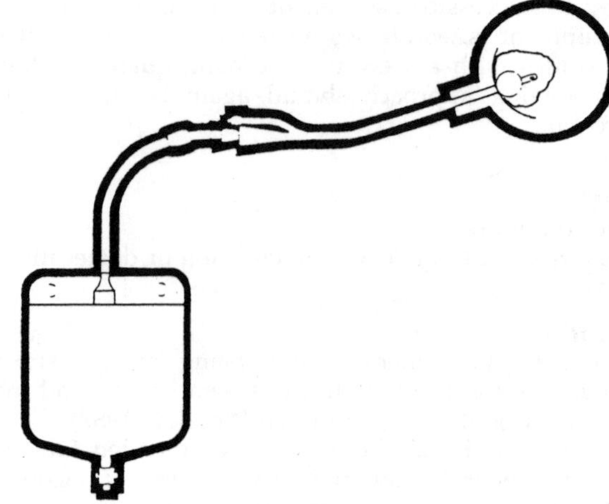

Fig. 24.6

Bladder lavage

Catheter and bladder lavages or washouts have enjoyed a vogue in recent years as a means of reducing urinary infection, catheter encrustation and debris and are often cited as preventive measures in the nursing of catheterised patients. Nurses should be clear that there is a difference between bladder irrigation and bladder lavage or washout. Strictly speaking, irrigation refers to the continuous washing out of the bladder (see Ch. 8). There is also disagreement as to whether these procedures should be carried out at all, as they disrupt the 'closed system' approach to management. Research findings suggest that bladder lavage is harmful (Elliott et al 1989, Bailey 1991) and should be carried out only where it is particularly indicated, never routinely (Roe 1990).

The use of prophylactic antibiotic therapy is also not recommended (Slade & Gillespie 1985). The intake of extra fluid to wash through the system is seen as the appropriate means of preventing infection and the accumulation of debris.

Nursing Care Plan 24.1 demonstrates the use of a problem-solving approach in identifying a patient's problems in caring for his catheter. It proceeds from identification of problems to setting goals with the patient and his relatives and then breaking down nursing interventions into their smallest components so that they can be carefully monitored and evaluated.

Supplying catheter equipment

Following the introduction of nurse prescribing it will be possible for certain qualified nurses working within the community to order the supplies required by catheterised patients. Patients should be given a list of all of their equipment, including sizes, types and capacity, as well as the name of a reliable chemist, retailer or mail order supplier. Appropriate details may be obtained by referring to the ACA's *Directory of Continence and Toileting Aids* (ACA 1990) and, in future, to the *Nurses' National Formulary*, which is to be updated bi-annually.

Emergency help and contact numbers. All catheterised patients in the community should be given a 24-hour contact number from which to gain help in an emergency. Practical advice on what to do in certain emergencies and on what constitutes a

Nursing Care Plan 24.1 Management of an indwelling catheter

Problem	Goal	Nursing action	Evaluation
2/7/92 Unable to manage catheter and urine bag due to lack of knowledge and lack of manual dexterity	2/7/92 To successfully and confidently manage care of his catheter and urine bags in as safe a manner as possible, by the time of his discharge: 9/7/92	2/7/92 Assess patient's ability to cope with buttons and zips	2/7/92 While dressing himself today, patient was able to manage zip, but was slow with buttons
		3/7/92 Change leg bag today and explain equipment and procedure	3/7/92 Took a great deal of interest in the management and asked how the catheter stayed in
		4/7/92 Discuss with patient and daughter the general management of the catheter	4/7/92 Married daughter visited, says she can visit him every day at home and phone him. She thinks he could cope if instruction was given
		4/7/92 Arrange a plan of teaching with patient and carer	4/7/92 Married daughter coming on 5/7/92 at 10 a.m. for a teaching session
		5/7/92 Display of equipment and information session. Provide written information	5/7/92 Patient and daughter took interest and a number of queries were raised
		5/7/92 Extra leg bag change Patient to change leg bag and put on night 'add-on' bag with supervision	5/7/92 Managed leg bag Night-time bag put on correctly but forgot to open valve
		6/7/92 Night nurse to supervise night-time add-on bag application	6/7/92 With prompting remembered to open valve
		7/7/92 Night nurse to supervise removal of night-time bag	7/7/92 Remembered to close valve. Successful in removal, drainage and disposal
		7/7/92 Liaison with district nurse for supervision at home	7/7/92 Contacted Sr G. Discussed patient's progress. Will visit 8/7/92 p.m.
		7/7/92 Supply patient with all equipment, written instructions and phone numbers for emergencies	7/7/92 Patient read all the information and was able to identify each piece of equipment and how used. Given DN's number and info on visit
		8/7/92 Discussion with patient and daughter on diet, emergencies, care and storage of equipment	8/7/92 Daughter and patient happy about discharge on 9/7/92. Able to change add-on bag successfully this morning
		9/7/92 Discharge 10 a.m.	9/7/92 Patient discharged, confident about catheter management. Has two weeks' supply. Daughter thanked staff for teaching session

real problem should be given in writing to patients and carers. Roe (1987) suggests that the patient should be advised to notify his district nurse or doctor if any of the following occurs:

- catheter falls out
- urine is not being drained
- persistent pain
- fever
- blood in the urine.

Sexuality

Incontinence does not suddenly remove sexual desire (Broomhead 1986) even if it often causes people to refrain from sexual activity. Although many professionals may not see this aspect of their patient's well-being as a priority, patients who have been sexually active and are suddenly faced with incontinence caused by injury, child birth or disease, as well as those who are facing progressive incontinence as a result of chronic disease will have to make a difficult adjustment to changes in their sexual life.

Problems of sexuality and incontinence affect the young and the old. An unmet need was clearly identified when various readers of *Woman* magazine voluntarily replied to a questionnaire on incontinence (Glew 1986). One in three of the respondents had never mentioned their problem to their husbands and 25% of those aged 25–34 had told no one at all, including their own doctor. 38% found the subject of incontinence too difficult to discuss with family and friends — 1 in 5 because they were embarrassed, and 1 in 5 because they worried what others would think.

Of the respondents 65% had suffered from incontinence for more than 2 years; 57% said their problem started with childbirth while 17% reported that intercourse produced leakage. The respondents identified anxiety in their sexual relationships as the main effect of incontinence; this included the difficulty of explaining the problem to a partner and the embarrassment of accidents that occurred during intercourse. These problems were severe enough to cause marriages to break up; yet a quarter of the women accepted their situation as 'a woman's lot'.

Gloves et al (1986) conducted a study in four London boroughs to determine how many patients with urinary symptoms due to bladder neuropathy experienced difficulties with sexual intercourse; this formed part of a larger study of the management of urinary symptoms in neurological disease. Of the 252 patients interviewed, 216 (86%) were questioned about sexual intercourse, 86% of whom answered the complete questionnaire. Difficulties with intercourse were reported by 48% of those with multiple sclerosis and 63% of those with other neurological diseases. Difficulties were more commonly reported by men (71%) than by women (40%). A further 12% were refraining from sexual intercourse.

The nurse's attitude

Following a review of the nursing literature on human sexuality, Brower & Tanner (1979) concluded that most nursing authors are not concerned with the sexuality of their patients and its implications for nursing care. Booth (1990) confirmed that this is especially the case with respect to older people.

These findings serve to remind us that nurses involved in counselling must examine their own attitudes and feelings relating to the subject of sexuality. Counselling with regard to the implications of incontinence for the individual's sexuality should be initiated only when the patient signals that he is ready to address the issue. However, the nurse may need to introduce the subject and thereby give the patient 'permission' to voice his concerns. Nurses may be prevented by inexperience and embarrassment from discussing questions of sexuality comfortably with their patient. Nelson (1977) argued that this difficulty is related to the fact that it can take individuals, including nurses, many years to form personal values regarding sex.

Practical problems and solutions

Certain issues concerning sexuality and incontinence may be dealt with in a practical manner, as outlined in the following.

Nocturnal enuresis is likely to inhibit both social and sexual intercourse and should be treated. The numbers of adults who are afflicted with this problem is uncertain; one indicator of its prevalence in the UK is the finding that it may affect in the region of 1% of entrants to the armed forces (De Jonge 1973).

It is important to chart the patient's pattern of enuresis before treatment is commenced. Often a form of bladder training is tried initially whereby the patient learns to hold on to urine longer during the day. The main treatment for nocturnal enuresis in the teenager and adult is to introduce the use of a personal alarm system. A small electrode attached to a battery alarm system about the size of a matchbox is pinned to the patient's nightgown or pyjamas. When the first drop of urine touches the electrode a signal is activated and wakes the patient.

The prescription of desmopressin is helpful but does not cure the problem. This drug is available as a spray and consists of a form of the antidiuretic hormone vasopressin. A single intranasal dose taken at night lasts for 10–12 hours; this affords control of enuresis without affecting daytime urine production. Prolonged use is not recommended.

An excellent resource centre dealing with all aspects of enuresis is the Enuresis Resource and Information Centre (ERIC; see Useful Addresses). Many helpful pamphlets are available from the Centre for adults as well as children.

Cystitis involves either an infection or an inflammation of the bladder. The causal bacteria is usually Escherichia coli. It occurs most commonly in women, because of the anatomical closeness of the urethra, vagina and anus and in some women may be linked to sexual intercourse. Incontinence rarely develops but frequency and pain are present. When this occurs many couples curtail their sexual activity, which may lead to tension in the relationship (Vosti 1975).

Careful hygiene, wiping the vulval area from front to back and avoiding contact by the penis or fingers with the anus during intercourse may prevent problems. Passing urine before and after intercourse has been found to be effective. Drinking copious amounts of water to flush the bladder can help when an attack occurs. Its management can also involve antibiotic therapy or self-help techniques (Shreeve 1986).

Preparation for intercourse

For many women who are incontinent, orgasm produces further episodes of urine loss. Passing urine before sexual intercourse may help. Protecting the bed and discussing the problem with one's partner can help to make the wetting less of an issue.

Catheterised patients need not avoid intercourse. For men the catheter may be strapped to the underside of the penis, and may in some individuals with a degree of impotence also help rigidity. In women the catheter may be strapped to the inner thigh (Broomhead 1986).

Counselling. Open and reflective counselling will help to reveal the extent of any problems that the incontinent patient is having sexually. Chapter 26, will help those who need to develop their skills in this area further. If the patient's difficulties are not easily resolved, he should be referred to experts in sexual counselling who are available either in the hospital or in the community, or to other appropriate agencies such as the Association to Aid the Sexual and Personal Relationships of People with a Disability (SPOD). The nurse should be prepared to furnish information on these organisations and details of how to obtain an appointment.

The reader is referred to Fairburn et al (1983) and Webb (1985) for discussion of the issues surrounding the management of sexual problems.

FAECAL INCONTINENCE

While urinary incontinence is more prevalent in the population than faecal incontinence, the latter is the more distressing problem. Faecal incontinence is socially even more unacceptable than urinary incontinence and raises strong emotions among carers who have to deal with it. It is a source of discomfort and acute embarrassment for the sufferer, and contributes to feelings of helplessness and a loss of self-esteem.

Thomas et al (1984) found that 1 in 200 adults (0.5%) experience regular faecal incontinence. It is especially prevalent among elderly people requiring long-term care. Most cases, however, can be cured and the remainder can be made more manageable with proper care (Henry 1983).

Normal defaecation

Defaecation is the expulsion of faecal matter from the rectum with the aid of peristaltic movements of the muscular walls of the intestine (see Ch. 4). The rectum is stimulated to empty from impulses received from mass peristalsis, often starting from the gastrocolic reflex. The need for defaecation is felt as a response to distension of the sigmoid colon and the stimulation of the receptors. Further information on normal bowel function can be found in Ch. 4.

Anxiety can produce an urge to defaecate more often and in situations of extreme crisis faecal control can be temporarily lost.

The causes of faecal incontinence must be determined before treatment is instigated. Other than simple constipation and impaction, the cause of faecal incontinence is usually damage to the pelvic floor and anal sphincters, resulting in an inability to recognize that the rectum is full or to distinguish between flatus and faeces. The resulting incontinence may be due to constipation, faecal impaction, diarrhoea or spurious diarrhoea (see p. 728). The causes of faecal incontinence vary from an episode of diarrhoea or severe constipation, which is within normal limits, to underlying pathological disease or injury.

Constipation

The constipated patient may complain of headache, general malaise and lack of appetite. Abdominal discomfort, rectal fullness and cramps may also be reported. During examination the abdomen can be measured for signs of increasing distension (Bishop 1982).

In people with a normal bowel constipation may be caused by any of the following:

- a low fibre diet
- low fluid intake
- ignoring the signals to defaecate
- pain in the anorectal region from haemorrhoids or fissures, or inability to position oneself comfortably in the necessary position, leading to avoidance of defaecation
- mouth pain leading to intake of soft foods only
- dental problems leading to inability to cope with foods that need to be chewed
- intake of narcotic analgesics, sedatives or hypnotic drugs
- unacceptable toilet conditions
- unfamiliar surroundings or circumstances leading to loss of habit
- inability to recognise social expectations, as in some cases of mental handicap, senile dementia or excessive consumption of alcohol.

Where constipation is not relieved by the regime described earlier in the chapter (see p. 732), or where no obvious cause is found, the problem may be due to damage to the pelvic floor and anal sphincter or to some other pathology, such as loss of rectal sensation as a result of surgery, injury or tumour. Other contributory problems include endocrine and metabolic reasons for dehydration and neurological damage.

Diarrhoea can also occur within normal limits; common causes are infection, inflammation in the bowel or rectum, excessive use of laxatives and the ingestion of certain foods or drugs. Parasitic infection can also cause diarrhoea.

Abnormalities resulting in faecal incontinence

The most common cause of faecal incontinence is damage to the puborectalis muscle and nerves, resulting in a failure of the valve at the anorectal flap or angle and associated lack of control and sensation. This may have been caused by straining at stool (Snooks et al 1985), trauma in childbirth (Swash 1988), congenital abnormalities and by damage sustained during surgery. Atonic muscles may also preclude adequate pushing to expel the faeces.

In the assessment of faecal incontinence a history of the complaint and an explanation of what previously constituted a normal habit should be obtained in order to establish the specific type of faecal incontinence that the patient has. Bleeding, loss of sensation and the presence of mucus are all symptoms that should be investigated. A full description of the incontinence and its frequency are also important to the diagnosis. Liquid leakage is quite different from true diarrhoea.

Following a rectal examination, referral for a Plain X-ray, proctoscopy, barium enema and stool culture may be necessary (see Ch. 4 'The Gastrointestinal System').

Interventions may be quite conservative involving such mea-sures as changing the diet and making toilets more accessible. In some cases, however, surgery will be indicated. For a full account of the operations currently used to correct problems with the anorectal flap, see Parks (1986), pp. 88–90. Gastrointestinal treatments for diarrhoea are fully described in Chapters 4, 20 and 21.

GLOSSARY

Anticholinergic. Inhibitory to the action of a cholinergic nerve by interfering with the action of acetylcholine.

Biofeedback. Presentation of immediate visual or auditory information about usually unconscious body functions.

Bulbospongiosum. Muscle that evacuates the bulb of the urethra. Responds to manual compression of the urethral bulb to prevent post-micturition dribbling in men.

Desmopressin. Artificial anti-diuretic hormone. Spray used intranasally for short relief of symptoms of nocturnal enuresis.

Faridism. Electrically induces a pelvic-floor contraction; mostly superseded by interferential treatments.

Gastrocolic reflex. Sensory stimulation arising on entry of food into stomach, resulting in strong peristaltic waves in the colon.

Interferential. Electrically induced impulses that can be used to strengthen the muscles of the pelvic floor.

Nulliparous. A woman who has not borne a child.

Marsupial pants have an external pouch, with a pocket to contain a pad.
Parous. Having given birth to a child.
Patulent. The external sphincter lacks tone and is open, due to a grossly overloaded rectum.
Perineometer. Pressure gauge inserted into the vagina or rectum to register the strength of contraction of the pelvic floor.
Piston effect. Movement of catheter up and down within the urethra.
Portage. Pre-school training programme, which takes place in the home, aimed at improving the child's abilities. Often aimed at a mentally handicapped mother or child.
Quality assurance. An ongoing process of assuring the client of a specific standard of excellence through measurement and evaluation of a product or service.
Quality audit. A systematic and independent examination of the effectiveness of the quality system or its parts.
'Sounds'. Medical probes of different sizes used to explore or expand a cavity, in this case, dilatation of the urethra.

REFERENCES

Armstrong D 1980 An outline of sociology as applied to medicine. John Wright, Bristol
Association for Continence Advice 1985 Guidelines on the role of the continence advisor. ACA, London
Association for Continence Advice 1990 Directory of continence and toileting aids. ACA, London
Badger F J, Drummond M F, Isaacs B 1983 Some issues in the clinical, social and economic evaluation of new nursing services. Journal of Advanced Nursing 8(6): 478–494
Bailey S 1991 Using bladder washouts. Nursing Times 87(24): 75–76
Bard 1984 Guidelines for the management of catheterized patients. Bard, Crawley
Bard 1987 You, your patients and urinary catheters. Bard, Crawley
Bielski M 1980 Preventing infection in the catheterized patient. Nursing Clinics of North America 15(4) Dec: 703–715
Bishop F K 1982 Notes from a district nurse. Community Outlook Nursing Times July 14: 195–196
Booth B 1990 Does it really matter at that age? Nursing Times 86(3): 50–52
Broomhead L 1986 Incontinence: a personal account. Nursing 10 Oct: 11
Brower H T, Tanner L A 1979 A study of older adults attending a programme on human sexuality: a pilot study. Nursing Research 28(1): 36–39
Cheater F, Hawthorn P 1987 Incontinence: a nursing perspective. Short Report Nursing Times 83(46): 46
Clegg 1980 Report on the standing commission on pay comparability. HMSO, London
Coloplast Foundation 1987 Objective: continence. Coloplast, Huntingdon, Cambs
Copperwheat M 1985 Putting continence into practice. Geriatric Nursing 5(3): 4–8
DHSS 1977 CNO (SNC) (77)1 HMSO, London
De Jonge G A 1973 Epidemiology of enuresis. In: Kolvin I, Mackeith R C, Meadows S R (eds) Bladder control and enuresis. Heinemann, London
Dept of Health 1991 Agenda for action on continence services. DOH, London
Devlin R 1985 Are they being served? Community Outlook Nursing Times June: 25–26
Dobson P 1990 Update on ERIC. Nursing Times 86(7): 75
Donaldson L J 1983 Survival and functional capacity. Journal of Epidemiology and Community Health 37: 176–179
Dove D 1987 The five second flow test in urinary assessment. The Professional Nurse March 2: 171
Edgington A, Shepherd A, Bainton D 1986 'D' is for dignity. Health and Social Services Journal Jan 13: 50–51
Egan M, Playmet K, Thomas T, Meade T 1983 Incontinence in patients in two district general hospitals. Nursing Times 79(5): 22–24
Egan M, Thomas T, Meade T 1985 Mix and match. Community Outlook Nursing Times June: 32–37
Elliott T J J, Gopal Rao G, Rigby R C et al 1989 Bladder irrigation or irritation? British Journal of Urology 64(4): 391–394
Ewles L, Simnett I 1985 Promoting health. Wiley, Chichester
Fader M J, Barnes K E, Malone-Leed et al 1986 Incontinence garments: results of a DHSS study. Health Equipment Information 159. DHSS/King's Fund, London
Fairburn C G, Dickerson M G, Greenwood J 1983 Sexual problems and their management. Churchill Livingstone, Edinburgh
Feneley R C L 1987 Enuresis at twenty-five. British Medical Journal 294 (Feb 14): 391–392
Fielding P 1986 Attitudes revisited: an examination of student nurses' attitudes towards older people in hospital. Royal College of Nursing, London
Freidson E 1970 Profession of medicine. Dodd Mead, New York
Glover D, Thomas T, North W et al 1986 Urinary symptoms and sexual difficulties. Nursing Times 85(15): 72–75
Glew J 1985 Incontinence: what every woman should know. Woman Magazine March 9th: 30–32
Glew J 1986 A woman's lot. Nursing Times 82(15): 69–71
Gilleard C J 1981 Incontinence in the hospitalized elderly. Health Bulletin 391: 58–61
Hatten J 1977 Nurses' attitude towards the aged: relationship to nursing care. Journal of Gerontological Nursing 3(3): 21–26
Heenan A 1990 Indications for long term catheterization. Nursing Times 86(14): 70–71
Henry M M, Parks A G, Swash M (1982) The pelvic floor musculature in the descending perineum syndrome. British Journal of Surgery 69: 470–2
Henry M 1983 Faecal incontinence. Nursing Times 79(33): 61–62
Holmes P 1990 Mind over bladder. Nursing Times 86(4): 16–17
Horsfield M 1986 Incontinence: a young woman's problem. She Magazine October: 86–87
International Continence Society (ICS) 1984 The standardisation of terminology of the lower urinary tract function. ICS, London
Keister K J 1989 Medication of elderly institutionalized incontinent females. Journal of Advanced Nursing 14(11): 980–985
King's Fund 1983 Action on incontinence. Report of a working group No 43 King's Fund, London
Laycock J 1987 Graded exercises for the pelvic floor muscles in the treatment of urinary incontinence. Journal of Physiotherapy 73(7): 371–373
Laycock J, Green R J 1988 Interferential therapy in the treatment of incontinence. Physiotherapy 74(4): 161–168
Lipedes J, Diokno A C, Silver S J et al 1972 Clean intermittent self-catheterization in the treatment of urinary tract disease. Journal of Urology 107: 458
McGrother C W, Castleden C M, Duffin H, Clarke M 1987 Provision of services for incontinent elderly people at home. Journal of Epidemiology and Community Health 40(2): 134–138
McLaren S M, McPherson F M, Sinclair F et al 1981 Prevalence and severity of incontinence among hospitalised female psycho-geriatric patients. Health Bulletin 38: 62–64
Meers P C, Ayliffe G A, Emmerson A M et al 1980 Report on the national survey of infection in hospital. Journal of Hospital Infection 2 Supplement: 1–11
Miller A 1984 Nurse–patient dependency. Journal of Advanced Nursing 9: 479–486
Miller A 1985 Nurse–patient dependency: is it iatrogenic? Journal of Advanced Nursing 10: 63–69
Montgomery E 1986 Pelvic power. Community Outlook Nursing Times Sept: 33–34
Mulhall A B, Chapman R G, Crow R A 1988 Bacteriuria during indwelling urethral catheterization. Journal of Hospital Infection 11: 253–262
Murray K, Lewis P, Blannin J et al 1984 Clean intermittent self-catheterization in the management of adult lower urinary tract infection. British Journal of Urology 56: 379–380

Nelson S E 1977 All about sex for students. American Journal of Nursing 77(4): 611–612
NHS and Community Care Act 1990 HMSO, London
Nursing Practice Research Unit (NPRU) 1986 A study of patients with an indwelling urethral catheter and related nursing procedures. NPRU Division of Nursing Studies, University of Surrey, Guildford
Parks A G 1986 Faecal incontinence. In: Mandelstam D (ed) Incontinence and its management. Croom Helm, Beckenham
Patrick D S, Scambler G (eds) 1986 Sociology as applied to medicine. Baillière Tindall, London
Peattie A B, Plevnik S, Stanton S L 1988 Vaginal cones: a conservative method of treating genuine stress incontinence. British Journal of Obstetrics and Gynaecology 95: 1049–1053
Pomfret I 1990 All shapes and sizes. Journal of District Nursing June 8(12): 9–10
Ritch A E S 1988 The use of oestrogen in incontinence in the elderly. Measuring and managing incontinence. Geriatric Medicine and Kabivitrium Ltd
Robb B 1967 Sans everything: a case to answer. Nelson, London
Roe B, Chapman R, Crow R 1986 Checking catheter care. Nursing Times 82(48): 61–63
Roe B 1987 Catheter care. A guide for users and their carers. Wallace, Colchester
Roe B 1990 Catheter prescribing and the use of antimicrobials. Nursing Times 86(14): 65–68
Ryan-Woolley B 1987 Aids for the management of incontinence. King's Fund, London
Scambler G 1986 Illness behaviour. In: Patrick D L, Scambler G (eds) Sociology as applied to medicine. Baillière Tindall, London
Schreiter F 1985 Bulbar artificial sphincter. European Urology 11: 294–299
Seth C 1987 Incontinence: doing it yourself. Nursing Times Community Outlook October
Shapiro R 1989 A shameful secret. Community Outlook Nursing Times Sept: 21–23
Shreeve C 1986 Cystitis: the new approach. Thorsons, Northamptonshire
Shuttleworth K E D 1970 Urinary tract diseases: incontinence. British Medical Journal 4: 727–729
Sibley L 1988 Confidence with incontinence. Nursing Times 84(46): 42–43
Slade N, Gillespie W A 1985 The urinary tract and the catheter: infection and other problems. Wiley, Chichester
Snooks S J, Barnes P R H, Swash M et al 1985 Damage to the innervation of the pelvic floor musculature in chronic constipation. Gastoenturology 89: 971–981
Southern D, Henderson P 1990 Tackling incontinence. Nursing Times 86(10): 36–38
Sutherst J R, Brown M C, Richmond D 1986 Analysis of the pattern of urine loss in women with incontinence as measured by weighing perineal pads. British Journal of Urology 58: 273–8
Swash M 1988 Childbirth and incontinence. Midwifery 4: 13–18
Syred M E J 1981 The abdication of the role of health education by hospital nurses. Journal of Advanced Nursing 6: 27–33
Taylor K, Henderson J 1986 Effects of biofeedback and urinary stress incontinence in women. Journal of Gerontological Nursing 12(9): 25–30
Thomas T M, Plymet K R, Blannin J et al 1980 Prevalence of urinary incontinence. British Medical Journal 281: 1243–1245
Thomas T M, Egan M, Walgrove A et al 1984 The prevalence of faecal incontinence. Community Medicine 6: 216–220
Townsend P 1964 The last refuge: a survey of residential institutions and homes for the aged in England and Wales. Routledge and Kegan Paul, London
Trounce J 1990 Clinical pharmacology for nurses, 13th edn. Churchill Livingstone, Edinburgh
UKCC (1984) Code of professional conduct for the nurse, midwife and health visitor, 2nd edn. UKCC, London
Vosti K 1975 Recurrent urinary tract infections. Journal of the American Medical Association 231(9): 934–940
Walker I 1987 The one problem we still can't talk about. Living Magazine May: 102–104
Webb C 1985 Sexuality, nursing and health. HM and M, Chichester
White M 1990 Independence for the handicapped child. Nursing Times 86(7): 69–72
World Health Organization 1975 Education and training in human sexuality: the training of health professionals. WHO, Geneva
Wysocki R 1983 Urinary incontinence and the older adult. Aust. Nurses' Journal 12(11): 49–50, 52
Zola I 1973 Pathways to the doctor: from person to patient. Society of Scientific Medicine 7: 677–689

VIDEO CASSETTES

DHSS 1987 Understanding urinary incontinence

USEFUL ADDRESSES

ACA (Association for Continence Advice)
The Basement/
2 Doughty Street
London WC1N 2PH
Tel. 071 404 6821

ERIC (Enuresis Resource and Information Centre)
65 St Michael's Hill
Bristol BS2 8DZ
Tel. 0272 26 4920

SPOD (Association to Aid the Sexual and Personal Relationships of People with a Disability)
286 Camden Road
London N7 OBJ
Tel. 071 607 8851

CHAPTER 25

Sleep

S. José Closs

CHAPTER CONTENTS

Introduction 743

The importance of the sleep–wake cycle 743

Describing sleep 744
The structure of sleep 744

Physiological control of sleep 746
Neurological control 746

Functions of sleep 746
SWS and restorative processes 746
REM sleep 747
Effects of sleep deprivation 747

Normal sleep 747
Factors affecting normal sleep 747

Common sleep disorders 749
Factors disrupting normal sleep: DIMS and DOES 749
Parasomnias 752

Methods of assessing sleep 752
Nursing assessment of sleep 753

Helping patients to sleep 753

Pharmacological treatments for insomnia 753
Hypnotic drugs 753
Herbal remedies 754

Psychological and behavioural treatments for insomnia 755

Conclusion 755

References 755

INTRODUCTION

The intriguing subject of sleep has been much written about. What happens when we fall asleep? Despite hundreds of years of observations of sleep and, more recently, extensive and systematic research, the mechanisms and functions of sleep are still poorly understood. Many theories, both physiological and behavioural, have been postulated, but there is still much to discover. Nevertheless, sleep is something that everyone does, and from which 'beggars in their beds take as much pleasure as kings' (Thomas Dekker 1604)*. Although there have been individuals who maintain that they never sleep, such claims have always been discredited after careful monitoring.

Ageing both exacerbates existing sleep disorders and introduces new ones. Given that the numbers of elderly people are rapidly rising, this is an area which is of increasing concern in nursing practice. An understanding of the structure and probable functions of sleep should allow nurses in all fields of care to help patients to get the best possible sleep, both at home and under the rather more difficult conditions in hospital. This chapter aims to provide both theoretical and practical information about sleep which is relevant to nurses working both in hospital and in home care settings.

THE IMPORTANCE OF THE SLEEP–WAKE CYCLE

Primarily, it is our circadian rhythms which dictate when it is time to sleep. The word circadian is derived from the Latin *circa*, 'about' and *dies*, 'a day', and refers to the physiological and behavioural patterns that repeat every 24 hours. Under normal circumstances these rhythms are synchronised by external time cues, such as the light–dark cycle, and by social time cues, such as mealtimes. These synchronising cues are known as Zeitgebers ('time-givers'). It seems, however, that there are internal as well as external synchronisers. Many studies have confirmed that endogenous 'clocks' govern the function of every living tissue. These clocks are coordinated directly or indirectly by the brain. It is probable that the 'pacemaker' controlling the sleep–wake cycle is situated in the suprachiasmatic area of the hypothalamus, since bilateral lesions in this area abolish the normal circadian pattern of rest and activity. When humans are placed in an environment free of time cues their circadian rhythms usually take on a 'natural period', which occasionally lasts fewer than 24 hours but is usually about 25 hours or sometimes more. Following this natural period is known as free-running.

* Thomas Dekker (c. 1572 – c. 1632), English playwright

The sleep–wake cycle coincides with other circadian rhythms, such as 24-hour fluctuations in body temperature, heart rate, and plasma levels of anabolic and catabolic hormones. Catecholamines and cortisol potentiate stress responses (see Ch. 17, p. 580), which are likely to be high among patients in intensive care units (see Ch. 29). If subjects are allowed to free-run, i.e. they are isolated from all cues signalling the time of day, then their various circadian rhythms tend to become dissociated from one another. For example, it has been demonstrated that in the absence of time cues the rest–activity cycle may have a period of, say, 33 hours, whereas body temperature might have a 24.5-hour cycle.

Desynchronisation of circadian rhythms has been shown to disrupt not only temperature and sleep–wake patterns, but also pulse rate, respiration, arterial pressure, diuresis and excretion of electrolytes. This acute desynchronisation can produce symptoms such as fever, alcohol hangover, migraine, and some mental disorders. Weitzman et al (1970) showed that EEG recordings of subjects following a phase shift of the sleep–wake cycle revealed changes in sleep structure similar to those found in endogenously depressed individuals. These included an increased time before the onset of rapid eye movement (REM) sleep (see p. 747) and more night-time awakenings. It has been suggested that endogenous depression might result from a long-term mismatch between metabolic rhythms and the sleep–wake cycle.

People have highly individual 24-hour routines. Many rise in response to an alarm clock at a specific time that allows them to arrive at work punctually. Patterns of activity tend to be dictated by work, family and social commitments, as well as by the individual's particular requirements for sleep. The propensity to fall asleep peaks twice during the day. The first peak is at the usual bedtime and the second after lunch (whether or not lunch has actually been eaten), when people in some countries customarily take a siesta.

Normal sleep–wake cycles may be disrupted by many different events. For example, new parents may find that 'night is turned into day' for the first three months or so of their baby's life.

It is not only the young whose sleep patterns differ from those of the normal adult. The circadian rhythms of elderly individuals tend to weaken as they get older. This results in less night-time sleep, more awakenings at night and sometimes more daytime napping. This has implications for those who care for the elderly, both in hospital and at home (see Ch. 36). In hospital, routines should be relaxed in order to accommodate the relatively irregular sleeping habits of elderly patients. At home, carers who have to get up several times throughout the night in order to attend to the needs of an elderly relative often find that fatigue reduces their ability to cope effectively, particularly if they also have to work during the day.

Shift-work is another common cause of disruption to the sleep–wake cycle. Student nurses working night-shifts for the first time may be surprised at their difficulty in adjusting to a new pattern of rest and activity. The degree of difficulty is highly individual, some nurses finding it relatively easy to adjust while others find it virtually impossible to get enough sleep during the day, when there is usually more noise and Zeitgebers which normally prompt night-time sleep are absent. Those nurses who do not sleep adequately may not be able to function efficiently throughout the night, resulting in a reduction in the quality of care that they give. The possibility of dangerous errors, such as in the administration of drugs, also becomes more likely.

Since the average free-running day is about 25 hours (see p. 743), changes in the rest–activity cycle tend to be adjusted to more easily when the cycle is being lengthened. Travelling west rather than east, and changing one's work-shift to a later rather than earlier period in the day, are easier to adjust to than the alternatives (Czeisler, Moore-Ede & Coleman 1982).

The circadian disruptions which occur upon the patient's admission to hospital may result from the absence or adjustment of the Zeitgebers normally responsible for synchronisation, as well as from stresses such as pain and anxiety. Of necessity, hospitals impose unfamiliar lighting conditions, and altered times for meals (or their absence) and awakening. Floyd (1984) found that psychiatric hospital inpatients slept less than a matched group of outpatients and that their normal times of sleeping and activity appeared to be altered by the hospital's rest–activity schedule. However, psychiatric pathology itself may interfere with sleep patterns, a point which will be discussed later (see p. 749).

Although much of the experimentation on desynchronisation has been conducted under tightly controlled circumstances, some of its findings may be applicable to daily life. It appears that the disruption of normal circadian rhythms (and, in particular, of the sleep–wake cycle) leads to numerous adverse physiological and psychological consequences. These are detrimental to patients in the community and particularly undesirable for hospital patients, who are subject to many additional stresses. Since the two major synchronising rhythms appear to be those of sleep and body temperature, nurses should try to maintain an awareness of these and attempt, where possible, to synchronise them with the patients' normal patterns.

?	**25.1** Discuss with your colleagues how nurses can use the notion of circadian rhythmicity to help patients to sleep better, both in hospital and in the community.

DESCRIBING SLEEP

For the most part, modern researchers have tended to use objective criteria to describe sleep, usually in terms of physiological events occurring during specific stages of sleep. These include changes in the electrical activity of the brain and fluctuations in the secretion of various hormones. It is important to bear in mind, however, that it is the individual's subjective experience of sleep which is of greatest importance in an assessment of the quality of his sleep. Even when an EEG indicates that sleep has been long and continuous, if the individual feels that he has slept badly he cannot be contradicted. Conversely, if a patient habitually sleeps for only two hours a night, but claims that this amount is adequate, leaving him rested and refreshed, then there is nothing wrong with his sleep.

In addition to recognising the importance of sleep as a subjective experience, it is also useful to have some basic knowledge about the structure and function of sleep. This may be put to good use in attempting to understand patients' sleep difficulties and their implications and in planning interventions.

The structure of sleep

Electroencephalography is a relatively new technology which has enabled researchers to describe the structure of sleep in terms of types of gross electrical activity which take place in the brain. This is achieved by attaching electrodes to the scalp which then conduct the electrical current generated by various areas of the brain to a device which allows them to be viewed. Usually this is either a TV monitor or an electroencephalograph, which inscribes a permanent trace of brainwaves on paper (i.e. an electroencephalogram, or EEG), in a manner similar to the recording of the electrical activity of the heart by an electrocardiograph (see Ch. 2, p. 12). EEGs and other recordings have shown that there are two distinct types of sleep.

NREM sleep

NREM (non-rapid eye movement, or orthodox, sleep) is comprised of four stages, as described by Rechtschaffen & Kales (1968). In each stage electrical activity of the brain progressively slows and increases in amplitude (see Fig. 25.1).

Stage O or W (wakefulness). During wakefulness the EEG is characterised by generally low voltage activity at 4–25 Hz. Sinusoidal alpha waves are present when the subject is awake with his eyes closed.

Stage 1 (drowsing). The alpha rhythm (8–12 Hz) begins to fluctuate and slow, rolling eye movements appear on the electro-oculogram (EOG). The EOG records electrical activity associated with eye movements. During stage 1 the pupils constrict and dilate at roughly 1–3 second intervals. The EEG shows mostly low-voltage, mixed-frequency activity at 2–7 Hz. This is the lightest stage of sleep. If asked, the subject may report that he felt drowsy but was awake. Even though the subject may feel fully alert, it is likely that observers will note his reduced attentiveness. Some simple perceptual distortions (i.e. daydreams) may occur during stage 1 sleep.

Stage 2 (light sleep). The alpha rhythm disappears and 'sleep spindles' of 12–14 Hz, lasting at least 0.5 seconds, appear. These spindles are the most consistent characteristic of stage 2 sleep. This phase of altered consciousness is such that, if awakened, most people recognise that they have been asleep. It is in stage 2 that body movements begin to diminish, and dreams involving a story line first appear. Dream recall on waking, however, is far less vivid than for REM sleep.

Stage 3 (slow wave sleep). The amplitude of the EEG increases, and 20–49% of the trace records delta activity (i.e. less than 2 Hz with amplitudes greater than 75 μV from peak to peak). Spindles are rarely seen. Body movements continue to diminish. The distinction between stages 3 and 4 is somewhat arbitrary, since the increase in the proportion of delta waves occurs gradually.

Stage 4 (slow wave sleep). Over 50% of the EEG shows delta activity. High amplitude slow waves are indicative of this stage. There is a high degree of immobility and intense external stimuli are required to arouse the subject. Large increases in the secretion of growth hormone occur. There is therefore some scientific support for the parent's injunction to the child, 'You must get your sleep if you want to grow'.

By convention, and throughout this chapter, stages 3 and 4 are considered together and termed slow wave sleep (SWS). The distinctions between wakefulness, stage 1, stage 2, SWS and REM are qualitative, involving clearly observable physiological differences, while the distinction between stages 3 and 4 seems arbitrary.

REM sleep

The second type of sleep is known as rapid eye movement (REM) or paradoxical sleep and is characterised by dreaming, muscular relaxation and high levels of physiological arousal. In order to identify this phase of sleep extra electrodes can be applied to the face to detect electrical activity due to eye movement, and below the chin to detect muscle tone. These may then be recorded as an EOG and EMG (electromyogram) to augment the information gained from the EEG. If all these electrical signals are recorded overnight, the result is a complex series of parallel traces known as a polysomnogram. From this, the most reliable indicator of REM, i.e. the disappearance of skeletal muscle tone, can be visualised. The EEG recorded during REM sleep is virtually indistinguishable from that taken during wakefulness, showing low-amplitude, mixed frequency activity. During REM sleep muscle tone is lower than in any other sleep stage. Blood pressure fluctuates, pulse and respiration rates increase and may become irregular, oxygen consumption increases, premature ventricular contractions may occur and there is penile tumescence in men and increased vaginal secretion in women. The eye movement which occurs in REM sleep usually consists of rapid darting movements of the eyes under closed lids, occurring in bursts of 3–10 seconds at intervals of 30–40 seconds. These do not always occur, and if they are absent this is most likely to be during the first REM period of the night. If subjects are woken up they frequently report that they have been dreaming; consequently, REM sleep is frequently referred to as dreaming sleep.

During a night's sleep, both REM sleep and all four NREM stages may occur many times, usually in a cyclical fashion (see Fig. 25.2). Sleep usually begins with stage 1 (drowsing) and progresses through stage 2 to SWS. This 'deep' sleep is frequently followed by a brief return to stage 2 before an

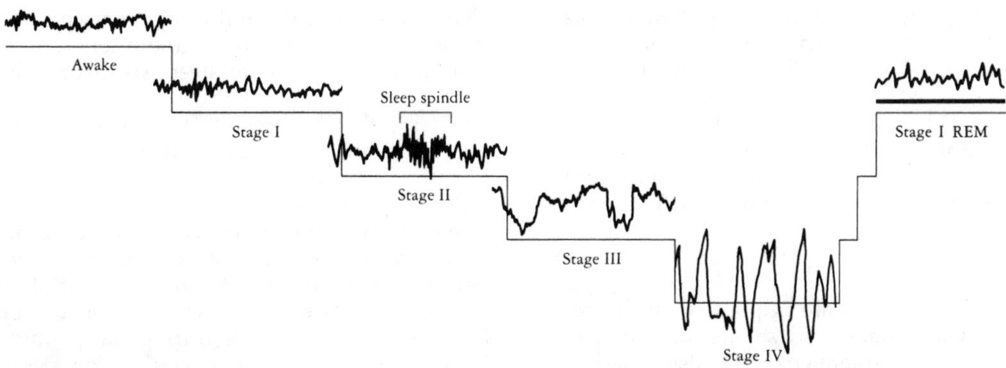

Fig. 25.1 Progressive changes in the EEG following the onset of sleep. (From SLEEP, by J. Allan Hobson. Copyright (c) 1989 by J. Allan Hobson. Reprinted by permission of W. H. Freeman and Company.)

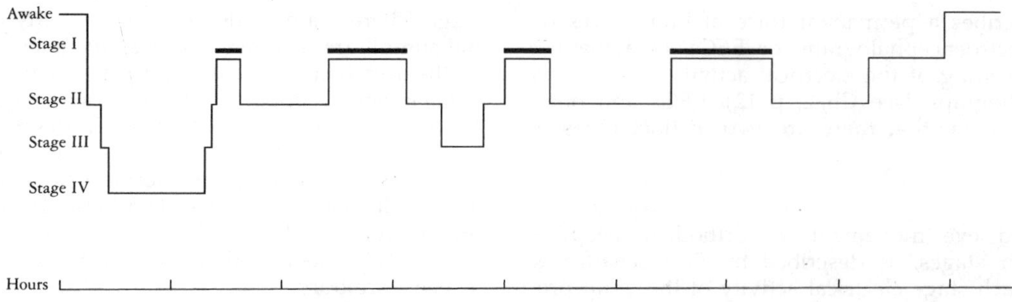

Fig. 25.2 Sleep architecture showing one night's progression of sleep cycles. (From SLEEP, by J. Allan Hobson. Copyright (c) 1989 by J. Allan Hobson. Reprinted by permission of W. H. Freeman and Company.)

episode of REM. The pattern then repeats, usually starting from stage 2. The duration of this cycle may vary considerably according to age and other factors, but in young healthy adults it lasts approximately 100 minutes.

The first part of the night tends to contain more SWS, while the latter part of the night contains a higher proportion of REM. Interestingly, even during the day people undergo 100-minute cycles of alertness and drowsiness, though they are usually unaware of these. During sleep, shifts from stage to stage tend to accompany body movements. Shifts to light sleep tend to occur suddenly, whereas shifts to deep sleep tend to be gradual.

Normally, sleep in healthy young adults comprises 4% stage 1, 50% stage 2, 23% SWS and 23% REM sleep (Johns 1984).

PHYSIOLOGICAL CONTROL OF SLEEP

Precisely how and why people sleep remains the subject of much research. At present it appears that the brain has several interlinked sleep centres. Some relate to the onset and timing of sleep, some to REM sleep, others to NREM sleep and others to wakefulness. In addition, there are several putative, naturally occurring sleep substances which seem to be diffused throughout the brain.

Neurological control

The neurological control of sleep is complex and is not yet completely understood. The medulla, pons and midbrain comprise the brainstem (see Ch. 9, p. 329) and accommodate many of the anatomical structures which govern sleep and wakefulness. The cell network known as the reticular formation is located within the brainstem and contributes to several aspects of brain function. Implicated in the regulation of sleep and wakefulness is the reticular activating system (part of the reticular formation), which describes collectively specific structures within the brainstem and the thalamus.

NREM sleep mechanisms in the basal forebrain interact with reticular systems, producing characteristic slow wave electrical activity in the cerebral cortex. The REM sleep generator in the pons interrupts this process periodically, reactivating the brain.

Neurotransmitters

Three different neurotransmitters are implicated in the regulation of sleep and wakefulness. These are noradrenaline, acetylcholine and 5-hydroxytryptamine (5-HT, also called serotonin), each produced by different sets of cells within the pons. Noradrenergic neurones are responsible for the arousal of the cortex observed during wakefulness and REM sleep. Cholinergic cells facilitate REM sleep, while cells producing 5-HT appear to be responsible for the maintenance of NREM sleep and to play an important role in the regulation of REM sleep.

Sleep substances

Theories claiming the existence of sleep substances have gained popularity from the beginning of this century. These are claimed to be naturally occurring substances which accumulate in the central nervous system and cause sleep. Several sleep substances have been isolated, but it is not known whether they are central to the regulation of sleep or part of a larger and more complex system.

FUNCTIONS OF SLEEP

Despite enormous research efforts, the only universally agreed reason for sleeping is to avoid being sleepy. Interpretations of research findings vary, but it is generally considered that sleep is a restorative process. It has also been suggested, however, that sleep is merely an instinctual behaviour, a genetic remnant of earlier days when immobility at night aided survival. Horne (1988) proposed a combination of these two explanations, with some sleep being obligatory (SWS and about two thirds of REM), and some optional (stages 1 and 2 and one third of REM). He concluded that the obligatory portion of sleep is essential only for the functioning of the brain and that other organs may require only physical rest and feeding for restitution. However, according to Oswald (1984) there are 'over 100 research reports showing that the protein synthesis and cell division for the renewal of tissues like the skin, bone marrow, gastric mucosa, bone or brain take place predominantly during the time of the 24 hours devoted to rest and sleep'. Therefore it would appear necessary for patients who have been ill or who have undergone any type of surgery or trauma to get adequate sleep. In theory, this would enhance healing processes and also help to prevent the psychological problems that can result from inadequate sleep (see p. 747) and which might hinder recovery.

SWS and restorative processes

The direct study of sleep and healing in human subjects presents practical and ethical difficulties. Consequently, there is very little evidence for the involvement of sleep in healing for humans. It has been shown that cell proliferation in human bone marrow increases during sleep, and that the rate of bone growth in boys increases during sleep as well. In addition, the highest rate of human skin mitosis has been shown to occur at night. Even though there is relatively little evidence that anabolic processes occur during human sleep, there are numerous animal studies which have produced findings that support the proposition that sleep coincides with restorative processes.

A rather less direct way of investigating body restoration is to study circadian variations in the levels of anabolic and catabolic hormones. These regular fluctuations suggest that anabolic processes occur during the sleep period. In man, protein synthesis is inhibited by hormones such as cortisol, glucagon and catecholamines, which reach their highest levels during the day. During sleep, energy expenditure in the tissues falls and the energy stored within the cells as adenosine triphosphate (ATP) rises to levels which become sufficiently high for protein synthesis to occur. Growth hormone, which stimulates protein and RNA synthesis and amino acid uptake, reaches peak secretion rates during SWS, the sleep state which has the highest positive correlation with the length of prior wakefulness and therefore appears to have restorative properties. All this evidence supports the assertion that sleep, and in particular SWS, is essential for tissue restoration.

REM sleep

The function of REM sleep is more difficult to explain. Babies have large amounts of REM sleep, whereas elderly sufferers of chronic brain degeneration have a reduced duration of REM sleep compared with age-matched controls (Hobson 1989, p. 77). This implies that REM sleep has a possible role in brain metabolism. Human studies of REM sleep deprivation have not yet produced a clear picture of its effects. There have been tentative suggestions that REM sleep is involved in the integration of emotional experiences and entirely new material, but does not affect tasks such as learning word lists or the assimilation of familiar sorts of experience. It seems possible that REM sleep is involved in learning and memory, but research has so far failed to provide convincing evidence to support these ideas. Individuals who take antidepressant drugs on a long-term basis may sustain a complete loss of REM sleep without any appreciable ill effects, a finding which suggests that REM sleep is not essential to normal functioning.

Effects of sleep deprivation

Total sleep deprivation has been shown to result in clear signs of central nervous system (CNS) impairment and there is evidence of physiological damage as well. Rechtschaffen et al (1983) deprived rats of sleep for 5–33 days and found that they suffered 'severe pathology and death' whereas control rats did not. The causes of death were not uniform, rendering the mechanism of sleep deprivation in causing such damage unclear. Total sleep deprivation for 48 hours in humans results in changes in CNS function, such as behavioural irritability, suspiciousness, speech slurring and minor visual misperceptions (Horne 1983). These may be accompanied by increased suggestibility and/or a reduction in motivation and willingness to perform tasks. In hospital this could impede mobilisation and other aspects of self-care. For patients in the community this could reduce efficiency at work and affect social and family relationships. Detrimental psychological effects of sleep deprivation observed in hospital patients include lethargy, irritability, confusion and, in more extreme cases, delusions and paranoia. Both acute and prolonged sleep disturbances, including delirium, have been observed following open heart surgery (Orr & Stahl 1977). Hartmann (1973) assessed sleep requirements by interview and questionnaire and found that stress and illness were virtually always accompanied by an increased subjective sleep need. Studies of coronary care patients have shown generally disturbed sleep, but suggest increased total sleep time (Karacan et al 1974, Broughton & Baron 1978). These observations support the hypothesis that sleep aids healing, suggesting that conditions favourable to sleep should be encouraged in all areas where patients are suffering from infection or trauma or are recovering following surgery.

> ? **25.2** Given that postoperative patients require frequent observation and attention, how can nurses help to ensure that these patients get adequate sleep in the period immediately following surgery?

NORMAL SLEEP

No matter what objective recordings of sleep might indicate about its duration, continuity or 'architecture', if the sleeper is satisfied with his sleep, then it may be considered to be normal. A good, restful, night's sleep and a good day's refreshed and efficient wakefulness are, of course, interrelated. Even though their relationship is not one of simple cause and effect, each depends on the quality of the other.

Individual requirements for sleep vary enormously. A range of 3–12 hours sleep per night has been cited as a normal range by Johns (1984). The average duration is about 7.5 hours, though the duration of sleep has a normal distribution (see Fig. 25.3).

Some people habitually take a nap during the day, while many do not. In addition, some people are early risers while others are more active in the evening and tend to go to bed late. The tendency of individuals to 'morningness' or 'eveningness' was first described by Horne & Ostberg (1976). Hospital routines tend to override these individual variations in behaviour, with a possible outcome of disturbed sleep patterns for some.

Factors affecting normal sleep

There are many factors which may affect normal sleep, including age, gender, diet and ambient temperature. These influences should be taken into account in nursing assessments of patients' sleep, since the normal habits and needs of individuals may bear little resemblance to one another.

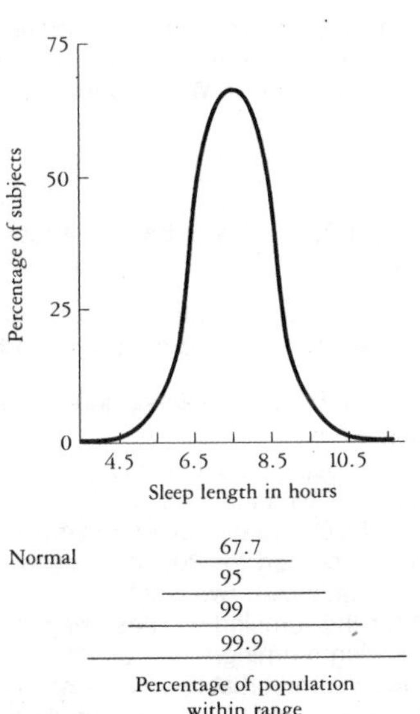

Fig. 25.3 Normal frequency curve of sleep durations. (From SLEEP, by J. Allan Hobson. Copyright (c) 1989 by J. Allan Hobson. Reprinted by permission of W. H. Freeman and Company.)

Age

The changes in sleep patterns associated with ageing are well documented (see Fig. 25.4). While neonates may spend 18 out of 24 hours asleep, young adults may sleep for 8 hours, while elderly individuals might sleep for 6. Elderly people tend to sleep less, to spend more time in bed, to have comparatively less stage 4 and REM sleep and to have more shifts between sleep stages than younger people (Williams et al 1974). McGhie & Russell (1962) found a significant increase in the proportion of patients over 65 years claiming to sleep for 5 hours or less compared with younger age groups.

These changes have been attributed to age-related loss of neurones and progressive fragmentation of circadian rhythmicity. Elderly people have increased amounts of wakefulness after sleep onset. Ancoli-Israel et al (1989) found that 41% of a sample of patients in a nursing home woke frequently due to apnoeic disturbances and leg jerks (see Research Abstract 25.1). Webb & Swinburne (1971) attributed 38% of night-time awakenings among elderly people to pain and physical discomforts such as bladder distension and urinary urgency. Awareness of such problems should prompt nurses to alleviate discomfort as far as possible and to encourage regular bowel and bladder habits (see Ch. 36).

Elderly people sustain an absolute and a relative reduction in time spent in stage 4 sleep, which may even disappear in a quarter of those in their sixth decade of life. Concurrently, they have an increased total duration of stage 1 sleep and an increase in the number of shifts into stage 1. The total sleep time (TST) is either reduced or unchanged in elderly people as compared with younger groups, though the time in bed tends to increase. This appears to be because older people spend more time lying in bed at night without attempting to sleep, or while unsuccessfully trying to sleep, and lying in bed resting or napping during the day. Obviously, these sleep patterns would be considered abnormal in a younger age group, but should cause no concern amongst the elderly; wards with large proportions of elderly patients should consequently adjust their routines in order to accommodate such sleep habits.

Zepelin et al (1984) studied subjects aged 18–71 years and found a correlation between a decline in the intensity of noise required to arouse individuals from sleep and increasing age. This reduction was present in all sleep stages but was greatest in stage 4. Since noise disturbs normal sleep stage progression and increases frequency of awakening, it may be that noise reduction in hospital is of particular importance in optimising the sleep of the elderly.

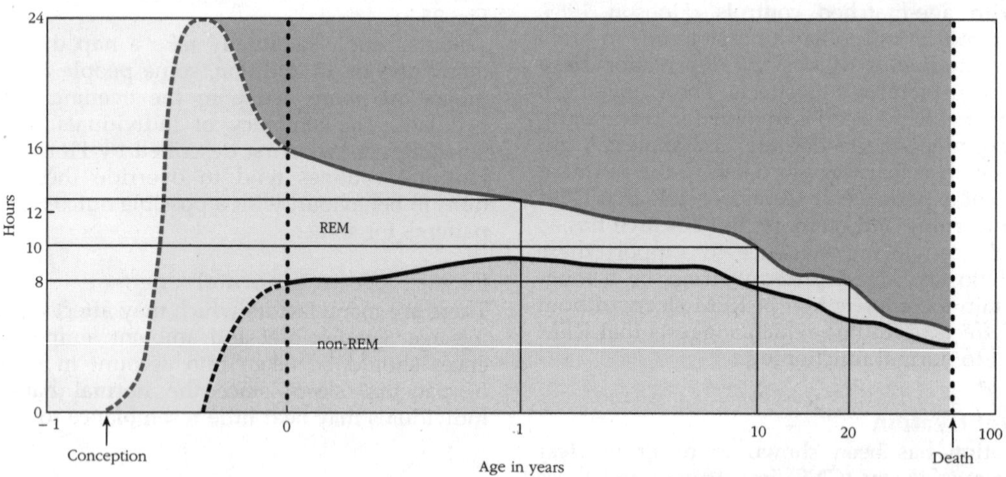

Fig. 25.4 Relative proportions of each 24-hour day spent awake, in REM sleep and in NREM sleep over a lifetime. (From SLEEP, by J. Allan Hobson. Copyright (c) 1989 by J. Allan Hobson. Reprinted by permission of W. H. Freeman and Company.)

Research abstract 25.1 Sleep fragmentation in patients from a nursing home

It is well known that elderly people tend to sleep poorly. Many try to lengthen their sleep by spending more time in bed. This then has a detrimental effect on sleep: increased time in bed makes sleep more fragmented and chronic bedrest interferes with the circadian sleep–wake rhythm.

The sleep of a group of institutionalised patients was monitored in order to compare it with that of similar elderly people in the community. Sleeping EEGs, respiratory movements and general body movements were recorded for 200 institutionalised elderly people. Recordings were made over two nights for 62% of the patients, and over one night for the remainder. These began at about 16.30 and finished the following morning.

Findings showed a remarkable amount of sleep disturbance and related daytime sleepiness. The average duration of time in bed was 15.5 hours, in which patients were asleep for about 8 hours and awake for 7.5 hours. In order to obtain that amount of sleep, the patients spent an extended amount of time in bed during the day, since they averaged no more than 39.5 minutes of sleep per hour in any hour of the night. Of the group studied, 50% woke up at least two or three times each hour; 41% had frequent disturbances due to sleep apnoea.

Although nursing home residents slept on average only one hour longer than elderly patients living independently, they had to spend substantially more time in bed to obtain the same amount of sleep.

Recommendations were made by the authors of the study to improve the sleep of elderly people by restricting time in bed, encouraging activity during the day and reducing daytime napping.

Ancoli-Israel S, Parker L, Sinaee R, Fell R L, Kripke D F 1989 Sleep fragmentation in patients from a nursing home. Journal of Gerontology 44(1): M18–21

For an elderly person the knowledge that degenerative changes in sleep patterns are commonly experienced and are therefore not necessarily pathological might be quite reassuring. Although some caution should be exercised lest treatable problems relating to sleep are overlooked, nurses have an important role to play in educating their patients about the predictable changes that occur in sleep habits with advancing age.

Gender
Research has shown that there are some interesting differences between the sexes in terms of their satisfaction with sleep. Men have more disturbances in sleep than women from early adulthood onward (Webb 1982), frequently due to nocturnal penile tumescence occurring during REM sleep. Wever (1984) found that women sleep significantly longer than men, although it is well recognised that women complain of problems with sleeping more than men do and that they consume far more sleep-inducing drugs. While this difference is evident from early adulthood, it becomes clearly marked in middle age.

Body weight
Crisp & Stonehill (1971) reported that weight gain is associated with an increased duration of sleep, while weight loss is associated with shorter sleep. This has been confirmed by several studies of anorexic individuals. As body weight falls, so does total sleep, which also becomes more broken and is interrupted by earlier waking. A small-scale study by Adam (1977) found a significant positive correlation between body weight and REM whereby the greater an individual's weight the more REM sleep he has. A larger study of 36 subjects by the same author (Adam 1987) confirmed that both total and percentage REM correlated with body weight, although the reasons for this were not clear.

Exercise
The effect of exercise on normal sleep is not straight-forward. Research studies have produced conflicting evidence: some have shown that exercise increases the duration of SWS, while some have found no effect and others a negative effect on sleep. It does appear, however, that exercise is *perceived* as having a sleep-promoting effect for many people (Vuori et al 1988) provided that it is not taken late in the evening.

Heredity
Finally, sleep quality and length appear to be influenced by genetic factors. This was demonstrated by Partinen et al (1983), who studied the sleep of 2238 monozygotic and 4545 dizygotic twin pairs. Familial clustering of narcolepsy (see p. 750) and idiopathic insomnia has also been observed. It may be worth noting a family history of sleep difficulties when assessing a patient, since it may not always be possible to remedy inherited sleep problems by means of nursing interventions.

?	**25.3** Discuss with your colleagues any changes in sleep patterns that have been experienced by elderly patients in your care.

COMMON SLEEP DISORDERS

Although the existence of sleep disorders has long been recognised, it is only in the past few decades that the seriousness of these has been acknowledged and a greater understanding of them has developed. Epidemiological studies in Europe and the USA have indicated that 14–40% of the population of Europe and the USA report difficulties in sleeping, with about 17% considering the problem to be serious. Insomnia is the most common complaint and may be defined as 'a subjective problem of insufficient or nonrestorative sleep despite an adequate opportunity to sleep' (Gillin & Byerley 1990). General practitioners have reported that one third of the subjective complaints made by their patients are of difficulties in sleeping.

Researchers have investigated sleep difficulties for patients at home and in hospital. A large multinational study of about 8000 patients in the community who had attended sleep clinics showed that 25% suffered from various insomnias, while 39% suffered from excessive daytime sleepiness (Coleman 1983). Smirne et al (1983) investigated sleep disorders of patients in general hospital wards, asking them about their sleep prior to admission. Of 2518 people, 25% reported some kind of sleep disturbance. These figures indicate that sleep presents difficulties for about a quarter of the population, posing a challenge to nurses in all fields of care.

There are different ways of grouping sleep disorders, but in 1979 the Sleep Disorders Classification Committee (Roffwarg 1979) produced a system which uses four basic categories based on sleep behaviour (see Box 25.1). These categories are not mutually exclusive; disorders of the first group, i.e. disorders of initiating and maintaining sleep (DIMS) often result in disorders belonging to the second group, i.e. disorders of excessive somnolence (DOES). DIMS and DOES will therefore be considered together in the following discussion.

Factors disrupting normal sleep: DIMS and DOES

Anxiety and depression
Anxiety and depression frequently interfere with sleep, and each of these is relatively common among the general population. Most people suffer at some time from occupational stress, family tension, bereavement, divorce, illness and so on. Admission to hospital may be a major cause of anxiety, with all the accompanying worries with regard to illness, investigations, surgery and so forth.

The increased activity of the sympathetic nervous system due to anxiety results in an increase in plasma noradrenaline levels. This in turn results in sleep changes similar to those seen in normal elderly adults (less stage 4 and REM sleep, and more stage shifts and awakenings), who also undergo elevations of daytime and night-time plasma noradrenaline.

Box 25.1 Sleep disorders classification (Roffwarg 1979)

1. Disorders of initiating and maintaining sleep (DIMS or insomnias)
Includes psychophysiological and psychiatric causes, problems relating to drug and alcohol use, sleep-induced respiratory impairment, sleep-related myoclonus and restless legs, medical, toxic and environmental causes, and others.

2. Disorders of excessive somnolence (DOES)
As above, plus narcolepsy and idiopathic CNS hypersomnolence.

3. Disorders of the sleep–wake schedule
Transient (due to jet lag/shift-work) and persistent.

4. Dysfunctions associated with sleep, sleep stages or partial arousals (parasomnias)
Includes sleepwalking, sleep terrors, sleep-related enuresis, bruxism (teeth-grinding), nightmares, sleep paralysis and others.

Insomnia due to depression has been associated with raised levels of monoamine oxidase, which catabolises the neurotransmitters noradrenaline and 5-HT, each of which is involved in sleep onset and maintenance. Depressed patients, therefore, tend to experience difficulty falling asleep; an increased number of awakenings during the night and early morning waking. Nursing staff should encourage depressed and anxious patients to discuss their feelings and, if possible, assist them to deal with underlying difficulties (see Ch. 17). Alerting medical staff to the apparent existence of anxiety and depression should ensure that the patient receives appropriate medical or psychological treatment.

Physical illness

Cardiac and pulmonary diseases often worsen during the night. The incidence of asthma attacks increases during the latter half of the night, while angina, cardiac dysrhythmias and nocturnal dyspnoea are all likely to worsen during sleep (see Ch. 3 and Ch. 2).

Metabolic disorders such as Cushing's disease, Addison's disease and diabetes mellitus may disrupt normal sleep patterns. Hyperthyroidism may reduce sleep time and hypothyroidism increase it (see Ch. 5). Diseases which mobilise the immune system, whether viral, bacterial or fungal, may result in increased sleepiness (see Ch. 16).

Since many areas of the brain are implicated in sleep regulation, any pathology impinging on these sites can cause problems. A rise in intracranial pressure from whatever cause increases sleepiness, while interference with the brainstem or hypothalamus may affect the onset and maintenance of sleep (see Ch. 9 and Ch. 30).

Sleep-induced nocturnal myoclonus

This condition is characterised by repetitive twitching of the legs occurring at regular intervals of 20–60 seconds. These episodes may last anywhere from a few minutes to several hours. Either or both legs may twitch. This does not always disturb the individual, unless he is a light sleeper or the twitching is severe enough to arouse him from 'deep' sleep. Associated with this condition is restless-legs syndrome, where an unpleasant, crawling sensation is experienced in the calves or thighs. Nocturnal myoclonus has been associated with the use of tricyclic antidepressant drugs (see Ch. 17, p. 589) and chronic uraemia (see Ch. 8, p. 321).

Narcolepsy

This disorder occurs in about 4 per 10 000 people and can be described as an imbalance between wakefulness, REM sleep and NREM sleep. Sleep frequently intrudes into wakefulness, and this change in conscious state is often triggered by strong emotions such as anger or laughter. It is REM sleep which intrudes, either partially or totally, producing the possibility of four different symptoms, as follows:

- excessive daytime sleepiness
- cataplexy, when only the muscular paralysis of REM occurs: the sufferer may be awake but is paralysed
- sleep paralysis, a type of cataplexy which occurs at sleep onset. Paralysis which occurs on waking from REM is benign
- REM dreaming during wakefulness: hypnagogic hallucinations.

Pain

Sleep problems are commonly experienced by people who live with chronic pain. Such pain may be due to arthritis, cancer and low back injury and is often described as intractable. Some types of chronic pain, such as that from gastric ulcers or dyspepsia, have a circadian rhythm of increasing intensity at night. GPs tend to manage such pain pharmacologically, sometimes by aiming to relieve the cause but more often providing symptomatic relief by means of analgesics. Sometimes the use of antidepressant drugs is successful, since some chronic pain syndromes can be associated with depression.

Nurses are closely involved in the delivery of pain relief in hospital because of their 24-hour contact with patients. Jones et al (1979) studied intensive care patients and found that pain was ranked second to discomfort as contributing to sleep loss. Pain has been shown to be a major cause of sleep loss in the postoperative period (see Research Abstract 25.2; Seers 1987). Subsequent research (Closs 1991) showed that postoperative patients had strong views about sleep and pain (see Box 25.2). If nurses are to be able to help patients cope with pain, they must perform an accurate nursing assessment of their quality of sleep (see p. 752).

Diet

There has been much research into the effects of diet on sleep. Brezinova & Oswald (1972) investigated the reasons why Horlicks malted beverage seems to enhance sleep. A link was noted between habitual bedtime practices and sleep: those who normally ate little or nothing before bedtime had no improvement in sleep after having Horlicks, while those who usually did have a bedtime drink slept better after Horlicks. Hot milky drinks are usually provided in hospital in the late evening, but these may not suit everyone. It should

Research abstract 25.2 A nursing study of sleep on surgical wards

In this study, 200 surgical patients were interviewed about their sleep. Reports of usual sleep patterns at home and matched questions about a specific night in hospital were recorded. Sleep habits and environmental factors were also taken into account. Nurses' recordings of sleep were examined.

Most patients felt that their sleep was worse in hospital than at home. They reported that both their time of settling down to sleep and their time of morning waking had been brought forward by almost one hour. Significantly less time was spent asleep at night and more night-time awakenings occurred.

A large number of factors disturbing sleep during the night were cited by patients; pain or discomfort was the most common, followed by noise, environmental temperature and dissatisfaction with beds. Other factors affecting sleep indices included gender, living alone, ward designs, type of mattress and use of hypnotic drugs.

Nurses' recordings of patients' sleep tended to be brief, usually offering a qualitative description. In many cases no mention of patients' sleep was made.

On the basis of these and other findings, several recommendations were made for nursing practice, education, management and research.

Closs S J 1988a A nursing study of sleep on surgical wards. Nursing Research Unit report. Dept of Nursing Studies, University of Edinburgh

Box 25.2 What patients say about postoperative sleep and pain (From Closs 1991)

- Effects of tiredness on postoperative pain:
  'The pain is more nagging and it's harder to put up with if you're tired.'
  'If you're tired, the pain's more draining, more severe, a down-puller. It can actually make you feel depressed.'
  'If you're tired and in pain you want to give up quicker. You could have shot me yesterday for all I cared.'
- Effects of sleep on pain intensity:
  'If you've slept well the pain isn't as bad a blow when you waken. If you don't sleep you wonder when it'll ever end. It's a vicious circle.'
  'If you're tired you're narky, if you're narky it hurts worse.'
  'Sleep makes you relax and takes away some of the pain.'
- Effects of sleep on coping with pain:
  'It's essential — you can't cope with anything unless you've slept, especially pain.'
  'You're not so well able to cope if you're tired, you have a good attitude if you're rested.'
  'It's impossible to cope properly if you haven't slept well.'
- Effects of sleep on recovery:
  'Sleep is the best healer in the world. You know it's going to take longer to get better if you can't get your sleep.'
  'You've got to get a good sleep before you get anything else. You feel fresh and don't get crabby, you can deal with the pain and everything else and it speeds up your recovery.'
  'Sleep is a great healer — that's why I don't understand why they wake you up early in the morning. I think why? What is it for? Certainly not for the patient. It makes you agitated. It's all done to their rules.'

be remembered that many people take an alcoholic 'nightcap' at home, and if they are normally heavy drinkers they will suffer from withdrawal symptoms in hospital if they are not permitted to drink.

Withdrawal from alcohol will result in disturbed sleep, as will withdrawal of hypnotics (sleep-inducing drugs). It should be noted that alcohol is not a good hypnotic, since although it accelerates sleep onset it disturbs sleep patterns later on in the night (Williams et al 1983) and can cause early waking due to a full bladder. Drinks such as tea, coffee and cola contain caffeine and therefore act as stimulants, disturbing normal sleep patterns. Karacan et al (1976) showed that coffee disturbed sleep even in those who felt unaffected by it.

In recent years there has been some controversy over the role of tryptophan, the amino acid precursor of 5-HT. Tryptophan is found in small amounts in most food proteins. It has been suggested that a high tryptophan diet enhances sleep, but as yet there is no convincing evidence to support this hypothesis. Little information is available regarding the effects of other nutritional substances, though Vitiello et al (1983) found that for a group of 10 healthy adult males a low sodium diet decreased REM and SWS and increased wakefulness.

The biochemical effects of diet on sleep are unclear, but avoiding stimulants and adhering to routines appears to enhance sleep. Although research in this area has so far been inconclusive, community nurses might be able to help poor sleepers simply by giving them dietary advice, while hospital nurses should allow patients to eat or drink as they would at home prior to bedtime, as far as that is feasible.

Drugs

There are many drugs which affect sleep, hypnotics being perhaps the best known. In addition there are many others which have side-effects on sleep; these include antidepressants, antihistamines, anticonvulsants and alcohol. L-dopa and beta blockers may produce vivid dreams and nightmares, while diuretics produce bladder distension and therefore nocturia. Other drugs such as amphetamines and caffeine stimulate the CNS, delaying sleep onset and reducing total sleep time.

Sleep position and bedrest

Sleep positions have been associated with objective and subjective sleep quality. Poor sleepers appear to spend a greater proportion of their time on their backs with their heads straight and to change position more frequently than better sleepers (Koninck et al 1983). Snoring and sleep apnoea have been associated with subjects who sleep flat on their backs. Since these symptoms are undesirable for the sleeper himself, and snoring may disturb others sleeping within earshot, nurses could perhaps encourage and assist poor sleepers to adopt alternative positions for sleeping.

Long periods of bed-rest have been shown to disrupt other aspects of circadian rhythmicity. Winget Deroshia, Markley & Holley (1984) found that after 56 days of bedrest the body temperature waveform remained the same but was at a lower level. This 'low-grade hypothermia' occurred in conjunction with a gradual increase in heart rate. According to Selye (1950) these changes are characteristic of acute stress, regardless of its cause.

Respiration

Hypoventilation and breathing irregularities are common during normal sleep but may sometimes be clinically important. Normal changes include the hypoxaemia and hypercapnia due to the slight reduction in metabolic rate which occurs during NREM sleep; in REM sleep irregular breathing is the norm.

Total sleep deprivation appears to reduce the hypercapnic ventilatory response by about one fifth and the hypoxic response by almost one third. Conversely, animal studies have shown that hypercapnia and hypoxaemia increase sleep onset latency, decrease total sleep time, increase the duration of episodes of wakefulness and prolong episodes of REM (Winget, Deroshia, Markley & Holley 1984). Although these experiments did not involve humans, the suggestion that hypoxia and hypercapnia interfere with normal sleep patterns could be seen to have implications for nursing. Patients at home who have respiratory difficulties might benefit from advice regarding sleep position and the use of pillows to prop themselves up in order to maximise lung expansion. In hospital, nurses should ensure that any patients with respiratory difficulties (such as postoperative patients or those with respiratory tract infections) receive adequate support and assistance, particularly regarding oxygen administration, posture, deep breathing and coughing.

Sleep apnoea syndrome

This problem was first recognised about 20 years ago. The literal meaning of sleep apnoea is cessation of breathing during sleep. Often these episodes are repetitive and each may last up to a minute or even longer. Such apnoeas frequently cause the sleeper to wake, in some cases many times during the night. The main symptom resulting from this disorder is usually daytime sleepiness, though some sufferers complain of insomnia.

There are two main types of sleep apnoea. Central sleep apnoea is caused by impaired neurological control of breathing, so that the intercostal muscles fail to contract. Obstructive apnoea is the result of obstruction of the airway, such as by large tonsils, a large or oedematous soft palate, fat deposits around the airway, retrognathia or micrognathia (see Ch. 15). The cause may be treated if the problem becomes severe. Obesity is common among these patients, in which case weight loss is usually the first approach to relieving the problem. Corrective surgery may be required in other cases.

Temperature

Even slight changes in ambient (room) temperature may affect an individual's normal sleep–wake cycle. Kendel & Schmidt-Kessen (1973) pointed out that unclothed and uncovered subjects awoke from cold at 26 °C and below. Total sleep deprivation has been shown to decrease the mean daily body temperature and to increase subjective feelings of cold (Horne 1985). Fever is associated with a greater number of awakenings, increased total waking time and reduced amounts of SWS and REM sleep. Elevated ambient temperature produces similar results (Karacan et al 1978). The duration of the REM phase is shortened in artificially induced fever as well as at high ambient temperature. Zulley (1980) found that the higher the body temperature at sleep onset the longer the duration of sleep, while REM sleep was negatively correlated with body temperature. These findings suggest that active management of pyrexial patients, perhaps by giving antipyretic drugs such as aspirin (or paracetamol for children), might improve their sleep.

Room temperature should be carefully monitored on general wards so that it may be maintained at a comfortable level, and patients should be encouraged to request more or fewer bedclothes as required. Elderly people are particularly vulnerable, especially at home, since their ability to perceive temperature changes is often diminished. Community nurses are well placed to identify at least some of those individuals susceptible to hypothermia, and have a useful role in advising them about adequate clothing, bedding and so on (see Ch. 22, p. 685).

Noise

Noise can disturb sleep under all sorts of circumstances. In the home, mothers may wake at the slightest whimper from their children, while others successfully adjust to the difficulties of living under noisy flight paths near airports. Although noise is often detrimental to sleep, there are occasions when the opposite is the case. People often become used to noise at night. For example, those who live near a busy main road may have great difficulty sleeping in a quiet environment. Similarly, town dwellers might have problems sleeping for the first few nights of a quiet country holiday, or a patient who has a long stay in a noisy hospital ward might have some difficulty readjusting to the quietness of his home environment. Individuals become habituated to the normal circumstances surrounding their sleep.

In hospital, noise poses a considerable problem, particularly in acute areas (Hilton 1985, Soutar & Wilson 1986). Closs (1988a) found that patients' sleep was disturbed by a wide variety of sounds, including noise made by other patients, nurses talking, footsteps, telephones, traffic, equipment alarms, squeaky doors, trolleys, rattling windows and many others. If possible, nurses should acquaint their more long-term patients with the unfamiliar sounds on the ward. This may help them to become accustomed to these noises and develop the ability to sleep through them. While some noise is unavoidable at night, careful maintenance of equipment and precautions such as wearing soft-soled shoes can considerably improve the night-time hospital environment.

?	**25.4** Mr B is a 47-year-old man who had an appendicectomy three days ago. His physical recovery has been straightforward, but he is feeling very tired and has been finding it difficult to sleep at night. Consequently, he has been reluctant to mobilise and has been taking short naps throughout the day. Construct a care plan, giving possible reasons for Mr B's inadequate sleep, suggesting possible nursing interventions and stating the expected outcome of these.	A

Parasomnias

Sleepwalking

This behaviour, when it occurs, commences during SWS, although the somnambulist appears to be in a part-sleeping, part-waking state. It can be very dangerous: sufferers have been known to walk out of windows and to attack family members. During an episode of sleepwalking the individual is usually uncommunicative and returns to bed spontaneously, rarely remembering the event the next morning. Sleepwalking is difficult to treat, so it is advisable to take precautions such as locking windows at night.

Night terrors and nightmares

Night terrors also arise during SWS and occur mostly in children. The sufferer often screams and shows signs of panic, such as a dramatic rise in heart rate, respiratory distress and sweating. He may be very difficult to arouse, but usually calms down within a few minutes, usually without waking up. Most people remember nothing about the incident. Nightmares occur during REM sleep and are often remembered very vividly on waking.

METHODS OF ASSESSING SLEEP

Assessing a patient's sleep is not an easy task. Inadequacies in the assessment of sleep appropriate to nursing practice persist, since as yet there are no valid and reliable methods available. While sleep assessment in clinical settings has been attempted by many researchers, the methods used have not always been suitable for general use by nurses (Closs 1988b). In general, these methods of assessing sleep can be classified into groups: those which rely on patients' subjective reports of their sleep, and those which obtain objective measurements of either physiological events which coincide with sleep or psychological attributes reflecting the effects of sleep (see Box 25.3).

Many of the objective methods of sleep assessment available involve the use of expensive and sometimes unwieldy equipment. In most cases nurses would neither have access to such equipment nor the expertise to use it. In addition, although these methods may be suitable for relatively healthy, stress-free individuals, most hospital patients would pro-

Box 25.3 Approaches to the assessment of sleep (Closs 1988b)

Subjective assessment of sleep
- Visual analogue scales
- Subjective rating scales
- Questionnaires
- Interviews
- Daily sleep charting (sleep diary)

Objective assessment of associated physiological/ psychological events
- Polysomnography
- Observation of sleeper
- Arousal thresholds
- Body movements
- Vigilance and sleepiness
- Electrodermal activity

bably find such monitoring anxiety-provoking, restrictive or uncomfortable.

Nursing assessment of sleep

The assessment of sleep is an important part of the general assessment of patients. While it is appropriate for researchers and clinicians in other disciplines to use sophisticated monitoring equipment, nurses must rely on their communication skills, i.e. on what patients tell them. Although people are unable to give accurate reports of the actual time it takes them to fall asleep, or how long they lie awake in the small hours, they can give reliable accounts of changes in their sleep patterns. For example, people suffering from insomnia will generally overestimate how long it takes them to fall asleep, and underestimate how long they spend asleep, but will nonetheless give realistic reports of changes in their sleep habits.

Although in hospital it is possible for nurses to observe patients during the night, this is a notoriously inaccurate way to determine the quality or quantity of someone's sleep (Aurell & Elmqvist 1985). In a home care setting, patients' reports of sleep are all the nurse has to go on. Consequently, the ability of nurses to make useful assessments of sleep depends on the acquisition of good communication skills. As Morgan (1987) points out, the only realistic method of assessing the quality of a patient's sleep is to ask him about it. Not all patients, of course, will be able to give their own account. In such cases, information might be gained from non-verbal clues, the descriptions provided by relatives and carers, and from nursing and medical records.

Communication skills in the assessment of sleep

Communication between patients and nurses in hospital wards has been studied by Faulkner (1979) and Macleod Clark (1983), who both found that patients' queries were frequently blocked by nurses, that communications were often discouraged and that patients were typically asked questions which were closed or leading. If patients are to communicate their concerns they must be given clear opportunities to do so. This applies to community nurses as much as to hospital nurses, although the former are more likely to identify chronic rather than acute problems. Encouraging patients, where possible, to talk about themselves, their feelings and their needs is vital. The use of open-ended questions and prompts can facilitate disclosure. For example, a closed question such as 'Did you sleep well last night?' is more likely to produce a polite and possibly meaningless 'Yes, thank you' than the question, 'How did you sleep last night?' The latter query provides a clearer invitation for the patient to inform the nurse of any difficulties. If the patient appears reluctant to complain, it could be helpful to follow up such a question with gentle prompting.

Body language is also important here: patients are less likely to be forthcoming if the nurse speaks from an uncomfortable distance, looking as if she is about to leave for some more important task. Planned nurse–patient interactions can provide ample opportunities for discussion and nursing assessment. In addition to general questioning about sleep, nurses might ask some specific questions. These could include details such as time of settling down to sleep, time of morning waking, duration of sleep, night-time disturbances, diet, medication, pain, anxieties and so on. The patient's disclosures should be recorded in nursing notes so that each nurse participating in his care is aware of his needs (see Ch. 26, p. 769).

Once an assessment of the patient's sleep has been made, nursing care relevant to sleeping habits may be planned. Nurses can help by providing information about sleep that enables patients to have realistic expectations. In addition, they can give basic guidelines for improving sleep through attention to sleep hygiene, i.e. behaviour and attitudes conducive to healthy sleep patterns. Among the factors concerned are attitudes towards sleep, the sleep environment, attention to diet, sleep scheduling, pre-sleep activities and daytime behaviours. If the patient requires specialised help, it is up to the nurse to alert the appropriate professionals. In the community this may be the GP or clinical psychologist, while in hospital it is usually the house officer.

HELPING PATIENTS TO SLEEP

The points listed in Box 25.4 should be borne in mind by nurses as they assist patients to cultivate healthy sleep patterns.

?	25.5 A middle-aged woman complains to a community nurse that she is having great difficulty in getting to sleep at night. She says that as a result she needs to take naps during the day. In addition she has found no help from taking drinking chocolate immediately before going to bed. What advice could the nurse give?

PHARMACOLOGICAL TREATMENTS FOR INSOMNIA

Hypnotic drugs

The major treatments available for insomnia are pharmacological. The majority of hypnotics which are currently prescribed belong to the benzodiazepine group, and include temazepam, triazolam, nitrazepam and others. These provide temporary, symptomatic relief and are not a cure. The sleep produced by these drugs does not resemble natural sleep: the duration of stage 2 sleep is increased at the expense of REM sleep and SWS. Adam (1984) pointed out, however, that even though the structure of sleep is changed by these drugs, most physiological processes associated with SWS continue as usual. It is difficult, therefore, to comment on the difference between the quality of sleep induced by hypnotics, and that of normal sleep.

The effects of benzodiazepines vary, particularly with regard to their duration of action. Nitrazepam has quite long-lasting

Box 25.4 Basic information and advice for poor sleepers

1. Patients' expectations of sleep should be realistic. Many people think that there is something wrong with their sleep if they do not get 8 hours every night. Such incorrect assumptions may in themselves cause anxiety and sleep disturbance. The great individual differences in sleep requirements and the normal effects of ageing should be clearly explained in order to instil realistic attitudes towards sleep.

2. Most people experience short episodes of poor sleep for which no particular treatment is needed. There is no evidence that transient insomnia has a detrimental effect on health. Chronic insomnia (lasting for at least 3 weeks) may require detailed assessment and treatment. If it is clear that the insomnia is transient, nurses may be able to reassure their patients on this point, and in so doing help them to overcome insomnia by reducing their anxiety about sleep loss.

3. People suffering from insomnia tend to stay in bed even when they are unable to sleep. This interferes with their sleep by reducing the psychological association between bed and sleep. They should, if possible, avoid going to bed until they are sleepy, and if they cannot sleep, they should then get up and do something else. For example, they might read, watch television or engage in any other activity they enjoy, preferably something relaxing.

4. It helps to establish a regular time of waking up in the morning, even if the previous night's sleep was unsatisfactory. This strengthens the circadian rhythm, and should be adhered to at weekends as well as weekdays. A reliable alarm clock or perhaps the assistance of a relative can help to ensure a regular waking time.

5. Patients who have difficulty sleeping at night may reduce their night-time sleep drive if they take daytime naps. Avoiding daytime naps also helps to reinforce circadian rhythmicity. Naps may be avoided by planning activities that can coincide with the times that naps are desired, so that there is always an alternative to napping available. If a post-lunch nap is to be missed, for example, the individual could plan to walk the dog or fetch a newspaper at that particular time.

6. Poor sleepers should try to reserve the evening hours for relaxation and leisure activities. They should avoid strenuous mental or physical exertion immediately preceding bedtime, with the exception of sexual activity, which may increase relaxation and encourage sleep. The development of calming pre-sleep rituals such as reading can help patients drift off to sleep.

7. Hunger and thirst can disturb sleep. If this is a problem, a light snack should be taken at bedtime. This may be anything, provided that it does not contain stimulants. A milky drink and a biscuit, or a piece of fruit may be appropriate. There is no evidence to suggest that eating cheese before going to sleep has any adverse effects. Some may wish to keep a drink beside the bed in case they wake up during the night feeling thirsty.

8. Many poor sleepers are sensitive to the stimulants found in some foods. It takes at least 8 hours to metabolise caffeine, so caffeine-containing beverages and foods should be omitted from the diet after midday. This includes tea, coffee, cola and chocolate. It is possible to buy caffeine-free tea and cola as well as coffee, for those who wish to take such drinks in the evening.

9. Sleep is disturbed by the use of nicotine as well as by withdrawal from nicotine. Thus the prevention of disturbed sleep is yet another good reason for not smoking. The role of the nurse as health educator is important here since many people are unaware of any connection between smoking and poor sleep.

10. Although small amounts of alcohol hasten sleep onset, larger amounts disturb sleep later on in the night. The detrimental effects of alcohol on sleep can therefore outweigh any benefits. Again, the nurse may have an opportunity to provide health education in this regard, as it is a common misconception that alcohol enhances sleep.

11. The sleep-disturbing side-effects of drugs such as antihypertensives and antiasthmatics should be understood. It might be that the patient has not linked his sleep difficulty with his medication. An explanation of such a connection could provide valuable reassurance. If disturbed sleep is accounted for in a rational manner in this way, the patient may perceive it as less of a problem.

12. Sudden noises are more disturbing than constant ones. If occasional loud noise is inevitable, using earplugs or masking the disturbing noise with a monotonous background sound such as that made by an electric fan can help.

13. Nurses should endeavour to create conditions favourable for sleep. Most people sleep best in a quiet, darkened room on a firm mattress which is large enough to allow movement and stretching. Individual preferences, however, should be respected as far as is feasible.

14. Being too hot or too cold can disturb sleep. Ambient temperature should be comfortable, and the amount and type of bedding adjusted to suit the individual.

effects and is used less commonly than other forms, particularly among the elderly, in whom the drug's 'hangover effect' may cause loss of balance resulting in falls. Triazolam has effects of very short duration, while those of temazepam last for a moderate period. Short-acting hypnotics tend to be favoured, since they are less likely to produce hangover effects during the day.

While these drugs are initially effective in inducing sleep, their regular use produces 'tolerance'. As time goes on the body requires increasingly large doses of the drug to achieve the same effect. It has been suggested that the effectiveness of most hypnotic drugs is diminished after 3–14 days of use (Committee on the Review of Medicines 1980). This should be borne in mind when such hypnotics are to be used as premedication.

Although benzodiazepine hypnotics can provide short-term improvement in sleep, long-term use can result in more problems with sleep. After an initial improvement, hypnotics may actually cause tiredness because of the reduction in SWS and REM sleep. When hynotics are withdrawn the patient may suffer from rebound insomnia. This involves extreme feelings of edginess, greater difficulty in falling asleep and more intense dreams and nightmares. These symptoms gradually diminish over time. In spite of these drawbacks the short-term use of hypnotics can be highly beneficial. For example, an anxious patient due to have surgery may greatly benefit from the limited use of hypnotics over, perhaps, 3 or 4 perioperative nights.

A new hypnotic drug, zopiclone, has been shown to be as effective as the benzodiazepines while producing far fewer side-effects (Goa & Heel 1986). It belongs to a group of drugs called the cyclopyrrolones, a new class of psychotherapeutic agents. The main drawback of zopiclone is its prohibitive cost; otherwise, it appears to have considerable potential for widespread use. Other hypnotics presently used include chloral hydrate and its derivative, dichloralphenazone, which are prescribed mainly for the elderly.

Herbal remedies

Although several herbs are claimed to have sleep-inducing properties, valerian is the only one whose use has been scientifically evaluated. Valerian taken in capsules has been shown to reduce significantly the time taken to fall asleep. However, other, unproven herbal remedies may be effective by virtue of a placebo effect (see Ch. 19, p. 628).

PSYCHOLOGICAL AND BEHAVIOURAL TREATMENTS FOR INSOMNIA

While pharmacological treatments of insomnia are palliative, psychological treatments aim to deal with the cause of the sleeplessness. In some cases insomnia may be attributed to physiological or psychological over-activity. Stress is a common cause of sleep disturbance and can be dealt with by a variety of techniques (see Ch. 17, pp. 587–590). However, some individuals who suffer from insomnia are constitutionally poor sleepers who are unlikely to respond to any treatment. These people usually have difficulties sleeping throughout their lives, and the process of ageing is likely to further reduce the quality of their sleep. For those whose sleeplessness is asso-ciated with physiological or psychological hyperactivity, many non-pharmacological methods of treating insomnia have been attempted, with varying degrees of success. Four of the most widely known are discussed below. These are relaxation therapy, paradoxical intention, associative learning technique and cognitive therapy. The choice of strategy depends on the cause of the sleeplessness, individual temperament and personal preference.

Relaxation techniques

Emotional problems such as anxiety can be modified using various types of relaxation therapy, which aims to reduce physical and mental tension. Autogenic training teaches people to concentrate on sensations of warmth and heaviness in their limbs by repeated suggestion. Progressive muscular relaxation achieves a similar effect by the alternate tensing and relaxing of a series of muscles. These methods have been successful in helping people fall asleep and increasing their satisfaction with sleep (Borkovec 1982, Lacks 1987).

Paradoxical intention

Paradoxical intention has been used with success in the treatment of patients who are particularly anxious about their difficulty in falling asleep. This anxiety produces the opposite of the desired effect, making patients too tense to fall asleep. When such individuals are instructed to stay awake all night their anxiety about falling asleep is reduced, paradoxically allowing them to relax and fall asleep (Ascher 1980).

Associative learning technique

This is a useful technique where the bed and the bedroom have become associated in the patient's mind with sleeplessness. For such people going to bed is an aversive stimulus which produces an aroused state. Bootzin (1972) devised a method of avoiding all behaviours in the bedroom not associated with sleep, such as reading, eating, watching television, or just lying awake. Individuals are instructed to go to bed only when they are sleepy, and to get up if they lie awake for more than 10 minutes. Eventually this re-establishes the psychological association between bed and sleep.

Cognitive therapy

The techniques embraced by the term cognitive therapy include meditation and guided imagery (see Ch. 17). A third technique, cognitive refocusing, can be used by an individual who is plagued by intrusive and repetitive thoughts which keep him awake. Usually these are problems and worries which the individual can learn to control, first by recognising that he cannot solve his problems by turning them over and over in his mind at night. Second, the individual learns to suppress the troubling thoughts, often by concentrating on alternative, benign thoughts.

For the most part, therapies for helping individuals to overcome sleeping difficulties are currently provided by clinical psychologists. While in some areas of the UK it may be possible for community patients to be referred to such specialists for help, clinical psychologists are a rare commodity in most general hospitals. If nurses could be educated in some of the simpler techniques (such as relaxation therapy) they might well be able to make a significant contribution to helping patients to sleep. Since sleep is such a fundamental activity of life, this extension of the nurse's role would seem perfectly legitimate.

CONCLUSION

Sleep is a complex and universal behaviour which is prone to disruption by numerous internal and external influences. Since everyone needs sleep, every nurse needs to understand it, and to know how patients may be helped when problems arise. This chapter has offered basic information on the structure and function of sleep, the importance of the sleep–wake cycle, normal and abnormal causes of sleep disturbance and strategies for treating patients' problems. The most crucial point to remember is that everyone is different: behaviours, attitudes and problems are highly individual. Consequently, nursing care both in hospital and in the patient's home should include careful assessment of sleep, since many difficulties can be overcome by simple changes in lifestyle and by adjustments to the individual's expectations of sleep. Where more serious problems occur, help from other health care professionals may be needed.

REFERENCES

Adam K 1977 Body weight correlates with REM sleep. British Medical Journal 1: 813–814

Adam K 1984 Are poor sleepers turned into good sleepers by hypnotic drugs? In: Hindmarch I, Ott H, Roth T (eds) Sleep, benzodiazepines and performance. Springer-Verlag, Berlin, pp 44–45

Adam K 1987 Total and percentage REM sleep correlate with body weight in 36 middle-aged people. Sleep 10(1): 69–77

Ancoli-Israel S, Parker L, Sinaee R, Fell R L, Kripke D F 1989 Sleep fragmentation in patients from a nursing home. Journal of Gerontology 44(1): M18–21

Ascher L M 1980 Paradoxical intention. In: Goldstein A, Foa E B (eds) Handbook of behavioural interventions: a clinical guide, p 266–321. Wiley, New York

Aurell J, Elmqvist D 1985 Sleep in the surgical intensive care unit: continuous polygraphic recording of sleep in nine patients receiving post-operative care. British Medical Journal 290: 1029–1032

Bootzin R R 1972 Stimulus control treatment for insomnia (summary). Proceedings of the 80th annual convention of the American Psychological Association 7: 395–396

Borkovec T D 1982 Insomnia. Journal of Consulting and Clinical Psychology 50(6): 880–895

Brezinova V, Oswald I 1972 Sleep after a night-time beverage. British Medical Journal 2(5811): 431–433

Broughton R, Baron R 1978 Sleep patterns in the intensive care unit and on the ward after acute myocardial infarction. Electroencephalography and Clinical Neurophysiology 45: 348–360

Closs S J 1988a A nursing study of sleep on surgical wards. Nursing Research Unit report. Department of Nursing Studies, University of Edinburgh

Closs S J 1988b Assessment of sleep in hospital patients: a review of methods. Journal of Advanced Nursing 13: 501–510

Closs S J 1991 A nursing study of patients' night-time sleep, pain and analgesic provision following abdominal surgery. Nursing Research Unit report. Department of Nursing Studies, University of Edinburgh

Coleman R M 1983 Diagnosis, treatment and follow-up of about 8000 sleep/wake disorder patients. In: Guilleminault C, Lugaresi E (eds) Sleep/wake disorders: natural history, epidemiology and long term evolution. Raven Press, New York, pp 87–97

Committee on the Review of Medicines 1980 Systematic review of the benzodiazepines. British Medical Journal 282: 910–912

Crisp A H, Stonehill E 1971 Aspects of the relationship between psychiatric states, sleep, nocturnal motility and nutrition. Journal of Psychosomatic Research 15: 501–509

Czeisler C A, Moore-Ede M C, Coleman R M 1982 Rotating shift work schedules that disrupt sleep are improved by applying circadian principles. Science 217: 460–463

Floyd J A 1984 Interaction between personal sleep–wake rhythms and psychiatric hospital rest–activity schedule. Nursing Research 33(5): 255–259

Faulkner A 1979 Monitoring nurse–patient conversation in a ward. Nursing Times Occasional Paper 75(35): 95–96

Gillin J C, Byerley W F 1990 The diagnosis and management of insomnia. The New England Journal of Medicine 322(4): 239–248

Goa K L, Heel R C 1986 Zopiclone: a review of its pharmacodynamic and pharmacokinetic properties and therapeutic efficacy as a hypnotic. Drugs 32: 48–65

Hartmann E L 1973 The functions of sleep. Yale University Press, New Haven & London

Hilton B A 1985 Noise in acute patient care areas. Research in Nursing and Health 8(3): 283–291

Hobson J A 1989 Sleep. Scientific American Library, New York

Horne J A 1983 Human sleep and tissue restitution: some qualifications and doubts. Clinical Science 65: 569–578

Horne J A 1985 Sleep function with particular reference to sleep deprivation. Annals of Clinical Research 17(5): 199–208

Horne J A 1988 Why we sleep: the functions of sleep in humans and other mammals. Oxford University Press, Oxford

Horne J A, Ostberg O 1976 A self-assessment questionnaire to determine morningness – eveningness in human circadian rhythm. International Journal of Chronobiology 4: 97–110

Ioffe S, Jansen A H, Chernick V 1984 Hypercapnia alters sleep state pattern. Sleep 7(3): 219–222

Johns M W 1984 Normal sleep. In: Priest R G (ed) Sleep: an international monograph. Update Books, ch 1.

Jones J, Hoggart B, Withey J, Donaghue K, Ellis B W 1979 What the patients say: a study of reactions to an intensive care unit. Intensive Care Medicine 5: 89–92

Karacan I, Green J R, Taylor W J et al 1974 Sleep in post myocardial infarction patients. Cited in: Eliot R S (ed) Contemporary problems in cardiology: stress and the heart. Futura Publications, pp 163–195

Karacan I, Thornby J I, Anch M, Booth G H, Williams R L, Sallis P J 1976 Dose-related sleep disturbances induced by coffee and caffeine. Clinical Pharmacology and Therapeutics 20: 682–689

Karacan I, Thornby J I, Anch A M, William R L 1978 The effects of high ambient temperature on sleep in young men. Sleep Research 7: 171

Kendel J, Schmidt-Kessen W 1973 The influence of room temperature on night-time sleep in man (Polygraphic night-sleep recordings in the climate chamber). In: Koella W P, Levin P (eds) Sleep. Karger, Basel, pp 423–425

Koninck J, De Gagnon P, Lallier S 1983 Sleep positions in the young adult and their relationship with the subjective quality of sleep. Sleep 6(1): 52–59

Kreuger J M, Bacsik J, Garcia-Arraras J 1980 Sleep promoting material from human urine and its relation to factor S from the brain. American Journal of Physiology 238: E116–123

Lacks P 1987 Behavioural treatment for persistent insomnia. Pergamon Press, New York

MacLeod Clark J 1983 Nurse–patient communication in surgical wards. In: Wilson-Barnett J (ed) Nursing Research: ten studies in patient care. Wiley, Chichester

McGhie A, Russell S 1962 The subjective assessment of normal sleep patterns. Journal of Mental Science 108: 642–654

Monnier M, Gaillard J 1980 Biochemical regulation of sleep. Experientia 36: 21–24

Morgan K 1987 Sleep and ageing, 12. Croom Helm, London & Sydney

Orr W C, Stahl M L 1977 Sleep disturbances after open heart surgery. American Journal of Cardiology 39: 196–201

Oswald I 1984 Good, poor and disordered sleep. In: Priest R G (ed) Sleep: an international monograph. Update Books, ch 2.

Partinen M, Kaprio J, Koskenvuo M, Langinvainio H 1983 Genetic and environmental determination of human sleep. Sleep 6(3): 179–185

Rechtschaffen A, Kales A 1968 A manual of standardised terminology, techniques and scoring system for sleep stages of human subjects. US Dept of Health, Education and Welfare, Bethesda, M D

Rechtschaffen A, Gilliland M A, Bergman B M, Winter J B 1983 Physiological correlates of prolonged sleep deprivation in rats. Science 221: 182–184

Roffwarg H P (ed) 1979 Diagnostic classification of sleep and arousal disorders. Sleep 2: 1–137

Ryan A T, Megirian D 1982 Sleep-wake patterns of intact and carotid sinus nerve sectioned rats during hypoxia. Sleep 5: 1–10

Seers C J 1987 Pain, anxiety and recovery in patients undergoing surgery. PhD thesis, University of London.

Selye H 1950 The physiology and pathology of exposure to stress. Asta, Montreal

Smirne S, Franceschi M, Zamproni P, Crippa D, Ferini-Strambi L 1983 Prevalence of sleep disorders in an unselected in-patient population. In: Guilleminault C, Lugaresi E (eds) Sleep/wake disorders: natural history, epidemiology, and long term evolution. Raven Press, New York, pp 61–71

Soutar R L, Wilson J A 1986 Does hospital noise disturb patients? British Medical Journal 292: 305

Vitiello M V, Prinz P N, Halter J B 1983 Sodium-restricted diet increases night-time plasma norepinephrine and impairs sleep patterns in man. Journal of Clinical Endocrinology and Metabolism 56(3): 553–556

Vuori I, Urponen H, Hasan J, Partinen M 1988 Epidemiology of exercise effects on sleep. Acta Physiologica Scandinavica 133, supplement 133: 3–7

Webb W B 1982 Sleep in older persons: sleep structures of 50 to 60 year old men and women. Journal of Gerontology 37: 581–586

Webb W B, Swinburne H 1971 An observational study of sleep of the aged. Perception and Motor Skills 32: 895–898

Weitzman E D, Kripke D F, Golmacher D, McGregor P, Nogire C 1970 Acute reversal of the sleep–waking cycle in man. Archives of Neurology 22: 483–489

Wever R A 1984 Properties of human sleep–wake cycles: parameters of internally synchronised free-running rhythms. Sleep 7: 27–51

Williams D L, McLean A W, Cairns J 1983 Dose-response effects of ethanol on the sleep of young women. Journal of Studies on Alcohol 44: 515–523

Williams R L, Karacan I, Hursch C J 1974 EEG of human sleep. Wiley, New York, pp 52–64

Winget C M, Deroshia C W, Markley C L, Holley D C 1984 A review of human physiological and performance changes associated with desynchronosis of biological rhythms. Aviation, Space and Environmental Medicine 55(12): 1085–1096

Zepelin H, McDonald C S, Zammit G K 1984 Effects of age on auditory awakening thresholds. Journal of Gerontology 39(3): 294–300

Zulley J 1980 Timing of sleep within the circadian temperature cycle. Sleep Research 9: 282

CHAPTER 26

Communication

Pat Webb

CHAPTER CONTENTS

Introduction 757
Theories of communication 757

Types of communication 758
Verbal communication 758
Non-verbal communication 760
The communication setting 761
Written and audiovisual communication for nurses 761

Nursing management of physiological disorders affecting communication 762
Disorders affecting verbal communication 762
Disorders affecting non-verbal communication 763

Communication in nursing practice 764
Effects of the health care context upon communication 764

Communication skills 765
Attending 765
Active listening 766
Communication skills in practice 766

Counselling 767

Communication among colleagues 767
The multidisciplinary team 768

Patient education 769
Giving information 769

Conclusion 769

References 770

Further reading 770

Useful addresses 770

INTRODUCTION

Communication is the basis of life, from birth to death, and in all circumstances. (Hockey 1984, p. 167)

Communication is the imparting or exchange of information, ideas or feelings. Such messages can be transmitted directly or indirectly through a wide range of media and with varying degrees of involvement of the 'sender' and the 'receiver'. For example, a target audience takes an essentially passive role in the impersonal communication carried out through the mass media of broadcasting and advertising, whereas personal communication between two individuals in face-to-face interactions, telephone conversations or letters demands the more active involvement of the participants. Nonetheless, it is possible in the course of personal interactions for messages to be communicated of which the sender is unaware: individuals convey information about themselves through their dress, posture and manner of speech of which they are often largely unconscious. These non-verbal messages may be at odds with the individual's explicit verbal statements and may, as this chapter will discuss, provide important clues about his state of mind.

Despite the rapid technological advances that have enhanced communications in all areas of human activity, interpersonal communication is still problematic for many people — and health professionals are no exception. Effective communication is fundamental to good practice in all areas of health care, and the challenge of attaining good interpersonal skills must be taken seriously. This chapter considers the particular challenges faced by the nurse in her role as communicator, a role which encompasses giving support, relaying information, promoting health, counselling, and liaising with colleagues. The physiological systems necessary for speech and for gestural communication are described, with particular attention to the implications for the individual of any loss of function which affects speech. Both the verbal and the non-verbal components of interpersonal communication are described to assist the nurse to sensitively interpret each patient's expressed and verbally unexpressed needs and to be more aware of the messages that she herself is sending. The kind of nurse–patient communication encouraged by this chapter is that in which both parties are active participants working toward agreed goals based on the patient's own priorities and values.

Theories of communication

Theories and models within any discipline are useful only when they provide a rationale for practice. If rigid adherence to theoretical notions and complicated models detracts from effective action, then such constructs are counterproductive. However, a carefully constructed theory may help to explain a set of existing phenomena and to predict future events. Theories of communication can thus help health professionals to understand the elements essential to effective communication and to achieve greater control over the outcome of interactions with patients.

Three of the most influential ways in which the process of communication has been conceptualised will be outlined here. These are:

- the mechanical theory
- the behavioural theory
- the response-oriented model.

For more-detailed information on these theories of communication see Ceccio & Ceccio (1982).

The mechanical theory. This model of communication, put forward by Shannon & Weaver in 1949, developed out of a study by the Bell Telephone Laboratories on the effects of telecommunications (Ceccio & Ceccio 1982). According to this theory, the transmission of a message involves the following ten elements:

- information source (encoder)
- initial message
- transmitter
- signal
- channel
- noise (random disturbance of the signal)
- received signal
- receiver (decoder)
- response message
- destination.

Although this theory has certain useful applications (the context of telecommunications is obvious), it includes no notion of feedback and does not describe how the receiver can also become a sender of messages.

The behavioural theory. This model, first described in 1960 by David Berlo, is more relevant to interpersonal interaction, as it takes into account the cognitive, emotive and behavioural elements of communication. Here, the act of communication is broken down into four elements (Berlo 1960):

- source
- message
- channel
- receiver.

As in the mechanical model, feedback is not explicitly considered and it is implied that communication moves in one direction only, from sender to receiver.

The response-oriented model (Ceccio & Ceccio 1982) was devised in an attempt to enhance understanding of the complexities of effective communication in nursing. This model divides the act of communication into four key elements:

- sender
- message (verbal and/or non-verbal)
- receiver
- feedback from receiver to sender.

In addition, this model describes communication as being context-dependent. That is, the context of an interaction influences the dynamic process of communication and may produce 'noise' or barriers to communication, which can distort the message at any point on the loop illustrated in Figure 26.1. One of the most common barriers to nurse–patient communication is fear and anxiety.

?	**26.1** Have you ever consulted your doctor about something you were very anxious about, and come out from the consultation wondering just exactly what it was he had said to you? Have you ever had a patient say to you, soon after the consultant's ward round, that he could not remember anything the consultant had said and so could you please explain? Can you think why this might be?

This chapter will place particular emphasis on developing an awareness of the many potential barriers to communication that may arise in the nurse's interactions with patients, nursing colleagues, and other members of the health care team. Strategies which can be used by the nurse to reduce or eliminate such barriers and to enhance the effectiveness of professional communication in all practice settings will be described.

TYPES OF COMMUNICATION

Verbal communication

Speech is a faculty unique to human beings. The loss of speech, whether temporary or permanent, curtails effective communication to an extensive degree and can cause considerable anguish to the individual. Most people take the capacity for speech for granted and have little awareness of the highly complex physiological mechanisms and mental processes upon which our use of oral communication depends.

Anatomy and physiology of verbal communication

The speech-producing systems. The following body systems are all involved in the production of meaningful speech sounds:

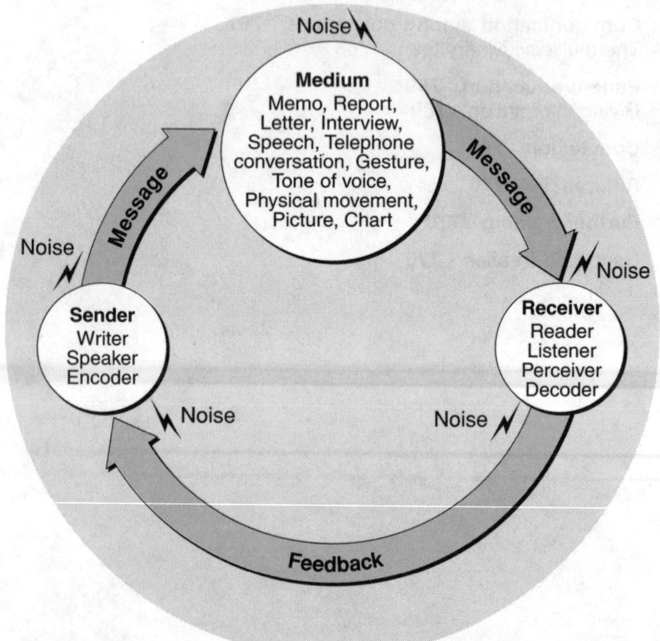

Fig. 26.1 A model of the communication process, including noise and feedback. (Adapted from Ceccio & Ceccio 1982.)

- the psychomotor system
- the musculoskeletal system
- the respiratory system.

The psychomotor system. The motor centre for speech in the brain is in the frontal lobe just above the lateral sulcus and is sometimes called Broca's area (see Fig. 26.2). It is dominant in the left hemisphere for right-handed people and vice versa. The sensory speech area is in the lower part of the parietal lobe and extends into the temporal lobe. Here, the spoken word is perceived. The dominant areas are as before: the left hemisphere for right-handed people and vice versa.

The musculoskeletal system. The upper jaw or maxilla, the anterior part of the roof of the mouth and the lateral walls of the nasal cavities are all involved in speech formation and tone. The mandible or lower jaw articulates with the temporal bone to form the temporo-mandibular joint and enables movement of the jaw for speech, mastication and so on.

The mouth or oral cavity is surrounded by muscles, bones and tissue, all of which are involved in speech production and quality. Superiorly, the bony hard palate and muscular soft palate are bonded laterally by the muscles of the cheeks. The soft tissues of the floor of the mouth and the muscular tongue form the inferior aspect. The back of the mouth is continuous with the oral part of the pharynx. In the anterior, the lips form the entry to the oral cavity and are involved in the formation and projection of speech. The teeth are embedded in the alveolar ridges of the mandible and maxilla. Absence of natural teeth and substitution with dentures can also alter the sounds produced in speech (see Ch. 15).

The respiratory system (see Chs 3 and 14), including the nasal cavity, pharynx, larynx, trachea, bronchi and lungs is significantly involved in sound production. The diaphragm is continuous with the organs of respiration and is involved in the expiration of air. The larynx (voice-box) provides a route for air to pass between the pharynx and the trachea. The functions of the upper respiratory tract of warming and moistening the inhaled air are continued in the pharynx, larynx and trachea. The two vocal cords of the larynx produce sounds of varying loudness and pitch.

The pitch of the voice depends upon the length and tightness of the vocal cords; thus men, whose vocal cords are longer, generally have lower voices than women.

The loudness of voice depends upon the force produced by the expired air which causes the cords to vibrate. The greater the vibration, the louder the sound. Quality and resonance of voice depend upon the shape of the mouth, the position of the tongue and lips, the facial muscles and the air sinuses in the bones of face and skull.

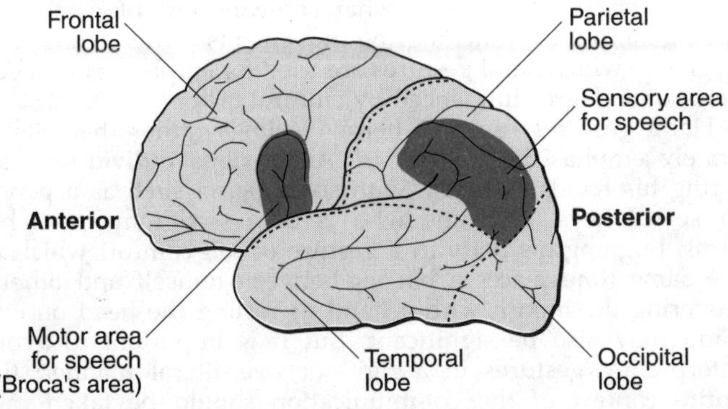

Fig. 26.2 The lobes of the cerebrum and centres for speech.

Psychological factors

While physiological systems play a vital role in the production of speech the psyche is also intimately involved. Mood changes and personality traits may affect the production and quality of speech and may lead to a reluctance to speak at all. The acquisition of speech in childhood involves intellectual as well as physiological maturation, and speech is one of the principal means by which the psyche is expressed. But while human beings need language to fully express their intellect, the loss of the capacity for speech does not necessarily mean that the intellect is impaired — a consideration which must be borne in mind in all interactions with dysphasic patients.

The use and interpretation of words

Jargon. It is important for health care professionals to continually scrutinise their choice of words, as a given term may have different nuances, and indeed entirely different meanings, for different people. It is especially important that health professionals realise that the use of jargon may confuse and alienate patients and relatives. Jargon can widen the distance between the practitioner and the client, reinforcing the mystique surrounding a profession.

Nurses should guard against this exclusion of the patient by making a conscious effort not to use unexplained jargon and abbreviations with patients and their relatives. Technical and medical words should be defined as they are needed, and incorporated into the patient's vocabulary in preference to the use of imprecise lay words. The patient's use of correct medical terminology will enhance his sense of control and confidence and thereby increase his empowerment within the health care setting. Those involved in developing health education materials have invariably noted patients' preference to learn and use correct terminology (Patient Information Service 1988).

Euphemism. The use of euphemism should also be avoided, as it serves only to create confusion and uncertainty. Euphemisms most frequently emerge in communications where 'bad news' must be related to the patient. Although euphemisms might be thought to 'soften the blow' and thus lessen the patient's distress, they in fact have the reverse effect by sending ambiguous messages and widening the gap between perception and reality. Eventually, such vague language will serve only to erode the patient's trust in the doctor or nurse.

The use of euphemism may also be a mechanism by which the professional distances himself or herself from the painful situation at hand, reducing the stress of being the bearer of bad tidings. This can be particularly damaging, however, if the different members of the health care team do not present the situation to the patient in the same way. The patient may question these conflicting messages, and the loyalties of team members will be divided as they grapple with the decision whether to tell the patient the truth. The patient will ultimately not know whom to believe. Health professionals should agree among themselves how to present the situation before the patient is involved. In this way the patient can be spared unnecessary confusion and stress.

Language and dialect. Health professionals should be aware of the potential difficulties posed by the diversity of languages and dialects in our multi-ethnic society (Elliott & Fuller 1991). Health professionals should establish contact with networks of interpreters who can translate information to patients in their own language.

Even within the English language differences in regional dialect can present barriers to communication. In such cases health professionals can ensure mutual understanding by speaking clearly and carefully and by taking the time to ask for clarification; care must be taken, meanwhile, to avoid adopting a patronising tone.

Local Community Relations Councils may be able to offer help and information on some of these issues. Interpretation services are available through these organisations and through certain Health Education Departments. Some organisations have also produced publications and audiovisual materials.

Tone of voice. The tone of voice should be appropriate to the message that is being conveyed. To relay bad news in a jolly tone will irritate the patient and may appear to make light of his real distress. Similarly, words of welcome spoken in a cold or menacing manner will hardly be convincing. The nurse should also be alert to the danger of betraying, through her tone of voice, emotions and attitudes which may intimidate or diminish the patient.

Non-verbal communication

Bodily or non-verbal communication plays a central part in human social interaction. It is a powerful means by which people convey information about themselves and should be given careful attention in all professional interactions. Patients will make certain assumptions about the nurse on the basis of non-verbal clues, just as the nurse will gather information about a patient and his family members even before words are exchanged. Non-verbal messages are often conveyed unintentionally, and can be especially revealing when they fail to match the explicit verbal message that is being offered.

An understanding of non-verbal communication will both enable the nurse to present herself more effectively and help her to interpret the patient.

Non-verbal communication may be considered in relation to the following elements:

- facial expression
- eye contact and gaze
- posture
- appearance
- gesture
- personal space
- bodily contact
- stigma.

Facial expression

The nurse should consider the messages that are conveyed by the expression of her eyes and mouth as she interacts with a patient. Is her smile welcoming or false? Does it match the expression in her eyes, and the bodily contact, such as a handshake, that she makes?

Eye contact and gaze

Impediments to effective eye contact may include pupil deviation, as in uncorrected squint, glass eyes, or dilatation of the pupil from whatever cause. Other factors that influence eye contact include the nature of the relationship between the nurse and patient. While a prolonged gaze may comfort a patient who has a long-standing, trusting relationship with the nurse, it may unnerve a new patient on a first meeting, making him feel exposed and challenged. On the other hand, the failure to maintain eye contact may be interpreted as withdrawal or evasion. Moreover, a patient who is insecure or perplexed by his own feelings may fix his gaze upon the nurse in order to elicit much-needed reassurance and feedback.

The expression of the eyes can convey warmth or, where necessary, widen the distance between the nurse and the patient, asserting that the relationship, although a caring one, is professional rather than social.

Posture

An individual's posture and general bearing may convey a number of non-verbal messages. For example, the person's involvement in an athletic or other discipline (such as dance) may be evident in the body's form and tone. An upright and erect posture may indicate such attributes as self-confidence, high social status, pride in appearance and self-discipline. A lack of tone evident in rounded shoulders and a slumped posture may indicate general apathy, poor self-concept or a lack of interest in the immediate surroundings.

Appearance

Clothing and general appearance may give helpful and accurate information about an individual. A widower living on his own and still mourning the death of his wife may appear to be neglectful of his appearance, but this may be a temporary deviation which misrepresents his normal habits. Individuals do not always convey the same impression by their appearance from one day to another. For example, at a planned first meeting in a clinical setting, a practice nurse may observe that the patient is neat and well groomed and assume that he has his life well in control. Visiting the patient's home at short notice, a district nurse may receive a very different, and perhaps more accurate, impression.

For nurses, questions of dress may centre upon the advantages and disadvantages of wearing a uniform. This issue is currently a controversial one and has been the subject of some debate in the letters and editorial columns of many nursing journals. Hawkey & Clarke (1990) present results of a study in a Nursing Development Unit where staff decided to wear mufti. Smith (1990) reports on the evidence in the literature for and against the wearing of uniforms by nurses working in psychiatric settings; he concludes that 'uniform-wearing should be optional' in such settings (p. 32).

> ? **26.2** Discuss with your fellow students what you perceive to be the effects of wearing a uniform, both for nurses and for patients. Why do you think uniforms have been retained for some areas of work and discarded for others? Why do you think the issue of whether female nurses should wear a cap has been the cause of so much controversy?

Gesture

People can convey a great deal about their personalities through their use of gesture. Most people use their hands to underscore their meaning as they speak; indeed, it is sometimes possible to imagine what someone out of earshot is saying simply by watching the movements of his hands. The degree to which hand gestures are used for emphasis in speech is to some degree influenced by cultural factors.

Hand gestures can also betray feelings rather than deliberately emphasising meanings. An anxious individual may wring his hands or fiddle with some object such as a pencil or set of keys. Someone who is depressed may cross his arms, hugging his body in a gesture of self-comfort which at the same time places a barrier between himself and others. Covering the mouth with a hand or resting the head on one hand may also be significant. But it is important to avoid interpreting gestures in a rigid or over-literal manner; the entire context of the communication should be taken into account, and all of the elements of verbal and non-verbal communication considered together to form a composite picture.

The use of hand gestures is, of course, extremely important for those individuals who have lost, for whatever reason, the use of the voice, the most extreme example being the use of sign language by deaf and dumb people. The psychological effects of being unable to gesture with the hands when this has been an integral part of the individual's conversational style will be considered later in the chapter (see p. 763).

Personal space

This may be defined as a zone around the body, of variable extent, which excludes most other people. Individuals use a variety of tactics to prevent the invasion of this space. For example, some people who are disturbed by the loss of personal space avoid going to parties, being in public places, or travelling on public transport. In some, the need to preserve personal space is so extreme that mental disturbances such as claustrophobia may develop, with disruptive consequences for day-to-day life. Phobias may also indicate the presence of a more general anxiety state. This possibility should not be excluded if phobic behaviour is described during the course of a patient's assessment (see Ch. 17).

In both intimate social contact and in other interactions individuals may allow their personal space to be encroached upon. The violation of personal space presents a particular problem for the person in a health care setting, where touch is necessary to clinical examination. Health professionals should acknowledge the potential discomfort of the situation, without overstating it and thus creating more embarrassment or irritation.

Nursing staff should be sensitive to the patient's need for space and should accommodate individual preferences to whatever degree is possible. For example, for someone who enjoys privacy, being in the middle of a row of beds on a ward is not ideal; an end position or a quieter, corner position may be a more tolerable compromise.

Territorial space is the extension of the individual's personal space in the home, workplace, and so forth. Nurses must have respect for the patient's territorial space when negotiating and carrying out home visits. The patient may accept but still be uncomfortable about the encroachment upon his domestic space by the health professional. It is therefore important to negotiate the terms of a visit, arranging a date and time that is acceptable to the patient and that will minimise the effects of intrusion.

Bodily contact

This is the most primitive form of social communication. Infants cling to their mothers and will often cry simply because they want bodily contact. Most babies will respond to being cradled, caressed and rocked. Among children, most touching occurs between members of the same sex until, from adolescence onwards, bodily contact with the opposite sex becomes important.

There are enormous cultural variations in norms of bodily contact. There are also significant variations between individuals, as determined by such factors as personality type, age and social status.

Touch. In most cultures, social interaction includes the use of touch, ranging from shaking hands to hugging, kissing and even rubbing noses. In formal or professional contexts, expectations concerning the use of touch tend to be quite fixed; for example, a handshake would be an expected greeting at an initial meeting with a solicitor or accountant, but is generally not expected at a first meeting with a health professional.

Given the fact that the use of touch in a health care setting is often at variance with the expectations of 'normal' social context, the nurse must exert some sensitivity in determining whether and when some forms of touch are appropriate. The nurse should take her cue from the individual's response, whether this is one of acceptance, giving permission to retain or extend touch, or of withdrawal, indicating that touch is not wanted and should be withdrawn.

Stigma

Individuals with particular conditions or who have suffered a change in body structure, function or image may experience some degree of social stigma, either real or imagined. Such individuals may assume that others are aware of the physical changes they have undergone and will consequently not want to touch them. Such feelings may arise, for example, in a woman who has had a mastectomy. She may have already felt stigmatised as a result of her breast cancer (see Ch. 7. p. 271), only to find that her feelings of isolation are increased after the surgery that was intended to resolve her situation.

The communication setting

Hospitals and other institutional environments can pose certain barriers to effective communication. The noise in a busy ward or department can be distracting and the lack of privacy a source of frustration for all concerned. Every attempt must be made to minimise these obstacles, and practical suggestions for doing so are made later in this chapter (see p. 765).

The home setting can have both drawbacks and advantages for effective communication; these should be observed and acknowledged by the health professional. Background noise from a radio or television can be distracting, as can interruptions caused by family members and household pets. On the other hand, the patient's home may afford a quiet and private place for consultation and discussion. The individual may feel more secure in his own environment than in an institutional setting and thus less threatened by professional communication.

Written and audiovisual communication for nurses

Nurses are increasingly becoming involved in health promotion and patient teaching. As this may include the production of information leaflets and audiovisual resources, the following discussion briefly outlines considerations of clarity and presentation that should be borne in mind in the preparation of such materials.

Readability

During the Second World War, the reading-ease of written material became an academic concept. Two pioneers in adapting readability formulas (as they became known) for newspapers, business and law firms were Rudolf Flesch and Robert Gunning (Flesch 1974, Gunning 1968). Flesch emphasised the need to replace prepositions, conjunctives and connectives with simpler, more easily understood words, such as 'so' instead of 'consequently' or 'accordingly'. Gunning was more concerned with the use of simple, non-technical words. These researchers devised indices or scoring systems whereby a sample of text could be tested or analysed for its readability. Such indices are regularly used today as a final check of the reading-ease of written materials.

Audiovisual material

Devising material for audio or visual presentation requires

thoughtful preparation and specialised skills; help can be obtained from individuals who regularly produce such materials for advertising or for education in various fields. Health professionals should not hesitate to seek help from those with greater expertise in the areas of language and communications. Moreover, colleagues in health promotion will have experience in the context of health and illness, and every Health Authority/Health Board has a health promotion and education unit that offers advice in this area of communication.

NURSING MANAGEMENT OF PHYSIOLOGICAL DISORDERS AFFECTING COMMUNICATION

Disorders affecting verbal communication

Abnormality in any of the systems involved in the production of speech (see p. 758) can impair verbal communication. Specific details of pathophysiology can be found elsewhere in this text (see Ch. 3, Ch. 9, Ch. 15.); the following discussion will be restricted to a brief outline of the major possibilities for speech disturbance.

Failure of language development. Perinatal brain damage may affect the centres responsible for speech in the frontal and parietal lobes. In mentally subnormal or emotionally disturbed children, the development of speech may be delayed or severely impaired. Specific learning problems may have an impact on language use and thereby impede effective communication. Health visitors routinely assess developmental progress in several areas, i.e. posture, large movements, fine motor skills, vision, hearing, speech, social behaviour and play (Sheridan 1981). In the area of speech development, assessment will combine skilled observation and testing of the child with detailed questioning of the parents about the child's behaviour and his use of language. In this way problems can be detected early and appropriate specialist help sought.

Airways obstruction. Enlargement of the tonsils and/or of the adenoids is a common childhood condition which, although it may not prevent speech, can cause alterations in the sound and resonance of the voice. Frequent and prolonged sinusitis can also affect the quality of speech sounds.

Accidents. There is still a high incidence of accidents among children and young adults, and these account for a significant percentage of speech problems in these two groups. Road traffic accidents causing head injury are especially likely to result in speech difficulties.

Brain disease. A cerebral tumour, whether primary or secondary in nature, affecting either the motor or the sensory speech centre of the brain (see p. 759) can have a devastating effect upon the individual's capacity for verbal communication. Even space-occupying lesions in the skull not directly affecting the two speech centres may cause a shift of structures due to increased intracranial pressure and so indirectly affect speech function. Senile and other dementias may also affect speech either because of organic brain disease or as a result of the emotional disturbance caused by it. (See Ch. 9.)

Ageing cerebral blood vessels. The ageing of cerebral blood vessels leading to minor infarctions or complete occlusion of part of the cerebrum, as in a cerebrovascular accident (CVA), will impair speech if it affects either the frontal or the parietal speech centre. The consequence of a CVA is that affected parts of the body refuse to obey the commands of the central nervous system. The patient may not be able to make himself understood even though in most cases his own understanding is not impaired. The effects of a CVA will vary, of course, depending on which side of the brain is affected. The right hemisphere of the brain governs the individual's body image and spatial judgement. Damage to this hemisphere governs functions concerned with logic, mathematics and communication. Speech and writing difficulties will thus be among the effects of a CVA on this side. This can be extremely frustrating for individuals who have previously been articulate. Sensitive, careful work on the part of a speech therapist and understanding from all health professionals involved are vital. It must always be remembered that a breakdown in the patient's ability to express himself does not always signal a loss of comprehension. (See Ch. 9, pp. 344–349.)

Respiratory tract disease. Disease or injury to any part of the respiratory tract or the head and neck in either children or adults may cause speech disruption or permanent impairment. An example of the latter would be where a total laryngectomy is needed to treat cancer of the larynx, or where that organ has been injured and must be bypassed by the raising of a tracheal stoma (tracheostomy). (See Ch. 14, pp. 515–517.)

Deafness. In addition to all the above potential disturbances to speech, nurses may come into contact with those who are profoundly deaf or dumb or both. These disabilities may have nothing to do with a current illness or injury but will need to be considered as part of the total care of the individual.

Dealing with problems of speech

Clearly, specific medical and nursing interventions will be necessitated by some of the problems outlined above. The present discussion will deal only with general considerations and strategies that apply to most situations.

Whenever the patient's capacity for verbal communication is lost, a key role of the nurse is to facilitate other means of communication. If the patient has adapted to a permanent speech deficit or loss, he may have devised personal ways of overcoming his handicap. A nurse visiting a patient at home or in hospital will need to discover these as part of her initial assessment.

Eliciting information may be a difficult task in itself and will require time, patience, understanding and good interactive skills. It seems to be a natural instinct to raise the voice when speaking to those who cannot speak themselves. However, this is not usually helpful and may only increase the degree of frustration and perhaps humiliation felt by the patient.

If no method of communication has already been established to compensate for speech loss, the nurse must show enterprise in introducing the best method for the particular need. This will depend to a great extent on any other functional problems the patient may have. Encouraging a patient to write messages would be impractical if he were illiterate or had a broken wrist, for example.

For those living at home alone who rely heavily on the telephone, special arrangements may need to be made. The most usual example in this context is that of an elderly man who has had a laryngectomy for cancer of the larynx. The isolation he already feels as a result of losing his most powerful means of communication will be compounded if he is unable to make contact with the outside world. There are various mechanical devices that can assist the individual to communicate by telephone. In some cases, consistent work with the speech therapist will restore a degree of speech to enable reasonable function.

It is vital that nurses are aware of the expert help that is available and have access to sources of information. Every Health Board or District has a speech therapy service for which medical referral is not required; the nurse may refer the patient or he may access the service on his own. Whatever the cause or duration of the speech loss, assessment by a speech therapist is essential. In addition, there are many organisations offering practical and emotional help to anyone with speech difficulties. The umbrella charity coordinating these organisations is called Voluntary Organisations Communication and Language (VOCAL). (See Useful Addresses, p. 770).

Disorders affecting non-verbal communication

Non-verbal as well as verbal communication can be adversely affected by illness or injury. The psychological and social impact of any impairment of the individual's non-verbal modes of communication should never be underestimated. Especially in conjunction with speech impairment or loss, problems with non-verbal communication can lead to an acute sense of isolation. Various ways in which non-verbal communication can be affected are considered in the following sections.

Facial expression, eye contact, gaze

Functional problems which affect the individual's facial expression, use of eye contact and gaze may be particularly obvious and may be a source of embarrassment and frustration, seriously affecting the quality of face-to-face interactions. Conditions and illnesses which may come into play include:

- facial injury, such as a fracture of the maxilla or mandible requiring fixation in order to heal. This will affect smiling and indeed the movement of most facial muscles.
- CVAs or space-occupying lesions in the brain. These may temporarily or permanently impair the function of facial muscles.
- Bell's palsy, i.e. facial hemiparesis resulting from oedema of the 7th cranial nerve.
- myasthenia gravis, a disorder caused by a biochemical defect involving the abnormal behaviour of acetylcholine at neuromuscular junctions. This condition causes weakness of voluntary muscles, especially those of the face and eye. Although a rare disease it is readily apparent when it occurs and will certainly affect the character of facial expression.
- Parkinson's disease (see Ch. 9, p. 360).
- tetanus, often called lockjaw, which is caused by anaerobic bacteria found in soil and manure. This disease restricts movement of the jaw and causes the typical spastic grin known as risus sardonicus. It also temporarily prevents effective speech and is a very frightening experience for the patient. Cuts and abrasions occurring in gardens or rural areas or at the sea should be properly cleaned and dressed. If required, the individual should be given a tetanus toxoid injection (TT) for active immunity to the organism. Those who regularly work on farms or in gardening or in similar activities are advised to be well protected with antitetanus serum (ATS), which contains tetanus antibodies and so produces an artificial, passive immunity.
- tetany, a condition caused by metabolic alkalosis and parathyroid gland disorders in which blood calcium levels are disturbed (see Ch. 5, p. 147). It causes generalised muscular hyperexcitability which usually includes the facial muscles.
- abnormal structure or anatomy of the head and face may also affect facial gestures. For example, in acromegaly (an enlargement of the hands, face and feet caused by an excess of growth hormone) a significant imbalance occurs in the proportions of the face and may compromise normal movement of facial muscles.
- abnormal pigmentation of the skin may distract the gaze of the onlooker and so block effective communication. Naevi, large moles, warts or petechial haemorrhages may be examples of these. Burns, scalds or other injuries may, by permanently damaging facial tissue and restricting muscular movement, give an impression of a fixed stare which bears no relation to the mood or personality of the individual.

Posture, gesture and appearance

Poor posture may be a result of lack of muscle tone, disease or injury of the skeleton, low morale, or psychiatric disturbance. Disease or injury of the hands, arms or shoulders may restrict the use of gestures and thus inhibit the individual's normal communication style. Nurses may encounter this in women who develop lymphoedema of the arm as a condition secondary to breast cancer (see Ch. 7, p. 280).

Nurses should be sensitive to the social and psychological effects that the loss of gestural expression can have upon individuals, especially those who belong to a culture in which gesticulation is an important aspect of conversational style.

Personal space

There will be times when normal personal space will have to be invaded in order for examinations to be carried out or for care to be given to dependent patients. The irritation, embarrassment and low morale that this might cause the individual should be handled with sensitivity on the part of the nurse. In many cases it will help to acknowledge and address the problem, thus reassuring the patient that such procedures are necessary and imply no loss of respect.

Bodily contact

Some degree of physical contact may be desired by the patient who needs reassurance or comfort, and for a patient with low self-esteem being touched on the hand or arm may indicate to him that he is being accepted. In some cases, the nurse may find it difficult to offer such bodily contact, possibly because she is not comfortable with this kind of communication, or because of some attribute of the individual, as discussed in the following.

Body/wound odour. One of the most difficult problems to deal with in nursing is that of offensive odour. In many cases odour is related to microorganisms infecting wounds or body cavities (see Ch. 34, p. 935) or to stomata such as colostomies and ileostomies. The strategy of most help to both parties is either to treat the cause of the offending odour or, where the problem is intractable, to use one of the several preparations now on the market in the form of dressings and solutions to remove or mask the odour (David 1986). If the problem cannot be entirely resolved, it is best acknowledged by the nurse and the patient rather than ignored, as the stress of behaving as if it does not exist will help neither the patient's recovery nor his self-esteem.

Disfigurement. Certain skin diseases may affect aspects of communication related to appearance and to touch. Psoriasis, for example, can cause severe excoriation and scarring of the skin and may affect wide areas of the body. Such disfigurement, even if temporary, may make extraordinary demands upon those caring for patients (see Ch. 12, p. 449). For the patient, feelings of being rejected by others will contribute to low self-esteem and reinforce a sense of isolation.

? **26.3** Think of a patient whom you have found it difficult to be near, for whatever reason. Why was that? How might you approach the care of that patient now? Try to write the relevant section of that patient's care plan, including patient outcome statements.

COMMUNICATION IN NURSING PRACTICE

Effects of the health care context upon communication

The health care setting and the nature of the relationship between the health professional and the patient may in themselves impede effective communication (Ley 1988) (see Box 26.1). It has been suggested that a potential communication gap exists from the very beginning of the patient's interaction with a health professional by virtue of the 'social distance' between the two parties (Macleod Clark & Webb 1985, Ashley 1987). See Fig. 26.3. In general, when a patient first presents with a problem — usually to his general practitioner — the learned roles of 'professional' and of 'patient' are established. Typically, both will behave in a way that endorses these roles, the professional taking control and the patient responding to questions and submitting to clinical examination or assessment. The professional's knowledge-base, and the position of power which this accords him, will be played against the patient's lack of specialised knowledge and his position of relative vulnerability.

Research has also indicated that the patient sometimes thinks it is inappropriate for him to initiate certain interactions (Webb 1989, Crotty 1985). This may derive from his perception of the professional's and of his own role. He may view the professional as a very busy person with important, life-saving tasks to perform, or assume that the professional will not deem his feelings and reactions to be important enough to devote time and attention to.

It is important for the nurse to counteract any hesitation the patient may have to voice his worries and concerns by creating opportunities for him to express himself. For example, an open question such as 'How are you feeling today?' will give the patient a chance to raise any issue that is troubling him. The patient who does not wish to pursue certain subjects may close the conversation or digress. The nurse should be sensitive to such cues and allow the patient to make the choice whether to disclose feelings or keep them private.

Box 26.1 Aspects of communication and the professional–patient role

- Communication is an important part of all clinical teaching.
- Sometimes doctors talk to each other, or to a nurse, across patients' beds almost as if they were inanimate objects.
- A barrage of routine questions can inhibit communication.
- Anxiety inhibits recollection of information.
- Patients tend to assume that no news is bad news.
- Few patients can understand medical jargon.
- Patients who have had tests that reveal nothing abnormal want to know why they feel ill.
- Without video training, students may not learn how to listen, notice and use non-verbal communication.

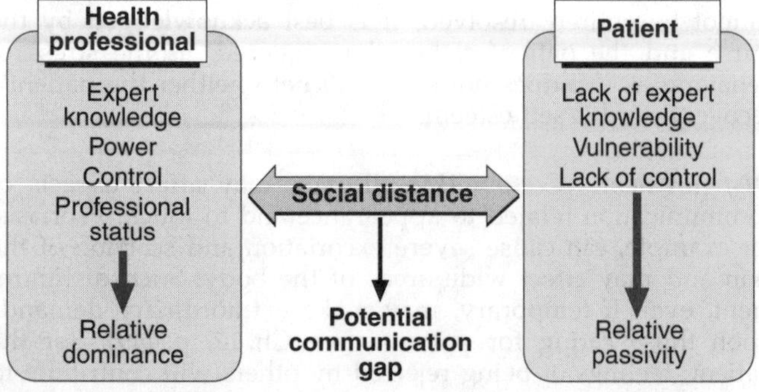

Fig. 26.3 The professional–patient relationship.

Patient dissatisfaction

There is much evidence to suggest that communication between health professionals and patients is poor. Patients have themselves described their dissatisfaction with the communications they receive from all health professionals (Raphael 1977, Reynolds 1978). Frustration at a lack of information is compounded by other emotions and may lead patients to complain through statutory structures (Health Service Commission 1986). The largest single complaint from patients and relatives is that they are given insufficient time to be heard, to ask questions and to benefit from useful and relevant information.

Nurses' communication skills

Research studies have documented a lack of effective communication skills within the nursing profession and the need for training to put this right. Menzies (1970) endorsed some of Jourard's (1960) observations by describing the defence mechanisms nurses use to conceal a lack of confidence in opening up conversations with patients and a fear of handling what may be disclosed. Several studies have attempted to monitor the quality and quantity of nurses' communication with patients. Research methods have included non-participant observation and the use of radiomicrophones, audiotapes and videotapes (Faulkner 1979, Crotty 1985, Macleod Clack 1981; see Research Abstract 26.1).

The importance of good communication skills in clinical teaching is highlighted in Box 26.1.

There is a continuing effort to include the teaching of communication skills in education programmes for health professionals. The Communication in Nurse Education project (CINE) devised ways of teaching communication skills to nurses and attempted to evaluate the outcome (Neeson et al

Research Abstract 26.1

The theoretical framework known as Six Category Intervention Analysis has been used in teaching interpersonal skills in various settings. There is little empirical work to test the theory but Morrison & Burnard (1989) devised an instrument for assessing student nurses' perceptions of their interpersonal skills based on the category analysis. A quantitative comparison was made with the results of an earlier study of trained nurses' perceptions. The key trend to emerge was the nurses' lack of skill in facilitating their communication with patients and their tendency to be authoritative instead. There were considerable similarities in findings between the student and trained nurse groups, demonstrating that skills did not increase with seniority.

Morrison P, Burnard P 1989 Students' and trained nurses' perceptions of their own interpersonal skills: a report and comparison. Journal of Advanced Nursing 14: 321–329

1984). Other projects have included teaching these skills to specific groups. For example, health professionals working with cancer patients and the dying have identified particularly difficult problems. Maguire & Faulkner (1988a–c) continue to address these issues through multidisciplinary workshops and evaluation of the outcome of these.

The Health Education Board for Scotland has worked in a more general way with the training of nurses, midwives and health visitors in communication skills and has developed a wide variety of resource materials (see Useful Addresses).

Effects of environment

Good interpersonal skills are not always sufficient in themselves for successful communication. The specific setting of an interaction can have both positive and negative effects upon the quality of communication that is achieved.

The patient's home. While home visits impinge upon the patient's territorial space, he will have requested (or at least not refused) the health professional's presence. The encounter is, of course, primarily a professional rather than a social one and the ground rules for the interview need to be established so that both parties are quite clear about what is expected of them. The professional might begin by restating the reason for the visit and confirming with the patient that this is understood and accepted. The patient may try to move away from the negotiated agenda by engaging in social chat. This may be a symptom of loneliness and the professional may have to spend several minutes participating in this type of conversation, perhaps also talking about her own home and family, before tactfully steering the patient back to the real purpose of the visit.

?	**26.4** How much can a degree of self-disclosure foster effective communication between patient and nurse? Can 'social chat' be a positive part of professional interaction?

The hospital and clinic. In an institutional setting patients consider that health professionals are in their own territory and expect them to be in control. Nonetheless, the reason for an assessment, bedside visit, or other interaction must be negotiated and clearly defined. Social chat may, of course, form part of an interaction, but if the encounter is to be of value the practitioner must maintain a professional relationship with the patient.

Environmental factors such as lack of privacy, noise, uncomfortable furniture and poor institutional design may undermine serious attempts at effective communication. Social factors may also intervene: a patient confronted by a group of health professionals during a consultation or ward round may feel especially powerless and vulnerable, especially if he is in bed wearing nightclothes while the others are standing, dressed in their usual work clothes. Eye contact can be difficult to maintain comfortably when the patient is in bed, and the health professional may need to make an effort to minimise the distance and the difference in eye level between herself and the patient.

COMMUNICATION SKILLS

The skills necessary for effective communication can be learned and are currently being given increased emphasis in the training of health care professionals. There are sufficient models and resources now available to allow communication skills training to be incorporated into any medical or nursing education programme (see, for example, Maguire & Faulkner 1988a–c, Tschudin 1987).

Communication skills are not ends in themselves but tools for achieving positive outcomes for patients and their families. Preoccupation with technique at the expense of genuine caring will be counterproductive and reduce the act of communicating to an academic exercise. If the nurse's role as communicator is to be used to help patients and their families cope with illness or disability more effectively, professional skills must be employed in combination with a sincere respect for the individual and his values and priorities.

Two fundamental skills are required to achieve good communication. These are:

1. Attending: giving attention
2. Active listening: indicating involvement and interest in what the person is saying.

Attending

Giving individual attention to the patient and acknowledging his current situation or difficulty is the first step in the process of successful communication. In her initial assessment and in any subsequent interactions, the nurse must both hear and see what the patient is 'saying' about himself through both verbal and non-verbal clues, building up a balanced picture of where the patient is located in his world and how he feels about his current situation. The nurse should avoid making assumptions about how the patient is feeling; he may not feel the same way that she would in a similar set of circumstances. An individual's personality, past experience and current values will contribute to his response to a given situation; his reaction will therefore be unique. Issues that seem important to the nurse may not be of primary concern for the patient. The nurse must elicit how the patient is *actually* feeling at any given time and work with him on the basis of that knowledge.

Attending skills relate to the way that the interviewer is orientated physically and psychologically to the patient. The nurse's manner and her choice of words can invite trust and openness on the one hand or distrust and a reluctance to disclose personal information on the other. The quality of the nurse's attending will affect the quality of subsequent interactions, for skilled attending will permit the collection of sound data upon which future action can be based. Finally, skilful attending is a prerequisite to active listening. Strategies that will enhance the quality of attending in a nurse–patient interaction may be described as follows:

1. The nurse should tell the patient who she is and the purpose of the interaction, for example: 'I am Nurse B, and I will be caring for you during at least the first few days of your stay in hospital. I would like to hear your own story of why you are here, so that we can plan your care together.'

2. The nurse should position herself in such a way as to facilitate comfortable and effective interaction, giving attention to eye level, distance and the effect of intervening objects such as desks or tables (see Fig. 26.4).

3. During the course of the conversation, the nurse may need to incline toward the patient to convey her active attention. This may be effected with the whole body, the head or with hand gestures. The patient may withdraw, indicating through body language that the nurse is moving in too closely and is not allowing him the personal space he needs in order to cope.

4. A relaxed, open posture will indicate the nurse's willingness to listen. Rigid folding of the arms, a tense posture and undue distance from the patient may indicate such negative attitudes as disapproval or lack of interest. Eye contact should

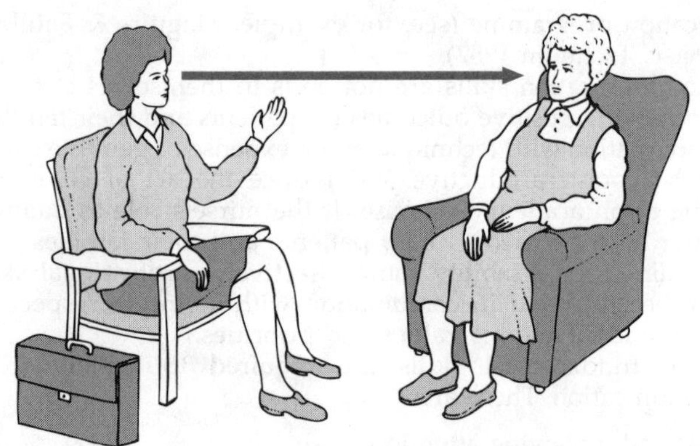

Fig. 26.4 Positioning conducive to effective interaction.

be maintained, but within the provisos discussed earlier (see p. 763). If a steady gaze is responded to with unease, it may be appropriate for the nurse to avert her eyes frequently until her gaze becomes accepted. The nature of facial expressions and of gestures will also indicate the degree of the nurse's interest. For example, nodding in recognition of a point made will help to signal her involvement in the interaction.

5. A lack of interest may inadvertently be communicated by repetitive gestures or by the habit of fiddling with objects such as a pen or paperclip. Such behaviour may convey to the patient that the nurse is anxious on her own behalf — that she is preoccupied, for example, or is worried about the time — and is therefore not giving him her complete attention.

?	**26.5** Ask your fellow-students, peers or family if you have a repetitive gesture or habit which they feel can indicate disinterest or lack of attention on your part to what they are saying.

Active listening

This aspect of communication involves the following strategies:

1. Listening to the patient's verbal communication and observing non-verbal clues to determine if these two components of his message match. The nurse may observe, for example, that a patient says he feels fine but is neglecting his home or his own appearance, and conclude that further assessment for depression is indicated.
2. Indicating one's interest and encouraging the patient to continue with his story with nods, gestures, and such interpolations as 'Yes' or 'Go on'.
3. Paraphrasing the patient's statements and asking for clarification, thus indicating a desire to understand him correctly.
4. Expressing empathy for the patient by acknowledging his feelings and the difficulty of his situation without presuming to know exactly how he feels.
5. Using silence when appropriate to convey empathy or to give the patient a chance to reflect on what has been said. Silence used in this way is constructive, not evasive; it is not a means of avoiding serious discussion.

Communication skills in practice

Nurse – patient interviews are generally of two types:

1. Planned interactions for assessment or counselling
2. Unplanned interactions in which the patient asks a question or makes a comment that requires immediate response and / or subsequent action.

Communication strategies appropriate to these two forms of interaction are outlined in the following sections.

The planned interview

Planned interviews occur during an initial meeting with a patient and often on several subsequent occasions when evaluation and reassessment are required. The intention of these interactions is to elicit information from the patient and to determine how he sees and feels about his situation.

Opening the conversation. The nurse should introduce herself, giving her name and specifying what role she will be playing in the patient's care; the latter information will help to orientate the patient to his new situation, whether at home or in hospital. At this stage the nurse should ascertain how the patient prefers to be addressed.

Stating aims. The aims of the interview should be clearly stated and a check made that the patient understands and agrees to these. The patient may indicate that the timing of the interview is inconvenient or that he is unable to concentrate; if this is the case, it may be better to settle upon an alternative time.

Setting a time limit. Although some nurses are uncomfortable with the notion of setting a time limit for an interview, it is often found that patients feel more comfortable when they know how much time they have to relate their story. A failure to specify time limits is also unrealistic, as nurses must divide their time fairly between patients. It may be necessary to arrange additional meetings so that all concerns that come to light are addressed.

Questioning. As questions are the key to any interview, it is important for the nurse to understand different question types and how they can best be used.

Open questions are generally the most useful. They usually begin with words such as 'what', 'why', 'where', 'how', 'which' and 'when', and help to place emphasis on the patient's, rather than the nurse's, perspective of the situation.

The actual question used to open an interview will be determined by the actual circumstances of the patient and should reflect the nurse's desire to ascertain the patient's concerns and anxieties. It is helpful at an early stage to ask the patient to verbalise his own understanding of the reason for his admission to hospital (or whatever the case may be). Establishing the patient's understanding of the situation can be a good start to building up a picture to which he and the nurse contribute.

Closed questions can be very useful in obtaining factual information quickly. An example of a closed question used in preparing a patient for surgery is 'Have you eaten anything since midnight?' Such questions are designed to elicit the basic responses 'Yes', 'No' or 'I don't know'. Such questions may be vital but leave little opportunity for the patient to influence the direction of the conversation.

Directed questions state the subject to be discussed and encourage the patient to give more detailed information; like closed questions, they do not make room for the patient to impose his own agenda upon the discussion. An example of a directed question is 'Can you tell me a little more about the last time you were in hospital?'

Structuring an assessment interview. The nurse may employ a number of strategies in the course of an assessment interview to elicit information, gain insight into the patient's feelings and reactions, and identify significant problems. Certain key areas are likely to create a framework for a comprehensive assessment; the emphasis given to these will vary according to the circumstances prompting the assessment (e.g. admission to hospital). These key areas are likely to include:

- the patient's current perception of his situation and his reaction to it
- the patient's view of the future, i.e. the outcome he anticipates. This will yield important information about the patient's psychological state and the strategies he might use to achieve health or cope with illness
- the actual and potential impact of the illness and its treatment on the patient's day-to-day life, mood, key relationships and participation in social life.

In order to ensure that each relevant area is addressed it may be helpful to direct the interview in accordance with an appropriate, predetermined structure. Such frame-works (Maguire & Faulkner 1988b) can be learned and have been incorporated into the practice of many health care professionals. However, in a collaborative study of health assessment of elderly people in their homes Runciman (1989) cautioned against the rigid imposition of interviewing frameworks or structures and devised a 'prompt list' which identified key areas of relevance in assessing the health of elderly people.

?	**26.6** Look up the article by Runciman (1989) and when you are on a community placement ask the Health Visitor or District Nurse who is your mentor for her views on the prompt list. Ask if together you might use it to assess an elderly person on your caseload.

Key interviewing strategies. It is generally advisable for the nurse to deal with the patient's concerns before her own professional agenda. This may be achieved by beginning an assessment interview with a review of the patient's health and illness background, ensuring that each topic is covered fully before a new one is introduced, and obtaining a list of key problems to work with. The nurse's professional agenda may then be introduced if it is found that an important area has not been addressed by the patient's expressed agenda. Key strategies that should be applied in patient-centred interviewing are listed in Box 26.2.

Interviewing and assessment skills will improve with practice provided that the nurse makes regular checks, perhaps with the help of a colleague, that she is communicating effectively. Without regular self-assessment inadequate or unsatisfactory modes of practice may become entrenched.

Box 26.2 Summary of interviewing assessment techniques

- Acknowledging the patient's situation and perceptions
- Organising information
- Encouraging specificity and precision in the patient's account
- Clarifying the messages received from the patient
- Exploring key verbal and non-verbal clues
- Keeping the patient to the point
- Using time well
- Encouraging the expression of feelings

Unplanned interactions

On some occasions the nurse will be called upon to give a spontaneous response to an unforeseen question. For example, she may be approached in an outpatient department by a patient whom she has not met before, who asks: 'Nurse, the doctor says I may need major surgery. What does this mean?' A surprise question such as this should not be evaded, but the nurse may need time to collect her thoughts in order to give an appropriate and helpful response. She may gain a little time by first responding with a question such as 'You say the doctor has just told you this — which doctor did you see and what exactly did he say?' The patient's response may again be followed by a query such as 'And did you find this news surprising?' Such preliminary questions may help the nurse to gain data on which to base a decision as to whether she should find out more, refer the question on, or handle it herself. By considering the patient's question in this way the nurse will communicate her concern and lay a foundation of trust for future interactions.

COUNSELLING

It is not within the remit of this chapter to explore fully counselling models and their use, as counselling is a highly skilled role which demands specialist training. However, the nurse's role may encompass some element of counselling, developing naturally from her involvement in identifying the patient's problems and helping him to find and implement ways of solving them.

The aim of skilled, supportive counselling conducted by an appropriately qualified specialist is to assist the patient to find his own solutions or coping strategies (Egan 1990). If the patient is unable or unwilling to do so, more direct intervention and advice may be appropriate. However, imposing solutions upon the patient is generally less than ideal, for it is the patient who will ultimately have to deal with his difficulties in day-to-day life (see Ch. 17, p. 585).

Counselling will involve helping the patient to verbalise his feelings about his problems and to generate possible solutions. Issues may need to be prioritised, and it may also be necessary to screen for any remaining difficulties and concerns. Subsequent interviews can then deal with each problem in turn. The patient should be made to feel confident that no issue has been forgotten, and that this situation can be made more manageable by establishing overall priorities and setting appropriate short-term goals to address each specific problem.

Typically, each counselling session will conclude with a check that the relevant issues have been satisfactorily explored. A date and time for the next interview is usually set, although in some cases it will be appropriate for the counsellor to leave it up to the patient to contact her when he feels he needs to consult her again.

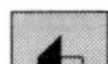
For further information see Egan (1990).

COMMUNICATION AMONG COLLEAGUES

Communication among professional colleagues, whether of the same or of different disciplines, presents special challenges. Within organisations and institutions communication difficulties may arise as a result of hierarchies of authority and seniority. The defence mechanisms described by Menzies (1970) and referred to earlier in the chapter (see p. 764) are part of an overall reaction to a professional culture which has not always encouraged open communication among colleagues. There does seem to be some improvement, however, in certain settings.

The multidisciplinary team

Nurses do not and should not work in isolation. Today's nursing practice involves working with other professionals in a multidisciplinary team, whether the care setting is a hospital, clinic, or the patient's home.

The potential difficulties encountered in multidisciplinary communication derive from the real or perceived power structures within the team. For example, if the student nurse is overawed by the medical consultant's experience and knowledge, she may find it difficult to contribute fully to team discussions. If, however, the consultant's personality and attitude allow the nurse to feel very much an active and valued member of the care team who can contribute important data relating to her patients she is more likely to feel comfortable in communicating freely with the doctor and other team members.

The ward sister is often seen as the leader of the ward team, setting the tone of the work environment and playing a central role in facilitating good communication among team members (Pembrey 1980, Fretwell 1982, Orton 1981). Of course, all members of the team must make a conscious effort to promote effective communication within the team, and frequent review will be required to ensure that an optimal level of communication is maintained (see Dingwall 1980, Evers 1981).

The primary health care team

Most members of the primary health care team do not stay in a central workplace for most of the day, but spend their time visiting patients in their homes or running screening, immunisation or other clinics in the local community. Special communication procedures may have to be developed to overcome the difficulties inherent in the lack of centralisation in this approach. For example, meetings of the whole team may be difficult to schedule, and may have to take place less frequently than would be the case with a hospital ward team. It may be necessary to subdivide the team into smaller groups, with one key worker in each; in such an arrangement, good record-keeping will be essential to keep all team members fully informed about each patient.

Accessibility to records may be another problem deriving from decentralisation, as a given patient's records may need to be consulted by the district nurse, by the patient in his own home, and by the doctor in the surgery or health centre. Apparently, several district nurse teams have tried to devise ways of making records more accessible. Portable hand-held computers are being used by some teams; these use compatible software to allow access to information in each of the relevant centres, while the written record remains in the patient's home as before.

Hospital-home liaison

Liaison sheets have been devised in several areas of nursing practice to overcome problems of staff communication between different care settings. Recent policies encouraging early discharge of patients from hospital and the provision of more complex and varied treatments in the patient's home will increase the need for accurate and flexible communication systems (Jowett & Armitage 1988; see Research Abstract 26.2). It is becoming common practice to input at least a summary of each inpatient's and outpatient's record on computer so that quick access to relevant points may be made from anywhere within the hospital. Such record-keeping policies require, of course, an up-to-date understanding of guidelines for confidentiality and copyright. Nurses should become familiar with the current legislation relating to both written and computerised patient records.

?	**26.7** Consult the Data Protection Act (1984) in your local library. What does it say with regard to patient records such as you use regularly, and in relation to the issue of confidentiality?

Nurse-to-nurse communication

If nurses fail to communicate with one another effectively, patient care may suffer. Procedures and policies for communication are designed to meet the specific needs of a given care setting, and range from lengthy meetings describing the

Research abstract 26.2

In an exploratory study of the structure and process of the liaison role, Jowett & Armitage (1988) interviewed 196 nurses, including liaison nurses, nurse managers, hospital sisters, district nursing sisters and health visitors.

Different models of liaison between nurses working in hospitals and nurses working in the community were identified. Liaison could be direct (no liaison nurse involvement), or indirect (with liaison nurse involvement).

The two key variables found to be crucial to liaison were communication and discharge planning. For example, where there was no liaison nurse involvement, communication on discharge tended to be unsatisfactory. Community nurses often felt that patients were inappropriately referred, that some patients were completely missed and that information was often scant or of poor quality. District nurses received little warning of discharges and, overall, discharges tended to be poorly planned.

When a liaison nurse was involved, the information received was felt to be more comprehensive and appropriate. However, community nurses also felt that information could become 'distorted' in transfer and could lose 'richness' compared to that available directly from the hospital nurses.

The effectiveness of communication and discharge planning was influenced by beliefs of nurses about the concept of continuity of care, and by the 'community awareness' of hospital staff — that is, by their knowledge of community services, perception of the roles of community nurses and understanding of the effects of patients' home backgrounds upon progress and recovery.

The study suggests:

1. that the role of the liaison nurse should be developed in an 'advisory' capacity, supporting effective, direct liaison between hospital and community nurses
2. that the concept of continuity of care and aspects of community care should be stressed as core elements throughout all basic nursing education.

Jowett S, Armitage S 1988 Hospital and community liaison links in nursing: the role of the liaison nurse. Journal of Advanced Nursing 13(5): 579–587 patient's past history, current problems and future needs to a one-to-one handover at the bedside. It is important to devise methods that work well for the team. If traditional reporting methods prove to be ineffective, new strategies should be explored.

?	**26.8** Compare with your fellow students your experiences of the handover report. Afterwards, look up Lelean's (1973) research monograph and discuss what, if any, changes have taken place and why.

Written records are often problematic. Despite the introduction in recent years of an increasing number of forms intended to support systematic and individualised care, written communication generally remains poor. Irrelevant information is often recorded while important details are omitted. Such deficiencies are significant not only in the day-to-day management of patient care but in circumstances where nursing activities must be reconstructed, as in a court of law.

A good rule of thumb to apply when documenting an inpatient's care is to imagine what a new member of staff or an agency nurse would need to know in order to form a clear, accurate picture of the patient's situation and thus be prepared to intervene appropriately. Needs or problems can be recorded in list form together with any actions taken; this information can then be scanned more quickly than pages of continuous prose. Notes on the patient's psychological well-being should not be omitted. All items must be dated.

Shared records. In some hospitals health professionals other than nurses are now recording their interventions in the nursing records as appropriate. Thus nursing records may summarise the advice given by the dietitian, any speech therapy given, or any prostheses fitted by a nurse specialist or appliance officer. Key staff may write notes in different coloured inks or on colour-coded paper to facilitate quick identification or location of particular types of information.

PATIENT EDUCATION

There is a sizeable body of research which affirms the value of teaching patients about healthy lifestyles and the management of ill-health. Some studies have demonstrated a reduction in distressing symptoms among patients who were given adequate information (Hayward 1975, Raphael 1977, Wilson-Barnett 1983, Webb 1989), while others have been concerned with the patient's sense of independence and personal control that goes along with being well informed about his condition.

Educating patients and their carers with a view to helping them to maximise independence must be seen as one of the prime goals of nursing. The nurse's role as educator requires good skills in communication whether she is working with individual patients and their families or within a more general health promotion programme (see Ch. 26).

Giving information

Information-giving is an important activity in itself and must be carried out in a systematic way. Many patients find that the need for information is particularly acute during waiting periods of various kinds, for example after tests have been completed but before a diagnosis has been confirmed. Although it may be impossible to provide the patient with specific information at such times, saying nothing may have the effect of increasing anxiety and allowing the patient to imagine the worst.

The period of discharge from hospital has also been identified as a time when the need for information is especially marked (Bond 1982, Hinds 1985). It would be wrong to assume that patients will be able to manage when they are back at home without being given specific, practical information on how to cope with an ongoing condition or during a period of rehabilitation.

Once the kind of information needed or wanted by the patient has been established, the nurse's role will include the following:

- discussing each item with the patient and with those family members or friends whom he wishes to involve
- planning and implementing a teaching programme, giving the patient short-term, achievable goals
- evaluating the effectiveness of the programme, reassessing needs and teaching strategies.

The nurse should remember that everyone learns at his own pace. Patients should be encouraged with praise when they do well and instruction should be reinforced in areas where improvement is needed. At all times, however, the nurse should avoid being patronising. It should also be borne in mind that illness can disrupt the psyche as well as affect the body; the nurse should therefore be sensitive to the depressed and labile moods that often accompany illness.

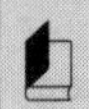

For further information see Webb 1989.

Information agencies

There are several voluntary and statutory bodies of which patients should be made aware that will provide information on such topics as illness, coping in the home, relaxation techniques and obtaining aids and benefits. Directories of help agencies can be found in public, medical and nursing libraries. Community Health Councils and Citizens' Advice Bureaux provide a useful service for consumers on all aspects of dealing with illness and its consequences. In addition, the Wessex-based organisation Help for Health has a database of all national and local agencies that may offer general help or support related to specific illnesses. Similarly, Health Search Scotland, provided as a service of the Health Education Board for Scotland, makes information available on all aspects of health. Specific directories of services can also be obtained through a range of voluntary organisations concerned with particular illnesses.

?	**26.9** Build up a resource file on local help agencies and information services which will be easy to access and available to patients and carers. Check with your local Health Promotion or Health Education Department and Citizens' Advice Bureaux to see what information they hold on voluntary or other help agencies.

CONCLUSION

Effective communication is one of the most challenging aspects of today's nursing practice. The acquisition of good communication skills requires thought, practice and continuing self-evaluation. The importance to the outcome of treatment of successful communication with colleagues, patients and carers should not be underestimated: failure to communicate well in any area of nursing intervention is a failure of professionalism and can result in unnecessary distress to patients and their families.

REFERENCES

Ashley Y 1987 Sharing and learning: the experience of health education in women's self-help groups and its implications for nursing, midwifery and health visiting. In: Health Education Board for Scotland, Developing health education in nursing, midwifery and health visiting. HEBS, Edinburgh

Berlo D 1960 The process of communication: an introduction to theory and practice. Holt, Rinehart & Winston, New York

Bond S 1982 Communicating with families of cancer patients: Relatives and doctors. Nursing Times 9 June 962–5

Cartwright A 1964 Human relations and hospital care. Routledge & Kegan Paul, London

Ceccio J F, Ceccio C M 1982 Effective communication in nursing: theory and practice. Wiley, New York

Crotty M 1985 Communication between nurses and their patients. Nurse Education Today 5: 130–144

David J A 1986 Wound management: a comprehensive guide to dressing and healing. Practical Nursing Health Books Series. Martin Dunnitz, London

Egan G 1990 The skilled helper: a systematic approach to effective helping, 4th edn. Brooks/Cole, Pacific Grove, CA

Elliott K, Fuller J 1991 Health education and ethnic minorities. British Medical Journal 302(6786): 802–803

Faulkner A 1979 Monitoring nurse–patient conversation in a ward. Nursing Times 75(35) Supplement 23: 95–96

Flesch R 1974 The art of readable writing, 2nd edn. Harper & Row, New York

Fretwell J E 1982 Ward teaching and learning: sister and the learning environment. Royal College of Nursing, London

Gunning R 1968 The techniques of clear writing, 2nd edn. McGraw Hill, New York, p 190

Hawkey B, Clarke M 1990 Dress sense or nonsense. Nursing Times 86(3): 28–29, 31

Hayward J C 1975 Information: a prescription against pain. Royal College of Nursing, London

Health Service Commission 1986 Selected investigations April–October 1986. HMSO, London, 13–14

Hinds C 1985 The needs of families who care for patients with cancer at home: are we meeting them? Journal of Advanced Nursing 10: 575–81

Hockey L 1984 Conclusions. In: Faulkner A (ed) Communication. Churchill Livingstone, Edinburgh

Jourard S M 1960 The bedside manner. The American Journal of Nursing 60(1): 63–66

Jowett S, Armitage S 1988 Hospital and community liaison links in nursing: the role of the liaison nurse. Journal of Advanced Nursing 13(5): 579–587

Lelean S 1973 Ready for report, Nurse? RCN, London

Lorenz K 1952 King Solomon's ring. Methuen, London

Ley P 1988 Communicating with patients. Croom Helm, London

Macleod Clark J 1981 Communication in nursing. Nursing Times 77(1): 12–18

Macleod Clark J, Webb P A 1985 Health education: a basis for professional nursing practice. Nurse Education Today 5: 210–214

Maguire P, Faulkner A 1988a How to do it: improve the counselling skills of doctors and nurses in cancer care. British Medical Journal 297: 847–849

Maguire P, Faulkner A 1988b How to do it: communicate with cancer patients. 1: Handling bad news and difficult questions. British Medical Journal 297: 907–909

Maguire P, Faulkner A 1988c How to do it: communicate with cancer patients. 2: Handling uncertainty, collusion and denial. British Medical Journal 297: 972–974

Menzies I E P 1970 The functioning of social systems as a defence against anxiety. Tavistock Institute of Human Relations, London

Morrison P, Burnard P 1989 Students' and trained nurses' perceptions of their own interpersonal skills: a report and comparison. Journal of Advanced Nursing 14: 321–329

Neeson B, Faulkner A, Bridge W, Macleod Clark J 1984 Teaching communication skills to nurses. Part II: Evaluating the development of communication skills. Nurse Education Today 4(3): 54–57

Orton H D 1981 Ward learning climate and student nurse response. Nursing Times (Occasional Paper) 77: 17

Pembrey S 1980 The ward sister: key to nursing. Royal College of Nursing, London

Raphael W 1977 Patients and their hospitals. King Edward's Hospital Fund, London

Reynolds M 1978 No news is bad news: patients' views about communication in hospital. British Medical Journal 1: 1673–1676

Patient Information Service 1986 Patient information series. Royal Marsden Hospital, London

Runciman P 1989 Health assessment of the elderly at home: the case for shared learning. Journal of Advanced Nursing 14(2): 111–119

Sheridan M 1981 Children's development progress from birth to 5 years: the STYCAR sequences. NFER, London

Smith D 1990 Worn out. Nursing Times 86(3): 32, 34–35

Tschudin V 1987 Counselling skills for nurses, 2nd edn. Baillière Tindall, London

Webb P 1989 Patient teaching. In: Faulkner A (ed) Nursing the patient with cancer. Scutari Press, London

Wilson-Barnett J (ed) 1983 Keeping patients informed. Nursing 31: 1357–1358

FURTHER READING

Argyle M, Henderson M, Furnham A 1985 The rules of social relationships. British Journal of Social Psychology 24: 125–139

Dingwall R C 1980 Problems of teamwork in primary care. In: Lonsdale S, Webb A, Briggs T L (eds) Teamwork in the personal social services, ch 7. Croom Helm, London

Evers H K 1981 Multidisciplinary teams in geriatric wards: myth or reality? Journal of Advanced Nursing 16: 205–214

Hayduk L A 1983 Personal space: where we stand now. Psychological Bulletin 94: 293–335

Heslin R, Alpin T 1983 Touch: a bonding gesture. In: Wiemann J M, Harrison R P (eds) Non-verbal interaction. Sage, Beverley Hills

Kleck R 1969 Physical stigma and task oriented interaction. Human Relations 22: 51–60

Nuffield Provincial Hospitals Trust 1988 Talking & listening to patients: a modern approach. NPHT, London

Roy C 1964 Introduction to nursing: an adaptation model, 2nd edn. Prentice-Hall, Englewood Cliffs, NJ

USEFUL ADDRESSES

Health Education Board for Scotland
Woodburn House
Canaan Lane
Edinburgh EH10 4SG
Tel. No. 031-452 8989

Help for Health
Health Information Centre
Grant Building
Southampton General Hospital
Southampton S09 4XY
Tel. No. 0703–779091

Patient Information Service
Royal Marsden Hospital
Fulham Road
London SW3 6JJ

VOCAL (Voluntary Organisations Communications and Language)
336 Brixton Road
London SW9 7AA
Tel. No. 071-274 4029

SECTION 3

Nursing patients with special needs

SECTION CONTENTS

27 The patient facing surgery 775

28 The patient who experiences trauma 809

29 The critically ill patient 827

30 The unconscious patient 839

31 The patient with burns 859

32 The patient with cancer 875

33 The chronically ill patient 905

34 The terminally ill patient 921

35 The patient in need of rehabilitation 943

36 The older person 959

37 The person with dependency problems 973

38 The person with HIV/AIDS 991

The final section of the book explores some of the most challenging areas of practice. The range of topics illustrates the broad spectrum of adult nursing. Stereotypes are challenged and established values and beliefs are examined.

This provides an appropriate end to the book, as it highlights how essential it is for nurses to be willing to adapt their practice in response to new and ever-changing health needs.

CHAPTER 27

The patient facing surgery

Sheila E. Rodgers

CHAPTER CONTENTS

Introduction 775
Changing patterns of surgical care 775

Presurgical care 776
Classification of surgery 776
Presenting for surgery 776

Informed decision-making 778
The decision to operate 778
Informed consent 780
The role of the nurse 780
Resolving dilemmas 781

Preoperative preparation 781
Assessment 781
Giving information 781
Safe preparation for anaesthesia and surgery 782

Perioperative safety 786
Caring for the patient in theatre 786
Anaesthesia 789
Recovery from anaesthesia 791

Postoperative care 792
Shock and haemostasis 792
Fluid balance 794
Metabolic and stress responses 796
Pain 796
Nausea and vomiting 798
Sleep 798
Elimination 799
Wound care 799
Potential complications 802
Communication 802
Body image 804
Discharge teaching 804
Discharge planning 804

Rehabilitation 805

References 805

Further reading 807

INTRODUCTION

This chapter aims to give an overview of the nursing care required by patients facing surgery. Discussion will include not only those interventions relevant to the period of hospitalisation, but also the support needed by patients during the diagnostic process and during their eventual rehabilitation at home. Patients undergo many types of surgery for a wide range of reasons, but the principles of care can to a large degree be generalised with reference to particular types of procedure. It should be stressed, however, that individuals often react quite differently to a given disease or treatment. What one person may regard as a 'minor' procedure may cause extreme anxiety in another. Nursing staff must be sensitive to each patient's individuality and try to appreciate the significance of the experience of surgery from the patient's own perspective.

?	**27.1** Think of an intervention or form of treatment you have experienced, such as removal of wisdom teeth, a cervical smear, or suturing of a cut. What sort of fears did you have, however irrational they might seem now?

No attempt has been made to apply any one model of nursing throughout the chapter, although it might be suggested that appropriate models can be selected according to the nature of the patient's illness and the care required. The present chapter does, however, highlight advances in care that are made possible by the use of primary nursing (see Allsopp 1991, Ersser & Tutton 1991, Manthey 1981, Pearson 1988, Wright 1990).

Changing patterns of surgical care

Advances in surgical technology have had a dramatic effect in recent years on the experience of patients undergoing surgery. Interventions now available range from laser treatment to shatter (ablate) renal stones (lithotripsy) to stapling and suturing of the bowel to restore continuity. Laparoscopic angiographic catheterisation, endoscopy and laser techniques are now advancing rapidly to incorporate treatment often at the time of investigation, and as treatments in their own right are replacing many standard invasive surgical techniques (Frost 1993). Arthroscopy is now the method of choice in managing tears of the menisci in the knee. Many gynaecological procedures can be carried out laparoscopically, e.g. excision of ovarian cysts and tubal ligation. Laser therapy for endometrial ablation, with a one-night stay in hospital as opposed to 10 nights for a standard hysterectomy, is being developed (Nursing Standard 1991).

There have been recent developments in laparoscopic cholecystectomy, which for some patients can now be done as day surgery with a local anaesthetic (Dubois, Berthelot & Levard 1989). In the UK, however, patients usually undergo this procedure under a general anaesthetic. Nonetheless, it only takes 40–90 minutes in experienced hands, leaving the patient with very little scarring or pain, and requiring only a 2-day stay in hospital. Many patients return to work within one week (Dubois et al 1990). In comparison, the standard treatment for gallstones — cholecystectomy — involves scarring, postoperative pain, a 7–10 day stay in hospital and 6 weeks off work (Cheslyn-Curtis & Russell 1991).

Day surgery has become possible for many general surgical patients. The trend is also apparent in surgical specialities: in Scotland, day cases for gynaecological surgery have grown from 6 324 in 1981 to 14 433 in 1990 and in plastic surgery from 1 432 in 1981 to 7 810 in 1990 (Common Services Agency, 1990). The effects of this trend include decreasing morbidity, shorter length of stay and increased patient turnover. This in turn has increased the responsibilities of informal carers and district nurses.

There are increasing numbers of elderly people in our society. In 1996, it is estimated that there will be 10.1 million people in the UK aged 65 and over, constituting around 16% of the population (Office of Health Economics 1989). With advances in medical and nursing care, the elderly are more likely to survive and achieve a good quality of life following surgery. Surgeons are now able to offer procedures to people who in previous years would not have been considered fit for surgery.

The nature of surgical services is changing rapidly to keep pace with technology and with advances in knowledge and skills. Not least among the factors affecting surgical care are changes in the overall approach to nursing practice. A study of one surgical ward demonstrated that many improvements in nursing practice, including the introduction of primary nursing, could be made without any need for increased staffing levels. During this time there were no obvious changes in medical practice, but a significant fall in postoperative complications, reduced length of stay, and an increase in patient satisfaction were noted. These effects were attributed to changes in nursing practice (Malby 1991).

The nurse's role in surgical care will continue to evolve rapidly in response to the shift toward day case surgery, which will intensify the needs of patients during their time in hospital and put increased emphasis on pre- and postoperative care in the community.

PRESURGICAL CARE

Classification of surgery

Some patients experience a long period of ill-health or disability before undergoing an operation; others experience a sudden illness or injury that necessitates immediate surgery. The degree of urgency of a surgical intervention is a useful criterion for its classification and prioritisation. An elderly patient with osteoarthritis of the hip who requires a total hip replacement operation would normally not be classified as an urgent case, but would be put on a waiting list and admitted 'electively'. However, if the same patient had fallen and fractured the neck of the femur, repair or (more commonly) total replacement of the hip to prevent further deterioration and ensure a speedy recovery would be regarded as 'essential'.

A given operation may be performed for different classifications of surgery. Surgery for a strangulated hernia will be handled as an emergency, whereas surgery for an irreducible hernia will be considered as essential, and for a reducible one as elective. Patients requiring essential surgery will be admitted to hospital within a week or two, but elective patients may have to wait for some considerable time. In 1990 there was a total of 50 719 patients waiting for general surgery in Scotland (Common Services Agency 1990); in 1989 the total in England was 876 009 (Connah & Pearson 1991).

Waiting times for surgery are among the issues addressed in the Patient's Charter (Scottish Office 1991). Patients are guaranteed a maximum waiting time for elective surgery of 18 months in Scotland and 2 years in England. There has been some debate as to the usefulness of this focus on waiting times. To say that all patients receive surgery within 2 years may meet a standard, but for an individual who requires surgery within several weeks the standard cannot apply. For those waiting for some types of surgery such as hip replacement a 2-year wait may be intolerable. However, within the guarantees of the Charter medical staff can no longer delay non-urgent surgery beyond 2 years in order to treat more urgent, but not immediately life-threatening, cases.

Presenting for surgery

> ? **27.2** In your surgical ward placement, ask your patients what signs and symptoms first brought their attention to their illness. What was it that made them seek out treatment? How do they define ill-health?

Personal definitions of health and ill-health and the decision to seek treatment are influenced by a range of factors such as previous experience, social context, perceived severity of the illness and judgements as to whether treatment would be beneficial.

In Case History 27.1(A), Mr W was reluctant to take time off work to seek treatment but eventually came to a point where pain and discomfort made it impossible for him to carry on. In Case History 27.2(A), Mrs B was very reluctant to seek help, partly due to her fear of having cancer, and partly due to what she felt was an embarrassing symptom. She had also convinced herself that she merely had haemorrhoids and could treat the condition herself.

In Case History 27.3(A), Mr L's community nurse had been alerted to problems developing and had contacted his general practitioner (GP) to initiate treatment. However, she remained worried about Mr L, as although the abscess was small it was not reducing. She knew Mr L well and was sensitive to the deterioration in his general condition. She pursued her reassessment of Mr L and liaised with the GP, the consultant, the patient's wife and the surgical ward nurse in providing care.

Pathways and progress

Patients may be referred for surgery by different paths. Figure 27.1 represents the progress of Mr W and Mr L through the health care system, and Figure 27.2 that of Mrs B. Patients might enter these pathways at various points; Mrs B for example, was taken straight to Accident and Emergency (A & E) by ambulance without seeing her GP about the illness. Patients may also be transferred from other wards. For example, a patient on a medical ward may undergo investigations which lead to a diagnosis that necessitates surgical treatment and therefore transfer to a surgical ward. A few patients admitted as emergencies may go straight to theatre from A & E and be admitted to the surgical ward following the operation. Some patients may need to go back to theatre or the intensive

Case History 27.1(A) Mr W

Mr W was a 42-year-old man who worked for a large construction company. He was married and had three young children. They enjoyed a comfortable lifestyle and had bought their own home that year. Mr W had been able to get some overtime work and this helped considerably with the mortgage repayments.

Mr W had been having some pain and swelling in his groin for some time, but it usually resolved on its own over time. However, over the past few weeks the swelling had got worse and was limiting the range of work he could do. One day when he was in obvious discomfort he was told by the foreman to see the occupational health nurse.

The nurse quickly assessed the extent of his inguinal hernia and rang Mr W's GP to make an urgent appointment. Before leaving the treatment room, she fitted him with a scrotal support and gave him some simple analgesia.

Mr W returned to light duties after a couple of days' sick leave. He thanked the nurse and returned the support she had given him. She was pleased to see Mr W looking relaxed and comfortable. She instructed him to continue to wear the support and gave him an extra one to help with laundering. He told her that his GP was referring him for surgery, but he was worried about taking time off work and being able to carry on with his job. The nurse reassured him that he would eventually be able to return to a full range of duties once he had completely recovered. She also suggested that if he were able to give up smoking he would have less of the cough that was partly exacerbating his hernia, and that he would have a better chance of a quick recovery after the anaesthetic. Mr W had always found he put on weight when he stopped smoking and was already moderately overweight. They discussed a plan of how he might give up smoking, including the use of chewing gum and nicotine patches. He knew his wife would be very supportive but was less sure of his mates, whom he met in the pub on Friday nights. The nurse also gave him a booklet on healthy eating to take home and look at with his wife. He quickly identified that his fried breakfasts and love of chips and beer was a major source of imbalance in his diet.

Several weeks later, the nurse spotted Mr W as she was touring the shop floor. He called her over to tell her that he had not had a cigarette for three weeks. He had saved the money he would have spent on cigarettes, which he felt would go some way towards keeping the family solvent during his sick leave. He also told her that he had a date for his operation at the end of the month. They talked about what sort of work he would be able to do after the operation. Mr W felt he knew the nurse well enough now to ask her about the effect of the operation on his ability to have sex and whether it would make him sterile. She reassured him on these points and explained that the operation would tighten a track through to his scrotum and would not affect his genitals. She did warn him, however, that he might be a little tender in the groin for the first week.

Case History 27.2 Mrs B

Mrs B was a 78-year-old woman who had lost her husband several years ago. Her eldest daughter lived nearby and was very supportive. Mrs B now lived in sheltered housing, which was a relief to her daughter, as she had previously lived in an isolated country cottage. Her sight had gradually deteriorated in recent years and the arthritis in her fingers and knees limited what she could do. At the time Mrs B became ill, she was pleased to have her own home still, and enjoyed going to the local day centre twice a week.

One of the care assistants at the day centre was a little concerned that Mrs B did not seem to be enjoying the singing quite so much as before and spent much of the afternoon dozing. Mrs B being an independent and spirited lady, thanked the young girl for her concern and joked that she wasn't getting any younger and that there was no need to worry about her.

Mrs B thought long and hard that evening. She had been constipated for some time but had put it down to old age. Now she was also passing blood and although she was frightened that it might be 'something nasty', she had decided that it must be piles. She had bought some ointment and laxatives from the chemist, but was reluctant to go to her GP, who had visited her when she just moved into the area. He was a nice young man, but she did not want him to examine her.

Several weeks later, the driver of the day centre minibus got no reply at Mrs B's door when he called to collect her. Worried that she might have fallen, he called the warden, who had a key to the flat. Mrs B was found still in her bed, in obvious pain and sweating profusely. The warden called an ambulance immediately and then phoned Mrs B's daughter. Mrs B was then taken to the A & E department of the local hospital.

Case History 27.3(A) Mr L

Mr L was a 56-year-old man who had suffered from multiple sclerosis for many years. He lived at home with his wife, and with the help of the community nurses, normally coped well with his disability. He now had no sensation or power in his legs, but was able to transfer to and from and get about in his wheelchair. He was extremely knowledgeable about his illness, and had a very positive approach to living with his disability.

The community nursing sister had worked out a plan of care with Mr and Mrs L to ensure that they received appropriate help and care and that the necessary equipment and aids were provided. She would visit every second day to give bowel care, as Mr L had no voluntary control over his bowels. Recently, she noticed a small red area developing on Mr L's buttock. She checked the inflation pressure in his Rohoe cushion and with Mr L decided to increase the frequency of pressure relief (i.e. raising himself off the seat of his chair).

The next time the nurse visited, a small abscess had begun to form with some obvious pus, and she phoned Mr L's GP, who then arranged to visit him at home the following day. The GP lanced the abscess with a scalpel and took a specimen of pus to send to the laboratory for culture and sensitivity. As the result could take several days to come back Mr L was started on a course of antibiotics which would be appropriate for common skin infections.

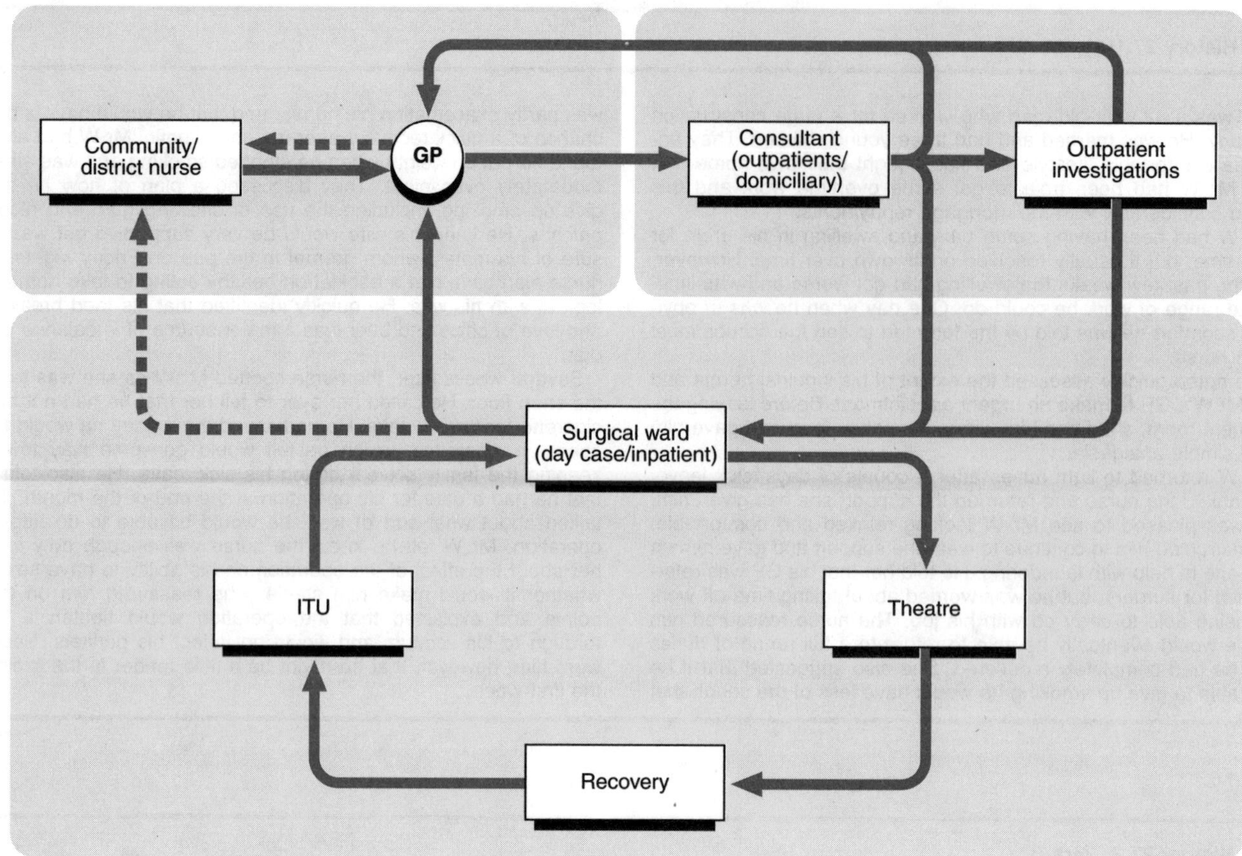

Fig. 27.1 Pathways to essential and elective surgery.

therapy unit (ITU) if their condition deteriorates or requires further intervention. Occasionally, a lengthy convalescence or rehabilitation may be required in another ward or hospital.

There are a number of patients, such as M in Case History 27.4(A), whose illness is of a chronic nature, and who will be readmitted to the surgical ward on one or more occasions. Patients with Crohn's disease can present at an early age, and may require repeated interventions and admissions to hospital throughout their lives. In a busy surgical ward these patients require a sensitive approach. One must not assume that because a patient has been through a procedure before she will need less support or information than she did the first time.

The vast majority of patients are admitted to hospital from home and return to their own homes. The GP can be seen as the gatekeeper to services, as unless the illness is a sudden emergency or an accident, he is the one who will refer the patient for further care under the hospital consultant. However, as with Mr L and Mr W, community nurses can be the first point of contact for the patient, referring the patient to the GP or seeking the GP's advice for further treatment. Community nurses have established lines of communication with the wards but these tend to be unidirectional, moving from ward to community nurse. However, in at least one centre, community nurses have been successfully included routinely in the preoperative assessment of patients for their suitability to have day surgery for varicose veins and hernias. To maintain continuity of care these same community nurses carry out the postoperative visits (Hart 1982).

A substantial morbidity exists among patients on waiting lists for surgery. Those waiting for hip surgery, for example, may suffer restricted activity and constant pain. Those awaiting gallstone surgery may suffer recurrent bouts of severe abdominal pain. Mr W is fortunately supported by his occupational health nurse, who institutes measures to reduce discomfort and prevent further injury while he waits for treatment.

?	**27.3** What actions might a community nurse take to improve the health of these patients awaiting surgery?

INFORMED DECISION-MAKING

The aim of this section is to introduce the issue of informed consent for surgery by discussing nursing responsibilities and highlighting some areas for ethical debate. (For a wider discussion on the ethical aspects of consent, see Rumbold 1986.)

The decision to operate

Once the outcome of investigations are known and have been considered in the light of the patient's presenting signs and symptoms, the surgeon can make a definite or provisional diagnosis and recommend a course of action. This may involve diagnostic, curative or palliative surgery, a combination of these, or no surgical intervention at all. If the patient can be treated as successfully without surgical intervention, then the relevant alternatives will be pursued. Consider the following examples:

- A middle-aged woman is found to have stage 2A cervical

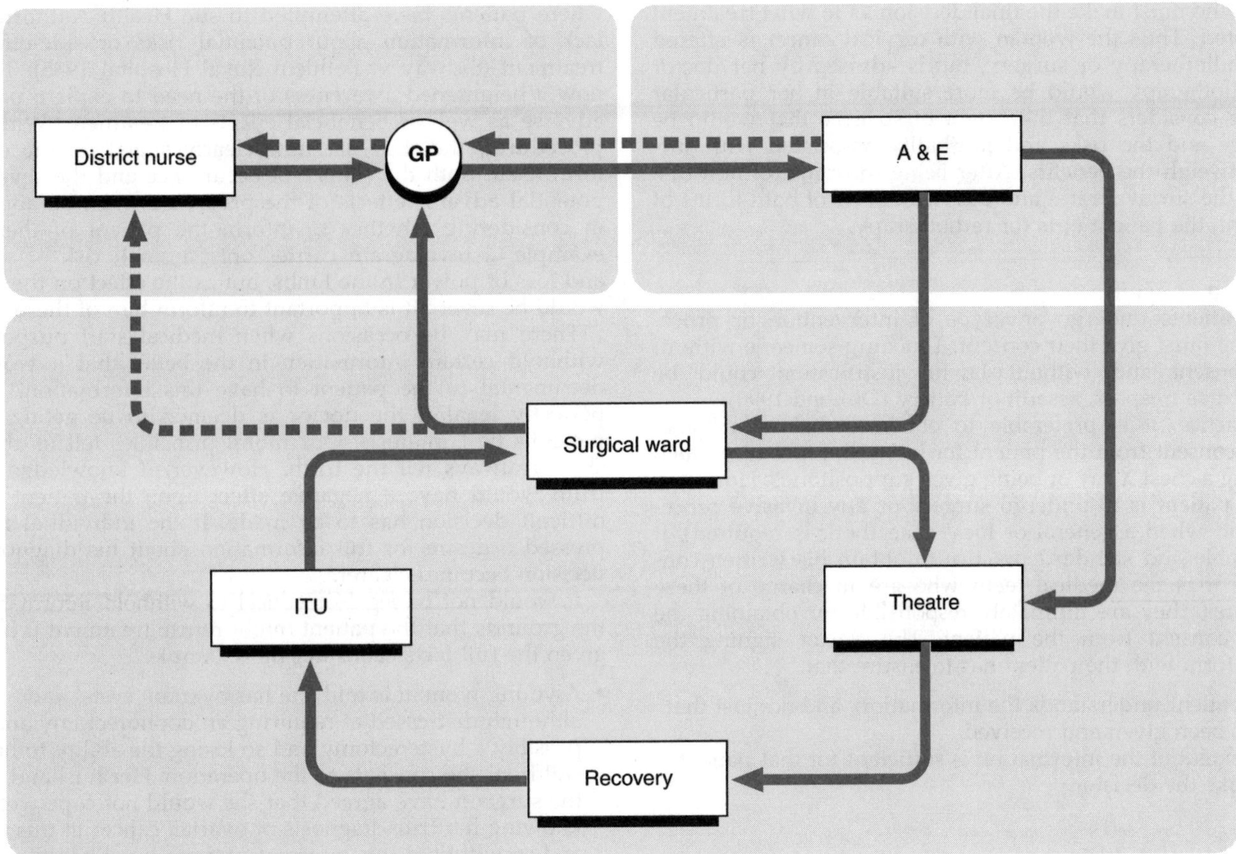

Fig. 27.2 Pathways to emergency surgery.

cancer (see Ch. 32) with infiltrating lymph nodes when she undergoes examination under anaesthesia (EUA). It is decided that surgery is not appropriate. She is referred to an oncologist, who prescribes a course of radical radiotherapy.

- Another patient has been referred to hospital for an oesophagoscopy and gastroscopy after complaining of heartburn. He is found to have a hiatus hernia and is prescribed an antacid and gelling agent (Gaviscon). The nurse in outpatients gives the patient advice on sleeping propped up at night, avoiding certain foods and on how to take his medication.
- M (Case History 27.4(A)) has been making frequent visits over the last few months to see her medical consultant about her vaginal fistula. Despite enteral diets, anti-inflammatory agents and antibiotics, the fistula does not resolve. She is referred to the surgeon and subsequently admitted to the surgical ward.

It might appear from these brief descriptions that it is the medical staff who take the decision on the course of treatment to be given. However, whereas the doctor decides what treatment appears to be the most appropriate, it is the informed

Case History 27.4(A) M

M was a 23-year-old hotel receptionist who had suffered from Crohn's disease for as long as she could remember. She had been in and out of hospital on account of her condition on many occasions. This time she was sent straight up to the ward after her appointment in the outpatients' department. The primary nurse who had looked after her on two earlier occasions felt a real friendship with her. When the nurse greeted her on the ward, M burst into tears. M told her how she had developed a horrible faecally discharge from her vagina and that she had been admitted for more investigations. She was pyrexial, looked pale, and with her small frame appeared extremely fragile. The primary nurse offered her a single room as she was obviously distressed by her uncontrolled diarrhoea.

Once M had telephoned her boyfriend, with whom she had been living for the past year, and had taken time to collect her thoughts, she was visited by the consultant. He suggested that a fistula was the cause of the current problem and that the best plan of action would be to close it surgically. M was informed that there was a chance that she would need a defunctioning stoma and spent some time talking to the primary nurse and the night staff about it.

The next day M started her bowel preparation. This consisted of 4 l of Go-lytely to be taken over the next 24 h. She was not allowed to eat that day but could take extra drinks of clear fluids if she wanted. She discussed with the primary nurse the use of large pads to absorb leakage from her vagina. She was also given some soft wipes and a tube of barrier cream to avoid excoriation of the perianal area by the diarrhoea.

patient who must make the final decision as to what treatment is accepted. Thus the woman with cervical cancer is offered either radiotherapy or surgery, but is advised by her doctor that radiotherapy would be more suitable in her particular case. He considers that the extent of surgery that would be necessary and the risks and morbidity associated with surgery outweigh the benefits. After being informed of and discussing the survival rates and adverse effects of both forms of treatment, the patient opts for radiotherapy.

Informed consent

When patients undergo any type of intervention or procedure they must give their consent. Touching someone without their consent and without lawful justification could be construed as trespass, assault or battery (Dimond 1990).

In practice, it is preferable to obtain verbal rather than written consent from the patient for low-risk procedures such as having a chest X-ray or being given suppositories. However, when a patient is to undergo surgery or any invasive procedure (and when a general or local anaesthetic is required), it is advisable and standard practice to obtain his written consent. As it is the medical team who are in charge of these procedures, they are ultimately responsible for obtaining the written consent from the patient. The doctor signing the consent form with the patient has to ensure that:

1. The patient understands the information, and not just that it has been given and received
2. The extent of the information is sufficient for that patient to make the decision.

The role of the nurse

The nurse has an important role to play in obtaining consent prior to surgery. For a patient to give a valid consent, he must comprehend fully what he is consenting to; that is, his consent must be informed. The nurse can provide the team with a knowledge of her patient's individual need for information and his comprehension of the information given.

The nurse will also provide the patient with information about the procedure and the recovery period and may be able to clarify points previously discussed between patient and doctor. However, the nurse cannot and must not be the provider of information in order for the doctor to obtain informed consent for surgery. This is a medical staff responsibility.

There may be occasions when the nurse considers she needs to obtain written consent from her patient for a particular nursing procedure or treatment. In this instance, providing the information for consent is the nurse's responsibility, as she is in charge of the procedure.

The need for informed consent raises several legal and ethical issues for nurses and patients. The current social climate emphasises consumerism and patients' rights. Patients have an increased desire to be 'partners in care', that is, to be well informed and to take responsibility for their own health. The established rights of the individual to be given an adequate explanation of proposed treatment (including any risks and alternatives) and to have access to health records have been reiterated in the Patient's Charter (Scottish Office 1991) and should be encompassed in local standards of care. (For discussion of the legal aspects of consent see DOH (1990) and Young (1991).)

However, there may be occasions when the patient is less than fully informed. The depth and complexity of information held by medical staff may be overwhelming for a lay person. This consideration must be balanced against individual needs and consumer demands. There have been some instances where patients have attempted to sue Health Authorities for lack of information about potential risks or side-effects of treatment (Sidway v. Bethlem Royal Hospital 1985). There is now a heightened awareness of the need to explain potential adverse as well as beneficial effects of treatment. With some procedures, the risks are now clearly stated on the consent form itself. Both the chance of occurrence and the severity of potential adverse effects of the procedure must be addressed in considering whether to inform the patient of them. For example, a myelogram carries only a small risk of seizures and loss of power in the limbs, but as the effect on the patient would be severe it is important to inform him of these risks.

There may be occasions when medical staff purposefully withhold certain information in the belief that it would be detrimental to the patient to have this information. This is perfectly legal if the doctor is deemed to be acting in the patient's best interests. Our moral principles tell us that one should always tell the truth. However, if knowledge of the truth would have a negative effect upon the patient then a difficult decision has to be made. If the individual has expressed a desire for full information about his diagnosis the decision becomes clearer.

It would not be legal or ethical to withhold information on the grounds that the patient might refuse treatment if he were given the full facts. Consider this example:

- A young woman is told she has ovarian 'cysts' and although distressed at requiring an oophorectomy and possibly a hysterectomy and so losing the ability to have children, she consents to the operation. Her husband and the surgeon have agreed that she would not cope well with knowing her true diagnosis of ovarian cancer at this time, and so withhold this information from her. She then questions the ward nurses, at first indirectly and then directly with questions such as 'It's cancer, isn't it?' and 'This is going to be the end of me, isn't it?'

?	**27.4** What might you do or say if faced with such a situation in the ward? How might the patient react if you told her you were not able to answer her questions? Discuss the example with your nursing and medical colleagues.

In theory, a nurse could face disciplinary action or even dismissal if she were to go against the surgeon's expressed wish to withhold information. This is highly unlikely if the nurse were clearly acting in the patient's best interests. In practice, it is more usual for nursing and medical staff to be sensitive to the individual needs of the patient and to work collaboratively with the patient and his family to resolve any such moral dilemmas (for further reading see Thomson et al 1988).

In some cases the patient may be too ill to comprehend what is proposed sufficiently well to give informed consent. When an adult patient is unable to give informed consent, e.g. when he is unconscious or mentally unfit, his relatives have no legal right in giving or, perhaps more importantly, in *refusing* consent. Good practice would dictate that relatives are consulted and a decision made in the patient's best interest. However, the ultimate decision in this case is the doctor's. (For further reading see Brennan 1989.)

Similarly, relatives have no legal rights in determining whether information should be given to or withheld from the patient. In fact, the doctor or nurse would be in breach of confidentiality if he or she were to tell the relatives first, or to tell them at all, without the patient's expressed consent. But if the patient is withheld the information how can he consent to it being divulged? (Young 1991).

Resolving dilemmas

When a patient is too ill to be told, or cannot give informed consent, then medical and nursing staff must carry out their professional duty to act in the patient's best interests, whilst considering the wishes of the relatives.

The UKCC Code of Professional Conduct (UKCC 1992) provides nurses with guidelines on professional practice and on exercising accountability (UKCC 1989). The nurses caring for the patient described above followed the code in terms of acting to safeguard his interests and in working in a collaborative and co-operative manner with other health care professionals. It is essential that nurses are familiar with the Code and apply it in everyday practice. Guidelines on informed consent have also been produced for doctors and nurses (DOH 1990, Medical Defence Union 1986).

PREOPERATIVE PREPARATION

Preoperative preparation might begin long before the patient is admitted to a hospital ward. Mr W's occupational health nurse and Mr L's district nurse were both involved in preparing their patients for surgery. As this aspect of care has already been considered, this section refers to the immediate preoperative period following admission to hospital.

Patients arrive for admission having experienced very different types of preparation. Mrs B had no preparation at all, being taken to A & E as an emergency. Mr L had already seen his consultant surgeon at home the day prior to admission and had discussed the need for hospital admission and possible surgery with him and the district nurse. Mr W had visited the ward one week earlier and met his primary nurse. She had talked to him along with a small group of patients coming in for 'minor' (short-stay) surgery over the next couple of weeks. He had received a short booklet about the ward and had some blood tests, a chest X-ray and an ECG. He arrived on the ward on the morning of admission having had nothing to eat or drink since going to bed the night before. The primary nurse showed him to a chair where he could wait for a bed to become available. It would be a busy day for the primary nurse. She had received a phone call to say that Mrs B was to be admitted from A & E as an emergency, and was also aware that Mr L would be arriving in time for the consultant's round later that morning.

All of these patients, whether emergency, essential or elective admissions, would require appropriate preoperative assessment, information about their care, and safe preparation for anaesthetic and surgery.

Assessment

Assessment of the patient is required in order to identify any special needs, to highlight potential problems, and to provide a baseline against which to measure postoperative progress. Ideally, the primary nurse would admit the patient herself in order to establish a relationship and to enable her to directly observe and question the patient. She may also use other sources of information, such as existing medical or nursing records, the patient's relatives, and other health care professionals to form a complete picture. The way a nurse assesses a patient will vary according to the model used. This might be one developed by the ward nurses or an established model such as Roper, Logan & Tierney's activities of daily living model (1990) or Johnson's behavioural system model (1980). But while each nurse's approach to, and description of, the delivery of care may be different, the needs of the patient remain essentially the same.

Giving information

Giving the patient information and emotional support preoperatively has been shown to substantially reduce pre- and postoperative anxiety (Mumford et al 1982). Reducing preoperative anxiety and stress is not only desirable on humanitarian grounds, but also promotes recovery. High levels of preoperative anxiety have been associated with an increased need for anaesthetic agents (Williams et al 1972), an increased need for analgesia postoperatively (Hayward 1975), a greater incidence of postoperative complications (Jarvis 1958) and a longer postoperative hospital stay (Egbert et al 1964). Giving information and support not only reduces anxiety but has a direct effect on reducing postoperative complications, partly by increasing compliance.

An increase in postoperative ventilation capacity has been clearly demonstrated with preoperative teaching (Lindenman & van Aeinman 1971). Teaching patients breathing exercises prior to theatre is now standard practice for almost all surgical patients. A study by Wong & Wong (1985) demonstrated that patients were more satisfied and more compliant with postoperative activities when they were given a structured and complete preoperative education programme.

It is important that patients receive information at an appropriate level and on matters that do in fact concern them — not simply on what the nurse assumes they will be anxious about. Inappropriate information not only fails to resolve existing anxieties but may create even more worries for the patient (Johnson 1982). Biley (1989) compared nurse and patient perceptions of issues causing anxiety in preoperative patients. There were some notable differences in the ranking of some items: being away from home and work, being away from relatives, and unsuitable/unsatisfactory food were all ranked much higher by patients than by nurses. Nurses incorrectly perceived that having drips, injections and tests, and being discussed by staff, would be rated high as sources of anxiety. Patients reported being in pain, not understanding instructions, not knowing test results, being away from home and work and not having enough information as their top five worries (in descending order).

?	**27.5** How will this knowledge change the way you would approach giving information to your preoperative patient?

Skilled, systematic and sensitive assessment is essential in determining what is important for the individual.

Sensitive, open questioning can determine what the patient already understands and what he would like to know more about. Simply giving a factual account of what will occur is insufficient. Patients want to know what to expect and how it will feel. They also need the opportunity to discuss their fears and worries. Factual and sensory information, coping strategies and counselling are then the essential components of preoperative education. During the admission procedure Mr W told his primary nurse that he was afraid of feeling pain during the operation, as he knew he could be awake throughout the procedure. The nurse then described to him what kind of sensations he might expect:

> Once all the checks and preparations have been completed in the ward, you will be given a tablet that will make you feel a little drowsy and more relaxed. The checks will take place again when you get to theatre and a nurse will stay with you at all times. When you go into theatre, the doctors will put up a screen with green cloths so you won't have to watch what is happening. They will also give you an injection around the top of your leg to begin to numb the area. It feels like a scratch under the skin as they make sure the skin is numb

before giving you a deeper dose of anaesthetic. You will probably feel quite sleepy during the procedure, but you may feel the doctor pressing around the area, although there should be no pain or discomfort. You will never lose consciousness and would always be able to tell the doctor if you felt anything. If you would like to listen to some music on the headphones when you are in theatre, let me know before you go up and I can show you what tapes we have. A lot of people find it takes their mind off things and helps them relax. Remember there is always a nurse with you whom you can talk to or ask about things whilst you are in theatre. How do you feel about things now?

?	**27.6** Can you identify the information given here in terms of knowledge, sensory information and coping strategies?

When and how information is given will influence its effectiveness. Many patients have difficulty in remembering verbal information; while a personal, verbal explanation is invaluable in that it allows for feedback from the patient, it has a poor recall over time. This is especially so when the information is given in a high-stress situation, such as the outpatients appointment at which the patient is told that he needs an operation, or in the days prior to the operation in hospital (Baskerville et al 1985).

Recall of information is improved when information is given in a relaxed setting (Reading 1981). One way of achieving this is by giving the patient written information prior to admission. In one study of surgical patients a constant preference for preoperative preparation in *advance* of admission to hospital was shown (Wallace 1985). The patients reported feelings of anxiety beginning at the time of the outpatients appointment. Preadmission information also allowed for emotional adjustment over a longer period, and enabled patients to share information with and seek support from their families. Rice & Johnson (1984) also found that there was increased learning and better surgical outcomes when information was given prior to admission rather than on admission or later. The patients were not in a high-stress situation and were able to reread the information and so assimilate it more easily.

Preadmission booklets for surgical patients can be beneficial in reducing patient anxiety and improving outcomes, but they are not a substitute for personalised explanation. They can, however, prepare patients to use this contact time more effectively. This allows the nurse to focus on areas of concern and to devote more time to counselling than to information-giving, as in reality it is often difficult to complete both tasks well in the busy preoperative period. Thus, in the example given above, the primary nurse is able to spend some time providing more detailed information and coping strategies as Mr W had already read about his operation and visited the ward to familiarise himself with the environment.

Preoperative information booklets should be easy to read without being patronising. Print size, reading ease and vocabulary should all be considered and the use of jargon avoided. A booklet must also be comprehensive, as this improves recall and compliance with instructions (Bradshaw et al 1975). Many wards produce their own booklets about the ward and general information about surgery. Some also have leaflets about specific operations which can be sent or given to the patient with the ward and/or hospital booklet prior to admission.

Preoperative education aims to produce a well-informed consumer, to promote healthy choices and to reduce anxiety. The informed patient is better equipped to make good decisions about his care and to discuss his treatment fully and openly with staff. In this sense, information also serves to produce a more autonomous patient (Ewles & Simnet 1992). One must then respect the view that the well-informed patient has the right to reject advice or treatment against professional judgement for personal reasons (Fahrenfort 1987). What the professional advocates may conflict with what the patient wants. Simply informing someone of an objective fact that appears rational (e.g. smoking causes lung cancer) will be insufficient in some cases to promote healthy behaviour or coping mechanisms (Galvin 1992). (For further reading on patient education see Coutts & Hardy 1985.)

Safe preparation for anaesthesia and surgery

In the admission assessment the patient's specific needs and potential problems may be identified. The general risks associated with anaesthesia and surgical intervention will also be taken into account in any related medical or nursing procedure. Patients undergoing surgery require medical assessment, the nature of which will depend on the extent of surgery, the age of the patient and on any pre-existing medical conditions. Mr W was given a chest X-ray to screen for any abnormalities of the lungs, a blood test for urea and electrolytes and a full blood count. An ECG was performed to rule out cardiac dysfunction, as it is important to ensure that a patient has no gross abnormalities of the cardiovascular and respiratory systems prior to the administration of an anaesthetic. The anaesthetist was pleased that Mr W had managed to stop smoking, and relieved that he no longer had a productive cough. Smoking considerably increases the risk of chest infection and atelectasis postoperatively.

Risk of chest infection

All patients receiving a general anaesthetic are at risk of developing a chest infection; this is one of the most common complications after surgery (Webb 1975). Drugs and gases used in anaesthesia are drying to the respiratory tract and inhibit the action of the cilia. Secretions of mucus become thick and tenacious, causing partial obstruction of the lower airways. Cigarette smoking also damages and paralyses the cilia and leads to excess mucus production. The secretions eventually pool in the base of the lungs and plug the bronchioles. The retained secretions obstruct the lower airways, inhibiting gaseous exchange and providing a source of bacterial infection.

Artificial ventilation during the operation is at tidal volume and does not fully inflate the lung (see Ch. 3, p. 61). Normally, a person will sigh intermittently or increase demands for oxygen by activity, so fully inflating the lungs and preventing stagnation and atelectasis. Changes of position, movement and coughing all serve to dislodge excess mucus or fluid, which is then expelled from the lungs as sputum. The patient will be lying still and unable to cough or sigh throughout the operation when under a general anaesthetic. There will also be a period of inactivity postoperatively and perhaps a reluctance to breathe deeply or cough if there is abdominal or thoracic pain.

Patients should be advised to stop smoking, at least for two weeks prior to surgery (Webb 1975) if not for good. They must be taught deep breathing exercises and coughing. It can be difficult to teach a patient to contract the diaphragm in order to deep-breathe preoperatively, let alone postoperatively. The tendency is to use intercostal and accessory muscles to lift the ribcage and draw the abdomen in. Although instruction may be the responsibility of the physiotherapist in some wards, it will still require reinforcement from the nursing staff. In this context, the need for early mobilisation can be described to the patient. (For further reading on deep breathing exercises see Webber & Pryor 1994.)

> **?** **27.7** Try some deep breathing exercises yourself. Did you draw your abdomen in and lift the ribcage? Try to breathe using the diaphragm. Place one hand on your abdomen. Breathe in through your nose while you try to feel your abdomen pushing your hand out (as the diaphragm moves downwards and displaces the stomach).

Risk of deep vein thrombosis (DVT) and pulmonary embolism (PE)

An intravascular clot or thrombus is most likely to occur when the following three conditions (known as Virchow's triad) exist:

- trauma: damaged endothelium
- stasis: slow blood flow
- hypercoagulable blood.

Thrombus formation is initiated by the activation of Factor XII in reaction to exposure to collagen filaments in the damaged endothelium. This results in platelet aggregation, formation of thrombin from circulating prothrombin, and stimulation of the production of insoluble fibrin from fibrinogen (see Ch. 11, p. 409).

It has been found that during surgery, the veins of the lower leg distend by up to 48% (Coleridge Smith et al 1991). This distension leads to subluminal endothelial damage, which can provide a site for clot formation. In the soleal and gastrocnemius veins, the blood flow is highly dependent on exercise, and so these are often the site of initial thrombus formation following prolonged periods of inactivity and lack of calf muscle pressure to assist venous return. The general adaptation reaction to the stress of surgery (see Ch. 17, p. 580) results in reduced levels of the coagulation inhibitors protein C, protein S and antithrombin III. Fibrin clots may be gradually broken down by the enzyme plasmin in a process called fibrinolysis. However, the thrombus may persist, causing some degree of venous obstruction. In a small proportion of cases a fragment of the clot breaks away, forming an embolus. The embolus may travel through the venous system, through the right side of the heart and into the pulmonary arteries. Here it becomes lodged at a point where the arteries become too small to allow the embolus to pass through. The extent of the resultant pulmonary infarct depends on the size of the vessel occluded. Some patients may have no signs and symptoms of either DVT or PE if thrombi are small and infrequent (see p. 54 for signs and symptoms). However, large thrombi can be devastating, causing sudden death in 50% of patients with pulmonary embolism.

All surgical patients are exposed to a number of risk factors for DVT. It is not surprising, then, that the incidence of DVT in patients over 40 years of age is around 30% where no preventive measures are taken (National Institutes of Health 1986). During the preoperative assessment the nurse should assess the patient for the presence of other known risk factors. Caprini et al (1988) have categorised risk of thrombosis into low, moderate and high risk categories (see Fig. 27.3).

The preventive measures taken by medical and nursing staff will depend on the level of risk for DVT and potential bleeding complications in individual patients. It is now generally accepted that patients in *all* risk categories should use

Risk factors

Age			
40–60 yrs = 1 point	☐	Trauma	☐
61–70 yrs = 2 points	☐	Theatre time = 2 hours +	☐
70+ yrs = 3 points	☐	Total joint replacement	☐
History of DVT/PE = 3 points	☐	Pelvic long bone fracture	☐
Immobilisation	☐	Leg: oedema, ulcer, stasis	☐
Varicose veins	☐	Malignant disease	☐
Obesity	☐	Pregnancy	☐
Myocardial infarction	☐	Inflammatory bowel disease	☐
Congestive heart failure	☐	Sepsis	☐
Stroke	☐	Oestrogen therapy (including contraceptive pill)	☐
Hypercoagulable states	☐		

Score one point for each risk factor except where noted. Calculate degree of risk as follows:

1 point = low risk
2–4 points = moderate risk
4+ points = high risk

Fig. 27.3 Assessing the risk of deep vein thrombosis in surgical patients. Score one point for each risk factor except where noted. Calculate degree of risk as follows: 1 point = low risk; 2–4 points = moderate risk; 4+ points = high risk. (Adapted from Caprini et al 1988.)

graduated compression stockings. (Jeffery & Nicolaides 1990, Caprini et al 1988). These stockings create a decreasing pressure gradient in the leg from around 18 mm/Hg at the ankle to 8 mmHg at the thigh (full length) or to 14 mmHg at the calf (below-knee length). The gradient increases blood flow in the femoral vein and prevents the venous distension that causes endothelial damage (Coleridge Smith et al 1991). Graduated compression stockings reduce the incidence of postoperative DVT by approximately 60% (from 30% to 11%) in general surgical patients. Reductions in incidence among orthopaedic and gynaecological patients have also been demonstrated (Turner et al 1984).

The nurse should ensure that a well-designed and well-fitting stocking is applied. Stockings are fitted according to calf size and leg length and are available in a wide variety of sizes. If stockings roll down, a constricting band is created which may create higher pressures leading to an inverse gradient and delayed venous emptying. For this reason, below-knee stockings have been found to be more comfortable for low-risk patients who are ambulant. Knee-length stockings have been shown to be as effective as full-length in increasing blood flow in the deep veins (Lawrence & Kakkar 1980), resulting in no significant difference in the incidence of DVT in patients wearing above- or below-knee stockings (Porteus et al 1989). It is, however, recommended that full-length stockings are used for patients in moderate and high risk categories. The patient should wear the stockings from admission to discharge unless he is in a low risk category *and* fully ambulant in the preoperative period, when the stockings can be applied prior to theatre.

Other measures that should be encouraged where possible are early activity and hourly leg exercises. The patient should be taught to dorsiflex the foot preoperatively. This will assist venous return by the action of the calf muscle compressing blood in the deep veins. Deep breathing exercises will also aid the respiratory pump as deep inspiration reduces intrathoracic pressure, and hence increases venous return. In addition, of course, ensuring adequate hydration will reduce hypercoaguability.

For high-risk patients, sequential pneumatic compression of the legs has been shown to be effective (Caprini et al 1988). This can be achieved by two plastic sleeves fitted over graduated compression stockings. The sleeves have small separate pockets at different levels up the leg. A pump inflates the pockets in order from ankle to thigh so that a wave-like action passes up the leg, 'milking' the blood up towards the heart (see Fig. 27.4). Teaching leg exercises and applying graduated compression stockings and/or sequential pneumatic compression devices (SCD) prevents DVT by their action on two aspects of Virchow's triad, namely stasis and endothelial damage. Hypercoaguability can be avoided to some extent by adequate hydration but will be stimulated in any event by the general adaptation to stress response and by the effects of surgery initiating clotting mechanisms. Medical staff will seek to minimise hypercoaguability with the administration of anticoagulants (with all but low-risk patients). The value of prophylactic low-dose heparin to prevent DVT and PE in general surgical patients is well known. To be effective it must be given at least 2 h prior to surgery (Collins et al 1988). The risk of bleeding complications are minimal unless the patient has a clotting disorder; in such a case administration of anticoagulants would have to be monitored closely and its value judged carefully against the risk of DVT. Small wound haematomas may be more likely to occur in the patient receiving low-dose heparin, but when cared for correctly do not usually pose a threat.

?	**27.8** Mr W is going to theatre later that morning to have a hernia repair under a local anaesthetic. Mrs B is to go straight from A & E to the operating theatre as her abdominal X-rays and clinical findings show that she has peritonitis due to perforation of the bowel. Mr L is scheduled for theatre the following day to excise and debride his perianal abscess. M is due to go to theatre for repair of her vaginal fistula in 2 days when she has completed her bowel preparation. Work out the risk of DVT in these four patients. Plan care appropriate to each individual in order to prevent DVT.

Preoperative fasting

Patients who are to receive a general anaesthetic, heavy sedation or a local anaesthetic with the possibility of proceeding to a general anaesthetic are all at risk of aspiration pneumonia (sometimes termed Mendelson's syndrome). When a patient is anaesthetised or unconscious, the swallowing reflex is absent. From the point of induction of the anaesthetic there is a risk that stomach contents may reflux and be inhaled through the open larynx into the lungs. This inevitably causes respiratory embarrassment and leads to the development of a diffuse chest infection. The risks are minimised partly through the administration of certain drugs (see p. 785) but also by fasting the patient of both diet and fluids.

Different foodstuffs pass through the stomach at different rates. Gastric emptying is usually complete for most meals in 4–5 hours. Even fasting patients may have up to 200 ml in the stomach (Pritchard & Walker 1984). Taking this into account, the minimum preoperative fasting period is 4 h for fluids and 6 h for food.

A study by Hamilton Smith (1972) found that patients were fasted preoperatively for varying periods of time, and often much longer than necessary. A small replication study by Thomas (1987) found that little had changed since the earlier research. Patients on the morning list for theatre were fasted for 10–18 hours whilst those on the afternoon list were fasted for 5–22 hours. Only 2 out of 21 were fasted for 6 h or less; 46% of the patients had no explanation of why they were being fasted and 62% did not know how long they should fast for.

The undesirable results of prolonged fasting are mainly dehydration and electrolyte imbalance. (The liver has glycogen stores sufficient to maintain blood sugar levels for about 18 h.)

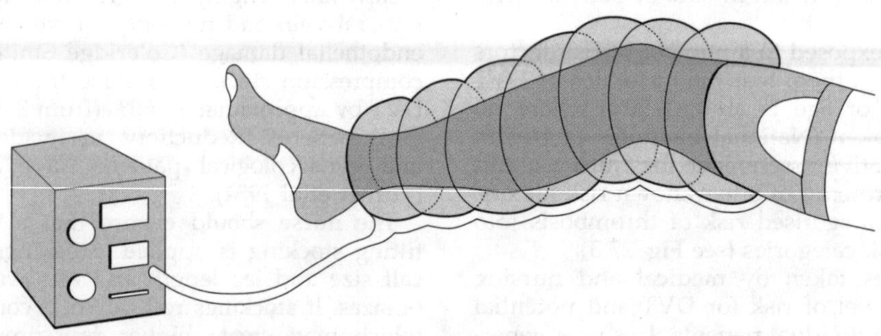

Fig. 27.4 Sequential pneumatic compression.

In elderly patients this occurs more rapidly and can lead to confusion. All patients experience to some extent feelings of starvation and a dry mouth. Some might not understand the reasons for fasting and eat or drink against advice.

Doctors and nurses are not unaware of proper fasting times, but tend to set a wide margin of safety and fast patients for at least 6 h. Theatre times are always approximate, apart from that of the first person on the list, as one cannot be entirely sure how long each operation will take. Surgeons may decide to alter the order of patients on the list, but this should not form part of everyday practice. Nurses work to the earliest likely time for theatre, but this often proves to be much later. A lack of individualised care leads to the imposition of one fasting time for all patients on the theatre list. A patient on the morning list is then fasted from midnight, but if he is last on the morning list he may not go to theatre until 2 p.m. and thus will have fasted for 14 h. Individual fasting times and close liaison with the anaesthetist can resolve such problems.

Patients must be given adequate information in order to understand what they cannot eat or drink, for how long, and how to care for a dry mouth in the meantime. If the patient has oral medication prescribed during the fasting time it should not be routinely withheld; rather, medical staff should be consulted as to whether the drug should be given or not. Tablets can be taken with 30–60 ml of water.

To return to our examples, Mrs B was to go to theatre as an emergency, so it was not possible to ensure she had fasted for at least 4 h. In this case her stomach was emptied by aspirating the contents through a nasogastric tube. Mr W had come into hospital on the morning of theatre but had received instructions about fasting in his booklet from the ward the week before. He was not sure whether he could have an early morning cup of tea and had asked his primary nurse about this during his visit. As theatre would not start until 9.30 a.m. she advised him he might have a drink at 6 a.m. but nothing after that. In fact Mr W was third on the list and did not go up to theatre until 11.30 a.m.

?	**27.9** Observe how long patients are fasted preoperatively in your ward experience. How would you explain the necessity for fasting prior to theatre to a patient?

Skin preparation

Preparation of the skin before theatre can help to reduce the incidence of postoperative infections. Another important factor is the exposure to nosocomial pathogens. The risk of infection can be reduced by shortening the length of preoperative stay. It has already been proposed that by reducing preoperative anxiety, psychological and physiological stress can be reduced and the incidence of postoperative infection lowered (Boore 1978).

Preparation of the skin formerly included shaving the site of the operation. However, shaving leaves small cuts and abrasions that can give rise to infection. Research has demonstrated that shaving delays discharge on average from 7.3 to 9.1 days (Lancet 1983). However, if sticking plaster is to be used, hair removal may be justified on humanitarian grounds. Hair removal may also be necessary if the hair occludes the surgeon's vision of the operation site, or if adhesive leads are to be applied, requiring a good skin contact. For example, a patient undergoing angiographic surgery may have the cannula inserted via the femoral artery in the groin. A pressure dressing is essential postoperatively which necessitates the use of strong adhesive tape in the groin.

If hair removal is necessary then hair clippers or depilatory cream can be used. A patch test for sensitivity to creams must be carried out before use. Application of depilatories must also be avoided around sensitive mucous membranes in the genital area. When creams cannot be used and clippers are not available, a well-lubricated shave with a sharp razor immediately prior to theatre may be sufficient. This does, however, carry a higher risk of infection than the use of creams or clippers. In some centres the shave may be carried out by the theatre orderly once the patient is anaesthetised.

The bacterial count on the skin can be actively reduced by having the patient shower prior to theatre with a skin antiseptic such as Hibiscrub, a chlorhexidine-based skin antiseptic (Brandberg & Anderson 1980). Bathing should be avoided where possible, as bacteria may multiply in the warm water and there may be a risk of crossinfection from organisms already present in hospital baths. The patient should be asked to shower several hours prior to theatre and to dress in a fresh theatre gown. It is unnecessary to change bed linen that is clean.

Specific measures

Premedication (premed) is the term used for drugs given to the patient before leaving the ward for theatre. They constitute part of the anaesthetic and are used to prepare the patient to receive a general or local anaesthetic. They are often also used to relax the patient and relieve anxiety (see Table 27.1). The premed is prescribed by the anaesthetist after he has assessed the patient for the administration of the anaesthetic. The prescription may be made at a set time or 'on call', i.e. the anaesthetist will phone the ward to ask the nurse to administer the prescribed drug when he is sure how long it will take for the patient to be called to theatre.

The nurse must ensure that the consent form has been signed and that all other preoperative checks are complete before giving the premed. The patient should then be instructed not to get out of bed unsupervised if the premed contains a strong sedative or narcotic agent. A quiet rest time should then follow to ensure the patient is as calm as possible prior to theatre.

Some patients will require very specific types of preoperative preparation as ordered by medical staff. The most commonly seen is that of bowel preparation prior to surgery on the gastrointestinal tract or pelvic organs. If a paralytic ileus is anticipated, or the bowel to be opened (resulting in risk of infection), then some sort of bowel preparation is usually necessary. This generally consists of oral laxatives and purgatives, or suppositories and enemas to clear the bowel, with oral antibiotics to reduce bacterial flora.

Again returning to our examples, Mr W's anaesthetist prescribed him a sedative (diazepam 5 mg) as a premed as he was aware that Mr W was particularly anxious. Mr W had also borrowed one of the personal stereos from the ward and was enjoying listening to a Simon & Garfunkel tape.

M received Go-lytely solution to cleanse her colon prior to theatre. This type of polyethylene glycol electrolyte lavage solution causes less electrolyte disturbance than purgatives and carries less risk of irritation and perforation than enemas. Go-lytely produces results equal to those of standard types of bowel preparations and has been shown to be acceptable to patients (Borkje et al 1991). However, some patients may find the solution unpalatable and have difficulty taking such a large volume of fluid.

A paralytic ileus was not anticipated with Mr W or Mr L and therefore no bowel preparation was given. Mr W did, how-

Table 27.1 Common premedications

Drug	Usual adult dose	Route	Effects
Diazepam (Valium)	2–10 mg	Oral	Sedative: reduces tension and anxiety. Decreases muscle tone and potentiates non-depolarising muscle relaxants. Induces mental detachment and amnesia
Temazepam	10–20 mg	Oral	Sedative: reduces tension and anxiety. Induces drowsiness
Morphine sulphate, papaveretum* (Omnopon)	5–15 mg 10–20 mg	i.m. i.m.	Narcotic analgesic: induces drowsiness, reduces anxiety, induces mental detachment, respiratory depression†, nausea†
Atropine	0.6 mg	i.m.	Anticholinergic: reduces smooth muscle tone, reduces bronchial and salivary secretions; blocks vagus nerve, preventing bradycardia due to vasovagal stimulation (from passage of endotracheal tube)
Hyoscine (Scopolamine)	0.2–0.4 mg	i.m.	Anticholinergic: reduces smooth muscle tone, reduces bronchial and salivary secretions and blocks vasovagal stimulation (as atropine). Depresses CNS. Antiemetic. Causes restlessness and delirium in elderly patients†

†Unwanted/undesirable effect.
*Papaveretum must not be used in women of childbearing potential (Committee on Safety of Medicines 1991).

ever, have the side of the inguinal hernia marked by the doctor before theatre, as when the patient is lying down on the operating table it can sometimes be difficult to assess which side of the body requires surgery. Similarly, a patient will have the breast or leg marked with indelible ink prior to theatre to avoid any mistakes in theatre.

Mrs B's operation was so urgent that her condition did not allow any time for bowel preparation.

Theatre safety

The nurse must ensure that certain preoperative checks are carried out before the patient receives the premed and leaves the ward to go to theatre. Preoperative checks should be completed prior to administration of the premed as the results of the checks may necessitate a delay in going to theatre. Moreover, the patient should not have received sedative or narcotic agents before signing the consent form. Many hospitals have created their own checklists to complete. Examples of criteria for checklists are given in Table 27.2.

In order for patients to understand and cooperate with preoperative procedures, adequate explanation and reassurance must be given. However, the nurse should also be aware that some information might cause unnecessary distress. For example, Mrs B did not want to remove her wedding ring. The nurse offered to tape this for her, but Mrs B said that she had never taken if off and that it would be secure. The nurse did not want to frighten her by telling her that it was to protect her from being burnt by the use of electric current to seal blood vessels during the operation. Many patients would have visions of being electrocuted. Instead the nurse said that if she didn't lock all the patients' valuables away, she had to secure them with tape for security, and to protect items from any antiseptics that might be spilt. Mrs B happily agreed to this and was relieved that she could continue to wear her ring.

There may be some patients who greatly rely on their hearing aids and/or glasses. In such cases, glasses or hearing aids can be labelled with adhesive tape and worn by the patient until he is anaesthetised. A note should be made to this effect on the checklist or anaesthetic form.

During the immediate preoperative period, the patient may feel extremely vulnerable and afraid. He will be wearing a flimsy gown with nothing underneath; he may have removed his dentures and be unable to see well without his glasses; and he will feel drowsy from the premed. Anxiety about the impending operation can be high. Reassurance by the nurse and sometimes distraction can be helpful. Otherwise, the patient should be encouraged to rest. Nursing Care Plan 27.1 (p. 788) summarises the preoperative care given to Mr W.

PERIOPERATIVE SAFETY

Caring for the patient in theatre

The patient arrives in the operating theatre accompanied by a nurse from the ward and a porter or operating department assistant (ODA). Patients may be brought to the theatre on a trolley or, in some cases, on the bed from the ward. (Once the patient transfers to the theatre table the bed is taken to a holding area. The patient is then transferred straight back onto his bed at the end of the operation. This reduces the discomfort of transferring from a trolley to the bed in the ward, and reduces the amount of patient lifting by nurses, porters and ODAs.)

The anaesthetic or theatre nurse receiving the patient goes through the preoperative check (as in Table 27.2) again. Once this is complete, the ward nurse will usually return to the ward. If the patient is especially nervous or a little confused, it can be comforting if a nurse who knows him well can stay with him until the induction of anaesthesia. All patients must be supervised by a nurse in this pre-induction time, as the patient may have received premedication and is in an extremely stressful and unfamiliar environment. It is now common practice for theatre nurses to visit their patients preoperatively to carry out a nursing assessment and to introduce themselves to patients and give any information required about their care in theatre (Roberts 1991).

In emergency cases the theatre nurse may continue the preoperative preparation. For example, Mrs B's daughter arrived at the hospital just as these preparations were being carried

Table 27.2 Preoperative checks

Criteria	Action	Rationale
Identification	Prepare 2 name bands with patient's full name, hospital unit number, date of birth, home address (as a minimum), plus ward and consultant Clearly note allergies on the anaesthetic sheet and on wrist bands as well as the drug Kardex Ensure site is correctly marked with indelible ink	Correct identification of patient Avoidance of all allergens Correct identification of site
Documentation	Ensure that medical notes, nursing notes, signed consent form, X-rays and anaesthetic sheet accompany patient to theatre	Ready availability of all necessary information
Fasting	Check with patient when he last had anything to eat or drink	Prevention of aspiration pneumonia
Empty bladder	Ask patient to pass urine prior to administering premed	To prevent damage to full bladder during surgery To enable complete bedrest after premed To prevent postoperative discomfort due to a full bladder
Risk of diathermy burns	Ask patient to remove all jewellery, hair pins and other items containing metal. (Wedding rings may be covered with tape.)	To remove all metal that may concentrate the diathermy current
Prostheses	Ask patient to remove all prostheses, e.g. dentures, hearing aids, contact lenses, false eyes, glasses, etc.	To prevent harm caused by prostheses To prevent loss
Care of valuables	Offer to receive valuables into safekeeping for the patient	Patient will be away from the ward and unfit to be responsible for his valuables
Circulatory assessment	Ask patient to remove all make-up, lipstick and nail varnish	To facilitate observation of colour of skin, lips and nail beds

out. She was escorted to theatre by the A & E nurse, and saw her mother for a few minutes in the anaesthetic room before she was anaesthetised. The theatre nurse briefly explained what was happening, and once her mother was asleep made her a cup of tea and let her make a phone call from the sister's office. She then phoned the primary nurse, who sent an auxiliary to bring Mrs B's daughter up to the ward where she was waiting to meet her.

The roles of the theatre staff are summarised in Box 27.1 (p. 789). The anaesthetist will visit the patient preoperatively in the ward, not only to assess the patient's ability to tolerate the anaesthetic, but also to introduce himself to the patient and give information and reassurance. He will also prescribe a premedication if one is to be given.

If the patient has minimally invasive surgery or investigations, e.g: colonoscopy, endoscopic retrograde cholangiopancreatography (ERCP) or cardiac catheterisation, a general anaesthetic may not be used. Instead, the patient may be sedated by drugs such as diazepam or midazolam, which also have amnesic properties. (This helps the patient to be less aware of what is happening and to remember less about the procedure.) In this situation, an anaesthetist may not necessarily be present but would be available should the need arise to proceed to a general anaesthetic or should other supportive treatment be required. The nurse may act as the surgeon's assistant and will take part of the responsibility for monitoring the patient's condition.

In main theatres at least two nurses as well as the anaesthetist and surgeon will be present. One nurse acts as the circulating nurse whilst the other is the scrub nurse. The scrub nurse wears sterile gloves and will provide instruments for the surgeons, assist where necessary and ensure safety with equipment during the operation. The roles of these nurses are summarised in Box 27.1.

The emphasis of the nursing role in theatre is on patient safety and on teamwork. Each professional has an important part to play in the patient's passage through theatre. As the team members develop trust and understanding amongst themselves it may be difficult initially for the student to appreciate the communication links in place, especially when staff have half their faces covered with a mask!

Environmental safety

The environment in the operating theatre is designed to minimise the risk of exogenous infection to the patient. Some of the measures used to ensure safety are as follows:

- Clean filtered air is pumped into clean areas. Air pressure is higher inside the theatre than out to maintain an air flow from the theatre to the outside. This prevents dirty air from the rest of the hospital moving into the theatres.
- Humidity is also controlled through the ventilation system to prevent static electricity build-up and the risk of sparks, as flammable gases may be in use. Staff are required to wear antistatic shoes (clogs or boots are usually worn). All equipment must have antistatic rubber wheels or covers.
- Clean and dirty areas are delineated by doors or a line on the floor. All personnel moving into clean areas must be clean and appropriately dressed (see below). All items brought into clean areas must be clean. All dirty items leaving theatre should do so via dirty areas. It is essential that staff are aware which are the dirty and the clean areas

Nursing Care Plan 27.1 Preoperative care for Mr W (see Case Histories 27.1(A) and (B))

Nursing considerations	Action	Rationale	Evaluation
Anxiety due to: • hospital environment • diagnosis/prognosis • anaesthesia and surgery	❒ Ensure Mr W is informed of and understands diagnosis, procedure, likely postoperative progress ❒ Provide opportunity to discuss fears and anxieties ❒ Enhance or supplement coping mechanisms (e.g. use of personal stereo)	To reduce anxiety and promote recovery	Anxiety is reduced to an acceptable level
Haemorrhage and shock*	❒ Record vital signs as baseline ❒ Encourage intake of fluids until 4 h before theatre ❒ Ensure blood tests and blood grouping completed	To make data available for postoperative comparison To maintain good fluid balance To ensure availability of blood products in case transfusion is necessary To ensure good haemoglobin status	Staff are prepared to deal with bleeding and shock is prevented
Wound infection*	❒ Have Mr W shower with Hibiscrub ❒ Provide clean theatre gown ❒ Remove hair in the groin area with depilatory (patch test should be done at preoperative visit)	To reduce skin flora To prevent obstruction of surgeon's view and prevent pain on removal of adhesive dressing	No infection occurs
Chest infection*	❒ Teach deep breathing and coughing exercises ❒ Continue to support Mr W in not smoking	To fully inflate lungs and clear stagnating secretions Patient is under stress and may return to inappropriate coping mechanisms	No infection occurs
Deep vein thrombosis*; pulmonary embolism*	❒ Teach leg exercises and stress importance of early mobilisation ❒ Fit and apply graduated compression stockings ❒ Teach deep breathing exercises (see above)	Contraction of calf muscle and graduated external compression increase blood flow in the femoral vein and promote venous return	Thrombosis and embolism are prevented
Aspiration pneumonia*	❒ Have Mr W fast 4 h (fluids) and 6 h (food) preoperatively from 06.00 h	Stomach must be empty prior to anaesthesia; Mr W. may need general anaesthetic	Vomiting is prevented
Theatre safety	❒ Complete checklist prior to administration of premed (see Table 27.6)	See Table 27.6	Patient is safely prepared for anaesthetic and surgery

* Potential problem

and corridors. The use of sticky mats at the main entrance to theatre was thought to reduce contamination from the feet of staff entering theatre. This has now been shown to be ineffective and the practice should be discontinued. Similarly, the use of overshoes has been questioned, as there is a risk of contaminating the hands by handling the overshoes to take them off which may outweigh the benefits of wearing them (Carter 1990).

- The numbers and movement of staff inside theatres are kept to an absolute minimum to reduce the number of skin scales shed and mixing of air.
- All staff entering clean areas are appropriately dressed. Clean theatre dresses or trouser suits are worn. Hair is completely covered by a bonnet-style cap and all jewellery, especially on the hands, is removed. Masks are worn inside the theatre itself to reduce airborne organisms. (Masks should be handled only by the tapes once applied, as the main fabric of the mask becomes contaminated with moisture and microorganisms that can then be transmitted on the hands.)
- Staff do not leave the theatre area when dressed in theatre clothing as the clothing can become contaminated.

Box 27.1 The roles of the theatre staff

The anaesthetic nurse
- Receives the patient in the reception area of the anaesthetic room
- Checks patient in, deals with any irregularities
- Helps to relieve patient anxiety
- Assists in the induction (and maintenance) of anaesthesia
- Performs emergency preparation of patients for theatre
- Uses and checks anaesthetic equipment
- Maintains patient safety and comfort

The anaesthetist
- Visits the patient preoperatively:
  — to assess fitness for anaesthesia
  — to provide information and reassurance
  — to prescribe a premedication
- Induces and maintains anaesthesia
- Monitors patient's condition during surgery
- Provides supportive treatment, e.g. fluid replacement, PO_2 level maintenance, correction of arrhythmias
- Initiates postoperative analgesia

The circulating nurse
- Assists with the provision of equipment
- Maintains nursing records
- Positions the patient
- Ensures safety with regard to instruments and swabs
- Cleans and sterilises equipment
- Observes, measures and records vital signs

The scrub nurse
- Positions the patient
- Provides appropriate sterile equipment
- Assists the surgeon
- Protects the patient's dignity
- Prevents diathermy and pressure injuries
- Ensures safety with regard to instruments and swabs
- Manages the high-risk patient

The recovery room nurse
- Maintaining patency of the airway
- Observing patient for level of consciousness and safety
- Observing vital signs: colour, respiration, temperature (core and peripheral), pulse, blood pressure, fluid intake and output, wounds and drainage, specific checks as required
- Assessing pain and nausea and administering analgesics and antiemetics
- Reassuring the patient and providing a quiet environment
- Providing total patient care
- Providing documentation and facilitating communication

- A sterile field is created around the patient. The patient and trolleys in this area are all covered with sterile drapes. The surgeon and scrub nurse wear sterile gloves and gowns to work within the sterile field.

Safety of the patient

The patient's safety in theatre is further ensured by the following precautions:

- Transfer to operating table and positioning is carried out with extreme care. The preoperative visit by the theatre nurse enables her to assess for any potential problems, especially in relation to joint mobility and the risk of developing pressure sores. Special types of ripple mattresses can be used with high-risk patients. Once patients are anaesthetised they may lose muscle tone. Care should be taken with all limbs; for example, if the arm is left to dangle off the edge of the table irreparable damage to the brachial plexus may result. The nurse must also be aware of the risk of back pain to the patient, which may require special supports to the lower back (Rafferty 1988).
- The diathermy pad is carefully positioned. A self-adhesive pad may be used and the pad is usually placed under the buttocks or strapped to the thigh to ensure good contact over the entire surface. A poor contact by only part of the surface may concentrate the current, causing it to leave a burn.
- Swabs, needles and instruments used during theatre are counted and checked throughout and at the end of the operation by the scrub and circulating nurse. This ensures that all items used are accounted for and none left inside the patient.
- Allergies to drugs, skin antiseptics and dressings are assessed preoperatively by the theatre nurse and anaesthetist so the use of any allergens can be avoided.
- The patient's skin is cleaned at the start of the procedure with an antiseptic solution to reduce skin flora and the risk of endogenous infection. Some surgeons also use a sterile plastic adhesive drape over the skin (Incisa-drape) through which to make the incision. This prevents the surgeons' and nurses' sterile gloves being contaminated with the patient's skin flora.
- Prophylactic antibiotics may be given (usually intravenously) during the operation, or the site of the surgery may be irrigated with an antibiotic solution. These measures are usually taken only if there is a specific risk of contamination, or if contamination from an abscess or the gastrointestinal tract is already present.
- During surgery the patient is at risk of primary haemorrhage. When an incision is made, the patient will bleed until a clot is formed or the pressure within the vessel and the cavity into which it is bleeding has equalised. Bleeding during surgery is minimised by the use of clamps and ligatures, local pressure, or diathermy to seal small vessels. Topical haemostatic agents such as cellulose and collagen may also be used. To facilitate the surgeon's vision, the site of operation is kept free of blood by swabs or suctioning. The circulating nurse may weigh the swabs to estimate blood loss and note the volume of blood in the suction bottle to estimate 'total blood loss'.
- Special procedures must be followed for the care of the patient identified as at high risk of carrying certain infectious diseases — commonly blood-borne diseases with a high morbidity and mortality. (See Ch. 11.) To prevent crossinfection and to reduce risks involved with cleaning and spillages, disposable equipment may be used where possible (see Ch. 16, p. 548). The surgeon and scrub nurse will wear two pairs of gloves, and the patient will not be taken into the recovery room after the operation in case of further blood loss but will be recovered in theatre instead. The high-risk patient should be at the end of a theatre list to enable recovery in theatre and thorough cleaning and disinfection before the theatre is used again.

In summary, the safety of the patient in theatre is the prime responsibility of all members of the theatre team. The Royal College of Nursing and the Medical Defence Union both have codes of practice for operating department safety; these might be consulted as further reading (National Association of Theatre Nurses 1983).

Anaesthesia

An anaesthetic is used to block any sensations of pain during surgery. It may be applied locally or regionally to the area of surgery or generally throughout the body. A brief introduction to the use of anaesthetics is given here. For further information please consult Trounce (1990) or Neal (1990).

Local anaesthesia
Local anaesthesia blocks transmission of pain from the region operated upon. In some cases, only the sensory receptors may be blocked; this is more correctly termed local analgesia. A local anaesthetic is often combined with adrenaline to constrict blood vessels and delay absorption of the anaesthetic into the bloodstream. This reduces the amount of local anaesthetic required and prolongs its action. Types and common uses of local anaesthetics are summarised in Table 27.3. Epidural or spinal anaesthetics may be used when a general anaesthetic could be harmful or is undesirable, e.g. in elderly patients with arteriosclerosis or diabetes, in patients with respiratory disorders, and in patients with hypertension. The procedure causes hypotension and so should be avoided in patients with this condition. Care must be taken to prepare the patient psychologically in order to reduce anxiety and ensure cooperation. Psychological support continues throughout the operation and the nurse should ensure that the patient's vision of the procedure is adequately screened.

Both Mr W and Mr L were conscious during their operations. Mr W had his operation under a local anaesthetic, but Mr L had such extensive demyelinisation that he had no motor or sensory function below the waist. The anaesthetist had fully assessed the sensation around Mr L's sacrum and was satisfied that the area was already anaesthetised and Mr L would feel no pain. He did prescribe a sedative for both patients and the nursing staff ensured that their vision was screened. Both patients were reassured and informed of progress throughout the operation by the surgeon and the nurse.

General anaesthesia
General anaesthesia is characterised by loss of consciousness, analgesia and muscle relaxation. These effects occur according to the stage of anaesthesia, as follows:

Stage 1: the pain is reduced or relieved, but the patient is still conscious. Heavy sedation can produce 'dissociative anaesthesia' and some muscle relaxation, whilst local analgesics supplement pain control as necessary. The patient may remain drowsy but conscious throughout the procedure.

Entonox (50% oxygen with 50% nitrous oxide) can be self-administered during childbirth or painful procedures to achieve Stage 1 anaesthesia for pain control. This application is discussed with other methods of pain relief in Ch. 19.

Stage 2: consciousness is lost, but the patient may exhibit wild movements and irrational behaviour. With intravenous induction of anaesthesia, this stage is passed through very quickly and may be more in evidence when the patient is *recovering* from anaesthesia.

Stage 3: breathing becomes regular and there is relaxation of the muscles along with loss of reflexes. This is the level of surgical anaesthesia. The degree of muscle relaxation required to facilitate surgery can be achieved by deepening this stage but this has undesirable side-effects such as fall in cardiac output, respiratory depression and liver damage. To overcome this problem, muscle relaxants can be administered to enable a relatively light anaesthetic to be used and so reduce the risks of anaesthesia in the elderly and those with cardiovascular and respiratory complications. This has also aided the development of day case surgery.

Premedication can be used to relieve anxiety, induce a state of analgesia, reduce bronchial and salivary secretions, prevent vasovagal stimulation (bradycardia, chiefly) and make the patient less aware and somewhat drowsy. Usually, a sedative or anxiolytic is given orally, or a narcotic analgesic with an anticholinergic agent is given as an intramuscular injection (see Table 27.1).

The induction of anaesthesia is usually achieved with a short-acting intravenous agent administered with a short-acting muscle relaxant (see Tables 27.4 and 27.5). This rapidly produces surgical anaesthesia, in which the patient is unable

Table 27.3 Local anaesthetics

Method of administration	Effect	Example of drugs and their uses
Topical: solution or cream applied to skin or mucous membranes	Blocks local sensory nerve receptors	Lignocaine, benzocaine Minor ENT procedures Insertion of cannulae
Infiltration: injection into surgical site	Blocks local sensory nerve receptors	Lignocaine, procaine Removal of skin moles Insertion of Hickman line Drainage of abscess
Nerve block: injection close to relevant nerve trunk	Blocks conduction of sensory impulses to central nervous system	Lignocaine with adrenaline Brachial plexus procedures on the arm (Bier's block) Intercostal blocks for pain relief
Epidural: injection into space outside the dura	Blocks nerves as they enter the spinal cord	Lignocaine, bupivacaine Rectal or pelvic surgery Caesarean section
Spinal: injection into the subarachnoid space below the 2nd lumbar vertebra	Blocks preganglionic fibres (motor and sensory) Position of patient determines distribution of drug and spinal nerves affected	Bupivacaine, lignocaine Amputation Abdominal surgery

Table 27.4 General anaesthetics

Method of administration	Effect	Example of drugs and their uses
Intravenous: for induction	Sedation, surgical anaesthesia Respiratory depression Some cause hypotension	Thiopentone, methohexitone, ketamine, propofol Induction of anaesthesia Short surgical procedures, EUA, dental extraction
Inhalation: for maintenance of anaesthesia	Surgical anaesthesia Some cause hypotension, nausea and vomiting	Halothane, nitrous oxide, isoflurane Maintenance of anaesthesia Wide range of surgical prodedures

to maintain his own airway (due to lack of reflexes) and the muscles of breathing are paralysed. An endotracheal tube is passed through the relaxed larynx and artificial ventilation is maintained throughout the operation. Anaesthesia can be maintained during surgery, usually by means of inhaled anaesthetics and a longer-acting muscle relaxant. At the end of the operation, the anaesthetic gas is discontinued and the effects of the muscle relaxant are reversed with the appropriate drug. The patient gradually regains consciousness, passing through Stages 2 and 1 of anaesthesia and regaining muscle tone, which enables him to breathe independently. During this time, the patient is transferred to the recovery room.

Recovery from anaesthesia

Once surgery is completed, the patient will normally be kept in the recovery room until the immediate effects of the anaesthetic have worn off. The patient should be able to maintain his own airway and be considered stable before transfer back to the ward. In some cases the patient will be transferred directly to the intensive therapy unit whilst he continues to be intubated and his respiration is maintained by artificial ventilation.

Whilst the patient is still unconscious the nurse must ensure that the airway is kept open. This can be achieved by placing the patient in a lateral or semi-prone position, tilting the head backward and pulling the mandible forwards, or inserting a Guedal airway. If a Guedal airway is used, it can be left in position until the patient expels it spontaneously as reflexes return. There is a risk of aspiration pneumonia should the patient vomit whilst regaining consciousness; therefore, suction equipment must be available. Anaesthetics, muscle relaxants, narcotics and severe pain itself can cause nausea and vomiting. Pain must be adequately controlled and antiemetics may be required.

The nurse should observe the patient's level of consciousness and be aware that a stage of excitement (Stage 2) may occur. Close observation and the use of side rails may be required. Many patients will be prescribed oxygen until fully awake, to maintain PO_2 whilst there is still some respiratory depression due to anaesthesia. The patient should be encouraged to commence deep breathing and leg exercises as soon as he regains consciousness.

As the patient regains consciousness the nurse should bear in mind that hearing is usually one of the first senses to return. Verbal reassurance that the operation is over should be given. It may be appropriate to return hearing aids and spectacles at this point. The patient should be allowed to rest as quietly as possible during this period and will usually fall asleep after regaining consciousness. Close and frequent observation of vital signs is required for the early detection of changes in the patient's condition. During the recovery period the patient is especially at risk of reactionary haemorrhage as his blood pressure rises (hypotension is often induced during surgery due to anaesthetic agents). A ligature or clot may become dislodged, leading to signs of haemorrhage and hypovolaemic shock (see p. 792). Observation of wound dressings and wound drainage will also aid assessment of the patient in the recovery period.

In surgery, the patient may have had a large surface area exposed, leading to loss of body heat. Shivering will have been suppressed, due to the use of skeletal muscle relaxants. The environmental temperature in theatres is therefore kept fairly high, but patients may still have a low body temperature and complain of feeling cold. Extra blankets and 'space blankets' can be used, but the nurse must be wary of warming the patient too quickly, as this can lead to peripheral vasodilation and a fall in blood pressure.

Pain control begins before or as the patient regains consciousness. A patient such as Mr W may have the operation site infiltrated with more lignocaine (with adrenaline) at the end of surgery to provide local anaesthesia. The anaesthetist may also prescribe some narcotic analgesia and some simple oral analgesia for the patient's return to the ward.

Some patients may have an epidural infusion commenced at the end of the operation or, as with Mrs B, be commenced on an i.v. infusion of morphine. Some patients may be able to administer a type of i.v. infusion of a narcotic drug themselves (see p. 797). Many patients will receive their first dose of intramuscular analgesia in the recovery room. The patient's pain should be controlled before he leaves the recovery room.

Table 27.5 Muscle relaxants

Name of drug	Effect	Use
Suxamethonium (depolarising): binds and blocks acetylcholine receptors	Skeletal flaccid paralysis Increased K^+ release Rarely: prolonged apnoea and malignant hyperpyrexia	Short-acting (15 min) Induction, manipulations, ECT No drug available to reverse effects
Tubocurarine and pancuronium (non-depolarising) Prevents acetylcholine gaining access to receptor site	Skeletal flaccid paralysis Can cause hypotension	Longer-acting (30–45 min) Maintenance of relaxation during anaesthesia or controlled ventilation Reversed by neostigmine (anticholinesterase — raises levels of acetylcholine)

In a partly conscious patient, a sudden rise in blood pressure and restlessness may indicate the presence of pain. The nurse must also be aware that narcotic analgesia may cause a fall in blood pressure and respiratory depression, but also that severe pain in itself can lead to shock and shallow breathing.

The patient may spend several hours in the recovery room and will in many aspects require the same care as an unconscious patient (see Ch. 30). Most patients will require attention to at least the mouth (mucous membranes will be dry due to anticholinergic drugs, fasting and perhaps dehydration) as well as pressure area care. The recovery room nurse will document the care given and provide a summary to the ward nurse who collects the patient. In this way, continuity of care can be achieved. The role of the recovery room nurse is summarised in Box 27.1.

POSTOPERATIVE CARE

All patients require close observation during the immediate postoperative period in order to detect any complications early on. This close observation may be continued for hours or days for the patient requiring intensive nursing care, or perhaps for an hour or two if a local infiltration of anaesthetic or a very light general anaesthetic has been used. The next stage of postoperative care focuses on recovery and repair along with the active prevention of complications. Rehabilitation will be achieved at a different pace and to differing levels by each patient. The patient having a hip replacement may find that his joint pain is almost immediately reduced postoperatively and that his functional ability is far better than before the operation. Some patients may not be able to achieve the desired level of recovery and others may be aiming for palliation rather than cure.

For purposes of clarity, this section will focus on the postoperative recovery, repair and rehabilitation most commonly experienced during the hospital stay whilst the next section entitled 'Rehabilitation' focuses on continued care after discharge from hospital. It is recognised, however, that many patients will still be recovering from the effects of the anaesthetic, which can take up to 24 h to be eliminated from the body, after discharge following day surgery. Examples of postoperative care are given in Nursing Care Plans 27.2 and 27.3.

Shock and haemostasis

Shock is discussed here with specific application to the care of surgical patients. For a wider discussion of the types and mechanisms of shock and their signs and symptoms see Ch. 18.

When the patient returns from theatre to the ward, he requires frequent observations for signs of impending shock or haemorrhage. As blood pressure continues to rise there is a continued risk of reactionary haemorrhage for the first 24 h. Hypovolaemic shock may also occur due to a slow, continuous loss of fluid; this might be a slowly bleeding vessel or the pooling of fluid in the gastrointestinal tract during the paralytic ileus that occurs as a consequence of surgery. The loss of fluid may be detected as soakage on the dressing or blood in the wound drains, but if the patient is bleeding into a body cavity or losing fluid into the gut it may be less obvious. Distinction should also be made between hypovolaemic and other forms of shock, i.e. cardiogenic, septicaemic, anaphylactic and neurogenic.

Cardiogenic shock is caused essentially by failure of the heart to pump and maintain adequate cardiac output. Possible causes following surgery may be pulmonary embolus causing massive resistance to the output of the right side of the heart, fluid overload and concomitant heart failure, anaesthetic depression of cardiac output, or myocardial infarction. Patient signs and symptoms, and measurement of central venous or pulmonary wedge pressures along with other vital signs can help the nurse to distinguish between hypovolaemic and cardiogenic shock.

Secondary haemorrhage can occur 1–7 days postoperatively due to vessel erosion by infection or tumour growth, or from a long, slow bleed. The patient may collapse suddenly and will usually need to return to theatre. Fortunately, this is not a common problem.

The patient may also be at risk of neurogenic shock (usually due to severe pain), anaphylactic shock (usually due to drug reactions) and septicaemic shock (from infections occurring following surgery).

The aim of nursing observations in the first 24 h following surgery is to detect changes that might indicate the initial stages of compensation to hypovolaemic shock. As the circulating volume falls, the nurse may see increased loss of blood on dressings or in wound drainage bags or bottles. There will be a slight rise in heart rate to maintain cardiac output but no change or a slight rise in systolic blood pressure. Peripheral vasoconstriction to conserve blood supply to vital organs (brain, heart, lungs, liver, kidneys) may lead to a clammy, sweaty appearance. The vasoconstriction of the veins maintains diastolic (end) volume and therefore increases stroke volume. This, along with increased cardiac contractility, maintains blood pressure to at least pre-shock levels. As the brain is extremely sensitive to hypoxia, the patient may also appear restless.

If the blood or fluid loss continues, then these mechanisms may eventually fail to compensate effectively. There may then be further vasoconstriction of the arterioles to increase peripheral resistance. There is also reduced parasympathetic activity to increase heart rate and stroke volume, resulting in increased cardiac output. At this point the heart rate increases further and blood pressure begins to fall. Urine output decreases rapidly (due to decreased renal perfusion over and above the effects of increased antidiuretic hormone (ADH) and aldosterone (see p. 795)) as blood flow is conserved to maintain the brain, heart and lungs as a priority. The patient appears breathless, centrally cyanosed and may be quite confused due to hypoxia. The signs and symptoms of the initial compensation and failing compensation are summarised in Box 27.2.

Box 27.2 Signs and symptoms of shock, by stages

INITIAL COMPENSATION

- Appears sweaty, clammy, pale
- Peripheral cyanosis
- Appears restless; may complain of feeling generally unwell
- Falling urine output but may remain above 30 ml/hr
- Increase in pulse rate
- Slight rise in systolic blood pressure
- Increased soakage of blood on wound dressings and in wound drains

FAILING COMPENSATION

- Appears cold, sweaty
- Central cyanosis
- Appears confused, often agitated, and then increasingly drowsy
- Urine output falls below 30 ml/hr
- Tachycardia
- Fall in blood pressure
- Large volumes of blood may be lost

Nursing Care Plan 27.2 Care for Mrs B on 6th postoperative day (see Case History 27.2)

Nursing considerations	Action	Rationale	Evaluation
Abdominal pain	❒ Administer i.v. analgesic pump as prescribed ❒ Increase rate 30 min prior to activity as prescribed ❒ Record respiratory rate hourly ❒ Ensure that Mrs B is positioned comfortably ❒ Encourage her to support wound on moving ❒ Apply heating pad to abdomen for 'wind' pains	To prevent pain and foster recovery by enabling Mrs B to cough, exercise, rest and sleep comfortably	Mrs B is sufficiently pain-free to cooperate with therapy
Fluid and electrolyte imbalance*	❒ Administer i.v. infusion as per chart (change giving set at 24 h) ❒ Observe pulse and BP 6 hourly ❒ Observe for dyspnoea ❒ Record all fluid intake and output ❒ Observe for nausea, vomiting and diarrhoea	To detect any signs of dehydration and electrolyte imbalance early	Fluid and electrolytes maintained at satisfactory levels
Paralytic ileus	❒ Observe for passage of flatus/faeces in stoma bag ❒ Administer antiemetics as prescribed ❒ Give oral fluids: water 60 ml/h	To detect return of normal peristalsis To prevent nausea and dehydration	Mrs B is comfortable until normal peristalsis returns
Retention of urine*	❒ Remove urinary catheter ❒ Take catheter specimen of urine for culture and sensitivity ❒ Observe urine output	To prevent retention of urine and related infection	Diuresis is adequate
Wound infection*	❒ Check wound daily for colour, exudate and temperature ❒ Record axillary temperature 6 hourly ❒ Observe exudate from wound drain; shorten drain according to medical staff's instructions	To detect early signs of infection and promote healing	Wound is kept free of infection
Pressure sores*	❒ Nurse Mrs B on low air loss mattress ❒ Change her position ½ hourly in bed; do not have her lie on left shoulder ❒ When Mrs B is sitting, have her stand hourly to relieve pressure ❒ TPN as prescribed (see Ch. 21)	To prevent loss of skin integrity	Mrs B does not develop pressure sores
Chest infection*	❒ Administer antibiotics as prescribed ❒ Keep Mrs B as upright as possible in bed ❒ Assist her with hourly deep breathing exercises with Triflo ❒ Assist with chest physiotherapy twice daily ❒ Encourage coughing and expectoration ❒ Observe temperature and respiration	To provide prophylaxis against infection and to prevent the build-up of secretions	No shortness of breath; sputum is clear

Nursing Care Plan 27.2 (cont'd)

Nursing considerations	Action	Rationale	Evaluation
Deep vein thrombosis and pulmonary embolism*	❒ Assess daily for calf tenderness and inflammation ❒ Use TED stockings, full length ❒ Encourage hourly leg exercises ❒ Administer Minihep as prescribed ❒ Encourage early mobilisation, e.g. walking to toilet and back twice daily with nurse; sit out 1–2 hours as able	To detect early signs of thrombus or embolus and encourage good circulation	No detection of DVT
Pain in knees and left shoulder	❒ Ensure Mrs B's position is comfortable ❒ Administer analgesia as prescribed ❒ Apply heating pad ❒ Assist with passive exercise and gentle massage	To alleviate pain and prevent stiffness	Mrs B's comfort is maintained at acceptable level
Inability to maintain own hygiene	❒ Encourage Mrs B in self-care tasks ❒ Assist with washing only for areas she cannot reach, i.e. back and lower half ❒ Assist with oral hygiene as required ❒ Encourage use of talcs and perfumes as desired ❒ Change and wash TED stockings daily ❒ Give psychological support when Mrs B changes nightclothes in view of stoma's effect on body image (see Nursing Care Plan 27.3)	To promote return to independence To help Mrs B maintaindignity	Mrs B is able to resume self-care and to cope with changed body image

* Potential problem

Shock must be detected at the first level of compensation and not when the classic picture of the falling blood pressure and rising pulse occurs and a crisis ensues. If a patient is allowed to continue at the first level of compensation, all but the vital organs will be deprived of oxygen and newly anastamosed tissue will have an increased tendency to breakdown and infection due to prolonged vasoconstriction and hypoxia.

The nurse should report any significant changes to the nurse in charge of the patient's care, who may then decide to call in the medical staff. Actions to correct shock must be taken swiftly and must be appropriate to the type of shock diagnosed. Raising the foot of the bed to aid venous return could have disastrous effects in patients undergoing gastrointestinal surgery. If there is bleeding or large volumes of fluid due to paralytic ileus or obstruction in the abdomen, these contents would fall against the diaphragm, impeding respiratory and cardiac funtion.

Aggressive fluid replacement in elderly patients can lead to heart failure, arrhythmias and cardiogenic shock. Needless to say, increasing the i.v. infusion rate would not help to maintain circulating volume.

Once the doctor has assessed the patient, oxygen therapy may well be started or increased to reduce hypoxia. In hypovolaemic shock the lost fluid must be replaced or returned to the circulation. (Some patients may have large amounts of fluid available in the body — as in paralytic ileus or peripheral oedema — but in the wrong body compartment. This fluid can be drawn back into the circulation by treating the cause, and by raising the osmotic pressure of the circulation.)

Crystalline fluids can be given intravenously but are soon lost from the circulation. Plasma protein substitutes (PPS and Haemaccel) can be given as plasma expanders. These raise the osmotic pressure and draw extracellular fluid into the circulation. Interstitial fluid also moves into the capillaries as hydrostatic pressure falls in response to lowered blood pressure and arteriolar constriction. In haemodynamic shock, rapid transfusion of blood may be required and should be given through a blood warmer. Central venous pressure measurements are of great value in assessing the volume of blood returning to the heart and the heart's ability to pump. A central venous line may be inserted as an emergency in a patient whose shock proves difficult to manage. Nursing Care Plan 27.4 (p. 796) illustrates the type of nursing care required to detect the early signs of shock.

Fluid balance

Most patients experience some loss of fluid during surgery

Nursing Care Plan 27.3 Stoma care plan for Mrs B (see Case History 27.2)

Nursing considerations	Action	Rationale	Evaluation
Patient's lack of knowledge about her colostomy	❒ Explain the reasons for the colostomy, liaising with medical staff ❒ Assess Mrs B's level of understanding and her wish for knowledge ❒ Include Mrs B's daughter in teaching ❒ Provide a colostomy booklet for Mrs B to read and to use as a guide for teaching ❒ Give basic information about appliances ❒ Discuss the effects of colostomy on lifestyle ❒ Check Mrs B's retention of information from previous sessions	To provide a sound basis for good stoma care	Mrs B acquires an understanding of the rationale of stoma care
Anxiety about stoma formation and change in body image	❒ Encourage Mrs B to voice fears; provide reassurance in the form of accurate information ❒ Introduce Mrs B to a suitable visitor with a colostomy ❒ Support Mrs B in her grief, provide privacy, passive listening, counselling, touch ❒ Provide support for daughter	To provide an outlet for anxiety	Mrs B is better able to adjust to her new situation
Lack of skill and confidence to care for the colostomy	❒ Implement the following stages: • encourage Mrs B to look at stoma; give reassurance • show her how to check and clean stoma, then supervise as she does this • discuss the range of appliances available, and guide her in making a suitable choice • show Mrs B how to fit appliance and teach skin care • encourage her to fit appliance under supervision, and to check and clean stoma independently • encourage her to care for stoma independently	To build confidence by helping Mrs B to succeed at each stage	Mrs B achieves independence in colostomy care
Inability to cope with the stoma at home*	❒ Refer Mrs B to a community stoma nurse at least one week prior to discharge ❒ Give advice and information on the following as appropriate: diet, fluid and electrolyte balance; alcohol consumption; clothing; prescriptions; flatus control; disposal of appliances; travel; pursuing hobbies and interests; intimate relationships; local colostomy association; attitudes of loved ones ❒ Provide on discharge: supply of equipment; prescription care; prescription exemption form	To prepare Mrs B for her discharge home	The transition from hospital to home care is smooth; Mrs B feels that she is able to cope

* Potential problem

Nursing Care Plan 27.4 Immediate postoperative care plan for M (see Case History 27.4(A) and 27.3(B))

Nursing considerations	Action	Rationale	Evaluation
Shock due to haemorrhage and pain*	❐ Observe TPR and BP ½ hourly ❐ Observe for pallor, sweating and confusion ❐ Record urine output hourly ❐ Give O_2 therapy at 4 l /min as prescribed ❐ Implement pain control (see below) ❐ Check wound and drains ½ hourly ❐ Maintain circulatory volume as prescribed	To ensure pulse is maintained at 65–90, BP at 100/65 to 140/95, urine output at ≥ 30 ml/hr	Shock does not develop
Abdominal pain	❐ Provide patient controlled analgesia as prescribed ❐ Record respiratory rate hourly ❐ Assess effectiveness of analgesia using appropriate assessment tool ❐ Ensure comfortable positioning ❐ Encourage M to support wound while moving	To control pain and enable deep breathing exercises to be performed	Pain is kept at an acceptable level
Fluid and electrolyte imbalance*	❐ Provide i.v. infusion as per chart; change giving set after 24 h ❐ Observe for dyspnoea, irregularities in CVS ❐ Record all fluid intake and output ❐ Observe for nausea, vomiting and diarrhoea	To maintain circulatory volume	Fluid and electrolytes maintained at satisfactory levels
Paralytic ileus	❐ Allow nil by mouth, provide oral hygiene hourly ❐ NG tube, free drainage: aspirate hourly ❐ Observe for flatus ❐ Administer antiemetics as prescribed	To accommodate loss of normal peristalsis To detect return of peristalsis	M is comfortable until peristalsis returns
Loss of bladder tone	❐ Observe and record urine output; urinary catheter with 10 ml balloon inserted in theatre ❐ Perform catheter care morning and evening ❐ Maintain asepsis of closed drainage system	To prevent urinary retention and infection	Diuresis satisfactory Urinary tract does not develop infection
Wound infection*	❐ Check wound and drains ½ hourly ❐ Do not disturb dressing until 48 h postop ❐ Observe vaginal loss twice daily	To promote healing and prevent infection	Wound begins to heal normally
(Cont'd)			

? **27.10** Make a list of factors that might delay wound healing for Mrs B and M (see Case Histories 27.2 and 27.4). What actions might be taken to minimise these predisposing factors? Now turn to Box 27.4 (p. 802), where the main predisposing factors for these two patients are given. What specific factors might you note for Mr L (see Case History 27.3).

Nursing Care Plan 27.4 (cont'd)			
Nursing considerations	**Action**	**Rationale**	**Evaluation**
Pressure sores*	❒ Change M's position according to comfort needs and prior to hyperaemia of skin ❒ Observe for reddening of pressure areas ❒ Ensure skin is clean and dry ❒ Use Spenco mattress	To safeguard skin integrity	M does not develop pressure sores
Deep vein thrombosis and pulmonary embolism*	❒ Administer Minihep as prescribed ❒ Use TED stockings below knee ❒ Assist with leg exercises hourly ❒ Have patient sit out for bedmaking on 1st morning postop	To encourage good circulation, especially venous return	No thrombosis or embolism
Chest infection*	❒ Nurse M as upright as possible ❒ Assist with deep breathing exercises hourly ❒ Encourage coughing and expectoration ❒ Assist with chest physiotherapy	To prevent buildup of secretions and resulting infection	Chest remains clear
Inability to maintain own hygiene	❒ Assist M to wash and change into own nightclothes when appropriate ❒ Provide bed bath with complete assistance on 1st day postop ❒ Provide oral hygiene as required ❒ Change and wash TED stockings daily	To assist M in maintaining dignity and regaining independence	M's comfort and hygiene maintained
Anxiety about outcome of surgery	❒ Reassure M about the outcome of the operation ❒ Repeat information as required if she is drowsy post anaesthetic	To reduce anxiety	M is encouraged about prospects for the future

* Potential problem

which may be compounded by electrolyte disturbances resulting from the illness itself or trauma during surgery. Preoperative dehydration due to excessive fasting should be avoided (see p. 784). Patients having a general anaesthetic will be fasted postoperatively until they are fully conscious and the cough and swallowing reflex has returned. Some may be required to fast for longer than this when there is a paralytic ileus or after facial or laryngeal surgery. These patients require fluid and electrolyte replacement via the i.v. route to meet normal demands. (Some require over and above this volume to replace fluid lost at theatre.)

Fluid balance can be significantly affected by the physiological response of the body to the stress of surgery. Glucocorticoid secretion increases reabsorption of sodium and water in the renal nephrons with a reciprocal loss of potassium and hydrogen ions. Elevated levels of antidiuretic hormone (ADH) also increase water reabsorption and high aldosterone levels increase sodium reabsorption further. The net effect is to increase the extracellular fluid volume and reduce urine output. Consequently, it would not be unusual for a well-hydrated patient to retain fluid and have a high positive fluid balance for the immediate postoperative period.

As a result of trauma to the tissues during surgery, the intracellular electrolyte potassium is released. This is excreted in part exchange for retained sodium. Potassium levels will be closely monitored by medical staff in patients who have undergone major surgery and appropriate replacement with i.v. fluids given.

Many surgical patients complain of thirst and a dry mouth postoperatively. This is due partly to dehydration and partly to the anticholinergic drugs given during the operation to reduce salivary secretions. Until the effects of the anaesthetic have fully worn off, thirst is therefore an unreliable measure of hydration.

Metabolic and stress responses

Surgery and general anaesthesia are major stressors which result in the 'general adaptation syndrome' (Seyle 1976). The psychological effects of stress are often seen as anxiety and withdrawal in surgical patients and are addressed in detail in Ch. 17. The importance of adequate preoperative education and counselling in minimising stress is discussed in this chapter on page 781.

The physiological effects of stress can be reduced by controlling anxiety preoperatively and continuing this postoperatively.

In the immediate postoperative period (and up to 4 days after a major operation) the patient utilises protein as a source of energy along with fats and carbohydrates. The amino acids act as a source of glucose for the brain. Blood glucose levels can be elevated to cause glycosuria. This will be a cause for concern and careful monitoring in diabetic patients and in patients receiving parenteral nutrition. It is important that patients are in a nutritional state sufficient to withstand this period of catabolism and negative nitrogen balance. The loss of nitrogen can also be reduced by administration of amino acid solutions (e.g. Vamin) but requires administration of glucose as an energy source to allow amino acids to be used for protein synthesis. (This solution is similar to that used in total parenteral nutrition (TPN) but omits lipids. It contains less glucose, and can be administered peripherally.) If the patient has a poor nutritional status, and/or is undergoing major surgery with or without prolonged fasting, TPN is generally indicated.

Most patients can tolerate catabolism and some starvation for approximately one week after major surgery (Canizaro 1981). Many become anabolic after a couple of days and begin to rebuild proteins, while hormones released in stress decrease. A large diuresis and negative fluid balance may be seen at this point. Chapter 21 describes nursing interventions to improve the nutritional status of the patient and provides a complete discussion of TPN.

Pain

Despite advances in methods of pain control, 75% of surgical patients in a recent study suffered severe pain (Royal College of Surgeons 1990). Thoracic and abdominal operations tended to cause the most pain but minor procedures could also cause severe pain. Firth (1991) found that 53% of patients having day surgery suffered moderate to excruciating pain. Being in pain was rated as *the* most anxiety-provoking issue for surgical patients in a study by Biley (1989). Clearly, postoperative pain deserves close attention in nursing practice, research and education. The issues relating to pain specifically in the postoperative period are discussed here. The reader is also referred to Ch. 19, where broader but equally pertinent issues are addressed.

Pain control after surgery is a prime concern on humanitarian grounds alone. It also has significant effects on other aspects of the patient's recovery.

Good pain control also allows for early activity, so minimising problems of immobility such as chest infections, urinary tract infections, deep vein thrombosis, pressure sores and muscle wasting. Pain after surgery has also been cited as one of the main reasons for poor sleep (Closs 1988). Elderly patients are at an increased risk of the complications described above. It should not be assumed that they have higher pain thresholds, but they may receive slightly lower doses of analgesics as the clearance and metabolism of analgesics is slower. Care must also be taken with patients already regularly using narcotic analgesics as they will have gained tolerance to these drugs and often require higher doses than normal. Accurate and systematic assessment of pain is essential. Seers (1987) found that nurses in her study consistently underestimated the intensity of patients' postoperative pain. She states; 'Patients' ratings of pain cannot be predicted by the type of operation or time since surgery' (p. 39).

One source of controversy in pain management concerns the assessment of pain as part of the diagnostic process. The nature of the pain (especially in abdominal pain) is an important diagnostic sign, which often results in medical staff withholding analgesia until a full assessment and provisional diagnosis is arrived at. The nurse then has to deal with the complaints or signs of obvious and sometimes severe pain from the patient whilst the doctor refuses to prescribe analgesia. The need for urgent examination of the patient followed by administration of a short-acting analgesic such as pethidine or Entonox should be stressed. Meanwhile, the nurse will require all her skills to comfort and reassure the patient physically and emotionally and will need to be assertive in ensuring that medical staff are kept fully informed of the patient's condition.

Postoperative pain can vary according to the site of the incision, being greater with midline, subcostal and intercostal incisions (see Fig. 27.5). The small incisions made by lapriscopes usually cause the least discomfort.

Controlling pain in the immediate postoperative period is the responsibility of the anaesthetist. The anaesthetist visits the patient preoperatively and will usually discuss pain control with him. This not only reduces one of the patient's main anxieties, but allows the anaesthetist to make a full assessment of that individual's needs. Narcotic analgesics are the mainstay of postoperative pain control. Some commonly used analgesics are given in Table 27.6. Intramuscular injection is the most commonly used method of administration, but is not always the most effective. The patient must understand that the drug is not absorbed to therapeutic levels immediately, so he will need to be informed to ask for analgesia as the pain starts to build up. Otherwise he may wait until the pain is unbearable (suffering the ill-effects of this pain) and continues to suffer for a further 15–20 minutes whilst the injection takes effect. Good cooperation with this method is essential to prevent long periods of severe pain. Plasma drug levels can vary enormously and drugs are often short lived, requiring administration every 4 h or so. Nurses should bear in mind that patients may fear the discomfort of the injection itself.

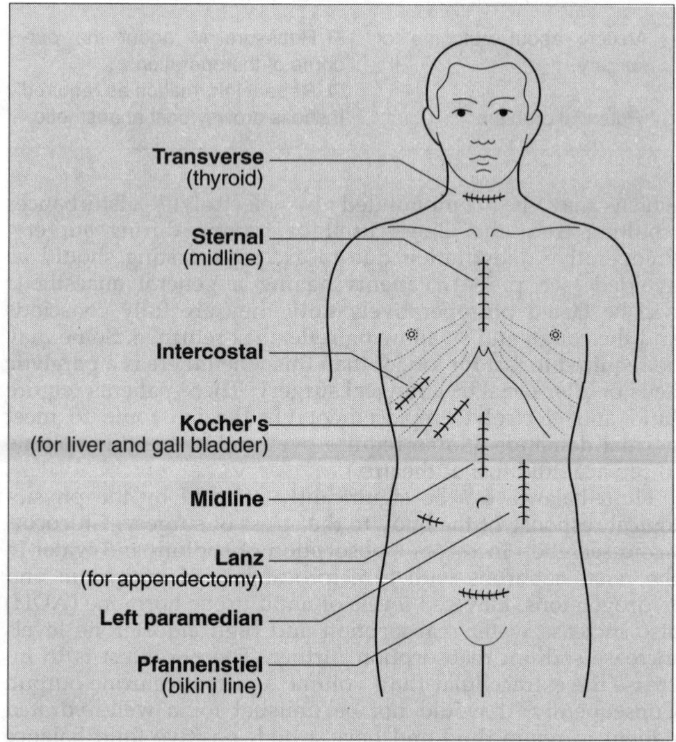

Fig. 27.5 Some incision lines used in surgery.

Table 27.6 Analgesics commonly used in postoperative pain control*

Method of administration	Example of drug used	Example of types of surgery
Epidural infusion	Bupivacaine and lignocaine	Major pelvic or lower abdominal, e.g. colectomy
Intravenous or subcutaneous infusion	Diamorphine, papaveretum† (Omnopon)	Major pelvic or abdominal, e.g. gastrectomy
Intramuscular injection	Morphine sulphate, pethidine, papaveretum†, codeine	Many types, e.g. total hip replacement, Specifically used in neurosurgery
Nerve blocks and local anaesthetic	Lignocaine with adrenaline	Thoracic surgery, wound areas can be infiltrated after surgery
Sublingual	Buprenorphine	Many types of major and minor surgery
Oral	Meptazinol, diclofenac sodium (Voltarol), co-proxamol, co-dydramol, paracetamol	Many products are available. Used in continued recovery and rehabilitation or alone after minor surgery

*For further reading see Trounce (1990).
†Papaveretum must not be used in women of childbearing potential (Committee on Safety of Medicines 1991).

Some newer methods of pain control aim to prevent such large fluctuations in plasma levels. Continuous infusions of narcotic agents can be given through the intravenous, subcutaneous or epidural routes. Intravenous infusion can be advantageous as it enables the rate of infusion to be altered immediately, according to the patient's respiratory rate as narcotic drugs may depress respirations if too large a dose is given. Patient controlled analgesia allows the patient to control the administration of small boluses of intravenous narcotic. A special infusion pump is set to give a specific volume of solution (and therefore a set dosage according to the dilution of the drug) when the patient presses a hand held button. The machine is programmed to provide a bolus only after a certain length of time has elapsed (lock out) and a maximum total number of boluses over a time period. This method of pain control is extremely effective with a cooperative patient (Hunter 1991).

All narcotic agents have similar side-effects, that is, central nervous and cardiovascular depression, and can lead to addiction. Some may induce nausea and vomiting (see Trounce 1990 for further detail). Fear of respiratory depression and of causing addiction often leads to doctors under-prescribing and nurses under-administering. Seers (1987) found that 85% of nurses in her study overestimated the risk of addiction to narcotic analgesics. The major narcotic agents (except buprenorphine) can be reversed with naloxone should respiratory depression occur. It should also be remembered that respiration will in fact be hindered by inadequate pain control (see p. 790). Addiction is unlikely when narcotics are administered only in the postoperative period.

The variety of causes of postoperative pain and discomfort and the wide range of nursing interventions available (see Box 27.3 and Case Histories 27.1 (B), 27.3 (B) and 27.4 (B)) clearly demonstrate that the nurse has a key role to play in alleviating postoperative pain. Primary nursing may also improve the quality of care in postoperative pain, as one experienced nurse and her team of associates can get to know the patient well. Detailed knowledge of the patient and his reaction to pain assists in planning and evaluating care, whilst the close relationship between nurse and patient instils trust and confidence. This not only reassures the patient, but also has a placebo effect that supplements the analgesia administered.

The therapeutic contribution of the nurse in relation to pain control is fully addressed in Ch. 19. The nurse's knowledge base with regard to pain assessment, measurement and relief, her assertiveness and communication skills, her knowledge of the psychological impact of surgery and pain, and her use of complimentary therapies such as relaxation and massage are all vital elements of her ability to provide effective postoperative pain control.

Nausea and vomiting

These problems are now less common as modern-day anaesthetics have fewer side-effects than drugs used formerly. However, some patients will experience nausea and vomiting due to inadequate pain relief, as a side-effect of narcotic analgesia or due to the collection of secretions in the stomach. The premedication atropine (see Table 27.1) reduces gastric motility and can slow stomach emptying. Paralylic ileus can lead to the accumulation of a large quantity of gastrointestinal secretions. Some patients may have some bleeding into the stomach postoperatively which can induce nausea (e.g. in partial gastrectomy).

Nausea and vomiting can be relieved by reducing anticipation and anxiety through preoperative teaching (Davis 1984). Antiemetics may be given as prescribed and nasogastric tubes may be used to relieve gastric distension or irritation due to the accumulation of secretions or blood. Note: metoclopramide should be avoided in patients with a gastrointestinal anastomosis or paralytic ileus, as its mode of action is by increasing gastric mobility.

Sleep

Recent research has demonstrated that surgical patients have greatly disrupted sleep patterns (Closs 1990). As well as the factors affecting the sleep of all hospital patients, surgical patients are exposed to many others. In addition to pain, general discomfort and restricted positioning can cause disturbed sleep. Postoperative patients may experience hypoxia and hypercapnia due to anaesthesic sedation or shock severely compromising CNS control of sleep (see Ch. 25). Aurell & Elmqvist (1985) have suggested that surgery itself can lead to disturbed sleep.

In the postoperative period, frequent observations and recordings are necessary, often into the first postoperative night. These disturbances, along with the general noise generated by procedures, new admissions and emergency action necessary at night all add to the disruption of patients' sleep. Sleep is especially important for the postoperative patient as protein synthesis takes place predominantly during sleep and rest. Growth hormone is secreted during periods of REM sleep. Sleep and rest are essential not only for a feeling of well-being but also for anabolism and tissue repair.

Pain control and general comfort measures are paramount in promoting a good night's sleep. Pulse oximeters can be useful to indicate hypoxia at night in vulnerable patients; however, they require careful use to prevent undue disturbance. Nursing

Box 27.3 Some specific causes of postoperative pain and discomfort

CAUSE	SUGGESTED NURSING ACTION
Joint, neck and back pain and stiffness	Prevent overextension of the neck at intubation point. Exert care in assessment and positioning of patients with rheumatoid arthritis and osteoarthritis. Assist with frequent change of position and passive exercises. Administer analgesics (NSAIDs can be given as suppositories as well as orally). Provide massage, heat pads.
Anastomatic leak (in GI surgery)	Observe for signs and symptoms of peritonitis, gradual or sudden onset of abdominal pain and shock, pyrexia, shallow breathing, abdominal distension, obvious change in drain output. Alert nurse in charge of the patient and/or medical staff immediately.
Nasogastric tube	Keep nasal passages clean, lubricate with petroleum jelly. Ensure tape is secure, clean and does not obscure view. Support the weight of the tube and/or bag by taping or pinning it to nightclothes (this also helps to prevent the tube being pulled out by sudden movement). Pass NG tubes while the patient is under anaesthetic where possible (see Ch. 21, p. 669).
Wound drains	Wound drains and softer tubes cause less pain. Sudden or severe pain at a drain site should be reported. (In case of anastomatic leak or haemorrhage, relieve weight of drainage bags by regular emptying, if appropriate.) Secure drains well with tape to prevent pulling on the securing suture. Label tubes if there is more than one. (The exit may become obscured from view by securing tape.) See p. 801. Provide analgesia cover prior to drain removal. Encourage patient to use relaxation techniques to reduce muscle tension.
Sutures, clips, staples	Sutures should not normally be a cause of pain. Deep tension sutures, wounds under tension (e.g. perianal) or clips catching on nightclothes can cause discomfort. Check wounds daily for signs of infection. Teach patient to support wound when coughing and moving. Cover clips with a light dressing to prevent catching. Provide reassurance and encourage use of relaxation techniques on suture removal. (See p. 804 for care of wounds.)
Dressing changes	These should not be painful for the vast majority of patients, provided good practice is followed. Irrigate wounds with warm saline to clean and use non-adherent wound care products. Wounds tend to become painful when granulating, as nerve endings are exposed. Any adherent dressings should be soaked to aid removal. Adhesives and strong chemicals such as eusol cause pain. Excess hair should be removed at operation site prior to surgery (see p. 785). Analgesics ranging from paracetamol to a general anaesthetic may be required for some dressings. Entonox can be extremely useful in providing short-acting pain relief during dressing changes.
Urinary retention	Observe urine output in uncatheterised patients having pelvic or abdominal surgery, or reduced mobility postoperatively. (Urinary catheters should be inserted in theatre if their need can be predicted.) Observe for a palpable bladder and rising blood pressure. (These signs may also be present in a catheterised patient if the catheter blocks up; measurement of specific gravity of the urine indicates if urine output is truly falling as urine becomes more concentrated.) Ensure privacy and comfortable positioning of patient when bedpans or bottles are being used. Discuss continued retention with medical staff and perform residual catheterisation if necessary, leaving the catheter in situ. Blocked catheters should be irrigated or changed. (See Ch. 24, p. 736 for care of patients with urinary catheters.)
Colic and wind pains	When the patient's paralytic ileus is strong spasmodic muscle contractions may be experienced. Pockets of gas may also have collected in the GI tract and may cause distension. Early and frequent mobilisation can reduce these pains. With approval of medical staff, peppermint water can be given, or, if appropriate, peppermint oil can be used in aromatherapy. Antispasmodic drugs are not usually prescribed, as they can cause a return of the ileus and constipation. Heat pads and gentle massage (by experienced hands) can be helpful.

observations should be minimised to safe levels and noise reduced where possible.

Elimination

Constipation is a common problem which arises as a consequence of immobility, the use of narcotic analgesia and dehydration. Conversely, diarrhoea can occur as postoperative paralytic ileus resolves. Patients may experience colicky pain due to flatus and muscle spasm; this can be reduced by increasing mobility and administering peppermint water (see Box 27.3). Ensuring adequate hydration and early mobilisation help prevent constipation before it becomes necessary to resort to oral laxatives. Diarrhoea following paralytic ileus will resolve spontaneously in a couple of days. Oral fluids and diet may be introduced gradually to prevent nausea and vomiting.

Urinary retention may occur due to immobility or the relaxation of bladder muscle tone by anaesthesia, or as the result of paralytic ileus following abdominal or pelvic surgery. When urinary retention is anticipated, the patient should be catheterised in theatre to minimise discomfort. Otherwise, patients should be given the opportunity for privacy and assistance to assume a normal position to pass urine where possible. If retention leads to distension of the bladder and discomfort, or is a cause for concern, a residual catheterisation may be done. The catheter can then be left in situ should the residual exceed approximately 300 ml.

Once the paralytic ileus resolves (as detected by return of bowel sounds or passage of flatus or faeces) the urinary catheter is usually removed. If the catheter is used for monitoring in haemodynamic shock, or in retention due to immobility, the catheter can be removed when monitoring is no

Case History 27.1(B) Mr W (cont'd from Case History 27.1 (A), p. 777)

Mr W had had his incision site for inguinal hernia repair infiltrated with lignocaine at the end of the operation. He did not experience any pain on return to the ward and was up and about that evening. He had some difficulty with lower back stiffness and pain, but found some relief from a gentle back massage by an associate of the primary nurse who had taken a course in this technique. She also used some aromatherapy oils to help him relax and get to sleep that evening. Mr W did not require any analgesia until the following morning, when he took some co-proxamol before getting up. After being seen by medical staff he got ready to go home. He had already bought some paracetamol to take at home as instructed in his preadmission booklet.

Case History 27.3(B) Mr L (cont'd from Case History 27.3(A), p. 777)

Mr L had no sensory perception in his lower back or perianal area, and therefore experienced no pain from the wound. He did, however, experience some considerable discomfort from the removal of the Elastoplast securing his i.v. cannula. A large piece of tape had been stuck onto his very hairy arm. Fortunately, the tape was not waterproof and could be soaked with plaster remover to dissolve the adhesive. The primary nurse shaved his arm around the new cannula and applied a sterile dressing film. She also made a mental note to mention the incident to the house officer responsible for the previous cannula dressing.

Case History 27.4(B) M (cont'd from Case History 27.4(A), p. 777)

M had had a couple of operations over the last few years for her Crohn's disease. She did not like having injections to control the pain, and had become more frightened and anxious about pain with each operation. The anaesthetist decided she would be a good candidate for patient-controlled analgesia (PCA) and spent some time teaching her about this preoperatively. M kept her infusion until she was able to manage her pain control with a simple compound analgesic. She made a quick postoperative recovery and said she had experienced far less pain than with her previous operations. She had also felt reassured that pain relief would be there as soon as she needed it.

longer required or the patient is mobile enough to pass urine successfully.

Use of urinary catheters should be avoided where possible due to the associated risk of infection (Crow et al 1986, Wilson 1990). The postoperative patient may also be at risk of urinary infection without catheterisation, as a result of immobility. A small volume of concentrated urine will remain in the bladder for prolonged periods, providing a medium for the growth of bacteria.

Following some surgical procedures on the bladder, continued blood loss and clot formation may obstruct the urethra. To prevent this, patients are catheterised with a three-way catheter (sometimes called a 'triple lumen') and continuous irrigation given to the bladder to wash out potentially obstructing clots or debris.

Wound care

Wound care is given with the aim of promoting healing and minimising the risk of infection (see Nursing Care Plan 27.4). Methods of promoting healing depend very much on the individual patient's circumstances. Factors that need to be considered, especially with the surgical patient, are: prolonged hypoxia due to shock, dehydration or local pressure; protein calorie malnutrition; and the local wound dressing. Factors to be considered with all patients with regard to wound healing are discussed in Ch. 23. Prevention of infection begins in the preoperative period with reduction of anxiety and skin and bowel preparation (see pp. 781–786). Asepsis in theatre reduces the threat of exogenous infection (see p. 787). The use of wound drains, prophylactic antibiotics and aseptic technique along with precautions against haematomas will help to reduce wound infections postoperatively. However, some patients will be more at risk of infection than others depending on the type of surgery and on exposure to endogenous bacteria (see Table 27.7 on p. 802).

In the immediate postoperative period, the wound and any drains to the operation site must be checked frequently for signs of bleeding. To assess the degree of soakage on a wound dressing, a ball point or felt-tip pen can be used to mark the margin of the soakage. Any advancing margin of soakage can then be easily detected. Volume markings on drainage bottles and bags give a clear indication of the amount of blood or fluid lost. (Large volumes of weakly blood stained fluid may be due to the fluid used to wash out a cavity but this should still be reported.) Wound dressings should not be changed as they become soaked with blood; instead fresh pads should be added on top to promote clot formation under both dressings. Disturbing dressings in the first or second postoperative day also increases the risk of infection.

The aim of wound drains is to drain blood and inflammatory exudate to prevent haematoma formation and give an indication of blood loss. Some drains may have suction applied to collapse the space left in the tissues after an operation. Drains can also indicate when an anastomosis has broken down (discharging blood, digestive or faeculent fluid) and when an abscess has resolved (cessation of discharge of pus). Some examples of the more common types of wound drain are given in Figure 27.6 (p. 803).

To prevent infection the entry site should be dressed aseptically and a closed drainage system maintained. If bags or bottles need to be changed (when the vacuum is lost or the receptacle is full or heavy) then asepsis should be maintained and sterile equipment used. The decision to remove the drain is made by the doctor when there is minimal or no further drainage. Non-vacuum drains may be shortened before removal to encourage the space left behind to collapse and granulate. Otherwise a cavity might be left that could fill with fluid and give rise to an abscess. Before a drain is removed, the patient will require an explanation and reassurance, and often analgesic cover. Vacuum drains should have their suction released and securing sutures will need to be removed. Relaxation exercises can help reduce the patient's anxiety and muscle tension. Drains that do not move smoothly may be eased by rotating the tube slightly. Traction should not be applied to drains if they are stuck. Such cases must be referred to the medical staff.

Drains that are shortened require securing to prevent them

Table 27.7 Risk of infection in different types of surgery*

Type of surgery	% of patient with infected wounds (% risk)	Examples of types of operations
Clean: hollow organs not opened, no preoperative inflammation or infection	2–5%	Inguinal hernia repair, mastectomy, total hip replacement
Clean contaminated: hollow organs (not bacteriologically clean, e.g. respiratory and urinary tract) opened	5–10%	Transurethral resection of prostate, pneumonectomy, elective cholecystectomy
Contaminated: in areas known to be heavily contaminated, e.g. lower GI tract or in the presence of infection	10–50%	Large bowel surgery, traumatic wounds, abscesses

*For further reading see Hare & Cooke 1991, Ayliffe et al 1990 and Richold (1990).

Box 27.4 Examples of factors that may predispose patients to delayed wound healing

Mrs B (see Case history 27.2(A))
- High risk of wound infection due to:
  - — perforated bowel
  - — unprepared bowel
- Anaemia (preoperative)
- Malnutrition (preoperative) and fasting (postoperative)
- Prolonged shock (postoperative)
- Immunosuppression (due to cancer and prolonged stress)
- Lack of preoperative skin preparation
- Age

M (See Case History 27.4(A) and 27.3(B))
- Steroid therapy (pre- and postoperative)
- Contamination of wound (bowel opened and infection present)
- Low body fat/protein reserves
- Pre-existing inflammatory condition

falling back into the patient as the securing suture has been removed. A large, sterile safety pin can be passed through the tube to prevent this from occurring. As the weight of a Penrose drain may pull out the entire length of the tube these are usually cut and a pin inserted through the end of the tube, which is then sealed inside a drainage bag applied over the drain site (see Fig. 27.6D). This also enables the patient to be more mobile, as a long drainage bag is not needed. It also is often more comfortable as the extra weight of the long tube is removed.

After the first 24 h, the wound and drains should be checked for signs of infection. As stated previously, wound dressings should not be disturbed for the first 48 h to reduce the risk of infection. However, most infections typically do not appear until at least 3 days postoperatively. Regular temperature monitoring may also detect signs of infection. Patients discharged home within the first 2 days after an operation should be taught how to recognise a wound infection and know whom to report it to. Community and practice nurses often continue checks on patients with wounds who have been discharged home early.

After 48 h, wounds healing by 'primary intention' have laid down a top layer of epithelium across the top of the wound. The wound is effectively sealed from exogenous infection and may be exposed to air, which also allows for easy observation. Dressings are not necessary unless the patient has clips or staples that may catch on clothing or there is continued discharge from the wound. Some wounds may be left to heal by 'secondary intention' due to lack of tissue to close the wound, or the presence of infection in the tissues where closure may well lead to abscess formation. Care of these types of wounds is discussed in Ch. 23.

Wounds heal at different rates according to growth rate and blood supply of the local tissues and the patient's general physical condition. Clips would be removed from a thyroidectomy incision line at 2–3 days postoperatively, whilst Mrs B's abdominal sutures were not removed until 12 days postoperatively. There is an increasing trend to use absorbable continuous sutures where good healing is expected. This is especially useful when the patient is to be discharged home in the first few days. Most patients are also relieved to hear that they do not have sutures to be removed. Some types of sutures and their removal are shown in Fig. 27.7. Patients discharged home with non-absorbable sutures in situ may be referred to the community or practice nurse for their removal. For further reading on sutures see Nightingale (1990).

Potential complications

Virtually all surgical patients will be at some risk of developing deep vein thrombosis (DVT), pulmonary embolism (PE), chest infection and atelectasis. Prevention is the mainstay of care and is described on pages 782–784. Preventive measures such as leg and breathing exercises, thrombo-embolic deterrent (TED) stockings and subcutaneous heparin are all continued throughout the postoperative recovery. Early mobilisation contributes significantly to the prevention of not only the complications just mentioned, but also the risks of immobility to which many patients are exposed. Mrs B's care exemplifies the type of proactive preventive measures required (see Nursing Care Plan 27.3).

Communication

When the patient recovers from a general anaesthetic, the first sense to return is that of hearing. Care of the patient in the recovery room can be enhanced by having aids to communication such as hearing aids and glasses available (see p. 791). A number of patients, especially the elderly or the very ill, become and remain confused postoperatively (Carter 1989). This may be due to the effects of the anaesthetic or to systemic illness. Efforts must be made to treat the cause, and nursing measures to reorientate and minimise confusion should be taken. The use of anticholinergic drugs that cross the blood–brain barrier, such as atropine and hyoscine, should be avoided in the elderly as they may cause confusion. Narcotic analgesics are undoubtedly the cause of delirium in some patients. Alternative non-narcotic analgesics such as diclofenac sodium (Voltarol) might be employed.

Patients with provisional diagnoses are often anxious to speak to the doctor about findings in theatre and their prognosis. When information is withheld, a moral dilemma may

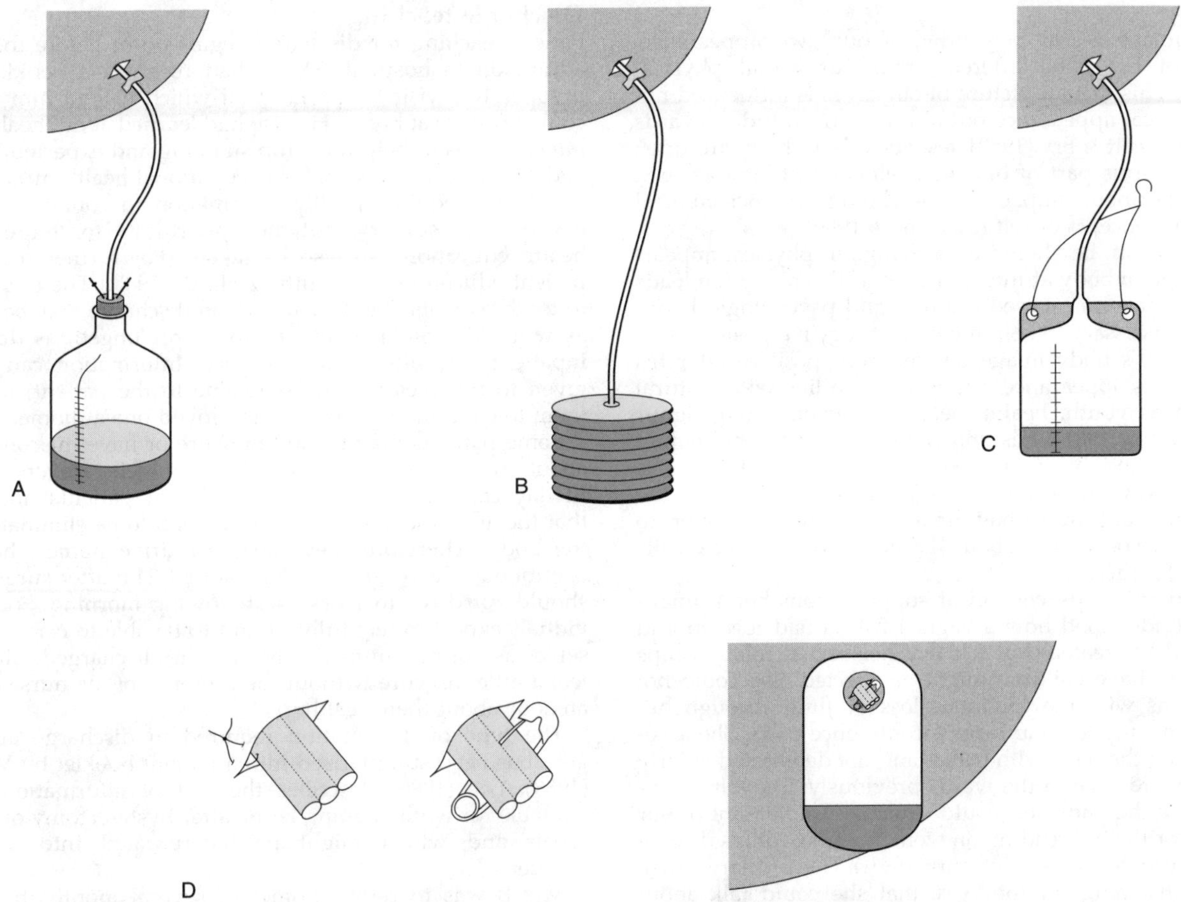

Fig. 27.6 Some types of wound drain. (A) Redivac drain (prongs come together as vacuum is lost) (B) Concertina-type drain (C) Simple tube/Penrose drain (D) Corrugated drain: secured by a suture then safety pin as drain is shortened to prevent it from falling back into the patient. Fluid drains down the channels and into a bag.

exist for nursing staff (see p. 780). Patients are often reluctant to raise all their concerns with the consultant or registrar surrounded by his or her entourage of juniors on ward rounds. The nurse has an important role to play in clarifying the patient's understanding and answering or referring on questions. The patient can experience an anxious time waiting to learn of his diagnosis if samples have been sent to the pathology labs for examination. Support for the patient will be required from the nurse and the patient's family (who themselves may require support), and is often gained informally from other patients.

Good communication among professionals in the postoperative period is essential. Medical and nursing staff must rely on one another for information and advice in order to provide a coordinated plan of care. In primary nursing, one nurse can become extremely knowledgeable about her patients, and is the central focus for channelling information among health care professionals. This is equally true in the case of short-stay patients, who require intensive discharge planning and a highly coordinated plan of care (Sutherland 1991).

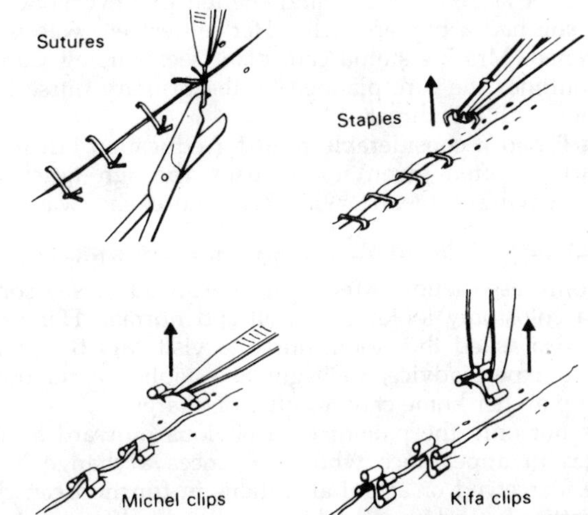

Fig. 27.7 Some common types of sutures and their removal. (Reproduced with kind permission from Jamieson, McCall & Blythe (1988).)

Body image

Our body image is our perception of our own appearance, which might be quite different from our actual physical appearance. This mental picture of ourselves is influenced not only by physical appearance but also by our attitude towards ourselves. Fawcett & Fry (1980) describe this as 'body attitude'. Body image forms part of our total self-concept, and as such can have enormous impact on psychological, sociocultural and physical concepts of self (Blackmore 1989).

Body image can be altered by a change in physical appearance, a change in body attitude, or both. If this alteration leads to a negative self-concept, educational and psychological support will be necessary to help the patient regain a positive self-concept. Mr W's body image became very positive after his operation as his appearance was restored in line with cultural values such as youth, health, beauty, intactness and vigour (see Smitherman 1981). His ability to provide for his family was restored, and he would be seen by his workmates as able to cope with all aspects of his job again. Fortunately, the occupational health nurse had already provided education to correct his misconception about the operation's effect on his sex life and fertility.

M needed much psychological support from her primary nurse. She understood how a vaginal fistula had formed and how it could be treated, but felt that her sexual relationships and ability to have children might be affected. She could not come to terms with the continous loss of fluid through her vagina and having to wear large incontinence pads. She associated wearing the pads with babies and the debilitated elderly patients she had seen in the wards previously. She felt everyone could see the pads and could detect an unpleasant odour from her. (For further reading on women with Crohn's disease and sexual problems see McHenry 1991.) The primary nurse provided a listening ear for M so that she could talk about her fears and her new relationship with her boyfriend. She also comforted and reassured her.

Mrs B recovered from the anaesthetic to find herself attached to tubes, loosely draped in a hospital gown and, worst of all, wearing a colostomy bag. As Mrs B went to theatre as an emergency, there was no time to prepare her for this. At first, she was totally disgusted by the stoma and refused to look at it. She was only able to begin to accept it and learn about it once she learned that it could be reversed in several months' time. Her attitude towards her body was also influenced by knowing that she had had cancer. Mrs B saw cancer as stigmatising, and she felt that everyone would know she had a bag and why. Her self-esteem was severely threatened. Mrs B's stoma care plan (see Nursing Care Plan 27.2) outlines the care planned by the primary nurse to help her cope with this threat.

Mrs B had a considerable need for education but required support — often given non-verbally through touch or by simply having someone with her before she was able to usefully receive any information. Her body image and self-esteem were helped enormously by a visitor from the colostomy association. Mrs B was surprised to see someone with a colostomy looking so well and normal. Her primary nurse also asked the stoma nurse to visit Mrs B in hospital to offer expert advice, to begin to establish a relationship, and to plan her home care for after discharge.

It is not only the patient with obvious outward structural changes in appearance who experiences a change in body image. Perceived or actual alterations in function can change body attitude and thus body image and self-concept. Some may be positive, others negative, but it is certain that all surgical patients are affected to some extent. For further reading see Salter (1988), Dewing (1989) and Hughes (1991).

Discharge teaching

Patient teaching for discharge begins on or before the day of admission to hospital. Mr W had received a booklet at his preoperative visit to the hospital which helped him plan for convalescence at home. He also had learned about healthy diet, interventions to help him stop smoking and expected function and return to work from his occupational health nurse.

Patients require specific information to continue their recovery from surgery, but the opportunity for more general health education can also be taken. (For further reading on patient education see Coutts & Hardy 1985.) The opportunity to teach patients about their care on discharge may be limited, as with day case patients, or more prolonged, as during an inpatient stay after major surgery. Information can also be given to relatives (when acceptable to the patient) to enable them to continue to support their loved one at home.

Some patients may be quite unsure or have misconceptions about how they should progress during their recovery at home. In day case surgery it is essential that patients understand that the anaesthetic may take a full 24 h to be eliminated from the body. Therefore they must *not* drive home, should be continuously accompanied for the first 24 h after surgery, and should *not* drive to work the following morning. Some individuals expect to feel fully fit and to be able to care for themselves as normal immediately they are discharged. Many will feel a little insecure without the presence of the nurse and feel anxious about their health.

The type of information required in discharge after surgery has been summarised into a patient booklet by Vaughan (1988). Lee (1989) describes the sort of information that is valuable for women going home after hysterectomy or vaginal repair and which might be incorporated into a patient booklet.

Mrs B was to return home for several months before the surgeon would consider reversing her colostomy. She had to be independent in caring for her stoma and so required staged teaching and much support (see Nursing Care Plan 27.2). She had a booklet to reinforce the teaching given by the nurses, which also acted as a focus for discussions of the stoma with her daughter. Mr and Mrs L were shown how to use the low air loss mattress they had hired for Mr L to use at home. The primary nurse also explained to Mr L how to use a urinary sheath and pointed out how to avoid common problems with it. Mr L quickly became independent and proficient in using the sheath.

All patients should be clear about seeking advice or treatment from the most appropriate source on discharge. Referral to community nurses and GPs, when possible, establishes continued support and may be preferable to telling patients just to ring the ward.

Discharge planning

Discharge plans aim to provide a smooth transition from hospital to home for continued patient care. There are many research studies to highlight the problems experienced in discharge planning (e.g. Skeet 1983, Littlewood 1984). However, there are also some examples of good practice in discharge planning for surgical patients. Hart (1982) describes a scheme in which the community nurse visits and assesses day case patients prior to admission and plans postoperative visits. In another setting nurses have found great value in the care and discharge planning of a patient all being coordinated by one nurse (Sutherland 1991). Continuous responsibility is a feature of primary nursing that facilitates this approach (Hegavary 1982). Ersser & Tutton (1991, p. 179) state:

> the primary nurse is in a position to develop a greater knowledge of

a smaller number of patients and . . . to engage in direct communication with all those involved in a patient's care. This would also suggest that practices which rely on careful co-ordination, such as discharge planning, may improve under this system.

Wilson-Barnett & Fordham (1982) suggest that a lack of discharge planning is one of the factors responsible for a delayed recovery at home. In a busy surgical ward there is often an urgent need for beds which can lead to a hasty and poorly planned discharge. All patients are referred to their GP on discharge from hospital by the surgeon (see Fig. 27.1, 27.2). The primary nurse will decide whether the patient needs to be referred to the community nurse as well. Referrals can be made for nursing interventions ranging from wound care — checking for signs of infection, changing dressings or removing sutures — to providing psychological support for the patient and his family, especially where cancer has been diagnosed with a poor prognosis. If patients are able to attend the health centre or clinic for wound dressing procedures, then arrangements for an appointment can be made before discharge. It should be remembered when starting a patient on a course of treatment that not all wound dressing materials are available in the community. District nurses often find the information given in a referral task-centred and inadequate (Parnell 1982). Information should also be included with regard to mental state, mobility, social circumstances, and what the patient has been told.

When there is extensive information to communicate to the community nurse, a personal phone call, a copy of the care plan on discharge, or a visit by the community nurse to the ward can all be useful. Mrs B's stoma nurse had visited her in hospital on several occasions prior to discharge and had liaised closely with her primary nurse to ensure she was well prepared to go home. Mr L's community nurse called into the ward to see him and the primary nurse, who was able to discuss the discharge arrangements and to ensure that the community nurse had a copy of Mr L's care plan and was familiar with the low air loss mattress. She also provided enough dressing material for Mr L's wound for the first week at home.

Liaison posts have been established to assist in the discharge of patients. These community nurses visit the wards and can advise on whether a patient may be ready for discharge and on the type of information required by the receiving community nurse, and will contact the relevant services on the ward's behalf. This system can be extremely useful but can also restrict the quality of information by the use of an intermediary (Age Concern 1980). The liaison sister and ward nurse must use their intimate knowledge of the individual patient to determine when a direct contact from the primary nurse to the community nurse (or vice versa) would be beneficial.

Discharge planning is becoming increasingly important as the decreasing length of stay means that less time is available for preparation. Forward planning and continuous responsibility as an element of primary nursing may help nurses to achieve the goal of effective discharge preparation.

REHABILITATION

Rehabilitation of the patient does not take place exclusively in either hospital or home, but is nonetheless an increasing focus of care in the community setting. The needs of patients in terms of recovery from surgery do not differ dramatically from the time they leave hospital to their arrival at home. Armitage (1985) sees discharge from hospital as a stage in patient care, involving transfer from one setting to another. The plan of care for the discharged patient may thus address similar problems to that of the patient who continues his recovery in hospital. Many interventions described in the sections on postoperative care will be equally relevant to the patient in hospital or at home.

Rehabilitation can be a lengthy process, requiring continued support by community nurses, or a short event with minimal professional intervention. Mrs B was visited by the community nurse at home to assess her self-care deficits using Orem's model (Orem 1980). She was also visited regularly by the stoma care nurse whom she had first met in hospital. Mr L's district nurse continued to care for his wound on discharge, following a very similar pattern of care to that given in hospital. M saw her practice nurse once to make sure that her abdominal wound was healing well, and Mr W talked to his occupational health nurse about resuming a full range of duties.

The demands made by postoperative patients in the community have increased enormously in recent years. This is partly due to an ageing population making greater demands on the service. The elderly are known to be vulnerable on discharge and are more likely to have contact with community nurses (Ross 1987). The trend towards day case surgery and early discharge (see p. 776) places more responsibility for postoperative care in the hands of community health care workers.

Williams (1985) describes a scheme in Peterborough by which the early discharge of hysterectomy, nephrectomy and hip replacement patients was found to be cost-effective and to shorten waiting lists. These trends have also been driven partly by public demand. Ruckley et al (1978) found that patients preferred day case surgery with postoperative care by the community nurse and GP to care in the surgical ward or the convalescent ward. The result is that community nurses have over the last 20 years almost doubled the number of visits they make, with an increasing proportion of these visits being made to elderly patients (Common Services Agency 1990). It is also noteworthy that there has been no real increase in the *numbers* of community nurses during this time.

The contribution that community nurses can and do make to the patient's recovery tends to be underestimated. There is a focus on performing tasks, such that referrals are made only for patients requiring specific nursing interventions — often the care of wounds. However, psychosocial needs must not be ignored and should also be communicated in handing over patient care to community staff (Parnell 1982).

REFERENCES

Age Concern 1980 Discharge from hospital: the social worker's view. Age Concern, London

Allsop C 1991 Primary nursing in a surgical unit. In: Ersser S, Tutton E (eds) Primary nursing in perspective. Scutari, London

Armitage S 1985 Discharge referrals: who's responsible? Nursing Times 81 (8): 26–28

Aurell J, Elmqvist D 1985 Sleep in the surgical intensive care unit. British Medical Journal 290: (6474): 1029–1032

Baskerville P A, Meddle R M, Jarrett P E M 1985 Preparation for surgery: information tapes for the patient. The Practitioner 229 (July): 677–678

Blackmore C 1989 Altered images. Nursing Times 85 (12): 36–39

Biley F C 1989 Perceptions of stress in preoperative patients. Journal of Advanced Nursing 14 (7): 575–581

Boore J R P 1978 Prescription for recovery. Royal College of Nursing, London

Borkje B et al 1991 Effectiveness and acceptability of three bowel

cleansing regimes. Scandinavian Journal of Gastroenterology 2 (Feb 26): 162–166
Bradshaw P W, Ley P, Kinnay J 1975 Recall of medical advice, comprehensibility and specificity. British Journal of Sociology and Clinical Psychology 14: 55–62
Brandberg A, Anderson I 1980 Whole body disinfection. Royal Society of Medicine International Congress and Symposium, Series 23. Royal Society of Medicine, London Academic Press
Canizaro P C 1981 Methods of nutritional support in the surgical patients. In: Yarborough M F, Curreri P W (eds) Surgical nutrition. Churchill Livingstone, Edinburgh
Caprini J A, Scurr J H, Hasty J M 1988 Role of compression modalities in a prophylactic program for deep vein thrombosis. Seminars in thrombosis and haemostasis (Supplement) 14: 77–87
Carter M 1989 Effects of anaesthesia on mental performance in the elderly. Nursing Times 84 (4): 40–42
Carter C 1990 Ritual and risk. Nursing Times 86 (13): 63–64
Cheslyn-Curtis S, Russell R C G 1991 New trends in gallstone management. British Journal of Surgery 78 (Feb): 143–149
Closs S J 1988 A nursing study of sleep on surgical wards. Nursing Research Unit, University of Edinburgh
Closs S J 1990 An explanatory analysis of nurses' provision of postoperative analgesic drugs. Journal of Advanced Nursing 15 (1): 42–49
Coleridge Smith P D, Hasty J H, Scurr J H 1991 Deep vein thrombosis: effects of graduated compression stockings on distension of the deep veins of the calf. British Journal of Surgery 78 (June): 724–726
Collins R, Scrimgeour A, Yusuf S, Peto K 1988 Reduction in fatal pulmonary embolism and venous thrombosis by perioperative administration of subcutaneous heparin. New England Journal of Medicine 318: 162–173
Committee on Safety of Medicines 1991 Genotoxicity of papaveretum and noscapine. Current Problems 31 (June)
Common Services Agency 1990 Scottish Health Statistics. ISD Publications, Edinburgh
Connah B, Pearson R (eds) 1991 NHS Handbook, 7th edn. Macmillan, London
Crow R A et al 1986 A study of patients with an indwelling urethral catheter and related nursing practices. Nursing Practice Research Unit, University of Surrey
Davis B D 1984 Preoperative information giving and patients' postoperative outcomes. Nursing Research Unit, University of Edinburgh
Department of Health (NHS Management Executive) 1990 A guide to consent for examination or treatment. DHSS Health Publications Unit, London
Dimond B 1990 Legal aspects of nursing. Prentice-Hall, Hemel Hempstead
Dubois F, Berthelot G, Levard H 1989 Cholecystectomie par coelioscope. La Presses Medicale 18: 988–992
Dubois F, Icard P, Berthelot G, Levard H 1990 Coelioscope cholecystectomy: preliminary report of 36 cases. Annals of Surgery January 211: 60–62
Egbert L D, Battit E W, Welch C E, Bartlett M K 1964 Reduction of postoperative pain by encouragement and instruction to patients. New England Journal of Medicine 270: 825–828
Ersser S, Tutton E 1991 Primary nursing in perspective. Scutari, London
Ewles L, Simnett I 1992 Promoting health: a practical guide. Scutari, London
Fahrenfort M 1987 Patient emancipation by health education: an impossible goal? Patient Education and Counselling 10 (1): 25–37
Fawcett J, Fry S 1980 An exploratory study of body image dimensionality. Nursing Research 29 (15): 324–327
Firth F 1991 Pain after day surgery. Nursing Times 87 (40): 72–76
Franklin B L 1974 Patient anxiety on admission to hospital. Royal College of Nursing, London
Frost J 1993 Clinical application of lasers. Professional Nurse 8 (5): 298–303
Galvin K T 1992 A critical review of the health belief model in relation to cigarette smoking behaviour. Journal of Clinical Nursing 1: 13–18
Hamilton Smith S 1972 Nil by mouth. Royal College of Nursing, London
Hart C 1982 Back home to nurse. Nursing Mirror (Supplement) Community Forum 154 (10): ii–vii
Hayward J 1975 Information: a prescription against pain. Royal College of Nursing, London
Hegavary S T 1982 The change to primary nursing: a cross-cultural view of professional practice. Mosby, St Louis
Hughes A 1991 Life with a stoma. Nursing Times 87 (25): 67–68
Hunter D 1991 Relief through teamwork. Nursing Times 87 (17): 35–38
Jamieson E M, McCall J M, Blythe R 1988 Guidelines for clinical nursing practice. Churchill Livingstone, Edinburgh
Jarvis I L 1958 Psychological stress: psychoanalytic and behavioural studies of surgical patients. Wiley, New York
Jeffery P C, Nicolades A N 1990 Graduated compression stockings in the prevention of deep vein thrombosis. British Journal of Surgery 77 (4): 380–383
Johnson D E 1980 The behavioural system model for nursing. In: Riehl J P, Roy S C (eds) Conceptual models for nursing practice, 2nd edn. Appleton-Century-Crofts, New York
Johnson M 1982 Recognition of patients' worries by nurses and by other patients. British Journal of Clinical Psychology 21: 255–261
Lancet 1983 Editorial: preoperative depilation I (June 11): 311
Lawrence D, Kakkar W 1980 Graduated static external compression of the lower limb: a physiological assessment. British Journal of Surgery 67: 119–121
Lee T 1989 Patient information: the key to increased autonomy — what shall I do when I get home (Advice for women who have had hysterectomy or vaginal repair). Professional Nurse 5 (1): 43–47
Linden man L A, Van Aeinman B 1971 Nursing intervention with the pre-surgical patient. Nursing Research 20: 319–333
Littlewood J 1984 Unmet needs of the elderly. Report Centre for the Study of Primary Care, London
Malby R 1991 Audit audibility in a nursing development unit. Nursing Times 87 (19): 35–37
Manthey M 1981 The practice of primary nursing. Blackwell Scientific, Boston
Medical Defence Union 1986 Consent to treatment. Medical Defence Union, London
Mumford E, Schlesinger M, Glass G 1982 The effects of psychological intervention on recovery from surgery and heart attacks: an analysis of the literature. American Journal of Public Health 72 (2): 141–151
National Institutes of Health 1986 Prevention of deep vein thrombosis and pulmonary embolism. National Institutes of Health Consensus Development Conference Statement 6 (2)
Nightingale K 1990 Making sense of wound closure. Nursing Times 86 (14): 35–37
Nursing Standard 1991 Endometrial ablation. (Editorial) Nursing Standard 5 (12): 15
Office of Health Economics 1989 Compendium of Health Statistics, 7th edn. Office of Health Economics, London
Orem D 1980 Nursing: concepts of practice, 2nd edn. McGraw-Hill, New York
Parnell J 1982 Continuity and communication. Nursing Times 78 (9): 33–40
Pearson A 1988 Primary nursing. Croom Helm, London
Porteus M J et al 1989 Thigh length versus knee length stockings in the prevention of deep vein thrombosis. British Journal of Surgery 76: 296–297
Pritchard A P, Walker V A 1984 The Royal Marsden Hospital manual of clinical nursing policies and procedures. Harper & Row, London
Rafferty A 1988 Postoperative backache. Nursing Times 84 (46): 32–35
Reading A E 1981 Psychological preparation for surgery: patient recall of information. Journal of Psychosomatic Research 25: 57–62
Rice V H, Johnson J E 1984 Preadmission self-instruction booklets. Nursing Research 25: 57–62
Roberts S 1991 Operation reassurance. Nursing Times 87 (40): 70–71
Roper N, Logan W, Tierney A 1990 The elements of nursing, 3rd edn. Churchill Livingstone, Edinburgh
Ross F 1987 District nursing. In: Littlewood J (ed) Recent advances in nursing: community nursing. Churchill Livingstone, Edinburgh
Royal College of Surgeons of England and the College of

Anaesthetists 1990 Pain after surgery. Royal College of Surgeons, London
Ruckley C V, Cuthbertson C, Fenwick N, Prescott R J, Garraway W M 1978 Day care after operations for hernia or varicose veins: a controlled trial. British Journal of Surgery 65: 456–459
Scottish Office (National Health Service in Scotland) 1991 The patient's charter: a charter for health. HMSO, Edinburgh
Seers K 1987 Perceptions of pain. Nursing Times 83(48): 37–39
Seyle H 1976 The stress of life, 2nd edn. McGraw-Hill, New York
Sidway Versus Bethlem Royal Hospital Governors and others 1985 1, ALL, ER 643
Skeet M 1983 Continuity of care. In: Clark J, Henderson J (eds) Community health. Churchill Livingstone, Edinburgh
Smitherman C 1981 Nursing actions for health promotion. Davis, Philadelphia
Sutherland E 1991 All in a day's work. Nursing Times 87 (11): 26–30
Thomas E A 1987 Preoperative fasting: a question of routine. Nursing Times 83 (49): 46–47
Thompson I E, Melia K M, Boyd K M 1988 Nursing ethics, 2nd edn. Churchill Livingstone, Edinburgh
Turner G M, Cole S E, Brooks J H 1984 The efficacy of graduated compression stockings in the prevention of deep vein thrombosis after major gynaecological surgery. British Journal of Obstetrics and Gynaecology 91 (June): 588–591
UKCC 1992 Code of professional conduct for the nurse, midwife and health visitor, 3rd edn. UKCC, London
UKCC 1989 Exercising accountability. UKCC, London
Vaughan B 1988 Discharge procedures: discharge following surgery. Nursing Times 84 (15): 28–33
Wallace L 1985 Surgical patients' preferences for preoperative information. Patient Education and Counselling 1 (4): 377–387
Webb W R 1975 Postoperative pulmonary complications. In: Artz C P, Hardy J D (eds) Management of surgical complications. Saunders, Philadelphia
Williams B, Williams J G L, Jones R 1972 The measurement and control of postoperative anxiety. 12th annual meeting of the Society for Psychophysiological Research, November 1972
Williams P 1985 Hospital at home. Journal of District Nursing 4 (2): 4–6
Wilson M 1990 Catheterisation under scrutiny. Nursing Times 86 (49): 71–72
Wilson-Barnett J, Fordham F 1982 Recovery from illness. Wiley, Chichester, pp. 88–102
Wong J, Wong S 1985 A randomised trial of a new approach to preoperative teaching and patient compliance. International Journal of Nursing Studies 22 (2): 105–115
Wright S G 1990 My patient my nurse. Scutari, London
Young A P 1991 Law and professional conduct in nursing. Scutari, London

FURTHER READING

Ayliffe G A J, Collins B M, Taylor L J 1990 Hospital-acquired infection: principles and practice, 2nd edn. Wright, London
Brennan A 1989 Clinical conundrum. Nursing Times 87 (20) May 17: 48–9
Coutts L C, Hardy L K 1985 Teaching for health: the nurse as health educator. Churchill Livingstone, Edinburgh
Dewing J 1989 Altered body image. Surgical Nurse August 2 (4): 17–20
Hare R, Cooke M 1991 Bacteriology and immunology for nurses, 7th edn. Churchill Livingstone, Edinburgh
Hughes A 1991 Life with a stoma. Nursing Times 87 (25) June 19: 67–68
McHenry C 1991 Silent suffering. Nursing Times 87 (46) Nov 13: 21
National Association of Theatre Nurses 1983 Code of practice: guidelines to total patient care and safety in practice in operating theatres. National Association of Theatre Nurses. Harrogate.
Neal M J 1990 Medical pharmacology at a glance. Blackwell Scientific, London
Richold J C 1990 Postoperative surgical wound infection. Nursing Times April 25 86 (17): 56
Rumbold G 1986 Ethics in nursing practice. Baillière Tindall, London
Salter M (ed) 1988 Altered body image: the nurse's role. Wiley, Chichester
Trounce J 1990 Clinical pharmacology for nurses. Churchill Livingstone, Edinburgh
Webber B A, Pryor J A 1994 Physiotherapy for respiratory and cardiac problems. Churchill Livingstone, Edinburgh

CHAPTER 28

The patient who experiences trauma

Teresa Barr

CHAPTER CONTENTS

Introduction 809
What is trauma? 809
Reception of patients in the A & E department 810

Immediate treatment of emergencies 811
The resuscitation room 811
Maintenance of the patient's airway 811
Maintenance of the patient's breathing 811
Maintenance of the patient's circulation 811
Organisation of resuscitation facilities 812

THE NURSING PROCESS IN A & E CARE 813

A patient with multiple trauma 813
Assessment and immediate treatment 813
Care of relatives 816
Diagnosis and further treatment 817
Admission 817

Death in A & E 818
Organ donation 818
Spiritual needs 818
Care of relatives following a patient's death 818
Staff grief 819

A patient with minor trauma 819
Assessment and treatment 820
Assessment of home circumstances and organisation of community services 821
Discharge 821

Aggression and violence in A & E 822
Our changing society 822
Defusing potential aggression 822
Body language 822
Listening to aggressive patients 822
Avoiding physical danger and attack 822
Documentation and the law 822

Major disasters 823
What is a disaster? 823
Disaster planning 823
Post-traumatic stress disorder 823

Health promotion in A & E 824

References 824

Further reading 825

Useful addresses 825

INTRODUCTION

This chapter examines what is meant by trauma and highlights the range of injuries and conditions which may be encountered by the nurse working in an accident and emergency (A & E) department. Innovations in trauma care such as nurse triage are detailed, and reference is made throughout to relevant research. As well as outlining procedures for resuscitation and the emergency treatment of physical injury, the chapter considers the emotional impact of the sudden injury or death of a loved one and discusses ways of helping relatives to cope with anxiety and grief.

Miscarriage and sudden infant death syndrome (SIDS), although not usually classified as trauma, are also considered here, as they are often handled by the A & E department and require, as any form of bereavement, sensitive and knowledgeable intervention.

The nursing process as it is practised in A & E nursing is demonstrated by means of two extended case histories: one dealing with a patient who has sustained major injuries in a motorcycle accident, the other dealing with an elderly person who has suffered a minor but nonetheless incapacitating injury in her home. These two studies illustrate how the four stages of the nursing process — assessment, planning, intervention and evaluation — can be implemented within the context of an emergency, and how nursing interventions may include family members both as vital members of the caring team and as individuals with needs in their own right.

An effort is made to relate the practical and ethical challenges faced by A & E staff to wider sociological and political issues. Strategies that may be adopted to prevent incidents of aggression and violence in the A & E department are discussed in some detail. A section is devoted to the key aspects of the A & E department's response to disasters in which large numbers of casualties have occurred. In conjunction with this, the psychological impact of disasters on survivors, onlookers, rescue workers and health care staff is examined. Finally, the important contribution that A & E nurses can make in promoting health in their day-to-day work is explored.

What is trauma?

Trauma may be defined simply as any bodily injury or wound ranging from a graze easily self-treated at home, to a major insult involving several body systems and resulting in death or permanent disability. Trauma usually results from various types of accidents, but it may be self-inflicted or caused by violence.

In the United Kingdom in 1989, 3.5% of all male deaths and 2.2% of all female deaths were caused by accidents or violence (Central Statistical Office 1991). In 1987, 70 718 people were killed or seriously injured in road traffic accidents (RTAs) in the UK, while 34 682 were killed or seriously injured at work, and 127 786 suffered fatal or serious injuries in the home (ROSPA 1989). These figures include only those patients who died or spent more than three days in hospital as a result of their injuries. In the same year, 12 797 000 people attended A & E departments in the UK. Not all of these patients suffered physical trauma. In fact, the vast majority had serious medical, surgical or psychiatric disorders, incidents of serious trauma accounting for only a small proportion of the A & E workload throughout the country. Others presented with conditions which do not, in fact, fall into the category of either an accident or an emergency.

Within the National Health Service, the general practitioner (GP) is identified as the source of primary medical care through whom patients are referred to hospital facilities and specialist practitioners. However, through A & E departments patients can gain immediate access to hospital facilities without GP referral. It is estimated that almost 80% of any A & E department's workload is made up of these self-referred patients. This is particularly the case in those departments with inner city locations, where GP practices are usually found in 'lock-up' premises (IHSM 1988). While 80% of A & E patients present with non-urgent problems, 20%, or around 2.5 million patients, are seriously ill or injured. These patients will usually arrive singly by ambulance, but sometimes several will arrive together, either coincidentally or because they have all been involved in the same accident. This will obviously be the case in the event of a disaster, which may involve hundreds of casualties. How then can A & E departments best cope with dramatic fluctuations in patient numbers, and with the diversity of conditions with which patients present?

Reception of patients in the A & E department

A & E departments cannot follow a 'first come, first served' policy. Those who need immediate treatment must have it immediately. Therefore, some means of establishing priorities is required.

In many departments prioritisation is facilitated by the physical division of available space. Most will have a designated resuscitation area and others will assign certain cubicles to 'major' and 'minor' trauma. Larger departments may have separate dressing rooms, plaster rooms and even cubicles specially equipped to assess and treat patients with, for example, eye injuries or dental problems. It has also been recommended that where children are treated in A & E departments, separate waiting areas and treatment rooms should be provided (DHSS 1971).

Every A & E facility will have a reception area and waiting room. Many have two points of access: one for ambulance patients, leading directly to the treatment area, and another for other patients, leading to the reception area. This may be the first means by which patients are categorised. Those patients arriving by ambulance will be received immediately by a nurse and those who walk in will usually approach the receptionist first. Protocols established between medical, nursing and clerical staff will ensure that patients with certain conditions are not kept waiting. These may include: all children; adults complaining of chest or abdominal pain; patients who have suffered a head injury; patients who are bleeding profusely; and patients who are in severe pain. Receptionists may also use their discretion to refer patients directly to nursing staff. In recent years much concern has been expressed about this method of identifying priority patients (Blythin 1988). Large attendances at A & E departments may mean that seriously ill or injured individuals may not see a professional for a long period of time. In order to rectify this unacceptable situation, many departments have introduced nurse triage systems.

Triage

This system involves the reception of all patients by a trained nurse before, or as soon as possible after, registration with the receptionist. The triage nurse assesses each patient's condition and assigns a priority rating to him. Rating scales may have as few as three or as many as seven divisions, but generally range from 'life-threatening' to 'delay acceptable'. The categories may be either numbered or colour-coded (e.g. red for 'life-threatening', green for 'delay acceptable'). An example of such a rating scale is given in Table 28.1.

The triage nurse may take a history of the illness or accident, record vital signs and examine the injured part of the patient, as appropriate. She does not diagnose conditions or prescribe treatments, although she may give first aid to those patients who will have to wait to see the doctor. She may request old notes or X-rays to be made available in order to reduce waiting times. If the patient is accompanied by relatives or friends these individuals may also be included in the assessment interview, with the patient's consent. In this way the nurse may gain additional information about the patient's condition and assess the relative's ability to support the patient if he is discharged home. When the patient is a child the accompanying adult is included in the assessment as a matter of course.

Those patients who are waiting are regularly reappraised by the triage nurse. If their condition deteriorates they may be moved to a more urgent category. If, because of an influx of seriously ill patients, waiting times become unacceptably long, the triage nurse may decide to admit lower-category patients to the doctor in a set ratio, e.g. one category 5 patient to every three category 4 patients. The system should be explained to the patient when he is being assessed and he should be told which group he is in and why. Patients readily understand that seriously ill people must take priority and are

Table 28.1 Triage rating scale (after Blythin 1988)

Rating	Examples
Life-threatening	Severe head injury with unconsciousness Crush injury to the chest Cardiac arrest
Urgent	Severe central chest pain Fracture dislocation of the ankle with absent pulses Lime burns to the eye
Semi-urgent	Closed fracture Deep laceration Abdominal pain
Non-urgent	Soft tissue injury, e.g. sprained ankle Superficial laceration Foreign body in the ear
Delay acceptable	Longstanding condition, e.g. ganglion Dog bite where skin is unbroken Sore throat

Research Abstract 28.1 Triage

Bailey et al (1987) hypothesised that patient satisfaction with A & E services is closely associated with length of waiting times. Since triage is believed to reduce waiting times, it follows that the introduction of such a system should increase patient satisfaction. This hypothesis was tested by means of a short patient questionnaire to elicit satisfaction levels, along with data collection relating to waiting times. This was undertaken both before and after the introduction of triage to the A & E department in order to obtain comparative data.

The pre-triage data demonstrated a strong relationship between waiting times and patient satisfaction: the longer a patient waited, the more dissatisfied he became.

The post-triage data showed that waiting times were indeed reduced by 24%. Although patients had been satisfied with their treatment before triage, satisfaction levels were further increased with the introduction of the system.

Bailey A, Hallam K, Hurst K 1987 Triage on trial. Nursing Times 83(44): 65–66

content to wait their turn once the system is explained to them (see Research Abstract 28.1).

In order to undertake this role, the triage nurse must possess good interviewing skills, knowing when to listen and when and how to ask questions (see Ch. 26).

Departments which employ the triage system will benefit from an ongoing training programme to allow new staff to develop these skills and experienced triage nurses to update their knowledge (Blythin 1988).

IMMEDIATE TREATMENT OF EMERGENCIES

The resuscitation room

Patients in the 'life-threatening' category will be taken immediately to the resuscitation room which must always be in a state of readiness. There should be space for at least two accident trolleys, with the equipment necessary to resuscitate two patients ready to hand. Unfortunately, lack of space or resources sometimes makes this impossible. The room should be set up so that the 'ABCs' of resuscitation — i.e., maintenance of airway, breathing and circulation — may be quickly and easily followed with no delays related to finding or assembling equipment.

Maintenance of the patient's airway

The airway must be checked for obstruction and appropriate steps taken to clear it if necessary. This may be done manually by using the fingers or with a rigid suction catheter. Until a full assessment is completed it is inadvisable to extend the neck to clear the airway. If the patient has an injury to the cervical spine extension of the neck may do added damage.

The resuscitation room should have a supply of oropharyngeal airways and endotracheal (ET) tubes in a variety of sizes. In some cases (for example, where there are severe facial injuries) it may not be possible to pass an ET tube, and so nasal tracheal tubes should also be available. Tubes should be fitted in advance with the appropriate mounts so that they can be connected to an anaesthetic machine quickly and easily. The resuscitation room should also have laryngoscopes and a ready supply of replacement batteries and bulbs, a syringe to inflate the tracheal tube cuff, forceps to retain the air in the cuffed portion of the tube, and scissors in case the tube needs to be shortened. Tape cut in appropriate lengths to tie the tube in place should be ready to hand. This equipment must be checked every morning and after each use to ensure that it is in place and in working order. Damaged equipment should be replaced immediately. Dim laryngoscope bulbs should be changed and failing batteries transferred to less vital pieces of equipment. At least one prepacked, sterile tracheostomy set should be in the department and others readily available, perhaps from an emergency store.

Those departments which also treat children should have infant and child sets of this equipment. These are perhaps best stored in separate, clearly labelled cases and should also be checked daily to ensure patency of the tubes and properly fitting connections. Children's ET tubes are normally uncuffed, whilst adult tubes are generally cuffed. A child's airway narrows naturally at the cricoid ring and this creates a seal.

Suction apparatus should be available, with tubing and catheters of various types and sizes. This may be connected to a central wall or ceiling point, but there should also be a portable suction machine for use while the patient is being transferred from the A & E department.

Maintenance of the patient's breathing

The resuscitation room should be equipped with an anaesthetic machine fitted with a ventilator in case the patient requires intermittent positive pressure ventilation (IPPV). The appropriate gases may be piped from a mains supply. Bottles of these gases should be fitted to the anaesthetic machine for use during patient transfer. These bottles should be checked regularly to ensure that they contain an adequate supply. Face masks in a variety of sizes, including those suitable for children, should be available.

Patients with chest injuries may have haemothorax, pneumo-thorax or both, in which case they will require the insertion of chest drains to reinflate their lungs (see Ch. 3, p. 72) (Jamieson et al 1992). The equipment necessary for this procedure must be available. This includes a sterile chest drain set, chest drains in various sizes and an underwater seal drainage system.

Maintenance of the patient's circulation

In severely traumatised patients the most common circulatory problem is hypovolaemia (see Ch. 18, p. 600). Emergency treatment consists of restoring circulating volume as rapidly as possible by the infusion of intravenous (i.v.) fluids. It may be necessary to erect more than one i.v. line and in order to infuse the fluid quickly a pump may be used. By the time the patient reaches hospital his peripheral circulation may be 'shut down'. This occurs in hypovolaemia as a result of the body's attempt to preserve the vital organs by constricting the peripheral blood vessels and redirecting the available blood to the major organs. Therefore it may be impossible to insert an i.v. cannula in a surface vessel, and it may be necessary to perform an i.v. cut-down. This involves making an incision in the skin and subcutaneous tissues and locating a deeper vein in which to insert a cannula. Again, the necessary equipment should be ready. Wide-bore cannulae should be used so that fluids may be rapidly infused. Initially, a plasma-expanding fluid may be chosen until the patient's own blood can be grouped and crossmatched. A central venous line may be inserted to enable close monitoring of the circulating blood volume, so that hypervolaemia does not result.

In order to assess the patient's condition, certain blood tests will be ordered. Sample bottles, forms and large syringes should be prepared and a policy should be in place for the quick transport of samples to the laboratory. The appropriate charts should be available for the recording of fluid balance and vital signs.

Organisation of resuscitation facilities (see Fig. 28.1)

Equipment

A policy of keeping 'a place for everything and everything in its place' should be followed, so that staff can learn the location of every item and find anything that is needed immediately.

Certain items may be prepared in advance. For example, the ECG monitor may have its chest electrodes attached, and receivers with the most commonly used blood sample bottles, corresponding forms and large syringes may be kept ready. Clipboards with the usual documentation may also be prepared in advance.

Emergency drug boxes may be stocked by the hospital pharmacy with the drugs commonly used in the A & E department. These boxes should be returned to the pharmacy as soon as they are used and replaced immediately.

The arrangement of the resuscitation room and its cupboards should not be changed unless all staff are informed. Moreover, staff must continually update their knowledge of the procedures which may be performed. It is easy to forget skills which are used infrequently, but patients' lives may depend on the rapidity with which certain measures are undertaken.

Staff

Effective staffing is as important as the organisation of equipment. Having too many people in the resuscitation room may be as dangerous as having too few, as overcrowding can lead to confusion and delays. There should be a system of identifying from the total nursing staff in the department a group of perhaps three or four nurses who will make up the resuscitation room nursing team. In order to give everyone this experience the team can be changed on a daily, or shift, basis. As well as the designated nurses there will be either an A & E consultant or a senior doctor from A & E and an anaesthetist and surgeon on call.

The nursing staff may be organised around the medical team such that each nurse's responsibilities are defined according to the medical staff member whom she assists. Thus, one nurse will assist the anaesthetist in intubation or ventilation of the patient. She may also be responsible for recording vital signs. A useful piece of equipment is one that automatically records pulse and blood pressure and thus frees the nurse for other duties. The anaesthetic nurse will also be responsible for getting and recording any drugs used.

A second nurse will assist the A & E doctor, first in assessing and then in treating the patient. Injured patients should have all clothing removed in order to be fully assessed. If necessary, clothes should be cut off so as to avoid unnecessary movement (see p. 813). This prevents further damage to a possibly injured spinal column or to the limbs and conserves the patient's energy when further demands on the circulatory and respiratory systems are best avoided. The patient's dignity should, of course, be preserved as much as is possible. The patient's body is examined from head to toe, front and back, so that no injuries are missed. Assessment must be rapid and may take place at the same time as the life saving resuscitative measures already mentioned.

An initial history will have been received from the ambulance crew, but further information may become available with the arrival of relatives or friends. Collecting this information may, in the absence of a triage system, be the responsibility of the third nurse. This 'runner nurse' may also be responsible for organising initial documentation such as the A & E record card. She will also get and assemble necessary equipment and communicate with other departments, e.g. the laboratory, X-ray, or portering services. It may be best for the runner to be a senior nurse who has the experience and ability to anticipate needs and requests. If the department operates a triage system, the triage nurse will act as liaison between the trauma team and the patient's family or friends. Otherwise, a fourth nurse may be allocated to this role.

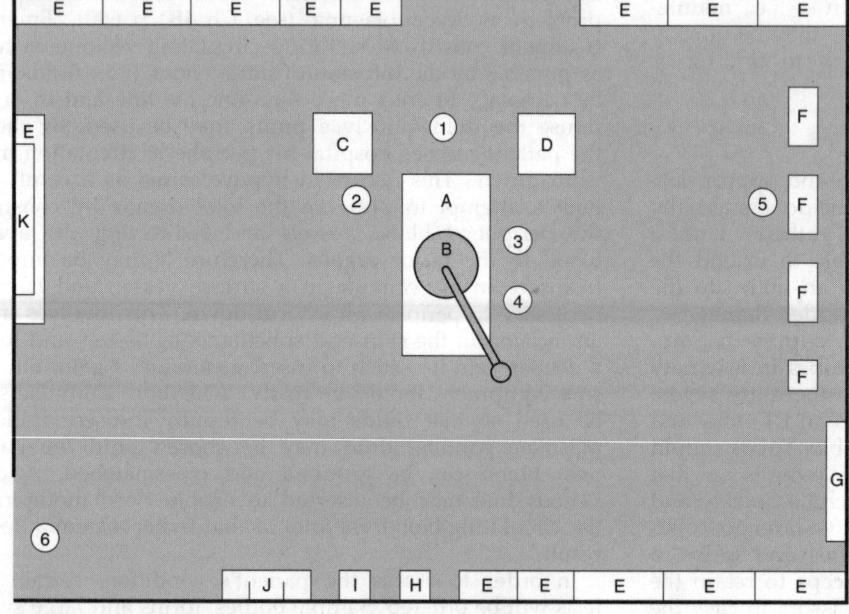

Equipment
- A Patient's trolley
- B Overhead operating lamp
- C Anaesthetic machine
- D Trolley with ECG machine and automatic vital signs recorder
- E Cupboards and drawers of various sizes
- F Trolleys set up for various procedures
- G Notice-board for recording trauma team or other information
- H Blood refrigerator
- I Drug refrigerator
- J Scrub-up sink
- K Large X-ray viewing box

Staff
1. Anaesthetist
2. Anaesthetic nurse
3. A & E doctor
4. Nurse assistant
5. Runner nurse
6. Triage or liaison nurse

Fig. 28.1 Organisation of the resuscitation room.

THE NURSING PROCESS IN A & E CARE

The nursing process approach is reflected in the systematic care of the traumatised patient. Assessment and prediction of actual and potential problems is the first stage. Planning, to meet present needs and avert future complications, is followed by the implementation of the planned strategies. These are then evaluated for their effectiveness. In the care of severely injured patients the components of the nursing process are necessarily contracted into a short period of time and may run concurrently, certain procedures being implemented whilst assessment is still ongoing and some treatments being evaluated before further planning is attempted. In the exigencies of an emergency situation, the roles of nurse and doctor may become blurred and even overlap.

In order to use the process of nursing in the A & E department effectively, it is helpful to base practice upon an agreed model of nursing. Dorothea Orem's model of nursing (Orem 1991), which is centred on the concept of self-care, has been chosen for this chapter because it allows for the rapid physical assessment which is of critical importance in emergency situations. Orem's model also allows for the inclusion of the patient's family in the plan for care, both as a resource in the treatment of the patient and as individuals with their own needs.

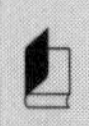

Readers are directed to Walsh 1989, which presents a comprehensive argument for the use of Orem's model in A & E care.

In order to facilitate the rapid assessment of the patient's condition a pre-printed care plan may be used. This does not mean that all patients are treated in the same way or that their individuality is ignored. These plans act only as a basis for assessing needs and planning care with a minimum of delay. A common complaint about the use of the nursing process in A & E departments is that it takes too much time to write up the care plans. If standardised core plan forms are used this need not be the case. It is essential to keep adequate records of the patient's initial condition, the actions performed and the outcomes of these actions. Nursing records are extremely important and (although this is not their primary purpose) often form the basis for medical notes. Nursing records may be the only written source of information about a patient's treatment and for medico-legal reasons as well as for the patient's benefit should be meticulously kept.

A PATIENT WITH MULTIPLE TRAUMA

Assessment and immediate treatment

In Case History 28.1, on J's arrival at the A & E department the receiving nurse first obtains a history from the ambulance crew, who report that J was unconscious when they arrived. They also report that identification was made by the police and that J's relatives are being contacted. J's airway is checked while this report is being given. It is found to be patent and J is transferred to an A & E trolley which has a sliding plate under the mattress to allow for X-rays to be taken without J being moved.

Case History 28.1 J

J, an 18-year-old man, has been knocked off his motorcycle while travelling at high speed. He was wearing a crash helmet, but is brought to the department unconscious by ambulance. He has an oropharyngeal airway in situ and has been given oxygen by the ambulance crew. His left leg is splinted from groin to toes, as the ambulance personnel suspect a closed fracture of the femur. The police, who were called to the accident site, succeeded in finding identification and are now trying to contact J's family.

Because of the nature of the accident and J's unconscious state, spinal injury must be presumed until disproven. Therefore, he has a backboard applied before he is lifted. In the absence of a backboard, a rigid cervical collar would be applied and J lifted with his back straight and someone applying gentle but steady traction to his neck. Once he is transferred safely to the A & E trolley, J's clothes are removed by cutting.

(**Note:** Motorcyclists often wear expensive leather protective clothing. Conscious patients will frequently forbid this clothing to be cut, preferring to suffer pain rather than have their leathers damaged. In a situation such as the one described here, the clothing *must* be cut to prevent further injury. Care should be taken, however, to cut clothing along the seams if at all possible, so that it can later be repaired. However, the patient's condition will dictate the urgency with which clothing should be removed.

Sometimes the patient will still be wearing a crash helmet. The ambulance crew may not have removed it for fear of damaging the cervical spine. If the helmet is still on, great care must be taken in removing it. A hard cervical collar should be applied before the helmet is taken off. If this is not possible a doctor should maintain traction on the neck while the helmet is removed. It should then be examined for cracks which might indicate a severe blow to the head.)

During the removal of J's clothes a rapid assessment is made. This follows the standardised form reproduced in Figure 28.2, beginning with an assessment of the patient's ability to meet 'universal self-care demands' (Orem 1991). This provides a basis for urgent intervention. A more in-depth assessment of 'human function' incorporating the ABCs of resuscitation is then recorded. Where there are life-threatening deviations in any of these functions, immediate action will be taken.

J's respirations are counted, and their rhythm and depth observed and recorded. His breathing appears laboured and, on inspection, it is found that one side of his chest is not inflating. Palpation of the chest wall reveals swelling and crepitus on the left side, indicating fractured ribs which have penetrated the lung. In order to reinflate the lung, thus allowing adequate gaseous exchange and tissue perfusion, two chest drains must be inserted (see Ch. 3, p. 72). This will also prevent mediastinal shift. The equipment is prepared and the drains inserted under strict asepsis. Local anaesthesia is used, even though J is unconscious, since he may still feel pain.

The amount of blood drained from the chest is carefully measured and recorded. Continued observation of respiratory rate, rhythm and depth, as well as the patient's colour and the oscillations of the drainage tubes, is required.

J's pulse is rapid (120 beats/min.) and thready. He is also hypotensive, having a blood pressure of 70/30 mmHg. These recordings show evidence of hypovolaemia (see Ch. 18, p. 600). His pupils are equal and reacting to light. He is unresponsive to verbal commands but has a slight reaction to painful stimuli. These observations are recorded on a Neurological Observation Chart (see Ch. 30, pp. 841–843) because J is unconscious and serious head injury is suspected.

Because of J's poor cardiovascular condition, two peripheral i.v. lines are inserted. The object of this early treatment of hypovolaemia is to restore circulating volume as rapidly as

Universal self-care demands				
Self-care demand	Ability of patient to fill demand			Reason for patient being unable to meet demand for self-care
	Fully able	Partially able	Not able	
Patient can provide for intake of :-				PENETRATING INJURY TO LEFT LUNG
air		✓		
water			✓	UNCONSCIOUS
food			✓	
Patient can provide for adequate and controlled excretion of :-				AS ABOVE
air		✓		
urine			✓	UNCONSCIOUS
faeces			✓	
other, e.g. sputum			✓	
Patient can achieve balance between activity and rest :-				UNCONSCIOUS + # LEFT FEMUR + RIGHT WRIST
ambulant			✓	
uses hands/arms			✓	
sleeps normally			✓	
Patient can achieve balance between solitude and socialisation. Is patient able to make adequate social contact at home?				OMIT FOR PRESENT
Patient can prevent hazards to life/safety at home?				"
Patient can achieve normalcy in :- hygiene, clothing, mental state, home environment				" "

Health deviancy and self-care			
A. Is the patient displaying a health deviancy in any of the following areas?			
1 Human functioning	Present	Suspected	Not present
i Airway			
Respiratory arrest			✓
Airway obstruction			✓
ii Breathing			
Paralysis due to spinal trauma			✓
Difficulty in breathing	✓		
Respiratory depression	✓		
Chest trauma	✓		
iii Circulation			
Cardiac arrest			
Shock	✓		
Abnormal pulse rate/rhythm	✓		
Chest pain		✓	
iv Mental function			
Unconscious	✓		
Diminished level of consciousness			
Head/facial trauma			✓
Unequal pupils			✓
A. What is the health deviancy relevant to the specific complaint of the patient?	PERFORATED LEFT LUNG DUE TO # RIBS		

2 Human structure			
Code	Structure	Present	Comment
1	Laceration	✓	PATIENT HAS BEEN IN RTA
			HAS GRAZES TO BOTH LEGS
2	Deformity	✓	SWELLING, DEFORMITY OF (L) FEMUR + (R) WRIST
3	Burn	—	BRUISING, SWELLING TO (L) CHEST WALL
4	Swelling	✓	
5	Bruising	✓	
6	Broken skin	✓	
7	Rash	—	
8	Pressure sore	—	
9	Amputation	—	
10	Other, e.g. foreign material	—	

3 Human behaviour (underline as appropriate)

i Vocal : <u>nil</u>/moaning/crying/talking (confused)/talking (orientated) shouting
ii Non-vocal : <u>still</u>/restless/agitated/very active/walking/running/limping.
iii Mood : relaxed/cheerful/quiet/<u>uncommunicative</u>/tense/anxious/aggressive.

4 History of event and why patient thinks he or she is in A & E unit

RTA. NO COMMUNICATION FROM PATIENT

Fig. 28.2 Standard nursing assessment: a patient with major trauma. (Adapted from Walsh 1989, with kind permission from Butterworth Heinemann.)

possible. J's arms are inspected; his right wrist appears swollen and deformed. The left arm is therefore chosen as the first i.v. site and a wide-bore cannula is inserted into the antecubital fossa. It is decided to infuse 500 ml of a colloid plasma expander rapidly. Since this fluid may interfere with cross matching, blood is drawn before the infusion is commenced. Samples are sent for grouping and cross matching, full blood picture, and urea and electrolyte analysis. These tests being urgent, the laboratories are notified and a porter called to deliver the sample immediately.

It is decided to obtain an arterial blood sample for analysis of blood gases. This will indicate the ability of J's lungs to exchange oxygen and carbon dioxide. The brachial, radial or femoral arteries are most commonly used for this procedure. The nurse provides a syringe containing 1 ml of heparin (5000 iu/ml) and prepares a sealable plastic bag with ice in order to keep the blood cool in transit. The bag is labelled carefully and it is ascertained that the porter is waiting in the department before the blood is taken, as delays may cause inaccurate results. Venous blood could also be analysed for blood gases if there were difficulty in obtaining an arterial sample; however, this would provide a less reliable indicator of pulmonary function. Four units of blood are ordered initially and the laboratory is informed that more may be necessary.

Although J's right wrist appears damaged, it is decided to insert the second wide-bore cannula here. Spinal injury has not yet been excluded, so the neck veins are not suitable. Abdominal injuries have not been ruled out, so it is not wise to use the legs for infusion sites, as the fluid may escape into the abdominal cavity. Once J's condition has been stabilised the cannula can be removed to allow the wrist to be treated. Another 500 ml of the plasma expander is erected and rapidly infused. In some circumstances a central line would be inserted. This decision would be made by the anaesthetist on the basis of the patient's cardiovascular status.

Assessment continues using the 'human structure' form shown in Figure 28.2. It has already been noted that there is swelling and bruising of the chest wall and that the right wrist is swollen and deformed. Further examination proceeds head-to-toe. The scalp is examined for lacerations (none are found) and the skull gently palpated for loss of continuity which might indicate a depressed fracture. Again, none is found. The face is inspected for swelling, bruising or broken skin. No abnormalities are noted. The upper limbs are palpated from shoulder girdle to fingers. The right wrist shows the only abnormality.

J's chest trauma has already been noted and treated. The abdomen is examined for bruising, distension and other marks. This is particularly important in vehicle drivers and passengers, as seat belts may have marked the skin, indicating the force which has been applied to the chest and abdomen. Internal bleeding will be indicated by the signs of hypovolaemia, but where there is multiple trauma it is not possible to rely solely on these signs. Abdominal girth may be measured to indicate bleeding from an abdominal organ. This measurement should be taken by the same nurse, at the same place, every 10–15 minutes, the site being marked with a pen. Measurement of abdominal girth is not completely reliable, as it may take some time for the girth to increase enough to be noticeable. If abdominal injury is strongly suspected, peritoneal lavage should be performed as a more reliable diagnostic procedure (see Box 28.1).

Muscle spasm and rigidity are found in the left upper quadrant of J's abdomen. A ruptured spleen is suspected, as this is often associated with left lower rib fractures. As the spleen is a highly vascularised organ, the likelihood is that J has lost a considerable amount of blood into the abdominal cavity. A nurse goes to contact the general surgeon on call. Given J's rib fractures, the severe degree of hypovolaemia, and the abdominal spasm and rigidity, the diagnosis of ruptured spleen is almost certain. Peritoneal lavage is not considered necessary or appropriate, especially in view of the risk associated with this procedure. While the blood is contained within the abdominal cavity it is, to a certain degree, self-limiting. However, once it begins to drain out it may be very difficult to staunch the flow without surgical intervention.

Further assessment is carried out while the team waits for the surgeon. The pelvis is examined by manipulation of the pelvic bones. Any unnatural movement or crepitus would

Box 28.1 Peritoneal lavage

Peritoneal lavage is carried out in order to diagnose intra-abdominal bleeding, and thus trauma to the abdominal organs. The equipment necessary for the procedure includes:

- resuscitation equipment
- trolley
- sterile dressing pack
- cleansing lotions, including alcohol-based and iodine
- local anaesthetic and equipment for administration
- peritoneal dialysis catheter with trocar
- 20 ml syringe
- 1 L normal saline for i.v. infusion at room temperature
- i.v. giving set
- suture material
- dressings.

In order to avoid bladder perforation, the patient is asked to void his bladder in advance of the procedure. If he is unconscious, a urinary catheter is passed.

Following thorough cleansing of the skin, local anaesthetic is injected to a site usually 2–3 cm below the umbilicus. When the area is adequately anaesthetised, a small skin incision is made. It is essential that any bleeding from this incision is arrested before continuing, as it may confuse the outcome. When haemostasis is accomplished the catheter is inserted. If a trocar or introducer is used to facilitate the catheter insertion, it is then removed. 20 mls of peritoneal fluid is then aspirated. If the fluid is grossly blood-stained the diagnosis is immediately made and the procedure discontinued. If the aspirate is less obviously blood-stained or appears clear, the procedure is continued by infusing the normal saline over a period of 15–20 minutes. Too rapid an infusion may cause sudden, excess pressure on the diaphragm and adversely affect respiration. The patient may be gently rolled from side to side, in order to mix the solution with the peritoneal fluid. The infusion bag is then placed below the level of the patient's abdomen so that gravity will siphon off the fluid. When the return is complete, the catheter is removed, the wound sutured and a dressing applied.

The lavage fluid is examined for blood-staining. If it is obviously blood-stained or cloudy a laparotomy is performed. Even if the fluid appears clear a sample should be sent to the laboratory for microscopic examination.

It is imperative that resuscitation equipment is prepared before the procedure is commenced. Patients may lose large quantities of blood and become severely shocked.

indicate fracture of the pelvic bones, or, less commonly, dislocation of the pelvic joints. Fracture of the pelvis may be associated with rupture of the bladder or transection of the urethra. For this reason urinary catheters should not be inserted until damage to these structures is excluded. Blood around the external urinary meatus may indicate transection of the urethra, which is more common in male patients.

A ruptured bladder would be indicated by bruising of the lower abdomen and swelling in the suprapubic region. Foley catheters should *not* be passed on these patients. Where the bladder is ruptured the urethra may also be damaged, so it is wiser to insert a suprapubic catheter if urinary drainage is urgent. Safest of all is to call a genito-urinary surgeon if one is available.

J does not appear to have any pelvic damage. His lower limbs are now examined from hips to toes, beginning with the unsplinted leg being inspected first. There are some minor abrasions on his knee and shin, but no obvious injury to the bone. The splint applied by the ambulance crew to the left leg is gently removed. It is necessary to do this in order to inspect the leg for lacerations as well as to determine the level of the fracture and any associated soft tissue damage e.g. to nerves or blood vessels. The lower third of the femur is extremely swollen and deformed, but the dorsalis pedis pulse is present.

?	**28.1** If the dorsalis pedis pulse were absent, what might this indicate? Refer to Chapter 2, p. 51.

J now begins to moan. His name is called and he opens his eyes. His blood pressure has increased to 90/50 mmHg and his pulse has decreased to 100 beats/min. It appears that his altered consciousness level was due to hypovolaemic shock rather than to head injury, but this cannot yet be assumed. Patients may have a period of lucidity following serious head injury and so the coma scale is still followed.

Although J is now conscious and is obviously in pain, he is not yet given analgesics as this may mask the symptoms or signs of his abdominal injuries. This is explained to him and he is told that he will be given pain relief as soon as the examination is complete.

(**Note:** Withholding analgesics is also necessary for patients who come to the A & E department complaining of abdominal pain. This can be most distressing, both for patients and relatives, who have come to hospital expecting immediate pain relief to be available. This situation requires the nurse to use her communication skills to explain to the patient and his relatives the rationale behind this action.)

In some circumstances Entonox may be used. This is a mixture of 50% nitrous oxide and 50% oxygen used as an inhalant analgesic. It produces pain relief without reduction of consciousness levels and is short-acting, so that it does not mask pain symptoms. However, it should not be used for patients with pneumothorax, since the nitrous oxide may diffuse into the space created by the pneumothorax, thus enlarging it and further compromising respiration.

J is now 'log-rolled' so that his back and spinal column can be examined. Since his known major injuries are on the left side, he is rolled to the right. Spinal injury has not yet been ruled out, so great care is taken to keep his spine in anatomical alignment. The spinal column is palpated for loss of normal continuity and abnormal curves or 'dips'. Now that J is conscious, he is asked to indicate any areas of pain. No abnormality is detected and no back pain is reported by J.

The blood has now arrived and two units are commenced, running quickly. Vital signs continue to be recorded and observation is made for signs of incompatible blood matching (see Ch. 11, p. 417).

The radiographer has already been alerted to the fact that portable X-rays may be needed, or that the radiography department may need to be available at short notice, depending on the patient's condition. X-rays will be taken of J's skull, chest, abdomen, left femur and right wrist. Although J has denied any pain in his neck or back, his cervical spine will also be X-rayed. It is decided to take portable X-rays of his chest and abdomen initially. When J has been examined by the surgeon the other areas will also be X-rayed.

Care of relatives

J's mother, Mrs S, has now arrived in the department. She has been met by the triage nurse and brought to the relative's room.

Ideally, each department should have a quiet room where the family and friends of seriously ill or injured patients may wait. This room should have comfortable chairs (waiting may often be long), facilities for making tea or coffee, and a telephone, so that other family members or friends can be contacted. Not every department has sufficient space for this facility, but some area other than the main waiting room should be found for these usually very distressed people. A sister's or doctor's office or the staff rest room, for example, might be used. A nurse should, if at all possible, stay with the relatives. People who are in a strange and, in this case, threatening environment are often unsure of how to behave and what is expected of them. They may have questions to ask, such as where the toilets are located, but may be reluctant to leave the room they have been shown into in case they miss some vital information about their loved one. They may also feel that if they come out and ask questions they are depriving their relative of a key member of staff who is essential to the team. Clearly, much anxiety and distress can be avoided if a member of staff remains with the family. Where pressures of work or staff shortages make this impossible, the family should be reassured that their relative is being constantly monitored and is never left alone. They should also be introduced to a nurse who will act as their contact, told where she can be found, and encouraged to approach her with any queries or problems. This nurse should be responsible for seeing the relatives every 15 minutes or so in order to bring them up-to-date with developments.

Mrs S has not had the opportunity to contact her husband, as she has come straight to the hospital with the police. She is offered the use of a telephone to get in touch with him but requests that a member of staff do this for her instead. She is given details about her son's condition. These details are truthful, conveying the seriousness of J's condition.

It is neither helpful nor compassionate to falsely reassure people in such circumstances. They need time to adjust their feelings in order to cope with what may be very bad news. If relatives are falsely reassured that everything will be all right they will, understandably, feel cheated if the outcome is not a happy one. Also at issue here is a question of rights: if relatives or patients are to make informed choices about treatment they must be furnished with adequate knowledge to do so. To deny people knowledge is to deny them the power to make necessary decisions (Thompson et al 1988).

At the same time, all hope should not be destroyed. In encounters such as this it is essential that the nurse is an experienced communicator, since there is a fine line to be drawn between giving false hope and causing unnecessary anguish. Relatives also have needs at such a stressful time which the nurse must assess before embarking on lengthy explanations. Mrs S, for example, may have preferred to wait until her husband arrived before being given any information.

Breaking bad news thus requires distinct skills, which nurses must learn and practise (see Ch. 32, pp. 900–902).

J's mother has already been told of the circumstances of the accident by the police. She wishes to 'know the worst' about his condition and is now informed of his injuries and the treatment he has received so far. The fact that he has a chest drain and is receiving i.v. fluids is explained, so that she is not alarmed by the presence of this equipment. Mrs S is told that a surgeon has been called and that J is at present being X-rayed, but that she may see him, if she wishes, as soon as this is completed.

The trauma team need not interrupt their treatment of J to allow his mother to see him. The team's first priority is, obviously, the patient's physical condition, and they may become so caught up in this that other considerations are forgotten. Often, all that is necessary to reassure relatives and patients is that they see each other briefly. Family members will be more content if they can see that the patient is actually alive and the patient will be comforted by knowing that his family is present. Mrs S is also told that J has not yet received analgesics, and why.

Mrs S is taken to the resuscitation room after the X-rays have been taken. She speaks briefly to her son while the X-ray machine is being removed. The surgeon has now arrived and J's mother returns to the relative's room with the nurse to wait for her husband. She asks if J's brother, sister and girlfriend should be contacted, and is told that it may, in fact, do everyone good if they are all together at this time of family crisis (Manley 1988).

Diagnosis and further treatment

The surgeon agrees that J has most probably ruptured his spleen. The abdominal X-ray confirms this, showing an enlarged spleen with medial displacement. Other abdominal organs may also be damaged, and so an emergency laparotomy is needed.

The theatre staff are informed, as are the staff on the ward to which J will be transferred postoperatively. He is now given analgesics; since the aim is to relieve his pain as quickly as possible, the i.v. route is chosen. He will also be given i.m. antibiotics and, because of the abrasions on his body, tetanus toxoid (see Box 28.2).

J's vital signs continue to be recorded at regular intervals. It is found that his pulse and blood pressure have stabilised, remaining at 100 beats/min. and 90/50 mmHg respectively. It is decided to take him to the X-ray department to complete the necessary range of X-rays. A nurse will accompany him and continue to take and record vital signs. Any deterioration will be immediately reported and the necessary action taken.

The doctor now has time to see J's mother. Some other family members have arrived and everyone is brought up-to-date about J's condition, the treatment he has already received, and the likely course of future events.

The orthopaedic surgeon has been informed of J's fractures. He views the X-rays and confirms the wrist and femoral fractures. Fortunately, he finds no fracture or dislocation of the cervical spine. Following a discussion with the general surgeon, it is decided that after the laparotomy is completed the orthopaedic surgeon will be called to reduce and immobilise the fractures while J is still anaesthetised. In the meantime, the temporary splintage will be sufficient to immobilise the femur and wrist. Further delays to apply plaster of Paris to the wrist and a Thomas's splint to the femur are not desirable. The fractures are not life-threatening and their treatment can wait.

Admission

All documentation is assembled and a family member is asked to give details for an admission form to be completed. J's clothing and valuables have already been placed in property bags and are now given to his mother. Departments differ as to policy for dealing with property; some record details in a property book, while others leave this task to the admitting ward.

(**Note:** In certain circumstances, notably in cases of violent assault such as shootings, stabbings or rape, the victim's clothes should be carefully bagged, recorded and given to the police for forensic examination. This may also apply in the case of hit-and-run accidents. It is preferred that items are bagged separately, so that one item does not contaminate another. If property is given to the police, it is important that a police officer signs the property book as receiver of the property, and that the nurse who hands it over also signs so that future queries from any source can be readily answered.)

J is now ready to be taken to theatre (see Ch. 27). His family and girlfriend are called to accompany him. They will be able to talk to him along the way and to say their goodbyes when he reaches theatre. The theatre staff are informed that J's family are going to wait, so that they can be kept informed of his progress and notified when he is returned to the recovery ward. The family are taken to a relative's room beside the wards and theatre staff are told where they can be contacted.

It is likely that J will make a full recovery, but what would have happened if he had died in the A & E department? The following section deals with the nurse's role in supporting

Box 28.2 Adsorbed tetanus vaccine

Adsorbed tetanus vaccine induces an active artificial immunity by introducing inactivated bacteria into the body. This provokes the body to produce the protective antitoxin to the disease. Tetanus vaccine is given with diphtheria and/or pertussis vaccines as part of the primary immunisation scheme for infants and children. Booster doses of the vaccine should be given at roughly 10-yearly intervals throughout life.

Patients with deep, contaminated wounds whose active immunity is unsure or unknown should be given antitetanus immunoglobulin of human origin (HTIG or Humotet). This provides immediate passive immunity, but a course of adsorbed tetanus vaccine should be commenced at the same time or as soon as is practicable afterwards. Where both are being given at the same time, separate syringes and injection sites in different limbs should be used. Otherwise, severe reactions may result.

In addition to administration of the vaccine, wounds should be thoroughly cleansed, irrigated or debrided as necessary. Special care should be taken with puncture wounds or wounds contaminated by garden or farm material. *Clostridium tetani* is an anaerobic organism whose spores may survive for many years in soil. Even minute pricks from rose thorns have been responsible for the contraction of tetanus, a frequently fatal disease. Patients and staff should be encouraged to maintain their immunity by receiving regular booster doses from their GP.

relatives who are bereaved by the sudden death of a loved one.

DEATH IN A & E

All bereavement is traumatic, but sudden bereavement is perhaps especially so. The deceased was usually last seen alive and well and the fact that he is now dead is very difficult for loved ones to comprehend. If the last parting happened to have been an angry one the survivor may be overcome with guilt. Feelings of guilt may also prevail if the bereaved person begins to reflect upon things he failed to say or do when the loved one was still alive. When breaking the news of a sudden death to relatives, it is wise to be prepared for a wide range of emotional reactions (Solursh 1990).

Whether or not relatives should see the body of their loved one is open to debate. It is sometimes suggested that viewing the body can help the grieving process, but there is little firm evidence to support this claim. Limited research in this area suggests that relatives should be encouraged to view the body, but that those who are reluctant should not be pressed (Cathcart 1988).

When relatives do decide to see the body, nurses can do much to help. If possible, those parts of the body which are exposed should be washed and cleaned of blood. One or, if possible, both of the deceased's hands should be left outside the sheets. The head of the trolley should be slightly raised, otherwise the face may seem distorted when the family first sees the body. False teeth should be replaced for the same reason and the hair combed or smoothed. Where there are severe head injuries, bandages should be left in place and perhaps covered with a clean outer layer. A nurse should initially accompany the relatives and indicate that it is all right for them to touch the body, perhaps by doing so herself, or by asking the family if they wish to hold the loved one's hand. The nurse should then offer to withdraw. Not everyone will want to be left alone, but some may have private words of parting to say and should be given the opportunity to do so. Where a whole family is present, this chance should be given to each person individually. One family member may not feel able to ask for this for himself, but when it is suggested by the nurse may gratefully accept. Relatives should also feel free to hug or kiss the body; in the case of a dead child, the parents should be able to take the child in their arms. This seems to help people to cope with the denial stage of grieving, especially in cases of sudden death (Kubler-Ross 1984).

A very difficult dilemma for A & E staff may arise when they begin to realise that resuscitative measures are not going to succeed. Should the team continue until the last possible moment, or should the family be allowed to take their leave while the loved one is still alive? There can be no definitive answer to this question. Each situation will be different, and in some cases time may be too short to do anything but inform the relatives of the death. In other instances it may be possible to offer this opportunity to relatives and serious consideration should be given to this question.

Organ donation

If it has become clear that resuscitation will not be successful, it may be possible to approach the family on the question of organ donation. Although the patient will usually be admitted to an intensive care unit until brain stem death tests (see Ch. 30, pp. 855–857) are completed, the subject may be broached initially in A & E, so that the family have time to consider their decision. This may seem a cruel intrusion at a time of great grief, but in the long term the donation of the organs of the deceased may help the family to come to terms with their tragedy. By helping someone else to live, their loved one's death may come to seem less futile (Solursh 1990).

This is not, of course, the only ethical dilemma which may face A & E staff. As in any other clinical setting, questions concerning patient autonomy in respect of informed consent, the right to refuse treatment and the right to confidentiality may arise. This is by no means a comprehensive list (Bell 1990). An added difficulty is that A & E staff usually do not have time to form a relationship with patients or their relatives in advance of facing some of these dilemmas.

Spiritual needs

Relatives should be asked if they wish to have a minister of religion contacted. Roman Catholics may ask for a priest to be present before the patient dies, so that he can be given the Sacrament of the Sick (last rites). The priest will in no way obstruct the resuscitation team, and usually stands at the bottom of the trolley, where he administers the sacrament as quickly as possible. Access to the patient should be given to all ministers of religion if the family wishes prayers to be said for or with the patient. The minister of religion may also be of great comfort to the bereaved, as well as to staff.

It is very difficult for staff to have worked hard to save a life without succeeding. Feelings of inadequacy and failure may arise, especially when the patient is young or when the circumstances of the accident seem senseless. It is also very hard for the nurse who has remained with the family and developed, albeit over a brief period, a relationship with them. In listening to the relatives she may have built up a picture of the patient which is not apparent to the other staff. Relatives may respond with anger and aggression, and it is difficult for the professional who has done her very best not to feel aggrieved that this hard work is ignored or even questioned or ridiculed (Manley 1988). Staff must remember that these reactions are natural and are not directed at them personally. Rather, they are a cry against the loss of a loved one.

Care of relatives following a patient's death

Unaccompanied relatives should not be left to make their own way home: other relatives or friends should be contacted to escort them. This has the added advantage of making someone available to be given details which the bereaved may not take in. People in emotional distress often appear to be listening but, in fact, cannot remember afterwards what has been said.

Relatives should be made aware that where death has occurred as the result of trauma, a postmortem is always required. The body will therefore be retained in the hospital mortuary. There will also be an inquest at a later date (IHSM 1986).

The parents of babies who have died from sudden infant death syndrome (SIDS) are particularly vulnerable. They will be asked to identify their baby in the presence of a police officer, before the postmortem examination. This may produce great anxiety and distress, as the parents may feel that they are being accused of causing their child's death. The police are very sensitive to this situation and extremely supportive of parents, but if staff forewarn the parents of this formality they can be saved much anguish. A further supportive measure which may be offered to these parents (and indeed to any bereaved person) is to take a photograph of the baby or deceased person. Most parents will have many snapshots showing their baby at different stages of development, but some, especially if the baby is very young, will not have had the time to do this and will greatly appreciate a photograph.

One area which has perhaps been neglected in the past is that of miscarriage (Oakley et al 1990). Women will often come to the A & E department if they start to bleed during pregnancy, particularly if the bleeding begins at night or over the weekend. The loss of a baby before birth is just as much a bereavement as any other death (Beard 1988), and women who have suffered a miscarriage must be treated with as much sensitivity as any grieving parent. Moreover, it is all too easy to forget the father in these circumstances. The mother is seen as the patient because she requires medical treatment, while her husband, who is also worried about his wife, is often overlooked as a bereaved parent (Campbell 1988).

Many departments now invite relatives to return at a later date so that they can ask questions which may not have occurred to them at the time of the death. They may have enquiries about the patient's last words or want to know if he had been in pain or had died peacefully. Those staff who were involved should be available to answer questions. Families may also be directed to a variety of support groups such as CRUSE or Compassionate Friends (see Useful Addresses). Most groups have local branches and it is helpful if the department can supply their addresses and telephone numbers. Many organisations produce leaflets or other information which may be beneficial to the bereaved. They may also be willing to speak to staff and give advice about coping with sudden death. A useful resource is a directory of voluntary organisations which gives the addresses and telephone numbers of all local and national associations (e.g. the Voluntary Agencies Directory (1991)).

Staff grief

It is important to consider the grief that will be felt by staff who have been involved with the patient or his relatives. There should be a forum for expressing feelings and anxieties within the department. This need not be a formal meeting but may simply involve releasing the relevant personnel after the event so that they can talk with one another about the experience in a relaxed atmosphere. This ventilation of feelings and re-run of events can be of benefit in two ways: it can allow staff to express their emotions, and it can highlight defects in the system or ways of improving practice in the future. This should not be conducted as a destructive exercise but rather as a mechanism by which staff can show support for one another and improve their practical and interpersonal skills. Staff may also find it difficult to cope with the grief of relatives and may need help in this area (Wright 1990). In some instances staff may feel the need for professional counselling. This will be discussed later under the heading of 'Disasters', on p. 823.

A PATIENT WITH MINOR TRAUMA

Assessment and treatment

In Case History 28.2, Mrs N is seen by the triage nurse, who assesses her condition using the standard assessment forms shown in Figure 28.3. She is fully able to meet most of her self-care demands, but because of the pain in her leg she cannot achieve equilibrium between activity and rest, as she cannot walk properly. The pain may also prevent her from sleeping. Due to this incapacity she may experience difficulty in other areas, such as hygiene. Wound dressings will make it impossible for her to have a bath and her lack of mobility may prevent her from shopping and cooking. Mrs N may also have difficulty in achieving a balance between solitude and socialisation, since her married daughter, son-in-law and three teenage grandchildren live across town. Her daughter visits at least one evening a week, but works full time. Mrs N spends Sundays with her daughter and family. Other social contacts are with neighbours, shopkeepers, and at church and church socials.

> **Case History 28.2 Mrs N**
>
> Mrs N, a 70-year-old widow who lives alone, arrives at the A & E department in a taxi, having tripped at home and 'barked' her shin on a coffee table. This has produced a V-shaped pretibial laceration, with the skin flap rolled under.

In her assessment of Mrs N's 'human functioning' (see Fig. 28.3) the triage nurse finds no deviancy in any area. In the 'human structure' component of the assessment the laceration is noted and described. There is a little swelling around the area but no bruising as yet. Mrs N is now assessed following the 'human behaviour' form. The nurse notes that Mrs N's remarks indicate no disorientation, and that although she seemed anxious on arrival, she now appears more relaxed and quite cheerful.

Mrs N is placed in a wheelchair and taken to a treatment area. Although there is no great urgency about her condition, the laceration must be cleaned and her leg needs to be elevated to prevent undue swelling. Also, the waiting room is not very warm, as the doors are constantly opening and closing, and Mrs N is an elderly lady who has suffered some distress and is feeling the cold more than usual.

Mrs N is helped onto a trolley and her leg elevated with pillows. It will take some time to clean and dress the wound, and it will be more comfortable for the nurse if the leg is at waist height.

(**Note:** In A & E departments nurses often forget about their own comfort and safety. Patients come and go so quickly that it often seems easier to have them seated on chairs to do certain tasks, such as applying dressings and bandages. However, the cumulative effect of bending and stooping, often in unnatural positions, places unnecessary strain on the back muscles and may eventually cause damage to the spine, even to the extent of necessitating a career change. It is also safer for patients to lie down. They may feel fine, but as soon as the doctor or nurse begins to inspect an injury, they may feel faint, falling from the chair and suffering further injury.)

Mrs N's wound is cleaned with sodium chloride solution. The wound is not contaminated and does not require extensive cleansing. Wounds sustained in other conditions (for example outdoors) may be heavily contaminated and need more aggressive cleansing or even surgical debridement (see Ch. 23, p. 708). The doctor examines the wound and prescribes the appropriate treatment.

Suturing is not a suitable treatment for this type of wound. The skin at the front of the shin is thin, with little subcutaneous tissue. In the elderly the skin is comparatively fragile and sutures may cause further traumatisation (see Research Abstract 28.2).

The skin flap is gently unrolled and cleaned underneath. It is then brought down to fit into the gap it has caused, but no pressure is exerted on the flap to make it fit exactly. The skin around the flap is painted with tincture of benzoin. This has a dual effect. It makes the skin slightly sticky, so that paper adhesive strips (Steri-Strips) will adhere more easily. It also forms a protective coating and prevents allergic reactions to the strips. These are laid across the laceration, again without exerting pressure. Any gaps between the skin flap

Universal self-care demands

Self-care demand	Ability of patient to fill demand: Fully able	Partially able	Not able	Reason for patient being unable to meet demand for self-care
Patient can provide for intake of :-				
air	✓			
water	✓			
food	✓			
Patient can provide for adequate and controlled excretion of :-				
air	✓			
urine	✓			
faeces	✓			
other, e.g. sputum	✓			
Patient can achieve balance between activity and rest :-				LACERATION TO PRETIBIAL AREA OF RIGHT LEG
ambulant		✓		
uses hands/arms	✓			
sleeps normally	✓			
Patient can achieve balance between solitude and socialisation. Is patient able to make adequate social contact at home?		✓		WILL NOT BE ABLE TO GO OUT FOR A FEW DAYS DUE TO INJURY
Patient can prevent hazards to life/safety at home?		✓		MAY NEED SOME HELP – CLIMBING STAIRS
Patient can achieve normalcy in :-				WILL NOT BE ABLE TO HAVE A BATH DUE TO DRESSING, BUT WILL MANAGE WITH SOME HELP
hygiene		✓		
clothing	✓			
mental state	✓			
home environment	✓			

Health deviancy and self-care

A. Is the patient displaying a health deviancy in any of the following areas?

1 Human functioning	Present	Suspected	Not present
i Airway			
Respiratory arrest			✓
Airway obstruction			✓
ii Breathing			
Paralysis due to spinal trauma			✓
Difficulty in breathing			✓
Respiratory depression			✓
Chest trauma			✓
iii Circulation			
Cardiac arrest			✓
Shock			✓
Abnormal pulse rate/rhythm			✓
Chest pain			✓
iv Mental function			
Unconscious			✓
Diminished level of consciousness			✓
Head/facial trauma			✓
Unequal pupils			✓
A. What is the health deviancy relevant to the specific complaint of the patient?	NONE		

2 Human structure

Code	Structure	Present	Comment
1	Laceration	✓	PRETIBIAL TO RIGHT LEG
2	Deformity		
3	Burn		
4	Swelling		
5	Bruising		
6	Broken skin		
7	Rash		
8	Pressure sore		
9	Amputation		
10	Other, e.g. foreign material		

3 Human behaviour (underline as appropriate)

i Vocal : nil/moaning/crying/talking (confused)/<u>talking (orientated)</u> shouting

ii Non-vocal : still/restless/agitated/very active/walking/running/<u>limping</u>.

iii Mood : relaxed/cheerful/quiet/uncommunicative/tense/<u>anxious</u>/aggressive.

4 History of event and why patient thinks he or she is in A & E unit

BARKED SHIN ON COFFEE TABLE – LEG IS CUT + BLEEDING AND NEEDS TREATMENT

Fig. 28.3 Standard nursing assessment: a patient with minor trauma. (Adapted from Walsh 1989, with kind permission from Butterworth Heinemann.)

Research Abstract 28.2 Steri-Strips

In a study by Sutton & Pritty (1985) 76 patients with pretibial lacerations were randomly allocated to one of two groups. One group had primary closure achieved by the use of 4/0 ethilon sutures, while the second group had the wounds closed by the use of Steri-Strips applied on tincture of benzoin. In both methods tension was avoided and all wounds were dressed in the same manner, with paraffin gauze, dry gauze squares held on by adhesive tape and tubular gauze from toes to knee.

Data were collected relating to the incidence of necrosis and infection, mean healing time, and other criteria. Sutures appeared to be associated with increased necrosis of the wound and slower healing than adhesive tapes. The mean healing time for the sutured wounds was 53 days as compared to 39 days for the taped wounds. It would appear from this small study that adhesive tapes are to be preferred over suturing for the primary closure of pretibial lacerations.

Sutton R, Pritty P 1985 Use of sutures or adhesive tapes for primary closure of pretibial lacerations. British Medical Journal 290: 1672

and wound edges are ignored as these will gradually diminish as healing takes place and fibrous tissue is laid down.

Patients may require some pain relief during a procedure of this type. Oral analgesia may be given 15–20 minutes in advance of the dressing. Alternatively, Entonox via a self-regulating valve may be used in some procedures such as the packing of deep wounds.

Mrs N's wound is covered with a paraffin gauze and a non-adherent dressing. The leg is then bandaged from toes to knee with an elastic crepe bandage; a tubular bandage could also be used, the object being to apply an even pressure.

Mrs N is given the first injection of a tetanus toxoid course, as she cannot remember ever having been vaccinated. With such a shallow wound tetanus is an unlikely complication, since Clostridium tetani is an anaerobic organism. However, there may be deep areas within the wound where the organism may thrive. Also, this presents a good opportunity to vaccinate the patient in case of future injury.

Assessment of home circumstances and organisation of community services

During this time, preparations are made for Mrs N to go home and for her treatment to be continued by the community nursing services. Her daughter has been contacted at work. Mrs N has insisted on going home to her own house as her dog is there and she cannot leave him alone. Moreover, she does not want to be a 'burden' to her daughter. She is given various instructions about how to care for her injury. These include the elevation of her leg for 48 hours, following which time she may use her leg normally. She is advised, however, to continue to elevate the leg when seated. It is important to explain in such cases that 'elevation' involves raising the ankle above the knee and the knee above the hip. A diagram may be very useful in explaining what is meant.

Mrs N is told that the extent of her activity should be dictated by pain. If she is unable to do her normal activities because of pain, she should rest. She is also instructed not to get the dressing wet, as this may encourage infection. If there should be any ooze or unpleasant smell from the wound she is told to return to hospital or contact her GP.

It is important to ensure that patients have absorbed all the necessary information for home care. The nurse should ask the patient to repeat her instructions to make sure that they are remembered and understood. Alternatively, instructions should be written down so that the patient has something to refer to at home.

Mrs N is not prescribed prophylactic antibiotics, as there seems no reason why the wound should become infected. She is given a note for her GP informing him of the injury, the treatment undertaken and asking him to prescribe analgesics.

As it is now late afternoon, it is arranged for Mrs N's daughter to leave work a little earlier and collect her mother on her way home. She will see to her mother's evening meal and help her to bed. They will call at the GP's surgery on the way home and collect the prescription. As the chemist will probably be closed, they are given a bottle of six tablets to provide pain relief until next morning. Many A & E departments have these 'six-packs' of the most commonly prescribed analgesics and antibiotics, prepacked by the hospital pharmacy and labelled with the relevant instructions. For elderly patients, it may be necessary to ask the doctor to rewrite these instructions in larger writing, so that the patient can read them.

The community nursing sister is also contacted and asked to arrange for Mrs N to be visited in the morning for the dressing to be inspected. A report of the injury and treatment is given by telephone, but Mrs N is also given a written account to pass on to the nurse. Some departments have a special form for this purpose, but it is also possible to photocopy the A & E nursing notes to enhance continuity between the hospital and community services. These notes will include the care plan constructed for the patient. A copy of the A & E notes will also be sent to Mrs N's GP.

Mrs N does not have a home help, and does not want one. Without probing into the patient's private affairs, the nurse may suggest he or she have a chat with the social worker, who may give advice and information or may contact community social services or voluntary groups, such as Age Concern, who may provide a local visiting service. Alternatively, if she wishes, Mrs N's church could be contacted so that friends who may wish to visit can be informed. Nothing should be imposed on the patient, as many people value their privacy and prefer to make their own arrangements. However, it can be very helpful for the nurse to mention services that are available and to show her willingness to help the patient make the initial contact.

Discharge

Mrs N is given a cup of tea and is made comfortable while she waits for her daughter. A & E cubicles are fairly boring places and may even be disorientating to patients, who behind closed curtains and with nothing to look at may find it difficult to gauge the passage of time and become frustrated and even frightened. Mrs N is placed where she can see and talk to people if she wishes, and is wrapped in a blanket to guard against the draught. She is reminded that she should not leave until a nurse has spoken to her daughter and reassured that she will not be forgotten about just because her treatment is completed. Mrs N is still the responsibility of the department until she leaves with her daughter, and her safety must be ensured. She may need to go to the toilet and will need some help to do so, or her wound may begin to bleed and require further treatment. If the triage nurse finds that she is unable to keep an eye on her because she is busy with new arrivals someone else should be allocated to look after Mrs N until her daughter arrives.

It has been arranged that Mrs N will have her dressing changed by the community nurse in a week to 10 days. This will involve the removal of the outer dressing, leaving the Steri-Strips in position. If any are loose, they will be replaced.

This will be repeated after a similar period has elapsed. Mrs N may be asked to return to the department in 3 weeks' time for the wound to be inspected. This is not absolutely necessary, but provides an opportunity for treatment to be evaluated. Alternatively, the community nurse may be asked to provide a written report for inclusion in the patient's notes. A recent innovation is the use of computerised discharge plans for A & E patients; these, whilst being quick and easy to use, allow patients to be given printed, individualised instructions (Dutton & Wood 1991).

AGGRESSION AND VIOLENCE IN A & E

Our changing society

A & E work is usually very enjoyable and rewarding. This area of practice affords the opportunity to practise a wider range of skills than is possible in other clinical settings. However, like every job, it has its drawbacks, of which aggression and violence towards staff is one of the most serious. A & E nurses perhaps face more verbal and physical abuse than any other nursing group (DHSS 1988). The nature of the work is such that patients are encountered at a time of great stress and uncertainty. Their condition is undiagnosed and aggression may be a direct result of that condition, e.g. a mental disorder such as schizophrenia or a physical state such as in the postictal phase of an epileptic attack. More common than these conditions and more difficult to deal with are the effects of alcohol or drugs.

Our society is becoming increasingly violent. In 1971 the number of offences recorded by the police under the heading of 'Violence against the person' amounted to 53 400 throughout the UK. In 1988 these had risen to 175 400 and one year later, in 1989, to 194 200. These are only the incidents of which the police have knowledge and which have been recorded by them. There are many more which are unreported and/or unrecorded (Central Statistical Office 1991).

Most patients come to A & E because they need help — in their view, urgent help. Some of the aggression manifested by patients, and perhaps more frequently by their worried relatives, arises because they are kept waiting for what they believe is an unnecessary length of time before being seen by a doctor.

Defusing potential aggression

Frustration provoked by the system may be circumvented by *changing* the system.

Good communication is also a key to preventing aggressive or violent outbursts. Nurses should remember that aggression is often a result of fear and frustration, and is a normal coping mechanism in response to a threat. If fear is lessened and frustration recognised and acknowledged, the situation will usually be defused. Aggression is seldom directed towards the nurse personally.

Body language

It is extremely difficult not to take up a stance which reflects that of the aggressor, for it is a natural human response to mirror the posture, whether friendly or belligerent, of those we are speaking to. This also holds true for patients: if the nurse adopts an aggressive stance this will be mirrored by the patient. Conversely, if the nurse's posture is non-aggressive, the patient will, in turn, find it difficult to maintain a belligerent stance. Constantly maintaining eye contact may be provoking, but completely avoiding eye contact is, again, suggestive of disinterest. If the patient is shouting, it is difficult not to shout back, but again the principle of mirrored behaviour may be used. If the nurse speaks in a normal tone, it will be hard for the aggressor to continue in a loud voice.

Listening to aggressive patients

It is essential that the nurse is sensitive to the patient's circumstances. If his frustrations are dismissed as being unimportant, he will feel humiliated and even more defensive. Aggressive confrontation will often be avoided by lending a sympathetic ear to the patient's concerns.

Avoiding physical danger and attack

It is well for the nurse to keep at the back of her mind that physical attack is a possibility in all encounters with abusive individuals. It is to be hoped, but never presumed, that all such situations will be amicably resolved. A nurse should not allow herself to become trapped in a room or cubicle and she should never be alone with an aggressive individual in a room with a lockable door. Most A & E cubicles will have curtains rather than doors and all should have panic buttons so that help can be summoned quickly in a medical emergency or during an attack. If a patient or relative looks as if he is going to attack, the best thing to do is to back away slowly, and then turn and run to a more populated part of the department where help is available.

Sometimes the department will be invaded by a gang, one of whose members may require treatment. No patient can be denied attention, but if it is suspected that the group will disrupt other patients or become threatening, they should be asked to leave. If the patient wishes to leave with them, that is his choice. Before asking such individuals to leave, the nurse should have as many security guards as possible escort them off the premises. Some departments with a history of violent attacks have a direct line or panic alarm to the nearest police station. The police should in any case be contacted if harm is done to staff or property.

> **?** **28.2** Find out about the procedure in your hospital/health centre to follow should a member of staff be injured. What documentation is required? Who should complete it and where should any forms be sent?

The safety of staff and other patients is of paramount importance. If a violent person threatens to break windows or damage equipment, he should not be restrained unless there are enough people present to do so effectively and with the minimum of force. Staff are, of course, subject to laws against assault and should not use unnecessary force on members of the public. In these situations it is best to withdraw all personnel, patients and relatives and telephone the police. It is better for property to be damaged than for people to be hurt. Again, if staff are threatened by addicts demanding drugs, they should hand over the drugs and telephone the police. They should not attempt to argue with these people, who may be armed with knives or other weapons.

Documentation and the law

It is important that a record be kept of abusive incidents. This serves a variety of purposes. Firstly, patterns may emerge which will allow preventive strategies to be formulated. For example, if it is found that more episodes occur at certain times extra staff may be assigned to duty at those hours. If such incidents appear to be on the increase, statistical evidence will be useful in making a bid to management for more security staff or better protection.

Such records may also be used for staff development, pointing out the reasons for an outburst, how staff managed the situation, and how it might have been better dealt with. The intention should not be to lay blame, but to help in the future prevention or management of violent episodes. Guidelines should be drawn up in advance to assist staff in dealing with this difficult and frightening aspect of A & E work.

Equally difficult situations occur when victims of violence and their assailants arrive in the department at the same time. It is not uncommon for a husband and wife to present following a violent argument in which both parties have been injured. It is difficult for staff to be caught in the middle of such conflict, but the patient must always be given first priority. In some cases, it may be relevant for the nurse to provide information relating to shelters for battered women. Where there are children involved, however, it may be necessary to refer the family to their local health visitor, social services or GP since even when the children have not been brought for treatment there is a danger that they are also victims of abuse.

In certain circumstances, e.g. where firearms have been used, the police must be informed. Patient confidentiality takes second place to the law and doctors and nurses are obliged to report gunshot wounds to the police. Staff who have been attacked may put in a claim for criminal injuries compensation. This does not involve prosecuting an individual for assault, but staff may feel that this is also appropriate.

MAJOR DISASTERS

What is a disaster?

A disaster may be defined as 'an incident with so many casualties as to require extraordinary mobilisation of emergency services' (Rutherford 1989). This definition is deliberately unspecific as to numbers of injured. What constitutes a disaster in a small, rural hospital may hardly make a ripple in a large, urban facility. Similarly, a disaster may affect only one hospital, or all the hospitals in a city, region or entire country.

Disaster planning

It is essential that every A & E department has a disaster plan. It is too late to wait until disaster strikes before protocols and procedures are agreed. The essence of any plan is that it is workable and flexible, so that any and all situations may be coped with. Routines should be as close as possible to what happens every day; otherwise, staff may become confused about their roles and responsibilities. A disaster does not affect the A & E department alone, and for this reason all hospital departments must be involved in drawing up the plan. All those providing services, including portering, cleaning, catering and clerical support, should also be included. Of major importance in a disaster situation is communication. It is essential that switchboard staff know exactly whom to contact and in what sequence.

Each hospital and district will design its own plan, taking into consideration the available resources of personnel and facilities. With the rationalisation of many services, it may be necessary to have joint plans between a number of hospitals or, where boundaries encroach between districts.

Disaster practices should be frequent so that routines are not forgotten. The disaster plan should be kept in a prominent place in every ward and department and should form part of the orientation programme of each member of staff.

?	**28.3** Where is the disaster plan held in your hospital? Ask your tutor if you may see it, and discuss it during a seminar.

A feature common to many disasters is the arrival of the 'walking wounded' in advance of the seriously injured. Many injured people will be brought to hospital by uninjured friends. Most will be only slightly hurt, although this cannot be presumed. Those who have only minor injuries should not be kept waiting in anticipation of an influx of seriously hurt patients. It may be some time before the severely injured are evacuated from the site and their condition stabilised enough for them to be transported to hospital. In the meantime, the less seriously hurt patients may be treated and discharged. As well as it being better for these patients not to be kept waiting, more space will be freed in the department. Staff will also gain valuable information about the numbers and types of injuries to expect, e.g. burns, crush injuries or high impact injuries.

Post-traumatic stress disorder

It has become apparent in recent years that the survivors of disasters and major incidents may suffer from a range of long-term psychological and physical symptoms unrelated to injuries sustained at the time. These may include feelings of desperation, helplessness, guilt at having survived where others have died, and shame at the loss of control. The survivors may also experience anger, feelings of loss, and profound sadness, and may be unable to put the incident out of their minds. Physical symptoms may include insomnia, nausea, diarrhoea, dizziness and palpitations, to name only a few (Johnston 1989; see also Ch. 17, p. 584). It is important for survivors to realise that these manifestations are normal reactions to a terrible tragedy and that they are not 'losing their minds'. Many will require prolonged counselling in order to come to terms with their feelings and anxieties, and members of their families may also need to be included in counselling sessions.

Witnesses of disasters may also be deeply affected. More than 100 residents of the village of Lockerbie in Scotland were referred to community psychiatric nurses following the Pan American Airways crash. O'Byrne (1989) reports: 'The brush with death had forced many of the town's inhabitants to re-evaluate what they were doing with their lives'. Close media coverage of such events may give those who were not involved but who were bereaved as a result of the incident the feeling that they were present when it happened. These people may also experience the feelings of guilt suffered by the actual survivors. This will naturally involve the families of the victims but may also include a much wider range of people. In the Zeebruge ferry disaster, 160 off-duty crew members of the *Herald of Free Enterprise*, some of whom had swapped duties with their shipmates, were among the circle of people requiring counselling and support (Johnston 1989).

Rescue workers and A & E personnel are also vulnerable to serious emotional disturbances following such incidents (Owen W 1990). Even with good deployment of staff, disasters provoke an 'all hands on deck' situation. Staff may need to be called in from off duty, and others will volunteer after hearing about the incident on the news. Staff will be required to work long hours under difficult conditions, especially if they are part of an on-site team. Some victims will not be saved and this may produce feelings of inadequacy or guilt. Because of the need for the department to return to normality as soon as possible so that it can deal with other patients, there may be insufficient time for staff to rest before returning to more mundane jobs. A rush of adrenaline will keep everyone going at the time, but afterwards they may display emotions ranging from anger to guilt or deep sorrow.

It is apparent that following major incidents support facilities must be made available to staff. The nature of these facilities may differ from place to place. Several authors (Owen G 1990, Owen W 1990, O'Byrne 1989) suggest that bringing in independent, professional counsellors after the event may not be the most effective way of assisting staff. Some staff who were surveyed felt that anyone who had not been involved would not be able to understand their feelings (Owen W 1990). Others seemed to be reluctant to accept professional counselling, fearing that this would amount to an acknowledgement of weakness or inability to cope (Owen W 1990). It is suggested that a range of facilities may be more appropriate. This should include educational programmes and a support network for all staff, and should, ideally, be in place before any such incidents occur. Where these networks are available and accepted, staff may be less inclined to feel stigmatised if they make use of them when the occasion arises.

Now that it is recognised that staff of all disciplines who are involved in disaster situations may suffer from post-traumatic stress disorder, it is essential that provision should be made in disaster planning for the support of these carers following a traumatic event.

HEALTH PROMOTION IN A & E

The waiting room of the A & E department is an ideal place to promote health. Many commercial companies may be willing to instal and maintain video equipment on which health education films may be shown. As well as providing useful information about various aspects of health, they can serve as a welcome distraction. Caution must be used, however, as the constant repetition of a limited number of such films may become irritating and, as a result, counter-productive. Furthermore, some patients may find certain topics embarrassing. A small-scale survey carried out following the installation of such equipment on which a film on cervical screening was featured found that many female patients were embarrassed by the film. Many had small children who asked questions about the video, and they felt uncomfortable because of the men who were present. Other patients commented that if they heard the commentator's voice again, they would be driven to violence! (Botham 1990.)

Posters concerning various aspects of health may be displayed in the waiting room and treatment cubicles, as can leaflets which patients and others may take home to read. These can be provided by local health education departments. These are, however, extra to the work of the nurse in educating patients and others with regard to maintaining and improving health. As well as needing good teaching and communication skills, she must be able to identify appropriate opportunities for patient education. If someone is frightened or in distress from an injury or illness he may not be receptive to advice about diet or smoking (Ewles & Simnett 1985). An overweight smoker who comes to the department complaining of chest pain may not respond to dietary advice while he thinks he is having a heart attack. All he wants is to be examined and treated. When he is told that he had indigestion, is given an antacid and begins to feel more comfortable, he may well be receptive to such advice. When the memory of his pain and fear is fresh and he is relieved and grateful that nothing is seriously wrong, he may feel that he has had a lucky escape and be willing to change his lifestyle. Much may also depend on the patient's personality (Coutts & Hardy 1985). The A & E department is not the best venue for the education of all individuals, as some will need long-term programmes to help them change their lifestyles. This should be acknowledged and patients referred to those professionals or agencies who will be able to help them, e.g. GPs, health visitors and voluntary organisations such as ASH (Action for Smoking and Health).

Nurses are in a position to encourage the wearing of safety clothing, helmets and goggles in the workplace. When a patient has had an accident at work, the nurse may enquire about the provision of safety gear at his place of work and urge its use.

Patients who have had accidents may be receptive to advice about home safety measures. A simple leaflet from the Royal Society for the Prevention of Accidents (ROSPA 1989) shows the hazards which exist for children in the home and how these may be removed or reduced.

A & E staff may also become aware of particular hazards related to consumer products. For example, children may present with injuries received from particular toys. Individual parents may not be aware that their child is not the only one to have been injured in this way, and there may be a case for the department to inform the relevant body, such as the British Standards Institution. It would certainly be wise to inform the department's liaison health visitor, who through her network of colleagues can draw the attention of the public to the hazard in question.

REFERENCES

Bailey A, Hallam K, Hurst K 1987 Triage on trial. Nursing Times 83(44): 65–66

Beard P 1988 When life ends before it has started. Nursing 3(32): 16–18

Bell N K 1990 Ethical dilemmas in trauma nursing. Nursing Clinics of North America 25(1): 143–154

Blythin P 1988 Triage in the UK. Nursing 3(31): 16–20

Botham L 1990 Promoting health in A/E. Unpublished research project

Campbell C 1988 The impact of miscarriage on women and their families. Nursing 3(32): 11–14

Cathcart F 1988 Seeing the body after death. British Medical Journal 297: 997–998

Central Statistical Office 1991 Social trends. No. 21. HMSO, London

Coutts L C, Hardy L K 1985 Teaching for health: the nurse as health educator. Churchill Livingstone, Edinburgh

DHSS 1971 Hospital facilities for children. HMSO, London

DHSS 1988 Advisory committee on violence to staff. HMSO, London

Dutton J, Wood I 1991 Computerised discharge instructions. Nursing 4(32): 26–30

Ewles L, Simnett I 1990 Promoting health: a practical guide to health education. Wiley, Chichester

Institute of Health Services Management 1986 Procedures following deaths in hospitals, 2nd edn. IHSM, London

Institute of Health Services Management 1988 Managing A & E. IHSM, London

Jamieson E M, McCall J M, Blythe R 1988 Guidelines for clinical nursing practices. Churchill Livingstone, Edinburgh

Johnston J 1989 Haunted by memories. Nursing Times 85(11): 56–58

Kubler-Ross E 1984 On death and dying. Tavistock, London

Manley K 1988 The needs and support of relatives. Nursing 3(32): 19–22

Oakley A, McPherson A, Roberts H 1990 Miscarriage. Penguin, London

O'Byrne J 1989 Talking through the pain. Nursing Standard 3(25): 12

Orem D 1991 Nursing: concepts of practice, 4th edn. Mosby, St Louis

Owen G 1990 Support networks in health care. Nursing Standard 4(38): 31–34
Owen W 1990 After Hillsborough. Nursing Times 86(25): 16–17
ROSPA 1989 Published statistics. Home safety topic guide: child safety in the home. ROSPA, London
Rutherford W (ed) 1980 Accident and emergency medicine. Churchill Livingstone, Edinburgh
Solursh D S 1990 The family of the trauma victim. Nursing Clinics of North America 25(1): 155–162
Sutton R, Pritty P 1985 Use of sutures or adhesive tapes for primary closure of pretibial lacerations. British Medical Journal 290: 1672
Thompson I E, Melia K M, Boyd K M 1988 Nursing ethics, 2nd edn. Churchill Livingstone, Edinburgh
Voluntary Agencies Directory 1991 12th edn. Bedford Press, London
Wright B 1988 Sudden death: aspects which incapacitate the carer. Nursing 3(31): 12–15

FURTHER READING

Dennis N 1984 Voting with their feet. Health and Social Services Journal 93: 465
Farmer R 1984 Patients like to be an emergency. Health and Social Services Journal 93: 466
Head S 1988 Nurse practitioners: the new pioneers. Nursing Times 84(26): 27–28
Lewis B, Bradbury Y 1981 Why patients choose A/E. Health and Social Services Journal 91: 1139–1142
Walsh M 1989 Accident and emergency nursing: a new approach. Heinemann, Oxford

USEFUL ADDRESSES

Compassionate Friends
6 Denmark Street
Bristol BS1 5DQ
Tel: 0272 292778

Cruse (National Organization for the Widowed and their Children)
Cruse House
126 Sheen Road
Richmond, Surrey
TW9 1UR
Tel: 081-940 4818

CHAPTER 29

The critically ill patient

Pat M. Ashworth

CHAPTER CONTENTS

The person 827

Environment 828

The physical environment and activity 828

Infection 829

Chemical hazards 829

Environmental–mechanical hazards 830

Physical hazards 830

Noise 830

Radiation 830

The sensory environment 831

The human environment 831

Health 833

Nursing 833

Meeting the needs of critically ill people 834

Physical needs 834

Biological rhythm 835

Identity 835

Self-esteem 835

Control and interdependence 835

Information and communication 836

Territoriality 836

Spiritual health 836

Care of relatives/friends 837

Summary 837

References 837

Further reading 838

'Critically ill patients' is the term usually used to describe people who have acute life-threatening conditions, but who might recover if given appropriate, effective and often 'high-tech' nursing and medical care. This definition does not include people who are dying from a known condition, who are terminally ill, and for whom appropriate care and treatment may be quite different. However, people who have a long-term condition such as cardiac disease or chronic obstructive airways disease may have repeated episodes of acute and critical illness as the condition progresses; and it may sometimes be difficult for all concerned to agree when the time comes to recognise that the stage of terminal illness has arrived and it is no longer appropriate to maintain physiological functions artificially at great human and financial cost.

Critically ill patients, the conditions from which they suffer, and the care and treatment they need are so varied that at least some of every chapter in this book is relevant to their care. The appropriate chapter should be consulted for detailed care and treatment related to a particular condition. This chapter is concerned with critically ill people, the often complex and technical care and treatment they receive, the environment in which it is provided and the other human beings involved — patients, families, friends and staff (particularly nurses) — and the interaction between all of these. An understanding of all the factors is necessary to provide optimal nursing.

It is now widely accepted that an understanding of:

- person
- environment
- health
- 'nursing'

is essential to any overall consideration of nursing. What nurses believe and understand about each aspect, whether it is made explicit or not, is likely to shape their practice. So each merits consideration in the context of nursing people who are critically ill.

THE PERSON

Everyone who becomes critically ill is first and foremost a person. 'Patient' is only one of their current subsidiary roles in life. It is sometimes difficult to remember this when immersed in performing life-saving procedures on the body of someone unknown. Mrs Jones, part-time teacher, wife and mother of four children, who competently fulfils these roles, is still the same person after being involved in a road accident and being admitted to hospital, dishevelled, and not entirely coherent.

Critical illness may be caused by trauma, infection or other pathophysiological states, possibly complicated (at least initially) by major surgery, and may affect any or all of the body systems and vital functions. Malfunction of one organ or system is likely to affect others, and may progress to multiple organ failure. Patients may be fully conscious and able to talk and move or totally unconscious and/or paralysed.

While common principles apply in the care of critically ill people, the individual people are often very different (see Box 29.1). Each person has a unique combination of age, sex, personality, ethnic origin, social and cultural background, general health and other experiences, which may result in different physical and psychological responses (Clark 1987).

? **29.1** Read the case details in Box 29.1. What further information do you need to nurse these patients? What are their major nursing needs?

? **29.2** If you were to have a serious road accident on the way to work tomorrow and be admitted, seriously injured but conscious, to an intensive or critical care unit, what might be your main thoughts and concerns about:

- current experiences in the unit
- the activities and people in the active independent life from which you have just been separated
- the future?

What support could you draw on and what might be your coping responses?

If you think of three other people who are different in some ways from you, what are the differences? If these people were in the situation described above, in what ways might their thoughts, concerns and resources be different? If possible, validate your answers by putting these questions to the people concerned.

Box 29.1 Four patients requiring critical care (See question 29.1.)

B, aged 18, crashed his motorbike 2 weeks ago on his way to college. He has multiple fractures and is just recovering from acute renal failure with the aid of ultrafiltration, but he still shows only slight signs of response to stimuli. His anxious mother sits by his bed. Another of her sons died from head injury 2 years ago.

Mrs S is 75 years old and has just had an operation to relieve intestinal obstruction, which she developed while on holiday. She was extremely dehydrated and ill on admission and is rather overweight. She is on assisted ventilation for a short time until she is able to maintain adequate independent breathing, and proceed towards recovery and the active and independent life she led until a few days ago, despite her arthritis. She is regaining consciousness, but seems frightened and bewildered as she becomes aware of strange sights, sounds and sensations.

Mr A, a 45-year-old businessman, was in the middle of a busy morning at the office when he felt terrible pressure and pain in his chest, and collapsed. After some commotion in the office and an ambulance journey with the siren screaming he has been admitted to hospital. Despite the morphia he has been given he lies looking around, thinking what has happened, worrying about work affairs, and anxiously eyeing the cardiac monitor.

M, aged 30, has little ability to move her arms and legs, and has now been artificially ventilated for 2 weeks, because of Guillain–Barre Syndrome. She sees her two children most days when they visit.

Much can be learned from reading the single or collected accounts of people who have been patients in critical care units, for example, Clark (1985), Heath (1989), Douglas (1982), Bergbom-Engberg & Haljamae (1988). There is increasing evidence of the physiological effects of psychological states, and the mind–brain–body connections which mediate them. The cardiovascular, endocrine and other physiological changes that constitute the 'fight or flight' response to stress (see Ch. 17) have been known for many years. There is now increasing evidence that:

> ... our immunity is affected by what goes on in our heads, by hormonal changes that are brought about from poor coping or by direct effects of our central nervous system. Indeed our cognitions (thoughts, beliefs, attitudes) and the social support perceived in our lives can alter the levels of our hormones and neurotransmitters, the chemical messengers that carry on communication between our cells and largely govern the activity of our physical processes. (Nguyen 1991)

Even in health, people's emotions and thus their perceptions and general well-being are affected by their environment. This is even more true of critically ill patients, who need an environment that promotes and supports recovery through effective care and treatment, and engenders trust, confidence and healthy coping responses.

ENVIRONMENT

On being admitted to hospital, someone who is critically ill will be transferred as soon as possible to an intensive care or critical care unit. Although intended to provide patients with the best possible chance of recovery; certain features of these units, such as the physical environment and activity, the sensory environment, and the human environment may impede recovery.

The physical environment and activity

In many general, and some cardiothoracic, surgical intensive care units patients are attached to numerous tubes and wires, and surrounded by machines which monitor, display or support their various physiological functions. Often there are several patients in an open area, so that constant surveillance is easier to maintain with a limited number of qualified and experienced nurses. Single rooms can also be used for patients who are heavily infected or particularly vulnerable to infection.

In specialised units, such as coronary care units, there is often less equipment, and all patients may be nursed in rooms or cubicles with one or two beds; a more normal environment for most people. Although such patients may be alert and anxious, they are less at risk of some of the environmental hazards that are described below.

Patients are admitted to critical care units to ensure that:

- measures to combat the ill-effects of disease, abnormality or trauma, and to support failing physiological functions, can be used safely and effectively under the management of skilled personnel
- any adverse changes in a patient's condition and response to treatment will be noticed quickly, leading to prompt and appropriate action designed to overcome the problem.

Electronic and mechanical equipment is needed for both these purposes.

Treatment, support or restoration of vital functions may include the use of:

- a ventilator to maintain adequate respiratory function
- an intra-aortic balloon pump (IABP) or other cardiac assist device to support cardiovascular function

- electronically controlled infusions of fluids and powerful drugs
- intravenous or intragastric fluids and nutrition
- haemofiltration or dialysis to complement or substitute for failing kidneys
- a ripple mattress or other special bed to compensate for inability to move enough to maintain intact skin at pressure areas.

In addition, there may be more commonly used equipment, such as traction (or a plaster cast) to maintain stability of broken bones, suction equipment, or drainage tubes from wounds or body cavities.

Developments in technology have now made it possible to measure and record a variety of physiological parameters and to display them in numerical or graphic form, so that abnormalities and changes can be detected very quickly (Box 29.2). The value of being able to see the heart rhythm continuously, as well as the heart rate, became evident with the discovery of external cardiac compression as a means of maintaining circulation when cardiac arrest or ventricular fibrillation had occured (Kouwenhoven, et al 1960). Coronary care units were opened with high ratios of nurses to patients so that nurses could watch the ECG displays and initiate cardiopulmonary resuscitation promptly when necessary, or give drugs according to predetermined protocols to deal with life-threatening dysrhythmias.

High technology has disadvantages as well as benefits (Box 29.3), however. Attention to the machines in addition to the treatment and care of patients often results in constant activity around the beds, particularly since there may be many people involved in multidisciplinary care. In units that were not designed for this purpose there may be little space around patients, which increases disturbance to them as well as impeding staff in their work.

Some of the hazards to nurses in ICUs are identified by Rogers & Travers (1991).

- infection
- chemical
- environmental–mechanical
- physical
- noise.

Box 29.2 Parameters that may be monitored

- cardiac rate, rhythm, and any changes or abnormalities in the electrocardiogram trace (ECG)
- cardiovascular pressures using a balloon flotation catheter (often a Swan–Ganz) and other arterial and venous lines connected to transducers
- respiratory rate, rhythm, tidal and minute volume, and pressures required to ventilate the lungs artificially; and the frequency and strength of voluntary respiratory effort when assisted ventilation is in progress
- body temperature, possibly at core and peripheral sites, as a crude indicator of peripheral blood flow
- fluid intake and output, possibly including osmolarity or osmolality, and some urine constituents
- blood gases (which may be monitored continuously or intermittently) and acid base and electrolyte balance
- intracranial pressures
- other factors, such as pain levels, or pressure sore risk
- other physiological functions
- indicators of function of machines in use, to detect any changes or malfunction (safety must be a consideration at all times)
- bacteriological factors.

Box 29.3 Advantages and disadvantages of high technology (Adapted from Ashworth 1990, p. 151.)

Benefits
High technology and machines can:

- substitute for some human functions
- save time
- measure accurately
- measure physiologic variables not directly perceptible by humans
- avoid frequent patient disturbance.

Problems
High technology and machines:

- are not infallible
- can depersonalise activities and people
- can cause iatrogenic harm
- output is only as good as input (programming and maintenance)
- have no intuition

High technology is as good as those who use it.

These are also hazards to patients.

However, specific hazards within each category are often different for patients.

Infection

Infection is a major threat to critically ill patients, because the numerous invasive lines and procedures provide potential entry routes for infection. Venous and arterial lines pass through the skin. Endotracheal tubes bypass the nose and mouth where air is normally warmed, moistened and to some extent filtered, and suction catheters damage mucous membranes. Urinary catheters provide an open, direct route from outside the body into the bladder. The equipment to which the various tubes are attached often provides sites where bacteria, viruses, fungi or other infective agents may grow and multiply (Yannelli & Goverich 1988, Massanari 1989). Pseudomonas aeruginosa may thrive in humidifiers or nebulisers, for example, (Woodrow 1992).

The most hazardous organisms in such an environment are those that are resistant to the more common antibiotics. Critically ill patients have often been treated with powerful antibiotics and resistant strains have developed, particularly if the patients have a long-term condition. They are also highly vulnerable to infection by virtue of their illness and the effects of the physical response to stress. Both physical and psychological stress may decrease the level of body immunity (Houldin et al 1991) (see Ch. 16). Inadequate nutrition may also reduce resistance to disease in hospital (Hill et al 1977) and even in critical care units insufficient attention is sometimes paid to ensuring that patients are well nourished (Dougherty 1988).

Adequate hand washing by staff appears to be the most important factor in avoiding nosocomial infections (EPIC 1992). Sterilisation of equipment, gentle and aseptic techniques, cleanliness and careful use of antibiotics, combined with maintaining the patient's immunity by adequate nutrition and stress reduction are also important.

Chemical hazards

Many potent agents are used to influence patients' physiological function and these may be harmful if given in inappropriate dosage or at an inappropriate site, or if side effects occur. For example, when an infusion of isoprenaline is in progress, an error in the infusion rate of even two or three drops per minute may have adverse effects. A vasoconstrictor such as noradrenaline may cause gangrene if it runs into the tissues, while a drug inadvertently given into an arterial rather than a venous line may have very severe local or general effects. The more ill the patient is, the more treatment may be needed and the more tubes, taps and wires there may be. Labelling of lines so that they can be easily distinguished is essential, as well as careful checking when administering any substance. Although many solutions are now prepared in the pharmacy, the nurse should check her calculations carefully as these are not always accurate (Pirie 1987). When staff are under pressure, mistakes are more likely to occur. Side effects of drugs may be difficult to detect in a patient whose condition is already unstable, but should always be considered if changes in a patient's condition occur.

Environmental–mechanical hazards

These are inevitable if there is much equipment in use. Equipment may become disconnected, may malfunction or fail to function altogether. For example, an arterial line which becomes disconnected, or a ventilator that fails to function may have serious or even life-threatening effects if not dealt with promptly and effectively. Any nurse responsible for a patient who is dependent on mechanical or electronic equipment should have thought through, 'What can go wrong? How will I know if it does? What must I do then?'. Often the answers are quite simple, but knowing them in advance provides safety for the patient and confidence for the nurse. Many machines have built-in alarm systems but sometimes staff may turn these off; for example, the ventilator alarm may be turned off during tracheal suction, but staff may then forget to switch it on again. It is always wise to check that an alarm is active.

Physical hazards

Hazards such as those related to electrical current, pressure and extremes of temperature may all be prevalent in critical care units.

Electrical current. 'Metal, water and the human body are all excellent conductors of electrical current. Should the nurse or patient inadvertently provide the conductive path between a faulty piece of equipment and good ground, an electrical shock may occur.'(Rogers & Travers 1991). Even small currents, such as 100 mA alternating current at 60 Hz frequency passing through the chest cavity can cause ventricular fibrillation (Cooper 1983), so all equipment must be electrically safe and taken out of use at the first indication of a fault.

Pressure. Tissue damage from pressure is a very real risk for critically ill patients, who are usually relatively or totally immobile and have many of the other risk factors known to be associated with pressure sores (Barratt 1990). In addition, there is a risk of tissue damage due to pressure from equipment, such as an endotracheal tube pressing on the lip, a tightly taped tap or tube pressing on skin, or even an over-inflated tracheal tube cuff, which has been known to cause necrosis through the tracheal wall into the oesophagus. It is easy to forget relief of pressure areas when the patient is critically ill and needing more dramatic life-saving measures but this is when it is most important. Pressure sores may delay recovery, pose increased infection risks and entail much discomfort for the patient.

A number of scales can be used to assess the risk of pressure damage occurring, but the most important factor is a constant awareness that preventive action can be taken even before full formal assessment is possible. For example, it is quite easy and quick to lift a foot a little to check the heel and allow more circulation to the affected area, but it may be very important when the patient has been lying on an operating table for some hours. It is also important to know enough about available pressure-relieving aids to be able to choose what is most appropriate if a patient needs one, and there have been a number of comparative studies (see for example, Neander & Birkenfeld 1991 and Bliss & Thomas 1993).

Extremes of temperature. Patients may be exposed to extremes of temperature, either deliberately or accidentally. Sometimes patients are deliberately cooled, for example, on cooling mattresses or by ice and fans, either to reduce the body temperature to within the normal range or to induce hypothermia and thus reduce the tissue oxygen demand. (This may be useful in preserving tissues when oxygen supply is low.) It is important to recognise that patients may find such cooling uncomfortable, even if they have been sedated or paralysed, to prevent shivering, which might increase body temperature and tissue oxygen consumption. As one nurse–patient later said; 'I felt perishing cold, but they kept saying, "Put more ice on", and I couldn't tell them how I felt'. Sometimes cooling may be accidental if the unit is cool and the patient is frequently uncovered.

On the other hand, patients may suffer from excessive heat, for example, if lying near a window when the sun beats through. Occasionally, malfunction of a heated humidifier may result in excessively heated air being blown into the trachea by a ventilator, although most modern equipment is designed to avoid such accidents.

Noise

According to a number of review papers and individual studies, noise is a well-confirmed but often little-considered hazard in critical care units. It is also mentioned by a number of ex-patients (Heath 1989). McCarthy et al (1991) indicate in their review that:

- recommended noise levels in hospital should be less than 45 decibels (dB) by day and below 35 dB at night (normal conversation is 50 dB — 'subjectively, an increase of 10 dB makes a sound perceived as twice as loud' (McCarthy et al 1991))
- average levels of 50–80 dB have been found in critical care units
- noise stress can have actual or potential adverse effects on physiological function, such as raised heart rate, disturbed sleep and delayed wound healing, and may also increase demand for analgesic administration
- nurses can usefully intervene by monitoring and reducing unnecessary noise, providing uninterrupted periods of rest for patients, and teaching relaxation, possibly with guided imagery or music therapy. (See Ch. 19 and Ch. 25.)

In a survey of psychosocial factors affecting patients in a surgical cardiovascular unit, Williams & Murphy (1991) identified noise as a major quality control issue that required attention. A further small study of 29 patients over 3 months identified personnel, and chairs squeaking across the floor as the main offenders. Actions taken to control noise included a successful application to the hospital board for new chairs of a type that were known to cause minimal noise. Although this study was undertaken in North America, the current emphasis on consumer satisfaction and quality assurance in the UK and other countries suggests that it has wider relevance. Well over 100 years ago, Florence Nightingale (1860) wrote at length about noise affecting sick people and described unnecessary noise as 'the most cruel absence of care'; yet it still remains a problem in many intensive care units.

Radiation

Radiation should not pose much of a hazard, even to critically ill patients, if modern and well-maintained equipment is used, with lead screening to protect the gonads when X-rays are taken. However, unnecessary X-rays should be avoided, despite the temptation to X-ray all the patients in critical care units frequently 'to see that everything is all right'.

The sensory environment

The variability and perceived meaning of auditory and other stimuli are important. Conscious human beings constantly receive stimuli through hearing, sight, touch, smell and, intermittently, taste. However, when stimuli are received, perception is selective. 'Human beings are able to perceive a stimulus only when the nervous system is oriented and appropriately receptive towards it, and it is the neurones of the reticular activating system that arouse the brain and facilitate information reception by the appropriate neural structures' (Vander et al 1975). People use the information they receive to orient themselves and make sense of their environment. Familiar sounds or other stimuli may be ignored; the individual responds only to those stimuli that are unfamiliar or perceived as significant. Lindsley (1965) suggests that the reticular activating system in the brain becomes accustomed to certain levels of activity and can adapt, but only within certain limits.

The sensory environment in an ICU is often highly abnormal, compared with the environment in which people usually live, and can be disturbing even to those who are healthy. In the USA, 17 nurses took it in turns to experience such an environment by lying for 1½ hours in one of the beds in their coronary care unit, dressed in a patient's gown, attached to a monitor and with infusions taped to each arm (Lindenmuth et al 1980). Even though the environment was familiar to them they were surprised at the negative emotions they experienced, such as loneliness, isolation, resentment, anxiety, loss of control, rejection, restlessness and agitation.

?	**29.3** In an acute care area, preferably an ICU, close your eyes and listen. Or, better still, tape record the sounds in an ICU and, using a time switch, set the sounds to come on as you wake in the morning, instead of an alarm clock or radio. This activity was suggested by a nurse who had experienced intensive care (Smith 1987).

The hiss of oxygen or ventilators, the sound of tracheal aspiration, the 'bleeps' or other warning signals of monitors or other equipment, the movement of trolleys or X-ray machines, the sound of voices, sometimes saying unintelligible things, and other noises all combine to provide an auditory environment which may be bewildering and provoke anxiety.

In addition to sound, patients may experience many other unusual stimuli. For example, there are often bright lights; strange equipment or procedures involving other patients can be seen; there are sensations of heat or cold; strange sensations from being handled by other people, or being attached to tubes and wires; fear of falling off the bed during a change of position while paralysed; discomfort from wet tapes holding the endotracheal tube (due to dribbling of saliva); and pain (Smith 1987). There may be lack of body privacy and a sense of humiliation (Ruiz 1993). Sensations of boredom, powerlessness, and fear that essential machinery might fail are commonly reported (Uprichard et al 1987).

Not only are patients assaulted by many unusual and often unpleasant stimuli, but also sensory perception may be altered:

- a lack of visual aids (spectacles or contact lenses), paralysis or eye dressings may impede sight
- blood in the ears, dressings, a missing hearing aid or other factors may impede hearing
- there may be other impediments to normal use of the senses, including drugs that can alter all sensory perception.

Critically ill patients may suffer sensory overload, sensory deprivation (some critically ill people receive little active intervention, needing mainly monitoring), or a combination of these. Many years ago Goldberger (1966) identified five areas of investigation related to sensory alteration:

- reduction of stimulus input variables; an absolute reduction in the variety and intensity of stimuli
- reduction of stimulus variability; the quantity of stimuli is the same but there is reduced patterning, imposed structuring, and homogeneous stimulation. When light is diffuse, sound muffled, and bodily sensations are non-distinct and difficult to interpret, this is referred to as perceptual deprivation
- social deprivation; isolation from people and a familiar environment
- confinement, immobilisation or restriction of movement
- increased sensory input; input via a number of senses at greater intensity than normal.

All of these can be found in individual or collected accounts of the experience of critically ill patients, as can accounts of the 'nightmare' auditory and visual hallucinations, delusions and paranoid feelings about staff and the environment (see, for example, Heath 1989, Bergbom-Engberg & Haljamae 1988, Douglas 1982). Patients may also experience depersonalisation (Roberts 1986), disturbed body image and extension of body boundaries so that they regard machinery such as a ventilator as part of themselves (Smith 1989). Patients may respond to sensory overload or deprivation with a variety of regulatory behaviours and physiological responses (Boxes 29.4 and 29.5). One factor which is important in determining a patient's responses to a critical care unit environment is the nature of the human environment.

The human environment

Psychological, as well as physical stimuli can be stressful and

Box 29.4 Nursing assessment of sensory overload (Reproduced with kind permission from Roberts 1986.)

Regulatory behaviours
Sweating hands
Constriction of peripheral blood vessels
Flutter in chest
Fidgetiness
Tachycardia
Increased cerebral blood flow
Numbness
Anorexia
Hyperventilation
Galvanic skin response
Increased blood cortisol and cholesterol.

Cognitive behaviours
Perceptual disorders:
  hallucination
  sound distortion
Disturbed sense of time:
  time expansion
Otherworldly feelings:
  unpleasantness
  floating in space
Feelings of loss of control
Somatic effects
Diminished reality testing:
  paranoia.

Box 29.5 Nursing assessment of sensory deprivation (Reproduced with kind permission from Roberts 1986.)

Regulatory behaviours
Increased galvanic skin response
Minor itching
Increased catecholamines
Altered electroencephalogram patterns
Feeling warmer or colder
Muscle movement
Numbness in fingers and toes.

Cognitive behaviours
Visual and auditory hallucinations and illusions
Temporal and spatial disorganisation
Inability to think clearly or to concentrate
Anxiety
Loss of sense of time
Delusions
Restlessness
Psychotic behaviour
Noncompliance behaviour
Confusion.

cause physiological reactions that may be harmful to critically ill patients. Such stimuli may result from deficiencies in the human environment. Nurses are an important part of the sensory and human environment of patients, and vice versa. Nurses affect the internal environment and responses of patients, and are in turn affected by them (Ashworth 1980) (Fig. 29.1). Many ex-patients say that a caring staff member (usually a nurse) whom they trusted was essential to their confidence and sense of security (Heath 1989, Smith 1987, Douglas 1982).

From the patient's perspective, technical competence is an important part of caring (Rosenthal 1992), but human aspects are important too. Caring includes being genuine, available, paying attention to the person, and communicating, including interest, acceptance, empathy and touch (Ray 1981). (See Ch. 26.) Patients have said that they need nurses whose names they know, who they feel understand and accept their behaviour even if they cannot cooperate, and who plan for periods of rest and sleep, and for some choice where possible (Adler 1976).

Both verbal and non-verbal methods are used by people to convey information, emotions, needs and, particularly, recognition and respect for the person with whom they are communicating. Critically ill patients may find it difficult or impossible to use effectively any of the usual verbal or non-verbal means of communication, due to tracheal intubation or paralysis. Nurses, however, inevitably communicate something to any conscious patient with whom they are in contact. Even lack of deliberate communication conveys a message that the patient, as a person, is not considered. A number of studies indicate that nurse–patient communication is sometimes inadequate, particularly with patients who are unable to talk (Ashworth 1980, Clark 1981). Characteristics of the nurse and patient, personal or other factors that affect them, and situational factors may all interfere with communication, for example by touch (Estabrooks 1989). Even nurses who would

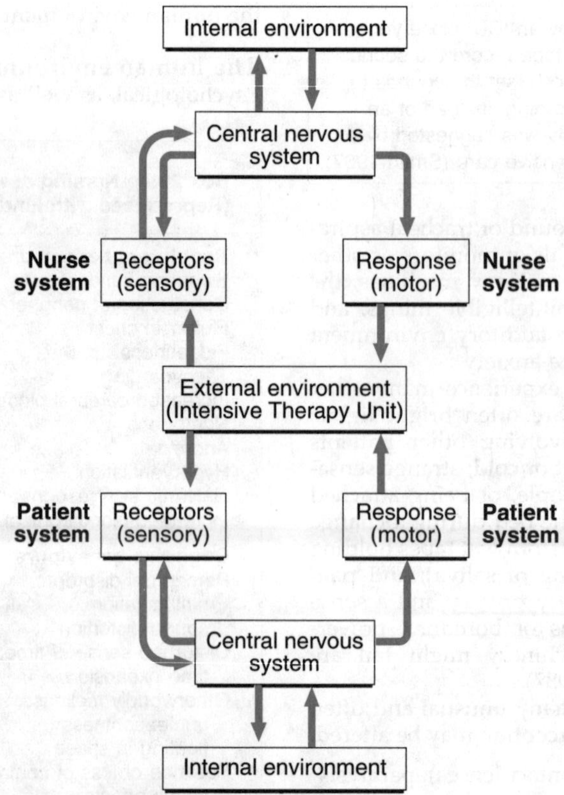

Fig. 29.1 Nurse–patient interaction in the intensive therapy/care unit. (Modification of Maron, Bryan-Brown & Shoemaker's model (1973) cited in Ashworth (1980, p. 39).

normally talk to patients may find it difficult to do so when they do not know a patient who appears unresponsive. Yet, without communication from nurses, patients may suffer social isolation even when surrounded by people.

Family and friends play an important role in relieving social isolation, depersonalisation and disorientation for patients. A number of ex-patients have emphasised the importance of this (Clark 1985, Van Lint 1975, Chen 1990, Heath 1989). Yet family and friends are unable to be of maximum help to patients unless they receive help from nurses in the form of access, information and activity, and emotional comfort. In both the UK and the USA, studies indicate that access for visitors may be restricted, ostensibly for patients' benefit, but apparently more for organisational reasons and service convenience (Biley et al 1993, Kirchoff et al 1993). It is important for nurses to recognise that their subjective feelings about patients and their families may influence their involvement with the family members, with the result that families who show negative behaviour may receive less support, even though they need more (Hickey & Lewandowski 1988). Lack of confidence in their ability to meet families' psychosocial needs, and the need to protect themselves from excessive emotional demands in stressful circumstances may also limit the success of nurses' interactions with family and friends (Hickey & Lewandowski 1988), as well as with patients.

Nurses act as 'gate keepers' and 'communicators' as well as providers of care (Boykoff 1986). Even when there is said to be an open visiting policy there are often restrictions on who may visit, particularly for children (Biley et al 1993), yet the literature suggests that there is little evidence to support these restrictions. One small study indicates that visiting by children may be a positive rather than a harmful experience for both visitors and patient, if there is good nursing support (Nicholson et al 1993).

Nurses have a great influence on the extent to which family and friends can support the sick person during intensive care, and after transfer to a ward and then home. A nurse, who is the mother of two children requiring intensive care, wrote:

> By becoming involved with us, talking long and deeply, sharing our grief, our worries and our joys, taking the brunt of our anger, the staff came to know us, and only by doing this could they help us to come to terms with our tragedies and gradually help us to gain that confidence required to enable us to happily take our children home, for whatever time was given. (Martin 1986)

The human environment also includes the relationships and interactions between nurses and doctors. There is now evidence that the interaction and communication between staff in ICUs directly and measurably influences the outcome for patients. For example, one of the differentiating characteristics of a unit which had a significantly lower death rate than expected (given the measured severity of the patients' illness and risk of death) was respect and excellent communication between the doctors and nurses to ensure that all patients' care needs were met (Knaus et al 1986, Baggs et al 1992).

Such communication and mutual respect must include dealing with the ethical dilemmas that inevitably arise. For example, patients designated 'not for resuscitation' may not only continue to receive high levels of nursing care but also aggressive medical treatment. 'Ethical decision-making is one of the most perplexing yet challenging areas in health care; . . . especially . . . about the limitations of life-sustaining medical treatment.' (Lewandowski et al 1985)

?	**29.4** Should ventilatory support ever be withdrawn from a live patient? Why and how? Or why not?

Considered, stated, ethical principles and guidelines For withdrawal of ventilator support for respiration, including the involvement of patients and their families, can help to provide a basis for such decision making, and good practice when the need arises (Daly et al 1993). However, there are many less dramatic aspects of intensive care which have ethical implications, including respect for the beliefs and values of patients and their families, informed consent and the giving and withholding of information.

HEALTH

It may seem strange to discuss health in relation to critically ill patients, but health can be defined in many more ways than as the mere absence of disease. Theories of health include ideas of responding appropriately, power to overcome disease when it occurs, achievement of human potential, and ability to respond positively to the challenges which arise (Seedhouse 1986). Nurse theorists have defined health in a variety of ways. Andrews & Roy (1986), for example, define health as 'a state and process of being and becoming an integrated and whole person'. Even critically ill people may function in more or less healthy ways within the limits of their situations. Patients' experience of critical illness, and possibly the extent and speed of recovery, are likely to be affected by the extent to which they are enabled to maintain healthy functioning. Nurses have an important part to play in dealing with obstacles, which may be biological, environmental, societal, familial or personal (Seedhouse 1986), and supporting critically ill patients so that they can function in as healthy a way as possible until they move on to recovery or death. However, this is very demanding and requires that nurses are aware of their own physical, social and spiritual needs. Nurses in critical care units, particularly, invest much in their work and can experience exhaustion, 'burnout' and what has been described as co-dependence, 'a disease of lost selfhood' (Snow & Willard 1989).

NURSING

Critically ill patients require good interdisciplinary care, communication and teamwork, and sometimes roles may overlap. Nurses may take on activities usually performed by doctors, physiotherapists or other staff, according to patients' needs. Doctors or other staff may sometimes take part in what are normally regarded as nursing activities. However, critical care nurses have their own areas of expertise and accountability, which can be summarised as meeting patients' needs by:

- maintaining support or substituting for patients' deficits in ability to perform the essential activities of living, and reducing demands to match capacity, for example by reducing activity and energy consumption when supply of oxygen to tissues is deficient
- constantly monitoring progress and condition so that appropriate care and treatment can be given and evaluated for efficacy and any side effects, with prompt action to initiate change according to patients' needs
- providing thoughtful, knowledgeable and personal support for each critically ill person during the illness experience, helping him or her to use healthy coping responses, and supporting healthy functioning with a view to the future as well as the present
- promoting an effective support system for patients by working with and sustaining their social support systems (family members and friends), and collaborating with other staff to provide excellent care and treatment in an environment conducive to human well-being.

Critically ill patients are very susceptible to the effects of the quality (good or bad) of care, which may considerably influence well-being and even prognosis.

> ? **29.5** In what ways may acts or omissions in basic nursing care affect a patient's physical condition?

Some examples of poor quality of nursing care are:

- allowing a patient to become chilled whilst attending to personal hygiene, causing peripheral vasoconstriction and increased peripheral resistance and discomfort
- failing to give the information and explanations necessary to relieve a patient's anxiety, resulting in tachycardia with increase in myocardial oxygen consumption and decrease in myocardial oxygen supply
- sitting a patient up too suddenly.

All of these may have harmful effects on a patient with borderline cardiovascular function. The second example illustrates the importance of mind–body interactions. Critical care nursing, therefore, includes care to meet all the current health-related needs of the critically ill person, as well as using safely and effectively any equipment that may be needed.

Systematic and planned nursing care is essential, but each stage of the nursing process may provide particular challenges in critical care. For example:

- Good nursing assessment, including information about the physical condition, the person who is ill, their usual way of functioning, and their personal support systems, is an important foundation for planning effective care. But much of this information may be difficult to obtain when confronted with an unknown patient in a hospital gown, who may be intubated or unconscious and unable to talk. Relatives or friends can be very helpful, if they are available, in providing a picture of the person as he or she was before illness or injury. Immediate life-sustaining action may be necessary after only brief assessment, and it is often necessary at first to do the best possible with very limited information.
- It is essential not only to identify accurately the problems requiring nursing intervention, but also to set priorities, since often such patients have many problems and it is impossible to deal with all of them simultaneously. Nevertheless, it is necessary to consider the consequences of delay. For example, postponing attention to pressure areas, such as heels, may cause pressure sores; putting off giving information may lead to psychological overload and disturbances which cause distress and delay recovery.
- Setting realistic and appropriate objectives is important to provide direction, facilitate evaluation and give encouragement to patient and staff when the objectives are achieved. Objectives may be difficult to set, however, when there is uncertainty about physical progress, lack of information about usual function, and the patient cannot take part.
- Care activities for each patient must be planned by a nurse to ensure that everything essential is covered, including periods of undisturbed rest. This requires diplomatic assertiveness in an open unit, where many other staff may be involved in treatment and care, and an emergency or unexpected situation may occur.
- Patient outcomes may be affected by many factors other than nursing. It is encouraging that the influence and effects of critical care nursing are often recognised not only by patients, their families and friends, and nurses, but also by other staff, but more research is needed to clarify the effects of nursing. The display of many indicators of physiological function, such as heart rate and rhythm, cardiovascular pressures, core and peripheral temperature, and PO_2, in many intensive care situations can be very useful in evaluating the effects of nursing, but these data are not always used for this purpose.

Meeting the needs of critically ill people

Given the wide range of age, medical diagnosis, situation and other characteristics of critically ill people, there is obviously wide variation in their individual needs. A number of common needs may not be met as well as they might be in critical care situations, however, unless the nurse takes them into consideration. These are:

- physical needs
- needs related to
  - biological rhythm
  - identity
  - self-esteem
  - control and interdependence
  - information and communication
  - territoriality
  - spiritual health with hope, meaning and purpose (Ashworth 1987).

Physical needs

The nursing requirements for meeting the physical needs of critically ill people are to a large extent covered in other chapters of this book. However, two points need emphasis.

1. Because patients are already so ill, so dependent on others, and often in an environment which poses hazards as well as benefit, it is particularly important that nurses use the best and most up-to-date knowledge available to guide care activities. Technical activities such as endotracheal suction and dressing arterial lines require constant review (Fiorentini 1992, Haglund & Wilkinson 1993) and one way of achieving enduring change may be by setting research-based standards. Basic preventative measures to avoid pressure sores require the selection of an appropriate way of assessing the risk of occurrence (Barratt 1990, Cubbin & Jackson 1991) and the choice of suitable aids to relieve pressure, particularly for patients whose condition does not allow much change of position. Collaborative development of a research-based sleep protocol, for example, can help to ensure that patients do not suffer the sleep deprivation that is a common problem for critically ill patients (Edwards & Schuring 1993). (See Ch. 25.) Help from other professionals may be necessary to keep up-to-date on physiotherapy or other areas where there are possible overlaps in care (Daber & Jackson 1987, Pearson & Parr 1993).

   Nurses are increasingly developing measures to increase precision in assessment, such as a 'Pain-o-meter' which measures affective as well as sensory aspects of pain (Gaston-Johansson et al 1991) and a sedation scale (Laing 1992). (See Ch. 19.) However, the quality of information produced is necessarily dependent on those who use such scales, as well as the validity and reliability of the scale. There can be problems of accuracy even with the well-known Glasgow Coma Scale, for example (Ellis & Cavanagh 1992).
2. Patients' immune defences are altered during critical illness. Nurses' responsibilities include not only maintaining up-to-date infection control techniques (Kingsley 1992), but also:

   - detecting alterations in immune response
   - preventing or limiting exposure to antigens
   - maintaining the body's first line of defence
   - enhancing defence mechanisms by reducing stress
   - maintaining an adequate level of comfort

- assisting the patient and significant others to gain cognitive control (Esperson 1986).

Biological rhythm

Human beings have biological rhythms that affect changes in body temperature and blood pressure (which tend to be lower at night) and cortisol and growth hormone levels (which tend to be higher at night) and other factors (Campbell et al 1986). The rhythmic routines of daily activities which occupy most people's lives interact with non-voluntary functions. At a more subjective level, many people recognise that they are 'owls' who function better later in the day and go to bed late, or 'larks' who feel at their best and brightest early in the day.

In critical care units, there is always the danger that activity and lighting may be more or less constant, because of the need for constant observation and frequent treatment, leading to lack of sleep, disturbance of biological rhythms and contributing to the sensory–perceptual alterations and delirium known to affect a considerable proportion of critically ill people, 12–38% according to some authorities (Easton & MacKenzie 1988). One small study indicated a significant increase in disorientation in patients aged 65 years or over after 4 days in an acute medical–surgical unit (Roslaniec & Fitzpatrick 1979), so it is possible that elderly patients in critical care units may be even more at risk.

Learning about and conforming, as far as possible, to each patient's usual daily routines, and maintaining a day–night routine, with diminished light, noise and disturbance as far as possible at night, can help to diminish such problems. Windows and natural light are also helpful (Easton & MacKenzie 1988), as well as a visible clock and calendar.

Identity

Self-image, a sense of identity and social integrity are maintained to a large extent by perceived stimuli from the world around and human responses to the person concerned. When patients are in a critical care unit, bombarded by unusual stimuli, deprived of their usual clothes, hairstyle and other chosen personal characteristics, and unable to talk or even maintain other functions independently, it may be very difficult to maintain a sense of identity and social integrity. Many might feel that their plight is symbolised by a man with neurological problems who said, 'Who am I? Where am I? Why do I hurt so much?' (Anon, 1981).

Much can be done to meet the need for recognition of individuality by seeking information about each patient and using it in planning and giving care; putting something personal such as a treasured photograph in sight; using the person's preferred name; and talking to, rather than over, him. Often, the most important focus is on helping family and friends to help the patient. As they are part of the person's usual social environment and support system, they are likely to be even more essential in a strange and anxiety-provoking situation.

Family and friends can only provide optimum support if their own needs are met, and nurses have an important role to play here. Some of the major needs that have been identified from a number of studies are:

- the need to reduce anxiety
- the need for information
- the need to be near the patient
- personal needs
- the need for support
- the need to be helpful (Millar 1989).

However, careful assessment is important (Coulter 1989, Dyer 1991), since nurses may be only moderately accurate in their assessment of the needs of family members (Forrester et al 1990). Research has also indicated that it is important to arrange visits to match patients' preferences by considering the characteristics of the person and the illness (Simpson 1991). Support for each patient is most likely to be optimal when nurses, visitors and patients collaborate to achieve it. A record of which visitors have been told what and by whom can be helpful in this (Hayes 1990).

Self-esteem

The self-concept has been defined as consisting of two components:

- the physical self, including body sensation and body image
- the personal self, including self-consistency, self ideal, and moral–ethical–spiritual self.

Inherent in each of these is the individual's perception of his or her own worth; the person's self-esteem (Andrews & Roy 1986). When someone is critically ill, there are likely to be changes affecting many of these components, which may result in low self-esteem.

It is difficult to maintain self-esteem when wearing a hospital gown, attached to equipment to which everyone pays great attention, unable to do anything voluntarily to maintain one's usual appearance and behaviour, and possibly unable even to control basic functions, including communication. The level of self-esteem can profoundly affect a person's thinking and behaviour (Brandon 1969).

It is important to support a patient's self-esteem by:

- showing respect when handling or communicating with the person; paying attention to his or her wants, preferences and appearance
- paying attention first to the person, then to the equipment
- using comfort measures, which may include massage of hands and feet (Hill 1993) or aromatherapy
- providing pleasant stimuli such as music (O'Sullivan 1991) and positive feedback to counteract some of the necessary but less pleasant stimuli in the environment.

Anything which conveys that the person is regarded as worthy of attention and respect can help to raise or support self-esteem.

Control and interdependence

An important part of human development in childhood is gaining increasing control of bodily functions and behaviour, and to some extent the surroundings. Adults usually have a considerable measure of control over their personal behaviour and activities, including the expression or control of emotions. Critically ill people, even those who are still able to talk and move are to a great extent dependent on others.

?	**29.6** Think of an occasion when you were in a critical care area for the first time, where you did not know anyone, did not understand much of what you saw or heard around you, did not know what people expected of you, and were anxious as to whether you could meet those expectations. What helped you most?

This question has asked nurses to think of their own feelings about control, or the lack of it. For patients it is, of course, much worse, because of their illness/injury, perhaps fear for life, discomforts, and even greater dependence on other people. In addition, patients may be aware of being unable to avoid what they regard as undesirable behaviour. For example, Douglas (1982) knew that she was giving the wrong answers when nurses tried to check her orientation, yet she could not stop herself. Ruiz (1992) writes:

Going into intensive care means 'not being me', not even in one's own body, when the theophylline begins to take effect and one has to call to be taken to urinate 20, 30 times, night and day; when one cannot even eat or wash without help, the need to call again with the fear that one is being a bother — that shame once more.

When possible, offering patients some choice and control by contracting for some aspects of care can reduce their perceived stress, hostility and depression (Ziemann & Dracup 1989) and lessen fatigue, anxiety and anger (Kallio & Sime 1980). But the choice offered must be a real choice, and it is important to convey to patients that 'personal control is an opportunity not an expectation' (Sime & Kelly 1983). Activities for personal control should:

- be clear, circumscribed and made explicit
- be personally relevant
- not require complex judgements or the expenditure of too much energy (Sime & Kelly 1983).

Once patients perceive that they are not totally helpless they are more likely to have the motivation to collaborate actively in their care and feel 'part of the team' working for their recovery.

Studies such as that by Lange et al (1988) show, for example, that patients who are enabled to control their own analgesia postoperatively may have fewer complications and use less medication. While the same principles are likely to apply in the care of all critically ill patients, involvement and choice may be more difficult to achieve for some than for others. However, establishing a relationship where the nurse is trusted and perceived as reliable and available to help when necessary is one way in which nurses can reduce the stress of dependence. Even totally dependent patients can be offered at least some sense of mental control through understanding, as a result of being given information.

The right of patients to refuse treatment must also be considered (Hunka 1993).

Information and communication

Nichols (1993) has identified informational care, emotional care, and counselling as the essential components of good psychological care in physical illness. All are dependent on communication. Similarly, 'reassurance' is often identified as an important part of nursing, particularly in intensive care, but it is often not defined in practical terms. The reassuring actions of nurses in one small study (Boyd & Munhall 1989) were aimed at enabling clients to experience themselves as capable of:

- identifying options and feeling themselves influential in determining their own experiences
- making decisions based on correct, pertinent information
- enduring difficult times in the presence of a caring and supportive person
- taking good care of themselves and comforting themselves, so facilitating recovery
- evaluating their responses in the context of 'normal' external expectations
- communicating effectively and influencing the responses of others.

It can be difficult to establish and maintain good nurse–patient communication in intensive care because of difficulties on the part of the nurse, the patient, or both. Sometimes a speech therapist may be helpful in advising on ways to overcome physical difficulties in communication (Easton & MacKenzie 1988), though a number of different methods have been used and tested by nurses. The most important factor is careful assessment by the nurse in order to identify impediments to good communication, so that efforts can be made to overcome them, using all possible verbal or non-verbal means.

The difficulties of communicating with intubated patients, and the theoretical reasons why communication is essential have long been known (Ashworth 1980). Good communication may enable patients to see monitoring equipment as helpful rather than frightening, even if they do not always remember being told about it (Thompson et al 1986). There are many studies showing the benefits to patients of information given by nurses, and there is increasing evidence that communication can influence patient outcomes in critical care. For example, short periods of counselling by nurses have been shown to increase knowledge and satisfaction and decrease anxiety and depression in coronary care patients and their wives (Thompson 1990).

Families also need open two-way communication. It can be useful to carry out a formal check on this, intermittently, as well as ongoing assessment (Dyer 1991). Helping the visitors can help the patient in many ways. For example, as one nurse who had been a patient said, 'I desperately wanted to reassure and educate my family. It was simply wonderful when my nurses did that job for me.' (Andre 1991)

Communication, however limited, can often be experienced by patients as a lifeline. Not only serious communication but even friendly teasing and humour may sometimes have a place in restoring a sense of normality (Uprichard et al 1987).

Territoriality

Everyone needs some 'personal space', and territoriality is a universal human need (Hayter 1981); it may, indeed, be stronger in the Western world, where people often have more space. Patients in critical care units are often unable to control their personal space and have little privacy. Not only may their bodies be exposed, at least intermittently, but strangers touch, move, and insert things into their bodies. Vital and usually private functions such as urination (by catheter) or changes in heart rate are fully visible to others in the unit. Not surprisingly, patients may have psychological disturbances associated with lack of privacy and lack of control of personal space (Margolis 1967) or may show signs of violence (Maagdenberg 1983).

Enabling some personalising of the patient's bed area, showing respect for the person's privacy, and seeking permission or at least warning patients of activities are important and possible. Creating a warm and friendly environment where the person feels safe and cared for, even though sometimes exposed, can considerably reduce distress (Ashworth 1989).

Spiritual health

This concept includes a sense of meaning, hope and purpose, not simply whether the patient has a religious faith. Cultural and personal values are very relevant to purpose in life and should be considered in assessment and care (Parfitt 1988, Lanara 1988).

Some critically ill patients lose hope and 'give up', ceasing to fight for life, particularly when ill for days or weeks, and this can contribute not only to their current physical and emotional experience but also to the outcome of the illness. Many nurses feel helpless, not knowing how to help to relieve the patient's suffering (Engberg 1991).

Anything a nurse can do, either directly or with the help of the patient's family or close friends, to help the patient to draw on his or her usual sources of support may be helpful. Simsen (1986) found that medical–surgical patients needed to learn the skills of 'knowing', 'hoping' and 'trusting' in order to make sense of the experiences of illness and in order to 'get through it'. Helping people to continue the practices usually important to them in life can enable them to do so, and there are a variety of ways of doing this. Many ex-patients have indicated that a person's faith may be an important part of their life and a comfort in crisis experience (Ashworth 1987).

Care of relatives and friends

Nursing care of family members does not automatically stop when the patient dies. Telling or talking to them about death (Dyer 1993), support in relation to organ donation (Johnson 1992), and even bereavement care (Jackson 1992) can all be a part of nursing critically ill people.

SUMMARY

Nursing critically ill people is often regarded as a highly technical affair, particularly in a critical care unit, but the same principles apply at home or in a general hospital ward. To be effective, nurses must have knowledge and understanding of physiology and other sciences, and of how the body works in health and illness; of technical equipment and its functions; and of how people function both in common and individually in health, and in illness and crisis. Equally important is to use this knowledge and put it into practice through skills, using 'head, heart and hands' to achieve the best possible experience and outcomes for patients, and also for their family and friends and for staff, so that they continue to care.

REFERENCES

Adler D 1976 Critical care nursing. Nursing Mirror 143(2): 54–55

Andre J A 1991 Being on the 'wrong end' of critical care. Focus on Critical Care 18(5): 392–393

Andrews H A, Roy C 1986 Essentials of the Roy Adaptation Model. Appleton-Century-Crofts, Connecticut

Anon 1981 Who am I, where am I? Nursing Times 77(15): 633–635

Ashworth P 1980 Care to communicate. Scutari, Harrow

Ashworth P 1987 The needs of the critically ill patient. Intensive Care Nursing 3(4): 182–190

Ashworth P 1990 High technology and humanity for intensive care. Intensive Care Nursing 6(3): 150–160

Baggs J G, Ryan S A, Phelps C E 1992 The association between interdisciplinary collaboration and patient outcomes in a medical intensive care unit. Heart and Lung 21(1): 18–24

Barratt E 1990 Pressure sores in intensive care. Intensive Therapy and Clinical Monitoring 11(5): 158, 160, 162–164, 167

Bergbom-Engberg I B, Haljamae H 1988 A retrospective study of patients' recall of respirator treatment (2): nursing care factors and feelings of security/insecurity. Intensive Care Nursing 4(3): 95–101

Biley F C, Millar B J, Wilson A M 1993 Issues in intensive care visiting. Intensive and Critical Care Nursing 9(2): 75–81

Bliss M R, Thomas J M 1993 An investigative approach. An overview of randomised controlled trials of alternating pressure supports. Professional Nurse 8(7): 437–38, 440, 442, 444

Boyd C O, Munhall P L 1989 A qualitative investigation of reassurance. Holistic Nursing Practice 4(1): 61–69

Boykoff S L 1986 Visitation needs reported by patients with cardiac disease and their families. Heart and Lung 15(6): 573–578

Brandon N 1969 The psychology of self-esteem. Nash, Los Angeles p. 104, as cited in Taylor M C 1982 The need for self-esteem. In: Yura H, Walsh M B 1982 Human needs and the nursing process. Appleton-Century-Crofts, Connecticut pp. 117–153

Campbell I T, Minors D S, Waterhouse J M 1986 Are circadian rhythms important in intensive care? Intensive Care Nursing 1(3): 144–150

Chen Y-C 1990 Psychological and social support systems in intensive and critical care. Intensive Care Nursing 6(2): 59–66

Clark J M 1981 Communication in nursing: analysing nurse-patient conversations. Nursing Times 77(1): 12–18

Clark K J 1985 Coping with Guillain–Barre Syndrome (a personal experience). Intensive Care Nursing 1(1): 13–18

Clark S 1987 Nursing diagnosis: ineffective coping, I A theoretical framework: II Planning care heart and lung 16(6): 670–685

Cooper K 1983 Electrical safety: the electrically sensitive ICU patient. Focus on Critical Care 9: 17–19

Coulter M A 1989 The needs of family members of patients in intensive care units. Intensive Care Nursing 5(1): 4–10

Cubbin B, Jackson C 1991 Trial of a pressure area risk calculator for intensive therapy patients. Intensive Care Nursing 7(1): 40–44

Daber S E, Jackson S E 1987 Role of the physiotherapist in the intensive care unit. Intensive Care Nursing 3(4): 165–171

Daly B J, Newlon B, Montenegro H D 1993 Withdrawal of mechanical ventilation: ethical principles and guidelines for terminal weaning. American Journal of Critical Care 2(3): 217–223

Dougherty S 1988 The malnourished respiratory patient. Critical Care Nurse 8(4): 13–22

Douglas A M 1982 Ch. 10 Where am I? In: Noble M A (ed) The ICU environment: directions for nursing. Reston Publishing, Reston

Dyer I D 1991 Meeting the needs of visitors: a practical approach. Intensive Care Nursing 7(3): 135–147

Dyer I D 1993 Breaking the news: informing visitors that a patient has died. Intensive and Critical Care Nursing 9(1): 2–10

Easton C, MacKenzie F 1988 Sensory–perceptual alterations: delirium in the intensive care unit. Heart and Lung 17(3): 229–235

Edwards G B, Schuring L M 1993 Sleep protocol: a research-based practice change. Critical Care Nurse 13(2): 84–88

Ellis A, Cavanagh S J 1992 Aspects of neurosurgical assessment using the Glasgow Coma Scale. Intensive and Critical Care Nursing 8(2):94–99

Engberg I B 1991 Giving up and withdrawal by ventilator-treated patients: nurses' experience. Intensive Care Nursing 7(4): 200–205

EPIC (1992) Nosocomial infection in ICU in 1992 (Report from the EPIC study). Intensive Care World 9(1): 24–25

Esperson S 1986 Nursing support of host defenses. Critical Care Quarterly 9(1): 51–56

Estabrooks C A 1989 Touch: a nursing strategy in the intensive care unit. Heart and Lung 18(4): 392–401

Fiorentini A 1992 Potential hazards of tracheobronchial suctioning. Intensive and Critical Care Nursing 8(4): 217–226

Forrester D A, Murphy P A, Price D M, Monaghan J R 1990 Critical care family needs: nurse–family member confederate pairs. Heart and Lung 19(6): 655–661

Gaston-Johansson F, Hofgren C, Watson P, Herlitz J 1991 Myocardial infarction pain: systematic description and analysis. Intensive Care Nursing 7(1): 3–10

Goldberger L 1966 American Journal of Psychiatry 122, 774–782, as cited in Ashworth P 1979 Sensory deprivation. The acutely ill. Nursing Times 75(7): 290–294

Haglund M, Wilkinson B 1993 A flexible path to permanent change. Implementing standard setting in an intensive therapy unit. Professional Nurse 6(9): 578, 580–582

Hayes E 1990 Needs of family members of critically ill patients: a Northern Ireland perspective. Intensive Care Nursing 6(1): 25–29

Hayter J 1981 Territoriality as a universal need. Journal of Advanced Nursing 6: 79–85

Heath J V 1989 What the patients say. Intensive Care Nursing 5(3): 101–108

Hickey M, Lewandowski L 1988 Critical care nurses' role with families. Heart and Lung 17(6): 670–676

Hill C 1993 Is massage beneficial to critically ill patients in intensive care units? A critical review. Intensive and Critical Care Nursing 9(2): 116–121

Hill G L, Blackett R L, Pickford I et al 1977 Malnutrition in surgical patients: an unrecognised problem. Lancet (8013): 689–692

Houldin A D, Lev E, Prystowsky M B 1991 Psychoneuro-immunology: a review of the literature. Holistic Nursing Practice 5(4): 10–21

Hunka S A 1993 The right to refuse treatment — an ethical case study. Intensive and Critical Care Nursing 9(2): 82–86

Jackson I 1992 Bereavement follow-up service in intensive care. Intensive and Critical Care Nursing 8(3): 163–168

Johnson C 1992 The nurse's role in organ donation from a brainstem dead patient: management of the family. Intensive and Critical Care Nursing 8(3): 140–148

Kallio J T, Sime A M 1980 The effect of induced control on the

perceptions of control, mood state and quality of care for clients in a critical care unit. Advances in Nursing Science 2: 105–107
Kingsley A 1992 Infection control in the intensive care unit. Intensive and Critical Care Nursing 8(4): 212–216
Kirchoff K T, Pugh E, Calame R M, Reynolds N 1993 Nurses' beliefs and attitudes towards visiting in adult critical care settings. American Journal of Critical Care 2(3): 238–245
Knaus W A, Draper E A, Wagner D P, Zimmerman J E 1986 An evaluation of outcome from intensive care in major medical centers. Annals of Internal Medicine 104: 410–418
Kouwenhoven W B, Jude J R, Knickerbocker G G 1960 Closed chest cardiac massage. Journal of the American Medical Association 173: 1064–1067
Laing A S M 1992 The applicability of a new sedation scale for intensive care. Intensive and Critical Care Nursing 8(3): 149–152
Lanara V 1988 Cultural value — influence on the delivery of care. Intensive Care Nursing 4(1): 3–8
Lange M P, Dahn M S, Jacobs L A 1988 Patient-controlled analgesia versus intermittent analgesia dosing. Heart and Lung 17(5): 495–498
Lewandowski W, Daly B, McClish D K 1985 Treatment and care of 'do not resuscitate' patients in a medical intensive care unit. Heart and Lung 14(2): 175–181
Lindenmuth J E, Breu C S, Malooley J A 1980 Sensory overload. American Journal of Nursing 80(8): 1456–1458
Lindsley D 1965 Common factors in sensory deprivation, sensory distortion and sensory overload. In: Sensory Deprivation. Harvard University Press, Harvard, pp. 193–194
McCarthy D O, Ouimet M E, Daun J M 1991 Shades of Florence Nightingale: potential impact of noise stress on wound healing. Holistic Nursing Practice 5(4): 39–48
Maagdenberg A A 1983 The 'violent' patient. American Journal of Nursing 83(3): 402–403
Margolis G J 1967 Post-operative psychosis on the intensive care unit. Comprehensive Psychiatry 8(4): 227–232
Martin M 1986 Confidence not courage. Intensive Care Nursing 2(1): 20–22
Massanari R M 1989 Nosocomial infections in critical care units: causation and prevention. Critical Care Nursing Quarterly 11(4): 45–57
Millar B 1989 Critical support in critical care. Nursing Times 85(16): 31–33
Neander K–D, Birkenfeld R 1991 The influence of various support systems on contact pressure and percutaneous oxygen pressure. Intensive Care Nursing 7(2): 120–127
Nguyen T V 1991 Mind, brain, and immunity: a critical review. Holistic Nursing Practice 5(4): 1–9
Nichols K 1993 Psychological care in physical illness, 2nd edn. Chapman & Hall, London
Nicholson A C, Titler M, Montgomery L A 1993 Effects of child visitation in adult critical care units: a pilot study. Heart and Lung 22(1): 36–45
Nightingale F 1860 Notes on nursing, 1952 edn. Camelot Press, London
O'Sullivan R J 1991 A musical road to recovery: music in intensive care. Intensive Care Nursing 7(3): 160–163
Parfitt B A 1988 Cultural assessment in the intensive care unit. Intensive Care Nursing 4(3): 124–127
Pearson S, Parr S 1993 Physiotherapy in the critically ill patient. Care of the Critically Ill 9(3): 128–131
Pirie S 1987 Nurses and mathematics. Royal College of Nursing, London
Ray M A 1981 A philosophical analysis of caring within nursing. In: Leininger M (ed) 1981 Caring: an essential human need. Slack, New Jersey
Roberts S L 1986 Behavioural concepts and the critically ill patient, 2nd edn. Appleton-Century-Crofts, Connecticut
Rogers B, Travers P 1991 Overview of work-related hazards in nursing: health and safety issues. Heart and Lung 20(5): 486–499
Rosenthal K A 1992 Coronary care patients' and nurses' perceptions of important nurse caring behaviours. Heart and Lung 21(6): 536–539
Roslaniec A, Fitzpatrick J J 1979 Changes in mental status in older adults with four days of hospitalization. Research in Nursing and Health 2: 177–187
Ruiz P A 1993 The needs of a patient in severe status asthmaticus: experiences of a nurse–patient in an intensive care unit. Intensive and Critical Care Nursing 9(1): 28–39
Seedhouse D 1986 Health. The foundations for achievement. Wiley & Sons, Chichester
Sime A M, Kelly J W 1983 Lessening patient stress in the CCU. Nursing Management 14(10): 24–26
Simpson T 1991 Critical care patients' perceptions of visits. Heart and Lung 20(6): 681–688
Simsen B 1986 Nursing the spirit. Nursing Times 84(37): 31, 33
Smith C 1987 In need of intensive care: a personal perspective. Intensive Care Nursing 2(3): 116–122
Smith S 1989 Extended body image in the ventilated patient. Intensive Care Nursing 5(1): 31–38
Snow C, Willard D 1989 I'm dying to take care of you. Professional Counsellor Books, Redmond
Thompson D R 1990 Counselling the coronary patient and partner. Scutari, Harrow
Thompson D, Bailey S, Webster R 1986 Patients' views on cardiac monitoring. Nursing Times Occasional Paper 82(9): 54–55
Uprichard E, Martin A, Evans S 1987 Guillain–Barre Syndrome: patients' and nurses' perspectives. Intensive Care Nursing 2(3): 123–134
Vander A J, Sherman J H, Luciano D S 1975 Human physiology. Tate, McGraw–Hill, New York
Van Lint J 1975 My new life. Neyensch Printers, San Diego
Williams M, Murphy J D 1991 Noise in critical care units: a quality assurance approach. Journal of Nursing Care Quality 6(1): 53–59
Woodrow P 1992 An opportunist to keep at bay. Pseudomonas in ITU. Professional Nurse 8(2): 100–102, 104
Yannelli B, Gurevich I 1988 Infection control in critical care. Heart and Lung 17(6): 596–600
Young M E 1988 Nutritional problems in critical care. Malnutrition and wound healing. Heart and Lung 17(1): 60–69
Ziemann K M, Dracup K 1989 How well do CCU patient–nurse contracts work? American Journal of Nursing 89(5): 691–2, 694

FURTHER READING

Cooper B, Larson 1992 Infection control issues for critical care units: an overview and a challenge — physician and nurse perspective. Heart and Lung 21(4): 317–321
Dobree L 1993 How do we keep time? Understanding human circadian rhythms. Professional Nurse 8(7): 446–449
Gould D 1993 Assessing nurses' hand decontamination performance. Nursing Times Occasional Paper 89(25): 47–50
Jowett N I, Thompson D R 1988 Basic life support: the forgotten skills. Intensive Care Nursing 4(1): 9–17
Knebel A R 1991 Weaning from mechanical ventilation: current controversies. Heart and Lung 20(4): 321–331
McClintock T T C, Hodsman N B A 1987 Patient controlled analgesia. Intensive Care Nursing 3(1): 8–13
Mitchell P H, Armstrong S, Simpson T F, Lenz M 1989 American Association of Critical Care Nurses Demonstration Project: profile of excellence in critical care nursing. Heart and Lung 18(3): 219–237
Narayanasamy B 1991 Spiritual care: a resource guide. Quay Publishing, Lancaster
Omery A 1991 A healthy death. Heart and Lung 20(3): 310–311
Puntillo K A 1988 The phenomenon of pain and critical care nursing. Heart and Lung 17(3): 262–271
Smith C E, Mayer L S, Parkhurst C 1991 Adaptation in families with a member requiring mechanical ventilation at home. Heart and Lung 20(4): 349–356
Stovsky B, Rudy E, Dragonette P 1988 Comparison of two types of communication methods used after cardiac surgery with patients with endotracheal tubes. Heart and Lung 17(3): 281–289
Thomas V M, Ellison K, Howell E V, Winters K 1992 Caring for the person receiving ventilatory support at home: care-givers' needs and involvement. Heart and Lung 21(2): 180–186

CHAPTER 30

The unconscious patient

Anne E. Murdoch

Douglas Allan (Additional material and advice)

CHAPTER CONTENTS

Introduction 839
Defining consciousness 839

Anatomical and physiological basis for consciousness 840
The reticular formation 840
The content of consciousness 841

States of impaired consciousness 841
Acute states of impaired consciousness 841
Chronic states of impaired consciousness 844

Assessment of the nervous system 844
The Neurological Observation Chart 844
The Glasgow Coma Scale 844
Recording other measurements 846

Causes of unconsciousness 846
Hypoglycaemia 847
Epilepsy 847
Drug overdose 847

Emergency care of the unconscious patient 847
A hospital emergency 847
A planned admission 848
Priorities of nurse management 848

Nursing management of the unconscious patient 849
Breathing 849
Communicating 851
Rest and sleep 852
Eating and drinking 852
Elimination 853
Personal cleansing and dressing 853
Maintaining a safe environment 853
Mobilising 854
Controlling body temperature 855

Dying 855

Glossary 857

References 858

Further reading 858

INTRODUCTION

The unconscious patient presents a special challenge to the nurse. His medical management will vary according to the original cause of his condition but his nursing care will be constant. The unconscious patient has no control over himself or his environment. He is, therefore, dependent upon the nurse to accept responsibility for the management of his activities of living and for monitoring his vital functions.

The quality of nursing care is of crucial importance if the patient is to relearn to perceive himself and others, to communicate, to control his body and his environment and to care for himself.

The responsibility placed on the nurse is considerable and can be a source of anxiety, even for experienced nurses (see Ch. 17). It is therefore essential that the nurse has a firm understanding of the mechanisms causing altered states of consciousness as well as a sound knowledge of the potential and actual physiological, psychological and social problems that these patients face. Skills training, exploring attitudes and using support systems can all help the nurse to overcome her anxiety and take up the challenge.

To nurse an unconscious patient back to recovery must be one of the most rewarding aspects of nursing; however, even with all the medical advances made recently, not all patients can hope for complete recovery. Some may not survive and others may be left with a residual mental or physical handicap. These patients and their families will need strong emotional support and reassurance. The nurse, who is with the patient more than other members of the multi-disciplinary team, is often in the best position to give this support.

Defining consciousness

Normal conscious behaviour is dependent on an intact brain function. Impaired, reduced or absent consciousness implies the presence of brain dysfunction and demands urgent medical attention if potential recovery is to be expected. In order to appreciate the importance of *altered* states of consciousness an understanding of consciousness itself is required.

Plum and Posner (1980) define consciousness simply as 'a state of awareness of the self and the environment'. The individual is wakeful, alert and aware of his personal identity and of the events occurring in his surroundings. 'Coma' is defined as the opposite, 'the total absence of awareness of self and environment even when the individual is externally stimulated'. The difference between sleep and coma is that in sleep the individual can be fully aroused by external stimuli whereas in a coma he can not (Williams 1970). Consciousness therefore depends on whether the person can be aroused.

It has been pointed out by several writers that consciousness is notoriously difficult to define (Bell et al 1972, Trimble 1979 and Myco & McGilloway 1980).

ANATOMICAL AND PHYSIOLOGICAL BASIS FOR CONSCIOUSNESS

The reticular formation

The reticular formation is a diffuse net-like aggregation of neurones located in the central core of the brain stem. It extends from the medulla at its junction with the spinal cord to the thalamus in the forebrain (Fig. 30.1). It is involved in the coordination of skeletal muscle activity, including voluntary motor movement and the maintenance of balance. It also assists in the regulation of activity controlled by the autonomic nervous system such as cardiovascular, respiratory and gastrointestinal activity (Wilson 1990).

The reticular activating system (RAS)

A particular feature of the reticular formation is the reticular activating system (RAS). This system occupies an anatomically restricted, although not defined, zone (Adams & Victor 1985) and extends from the upper pons to the thalamus and hypothalamus. The RAS has a large number of projections or radiations to the cerebral cortex (Fig. 30.1).

The RAS was first described by Moruzzi and Magoun (1949). Animal experiments demonstrated that marked alterations in the conscious level could be produced by cutting the brainstem at various levels. Later experiments demonstrated that stimulation of the RAS would awaken an animal, whereas destruction led to coma. Thus it was postulated that the RAS was involved in the regulation of consciousness.

Two separate parts of the RAS have been identified (Guyton 1991):

- the mesencephalon
- the thalamus.

The mesencephalic area is composed of grey matter in the upper pons and midbrain. Stimulation causes a very diffuse flow of impulses which project upwards throughout the thalamus. The impulses then fan out to wide regions of the cerebral cortex (Fig. 30.1). This causes a generalised increase in cerebral activity leading to general wakefulness.

The thalamic area is composed of grey matter within the thalamus (Fig. 30.1). It differs from the mesencephalic part in that stimulation of this area activates localised areas of the cerebral cortex. Signals from specific parts of the thalamus initiate activity in specific parts of the cortex, rather than activating the whole cortex. It is postulated that this process of selection is carried out by discriminatory receptor neurones (Milner 1970). These act as a 'gate', letting through inputs that are to continue to the cortex and inhibiting or rejecting extraneous inputs. If this process did not exist the cortex would be inundated with information that it could not process and confusion would result.

The arousal reaction

In order to function, the RAS must be stimulated by input signals from a wide range of sources via the spinal reticular tracts and various collateral tracts, such as the specialised auditory and visual tracts and therefore all the modalities of sensation (see Ch. 9). The RAS is also stimulated by signals from the cerebral cortex, that is the RAS may first stimulate the cerebral cortex and the cortical areas responding to reason and emotion may 'modify' the RAS either positively or negatively according to the 'decision' of the cerebral cortex. The RAS transmits and filters (habituation).

For instance, when an individual is in a deep sleep, the RAS is in a dormant state. Almost any type of sensory signal, however, can immediately activate the RAS and waken him, for example, pain stimuli or unaccustomed noise. This is called the 'arousal reaction' and is the mechanism by which sensory stimuli wake us from deep sleep (Guyton 1991).

The RAS is also stimulated by signals from the cerebral cortex. There are numerous pathways to both mesencephalic and thalamic portions from the sensory and motor cortex and from cortical areas that deal with the emotions. Whenever any

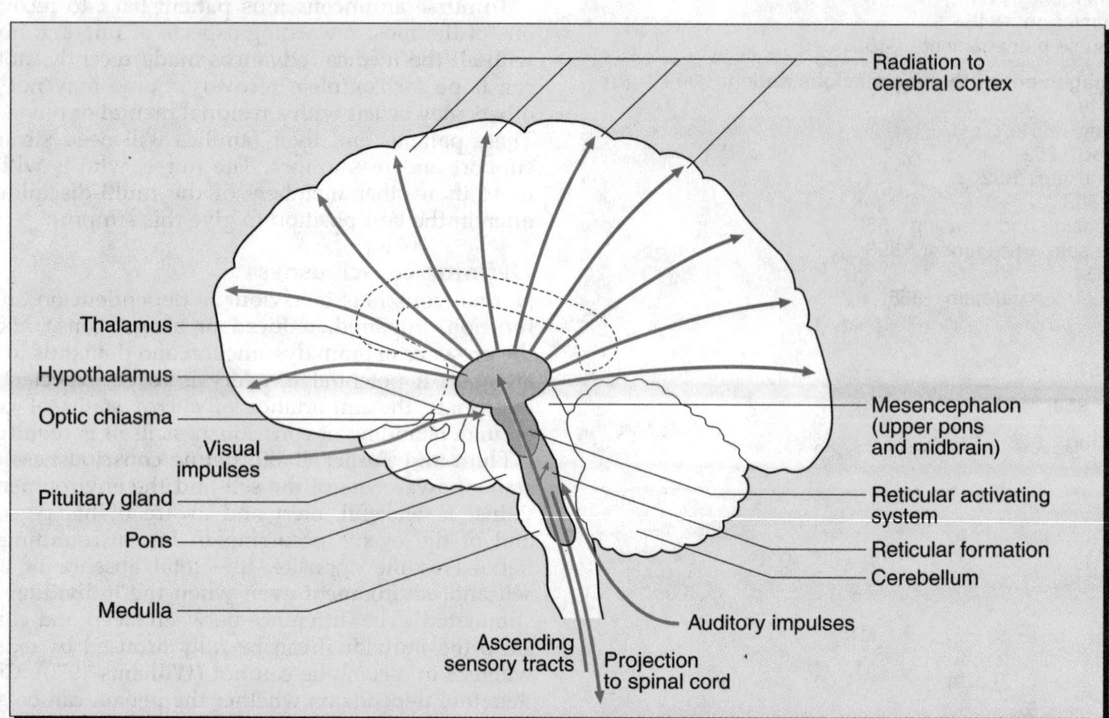

Fig. 30.1 The mid-sagittal section of the brain, showing the reticular activating system and related structures.

of these areas becomes excited, impulses are transmitted into the RAS, thus increasing the activity. This is termed a 'positive feedback response' (Spence & Mason 1987).

The feedback theory

Magoun (1963) claimed that the cerebrum regulates incoming information by a positive feedback mechanism (Fig. 30.2). A second feedback cycle that stimulates proprioceptors is also shown in Figure 30.2.

After a prolonged period of wakefulness, the synapses in the feedback loops become fatigued, the RAS becomes dormant and sleep is induced (Spence & Mason 1987). The degree of wakefulness and consciousness is normally dependent on the number of feedback loops activated (Guyton 1991). Figure 30.2 illustrates a number of activating pathways passing from the mesencephalon upward through the thalamus to the cortex. If only one of these becomes activated the degree or level of consciousness is minimal. Conversely, if all pathways are activated simultaneously, a high level of consciousness ensues.

The return to consciousness demonstrates that the RAS is still functioning and capable of screening and discrimination.

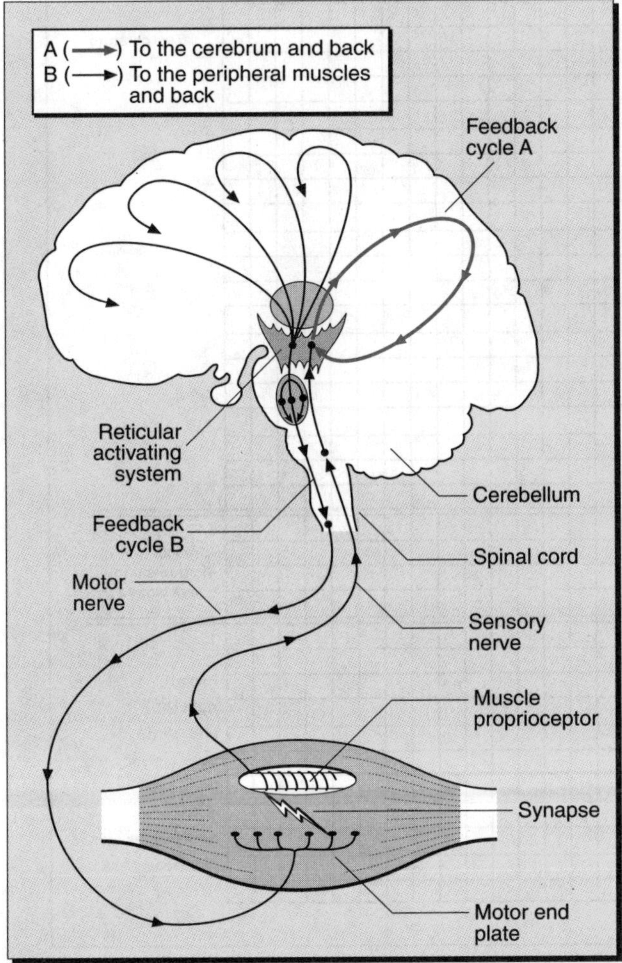

Fig. 30.2 The feedback mechanism, showing two feedback cycles passing through the RAS. In cycle A, the RAS excites the cerebral cortex and the cortex in turn re-excites the RAS. This initiates a cycle that causes continued intense excitation of both regions. In cycle B impulses are sent down the spinal cord to activate skeletal muscles. Activation of the muscle stimulates proprioceptors to transmit sensory impulses upward to re-excite the RAS. Consciousness results when the RAS, in turn, stimulates the cerebral cortex.

The content of consciousness

The content of consciousness refers to the sum of cognitive and affective mental functions. It is dependent upon relatively intact functional areas within the cerebral hemispheres that interact with each other as well as with the RAS.

Injury to, or disease of, the cerebral hemispheres, resulting in diffuse damage, can inhibit or block the signals from the RAS and consciousness cannot be completely maintained. The damaged cortex is unable to interpret the incoming sensory impulses and therefore cannot transmit them to other areas for action.

Localised damage to the cerebral hemispheres can also diminish the content of consciousness to a lesser degree (Plum & Posner 1980). For example, a patient who has suffered a stroke causing aphasia may appear awake and alert. His inability to understand or to use language, however, decreases his full awareness of himself and his environment. Such localised defects are not generally regarded as a true altered state of consciousness, but this example highlights the difficulties in defining true conscious behaviour.

STATES OF IMPAIRED CONSCIOUSNESS

Various states or levels of consciousness exist between full consciousness and coma. Decreasing consciousness is usually considered on a continuum ranging from full alertness through sleep, clouding of consciousness, stupor and coma to death (Trimble 1979). This order is generally consistent but not all patients behave in exactly the same way. The definitions of the impaired states given in this section are therefore intended to be used as broad guidelines. (Sleep is considered a normal phenomenon and is discussed in Chapter 25.)

The impaired states of consciousness can be divided into the categories of acute and chronic. Acute states are potentially reversible, whereas chronic states tend to be irreversible as they are caused by destructive brain lesions.

Signs of deterioration in a patient's conscious level demand urgent attention if further brain damage is to be avoided. The ability of the nurse to accurately assess the patient's conscious state is therefore of the utmost importance. The Glasgow Coma Scale (see Fig. 30.3) provides a useful assessment tool which eliminates subjectivity and this will be described on pages 844–846.

Acute states of impaired consciousness

The acute states are caused by intracranial diseases and metabolic upsets, such as alcoholic coma or drug overdose, which alter brain function. The acute states are:

- clouding of consciousness
- delirium
- illusions
- hallucinations
- delusions
- stupor
- coma.

Clouding of consciousness

Clouding of consciousness refers to changes of conscious activity where the patient's awareness is reduced. It reflects generalised brain dysfunction, as seen in systemic and metabolic disorders (see Fig. 30.4). These have interfered with the integrity of the RAS, thus affecting the arousal response.

In its early stages, clouding may include hyperexcitability and irritability, alternating with drowsiness (Plum & Posner 1980).

More advanced clouding produces a confused state in which stimuli are more consistently misinterpreted. The patient is bewildered and often has difficulty in following commands.

NAME

HOSP. No.:—

AGE:—

OBSERVATION CHART

CONSULTANT:—

DATE:—

TIME

COMA SCALE

Eyes open: Spontaneously; To speech; To pain; None — Eyes closed by swelling – C

Best verbal response: Orientated; Confused; Inappropriate Words; Incomprehensible Sounds; None — Endotracheal tube or tracheostomy – T

Best motor response: Obey commands; Localise pain; Flexion to pain; Extension to pain; None — Usually record the best arm response

Pupil scale (m.m.): 1, 2, 3, 4, 5, 6, 7, 8

Blood pressure and Pulse rate: 240, 230, 220, 210, 200, 190, 180, 170, 160, 150, 140, 130, 120, 110, 100, 90, 80, 70, 60, 50, 40

Respiration: 30, 20, 10

Temperature C: 40, 39, 38, 37, 36, 35, 34, 33, 32, 31, 30

PUPILS: right — Size, Reaction; left — Size, Reaction — + reacts; – no reaction; c eye closed

LIMB MOVEMENT

ARMS: Normal power; Mild weakness; Severe weakness; Spastic flexion; Extension; No response

LEGS: Normal power; Mild weakness; Severe weakness; Extension; No response

Record right (R) and left (L) separately if there is a difference between the two sides

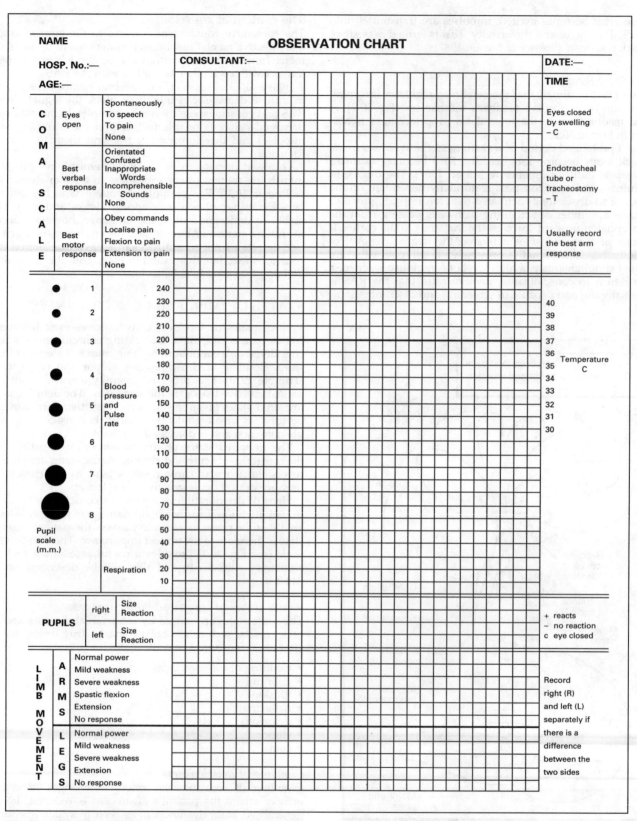

Fig. 30.3 The Neurological Observation Chart, including Glasgow Coma Scale. (Reproduced with kind permission from Nursing Times where this figure first appeared on 19 June 1975.)

The signs of clouding are therefore reflected in subtle changes in the patient's behaviour. Minor disturbance of consciousness can easily go undetected if attention is not paid to what the patient says and does. If a normally placid and cooperative patient becomes irritable and aggressive, this should denote a behaviour change that requires further investigation. Similarly, comments from a relative, such as, 'he does not seem to recognise me today' should alert the

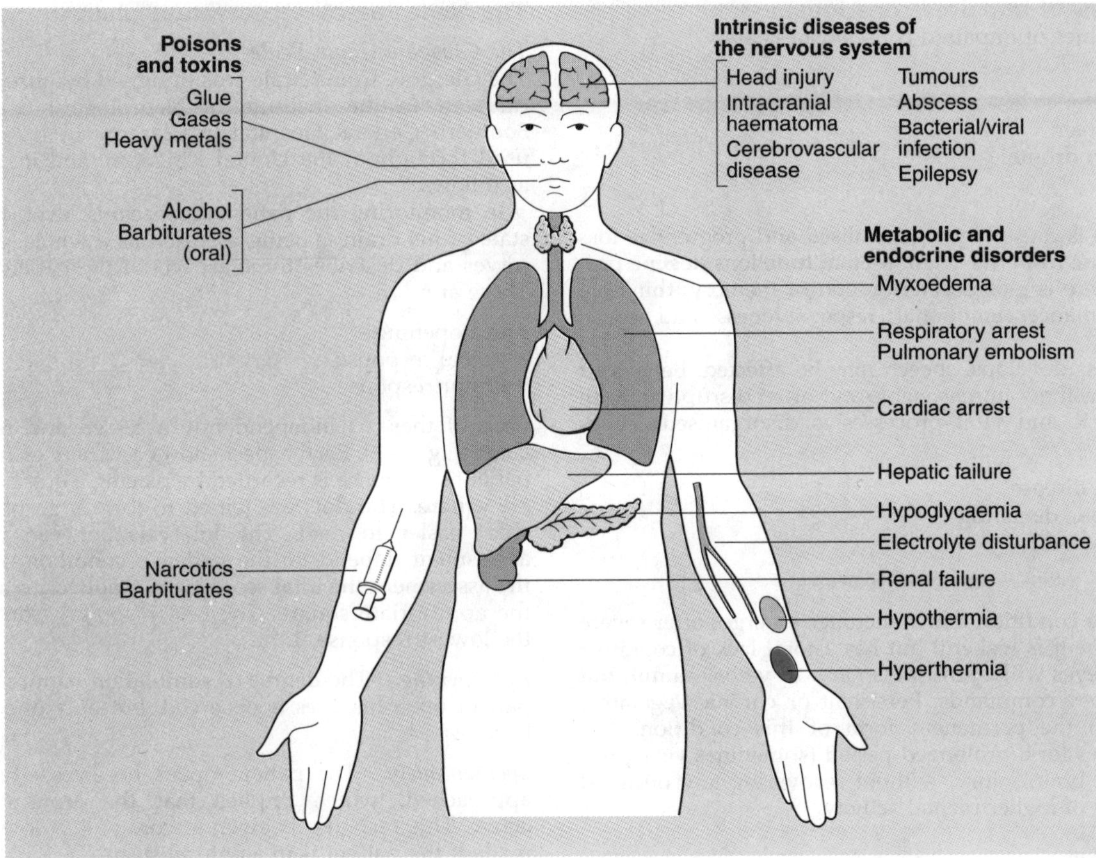

Fig. 30.4 Common causes of unconsciousness.

nurse to the fact that something is not quite right with the patient.

Any change in the patient's behaviour must be reported to the appropriate nursing or medical staff, particularly if he has not previously experienced any of these signs. The patient's nursing care plan will also need to be evaluated and a new goal for care set.

Delirium

Delirium is often described as a form of clouding. If refers to a fluctuating noticeable mental state characterised by confusion, disorientation, fear and irritability. The patient is usually loud, talkative, offensive, suspicious and agitated (Plum & Posner 1980). This behaviour reflects generalised brain dysfunction due to interference with the RAS, affecting arousal. The causes of delirium are listed in Box 30.1.

Illusions are defined as misinterpretations of sensory material in the patient's environment. A shadow on the wall is seen as an animal or person, for example, or noises are misinterpreted as voices of strangers who have come to do harm.

Hallucinations are normally defined as seeing or hearing something in the absence of any sensory stimuli, for example, the patient will hear voices when no-one is present or see objects that do not exist in his environment (Trimble 1979). Other senses, such as touch, taste or smell, can be affected but with acute disorders of the brain hallucinations are usually visual (Plum & Posner 1980).

Delusions are defined as persistent misperceptions that are firmly held by a person, even although they are illogical. In some forms of schizophrenia, for example, the patient suffers from a delusion that his feelings, beliefs, thoughts and actions are controlled by some outside force.

Stupor

The term stupor describes a state whereby the patient can be aroused only by vigorous and repeated noxious stimuli (Plum & Posner 1980).

Coma

Coma is an impaired state where the patient is totally unaware of himself and his environment. It may vary in degree and in its deepest stages no reaction of any kind is obtainable (Adams & Victor 1985).

Box 30.1 Causes of delirium

Toxic disorders of the nervous system, for example,
- acute poisoning by:
  - metals
  - gases
  - drugs
  - alcohol.

Metabolic disorders, such as:
- renal failure
- hepatic failure
- encephalitis.

Severe head injury.

Psychological manifestations:
- illusions
- hallucinations
- delusions.

Chronic states of impaired consciousness

The chronic states of impaired consciousness are:

- dementia
- vegetative
- akinetic mutism
- locked-in syndrome.

Dementia

This condition is caused by a generalised and progressive loss of cortical tissue from the brain. Mental functions decline progressively. There is global deterioration of memory, thinking, motor performance, emotional responsiveness and social behaviour.

As the illness develops, speech may be affected. Behaviour becomes increasingly unreasonable and often disruptive, until control of basic and vital processes is disorganised. Types include:

- Alzheimer's disease
- arteriosclerotic dementia
- pre-senile dementia.

Vegetative

This refers to a condition that sometimes emerges after severe coma. The patient is wakeful but has a total lack of cognitive function. His eyes will open in response to verbal stimuli but he will not obey commands. Persistent or chronic vegetative state refers to the permanent form of this condition. The patient survives for a prolonged period (sometimes years) following severe brain injury, without recovering any outward manifestations of higher mental activity.

Akinetic mutism

This describes a condition of silent immobility, where the patient retains periods of apparent wakefulness. He gives the appearance of vigilance but there is little or no vocalising. He is doubly incontinent and makes only the most rudimentary skeletal muscle movements, even in response to painful stimuli.

Damage to the RAS, cerebral frontal lobes or basal ganglia is held to be the pathological basis for this condition.

Locked-in syndrome

This condition produces paralysis of all four limbs and the lower cranial nerves, without interfering with consciousness. The patient is unable to speak and is dependent on vertical eye movements or blinking in order to communicate.

The pathological basis for this condition is damage to the pons, predisposed by cerebral vascular disease or trauma.

It is important to remember that the patient is aware of his surroundings, even although he appears to be physically and mentally inert.

ASSESSMENT OF THE NERVOUS SYSTEM

Nurses frequently need to monitor the conscious level because impairment may complicate not only intracranial conditions but those affecting other areas of the body, such as cardiac arrest, hepatic and renal failure, diabetic coma and drug overdose. The need to assess conscious level may arise in any ward in any hospital. Ambiguities and misunderstandings can result when passing on information about the patient's state to other staff (Teasdale 1975). There is clearly a need for a standardised system of assessing the conscious level, so that different nurses and doctors will make similar observations on the patient at any one time. The system must however encompass enough detail to determine changing status so that appropriate action can be taken.

The Neurological Observation Chart

The Glasgow Coma Scale

The Glasgow Coma Scale was designed by nursing and medical staff in the Institute of Neurological Sciences of the Southern General Hospital in Glasgow in 1975. It is widely used throughout the United Kingdom, and its application is as follows.

In monitoring the patient's conscious level, the functional state of his brain is being assessed as a whole. The nurse observes and describes three aspects of the patient's behaviour. These are:

- eye opening
- verbal response
- motor response.

Each of these is independently assessed and recorded on a chart (Fig. 30.3). Each aspect shows a variety of responses. The patient's response is recorded by placing a dot in the appropriate square. The dots are joined to form a graph, making the chart easier to read. The intervals between recording the assessment depend on the patient's condition. At the end of the assessment the total score may be added up and written in the appropriate square. The best response scores 4 or 5 and the lowest response, 1.

Eye opening. The degree of stimulation required to make the patient open his eyes is observed, but only one eye needs to be assessed.

Spontaneously. The patient opens his eyes when he is first approached, which implies that the arousal response is active. This response is given a score of 4. Allowance must be made if the patient is in a natural sleep.

To speech. The patient's eyes are not open when he is first approached. The nurse should speak to him by calling his name and then ask him to open his eyes. It may be necessary to shout. A successful response scores 3.

To pain. A painful stimulus is applied if the patient fails to open his eyes spontaneously or to speech. Pressure is applied to the proximal side of the patient's fingernail by a pen or pencil (Fig. 30.5). This response scores 2 on the coma scale. Care must be taken not to exert pressure on the patient's cuticle as this will damage the nail bed.

None. If the painful stimulus does not cause the patient to open even one eye, then he is recorded as having no eye-opening response. This indicates a deep depression of the arousal system and is scored as 1 on the scale.

Possible assessment problems. The patient who is in a deep coma with flaccid eye muscles will show no response to stimulation. If the eyelids are drawn back, however, his eyes may remain open. This is very different from spontaneous eye opening and should be recorded as 'None'.

After trauma or surgery, eyelid swelling occasionally prevents eye opening. A condition such as ptosis (nerve palsy) will also have this effect, although this seldom results in complete closure of both eyes. Enforced closure of the eyelid(s) should be recorded as 'C' on the chart.

Opening of the eyes implies arousal but it must be remembered that this does not necessarily mean that the patient is aware of his surroundings. This can be misleading and be a source of false optimism in relatives.

Verbal response. The patient's best achievement in respect of verbal response is observed.

Orientated. The patient is recorded as orientated if he can state his name, where he is and what the year and month are.

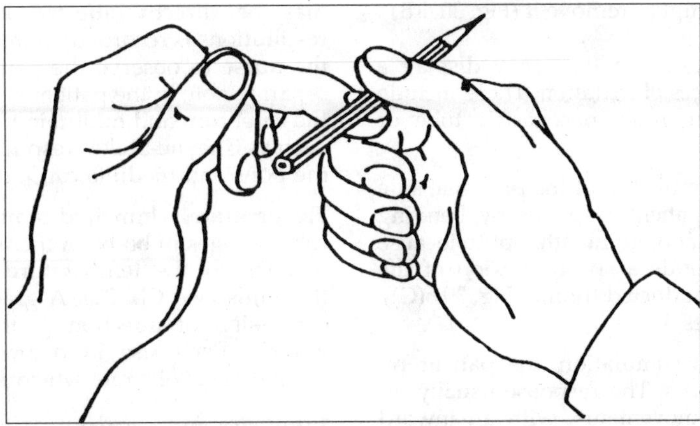

Fig. 30.5 Applying a painful stimulus: fingertip stimulation. (From Teasdale 1975. Reproduced with kind permission from Nursing Times where this figure first appeared on 12 June 1975.)

This is orientation in person, place and time, respectively, and is given a score of 5. Questions can be varied but they must be kept simple; for example, the date and even the day are not easily remembered; especially after a period in hospital.

Confused. If the patient is capable of producing phrases or sentences but the conversation is rambling and inappropriate to the questions about orientation, it is a confused verbal response and scores 4.

Inappropriate words. The patient will only speak one or two words, usually in response to physical stimulation. The words are usually obscenities. On occasions, the patient will shout out obscenities or call a relative's name for no apparent reason. These all indicate a lower level of responsiveness and score 3.

Incomprehensible sounds. The patient will moan or grunt in response to physical stimulation. The verbal response may contain indistinct mumbling but no intelligible words. The response scores 2.

None. The patient will not produce any verbal response even when prolonged and repeated stimulation is given. This scores 1.

Possible assessment problems. The patient may be unable to understand the nurse's commands because he does not understand the language or has a hearing defect. The patient's verbal response may be impaired as a result of a speech defect such as dysphasia. If appropriate, written instructions and replies can be used to assess the patient's language ability. As well as noting the level of the response, the chart should be marked 'D' where the impairment is thought to be due to dysphasia.

The verbal response may also be compromised by the presence of an endotracheal or tracheostomy tube. This is indicated on the patient's chart as 'T'.

Motor response. The patient's best motor response is observed (see Fig. 30.6). Only upper-limb responses are recorded, as leg responses to pain are less consistent and inappropriate spinal withdrawal reflexes occur more readily in many patients who would otherwise show a total absence of brain function.

Obey commands. The patient has the ability to appreciate instructions (Fig. 30.6(A)). These are usually given by verbal commands such as, 'Put out your tongue, please' or 'Hold up your arms, please'. If the patient obeys these instructions he is given a score of 5.

Localise pain. If the patient does not obey commands, a pain stimulus is applied. Using the trapezium pinch is the safest method. The patient's shudder is partially exposed and the trapezius muscle is grossly pinched (Frawley 1990). The patient is recorded as 'localising to pain' when he moves his

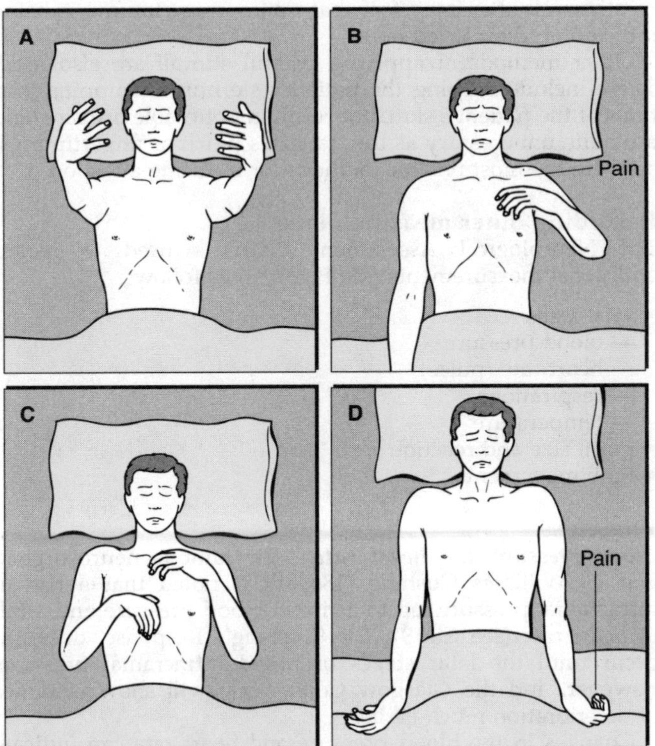

Fig. 30.6 Motor responses.
(A) Obeys commands ('Lift up your arms.')
(B) Localising to pain.
(C) Flexing to pain.
(D) Extending to pain.

arm to locate the pain, in an attempt to remove it (Fig. 30.6(B)). This response scores 4.

During the course of the day, the patient may display a localising response to other sources of irritation. These include attempts to remove his oxygen mask, nasogastric tube or urinary catheter.

Flexion to pain. After painful stimulation of the proximal side of the patient's fingernail, the patient responds by bending his elbow and withdrawing his hand but no attempt to localise is made. The response may include a spastic flexion of the wrist and finger joints across an adducted thumb (Fig. 30.6(C)). This is 'flexion to pain' and scores 3.

Extension to pain. After painful stimulation, the patient responds by straightening his elbows. The response usually includes spastic hand and wrist movements, with an inward rotation of the shoulders and forearms (Fig. 30.6(D)). The legs are generally straight, with the feet pointing outwards. This posture may be adopted without stimulation (Teasdale 1975). The response scores 2.

None. This response is recorded when repeated and varied stimulation provokes no detectable movement of or change of tone in the limbs. It scores 1.

Possible assessment problems. Variations in the motor response may occur during the assessment; therefore, it is the best response that should be scored; for example, if the patient localises to pain on his left side but flexes to pain on his right, the localising response is recorded. Asymmetrical responses are significant, indicating that a focal neurological deficit is present, but overall brain function is more accurately reflected by the level of best response on the better side.

When applying a painful stimulus, it is important to explain to relatives what you are about to do and why you are doing it, otherwise they may feel that unnecessary trauma is being inflicted on their loved one.

Other methods of applying painful stimuli are also used. These include rubbing the patient's sternum or nipping portions of the patient's skin, but result in noticeable bruising and are quite unnecessary as the trapezius pinch or fingertip pressure are the most reliable methods for inducing a response.

Recording other measurements

The Neurological Assessment Chart is used to record additional measurements (see Fig. 30.3) as follows:

- vital signs
  - — blood pressure
  - — heart rate (pulse)
  - — respirations
  - — temperature
- pupil size and reaction
- limb movements.

Vital signs

Blood pressure and heart rate. The famous neurosurgeon Harvey Williams Cushing (1869–1939) noted that a rise in intracranial pressure led to a rise in blood pressure and a fall in heart rate (see Ch. 9). The 'Cushing's Response' does not occur until the later stages of raised intracranial pressure, however, and the Glasgow Coma Scale will show evidence of deterioration much earlier.

Changes in the blood pressure and heart rate can indicate injury or disease elsewhere in the body; for example, falling blood pressure and a rapid and weak heart rate are indicative of haemorrhage and shock.

Respirations. Conditions that impair consciousness may also cause respiratory changes. The pattern and rate of respiration may be directly affected by brain damage. The rate of respirations is recorded on the chart, but it is also important for the nurse to observe the pattern of respirations by making a separate note in the patient's nursing care plan. Deep lesions in the cerebrum and midbrain tend to produce a periodic pattern such as Cheyne-Stokes respiration (see Ch. 3). Lesions affecting the pons and medulla cause more irregular patterns.

Temperature. Impaired brain function seldom causes significant changes in body temperature unless there has been direct damage to the temperature-regulating centre in the hypothalamus (see Ch. 22). A gradual elevation is likely to be an early sign of infection in the lungs or urinary tract, or a wound. Each rise in degree of temperature increases the brain's metabolic rate which further affects the injured organ.

Pupil size and reaction

The size of both pupils is measured by comparing them with a series of circular millimetre measures on the chart (Fig. 30.3). Reaction to light is scored by a plus (+) whereas no reaction is recorded by a minus (–). Pupil reactions should be assessed in dim surroundings, using a bright flashlight. To elicit the direct-light reflex, the nurse holds each of the patient's eyelids open in turn and shines the light directly into the eye. This should cause a brisk constriction of the pupil. The size and reaction are observed and recorded on the chart.

A widely dilated and non-reactive pupil on one side is indicative of pressure on the oculomotor (IIIrd) nerve. As intracranial pressure increases, the uncus of the temporal lobe herniates through the tentorial hiatus comprising the midbrain and IIIrd nerve (see Ch. 9). An aneurysm on the posterior communicating artery will have the same effect on the pupil. Pinpoint pupils are indicative of lesions of the pons. Haemorrhage and ingestion of opiates usually have the same effect.

Limb movement

Disturbances of limb movement indicate local brain damage and vary according to the site and extent of the damage; for example, the right arm and leg will be affected by a lesion in the left cerebral hemisphere. More diffuse brain damage will result in a greater disturbance of movement.

When no localised brain damage is suspected, such as in metabolic or drug coma, the best motor response on the coma scale is usually sufficient for monitoring responses. When localised brain damage is suspected an additional detailed assessment of each limb is necessary. The nurse observes the limbs for normal power; mild weakness; severe weakness; spastic flexion (arms only); extension; or no response (Fig. 30.3).

The nurse examines the arms and legs for movement and strength, and compares the right and left sides. When the two sides are the same recordings are made in the standard manner (see p. 844). When differences exist, right and left are recorded independently, using 'R' for right and 'L' for left. Responses can be elicited by verbal commands, such as asking the patient to grip the nurse's hand as tightly as possible, to lift up his arms or to bend his knees. To test strength, the nurse may need to provide some form of resistance, such as pressing down on the knee when the patient is trying to bend it.

Painful stimuli may be applied to the appropriate limb if verbal comments fail to elicit a response.

CAUSES OF UNCONSCIOUSNESS

The major causes of unconsciousness are shown in Fig. 30.4.

Unconsciousness occurs when the RAS is damaged or its function depressed so that there is an interruption of the normal arousal mechanisms. This may be caused by a primary or secondary insult to the nervous system. Primary insults are commonly caused by intrinsic diseases of the brain. Secondary involvement is most often caused by metabolic, endocrine or toxic conditions, where the critical insult is manifested elsewhere in the body.

The following conditions have been selected for brief discussion because they can occur in almost any situation, at home, in the street, in the workplace or in hospital:

- hypoglycaemia
- epilepsy
- drug overdose.

Hypoglycaemia

In hypoglycaemia, too much insulin is circulating in the bloodstream (see Ch. 5). The causes are variable, the commonest being:

- insufficient food after insulin has been administered
- miscalculation of the dose or strength of insulin
- unusual physical exertion
- mental stress.

The energy of the central nervous system (CNS) is reliant on glucose metabolism (Mahon 1979). An increased amount of insulin in the bloodstream will cause the blood glucose level to fall. The metabolism of the CNS therefore becomes depressed. Initially the CNS becomes excitable, which is manifested by hallucinations or illusions and extreme nervousness. Loss of consciousness occurs when the blood glucose levels fall to between 50% and 20% of normal values.

Epilepsy

Epilepsy is caused by an abnormal electrical discharge from an unstable group of nerve cells in the brain (Markham 1979). It is a symptom of disturbed cerebral function which consists of episodes where there is a disturbance of movement, sensation, behaviour or consciousness.

During the tonic phase of a grand mal epileptic seizure, unconsciousness is profound, with rigid contractions of all muscles, causing apnoea and cyanosis (see Ch. 9). Unconsciousness is also a feature of the chronic phase of a seizure. Status epilepticus is a medical emergency which is manifested by a series of fits where one seizure follows the other without the patient regaining consciousness.

Drug overdose

Impaired consciousness is often a characteristic of drug taking. Sometimes it is a side effect but more often it is the reason for self-medication and illegal drug use (Woollatt 1979).

Barbiturates have played an important part in anaesthesia and in the treatment of epilepsy. (**Note:** There is now a new generation of anti-epileptic drugs which do not have a sedative effect. See Ch. 9.) It is, however, the effectiveness of barbiturates as sedatives that has made them both popular and contentious. Barbiturates act by depressing the RAS. The action of barbiturates is often potentiated by alcohol. Consumption of large amounts of alcohol also tends to produce disinhibition and depression.

Ghodse (1977) showed that barbiturates were the drug of accidental overdose in over 50% of drug-dependent individuals treated in London casualty departments. Drug addicts also tend to dissolve barbiturate tablets in water and inject the preparation into their veins. This crude and often unsterile technique increases the incidence of systemic diseases such as septicaemia.

EMERGENCY CARE OF THE UNCONSCIOUS PATIENT

Whatever the cause of unconsciousness and wherever the event occurs, the patient's life depends on the knowledge and skills of those who find him. The first aid and care that he receives until he regains consciousness (if this is achievable) will predict the outcome for the patient (see Boxes 30.2 and 30.3).

A hospital emergency

In a hospital ward or department, a patient can be rendered unconscious by any of the causes shown in Fig. 30.4. The victim does not necessarily need to be a patient; visitors or members of staff are also at risk from events such as cardiac arrest, cerebrovascular accident or falls, resulting in head injury. The measures a nurse should take if she finds a collapsed patient are as follows.

1. Shout for assistance and press the nurse call button.

Box 30.2 First aid for an unconscious patient

1. Check the victim's breathing and pulse. If he is not breathing and a pulse is not felt in the carotid artery, turn him onto his back and initiate cardiopulmonary resuscitation (see Ch. 2). If possible, get help to do this.
2. Send someone to telephone for an ambulance. Make sure that the person knows the location and has some details of the victim.
3. If the victim is breathing and has a pulse, loosen his clothing at the neck, chest and waist. Try to ensure plenty of fresh air by opening windows and doors or keeping bystanders away from the victim.
4. Clear the victim's airway with your finger. Remove dentures or dental plates, if possible, and keep them in a safe place.
5. Check for any other injuries or bruises and stem any bleeding.
6. Place the victim in the unconscious or recovery position, as follows.
   a) Kneel beside him and place his arms alongside his body.
   b) Cross the ankle furthest away from you over the one nearest to you.
   c) Turn him over, cushioning his head with your hand.
   d) Place your other hand on the hip furthest from you and roll him gently towards you by resting him on your thighs.
   e) Maintain a clear airway by grasping under his jaw and moving his chin upwards and backwards. This extends his neck and prevents his tongue from falling back into his throat.
   f) Pull up the arm nearest to you so that the point of the elbow is in line with the victim's shoulder.
   This position prevents the victim's tongue from falling into the back of his throat and choking him. It also allows fluid, such as blood or vomit, to drain from his mouth.
   The position is *contraindicated* in victims with suspected *spinal injury*, when movement risks further damage to the spinal cord (see Chs 19 and 28).
7. Stay with the victim until the ambulance arrives. If possible, accompany him to hospital. Failing this, give a detailed account of events to the ambulance attendants. This should include how the victim was found and what resuscitative measures were taken.

Box 30.3 Additional first-aid considerations in hypoglycaemic coma, epileptic seizure and drug overdose

HYPOGLYCAEMIC COMA

1. Initiate cardiopulmonary resuscitation (CPR), if necessary.
2. Place the victim in the unconscious or recovery position.
3. Look for medical-alert jewellery or a diabetic card.
4. Transport to hospital as quickly as possible.

EPILEPTIC SEIZURE

1. **Do not** place a wedge in the victim's mouth. It is preferable for the victim to have a bitten tongue than broken teeth, which could obstruct the airway.
2. Place the victim in the unconscious or recovery position, if possible. Remove any objects that could cause further injury.
3. Gently restrain the victim to prevent further damage, particularly by the drumming of heels on the ground.
4. **Do not** attempt to restrain all movements, as this requires too much force.
5. Transport to hospital as quickly as possible.

DRUG OVERDOSE

1. Initiate CPR, if necessary.
2. Place the victim in the unconscious or recovery position.
3. Keep any vomit, tablet bottles or containers to help identify the drug taken.
4. Transport to hospital as quickly as possible.

Note: Addicts who inject drugs will have visible needle marks on their arms. If alcohol has been ingested there will usually be a distinct odour from the victim's breath.

2. Move the patient into a wider space if this is possible.
3. Initiate CPR if the patient is not breathing and the carotid pulse is absent. The cardiac arrest team should be called at this point.
4. If the patient is breathing and a pulse is present, place him in the unconscious or recovery position. Stay with the patient until assistance arrives and he can be moved to his bed for further treatment and investigation.

Planned admission

When an unconscious patient is to be admitted to a ward or department, the following measures must be taken.

1. Remove the top bedclothes and the head of the bed to facilitate easy access to the patient.
2. Check that the oxygen supply and suction apparatus is functioning and that there is an adequate supply of suction catheters.
3. The necessary equipment should be available for immediate use.
   1. A resuscitation trolley containing the following:
      a) Guedel airways (usually size 3 or 4 for an adult)
      b) Ambu resuscitator (commonly called an 'ambu bag') with universal catheter mount
      c) laryngoscope and selection of endotracheal tubes
      d) lubricating jelly; strapping or tape; 5 ml syringe to inflate the endotracheal tube
      e) emergency drug box or pack
      f) a mechanical ventilator, if possible. (Not all wards will have this facility. If the patient is unable to breathe on his own, he is ventilated manually via an endotracheal tube, using an Ambu resuscitator until he can be transferred to an intensive care unit.)
   2. An intravenous infusion stand.
   3. Equipment for the passage of a nasogastric tube to aspirate the stomach contents.
   4. A neurological examination tray.
   5. The appropriate charts and routine admission forms.

Priorities of nurse management

The following checklist itemises the priorities of nurse management in an emergency situation, in order to sustain the patient's vital functions.

1. Maintenance of a clear airway:
   a) the patient's position
   b) artificial airways
   c) suction
   d) oxygen
   e) nasogastric tube.
2. Assessment of the central nervous system:
   a) Glasgow Coma Scale
   b) vital signs
   c) pupillary reactions
   d) limb movements.
3. Maintenance of fluid balance:
   a) intravenous infusion
   b) catheterisation of the urinary bladder.
4. Care of relatives.
   Measures to sustain the vital functions of the patient must take priority over anything else. Relatives of the patient must also be considered, however, and a nurse who is not involved in the immediate care of the patient should be allocated to take care of them. She should provide them with written information regarding hospital procedures and explain the investigations related to the patient's condition. At the same time she will be able to gather the patient's biographical data and other information to help in planning the patient's nursing care.

MEDICAL MANAGEMENT

An unconscious patient is a medical emergency, unless the unconscious state represents the terminal state of a progressive and not specifically treatable disease (Haerer 1976). The cause of the unconscious state must be determined before the appropriate treatment can be given, although life support measures have priority over anything else. These measures include establishment of an adequate airway, control of haemorrhage, and fluid or blood replacement. Stomach lavage is indicated when the victim has ingested an overdose of drugs.

The medical history

The doctor will need to ask certain questions about the patient. It is therefore important that the people who accompanied the patient to hospital do not leave until the doctor has had an opportunity to question them. He will need to find out as much as possible about the medical history and the circumstances preceding and surrounding the onset of the unconscious state. Questions he may ask are listed in Box 30.4.

The physical examination

The general physical examination of the unconscious patient will include special attention to the patient's:

- vital signs
- pattern of respirations

Box 30.4 Questions to ask about the patient

CIRCUMSTANCES PRECEDING THE ONSET OF UNCONSCIOUSNESS (Haerer 1976)

Mode of onset of unconscious state (gradual or abrupt)
Duration of unconscious state
Trauma sustained
Exposure to extremes of temperature
Exposure to electric shock
Exposure to toxins
Drug abuse
Alcohol abuse.

MEDICAL HISTORY

Use of prescription drugs
Exposure to other sick persons
Fever, nausea or vomiting prior to onset
History of heart disease or hypertension
History of respiratory disease
History of diabetes
History of renal or hepatic disease
History of headaches (type and severity)
Major psychiatric illness
Complaints immediately prior to onset.

- signs of trauma
- skin colour and texture
- breath odour.

The symptoms listed in Table 30.1 can provide clues to the cause of the unconscious state.

The doctor will also carry out a neurological examination of the patient. This will involve assessment of the cranial nerves and motor and sensory function. The patient's reflexes will also be tested. The reader is referred to Chapter 9 for a more detailed account of neurological examination.

Laboratory tests

Laboratory tests in unconscious patients usually include a complete blood count, blood glucose levels and blood urea, and electrolyte estimation. Blood gas analysis is obtained when the patient's cardiovascular state is compromised. Screening tests of blood and urine are carried out if drug intoxication, including alcohol, is suspected. The patient's urine is normally checked for glucose, acetone, blood and infection.

Radiological studies

Radiological tests are carried out once the patient has been resuscitated and his condition is stabilised. Chest X-rays and electrocardiograms are routine requirements. Skull and cervical spine X-rays are obtained when head trauma is obvious or suggested from neurological signs (possible injury to the cervical spine should always be suspected in cases of head trauma).

If the diagnosis remains in doubt, computerised axial tomography (CAT scan) may be necessary. The results of an electroencephalogram (EEG) will support the diagnosis of possible causes determined by symptoms, history and clinical examination.

NURSING MANAGEMENT OF THE UNCONSCIOUS PATIENT

The activities of living model described by Roper, Logan and Tierney (1990) is used to illustrate the nursing management of the unconscious patient. This model is based on 12 activities of living. The author has expanded this to include a thirteenth activity, spiritual care, which is taken from the work of Virginia Henderson (1960).

Breathing

Oxygen is essential for the survival of all body cells. Irreversible damage to the brain cells will occur if they are deprived of oxygen, even for a few minutes. Consequently all activities of living and life itself are entirely dependent on breathing and the establishment and maintenance of a patient's airway is essential for the unconscious patient.

Position of the patient

Any obvious obstructions such as dentures or dental plates should be removed. The nurse also needs to be aware of the presence of loose teeth as these could become detached and

Table 30.1 Clues to the cause of unconsciousness on general physical examination

Sign or symptom	Possible cause
Elevated temperature	Infection Heat stroke
Subnormal temperature	Dehydration Alcohol Barbiturate intoxication Myxoedema
Bleeding from the mouth	Epileptic seizure Trauma
Pulse irregularities	Hypoxia from inadequate cardiac output
Slow, regular respirations	Myxoedema Morphine or barbiturate intoxication
Cheyne-Stokes respiration	Bilateral cerebral dysfunction Late stages of increased intracranial pressure Severe cardiopulmonary disease
Ataxic, irregular (cluster) respirations	Lesions of the brain stem — signifies impending apnoea
Breath odour	Alcohol abuse Hepatic dysfunction Renal dysfunction Ingested poisons
Skin	Jaundice Cyanosis Rashes indicating infection Drug abuse
Hypertension	Raised intracranial pressure — Intracranial haemorrhage
Hypotension	Blood loss Septicaemia Myocardial infarction Pulmonary embolism

obstruct the airway. Obstruction may also be caused by bleeding into the oropharynx from head or facial injuries. Vomiting presents another hazard. The insertion of a nasogastric tube in the initial stages of coma will facilitate the emptying of the stomach, thus helping to avoid the potential aspiration of gastric contents into the respiratory tract.

The patient should be nursed in a semi-prone position with the head of the bed tilted slightly upwards (10–30°). This prevents the tongue from obstructing the airway, encourages the drainage of respiratory secretions and saliva and therefore reduces the danger of aspiration into the lungs. Pillows positioned at the patient's back and between his knees help maintain the position. At no time should an unconscious patient be flat on his back, except to facilitate medical procedures, for example, intubation or radiological studies.

Artificial airways

The unconscious patient's cough reflex is depressed, so he is unable to cough and clear his own airway. The use of artificial airways may therefore be required.

Oropharyngeal airway. The Guedal Airway is the oropharyngeal airway most commonly used in UK hospitals. These have the advantage of relatively easy insertion and are available in varying sizes to facilitate the needs of individual patients. The airway is designed to lie over the tongue and permit the passage of air into the pharynx (Fig. 30.7). It keeps the patient's tongue from obstructing his throat and it has a passage that allows the patient to breathe through the device. It also allows easier access to facilitate suction of the mouth and throat.

Endotracheal tube. An endotracheal tube is indicated if the Guedal Airway proves inadequate. The tube is usually made of plastic and has an inflatable cuff (Fig. 30.8). The tube is inserted by a doctor through the mouth or nose. It is then passed into the trachea to a point above the bifurcation of the trachea which is proximal to the bronchi. This permits deep suctioning. Breath sounds are determined immediately after insertion to make certain that the tube is properly positioned and is not obstructing one of the primary bronchi. The tube is then inflated with air. It is recommended that this be the smallest volume of air needed to inflate the cuff to barely occlude the trachea (Mulvaney 1976). The inflated cuff provides an airtight seal, particularly when mechanical ventilation is required. It also prevents the aspiration of material from the digestive tract. The tube is secured in position by zinc oxide tape or tied with ribbon gauze. It is the nurse's responsibility to check the patency and position of the tube.

In some hospitals the practice of deflating the cuff for a few

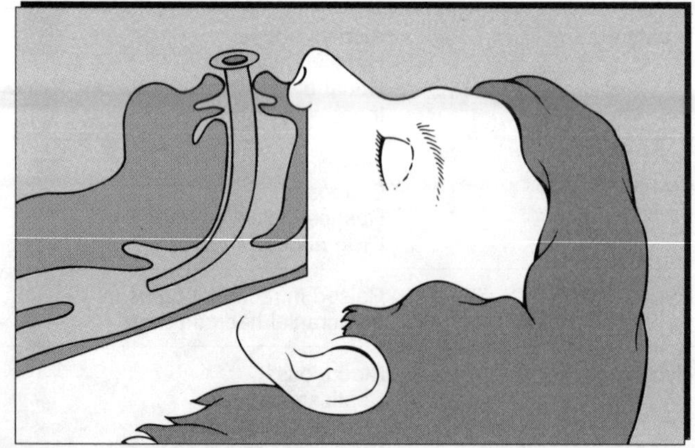

Fig. 30.7 A Guedal airway in situ.

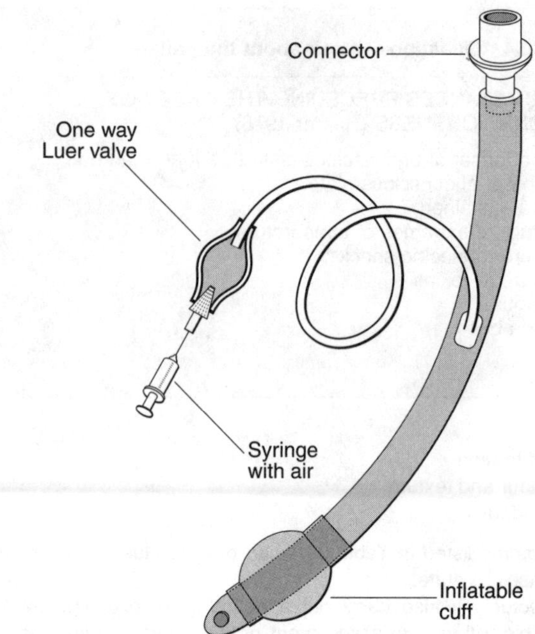

Fig. 30.8 Endotracheal tube.

minutes each hour is employed in order to minimise the occurrence of erosion of the tracheal wall. The value of this practice is questionable (Bryant et al 1971; Powaser 1976). Hourly five-minute cuff deflations did not lessen tracheal damage and when periodic cuff deflats were ordered there was a tendency to over-inflate the tube. The nurse must be aware of the local policy on this practice.

Tracheostomy tube. The tracheostomy bypasses any obstructions in the upper airway and facilitates suctioning of bronchial secretions. Tracheostomy is usually indicated if endotracheal intubation is to be prolonged. An endotracheal tube is not usually left in situ for more than 3–4 days.

An incision is made into the trachea through the second and third, or third and fourth, tracheal rings. The tube is inserted and secured with tape. The tubes are made of silver, plastic or nylon and may be cuffed or uncuffed (see Ch. 14).

Most tubes consist of three parts: an obturator to insert the tube, an outer cannula and an inner cannula. The advantage of a tube with an inner cannula is that this can be removed every 2–4 hours for cleaning, and then replaced. This prevents the potential danger of obstruction with secretions. The procedure can also be carried out without disturbing the outer tube. This reduces the frequency of outer tube changes, thus minimising the risk of trauma to the stoma and trachea.

Infection is a potential problem and the tracheal stoma should always be treated like an open wound. The incidence and severity may be minimised by keeping the wound area free of secretions that collect around the tube. Using an aseptic technique, the nurse cleanses the stoma according to local policy. A sterile absorbent, non-adherent dressing may be applied. It is, however, usually better to dispense with any dressing around the tracheostomy tube after initial bleeding has stopped (De Young 1983). The dressing may hide secretions and act as a culture medium for bacteria.

The policy with regard to inflation and deflation of the cuffs of endotracheal tubes also applies to tracheostomy tubes.

Suctioning

The nurse carries out suctioning to remove potentially dangerous secretions from the oropharynx, trachea and bronchi. The nurse's assessment of the patient's colour, his respiratory rate and pattern will indicate how often this is required. Specific indicators include one or more of the following:

- signs of cyanosis
- increased and irregular respirations
- noisy, gurgling respirations.

The following equipment is required:

- a piped source of vacuum pressure, indicating calibrated pressures, or a portable suction device
- a collection jar and disposable connecting tubing
- disposable plastic sterile suction catheters of the correct size for the patient (usually 12–14 French gauge for an adult)
- disposable plastic gloves
- bowl of sterile normal saline
- masks (optional).

Procedure. Each ward will have its own policy regarding suctioning but the procedure described by Allan (1988) provides a general example.

- Explain the procedure to the patient.
- Assemble the equipment needed (masks are advocated in some units for the nurse's protection). Turn on the suction device to 100–120 mmHg.
- Wash hands and pour the saline into a sterile bowl.
- Administer oxygen to the patient, if necessary.
- Break open the packet containing the sterile catheter and put the glove on the dominant hand.
- Attach the catheter to the connecting tube, taking care not to contaminate the catheter.
- Insert the catheter into the airway without applying suction, that is, leaving the side porthole uncovered.
- Advance the catheter as far as it will easily pass.
- Withdraw the catheter a few centimetres and apply suction by occluding the side porthole. Suction is applied intermittently as the catheter is slowly withdrawn, using a rotating action.
- As many secretions are removed as possible within a time limit of *15 seconds*.
- The catheter is removed and discarded and the tubing is rinsed through with saline. The patient is given at least 60 seconds to recover before suctioning again. Oxygen is given, if required.
- If all the secretions have not been removed, the procedure is repeated using a new sterile catheter.
- Using a separate catheter, the patient's mouth and nose are suctioned at the end of the procedure. Nasal suction is contraindicated if the patient has sustained a frontal skull fracture or has cerebrospinal fluid (CSF) rhinorrhoea. The passage of a suction catheter through the nose could lead to damage to brain tissue and infection.
- Collection jars should be emptied and disinfected at least once every 24 hours during regular use.

Immediately before suctioning some units advocate the instillation of 5–10 ml of sterile, normal saline into the airway in order to loosen the secretions. The value of this technique is, however, questioned (De Carle 1985, Ackerman 1985). Ackerman argues that this practice can irritate the mucosa and has little or no value in thinning, mobilising or removing dried secretions.

Humidification

Normally the air drawn into the lungs is warmed, moistened and filtered through the nose and upper respiratory tract. If the patient has an endotracheal or tracheostomy tube, the air is dry so a humidifier must be used, otherwise irritated mucous membranes and dried tenacious secretions soon result.

The humidifier is attached to the oxygen supply and filled with sterile water that is heated to a temperature of 35–40 °C. This allows for a drop to body temperature by the time the air reaches the patient. The nurse checks the temperature and water level at frequent intervals and adjusts as necessary.

Oxygen

The amount of oxygen prescribed depends on the respiratory status of the patient and the laboratory evaluation of his arterial blood gases. A specimen of arterial blood is taken to ascertain the pH, partial pressure of oxygen (pO_2) and carbon dioxide (pCO_2). Deviations from normal values may be corrected by an increase or decrease in the amount of oxygen delivered. Mechanical ventilation may be indicated to assure adequate oxygenation.

There are various methods of administering oxygen and the doctor's prescription will include instructions about the rate of flow, duration of therapy and type of equipment to be used. It is within the remit of the nurse to monitor the administration of oxygen and to observe the patient for complications. The reader is referred to Ch. 3 for a more detailed account on the administration of oxygen.

Role of the physiotherapist

The prevention of respiratory complications is a priority in the nursing management of the unconscious patient but infection may occur despite every precaution being taken. Antibiotics are effective against organisms but the patient could drown in his own purulent secretions unless these are removed. The patient is, therefore, even more dependent on the skill and cooperation of the nurse and physiotherapist.

The physiotherapist will visit the patient regularly each day to assist in chest care by 'clapping', shaking and suction. 'Clapping' is a method of loosening sputum within the lungs by externally beating the chest wall. The physiotherapist uses her cupped hands alternately in a gentle, relaxed, rhythmic manner. The procedure is performed over the whole chest wall, starting at the base and working towards the bronchi. This is followed by shaking the chest to dislodge sputum and stimulate coughing (Verran & Aisbitt 1988).

Communicating

The patient

There is evidence of patients recalling, with startling accuracy, conversations they have overheard whilst unconscious. Conversations not intended for the patient should not be held in his presence as unguarded or misinterpreted expressions can cause distress.

It is imperative that the nurse explains clearly and simply to the patient every aspect of his care, whether it is related to the associated equipment or the patient's progress. The explanations and reassurances need to be repeated whenever a procedure is carried out.

Research (Allan 1986) has indicated that recovery from certain types of coma is faster when all the patient's senses are bombarded, for example with common smells, distinctive flavours, soft or harsh fabrics, visual stimuli, for example, a torch, and certain types of sound, such as favourite music. The BLAT (British Life Assurance Trust) Centre for Health and Medical Education have devised a COMAKIT (a programme of intense stimulation) which it supplies to relatives. They must obtain permission from the patient's doctor, before using the kit.

The family

Relatives and other visitors will be bewildered when they see the unconscious patient with his associated equipment, particularly for the first time. Time should be spent with them before they see the patient in order to explain what is happening, and what the patient looks like. A brief explanation of the immediate environment and the function of any equipment is provided and the relative should be encouraged to speak with and touch the patient. The family should be provided with an opportunity to ask any questions and should be able to speak with the doctor or nurse in charge about the patient's progress. Many misconceptions have developed, particularly through the media, about coma and these should be corrected.

?	**30.1** Can you think of any of these misconceptions? How might you correct them?

Rest and sleep

Providing rest for a patient is one of the most difficult problems confronting the nurse and it is doubtful whether it is ever achieved with the associated hospital background noise. Rest is said to occur when the person:

- is in control of his environment
- is accepted by himself and others
- understands his current situation
- is free of physical or mental discomfort
- is involved in purposeful activity
- is aware that help is available if needed (Narrow 1967).

Eating and drinking

The unconscious patient will be unable to eat or drink in the normal way and will need to receive nourishment and fluids by an alternative method. An adequate fluid intake also helps to prevent dehydration, which can result in the drying and thickening of secretions, making suctioning difficult and creating a breeding ground for bacteria.

Fluids

The usual method of administering fluids to an unconscious patient is intravenously and usually peripherally. The fluids are sometimes administered via a central line, usually placed in the subclavian vein. Intravenous (i.v.) fluids are also given to:

- administer medications, such as antibiotics
- administer additional electrolytes, such as potassium, to correct imbalances.

Fluid intake is normally prescribed by medical staff on the patient's fluid balance chart, following scrutiny of the patient's serum electrolyte levels which are drawn on a daily basis. Fluids are usually prescribed for the following 24 hours although in seriously ill patients it may be for a much shorter period. It is essential that the correct fluids are administered at the prescribed rate to maintain fluid balance.

Care of the intravenous cannulae will be in accordance with local policy. Cannulae and their insertion sites will require closer attention than usual. The likelihood of problems such as thrombophlebitis developing is increased due to the presence of potentially irritant substances such as drugs. The failure of the intravenous infusion at a crucial moment, for example, when an anticonvulsant is quickly needed, could be disastrous for the patient. To avoid this situation there is usually more than one cannula in place, but the presence of multiple intravenous infusions increase the likelihood of infection.

Lines and ports can be labelled with different colours to distinguish them. An additional problem is that the patient may also have in place an arterial line, which looks very similar to an intravenous cannula and could be easily mistaken for one. Strict rules exist for the identification of arterial lines.

Observations. During the course of the infusion the following observations are required.

1. Possible fluid (circulatory) overload, indicated by overdistended neck veins. Overhydration can occur, particularly if the patient is prone to right-sided heart failure. These patients are sensitive to fluid shift and the excess fluid has a tendency to accumulate in the lungs, further adding to the patient's respiratory problems.
2. Reactions to medications which may be incompatible. In departments likely to administer mixtures of intravenous medications, information should be readily available detailing known drug interactions. This is backed up with support and guidance from hospital pharmacy services. In some centres the intravenous drugs are prepared by the pharmacy and this can act as a secondary checking system.
3. Urinary output should be measured hourly. A decrease could result in circulatory overload and electrolyte imbalances.
4. The infusion site should be observed for:
   a. signs of infiltration
   b. signs of thrombophlebitis.
5. The cannulae should be checked to ensure that they are securely attached to the giving set (Luer Lok connections are the safest) and that the tape fixing it to the patient's skin is intact.
6. The intravenous tubing should not be kinked or the flow impeded in any other way.
7. Ensure that the correct fluids are infusing at the prescribed rate. An infusion pump may be used to ensure accurate flow rates in the seriously ill patient.

Nutrition

Provision of adequate nutrition is important in the unconscious patient. Malnourishment will result in loss of muscle mass and energy, both essential for recovery, and weakening of the body's immune system.

Intragastric tube. The easiest and most economical way to provide an alternative means of feeding is with an intragastric tube, passed either nasally or orally. These were traditionally wide bore but newer fine-bore tubes are said to be more comfortable for the patient (James 1982). Intragastric tube feeding is the most frequently used method in the unconscious patient and, if the patient's alimentary tract is functional, is the preferred method to provide total nutritional support. The patient's nutritional requirements should be assessed and the appropriate dietary solutions prescribed with the help and advice of the dietitian. Examples of proprietory feeds are Ensure and Clinifeed. The patient's nutritional status will require to be reappraised at regular intervals.

Daily nutritional requirements are usually calculated on the basis of body weight.

Complications include:

- misplacement of the feeding tube
- diarrhoea.

A misplaced tube could result in the feed being administered into the trachea instead of the oesophagus, resulting in aspiration and serious deterioration of the patient's respiratory status. Feeding the patient in a slight head up tilt or sitting position is recommended to reduce this risk, although this is not always possible. This problem can be prevented by frequently checking the position of the feeding tube, to ascertain that it is in the stomach. If aspiration is suspected, indicated by obtaining feed on trachea suctioning, then it can be tested with a reagent dipstick. This will prove positive if there is feed present as normal respiratory tract secretions do not contain sugar.

Diarrhoea is commonly due to the too-rapid introduction of concentrated hyperosmolar nutrient solutions into the alimentary tract. This is the main reason for using a slow continuous-drip method for tube feeding rather than the more traditional bolus method. Antibiotic therapy may also be the culprit. Diarrhoea is profoundly distressing to a fully dependent patient and if it occurs the feeding method and regime should be scrutinised (see Ch. 21 and Ch. 20).

Parenteral feeding, a more complex method, may be indicated in patients who are unable to tolerate any other method. It requires the placement of a central line as the feeding solutions irritate the peripheral blood vessels. Total parenteral nutrition (TPN) should only be administered under very careful conditions and in departments familiar with the routine.

Complications of TPN are:

- pneumothorax
- infection
- metabolic complications.

During placement of the central catheter, a lung may be accidentally pierced, resulting in a pneumothorax, which will compromise the patient's respiratory system and necessitate the insertion of a chest drain.

Infection may occur if a suspect aseptic technique is used during insertion of the central catheter, giving nutrient solutions. It is recommended that feeding solutions are prepared under a laminar flow by an experienced pharmacist.

Metabolic complications are usually due to too rapid administration of hypertonic dextrose solutions, causing hyperglycaemia. Routine monitoring of blood sugar will detect this. In some instances, a slow continuous infusion of insulin is given.

As the patient begins to gain strength it may be possible, even with a tube still in place, to allow the patient to taste some soft ice-cream. This will give the patient positive sensory stimulation and indicate to him that some progress is being made.

A gradual return to a more substantial diet is then undertaken according to the patient's progress.

Elimination

Confinement to bed requires alterations to the normal means of elimination and the ability of the patient to urinate or defecate is impaired by his altered level of consciousness.

The patient will not be able to indicate when he requires the toilet so catheterisation is the usual recourse for urinary elimination. Despite the acknowledged dangers, if the patient is unconscious for more than 24–36 hours catheterisation should be considered. It helps to retain the patient's dignity and avoid the embarrassment of incontinence. An accurate measurement of urinary output is also often required and a closed collection system provides this.

Not all unconscious patients require to be catheterised. Many male patients can be managed with external penile collection devices such as uri-sheaths. This is useful once the initial acute period is over and the patient is stabilising.

There is no ready solution for the management of defecation. The patient's bowel movements ought to be monitored, particularly if receiving tube feeding. If necessary, prophylactic stool softeners may be needed in order to produce a stool every other day. It is important for the patient to avoid straining as this will raise intracranial pressure.

Personal cleansing and dressing

The unconscious patient is dependent upon the nurse to attend to all aspects of personal cleansing and dressing, but still has the right to have these procedures performed in privacy. This is especially important when performing intimate procedures such as the provision of personal hygiene in the menstruating female or in giving urinary catheter care.

Bathing in bed is normal for any dependent patient but when turning the unconscious patient to wash his back there is a danger that the airway may become compromised and the patient's chest movement may be impeded. To avoid this, turning should be planned and requires a minimum of two nurses to execute it safely. Bathing, hair and nail care should all be performed as often as necessary. Hair washing can be difficult and, if the use of wet shampoos is impossible, a dry shampoo could be used. Nails should be kept short and clean.

Eye care is carried out on a regular basis to prevent damage caused by dryness of the patient's corneas. In the deeply unconscious patient the unresponsive eye, particularly the cornea, can also be damaged.

The eye and the immediate surrounding area is cleansed with sterile saline, followed by artificial tear drops. If the patient's eyelids will close naturally, this should be done but, if not, perhaps because of swelling, tape may need to be applied. If tape is used, the delicate skin of the eyelid will need to be closely observed for excoriation. This can be minimised by regularly altering the position of the tape.

Oral hygiene can cause difficulties as the presence of an artificial airway prevents the usual access to the mucosal lining of the mouth. The objective of good oral hygiene is a mouth which is clean, comfortable for the patient, and moist and free of infection (Gibbons 1983). Gibbons further recommends that a small multi-tufted, child's toothbrush should be used with a fluoride-based toothpaste or, if indicated, a chlorhexidine-based gel, which will reduce plaque and the incidence of gingivitis. Brushing of teeth can still be performed by manoeuvring around the artificial airway, using the toothbrush to reach as far back as possible in the mouth.

A sodium bicarbonate solution is the most appropriate for a dry, encrusted mouth and vaseline should be applied to dry lips. Some patients may benefit from chlorhexidine mouthwashes. The importance of brushing the whole mouth is stressed.

The prevention of pressure sores is also important for good practice. Regular alteration of the patient's position is the main factor. Other causative factors have been identified in the literature and the reader is referred to these for further information.

Maintaining a safe environment

The unconscious patient is vulnerable to many threats and maintaining a safe environment can pose problems for nursing staff.

Infection

The unconscious patient is at risk of infection occurring in the chest and bladder. The most commonly acquired infection associated with respiratory therapy is Gram negative bacillary pneumonia, which is constantly present in the environment. Most people are resistant to it, but certain factors contribute to the breaking down of our physiological and immunological defences and the unconscious patient fulfils many of these, including endotracheal intubation and the presence of invasive lines such as intravenous cannulae and urinary catheters.

The mechanism of infection. Infection will occur if a sufficient number of microbes reaches the lower respiratory tract or urinary bladder. The likelihood of infection occurring depends on the virulence of the organism and the susceptibility of the patient. Ironically, the original source of the Gram negative bacilli is often the patient himself. It can spread from the digestive tract, its usual home, into the lungs or bladder, given the correct conditions. Endotracheal or tracheostomy tubes which bypass the normal protective mechanism of the nose, encourage the spread of infection and a depressed cough reflex encourages pooling of secretions within the lungs, resulting in stasis. Urinary bladder catheterisation provides a ready entry route to the bladder. Preventative measures, in which the nurse plays a major role, include:

- unit design
- a control-of-infection policy
- aseptic techniques.

Medication

The hazards of administering medication to patients are well documented but the risks are increased in the unconscious patient for two reasons.

1. The routes that require to be used carry a greater risk for the patient. The simpler, and safer oral route is usually contra-indicated. Other methods of administration require to be utilised including intramuscular injections, intravenous infusions, via an intragastric tube, and per rectum.
2. The patient cannot confirm his identity so the nurse must be vigilant in ensuring that the medication is being given to the correct patient.

The types of medications most commonly used in the unconscious patient include analgesics, anticonvulsants, antibiotics and laxatives.

Motor and sensory loss or impairment

The motor and sensory loss experienced by unconscious patients may be drug induced or it may be part of the underlying disease process. Whatever the cause, the nursing intervention remains the same.

Motor loss. See the section on 'Mobilisation'.

Sensory loss. The sensory system is part of the body's defence system and the unconscious patient is unable to process sensory information. It is imperative that the patient is not exposed to extremes of temperature, particularly in a localised area of the skin, for example, if heating or cooling devices are used.

Seizure

The role of the nurse (or onlooker) when a patient has a seizure is to ensure that the patient does not harm himself (see Box 30.5).

Recording an observed seizure. Detailed record of seizure activity is crucial to effective treatment. One suitable approach to observation is as follows.

1. Did the person cry out or attract the nurse's attention in any way?
2. What was the patient doing when the seizure started?
3. Did the position of the body change after the onset of the seizure?
4. Did the eyes deviate in one direction? Did the pupils change in size, were they equal or did they react to light during the attack or after?
5. Did the face and lips change colour?
6. Was there frothing at the mouth or flecks of blood?
7. Was there a tonic phase? How long did it last and what parts of the body were involved?
8. Was there twitching or jerking of any particular part of the body? Where did it begin? How did it spread and how long did it last?
9. Was the patient unconscious, and for how long?
10. How was the patient after the attack? Was he confused or did he have difficulties with speech, or complain of having a headache?
11. How long did the attack last?
12. Did the patient have incontinence of urine or sustain any injury from the attack?

Mobilisation

The nursing management of mobilisation and activity remains the same whatever the cause of the unconsciousness, whether it is drug-induced or part of the disease process. Lack of attention to mobilisation could lead to the development of:

- contractures
- muscle atrophy
- pressure sores
- postural hypotension
- deep-vein thrombosis
- hypostatic pneumonia.

Any one of these hazards will delay the patient's rehabilitation and result in additional pain.

Range-of-movement (ROM) exercises

Whilst the patient remains dependent, the nurse is responsible,

Box 30.5 Dealing with a seizure (from Lindsay 1988)

WHAT TO DO WHEN SOMEONE HAS A SEIZURE

- Stay calm. Do not try to restrain or revive the person.
- Help the person into the recovery position on the floor (or in bed) and put something soft under their head.
- Remove glasses and loosen any tight clothing. Remove hazards, such as hard objects that could cause injury if the person falls or knocks against them.
- If respiration continues to be laboured after the movements have stopped, gently check that saliva, vomit or dentures are not blocking the back of the throat.
- There will be no memory of the seizure and the person should not be left alone until fully alert. Some people are quite able to resume their normal routines after a period of sleep or quiet rest. Calm reassurance is needed as the person may feel embarrassed or disorientated after an attack.

WHAT NOT TO DO

- Do not try to revive the person. A seizure cannot be stopped once it has begun.
- Never attempt to force anything between the teeth. It is impossible to swallow the tongue, and cut tissue on lips and tongue heals but broken teeth are a social embarrassment.
- There is no need to call the doctor if the seizure ends in under 15 minutes, if consciousness returns without further incident and if there are no signs of injury, physical distress or pregnancy.
- Do not give anything to drink until the person is fully awake.

along with the physiotherapist, for ensuring that the patient's limbs are put through a range-of-movement (ROM) exercise programme, which exercises each joint through its full movement range.

Stages of ROM exercise. There are three levels:

- passive
- active–assistive
- active.

Passive. Initially the nurse makes all the effort during ROM exercises, that is, without the cooperation of the patient. These are 'passive' ROM exercises.

Active-assistive. As the patient progresses he may be able to cooperate. The exercises then become 'active–assistive', that is, the movement is initiated by the patient but with the assistance of another person.

Active. The final stage is 'active', with the patient making all the effort against some resistance.

Procedure. ROM exercises should be performed at 4-hourly intervals, over a 24-hour period. They are not just performed by the physiotherapist; a schedule should be agreed for each individual patient and implemented by all concerned with the patient's care. The exercises should not be performed if the affected limb is injured or if contra-indicated by medical treatment.

To perform ROM exercises, one hand is placed above the joint to provide support against gravity and prevent any unwanted movement. The joint is then exercised by smooth, slow, rhythmical movement through its range. The movement should stop at its normal extreme but sooner if the patient expresses pain or the nurse feels resistance. To carry out the procedure proficiently, the nurse should adopt a good upright stance to maintain her own posture. The usual pattern of exercises consists of five repetitions of movement for each limb, gradually increasing to a maximum of 10 as the patient's toleration increases. Relatives sometimes learn to carry out these exercises for the patient as a way of becoming involved in his care.

Recovery from coma

Patients who have been nursed in bed for just a few days often experience dizziness and light-headedness when they sit up for the first time and the patient recovering from coma, who may also have some motor weakness, is no exception. It is advisable to nurse the patient in a sitting position in bed for a couple of days, before progressing to sitting in a chair. This will help the patient to get used to the position and will give a psychological boost.

The nurse should check the patient's vital signs and colour, and ask whether he is experiencing any untoward symptoms. If he is, the mobilisation programme should be implemented at a slower rate.

The patient will be very unsure and frightened of altering his position so repeated explanations of what is expected of him will provide the necessary reassurance.

If the patient has not suffered any ill efects, he can progress to sitting on the edge of the bed. This will require the full co-operation of the patient and the assistance of two, preferably three, nurses. On the first occasion, the patient should sit for no more than 10 minutes. The patient's colour and vital signs should be observed, as outlined earlier. If the patient's respiratory status is not compromised, the length of time and frequency of sitting can be gradually increased.

Sitting up in a chair is the final act of mobilisation. The procedure is as already outlined, ensuring that the patient does not suffer any ill effects. The patient with motor loss or impairment can sit up if given a high-backed chair, provided that adequate support is provided. Once in the chair any equipment which the patient is able to use, such as call bells, drinks, radio or newspapers should be readily available to him. The amount of time that the patient is up sitting should be noted; it is more beneficial for the patient to sit up for several short intervals in one day rather than one long period.

Controlling body temperature

Body temperature requires to be maintained within a relatively constant range to sustain life, that is, 36–37.5 °C. It is controlled by the heat regulating centre in the hypothalamus, which acts like a thermostat. Pyrexia, an abnormally high temperature, is more commonly seen in the unconscious patient than hypothermia, an abnormally low temperature.

Pyrexia may be due to damage to the heat-regulating centre in the hypothalamus or to an infective process or metabolic disorder (see Ch. 22). The danger is that for each degree of temperature over the normal range a proportionately greater amount of oxygen is utilised from the patient's often diminishing reserves, which may have serious implications for recovery.

The nursing interventions remain similar irrespective of the cause of pyrexia.

Measurement of temperature

The most popular method of temperature measurement is the mercurial thermometer, placed in the axilla or anus. The use of oral measurements in the unconscious patient is contra-indicated. The usual precautions and limitations of these methods should be borne in mind when undertaking this important procedure (see Ch. 22).

Dying

Care of the unconscious patient often saves life, but some patients will die despite all measures taken. Active treatment may have been continued right up until the last moment, or it may have been decided that no further active intervention will benefit the patient. The emphasis would then move from curative to terminal care. A third possibility is that the patient fulfils the criteria for brain-stem death.

Brain-stem death

Certain patients in apnoeic coma can suffer severe and irreversible brain damage but continue to have their blood pressure, heartbeat and respirations artificially maintained for a period of time by drug therapy and other life-support interventions. However, some of these patients will never recover and the brain-stem death criteria are designed to identify those patients in order that therapy can cease.

Brain-stem death may be clinically diagnosed following a set of guidelines issued by the Conference of Medical Royal Colleges and their Faculties (1976, with minor update in 1983). These consist of a number of tests that can only be applied after a series of pre-conditions have been fulfilled (see Fig. 30.9).

Pre-conditions. These include positively diagnosed structural damage that is irreversible, and loss of brain-stem function. The examiner must satisfy himself that any reversible causes of coma have been eliminated. These include:

- the ingestion of depressant drugs, for example, in an overdose
- the administration of a neuromuscular blocking agent such as Pavulon to facilitate passage of an endotracheal tube
- primary hypothermia
- metabolic imbalances such as uncontrolled diabetes (Allan 1987).

Diagnosis to be made by two doctors, one a Consultant and the other a Consultant or Senior Registrar.

Diagnosis should not be considered until at least 6 hours after the onset of Coma; 12–24 hours will be more usual.

NAME: .... **UNIT NO.** ....

PRE-CONDITIONS	**Time of event leading to coma**
Nature of irremediable brain damage	
Dr A	....
Dr B	....

Do you consider that Apnoeic Coma is due to:	**Dr A**	**Dr B**
Depressant Drugs		
Neuromuscular Blocking (relaxant) drugs		
Hypothermia		
Metabolic or Endocrine Disturbances		

TESTS FOR ABSENCE OF BRAIN STEM FUNCTION	**Dr A**	**Dr B**
Is there evidence of:		
Pupil reaction to light		
Corneal reflex		
Eye Movements with Cold Caloric Test		
Cranial Nerve Motor Responses		
Gag reflex		
Respiratory movements on disconnection from Ventilator to allow adequate rise in $PaCo_2$		

Date and time of First Testing ....

Date and time of Second Testing ....

Dr A	**Dr B**
Signature	....
Status	....

Fig. 30.9 Criteria for the diagnosis of brain death. (Reproduced with kind permission from Professional Nurse where this figure first appeared.)

Testing brain-stem function. Once satisfied that the pre-conditions have been fulfilled the testing of brain-stem function can be performed. There are six parts to this.

1. The pupillary response to light is tested, using a bright torch. Absence of response indicates loss of function, although the examiner should be satisfied that a non-responsive pupil is not due to the instillation of paralytic eye drops or damage to the third cranial nerve.

2. The integrity of the corneal reflex is tested by drawing a piece of cotton wool across the exposed cornea. Absence of a response indicates loss of function, although the examiner should be satisfied that the presence of corneal oedema is not preventing the normal blink response.

3. Cranial nerve motor responses are tested at several sites including the head and face, lest the patient have a cervical cord injury. Again, no response indicates loss of function, although spinal reflexes can remain intact even in a brain-dead patient (Ivan 1973).

4. The gag reflex is tested by moving the endotracheal tube back and forth or by applying suction and observing the patient's throat muscles for movement. No response would indicate loss of the pharyngeal and laryngeal reflexes.

5. Absence of the occulovestibular reflex rules out the existence of normal functioning anatomical pathways within the brain stem and is a very sensitive test of brain-stem function. It is tested by syringing 20 ml of ice-cold water into each of the patient's ears in turn and noting any eye movement in response. This is called 'cold caloric testing'. Before testing the examiner should look directly at the tympanic membrane to ensure that there is no obstruction preventing the water from making contact.

6. The final test is that for apnoea. This involves disconnecting the patient from the ventilator and providing a continuous flow of intra-tracheal oxygen. The patient's chest wall is observed closely for any respiratory movement and the pCO_2 is allowed to rise above threshold level to stimulate breathing, usually to at least 50 mmHg. The time taken to achieve this will vary, but is no more than 10 minutes for most patients. Blood gas analysis facilities, whilst not essential, are useful in determining the pCO_2 level (Allan 1987).

The entire process is repeated by another examiner to eliminate observer error and the patient is then declared brain dead. For medico-legal purposes the completion of the second testing determines the time of death and the patient is normally disconnected from the ventilator by medical staff (see Ch. 34). It may previously have been indicated that this patient wished to donate organs for transplantation and if so, following the usual preliminary procedures, the patient would remain ventilated until the organs were removed.

Physical and psychological care

The patient. The physical and psychological care of the dying unconscious patient is the same as that of the terminally ill patient (see Ch. 34).

The family. Psychologically, this is a traumatic and emotionally distraught period for the patient's family and friends. They have perhaps spent the last few days watching the patient in the technical surroundings often used to support the unconscious patient and may be relieved that some sort of ending has been achieved. Often the patient's appearance has changed so much that the relatives do not recognise him any more.

The support of a religious adviser may be appreciated. The nurse should ascertain if this is desired and arrange it if the relatives request her to do so.

A coherent strategy for caring for the relatives is needed. The nurse should know what information has been given to the relatives by other members of staff including doctors. This will enable her to reinforce what has been said and avoid confusing them at a time when their ability to process information is drastically reduced. Allan (1988) emphasises the need for the relatives to see the patient being treated as a person through a humane, caring attitude on the part of the nurse, despite the ever-present life-support machinery.

Some relatives may be helped by being encouraged to perform simple acts of care for the patient such as bathing or, providing his head is not shaved or bandaged, combing his hair. This reduces their feelings of passivity and helplessness in the strange, alien world of the hospital and in a situation in which they are unlikely to be able to draw on previous experience.

Inevitably, this chapter has focused on the care of unconscious people in hospital because, at the present time, only a very small minority are cared for at home. This may change, at least to a certain extent, in the future, as new technology is developed. Where the outcome is death, some families may cope more easily with the stress and sadness in the familiar surroundings of home. Wherever the location of care, it is important for nurses to be sensitive to the fundamental changes the unconscious patient has wrought in the lives of those who know him as a responsive being. Not only is the patient totally reliant upon the nurse, but the family or carers also often require a great deal of support.

As noted at the outset of this chapter, caring for the unconscious person is a major challenge for nurses. Whatever the outcome, whether death, permanent disability or complete recovery, meticulous attention to nursing observations and careful nursing care are vital.

GLOSSARY

Affective. Refers to affect, an outward manifestation of a person's feelings or emotions.

Auditory tract. Transmits impulses for hearing.

Cognitive. Refers to cognition, the mental process characterised by knowing, thinking, learning and judging.

Leminiscal tract. Transmits impulses for more disciminating touch and pressure sensations.

Mesencephalon. The midbrain, which is one of three parts of the brain stem, lying just below the cerebrum and just above the pons.

Proprioceptors. Any sensory nerve ending, as those located in muscles, tendons, joints and the vestibular apparatus, that respond to stimuli regarding movement and spatial positions.

Reticular. From the Latin word 'reticrius', meaning a Roman gladiator who fought with a net.

Spinothalmic tract. Transmits impulses for crude touch, pain and temperature sensations.

Synapse. The point of communication between two adjacent neurons.

Thalamus. A collection of grey matter located within the forebrain or prosencephalon.

Visual tract. Transmits impulses for seeing.

REFERENCES

Adams R D, Victor M 1985 Principles of neurology, 3rd edn. McGraw Hill, New York

Ackerman M H 1985 The use of bolus normal saline instillations in artificial airway: is it useful or necessary? Heart and Lung 14(5): 505–506

Allan D 1984a Patient care in hyperalimentation. Nursing Times, 80(18): 28–30

Allan D 1984b Patients with an endotracheal tube or tracheostomy. Nursing Times 80(13): 36–38

Allan D 1984c Glasgow Coma Scale. Nursing Mirror 158(23): 32

Allan D 1986 Nursing the unconscious patient. Professional Nurse 2(1): 15–17

Allan D 1987 Criteria for brain stem death. Professional Nurse 2(11): 357–359

Allan D 1988a Making sense of suctioning. Nursing Times 84(10): 46–47

Allan D 1988b The ethics of brain death. Professional Nurse 3(8): 295–298

Allan D 1988 Nursing and the neurosciences. Churchill Livingstone, Edinburgh

Allan D 1989 Assessment of the head injured patient. Nursing Review 7(3/4): 19

Allan D 1989 Brain Death. Nursing Times 85: 35, 30–32

Anthony C P, Thibodeau G A 1983 Textbook of anatomy and physiology, 11th edn. C V Mosby, St Louis

Bell G, Davidson N, Emslie-Smith D 1972 Textbook of physiology and biochemistry. Churchill Livingstone, Edinburgh

Bryant L R, Kent-Trinkle J, Dubilier L 1971 Reappraisal of tracheal injury from cuffed tracheal tubes. Journal of the American Medical Association 215: 4

Conference of Medical Royal Colleges and their Faculties in the UK 1976 Diagnosis of brain death. British Medical Journal 2: 1187

De Carle B 1985 Tracheostomy care. Nursing Times Occasional Paper 1981: 6

De Young S 1983 The neurologic patient — a nursing perspective. Prentice-Hall, Englewood Cliffs

Janes E M H 1982 Nursing aspects of tube feeding. Nursing 2(4): 101–104

Gibbons D E 1983 Mouth care procedures. Nursing Times 79(7): 30

Guyton A C 1991 Physiology of the human body, 5th edn. Saunders, Philadelphia

Haerer A F 1976 Coma: some differential considerations in diagnosis and management. Hospital Medicine April 1976: 68–83

Henderson V 1960 Basic principles of nursing care. International Council of Nurses, Geneva

Ivan L P 1973 Spinal reflexes in cerebral death. Neurology 23: 650

Lindsay M D 1988 Care of the patient with epilepsy. In: Allan D (ed) Nursing and the neurosciences. Churchill Livingstone, Edinburgh

Magoun H W 1963 The waking brain. Thomas, Springfield, Illinois

Mahon S 1979 Consciousness and diabetes. Nursing, 1st series 8(1): 363–364

Markham G 1979 Epilepsy. Nursing, 1st series 8(1): 356–359

Milner P 1970 Physiological psychology. Rhinehart & Winston Holtz, New York

Morruzi G, Magoun H W 1949 Brain stem reticular formation and activation of the EEG. Clinical Neurophysiology 1: 455–463

Mulvaney D 1976 Maintaining minimal occluding volume or use cuffs with care. Journal of American Nursing 2(5): 17–18

Myco F, McGilloway F A 1980 Care of the unconscious patient: a complementary perspective. Journal of Advanced Nursing 5: 273–238

Narrow B 1967 Rest is . . . American Journal of Nursing 67: 1646

Plum F, Posner J B 1980 The diagnosis of stupor and coma, 3rd edn. E A Davies, Philadelphia

Powaser M M 1976 The effectiveness of hourly cuff deflation in minimising tracheal damage. Heart and Lung 5: 5

Roper N, Logan W, Tierney A 1990 The elements of nursing, 3rd edn. Churchill Livingstone, Edinburgh

Spence A P, Mason E B 1987 Human anatomy and physiology, 3rd edn. Cummings, Menlo Park

Teasdale G 1975 Acute impairment of brain function: assessing conscious level. Nursing Times 71(24): 914–917

Trimble M 1979 Altered consciousness. Nursing, 1st Series (8): 344–348

Verran B A, Aisbitt P E 1988 Neurological and neurosurgical nursing. Edward Arnold, London

Williams M 1970 Brain damage and the mind. Penguin, Harmondsworth

Wilson K J W 1990 Ross & Wilson anatomy and physiology in health and illness, 7th edn. Churchill Livingstone, Edinburgh

Woollatt B 1979 Drug abuse and altered consciousness. Nursing, 1st series 8(1): 372–375

FURTHER READING

Frawley P 1990 Neurological observations. Nursing Times 86(35): 29–34

Ghodse H A 1977 Drug dependent individuals dealt with by London Casualty Departments. British Journal of Psychiatry 131: 278–280

Health Departments of Great Britain and Northern Ireland. Cadaveric organs for transplantation. London

Jones E 1986 Communication aids for the critically ill. Care of the Critically Ill 2(3): 117–122

LeWinn E B 1980 The coma arousal team. Royal Society of Health Journal 100(1): 19–21

Lloyd F 1990 Eye care for ventilated or unconscious patients. Nursing Times 86(1): 36–37

Lowthian P 1982 A review of pressure sore pathogenesis. Nursing Times 78(3): 117–121

Luria P R 1973 The working brain: an introduction to neurophysiology. Allan Lane, London

Manley K 1986 The dying patient in the intensive care unit. Care of the Critically Ill 2(4): 152–154

Mauss-Clum N 1982 Bringing the unconscious patient back safely. Nursing 12(8): 34–42

Shuldham C 1984 Communication — a conscious effort. Nursing 2(23): 673

Torrance C 1983 Pressure sores: aetiology, treatment and prevention. Croom Helm, London

Wilcock A C, Wan O C 1984 The unconscious patient — total patient care. Nursing 2(23): 675

CHAPTER 31

The patient with burns

Frances M. Davidson

CHAPTER CONTENTS

Introduction 859

Prevention of burn injuries 859
Assessment 859
Planning 860

First aid treatment of burns 861

Assessing the severity of burn injuries 862
Extent of burn 862
Burn depth 863
Burn-associated respiratory tract injury 865
Other injuries 865

The patient with extensive burns 865
Early problems and nursing care 865
The accident and emergency department 866
Transfer of the patient with extensive burns 866
Admission to a regional burns unit 866
The post-shock phase 868

The burn wound 869
Pain control 869
Wound cleansing and debridement 869

Psychological effects of burn injuries 872
The critical phase 872
Stabilisation 872
Recovery 872
The pre-discharge phase 873
After discharge 873

References 873

INTRODUCTION

Imagine for a moment having lost everything: your loved ones; your home and possessions, including mementoes from the past; your health and ability to function normally; your appearance; in other words, yourself. This not infrequently occurs to people who are victims of a house fire.

Most people are burned more than once in their lifetime but few have any conception of the horror associated with severe burns injury. The scenes depicted on national television networks showing recent fire-related disasters, e.g. at Manchester airport, Bradford football stadium, the Piper Alpha oil rig and King's Cross subway station were awesome to the observer, but to the victims the most devastating experience imaginable.

Extensive burns injury is catastrophic, both physically and psychologically, for the patient and his family. It is also one of the most challenging and arduous types of injury to treat. In order to help the patient and his family to achieve optimum function the responsibility of care must be distributed throughout the multidisciplinary team. However, the nurse, being the only professional in 24-hour attendance will play an especially important role. Nurses also attend to many patients whose burns are not extensive, providing care in the community, in accident and emergency (A & E) departments and in general surgical wards. This chapter aims to provide information which will help the nurse care for patients with burn injuries in any of these settings.

PREVENTION OF BURN INJURIES

Burns are frequently described in the literature as being among the most serious of injuries because of the long-term physical and psychological problems which are often associated with them. Advances in treatment and improved facilities have led to a reduction in mortality rates but the morbidity resulting from burns is such that prevention must be viewed as the responsibility of all health care personnel.

The first of the five aims stated in the Constitution of the International Society for Burn Injuries, formed in 1965, is 'To disseminate knowledge and to stimulate prevention in the field of burns' (ISBI 1979). Bouter, Van Rijn & Kok (1990) emphasise that in order to be effective a burn prevention programme must involve assessment of the incidence of burn injuries followed by the planning, implementation and evaluation of appropriate interventions.

Assessment

This includes identifying the extent of the problem, its causative agents and any predisposing factors.

The extent of the problem

In Great Britain in 1988 burning accidents comprised 4% of all home accidents treated in hospital (CSO 1991). Kemble & Lamb (1987) estimate that 150 000 people with burn injuries attend casualty departments each year and that of these 15 000 are admitted to hospital. Of the fires attended by fire brigades in 1988 915 resulted in fatal and 13 376 in non-fatal casualties. Although this shows a 17% reduction in the number of deaths caused by fire, the total number of non-fatal casualties was the highest annual figure ever recorded (CSO 1991). Linares & Linares (1990) point out that although statistical data on burn mortality is generally available, the incidence of burn morbidity is difficult to estimate. Bouter et al (1990) identify the problem as being 'substantial in terms of morbidity, medical consumption and absence from work'.

Case History 31.1 Mr M

Mr M (47) regularly abused alcohol and was a heavy smoker. One evening he fell into an alcoholic stupor, dropping his cigarette on the horsehair sofa on which he was resting. The material smouldered, but did not burst into flames or produce toxic fumes. Robert was lying on his left side with his right hand resting on the sofa. He was eventually found by his brother, who dragged him off the sofa, extinguished the flames and called for an ambulance. On admission to the burns unit Robert was found to have sustained full thickness burns of the left side of the face and chest. There was no circulation through his left hand and arm (which required above-elbow amputation) and the fingers of his right hand were burned down to bone. The total body surface involved was estimated at 20%.

Causative agents

A more or less equal number of studies report either that scalds or flame burns are the most common type of burn injuries (Darko et al 1986b). Contact burns (from touching hot objects) also have a high incidence. Chemical and electrical burns occur less frequently.

The Central Statistical Office (1991) identifies the most common cause of both domestic fires and non-fatal burn casualties as the misuse of equipment or appliances, most commonly cooking appliances. In the case of scalds, the electric kettle is recognised as a major cause of injury, usually in children of preschool age. Hot water in plumbing systems is also a considerable cause of concern in countries where there is no legislation governing the upper limit of plumbed water temperature. Davies (1985) found that this was the cause of 49% of burns in young British children and Adams et al (1991) have identified tap-water as an important cause of burn injury in the United States, particularly affecting children, the elderly and those with neurological impairment.

Predisposing factors

All epidemiological studies identify toddlers as being at greatest risk of burn injuries with scalds accounting for most of these. Adult high-risk groups include those of low socioeconomic status and poor education (Darko et al 1986a) and those with a long history of physical disorders such as diabetes or hypertension and psychological problems such as alcoholism and anxiety neurosis (Noyes et al 1979). Studies agree that males of all ages are at higher risk than females. Trier & Spaabaek (1987) found in their study group of elderly nursing home patients that most fires started when patients were unsupervised and alone in their rooms.

? **31.1** In what other ways might poor and uneducated individuals be disadvantaged when it comes to health care?

Scalds in young children are most commonly associated with the preparation and consumption of hot beverages (Van Rijn, Bouter & Meertens 1989). In the adult population altered consciousness levels resulting from the abuse of alcohol has been cited as a predisposing factor by many authors (Pegg et al 1978, McArthur & Moore 1975, Palmer & Sutherland 1987). Darko et al (1986b) found that alcohol abuse combined with smoking is a major risk factor in burn injuries and results in increased mortality rates. (See Case History 31.1.) Other causes of altered consciousness include the use of drugs, epilepsy, senility and cerebrovascular accidents (CVAs). The Central Statistical Office (1991) does not refer to the problem of altered consciousness but does identify the main cause of death in domestic fires as 'careless handling of fire and hot substances, mainly smokers' materials'.

? **31.2** Why does altered consciousness predispose people to burn injuries?

Planning

Planning for a burns prevention programme must be realistic. While Bouter et al (1990) accept that it is impossible to manipulate some of the risk factors, e.g. sex, socioeconomic status and age, they argue that having identified the groups most at risk it should be possible to alter some of the related predisposing factors.

In the past, most burn prevention programmes have been based on education of the public but recent studies indicate that this is not an effective method. Adams et al (1991) found that an awareness of danger did not alter the behaviour of high-risk groups. Linares & Linares (1990) claim that the reduction in burns-related mortality rates has in fact been less than expected and may, to some extent, be due to improvement in treatment rather than prevention. They suggest that education alone is not sufficient to change high-risk behaviour and that the enactment of new legislation based on sound motivational theory would be more effective.

Elberg et al (1987) reported that, following a burns prevention campaign involving the dissemination of information through the media and revision of legislation and regulations over a 10-year period in Denmark, there was a significant reduction in scalds and electrical and chemical burns in children but little change in the numbers of adult burn injuries.

? **31.3** Are adults more greatly motivated to prevent burns in children than in themselves?

There are already numerous health education campaigns aimed at persuading the public not to smoke and to drink alcohol only in moderation. It seems unlikely that those who do not comply would be influenced by the knowledge that smoking and drinking increase their risk of burn injuries. Tones et al (1990) point out that, unlike the promotion of commercial products, which is based on enhancing pleasure and promises immediate gratification, health promotion usually urges people to stop doing something which they find pleasurable in the hope of long-term gratification. They also state that the public have a right not to be 'unreasonably

Box 31.1 Reducing the risk of scalds

- Water does not have to be close to boiling point to cause severe injury.
- A cup of freshly made tea or instant coffee takes 20 minutes to reach a temperature which will not damage the skin and 15 minutes if milk is added (Mercer 1988). The same study found that the contents of a newly boiled kettle containing 1.5 litres of water will take one hour to reach a safe temperature.
- Water at a temperature of 66 ° C will cause a full thickness scald after 2 seconds' contact and, at 60 ° C, after 6 seconds (Moritz & Henriques 1947). Many authors advocate the reduction of plumbed hot water temperatures to 50–55 ° C (Baruchin et al 1982, Walker 1990, Adams et al 1991).
- Setting the hot water thermostat to a lower temperature will help to reduce fuel bills.

frightened'. Blatant shock tactics are therefore unacceptable and are only likely to make people 'switch off'. More subtle messages may be conveyed, e.g. by incidental reference in popular television series.

The information given in Box 31.1 may encourage some people to alter their behaviour.

The Child Accident Prevention Trust (1985) identifies the following logical steps in the prevention of flame burns:

- reducing the number of sources of ignition or promoting their safer use
- reducing both the amount and the flammability of the material ignited, and limiting the spread of the fire
- ensuring that people are warned of the existence of a fire
- ensuring their safety, e.g. by ensuring a means of exit from a home.

Since 1990 it has been against the law to sell new or reupholstered soft furnishings which are padded with foam which is not combustion-modified, or which are covered with fabric which does not resist ignition tests for both smouldering cigarettes and match-like flames. Previous legislation and regulations include the prohibition of the sale of highly flammable children's nightwear and the requirement that all new gas or electric fires and radiant oil-burning stoves are fitted with a fireguard which passes British Standards specifications. Few people seem to be aware that if a child under 12 years of age (under 7 in Scotland) is left alone in a house with an unguarded or inadequately guarded fire or heating appliance and, as a result, the child is injured, the parents are legally responsible.

Currently a great deal of interest is being shown in the use of smoke detectors. It is suggested that their installation into both new and established domestic properties may become legally required. Because of their sensitivity they may be set off by cooking fumes (e.g. burning toast) and there have been numerous reports of people consequently removing the batteries in Council-owned properties where they have been installed. Some detectors have a temporary 'silence' button which may solve the problem of false alarms unless the ceiling, which is the recommended site for mounting, is out of reach.

It must be accepted that the groups at highest risk of injury from burns — i.e. people who are elderly, disabled or in a lower socioeconomic bracket — will be less able than others to purchase the new, safer soft furnishings and heating appliances. Smoke detectors may be bought for as little as £5 but their fitting, although simple for the able-bodied, may be impossible for elderly or disabled individuals.

Health care workers therefore not only have a responsibility to disseminate information on the prevention of burn injuries but must also work closely with other interested groups such as the Fire Brigades, The Royal Society for the Prevention of Accidents and both local and national government offices in order to lobby for more effective legislation and regulations. Nurses working in the community have special opportunities to observe the environment and to give specific advice relating to burns prevention.

FIRST AID TREATMENT OF BURNS

Burn injuries result from the transfer of energy from a source of heat to vulnerable tissues. The higher the temperature of the heat source and the longer it is in contact with the tissues, the greater will be the destruction.

The first priority of first aid treatment is to remove the individual from the source of heat. If the causative agent is electricity it is important to switch off the supply if possible or to use a non-conductor to rescue the person. Frequently there is a continuing source of heat in the form of the individual's clothing, which may be on fire or saturated by a hot liquid. The most effective way to remove this continuing heat source is to throw cool liquid (which is neither flammable nor corrosive) over the affected material, thus dousing the flames or reducing the temperature of the scalding liquid. If no such cool liquid is immediately to hand, rapid removal of hot saturated clothing will arrest the heat transfer. Where clothing is on fire it is important to stop the person running around as this will fan the flames. The person assisting should lie the victim on the ground and use heavy material such as a coat or blanket to smother the flames. If chemicals are the causative agent prompt sluicing with copious amounts of water will dilute the strength of the agent and limit the penetration of the chemical into the skin, where it will continue to cause damage for many hours. Herbert & Lawrence (1989) emphasise the advantage of taking this universal first aid measure rather than taking time searching for specific neutralising agents. (In the clinical situation a useful means of identifying whether a chemical is acid or alkaline is to apply a Multistix, normally used for urine testing, as this will give a pH reading.)

Having taken steps to remove the heat source from the skin the next measure is to cool the superheated tissues. The easiest means of doing so is to place the affected part (obviously not the face, to which cold soaks should be applied) in cold water. Lawrence & Wilkins (1986) showed that when cold water was applied 5 seconds after experimental burning (by the application of a metal block at 100 ° C for 10 seconds) the subdermal temperature returned to normal in approximately 25 seconds compared with untreated tissue, which took approximately 4 min. The length of time that the cold water treatment should be continued is debatable. There is no doubt that continuing application helps to reduce pain from the burn wound but if a large area of the body surface is involved there is a risk of hypothermia. Lawrence (1987) recommends limiting the duration of cold application to 20 minutes in such cases.

Palmer & Sutherland (1987) advise against using cold soaks or ice packs during the transfer of patients to hospital, especially if the journey will take some time. In a recent case, a 10-year-old girl sustained 12% burns on her back when her shirt-tail came in contact with a gas flame. Her brother, with whom she was playing, threw the contents of a jug of lemonade over the flames; then she was placed in a bath by her mother, who repeatedly scooped cold water over the burned area. She then wrapped her daughter in a clean sheet and took her to the local hospital. From there the child was transferred to a specialist unit, a journey of more than 1 h. During the period of transfer she was lying prone on a stretcher lined with incontinence pads, absorbent surface up; the escorting nurse carried out her instructions, which were to continually irrigate the saline soaks which had been placed on the girl's back with cold saline from a cool-pack. When the patient arrived at the specialist unit rectal temperature was recorded at 34.8 ° C. Marichy et al (1989) and Steinmann et al (1990) have noted the high mortality related to trauma patients who have core temperatures of less than 35 ° C at the time of their admission to hospital. **Note:** Patients with extensive burns have problems in retaining body heat. The use of space blankets or other heat-retaining coverings is advised during the period of transfer.

Many burns units in the UK are now advising that the temporary wound dressing of choice is polyvinyl chloride film e.g. cling film (Lawrence 1987). The reasons for this are as follows:

- the film is sterile on the inner rolled surface
- it does not adhere to the wound surface and cause pain on removal
- it conforms closely to the body contours and excludes air, thus reducing pain
- a succession of personnel can view the wound without removal of the transparent film.

This kind of material is often available in the home but, if not, a clean cloth should be used as temporary cover. The use of ointments, lotions and powders should be avoided as they may change the appearance of the wound and thus cause difficulty in the assessment of wound depth.

Practice and Treatment Room nurses often see people with severe sunburn that has been unsuccessfully self-managed and has become infected. This can also happen with other types of burns, as in Case History 31.2.

To summarise, first aid treatment of burn injuries consists of:

1. Separating the individual from the source of injury
2. Immersion of the affected part in cold water for 10 min (cold soaks to face)
3. Application of polyvinyl chloride (cling) film or a clean cloth to the wound (cold soaks may be used for wounds which are not extensive).

ASSESSING THE SEVERITY OF BURN INJURIES

The majority of patients with burn injuries do not require hospital inpatient care. Phipps (1986) identifies the groups of patients for whom admission or referral to a regional burns unit is advisable:

- those whose burns exceed 5% of the body surface area
- those with small but deep burns which will require skin grafting
- those with infected wounds or evidence of infection
- most patients with burns of face, hands, feet or perineum
- those whose injury limits their capacity to care for themselves at home
- those with associated injuries e.g. smoke inhalation or electric shock
- those with other medical conditions, e.g. epilepsy.

For patients who come under none of these categories relief of pain and local treatment of the burn wound are generally all that is required. Both interventions will be described later in the chapter (see p. 869).

Assessment of the severity of the burn injury involves estimation of:

- the extent of body surface area involved
- the depth of tissue damage
- the probability of associated respiratory tract injury.

Knowledge of the circumstances of the accident (e.g. whether electricity was involved) and information about the individual's general health and domestic situation will help in deciding whether the patient may or may not be managed by the primary health care team.

Extent of burn

Whenever body tissues are traumatised the inflammatory response is stimulated, resulting in increased circulation to the area (hyperaemia) and increased movement of fluids from intravascular to interstitial compartments. If this occurs in a small area i.e. over less than 5% of the body surface, the effects are localised. However, when a larger percentage of the body surface is injured there is a massive shift of fluids into the tissues with a corresponding reduction in circulating volume (see Case History 31.3). It is generally accepted that children with burns greater than 10% of body surface area and adults with burns greater than 15% will suffer from hypovolaemic shock unless there is prompt intravenous replacement of fluid.

In order to estimate the percentage of body surface affected the simplest and most easily remembered method is the 'Rule of Nines' introduced by Wallace in 1951 (see Fig. 31.1). In this the head and each upper limb equals 9% whilst the anterior trunk, the posterior trunk and the lower limbs each equal

Case History 31.2 Miss K

Miss K (53) suffers from diabetes and lives alone. One morning she awoke to find that she had blistering on her left lower leg. She assumed that this had been caused by contact with her hot-water bottle. As there was no pain, she did not contact her doctor but dressed the burn herself, using an antiseptic cream and a bandage. A week later she attended the local hospital, as the wound was now very inflamed and producing pus.

Case History 31.3 Ms C

Ms C (24) returned home after a night out with her friends and, feeling hungry, decided to have some French-fried potatoes. She put the chip pan on the stove, leaving the fat to heat whilst she got ready for bed. Smelling smoke, she rushed back to the kitchen to find the saucepan in flames. In her panic she tried to douse the flames by smothering them with a dry towel, which promptly caught fire. She then remembered to put the lid on and turn off the stove. Her screams alerted the neighbours, who phoned for an ambulance. June was rushed to the nearest casualty department, where, on examination, she was found to have a total of 8%, mainly superficial, burns to her hands, forearms, chest and face.

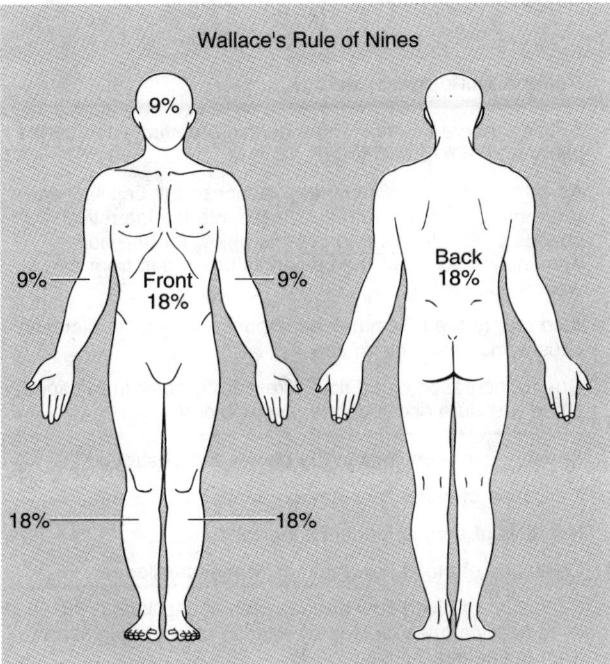

Fig. 31.1 Wallace's Rule of Nines.

18%. The remaining 1% is usually applied to the perineum. Another rapid approximation of percentage can be made by using the palmar aspect of the patient's hand (with fingers together) as 1% of the body surface area.

The Rule of Nines should never be used for estimating burn percentage in young children as it does not allow for the different proportions of head and lower limbs in infants and toddlers. Under the age of one year the child's head equals 19% of the body surface area and the lower limbs are correspondingly smaller. A more accurate chart which allows for the changing proportions of different age groups and which shows percentages applicable to smaller more specific areas of the body surface is the Lund and Browder (1944) burn chart (see Fig. 31.2). This is generally in use in specialist units and is available in A & E departments throughout the country.

Among adults, the greater the burn area and the older the patient the higher the mortality. Bull (1971) devised a sliding scale of mortality probabilities which indicates that in patients over 20 years of age if the person's age and the percentage of body surface area burned added together exceed 100 there is minimal possibility of survival unless the burn depth is superficial and healing is rapid.

The depth of a burn influences the rate at which the wound will heal spontaneously. The longer the wound takes to heal the greater the probability of infection and the worse the scarring and loss of function (see Ch. 23). There are a number of methods of classifying burn depth. In the UK the most popular is to differentiate between partial thickness and full thickness skin destruction. Partial thickness burns involve the epidermis and part of the dermis. Full thickness burns destroy the epidermis and all of the dermis. Full thickness burns may also involve deeper structures such as fat, muscle and bone. Partial thickness burns are classified as 'superficial' or 'deep', depending on the amount of dermis involved. As a general rule, deep partial thickness and full thickness burns require surgical enhancement of healing in the form of skin grafting.

As may be seen from Figure 31.3, the more superficial the

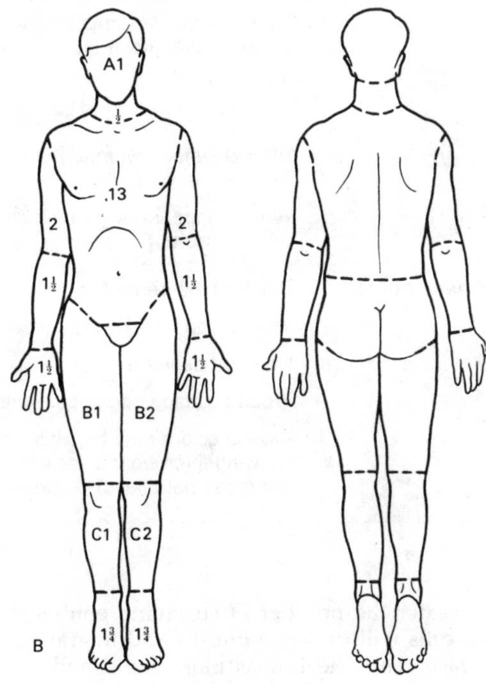

Percent of areas affected by growth

	0	1	5	10	15	Adult age
A = $\frac{1}{2}$ head	$9\frac{1}{2}$	$8\frac{1}{2}$	$6\frac{1}{2}$	$5\frac{1}{2}$	$4\frac{1}{2}$	$3\frac{1}{2}$
B = $\frac{1}{2}$ one thigh	$2\frac{3}{4}$	$3\frac{1}{4}$	4	$4\frac{1}{4}$	$4\frac{1}{2}$	$4\frac{3}{4}$
C = $\frac{1}{2}$ one leg	$2\frac{1}{2}$	$2\frac{1}{2}$	$2\frac{3}{4}$	3	$3\frac{1}{4}$	$3\frac{1}{2}$

To estimate the total of the body surface area burned, the percentages assigned to the burned sections are added. The total is then an estimate of the burn size.

Fig. 31.2 The Lund and Browder burn chart.

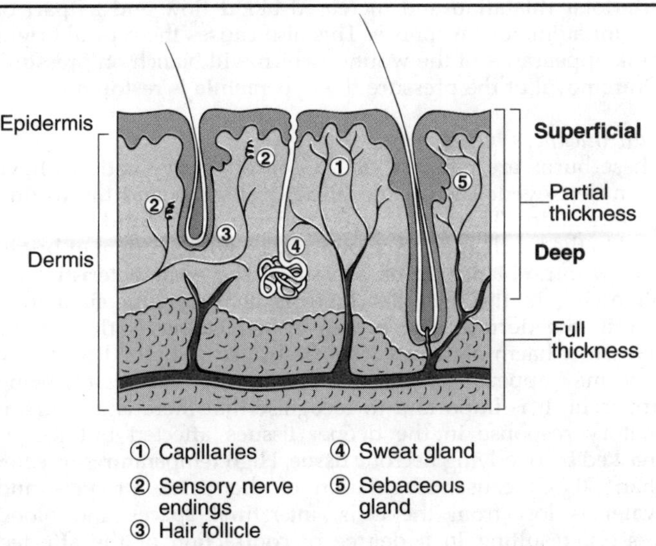

Fig. 31.3 Classification of burn depth.

Table 31.1 Indications of burn depth

Depth	Signs and symptoms	Related anatomy/physiology
Superficial partial thickness	Very painful	Sensory nerve endings in the dermis are stimulated by the injury and/or exposed to air
	Oedema, blister formation, serous exudate where blisters have burst	As a result of the inflammatory response the capillary walls are more permeable and fluid leaks into the interstitial spaces of the dermis and collects below the the non-germinating layers of the epidermis or exudes from the wound surface
	Wound surface warmer than unburned skin	Also due to the inflammatory response; arteriolar dilatation causes increased blood flow
	Wound appears bright pink and blanches with pressure	Due to increased blood flow. Pressure greater than capillary blood pressure occludes the flow of blood
Full thickness burns	Painless, no sensation	Sensory nerve endings in the dermis are destroyed
	Wound surface dry. No blistering	Cessation of blood flow through dermal capillaries
	No overt oedema	Necrosis of dermis renders it inelastic
	Wound surface cooler than unburned skin	Cessation of blood flow through dermal capillaries
	Wound colour may be white; brown; translucent showing thrombosed vessels; or bright red (does not blanch on pressure)	Cessation of blood flow through dermal capillaries. Brown or red appearance caused by release of haem pigments from destroyed red blood cells

injury the greater the number of surviving epithelial sources from which cells will undergo mitosis and migrate across the wound surface. Thus healing is more rapid and causes less wound contraction the more superficial the burn is. The effects of superficial partial thickness burns and full thickness burns are described below and in Table 31.1.

Superficial partial thickness burns
These burns are very painful as the sensory nerve endings are stimulated by the injury or exposed to air. They are characterised by oedema, blister formation and serous exudate where the blisters burst. The blistering results from the increased permeability of the capillary walls, with fluid leaking into the interstitial spaces and from the wound surface (this fluid collects into blisters beneath the non-germinating layers of the epidermis). Heat radiates from the wound surface due to arteriolar dilatation and increased blood flow and as part of the inflammatory response. This also causes the typical bright pink appearance of the wound, which will blanch on pressure. On removal of the pressure the hyperaemia is restored.

Full thickness burns
These burns are painless, as the sensory nerve endings have been destroyed. There is no blister formation and the wound surface is dry. There is no overt oedema, the wound surface is cool to the touch and the colour may be white, brown or bright red (with no blanching on pressure). These characteristics are all owing to the fact that there is no surviving circulation within the dermis. The brown or red colour is due to the release of haem pigments from destroyed red blood cells. The area may appear translucent with thrombosed vessels being apparent. It is important to recognise that there is an inflammatory response in the deeper tissues affected but this is masked by overlying necrotic tissue. High temperatures (greater than 60 °C) cause coagulation of the tissue proteins and water is lost from the cells, interstitial spaces and blood vessels, resulting in a degree of contraction of the affected tissues. Destruction of the dermis renders the skin inelastic and the texture becomes firm and leathery. This destroyed tissue is known as eschar (see Box 31.2).

Deep partial thickness burns
As the depth of destruction is between those of superficial partial thickness and full thickness the presenting signs and symptoms indicate moderation of the extremes in sensation, blistering, temperature and colour.

Problems in assessment
The assessment of burn depth is not an exact science although much work has been carried out to make it more so in recent years. The use of a hypodermic needle to test for pinprick sensation was first described by Bull & Lennard-Jones in 1949. Muir et al (1987) discuss the usefulness of positive pinprick reactions in view of the false conclusions which may be drawn from negative results obtained in body areas which are naturally low in sensitivity. Thermography has been used in relating burn depth to the temperature of the burn surface (Watson & Vasilescu 1972, Newman et al 1981, Cole et al 1991) but this requires the use of specialised equipment which is

Box 31.2 Escharotomy

Where full thickness burn injury occurs circumferentially around a limb the combination of a firm inelastic eschar and the covert inflammatory response in the subcutaneous tissues will cause compression of the deeper structures, especially the blood vessels. Incisions through the eschar to allow decompression are carried out by the surgeon and are termed **escharotomy.**

Escharotomy may also be carried out when full thickness burn injury of the chest and upper part of the abdomen inhibit rib or diaphragmatic movement, causing respiratory difficulty.

Nursing note: Monitoring of circulation to distal parts of limbs involved or of respiratory ease is required when full thickness burns are suspected in either site.

not generally available. Wyllie & Sutherland (1991) found that temperature sensors, which (with minor adaptation) are available in most anaesthetic departments, may be used successfully in aiding diagnosis of burn depth in some areas of the body. Frequently assessment of burn depth is dependent on the characteristics of the wound, the information given regarding the circumstances of the accident, the agent involved and the first aid measures carried out.

BURN-ASSOCIATED RESPIRATORY TRACT INJURY

Inhalation of smoke and hot toxic gases is frequently associated with burn trauma. The synergistic effects of burns and smoke inhalation are described by Heimbach (1984), who states that for victims of smoke inhalation who are unburned and conscious on arrival at the emergency room the mortality rate is low, whereas for those who are also burned the mortality rate associated with the extent of burn is approximately doubled.

The main causes of inhalation injury are:

- carbon monoxide poisoning
- thermal injury
- inhalation of toxic chemicals.

Carbon monoxide poisoning
Carbon monoxide (CO) is a colourless, odourless, non-irritating gas produced by the combustion of carbon and organic materials in a limited oxygen supply. Its affinity for haemoglobin is many times that of oxygen. Therefore, following inhalation of CO there is displacement of oxygen on the haemoglobin molecules and the production of carboxyhaemoglobin (COHb) with resulting generalised hypoxia. The symptoms of CO poisoning are related to the concentration of the inspired gas and of COHb levels and are recognised as mild headache, dizziness, confusion, irritability, nausea, vomiting and fainting. At higher levels there will be convulsion, coma, respiratory failure and death. Diagnosis is suggested by the typical cherry pink appearance of the patient and confirmed by checking COHb levels. The formation of carboxyhaemoglobin can be reversed by the administration of high concentrations of oxygen.

Thermal injury
Inhibition of respiratory function may result from thermal injury to the skin of the trunk and neck, or the mucosal lining of the airway, or both. Covert oedema formation below the leathery, inelastic eschar of circumferential full thickness burns (see p. 864) causes pressure on the deeper structures. In deep burns of the neck this may cause compression of the trachea, and, if there is involvement of the chest and upper abdomen, will inhibit expansion of the thoracic cavity. Decompression by escharotomy will be required (see Box 31.2).

The upper airway may be damaged by the inhalation of hot gases, hot vapours or combustible gas mixtures. Mucosal oedema will narrow the lumen of the airway. The diagnosis is suspected where there is a history of explosion, burns of the face, singed nasal hairs, erythema and ulceration of the oropharynx. Hoarseness and inspiratory stridor may present later. As signs of upper airway obstruction may take several hours to become apparent, constant supervision is advised.

Hot, dry air seldom causes burns of the airway below the level of the epiglottis as the respiratory tract has an excellent heat exchange capability. Injury to the lower airway is most commonly caused by inhalation of toxic chemicals.

Inhalation of toxic chemicals
The combustion of various materials produces a wide spectrum of toxic chemicals, including chlorine, ammonia, formaldehyde, phosgene and hydrogen cyanide. The extent of the resultant damage to the respiratory system will be determined by the density of the smoke and the duration of exposure. Patients who are asleep or under the influence of drugs or alcohol at the time of the fire will tend to have a longer exposure time, as will those who have restricted mobility, e.g. elderly or disabled individuals.

When toxic chemicals bound to carbon particles settle on the respiratory endothelium the following reactions occur:

- the inflammatory response, causing increased secretions and narrowing of the lumen of the trachea, bronchi and bronchioles. Inflammation of the alveolar capillary membrane will interfere with gaseous exchange and capillary exudate will leak into the alveoli
- bronchospasm, further narrowing the lumen of the airway
- clinical denaturation of all protein, leading to:
  - — necrosis and ulceration of the endothelial tissue, with an increase in cellular debris
  - — cessation of ciliary activity, inhibiting removal of secretions and cellular debris
- loss of surfactant production by specialised alveolar endothelial cells. Surfactant normally lowers the surface tension of the walls of the alveoli, thus preventing collapse, and also prevents the transudation of fluid from capillaries into the alveoli. Loss of surfactant production will therefore lead to atelectasis (see Ch. 3).

In summary, the pathophysiological results of inhalation of toxic chemicals may include tracheobronchitis, pulmonary oedema, atelectasis and airway obstruction. These are frequently compounded by infection.

In cases where the patient survives long enough for admission to hospital the respiratory damage related to inhalation of toxic chemicals may take several hours or even days to become manifest. Suspicion should be aroused where:

1. The fire occurred within an enclosed space, especially at night
2. There is a history of exposure to smoke, especially if the patient required bodily rescue
3. The patient's breath and clothing smell of smoke
4. There is inflammation of the conjunctivae
5. Carbon particles are present in clothing, wounds, nose, mouth and sputum.

Other injuries

The appearance of a patient with extensive burns may be so visually dramatic as to distract the assessor from checking for other, less obvious, injuries. Fractures, internal injuries and spinal cord damage may have been sustained, especially if the burn was a result of a road traffic accident, an explosion, or high tension electricity, or if the patient jumped from a burning building.

THE PATIENT WITH EXTENSIVE BURNS

Early problems and nursing care

The patient with extensive burns has multiple problems, the relative urgency of which will vary during the perhaps very extensive period following injury. During the first 36–48 h the most life-threatening problem (except where inhalation injury is present) will be burns shock. The subject of shock is covered in Ch. 18 but a summary of events which have

Table 31.2 Pathology and related clinical features of burn shock

Pathological condition	Clinical signs and symptoms
Hypovolaemia	Thirst Rapid, weak pulse Hypotension Peripheral and splanchnic vasoconstriction
Peripheral vasoconstriction	Pale skin and mucosa Extremities feel cold Patient complains of feeling cold
Reduced perfusion of kidneys	Oliguria, anuria Impairment of renal function Metabolic acidosis Renal failure may occur
Red cell haemolysis	Haemoglobinuria Renal failure may occur
Reduced perfusion of lungs	Rapid, shallow breathing Air hunger: gasping
Reduced perfusion of gastrointestinal tract	Reduced absorption and intestinal stasis Vomiting, loss of electrolytes Paralytic ileus, lack of bowel sounds
Hypoxaemia/electrolyte imbalance	Restlessness, disorientation, confusion May lead to coma and death

particular relevance to burns injury is given here (see Table 31.2).

The initial physiological response to a burn injury results in plasma loss from the circulation (see p. 862). This in turn is accompanied by:

1. gross oedema of the affected tissues
2. hypovolaemia. As in all types of shock, this results in decreased circulation of the skin, muscle, and internal organs. Cerebral and coronary perfusion, being of greatest priority, are temporarily maintained
3. haemoconcentration. Unlike the hypovolaemia which results from haemorrhage, the loss of plasma alone from the intravascular compartment causes an increase in the ratio of blood cells to plasma in the circulation (raised haematocrit). This increases the viscosity of the blood, further reducing the flow through the capillaries.

In addition to suffering from burn shock the patient may be emotionally shocked, in great pain, and have extensive destruction of the skin and, possibly deeper structures. There may be associated injuries, especially inhalation of smoke, and a pre-burn illness may be present.

Haemoglobinuria may develop in patients who have been badly burned. This is described in Box 31.3.

The accident and emergency department

Ellis & Rylah (1990) highlight the fact that, to those who are unfamiliar with burns, the patient with extensive burns may not appear to be critically ill. The loss of plasma from the circulation is less rapid than haemorrhage from ruptured vessels and the patient may appear quite well. Inexperienced staff should consult with the regional burns unit to ensure that treatment is appropriate to the severity of the injury.

Box 31.3 Haemoglobinuria

In patients with large areas of deep partial thickness or full thickness burns there can be a massive breakdown of the red blood cells subjected to high temperatures. This causes the release of degraded haemoglobin (and if there is muscle involvement, of myoglobin) into the circulation. These haem pigments are excreted by the kidneys and the urine appears black or dark red. This is known as haemoglobinuria. Barrett (1986) reports that there is evidence which indicates that normal, well perfused kidneys are not harmed by the pigment, but it is generally agreed that the combination of haemoglobinuria and poor renal perfusion, unless rapidly treated, will lead to renal failure (Barrett 1986, Settle 1986, Kemble & Lamb 1987).

Settle (1986) lists the following actions to be taken by medical staff assisting burn victims:

1. Make sure there is a clear airway
2. Obtain a brief history of the accident
3. Carry out a brief general examination of the patient
4. Set up a reliable plasma infusion
5. Take blood samples
6. Provide analgesia
7. Catheterise the bladder
8. Reassess the patient's general condition
9. Reassess the burn
10. Arrange admission or transfer.

The role of the nursing staff is to assist with the above procedures, to support the patient and his relatives and to keep meticulous records of fluid balance and of drugs given.

Transfer of the patient with extensive burns

The patient should be prepared for transfer with the application of a temporary wound dressing, preferably cling film, and covered with a space blanket or layers of ordinary blankets. As described earlier (see p. 861) there is a high risk of hypothermia, especially during transfer (Ellis & Rylah 1990) and wet dressings should not be used. The patient will need to be accompanied by an experienced nurse, as well as by a member of the medical staff if there are airway problems. Monitoring of vital signs and maintenance of the intravenous fluids is usually carried out by the nurse. The speed of travel is frequently rapid, which will make the task of monitoring and recording fluid balance and vital signs very difficult, nonetheless these records are important and should be given, along with the A & E file, to the staff of the burns unit on arrival.

Admission to a regional burns unit

The burns unit staff are usually informed in advance of the imminent admission of a patient with extensive burns. The time between their notification and the actual arrival of the patient, depending on the distance from the referral centre, is used to prepare the environment and to get the necessary equipment ready.

Reception of the patient

When the patient arrives at the unit he should be greeted and orientated as to place, as many regional burns units receive patients from a wide catchment area. One nurse should be designated to receive the patient from the escorting nurse. Where possible the patient should be reassured and given a simple explanation of what is being done at every stage of the admission procedure — and thereafter, throughout his stay in the unit. The appearance and smell of the burn wounds may be very upsetting for inexperienced staff, but it is important to appear calm and confident.

The receiving staff must wear protective clothing, e.g. waterproof gowns, plastic aprons or tabards and gloves. This is to protect staff against contact with wound exudate and desquamated skin, and the patient against wound contamination.

The patient should be received into a single room warmed to a temperature of 28 ° C, as heat loss from the inflamed wounds in addition to evaporative heat loss from the wound exudate can be extensive.

Maintaining the airway

If the patient has inhalation injury endotracheal intubation and assisted ventilation may have been instituted in the A & E department or may be required at the time of admission to the unit. In any case all nursing care and observations relative to this treatment must be carried out (see Ch. 29).

Constant observation of respiratory rate and ease and of the colour of unburned skin and mucosa must be carried out and recorded. Humidified air or oxygen administered by face mask or nasal catheter may be required.

Weighing the patient

If possible an accurate body weight in kilograms should be obtained as this is one of the baseline measurements on which the volume of fluid replacement is calculated. Estimation of weight is sometimes carried out but, unless the person doing so is experienced in this, gross over- or under-transfusion may result. In many units the patient is weighed still covered in the blankets and temporary dressings used for the transfer; these are then gently removed and the patient laid on and covered with sterile sheeting (linen, foam or cling film). The original coverings are then weighed and their weight subtracted from the total in order to get a naked weight. It is important to record the weight immediately as the exact figure may easily be forgotten if there is a great deal of activity in the room.

Wound assessment

The medical staff will estimate the depth of the burn wounds and chart their position and extent. Coloured photographs may also be taken for recording purposes. Whilst the wounds are exposed the nurse can take swabs for bacteriological examination from each wound site, e.g. right hand, left hand, chest, neck. This reduces the possibility of wound contamination and the discomfort and possible loss of dignity suffered by the patient during repeated removal of the coverings. The initial wound swabs usually show no bacteriological contamination but provide a useful baseline for further monitoring. The wounds are then covered with a temporary dressing. Specific care will be carried out once the patient's condition has been stabilised.

Bacteriology swabs from nose and throat are also obtained in order to identify commensals which may act as wound pathogens.

Any rings which the patient is wearing are best removed, as the hands, even if not burned, are liable to become oedematous.

Analgesia

It is unusual for patients to complain of pain at this stage, even if their wounds are of partial thickness. If pain is felt, however, analgesia, usually in the form of morphine, is given intravenously. The intramuscular route should never be used if the patient is shocked, as the drug will not be absorbed owing to the peripheral vasoconstriction.

Intravenous fluid replacement

Once an accurate body weight has been obtained and the percentage area of the burn estimated the medical staff will calculate the volume of intravenous therapy required. There are a number of different formulae in current use but most depend on these two parameters for calculation of the volume to be infused. Regulation of the rate of flow and recording of the volume transfused as well as care of the intravenous site is the responsibility of the nurse. It is usual to use a volumetric intravenous pump to aid accuracy in intravenous infusion as the volumes required in each period may be very large.

Monitoring urine

If this has not been carried out in the A & E department an indwelling urinary catheter is passed, the bladder emptied and the urine volume measured. A specimen is tested for specific gravity and analysed using a Multistix. The appearance is noted. A urimeter which allows hourly measuring and sampling whilst maintaining a closed system is attached to the catheter. Settle (1986) emphasises the importance of monitoring renal function through regular, frequent measurement of volume and composition of the urine. A volume of 0.5–1.0 ml/kg body weight is generally accepted as indicating that intravenous fluid replacement is satisfactory, although urine concentration (measured by specific gravity or osmolality) must also be estimated in order to assess renal function (Muir et al 1987, Kemble & Lamb 1987).

The appearance of the urine is monitored for indications of haemoglobinuria (see Box 31.3) and, if this is present, for indications that it is diminishing. It is important that the nurse inform the medical staff at the first indication of haemoglobinuria, as it is usual for an osmotic diuretic (e.g. mannitol) to be prescribed in order to clear the pigments. Kemble & Lamb (1987) state that if the haemoglobinuria persists for longer than 24 h there is a greater likelihood of renal failure occurring.

Monitoring vital signs

Pulse. If the patient is shocked the pulse will be rapid and weak; this, combined with generalised oedema, can make manual counting very difficult and mechanical aids such as the pulse-oximeter (see p. 42) are normally used. The pulse-oximeter can be clipped to a toe or fingertip and as well as giving a pulse rate will also indicate the state of peripheral perfusion and respiratory function by indicating oxygen tension.

Blood pressure. Where all four limbs have been burned it has not always been usual practice to record blood pressure. Indeed, even if one limb is unaffected it has been considered more important to ensure effective intravenous replacement rather than to repeatedly constrict the vessels with a blood pressure cuff. Bainbridge et al (1990), however, have found that it is possible to monitor mean arterial pressure by using oscillometric automatic blood pressure monitors with the cuff applied over bulky dressings around the upper limb. They postulate that this method would be useful for monitoring blood pressure in patients with burns.

The routine measurement of central venous pressure or of arterial pressure is not recommended in most British burns units because of the risk of systemic infection associated with such techniques, especially if the site of entry of the catheter is close to the burn wound (Bainbridge et al 1990, Cason 1981, Muir et al 1987).

Temperature. A good indicator of the state of peripheral perfusion is the difference between core and shell temperature. In the normal person under warm conditions the temperature of a toe is 1–4 ° C lower than rectal temperature, but in the patient suffering hypovolaemic shock the vasoconstriction is such that the difference may be as much as 15 ° C (Muir et al 1987). Temperature monitoring is usually facilitated by the use of thermistor probes in preference to the repeated insertion of a rectal thermometer. In some units a specially designed probe is inserted into the external auditory meatus in preference to using the rectum. If thermistor probes are not available it is possible to gauge the shell temperature by feeling the temperature of the peripheries, especially the toes or the tip of the nose.

In addition to monitoring the difference between a normal core temperature and changes in the shell temperature, measuring the core temperature will of course also indicate a trend towards hyperpyrexia or hypothermia (see Ch. 22).

Oral intake

Because of the reduction in gastrointestinal tract perfusion which results from hypovolaemia it is necessary to restrict the volume of oral fluids initially, even if the patient is very thirsty, until it has been established that there is no nausea or vomiting. If there is persistent vomiting a nasogastric tube is passed and is either allowed to drain freely or aspirated hourly before small amounts of water are given. In some units a tube is passed routinely in all patients with burns greater than 35% of the body surface.

Patient behaviour

In addition to recording clinical measurements as described above it is useful for the nurse to keep a record of the patient's behaviour, noting restlessness, confusion, distress, apathy, etc. as these along with the measured recordings will give a more complete picture of the patient's condition.

The post-shock phase

After the first 36–48 h following injury the fluid in the interstitial spaces is reabsorbed into the circulation and, although there is continuous fluid loss through exudate and evaporation from the wound surface, there is normally no longer a need for intravenous replacement of fluids. Unless complications arise (see Box 31.4), the intermediate stage of management will have been reached.

Nursing management during the intermediate stage of burn injury recovery follows the basic principles of burn care whatever the extent of body surface involved. Thus nursing priorities include:

- hydration and nutrition
- prevention of infection and local wound care
- pain relief
- psychosocial support for patients and relatives.

Hydration and nutrition

Until wound closure is complete there will be continuous loss of the water, protein and electrolytes which comprise the wound exudate. In addition, nutritional requirements will be increased because of the elevation in the metabolic rate resulting from trauma, as well as the cellular requirements of wound healing. In patients whose burn area is less than 20% of the body surface oral intake of a normal diet, perhaps supplemented with high-protein, high-calorie drinks, should be all that is required. Dietary intake should be monitored to allow assessment by the dietitian and the patient should be weighed weekly. The patient should be encouraged to take fluids when he is awake and fluid balance should be charted.

In more extensive burns metabolic requirements will be increased, making enteral nutrition via a nasogastric tube necessary. As a fine-bore tube is used to facilitate patient comfort and reduce trauma there may be difficulty aspirating gastric contents to ensure correct placement; X-ray confirmation may therefore be required. There are a number of proprietary preparations of enteral feeds available and the dietitian will prescribe the type, volume and rate of administration for each individual. Many manufacturers of enteral feeds produce their own giving sets and volumetric pumps; their instructions should be followed in the use of this equipment. Diarrhoea, nausea and vomiting may complicate enteral feeding. Henly (1989) advises that, rather than commencing with diluted feeds, patient tolerance is best developed by introducing the feed at a slow drip rate and gradually increasing until the required rate is reached. Parenteral nutrition is reserved for patients who are unable to achieve adequate nutrition by the enteral route because of the danger of infection associated with the introduction of central lines; peripheral lines are usually impractical because of the limited availability of peripheral veins.

Prevention of infection

Because of the large areas of skin destruction and the presence of exudate and necrotic tissue, burn wounds rapidly become colonised with bacteria. It has been found that most of the bacteria are acquired from other patients in the ward or unit (Lee et al 1990) and that meticulous attention must be paid to the prevention of cross-infection (see Ch. 16). When possible the patient should be nursed in a single room and isolation techniques implemented. Muir et al (1987) emphasise that once the patient's wound becomes colonised with an organism it will soon be found on his bedclothes, personal clothing and on the surface of dressings. Protective clothing must be worn whenever the patient is attended to; this normally consists of plastic aprons or water-resistant gowns. Disposable water-resistant gowns are expensive but are necessary in the care of patients with major burns, as bodily contact between nurse and patient extends well beyond the confines of an apron when lifting and turning procedures are carried out or when dressings are being changed. The wearing of masks and caps is usually not necessary except when the wound is exposed. Gloves should be worn during any direct contact with the patient and his immediate surroundings; clean (rather than sterile) gloves may be used for procedures other than wound

Box 31.4 Complications of burn injuries

In some patients with extensive burns recovery from the initial injury may be complicated by episodes of severe illness such as septicaemia, adult respiratory distress syndrome and/or disseminated intravascular coagulation, causing them to fluctuate between a satisfactory and a critical condition, perhaps for many weeks. This is especially distressing for the relatives who are trying to cope with the altered appearance of their loved one and who can be given no assurance of eventual recovery; their hopes are raised and dashed repeatedly by their own observations of the patient's condition. Less life-threatening complications include: gastrointestinal ulceration and haemorrhage; systemic infection of the respiratory system or urinary tract; wound infection; and wound contraction and scar formation.

care. Adherence to good handwashing practice requires frequent emphasis, as Lee et al (1990) found that compliance with the correct procedure declines over a period of time following education.

The bacteriological status of the wounds should be monitored regularly by obtaining wound swabs during dressing changes.

THE BURN WOUND

As for any wound, the aim of management is to provide the optimum environment for natural healing processes to take place (see Ch. 23). However, burn wounds differ from other types of wound in a number of ways, which Quinn et al (1985a) identify as follows:

1. Colonisation by potentially pathogenic organisms
2. Presence of large amounts of nonviable tissue
3. Exudation of large amounts of water, serum and blood
4. Remaining open for extended periods of time, thus not offering protection from pathogenic bacteria colonising the burn wound environment
5. Frequent requirement for tissue to be mobilised for its permanent closure.

These factors will be present to a greater or lesser extent, depending on the burn depth. In more superficial wounds the depth of tissue destruction is less and therefore there is less nonviable tissue; consequently the wound will heal more rapidly, reducing the likelihood of colonisation by pathogenic organisms and negating the requirement for mobilisation of tissue for permanent closure. In the case of full thickness burns the opposite is true.

One factor not included in the above list is the fact that most burn wounds involve larger areas of the body surface than is common in other types of wound; this in itself presents many problems in wound management.

Most burn wounds exude copious amounts of fluid. This is evident in superficial partial thickness wounds right from the start but in deeper wounds the surface is initially dry and, depending on the depth of tissue destruction, it may take days before the eschar becomes saturated with fluid leaking from the damaged capillaries in the deeper tissues. The volume of exudate has been calculated to be as much as 5200 $g/m^2/day$ in some burn wounds (Lamke et al 1977) and the evaporative water loss may be as much as 20 times the rate of normal skin (Quinn et al 1985a).

Unless the superficial partial thickness burn wound becomes infected or is subjected to further trauma it should re-epithelialise in 7–10 days. As migration of the epithelial cells occurs the exudate will gradually diminish. Bayley (1990) describes the major aim in burn wound care as obtaining wound closure as soon as possible. In order to meet this goal management must entail:

- meticulous cleansing and debridement of devitalised tissue in order to prevent infection
- facilitating re-epithelialisation, or granulation in preparation for wound grafting
- reducing contractures and scarring
- promoting patient comfort.

Pain control

It is generally agreed that patients with burns experience the greatest pain during therapeutic procedures (Choiniere et al 1989, Kinsella & Booth 1991). Pain-relieving strategies used in wound care include:

- the administration of morphine and other similar opioids timed to ensure optimum cover during the procedure
- patient-controlled analgesia by intravenous or inhalation methods
- relief of anxiety through explanation, hypnosis and other psychological coping strategies.

The degree of discomfort the patient experiences will be strongly related to the skill of the dresser and to her ability to recognise and appreciate the individual's pain tolerance level. Examples of useful pain assessment tools are given in Chapter 19, page 625.

Wound cleansing and debridement

The following procedures must be carried out using strict aseptic technique. If done correctly they may be very time consuming and, where wounds are extensive, will require a number of staff. In some units patients with extensive burns will have dressings changed under general anaesthesia with the involvement of a full surgical team.

A number of different methods are currently in use for burn wound cleansing. Depending on the size and site of the wound the method of choice may be to use saturated gauze or foam pads, irrigation via a syringe, showering or immersion in a special tub. The main debate is over the type of solution to be used. A great deal of research has been carried out on the use of antiseptics for wound cleansing (Morison 1990) and local policy is best adhered to. What is important for both patient comfort and to limit heat loss, especially when the wounds are extensive or on the trunk, is to ensure that the solution used is warmed to body temperature.

Following cleansing the wound is patted dry and loose devitalised tissue trimmed using sharp scissors. Specialists vary in their approach to the management of blisters: Bayley (1990) advises that they be left intact unless they appear contaminated or restrict joint movement; Kemble & Lamb (1987) advocate that blisters be punctured, allowing the 'roof' of the blister to come in contact with the wound surface and act as a biological dressing; Muir et al (1987) recommend removal of the overlying skin. The author's personal experience suggests that the middle road is best. Leaving the (devitalised) skin reduces the pain that would be experienced if the blister were removed totally, but if the blister is left intact it will burst whenever pressure, such as that caused by application of a dressing, is applied and the released fluid will add to the volume of exudate the dressing has to cope with.

As hair harbours bacteria, it should be clipped short in the area of the wound and a surrounding margin of about 5 cm. Shaving is not advised as it can be painful and cause further wound trauma. Long hair which may encroach on the wound should be restrained with elastic bands or adhesive tape.

Promotion of re-epithelialisation or granulation and the prevention of wound contamination may be facilitated either by exposing the wound or by applying dressings.

Exposing the burn wound

Exposure treatment of the burn wound was reintroduced in modern times by Wallace (1949) with the rationale that by producing a dry, cool surface exposed to light one will inhibit bacterial growth. This has been a popular method throughout the world but is currently most commonly used for burns of the face, burns of a single aspect of the trunk or limbs, burns of the perineum, and extensive, complicated burns which cannot be dressed properly (Muir et al 1987). The aim of the exposure method is to provide a dry, intact scab under which re-epithelialisation will take place. Relevant nursing management will be described in the section dealing with burns of the face (see below).

Dressing the burn wound

One of the main problems presented by the burn wound is the copious amount of exudate it produces. This strongly influences the choice of dressing material used. Queen et al (1987) found that the most common classification for burn wound dressings referred to the material involved, i.e. synthetic, biological or conventional.

Synthetic dressings include films, foams, composites, sprays, and gels. Many of these are in popular use for other types of wounds and some are especially designed to be highly absorbent (e.g. Granuflex E) or to allow rapid transmission of water vapour (e.g. Tegaderm, Opsite). These types of dressings can be used successfully in burns which are of a relatively small area but they require a substantial margin to be in contact with unburned skin to prevent leakage of exudate. Thus their use is often not feasible for large wounds.

Biological dressings are normally restricted for use on deep partial thickness or full thickness burn wounds. The ideal biological cover is the patient's own skin in the form of a graft (autograft) which 'takes' to provide wound closure. Other types of skin grafts, i.e. from other humans (allograft) or from animals (xenograft) provide only temporary cover except in the case of identical twins. Sheets of epidermal cells may be cultured from the patient's own skin but the technology required is not readily available. In concluding a review of the current status of skin culture, Donati (1992) emphasises the need for increased effort and financial input to develop this very promising area in the treatment of burns.

Conventional dressings are still the most widely used for all types of wounds (Queen et al 1987). These comprise: an inner layer of mesh, usually impregnated with paraffin or water-miscible cream, which may or may not provide a base for antibacterial agents; layers of cotton gauze; cotton wool or Gamgee; cotton conforming bandages. Unlike many of the synthetic and biological dressings these materials are available in large sizes suitable for extensive burn wounds. Conventional dressings should extend about 10 cm beyond the margin of the wound, and Quinn et al (1985a) suggest that they will remain in use because they are relatively inexpensive and are easily stored.

The aim of conventional dressings is to allow exudate to filter through the layers and for water to evaporate from the surface of the dressing, thus preventing maceration of the wound. It is important therefore that the surface of the dressing is not occluded with a non-porous material such as many of the adhesive tapes used to retain bandages. Other non-porous materials which may come in contact with the surface of the dressing include plastic mattress and pillow covers; such contact should be avoided by the use of foam wedges, slings and special mattresses or beds. If the outer surface of the dressing does become moist, the outer layers only are changed under aseptic conditions. To change the whole dressing unnecessarily exposes the burn to contamination from the atmosphere and may disrupt healing if the innermost layer has become adherent.

The frequency of scheduled dressing changes depends on the depth and state of the wound, and on the properties of any medication incorporated in the innermost layer. Superficial partial thickness burns may have their dressings left undisturbed for 7–10 days (estimated time of healing) unless there are indications for investigating the wound, such as signs of infection. More frequent changes (daily, every second day or twice weekly) are required in deeper burns as the presence of necrotic tissue increases the likelihood of bacterial growth. In such cases antibacterial agents are normally used.

Care of burn wounds prior to skin grafting

The necrotic tissue has to separate from the wound bed before granulation tissue, suitable for skin grafting, is produced. This process of separation may take many weeks and is aided by judicial trimming of loose slough at each dressing change. In small wounds the process may be speeded up through the use of chemical or enzymatic debriding agents such as Scherisorb, Aserbine and Varidase, which are effective but costly.

Surgical removal of necrotic tissue may be carried out, usually within the first 4 days following injury. The tissue is either excised with a scalpel or shaved down to a viable (bleeding) surface with a skin grafting knife. This procedure can result in extensive blood loss and multiple transfusion may be required. The freshly prepared bed is usually skin grafted immediately, but if the bleeding is difficult to control, the skin grafts will be harvested and stored in order that they can be applied without a second operation, usually within the following 48 h.

A skin graft 'takes' by the ingrowth of capillaries from the wound into the graft, a process which takes only a few days. This will be disrupted if there is any blood, serum or pus preventing contact between graft and wound. Other factors which can cause disruption of the graft include any shearing of the graft/wound interface and the presence of β-haemolytic Streptococcus, Lancefield group A (*Strep. pyogenes*) which produces a potent fibrinolytic enzyme (McGregor 1989). Sometimes the surgeon will choose not to apply a dressing to a newly grafted area; nursing staff will be responsible for ensuring there is no collection of fluid under the graft. This is done by gently rolling a rolled-up swab from the centre to the margins of the graft, thus expressing any blood or serum. An aseptic technique is employed and great care is required to prevent the graft shearing on its bed.

The skin graft donor area is a very superficial wound and as a result can be very painful. For the first 48 h or so it produces large amounts of blood-stained exudate and is usually dressed with a conventional dressing which is managed in the same way as that covering a superficial burn. The speed of re-epithelialisation depends on the depth of dermis removed along with the epidermis but is normally between 10 days and 2 weeks.

Ideally, the dressing is left intact until it falls off. Injudicious early investigation will cause further trauma and delay healing.

Care of special areas

The face. The most common method of managing facial burns is that of exposure. Bulky absorptive dressings which extend well beyond the wound margin are liable to encroach on the facial features, which should not be covered.

The face becomes very oedematous and the head should be elevated as soon as the patient's condition allows. Drying out of the exudate is encouraged in order to produce a thin scab. The longer the wound exudes the greater the build-up of serum; this will produce a thick crust which may never completely dry out and is more likely to crack. Rapid drying may be facilitated by regular aseptic application of well wrung-out saline swabs which quickly absorb the exudate and are then removed. (Barely damp material absorbs liquid more effectively than dry material.) Careful use of a hairdryer on a cool setting will also speed the drying process but care should be taken that the patient is able to achieve complete closure of the eyelids before such air-flow is directed at the face.

Once the scab has formed it will be similar to a cosmetic face mask and greatly restrict facial movement. Because of this it is usual practice in some units to apply a thin layer of liquid paraffin to the areas around the eyes and mouth as mobility of these areas is most important (Wilding 1990). The resultant stickiness may allow adherence of debris and it is important to cleanse these areas gently with saline on a regular basis.

Oedema of the periorbital region can cause closure of the eyelids. This is very frightening for the patient, who may think the blindness is permanent. The nurse should warn the patient that eyelid closure may occur and assure him that the swelling will reduce in a few days. Eye drops or ointment will be prescribed in order to reduce the possibility of conjunctivitis. The use of artificial tears will make the patient more comfortable.

Oedema of the lips may cause eversion of the oral mucosa, which should not be allowed to dry out. The skin of the lips should be kept lubricated with yellow soft paraffin and care must be taken when oral hygiene is being performed. The use of a small child's toothbrush, by patient or nurse, will help to maintain normal mouth care and, if the patient is unable to eat, regular mouthwashes should be given. If oral intake is allowed the patient may experience difficulty in drinking from a normal cup; a feeding cup with a spout is preferable to using a straw as the patient may find it difficult to exert just the right pressure to allow suction without collapsing the straw.

Oedema of the ears may cause them to jut out at right angles to the head, making them more susceptible to further trauma. If the pinna produces exudate this is liable to trickle into the external auditory meatus, where it will collect and dry out at the level of the eardrum, reducing the patient's ability to hear. This may not be detected until some time later in which case it may prove very difficult to evacuate the plug. It is easy to avert this problem by inserting a small piece of gauze just at the opening of the meatus to absorb the exudate and changing it as necessary. The ears may be dressed lightly with a conventional dressing or have gauze spread with an antibacterial ointment (e.g. Flamazine) gently applied. The ears will be very painful when touched and it is useful to elevate the head slightly off the pillow, using either a well-padded foam ring or a foam wedge, as this will reduce the possibility of the ears coming in contact with the pillow.

The lower nostrils should be kept free of exudate build-up by regular cleansing with a dampened cotton bud. If exudate dries on the nasal hairs the crust will occlude the nostrils and its removal will be very painful indeed. This problem may be prevented by the application of a light smear of soft yellow paraffin just inside the nostrils.

The beard in male patients also becomes incorporated in the crust as it grows. This does not usually present problems until the scab is separating from the newly epithelialised facial skin (in the case of deep burns the hair follicles will be destroyed and no hair growth will occur). Once the scab starts to lift it may be rehydrated using a moisturising lotion or hydrogel such as Scherisorb Gel; this causes swelling of the scab, which will then no longer fit the contours of the face, and softens it to allow painless removal. Many men prefer to keep their beard for a time but if they wish to be clean shaven the use of an electric razor is preferable as it causes less trauma to the skin.

Scab removal. As the scab lifts on the rest of the face loose areas should be trimmed with care. There may be a strong temptation on the part of both nurse and patient to remove as much as possible, as the satisfaction of revealing nice pink skin can prove irresistible. However, it must be borne firmly in mind that removing adherent crust causes trauma and may increase the possibility of scar formation. Newly epithelialised skin needs to be moisturised regularly with a bland cream to keep it from drying out (see Box 31.5).

Box 31.5 Care of newly healed skin

Care of newly healed skin consists of washing with mild soap, rinsing well, patting dry and applying a moisturising cream. Newly healed skin does not produce sufficient sebum to prevent it from drying out or cracking on the surface. Neither does it produce enough melanin to prevent burning if exposed to sunlight; it must therefore be protected by covering with clothing or by high protection factor sun creams for at least a year.

The hands. Burns of the hands are most commonly treated by the application of polythene bags or gloves in order to facilitate movement and thus prevent joint stiffness and allow the patient a degree of independence. Because the polythene does not allow evaporation of water the wound environment is very moist and the non-burned skin will become macerated. As large volumes of exudate will collect it is usual to apply several layers of gauze around the wrist before applying the bag to absorb some of the exudate.

The warm wet environment created is an excellent culture medium for bacteria and it is usual to use the bags in conjunction with an antibacterial cream such as Flamazine. Application of this cream directly to the hand can be difficult; it is much easier to drop some cream into the empty bag and rub the two surfaces together to give an even cover. The bag is then applied to the hand and secured at the wrist with a light bandage. The bags should be changed on a daily or more frequent basis, and the hand gently cleansed at each change.

In recent years there has been increased interest in the use of Gore-tex material, made into draw-string bags, for the treatment of burned hands. This material is semipermeable; therefore there is less maceration, less weight from the accumulated exudate to restrict mobility, and fewer problems associated with leakage of exudate. The material is much stronger than polythene and can be washed and autoclaved (Muddiman 1989). Terril et al (1991) have found that the opacity of the material is preferred by patients and their visitors and that the material allows a more secure grip.

Limbs. In order to reduce oedema formation burned limbs are elevated and exercised on a regular basis, unless freshly laid skin grafts preclude movement.

Wound contraction is an integral part of the healing process, but excessive contraction leads to dysfunction and deformity. As flexor surfaces are more liable to contract, joints must be correctly positioned, with compensatory hyperextension especially of the wrists and neck. Physiotherapy should be carried out regularly, with adequate analgesic cover, to maintain a full range of movements of all joints. However, splinting may be necessary to arrest or correct contracture formation.

Scar formation

Scar formation is part of the maturation phase of the healing process. In wounds healing by secondary intention the scar often appears red and is raised above the level of the surrounding skin (hypertrophic). Hypertrophic scarring is a well-known complication following burn injury and the resulting disfigurement causes great distress. The most common means of prevention is the application of external pressure, usually effected by the use of specially designed elasticated garments which can be made to fit any anatomical part. Cheng et al (1983) report that, generally, pressure therapy should be commenced within 2 weeks of skin grafting or complete re-epithelialisation of the wound; the garments should be worn, apart from bathing and skin care, for 24 h/day; treatment should continue for at least 9 months; and a pressure of at least 24 mm Hg is necessary for the treatment to be effective. Patients are provided with at least two sets of garments, which are alternately washed and worn.

Elastic garments are not very effective for applying pressure to concavities on the body surface, especially on the face around the nose and mouth. For treatment of these areas a rigid, or semi-rigid, transparent face mask can be made. Powell et al (1985) found the latter type to be especially acceptable to patients. One technique which does not rely on pressure to reduce the hypertrophy and redness of scars is the use of silicone gel sheets (Quinn et al 1985b). These need to be retained in place with light bandages or adhesive tape, and must be removed regularly for washing as they are reusable for a few applications. The sheets are relatively expensive and are usually used only when problems arise in pressure therapy.

PSYCHOLOGICAL EFFECTS OF BURN INJURIES

The disfigurement and impaired function which result from wound contracture and scar formation are generally accepted as the major sequelae of burn injuries, causing great distress and psychological problems for the patient and his loved ones. This, however, describes the long-term view and does not consider that for the patient and his family the psychological effects start at the time of injury.

Partridge (1990) gives a graphic account of his experiences when he sustained burns in a road traffic accident and notes that 'being on fire is unforgettable, you will recall those seconds with crystal clarity for the rest of your life'. Many patients voice their relief at being alive in the immediate period following the accident but as the implications of their injury sink in their emotions and behaviour may begin to go through a series of changes.

Bereni-Marzouk et al (1981) describe four psychological phases experienced by patients hospitalised following burn injuries:

- critical
- stabilisation
- recovery
- predischarge.

This categorisation will be adopted in the following discussion of the problems commonly encountered by individuals with burn injuries.

The critical phase

During the early stages of his treatment the patient will be preoccupied by bodily feelings and by the care provided by nursing and medical staff. If his wounds are extensive and complications arise he will require constant attendance, perhaps for lengthy periods of time, which may result in intensive care psychosis (see Ch. 29, p. 831). Briggs (1991) emphasises the need for nursing staff to be aware of the harmful effects of intensive care, providing communication and controlling environmental factors in order to promote sleep and sensory balance. Nightmares associated with the accident are common at this stage, as are fears of dying. Constant reassurance and reorientation will be necessary.

Stabilisation

When the patient reaches this stage anxiety related to survival is replaced with fears for the future, both short and long term. In the short term, stress is related to anticipation of pain and many patients become depressed or are hostile towards the nursing staff. They may regress in their ability to cope with activities of living and demand care and attention. This is perhaps the most difficult phase for the unit staff to cope with. Pain control helps to reduce patient anxiety related to wound care and physiotherapy and monitoring of pain should continue throughout the period of hospitalisation.

Although there is a tendency to expect that there will be more pain the greater the injury and that pain will reduce in time, in their study Choiniere et al (1989) found no correlation between pain scores and the time elapsed following injury, nor between pain scores and size of burn.

Longer-term anxieties include the fear of disfigurement and of losing function and former roles. Nursing staff can help the patient come to terms with his changed situation by being honest and supportive and allowing him to grieve. The first look in the mirror should not be accidental but a planned occasion with the patient making the choice whether to be alone or to be accompanied by nursing staff or loved ones. Although he may have some idea of his changed appearance from watching reactions of his visitors he will see the true extent of his disfigurement only when he first looks in a mirror. Some patients have glimpsed their reflection in the spectacles of attendant personnel, in darkened windows or in plate glass doors and later reported that they were able to deny their appearance, attributing it to a flaw in the glass. If his hands are not injured the patient may gauge contour and textural changes through touch, but the reality of his changed appearance will still be a great shock.

Manifestations of hostility may range from refusal to co-operate with treatment, through cursing and swearing, to actual bodily assault. Sometimes the hostility is directed only towards certain nurses and the patient may manipulate the situation to create discord among the staff. Care should be planned to ensure a consistent approach by all staff but, especially if primary nursing is practised, it may be necessary to reallocate staff. If the patient's behaviour is uncooperative to the extent that it will interfere with his recovery, behaviour modification techniques may be in order. A contract may be drawn up specifying the type of behaviour expected of the patient and describing the rewards which will be given or withheld accordingly. Many such contracts exist informally, e.g. the patient may be allowed a small whisky if he eats all his supper, but Wallace (1987) advocates a more formal agreement.

Regression in physical ability may also be managed by behavioural modification with the patient being set easily achievable tasks such as pouring a drink from his own water jug, and being encouraged to feel a sense of achievement when he does so. Many patients regress when there is a sudden, unexplained reduction in the amount of nursing care they receive. Explanation about their improving condition, and patient involvement in identifying needs and planning the reduction of care can help to alleviate this problem.

Recovery

This phase is marked by the patient beginning to rediscover former interests and pleasures. He may, for example, take more notice of the goings-on in the unit and of the other patients. When possible, mixing with the other patients should be encouraged; the patient's involvement in small tasks such as distributing newspapers will also aid independence and self-esteem. When disfigurement is highly visible, such as on the face and hands, the patient may not wish to mix with others and will require a great deal of support from staff as well as from visiting family and friends. Griffiths (1989) offers the following list of coping strategies which the nursing staff can explore with the patient:

1. Do not give in to fear
2. Learn to control fear and anxiety
3. Practise positive self-talk
4. Concentrate on relevant pieces of information
5. Do not interpret discomfort as rejection
6. Find your own way of acknowledging the disfigurement
7. Congratulate success.

The pre-discharge phase

Patients frequently experience ambivalence about leaving the safe confines of the unit where they are known and accepted. The actual discharge may be graduated by the introduction of progressively longer visits home and by giving the patient the opportunity to discuss the pleasures and problems he encountered. Williams & Griffiths (1991) emphasise the patient's need for practical advice in the form of staff-led discussions during the period prior to or immediately following discharge from hospital in order to reduce the psychological sequelae of burn injuries. Liaison with the primary health care team will ensure continuity of care and involvement of the social work department and occupational therapists in the community will provide financial and practical help in the resumption of home life.

After discharge

It is possible that the patient will need to return to hospital for clinic appointments and, later on, for plastic surgery to improve appearance and function — a process which may involve many operations over a span of years. Many patients suffer long-term psychological problems including depression, anxiety and other post-traumatic stress symptoms. Wallace (1988) found that the provision of continuing support is currently inadequate and that even two years following discharge from hospital most patients would like to receive a newsletter or to attend social meetings, self-help groups or a staff-led discussion group at the hospital. Many burns units do try to provide such services but the constraints of finance and time often make this impractical.

No matter how high the standard of care provided, the patient who suffers extensive burns may never return fully to his former physical or emotional functioning — a fact which can only serve to emphasise the need for greater effort in the field of burn prevention.

REFERENCES

Adams L E, Purdue G F, Hunt J L 1991 Tap-water scald burns: awareness is not the problem. Journal of Burn Care and Rehabilitation 12(1): 91–95

Bainbridge L C, Simmons H M, Elliot D 1990 The use of automatic blood pressure monitors in the burned patient. British Journal of Plastic Surgery 43: 322–324

Baruchin A M, Rosenberg L, Mahler D 1982 Burns caused by faulty water-heating systems (Waterloo scalds). Burns 10(2): 207–209

Bayley E W 1990 Wound healing in the patient with burns. Nursing Clinics of North America. 25(1): 205–221

Barrett A M 1986 Renal function following thermal injury. Care of the Critically Ill 2(5): 197–201

Bereni-Marzouk T, Giacalone L, Thieulard L et al 1981 Behavioural changes in burned adult patients during their stay in hospital. Burns 8(5): 365–368

Bouter L M, van Rijn O J L, Kok G 1990 Importance of planned health education for burn injury prevention. Burns 16(3): 198–202

Briggs D 1991 Preventing ICU psychosis. Nursing Times 87(19): 30–31

Bull J P 1971 Revised analysis of mortality due to burns. Lancet ii: 1133–1134

Bull J P, Lennard-Jones J E 1949 The impairment of sensation in burns and its clinical application as a test of the depth of loss. Clinical Science 8: 155

Cason J S 1981 Treatment of burns. Chapman and Hall, London

Central Statistical Office (CSO) 1991 Social Trends 21. HMSO, London

Cheng J C Y, Evans J H, Leung K S et al 1983 Pressure therapy in the treatment of post-burn hypertrophic scars. Burns 10(3): 154–163

Child Accident Prevention Trust 1985 Burn and scald accidents to children. CAPT, London

Choiniere M, Melzack R, Rondeau J et al 1989 The pain of burns: characteristics and correlates. Journal of Trauma 29(11): 1531–1539

Cole R P, Shakespheare P G, Chissell H G, Jones S G 1991 Thermographic assessment of burns using a non-permeable membrane as wound covering. Burns 17(2): 117–122

Darko D F, Wachtel T L, Ward H W et al 1986a Analysis of 585 burn patients hospitalized over a 6-year period. Part I: demographic comparison with the population of origin. Burns 12(6): 384–390

Darko D F, Wachtel T L, Ward H W et al 1986b Analysis of 585 burn patients hospitalized over a 6-year period. Part III: psychosocial data. Burns 12(6): 395–401

Davies J W L 1985 The incidence and causes of burns and scalds in children in the United Kingdom. Occasional paper No.7, Symposium on accidents in childhood, London

Donati L 1992 Conclusions. Burns 18 Supplement 1, S 32

Elberg J J, Schroder H A, Glent-Madsen L and Hall K V 1987 Burns: epidemiology and the effect of a prevention programme. Burns 13(5): 391–393

Ellis A, Rylah L T A 1990 Transfer of the thermally injured patient. British Journal of Hospital Medicine 44(September): 206–208

Griffiths E 1989 More than skin deep. Nursing Times 85(40): 34–36

Heimbach D 1984 Inhalation injury. In: Wachtel F (ed) Burns of the head and neck. W B Saunders, Philadelphia

Henly M 1989 Feed that burn. Burns 15(6): 351–361

Herbert K, Lawrence J C 1989 Chemical burns. Burns 15(6): 381–384

ISBI (International Society for Burn Injuries) 1979 Constitution.

Kemble J V H, Lamb B E 1987 Practical burns management. Hodder & Stoughton, London

Kinsella J, Booth M G 1991 Pain relief in burns. Burns 17(5): 391–395

Lamke L O, Nilsson G E, Reithner H L 1977 The evaporative water loss from burns and the water vapour permeability of grafts and artificial membranes used in the treatment of burns. Burns 3, 159–165

Lawrence J C 1987 British Burn Association recommended first aid for burns and scalds. Burns 13(2): 153

Lawrence J C, Wilkins M D 1986 The epidemiology of burns. In: Lawrence J C (ed) Burncare, a teaching symposium arranged by the British Burn Association. Smith & Nephew, Hull

Lee J J, Marvin J A, Heimbach D M et al 1990 Infection control in a burn centre. Journal of Burn Care and Rehabilitation 11(6): 575–580

Linares A Z, Linares H A 1990 Burn prevention: the need for a comprehensive approach. Burns 16(4): 281–285

Lund C C, Browder N C 1944 The estimation of areas of burns. Surgery, Gynaecology and Obstetrics. 79: 352–354

MacArthur J D, Moore F D 1975 Epidemiology of burns: the burn

prone patient. Journal of the American Medical Association 231, 259
Marichy J, Vaudelin T, Marin-Lafleche I et al 1989 Transportation of burn patients. Annals of the MBC 2(2): 66–68
McGregor I A 1989 Fundamental techniques of plastic surgery, 8th edn. Churchill Livingstone, Edinburgh
Mercer N S G 1988 With or without? A cooling study. Burns 14(5): 397–398
Morison M J 1990 Wound cleansing: which solution. Nursing Standard. 19 September, Supplement, p 4
Moritz A R, Henriques F C 1947 Studies of thermal injury: the relative importance of time and surface temperature in the causation of cutaneous burns. American Journal of Pathology 23: 695–699
Muddiman R 1989 A new concept in hand burn dressing. Nursing Standard, Special supplement (September 23): 1–3
Muir I F K, Barclay T L, Settle J A D 1987 Burns and their treatment, 3rd edn. Butterworths, London
Newman P, Pollock M, Reid W H R et al 1981 A practical technique for the thermographic estimation of burn depth: a preliminary report. Burns 8, 59
Noyes R, Frye S J, Slymen D J et al 1979 Stressful life events and burn injuries. Journal of Trauma 19: 141
Palmer J H, Sutherland A B 1987 Problems associated with transfer of patients to a regional burns unit. Injury 18: 250–257
Partridge J 1990 Changing faces: the challenge of facial disfigurement. Penguin, London
Pegg S P, Gregory J J, Hogan P G et al 1978 Epidemiological pattern of adult burn injuries. Burns 5(4): 326–334
Phipps A R 1986 The treatment of outpatient burns. In: Lawrence J C (ed) Burncare, a teaching symposium arranged by the British Burns Association. Smith & Nephew, Hull
Powell W E M, Haylock C, Clarke J A 1985 A semi-rigid transparent face mask in the treatment of post-burn hypertrophic scars. British Journal of Plastic Surgery 38: 561–566
Queen D, Evans J H, Gaylor J D S et al 1987 Burn wound dressings: a review. Burns 13(3): 218–228
Quinn K J, Courtney J M, Evans J H et al 1985a Principles of burn dressings: biomaterials. 6(6): 369–377
Quinn K J, Evans J H, Courtney J M et al 1985b Non-pressure treatment of hypertrophic scars. Burns 12(2): 102–108
Settle J A D 1986 Burns: the first five days. Smith & Nephew, Hull
Steinmann S, Shackford S R, Davis J W 1990 Implications of admission hypothermia in trauma patients. Journal of Trauma 30(2): 200–202
Terril P J, Kedwards S M, Lawrence J C 1991 The use of Gore-tex bags for hands. Burns 17(2); 161–165
Tones K, Tilford S, Robinson Y K 1990 Health education. Chapman & Hall, London
Trier H, Spaabaek J 1987 The nursing home patient: a burn-prone person. An epidemiological study. Burns 13(6): 484–487
Van Rijn O J L, Bouter L M, Meertens R M 1989 The aetiology of burns in developed countries: review of the literature. Burns 15(4): 217–221
Walker A R 1990 Fatal tapwater scald burns in the USA, 1979–86. Burns 16(1): 49–52
Wallace A B 1949 Treatment of burns: a return to basic principles. British Journal of Plastic Surgery 2: 232
Wallace A B 1951 The exposure treatment of burns. Lancet i: 501–504
Wallace L 1987 Behavioural contracts. Nursing Times 83(47): 33–34
Wallace L 1988 Abandoned to a social death. Nursing Times 84(10): 34–37
Watson A C H, Vasilescu C T 1972 Thermography in plastic surgery. Journal of the Royal College of Surgeons (Edinburgh) 17: 247
Wilding P A 1990 Care of respiratory burns: hard work can bring spectacular results. Professional Nurse (May): 412–419
Williams E E, Griffiths T A 1991 Psychological consequences of burn injury. Burns 17(6): 478–480
Wyllie F J, Sutherland 1991 Measurement of surface temperature as an aid to the diagnosis of burn depth. Burns 17(2): 123–128

CHAPTER 32

The patient with cancer

Catherine A. Crosby

CHAPTER CONTENTS

Introduction 875
Oncology as a specialty 876
Epidemiology of cancer 876
The cancer process 876
Tumour histology 877
The spread of cancer 877
The effects of cancer 877
The causes of cancer 880
Intrinsic factors 880
Extrinsic factors 880
Cancer prevention and screening 881
Primary prevention 881
Secondary prevention: screening 882
Medical intervention and the nurse's role 883
Diagnosis and staging 883
The TNM system 883
Psychological impact of diagnosis and staging 884
Aims of treatment 885
Response to treatment 885
Forms of treatment 885
Surgery 885
Radiotherapy 886
Chemotherapy 891
Non-cytotoxic chemotherapy 894
New developments in cancer treatment 894
Nursing practice in cancer care 896
The cancer nurse 896
Hospital — community liaison 896
Cancer care in the community 896
Choosing a nursing model for cancer care 898
Activities of living model 898
Roy adaption model 898
A combined model 898
Family coping 898
Eating and drinking 899
Expressing sexuality 899
Communicating 900
Acknowledgements 902
Glossary 902
References 903
Further reading 904
Useful addresses 904

INTRODUCTION

Cancer is a disease with a profound effect on every aspect of life, whether physical, psychological, social or spiritual. There are two principal reasons for this. First, cancer causes a great deal of suffering and is, after cardiovascular disease, the leading cause of death in the UK. Secondly, despite improvements in cure rates, many uncertainties persist concerning the nature and causes of cancer and methods of prevention and cure. This uncertainty serves to perpetuate various myths and fears surrounding the disease, some of which are described in Box 32.1.

?	**32.1** a. What words come to mind when you think of the word 'cancer'? b. Ask the same question of a few friends, or a member of your family. c. How do their responses compare with yours? d. Is their overall attitude one of optimism or of pessimism?

Indeed, cancer is a serious social problem, costing much in human and financial terms. One in 3 people in the UK will develop cancer in their lifetime, and 1 in 4 deaths are caused by cancer (Cancer Research Campaign 1990). Incidence appears to be rising; it has been estimated that if current trends persist, by the year 2050 1 in 2 persons in Europe will develop cancer during their lifetime (Einhorn 1989).

While statistics present a bleak picture, nurses and other health professionals should be aware that there are reasonable grounds for a positive approach that will foster realistic hope in their patients. Before reading further, consider your own knowledge about and attitudes towards cancer by carrying out the following exercise.

?	**32.2** Consider the following statements. Decide whether they are true, partly true, or false. a. Everyone with cancer dies from the disease. b. Cancer is the cause of the highest number of deaths per year in the UK. c. Cancer is the result of a person's lifestyle. d. Cancer is hereditary. e. Certain personality types are more prone to cancer than others. f. Some forms of cancer are contagious. g. Most persons with cancer are disfigured in some way by the disease. (cont'd)	A

? **32.2 (cont'd)**
h. Cancer patients can enjoy many years of normal, productive life.
i. A cancerous growth is a collection of cells that are foreign to the body.
j. The side-effects of all cancer treatments are particularly severe.
k. Everyone with cancer suffers pain at some point during the disease.

Oncology as a speciality

The idea that cancer patients should be cared for in separate units by specialised staff is a relatively recent one. In some parts of the UK, patients with cancer are still cared for largely on general wards. The increasingly technical nature of cancer treatment has created the need for centralisation and the development of cancer centres in large cities. The disadvantage of this approach is that some patients may have to travel long distances away from their own communities in order to receive treatment.

The establishment of such centres, however, has led to a development of expertise in the coordination and planning of treatment and supportive care. Equally important has been the development of nursing knowledge, specialist education, experience and research in the physical and psychological support both of patients undergoing treatment and of those requiring palliative care.

Cancer may occur in almost any part of the body and affects people of all ages and in all walks of life. Established cancers may present in a wide variety of ways and nurses will meet patients in many care settings who have cancer. As in other areas of health care, increasing emphasis is being given to the role of the health professions in screening for early-stage disease and in promoting awareness of cancer prevention.

Epidemiology of cancer

Epidemiological studies have given rise to theories about the possible causes of different forms of cancer and hence to strategies for cancer prevention and for the screening of high-risk population groups for early-stage, treatable disease. Figure 32.1 shows the incidence of the 10 most common cancers in the UK.

Cancer is mainly a disease of old age: 70% of all new cases occur in people over 60. Hence it is the ageing of the population that largely accounts for the steady increase in the incidence of cancer in the UK. Although cancer is very rare in children, it is the third most common cause of childhood death, despite the fact that childhood tumours respond to treatment far more readily than those of the adult.

See Oakhill 1985 for a specialist treatment of paediatric cancer care.

The incidence of cancer in the UK is one of the highest in the Western world. In Scotland, the incidence of lung cancer in women is the highest in the European Economic Community (Cancer Research Campaign 1988). Generally, people in Western developed countries appear to have a higher risk of cancer than those in the Third World. This may in part be explained by the fact that the West has more sophisticated screening, diagnostic and reporting procedures, and by the fact that since life expectancy is greater death is less likely from other diseases. However, this comparison is also thought to indicate that the rich Western diet, industrial pollution, and behaviours such as smoking and excessive alcohol consumption are the chief causes of cancer.

Geographical variations in the incidence of cancer provide fascinating clues to the causes of the disease. The Japanese, for example, have a low incidence of breast cancer but a high incidence of stomach cancer, thought to be related partly to the consumption of large quantities of salted food. Within one or two generations, Japanese immigrants to Hawaii show the American pattern of a high incidence of breast cancer and a moderate incidence of stomach cancer. The cause is thought to be the adoption of an American diet that is high in fat and protein. These and other similar studies indicate that geographical variations in cancer incidence are attributable to the environment rather than to genetic factors (Haenszel & Kurihera 1968).

The cancer process

The cancer disease process is an abnormal accumulation of altered cells which are out of the control of the body's normal mechanisms. These cells have no specific tissue function, but

Box 32.1 Sociohistorical perspectives

In medieval times cancer was believed to be contagious, caused by uncleanliness and even by a form of demon possession (Nery 1986).

Society

The cultural legacy of historical beliefs is the aura of fear and shame that surrounds the disease even today. Benner & Wrubel (1989) examine the phenomenon of cancer from a sociocultural rather than medical perspective and examine the highly metaphorical language in which the disease process is described — for example, in terms of 'decay' and 'disintegration' or of an 'invasion' by an 'alien army' of 'colonising' cells.

This tendency to view cancer symbolically is also evident in the causes to which many patients attribute their disease, ranging from divine retribution to a stressful life event, a fall or physical blow, dirt or, very commonly, personal failing (Walker 1990).

Cancer stigma

Fitzpatrick et al (1984) define 'stigma' as the disgrace associated with some condition or behaviour which 'breaks the rules' of society, even if unintentionally. Cancer, particularly in a younger person, is viewed as deviant in 20th-century Western society. It threatens the valued attributes of health and longevity and challenges the pre-vailing belief in the capacity of medical science to 'fix' any ailment.

In favourable circumstances most people are not conscious of these underlying social attitudes. However, a person with cancer may soon become painfully aware of the degradation and isolation which accompanies his disease. Family and friends may struggle to maintain a relationship with the person at the same time as they avoid confronting the crises precipitated by his illness.

Media coverage and the widespread availability of accurate information about cancer may be slowly replacing such negative attitudes with a more realistic and helpful public awareness. However, cancer remains a taboo subject, as anyone who tries to discuss it in social gatherings will discover.

Patients and their families bring these attitudes and beliefs into their cancer experience. Assessment of their perception of their situation is an essential first step in the provision of supportive care.

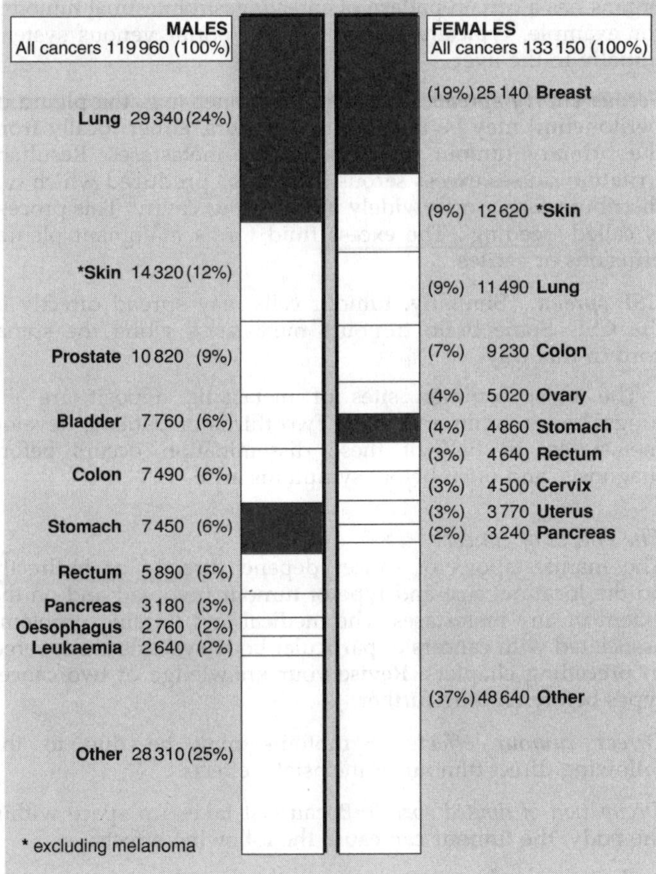

Fig. 32.1 Incidence of the ten most common cancers in the UK: numbers of new cases in 1985. (Reproduced with kind permission from the Cancer Research Campaign 1990.) Variations in the incidence of cancer between the sexes reflect, as well as anatomical differences, different behavioural and environmental factors. For example, the prevalence of lung cancer in men reflects the fact that many men began to smoke during the First World War; the result was a rapid increase in lung cancer in these men, who are now elderly. Women began to smoke in large numbers during the Second World War; hence, lung cancer in women has begun to overtake breast cancer in incidence. In Scotland this has already occurred.

are able to spread from the site of origin to distant tissues. There remain many unanswered questions concerning the steps in this process.

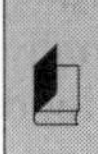

In order to understand what is now known about the cancer process a knowledge of the structure and function of cells and DNA, and of the cell cycle of division is necessary (see Marieb 1989, Ch. 3).

Malignant changes are thought to originate from a mutation or alteration in the DNA of a single cell, which then divides and multiplies to form a colony of altered cells, i.e. a tumour. Recent research shows that this DNA mutation may occur in certain genes, called oncogenes, which are involved in the production and regulation of growth factors. Growth factors are hormones that control cellular division and growth, ensuring that, in normal tissues, growth stops once a certain size has been reached or repair has occurred. Cancer cells, by comparison, grow in an erratic and uncoordinated way because of an alteration in the quality or quantity of these growth factors.

As tumours grow by repeated cell divisions, their rate of growth is often defined in terms of 'doubling time'. Tumours vary greatly in their doubling time but, contrary to popular belief, their growth is not as rapid as that of certain normal tissues. As a tumour grows, blood capillaries proliferate into it, possibly in response to substances produced by the tumour called angiogenesis factors (substances which stimulate blood vessel formation).

At any one time a tumour consists of a mixture of cells, some dividing or growing, some dying or dead. Tumour cells appear to have the capacity to develop various strains within one tumour, each with different properties and, unfortunately, different levels of resistance to anticancer treatments.

Tumour histology

Histology is the study of types of tissue, both normal and diseased. A definitive cancer diagnosis is usually made by histological examination of tumour cells under a microscope.

Histology reports often refer to the degree of differentiation of tumour cells. Well-differentiated tumour cells bear considerable resemblance to the host tissue in structure and function. These tumours are usually slower-growing and are less likely to metastasise (spread); they often respond well to treatment. Undifferentiated, or anaplastic, tumour tissue has lost all resemblance to the corresponding normal tissue. It grows and disseminates (spreads) more rapidly than differentiated tissue and usually responds poorly to treatment.

Malignant and benign tumours. The word 'cancer' is a general term used to describe all malignant neoplasms. A neoplasm is a new growth of tissue, often called a tumour. It may be benign or malignant, although this distinction is not always clear. Brain tumours, for example, may be benign in nature (e.g. meningioma) but because of their location within a limited space may prove to be fatal.

In general, benign tumour cells are well differentiated and slow-growing and do not invade surrounding tissue or form metastases in distant tissue. Once removed, they rarely recur. Malignant tumours have the opposite properties, albeit to varying degrees. A malignant tumour poses a threat to life mainly because of its ability to proliferate destructively into surrounding tissue and to metastasise to other parts of the body.

Tumours are named according to their tissue of origin (see Table 32.1). Tumours of one organ may be of various tissue types with varying behaviours and prognoses. For example, adenocarcinoma of the lung behaves in a much less malignant way than small cell carcinoma of the lung, which carries a very poor prognosis.

Cancer is therefore not one disease but many, each type behaving in a very different way. This must be taken into account in all discussions about cancer and in all relationships with cancer patients.

The spread of cancer (see Fig. 32.2)

The term 'carcinoma in situ' refers to cancer before it has become invasive. The exact manner in which invasion occurs is unknown, but is thought to be partly due to physiological changes occurring in tumour cell membranes which reduce their adhesion to other cells. Tumours also produce proteolytic (protein-dissolving) enzymes which may assist the invasion of normal tissue. Malignant cells also seem to lose 'contact inhibition', thus failing to cease growth on meeting a different tissue type. For example, tumours of glandular lung tissue may continue invasion through the pleura to the chest wall. Once local invasion has occurred to any degree metastases may

Table 32.1 Classification of malignant tumours

Tissue of origin	Malignant tumour
Epithelium	*Carcinoma*
Surface epithelium, e.g. skin, cell lining and covering, body cavities, organs and tracts	Squamous cell carcinoma, e.g. of the skin, lung, stomach
Glandular epithelium, i.e. glands or ducts in the epithelium	Adenocarcinoma, e.g. of the breast, lung
Basal cell layer of the skin	Basal cell carcinoma, often termed 'rodent ulcer'
Transitional cells, e.g. of the bladder lining	Transitional cell carcinoma, e.g. of the bladder
Connective tissue	*Sarcoma*
Bone	Osteosarcoma
Cartilage	Chondrosarcoma
Fatty tissue	Liposarcoma
Fibrous tissue	Fibrosarcoma
Muscle	*Myosarcoma*
Smooth muscle	Leiomyosarcoma
Striated muscle	Rhabdomyosarcoma
Endothelium	
Blood vessels	Angiosarcoma
Meninges	Meningioma
Mesothelium: cells covering the surface of serous membranes, e.g. of the pleura, peritoneum	Mesothelioma
Haemopoietic and lymphoid tissue	
Bone marrow	Myeloid leukaemias Multiple myeloma
Lymphoid tissue	Lymphocytic leukaemias Lymphoma
Nervous tissue	
Nerves	Neuroblastoma
CNS supporting tissue	Glioma, e.g. astrocytoma, oligodendroglioma
Germ cells	
Testes or ovary	Seminoma, teratoma

develop in distant tissue. Metastatic spread (dissemination) may occur in one of four ways:

1. Via the lymphatic system
2. Via the bloodstream
3. Via serous cavities
4. Via the cerebrospinal fluid (CSF).

Lymphatic spread. Tumour cells may invade the lymphatic vessels and grow in clumps and cords, establishing themselves en route in local lymph nodes. This is termed 'regional spread'. It causes lymph node swelling, which may be painful, and may prevent local tissue fluid drainage, causing lymphoedema. This is common in the arms of patients with breast cancer. Eventually, distant lymph nodes are also involved.

Arteriovenous spread. Tumour cells enter blood vessels near the primary tumour, or are shed into the blood via the thoracic lymph duct. They then become enmeshed in the next capillary network they encounter. Hence cancer of certain organs has a certain pattern of spread; gastrointestinal tumours, for example, typically spread via the portal venous system, initially to the liver.

Serous cavity spread. Serous membranes (e.g. the pleura or peritoneum) may be invaded by tumours, either locally from the primary tumour, or from nearby metastases. Resultant irritation causes excess serous fluid to be produced which can distribute cancer cells widely in the serous cavity. This process is called 'seeding'. The excess fluid forms malignant pleural effusions or ascites.

CSF spread. Similarly, tumour cells may spread directly in the CSF. Some brain tumours metastasise along the spinal cord in this way.

The most common sites of metastatic deposit are the lungs, bones, brain and liver. Two thirds of patients develop metastases; in half of these dissemination occurs before diagnosis, and often before symptoms arise.

The effects of cancer

The manifestations of cancer depend directly or indirectly on the location, size and type of tumour involved and on the extent of any metastases. The medical and nursing problems associated with cancers of particular body systems are covered in preceding chapters. Revise your knowledge of two cancer types before reading further.

Direct tumour effects. Symptoms may be due to the following direct tumour or metastatic effects.

Occupation of limited space. Because it takes up space within the body, the tumour can cause the following effects:

- obstruction of passageways, e.g. the oesophagus, causing dysphagia
- compression of major blood vessels; e.g. tumours at the apex of the lung or metastatic mediastinal lymph nodes may compress the superior vena cava, causing ischaemia, oedema of the head, neck and right arm, and dyspnoea
- compression of neighbouring tissues and organs; e.g. brain metastases may cause pressure and local oedema, which compromises brain function and consciousness, depending on the area of brain tissue involved
- pressure on regional nerves causing pain and/or paralysis; e.g. metastases of the spinal vertebrae may compress the spinal cord and result in pain or loss of sensation and paralysis from the level of the lesion downward
- invasion and replacement of normal tissue; e.g. gastric tumours often spread diffusely across the gastric mucosa, compromising its digestive function.

Haemorrhage. Tumours may invade small local blood vessels, causing chronic haemorrhage and anaemia. Occasionally haemorrhage may be sudden and fatal, as when a major blood vessel such as the carotid artery is eroded.

Ulceration. Tumour tissue growth may outstrip local blood supply, causing necrosis, or ulceration, of part of the tumour and adjacent normal tissue. This ulceration may be internal or external. Advanced breast tumours may cause surface ulceration. Due to their appearance, these lesions are often termed 'fungating'.

Infection. This is very common and has been calculated as the cause of death in 50% of patients with metastatic cancer. Increased susceptibility to infection is caused by malnutrition, cancer treatments and, sometimes, by metastatic invasion of the bone marrow, compromising haemopoiesis. Eroded or

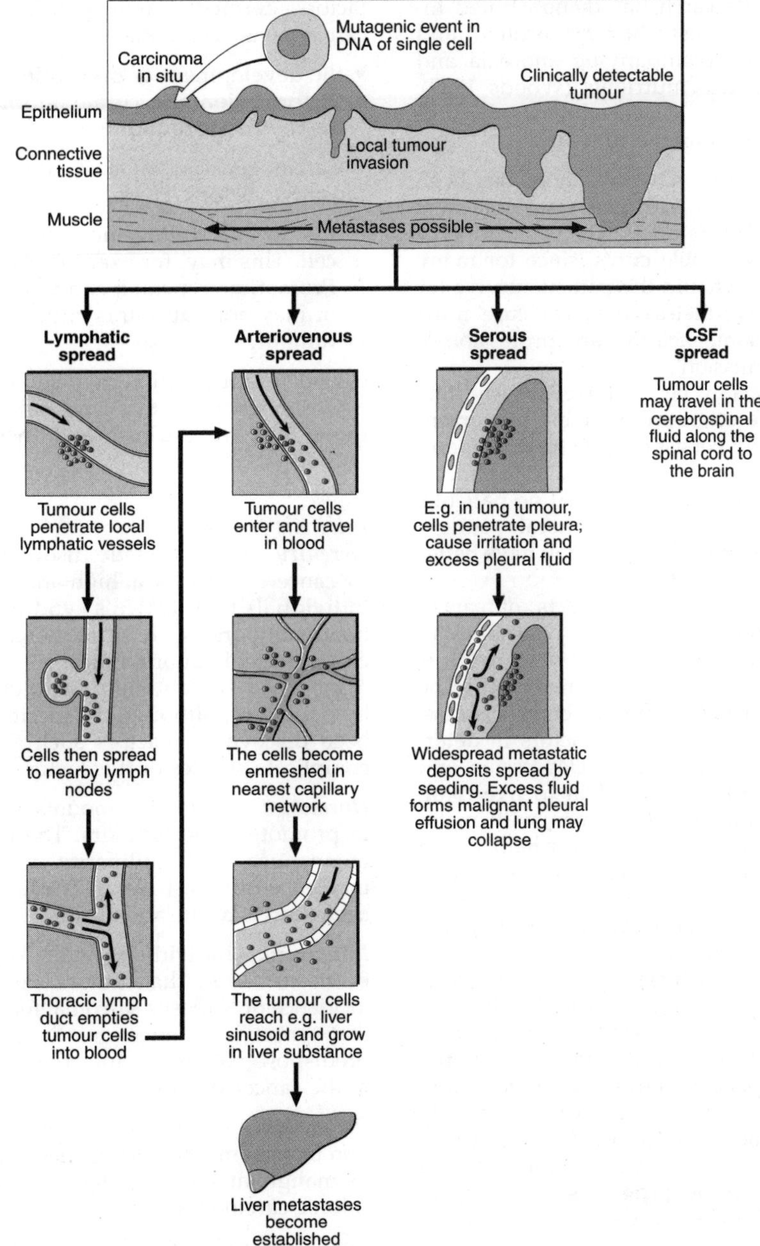

Fig. 32.2 The cancer process.

ulcerating tumours are prone to local infection, which may become systemic.

Metabolic imbalances. These are numerous, tumour specific, and may become widespread with advancing disease. Tumours of the pancreas may cause disturbance in glucose metabolism. Liver metastases may alter ability to metabolise essential drugs. Renal tumours cause progressive renal failure, leading to fluid and electrolyte imbalance. Hypercalcaemia is a com-mon and serious manifestation of advanced cancer of the breast, bone, lung and kidney and is caused by bone destruction due to metastases or by the tumour's production of substances causing bone dissolution.

Indirect tumour effects. These are sometimes termed 'paraneoplastic' effects. They may include skin changes, peripheral neuropathy and myopathy, cerebral degeneration, anaemia, white blood cell abnormalities, and generalised endocrine and metabolic disturbances. These effects are relatively common but vary with tumour type and are usually more marked with advanced cancer. The causes are often uncertain. Early detection is important as these symptoms can often be alleviated even when the primary tumour cannot be controlled.

Cancer cachexia. Approximately two thirds of cancer patients suffer some degree of cancer cachexia. This syndrome has been termed 'a physical fading of wholeness' (Costa 1977). It involves progressive and extreme weight loss and muscle wasting. The resulting weakness can be very severe and death may eventually ensue due to exhaustion of the respiratory muscles. This is most common in patients with gastrointestinal and lung tumours. The causes are many, some directly related to the tumour and some not. Research has demonstrated increased basal metabolic rate and disturbed fat, protein, and carbohydrate metabolism, with accompanying anorexia and altered digestion and absorption of nutrients (Woods 1989). Many of these effects are thought to be caused by a substance called cachectin which is produced by the tumour.

Prognosis and the cause of death. Overall, there has been little change in 5-year disease free survival rates for most common cancers (Souhami & Tobias 1986). The calculation of these rates is used to estimate possible cures, since for many tumours recurrence is less likely should the patient survive for 5 years following treatment. Nevertheless, the term 'cure' must be used cautiously; indeed, some health care professionals prefer the phrase 'complete remission'.

This bleak outlook can probably be explained by the fact that malignant cells, which are often undetectable by current diagnostic techniques, frequently persist despite treatment and in time cause local recurrence of the tumour and/or metastases. Many factors intervene, however, such that no patient's prognosis can be calculated with certainty. In general, younger patients in good health and with a positive outlook have better survival rates, whatever the tumour site.

It may seem obvious that any of the effects of cancer (described on pp. 878–880) may result in or contribute to death. While this is the case, the immediate cause of death is often uncertain, in which case it is generally presumed to be the subtle interplay of the failure of different body systems. The 'significance of psychological and social factors in determining prognosis cannot be underestimated. Depression and loss of hope may result in the loss of the will to live (Stoll 1979). Spiegel et al (1989) found that 50 women with metastatic breast cancer who were involved in a self-help group and were taught self-hypnosis for pain survived an average of 18 months longer than the control group. Such results may possibly be attributed to psychological factors affecting the immune defence system and hormone production, which in turn may influence the tumour growth rate. It should be borne in mind that it is almost impossible to prove this type of relationship; tumour progression could itself be the cause of psychological morbidity and it may be quite unfair to attribute physical deterioration to the patient's emotional state. However, research has indicated that social deprivation and life crises can have a negative impact on prognosis (Hughes 1987). It is therefore clear that the expected time of death is often uncertain; a specific prediction of prognosis is therefore unwise and may even lead to loss of hope.

?	**32.3** Consider patients you have cared for who have died with cancer. Do you know what the immediate cause of death was? Ask a doctor involved if you are unsure. Is he or she certain of this cause? Were psychological and social factors important?
?	**32.4** It is common for relatives to express the need to know the details and exact cause of death of the patient. Discuss with other students why you think this need is so common. Relate any experiences of being with the recently bereaved. What do you think is the nurse's role in the face of this uncertainty? What are the ethical issues involved?

The causes of cancer

Much remains to be discovered about the mechanisms involved in the cellular mutations that lead to cancer. However, epidemiological studies have identified certain causative factors, termed 'carcinogens'. A knowledge of identified carcinogens is essential for:

- the development of prevention and screening strategies
- the provision of accurate information for patients, allaying the myths surrounding cancer causation.

Carcinogenesis is at least a two-stage process and has several causative factors. These stages are:

1. Initiation: a mutagenic event occurs in the DNA of a single cell. This may, for example, be radiation-induced.
2. Promotion: repeated exposure to carcinogenic agents may, or may not, cause this initiated cell to proliferate to form a tumour.

Genetic predisposition may be important at both stages.

Carcinogenic factors and substances can be divided into those that are intrinsic and those that are extrinsic to the individual.

Intrinsic factors

Heredity. Some genetic disorders predispose the individual to cancer. There is a high incidence of acute leukaemia in individuals with Down's syndrome, for example. Most childhood tumours, such as retinoblastoma, are due to inherited chromosomal abnormalities.

Inherited susceptibility to adult cancers is also thought to be important, although no specific genetic mechanism has yet been discovered. Factors such as shared lifestyle in families complicate studies of this factor.

Hormones. Excessive amounts of certain hormones are thought to promote some tumours. The fact that early menarche, late menopause, and nulliparity are all associated with a high incidence of breast cancer implies that prolonged exposure to oestrogen is a causative factor.

Immunity. Individuals with impaired immunity are more prone to cancer than others. People with AIDS have a high incidence of Kaposi's sarcoma, for example. This does not mean that cancer is an infectious disease. Immunosuppression may predispose to certain infections, which may then contribute to the cancer process.

Pre-existing disease. Any tissue subjected to constant irritation or to some disease process has an increased susceptibility to malignant change. Hence, ulcerative colitis may precede colonic carcinoma.

Age. The rising incidence of cancer with age is thought to be attributable to:

- prolonged exposure to carcinogens
- decreased resistance to carcinogens
- hormonal changes that occur with age.

Stress. Increasing interest has been shown in the role of life-stress in cancer causation. For example, the number of deaths due to cancer was higher in a group of recently bereaved men (Parkes et al 1969). In general, however, evidence is limited, although there is some reason to believe that stress may alter the growth rate of a tumour (Hughes 1987). Hence, a particularly traumatic life-event may cause a tumour to increase rapidly in size to a clinically detectable stage.

Extrinsic factors

The fact that 70% of cancer occurs in epithelial cells that are constantly exposed to external, ingested, or inhaled substances implies that extrinsic factors related to lifestyle and the environment are by far the most important in carcinogenesis.

These factors may be considered under the following headings:

1. Physical agents
2. Chemical agents
3. Viruses
4. Diet.

Physical agents. Radiation is known to cause cellular mutations and cancer. Survivors of the atomic bomb explosions at Hiroshima and Nagasaki have a high incidence of leukaemia and skin cancer. Recent research has shown an apparent increase in the incidence of leukaemia among the children of fathers working in the nuclear industry, possibly due to germ cell mutations (Gardner et al 1990). Repeated exposure to therapeutic doses of radiation is not thought to be harmful, although stringent precautionary regulations should be followed for the protection of all exposed workers.

Exposure to ultraviolet light in excessive amounts may cause melanoma, a form of skin cancer. Fair-skinned or freckled individuals who are unable to manufacture sufficient protective melanin are particularly at risk. In the UK, a 50% increase in the incidence of melanoma occurred between 1974 and 1984; this is thought to be due to an increased popularity of sunbathing holidays in hot climates.

Chemical agents. Tobacco smoking causes 90% of all cases of lung cancer. It has been estimated that it is responsible for 35% of all cancer deaths, as it is also a contributing factor in cancers of the mouth, pharynx, larynx, oesophagus, bladder and cervix. High-tar cigarettes carry the highest risk, although risk is more dependent on duration of smoking than on consumption. Smoking 20 cigarettes a day for 40 years is 8 times more hazardous than smoking 40 cigarettes a day for 20 years. Risk is reduced by ceasing to smoke; within 10 years an ex-smoker's risk of cancer returns to almost that of a non-smoker. Recent research shows that non-smokers are at risk by exposure to other people's smoke: one quarter of lung cancer cases in non-smokers are estimated to be due to passive smoking (Cancer Research Campaign 1988).

Excessive alcohol, ingested over long periods of time, contributes to cancers of the mouth, pharynx, oesophagus and liver. Those who drink spirits as opposed to wine and beer and those who smoke as well as drink are particularly at risk.

Many other chemicals, whether inhaled, ingested, or absorbed through the skin, have been shown to cause cancer. Lung cancer in non-smokers is most prevalent in large cities where traffic fumes and chimney smoke raise atmospheric levels of polycyclic hydrocarbons, the same chemicals present in cigarette smoke.

Other carcinogenic chemicals present occupational hazards. Some of these, but by no means all, are now subject to government control or ban. These controlled substances, and associated cancer sites include:

- asbestos (lung)
- vinyl chloride (liver)
- certain chemical dyes (bladder)
- arsenic (lung and skin)
- some hardwood dusts (nasopharynx).

Viruses. Although cancer is not contagious, infection with some viruses does contribute to certain forms of cancer. The Epstein-Barr virus causes a systemic infection that may precede Burkitt's lymphoma, a malignant disease common in parts of Africa. Patients with chronic hepatitis-B are more susceptible than others to liver cancer. The human papilloma virus, which may be sexually transmitted, is associated with cervical cancer.

Diet. Epidemiological studies that isolate diet as a causative factor in the development of cancer are extremely problematic to undertake. Nevertheless, dietary factors have been implicated as the chief cause of the high incidence of cancer in the West. Diet may in fact be responsible for 35% of cancer cases (Cancer Research Campaign 1988). Countries where the average diet is high in fat and protein have a high incidence of breast cancer. Low-fibre diets are thought to contribute to bowel cancer. Some food additives have been found to be carcinogenic and have been removed from the market, although many others have not yet been fully investigated.

Cancer prevention and screening

A 15% reduction in cancer mortality by the year 2000, the target set for Europe by the Commission of the European Communities (CEC) in 1989, would result in 24 384 fewer deaths annually in the UK. The principal hope of achieving this target lies in the rigorous application of prevention and screening programmes. The goal of primary prevention is to reduce the risk of the healthy population developing cancer. Secondary prevention aims to detect early-stage, curable, cancer. Primary prevention is the most effective and economical method of controlling cancer.

The role of the nurse in disease prevention is receiving increasing emphasis, particularly in the community. Especially since the health reforms of 1989, community health centres have assumed greater responsibility for health promotion. Health visitors, district nurses, and some practice nurses have the appropriate skills and are ideally placed to carry out innovative health promotion programmes as well as screening for ill-health. Antenatal care, well-woman or well-man clinics, family planning centres and other health screening clinics all provide opportunities for the promotion of cancer prevention.

Primary prevention

Fear of cancer. Cancer prevention programmes that use fear of the disease to motivate compliance are counter-productive (Walker 1990). Cancer scares propagated by the media are common and add to the aura of fear and stigma surrounding the disease. Such media reports must be responded to cautiously, particularly by health care personnel, and should be put into perspective by reference to the original studies on which they are based. It is important to remember that substances that are carcinogenic in animals are by no means always so in humans. Moreover, everyday exposure to some of the substances implicated is so minimal as to make risk insignificant. Some of these media scares do little to promote health; fear of cancer, after all, is one of the most common reasons why people avoid screening or fail to present with symptoms.

Health promotion programmes. Box 32.2 lists 10 actions that people can take to reduce their risk of cancer. Obviously, observing this code will result in a healthy lifestyle with a low risk of many health problems other than cancer. Health promotion programmes should explore practical and realistic ways of assisting people to integrate such generally healthy behaviours into their daily lives.

Health education programmes have been shown to have a measure of success (Ewles & Simnet 1992). For example, anti-smoking campaigns seem to have contributed to the decrease in the percentage of male cigarette smokers from 65% in 1948 to 35% in 1985, with a resultant decline in the incidence of

Box 32.2 The ten-point European code against cancer (Adapted from CEC 1989)

CERTAIN CANCERS MAY BE AVOIDED

1. Do not smoke. Smokers, stop as quickly as possible. Do not smoke in the presence of others.
2. Moderate your consumption of alcoholic drinks.
3. Avoid excessive exposure to the sun. Tan slowly, avoid sunburn, and use sun-filter preparations. Take special care if you are fair skinned or burn easily.
4. Follow health and safety instructions, especially in a working environment, concerning the production, handling or use of any substances that may cause cancer.

THE RISK OF SOME CANCERS MAY BE REDUCED

1. Eat fresh fruit, vegetables, and high-fibre foods frequently. Cut down on fatty foods.
2. Avoid being overweight.

SOME CANCERS CAN BE CURED IF THEY ARE DETECTED EARLY

1. See a doctor if you notice a lump, a change in a skin mole, or any abnormal bleeding.
2. See a doctor if you have persistent problems, such as a nagging cough or hoarseness, a change in bowel habit, or unexplained weight loss.

FOR WOMEN

1. Have a cervical smear test every 3–5 years if you are, or have been, sexually active.
2. See a doctor if you notice any changes in your breasts, e.g. lumps, dimples, or skin puckering. Women over 50 should be screened regularly by mammography.

lung cancer (Cancer Research Campaign 1988). However, it is thought that success has not been greater because the dissemination of knowledge is not in itself sufficient to motivate changes in behaviour. A European survey showed considerable discrepancies between knowledge and action in relation to each item of the European Code Against Cancer (CEC 1989).

Attitudes. Many factors other than knowledge deficit are known to affect a person's health attitudes. Psychologists have developed a Health Belief Model (as summarised by Niven 1989) to predict an individual's preventive health behaviour and account for some of the factors which determine attitude.

The Health Belief Model states that an individual feels vulnerable to a disease if he believes himself susceptible to developing it and believes the disease to be serious. Furthermore, preventive action will be taken only after the individual has balanced the benefits of that action against its physical, psychological and financial costs.

Despite being taught about the risks of smoking, a teenage smoker may consider himself to be young and healthy and therefore not 'at risk'. Young people in general are motivated by short-term rather than long-term rewards. Smoking in some subcultures and families is associated with attributes such as maturity or rebelliousness which the young person and his peer group may value. Later, the physical addiction to nicotine becomes a mechanism for coping with the stresses of life and social deprivation. For such people, possible avoidance of lung cancer is not worth the cost of surrendering the immediate gratification and social status that smoking offers.

Clearly, consideration of the wider causes of individual behaviour would lead those involved in health promotion to an awareness of the social and political action necessary. Most cancers are more common in lower socioeconomic groups, yet uptake of preventive and screening services in these groups is also lower than among more affluent groups. The causes of social deprivation need to be considered alongside individual behaviour. Preventive services must be readily accessible and based on the expressed needs of the local community. Political action in the form of the control of tobacco sales, legislation concerning occupational exposure to carcinogens and regulation of food additives are also necessary.

? **32.5** Using the Health Belief Model, consider the factors that would be taken into account by a practice-based health visitor working in liaison with an area health promotion officer in devising a cancer prevention programme in the following community health centres:

1. An inner city practice, where 50% of the population are first and second generation immigrants from the Indian subcontinent. The other 50% consist of students in rented housing, young professional people in their first jobs and homes, and workers in a local petrochemical industry.
2. A new town practice which covers a large area of farmland. The new town housing estates accommodate a large percentage of single, unemployed parents. The nearest large hospital is 20 miles away.

Discuss this question as a group. Also consider how the community nurses in each centre might incorporate cancer prevention into their practice.

Secondary prevention: screening

The prognosis of patients with most types of cancer is very much improved if the tumour is detected at an early stage. Often, complete cure can be assured if precancerous tissue can be identified and treated, as in the case of cervical intraepithelial neoplasia (CIN).

Problems in cancer screening. The development of accurate and cost-effective methods of screening at-risk sections of the population is problematic for several reasons (Skrabanek 1990a). The test must have a high degree of sensitivity, reducing the risk of false negative results, and of specificity, reducing the psychological trauma and expense of treating false positive results. It must be possible to identify an at-risk group: otherwise, the cost of screening becomes prohibitive. Finally, and most problematically, it must be determined whether detecting the cancer type at an early stage will actually prolong life. In the case of small cell lung cancer, for example, early detection with existing tests would simply mean that patients would have an earlier knowledge of their diagnosis, but still live for the same number of years (see Ch. 3).

Two screening methods of proven worth both concern cancers affecting women. These are:

1. Breast cancer screening
2. Cervical screening.

Breast cancer screening. In large-sample studies in New York and Sweden, screening for breast cancer by mammography has been shown to reduce breast cancer by one third (Chamberlain 1988). The Forrest Report (HMSO 1986) led to the implementation of a nation-wide, 3-yearly breast screening service for women between the ages of 50 and 64. The denser breast tissue of premenopausal women makes mammograms difficult to interpret for this age group. Targeting 50–64-year-old women maximises the potential number of life-years saved, as the incidence of breast cancer rises sharply with age.

Cervical screening by the Pap (Papanicolaou) smear test has been available for over 20 years. However, reduction in mortality in the UK has not been achieved. This is due mainly to the following reasons:

1. Progression of cervical cancer is still not understood, hence the value of cervical screening is uncertain, and indeed is disputed by some (Skrabanek 1990b). It is ethically important that women are informed about this uncertainty and of the possibility of a false negative or positive result.

2. Uptake of the service by the group at highest risk, i.e. women over the age of 40 of lower socioeconomic status, has been poor. Research shows that two thirds of patients with cervical cancer have never been screened (Walker 1990). A South Tees–based study showed that many women and their partners hold negative attitudes towards cervical screening, based in part on the possible link between cervical cancer and multiple sexual partners (McKie & Gregory 1989). A similar study showed that resulting feelings of guilt and embarrassment may be exaggerated by judgemental attitudes of health professionals and a lack of privacy and supportive care in clinics. This research has resulted in a practical guide to cervical screening and the experience of a positive smear (Quilliam 1989). Staff working in screening services need training in communication skills, and clinic schedules should allow time for necessary counselling.

? **32.6** Consider the role of (a) school nurses and (b) occupational health nurses in the primary and secondary prevention of cancer. Try to arrange to spend a day with one of these practitioners, and identify the elements of her role which could be further expanded to fulfil this function.

MEDICAL INTERVENTION AND THE NURSE'S ROLE

Diagnosis and staging

Patients present with cancer in a wide variety of ways. Consider the different physical and psychosocial care needs of the three patients in Case Histories 1, 2 and 3.

Patients may present at any point in the disease process, ranging from the premalignant to the metastatic phase. Staging is the process whereby the extent of the disease is established; this involves a varied number of tests for each patient. (See Glossary and the chapter appropriate to a given tumour site.) Diagnosis and staging are carried out in a variety of settings, depending on the patient's presenting signs and symptoms. This process can be long, complex, and tedious for the patient.

Case History 32.1 (A) Mr D

D, a 22-year-old student, discovered a testicular swelling but chose to ignore it, initially because he misinterpreted it as a sports injury, and later because he felt embarrassed. Nine months later he presented to the student health centre because he was becoming breathless far more readily than usual and suffered a constant backache. These symptoms were due to lung metastases and referred pain caused by metastases in the para-aortic lymph nodes.

Case History 32.2 Mrs F

Mrs F is 54, married, and has three grown-up children. She is very health conscious and presents herself every two years for a cervical smear at the occupational health centre of her workplace. On this occasion, she is informed that her smear is positive. Subsequent colposcopy reveals carcinoma in situ, i.e. a preinvasive cancer of the cervical cells that is curable by cone biopsy or laser therapy.

Case History 32.3 Mr H

Mr H is a 76-year-old widower. A heavy smoker, he has suffered from chronic bronchitis for 30 years. His respiratory symptoms have seemed more troublesome lately, but it is pain in the ribs and back (due to bone metastases) which finally cause him to consult his GP. These pains are initially considered to be arthritic in nature, causing further delay in the eventual diagnosis of disseminated small cell bronchogenic carcinoma.

However, accurate staging of the extent of the disease is vital for the following reasons:

1. Certain modes of treatment are known to be effective at specific disease stages. For example, thoracic surgery for Mr H (see Case History 32.3) would be inappropriate given the dissemination of his disease. Staging spares the human and financial cost of inappropriate treatment.
2. The prognosis can be estimated according to the disease stage.
3. Staging information is valuable for cancer research, for statistical analysis, and in considerations of the patient's eligibility to enter a trial of a new treatment.

The TNM system

The most common internationally used method of defining disease stages is the TNM system, in which

- T denotes the size or extent of local invasion of the primary tumour
- N refers to the spread to local lymph nodes
- M refers to the presence of metastases.

Box 32.3 illustrates the use of the TNM system in non-small cell carcinoma of the lung. Some types of cancer — usually those that are disseminated at presentation — cannot be effectively staged with the TNM system and have necessitated the development of other systems. Box 32.4 shows the staging

Box 32.3 TNM staging system for non–small cell lung cancer (Adapted from UICC 1987)

T (primary tumour)
T1 Tumour ≤ 3 cm in diameter. No local invasion.
T2 Tumour >3 cm in diameter, or invading pleura.
T3 Tumour of any size with chest wall invasion, or tumour causing lung collapse or pleural effusion.

N (lymph nodes)
N0 Nodes negative.
N1 Positive nodes in hilum of affected lung.
N2 Positive mediastinal nodes.

M (distant metastases)
M0 No metastases
M1 Metastases present

The disease is then staged using the above information, as follows:

Stage I	T1	N0	M0
	T2	N0	M0
Stage II	T1	N1	M0
	T2	N1	M0
Stage III	Any	T3	M0
	Any	N2	M0
Stage IV	Any	M1	

system generally used in the UK for testicular tumours. During the course of their illness, patients may be restaged in order for their response to treatment, or the extent of disease recurrence, to be assessed. Case History 32.2 illustrates the experience of staging for a patient with testicular cancer.

Psychological impact of diagnosis and staging

Confirmation of diagnosis. It is very common for patients to be aware that they have cancer before they are told formally of their diagnosis. This awareness derives from their experience of symptoms, tests and, in some cases, surgery, and from the non-verbal communication of staff or relatives. Whether to inform patients in full of their diagnosis, and when and how this should be done, are issues of ethical debate (see Box 32.5).

Even if they suspect their diagnosis, patients often cling to hope, or use denial as a coping mechanism. These are the early emotional reactions experienced by people faced with any actual or potential life crisis or loss, as described by Kübler-Ross (1973).

Box 32.4 UK staging system of testicular tumours

Stage I Tumour confined to testes
Stage II Pelvic and abdominal lymph node involvement
Stage III Mediastinal and/or supraclavicular lymph node involvement
Stage IV Distant metastases, e.g. lung

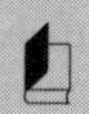

See Niven 1989 Health psychology: an introduction for nurses and other health care professionals. Churchill Livingstone, Edinburgh, Ch. 5.

For most patients, confirmation of their fears comes as a

Box 32.5 Informing patients of their diagnosis: ethical considerations

Two ethical principles are central to the discussion of whether it is always right to tell a patient the whole truth about his diagnosis: these are the principles of autonomy and of beneficence (for a fuller discussion see Thompson et al 1988).

Autonomy

Patients have a right to autonomy, or self-determination. They cannot make decisions about their treatment or the future if they are not fully aware of their diagnosis. Nevertheless, research implies that some patients adapt better if they can deny certain information about the seriousness of their disease (Haes 1989). Although there is some consensus that patients should be told of their *diagnosis*, discussion of *prognosis*, which is very often a medical uncertainty, should be considered individually. Stoll (1979) claims that prognostication may deprive patients of hope, and even give rise to self-fulfilling prophecies of death. Some patients demand to know their prognosis so that they can order their lives and affairs accordingly. Others make it clear that they do not want to know. Still others do not need to be told.

Beneficence

The principle of beneficence obligates health care professionals to prevent harm and 'do good' for their patients. It may seem obvious that to tell lies or withhold the truth is wrong. The patient may suffer severe psychological problems if he continues to feel unwell despite the optimistic messages he receives from others, and may even blame himself for his symptoms. He may also lose trust if and when he discovers the 'conspiracy'.

Discussion

The matter is seldom as simple as the choice between lying and truth-telling, and each case must be considered individually. Relatives may ask that their family member be protected from the whole truth. In most instances, respect for the patient's autonomy should override such a request, especially if the patient is able to ask direct questions of staff.

Tension can arise within the health care team when medical staff fail in their responsibility to disclose diagnosis and prognosis to those patients who clearly wish to know them. Other staff — nurses in particular — who spend more time with patients become frustrated in their attempts to meet the psychological needs of individuals who lack awareness of reality. There must be an open staff forum for the discussion of such problems.

In most cancer centres, the issue is not *whether* but *how and when* to inform patients of diagnosis and prognosis. A study by Walker (1990) showed that patients feel they need time to take in the full implications of what they are told, and then to be given a 'second chance' to ask questions of the doctor when they are less 'shell-shocked'. It would seem appropriate that a nurse is present at such discussions because she can follow up the conversation and help the patient to strike a balance between realistic hope and the acceptance of reality.

devastating shock; this is often followed for varying periods by a normal stress reaction, which may include anxiety, depression, insomnia and poor concentration. This stressful time is one of great emotional confusion, during which the patient attempts to adjust to a shattered world. Relatives and friends also experience a conflict between their desire to be supportive and their fear of impending change and loss. The following words summarise the feelings of one patient immediately after she was told of her diagnosis:

> Then he mentioned cancer. I suddenly went numb, rooted to the spot. The only thing that I could think of was that I was going to die. With that one word he had shattered my well ordered world. I felt my life was closing in on me. I wanted to cry but the tears would not come. I wanted to laugh but it was not funny. Shock and fear invaded my mind. Did I really hear correctly what he had said? I wondered what on earth I was going to do. I turned to my husband and looked into his eyes, hoping to find the much needed help and support. All I could see was my own disbelief, horror, and fear mirrored back at me. I knew I was on my own. (Evans 1989)

At the same time, this patient expressed relief at having a label for her symptoms and knowing that treatment could now proceed.

The discovery that the disease has recurred after a symptom-free period has been shown to provoke even greater psychological disturbance, for the patient's hopes of cure have been disappointed (Moorey 1988). In any event, most newly diagnosed or re-diagnosed patients will be anxious to proceed with treatment as soon as possible, and many will become frustrated with the staging process. The period of waiting for test results is one of great anxiety; the patient is often afraid of the verdict but nonetheless desperate to know it.

Psychological support. Aside from providing the necessary nursing care prior to and following each test, the nurse must act as communicator. It is important for her to know why each test is being performed and what it will entail for the patient so that she can provide explanations and reassurance. The nurse should also act as facilitator, ensuring that test results and their significance are explained to the patient by the doctor as soon as possible, preferably with a nurse present (see Box 32.5). Many fears for the future, both rational and irrational, arise at this time. These need to be discussed openly, and it is the nurse who is most suitably placed to do this.

? **32.7** a. Consider D's needs for information and emotional support during the staging process (see Case History 32.1(B)). Devise a care plan showing how you would meet these needs.

b. Mr H (see Case History 32.3) has been discharged home following palliative radiotherapy to his ribs and spine. One day he asks his district nurse how long it will be before his strength returns. Consider the other questions he may be implying by asking this. What information would the nurse need and how might she reply?

Aims of treatment

Cancer treatments can be described in terms of the following categories:

1. Curative: often termed 'radical' treatment
2. Palliative: given with the intention of controlling distressing symptoms.

The transition from radical to palliative therapy need not be presented to the patient as a major or sudden change of direction, as this may lead to feelings of abandonment and hopelessness. Often, several forms of treatment are given in combination; this is termed 'multi-modal therapy'. Usually one therapy is the primary therapy while the others are termed 'adjuvant' therapies, as in the case of adjuvant radiotherapy following breast surgery.

Response to treatment

Changes in the size of a tumour following treatment are termed 'response rates'. These may be complete, partial ($\geq 50\%$), minor, or absent (in which case the disease is termed 'progressive').

A good tumour response does not necessarily prolong the patient's survival, but it may, in any event, significantly improve quality of life. Unfortunately, cancer treatments can have considerable side-effects which may seriously reduce quality of life. Thus, the decision to treat a patient must be based upon a careful balancing of the costs and benefits of treatment and should, ideally, be taken jointly by the health care team and the patient.

Forms of treatment

The principal forms of cancer treatment are:

- surgery
- radiotherapy
- chemotherapy.

Surgery

Surgery is the oldest form of treatment for cancer and remains the most successful method of achieving long-term survival

Case History 32.1 (B) D (cont'd from Case History 32.1 (A), p. 883)

D was admitted to a surgical ward, where a biopsy under general anaesthesia was performed. A frozen section taken for histology showed a testicular teratoma. A left orchidectomy was then performed.

Following postoperative recovery, D was taken to an oncology ward for staging. D lived too far away to travel to the department each day; otherwise, the necessary tests could have been performed while he was an outpatient. The tests were carried out and their results were as follows:

- chest X-ray: showed multiple lung metastases
- thoracic CT scan: confirmed lung metastases
- abdominal CT scan: showed a large para-aortic lymph node
- liver ultrasound for liver metastases: negative
- blood samples for full blood count, urea and electrolytes, liver function and tumour markers.

These tests showed that D had stage IV testicular teratoma. But even in such extensive disease, the cure rate with **cisplatin**-based chemotherapy is approximately 70% (Souhami & Tobias 1986). Accordingly, this was the treatment course chosen.

A 24-hour urine collection for creatinine clearance and an audiogram were performed to establish baseline measurements for subsequent assessment of any **nephrotoxicity** or **ototoxicity** induced by cisplatin.

for patients with various types of localised tumour. Surgical removal of tumours of the skin (non-melanoma), thyroid gland, uterus, colon and rectum (early stage) are associated with an excellent chance of cure. Certain other tumours, particularly those disseminated at presentation such as small cell carcinoma of the lung, are inoperable.

Surgical procedures are not always performed with curative intent. Surgery may be used adjuvantly with other treatments, for example in the resection of diseased bone after radical chemotherapy for osteosarcoma. Palliative surgery can improve the quality of the patient's remaining life; for example, a bypass of the common bile duct can be performed to relieve jaundice in cancer of the head of the pancreas.

In the case of some cancers, diagnostic methods are not accurate enough for thorough staging; hence, 'second look' laparotomies may be necessary to assess response following chemotherapy in, for example, ovarian cancer.

Psychological support. Surgical techniques, pre- and post-operative nursing care, and the psychological problems associated with undergoing surgery are discussed in Ch. 27. The patient with cancer has all of the usual problems of the surgical patient to contend with, together with the stigma of cancer, and the fear and uncertainty of an unknown outcome. Frequently it is during the perioperative period on a general surgical ward that the patient is told of his diagnosis. There is a need for the nurses on these wards to be aware of the particular problems and needs of the cancer patient.

Radiotherapy

Approximately half of all patients with cancer receive radiotherapy during the management of their disease.

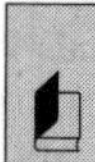

Radiation physics and biology are complex topics which are subject to intense research and development. More comprehensive accounts can be found in Groenwald (1987) and Holmes (1988).

There are two kinds of radiation:

1. Particle radiation, e.g. alpha particles and beta particles. Beta particles are electrons.
2. Electromagnetic radiation, i.e. gamma (γ) rays and X-rays. These are similar to light or radioactive rays, but have a very much higher energy level.

Alpha particles are of low energy; they can be absorbed by a sheet of paper and are too weak to kill cancer cells. Electrons are of higher energy and can penetrate anything up to the density of wood. They are occasionally used in radiotherapy, for example in the form of radioactive phosphorous. Gamma rays are short, very powerful waves that require lead or concrete to absorb them. They are widely used in radiotherapy due to their ability to penetrate deeply into the body tissues.

The most common form of radiotherapy is now the X-ray. These rays are artificially manufactured in an X-ray tube in which electrons are transmitted using a high voltage current. These electrons, on colliding with a tungsten target, emit energy in the form of electromagnetic rays. These rays are termed X-rays and behave in exactly the same way as gamma rays.

Radioactivity. Some knowledge of atomic structure is necessary for a practical understanding of radiation. All matter is made up of atoms, which consist of a central nucleus composed of positively charged protons and uncharged neutrons, orbited by negatively charged electrons (see Fig. 32.3). Strong nuclear forces, provided in part by the neutrons, are required to overcome the electrostatic forces which push the charged protons apart.

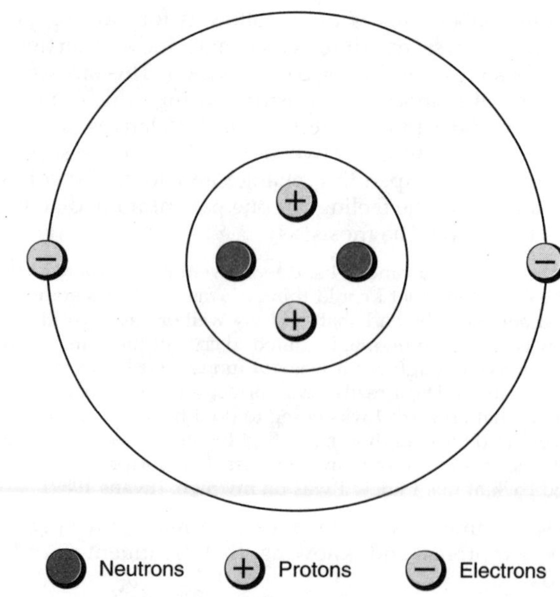

Fig. 32.3 The stable atom. The nucleus of this atom is stable because the number of neutrons and protons are in balance. The neutrons counteract the electrostatic forces pushing the protons apart.

The atom in Figure 32.3 is stable. However, as the number of protons increases, an excess number of neutrons is required in order to hold the nucleus together. This imbalance of neutrons and protons causes the nucleus to be unstable and liable to emit gamma rays and particulate radiation.

Some elements exist in a variety of states, depending on the number of neutrons in the nucleus. These are termed the isotopes of an element. Two isotopes of iodine, for example, are I^{127} and I^{131}. The latter is a radioisotope, i.e. is unstable, because the nuclei of its atoms have a disproportionate number of neutrons. Radioisotopes may be naturally occurring, such as radium-226 (R^{226}), which is now seldom used in radiotherapy, or artificially manufactured by bombarding elements with neutrons in a nuclear reactor, e.g. cobalt-60 (Co^{60}).

The effects of radiation. Cellular response to radiation is not yet fully understood. Radiation causes ionisation of atoms and molecules in living cells. During ionisation, electrons are 'knocked off' one atom and may be taken up by another, creating one positively and one negatively charged atom, both of which will be unstable. The main target of radiation is DNA, which is altered either by direct ionisation of its own molecules, or by changes in the chemical environment of the cell, caused by ionisation of other molecules, particularly water.

These chemical changes irreparably damage DNA, which retards cell metabolism and ultimately causes cell death. Cells are therefore most sensitive to radiation-induced damage towards the end of the G_1 phase, in the G_2 phase, and in the M phase of the cell cycle.

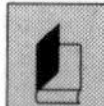

To revise your knowledge of the cell cycle, see Marieb 1989, Ch. 3.

As malignant cells are constantly dividing, they are all radiosensitive, although to varying degrees. Unfortunately, rapidly dividing healthy cells, such as those of the skin, the epithelium of the gastrointestinal and urinary tracts, the gonads and the bone marrow are also vulnerable to radiation damage; this accounts for the unwanted side-effects of radiotherapy. Figure 32.4 explains the difference between the radiation response of tumour cells and of normal cells. In theory, all tumour cells could be eradicated by radiotherapy, but some would require such high doses that normal cell damage would be irreversible; such tumours, for example, malignant melanoma, are termed 'radioresistant'.

Radiotherapy is prescribed as an 'absorbed dose'. The unit used is the Gray (Gy), where 1 Gy = 1 joule as absorbed by 1 kilogram of body tissue. The dose will vary for each patient, depending on whether he is receiving radical or palliative treatment and on the radioresponsiveness of the particular tumour.

Sources of radiation. Radiotherapy is given in a variety of ways, according to tumour type and stage and, occasionally, the patient's condition. Teletherapy (from the Greek tèle, 'far'), sometimes called 'external beam therapy', is the most common method of treatment. Brachytherapy (from the Greek brachys, 'short') is administered via radioactive sources placed within, or on the surface of, the body.

Teletherapy. External beam radiotherapy is administered by X-ray machines called 'linear accelerators', which function at very high voltages (mega-voltage) and in which X-rays are 'hitched' on to radiowaves and thus accelerated. Machines delivering lower voltages are still used to treat superficial lesions, such as skin carcinomas. The total prescribed radiation dose, if administered in one session, would be far too toxic to normal tissue and possibly even fatal to the patient. Hence treatment is administered in daily 'fractions' of the total dose, usually over a period of from 4 to 6 weeks.

The patient's initial visit to the department involves a planning session which may take several hours.

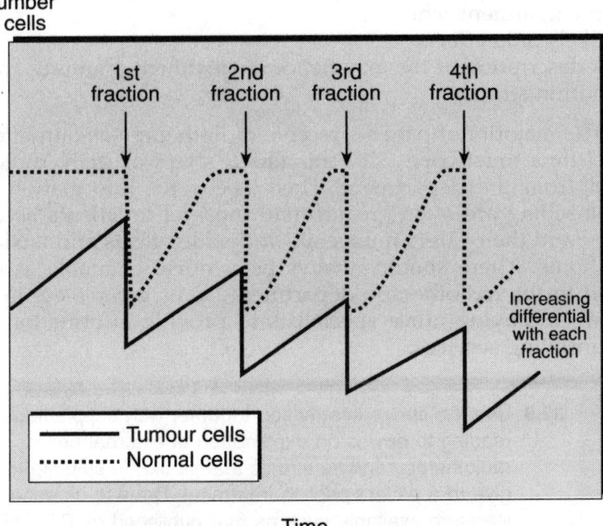

Fig. 32.4 The difference between normal and tumour cell kill and recovery in radiotherapy. Normal cells have the capacity to recover to their previous population level more rapidly than malignant cells. Therefore, successive treatments given after normal cell population recovery but before malignant cell population recovery will result in minimal damage to normal tissue, but successive reductions in tumour size.

Extreme accuracy in devising a unique individualised plan for each patient is vital, the aim being adequate dosage to the tumour and minimum exposure of healthy tissues and organs. Machine called a 'simulator' is used in planning. This mimics the treatment machine and is equipped with tumour visualisation facilities. The treatment field is marked out on the patient's skin using ink, which must not be washed off, or very small tattoos, which are permanent.

Radiation to the head or neck involves the manufacture of a Perspex shell, which can be fixed to the treatment table in order to ensure the accuracy necessary and to avoid marking the skin on the patient's face.

Brachytherapy. This form of treatment is less common than teletherapy, but is often used to treat cancer of the cervix and it is becoming more common for other conditions. Nurses caring for patients receiving brachytherapy are advised to use a specialist text (e.g. Groenwald 1987, Holmes 1988).

Types of radiotherapy treatment. Radiotherapy may be:

- radical
- adjuvant
- palliative.

Radical radiotherapy is used as a local treatment modality, and is often the treatment of choice for early-stage, localised malignant disease, such as tumours of the head and neck, early-stage carcinoma of the breast and cervix, and stage I and II Hodgkin's disease. Tumours vary in their radioresponsiveness, and therefore their curability. Approximately 80–90% of stage 1 and 2 Hodgkin's disease patients are cured by radiotherapy. The curability of early-stage seminoma (a germ cell tumour, usually testicular in origin), skin cancer and breast cancer (postoperatively), is also high. Later stage breast cancer, small cell lung cancer, and thyroid cancer have a poor response rate.

Adjuvant radiotherapy. Radiotherapy is commonly used as adjuvant treatment, usually either pre- or postoperatively, or, increasingly, with chemotherapy. Early-stage carcinoma of the larynx, for example, is treated by radiotherapy alone, with a cure rate of 95%. Later stage disease is treated by a combination of surgery and radiotherapy, i.e. either with emergency surgery followed by postoperative radiotherapy to ensure control of local lymph nodes, or with 4 weeks of planned radiotherapy followed by surgery.

Palliative radiotherapy is widely used and involves much lower doses than radical or adjuvant therapy. Its aim is to achieve symptom relief with minimum side-effects. Again, radiotherapy is effective primarily in the control of local problems, such as local recurrence of breast cancer, pain, compression of adjacent structures by metastases and bleeding, (such as haemoptysis in carcinoma of the lung or rectal bleeding in carcinoma of the rectum). Spinal cord compression and superior vena cava obstruction, for example, often present as emergencies, and the treatment is usually immediate radiotherapy.

Large field radiotherapy. Occasionally, radiotherapy is given to much larger areas of the body. Total body irradiation is used for some patients with leukaemia to irradicate all tumour cells from chemotherapy-resistant tissues. This treatment must be followed by bone marrow transplant to restore bone marrow function (see Ch. 11).

Hemi-body (half body) radiation provides effective palliation for patients with extensive bone metastases, as are common in prostatic cancer, for example.

Radiation protection. There is much fear and misconception amongst both professionals and laypersons about the dangers of radiation exposure. Indeed, radiation is potentially extremely hazardous, and exposure to high doses can cause all of the side-effects itemised in Table 32.2 together with cell mutations that may lead to carcinogenesis, or to congenital abnormalities if pregnant women are exposed.

Every institution dealing with radiation is legally obliged to appoint a Radiation Protection Officer and to follow stringent guidelines for radiation monitoring and protection. If these are adhered to, radiation damage risk is minimal. Staff at highest risk are those working constantly in the radiotherapy or X-ray department, and nurses caring for patients receiving brachytherapy, particularly from unsealed sources. These staff should wear badges in which radiographic film records the cumulative amount of radiation exposure per month.

?	**32.8** Arrange to visit a radiotherapy department. Where is it located in the hospital, how is it designed, and why? Ask what kinds of machines are in use and what kind of treatment each is used for. Ask who the Radiation Protection Officer is and ask to see a copy of the local policy. Try to imagine how a patient might feel, arriving at the department for his first treatment. Compare your impressions with that of another student.

Side-effects of radiotherapy. Side-effects occur when normal tissue is irradiated and subsequently destroyed. The management of side-effects forms a major part of the nursing role in the radiotherapy department (see Table 32.2). Manifestation of side-effects varies greatly from patient to patient, depending on the location and amount of tissue being irradiated, the dose and its fractionation, and the patient's physical and psychological state. Modern treatment techniques have greatly improved the accuracy of treatment and reduced its side-effects, particularly to the skin.

Patients may suffer from systemic side-effects such as fatigue, lethargy, nausea, anorexia and headaches. This syndrome, termed 'radiation sickness', may be due to the circulation of tumour breakdown products. In general, however, radiotherapy affects only those tissues in the area being irradiated. For example, a patient receiving treatment for bladder carcinoma will not lose the hair on his head.

Side-effects may be 'early', occurring 10–14 days after commencement of treatment, or 'late', usually presenting 18 months to 2 years after treatment. Acute problems manifest in areas of rapid cell growth and division and are usually reversible. The nursing management of the most common of these is discussed in Table 32.2. The effects of radiation on the bone marrow have not been included as it is rare for bone marrow to be irradiated to the extent of serious compromise of haemopoiesis, except in the case of total body irradiation.

Late side-effects occur as, due to DNA damage, slowly dividing cells fail to replicate. Problems are most often a consequence of damaged vasculature, and are usually permanent. Examples include fibrosis of the lung, chronic bowel inflammation, and lymphoedema resulting from lymph node damage.

Psychological support. Much research about radiotherapy has concentrated on the patient's emotional and social needs and on the kind of information he requires. The findings of most of these studies are in agreement with Peck & Boland's work (1977; see Research Abstract 32.1). Patients are frequently poorly informed about their disease and its treatment and as a result suffer a high degree of anxiety and depression (Eardley 1986, Lyon 1977, Johnson et al 1988). A recent British study concluded that psychological problems such as anxiety, sleep disturbance and worry about the treatment's effect on family members were of more concern to patients than their physical problems (Munro et al 1989).

Myths and fears. For many patients, the news that they are to receive radiotherapy comes soon after knowledge of their diagnosis and hence when they are already coping with multiple stresses and feelings of loss. Compounding these stresses are the many myths and fears that abound about radiotherapy (often instigated by exaggerated stories about the experience of others) and the connection of radiation treatment with nuclear power. Strohl (1988) lists some of these fears: being left alone in the treatment room, being strapped down, being crushed by the machine, being burnt, hair loss, sterility, cancer induction and receiving too much radiation. Some of these fears are founded on truth; others are irrational. The stress of the experience of radiotherapy must be seen in the context of a cancer diagnosis, and can be illustrated by the following comment: 'Left alone to stare into the source of this invisible and powerful force, patients relate that this experience exemplifies the loneliness and isolation of the entire cancer experience' (Strohl 1988).

The nurse's role. Nurses can do much to alleviate the patient's fears and make the experience of radiotherapy tolerable. In a study by Johnson et al (1988) 42 patients with prostatic carcinoma who were given systematic, descriptive explanations of all stages of their radiotherapy showed a significantly improved quality of life over a control group.

The patient's greatest need is for information. Nurses are responsible, therefore, for becoming accurately informed themselves about radiotherapy in general, and about each patient's individual treatment plan and likely side-effects in particular. A patient survey (Lauer et al 1982) found that the information most desired, in rank order, concerned:

- the purpose of the treatment
- the action of radiotherapy
- the treatment schedule
- likely side-effects
- a description of the experience of treatment planning and administration.

The majority of patients receive radiotherapy as outpatients, and thus must cope with the added stress of daily travel to and from the department. Their needs for information and counselling are often greater than those of inpatients because they and their carers must cope with side-effects and anxieties at home. There should always be a nurse available at each visit to the radiotherapy department; some centres are in fact now employing nurse specialists to provide information and counselling services.

?	**32.9** Use the above information together with supplemental reading to devise an explanation of external beam radiotherapy and its effects that would be suitable to give to a patient prior to treatment. Draw upon patient literature available such as that published by BACUP (British Association of Cancer United Patients) and your own impressions during your visit to the radiotherapy department. Avoid technical terms and emotive words such as 'burn' or 'blast', and bear in mind that patients need to know what they will actually *experience*.

Table 32.2 Nursing management of the side-effects of radiotherapy

Irradiated body part/organ	Radiation effect	Nurse intervention	Rationale
General	Fatigue	Reassure the patient that this is normal Encourage extra rest but also maintenance of as normal a life as possible	Patient may otherwise fear disease progression To prevent feelings of social isolation and depression
Skin, particularly thinner skin and/or moist areas, e.g. skin folds, axilla, groin. Fair skin is especially radiosensitive.	3-stage reaction: 1. Erythema: redness, heat, itchiness	No metal-containing skin preparations Washing, if permitted, must be with tepid water and gentle patting, not rubbing Avoid exposure to sun and extremes of heat and cold Encourage non-constrictive clothing in light, natural fabrics; no tight bras or elastic	Metal intensifies radiation reactions Friction causes irritation Ink marks must not be washed off, but there is no evidence that washing causes damage Ultraviolet light may intensify any reaction Reduces sweating and friction
	2. Dry desquamation; dryness, scaliness, tight feeling, pain on movement	Baby powder may be used Also 1% hydrocortisone or lanolin cream (centres vary in their recommendations) Expose skin to fresh air or cool fan	Soothing, reduces friction Soothing, emollient and/or anti-inflammatory Cooling, with an analgesic effect
	3. Moist desquamation: blisters, loss of surface epithelium, pain, susceptibility to infection. Occasionally progresses to necrosis	A break in treatment may be necessary Analgesia Observation for signs of infection; topical antibiotics as prescribed Absorbant, non-adherent dressing if area can not be exposed	Infection exacerbates skin damage and may become systemic To prevent exudate adhering to clothing and reduce friction to skin surfaces
Scalp	Alopecia (in treatment field only). Loss of any body hair occurs from week 2–3	Reassure the patient that hair will usually grow back in 2–3 months, though it may be of a different texture and colour. Organise provision of a wig. Assist patient to arrange remaining hair to cover bald patches Wearing of scarf/turban at night	Hair loss poses a very stressful threat to body image, especially for women Prevents distress of hair on pillow
Brain	Cerebral oedema (within week 1 of treatment): altered mental state, restlessness, irritability, headaches, nausea, ↑BP, ↓P, ↓respirations	Administer steroids Observe and report alterations in mental status Ensure patient safety	Anti-inflammatory Enables prompt medical intervention
Mouth	1. Mucositis due to damaged, sloughed oral mucosa. Opportunistic infection may ensue, e.g. candida albicans	Regular oral assessment. Teach and assist with frequent, gentle oral hygiene using a soft toothbrush. Use antibacterial/antifungal preparations prophylactically, e.g. chlorhexidene, nystatin. Analgesia: topical, e.g. benzydamine, and systemic; occasionally opiates are necessary. Observe for signs of dehydration and inadequate nutrition	To prevent further damage and infection which may become systemic Oral pain is excruciating and always to the forefront of consciousness Prompt parenteral hydration and dietary supplements or enteral feeding may be commenced

Table 32.2 Nursing management of the side-effects of radiotherapy (cont'd)

Irradiated body part/organ	Radiation effect	Nurse intervention	Rationale
	2. Xerostomia (dry mouth) due to altered salivary gland function. May be permanent. Causes difficulty in chewing, swallowing and talking	Frequent mouth rinses with water. Artificial saliva	Comforting, aids swallowing
		Avoid spices, alcohol, smoking, extremes of temperature	These are mucosal irritants
	3. Taste changes due to xerostomia and damaged taste buds	Assist patients to experiment with other foods	Only certain tastes are altered (see Holmes 1988 p. 88)
	4. Dental decay/due to xerostomia and radiation gingivitis	Pre-treatment dental referral	Any caries will be exacerbated by radiation and form foci for infection
Neck area	1. Pharyngitis, laryngitis, causing pain, hoarseness, loss of voice, dry cough, and occasionally respiratory stridor	Discourage smoking Encourage patient to rest voice	Mucosal irritant
		Observe respiratory status and colour	Medical intervention in the form of steroids or even a tracheostomy may be necessary
		Linctus as a cough suppressant	Prevents mucosal irritation caused by coughing
		Topical analgesia prior to food, e.g. aspirin gargles, anaesthetic throat spray; systemic analgesia	Promotes comfort and aids swallowing
	2. Oesophagitis (upper one third) causing dysphagia	Maintain nutrition. Soft diet and dietary supplements. Avoid irritant foods, strong alcohol and smoking	These patients are often already malnourished
Thorax	1. Oesophagitis (lower two thirds) causing 'heart burn' type pain	As above; also administer antacids prior to food (some antacids contain topical anaesthetics)	Lines oesophagus and prevents pain and trauma of swallowing and from gastric acid reflux
	2. Pneumonitis due to inflammation of bronchioles and alveolar lining. May cause dyspnoea, productive cough and haemoptysis	Discourage smoking Observe for signs of infection: pyrexia, purulent sputum Oxygen as prescribed (see Ch. 3)	Enables prompt commencement of antibiotics
	3. Dyspepsia, nausea and vomiting (less severe than with abdominal radiation)	(See below)	
Abdomen and pelvis	1. Nausea and vomiting. Due to inflammation of gastrointestinal epithelium; also a generalised radiation reaction	Encourage a small meal 3 h before treatment and light snacks after	Some patients are unable to eat after treatment due to nausea
		Regular antiemetics: systematically try various kinds and routes	Regular administration required to prevent and relieve nausea
		Distraction/relaxation techniques	There may be a contributing psychological factor in nausea (Holmes 1988)
		Monitor fluid and food intake	
	2. Diarrhoea, possibly accompanied by rectal bleeding	Maximise privacy Administer antidiarrhoeals as prescribed Low-residue, bland diet Observe for dehydration Maintain high fluid intake	
		Observe perianal skin: gently apply barrier cream after washing if necessary	To prevent skin excoriation
	3. Cystitis due to inflammation of urinary tract. Predisposition to urinary tract infection	Encourage high fluid intake (3 L daily)	Prevents stasis of urine and sloughed epithelium
		Encourage and/or assist with personal hygiene	Helps prevent ascending urinary tract infection
		Regular collection of urine specimens for microbiology	Enables prompt antibiotic treatment of urinary tract infection

Table 32.2 Nursing management of the side-effects of radiotherapy (cont'd)

Irradiated body part/organ	Radiation effect	Nurse intervention	Rationale
	4. Altered sexual function (degree depends on exact treatment site and dosage)	Psychological support and counselling (see Holmes 1988)	Loss of any degree of sexual function is very threatening to most people's self-image; opportunity to talk this through is vital
		Include partner in discussion if patient wishes	To gain understanding and support and minimise body image problems
	Men:		
	Impotence (usually temporary)		
	Sterility (usually permanent)	Offer pre-treatment sperm banking if appropriate	
	Women:		
	Sterility (if ovaries are irradiated. May be temporary or permanent)	Advise continued contraception during and for several months after treatment	Fertility is not always immediately affected and any pregnancy may not be viable
	Dyspareunia due to vaginal fibrosis and dryness	Advise use of vaginal lubricant	
		Discourage intercourse during treatment and for 2–4 weeks after	Intercourse would exacerbate vaginal inflammation
		Provide vaginal dilator after treatment, especially brachytherapy	Aids in preventing vaginal fibrosis, eases future intercourse and internal examination
	Loss of libido	Sensitively explain that this is not uncommon and is usually temporary	
	Premature menopause (if ovaries irradiated)	Inform of possibility	
		Administer hormone supplements if prescribed	To prevent menopausal symptoms

Chemotherapy

The word 'chemotherapy' literally means 'treatment with chemicals' and therefore can refer to any form of drug therapy. *Cytotoxic* (literally: 'poisonous to cells') chemotherapy involves the use of drugs to kill malignant cells. Other drugs, which are not necessarily cytotoxic, are also used in cancer management and will be discussed briefly on page 894.

How cytotoxic chemotherapy works. Cytotoxins are termed 'antiproliferative': like radiation, they are toxic to dividing cells, both healthy and malignant. There are many different types of cytotoxic agents, which have various modes of action, and therefore work at different phases in the cell cycle. (See Marieb 1983, Ch. 3, for a description of the cell cycle.) Cytotoxic drugs are usually classified according to their mode of action, for example:

- antimetabolites
- alkylating agents
- antitumour antibiotics
- spindle poisons.

The action of these types of cytotoxins is described in Box 32.6.

Modes of cytotoxic chemotherapy treatment. Cytotoxic chemotherapy differs from radiotherapy in that it is a systemic rather than localised treatment modality. It is therefore particularly useful for the treatment of haematological malignancies, which are by their very nature usually disseminated, and of metastatic disease. These drugs are a relatively recent development, the first being discovered in the 1940s, and their use has become widespread only in the last 25 years. Despite their great potential, results have been disappointing to date because it has been mainly the rarer tumours that have responded well. Childhood leukaemia is particularly responsive, with approximately 70% of children being cured. Complete responses are also being achieved in adults with Hodgkin's disease. Very few solid tumours are as responsive, the exception being some childhood tumours and testicular teratoma, in which cure rates of 80–90% have been achieved. Sadly, these potentially curable malignancies represent only 4% of patients with cancer.

Adjuvant and palliative chemotherapy. For the most part, chemotherapy is used as adjuvant or as palliative treatment, either pre- or postoperatively. Chemotherapy can be used to 'debulk' tumours, such as those of the head, neck and bladder, in order to make surgery or radiotherapy more feasible. Surgical removal of some tumours, such as those of the breast or ovary, frequently fails to eliminate the possibility of micrometastases, and adjuvant postoperative chemotherapy is commonly used to improve disease-free survival.

Chemotherapy, usually in lower doses, can be used as a palliative measure. Some tumours are partially chemoresponsive, so that treatment may relieve symptoms and improve the quality of, and possibly lengthen, life. Small cell cancer of the lung was formerly considered untreatable, frequently with a prognosis of weeks from diagnosis. It has recently been found to be relatively chemoresponsive, but as average survival is still only one year, such treatment is still termed palliative.

Combination chemotherapy, which uses a variety of agents, has been found to be far more effective than single agent chemotherapy. At any given time, the cells of one tumour will be

Research Abstract 32.1

This descriptive American research, carried out by psychologists, was the first study to examine the information that is given to radiotherapy patients, and how that information influences emotional response. Fifty patients, most of whom were receiving radical radiotherapy, were interviewed before and during radiotherapy. The majority had many unanswered questions about their disease and about radiotherapy and its side-effects. They also regarded the prescription of radiotherapy as bad news, rather than as a postoperative attempt at cure. The fear of losing the doctor's good will by asking questions was described by several respondents, and these particular patients reported a high level of anxiety and depression.

The anxiety level was found to be 60% before and 80% during treatment. Depression levels were similar. This is an American study, however, and the diagnostic definitions of 'anxiety' and 'depression' used in this research vary considerably from the application of those terms in the UK. Criticisms of the study include the fact that 74% of the sample were women, and 22% had a pre-existing psychiatric disorder, leading to some difficulty in making generalisations from these results.

Perhaps, with increasing awareness of patients' needs, the picture has changed since 1977, although a later British study indicates that provision of information and support for radiotherapy patients is still inadequate (Eardley 1986). While Peck & Boland imply that the problem lies with the doctor's lack of time, Eardley argues that information in written form is needed as soon as a patient discovers that he needs radiotherapy, rather than when he arrives, in an extremely anxious state, for treatment. Neither study considers the role of nurses, who, according to Strohl (1988), are ideally placed and skilled to provide the kind of support that radiotherapy patients need.

Peck A, Boland J 1977 Emotional reactions to radiation treatment. Cancer 40: 180–184

at different phases of the cell cycle: a combination of agents acting in those various phases will therefore kill more cells than a single agent. In this way, a lower dose of each agent can be given, thus reducing the side-effect of each. Tumour cells unfortunately have the capacity to acquire resistance to single agents, and so combination therapy partially compensates for this problem.

Administration of chemotherapy. Chemotherapy is usually given in 'intermittent' doses, sometimes called 'pulses' or 'cycles', the principle being similar to fractionation in radiotherapy. Chemotherapy is toxic to rapidly dividing healthy cells, although these have the capacity to recover more quickly than tumour cells. A graph similar to Figure 32.4 could be drawn to illustrate this principle. Hence, most chemotherapy is organised in 'regimes', which are sometimes called 'protocols' if the treatment is part of a research trial.

Most commonly, chemotherapy is given by intravenous injection or infusion, but it may also be given orally, subcutaneously, intrapleurally, as a bladder installation, or intrathecally (see Fig. 32.5 and Box 32.7).

Many patients receive chemotherapy as outpatients, on a day unit, and so need a considerable amount of support and teaching in order to be able to cope with the side-effects they experience at home. There is agreement that although this represents role extension, trained nurse specialists are the best people to fulfil this role and to give chemotherapy (Souhami & Tobias 1986).

Side-effects of chemotherapy. As seen in Table 32.3 each cytotoxic agent causes different side-effects, varying in intensity with dosage. Nursing care of chemotherapy patients is similar to that described in Table 32.2.

Physical and emotional responses to chemotherapy vary greatly with each patient in accordance with differing healthy cell sensitivity and the individual's capacity to cope with stress. The following describes some of the potential physical side-effects.

Infertility may occur, depending on the drug, its dosage, the patient's age and sex, and other, unknown, factors. Infertility may be temporary or permanent. This variability must be stressed when patients are informed about potential side-effects.

Myelosuppression, i.e. the suppression of the production of blood constituents by the bone marrow, occurs to varying degrees after almost all types of cytotoxic chemotherapy. The

Box 32.6 Types of cytotoxic drugs

ALKYLATING AGENTS

Alkylating agents join together or cross-link the two strands of DNA, preventing them from separating and therefore replicating. Cyclophosphamide acts in this way. A metabolite (breakdown product) of cyclophosphamide is acrolein, which is an irritant to the bladder mucosa and can cause haemorrhagic cystitis. This can manifest as mild cystitis, and occasionally as massive haemorrhage. With high doses, another compound, 'Mesna', can be given with the cyclophosphamide to prevent cystitis. In addition, large amounts of intravenous fluids are administered and the taking of oral fluids is encouraged to maintain a good flow of urine to dilute the acrolein.

ANTIMETABOLITES

These drugs prevent the synthesis of DNA by interfering with the various enzymes and precursors necessary for its formation. Methotrexate, for example, inhibits the enzyme necessary for the conversion of folic acid to folinic acid. Folinic acid is necessary for the formation of purines and pyrimadines, which are components of DNA. Folinic acid rescue (in the form of folinic acid replacement) is necessary 12–24 hours after the administration of methotrexate, to prevent the death of too many healthy cells. Other antimetabolite drugs include 5-fluorouacil (5-FU) and cytosine arabinoside.

SPINDLE POISONS

The action of the vinca-alkaloid drugs, vincristine and vindesine, involves interference with the microtubules of the spindle, which pulls the two daughter cells apart. Etoposide works in this way.

ANTITUMOUR ANTIBIOTICS

Some classes of antibiotic have been found to be cytotoxic. In general they act by intercalation or binding of the base pairs on the DNA molecule such that replication is impossible. The most widely used is doxorubicin because it has a broad spectrum of activity; others include mitoxantrone and bleomycin.

Cytotoxic drugs are constantly being researched and developed. There are several which do not fit into the above categories and whose action may not be fully understood; cisplatin, a platinum compound, is one such example.

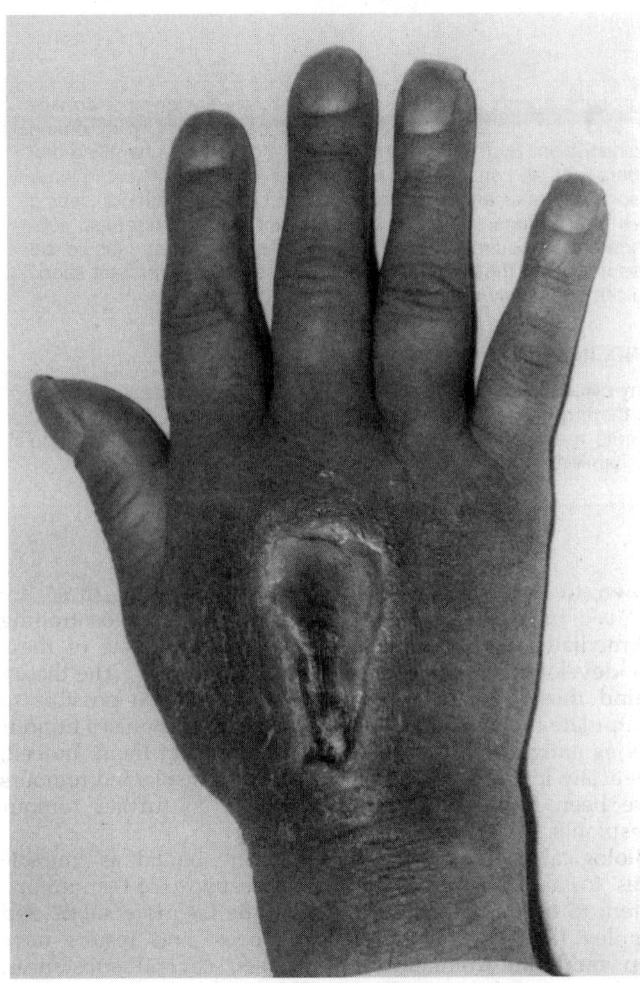

Fig. 32.5 Skin damage caused by extravasation of vesicant cytotoxins. This photograph shows a moderate degree of damage; in some cases there may be nerve and blood vessel damage, progressing to necrosis requiring skin grafting or even amputation. The key factor in avoiding this situation is vigilant, regular observation of cannulation sites during injection or infusion. The patient should also be asked to report any altered sensation in the area, e.g. wetness, coldness, heat, tingling, numbness or swelling.

Should extravasation occur, the infusion should be stopped immediately, the cannula removed, a doctor informed, and a pharmacist consulted for advice. There is a lack of research to guide treatment for extravasation; however, pharmacy departments usually issue local guidelines. It is most important to avoid concentrating only on the affected limb whilst ignoring the stress generated for the patient in this situation.

nadir (low point) in white and red cell and platelet count is reached on days 7–14 post-therapy. The resultant three problems of leukopenia, anaemia, and thrombocytopenia are far more severe in the case of chemotherapy for haematological malignancies (see Ch. 11). For all patients, myelosuppression may compound other side-effects such as stomatitis.

Stomatitis induced by chemotherapy is caused by a two-stage effect. First, some cytotoxic agents have a direct effect on the oral mucosa, causing thinning and ulceration within 4 to 7 days of administration. Nausea, vomiting and a reduced food and fluid intake compound this effect, making the mucosa an ineffective barrier to opportunistic infection. Within 10–16 days myelosuppression results in neutropenia and thrombocytopenia, causing the already compromised mucosa to be even more susceptible to infection and haemorrhage. Nursing care is similar to that for the patient with radiation stomatitis, described in Table 32.2. Patients who are also myelosuppressed require very thorough prophylactic oral assessment and care (see Crosby 1989).

Nausea and vomiting induced by chemotherapy can be particularly troublesome, especially with agents such as adriamycin and cisplatin. These drugs activate the chemoreceptor trigger zone in the brain, which in turn stimulates the centre in the brain stem which controls nausea and vomiting. It is important to remember that persistent nausea is often more unbearable than vomiting, which may relieve nausea. The problem may be severe enough to trigger 'anticipatory vomiting' at the sight of the hospital or anything concerned with chemotherapy. A considerable amount of research has been invested into this problem, and new approaches have arisen. These include the use of high-dose metoclopramide, a new antiemetic called ondansetron and sedatives such as lorazepam. Relaxation and meditation have also been found to be helpful for some patients.

Alopecia, caused by some agents (adriamycin and etoposide in particular), may be total and often includes thinning of all body hair. It usually occurs approximately 3 weeks after therapy, but is temporary. It has been discovered that cooling the scalp by means of various 'cold-cap' devices may prevent alopecia, although the methods are uncomfortable and the results inconclusive (Tierney 1987).

? **32.10** Choose a patient who is about to receive combination chemotherapy. Find out whether the doses or drugs in the regime are low or high. List the side-effects you may expect to see, and those that actually occur. For information, consult the manufacturers instructions, your hospital pharmacy manual and texts on chemotherapy, e.g. Holmes (1991).

Psychological support during chemotherapy. There is increasing recognition, supported by research, that chemotherapy, particularly the highly toxic regimes, can cause severe psychological distress (Hughes 1987). Postoperative adjuvant chemotherapy for breast cancer is associated with an increase in depression, anxiety and sexual problems, possibly because patients see no tangible improvement in their condition to outweigh the distress of the side-effects (Maguire et al 1980).

As with radiotherapy, the key to effective support for these patients is to provide written and verbal information in a suitable, individualised form. Nurses have more potential for involvement and support than radiotherapy department staff. A trusting, supportive relationship may be established if the same nurse is able to give the chemotherapy at each of the patient's visits.

The severity of the side-effects usually peaks when the patient is at home. Specific, preferably written, information on how to cope with these is vital, together with a contact phone number for information and assistance (see Box 32.8).

? **32.11** The patient receiving palliative chemotherapy often finds travelling exhausting and feels that staying at home is far preferable to spending precious time in hospital. Richardson (1989) describes a scheme in which Macmillan nurses give single-agent palliative chemotherapy in the patient's home. What problems can you foresee for the patient, the family, and the nurse? On balance, do you think this is a worthwhile scheme?

Box 32.7 Safe administration of chemotherapy

As with radiation, cytotoxic agents can be dangerous if they are not handled according to strict guidelines (e.g. RCN 1989).

EXTRAVASATION

Some cytotoxic agents, e.g. doxorubicin and vincristine, are termed 'vesicants' and can cause severe burns and tissue damage if they become extravasated from the vein into the tissue. Figure 32.5 shows the possible result of extravasation.

STAFF PROTECTION

As yet, research has not demonstrated adverse effects on staff who handle cytotoxic agents. It is known, however, that at therapeutic doses these substances can cause carcinogenesis, cell mutations and fetal damage. Therefore it is now recommended that chemotherapeutic agents are prepared in a specially designed pharmacy unit and that protective clothing and goggles are worn during administration. Staff should always wear gloves when handling oral preparations and should mop up spillages immediately, using large amounts of water and wearing protective clothing. Patients, seeing these precautions, may be alarmed that such dangerous substances are required to control their disease. They should be reassured that these measures are necessary to protect those who are constantly dealing with cytotoxics.

HANDLING BODY FLUIDS

Many cytotoxic agents are excreted unchanged in urine and faeces. It is therefore wise to wear gloves when handling the body fluids of patients receiving chemotherapy, and also to teach patients and their families to take precautions.

Non-cytotoxic chemotherapy

Agents other than cytotoxic drugs are used to control, but as yet not to cure, cancer. Tumours that arise in tissues under the control of hormones have been found to respond to hormone manipulation. This may mean surgical removal of the ovaries (oophorectomy) or testes (orchidectomy) to reduce the growth stimulus to tumours of the breast and prostate provided by oestrogen and testosterone, respectively. Recently, however, similar control has been achieved using drugs. Tamoxifen blocks the effect of oestrogen by binding to oestrogen receptor sites on tumour cells. Various forms of oestrogen can inhibit the production of testosterone by the testes. These drugs and their side-effects are discussed further in Ch. 7, p. 277.

Steroid hormones, such as prednisolone and dexamethasone, are also widely used, the former in conjunction with cytotoxic drugs as primary treatment (usually for lymphomas) and the latter for its anti-inflammatory action in symptom control.

Symptom control forms a major part of both the nursing and medical roles in oncology (see Ch. 34).

New developments in cancer treatment

Despite an enormous amount of worldwide investment in research, cancer remains on the whole an incurable disease. Most cancer centres are involved in multiple research trials, and nurses should be familiar with the format of these trials in order to understand the implications for patients and their nursing care, and to consider the ethical dilemmas which arise around all experimental therapy.

Following laboratory testing, new methods of treatment are tested using consenting patients by means of a series of trials termed phase 1, 2 and 3 trials. The maximum tolerable dose is established during phase 1; phase 2 trials discover which type of cancer is most responsive; finally, phase 3 trials discover the extent to which the treatment improves survival. In phase 3 trials patients from the target group are randomly selected to receive either the new treatment or the best established one. Survival rates are then compared.

New approaches to established radiotherapy and chemotherapy treatments are constantly being tested in this way. In addition, some centres are involved in trials of totally new modes of treatment; two of these are biological therapy and laser therapy.

Biological therapy involves the therapeutic use of substances known to occur naturally in the body. Most of these are involved in some way in the immune response, controlling cell-mediated and humoral responses; hence some of these new developments are termed 'immunotherapies'. The theory behind these new treatments is that it may be possible to manipulate the immune system such that it recognises tumour cells as antigens and causes the body to reject them. Indeed, genetically identical laboratory mice with transplanted tumours have been found to develop resistance to further tumour transplants.

Biological therapies were prematurely hailed as 'miracle cures' for all cancer types. In fact, the response of the immune system to tumours has been found to be far more subtle and complex than the response to microbes, and results have been far from dramatic. Nevertheless, several substances, mostly created by recombinant DNA technology, have been developed. Although research is still at a very early stage, tumour response, however transient, has been achieved for some cancer types.

Interferon, for example, is a substance that protects host cells against viruses. It has been found to maintain remission in a rare form of leukaemia called hairy cell leukaemia, and is being used with some success for certain patients with renal cell carcinoma. Side-effects include 'flu-like symptoms and can be very unpleasant. Other similar substances include tumour necrosis factor (TNF) and interleukin 2.

Granulocyte colony stimulating factor (GCSF) stimulates proliferation of leucocytes. In the future this may enable higher and more tumour-lethal doses of chemotherapy to be given without some of the problems of myelosuppression.

Although results in terms of tumour response are very limited, and occur mainly in rare tumours, research into biological therapy has yielded new knowledge that can be applied elsewhere in oncology. For example, tumours have been found to possess antigens on their surface. Antibodies to some of these can now be manufactured in laboratories. It is hoped that in time these antibodies, called monoclonal antibodies, can be attached to cytotoxic substances or radioisotopes and 'targeted' at the tumour tissue, minimising healthy tissue toxicity.

A useful summary of these new therapies can be found in Hall (1988).

Laser beam therapy. A laser beam is an intensified form of light that can be focused on a spot the size of a pinprick and

Table 32.3 Cytotoxic agents and common side-effects

Cytotoxic	Action	Common use	Side-effects
Methotrexate	Antimetabolite (folic acid antagonist)	Wide spectrum Acute lymphocytic leukaemia Non-Hodgkin's lymphoma Breast cancer Osteosarcoma	Myelosuppression Stomatitis Diarrhoea Renal failure (HD) Occasional nausea
5-fluorouacil	Antimetabolite	Breast cancer Colonic cancer	Myelosuppression Diarrhoea (HD) Stomatitis Vein discolouration Occasional nausea
Cytosine arabinoside (Ara C)	Antimetabolite	Acute myeloid leukaemia Acute lymphoblastic leukaemia (low dose often given subcutaneously)	Severe nausea and vomiting (HD) Myelosuppression 'flu like symptoms Stomatitis Corneal ulceration
Cyclophosphamide	Alkylating agent	Wide spectrum Small cell carcinoma of the lung Cancer of the breast, ovary and bladder Acute leukaemias	Nausea and vomiting (HD) Myelosuppression Haemorrhagic cystitis Alopecia (HD) Infertility (especially in men)
Melphalan	Alkylating agent	Myeloma Cancer of the breast, ovary	Nausea and vomiting (HD) Alopecia (HD) Myelosuppression
Doxorubicin (Adriamycin)	Antitumour antibiotic	Wide spectrum Lymphomas Small cell carcinoma of the lung Cancer of the ovary, breast, stomach, bladder	Severe stomatitis Severe nausea and vomiting Cardiotoxicity Myelosuppression Total alopecia Vesicant if extravasated
Mitoxantrone	Antitumour antibiotic	Similar to doxorubicin Metastatic breast cancer Leukaemias Lymphomas	Cardiotoxicity Mild nausea and vomiting Myelosuppression Minimal alopecia Green discolouration of urine (persists approx. 24 h)
Vincristine (Oncovin)	Vinca alkaloid Spindle poison	Acute lymphocytic leukaemia Lymphomas Small cell carcinoma of the lung Breast cancer	Peripheral neuropathy: numbness, tingling and loss of function. Constipation due to neurotoxicity Alopecia (HD) Vesicant if extravasated
Etoposide (VP 16)	Action uncertain Similar to spindle poison	Testicular cancer Small cell carcinoma of the lung Lymphomas Acute lymphocytic leukaemia	Myelosuppression Stomatitis (HD) Total alopecia Hypotension if infused rapidly
Cisplatin	Action uncertain; similar to alkylating agent	Small cell carcinoma of the lung Cancer of the testes, ovary, bladder Tumours of the head and neck Lymphomas	Severe nausea and vomiting Metallic taste during infusion Diarrhoea (HD) Myelosuppression Hearing changes and loss (due to damage to 8th cranial nerve) Peripheral neuropathy

HD = high dose

Box 32.8 Chemotherapy: the patient's perspective

The need for information and emotional support during chemotherapy varies according to the patient's perception of the treatment. The following responses by patients to the discovery that they required chemotherapy (cited in Tierney et al 1989) reflect this variability.

Negative feelings

I can't tell you how terrified I am . . . it's like being put into a dark room . . . you've no idea what to expect and you're really frightened.

The word "chemotherapy" sends shivers up my spine — you hear so much about how awful it is.

Mixed feelings

I do want it, but I don't. I feel really nervous . . . . Butterflies in my tummy all the time . . . . and then I tell myself not to be silly . . . . You'll manage, I say.

Positive feelings

I'm making myself feel positive because I intend to do everything possible to survive. That never occurred to me before . . . the idea of survival . . . but your priorities change when you are faced with a disease like this.

is capable of vaporising tumour tissue. Apart from its use in removing premalignant or neoplastic cells from the cervix, this treatment to date has mainly been used as a palliative measure, as tumour tissue tends to regenerate. Intraluminal tumours of the oesophagus, for example, can be reduced in size to relieve dysphagia and malnutrition.

Complementary therapy. The outcome of conventional medical cancer treatments is a matter of great uncertainty for patients. For many, cancer will become a chronic illness that affects every area of their lives. For these reasons there is increasing interest in complementary therapies, such as therapeutic touch, aromatherapy, relaxation techniques, yoga, hypnotherapy, and special diets.

No research exists to justify the use of any of these therapies as alternatives to orthodox treatments (British Medical Association 1986). Evidence for the value of complementary therapy is conflicting. Bagenal et al (1990) found that certain therapies, particularly extreme dietary control, may be detrimental to survival. However, a study of 86 patients with metastatic breast carcinoma showed that those who were taught self-hypnosis for pain control and were involved in supportive group therapy lived an average of almost 18 months longer than the control group, even though they received the same orthodox treatment (Spiegel et al 1989).

There may be a physiological basis for this finding in recent discoveries of neurotransmitters connecting the brain, body and immune system. It is also possible, however, that the extra time, attention and caring mediated by therapists in the course of complementary treatments is the crucial factor in the client's feeling of well-being. Many of these therapies also focus on the 'holistic' approach to health, in which the individual is encouraged to take control of his own life, mentally and physically. It is well established that when patients feel in control they have a positive attitude, comply more willingly with medical treatment, and, most importantly, experience subjectively a better quality of life.

Problems in complementary therapy. Problems associated with some complementary therapies include the fact that an overemphasis on 'taking control' may lead to feelings of guilt and failure when disease problems recur. Some therapies, such as hypnosis, must be practised by experts only. More basic techniques such as aroma-therapy and massage may be incorporated into the nursing care plan, but nurses practising these must be taught to do so by experts. Certain complementary therapies are contraindicated for some patients: all but the gentlest massage may be dangerous for those with bone metastases, for example. It is a good idea to discuss any planned complementary therapy with the whole health care team as well as the patient.

NURSING PRACTICE IN CANCER CARE

The cancer nurse

Cancer and its treatment have a unique impact on an individual's life. Although the physical problems experienced by cancer patients may be similar to those of patients with many non-malignant conditions, the combination of these problems with the chronic nature of cancer, the particularly toxic effects of treatment, and the profound psychological impact of the disease means that cancer nurses require specialised knowledge and skills. The key skills in cancer nursing are those that help the cancer patient and his carers to adapt to the reality of living with cancer while maximising quality of life.

Hospital–community liaison

Without proper coordination and integration of services the cancer patient's 'career' or 'journey' through the health care system can be a bewildering and demoralising experience. The example of Mr A in Case History 32.4 illustrates the need for good discharge planning and liaison between hospital and community nurses. The goal of care for all staff should be to maximise the patient's independence and quality of life. Usually this means facilitating care at home for as long as the patient and his carers can reasonably be expected to cope. The patient's and his carers' psychological adaption to the disease will be as important as physical and practical adaptions in the ongoing assessment of care provision strategies.

Community nursing has always involved 'primary nursing' whereby one nurse is responsible for all stages of the nursing process for each patient. The fact that the career of a cancer patient often involves repeated admissions makes primary nursing a particularly appropriate system for hospital care as well; it enables continuity of care, effective liaison between community and hospital, and the establishment of consistent and trusting relationships with the patient and his family.

Cancer care in any setting can be very satisfying; it may also be stressful and nurses working in this specialism will need to develop healthy and effective strategies for coping (see Box 32.9).

Cancer care in the community

Community nursing staff are involved in cancer care during three phases:

- preventive schemes
- rehabilitation following initial cancer treatment
- palliative care.

It is mainly practice nurses and health visitors who are involved in preventive schemes. Some health visitors also visit patients recently discharged from hospital in order to assess how they and their families are coping and their needs for care and emotional support. District nurses coordinate and carry out nursing care for patients throughout their time in

Case History 32.4 Mr A

Mr A, a 58-year-old head teacher, was married with two children: a daughter in Australia, and a married son who lived nearby and had two small children.

He presented to his GP with urinary hesitancy and frequency. Examination and subsequent referral to a urologist revealed a T3 adenocarcinoma of the prostate (a locally invasive tumour with no metastases). A biopsy of the tumour and a bone scan were performed with Mr A as outpatient. Mr A opted for 4 weeks of radical radiotherapy rather than a prostatectomy. Because he lived in a small town 50 miles away from the nearest radiotherapy department, he became an inpatient, going home at weekends. During his recovery at home a health visitor visited twice.

Two years later, one week after his retirement, rib pain necessitated a further bone scan. This showed metastatic deposits in the ribs and spine. At Mr A's local hospital a bilateral orchidectomy was performed to reduce hormonal stimulation of tumour growth. Mr A was then readmitted to the radiotherapy department. One week of palliative radiotherapy and the commencement of opiate analgesia enabled discharge and 6 months of reasonably independent life.

However, a fall whilst Mr A was gardening resulted in the collapse of the 3rd thoracic vertebrae, with resultant severe pain and paraplegia due to spinal cord compression. Emergency radiotherapy and intensive physiotherapy restored some function, but Mr A was now confined to a wheelchair and had no bladder or bowel control.

Mrs A was fit and was very determined to cope at home with the help of her son and his wife. Prior to Mr A's discharge, the community occupational therapy department oversaw the installation of a wheel chair ramp, bath aids and a hoist in the A's bungalow. District nurses visited daily, and the Macmillan nurse weekly.

Within 6 weeks a further admission, this time to the local hospital, was necessary due to hypercalcaemia. Following this, Mr A was generally too weak to get out of bed. District nurses now visited him twice a day, and the Macmillan nurse every second day as the control of pain and nausea became a problem. It was arranged for Marie Curie nurses to care for Mr A at night, in order to give the family a rest. Mr A died peacefully at home with his family, 10 days after discharge.

the community. However, usually towards the later stages of the disease, symptoms may become more problematic and place more strain on carers; at this stage Macmillan nurses become involved. Macmillan nurses have thorough knowledge of symptom control, additional training in counselling skills and time to assess each patient and to plan care in conjunction with the district nurse. The fostering of links with the Macmillan service as early as possible, when a patient is still able to discuss his hopes, fears and goals, assists in the establishment of a supportive relationship. The role of Macmillan nurses is further discussed in Ch. 34, p. 936.

The role of the district nurse. The role of community staff is one of partnership with the patient's family, who constitute the main 'unit of care'. Providing information, support and advice are often as important as assistance with physical care.

Another major role of the district nurse is one of coordination of the primary care team and integration of statutory and non-statutory services. Because of the nature of cancer, the need for these services is considerable. Statutory services available include all of those necessary for the care of the chronically ill in the community (see Ch. 33).

Non-statutory services in the community. Non-statutory services for cancer patients are particularly comprehensive in their provision. They include:

Support and self-help groups. Such groups can reduce the isolation of the cancer experience. The sharing of feelings and experiences provides emotional support, fosters hope and encourages a sense of self-worth and purpose. Many local groups exist for patients and/or their carers; a directory is published by Cancerlink (see Useful Addresses, p. 904).

Counselling services. Counselling may be necessary to assist the patient and his family to adapt emotionally to cancer and can help to relieve anxiety and depression. Cancerlink and BACUP provide this service by telephone and in person. Both also provide information on other local counselling services.

Box 32.9 Stress in cancer nursing

Speck (1988) states that the most important ethical choice made by cancer nurses is whether or not to engage in 'an intense, personalised involvement' with their patients in response to human need. A degree of emotional involvement is inevitable, and even necessary, to achieve excellence in cancer care. But such involvement, particularly as it may be terminated by the patient's death, results in considerable occupational stress. Community staff are particularly vulnerable because they often work in isolation and build up relationships with cancer patients over longer periods of time than hospital nurses do.

Bailey & Clarke (1989) describe 'indirect' coping methods as more constructive ways of dealing with this inevitable stress than 'palliative' methods (e.g. smoking, excess alcohol consumption, work absenteeism). Indirect coping involves achieving personal awareness and control under stress. Bailey & Clarke give practical guidelines to such methods, which include relaxation, desensitisation and assertiveness training.

The constructive expression of emotions is as important as stress control. A work atmosphere in which it is safe to admit to colleagues feelings of inadequacy, grief and guilt and even personal fears about cancer and death is beneficial in relieving stress. Such support should also be provided on an organised basis in the form of support groups and counselling services (Tschudin 1988). An active life and supportive relationships outside of work are also vital in maintaining a realistic perspective on life. Without external interests it may be easy for the nurse to imagine that cancer is far more prevalent than it is.

A study of cancer nurses by Wilkinson (1990) showed that feelings of inadequacy and lack of knowledge and skill, particularly in communication, were major stressors. A commitment to continuing education by nursing management is therefore essential in stress control. However, as Tschudin (1988, p. 47) concludes, 'nurses themselves need to take on more direct responsibility for their own psychological care', and in campaigning for support and education.

Areas of high stress in nursing often correlate with high job satisfaction (Bailey & Clarke 1989). Wilkinson's study (1990) confirms this: 96% of the sample claimed that they would chose cancer nursing as a career again.

Information services. Information promotes independence in decision-making and can be supportive in itself. Organisations for particular groups of cancer patients include The Breast Care and Mastectomy Association (BCMA) and The British Colostomy Association.

Financial aid. The Cancer Relief Macmillan Fund (CRMF) can provide financial aid to meet the cost of aids, appliances, heating, bedding, holidays and other special needs.

Nursing services. Macmillan nursing services are discussed above. The Marie Curie organisation provides nursing staff to allow carers some respite or sleep.

Choosing a nursing model for cancer care

No one model of nursing can be suitable for every cancer care setting. It is important to adapt and combine models and approaches to provide a workable framework of care for each patient group.

Activities of living model

Cancer may affect every activity of living. Because cure is often not possible, the emphasis in care is on maximising quality of life. This means promoting as much independence as possible. The basic framework of the Roper, Logan & Tierney activities of living model (1983) can be used here. This model focuses on three components of nursing activity, preventing, comforting and assisting, in relation to each of 12 activities of living (ALs). Each component may be relevant at different stages in the cancer process.

The AL model is not in every respect applicable to cancer care. Most people with cancer live with the disease as a chronic illness and many will find it impossible to regain or maintain independence in every AL. And yet, some of these individuals may be described at a given point as healthy because they have learned to cope with their limitations. Another shortcoming of the model is that 'communication', one of the ALs, is not a sufficiently comprehensive category to encompass the whole range of psychological and emotional needs and responses that the cancer patient will experience.

Roy adaption model

Some aspects of the Roy adaption model (Roy 1989) may be more applicable to the nursing care of cancer patients, particularly in a community or rehabilitative setting. Roy sees the cancer as a stimulus to which the patient and his family must be assisted to adapt. The nurse either manipulates the stimulus and its symptoms or promotes the coping abilities of the patient and his family. This inclusion of the family is especially important in any chronic disease.

A combined model

A suitable nursing approach for many cancer care settings would be to combine those aspects of both the AL and Roy models that are especially relevant, giving particular emphasis to the communication needs of the patient as these would now be defined more broadly. Whatever model is selected or devised will attempt to outline the nurse's unique contribution to care. It should be stressed, however, that in many situations, particularly those where cure is not possible, it would be artificial to think in terms of separate approaches by nursing and medical staff. Here, a teamwork model is required which will allow the nurse's role to overlap greatly with that of other team members, but which acknowledges and makes provision for the special contributions of the nurse, such as her role in ensuring continuity, consistency and coordination of care.

Cancer patients may have multiple nursing problems. Four such areas of potential difficulty have been selected for discussion in the following sections. The first, family coping, is a problem of adaption. The others — eating and drinking, expressing sexuality, and communication — are three of the ALs. For each, various considerations relevant to assessment are listed, followed by a set of possible nursing interventions to aid the patient in adapting to his situation.

Family coping

A cancer diagnosis can have a drastic effect on the patient's family and loved ones in the following ways:

- Cancer can disrupt patterns of familial and other interpersonal interaction. Those who are close to the patient are usually perplexed as to how to relate to him in the most helpful way. Reactions vary from overprotection and excessive vigilance to distancing behaviour and even the complete breakdown of relationships. Many patients, especially in the early stages of the disease, find they have to be the strong one emotionally, supporting and holding the family together (Evans 1989). Under such strain it is no wonder that cancer can and does precipitate partnership and marital breakdown. Those most at risk are those who already have an unstable relationship. In a study by Hughes (1987), however, a majority of married people actually felt closer to their partners in the few months following a cancer diagnosis.
- Cancer disrupts planning for the future. An experience with cancer may last for many years. The uncertainty involved disrupts family plans and dreams — for holidays, for retirement, for parenthood, and so forth. Roles within the family change, particularly if the patient is a breadwinner or parent. Such change is stressful and can undermine the patient's sense of self-worth and purpose. Loss of income and increased expenditure due to the illness can create financial strain.
- Cancer alters the interaction of the family with external groups. Patients and their families may easily become isolated as a result of the social stigma of cancer, financial hardship and any residual disability. For some, however, involvement in self-help groups and cancer charities expands social interaction.

Nursing interventions. Following assessment of family dynamics and needs, the following nursing interventions may help to alleviate some of the above problems:

- Providing regular information about the patient's status and plans for care, preferably with the patient and his family together to facilitate open communication. Studies show that relatives feel they may not be entitled to information, yet nurses usually leave it to them to take the initiative in asking for it (Bond 1982)
- Encouraging relatives to express their feelings of fear, loss, guilt, and exhaustion
- Encouraging realistic, mutual goal-setting, for example, the timing and planning of holidays
- Encouraging the family to adapt the patient's role within the family to maintain his sense of belonging and of worth; for example, by exchanging physical tasks for clerical ones
- Referring families promptly to the social work department for financial assistance and, if necessary, rehousing
- Recognising signs of exhaustion in carers; giving them 'permission' to take time off. Arranging respite care or hospital admission if necessary
- Encouraging continued social involvement, suggesting appropriate activities if necessary

- Suggesting referral to a psychologist or marriage guidance counsellor if a family is clearly breaking down.

Eating and drinking

Malnutrition accompanied by varying degrees of weight loss affects up to two-thirds of cancer patients at some stage in their disease; 40% of cancer patients have a deficient intake of protein and calories.

Cancer cachexia is described on page 879. Although not all patients suffer from this in the extreme, the associated weight loss can have a very negative effect on a patient's body image and sexuality, and serves as a constant reminder of their disease.

Malnutrition in cancer patients is associated with a poor prognosis, reduced response to anticancer treatments, and prolongation of side-effects (Holmes 1988). Causes of malnutrition and weight loss in cancer patients are numerous and interrelated. They include:

1. Reduced food intake due to:
   - anorexia: multiple causes, but possibly partly due to cachectin, a substance produced by some tumours
   - taste changes: may occur in any cancer patient (Stubbs 1989); commonest following radiotherapy to the head or neck due to destruction of salivary tissue. Usually involve:
     — lowered threshold for bitter tastes, and therefore aversion to meat
     — raised threshold for sweet tastes; therefore, many foods taste bland and 'cardboard-like'
     — alteration of the taste of tea and coffee
   - early satiety: a premature feeling of fullness, usually progressing over the day
   - other symptoms, such as pain, nausea, vomiting and drowsiness
   - physical difficulties due to the tumour or its treatment, e.g. stomatitis, or dysphagia due to oesophageal obstruction
   - anxiety and depression
2. Malabsorption due to:
   - tumours of the GI tract
   - impairment of nutrient absorption resulting from chemotherapy and abdominal radiotherapy
3. Excess expenditure of nutrients, due to:
   - (in many patients) raised basal metabolic rate, partly due to the demands of the tumour
   - excessive loss of body protein due to vomiting, diarrhoea, haemorrhage, oedema, and exudates from stomas, fistulae, and ulcerations.

Nursing interventions. Actions that the nurse can take to help the patient overcome or manage difficulties with eating and drinking include the following:

- Carrying out an initial assessment of the patient. This should include a thorough nutritional assessment repeated at regular intervals. Weekly weighing is adequate; more frequent weighing may cause the patient to become anxious about and demoralised by continued weight loss
- Identifying the major factors from the list above that contribute to the nutritional deficit
- Referring all at-risk patients to a dietitian
- Enlisting the help of relatives and friends in providing encouragement and supplying the patient's favourite foods. The nurse should explain, however, that there are very real reasons for the patient's reluctance to eat
- Being persistent in encouraging the patient to eat, whilst respecting the patient's autonomy. It may be necessary to encourage the patient temporarily to regard food as a necessary medicine
- Offering frequent, small, attractive meals. Negotiating with the catering department for flexibility in portion size and for a supply of nutrient-rich foods to be kept at ward level
- Encouraging patients to take fluids in the form of high-energy drinks. Discouraging drinking at mealtimes, to avoid early satiety
- Reassuring the patient that taste changes are normal and may disappear in time. Offering taste-enhancing herbs and spices and alternatives to tea and coffee
- Encouraging, if appropriate, consumption of a small amount of alcohol with meals as an appetite stimulant
- Controlling other symptoms. Antiemetics should be administered 30 min before meals. Patients with a painful mouth or throat may be given topical anaesthetic mouthwashes immediately before eating
- Providing dietary supplements in liquid form between meals and as powdered additives with meals. A study by Parkinson et al (1987) showed that Polycal and Protifar were the most palatable additives for a group of cancer patients. The use of these achieved a significant increase in calorie and protein intake in 30 patients
- Eliminating nauseating environmental stimuli at mealtimes, such as bedpans, odours, and disturbing procedures
- If intake is consistently inadequate and/or weight loss continues, commencing other forms of feeding: nasogastric if absorption is adequate; parenteral if not
- Once the patient is well, encouraging a healthy, well-balanced diet, similar to that recommended for preventing cancer (see Box 32.2). Discourage faddish or drastic diets, particularly those involving prolonged fasting.

Expressing sexuality

Following treatment for cancer, up to 50% of patients who were sexually active before the illness report some reduction in sexual interest or activity (Hughes 1987). Health care professionals in general fail to take the initiative in discussing their patients' sexual problems. Wilson & Williams (1988) demonstrated a discrepancy between nurses' attitudes toward the need for assessment of sexual problems and their actual behaviour. The reticence of some nurses may be due to embarrassment, but a lack of relevant knowledge and counselling skills was also reported.

Sexuality involves more than sexual intercourse. It includes self-image in relation to gender, role behaviour within a partnership, and many forms of love and affection between partners. A cancer patient's sexuality may be altered for many reasons, including:

- The physical effects of the tumour; e.g. lesions of the spinal cord may interfere with the nerve pathways necessary for sexual sensation or motor function
- Symptoms caused by the tumour; e.g. pain, immobility, and fatigue all decrease libido and performance
- The physical effects of treatment: hormone manipulation may alter sexual function; surgery may alter the anatomy (e.g. a prostatectomy may cause pelvic nerve damage resulting in impotence); pelvic irradiation may reduce vaginal lubrication causing dyspareunia (painful intercourse)
- Body image problems, e.g. post-mastectomy or following stoma formation. Less obvious changes may also contribute, e.g. mild degrees of weight loss or hair loss

- Anxiety and depression related to the cancer diagnosis resulting in low self-esteem.

Nursing interventions. The nurse can provide support for the cancer patient experiencing problems with the expression of sexuality in the following ways:

- Initiating discussion in order to give the patient 'permission' to voice his concerns. Once the discussion is initiated, the patient will indicate whether or not he wishes to pursue the topic
- Anticipating problems before treatment; explaining how long they will last and that they are normal. Describing measures that can be used to relieve them. See Table 32.2 for examples of interventions for radiotherapy patients
- Opening discussion with non-threatening subjects such as contraceptive advice or the alterations in partnership roles due to illness. This will aid progression to potentially more embarrassing issues
- Discovering and using the patient's own language in relation to his sexuality
- Ensuring that anxiety and depression are treated and body-image problems are addressed. Severe body-image problems may require desensitisation therapy by a psychologist
- Involving partners in discussion and physical care as appropriate
- Facilitating the privacy of couples in hospitals
- When appropriate, discussing ways in which a couple may share sexual pleasure that does not involve intercourse. Cancerlink provide information that describes these methods
- Referring patients and partners with severe problems to a psychologist or sexual counsellor as appropriate.

Communicating

From the cancer patient's perspective, communication can be the most important aspect of treatment, in part because of its capacity to exacerbate or allay the fear that often accompanies cancer (Thorne 1988). Communication can be divided into three areas of activity, which may be described as:

- cognitive: the giving and receiving of information
- emotional: the feeling and expression of psychological responses
- spiritual: the expression and feeling of thoughts relating to existential issues beyond the self.

Although this division can help us to identify specific nursing activities, the three areas are very much interrelated. Providing information in a sensitive, caring manner affords emotional support, and many people do not consciously make the distinction between the emotional and spiritual dimensions.

Cognitive activity. The patient's need for information in relation to diagnosis and treatment has been examined in earlier sections of this chapter. To this discussion the following observations may be added:

- Information is power: power to enable independence, autonomous decision-making, and realistic goal-setting for patients and their families. Information promotes the patient's sense of control over his life.
- Studies of patients' perceived needs rank information as the highest need (Peck & Boland 1977; Eardley 1986).
- Lack of information can deepen a depressive reaction to a cancer diagnosis.
- Cassileth et al (1980) showed that specific information about diagnosis and prognosis can encourage active participation by patients in their own care, and in fact generates rather than negates hope.
- Patients expect their needs for information to be met by doctors, and their needs for support to be met by nurses (Thorne 1988). Doctors, however, often do not have the time or the skill to present information in a simple, unhurried manner.
- Studies show that patients seldom take the initiative in seeking information, mainly because staff appear busy and unavailable (Bond 1982; Holmes & Dickerson 1987).
- A nurse who is behaving in an unavailable manner *may* be too busy to answer questions. She may also lack the information the patient is seeking, or fear that information-giving may lead to an emotional unburdening by the patient, for which she may lack the personal resources necessary to cope.
- Patients and their families need information on the cause of their cancer, the possible course of their disease, treatment options, the role of the health care team, available services, and sources of further information.
- Patients vary greatly in their desire for, and receptivity to, information. For example, patients who actively deny their cancer will not listen to information about community nursing support on discharge, and patients with a fatalistic attitude may not be interested in information about self-help groups or complementary therapy.

Nursing interventions. The following advice may assist the nurse as she strives to meet the patient's communication needs.

- Be equipped with the information that the patient needs. Be assertive in obtaining this information from other members of the health care team so that a consistent 'story' is given to the patient.
- Be present at as many interactions between the patient and the doctor as possible. Afterwards reinforce messages and ensure that the patient has understood.
- Find out what the patient already knows and has been told, and what he wants to know. In general, follow the patient's agenda.
- Discover the patient's principal fears and give information to allay these first. For example, the patient may think that all cancer patients develop severe pain whereas in fact only 20–40% of patients do and, of these, only 10% have pain that is difficult to control.
- Bear in mind that when receiving information most people remember only three specific points; the first three points made are those most likely to be remembered.
- Avoid jargon: 'your white cell count will fall', for example, will mean nothing to most patients. Information about how they will feel and what they will experience is most important to patients.
- Document information given together with an estimation of the patient's retention and reaction.
- Be prepared for the patient to forget or deny the information given.
- Reinforce verbal information with written information. BACUP and Cancerlink produce patient literature on a wide range of subjects.
- Be prepared for information-giving to lead to emotional issues. Allow time for this, or promise to return at an arranged time.
- Give the patient and his relatives the same information. Give each the opportunity to receive this information both together and separately, so that personal anxieties can be expressed privately and within the family group.

Emotional activity. Enabling patients and their families to cope with the emotional impact of cancer demands effective listening skills and is an essential component of counselling (see Box 32.10). The following considerations should be borne in mind by the nurse as she addresses the cancer patient's emotional needs.

- During any stage of the disease, the cancer patient is suffering the effects of various actual or potential losses. These may include loss of a body part or function, loss of self-image, loss of work or leisure activities, loss of family or social role, loss of control over one's life, loss of goals and dreams for the future, and, ultimately, loss of life itself. Loss is the predominant factor in all sadness and depression.
- There are many uncertainties involved in cancer; uncertainty leads to anxiety.
- While the majority of cancer patients adjust emotionally and cope reasonably well with loss and uncertainty, several studies document the prevalence of psychological distress and even psychiatric illness among this client group. For example, within the first 12–18 months of mastectomy, at least 1 in 5 patients develop an anxiety state or depressive illness. Even in the case of Hodgkin's disease, which has a good prognosis, up to one third of patients develop psychiatric morbidity, particularly if chemotherapy and/or radiotherapy are used (Maguire 1985).
- A great deal of this emotional turmoil, anxiety, and depression passes undetected and unrelieved. Maguire (1985) calculates that only one fifth of patients with severe emotional problems are helped effectively.
- Some studies show that this lack of emotional support is not related to inappropriate communication by nurses, i.e. to the saying of unhelpful things, but rather to their lack of availability or willingness to communicate at all (Bond 1982, Holmes & Dickerson 1987).
- Emotional support is not a luxury in nursing care. Emotional distress may result in somatic symptoms such as confusion, immobility, insomnia, and pain. Some research suggests that the patient's emotional coping ability and level of hope may even prolong life: patients who express their feelings of anxiety and anger, and who adopt a 'fighting spirit' with a degree of positive denial, have a better prognosis (Greer et al 1979).
- The growth of complementary therapies in cancer care represents a recognition that healing is a much wider concept than that of cure; indeed, healing can take place even in the absence of a medical cure (see p. 896). Healing involves psychological adaption to living with cancer, a process of coming to terms with one's situation.
- Patients' reactions to cancer vary greatly, depending on personality, past experience, and learned coping strategies.

Nursing interventions. The following strategies can be employed to give the patient support as he adjusts emotionally to his illness and treatment.

- Many patients cover up a great deal of their distress and assume that nurses do not have time to listen to them. Be alert to clues to this distress such as constant information-seeking, manipulative behaviour and unrealistic goal-setting.
- Give the patient 'openings' to state what is on his mind, for example, by concluding an information-giving session by asking him how he feels about the information, or by remarking upon a worried or sad expression.
- Do not be afraid of saying the wrong thing. A study by Thorne (1988) showed a strong association between 'perceived concern' and interpretation of a communication as helpful by patients. A desire to understand and an attitude of concern are what is important.
- Learn and apply interviewing techniques used in counselling, e.g. reflecting a patient's question or statement back to him. This gives the patient the chance to realise what he has said and to expand on it, and the nurse time to reflect on what is meant. Remember, however, that constant reflection of questions will irritate patients. Once the patient's main concerns have been established it may be time to give direct answers.
- Resist giving pat answers and false reassurances. Many of the dilemmas faced by cancer patients have no ready solution. Do not be afraid to admit that you cannot give an answer to all of the patient's questions about the future.

Box 32.10 Communication skills: an example

This is an example of how one nurse offered her support to a young woman with acute leukaemia and her family. Notice the importance of following the patient's agenda and responding to the situation as it developed rather than imposing a preconceived structure for communication.

While waiting for confirmation of the diagnosis, I did a lot of listening. I listened to the expression of shock, fear and guilt. I did not negate their concerns or try to offer false assurances.

It was clear that one of the most useful things I could do for this distraught family, who were in a strange and overwhelming place, was to assist them, little by little, in gaining control over their experiences. This involved helping them anticipate and be prepared for what was to come, for how it might feel or look physically or emotionally. It also involved helping them to continue in their usual roles as much as possible, and engaging them in the decisions affecting Lara's care.

Although she knew that she had less than a 50% chance of survival, she concentrated on the here and now; the pain associated with frequent i.v.'s, bone marrows and lumbar punctures; the embarrassment of hair loss, the isolation from her friends, and the nausea and vomiting associated with her chemotherapy. I followed her lead by responding to her immediate concerns.

I used a variety of approaches in working with her, depending on what kind of day she was having. Sometimes we would just joke around; other times we would talk about more serious issues — not just her illness but her personal life, as well as my own.

I was always open with her, accepted her feelings, and never made light of them. I did not assure her that 'it would get better soon' or that 'I knew how she must be feeling' because I truly did not know whether she would get better, or how she actually felt.

Lara was just plain miserable. All I could do with her was listen, acknowledge how awful it must be, and honestly say that she must feel like crying. Permission to cry was all she needed to let the tears flow. One day, she looked me directly in the eyes and said 'I'm so sick, am I going to die?' Although it was a matter of seconds before I answered, it seemed like hours as my mind groped for the right words. I did not avert my gaze and answered from my heart 'I'm afraid Lara, that you are so sick that you could die.' (Cited by Benner & Wrubel 1989, pp. 298–308)

Try, however, to leave the patient with some hope: help him to identify something positive in his situation to focus on.

- Assist the patient in identifying realistic goals in order to foster hope. These goals should originate from the patient, but often need an objective person to identify them. Examples may be the goal of fighting the disease, of living until a daughter's wedding, of returning to work part-time, and so on.
- A certain degree of worry and sadness is to be expected. Be alert to signs of disabling anxiety (somatic stress symptoms, lack of concentration, feelings of panic), or depression (a 'flat' mood, an exaggerated feeling of guilt and self-blame, suicidal ideation). If these are noted, refer the patient to a psychologist or psychiatrist. Anxiolytic and antidepressant drugs and various forms of psychological therapy may be required before other forms of counselling therapy can be effective (Moorey 1988).
- Patients may react to their disease with denial, anger, bargaining, depression and acceptance (Kübler-Ross 1975). Counselling cannot force the patient to move from one stage to another, but it does allow him to express feelings and perhaps make progress. The nurse should give the patient permission to express his feelings in any safe way he chooses and should not feel that she has failed when a patient becomes emotionally distraught. The expression of emotions is therapeutic and is an important part of psychological adaption.
- Supporting patients and their families through the cancer experience is very demanding emotionally. It is important for nurses to recognise the resultant stress in themselves and their colleagues and to seek and offer active support (see Box 32.9).

Spiritual activity. A full consideration of the cancer patient's quality of life must recognise the spiritual dimension of his experience, which we might describe, in the most basic terms, as his search for meaning and purpose. Cancer has been described as 'a modern metaphor for human confrontation with existential uncertainty' (Goldberg & Tull 1983). Because spirituality involves the contemplation of things that affect us but lie beyond our control, cancer has the capacity to precipitate a spiritual crisis.

For many in modern society the spiritual needs for love, hope, creativity and purpose are met in relationships with others and in their engagement with the material world. The person faced with a cancer diagnosis may feel such needs with particular acuteness and may be assisted by interventions similar to those described in the section on emotional activity (p. 901).

For some, whether or not death is likely, a cancer diagnosis creates a greater urgency to come to terms with concepts of God, the meaning of life, the problem of human suffering and the possibility of an afterlife. For a minority, religious conviction will provide a framework for such questioning and a vehicle for spiritual expression.

Nursing interventions. In acknowledging and addressing the cancer patient's spiritual needs the nurse should bear in mind the following considerations.

- Spiritual issues are often not expressed as such by the patient. They may be expressed as anger and disbelief, doubts about self-worth, feelings of guilt, and a fear of death. These feelings should be recognised as stemming from spiritual questioning. The nurse should listen non-judgementally to the patient's views and acknowledge that some questions can never be answered.
- Patients of all faiths should be assisted to worship according to their custom. Nurses who share the patient's faith may find that a few minutes of prayer with him may be of more benefit than an hour of counselling.
- Even the most religious patients may express feelings of doubt, despair, and anger against their God. This does not necessarily mean that they are losing their faith, but that they are grappling with it. The nurse should acknowledge the patient's distress, and, if the patient wishes, enlist the help of a spiritual counsellor or minister.
- Not everyone with cancer is dying. However, almost all cancer patients consider the possibility of death at some point. If the patient verbalises this possibility, and the timing is appropriate, he should not be denied the chance to begin the very necessary process of anticipatory grief. At the same time, all reasonable hope for the short-term future should be fostered and the patient's quality of life in the present should be enhanced by all means possible.

New directions for cancer care. Slevin et al (1990) indicate that those who do not have cancer, whether they are lay-persons or professionals, have very little concept of the experience of cancer or of how the cancer patient perceives his quality of life, his future, and the decisions that must be made. Experience and research, however, are pointing the way toward nursing approaches that are most likely to assist patients in the process of adapting to treatment and to living with cancer. Nursing research and interest in this field of care are rapidly growing/and standards are constantly being developed, re-evaluated and improved.

ACKNOWLEDGEMENT

The author wishes to thank Dr David Whillis, MB, BS, MRCP (UK), FRCR, Consultant Oncologist, Raigmore Hospital, NHS Trust, Inverness for reviewing the medical content of this chapter and for his many helpful suggestions.

GLOSSARY

Adjuvant therapy. Any therapy which is deliberately planned in conjunction with another form of therapy, e.g. adjuvant chemotherapy following surgery for breast cancer.

Cisplatin-based. Chemotherapeutic agents of similar chemical structure and use as cis-platinum, e.g. carboplatin.

Differentiation. The development process during which immature cells and tissues become more complex and specialised.

Disseminated disease. Disease which is distributed over a considerable area of the body, e.g. metastatic cancer.

Metastases. The transfer of disease from one organ or part of the body to another not directly connected with it. Most commonly used to describe secondary growth of malignant tumours.

Nephrotoxicity. The degree to which a substance may impair kidney function.

Ototoxicity. The degree to which a substance may cause damage to the ear.

Palliative therapy. Therapy used to treat distressing symptoms and improve quality of life where no cure is thought possible, e.g. radiotherapy to painful bone metastases.

Prognosis. A forecast of the probable course and outcome of a condition and the prospects of a recovery.

Staging. A process of identifying the stage of progression of a disease, e.g. the size of a tumour and the extent of any spread.

REFERENCES

Bagenal F S, Easton D F, Harris E et al 1990 Survival of patients with breast cancer attending the Bristol Cancer Help Centre. Lancet 336: 606–610

Bailey R, Clarke M 1989 Stress and coping in nursing. Chapman & Hall, London

Benner P, Wrubel J 1989 The primacy of caring: stress and coping in health and illness. Addison-Wesley, Menlo Park, C A

Bond S 1982 Communication in cancer nursing. In: Colhoon M C (ed) Cancer nursing. Churchill Livingstone, Edinburgh, ch 1

British Medical Association 1986 Alternative therapy: report of the Board of Science and Education. BMA, London

Cancer Research Campaign 1988 Factsheet on cancer. CRC, London

Cancer Research Campaign 1990 Factsheet on cancer. CRC, London

Cassileth B R, Zupkis R V, Sutton-Smith K et al 1980 Information and participation preferences among cancer patients. Annals of Internal Medicine 92 (6): 832–836

Chamberlain J 1988 Screening for early detection of cancer. In: Phylip Pritchard A (ed) Oncology for nurses and health care professionals, 2nd edn. Harper & Row, London, vol 1, ch 7

Commission of the European Communities 1989 Europe against cancer. CEC, Luxemburg

Costa G 1977 Cachexia: the metabolic component of neoplastic disease. Cancer Research 37: 2327–2335

Donovan C 1989 Approaches to advocacy. In: Phylip Pritchard A (ed) Cancer nursing: a revolution in care. Macmillan, London

Eardley A 1986 What do patients need to know? Nursing Times 82 (16): 24–26

Einhorn J 1989 Europe against cancer: a plan for action. In: Phylip Pritchard A (ed) Cancer nursing: a revolution in care. Macmillan, London, pp 5–7

Evans J 1989 The cancer experience: a patient's view. In: Phylip Pritchard A (ed) Cancer nursing: a revolution in care, Macmillan, London, pp 17–18

Ewles L, Simnett I 1992 Promoting health: a practical guide to health education, 2nd edn. Wiley, Chichester

Fitzpatrick R, Hinton J, Newman S et al 1984 The experience of illness. Tavistock, London

Gardner M J, Snee M P, Hall A J et al 1990 Results of case control study of leukaemia and lymphoma in young people near Sellafield nuclear plant in West Cumbria. British Medical Journal 300: 423–429

Gillon R 1986 Philosophical medical ethics. Wiley, Chichester

Goldberg R J, Tull R M 1983 The psychosocial dimensions of cancer: a practical guide for health care providers. Free Press, New York

Greer S, Morris T, Pettingale K W 1979 Psychological response to breast cancer: effect on outcome. Lancet 2: 785–787

Haenszel W, Kurihera M 1968 Studies of Japanese migrants: 1. Mortality from cancer and other diseases among Japanese in the United States. Journal of the National Cancer Institute 60: 545–571

Haes H 1989 Decision making in oncology: the role of patients and nurses. In: Phylip Pritchard A (ed) Cancer nursing: a revolution in care. Macmillan, London, pp 65–68

HMSO 1986 Breast cancer screening: a report chaired by Sir Patrick Forrest. HMSO, London

Holmes S 1988 Radiotherapy. Austen Cornish, London

Holmes S 1991 Chemotherapy. Austen Cornish, London

Holmes S, Dickerson J W 1987 The quality of life: design and evaluation of a self assessment instrument for use with cancer patients. International Journal of Nursing Studies 24: 15–24

Hughes J 1987 Cancer and emotion: psychological preludes and reactions to cancer. Wiley, Chichester

Johnson J, Nail L, Lauver D et al 1988 Reducing the negative impact of radiation therapy on functional status. Cancer 61: 46–51

Kübler-Ross E 1975 Death, the final stage of growth. Prentice-Hall: New York

Lauer P, Murphy S, Pavers M 1982 Learning needs of cancer patients: a comparison of nurse and patient perceptions. Nursing Research 31 (1): 11–16

Lyon J S 1977 Management of psychological problems in breast cancer. In: Stoll B A (ed) Cancer management: early and late. Heinemann, London

McKie L, Gregory S 1989 Wasted Lives. Nursing Times 85 (18): 22–23

Maguire P, Tait A, Brooke M et al 1980 Psychiatric morbidity and physical toxicity associated with adjuvant chemotherapy after mastectomy. British Medical Journal 281: 1179–1180

Maguire P 1985 The psychological impact of cancer. British Journal of Hospital Medicine 34 (2): 100–103

Melia K 1989 This house believes that the nurse is ideally placed to act as the nurse advocate. In: Phylip Pritchard A (ed) Cancer nursing: a revolution in care. Macmillan, London, pp 160–163

Moorey S 1988 The psychological impact of cancer. In: Webb P (ed) Oncology for nurses and health care professionals, 2nd edn. Harper & Row, London, vol 2, ch 2

Munro A J, Biruls R, Griffin A V et al 1989 Distress associated with radiotherapy for malignant disease. British Journal of Cancer 60 (3): 370–374

Nery R 1986 Cancer: an enigma in biology and society. Croom Helm, London

Niven N 1989 Health psychology: an introduction for nurses and other health care professionals. Churchill Livingstone, Edinburgh

Parkes C M, Benjamin B, Fitzgerald, R G 1969 Broken heart: a statistical survey of increased mortality among widowers. British Medical Journal 1: 740–743

Parkinson S A, Lewis J, Morris R et al 1987 Oral protein and energy supplements in cancer patients. Human Nutrition: Applied Nutrition 41 A: 233–243

Peck A, Boland J 1977 Emotional reactions to radiation treatment. Cancer 40: 180–184

Quilliam S 1989 Positive smear. Penguin, Harmondsworth

Richardson J 1989 The administration of chemotherapy in the patient's home: a new perspective. In: Phylip Pritchard A (ed) Cancer nursing: a revolution in care. Macmillan, London

Roper N, Logan W, Tierney A (eds) 1983 Using a model for nursing. Churchill Livingstone, Edinburgh

Roy C 1989 The Roy adaption model. In: Reihl-Sisca J (ed) Conceptual models for nursing practice, 3rd edn. Appleton & Lange, East Norwalk

Royal College of Nursing 1989 Safe practice with cytotoxics. RCN, London

Skrabanek P 1990a Screening for cancer. Update 15 February: 384–387

Skrabanek P 1990b Cervical cancer screening. Update 15 April: 868–872

Slevin M, Stubbs L, Plant H et al 1990 Choices in cancer treatment: comparing the views of patients with cancer with those of doctors, nurses, and the general public. British Medical Journal 300: 1458–1460

Souhami R, Tobias J 1986 Cancer and its management. Blackwell, Oxford

Speck P W 1988 Ethical issues in cancer care. In: Webb P (ed) Oncology for nurses and health care professionals, 2nd edn. Harper & Row, London, vol 2, ch 3

Spiegel D, Kraemer H C, Bloom J R et al 1989 Effect of psychosocial treatment on survival of patients with metastatic breast cancer. Lancet 2 (8668): 888–891

Stoll B (ed) 1979 Mind and cancer prognosis. Wiley: Chichester

Strohl R A 1988 The nursing role in radiation oncology: symptom management of acute and chronic reactions. Oncology Nursing Forum 15 (4): 429–434

Stubbs L 1989 Taste changes in cancer patients. Nursing Times 85 (3): 49–50

Thorne S E 1988 Helpful and unhelpful communication in cancer care: the patient perspective. Oncology Nursing Forum 15 (2): 1647–1672

Tierney A J 1987 Preventing chemotherapy induced alopecia in cancer patients: is scalp cooling worthwhile? Journal of Advanced Nursing 12: 303–310

Tierney A J, Taylor J, Closs S J 1989 A study to inform nursing support of patients coping with chemotherapy for breast cancer. Nursing Research Unit, University of Edinburgh, Edinburgh

Tschudin V 1988 Nursing the patient with cancer. Prentice-Hall, Hemel Hempstead, Herts

UICC (International Union Against Cancer) 1987 TNM Classification of malignant tumours. Springer-Verlag, Berlin

Walker A 1990 The problems of patients with cervical cancer. In: Faulkner A (ed) Excellence in nursing: the research route: oncology. Scutari, London, ch 3

Wilkinson S 1990 Nursing the patient with cancer. In: Faulkener A (ed) Excellence in nursing: the research route: oncology. Scutari, London, ch 6

Wilson M E, Williams H A 1988 Oncology nurses' attitudes and behaviours related to sexuality of patients with cancer. Oncology Nursing Forum 15 (1): 49–53

Woods M 1989 Tumour takes all. Nursing Times 85 (3): 46–47

FURTHER READING

Burnard P 1985 Learning human skills: a guide for nurses. Heinemann, London

Crosby C 1989 Method in mouthcare. Nursing Times 85 (35): 38–41

Groenwald S L 1987 Cancer nursing: principles and practice. Jones & Bartlett, Boston

Hall J 1988 Immunity and cancer. In: Phylip Pritchard A (ed) Oncology for nurses and health care professionals, 2nd edn. Harper & Row, London, vol 1, ch 5

Harrison S 1987 New approaches to cancer. Century, London

Lamb M, Woods N 1981 Sexuality and the cancer patient. Cancer Nursing 4: 137–144

Marieb E 1989 Human anatomy and physiology. Benjamin/ Cummings, Redwood City

Oakhill A 1985 The supportive care of the child with cancer. Wright, London

Open Tech 1987 The nature of cancer. Open Tech, London

Sellu D 1986 Why do people die from cancer? Nursing Times 82 (21): 32–35

Tiffany R (series ed) 1988 Oncology for nurses and health care professionals. Harper & Row, London, vols 1,2,3

Thompson I, Melia K, Boyd K 1988 Nursing ethics, 2nd edn. Churchill Livingstone, Edinburgh

USEFUL ADDRESSES

England & Wales
Cancerlink
17 Britannia Street
London WC1X 9JN
Tel. 071 833 2451

Scotland
Cancerlink
9 Castle Terrace
Edinburgh EH1 2OP
Tel. 031 228 5557

BACUP (British Association of Cancer United Patients)
121–123 Charterhouse Street
London EC1M 6AA
Tel. 071 608 1661

CHAPTER 33

The chronically ill person

Erica S. Alabaster

CHAPTER CONTENTS

Introduction 905

The nature of chronic illness 905
Terminology 905
'Illness' and 'disease' 905
'Impairment', 'disability' and 'handicap' 905

Societal attitudes towards illness and disability 906
Disability and unemployment 906
Stigma 906
Public awareness campaigns 907

The prevalence of chronic illness 907

Features of chronic illness 908
Chronic illnesses are long-term by nature 908
Chronic illness is uncertain 908
Chronic illnesses require proportionately greater efforts at palliation 909
Chronic diseases are multiple diseases 909
Chronic diseases are disproportionately intrusive 910
Chronic diseases require a wide variety of ancillary services 910
Chronic disease is expensive 911

A framework for understanding the experience of chronic illness 911
Key problems 911
Basic strategies 911
Agents 911
Organisational or familial arrangements 911
Consequences 911

Nursing intervention 912
Developments in the location and organisation of care 912
The foundation for the nursing role 912
Using models to guide practice 912
Orem's self-care model 913
Roy's adaptation model 913
The Roper–Logan–Tierney model 914

Applying the Roper–Logan–Tierney model using the process of nursing 916
Assessment 916
Planning 917
Implementation 917
Evaluation 918

Conclusion 918

Glossary 918

References 918

Further reading 919

INTRODUCTION

The care of people with chronic illness has long been of concern to nurses, presenting them with many challenges and opportunities and demanding the use of a broad range of skills. In seeking to articulate the concepts which underpin the process of care, nursing theorists now define health in terms of an integrated state of wellness within which the individual achieves optimal physical, social, psychological and spiritual balance. This holistic approach therefore regards ill-health as a state of disequilibrium. Further, it does not rely solely on the application of a medically-determined diagnostic label to legitimise nursing involvement and to dictate the direction this takes.

Chronic illness has significant consequences for the individual's social and psychological well-being. The nurse's role in caring for people who are chronically ill must be formulated within a broad context, which includes the nature of chronic illness, its impact on individual experience and functioning, its prevalence, and the relationship between patients, informal carers and health care agencies. Perhaps the best place to begin in considering this role is with a practical definition of chronic illness.

THE NATURE OF CHRONIC ILLNESS

Terminology

Dimond & Jones (1983) note that a number of terms have been employed to describe illness 'that is of long-term duration, is not curable, and/or has some residual features that impose limitations on an individual's functional capabilities' (p. 53). An analysis of such terminology is an essential starting-point for any discussion of chronic illness. The way in which key terms are applied may reveal the existence of certain assumptions about the causation and prognosis of chronic conditions and about the individuals who experience them. Along with many other North American authors they refer to the definition of chronic illness agreed by the Commission on Chronic Illness in 1956:

> All impairments or deviations from normal which have one or more of the following characteristics: are permanent, leave residual disability, are caused by non-reversible pathological alteration, require special training of the patient for rehabilitation, may be expected to require a long period of supervision, observation, or care. (Mayo, cited in Strauss et al 1984, p. 1.)

This statement is still considered to have currency despite its ambiguity and biological emphasis. How, for example, is a 'normal' state to be defined? What constitutes a 'disability'?

'Illness' and 'disease'

It is important to note that the definition cited above is orientated towards disease rather than illness. A distinction is made between these two terms by some writers such that 'disease' is a medical conception of pathological abnormality as indicated by its presenting features, whereas 'illness' is the subjective response by the individual to feeling unwell (Fitzpatrick 1982, Blaxter 1984). Field (1976) argues, however, that although it is possible to feel ill without having a disease and vice versa, 'illness' and 'disease' do not constitute discrete phenomena but, rather, operate at different levels of human experience. Their relationship is dependent on the nature and severity of the disease process and on coexisting psychosocial variables. Chronic illness is generally associated with the presence of a protracted disease process which is not amenable to treatment and which is responsible for impairment or disability and so has a sustained influence on the functioning and lifestyle of the individual. In this view, the relationship between disease and illness is characterised by its complexity.

'Impairment', 'disability' and 'handicap'

Anderson & Bury (1988) demonstrate that biomedical classifications of disease do not necessarily account for the psychological and social consequences which accompany the conditions identified. To support this idea they cite the work of Harper et al (1986) who conducted a study to investigate the problems experienced by people diagnosed as having multiple sclerosis. These writers concluded that psychosocial disabilities which could result in a reduction in the quality of life were not associated with the nature of the underlying disease.

The terms 'impairment', 'disability' and 'handicap' are commonly employed in the literature with reference to chronic illness and are applied in a variety of ways, whether their definitions are stated explicitly or merely implied. Dimond & Jones (1983) comment that the term 'impairment' is generally used to describe physiological or anatomical abnormalities caused by disease processes. Impairment may also be influenced by extrinsic factors such as the manner in which the presenting condition is managed. Pressure sores, constipation, urinary tract infections and other complications of restricted mobility are examples of these.

The word 'disability', on the other hand, can be used to identify any long-term or permanent incapacity which is due to disease, injury, innate defect or old age. This is related to functional limitation but may in addition be defined in terms of behaviour, such as that arising from the individual's inability to perform activities which are expected of him (Bury 1979, Roberts 1985). The level of disability experienced by an individual reflects the severity and duration of impairment, taking into account concurrent disease, illness and the effects of the ageing process.

Dimond & Jones (1983) argue that it is constructive for people interested in the study of chronic illness to consider the notion of disability since this presents an opportunity to discuss a range of behavioural *responses* without concentrating on the diseases concerned. They explain that the term 'handicap' may be applied when limitation of activity persists as a residual effect of impairment, even following rehabilitative efforts to restore function. Handicap is not, therefore, merely the presence of disability and impairment, but the social, economic and environmental consequences of these. The individual is considered to be disadvantaged in so far as he is unable to participate in socially prescribed roles and relationships. Further, Anderson & Bury (1988) suggest that handicap can have different implications for individual experience depending on the way in which social, cultural and economic values are applied to restricted role behaviour. In this way 'handicap' can be interpreted as both more and less than 'disability'.

Issues surrounding the concepts 'impairment', 'disability' and 'handicap' are also explored in Chapter 33.

SOCIETAL ATTITUDES TOWARDS ILLNESS AND DISABILITY

The literature suggests, however, that attention is still clearly directed towards drawing associations between aspects of lifestyle and some chronic illnesses; for example, smoking is linked with lung cancer and a high dietary intake of saturated fats with coronary heart disease. Neuberger (1987) contends that a general awareness of these relationships may result in the individual being judged to be the cause of his own disease and related suffering. There is also an implication that the individual has failed to respond to preventive health education campaigns. Attribution of personal blame is shown to have a strong moral influence where an association has been made between disease and sexual behaviour, such as that alleged between cervical cancer and promiscuity (Neuberger 1986).

Current beliefs concerning the origin of chronic illness and disability appear therefore to reflect a combination of moral ideology and scientific principles.

Disability and unemployment

The individual's economic survival in a pre-industrial society largely depends on his capacity to engage in physical labour. Those who are restricted by the effects of protracted illness or impairment will thus have a limited function within their social group. This, together with their likely dependency on others, can result in the perception that disabled people are of less value than their able-bodied counterparts.

In an industrialised society technological developments and diversification of working practices should create opportunities for people with a wide range of disabilities to gain employment. Nonetheless, discrimination is still encountered by disabled individuals seeking to enter the labour market (Oliver 1990).

Governmental response to poverty is influenced by the way in which poor people are viewed by other members of society. The assumption that those living with chronic illness experience economic difficulties because they are unable to obtain employment as a direct result of their incapacity is not held universally. Some may take the view instead that such individuals are malingerers who choose not to work (Scambler 1982). When this interpretation predominates, programmes for the alleviation of poverty concentrate on motivating individuals by reforming attitudes and offering retraining programmes and may appear to be punitive rather than benevolent.

Stigma

As Goffman (1963) points out, the word 'stigma' was originally used with reference to visible signs inflicted with the intent of branding individuals (including slaves or criminals) as unfit for participation in normal social interaction.

The stigma attached to a chronic illness depends on the part of the body affected, the degree to which effects of the condition are visible, the application of a diagnostic label and the likelihood of cure. People with a chronic illness may be so affected by the embarrassment or discomfort which their disorder creates in others that their stigmatising condition assumes primacy as they establish their social identity and manage relationships with others. Case History 33.1 gives some insight into the stigmatisation that may be suffered by an individual with an obvious skin condition.

Case History 33.1 Mrs I

Mrs I is 44 years old and is employed as a part-time receptionist. She lives in a terraced house with her husband and their three teenage children. Mrs I has had psoriasis for some years involving much of her body surface.

Although prescribed treatment has controlled features of the condition to some extent, Mrs I has periods of exacerbation. Reddened raised patches sometimes appear on her face, and her scalp is often affected. Medical opinion varies as to whether this is actually due to psoriasis or to seborrhoeic dermatitis. Mrs I feels this distinction to be largely academic because she believes that neither condition is curable and the outcome for her remains the same. At present her scalp is covered in a thick, hardened layer of scales. When these areas are detached her scalp surface weeps and becomes painful. Scales are also deposited continually on her clothing and in her immediate vicinity.

Mrs I finds that living with a skin condition is made more difficult by the reaction of others. She is often conscious that people stare at her and that they look at her affected skin rather than making eye contact during conversations. Mrs I remembers that when her children were small, one of them tried to prevent her from attending a school play. After a long discussion he admitted that it was because he was embarrassed by her appearance. Mrs I thinks that some people regard her condition to be contagious or to be caused by poor personal hygiene. She considers that this explains why passengers on the bus she takes to and from work rarely occupy space next to her until the vehicle becomes crowded. Such behaviour still makes her uncomfortable but she has learned to accept it as something she must live with.

Mrs I feels that she has developed effective methods of coping with the problems resulting from her disorder. Since her job involves meeting the public she has learned to project an outgoing and friendly image which she feels is stronger than the visual impression which her condition creates. She avoids wearing dark clothes likely to make her fallen scales more obvious and purchases her clothing by mail order or from shops which do not have communal changing rooms. She has learned by trial and error which chemicals or cosmetics irritate her skin and excludes them from the household. She takes her own prescribed shampoo to the hairdressers and never uses biological washing powder. Her friends and relations are aware that only selected toiletries are welcome as birthday and Christmas presents. Mrs I has also adapted her treatment regime to account for exacerbations of her condition. She applies some creams only when she feels that she needs to, rather than at prescribed intervals. As some preparations require careful application due to possible staining of clothes and localised burning (see Ch. 12) Mrs I tries to restrict their use to days when she is not rostered to work. To prevent unnecessary soiling she reserves specific bedlinen for occasions when she needs to leave scalp ointment on overnight.

? **33.1** Have you ever been aware of being embarrassed or uncomfortable when you were with someone with an obvious skin disorder? What were your reactions?

Public awareness campaigns

A variety of groups have been established to raise public awareness of the problems encountered by individuals with long-term illness and disability. Dimond & Jones (1983) recall that in the United States veterans of the First World War were successful in exerting large-scale efforts to obtain privileges and opportunities for disabled servicemen returning to civilian life. The amount of popular support such programmes receive is dependent upon whether the situations to which they are related are viewed positively. This can be illustrated with reference to American veterans of the Vietnam War, who endure stigmatisation by association with a controversial and unpopular conflict.

Other groups act to draw attention to named conditions and their effects on individual experience. These organisations function as a resource for sufferers and their families, campaign for issues such as open access to public buildings, and raise funds for facilities and research. It may be suggested that some groups encourage little active participation by disabled people themselves, and that aid programmes are consequently planned in relation to assumed more than actual need. In addition, activists within campaigns such as the British Council for the Organisation of Disabled People assert that national fundraising events merely serve to reinforce the notion that an automatic relationship exists between disabled people and charity. Members of these groups believe that sick and disabled people should avoid passivity and the socialised dependency which results. Their practice of self-advocacy, use of direct action and insistence upon parity rather than charity contrast sharply with the conventional image of disabled people as recipients of care.

THE PREVALENCE OF CHRONIC ILLNESS

The prevalence of chronic disease is difficult to establish in view of the many definitions and interpretations of these conditions offered by various agencies. Some indication of their prevalence may, however, be derived from a review of studies which take into account such variables as demography and disability.

Improvements in public health in the United Kingdom since the turn of the century have resulted in the near-eradication of some infectious diseases, whilst others have been largely controlled by vaccination programmes. In addition, once contracted, infectious diseases are amenable to treatment, with the possible exception of acquired immune deficiency syndrome (AIDS; Anderson 1988). Chronic rather than infectious disease therefore remains as the major cause of premature death and disability.

The decline in mortality from infectious disease is also reflected in an increased expectation of life for all age groups, a trend which is predicted to continue (Central Statistical Office 1990). This has implications for the number of people afflicted by chronic disorders. In a review of the literature McClymont (1985) concludes that the proportion of the population considered to be handicapped or impaired rises with advancing age. This reflects a similar analysis performed in the United States by Strauss et al (1984). Confirmation of this relationship can be found in a report published by the Department of Health (1990) using data from the annual General Household Survey (GHS) provided by a sample of 20 000 adults and 5000 children. In 1988, respondents were asked whether they had any longstanding illness, disability or infirmity and if so to name the source of their problem, stating whether it served to limit their activities in any way. A longstanding illness was reported by 33% of the respondents and a limiting longstanding illness by 19%. A comparative measure of acute sickness was obtained by enquiring whether participants had limited their usual activities as a result of illness or injury within the two-week period prior to the interview. Only 12% of the sample fell into this category. The report concludes that in the decade between 1979 and 1989 rates of longstanding illness seem to have increased whilst the incidence of acute illness remained virtually unchanged.

Musculoskeletal, circulatory, respiratory and digestive disorders were most frequently reported by respondents with longstanding illness. Among these disorders, musculoskeletal conditions were the most common. A similar finding was obtained in a study by Martin et al (1988). Circulatory problems were the second most common form of chronic illness identified in the GHS; these were reported by 2% of adults aged 16–44 years and approximately 25% of those aged 65 years or older. A summary of selected causes of death for the years 1951 and 1988 provides evidence to suggest that the incidence of circulatory disease is rising. Deaths from such disorders, including myocardial infarction and cerebrovascular accident (CVA) accounted for around one third of all deaths in 1951 and almost half of all deaths in 1988 (Central Statistics Office 1990).

The DOH report records a striking similarity between the proportions of men and women experiencing various forms of chronic illness, with the following two exceptions. Firstly, 22% of men aged 75 years and above stated that they had a longstanding musculoskeletal disorder, compared with 40% of their female counterparts. This is thought to be due in part to the higher proportion of very elderly women who fall into this age category. Secondly, 13% of elderly males considered themselves to be suffering from a respiratory disease, whereas only 8% of women in the same age group characterised themselves in the same way. Differences in smoking behaviour are felt to be reflected here, although occupational factors may also be significant.

Although the reporting of longstanding disorders rose from 24% of 16–44-year-olds to 71% of those aged 75 years or more, fewer elderly men were found in this category. The number of conditions identified per person increased with advancing age, being 1.2 for those aged 16–44 years and 1.7 for those aged 75 years and above. In this regard little variation was found between males and females.

The findings of this survey support the notion put forward by Anderson & Bury (1988) that whilst chronic illness is widespread and involves a variety of conditions, only a proportion of those affected are appreciably disabled. Anderson & Bury's review of a number of studies concerning the prevalence of specific diseases, including neurological disorders, reveals stroke, Parkinson's disease, rheumatoid arthritis, multiple sclerosis and cardiorespiratory problems to be the major causes of disability.

? **33.2** Given that chronic illness is so widespread, think again about the meaning of health for different people. Can people with chronic disease be 'healthy'?

FEATURES OF CHRONIC ILLNESS

Whilst an analysis of the prevalence of longstanding disease is useful in predicting the demand for support services it may be argued that it is of limited value in gaining an appreciation of the impact of such conditions on the daily lives of individual sufferers. An over-emphasis on diagnosis and disease entities is also felt by Strauss et al (1984) to conceal psychological and social problems shared by people who are chronically ill. These authors have therefore developed a framework to enable the experience of chronic illness to be understood more clearly, and in an empathic manner. To provide a basis for this, the seven features of chronic illness outlined below were identified. Only when she is aware of these features can the nurse appreciate the profound effect of chronic illness on individuals, their families and health care personnel.

Chronic illnesses are long-term by nature

The timespan for the treatment of acute illness contrasts markedly with that of chronic disease. Once contact with medical services is initiated and treatment commenced, the resolution of acute illness is generally achieved within a short period of time. The protracted nature of chronic illness results in repeated interactions between individuals and health care services, perhaps over a period of months or years. This leads to patients gaining familiarity with the organisations providing support and personnel with whom they come into contact, and has implications for the development of complex social relationships between patients and carers as the illness progresses.

Adulthood is a dynamic period usually associated with autonomy and control. It is a time of life in which the individual expects to nurture others, rather than to be nurtured. The need for protracted nursing care conflicts with these expectations and can be damaging to the individual's self-esteem. Once admitted to caring facilities people with chronic illness may be encouraged to relinquish whatever control they still possess in favour of the staff. Failure to do so may be regarded as active opposition to adopting the role of patient, and lead to the individual acquiring a reputation for being 'difficult'. Long-term admission to hospital does not necessarily enhance the relationship between patients and nursing staff, despite the opportunity it presents for interpersonal development in the course of continued interactions (Stockwell 1972).

Chronic illness is uncertain

The difficulty in establishing a prognosis for chronic illness with any degree of certainty is a source of stress for sufferers and their carers. Strauss et al (1984) note that only the progress of the disease itself gives sufficient information to suggest a likely timescale of events for a particular individual.

Adulthood is associated with the achievement of socially and culturally specified tasks such as leaving the parental home, finding a partner and rearing a family (McClymont 1985). The restriction, discomfort and possible dependence accompanying chronic illness may force the individual to forgo these roles and adopt an alternative lifestyle. Fear of dependence, which in itself causes uncertainty, is identified by Pinder (1990) as a fundamental human concern 'in a culture which values self-reliance and economic and physical independence' (p. 2). Her study demonstrates that following a diagnosis of Parkinson's disease this problem is shared to an extent by medical staff, who must decide how much information to give the patient regarding the likely course of the disorder and difficulties of treatment. Although it is seen as important to provide patients with sufficient data to enable them to exert maximum control over their new situation, doctors are shown to question their own professional commitment in situations where purely medical solutions have only a limited effect.

Uncertainty is also present because of the inherently episodic nature of many chronic illnesses, in which recurrent unpredictable crises occur followed by periods of remission or control. Since the onset and duration of these crises cannot be anticipated, patients and their carers must constantly be on the alert for indications of impending difficulty and must be ready to respond at any time. This results in the restriction and reorganisation of lifestyle in an attempt to accommodate the sudden changes in behaviour which may be imposed. Social uncertainty thus exists for people with chronic illness and their families, who find it difficult to plan their activities in either the long or short term, and may be excluded from full participation in community life as a result (Strauss et al 1984). (The difficulty that individuals with a degenerative illness may have in visualising the future is illustrated in Case History 33.2.)

In his study of the social context of multiple sclerosis, Robinson (1988) provides evidence to show that the occurrence of crises in chronic illness influences the way in which sufferers are perceived by others. People with multiple sclerosis felt that the consequences of living with a protracted disorder were largely ignored by others, who believed them to be directly affected by the disease only when it became visible through the exacerbation of physical symptoms. Variation in their ability to perform daily activities in periods of crisis and remission were therefore poorly understood.

Chronic illnesses require proportionately greater efforts at palliation

In view of the remote prospect of effecting a cure in chronic illness, the control of elements which influence the individual's quality of life assumes primary importance. More emphasis is placed on palliative measures, i.e. on alleviating pain and discomfort, providing symptomatic relief, and on addressing the problems created by the restriction of activity. Strauss et al (1984) contend that palliation is of greater significance here than in acute illness because people with long-term disease must learn to live with both the features of their condition and with the side-effects of treatment. The cooperation of patients, their families and close associates is necessary in order to achieve this. Since symptoms such as constant pain and nausea can compromise the ability of individuals to engage in a variety of activities, their treatment is seen to be desirable even though it will have little effect upon the disease process itself.

Decisions as to which palliative measures are selected for individual treatment are influenced by availability, their acceptance by the medical profession, their perceived benefit to the patient, and financial constraints. Improvements in quality of life following palliation are difficult to measure in an objective manner, and this has implications for the allocation of resources.

Individuals have considerable resources of their own and may first try to solve their health problems themselves before seeking professional and statutory help. Should statutory health services be unable to provide palliation, or if their efforts prove to be unsuccessful, people with chronic illness may seek alternative methods to resolve their symptoms. Coping strategies can be learned through experience and by sharing ideas with others through membership of support groups. The use of complementary therapies is increasingly common among people with intractable disease who feel that conventional medicine has no further treatment to offer them and is supported by writers such as Sharma (1990). This not only represents the individual's assumption of responsibility for his own well-being in the face of perceived medical impotence, but also reflects a desire to achieve control over an unpredictable illness (Montbriand & Laing 1991).

Chronic diseases are multiple diseases

According to Strauss et al (1984) the systematic and degenerative effects of a number of chronic diseases are such that in time the failure of one organ or physiological system leads to the involvement of others. In addition, long-term *disability* related to an existing chronic condition is likely to generate further *disease*. This can be illustrated with reference to complications associated with diabetes mellitus. Kelleher (1988) explains that these include vascular damage, which may result in renal and visual dysfunction and an increased risk of myocardial infarction. Impaired circulation to the lower limbs also predisposes to the development of gangrene, the onset of which is in turn influenced by degeneration of the nervous system and greater susceptibility to infection. Amputation of an affected limb results in further alteration of physical, psychological and social functioning. Clearly, the disabling effects of chronic conditions are not merely confined to the features of the disease process, but are compounded by the consequences of treatment used.

The patient's efforts to adjust to the reduction in activity imposed by chronic disease are complicated by the multiplication of symptoms and the increasing disability that results

Case History 33.2 S J

S J is 28 years old and works as a cook in an independent school for girls. She has been in this employment since leaving college and lives on the premises. Her social life revolves largely around sporting activities, an interest shared with her boyfriend, A.

S was diagnosed as having multiple sclerosis (MS) two years ago when she was admitted to hospital following a fall whilst playing tennis. She had been experiencing difficulty in focusing her eyes for some time, but had thought that this was due to overwork. She had also begun to find it difficult to coordinate her movements and became known for dropping and spilling things. These events were explained when the diagnosis was made and S found it strange that she had lived with the condition for so long without realising that something was seriously wrong.

After the diagnosis was confirmed S felt compelled to visit a library to find out more about the condition and what it would mean to her. She resolved that her approach would be to get on with living despite the disease. Within a short period, however, her balance deteriorated and walking became difficult. She also found that she tired easily. S responded by opting out of strenuous activities. Having valued her physical fitness she began to experience frustration at her loss of ability and function. She felt as though her body had betrayed her and she did not like to be seen walking with a stick. When S developed frequency and urgency of micturition she began to avoid visits to public places where toilets would be difficult to reach or where queues were likely.

In private, S found herself increasingly reduced to tears of frustration and despair, believing that no one else could understand her experience. She chose not to share these feelings. She had always been able to manage her life independently and wanted to appear to be continuing to do so. A tried to support S as much as possible but maintaining a positive stance at all times was hard. His friends advised him not to remain in the relationship purely because of his concern for S, and his feelings for her were sometimes confused. He wondered if her reluctance to visit public venues was actually her way of avoiding him because she wanted their relationship to end.

S was preoccupied by questions about her future. How long would she be able to continue in her present post? Would it be possible to seek alternative employment? Giving up her job would mean giving up her home. Her parents wanted her to live with them but S was anxious to retain her autonomy and knew that her mother would try to protect her too much. However, it was her future with A that was her greatest concern. S loved him and had hoped that their relationship would lead to marriage. She wanted children of her own and already felt that time was running out. S felt it impossible to confront A about such a commitment, fearing that he would perceive this as pressure to make an immediate decision, and that as a result she may lose him altogether. Her sad conclusion was that with MS she could no longer be sure of anything.

(Strauss et al 1984). To be confronted with the inevitability of his condition worsening is an important psychological challenge for the individual and acts as an additional source of stress. Individuals may fear the prospect of total disability and regard any development of their disease with anxiety and anger, directing these emotions towards close associates and health care personnel. Staff may be perceived by the individual to be incapable of resolving certain problems or of actually being responsible for them. This has obvious implications for the quality of nurse–patient relationships, which must be characterised by mutual trust and cooperation in order to be genuinely therapeutic.

Chronic diseases are disproportionately intrusive

People with chronic illness may direct much of their lives towards monitoring symptoms and adhering to treatment regimes (Gull 1987). Strauss et al (1984) comment that this prompts a fundamental reorganisation of lifestyle and of personal commitments. In episodes of acute illness it is both feasible and acceptable for individuals to gain temporary exemption from normal social obligations. This is not always possible, however, for those who are chronically sick and must structure daily life such that persistent features of their condition and periods of crisis can be accommodated. It may be difficult for these patients and their families to enjoy a sense of continuity in their lives, as their capacity to pursue various activities will vary unpredictably over time.

Dimond & Jones (1983) consider this idea as they question the application of the notion of the 'sick role' to long-term illness. They point out that the conceptualisation of the sick role by Parsons in 1951 forms the dominant framework within which health professionals work even though it has limited applicability to the management of protracted illness. The expectation implied in the concept of the sick role that individuals should be obliged to get well is not appropriate in the face of irreversible pathology.

Strauss et al (1984) assert that chronic illness often results in the imposition of changes to normal domestic routines to allow for physical limitations and requirements of the treatment regime. Structural alteration of accommodation may also be required; it may be necessary to install equipment and reassign room space to allow access to household facilities. These adaptations, together with alterations in appearance and behaviour associated with the long-term disease, will have an impact on other members of the household and their relationship with the patient.

Chronic illness will also have economic implications. Even if he is not totally disabled, the individual may be unable to continue employment because of the demands which his condition and its treatment make upon his time, strength and stamina. Difficulty in adhering to work schedules and periods of absence during more acute phases of the disease can give employers the impression that people with chronic illness are unreliable. Gaining employment may be problematic in itself; the prospect of incapacity and variable function may be seen by the employer to represent hidden costs, including lost production and redeployment of other workers. In a study of the consequences of living with renal failure Morgan (1988) reveals that people with kidney disease seeking new work were frequently unsuccessful in their applications. They alleged that prospective employers labelled them as 'kidney patients' and identified them as an employment risk.

Chronic illness may also affect the individual's ability to participate in a broad range of social activities. The degree to which these activities are impeded will depend to some extent on whether the individual has learned to deal with the features of the disease process. For example, Lambert & Lambert (1987) explain that fear of frequent episodes of loose stools and the presence of odour are major social concerns for people with ulcerative colitis. The management of these features is particularly difficult in settings where toilet facilities are not readily available. Individuals may respond either by withdrawing from interaction or by planning their outings carefully, using known routes and venues with accessible lavatories. The accidental emission of faecal odour or diarrhoea during sexual encounters is an additional source of anxiety, which can be met either by avoiding intimate relationships or by instituting coping strategies such as keeping an absorbent towel unobtrusively at the bedside. Spontaneous sexual engagements are felt to be preferable by some, as these provide little opportunity to become preoccupied with the manifestations of the disorder.

The nature of chronic disease is such that it impinges on domestic, work-related and recreational activities, and is liable to result in social isolation. This is recognised widely as a consequence of long-term illness and disability which affects both sufferers and their close associates (Roberts 1985). People who are chronically sick require sustained support from those around them to manage their conditions and treatment regimes. The daily activities of their families must therefore be centred around meeting these needs, and it may no longer be possible for them to pursue interests which they once enjoyed as a family. Anderson (1988) discusses this with regard to the quality of life experienced by patients and their supporters after a CVA. Carers found the restrictions placed on their social lives and use of free time distressing, and deeply regretted not being able to go for walks or enjoy holidays with the patient as they had previously.

Chronic diseases require a wide variety of ancillary services

McClymont (1985) comments that there is an abundance of statutory and voluntary agencies in the UK concerned with the care and support of people with long-term illness. Statutory support is provided in the main by the National Health Service, the Department of Social Security, the Department of Employment and the Local Authority Social Services. The responses of these agencies are not always effective, however, due to differences in priorities and administrative practices. Care within institutional and domestic settings requires the close collaboration of a wide range of representatives of these services, such as nurses, therapists, doctors, social workers, civil service employees and home care workers. This can be difficult to achieve given the number and variety of staff necessary to meet an individual's needs, and problems are sometimes compounded by poor interservice coordination and frequent transfers between care settings.

Roberts (1985) states that the relationship between disabled people, their families and public services stems from the claim which any citizen may make for collectively funded care or support when independence is not possible. The legal, bureaucratic and medical definitions adopted routinely by formal agencies in order to categorise individuals and allocate resources are not generally compatible with the experience of people with long-term illness. For example, assessment to determine eligibility for benefits and support services may fail to acknowledge variation in function during episodes of crisis; if the assessment is performed during a period of relative wellness the type and level of support required at other times may not be apparent to the assessor.

Roberts (1985) argues that some people either fail to obtain statutory support or decline the support to which they are entitled because they perceive the organisation of services to be complex or somewhat arbitrary. Ineffective communication can present an obstacle when individuals who are entitled to benefits lack information or have difficulty interpreting the information they are given. In addition, some families may be reluctant to seek or accept help from formal or informal agencies because to do so would be at variance with their cultural values regarding responsibility and self-sufficiency.

Roberts (1985) further asserts that provisions of the Chronically Sick and Disabled Persons Act (1970) intended to ensure support for disabled people living in their own homes have not been realised because implementation by local authorities varies in accord with economic and political pressures. Variation can again be found in criteria used to define need and eligibility. The literature indicates that the overall provision of statutory services is structured in terms of perceived need, and that individuals are expected to fit into the network of support already available. People with long-term illness and their families may not, therefore, receive the kind of help which they believe would be of greatest benefit to them in maintaining their desired way of life (Walker 1984, Pitkeathley 1991).

Chronic disease is expensive

The direct and indirect costs of chronic illness are high (Strauss et al 1984). While expensive technological intervention is not always required, any support that is given will be continuous and will increase in intensity as the illness progresses. The chronically ill individual will have to make repeated contact with health agencies to monitor the effectiveness of treatment and rehabilitation programmes. This may involve regular encounters with members of the primary health care team and frequent visits to hospital-based outpatient clinics. People with chronic illness are likely to experience multiple pathology as a result of systemic and degenerative disease; and since contemporary medical services are organised by area of specialisation, patients will frequently need to attend a variety of clinics. An individual with diabetes, for example, may require referral to a physician in renal medicine, an ophthalmologist and a vascular surgeon.

The long-term prescription of drugs to control or palliate features of chronic conditions has significant financial implications. Additional medications may need to be added to the regime as the illness evolves and to compensate for side-effects of treatment or drugs already prescribed. Changes in the treatment programme may be initiated by episodes of crisis. This, and the increased use of health and social services during such times, is a source of considerable expense.

Repeated periods of admission for acute hospital care in order to achieve management of crises may be necessary. Multidisciplinary involvement will be desirable in view of the effect which chronic illness has on all aspects of the individual's life.

The cost of chronic illness in comparison with that of acute illness is very high in respect to lost employment, reliance on state benefits and cessation of social activities. The onset of disability may also pose a threat to the stability of marital relationships (Roberts 1985).

A FRAMEWORK FOR UNDERSTANDING THE EXPERIENCE OF CHRONIC ILLNESS

The features of chronic illness detailed above are reflected in the framework subsequently presented by Strauss et al (1984) for understanding the experience of ongoing ill-health. This framework is built around the five components outlined in the following.

Key problems

Any disease has the potential to create multiple problems for individual sufferers, and these are liable not only to disrupt routine activities but also to lead to social isolation and attendant psychological and familial difficulties. For example, people with multiple sclerosis and their associates may have difficulty adjusting to the effects of variation in ability and fatigue experienced during swings to and from 'good' and 'bad' days or weeks. It may be difficult for them to make firm arrangements to attend social gatherings and friends may eventually hesitate to extend invitations when the affected individual repeatedly withdraws from events due to fatigue. Family members may begin to feel some resentment as outings and social activities are curtailed.

Basic strategies

Patients and their associates need to develop a repertoire of methods or techniques for overcoming key problems. For instance, an individual with diabetes can learn to adjust his behaviour and treatment regimen when attending social occasions where food and drink are offered. His selection from a menu or buffet table may be guided by his dietary regime rather than purely by desire in terms of the type and quantity of foods taken. If he does not wish to bring his condition to the attention of others at this time, he might avoid alcoholic drinks on the pretext of wanting to 'keep a clear head'; or he may choose to amend the timing and dosage of insulin injections to allow him to indulge in the food and drink which he actually prefers.

Agents

Any basic strategies employed require the assistance of family members, friends, acquaintances or strangers. These 'agents' may function in a variety of ways, for example, by assisting the individual to maintain a treatment regime or protecting him from harmful effects of the disorder. A person who has epilepsy may need help from colleagues such that should an unexpected seizure occur in the workplace he is eased to the ground and away from dangerous machinery.

Organisational or family arrangements

The strategies adopted to address key problems require the coordinated effort of the individual and agents involved. The establishment and maintenance of arrangements relies on trust, skilled interaction, sufficient resources and realistic negotiation of the roles, responsibilities and expectations of all concerned. Someone who is housebound due to long-standing arthritis may be able to enlist family members and neighbours to do shopping, pick up drug prescriptions and collect benefit monies. The continued success of such an arrangement will depend on each person involved having a clear appreciation of what the sufferer actually requires as well as an understanding of his or her own contribution to the well-being of the individual in the context of the help given by others.

Consequences

The strategies and arrangements adopted by people with chronic illness and their associates to manage key problems may be successful in resolving them but can have implications for the agents taking part, thus creating further problems. For example, the paced schedule of activities that enables individuals with chronic obstructive airways disease (COAD) to accommodate oxygen deprivation and recovery times between tasks may present little opportunity for flexibility. Events such as a visit to the hairdresser's can disrupt well-established routines, with implications for the sufferer and carer alike. Both parties are also faced with developing a lifestyle structured by demands of the presenting condition within which spontaneity has no place. See Research Abstract 33.1.

Research Abstract 33.1 Carers of the chronically ill

A survey conducted by the Carers National Association (CNA) to establish both perceptions and experiences of its members revealed the following (N = 2916)

- 72% are female and 66% are over 55 years old
- 38% have been caring for more than 10 years and 22% for more than 15 years
- 79% had no choice in taking on the caring role
- 39% did not talk to anyone about taking on the caring role
- 33% get no help or support at all with their caring responsibilities
- 20% have never had any break from their caring responsibilities
- 47% have experienced financial difficulties since becoming a carer
- 65% say their own health has suffered from their caring responsibilities
- people cease being carers mainly because those they care for die (61%)
- for only 1% had someone else taken over the caring responsibilities

Carers National Association 1992 Speak up, speak out: a survey of carers. CNA Publications, London

NURSING INTERVENTION

Developments in the location and organisation of care

Nurses will encounter adults with chronic illness in both community and institutional settings. These can include the person's own home, residential and nursing homes, or hospitals providing acute or continuing care. Acute hospital care occurs in relation to the establishment of diagnoses and periods of crisis during which features of the illness are exacerbated. Acute care is also necessary when the disease process necessitates revision of treatment regimes in order to achieve stabilisation or palliation. Such contact is therefore intermittent and recurrent.

In general terms, admission to a long-term care facility has always been seen as the last resort for people with chronic illness.

It could be argued that the pattern of care in long-stay facilities developed in response to the interests of the staff rather than to meet the needs of individual patients. A study by Clarke (1978) reveals that the completion of physical tasks assumes priority in the provision of care for elderly people who are mentally ill and that nurses expect their own worth to be judged purely in terms of the amount of energy expended whilst on duty. Echoing ideas first expressed by Coser in 1963, Clarke demonstrates that adherence to routinised methods of working is a strategy used by nurses working within an environment which cannot provide job satisfaction through the achievement of cure. Here, effort is diverted to aspects of housekeeping by which success is made visible and measured. Routine practices, however, can result in patients being socialised into dependency, and can undermine philosophies of care which place emphasis on promoting optimum independence.

People admitted for continuing care are deprived of their familiar social environment and accustomed lifestyle. The quality of their daily lives while in hospital will depend upon the extent to which nursing staff recognise their adult status, enable them to exercise choice in their activities, and help them to preserve their links with the wider social world.

An increasing commitment to the concept of community care by NHS management has been evident in recent years (DOH 1989). This policy is demonstrated by Schofield (1987) to be the only response by the health, social and voluntary services which can help to meet rising demands whilst taking into account the short comings of long-term institutionalisation as a means of providing a genuinely individualised service. The shift towards community care has resulted in the closure of a number of long-stay facilities; as a result, it is now more likely that nurses will come into contact with people with chronic illnesses who are being cared for in their own homes.

The foundation for the nursing role

It is important to recognise that formal health care personnel are of relatively little importance in the overall management of long-term illness. Whilst their contribution to care is crucial during periods of crisis and in the establishment of treatment regimes, the sufferer and his associates hold primary responsibility for day-to-day management of the condition (Strauss et al 1984).

McClymont (1985) explains that although the majority of people with chronic illness are able to manage their conditions with minimal and intermittent assistance from medical or nursing staff, a significant proportion are not able to function independently and require support from others. Responsibility for this level of caring for adults with chronic illness thus frequently rests with family members. The nursing role in relation to adults with chronic illness is therefore far from restricted to the delivery of direct care. For example, in order to develop effective self- and lay-care practices it is essential to investigate the capacity of individuals and their carers to take on this responsibility. It is also vital to ensure that the information that patients and their carers need in order to implement care regimes at home has been successfully communicated (see Case History 33.3). In pursuing the goal of optimum patient autonomy the nurse must also be prepared to adopt a flexible approach to care. During some phases of long-term illness it may be necessary to act for patients and carers, whilst on other occasions support will be focused on monitoring the performance of self-care activities, imparting knowledge or teaching practical skills to facilitate coping behaviour (see p. 585). This means that nurses need to be committed to the idea of forming and maintaining *collaborative* relationships with clients. This will present difficulties for a nurse who feels that sharing information constitutes a threat to her control of the caring situation or somehow undermines her professional role.

? **33.3** Look again at Chapter 26, 'Communication'. How could communication have been enhanced to prevent the problems which occurred when Mr P was learning about his diabetes? How might the use of an interpreter have helped?

The complexity of long-term illness and its impact on individual lifestyle and functioning have already been emphasised. It is all too easy for nurses to make assumptions about the problems experienced by individuals in their care on the basis of medical diagnosis alone. There are additional implications arising from the patient's classification as 'chronically ill'. The overuse of this label can leave the impression that people with longstanding illness or disability are members of an homogeneous group for whom care can be planned unilaterally.

Using models to guide practice

The case has already been made that whilst a variety of characteristics are shared by adults with chronic illness there is considerable diversity in the way in which individuals are affected by ongoing ill-health. It is therefore advantageous

Case History 33.3 Mr P

Mr P is 62 years old and lives with his wife and their son V in a suburban area of a large city. The family own and manage a successful video rental business and are active within the local Asian community.

Mr P usually enjoys good health but had been feeling unwell during recent months, experiencing frequency of micturition and an increased thirst. He was eventually persuaded to visit his general practitioner and was admitted to hospital on her advice. A diagnosis of diabetes mellitus was made and medical staff decided that control could be achieved through a combination of prescribed oral hypoglycaemic agents and a restricted carbohydrate diet (see Ch. 5). In the 10 days which followed, stabilisation of blood glucose levels was achieved. Nursing staff and the ward dietitian spent time with Mr P explaining the nature of his condition and his future role in its management. He seemed to listen carefully to what was said but did not ask questions of the staff. It was believed that this was an expression of his quiet and reserved nature which had been in evidence since admission. The dietitian was anxious to speak to Mrs P about her husband's dietary requirements, but the latter was not able to visit the hospital during office hours. Mr P said that he had discussed his condition with his wife and was confident that he would be able to cope after discharge. He was very much looking forward to returning home.

The responsibility for Mr P's nursing care was transferred to staff outside the hospital by way of the community liaison sister. When the community nurse, Susan, visited to assess the level of support which would be needed she was greeted by V. He told her that both he and his mother were concerned about Mr P, who now appeared to be little better than he had been before admission to hospital. Susan checked Mr P's blood glucose level and found it to be higher than expected. In an attempt to discover the likely cause of this problem she asked Mr and Mrs P what they knew of the condition and to describe the treatment regime.

It soon became clear that Mr P had not understood the information given to him in the hospital. He felt that the staff had been kind and concerned for his welfare, but he had observed them to be busy and did not wish to detain them unnecessarily by asking what he feared were trivial questions. He also confided that he was a little deaf and could not always hear what was said to him. The nurses had spoken quietly and quickly but Mr P had been too embarrassed to ask them to repeat all the information given. Although his working knowledge of English is good, Mr P uses this as his second language in daily life. Unfamiliar vocabulary presented during his admission had not enhanced communication with hospital staff. Susan discovered that Mr P believed he should reduce only the amount of sugar in his diet. Apart from this his food intake was unaltered, being predominantly based on rice and other foods high in carbohydrate. Susan recognised that the specific support she could give was limited and decided to offer the family contact with a community link worker.

to adopt an approach to the delivery of nursing care which recognises explicitly the uniqueness of each individual and enables the totality of his situation to be understood. The use of a formalised framework to guide practice is also valuable in that it presents a systematic prescription for action and encompasses a sound theoretical base.

A variety of nursing models have been constructed which serve to articulate beliefs about the essential components of nursing practice and the concepts and theories underpinning them. These conceptual models are intended to provide a descriptive representation of the reality of practice. Consideration of the individuals receiving nursing care, the environment in which they are placed, the meaning of 'health' and the role of the nurse is therefore central to any model of nursing practice (Fawcett 1984). The selection of a particular model by a team of nurses largely depends on the extent to which it reflects their own personal values and what they perceive their goals of work to be. Pearson & Vaughan (1986) note that several possible advantages can be gained when a nursing team achieves agreement as to their model of choice; not least among these are consistency and continuity of nursing action.

Whilst there are a number of models which have relevance for nursing adults with chronic illness, the three models discussed in the following may be of particular value and interest to nurses entering this field of care.

Orem's self-care model

It is likely that the model put forward by Dorothea Orem (1991) would be favoured by nurses who consider that its emphasis on client autonomy and motivation is consistent with the aim of helping individuals to accept responsibility for themselves. This may be seen as an appropriate choice in view of the limited role of formal health care personnel in the day-to-day management of longstanding disease. There may be a tendency, however, for nurses to select this model simply because they feel it to be synonymous with the concept of self-care (Cavanagh 1991). As a result, it is possible that some would fail to recognise fully that this concept forms only part of the model, and that it must be seen in the context of the other components in order for the underlying theory to be understood.

According to Eben et al (1986), Orem believes that self-care is the contribution made by adults to their own continued existence and involves the practice of activities to maintain health and well-being. The nurse acts to assist patients and their associates to achieve self-care in view of ability and need. Patient care is organised in terms of one of three nursing systems following negotiation involving all parties concerned. Intervention can be wholly compensatory, partly compensatory or supportive–educative; that is, the nurse may perform activities for the individual, assist the individual in carrying out shared activities, or help him to develop the ability to act on his own behalf. The decision to use a nursing system or a combination of systems is not static but changes in response to patient need over time.

Orem's model, therefore, presents some advantages for the care of people with chronic illness in both hospital and community settings. The importance of the role of the patient and his lay carers is acknowledged and their involvement in the planning of nursing interventions is considered essential. Attention is given to the notion that patients and their families are active in learning to live with the effects of the condition, and it is assumed that they are motivated to do so. The variation in nursing activity necessary to address the range of problems likely to be experienced during the course of long-term illness is also accounted for.

Roy's adaptation model

Another model which may be applied to the nursing care of chronically ill individuals is that devised by Callista Roy (1984). In Roy's view the behaviour of individuals is influenced by an interrelated set of biological, psychological and social systems. Each of these systems is directed towards achieving a state of relative balance which will, as far as is possible, promote the regularity of function and the ability of each person to adapt positively to environmental stimuli (Aggleton & Chalmers 1986). Roy identifies three types of stimuli to which individuals are exposed, i.e. focal, contextual and residual. A focal stimulus is something which has an immediate effect on the person. A contextual stimulus is a contributory circumstance. A residual stimulus arises from beliefs or attitudes relating to past experiences. Walsh (1991) comments that a focal stimulus should be present for each patient problem identified, but that contextual and residual stimuli are not necessarily present.

Where the effect of any stimulus exceeds the capacity of the individual to make a positive response maladaption is said to occur. This results in a threat to continued health and well-being. Roy's model accepts that each individual possesses a unique capacity to deal with stimuli, such that people react differently when faced with the same events. The ability to adapt thus varies from person to person.

Nursing intervention is needed when an individual's usual methods of coping with stressors prove ineffective. The role of the nurse centres on promoting adaptation both in maintaining health and during periods of illness, and is concerned with the manipulation of stimuli so that the patient is able to respond in a positive way. Roy emphasises that patients have an active responsibility to participate in their own care (Fawcett 1984).

This model would be of value in the treatment of long-term illness in a variety of care settings. Its focus is congruent with the idea that it is desirable for people with chronic illness to develop the ability to live with the effects of their condition. Nurses are encouraged to consider factors which influence the individual's total situation, not merely the immediate problems confronting him. In this way it is possible for them to appreciate the effects of the disorder on the patient's personal functioning over time and how he feels about this. The model assists nurses to identify successful coping mechanisms which have been used in the past and elements likely to impede future adaptation so that intervention may be planned with realisable goals. Care can therefore be tailored in relation to individual resources.

The Roper–Logan–Tierney model

A more detailed examination will be made here of the model for nursing put forward by Nancy Roper, Winifred Logan and Alison Tierney (1990). This model has been widely adopted to guide nursing education and practice in the UK, and is thus one with which many nurses are familiar. In addition, as Newton (1991) points out, it is based on ideas drawn directly from practice and is articulated in terms which may be readily understood. The representation of the reality of practice presented in the model by Roper, Logan and Tierney is such that it can be identified as being 'for real nurses, nursing real people' (Newton 1991, p. 193). Examples of how this model may be applied have already been given in earlier chapters.

The authors based their model for nursing on a model for living. This demonstrates that health status and lifestyle are closely related. It is also intended that an awareness of this relationship should assist nurses to perceive that their role is broadly concerned with health maintenance and is not merely disease-orientated. Their portrayal of an uncomplicated view of nursing is a deliberate attempt to provide a flexible framework which can be applied in a variety of settings. The stated purpose of this model for nursing is to equip practitioners with a means to plan and deliver individualised care. This refers mainly to nurse-initiated activity, but acknowledges the contribution of other members of the health care team. Roper et al (1990) explain that the model also offers a method of thinking about the beliefs, aims and practice of nursing in general terms.

The Roper–Logan–Tierney model for nursing has the following five components:

- the Activities of Living
- lifespan
- the dependence/independence continuum
- factors influencing the activities of living
- individualising nursing.

These will now be considered in turn with reference to the care of adults with chronic illness.

Activities of Living. Roper et al (1990) identify 12 Activities of Living as follows:

- maintaining a safe environment
- communicating
- breathing
- eating and drinking
- eliminating
- personal cleansing and dressing
- controlling body temperature
- mobilising
- working and playing
- expressing sexuality
- sleeping
- dying.

The authors incorporated these activities into their model of living in order to provide a description of behaviours involved in the process of engaging in daily life. Although Roper et al (1983) advise that the Activities of Living should be used as a framework for assessment when the model is applied to practice, there is a danger that some nurses may employ this component of the model simply as a checklist to guide the organisation of care, and that its other dimensions may be overlooked as a result (Price 1991). This would both restrict the model's usefulness and yield a limited understanding of the needs of patients and their families.

The focus of nursing intervention in this model is on assisting patients in the prevention, resolution and management of problems identified in relation to the Activities of Living. Problems are defined as actual or potential, as the nurse is not only concerned with problems which actually exist, but also seeks to prevent the development of others.

The performance of any of the Activities of Living requires the coordination of a complex pattern of behaviour. The ability to communicate, for example, relies on a number of skills, including the reception and interpretation of information and the formulation and transmission of appropriate verbal and non-verbal responses. This is influenced by many variables, such as the efficiency of physiological and psychological functions. There is thus considerable scope for errors to occur, and it is likely that people with chronic illness will experience a wide range of associated problems. For example, some individuals may discover that they cannot understand or express ideas verbally following a CVA, whilst others find no difficulty in this area but are unable to articulate words clearly. In either case sufferers will be limited in their ability to make their thoughts and feelings known, and this will cause frustration for all concerned. Speech deterioration also takes place in Parkinson's disease. In this condition, communication is further inhibited by memory impairment and loss of facial expression. The latter provides the listener with poor feedback and results in the absence of important non-verbal cues. Alteration in physical appearance can also present a barrier to communication. People may be embarrassed when they encounter disfigurement and avoid casual social contact with someone whose appearance disturbs them. In addition, they may make unfair assumptions about the individual's mental state. Wheelchair users often comment that people tend to speak over their heads to anyone who happens to be accompanying them, even when it would be more appropriate for them to be addressed directly.

It is common for people with long-term illness to find that disruption in the performance of one Activity of Living leads to difficulty in the performance of others. For instance, someone who has COAD and experiences shortness of breath may discover that his capacity to walk, eat and drink, communicate and attend to personal hygiene is also compromised. The restriction in mobility associated with arthritis can also interfere with the performance of workplace, domestic and recreational activities. For example, the purchase of food may prove problematic due to an inability to carry shopping and the preparation of meals may be made difficult by reduced physical dexterity.

Lifespan. This component of the model represents the passage of each person through life from conception to death. The progression along the lifespan is marked by continual change as the individual moves through a series of developmental stages, each of which is associated with the expression of different levels of physical, cognitive and social function. Roper et al (1990) acknowledge that adulthood is sometimes described in terms of three stages, i.e. young adulthood, the middle years and late adulthood.

As mentioned previously, adulthood is a period generally characterised by self-reliance which centres around occupational and family interests. There is, of course, great diversity in the lifestyle and behaviour exhibited by individuals in this stage of life. Awareness of an individual's chronological age does not give the nurse sufficient information to appreciate the likely impact of chronic illness. Rather, the nurse will need to gain an understanding of the developmental tasks which the individual has already achieved, those he aspires to and the value placed on them by the individual himself and those who are close to him.

This kind of information, obtained during assessment, would reveal the existence of actual or potential problems requiring nursing intervention. For example, a woman who has multiple sclerosis may have to come to terms with the fact that becoming pregnant would threaten her own health and that her functional impairment would present difficulties in meeting the needs of an infant. If despite her desire to become a mother she decides not to have children she may experience profound regret. Once the nurse identifies this as a source of emotional distress it can be accounted for in the subsequent planning and implementation of care.

The dependence/independence continuum. By including this element in their model Roper, Logan and Tierney acknowledge that individuals are not always able to perform each of the Activities of Living independently. Some people have yet to acquire the necessary skills or do not have the means to develop them, whilst others lose abilities which they once had, possibly as a result of illness or trauma.

According to Roper et al (1990) there can be no single measure which reflects the capacity for independent function in all Activities of Living, since it can be argued that few — if any — people are truly self-sufficient. In addition, they concede that the concepts of dependence and independence have meaning only when considered in relation to each other. For these reasons any form of assessment will have a subjective bias which is determined by the nurse's interpretation of the abilities of each individual in comparison with clinical, developmental and social norms (Newton 1991). Assumptions about the inevitability of global deterioration with age and chronic illness need to be questioned, for example. Health professionals must not fall into the trap of labelling or stereotyping the older person. Take, for example, the case of a health visitor who was asked to call on a frail elderly woman with chronic arthritis. She assumed her client would require support and services for health needs. To her astonishment she found herself being asked to find out about entrance requirements for the Open University. Her client was planning to gain a degree!

The interactive nature of the Activities of Living has been mentioned earlier with reference to the way in which difficulty in carrying out one activity can affect adversely the performance of others. This notion also has implications for the maintenance of independent action in chronic illness. For example, an individual with Parkinson's disease who cannot dress independently may need assistance with elimination in so far as he will need help with his clothing when using the toilet. In recognition of this it is essential that attention is paid to each of the Activities of Living when assessment is made of a patient's dependence/independence status.

Factors influencing the Activities of Living. Individual differences can be identified in the way in which the Activities of Living are performed, regardless of the point reached in the lifespan, or the level of dependence held. As an aid to describing these differences Roper, Logan and Tierney include five groups of factors in this component of their model, as follows:

- physical
- psychological — incorporating intellectual and emotional factors
- sociocultural — incorporating spiritual, religious and ethical factors
- environmental
- politicoeconomic — incorporating legal factors.

These factors, acting singly or in combination, influence each of the Activities of Living to some degree. It is not always easy to distinguish the influence of one group of factors from that of another since they are interrelated and share several areas of concern.

Consideration of this range of factors during assessment provides the basis for a deeper understanding of the cause of difficulties experienced by individuals as well as indicating likely outcomes. This has particular relevance for chronic illnesses in view of the time-scales involved, the multiple effects of these disorders and the cycle of deterioration that may be associated with them. For example, knowledge of normal anatomical structure and physiological function enables the nurse to appreciate the effects of disease processes. This is useful both in guiding immediate action to alleviate existing problems and in devising patterns of care to prevent the onset of anticipated complications. An exploration of psychological status will reveal what the individual comprehends about his condition. His capacity and motivation to acquire further information and develop the skills necessary for self-management can also be identified.

The behaviour an individual exhibits in everyday life in relation to the promotion of health and the management of chronic illness has strong social and cultural determinants. The nurse should attempt to understand how the individual's condition has affected his accustomed roles and in what respect this has influenced his relationships with others. A male manual worker who has multiple sclerosis, for instance, may perceive that his role as head of the family group is threatened when he is no longer able to continue employment and requires help from his partner to perform basic living activities.

Environmental factors such as noise, climate and atmospheric pollution can affect the performance of each of the Activities of Living in protracted illness. People with COAD experience worsening of their symptoms during periods of poor air quality. They may also find it difficult to obtain adequate rest and sleep if their home is located in a noisy neighbourhood or following admission to a busy hospital ward.

The structure and layout of buildings in which activities are performed are also of interest here. Someone who suffers from arthritis and lives in a top-floor flat without a lift may not be able to negotiate the stairs easily in order to leave the building. These circumstances would serve to further reduce his mobility, limiting opportunities for social interaction and activities such as shopping for clothes. Access to health centres can be made difficult if they are sited at some distance from available public transport or situated on a steep incline. This may deter individuals from attending appointments with members of the primary health care team and result in inadequate monitoring of treatment regimes and a lack of attention to some features of the disease. Lastly, admission to hospital is a source of anxiety to people for whom the environment is unfamiliar. The distance between facilities and the need to share bathing and sleeping accommodation may interfere with the individual's routine performance of a number of Activities of Living.

The organisation of all public services such as education, housing and social welfare is subject to political and economic influences, and these factors therefore have a significant effect on the manner in which people conduct their daily lives. Despite the high cost of chronic illness in both direct and indirect terms (see p. 911) long-term illness is not always given high priority in the allocation of health care funding. This has implications for staffing levels and the provision of equipment and hence for the quality of nursing support that can be offered to patients as they strive to attain optimum functioning and independence in the Activities of Living. Poor resourcing has additional implications for individual lifestyles. If a chair of a suitable height cannot be obtained for someone who has arthritis and he is unable to rise to a standing position as a result, it will not be possible for him to obtain exercise or travel to the toilet independently.

Individualising nursing. This component of the model reflects the fact that the way in which each individual carries out the Activities of Living is unique. This individuality arises from the complex interaction between the components described above and is apparent in the frequency, location and timing of activities, the rationale for the use of particular practices, and the knowledge, beliefs and attitudes of the person concerned. An appreciation of such variables provides the foundation for individualised nursing. Roper et al (1990) employ the nursing process as a vehicle to translate theory into practice and as a means of achieving the individualisation of care.

APPLYING THE ROPER–LOGAN–TIERNEY MODEL USING THE NURSING PROCESS

Assessment

This stage of the nursing process should be recognised as a dynamic and ongoing activity, rather than as a singular event associated with the first encounter between nurse and patient. In protracted illness an initial assessment is important because it presents the nurse with a structured method of data collection which will create a total picture of the individual and thus provide a baseline against which change can be measured (see Case History 33.4). It must be acknowledged, however, that in ongoing illness circumstances are seldom static and therefore continued assessment will be essential.

Roper et al (1990) advise that two forms of information should be gathered, i.e. that relating to biography and health and that concerning the Activities of Living. It might be suggested that these elements will be closely related in people who are chronically ill; for example, the perception which the individual and his lay carers have of his health status can shape the performance of some life activities. Efforts should therefore be directed towards obtaining a comprehensive assessment in any stage of the nurse–patient relationship.

A number of variables will warrant attention during the assessment of an adult with chronic illness, whether nursing care is to be delivered in an institutional or a domestic setting. Some are related directly to the disease process, and include the type and duration of the presenting condition, the methods already used for managing symptoms, and the extent to which strategies have been developed to cope with the uncertainty generated. Details of the treatment regime should also be collected to help the nurse to ascertain how the individual deals with incorporating this into daily life.

Case History 33.4

Tim H is a 19-year-old nursing student who was diagnosed in early adolescence as having epilepsy. Since leaving home to take up his studies Tim has become more acutely aware that he is in some way 'different' from other people. Although realising the importance of informing teaching and ward staff of his condition, should any seizures occur whilst he is working with equipment or patients, Tim feels as if he is introducing himself as an epileptic first and an individual second. He believes that people are more likely to remember him by his diagnosis rather than his personal qualities.

Tim's epilepsy had been generally well controlled by prescribed medication but recently he has become tired, vague and forgetful. He has experienced seizures in the student residences and in the hospital canteen and feels angry that he seems to be losing control of himself.

Although Tim's medication was changed following a visit to the outpatient department, the seizures have continued. Their onset is unpredictable and Tim finds that he is increasingly anxious about the uncertainty of his situation. He spends much of his time wondering when the next seizure will occur. He has not taken sick leave because he fears that this would detract from his image, which he considers to be already tarnished by his condition.

Tim has stopped riding his bicycle and limits his excursions to journeys within a small radius of the hospital campus. His friends do not seem to understand this change in behaviour. Tim had always been the first to suggest visits to the pubs and clubs in the city centre. They respond by going out without him and suggest that he is taking himself too seriously. Tim feels isolated and is annoyed by having to think before doing anything.

When he next visits the outpatient department Tim's unstable condition results in admission to hospital for monitoring of his seizures. Jayne E, Tim's allocated nurse, finds him to be aggressive during her initial assessment. As they talk, Tim tells her that he has always made every effort to take his medication at prescribed intervals and yet his difficulties persist. He thought that he had recognised the problems his current situation presents for his safety and had adjusted his activities accordingly. He now feels as though he were somehow being punished for this. Tim considers that he has done everything in his power to help himself and he expresses resentment towards hospital staff because he believes that they have failed him. Tim is also concerned that he will not be able to continue to cope with the demands of his studies. His sole ambition is to become a nurse. From what he says Jayne becomes aware that Tim has lost confidence and lacks self-esteem. Her assessment reveals that Tim's condition has more implications for his care than had at first been obvious.

In encouraging the review of biographical data Roper et al (1990) provide an opportunity for nurses to explore the individual's previous lifestyle and to appreciate the changes imposed by long-term illness in this context. The impact of these changes should be reviewed with reference to the Activities of Living while the other components of the model are borne in mind. It is suggested that all the activities should be considered so that for each individual their specific relevance can be established and the relationships between them identified. For instance, some people may be concerned that their disease presents them with the prospect of dying, while others may instead express profound grief at the loss of social function which has resulted from the gradual loss of personal and occupational roles.

The Roper–Logan–Tierney model prompts nurses to pay attention to the individual's abilities as well as disabilities in carrying out the Activities of Living through reference to the dependence/independence continuum. Any equipment used to assist independence in daily routines can be identified, and the involvement of statutory support services and of lay carers can be examined. This part of the assessment may well help to determine whether the individual has a realistic idea of his own abilities.

Although much of the data required for assessment may be obtained from the patient, other sources of information must not be ignored. The views of both formal and informal carers should be solicited in order to build up a more detailed impression of behaviour and events. For example, when a man who has motor neurone disease is admitted to hospital for respite care a community nurse might communicate her observation to the caring team that during recent months there has been a marked deterioration in the relationship between the patient and his spouse although the couple strenuously deny that this has taken place. This could then be interpreted with reference to the features of chronic illness and the key problems associated with these (see p. 908), and borne in mind as a plan for care is drawn up.

Planning

A plan for care is formulated to address the actual and potential problems identified in the course of assessment. The priority accorded to each problem depends upon the situation in which the individual is placed. Roper et al (1990) accept that life-threatening problems must assume precedence over those with a less immediate impact. Aside from this, priority-setting in chronic illness should always be negotiated by the nurse, patient and main lay carer. An open discussion is useful in clarifying the meaning of each problem to the individual, determining how problems are related to each other and creating a shared awareness that certain difficulties exist. This helps to foster a collaborative relationship and enhances the motivation of all concerned.

The aim of the care plan is to assist the patient in preventing, solving, alleviating or managing problems as far as is possible. Goals are set for each actual and potential problem and appropriate activities are devised to attain these goals. In chronic illness it is particularly important that the goals selected are realistic in view of the capacity of the individual to achieve them and their consistency with his own values and priorities. The patient and relevant lay carers should therefore be involved in this process.

> **?** **33.4** Sometimes a care plan has been well established prior to any nursing involvement at home or in hospital. What might the implications of this be for the patient and his carers when the nurse as a professional carer becomes involved?

Both short- and long-term goals can be specifed. However, given the instability of chronic illness the selection of broad objectives for future achievement, such as adaptation to the features of the condition and total self-management, may not be appropriate. It is preferable to simplify these by dividing them into a series of short-term goals related to the performance of relevant Activities of Living so that some progress can be achieved. Goals must also be expressed in measurable terms so that their attainment can be seen.

This information should be articulated in the form of a care plan with prescribed nursing interventions described in detail. This provides a means of ensuring continuity of care and is of particular value in long-term illness; for example, it can help to prevent confusion when a patient is learning to develop a routine for renal dialysis in a domestic setting. Activities initiated by other members of the multidisciplinary team can also be integrated into the care plan.

Implementation

The actions proposed in the care plan are realised in this phase of the nursing process. It is tempting to believe, as Roper et al (1990) point out, that as the majority of nurses are familiar with the idea of carrying out practical activities they will experience little difficulty in this area. Whilst there may be some truth in this assumption there is a tendency for ease of performance to conceal the depth of knowledge and the complex array of skills necessary to allow the nurse to meet the needs of an adult with chronic illness effectively.

The delivery of care in relation to the Activities of Living should be consistent with the way in which individuals usually behave, whether or not they normally require assistance. As in Orem's model this may require the nurse to act for the patient, or to supplement and develop his self-care capability, or to help him develop an understanding of the promotion of health (see p. 913). In order to determine the emphasis to be placed on each of these activities in a given situation, nurses must be sensitive to the individual's experience of chronic illness in the light of the factors considered in the first part of this chapter, whilst being aware of the possiblities of their nursing role.

The development of a therapeutic relationship with patients and lay carers is a sound base from which to work. It is important for the nurse to gain their trust and to recognise that under normal circumstances they have the responsibility for the management of daily life and features of the disease process. In both hospital and domestic settings nurses must be mindful of their role in enabling these individuals to retain control of their situation rather than expecting them to conform to alien norms and expectations.

In chronic illness nursing intervention is far from restricted to the delivery of physical care, although the value of this should not be underestimated. Assisting another person in carrying out any activity, such as washing and dressing, requires more than the ability to reproduce simple physical actions. Nurses working with people who are chronically ill need to be prepared to help patients to express their needs and, if necessary, to adopt the role of advocate in liaising with statutory and lay carers. The promotion of self-care capability requires an understanding of an individual's developmental level as well as effective teaching techniques. This involves the use of refined communication skills, as does the role of counsellor and supporter to both the patient and his family.

When helping an individual to adapt to the presence of a protracted degenerative disease and the difficulties which this can cause the nurse should present explanations honestly yet positively to foster realistic hope for the future. It is worth remembering that non-verbal communication, principally that of touch, can be a useful tool to strengthen a caring relationship. Some nurses consider it appropriate to extend their traditional skills in this direction. The provision of massage, for example, can be of value in assisting the individual to deal with stress, creating a sense of self-worth and obtaining a palliative effect.

Evaluation

The effectiveness of nursing interventions can be judged by evaluating whether or not goals have been achieved. This phase of the nursing process thus lends meaning to the phases which precede it. The extent to which goals have been achieved should be measured objectively where possible. For example, successful self-management of insulin-dependent diabetes can be demonstrated by a pattern of stability in blood glucose readings. It is also possible to identify movement on the dependence/independence continuum in response to teaching programmes or the handling of symptoms.

The evaluation of some aspects of care is, however, largely dependent upon subjective data. For instance, it is difficult to measure to what extent a patient has adapted to the idea of having a chronic disease. Evaluation in this area could be guided instead by questioning the individual and interpreting his responses in terms of known variables, such as evident interest in the management of the condition or avoidance of discussion of the illness and its related problems.

The achievement of any goal for care relies on a variety of situational variables. It is therefore sometimes difficult to identify whether nursing strategies have been successful or not. The contribution of staff and material resources, efforts made by lay carers and the emotional status of the patient can all influence outcome. Nurses should be prepared to recognise that not all interventions which they initiate will be effective for each individual, even if they have been used with success on previous occasions. This serves as a stimulus for reassessment, from which revised problem statements and new goals for care can be generated (Newton 1991).

The importance of the nurse's own self-evaluation must not be forgotten here. Caring for adults with chronic illness exerts considerable physical and emotional pressures on nursing staff as well as on principal lay carers. There are a number of reasons for this. Nurses sometimes find it difficult to work within the boundaries of their occupational role as their relationships develop with individuals and their families over time. They may find it difficult to accept the inevitability of the patient's decline in health and independence. It is also likely that they will identify with the experience of a patient if they occupy the same stage of the lifespan. Some nurses will be unable to form close protracted relationships with particular patients due to differences in personality and attitude. Individual nurses must recognise that they cannot give all things to all people. They should develop their own strategies for coping with the stress of caring and be prepared to share this burden with other members of the nursing team.

CONCLUSION

Nurses encounter people who are chronically sick in a variety of settings. Effective care requires a grounding in social and physical sciences so that the experiences of the individual and his family can be interpreted accurately. The nursing role is collaborative in nature and involves the expression of technological, clinical and interpersonal skills. In the long term, emphasis is placed on caring, a concept fundamental to the practice of nursing which has often been overshadowed by other considerations. Working with individuals with chronic illnesses presents nurses with the opportunity to reaffirm their unique contribution to health care.

Finally, it is suggested that a good foundation for this role is to avoid thinking about the person in need of nursing intervention as a chronically ill person, but to focus attention towards an individual who is a person with a chronic illness.

GLOSSARY

Advocate. An aspect of the nursing role essential to humanistic care whereby the nurse assists the patient to make decisions in a self-determined manner.

Autonomy. To act with self-determination.

Collaborative relationships. Relationships within which the nurse, patient and his significant others work together as a cohesive team with shared responsibilities.

Complementary therapies. Those methods of diagnosis and therapeutic practice which do not necessarily adhere to the principles which guide conventional scientific medicine, for example acupuncture, aromatherapy and homeopathy.

Demography. The study of statistics relating to population variables such as age gender, income and dependency.

Disability. An enduring incapacity arising from congenital defect, disease, injury or old age.

Handicap. The social, economic and environmental consequences of impairment and disability.

Impairment. Physiological or anatomical abnormalities caused by disease processes.

Mortality. A measure of causes of and age at death for a given population which can provide information on changes in life expectancy but may not indicate quality of life experienced.

REFERENCES

Aggleton P, Chalmers H 1986 Nursing models and the nursing process. Macmillan, Basingstoke

Anderson M P 1988 Stress management for chronic disease: an overview. In: Russell M L (ed) Stress management for chronic disease. Pergamon, New York, ch 1

Anderson R, Bury M (eds) 1988 Living with chronic illness: the experience of patients and their families. Unwin Hyman, London

Benoliel J Q 1983 Foreword. In: Dimond M, Jones S L Chronic illness across the lifespan. Appleton-Century-Crofts, Norwalk, CT

Blaxter M 1983 The causes of disease: women talking. In: Black N, Boswell D, Gray A, Murphey S, Popay J (eds) Health and disease: a reader. Open University Press, Milton Keynes, pp 34–43

Brocklehurst J C 1975 Geriatric care in advanced societies. MTP, Lancaster

Bury M 1979 Disablement in society: towards an integrated perspective. International Journal Of Rehabilitative Research, 2(9): 33–40

Cavanagh S J 1991 Orem's model in action. Macmillan, Basingstoke

Central Statistical Office 1990 Social trends 20. HMSO, London

Clarke M 1978 Getting through the work. In: Dingwall R, McIntosh J (eds) Readings in the sociology of nursing. Churchill Livingstone, Edinburgh, ch 5

Coser R L 1963 Alienation and social structure. In: Freidson E (ed) The hospital in modern society. The Free Press, New York

Department of Health 1989 Caring for people: community care in the next decade and beyond. HMSO, London
Department of Health 1990 On the state of the public health for the year 1989. HMSO, London
Dimond M, Jones S L 1983 Chronic illness across the lifespan. Appleton-Century-Crofts, Norwalk, CT
Eben J D, Nation M J, Marriner A, Nordmeyer S B 1986 Self-care deficit theory of nursing. In: Marriner A (ed) Nursing theorists and their work. Mosby, St Louis, MO, ch 11
Fawcett J 1984 Analysis and evaluation of conceptual models of nursing. Davis, Philadelphia
Field D 1976 The social definition of illness. In: Tuckett D (ed) An introduction to medical sociology. Tavistock, London, ch 10
Fitzpatrick R M 1982 Social concepts of disease and illness. In: Patrick D L, Scambler G (eds) Sociology as applied to medicine. Baillière Tindall, London, ch 1
Goffman E 1963 Stigma. Penguin, Harmondsworth
Gull H J 1987 The chronically ill patient's adaptation to hospitalisation. Nursing Clinics of North America 22(3): 593–601
Kelleher D 1988 Coming to terms with diabetes: coping strategies and non-compliance. In Anderson R, Bury M (eds) Living with chronic illness: the experience of patients and their families. Unwin Hyman, London, ch 6
King K (ed) 1985 Long term care. Churchill Livingstone, Edinburgh
Lambert C E, Lambert V A 1987 Psychosocial impacts created by chronic illness. Nursing Clinics of North America 22(3): 527–533
Martin J, Meltzer H, Elliot D 1988 The prevalence of disability among adults (OPCS surveys of disability in Great Britain: report 1). HMSO, London
McClymont M E 1985 Intervention and care. In: King K (ed) Long term care. Churchill Livingstone, Edinburgh, ch 4
Montbriand M J, Laing G P 1991 Alternative health care as a control strategy. Journal of Advanced Nursing 16(3): 325–332
Morgan J 1988 Living with renal failure on home dialysis. In: Anderson R, Bury M (eds) Living with chronic illness: the experience of patients and their families. Unwin Hyman, London, ch 9
Neuberger J 1986 When no-one's to blame. Nursing Times 82(25): 23
Neuberger J 1987 Prevention not punishment. Nursing Times 83(3): 25
Newton C 1991 The Roper–Logan–Tierney model in action. Macmillan, Basingstoke
Oliver M 1990 The politics of disablement. Macmillan, Basingstoke
Orem D E 1991 Nursing: concepts of practice, 4th edn. McGraw-Hill, New York
Parsons T 1951 The social system. Routledge & Kegan Paul, London
Patrick D L, Scambler G (eds) 1982 Sociology as applied to medicine. Baillière Tindall, London
Pearson A, Vaughan B 1986 Nursing models for practice. Heinemann Medical, London
Pinder R 1990 The management of chronic illness: patient and doctor perspectives on Parkinson's disease. Macmillan, Basingstoke
Pitkeathley J 1991 Seen but not heard? Nursing Times 87(42): 22
Price B 1991 Preface. In: Newton C The Roper–Logan–Tierney model in action. Macmillan, Basingstoke
Roberts I 1985 Social and economic implications of chronic illness: a British perspective. In: King K (ed) Long term care. Churchill Livingstone, Edinburgh, ch 5
Robinson I 1988 Reconstructing lives: negotiating the meaning of multiple sclerosis. In: Anderson R, Bury M (eds) Living with chronic illness: the experience of patients and their families. Unwin Hyman, London, ch 2
Roper N, Logan W, Tierney A J 1983 Using a model for nursing. Churchill Livingstone, Edinburgh
Roper N, Logan W, Tierney A J 1990 The elements of nursing, 3rd edn. Churchill Livingstone, Edinburgh
Roy C 1984 Introduction to nursing: an adaptation model. Prentice Hall, Englewood Cliffs, NJ
Sagan L A 1987 The health of nations: true causes of sickness and wellbeing. Basic Books, New York
Scambler G 1982 Deviance, labelling and stigma. In: Patrick D L, Scambler G (eds) Sociology as applied to medicine. Baillière Tindall, London, ch 15
Schofield M 1987 Dramatic change — but all in the public interest. Health Service Journal 97(5047): 472
Sharma U M 1990 Using alternative therapies: marginal medicine and central concerns. In: Abbott P, Payne G (eds) New directions in the sociology of health. Falmer, London, ch 9
Stockwell F 1972 The unpopular patient. Royal College of Nursing, London
Strauss A L, Corbin J, Fagerhaugh S, Glaser B G, Maines D, Suczek B, Weiner C L 1984 Chronic illness and the quality of life. Mosby, St Louis, MO
Walker A 1984 The care gap. Local Government Information Unit, London
Walsh M 1991 Models in clinical nursing: the way forward. Baillière Tindall, London

FURTHER READING

Ewles L, Simnett I 1992 Promoting health, 2nd edn. Wiley, Chichester, chs 1, 4
Hyde A 1990 What is health? Health studies in nurse education. Discussion paper 2. Health Education Board for Scotland, Edinburgh
Seedhouse D 1986 Health: foundations for achievement. Wiley, Chichester
Shanley E 1992 Health and chronic conditions. Health studies in nurse education. Discussion paper 6. Health Education Board for Scotland, Edinburgh

CHAPTER 34

The terminally ill patient

Margaret Kindlen

CHAPTER CONTENTS

Introduction 921
Nursing issues 921
Changing patterns of care 922

Organisational provision for palliative care 922
Developments in services 922
Teamwork in palliative care 922
Hospital care 922
Hospice care 923
Community care 923

Understanding loss and change 924
Responses to illness 924
Theories of loss 924

Quality of life and death 925
The disease process 925
The experience of terminal illness 925
Communication 926

Nursing management 926
Palliative care and the nurse 926
A framework for palliative nursing care 927

Nursing care of patients who are terminally ill 928
Assessment 929
Presenting symptoms 929
Other potential self-care deficits in terminal illness 932

Dying, death and bereavement 935
Support for carers 936
Death 936
Bereavement 938
Support for nursing staff 939

Conclusion 940

References 941

Video cassettes 941

Further reading 942

Useful addresses 942

INTRODUCTION

In this chapter, important issues relating to the care of terminally ill patients will be raised, drawing from the author's experience of nursing in community, hospital and hospice settings. Emphasis is placed on the challenge faced by patients and their carers in facing death and living with loss. Reference will be made to other chapters especially those dealing with pain management, the treatment of symptoms relating to cancer, and communication skills. The Orem model of nursing will be used to illustrate how principles of self-care can be applied in different settings.

The phrase 'terminal illness' refers to a range of advanced progressive disorders from which death is a certain but not necessarily imminent outcome. For an individual to be told that he or someone close to him has a terminal illness must be one of the most daunting experiences of his lifetime. Inevitably such an experience raises questions ranging from 'What is this all about?' and 'Why is this happening?' to 'When, where and how will death occur?'

For health care professionals, the challenge is to address these issues using their expertise, knowledge, and fundamental skills to ensure the best possible quality of life for the patient and his carers throughout the course of illness and bereavement. In recent years this area of care has become known as 'palliative care', but its aims are not new for health care professionals; indeed, they echo the philosophy of Hypocrites:

- to cure sometimes,
- to relieve often,
- to comfort always.

Nursing issues

The enormous advances in knowledge and technology of the last four decades have endowed the medical profession with impressive expertise in restoring health and prolonging life. But while illness is viewed by nurses as 'the human experience of sickness' (Kleinman et al 1978) it is seen by doctors primarily as a disease process. High expectations of obtaining a cure reinforce a sense of defeat when disease overtakes the recovery process. Consequently, death is viewed as failure.

Caring for dying patients brings into focus many issues for nurses. In addition to the likely physical distress caused by a terminal illness, the patient will have to face great emotional strain. The many dimensions of loss, both personal and social, will affect the entire network of family, friends and professionals involved in the care of the patient. The process of dying challenges the value systems of the individual as well as of his professional and lay carers, raising issues relating to personal autonomy, quality of life and dignity in dying. The nurse's view of these issues will affect her approach to the care of sick and dying patients. For the patient and his family, attitudes to living and dying will inevitably influence where they wish the last days of the patient's life to be spent.

Changing patterns of care

During the 1980s 60–70% of deaths occurred in hospital or other institutions. However, Doyle (1987) estimates that patients with advanced cancer spend up to 90% of the last year of their illness at home. It is for this reason that the needs of patients and their families must be considered together.

During the latter part of the 20th century, caring for terminally ill patients has been greatly influenced by the hospice movement. This has reinforced the philosophy of patient-centred care within an environment which best suits the needs of patients and families, be it hospital, home or hospice. Central to this is the concept of teamwork, which recognises that no one professional can be entirely responsible for the amount of emotional and social support that patients, families and indeed professionals themselves require when dealing with physical suffering, grief and bereavement.

In the 1990s greater emphasis is being placed on providing care outside of the hospital setting, especially for elderly and chronically ill patients. There has already been an increase in residential care establishments in the private sector. This may widen the choice for patients and their carers but may also mean that terminally ill patients will be cared for in settings where nursing input is widely variable. Patient Charters (see Ch. 27, p. 776) will provide some guide as to the quality of care to be expected; however, it could be argued that nurses have a responsibility to provide the appropriate information to help patients make informed choices about the environment in which they choose to die. Carers and patients themselves may have considerable insight to offer to professionals.

ORGANISATIONAL PROVISION FOR PALLIATIVE CARE

Development in services

The recent developments in hospice care have made an enormous contribution towards the care of terminally ill patients and their families. It would be a mistake, however, to regard hospices as providing sufficient resources to meet all palliative care needs in the future. Although many lessons have been learned from hospice care, there are also some important distinctions to be made in relation to the terminal phase of non-malignant diseases. Seale (1991) considers age to be an important factor. His findings suggest that people dying from cancer are younger, on average, than those dying from non-malignant disease. This has implications for informal carers in that cancer patients are more likely to draw on family and friends to assist them. Other differences were in the type and intensity of symptoms, showing that the period of suffering and dependency in cancer patients is relatively greater but of shorter duration than that of other illnesses. Seale also makes the important point that in the absence of cancer a diagnosis of dying is difficult to establish. This undoubtedly has implications for the place of death.

The range of services offered as an alternative to dying in hospital raises questions about the individual's freedom to choose a place to die. Although some attempt has been made to explore preferred versus actual place of death, there is an inevitable bias in the samples used in such studies towards cancer deaths. These studies do, however, indicate that irrespective of individual stated preference some 60% of people die in hospital, 10% in hospice and 30% at home (Dunlop et al 1989, Townsend et al 1990).

Teamwork in palliative care

Teamwork, be it uni- or multidisciplinary, is central to the philosophy of patient-centred care. It is especially important in palliative care that overlapping areas of practice are acknowledged and that professional responsibilities are distributed in the best interests of the patient and his family. The rationale for this becomes clearer as the disease progresses and the profile of different members within the team changes. Significantly, the doctor is often the most prominent person for the patient and family during the early phase of an illness. Nursing staff and other professionals may gradually be introduced. It is largely a matter of patient and family choice which team member becomes the key confidant(e). As death approaches, however, there is little doubt as to the high profile that nurses have in the patient's life. The team leadership role may consequently shift to allow nursing staff to coordinate resources according to the changing needs of the patient and his family. The professionals involved will also need the support of colleagues, mentors or friends in whom they can confide as part of the process of resolving personal and professional dilemmas (see Ch. 17, pp. 591–593).

> ? **34.1** Before reading further consider the following questions:
> a. What attitude, in general, prevails among professionals toward patients for whom care rather than cure has become the priority in management?
> b. Does this vary from ward to ward and hospital to community?
> c. Have you personally experienced conflict between your values and those of colleagues with whom you have worked?
> d. Is there a medium for resolving such conflict?

Hospital care

Nash's (1989) review of the literature suggests that when patients are in hospital relatives experience confusion, isolation, separateness from the dying patient and a reliance on professionals to provide care. It is suggested that when this induced helplessness is encouraged by professionals it undermines the relatives' desire to provide care and becomes a source of guilt. Implicit in this is a nursing role which is concerned solely with direct patient care of a physical nature and the resulting attitude that it is quicker and easier to take over this area of care than to allow relatives to participate. Nash refers to an investigation of family members' reactions when patients with dementia were admitted to hospital. She discusses how family members resolved their feelings of guilt through being supported by nursing staff and by being included in the care of their relative. In the same study, however, 22% of staff were found to be against relative involvement in patient care.

Among the reasons identified by Townsend et al (1990) for terminally ill people dying in hospital other than by choice are:

- the patient's unexpected deterioration whilst undergoing treatment
- waiting time for transfer to hospice care
- inability of informal carers to cope with home care.

This last point confirms Wilkes' (1985) earlier report that dying patients were admitted to institutions more often because of the needs of relatives and raises questions about the adequacy of the support offered to families by the primary health care team. Many district nursing sisters advocate early referral on the grounds that this would allow them access to patients before the end stage of life and give them time to build relationships with the whole family (Kindlen 1987, Hockey 1990).

The high profile of nursing was discussed by Lunt & Neale

(1987) when they compared the goal-setting of hospital staff with that of hospice staff. They concluded that doctors in district general hospitals should take account of the views of their nurse colleagues and should attend more positively to patients' rehabilitative and emotional needs, to patient–family relationships, and to the emotional needs of families.

There is much evidence to support the conclusion that through philosophies of care the hospice ethic has been adopted by nurses across a wide spectrum of hospital practice (Haigh 1990, Stott 1990, McGhee 1991, Williams 1991).

Elderly patients who are terminally ill

In his study of terminally ill elderly patients in hospital, Blackburn (1989) identified important practical differences between the care appropriate to this group of patients and that required by younger cancer patients in hospices. Elderly patients experience a range of problems such as sensory loss, impaired perception, confusional states and dementia which impede verbal and non-verbal communication. This may be compounded by poor social and family support networks. Consequently, elderly patients often need additional attention and support which may be beyond the scope of the resources available in hospital. Wilson et al (1987) reported that 32% of geriatric patients in long-term hospital care were distressed during the last week of life and that nursing staff were the first to recognise when a patient was dying.

Hospice care

Hospices have the potential to provide a greater degree of privacy and a more flexible plan for care than is possible in many hospitals. The philosophy of hospice/palliative care is practised throughout the United Kingdom in acute and long-term hospitals, in specialist and independent units, and through statutory and back-up domiciliary services, including day hospice care.

Evaluative research of hospice care in the 1970s identified the psychological support given to patients and carers as an important strength. Parkes (1985) highlighted the finding that where hospital doctors and nurses took advantage of the education programmes offered by staff at St Christopher's Hospice, London, their subsequent management of symptoms matched that in the teaching hospice environment. Whilst this was so of symptom control, there were gaps in the overall support offered to the spouses of patients. It has been suggested in a number of research studies that failure in communication between professionals is one reason for the ineffective support in some hospitals. The main difference which emerged, when comparisons were made between hospital, hospice and community teams was in the strength of the multidisciplinary teams (Ward 1985, Kindlen 1987, Hockey 1990).

Dunlop et al (1989) found distress in patients admitted to hospice care against their choice. This reinforces the findings of other investigations that patients, particularly those with non-malignant disease, have little choice concerning their place of death (Cartwright et al 1973, Cowley 1990).

A number of studies relating to hospices have been conducted in the UK. Higginson & McCarthy (1989) point out that much of this research concentrates on describing processes of care rather than on measuring outcomes. The challenge to hospices in the 1990s lies in assessment of the value of care provided. If hospice care is to continue to ensure quality for patients and their carers, then the way forward must include the development of clinical audit, the measuring of standards of care and the prediction of problem areas.

Community care

Although there has been a steady decline in the UK of the actual number of deaths occurring at home, there is evidence that people do spend longer periods at home during a terminal illness (Parkes 1985, Ward 1985, Lunt & Yardley 1986).

Cowley (1990) reported an artificial division between those at home dying from cancer and those dying from other causes. This division seemed to be largely in the minds of general practitioners, who saw no reason to refer patients with non-malignant disease to district nursing services for terminal care. Cowley points out that needs assessment and care planning are vital components of the nursing role for patients when death is the predictable outcome whether or not there is a diagnosis of cancer. When this is ignored, phenomenal pressures can build up, resulting in physical and stress illnesses for other family members. The evidence of case histories reported in the literature underlines the benefits for patient, family and professional carers when appropriate referral to district nursing services is made (Langlands 1991, Collinge 1990, Cowley 1990).

The role of the community nurse

The community nurse aims to provide initial care, to teach patients and relatives how to perform care tasks, and to support them in the continuance of that care and in any decisions that they need to make. This puts the family very much at the centre of care and enables them to sustain the patient at home until his death, if this should be their wish. Once a pattern of family-centred care is established, it should be continued in the event of the patient being admitted to hospital or hospice.

Palliative care home support services

There are few areas of the UK without a palliative care support service, whether that is provided by a hospice, Macmillan nurses, Marie Curie home care nurses or a day care facility. These services have grown to complement the services provided by primary health care teams, acting as a back-up to existing care and often providing a link with the local hospice service.

Voluntary support organisations

Many groups exist to provide information, advice, practical help, support and counselling appropriate to a wide spectrum of illness and disease. The organisation CancerLink, for example, began in a small way with a group of people with personal and professional experience of cancer. It is now associated with a major cancer charity, the Macmillan Cancer Relief Fund and offers support and guidance for patients, relatives and professionals. The same pattern of growth has been seen in other voluntary support organisations. Registers of these groups are held at local social services departments; nurses should consult these to find out what support groups are available for patients in their area of practice.

National networks

In 1991 two organisations were initiated to support cancer and palliative care services: The National Hospice Council (NHC) in England, Wales and Northern Ireland, and The Scottish Partnership Agency for Palliative and Cancer Care (SPAPCC). These organisations exist to provide links between national charities, the National Health Service (NHS), voluntary hospices, voluntary support agencies and professional associations. The centralisation of information within these organisations enables them to authoritatively advise the Government and local authorities and health boards on the changing needs within palliative care services.

UNDERSTANDING LOSS AND CHANGE

Responses to illness

An important influence in recent years has been the acceptance of a holistic view of illness. In this approach, vulnerability to illness and trauma, an inability to understand fully what is happening, and separation from significant people are all recognised as being among the causes of the emotional pain that can arise during illness and disability and which must be recognised by professionals in their delivery of health care.

Change in health status

A change in an individual's health status might be reflected in an inability to understand what is happening. This is likely to be accompanied by a corresponding change in other people's expectations and in the individual's perception of his own ability to adhere to social norms and accustomed roles. Such change has been defined by Benner & Wrubel (1989) as an experience of loss or dysfunction.

Theories of loss

A number of theories have been developed to account for the emotional impact of the experience of loss. Caplan (1961) described normal health as a state of equilibrium within which the introduction of any imbalance produces a stress reaction. Stress reactions have been compared with responses to loss, separation and bereavement. The process of coping with life's critical events is viewed as part of normal growth and development; consequently, stress, separation anxiety and mourning should be regarded as healthy responses. These are, of course, highly individual reactions which will be shaped by the person's individual life experiences and coping strategies (Benner & Wrubel 1989, Bowlby 1988, Parkes 1986).

Emotional responses to loss and change

The transition from loss (as in a change in health status) to readjustment is a gradual process. Bowlby (1969) described a sequence of responses associated with loss and change wherein an individual experiences internal feelings and displays external behaviours according to whether a state of protest, despair, detachment or readjustment exists (see Fig. 34.1). In his later work he identified the degree of response with the sense of security and confidence that the person experiences within relationships (Bowlby 1988).

Kubler-Ross (1970) also described responses to illness and impending death (see Table 34.1). Her conclusion was that people approach and deal with the crisis of illness and death in the same manner that they face other life crises; that is if an individual's normal response to a crisis event is anger then one should expect that he will be angry about dying.

Grieving. The individual nature of grieving can not be overstressed. Different members of a family will not only have different ways of coping, but will respond according to their different perspectives of a situation. Parkes (1986) urges that we should take care to identify the particular loss to which an individual is responding.

> **?** **34.2** Take a few moments here to think about what might influence a person's way of responding to critical events in his life. For example, pause here and consider how the different members of your family view your possession of a car. How would you and the other members of your family respond to your loss if this car was stolen?

Anticipatory grieving. There is agreement between research-

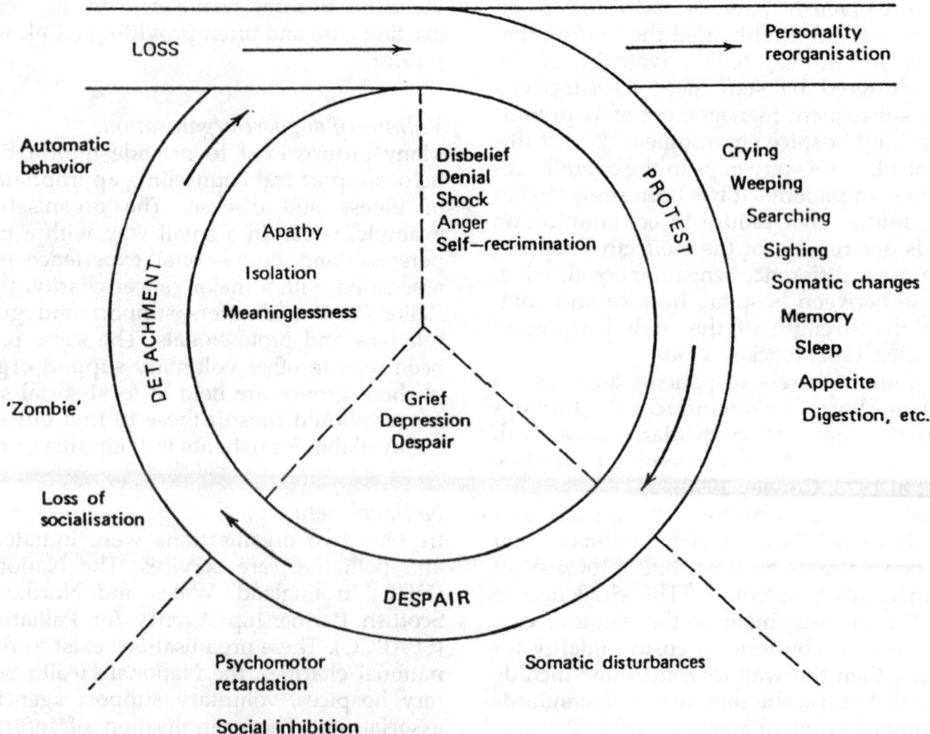

Fig. 34.1 Grief following object loss and loss of others. (Reproduced with kind permission from John Wiley & Sons, from Bowlby (1969). In: Bower F (ed) Nursing and the concept of loss. Copyright © 1980 John Wiley & Sons, Inc.)

Table 34.1 Emotional responses to illness and dying (After Kubler-Ross 1970)

Emotion stage	Typical responses
Denial	Stunned/dazed 'Oh no, not me!!' 'There must be some mistake!!'
Anger	'Why me?' Projected feelings of anger resulting in criticism and irritability
Bargaining	'Just this once?' 'If I'm cured I'll . . .'
Depression	Reminiscence over past sad and negative events Withdrawal
Acceptance	Open expression of feelings; person has experienced anger, envy, and longing and now recognises and accepts such feelings

ers that individuals will draw on a range of possible emotional and behavioural responses as they experience a variety of losses during a lifetime. The way in which individuals prepare themselves for expected life changes is referred to as anticipatory grieving. Speck (1978) argues that the more effective the preparation the more 'normal' the subsequent response will be to the eventual change or crisis. Preparation for an expected crisis event is not a new concept. In his crisis theory Caplan (1961) refers to anticipatory guidance as a means of 'preventative intervention'. This involves providing individuals with realistic information, reassurance, and the opportunity for active participation, thus allaying fears, anxieties and feelings of helplessness. This anticipatory guidance is, in fact, a large component of every nurse's role in the preparation of patients for admission to or discharge from hospital, or for the many aspects of clinical and nursing care which patients undergo. Speck (1978) strongly advocates that this familiar practice should be given particular emphasis in situations where there is a life-threatening illness as a way of preparing the patient, family and professional carers to cope with the experiences of loss that they may encounter.

Atypical grief. In contrast to the pattern of emotional responses and behaviours which have been described, atypical grief occurs when these usual responses are in some way inhibited, delayed, prolonged or distorted. Atypical grief may be characterised by physical illness, anger, bitterness, hostility, inappropriate behaviour such as drug or alcohol abuse, persistent low self-esteem, despair and the potential for suicide (Parkes 1986, Raphael 1984).

QUALITY OF LIFE AND DEATH

According to Benner & Wrubel (1989) terminal illness involves both a biological response to disease and an emotional response to an everchanging set of circumstances. The implications of these two aspects of illness for nursing care will be considered in the following discussion.

The disease process

Because of the multiple pathology associated with terminal illness the nurse may encounter a very wide range of symptoms among patients who are dying. It is important for the nurse to know whether each symptom experienced is a primary or secondary effect of the disease, or whether it is in fact secondary to an existing symptom. The situation may be further complicated when an acute episode of illness is superimposed upon existing disease or when an unrelated illness occurs. It is therefore essential for nurses to be familiar with the underlying disease processes and potential symptoms that may arise.

Malignant disease

There are three routes of metastatic spread involved in any malignant tumour. These are:

- local invasion of surrounding tissues
- through the lymphatic system
- through the circulatory system.

An understanding of these routes can help to predict the spread of, for example, breast cancer and the related symptoms that might arise (see Ch. 32).

Non-malignant disease

Cowley (1990) reports that many chronically ill patients receive inadequate care towards the end of their lives because they are not dying of cancer. As with cancer, the nurse's knowledge of the disease process of non-malignant conditions should be adequate to enable her to recognise symptoms.

Cardiovascular disease is the most frequently recorded single cause of death in persons over 65 years of age (see Ch. 2). Heart failure commonly occurs as a result of ischaemic heart disease or arterial hypertension. Heart failure has a direct effect on

- the heart
- the respiratory system
- the fluid and electrolyte balance of the body.

> ? **34.3** Pause here to reflect on the last paragraph. List the symptoms that you might anticipate in advanced cardiovascular disease (see Ch. 2).

Dementia. Jacques (1992) suggests that 'to understand dementia we need simply to think of all that the upper parts of our brains do, and that is the list of all the functions which are likely to decline' (p. 9). In dementia, the whole personality, all that has ever been learned, and all the basic controlling and organising functions of the brain are affected. Mental activities, sensory perception and the initiation and control of voluntary muscle contraction are eventually compromised.

Jacques further states that the functions of the brain which develop later in life are the first to deteriorate when widespread damage occurs. Bowel and bladder dysfunction, for example, comes much later than memory disturbance. This information is essential to enable nurses to recognise concurrent illness such as urinary tract infection in patients with mild to moderate degrees of dementia.

Physical symptoms of terminal illness

The list of symptoms experienced by patients who are terminally ill is a long and variable one and it has been noted that patients and their relatives report only about half of the symptoms which are truly distressing. Doyle (1987) points out that it is seldom realised that there are remedies for halitosis and other odours and that thirst and muscular pains can be relieved. Furthermore, it is unlikely that a dying patient will reveal fears and anxieties in the presence of physical symptoms (Doyle 1987).

The experience of terminal illness

In the video *Cancer Journey* Cassidy et al describe a number of emotional responses noted during patients' experiences of terminal illness. These include fear, loss, anger, powerlessness, alienation, sadness and depression. Each of these emotions will be considered here in turn.

? **34.4** This may be an appropriate place for you to take a few moments to consider some of the factors within your own working environment which might precipitate the following feelings in patients:

- fear
- loss
- anger
- powerlessness
- alienation
- sadness and depression

Think these over and then read on.

Fear

Fear is associated with previous distressing experience or with anticipation of the unknown. It is a natural response when the need to understand is blocked in some way and may arise when the person is unable to fully understand events or when information is either unclear or withheld. The fears that patients have will be associated with their own experience of illness and impending death but may well be compounded by some previous experience which they have either been involved in or witnessed.

Loss

Feelings of loss are associated with many of the changes which take place during a terminal illness. Such changes will involve a deterioration in health status resulting in, for example, a loss of self-image or independence. Inevitably, there will be changes in social and family relationships and those involved may regret the loss of 'what might have been'. Any change in an individual's capacity for self-care raises the possibility of a loss in privacy and personal dignity. Parkes (1986) stresses the importance of identifying the number of loss processes which might be experienced concurrently or sequentially in the course of a terminal illness. Bowlby (1988) points out that the intensity of an attachment must be considered as we try to understand the nature and depth of feelings that an individual has in response to a particular loss.

Anger

Contrary to common belief, anger is a natural and healthy response. Anger arises when a person has no control over his circumstances, as when he is faced with the fact that the illness he is experiencing will inevitably result in death. Questions and fears about the meaning and purpose of life may direct anger towards the spiritual self. Anger may also result from the individual's lack of involvement in decisions which affect his circumstances. How often do professionals think they know best and collude with families over matters which they think are too painful for patients to deal with?

Powerlessness

When angry feelings have been persistently suppressed or not permitted by others, an individual's motivation to take control of personal circumstances gradually diminishes. Powerlessness is a distortion of anger. It is linked with feelings of low self esteem, rage, hatred and a desire for revenge. A combination of fear and anger might in the first instance have been precipitated by

- poor communication
- lack of honesty
- poor symptom management
- lack of acknowledgement of the individual
- stereotyping.

Alienation

Another distortion of anger, grief, fear, love and envy is alienation or a state of extreme and self-induced loneliness. It is associated with low self esteem and a feeling of being constantly underestimated. The person consequently harbours hostile feelings within most, if not all, personal relationships.

Sadness and depression

Sadness and depression arise from the frustration of being unable to freely express feelings about one's self and to give and receive within relationships. This can happen when the individual distances himself or is kept at a distance from significant people, places or possessions. The potential for depression in people who are seriously ill has strong implications for assessment of needs, styles of listening and responding, and for the approach to breaking bad news. It also has an important bearing upon decision-making related to where patients might be nursed during the final days of life.

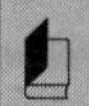

The reader will find it helpful at this point to view, if possible, the video *The Cancer Journey* by Cassidy et al.

Communication

Skill in both verbal and non-verbal communication is fundamental to good nursing practice. The quality of communication will to a significant degree determine the effectiveness of the nurse's interpersonal relationships with patients, family members, and colleagues. All nursing procedures are accompanied by some form of verbal and non-verbal communication. In verbal communication the skills of active listening and responding are employed. Although this also involves attention to non-verbal cues, the use of touch itself is a fundamental means of conveying both positive and negative feelings.

Touch

Through touch one enters into another person's personal territory. This is the area of personal security, privacy, autonomy and self-identity. Any change in a person's normal state of health is likely to alter the boundaries of this personal territory.

Touch as a form of communication has personal and cultural implications. McCorkle (1974) reported that through touch a rapport between nursing staff and seriously ill patients can be established within a very short period of time (see Research Abstract 34.1).

NURSING MANAGEMENT

Palliative care and the nurse

In their delivery of palliative care, nurses have many valuable opportunities to make and to strengthen relationships with patients and relatives. At the same time, nurses themselves have an opportunity for personal growth. All too often nurses

Research Abstract 34.1 Touch

Ashworth (1984) reports that the amount of touch offered by nurses working in intensive care units varied between patients whose reported condition was 'good' and those whose condition was 'poorly or critical', the latter group being less frequently touched. Ashworth asks if the lesser degree of touch offered is indicative of the technical nature of interventions in intensive nursing care, or if, on the other hand, it is associated with nurses' fear of death and their difficulties in providing emotional support.

Ashworth P 1984 Communication in intensive care units. In: Faulkner A (ed) Communication. Churchill Livingstone, Edinburgh claim that deficits in time, in staffing numbers and in skill mix impede their ability to provide patients and their families with adequate psychological support. On the other hand, as a group nurses have more patient contact hours than any other health care professionals. Perhaps, then, nurses need to examine how effectively they use their existing time. Are nurses truly identifying a deficit in resources, or might it be one of self-awareness?

An approach to care

Benner & Wrubel (1989) use the term 'care' to describe 'a wide range of involvements, from romantic love to parental love, to friendship, from caring for one's garden to caring about one's work to caring for and about one's patients' (p. 1). In nursing, where caring is essential for coping, involvement will generate loss and pain as well as joy and fulfilment. But stress and coping must be viewed as positive factors which provide the individual with opportunities for growth and challenge. Caring and coping, in Benner & Wrubel's view are grounded in attachment. Illness is the human experience of loss or dysfunction, whereas disease is an indication of tissue cell or organ destruction. The two are not synonymous.

In their clinical work nurses will encounter the emotional impact of bereavement, trauma, violence, marital separation and divorce. They will come across elderly people being admitted to residential situations and people with physical and mental disabilities and illnesses being integrated into community care settings. These are all critical events for the individuals concerned which demand an effective assessment of emotional needs (see Box 34.1).

In addition to providing a foundation for care for patients and their families, an understanding of the concept of loss should enable practitioners to appreciate the dynamics of professional relationships within the caring team and provide opportunities for staff support.

A framework for palliative nursing care

Orem's model of nursing

Dorothea Orem (1980, cited in Pearson & Vaughan 1986) used the concept of self-care deficits in her framework for nursing care. In her opinion, every individual has the right and the responsibility to attend to his own self-care requisites. The ability to maintain one's basic human needs is influenced by life cycle changes and life crises (see Box 34.2), and a person's state of well-being greatly influences his motivation for self-care. Consequently, when self-care demands exceed the person's ability to meet them a deficit exists. Orem thus implies that nursing is the act of assisting with those activities that an individual would normally perform independently. This suggests that nursing is complementary to the person's self-care ability and aims to compensate for any disability (Table 34.2). In Orem's model, nursing combines certain responsibilities. These are:

- acting for or doing for the patient
- teaching the patient
- guiding the patient
- supporting the patient
- providing an environment in which the patient can develop and grow.

The nursing approach presented here aims to promote optimum independence for patients and their carers. It combines the previously described concept of palliative care and an application of theories of loss and change with a model of nursing based on the concept of self-care.

Acting for or doing for the patient. The nurse has a responsibility to assess needs and to plan, implement and evaluate care, whether the source of distress is physical, emotional, spiritual or social. In doing so she must work alongside other professionals to enable symptom relief and social and emotional support for patients and their families.

Teaching the patient. The nurse has a responsibility to give information and to teach the skills involved in providing adequate personal and oral hygiene, nutrition, feeding, positioning, breathing and relaxation in order to enable patients and their families to become involved in care and achieve a sense of control over their own situation.

Box 34.1 Guidelines for assessing the emotional needs of individuals who are grieving

PERSONALITY TYPE

Consider the individual's personality type, i.e. his tendency towards introversion or extroversion (see Ch. 17, p. 585). This information will prove helpful in understanding the person's need for company or solitude. The patient, family and friends and perhaps members of the primary health care team will collectively supply this information.

SPIRITUALITY

Acknowledge that spirituality has a wider meaning than denominational religion. Listen to the patient's own thoughts about the meaning of life, of illness and of death. Offer appropriate resources. Be aware that cultural and religious practices are often interwoven and are not always indicative of the individual's strength of faith or of a search for inner peace.

CHANGE

Patients and family members need time to readjust. Observe the attitudes of professionals. Their behaviour can alter the patient's security and self-esteem. Emphasise the positive aspects of change. Offer explanation and listening time.

MOOD CHANGES

Consider whether the cause of a mood change is likely to be related to social, marital, family or other circumstances. Be aware of potential problems. Patients and family members should choose their own confidantes. Allow trust and honesty to develop in relationships between patients, their family members, friends and professionals. Be mindful of environmental factors and enable privacy when appropriate.

PHYSICAL DISTRESS

Establish the extent of physical distress. Anticipation and prevention of potential symptoms, and the provision of appropriate explanations and information will go a long way to help build confidence and trust in professionals.

INFORMATION SHARING

Is there any discrepancy in knowledge between patient, family and professionals? Watch and listen for cues and be aware that patients and families are also looking for cues. Provide opportunities for patients and family members to discuss and ask questions. Demonstrate trust and understanding through non-verbal behaviour. Most importantly, keep other team members updated.

Box 34.2 Factors influencing the individual's capacity for self-care (After Orem 1980)

BASIC HUMAN NEEDS

- Air
- Water
- Food
- Elimination
- Activity/rest
- Solitude/social interaction
- Prevention of hazards
- Promotion of normality

LIFE CYCLE CHANGES

- Intrauterine life
- Neonatal life
- Infancy
- Childhood
- Adolescence
- Early adulthood
- Pregnancy
- Adulthood
- Old age

LIFE-CRISES

- Environmental hazards
- Education deprivation
- Problems of social adaptation
- Loss of relatives/friends/associates
- Loss of possessions/job
- Sudden change in living conditions
- Change in social/economic status
- Disability
- Terminal illness/expected death

Guiding the patient. The nurse has the responsibility to offer, clarify and/or reinforce information as appropriate to patients and their carers, and to keep other professionals updated about the knowledge and perceptions held by the patient and different members of his family with regard to their situation.

Supporting the patient. The nurse has the responsibility to offer comfort to patients and relatives, to allay fears, and to anticipate and acknowledge loneliness, grief and other emotions which might cause distress.

Providing an environment in which the patient can grow and develop. The nurse must work with other professionals to ensure continuity in the delivery of care, in the advice offered and in the additional resources provided. This will facilitate the provision of optimum care and support for patients and their families within an environment which best suits their overall needs.

Table 34.2 Orem's classification of nursing care (Orem 1980)

System	Degree of self-care possible
Totally compensatory	Neither patient nor relatives can take responsibility for meeting the patient's self-care needs
Partially compensatory	The nurse teaches, supervises and/or assists to a lesser extent in meeting the self-care needs of the patient
Educative-supportive system	The patient or relative takes on full responsibility for meeting the self-care needs and the nurse works as the facilitator for care

This framework places an emphasis on needs assessment of patients and their carers and implies an understanding of the situations to which patients, carers and the professionals concerned are exposed. It highlights the importance of well-developed communication skills, that is, the ability to actively listen, to ask questions appropriately, to reflect on information gathered, and to observe, understand and respond to the verbal and non-verbal cues that arise in all interactions (see Ch. 26).

The framework presented here addresses the primary aim in palliative care, which is to anticipate the disease process so that plans can be made to deal with symptoms as they present. Such planning provides opportunities to prepare and teach carers in advance, thus allowing choices to be made about treatments, lifestyle, where the patient might be nursed and where he will die.

Teamwork is central to this framework. Nursing assessment often raises issues which must be referred to medical assessment and diagnosis. Members of the multidisciplinary team, along with the patient and his family, can thus set goals depending on whether an individual's self-care deficits can realistically be removed or reduced, or are likely to remain static or increase with the progress of illness. Priorities in goal-setting will of course vary according to an individual's overall well-being and his motivation towards self-care.

Within this framework the nurse faces many challenges; these include:

- upholding the individual's right to self-care
- including significant people in the provision of care
- fulfilling her multifaceted role as advisor, supporter, facilitator, teacher and carer.

The nurse–patient relationship must engender mutual respect, confidence and trust, in order that fears and anxieties can be freely expressed and the patient's needs can be sensitively and effectively addressed.

Self-esteem

An individual's level of self-esteem is a measure of his response to the perceptions that significant people in his life hold of him. These might be family, friends, colleagues and other social contacts. The reaction displayed by people in respect of an individual's personal circumstances will influence the value which that individual attributes to himself. Evans (1982) suggests that a low self-esteem promotes unrealistically low or high goals. This is especially important to bear in mind when caring for terminally ill patients.

Many physical changes can occur in the course of a terminal illness which are likely to affect the individual's self-esteem. These may include weight loss or gain, disfigurement following surgery, changes in appearance resulting from central nervous system disorders, and extreme weakness. In addition, changes in social and domestic roles and any negative attitudes displayed by family and friends can alter the patient's self-esteem. Throughout their interventions, nurses should pay attention to their own attitudes and the effect of these on the people in their care.

NURSING CARE OF PATIENTS WHO ARE TERMINALLY ILL

In order to link the theory already discussed to practice, the patient profile given in Case History 34.1 will be used to focus on nursing issues that might arise for patients in the last weeks of life.

Case History 34.1 Mrs M (see Table 34.3)

Mrs M is a mother and schoolteacher. She is 42 years old. Her husband, a business executive, has recently been rendered unemployed due to the collapse of his business. They have two teenage children: A, aged 18, is in his final year at school; D is 15 years old.

Mrs M has advanced disease following surgery and treatment for carcinoma of the breast diagnosed three years earlier. Both husband and wife know the diagnosis and the children are aware that their mother is seriously ill.

Mrs M is admitted to hospital subsequent to a deterioration in her condition. The district nursing sister supplies the hospital team with the information that Mrs M was devastated by the suddenness of her husband's unemployment and has felt unable to provide him with the support which she believes he needs. She is also angry and feels cheated out of her role as wife and mother.

Mrs M is unable to describe her pain, for which the current prescription of opiate analgesia is ineffective. Other symptoms include nausea and constipation. Over the last 48 hours she has become mentally confused and her balance is erratic. She has had a number of falls.

Assessment

Combined skills in observation, measurement and communication are demanded of nursing staff, Mrs M and her family in order to establish Mrs M's normal patterns of breathing, eating, drinking, eliminating, mobility, socialisation, maintenance of personal safety and normality. Likewise, identification of Mrs M's present ability to sustain these patterns and the amount of assistance she requires will establish her self-care deficits. The family will, initially, play a major role in supplying information about the changes which have occurred in Mrs M's lifestyle, her domestic social role, her physical appearance and her emotional state. For the family as a whole, huge adjustments will be needed in order that they can effectively deal with the potential changes and fluctuations that are likely to occur in Mrs M's self-care demands and deficits. These will range from removal of deficits to total support of them in relation to the pattern of symptoms and their subsequent management.

In Mrs M's case, admission to hospital is a statement that her self-care deficits are large enough to warrant intervention, whether partial or total. Her identified symptoms are pain, nausea, constipation, confusion, falls and poor balance. Once the source of these symptoms is identified and management implemented, assessment will be ongoing. This is in anticipation of potential changes in Mrs M's condition, her environment, and indeed, in the involvement that she, her family and the professionals concerned share in her care.

Presenting symptoms

Some of Mrs M's self-care deficits will be considered here in relation to her presenting symptoms. (A fuller assessment of her self-care deficits is given in Table 34.3.)

Pain. Mrs M is unable to describe her pain. By helping her to identify different pains, it should be possible to investigate the location, duration, pattern, intensity and character of each (see Table 34.4). In her assessment the nurse should consider the following questions:

1. Could Mrs M's inability to describe her pain be a consequence of her confusion, or might it be that she has not been asked to describe it, or is she unable to differentiate between a number of pains?
2. Mrs M is constipated: does she have abdominal discomfort?
3. From the history of Mrs M's falls, is there evidence of bruising or deformity suggesting either soft tissue injury or fracture or both?
4. Mrs M is confused and her balance is erratic. Is there evidence of intracranial pressure? Does she suffer headaches? If, so when do they occur?

See Ch. 7, Ch. 19 and Ch. 32.

Nausea. Mrs M is not interested in food. Here, the following factors should be considered:

1. Mrs M has been prescribed an opioid analgesic for her pain (see Table 34.5). The knowledge that nausea might be present for a few days following the initial prescription should raise questions: When was the opiate first prescribed? What dose is Mrs M taking and how often?
2. Nausea is associated with constipation. Is Mrs M's constipation thus a contributing factor?
3. Oral thrush produces nausea. Are there cracks at the corners of Mrs M's mouth? What is the general condition of her mouth?

Constipation. Mrs M's normal bowel pattern is disrupted. Here, nursing interventions should take the following concerns into account:

1. Constipation is the most frequently occurring symptom in patients with advanced disease and is an inevitable side-effect of opiates. An aperient is always prescribed concurrently.
2. Oral thrush may be present as a result of anorexia and a reduced fluid intake.
3. Compromised mobility, perhaps associated with fear of falling, might well be a precursor of constipation.
4. Mrs M's nausea will inevitably reduce her interest in taking fluids. This is another warning of the possibility for constipation.
5. The degree of constipation present needs accurate assessment to ascertain whether or not there is an associated faecal impaction (see Box 34.3).

Confusion. Mrs M is unable to take control of her everyday activities. Her confusion renders her partially or wholly dependent upon her family to help assess her self-care deficits. It should not be assumed, however, that Mrs M is without insight into her physical and mental condition. The nurse should consider these points:

1. Cerebral metastases and consequently raised intracranial pressure is a possible cause of Mrs M's confusion.
2. Confusion may be related to the dosage and timing of opiate therapy.
3. Confusion may be associated with other factors such as inadequate fluid intake.

Emotional symptoms. In addition to experiencing anger directed at herself and her sick role, Mrs M is attempting to cope with the sudden change in the social situation associated with her husband's business failure. Feeling unable to provide the support which she knows he requires is likely, along with her other losses, to compromise her self-esteem. Mrs M's entire family is extremely vulnerable.

?	**34.5** Pause for a few moments to consider the different losses which each member of this family has suffered.

Short-term considerations

Mrs M's physical symptoms at this time might readily respond

Table 34.3 An assessment of self-care deficits and care plan for Mrs M, using Orem's framework (see Case History 34.1)

Self-care requisites	Self-care abilities	Self-care deficits	Self-care actions	Potential self-care deficits	Self-care actions	Nursing actions	Nursing mode
Universal	Maintenance of intake of air	Able to manage own needs	None	Dyspnoea, respiratory infection, pleural effusion, pain: due to lung metastases	The patient will when not confused report any new symptom	❐ The nurse will observe for change in self-care ability	Act for Guide Support
	Maintenance of intake of fluid	When not confused is able to manage own needs	Is poorly motivated to drink	Dry mouth and poor oral hygiene due to inadequate fluid	When not confused: • be responsible for own fluid intake and oral hygiene • report episodes of nausea	❐ Monitor nausea/vomiting when patient is poorly motivated ❐ Encourage her to drink ❐ Supervise/assist with oral hygiene	Teach Guide Support
	Maintenance of intake of food	When not confused is able to manage own needs	Is poorly motivated to eat	Anorexia	When not confused: • inform nursing staff of dietary likes/dislikes • report episodes of nausea • aim to eat an adequate and nourishing diet	❐ Monitor nausea/vomiting when patient is poorly motivated ❐ Encourage small, nourishing snacks at frequent intervals	Teach Guide Support
	Management of elimination	Able to manage with support of medication	Normal bowel pattern is disrupted	Bowel impaction	When not confused: • inform nursing staff of the nature of bowel movement • inform nursing staff of new bowel or urinary symptoms	❐ Treat constipation as prescribed ❐ Alert patient to ongoing potential for constipation and importance of continuing medication	Act for Teach Guide Support
	Maintenance of balance between activity and rest	Variable because of confusion/ pain/erratic balance	Disturbed periods day and night with pain/ nausea and confusion	Exhaustion/ depression	When not confused: • report symptoms • ask for necessary assistance with mobilisation • keep herself occupied within her limitations	❐ Monitor symptoms ❐ Ensure medical staff are aware of symptoms either from patient or on her behalf ❐ Assist patient with mobilisation ❐ Ensure patient has adequate rest	Act for Teach Guide Support
	Maintenance of balance between solitude and social interaction	When not confused enjoys close relationships with family/ friends but also likes to be alone	Appears distant and preoccupied. Becomes easily irritated and sometimes angry with little or no provocation	Exhaustion due to distressing symptoms (irritation, sadness, anxiety) in relation to her knowledge/ insight	When not confused: • maintain relationships with family and friends • indicate her desire for time alone • indicate when tired	❐ Monitor patient's emotional responses ❐ Be aware of cues and offer listening opportunities ❐ Be a source of information and a resource ❐ Alert husband/ family to patient's emotional needs	Teach Guide Support Provide environment for growth
	Prevention of hazards to life, well-being and functioning	Limited due to erratic balance and confusion	Variable due to episodes of mental confusion	Injury from falls and possible fractures due to skeletal metastases. Pain	When not confused: • indicate need for assistance when balance is poor • report pain	❐ Monitor activities when Mrs M is confused and assist as appropriate	Act for Teach Guide Support
Developmental	Maintenance of lifestyle that promotes maturation	Mrs M's ambitions and expectations have been shattered in the realisation of her short life expectancy	She is frightenend and angry and unsure of how she and her family will cope in the face of her death	Powerlessness Despair		Provide positive reinforcement for Mrs M as a person Be honest and ensure clear and open communication	Support Provide environment for growth

Table 34.4 Pain diagnosis (After Doyle & Benton 1991)

Pain types	Description
Visceral	Dull, deep-seated and described as an aching over an organ such as liver or kidney
Bone (metastases)	A dull ache over a large area or a clearly localised area of pain and tenderness over the affected bone
Nerve compression (adjacent tumour)	An 'aching' or 'stabbing' pain localised to one or two dermatomes
Nerve/nerve root infiltration	A 'discomfort', 'burning' or 'numbness' localised over one or two dermatomes
Headache (cerebral metastases)	A 'dull', 'oppressive' and 'vice-like' pain which is worse in early morning or late evening
Muscular	Spasm

to treatment. The short-term goal for treatment at this stage may well be that she return home with an adequate compensatory support system (see Table 34.3). Priorities for symptom management would include the following.

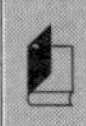

You may find it helpful to read Regnard & Davies (1986) or Doyle & Benton (1991) before or alongside the remainder of this section.

Pain control. Once Mrs M's pain is accurately identified and appropriately treated, preparation for going home would include teaching her and her family about:

Table 34.5 Principles for using opiates (Video: Twycross on cancer pain)

Response to opiates	Type of pain	Treatment modality
None	Muscular	Heat/massage Muscle relaxant
	Nerve destruction (a) burning hypersensitivity (b) stabbing	 Tricyclic analgesic anti-convulsant
Partial	Bone metastases	(a) Anti-prostaglandin plus opiate analgesia (b) Radiotherapy
	Nerve compression	(a) Corticosteroids plus opiate analgesia (b) Nerve block
Total		Analgesic step ladder

Use of morphine:

BY MOUTH
In most circumstances patients will tolerate the oral route of administration. Other routes need to be considered only if the patient is unable to swallow, has some problem with malabsorption of the drug, has a buccal fistula or requires a stat dose of analgesic to control unanticipated pain.

BY THE CLOCK
It is a well-established principle to anticipate and prescribe accordingly for chronic pain rather than allow such pain to become established.

BY THE LADDER
The use of the analgesic step ladder allows for a logical progression in strength and dose of an analgesic being prescribed.

Box 34.3 Guidelines for managing constipation (Doyle & Benton 1991)

1. When the rectum is found to be filled with hard faeces, a faecal expander will convert the hard mass into a large soft one which is impossible to expel. In such circumstances give an arachis oil retention enema at night on two successive nights, followed by two bisacodyl suppositories or a phosphate enema in the morning.
2. When the rectum is empty but ballooned, indicating faecal impaction around the rectosigmoid junction, use lactulose accompanied by a peristaltic stimulant (senna or bisacodyl). When a mass collects in the lower rectum a phosphate enema may be required to ease evacuation.
3. When the rectum is empty and collapsed, use oral medication such as faecal expanders (Normax) and peristaltic stimulants.

- the information which nurses and doctors need to help understand and effectively treat pain
- what 'breakthrough' pain is and how to deal with it in relation to an 'extra' dose of medication
- the importance of taking medication regularly and in advance of the experience of pain
- the anticipation of constipation
- the integration of non-invasive interventions such as relaxation, distraction, aromatherapy or massage.

Nausea/constipation. We will assume here that the nausea which Mrs M is experiencing is directly associated with constipation. In the first instance the degree of constipation should be assessed and a faecal softener and aperient prescribed. Mrs M and her family will need to be made aware of the importance of continuing with bowel treatment alongside opiate medication. With this treatment it is unlikely that Mrs M's nausea will persist; if it does, other possible sources of the nausea must be investigated.

? **34.6** Please read one of the following discussions of nausea and vomiting:

1. Regnard C, Tempest S 1992 A guide to symptom relief in advanced cancer 3rd edn. Haigh & Hochland, Manchester, pp. 26–27
2. Regnard C, Comisky M 1992 Nausea and vomiting in advanced cancer. Palliative Medicine 6: 146–151
3. Twycross R, Lack S 1990 Nausea and vomiting. In: Therapeutics in cancer care. pp. 57–62.

Now list the possible sources of nausea and/or vomiting which may present in a patient with advanced carcinoma of the breast.

Confusion. A likely cause of Mrs M's confusion, dizziness and consequent falls is increased intracranial pressure. Large doses of steroids will reduce this and restore her balance and mental state to some degree (Regnard & Davies 1986).

Mrs M and her family should be made aware that steroid therapy can alter appetite, compromise buccal mucosa and cause fluid retention. These may be additional factors affecting Mrs M's self-image. Dealing with Mrs M's physical and emotional well-being will draw upon the teaching, supervisory and supportive elements of the nurse's role. Providing an environment appropriate to her needs should also be kept in mind when discussing and planning discharge with Mrs M and her family. Both Mrs M's general practitioner and her community nurse should be consulted about the resources that they can marshal to help this family build up an effective support system.

Long-term considerations
It is likely that Mrs M and her family will face many changes in consequence of her illness. Some of these changes will be anticipated and others not. Nursing staff will be involved in interacting with Mrs M and her family in observing, measuring and documenting data about her symptoms and her ability to undertake the activities of daily living. It will also be important for nursing staff to observe the amount and the quality of interactions that Mrs M and her family engage in with one another and with members of the ward team. Such information will provide a basis for continuity of nursing and other professional care, whether in hospital, hospice, or at home.

Other potential self-care deficits in terminal illness

It should be emphasised that there are a number of other self-care deficits that might arise in patients suffering from advanced disease. These will be considered here in relation to the universal self-care requisites identified in Orem's model (see Table 34.3).

Intake of air
Breathlessness is an outstandingly distressing symptom. Sufferers fear death from suffocation and relatives feel powerless to help. The expertise and strengths of all team members are required to assist the patient. This will include:

- the doctor's clinical skills in relieving the distress with appropriate treatment
- the physiotherapist's expertise in initiating and teaching breathing exercises
- the nurse's skills in providing comfort and reinforcing measures introduced by colleagues.

Common to all is the need for quiet confidence and a commitment to teach and support the patient and her relatives.

Nursing care. Time and patience are essential. In an acute episode of breathlessness the fully conscious patient will be more comfortable in an upright sitting position. This allows for maximum expansion of the lungs. On the other hand, the distress of a semi-conscious or unconscious patient is best relieved when he is nursed in a lateral position with the affected lung uppermost.

Nursing the patient near an open window to allow cool air to circulate can also afford relief. Alternatively, a fan is useful. Staff may need to be reassured that in dealing with terminal illness the use of opiates is safe and is recommended. Unlike in acute respiratory illness, where opiate drugs depress the respiratory centre, in terminal illness a small dose of morphine will effectively slow down the respiratory rate and reduce anxiety.

The principles of managing breathlessness apply whether the patient is at home or in hospital. At home, the patient will rely heavily on family members for support. To this end, a strong back-up support from community nurses and perhaps specialist nurses will enhance the confidence of carers.

In hospital, patients will require a great deal of support and reassurance in order that they can build up confidence in a staff whose members are seen to change frequently during a 24-hour period. There is no substitute for sensitive reassurance from a confident attendant. The nurse's responsibility lies in either being that attendant or ensuring that the patient's family have such abilities (see Research Abstract 34.2).

Maintaining intake of food and fluid
In order for the patient to take in adequate food and drink, attention must be paid to potential problems in oral health.

Oral hygiene. A healthy mouth is a measure of a person's general state of physical and emotional well-being. The only effective remedy for a dry mouth is an adequate fluid intake. This makes exhausted, terminally ill patients especially vulnerable in view of possible reluctance to drink, pain, apathy and the effects of drugs. The potential for dry, cracked lips, ulceration of gums, halitosis, dental caries and infection, particularly oral thrush, is great (see Research Abstract 34.3).

Halitosis is a source of embarrassment and a barrier to communication and is distressing for both patients and relatives. Possible causes include poor oral hygiene, a delay in gastric emptying (e.g. in carcinoma of the stomach), diseases of the mouth and respiratory system, sinusitis, bronchiectasis, and tumours of the mouth, pharynx and larynx.

Intensive oral hygiene measures are called for, with particular attention to the teeth. Drugs can be prescribed to increase gastric emptying and to reduce the odour associated with bronchogenic carcinoma.

Nursing care. Initial assessment will establish the patient's physical ability to perform mouth care. Intervention might take the form of simply explaining to the patient his vulnerability to oral symptoms. Once the patient and his carers realise the importance of oral hygiene they can be encouraged and taught to regularly inspect the mouth.

Some patients with functional disorders of the upper arm (as might result from stroke or lymphoedema) may be assisted to regain some of their independence. Toothbrushes can be adapted or some other aid introduced. Other patients will need to have their oral hygiene performed by a family member or nurse.

When debris has to be removed, a soft child-sized toothbrush may be suitable along with the use of dental floss (Shepherd et al 1987). The use of mouthwashes is discussed in Box 34.4.

Eating and drinking are social activities of considerable sig-

Research Abstract 34.2 Breathlessness: a teaching programme

Brown & Mann (1990) developed a teaching programme to implement in anticipation of respiratory difficulties. Patients with chronic lung disease who were taught breathing exercises were able to control their breathing pattern, firstly at rest, and then during activity. The outcome included reduced anxiety about breathlessness and an improved quality of life.

Relatives were also included in this process as a way of ensuring support for the patient from confident attendants. Other interventions reported to assist in the management of breathlessness and enable the family unit to remain independent include relaxation and guided imagery therapies.

Brown S, Mann R 1990 Breaking the cycle: control of breathlessness in chronic lung disease. Professional Nurse 5(6): 325–328

Research Abstract 34.3 Oral thrush

Doyle (1987) reports that about 75% of terminally ill patients develop oral thrush. The incidence is greater among patients receiving treatment with steroids, antibiotics, cancer chemotherapy or radiotherapy. Such treatments render the host immunocompromised.

Doyle D 1987 Domiciliary terminal care: a handbook for doctors and nurses. Churchill Livingstone, Edinburgh

Box 34.4 Mouthwashes

While opinions vary as to the best solutions to use in mouth care, the choice should always be determined by ongoing assessment, the aim always being to restore and maintain an optimum standard of oral hygiene.

Chlorhexidine mouthwashes/sprays are effective in the treatment and prevention of oral infection (Gibbons 1983). Hydrogen peroxide (6%) diluted solution has long been found to be useful in dislodging and removing debris. Its unpleasant taste, however, limits its use when patients are reluctant to drink. From hospice experience, effervescent ascorbic acid has been found to be both effective in dislodging debris and pleasant to use. As an alternative to dissolving the ascorbic acid in water, small pieces of the ascorbic acid tablet can be placed on the patient's tongue.

The use of lemon and glycerin compounds should be discouraged. Whilst at one time this was thought to be a refreshing and soothing solution, it has since been established that the action of glycerin ultimately increases rather than reduces the problem of a dry mouth (Trenter & Creason 1987).

nificance in people's lives. Families share mealtimes as part of their everyday routine and on special occasions such as birthdays and religious feastdays a high value is placed on eating and drinking. It is therefore extremely important that nurses know the normal eating patterns of their patients. Observations in hospices have revealed that patients with terminal illnesses experience taste changes and food aversions. Anorexia is the most common disruption to eating and drinking experienced by these individuals.

Anxiety is known to increase or decrease appetite. Anxiety might be disease related, but can also be associated with other factors such as the individual's level of independence and the attitudes of others towards the person and his illness.

The presence of a dry mouth, thrush, or other infection affects the appetite, as does the experience of nausea and vomiting. Dysphagia, with its associated fear of choking, is yet another potential cause of reduced desire to eat.

Anorexia in its extreme form, cachexia, is an enormous source of distress for patients and carers. Cachexia occurs in approximately 50–60% of patients with advanced cancer. It is characterised by a progressive loss of body fat and is associated mainly with patients who have gastric or lung tumours, or where a fistula exists. Cachexia can also occur in non-malignant illness in patients who have experienced acute starvation (see Chs 21 and 32).

Management of anorexia and cachexia is directed at treating the primary cause, whilst problems of oral hygiene are addressed and the patient is encouraged to eat and drink. Steroids are often used and are extremely effective in boosting appetite (Regnard & Davies 1984).

Nursing care. Nursing management of patients with anorexia is centred on ensuring good oral hygiene, giving dietary advice and providing ongoing emotional support.

The patient who has a painful mouth is likely to prefer that drinks and food should be either very cold or very hot, and that food should be of a semi-solid consistency.

Explanation about taste change and food aversions will help patients and relatives to understand why certain foods are no longer preferred and why seemingly bizarre 'fancies' occur. This will also allay confusion and feelings of rejection when the ill person refuses special and carefully prepared meals.

Stubbs (1989) advises that patients and relatives be encouraged to regard food and fluid intake with the same importance as regular medication. It is quite usual for the patient's appetite to be at its best in the morning. For this reason it might be worth encouraging friends and relatives to regard breakfast as an important occasion and thus reduce distress when the patient feels unable to join in family meals at other times.

Overcoming the difficulties posed by taste changes is not easy and requires much trial and error. Freshly prepared snacks given in small enough portions to encourage the patient to ask for another helping does much for morale. Tackling anorexia presents a challenge to the patience and the imagination of carers.

?	**34.7** Bearing in mind that anorexia may be a primary or a secondary symptom, outline a plan of management for a patient who is in hospital and likely to go home. (See Ch. 21.)

Managing elimination

People feel devastated by the effects of urinary or faecal incontinence. It is damaging to self-esteem and can adversely affect relationships with others. Close family members may either shun the sufferer or share his embarrassment and sense of indignity. For patients facing these challenges, death may seem a happy release. Professional attitudes can either reinforce negative feelings or provide a basis for rebuilding self-esteem.

Urinary incontinence. The possible causes of this problem are many. Urinary incontinence may be an irreversible effect of the disease process, or symptomatic of a urinary tract infection, or due to the sedative effect of drugs (see Ch. 24).

Nursing care. A sensitive and discreet approach is essential. In the event of an unusual problem arising, a continence advisor should be involved in the overall plan for care and will have an important role in supporting and advising the patient and family members over lengthy periods.

In keeping with all clinical interventions, respect for the attitudes and feelings of the patient and his family is paramount. Catheterisation, for example, may seem the most obvious and effective way of dealing with urinary incontinence but may be unacceptable to a patient and his family. Furthermore, family members at home may not be prepared to apply a uro-sheath to a male relative.

When incontinence pads are used, the importance of good skin care cannot be overemphasised. This will involve a daily assessment of the required frequency for washing, drying and the application of suitable barrier cream. At home, patients and family members must know about disposal and replenishing arrangements for pads and about local laundry services.

Faecal incontinence. As with urinary incontinence the cause determines the management. Diarrhoea as a consequence of faecal impaction is common and can be resolved with appropriate bowel treatment. A warm arachis oil retention enema given 6–8 hours in advance of an evacuant enema is the treatment of choice.

A possible cause of faecal incontinence for some patients is an atonic colon resulting from extreme weakness. These patients are likely to feel helpless, depressed and embarrassed.

Colostomy. Sometimes a palliative colostomy may be performed when a rectal tumour or a recurrence exists. Provided that the patient and family members are emotionally prepared for this relatively minor operation, dealing with the colostomy can be much less embarrassing or difficult than the faecal incontinence, potential pain and rectal bleeding which might otherwise exist.

Nursing care. To ignore or deny the foul odour associated with incontinence will reinforce negative feelings and further isolate the patient. Sensitive acknowledgement of the smell, combined with an immediate attention to personal hygiene, a change of clothing, bedlinen and appropriate measures taken to freshen up the immediate environment will do much to restore morale.

Maintaining a balance between activity and rest

Mobility. Any threat to independent mobility has far-reaching consequences for terminally ill patients. Pain (see Box 34.5), paraplegia, bone fractures, lymphoedema and exhaustion feature largely in possible changes in mobility in these individuals.

Paraplegia. A failed response to treatment for vertebral collapse or spinal cord compression can result in paraplegia. When this happens much is demanded of professionals, the patient, and family members. With the goal of optimum independence in mind, sometimes extraordinary requests are made in respect of domiciliary assessment and intervention from the occupational therapy, physiotherapy, social work, and primary care teams to ensure that the patient has an opportunity to spend short or long periods at home.

Lymphoedema is caused by a degree of obstruction of the lymph channels. The resulting tension and swelling is uncomfortable and sometimes painful. Lymphoedema of the upper and lower limbs will have an effect on mobility and the patient's morale is likely to be affected when he discovers that clothes and shoes no longer fit.

The main features in treating lymphoedema are:

- prevention of skin infection
- maintenance of the flow of lymph.

The skin is vulnerable to breakdown and infection. Particular care is therefore needed when drying the skin and the application of a moisturising cream is an important preventive measure. When signs of inflammation appear, rest, limb elevation and antibiotic treatment should be promptly implemented.

Box 34.5 The effect of pain on mobility

Pain is a major cause of immobility in terminally ill patients. The nurse will need good communication and assessment skills in order to identify difficulties in mobilisation arising from pain. Medical intervention, by and large, will be the first line of treatment for pain. This will involve the nurse in administration of drugs and in observation during and following treatments such as radiotherapy and neurolytic procedures. Although certain nursing procedures will on occasion be the only remedy necessary to relieve pain, more often nursing care is an adjuvant to medical intervention.

The nurse can help to ease difficulties caused by painful mobilisation by offering the following:

- a sensitive and empathic approach to care
- touch and reassurance
- smooth, consistent and synchronised movement
- comfortable and logical positioning
- correct lifting techniques
- informed selection of equipment
- appropriate use of heat and cooling appliances and bathing
- gentle exercise
- massage
- relaxation and visualisation techniques.

McCaffery & Beebe's (1989) *Pain: A Clinical Manual for Nursing Practice* is an exceptionally useful source book.

The stimulation of undamaged lymph vessels can be aided through massage, normal exercise and the application of graduated support hosiery (Regnard et al 1988). Diuretics are used in the treatment of lymphoedema when the latter is associated with the use of corticosteroids or with cardiac disease.

In most situations a concerted effort by members of the multidisciplinary team and the patient will ensure successful management of lymphoedema. Referral to a specialist centre is recommended when there is gross lymphoedema in which fingers or the trunk are involved or in which persistent leakage, pain or episodes of acute inflammation occur.

Nursing care. Assessment of the individual's level of mobility relative to his previous ability should take account of restrictions in the environment, new physical deformity, defects of the upper or lower limbs caused by lymphoedema, neurological damage, emotional state and pain.

The goals in sustaining optimum mobility are to:

- encourage maximum muscle tone
- prevent joint stiffness
- prevent deformity, e.g. contractures.

Walking provides gentle exercise and helps to maintain circulation. Most importantly, it also prevents pressure area breakdown. Assistance from one or two attendants or the use of a walking aid might be necessary to implement an exercise plan.

For patients who spend a lot of time in bed, those experiencing extreme exhaustion, and those who are comatose, the physiotherapist may initiate a range of exercises, the management of which can be taken over by nurses and taught to patients and relatives. Alongside the exercise plan, correct positioning and support of joints will help to ensure patient comfort.

Maintaining a balance of solitude and social interaction

Extreme weakness. Exhaustion might be the penultimate stage of life or a symptom of emotional disturbance. Although sadness is to be expected when a person is approaching death, effective communication might reveal signs of an emotional disturbance which would benefit from some form of clinical or counselling intervention.

Nursing care. The link between tiredness and boredom is well accepted. There are strong implications here for the environment wherein a patient is nursed. Whether he is being cared for in hospital or at home the patient's lifestyle preferences have to be considered. This may be a prime consideration for the sideroom facility. A careful assessment of interests might lead carers to appreciate that minor adjustments in the daily routine are sometimes sufficient to stimulate some motivation for activity.

Promoting 'normalcy': developing and maintaining a realistic self-concept

Personal hygiene. An individual's attitude towards personal hygiene is a good indicator of the level of his self-esteem. Constant preoccupation with cleanliness might signify a high level of anxiety and/or an attempt to conceal incontinence or a malodorous wound. Alternatively, what appears in the first instance to be an inability to perform hygiene tasks consequent to extreme weakness may in fact be symptomatic of a depressive state.

Nursing care. The maintenance of the terminally ill person's hygiene is essential to ensuring his physical and emotional comfort. For those who are incontinent or have an unpleasant body odour or malodorous wound, a full daily wash is desirable. Whether this should take the form of a bath, shower or wash in bed ought to be negotiated between nurse and patient, and a mutually acceptable time should be agreed. This activity should be unhurried as it is often during the daily wash time that a patient seizes the opportunity to make an important disclosure. The daily wash is therefore not an activity to be routinely delegated to junior members of staff. Being with a patient in these circumstances provides a nurse with opportunities to develop observational, assessment, decision-making and communication skills.

Changes in mobility, or in a patient's ability to wash and dress, should be noted. The suitability of various aids such as wheelchairs, hoists, special baths and bathing aids can be assessed during wash time. This might be the most important activity in the patient's day. Even the most frail patients sometimes enjoy a soak in the bath.

Attention to hair, manicure, and make-up can provide a wonderful morale booster. In the absence of services provided within hospital settings it is seldom difficult to make private arrangements. This is an ideal way of including a family member or friend in the overall plan of care. Likewise, at home, a trip to or a visit from the hairdresser may provide a welcome distraction in the patient's day.

Ostomies. The majority of patients will be skilled in caring for their colostomy or ileostomy and should be encouraged to remain independent. The size of the stoma, however, may alter and require refitting with a new appliance.

Occasionally the ostomy will be recent and the patient less able to manage. A stoma care specialist nurse will be able to provide much support to the patient and his family. She will ensure that appropriate appliances are issued in respect of the actual and potential outcome for the patient.

Discharge planning. If a patient with a stoma is discharged home, adequate time should be allowed for teaching and supervising relatives. There is always a possibility that family members will be required to assist with or to take over the management of the colostomy. Teaching is a shared responsibility undertaken by the stomatherapist along with hospital and community nursing staff.

Ongoing assessment must take into account the consistency and frequency of bowel action, as this has implications for dietary advice (see Ch. 21). The patient and family, if at all possible, ought to be given the opportunity to meet and discuss home management with the community nurse. The benefits of this are many, and it is reassuring for the patient and family to know that the hospital and community staff work together. The community sister may wish to visit the family prior to the patient's discharge to ensure that adequate supplies of dressings and other essential aids and equipment are available in the patient's house.

Fungating wounds. Although usually associated with cancer a fungating wound may occur with benign disease. The principal aim in managing any wound is cleansing in order to create optimum conditions to allow healing. In fungating wounds the presence of blood, pus and sloughing and necrotic tissue make this a difficult task (see Chs 7 and 23). In practice, healing may not be a realistic goal, in which case the aim of management will be to minimise infection and to deal with odour, bleeding and discharge.

Odour. Dealing with odour has long been a difficult area of nursing practice. A number of odour-absorbing dressings containing activated charcoal are available. The charcoal dressing placed directly on the wound acts by drawing bacteria and toxins from the wound fluid, thereby removing the odour (Thomas 1989). The use of **metronidazole**, topically or systemically, has been found useful in the presence of anaerobic organisms. Clinical observation and experience show that non-conventional agents such as icing sugar and yoghurt can be effective. Although there appears to be conflicting evidence, it is generally believed that radiotherapy is effective in dealing with such wounds (Ivetic & Lynne 1990). In some cases, however, the noxious odour of a wound will persist despite any measures taken.

Bleeding can be a real source of anxiety for patients and nurses dealing with fungating wounds. In general, non-adherent and haemostatic dressings (e.g. Oxycel) have a prophylactic effect.

Wound discharge. Sometimes a colostomy bag is used to contain leakage from a draining sinus or fistula. In using colostomy bags the aim is to prevent skin maceration and odour. When this is not a suitable option scrupulous attention must be paid to the skin surrounding the orifice. A thorough wash with soap and water or a shower may be needed several times a day, followed by the application of a barrier cream, a secure padded dressing, fresh clothing and, where necessary, clean bedding. Advice about suitable clothing will go a long way to lessen any alienation that patients are likely to feel.

Psychological support. In the absence of healing, psychological support for patients with a fungating wound is essential. While this demands considerable sensitivity, honesty about the expected outcome of management, acknowledgement of the odour, and an explanation regarding efforts to neutralise it will be appreciated.

Discharge plans. Plans for discharge may be seriously affected by the presence of a fungating wound. Assessment of home conditions must take account of the fact that in confined spaces and where ventilation is poor the atmosphere will rapidly become impregnated with a noxious odour.

Preventing hazards to life, well-being and functioning

Pressure area care. Pressure area breakdown is a potential source of distress for terminally ill patients. Immobility due to pain, paralysis, incontinence, general weakness and poor nutritional state are but some of the predisposing factors. In addition, there is a slowing down of the healing process in patients receiving steroid treatment, radiotherapy and chemotherapy. Preventive measures are therefore not straightforward.

Nursing care. A patient who has had, or who is experiencing pain will be fearful of moving. Despite strenuous efforts to control pain, it may be that only one position offers relief. The nurse must provide explanations to ensure that the patient understands the potential for a pressure sore and to allow him to build trust in the decisions made by nursing staff (see Box 34.6).

Frequent change of position, as often as hourly, may be required where a patient is severely emaciated. On the other hand, the patient in the end stage of life might find repositioning intolerable. The benefits of moving such patients need to be weighed against the resulting distress. The question of positioning requires frequent reassessment throughout a 24-hour period. Very gentle massage can be beneficial and relaxing and may even provide the medium for aromatherapy should the patient so wish.

DYING, DEATH AND BEREAVEMENT

The patient's awareness that he is making poor or no progress together with his increasing weakness will reinforce any suspicion that death is impending. Patients will vary enormously in their desire and ability to talk through their anxieties about death, but it is likely that their feelings of helplessness will

Box 34.6 Nursing appliances

There are many appliances which can be introduced both at home and in hospital to reduce the risk of pressure sores. These range from sheepskin rugs to Spenco-type mattress and special beds. The Mediscus and the Mecabed both allow for a change of position and pressure relief to be achieved with minimum handling of the patient. The decision to use these special beds must be made with the consent of patients and families. Despite the benefits that can be obtained, it should be remembered that unusual-looking equipment may provoke fear and a sense of isolation in patients and family members, who may already be feeling alone with their situation. The remedy is in giving information and demonstrations and negotiating with the patient and his carers to give the equipment a trial run.

grow if their fears are mirrored in the manner or behaviour of relatives and friends.

Support for carers

Support for relatives is an important aspect of the overall care for patients. Everyone who has a significant relationship with the dying patient will experience a grieving process. For each, it will be different and unique. It is important to consider what nurses can do to facilitate the grieving process.

Relatives expect nurses to direct their care toward the patient, and in their desire to see the patient receive expert nursing care, they often accept a low priority for their own needs.

A number of researchers have identified increased levels of distress among relatives of dying patients when communication with staff is inadequate. Conversely, stress levels have been found to be manageable in instances where staff are approachable, friendly and have time to listen to their concerns (Stedeford 1984, Parkes & Parkes 1984). Lugton's (1988) research within a hospice highlights that even when staff are approachable and friendly, relatives may perceive them as busy people who are not to be disturbed. The onus is very definitely on nursing staff to initiate conversation, provide information and offer listening time.

Most people would agree that a lasting impression is created by the members of staff involved in the first and the final contact. The same is true whether the patient is at home, in hospital or in a hospice. Often, staff are eager to impart a great deal of information during the first meeting with relatives. In reality, very little new information can be absorbed in this situation, given the kind of anxieties that relatives have when meeting health care professionals for the first time. There is much to be gained by acknowledging this difficulty and inviting relatives to speak about their experiences and circumstances. In so doing, an openness is encouraged which will permit the professional and the carer to pursue or return to issues as appropriate.

Family-centred care

Enabling family members to work through their emotions can consume much more time and energy than simply facilitating physical care. Nonetheless, this aspect of the nurse's intervention is an extremely important one. Reinforcing information and giving reassurance will stimulate the confidence of relatives and allow them the freedom to make decisions — right or wrong.

Empathy and a non-judgemental attitude are essential when working alongside family members. Suffice it to say that nurses involved in the care of dying patients will be exposed to a range of relationships, some of which will be easily understood and others not. Previous experiences will enhance the nurse's understanding but cannot provide prescriptions for new situations.

Family involvement in care. The idea of the family being involved in patient care is incorporated into the framework for anticipatory guidance. This involvement is also a means of overcoming barriers in communication. Every day is precious in terminal illness; this is good reason in itself for family and friends to continue their involvement. Support, guidance, assistance and frequent evaluation by nursing staff will be crucial.

Home. At home there is a risk that family members will become deeply absorbed in patient care to the detriment of their own health. Additional support from specialist services, both voluntary and statutory, can ease the burden. Macmillan nurses have a dual role in supporting the professional and non-professional carer; at the same time, they can themselves draw support from the primary and home care teams with whom they work.

Hospital. In hospital it may be somewhat difficult to plan daily care tasks such that relatives can be involved in patient care. Nevertheless, relatives should be kept informed of events and encouraged to participate in care if they so wish, for example by giving the patient drinks, performing oral hygiene, or simply offering comfort (see Research Abstract 34.4). Certain features of the disease process, especially patterns of breathing, should be anticipated and explained to relatives.

Some relatives may wish to be at the bedside when death occurs. In spite of all efforts this may not be achieved. Sensitive reassurance may be required from nurses, who may indeed have supported the family in their decision to leave the bedside at a particular time. In such situations it is wise to forewarn the family of the possibility that the patient may die in their absence. It needs to be stressed for the benefit of these family members that their intention to be present at time of death together with the efforts they made are important.

Death

A patient's death affects many people. Where the patient has been nursed at home, the community nurse, home help, general practitioner and other professional carers will share in the family's grief. In hospital, the grief of family and friends will touch other patients and their visitors as well as the professionals who have been involved in the patient's care.

Immediate effects

Professional carers will find themselves in key positions for providing support immediately before, at the time of and after the death. This has implications for the knowledge required by nurses about different religious and cultural practices surrounding death.

Research Abstract 34.4 Symbolic feeding

The involvement of family members in providing oral hygiene was examined by Miles (1985), who discusses the concept of 'symbolic feeding'. Through the procedure of providing oral hygiene, the carer stimulates the sick person's sucking reflex. This serves to provide comfort in the way that an infant derives comfort and security through feeding. It therefore becomes a very important responsibility that can be shared with very close family members.

Miles S H 1985 The terminally ill elderly: dealing with the ethics of feeding. Geriatrics 40(5): 112–120

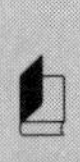

A comprehensive account of the practices of different religions and cultures surrounding death and bereavement is given in Green 1991 *Death with Dignity*. You may find it helpful to read this book alongside this section or at some time in the near future.

Last offices. The last sight of the patient will remain in the memory of relatives for a very long time. Nurses therefore have a responsibility to make sure that the appearance of the body does not disturb relatives and friends.

First, the body is given a general wash and, if male, the face is shaved. Any discharging orifices are sealed to guard against odour. If need be, eyelids can be temporarily taped. Dentures should be cleaned and replaced, using a dental fixing solution to hold them. Then the jaw is securely closed. Hair is then brushed into the deceased's usual style and, if necessary, attention is given to the fingernails.

A shroud or other preferred garment is placed on the body and the bed freshly made. In hospitals the practice is to fasten identification labels to the outer attire, and to wrap a sheet around the body before it is removed to the mortuary. Prior to this last step the relatives should be invited to view the body. Seeing their relative 'at peace' may be the memory which will ease some distress for a long time to come (Jamieson et al 1991).

Effects on other patients. The death of a patient undoubtedly affects other patients and raises the question of whether they should be told directly about a death or whether it should be assumed that they will not want to be upset. Consider, from a patient's viewpoint, the sequence of events described in Case History 34.2 surrounding the death of another patient who is in the same ward.

Effects on the family. The death of a patient takes the family members through another life change. Lindemann (1944) describes the initial experience of being bereaved as 'waves of distress lasting between 20 minutes and an hour' (p. 33). This intense reaction is characterised by a tightness in the throat and gasping short respirations. Should the family be present at the time of death, the onset of this reaction does not provide a good reason for rushing them away from the bedside. Neither does it provide an excuse for protecting other patients. A little time allows the reality of the situation to be absorbed — and this is as true for the rest of the patients.

Coping with the immediate responses of the bereaved. In general it is believed that the reality of a death is reinforced through sight and touch. Relatives, however, do not always feel able to look at the dead person. For those who refuse or are fearful, it is worth spending time, to explore their fears or the reasons why seeing the body is unacceptable to them.

Reassurance that the dead person looks peaceful and asleep is usually sufficient to assuage fears and anxieties. This is especially true when the last memory held by relatives is of a patient in physical or emotional distress. Once they have expressed a wish to see the body they should feel no restrictions on time or their expression of emotion.

The time immediately following a death is significant in some religions and cultures. Prior discussion will allow for any provisions to be made at ward level and so avoid unnecessary distress or embarrassment for family members. Every person's right to self-care should be acknowledged, including the right to grieve. There may be someone important (priest, minister, family member, friend or partner) missing from those present. Sensitive questioning will reveal if that person should be contacted and given the opportunity to join the other family members and view the body.

Following the initial reaction, relatives often become sufficiently composed to accept help. This a realistic time to invite them away from the bedside to an appropriately quiet area. Grieving relatives need physical and emotional comfort at this time. Given some privacy, they will console each other and may offer or be receptive to spontaneous hugs from members of staff. The non-verbal behaviour of staff members can convey more support than the most carefully chosen words. A non-imposing environment and a cup of tea will help the group of grieving people to sit and quietly compose their thoughts.

Explaining emotional reactions. Family members appreciate a little time being taken to help them understand what to expect of themselves physically and emotionally over the following days. The waves of distress mentioned earlier will continue intermittently, sometimes in response to meeting a new person or set of circumstances. These will certainly be most prominent at the funeral service and immediately after.

Because of the individuality of grief, these reactions may not happen simultaneously for all members of the family. Close relatives and friends will continue to provide each other with mutual support. In addition to this emotional reaction, those who are grieving should be alert to the fact that the distress they are experiencing might compromise their memory. Whereas sleep may not come easily before the funeral, often families are so exhausted following the service that their sleep patterns return to normal almost immediately.

Case History 34.2 Mr J

Mr J is dying. He will have made some impression on the other patients. He may have been particularly popular with everyone. On the other hand, he might have been so ill as to monopolise the nurses' attention. Some patients might have felt great sympathy and subsequently refrained from taking up the nurses' time. Others may have felt hostility, thinking that Mr J was being cared for to their detriment.

Perhaps a number of deaths have occurred recently. Other patients begin to wonder, even chat among themselves: 'What is going on around here?' For themselves, some patients might wonder: 'Is there something I have not been told about my illness? Am I also going to die? When?' Certain signals may become significant: all the people who have died appeared to be in pain; they became drowsy and drowsier; they were given a syringe pump; then the bed was moved.

There is an increase in activity at Mr J's bed. Screens are drawn; distressed sobbing is heard from relatives. A nurse ushers the relatives away from the bedside. The remaining nurses are very busy and just not able to give direct attention to patients in the immediate vicinity of Mr J.

There is more activity behind the screens. A nurse moves around the patients and asks, 'Do you mind if I pull your bed screens for a few minutes — we are busy with Mr J. There is a rumbling, like a trolley being wheeled into the ward, a noise like a door being shut, then the rumbling noise again! After another interval the screens, with the exception of those around Mr J's bed, are pulled back.

Later on in the day, when the final set of curtains are pulled back, an empty bed is revealed. The patients wonder: 'Where is Mr Jones?'

How would you answer this question?

Information. The family may still require information to help them understand the events of the last few hours, days or weeks of the patient's life. If they were absent at the time of death, the knowledge that a staff member was present, if this is the case, will provide some comfort. This can, in addition, forge a special link with that member of staff. As pointed out earlier, people in a state of numbness following the receipt of bad news do not always assimilate the information being presented to them. For that reason, relatives should be encouraged to seek reiteration or clarification from hospital or community staff if they are uncertain about any detail at a later date. Staff members must be sensitive to this need and prepared to answer the same questions many times.

Special requests. Relatives might express a desire to see the dead person dressed in specific attire, a wish to assist with the last offices, or a need for cooperation in the arrangement of a non-conventional funeral. Some requests may seem unusual. These are, however, choices which have been made by families, and sometimes by patients, prior to death. Every effort should therefore be made to comply. The nurse's role is to facilitate the grieving process, not to prescribe how it should be carried out.

> ? **34.8** Bereavement is a psychological process. Why should nurses be concerned with the consequences for families beyond the time of their involvement?

Death at home

If it is by choice that an anticipated death occurs at home, and provided that the community nurse has been involved early, there will have been discussions with the family about what to expect and what to do when the death finally occurs. A Macmillan nurse might also be involved. In such situations, these two professionals will arrange their day's schedule to ensure that one of them is available to provide whatever support a family requires. Families often talk about the security and confidence which is generated from the knowledge that 'help is only a phone call away'.

The knowledge, for example, that the death of the patient does not, in itself, necessitate an emergency call gives family members the opportunity for privacy. They can thus take all the time they need with their grief before making the necessary phonecalls to the doctor, nursing staff and funeral director. Usually there is a very special relationship between the community nurse and the family; often, the former is felt to be an integrated member of the family group immediately before and following the death.

Funeral arrangements

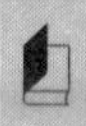

> A very useful handbook available (in Scotland) from local Citizens' Advice Bureaux is *What to do after a Death in Scotland* (SHHD 1992).

Arranging the funeral is an immediate source of anxiety, especially for those who have had no such experience. Some guidance may help in choosing a funeral director and in facilitating the first contact. A death certificate completed by the doctor (and in the case of cremation, a second certificate signed by two doctors) is required. Early preparation of this second certificate will avoid delay for the funeral director when he arrives to remove the deceased person from the hospital mortuary. Unless unavoidably prevented, the majority of doctors will personally hand over the death certificate to the family and answer their questions.

During his period of involvement, the funeral director will ensure that the family's wishes are respected and that no detail of the arrangements is omitted. It is advisable to suggest that relatives write down details of matters which require attention beyond the funeral.

Taking leave of the family in hospital

In hospital, there is a formal handing-over of the deceased's valuables. These need to be identified and signed for by the next of kin. This is a distressing process for all concerned and some relatives view it as a triviality amidst the personal loss they are enduring. Nevertheless, nurses cannot afford to minimise this responsibility. Apart from any monetary value, relatives may attribute a sentimental value to these possessions at a later date.

Travel arrangements. Relatives might not be prepared for the initial impact of leaving the hospital. The fact that they travelled to hospital by car is no reason to assume that the driver will feel able to drive home. The family may be relieved to discover that this is acknowledged and welcome the suggestion that the journey home be made by taxi.

Future contact. Finally, it may be reassuring for relatives and friends to be given contact numbers for community agencies should they feel inclined to ask for help in the future.

Withdrawing services in the community

Taking leave of relatives is a more gradual process in the community. Often a community nurse and Macmillan nurse will continue to visit the family over the period immediately following the funeral. Further contact or referral to other professionals such as the general practitioner, health visitor or social worker will depend on individual circumstances.

> ? **34.9** Find out what (a) statutory and (b) voluntary support is available locally for bereaved persons.

Bereavement

In Britain, a statutory compassionate leave of three days is granted to the immediate relatives of a deceased person. This usually covers the period from death to the funeral day. The question might be posed whether this perpetuates the notion that life should return to normal as soon as possible following a funeral. Bereavement has been described as a severe psychological stress, its nature and intensity being determined by the quality of the relationship which has previously existed between the dead person and those who are bereaved (Bowlby 1969).

Grieving people are sad, lonely and often confused by their own feelings, which can range from anger to frustration. Many people successfully work through the grieving process. For those who have difficulty in expressing or talking about their feelings, it can be a lengthy struggle to achieve a sense of purpose and value in their own lives. Helping the bereaved calls for effective communication and sensitive problem-solving skills.

Nurses have many opportunities to develop relationships with the families and friends of dying patients. Used effectively, such opportunities can affirm for relatives that their needs, as distinct from those of the patient, are recognised. The grieving person can thus begin to explore his own responses and raise questions about the ongoing and impending changes in his situation.

Building relationships

Machin (1990) provided guidelines, based on Worden's (1983) work, for professionals to aid bereaved individuals (see Table 34.6). Building a trusting relationship is the first step

Table 34.6 Helping the bereaved: tasks and goals (Worden 1983). Adapted with kind permission from Machin (1990).

Tasks of the bereaved	Goals of the professional	Interventions	Essential components of intervention
To accept the loss	To increase the reality of loss	Help bereaved focus on the reality of the loss by: talking of the last illness; death; funeral	1. Provide time to grieve 2. Interpret normal behaviour/ responses 3. Allow for individual differences and styles of coping 4. Offer continuing support 5. Identify abnormal grief and if necessary refer on
To experience the pain of grief	To help the client deal with his feelings	Help identify and express feelings by: exploring guilt; anger; anguish and allowing the client to emerge in rage, tears	
To adjust to life without the deceased	To help overcome problems in readjusting	Assist living without the deceased by looking at social and practical implications of bereavement and increasing self-confidence and self-esteem	
To withdraw energy from the past and reinvest in other relationships	To encourage the client to withdraw from deceased and look to new relationships	Facilitate emotional withdrawal by: exploring new sources of social and emotional gratification	

towards enabling grieving individuals to express themselves. Fears, anxieties, anomalies, hopes and disappointments might be voiced. Sensitivity and a non-judgemental response from a listener who understands will allow repeated accounts of situations whilst enabling clarification and exploration of feelings to take place.

Giving bereaved individuals the opportunity to focus on their grief in a protected environment will free their relatives and friends to provide support within their own limitations. This is extremely important, as it is the intensity of the bereaved person's grief in combination with the helplessness and embarrassment felt by relatives and friends that can isolate a grieving person.

Accepting reality. Active listening on the part of the professional enables the bereaved person to accept the reality of his situation. This is helped by the acknowledgement that grief is a natural healing response to a significant loss and by explanations about the nature, intensity and duration of the grieving process. Most importantly, the myth that life can and should return to 'normal' within a short time must be dispelled. The bereaved person needs to give himself permission to expose rather than suppress the feelings that he thinks might distress the non-professionals who are close to him.

Working through a bereavement

Bereavement as described by Bowlby (1969) is a process of adjustment to major change involving the person in the exploration of immediate and potential difficulties and in setting small goals. For some time to come the future should be viewed in terms of 'tomorrow', not in terms of weeks or months.

Bereaved people sometimes speak of induced helplessness resulting from constantly being the recipient of kindness, sympathy and assistance. When the bereaved person is able to invest energy in new pursuits the pain of grief will lessen. His sadness, however, will continue, as will periods of vulnerability.

The first year of bereavement. Doyle (1987) identifies specific periods of vulnerability during the first year of bereavement. Immediately following the death emotions will be strong; the bereaved person will be confused and unsure about his ability to cope in the future.

Within weeks, family and friends tend to withdraw, leaving the bereaved person feeling lonely and anxious. This withdrawal can result from the feeling of these individuals that they are unable to deal with the strength and depth of the bereaved person's grief.

Doyle recommends that general practitioners be alert to the increased physical and psychological morbidity, even mortality, for widowed elderly people during the first year of a bereavement. The first anniversary is a particularly painful day for a bereaved person which, sadly, is often forgotten by friends and even relatives. There is often a reluctance to raise the memory of the deceased person to the level of conversation.

People at risk. Certain people are especially vulnerable during bereavement; this includes individuals:

- who are isolated from family and friends
- with few social contacts
- with existing social problems
- who are harbouring intense guilt relating to the deceased
- with a history of psychiatric illness.

It is essential that nursing staff in hospitals and the community are aware of the grieving individual's vulnerability. A knowledge of any special risk factors should influence plans for future support. Family members sometimes have different general practitioners and it is conceivable that a family doctor could be unaware of the bereavement. It is therefore good practice to notify the bereaved person's doctor at the same time as the deceased person's general practitioner is informed.

Support for nursing staff

Nurses and bereavement

When the death of a patient occurs, there are two distinct groups of mourners: relatives and friends on the one hand, and staff on the other. Traditionally, nurses have been discouraged from admitting to or displaying feelings of sadness or distress. Indeed, they are strongly encouraged to 'control' their behaviour.

Nurses encounter many losses. This happens on a personal level and in relation to the involvement they have in helping patients, relatives and, often, their colleagues with varying degrees of grief. It would be a mistake to assume that all the grief experienced by professional carers is resolved without difficulty (see Research Abstract 34.5).

Research Abstract 34.5 Nurses' reactions to death

Popoff (1975 in Hurtig & Stewin 1990) reports that the level of anxiety felt by nurses when caring for dying patients is strongly related to the fear of their own death. The intensity of the nurse's involvement with a dying patient and her previous personal experience of loss will affect her response and the way she deals with the patient's relatives. Stoller (1980) suggests that, with increasing experience, nurses become less rather than more able to deal with relationships with dying patients and their relatives. Difficulties increase for nurses when the presence of grief in professional settings is not addressed.

Popoff D 1975 What are your feelings about death and dying? In: Hurtig W A, Stewin L 1990 The effect of death education on nursing students' attitudes towards death. Journal of Advanced Nursing 15(1): 29–34

Attachment and patient care. The period of acquaintance has no bearing on the strength of attachment which develops between nurses and the patient and families with whom they work. Attachment will vary according to the nature of the exchanges between people of different ages and personalities and the intensity of their involvement. Inevitably, the death of a patient and subsequent separation from the deceased's family will result in some degree of bereavement for the nurse. If this reaction is ignored or disallowed by colleagues (or indeed by the nurse herself) the need to work through the grief will still remain. Often, the root of this problem is not a lack of available resources, but rather, an unwillingness to use the most essential resources, i.e. the nurse herself and her colleagues. The resulting imbalance between need and utilised resources is a significant factor in producing stress (Caplan 1961). The nurse's mechanisms for dealing with this stress may include reducing and depersonalising her contact with patients (Menzies 1960). Patients and families can thus be deprived of listening time, of empathy and of a non-judgemental attitude, all of which facilitate communication. Undue stress can further result in the nurse becoming isolated from her colleagues when negative behaviour becomes apparent (see Ch. 17).

?	**33.10** Is it possible to provide nursing care without some degree of emotional attachment forming between you/patient/family?

Personal qualities. The unique qualities that each nurse brings to her interactions with terminally ill patients and their carers need to be acknowledged and valued as highly as her professional skills, for these inner strengths make a major contribution to 'caring'. In drawing upon her personal strengths the nurse requires a growing self-awareness, a positive belief in self, and secure perspective of the meaning of life. It is vital for nurses to be aware of the sometimes unclear boundaries of practice which exist between them and other professional carers, and of the strengths and limitations of various disciplines as applied to palliative care.

Nurses need encouragement and sufficient opportunity to build on their existing knowledge, to develop and sustain interpersonal relationships, to make the transition from curative to palliative care, to help patients, relatives and colleagues in similar situations, and, most importantly, to *be with* people when distress is evident. A sense of humour is important. It could be argued, however, that the latter will develop naturally as secure relationships are forged between members of a team.

CONCLUSION

Central to the approach to the care of terminally ill patients described in this chapter is a philosophy which acknowledges the right of individuals to self-care. While in the present discussion there has been a strong emphasis on caring for patients with end-stage cancer, it is hoped that students using this text will appreciate that the principles offered here are applicable to any group of patients. A sound knowledge of the disease process of terminal illness will assist the nurse in her assessment of the physical, emotional, social and spiritual needs of her patients.

Nurses very often report a high level of job satisfaction associated with caring for this group of patients and relatives (Kindlen 1987). This comes from providing individualised care for a family group and from the support received in return.

Perhaps the most difficult lesson for nurses is to apply this philosophy of care to themselves. Individuals have not only the right but also the responsibility for their own care. This is not to deny that nurses also have a responsibility to ensure that their colleagues' coping strategies are being facilitated. Sadly, the grieving response is often suppressed by nurses or regarded by many of their colleagues as a form of self-indulgence.

The demands of nursing terminally ill patients and caring for bereaved relatives carry a high risk of emotional and physical exhaustion. Perhaps by using the framework for anticipatory guidance outlined in Box 34.7, individual nurses might enhance their own well-being and, consequently, their effectiveness in caring for terminally ill patients.

Box 34.7 Anticipatory guidance for nurses

It is a fact of their professional life that nurses will encounter many situations of loss during a working day. Some of these will be directly related to the death of a patient, whilst others will be consequent to the amount of energy expended in facilitating the grieving process in others.

Reassurance comes in acknowledging the nurse's grief and allowing her the right to her response. Empathy and unconditional regard from colleagues will seal this understanding. In practical terms it takes a very brief encounter to convey understanding and empathy towards a colleague. Acknowledgement, whether verbal or non-verbal, grants the permission to grieve required by the nurse. This permission can revitalise and motivate the nurse to return to the working situation, in the knowledge that colleagues care and if necessary will provide listening time.

Involvement in care can be translated into building support strategies for oneself. It is every nurse's professional responsibility to care for herself. In an environment where acknowledgement and permission are given, there is every possibility that staff will develop positive professional and personal support strategies. Professional support strategies include efficient management of time within the working day, a responsibility for one's own professional development, uptake of available educational opportunities and the development of personal coping mechanisms in keeping with one's own personal strengths and interests.

REFERENCES

Ashworth P 1984 Communication in intensive care units. In: Faulkner A (ed) Communication. Churchill Livingstone, Edinburgh

Benner P, Wrubel J 1989 Primacy of caring: stress and coping in health and illness. Addison-Wesley, Menlo Park, CA

Blackburn A M 1989 Problems of terminal care in elderly patients. Palliative Medicine 3: 203–206

Bowlby J 1969a Attachment and loss. Vol 1: Attachment. Hogarth, London

Bowlby J 1969b Grief following object loss and loss of others. In: Bower F 1980 Nursing and concepts of loss. Wiley, Chichester

Bowlby J 1988 A secure base. Tavistock, London

Brown S, Mann R 1990 Breaking the cycle: control of breathlessness in chronic lung disease. Professional Nurse 5(6): 325–328

Caplan G 1961 An approach to community mental health. Tavistock, London

Cartwright A, Hockey L, Anderson J 1973 Life before death. Routledge & Kegan Paul, London

Collinge D 1990 The art of dying. Nursing Times 86(34): 34–35

Cowley S 1990 Who qualifies for terminal care? Nursing Times 86(22): 29–30

Doyle D 1987 Domiciliary terminal care: a handbook for doctors and nurses. Churchill Livingstone, Edinburgh

Doyle D, Benton F 1991 Pain and symptom control in terminal care, 2nd edn. St Columba's Hospice, Edinburgh

Dunlop R, Davies R J, Hockley J M 1989 Preferred versus actual place of death: a hospital palliative care support team experience. Palliative Medicine 3: 197–201

Evans P D 1982 Motivation. In: Chapman A, Gale A (eds) Psychology and people: a tutorial text. Macmillan, New York

Gibbons D E 1983 Mouth care procedures. Nursing Times 79(7): 30

Haigh C 1990 Adopting the hospice ethic. Nursing Times 86(41): 40–42

Higginson I, McCarthy M 1989 Evaluation of palliative care: steps to quality assurance. Palliative Medicine 3: 267–274

Hockey L 1990 St Columba's home care team: an evaluation study. Unpublished report, St Columba's Hospice, Edinburgh

Ivetic O, Lynne P 1990 Fungating and ulcerating malignant lesions: a review of the literature. Journal of Advanced Nursing 15: 83–88

Jacques A 1992 Understanding dementia, 2nd edn. Churchill Livingstone, Edinburgh

Jamieson E M, McCall J M, Blythe R 1992 Guidelines for clinical, nursing practice, 2nd edn. Churchill Livingstone, Edinburgh

Kindlen M 1987 The role of the hospice home care sister as perceived by district nursing sisters, health visitors and Macmillan nurses. Unpublished thesis, University of Edinburgh

Kleinman M, Eisenberg L, Good B J 1978 Culture, illness and care. Annals of International Medicine 88: 251–258

Kubler-Ross E 1970 On death and dying. Tavistock, London

Langlands M 1991 Dying with care. Nursing Times 87(7): 37–38

Lindemann 1944 The symptomology and management of acute grief. In: Bower F 1980 Nursing and concepts of loss. Wiley, Chichester

Lugton J 1988 Communicating with dying people and their relatives. Austin Cornish/Lisa Sainsbury Foundation, Croydon

Lunt B, Neale C 1987 A comparison of hospice and hospice support teams for the terminally ill. Cancer Care Research Unit, Royal South Hants Hospital, Southampton

Lunt B, Yardley J 1986 A survey of home care team and hospital support teams for the terminally ill. Cancer Care Research Unit, Royal South Hants Hospital, Southampton

Machin L 1990 Looking at loss and bereavement counselling pack. Longman, Harlow

McGhee J 1991 The old man's friend. Nursing Times 87(39): 44–45

McCorkle R 1974 Effects of touch on seriously ill patients. Nursing Research 23: 125–132

Menzies I 1960 A case study in the functioning of social systems as a defence against anxiety. Tavistock, London

Miles S H 1985 The terminally ill elderly: dealing with the ethics of feeding. Geriatrics 40(5): 112–120

Nash A 1989 Palliative care: improved services. Nursing Times 85(44): 43–44

Orem D 1980 Nursing concepts and practice. In: Pearson A, Vaughan B (eds) 1986 Nursing models in practice. Heinemann, Oxford

Parkes C M 1985 The dying patient: terminal care, home or hospital. Lancet 8421 (Jan 19): 155–157

Parkes C M 1986 Bereavement: studies in grief in adult life, 2nd edn. Penguin, Harmondsworth

Parkes C M, Parkes J 1984 Hospice versus hospital care: re-evaluation after 10 years as seen by survey sponsors. Post Graduate Medical Journal 60: 120–124

Popoff D 1975 What are your feelings about death and dying? In: Hurtig W A, Stewin L 1990 The effect of death education on nursing students' attitudes towards death. Journal of Advanced Nursing 15(1): 29–34

Raphael B 1984 The anatomy of bereavement. Hutchinson, London

Regnard C, Badger C, Mortimer P 1988 Lymphoedema: advice on treatment. Beaconsfield Publishers, Beaconsfield, Bucks

Regnard C, Davies A 1984 A guide to symptom relief in advanced cancer, 2nd edn. Haigh & Hochland, Manchester

Regnard C, Tempest S 1992 A guide to symptom relief in advanced cancer, 3rd end. Haigh & Hochland, Manchester

Seale C 1991 Death from cancer and death from other causes: the relevance of the hospice approach. Palliative Medicine 5: 12–19

Shepherd G, Page C, Salmon P 1987 Oral hygiene. Nursing Times 83(19): 25–27

Speck P 1978 Loss and bereavement in medicine. Baillière Tindall, London

Stedeford A 1984 Facing death: patients, families and professionals. Heinemann, London

Stoller E 1980 Impact of death related fears on attitudes of nurses in a hospital work setting. In: Hurtig W A, Stewin L 1990 The effect of death education on nursing students' attitudes towards death. Journal of Advanced Nursing 15(1): 29–34

Stott B 1990 Taking the final steps. Nursing Times 86(51): 29–31

Stubbs L 1989 Taste changes in cancer patients. Nursing Times 85(3): 49–50

Thomas S 1989 Treating malodorous wounds. Community Outlook (October): 27–30

Townsend J, Frank A O, Fermont D, Dyer S, Karran O, Walgrove A, Piper M 1990 Terminal cancer care and patients' preference for place of death: a prospective study. British Medical Journal 301: 415–417

Trenter P, Creason N 1987 Nurse administered oral hygiene. Is there a scientific basis? Journal of Advanced Nursing 11(3): 323–331

Twycross R, Lack S 1990 Therapeutics in terminal cancer, 2nd edn. Churchill Livingstone, Edinburgh

Ward A 1985 Home care services for the terminally ill: a report for the Nuffield Foundation. University of Sheffield

Wilkes E 1984 Dying now. Lancet I: 950–952

Williams C 1991 Preserving dignity through care. Nursing Times 87(3): 46–49

Wilson J A, Lawson P M, Smith R G 1987 The treatment of terminally ill geriatric patients. Palliative Medicine 1: 149–153

Worden W 1983 Grief counselling and grief therapy. Tavistock, London

VIDEO CASSETTES

Cassidy S, Burns G, Smearden K The cancer journey. Sponsored by British Gas, available from Meditec Books, Grantham

Twycross on cancer pain. Napp Laboratories, Cambridge

FURTHER READING

Bower F 1980 Nursing and concepts of loss. Wiley, Chichester
Bowling A 1983 Teamwork in primary health care. Nursing Times 79(48): 56–59
Green J 1991 Death with dignity. Macmillan, London
McCaffery M, Beebe A 1989 Pain: a clinical manual for nursing practice. Mosby, St Louis
Morison M 1989 Wound cleaning: which solution? The Professional Nurse 4(5): 220–225
Regnard C, Comisky M 1992 Nausea and vomiting in advanced cancer. Palliative Medicine 6: 146–151
SHHD 1991 What to do after a death in Scotland. HMSO, London

USEFUL ADDRESSES

The National Hospice Council
59 Bryanstone Street
LONDON W1A 2AZ

The Scottish Partnership Agency for
Palliative and Cancer Care
21a Rutland Street
EDINBURGH

CHAPTER 35

The patient in need of rehabilitation

Margaret Harris

CHAPTER CONTENTS

Introduction 943
What is rehabilitation? 943
Who needs rehabilitation? 944
Research awareness 944

The psychology of disability 945
Stigma 945
Grief 946
Stress 946
Control 946

The process of rehabilitation 946
Inter-disciplinary teams 946
Rehabilitation units 946
Statutory and voluntary bodies 946
Sport and leisure 947
Artificial aids 947
A process of modification 947
Outcome 947

Roles 947
Patient-professional roles 947
The role of the nurse 948

Activities forming the nursing role 948
Control of the environment 948
Holistic assessment 949
Communication 949
Meeting self-care needs 950
Mobility 951
Social, emotional and economic self sufficiency 952
Teaching 952
Preparing the patient for an unsympathetic environment 953

The role of the patient — an instrumentality model 953
Applying an instrumentality model 953

Quality of life in the community 954
Personal care 955
Physical activity 955
Role fulfilment 955
Mental health status 955
Medical status 956
Economic productivity 956

Conclusion 956

References 957

Further reading 957

Useful addresses 958

INTRODUCTION

The unique function of the nurse is to assist the individual, sick or well, in the performance of those activities contributing to health or its recovery (or to peaceful death) that he would perform unaided if he had the necessary strength, will or knowledge. And to do this in such a way as to help him gain independence as rapidly as possible.

Henderson 1966

This chapter devotes itself to a patient group for whom full recovery is not an option because, whether or not it has been possible to reverse the disease process, there are *consequences* which do not simply go away. For some, the development of these consequences is insidious; for many the onset will be sudden and traumatic; for all, there is a huge need for psychological adjustment.

The Henderson (1966) description of the function of the nurse suggests a causal link between the assistance given and the regaining of independence by the individual. The difference between 'I assist you because you cannot do it yourself' and 'I assist you in order that you may be able to do it yourself' lies in teaching and motivating in order to increase will and knowledge. These skills can be developed in rehabilitation nursing because time is not the enemy that it is in acute care. Often, the value of nursing interventions cannot be evaluated because the period of patient–nurse contact is too brief. In rehabilitation nursing, there is an opportunity for the nurse to function in a different and rewarding way.

The standard ingredients of scientific nursing practice are still required (see 'Meeting self-care needs', p. 950) but distinctive priorities derive from the inter-disciplinary approach to the tasks (see 'The process of rehabilitation', p. 946) and a different value system where wholeness as a human being involves looking forward to an adapted lifestyle rather than back to previous levels of health and achievement.

The nurse may require increased self knowledge and perhaps personal growth before she can cope with disability. There may be a need for a different theoretical model within which to function. Certainly, the meaning of professionalism comes under scrutiny.

Finally, an instrumentality model of achievement is presented (see p. 953) which reminds us of the value of feedback (or knowledge of results) in the motivation of all involved in the task of rehabilitation.

The chapter gives general, rather than prescriptive guidelines, so the final activities are important in guiding the students to apply the general principles to day-to-day practice.

What is rehabilitation?

It is about rebuilding lives. 'Acute care deals with a threat to life. Rehabilitation deals with a threat to living' (Pires 1989). Henderson and Nite (1978) defined rehabilitation as being the restoration of each 'individual to his or her optimum physical, mental, social, vocational and economic usefulness'. In medical terms rehabilitation means restoring people to their fullest physical, mental and social capabilities (Mair 1972).

The notion that one should *work* to get better, rather than wait for recovery to occur, is quite modern. During the mid 20th century, rehabilitation became a speciality in its own right, concerning itself with problems that cross many diagnostic boundaries, continue after discharge and require teamwork to achieve success.

Rehabilitation takes place in three stages:

- preventing complications
- promoting independence
- maintaining independence.

Preventing complications

Earlier chapters have emphasised how nurses should intervene early in the disease or injury process to prevent avoidable complications. This is the first stage or principle of rehabilitation.

Promoting independence

The second is the active promotion and restoration of independence. It is a post-acute phase when patients need help to decide what should be done, by whom, where and at what pace. In this phase, patients regain control of their own lives and exchange their sick role for a health-seeking role.

Parsons (1951) described the sick role as exempting the patient from:

- 'normal' social activities and responsibilities
- responsibility for his own condition.

The sick role is not compatible with rehabilitation, and the beginnings of successful rehabilitation occur when the sick role is abandoned in favour of self-determination. There is an unwritten contract between a professional who abandons paternalistic attitudes and a patient who abandons the sick role.

The focus of interest is no longer on disease but on an active person with health-seeking behaviour.

Maintaining independence

Once an acceptable level of functioning has been established and social integration achieved, the third stage of rehabilitation is entered: management of problems that might cause the person to become dependent again.

Beyond this are the goals of rehabilitation as a social movement. 'Its objectives include the education of all the professions involved in medical and supportive care in order to focus endeavours on human values rather than more technical success. They include the orientation of the public towards a fair deal for the disabled in opportunities to work and share the joys of living' (Hirschberg et al, 1976).

The disabled person may be required to adopt a different way of life, often comprising an uneasy alliance between:

- accepting the disability but fighting for independence
- wanting routines that are flexible but needing disciplines that are rigid.

Who needs rehabilitation?

Rehabilitation skills are inherent in sound, scientific nursing practice and will have been described for specific conditions elsewhere in this book. The purpose of this chapter is to focus on a particular client group whose disease or disorder causes continuing functional disability, requiring professional involvement.

WHO models and terminology

The World Health Organization (1980) provides a medical model of illness-related phenomena, which is adequate for the many diseases that are self limiting and are amenable to prevention or cure. The model encompasses a search for cause, that is *aetiology*, the identification of *pathology*, and the identification of signs and symptoms, that is, *manifestation*.

To accommodate chronic, progressive or irreversible disorders, the model has a different focus, encompassing the concept of disease, impairment, disability and handicap. This model gives more emphasis to the consequences of disease. Duckworth (1982) defines these consequences as follows:

Impairment is any loss or abnormality of psychological, physiological or anatomical structure or function. It does not necessarily indicate that disease is present or that the individual should be regarded as sick. Very few people are free of impairment, for example, missing teeth, short sight or scars.

Disability is any restriction or lack (resulting from impairment) of ability to perform an activity in a manner or within a range considered normal for a human being. The functional limitation expresses itself in everyday life.

Handicap is a disadvantage resulting from an impairment or a disability that limits or prevents the fulfilment of a role that is normal (depending on age, sex, social and cultural factors) for that individual.

Handicap is a social phenomenon and the state of being handicapped is relative to other people; for example, being unable to reach up to a cashpoint from a wheelchair is no handicap for someone who lives in a village without a cashpoint.

To summarise:

Impairment: parts that do not work
Disability: activities that can not be carried out
Handicap: roles that can not be performed (Duckworth 1982).

The main disorders resulting in a need for rehabilitation are listed in Box 35.1. This list is not intended to be exhaustive, and is continually growing. Advances in medical technology not only prevent death but provide challenges regarding quality of life. Lambert (1985), who suffers from tetraplegia, said, 'I died in 1981, to be resurrected and given life imprisonment by modern medicine'.

Successful rehabilitation

Many studies have sought to identify the factors that influence long-term success in rehabilitation. Those who deteriorate physically and have problems with psychological well-being are not those with the poorest medical prognosis (Lawes 1984, Belanger et al 1988). Work, marital status and high social support are associated with favourable outcomes, critical factors being the regular presence of another person in the home and significant others nearby.

Research awareness

Research provides the foundation for good practice in any field, but the speed of change in rehabilitation poses a particular challenge. The obligation is not necessarily to do research but to be influenced by the relevant work of nurses, pharmacologists, psychologists, bioengineers and others. The current trend is towards high technology, which has improved quality of life with, for example, phrenic nerve pacers as aids to breathing and sacral stimulators as aids to continence. Other developments, such as electronically assisted walking, can raise false hopes and actually hinder realistic adaptation.

Box 35.1 Some examples of disorders causing functional disability

NEUROLOGICAL
Paraplegia
Tetraplegia
Hemiplegia
Head injury

MUSCULOSKELETAL
Arthritis
Osteoporosis

CARDIOVASCULAR
Cerebrovascular accident (stroke)
Intermittent claudication

ENDOCRINE — METABOLIC
Diabetes mellitus

SENSORY
Visual impairment
Deafness

CONSEQUENCES OF MUTILATING SURGERY
Mastectomy
Stoma
Amputation

CONSEQUENCES OF PROGRESSIVE DISEASES (IN REMISSION)
Multiple sclerosis
Parkinson's disease
Malignancy
HIV/AIDS

Research awareness should also provide knowledge of the extent of disablement problems. Chamberlain (1989) found that:

- some 6 million adults in the UK (one in seven) have at least one disability
- current provision is documented as being chaotic, fragmented, and piecemeal, with most disabled people receiving little practical help
- disabled adults with rheumatological and neurological diagnoses constitute the largest group with disabilities.

The cost of *not* intervening to prevent handicap is probably high. Roy et al (1988) found increased independence and a reduction in the use of community staff among those who had used the Edinburgh Rehabilitation Medicine Department. Similarly Geddes et al (1989) found that 10 % of patients discharged from the Leeds Rehabilitation Unit to a Family Placement Scheme did not require the predicted institutional living thereafter.

There are great needs and opportunities with which nurses must identify (see Research Abstract 35.1). The role of the nurse has not been well described in the literature and needs more research. In particular, the role of the nurse specialist needs to be empirically described and evaluated.

THE PSYCHOLOGY OF DISABILITY

Anything that assists with widening perceptions of how emotional and psychological factors have such an enormous impact on the well-being of people with disabilities, has to be welcomed .... Expecting people to be grateful for whatever they receive or whatever options are put before them is unacceptable. People with disabilities not only want the same choice that those offering it would expect themselves, but they want a share in exploring those options and possibilities (Blunkett 1985).

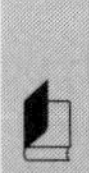

Chevigny (1962) previously a successful radio scriptwriter, reports how, after going blind, he was assured of a secure future making mopheads in a sheltered workshop! He had sufficient self esteem and confidence in his own abilities to resume his original career on his own terms.

An understanding of the psychology of disability provides the basis for the sustained therapeutic relationship which is crucial in the rehabilitation process (see Box 35.2). Understanding:

- promotes empathy
- predicts success
- analyses the effects on family members
- facilitates adjustment.

Stigma

In his review of research on handicap Richardson (1976) remarked that physical disability is a 'powerful and pervasive' disadvantage in initial social encounters. Goffman (1968) found that people view the person with a stigma as 'not quite human' and therefore accept treatment of the disabled that they would not tolerate for the able bodied.

Hahn (1983) suggested that disabilities arouse anxiety by reminding people of departures from standards of beauty and perceived competence. It is assumed that beauty is accompanied by traits of sensitivity, kindness and amiability. The able bodied may be embarrassed, made uncomfortable or even repulsed by the awkward or unusual. Rubin and Peplau (1975) point out that an encounter with a disabled person violates belief in a just world; for able-bodied people to maintain their belief in justice, people with disabilities are viewed as deserving the disability.

Research Abstract 35.1 Nurses' attitudes towards stroke patients in general medical wards

Gibbon's (1991) paper summarises a research study inquiring into the attitudes of qualified nursing staff and nursing auxiliaries towards stroke patients in general medical wards. The survey was undertaken on eight mixed-sex wards in a large teaching hospital. All wards were used for clinical nursing experience for nurses in training. Each of the wards, despite having a particular interest in one or more medical specialities, regularly admitted patients following stroke. All nurses were therefore familiar and in regular contact with this particular client group.

Results showed that nurses were largely ambivalent in their attitudes towards stroke rehabilitation. Nurses who had the more positive attitudes about stroke patients considered that they had a role in stroke rehabilitation and they valued the nursing contribution. Nurses with less positive attitudes, saw stroke patients as uncooperative and demanding. All nurses and auxiliaries believed that the more they learnt about stroke rehabilitation, the more motivated they became.

The findings suggest the need for specific education for the role of the nurse as a rehabilitator and for further research to explore the role.

Gibbon B 1991 A reassessment of nurses' attitudes towards stroke patients in general medical wards. Journal of Advanced Nursing 16 (11): 1336–1342

Box 35.2 Liberty, equality, disability: the facts.
(Reproduced with kind permission from *New Internationalist* (1992) 233: 18–19.)

SOME FACTS . . .

Poverty
In the US and UK over 60 per cent of disabled people live below the poverty line.

Education
In rich countries the majority of disabled children receive segregated education that does not enable them to reach their full potential.
In the UK only 0.3 per cent of higher-education students are disabled although disabled people are 10 per cent of the population.

Work
Disabled people in the US and the UK are three times more likely to be unemployed than any other group.
Disabled men in full time work in the UK earn almost a quarter less than non-disabled men, and disabled women earn a third less than disabled men.

Rights
Only one country in the world has anti-discrimination legislation – the United States which in July 1990 passed the Americans with Disabilities Act.
Many countries have equal opportunities laws but these are rarely implemented.
The UN Human Rights Declaration on Disability of 1975 would give disabled people rights internationally – if it were properly implemented, monitored and evaluated.

In a culture prizing competence and autonomy, people with disabilities also evoke strong anxieties about loss, vulnerability and weakness. For most people, the sick role is a temporary experience of incompetence and dependency. It is too short for them to become familiar with the methods used by people with permanent disabilities to accomplish tasks of daily living and work. They may consequently treat disabled people as though they have no ordinary functions and no capacity for making decisions.

Grief

The impact of sudden disability is similar to that of bereavement. Kubler-Ross (1974) noted that, for some, facing death is easier than facing life with a serious disability. Grief is a normal reaction to the loss of abilities and should not be mistaken for a depressive episode. Symptoms of grief include:

- preoccupation with the lost object (a limb, a function, a status)
- somatic distress
- inappropriate behaviour
- hostility
- denial.

Guttman (1976) said, 'It is a well-known fact that patients in the rebellious frame of mind against their disability curse not only God but also, naturally, their medical advisers'.

Fink (1967) describes four phases of adjustment to loss:

- shock
- defensive retreat
- acknowledgement
- adaptation.

There are two dangers in describing these phases in order. First, the assumption that each will pass and give way to the next, leading to eventual acceptance. This is not always the case. Second, that each phase is discrete and, having passed, is over and done with. Again, this is not so. The phases are likely to interact in a dynamic and sometimes erratic flow.

Gunther (1971) hypothesises a difference between the mourning associated with physical disability and bereavement for the dead. While patterned cultural rituals help to deal with mourning for the dead, there is no such established way to deal with the loss of a physical function.

Stress

Engel (1964) identified three broad classes of psychologically stressful events:

- loss or threat of loss of psychic objects, people, possessions, ideals or anything that is of great importance for that individual
- real or threatened injury to the body
- frustration of drives.

On all three counts, the newly disabled are stressed.

Control

The concept of control, or perceived control, is particularly relevant to disability. Seligman (1975) described how feelings of helplessness produce depression, inertia and inability to learn. De Charms (1968) described people as 'originators' or 'pawns'. Those who consider themselves to be mere pawns in the hands of fate will see little point in making much effort, but those who feel they can control the outcome of what they initiate are more likely to succeed.

THE PROCESS OF REHABILITATION

Inter-disciplinary teams

Rehabilitation is an inter-disciplinary endeavour. The challenge to the organisation is to create a client-centred team structure which involves family and other carers, and concerns itself with quality of life. This is very different from each profession providing therapy, however skilled, in isolated units. The patient can be seen as the pivot or hub of the structure, while the nurse coordinates management of the patient's day.

Leadership
Teamwork is facilitated by inter-disciplinary meetings. Team meetings are commonly chaired by the medical consultant, who also functions as team leader; however, it often happens that informal leadership occurs, particularly if the official leader is unpopular. In a well-integrated team, leadership will be shared according to the task and the organic growth of relationships around the patient. In some rehabilitation units, for example, The Royal Marsden, London, patients choose their own mentor. The person chosen will have leadership functions but always as a contributor to the strategic plan.

Rehabilitation units

Rehabilitation units or hospitals tend to specialise in one type or group of impairments so that resources are concentrated, research is facilitated and professionals become very expert. Demonstration Centres and Professorial Units are centres of excellence from which all can benefit. Many take on a formal educational role, for example, the Disabled Living Centre, Cardiff. All acknowledge that a key feature of the structure is adequate information resources. A great deal of help is available but people can only benefit if they know about it.

Statutory and voluntary bodies

For practically every form of disability there is a statutory or voluntary body, for example, the Partially Sighted Society, the Music Advisory Service, the Disabled Drivers Association, The Horder Centre for Arthritics and The Winged Fellowship Trust. A full list is obtainable from the Disabled Living Foundation and the Disability Rights Handbook (1993). See 'Useful Addresses', p. 958.

Many special training centres and colleges exist. Employment retraining centres provided one of the earliest forms of rehabilitation. Disablement Resettlement Officers now function under the auspices of the Manpower Services Commission and have considerable powers to help people realise personal ambitions.

Sport and leisure

Everyone has heard of the Paralympics, but the British Sports Association for the disabled tries to ensure that no-one is excluded from leisure pursuits due to disability. There is a charity called 'Holiday Care Service', and information is also provided by agencies such as Threshold Travel, The National Trust and British Airways (Care in the Air).

? **35.1** Are the Paralympics a good or a bad idea? Debate this in your group.

Artificial aids

There are over 40 Artificial Limb and Appliance Centres in the United Kingdom.

The manufacture of aids and appliances represents big business and mobility is a high priority. In the 1980s invalid cars were phased out in favour of adaptations to conventional cars.

Living accommodation ranges from ordinary housing, through purpose-built individual properties to residential hostels with full-time staff.

A process of modification

Evans (1982) described rehabilitation as a process of modification of:

- the disability by therapeutic management
- the environment for safety and optimum function
- attitudes in
  - the disabled
  - the carers, to prevent handicap
  - society.

Morris (1970) and Evans (1982) have found that prevailing attitudes to disability, dependency and incurability are at odds with the concept of rehabilitation. Many political decisions seem based on the notion that all institutionalisation is bad, and all rehabilitation to the community is good, yet many instances have been reported where the, admittedly impoverished, life of hospital has been exchanged for greater loneliness and isolation at home. Good rehabilitation is only possible if society is willing to undertake its responsibilities, and if human resources are shifted from medical care providing a quick cure to that dealing with lasting disability, until preventive medicine is improved or function can be restored to parts impaired by trauma, disease and the ageing process.

Outcome

The intended outcome is an optimal or an acceptable level of function. This will be highly individual but has been described by Kallio (1982) as:

- regaining premorbid function within the usual environment, or
- adapting function to enable the person to be effective in the usual environment, or
- modifying the environment to facilitate function, despite restricted abilities.

Measurement of the success of the rehabilitation process is problematic. A crude, though useful, measure is *lack* of need for re-admission to hospital (see Fig. 35.1).

Quality of life is not just a luxury. The Black (1980) report and other studies demonstrate that quality of life and health status are linked and have medical consequences. The objective of improved quality of life can be justified economically as failure in this area will lead to medical complications and readmission to hospital. This is not only disappointing, it is expensive.

ROLES

Patient – professional roles

Rehabilitation requires a well-integrated interdisciplinary team of people prepared to work together in the interests of the disabled person and his family.

The skills required by the patient will change and become redundant as the sick role is abandoned. The nurse, other professionals and the family must share the goals but tolerate movement of the goalposts. Professional input must be flexible, enabling change to occur.

Major problems are:

- the patient may have difficulty in setting goals and in coping with professionals who refuse to do it for him

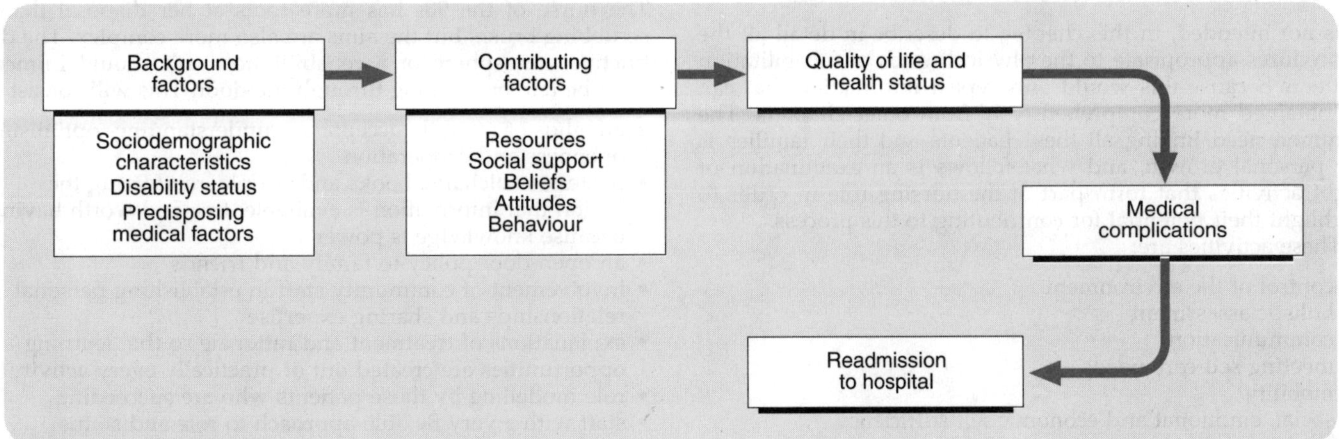

Fig. 35.1 A model of rehabilitation. (Adapted from Lawes 1984.)

- professionals may have difficulty in coping with an interdisciplinary team approach.

The patient
Recently disabled people usually have little experience of disability, or of the options and opportunities available to them. Decision making may be complicated by depression, hidden family dynamics and ambivalent feelings. Patients may try to avoid therapy sessions, for example, so staff may encourage, bargain with or even coerce patients into compliance. In the patient role, people are reassured and comforted by professional paternalism and professionals gain confidence from having their judgements respected.

The professional
In rehabilitation, professionals must learn to modify their judgements not only to allow for unpredictable patients but in order to achieve a consensus with other team members. Professionals bring their own values, moods and states of health to every situation. They must learn to separate their own needs from the patient's, and respect the patient's wishes if these seem well considered (Jennett 1987).

The role of the nurse
For knowledge to be useful, it must be *applied*. Care should mean active therapeutic management, which requires:

- *knowledge* of the therapeutic use of self
- *skill* in ensuring that the patient's self-care needs are met
- *attitudes* that adapt and progress with the patient's increasing independence.

The Orem model
Orem (1980) described a self-care model of nursing that can be applied in rehabilitation. The beliefs on which this model is based are:

- all individuals have self-care needs
- it is the right of individuals to meet these needs themselves, if possible
- self care is given by oneself for oneself
- self care is grounded in the belief that self maintenance and self regulation are valued as first-line strategies for effective human functioning in society (see Research Abstract 35.2).

It is not suggested that Orem provides the only, or even the best, model for rehabilitation nursing, but the model does have the virtue of emphasising the need for progressive attitudes and behaviour on the part of nurses.

ACTIVITIES FORMING THE NURSING ROLE

It is not intended, in this chapter, to describe in detail all the procedures appropriate to the physical needs of rehabilitation patients because this would only repeat information that can be obtained more comprehensively from other chapters. The common need linking all these patients and their families is for personal growth, and what follows is an examination of eight activities that form part of the nursing role in order to highlight their potential for contributing to this process.

These activities are:

1. control of the environment
2. holistic assessment
3. communication
4. meeting self-care needs
5. mobility
6. social, emotional and economic self sufficiency
7. teaching
8. preparing the patient for an unsympathetic environment.

Research Abstract 35.2

Patients who have had bowel surgery that results in the formation of a colostomy require to re-learn self-care skills in relation to elimination.

In this study, the nursing care provided for 12 such patients during changes of their colostomy appliance was observed and analysed within the framework of Orem's model of nursing. From the literature, nine elements of physical care which the patients had to accomplish in order to manage their appliance were identified. These were preparation of the equipment, preparation of the patient, removal of the old appliance, skin care, skin protection, selection of the new appliance, preparation of the new appliance, its application and the disposal of the old appliance.

The study, albeit on a small scale, demonstrated an uncoordinated approach to the process of preparing the patients for self-care and insufficient opportunities for these patients to practise all the steps in the physical management of their stoma. As a result, all were discharged without having demonstrated the necessary new self-care skills.

Given that containment rather than control of elimination is a key issue in the rehabilitation of such patients, the study concludes that, as the period of patients' post-operative hospitalisation becomes ever shorter, a planned approach to the development of self-care is required. Where continuation of self-care preparation is necessary after discharge, there should be an organised exchange of information between hospital and community staff.

Ewing G 1989 The nursing preparation of stoma patients for self-care. Journal of Advanced Nursing 14:5 411–420

Control of the environment
The nurse's role in the hospital setting is to care for whole people over a 24-hour period and to be responsible for the environment in which the activities of living take place. This is undoubtedly the most powerful tool she has at her disposal because the psychological change and personal growth required to cope with disability will only occur in a proper therapeutic milieu. Florence Nightingale's supreme aim was to provide an environment in which the body could heal itself. She may not have been familiar with the term 'model of nursing', but it is possible to produce a simple diagram (Fig. 35.2) of the approach she took.

?	**35.2** Identify ways in which the nurse could foster a therapeutic environment in the person's home and community.

The nurse of the 90s has more tools at her disposal than a scrubbing brush, but the aims are also more complex. The distinctive atmosphere of a rehabilitation unit should immediately be felt, on walking through the door. This will consist of:

- an ethos of warmth, acceptance, understanding, optimism, openness and cooperation
- posters, wallcharts, books and people, reinforcing the notion that information is available, free and worth having because knowledge is power
- an open-door policy to family and friends
- involvement of community staff in establishing personal relationships and sharing expertise
- explanations of treatment and rationale so that learning opportunities are created out of practically every activity
- role modelling by those patients who are succeeding
- staff with a very flexible approach to role and status
- adaptations of physical layout with aids and appliances as appropriate.

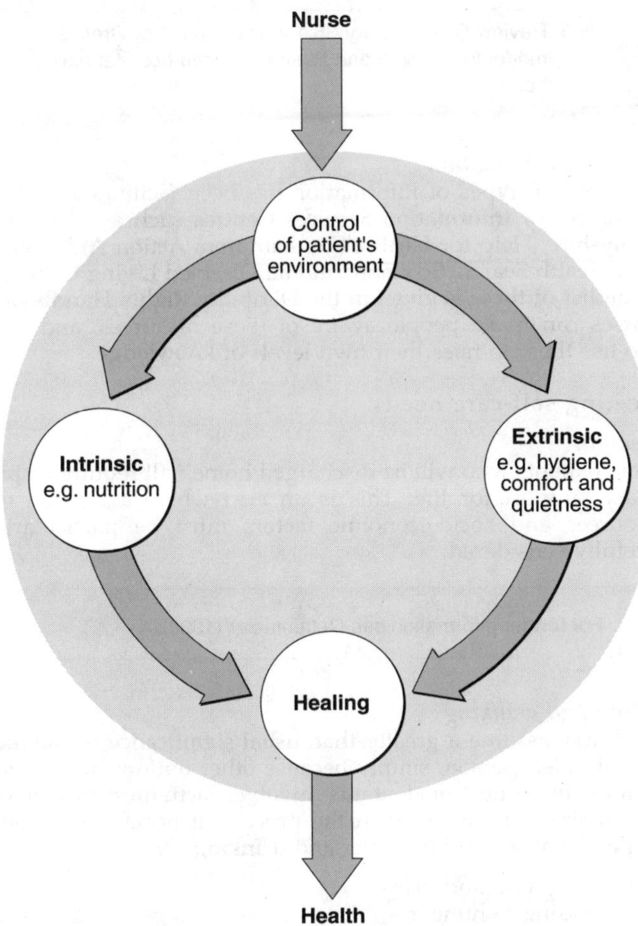

Fig. 35.2 A model of Florence Nightingale's approach to nursing.

Holistic assessment

Holistic assessment should consider the person both in hospital and at his or her own home. Assessment must adopt a counselling approach in order to be person- and family-centred, and individualised. Every nurse should attempt to be a good listener and sensitive to a patient's emotional state, but counselling is a high-level skill that requires long periods of training. Rehabilitation nursing is practised at several different levels by those who:

- are simply involved in such care
- have chosen to specialise in such care
- have been appointed to senior posts comprising advanced-level practice in consultancy, liaison, innovation and research.

The nurse may be the person best suited to make holistic assessment but, depending on the way in which the team functions, this may not be her role. Nevertheless, nursing assessment, planning and intervention must be in the light of the total rehabilitation assessment, however this is achieved.

The nursing plan

A plan that is coherent and integrated will only emerge from a functional profile of the patient to which the entire team have contributed. There are many frameworks for this, all basically similar since all must take account of the common major life activities. Halstead and Grabois (1985) use the acronym, PULSES.

P Physical condition, including visceral, cardiovascular, gastrointestinal, genitourological, endocrinological, and neurological disorders.
U Upper-limb function upon which *self-care* activities depend, for example, grooming, bathing, perineal care, drinking, feeding, dressing, applying braces and / or prostheses.
L Lower-limb function, upon which *mobility* depends, for example, transferring, walking, or negotiating stairs.
S Sensory components relating to *communication*, that is speech, hearing and vision.
E Elimination functions of the bladder and bowel.
S Supportive components:
— intellectual ability
— emotional adaptability
— support from family
— financial capability.

In each of these areas present abilities and limitations must be set against:

- previous level of functioning
- desired level of functioning
- predicted or realistic level of functioning.

Functional status and goals may be rated as:

1. dependent
2. requiring assistance
3. requiring supervision
4. independent.

Nurses are familiar with care planning that is compatible with the therapeutic plan prescribed by the doctor. Planning to meet the goals of the total rehabilitation strategy is much more challenging. It may be necessary for the therapists to adapt their day so that nurse and patient can work with, for example, an occupational therapist for dressing, a physiotherapist for walking, and a speech therapist for feeding and communication.

Last, it must be stressed that the PULSES framework does not present functional abilities in order of importance. The supportive components are as vital as the physical, so emotional status, mood and motivation must be monitored and taken into account.

People must be allowed to grieve, and given time and help to work through this process. Moments of optimism must be exploited. Motivation must be reinforced by positive feedback.

Communication

Brown (1954) wrote, 'They thought because I couldn't speak I had nothing to say.' No relationship, much less a therapeutic one, can get started without communication (see Ch. 26 and Research Abstract 35.3).

Every communication involves:

- a sender
- a message
- a receiver.

There may be problems at any or all of the stages. Among the many conditions that can interfere with communication are:

- confusion and disorientation
- hearing loss
- visual loss
- aphasia
- dysarthria
- loss of voice
- respiratory insufficiency.

There is also a tremendous mix of lay and professional people, all sending, interpreting and receiving messages.

Research Abstract 35.3

Nieuwenhuis (1989) established group activities in a ward for long-stay patients with neurological deficits. She demonstrated that their communicative potential was greater than it had previously appeared and intra-group awareness was greatly raised, with people making an effort to compensate for each other's disabilities.

Nieuwenhuis R 1989 Breaking the speech barrier. Nursing Times. 85(15): 34–36

Health-care professionals

Health professionals do not have good reputations as communicators. Many nursing studies have shown that patients want more information, that information is therapeutic in terms of reducing stress and pain, and that patients perceive themselves to have received less information than they have actually been given (Boore 1978, Hayward 1975).

When speaking, writing instructions, or interpreting those that already exist, it is important to recognise the patient's frame of reference. The nurse should restate, rephrase, and reinforce information that needs clarification. Non-verbal communication is very powerful.

It is a myth that speech therapists simply help people talk, and, as nurses cooperate best with the therapy if they know what is taking place, group activities, in the ward, use time efficiently by allowing staff and patients to learn together. They also build up confidence in social skills.

Patient choice

Good communication is also vital to patient choice and control and is essential to informed consent. Maguire et al (1978) have shown that up to one-third of women with breast cancer suffer from the 'post-mastectomy syndrome' of depression, inadequacy, anxiety and sexual difficulties; this correlates with the 25% of patients in his study who expressed dissatisfaction with the amount of information they received before surgery. Hames and Stirling (1987) argue that providing information and allowing choice of treatment can considerably lessen the trauma of mastectomy. It seems that active involvement of the husband is also very therapeutic, and those without close confidants are most vulnerable to post-operative distress. (See Ch. 7.)

Team liaison

Communication and liaison are fundamental to the success of the multidisciplinary team concept. For instance, pressure-sore care now benefits from nursing-assessment tools such as those researched by Norton et al (1975) or Waterlow (1985), but for high-risk patients such knowledge is less than adequate (see Ch. 23). Continence, nutritional status and mobility must be dealt with, but the critical factor is pressure and nothing will prevent pressure sores except lack of pressure. If bio-engineers are available consult them.

Liaison work is sometimes delegated to the ward sister but may be the responsibility of a specially appointed rehabilitation nurse who could be hospital or community based. If hospital based, early contact can be made with the community staff who will take over post-discharge care (see Case History 35.1). They can be encouraged to come into the hospital, meet their patient, get to know the family and learn specific skills. Patients who need long periods of rehabilitation may become institutionalised and anxious about discharge. Previous encounters with community staff will build up confidence in them.

? **35.3** Review Case History 35.1 in the context of Orem's model for nursing and liaison between hospital and home.

Access to information

Access to all types of information has been facilitated by the setting up of Information Services Centres such as Dial UK, Derbyshire; Help for Health, Southampton; Action Aid, Newport; Health Search, Scotland; and all Disabled Living Centres. A full list of these is given in the Disability Rights Handbook. Nurses can make people aware of these resources, and can also use them to raise their own levels of knowledge.

Meeting self-care needs

Breathing

Some patients who will be discharged home will require respiratory support for life. This is an area where allocation of resources and socio-economic factors must be particularly carefully considered.

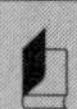

For further information see Dettenmeier (1990).

Eating and drinking

Food may assume a greater-than-usual significance in the life of a disabled person, simply because other options are fewer. Maintaining nutritional status involves activities that may be impaired at any point in the process of purchasing food, preparing meals and of eating and drinking:

- choosing food and drink
- responding to hunger
- balancing the diet
- gaining access to shops
- preparing food and drink
- conveying food and fluid into the mouth
- chewing and swallowing
- controlling weight.

? **35.4** How many modifications would be needed to help a young tetraplegic man to enjoy eating and drinking?

Pleasure and freedom in eating and drinking is an area of personal choice and control, certainly, but choice means having information, for example, that alcohol consumption increases the risk of epileptic attacks. Physically disabled people who gain weight, especially those in wheelchairs, increase the load on pressure areas and may reduce their mobility. Mutilating surgery, which can lead to comfort eating, may add obesity to an already-unacceptable body image. Stroke victims who do not master their eating impairments may choose to

Case History 35.1 A

A, an 18-year-old youth suffering from paraplegia, was totally unprepared emotionally for discharge when he was physically ready, but he was determined to go.

He was given over to the care of a skilled, motherly community nurse, but he did not want mothering. It was only after he and his girl-friend had been unable to cope with his rehabilitation programme, and he had nine pressure sores that he consented to receive care.

become socially isolated or may experience rejection in social encounters.

For further information see Gilbert S (1986) and Bender & Brookes (1987).

Eliminating

See Case Histories 35.2 and 35.3. Control of urinary and faecal elimination is not only a critical component of quality of life but is often vital to life itself. The regime for the spinally injured devised by Sir Ludwig Guttman, in the 1940s, meant that 80% of patients lived, whereas previously 80% had died within 2 to 3 years. The key differences were in the management of bladder, bowels and pressure areas in order to preserve the integrity of the renal tract and skin. Previously, there was a causal relationship between pyelonephritis or osteomyelitis, leading to renal failure and death. The nursing challenge was that if the urine could be kept sterile, life expectancy would be normal. This still holds good today (see Ch. 24).

Continence advisers refer to:

- education to maintain continence
- training to regain continence
- management to contain incontinence.

? **35.5** Consider Case History 35.2. Does P fit neatly into any of these categories? Does it surprise you that the leg bag was more of a problem than the wheelchair?

Personal cleansing and dressing

Together with management of bladder and bowels, self care in personal cleansing is the area where independence is likely to be most desired by the physically disabled. For effective rehabilitation, the combined expertise of the nurse and the occupational therapist is often needed, for example, in dressing techniques for stroke patients.

Hygiene and grooming are basic to self-respect and involve activities that are usually carried out in private. For those who cannot regain self-care abilities, a lack of attention to detail in areas formerly controlled by the patient greatly reduces self esteem. Personal care provides the basis for a therapeutic relationship because all such care has the potential for providing physical and psychological support.

? **35.6** Discuss the statement, 'The social dynamics of a bed bath are just as important as the social dynamics of a cocktail party'.

Whereas intimate care giving has probably always been the pivot of nursing activities it is only since Henderson (1966) that its value has been expressed in literature. In 1963 Lydia Hall abandoned the notion of a hierarchy of procedures ranging from highly complex technical tasks to what were regarded as simple and mundane tasks, such as giving bedpans. Hall instituted total patient care by trained nurses. She opened the Loeb Centre for nursing and rehabilitation in New York in 1963. There were two strands to Hall's philosophy:

1. professional nursing is a therapeutic force
2. people learn best in a non-directive environment.

Recent developments such as primary nursing are particularly appropriate for rehabilitation. Primary nursing increases the potential for the nurse to create and sustain a therapeutic relationship. However, the goals of the multi-disciplinary team concept must be upheld, and it cannot be assumed that the primary nurse will be regarded by the patient as the key person in his rehabilitation programme. Such a role will grow organically from any relationship in which empathy is demonstrated (see Case History 35.4).

Mobility

See also Ch. 36.

Mobility can be considered at two levels:

1. any change of position that aids physiological function
2. movement from one place to another, which is important for quality of life and also has benefits in terms of continence, shopping and travel.

Changing position

Prolonged inactivity results in serious deterioration in functional capacities, known as *'immobilisation syndrome'*, in which practically all organs and systems of the body suffer the consequences of immobilisation. This can be avoided if early rehabilitation nursing provides:

Case History 35.2 P

P, a 19-year-old man with paraplegia, adapted to his wheelchair more successfully than to his leg bag, which he felt was the ultimate indignity. Learning self-catheterisation techniques made a vast difference to his self image. Despite the discipline of 4-hourly catheterisation he now feels 'free'. He attaches a leg bag only for long-distance travel or trips to the pub, where he drinks beer in pints rather than halves.

Case History 35.3 J

J, a 50-year-old woman, had suffered from diverticulosis for many years. Her social life was handicapped by dietary restrictions, pain and embarrassment. A sudden, life-threatening episode of peritonitis resulted in gut resection and the fashioning of a colostomy. Within a few months she had learned self management and was particularly grateful for well-designed and individually prescribed stoma bags. She has no ambition to have the colostomy reversed.

The role of the hospital nurse in preparing the patient to live at home with a stoma is highlighted in Ewing (1989).

Case History 35.4 B

B, a 53-year-old woman suffering from paraplegia, expressed a desire to be totally self caring that is, free of the community nursing service. Despite having a husband and three supportive children she was determined not to impose a physical burden on anyone.

Her two principal problems were incontinence due to urine bypassing her indwelling catheter and an inability to wash the lower half of her body. Although she appreciated the weekly bath given by community nurses she wished to be able to shower herself. It required the efforts of the multi-disciplinary team to provide the necessary aids and adaptations, but it was the nurse's initial help with catheter management and access to a shower that allowed her to meet her own goals for quality of life.

- environmental stimuli
- regular passive movements of all limbs
- passive tilting
- regular turning and changes of position
- breathing exercises
- adequate nutrition and hydration
- skin care.

Movement

It is important for nurses to learn from and cooperate with other professionals in the training of patients and carers, as the effects on the patient are considerable, and there are so many techniques and aids available.

Nurses must have knowledge of different lifts and transfers, so that they can assess with the physiotherapist the best way to manage the patient, to gain maximum independence and prevent complications. For example, a 34-year-old man who had suffered a head injury was encouraged to put some weight through his legs by being continually transferred by two nurses, using a waist transfer, with one nurse at the front and one behind, rather than being passively lifted or hoisted.

In particular cases, for example with stroke patients, the use of a quadruped may encourage even further neglect of the patient's hemiplegic side. Unsuitable transfers can also cause complications; for example, one stroke patient developed a painful shoulder due to being transferred by nurses using a bear hug, with the hemiplegic arm being raised above waist level. This could have been avoided by using a waist transfer.

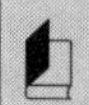
For further information see Jamieson, McCall & Blythe (1991) and RCN (1992).

Available techniques and aids include:

- lifting in a safe manner
- pivot transfers
- hoists
- walking with a stick
  - — crutches
  - — quadrupeds
  - — frames
- getting about in a wheelchair
  - — self propelled
  - — powered
- shopmobility schemes
- motability allowances
- adaptations that facilitate access and manoeuvre.

? **35.7** Assess ease of access to public buildings in your community.

Social, emotional and economic self-sufficiency

The nurse has a role in the sharing of information obtained from formal assessments and in the ongoing monitoring of interpersonal relationships, emotional status and future plans.

Family relationships

The onset of a disability is not only a crisis for the individual. It is likely to instigate a family crisis. It inevitably changes the nature of the marital relationship between partners. The spouse will feel the strain of assuming more family obligations. The range of sexual activities may be limited and fertility threatened. There are a number of barriers that impede the delivery of effective sexual rehabilitation to disabled people. Two of the most common are negative attitudes about sexuality and lack of information about normal sexual function in the presence of a specific impairment. Nurses often find themselves in the role of sexual counsellor because of their intimate care-giving functions, although social workers sometimes volunteer for the role, and doctors can advise on the functional limitations.

Misunderstanding by the patient and his family about the severity, prognosis and recovery process of the impairments can lead to high anxiety and impede progress. Consistency and openness in discussions foster realistic adjustment.

Employment

Economic self-sufficiency is usually dependent on employment, and many people obtain their self-image and primary sources of satisfaction from their work. The implications of disability for employment will depend on the previous employment and the types of impairment.

Social, emotional and economic self-sufficiency are fluctuating states that require empathy at all times; emotional support must be given as and when the need arises, rather than being parcelled out in hourly sessions. Very few units have psychologists on site, even fewer have family therapists, and the Disablement Resettlement Officer is usually only an occasional visitor. The nurse offers a more constant presence, enabling a therapeutic relationship to develop. Liaison with, and referral to, the appropriate experts can then occur as needed.

? **35.8** A young man of 17 years of age, and another of 41, have both suffered traumatic amputations, the former as a result of foolhardy behaviour and the latter due to an industrial accident. The youth may not have achieved independence from his parents, trained for a job or completed self-development. His self-image and intended lifestyle may be shattered. The middle-aged man may have a wife and family to support him, an offer of his job back or something lighter if preferred, and perhaps industrial compensation.

Consider whether one man's needs are greater than the other's. Is that too simplistic a viewpoint? Think about the differences in their rehabilitation needs.

Teaching

Teaching is ongoing and for all; professional knowledge must not be jealously guarded. Formal, informal, individual and group approaches can be used to educate the patient, family, friends and community carers. Preventable complications may be caused by episodes of depression, indiscretion or neglect but should not be allowed to occur because of ignorance.

Family

Whereas patient teaching will be viewed as a part of the rehabilitation process, the involvement of family and others must be timed and handled with sensitivity, since it represents an acknowledgement that the patient needs the help of others to manage or improve, and that the disability is not going to disappear overnight.

Planning a programme

The structure of educational programmes should be as carefully organised as any in a college of nursing. Individual educational needs should be assessed (using a counselling approach). Plans should take account of available:

- time
- place
- resources.

Implementation methods should be varied to include:

- demonstrations

- videos
- discussions
- experiential roles.

Evaluation should require feedback which demonstrates:

- understanding
- acceptance
- competence.

All nurses should be involved in the health-promotion aspects of rehabilitation. A study by Chow et al (1989) demonstrates the benefit of exercise in preventing osteoporosis. Pre-retirement courses take on the concepts of 'Fitness, Fun and Finance', all relevant to preventing disability in old age. Wright (1988) found that community nurses can provide relevant and useful information on the prevention and management of leg ulcers in the home setting.

For further information see Coutts & Hardy (1985) and Ewles & Simnett (1985).

? **35.9** During your community placement, assess how many patients have a leg ulcer. Select one of these patients, decide on a suitable model of nursing, and with the help of the district nurse plan a programme that includes short-term, intermediate and long-term goals.

Preparing the patient for an unsympathetic environment

The physical environment

Shearer (1981) says, 'What I feel the able-bodied person does not realise is the tremendous self discipline the disabled life entails . . . travel is limited, shopping difficult, entertainment has to be planned like a campaign. Just getting there in a wheelchair is a major hurdle.' (See Box 35.3.)

The social environment

Sutherland (1981) suggests that disabled people often find their attempts to be independent are frustrated by overprotection or stigmatisation. This will exacerbate the new experience of grief and loss that may be caused by discharge from the care of particular therapists.

For the individual, discharge from hospital can be very threatening rather than being a joyous experience. Visits home, gradually increasing in length from a few hours to a few days, help to prepare the patient by building up confidence and highlighting any problems, although, where home adaptations are necessary, it is rare for these to be finished before the discharge date.

Given that the environment is unsympathetic, or even hostile, it may be that more psychological training strategies should be built into rehabilitation programmes. These might include:

- assertiveness training
- relaxation
- cognitive therapy
- coping skills.

? **35.10** Discuss with your fellow students the pivotal importance of the loving support of family and friends in the rehabilitation of a severely disabled patient.

Box 35.3

During the International Year of the Disabled in 1981, Neil Slatter, who suffers from tetraplegia, did a 2000-mile sponsored wheelchair tour of the United Kingdom, in order to raise money to buy Meyra wheelchairs. A major side-effect of the tour was that 'a new version of the country emerged, defined not by antiquity, charm or the niceness of the people, but by its tolerance of the wheelchair'. It was shown that 70% of the town halls visited were inaccessible and the mayors who had agreed to support the project found themselves meeting Neil in the street (Hurley 1983).

THE ROLE OF THE PATIENT: AN INSTRUMENTALITY MODEL

In any rehabilitation programme it is the patient who must do the work. For this he will require the desire, the means, the ability and the opportunity to achieve his goals.

Possibly the first psychology lesson anyone learns is motivation, with sticks and carrots, or drives and incentives; where physical needs are paramount and self-actualisation the pinnacle. Maslow's (1954) theory that there is a hierarchy of needs is a useful reminder that, although physiological needs must take priority, security and acceptance must be present before the patient can feel self-esteem.

The limitations of Maslow's model derive from the fact that hierarchies do not acknowledge inter-relationships between the levels and, perhaps most important of all, the value of feedback. Porter and Lawler (1968) include all these concepts in a theoretical model of instrumentality (Fig. 35.3). This demonstrates that nothing is achieved without effort and that the effort will be moderated by both intrinsic and extrinsic constraints.

Applying an instrumentality model

The model can be used for any sort of achievement in life from a short-term goal such as getting up from a chair unaided when suffering from hemiplegia, to a long-term goal such as becoming a computer programmer. The model can, for example, be applied to the overall aim of rehabilitation, that is, maximum autonomy over one's own life, as follows.

Value of reward (desire)

- Is maximum autonomy what I want?
- Am I happy to be dependent on others?
- Would I prefer to die?

Two critical constraints seem to be age and sex. Young adults seem to be particularly vulnerable if they have not had opportunities to establish an independent lifestyle. People aged about 40 also have problems as they are too young to retire but too old to 'start again'. It seems that women are much better at coping with social isolation.

Effort to reward probability (means)

- Do I have the means, that is,
  — aids
  — adaptations
  — prostheses.

The critical constraint is money. The ability to buy whatever is needed is an enormous asset. People are entitled to a great deal of help from Social Services but there are often delays in receiving help.

? **35.11** Analyse possible reasons for delays. How might the nurse adopt an advocacy role for the person?

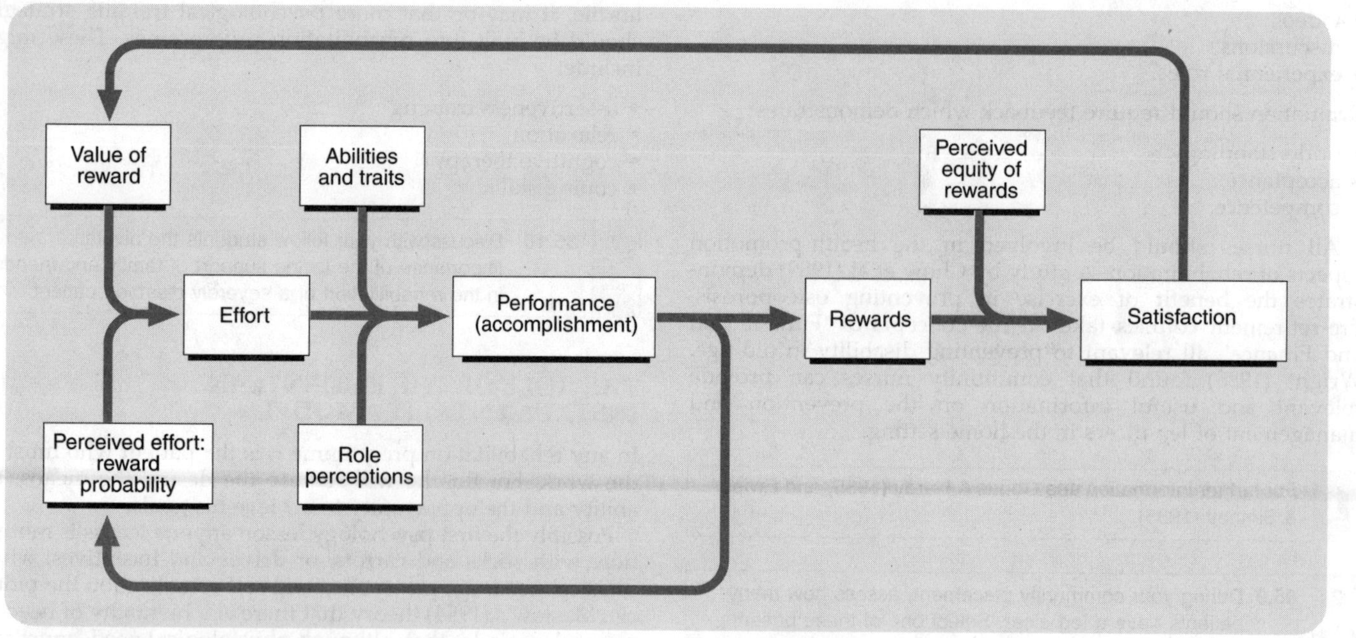

Fig. 35.3 A theoretical model of instrumentality. (Adapted from Porter & Lawler 1968.)

Abilities and traits

- What was my previous personality?
- What talents do I have?

The constraints are learning abilities, adaptability and type of impairment. Many people who were physically active previously complain of lack of aptitude for fine or intellectual skills.

Role perception (opportunity)

- How do I see myself?
  — breadwinner?
  — invalid?
  — a whole human being?
  — a useless wreck?

The perceptions here are strongly affected by external influences such as the attitudes of carers and society.

Interaction occurs between the boxes in Figure 35.3. As 'effort to reward probability' increases, the reward itself becomes more attractive. As people's abilities develop, their role perception is also modified. The usefulness of aids depends on the person's ability to use them and the value of reward is dependent on role. Success breeds success; if a goal is accomplished once, this increases the probability that it could happen again. 'Perceived equity of rewards' refers to the effort put in, and achieving the goal further motivates the patient.

This model could be used by the multidisciplinary team as an assessment tool to identify problems of non-achievement, as well as reasons for successful rehabilitation.

QUALITY OF LIFE IN THE COMMUNITY

For each patient, specific goals will need to be set, and outcomes defined and measured prior to discharge but this should only be regarded as an interim assessment. Rehabilitation is rarely completed in hospital and adjustment to disability may be a painful and difficult process. The self-image of a mastectomy patient, the sex life of a crash victim and the employment status of a person following a stroke can only be monitored over a period of time.

For some patients, for example, those with severe head injury or with paraplegia, follow-up is particularly important as they can improve very slowly over a long period of time. They may plateau for a period, but may then progress again later. The possibility of further improvement should never be forgotten.

Following discharge, disability may improve, deteriorate, or may fluctuate slightly. The goals of care are:

- to prevent deterioration
- further improvement of functional status
- possible discharge from professional care.

Belanger et al (1988) found that, whereas 73% of stroke patients were able to return home and over 60% were autonomous in self-care and mobility, many had deteriorated after 6 months. About 25% had problems with psychological well-being and complained that these had not been addressed during their rehabilitation programme.

This is a complex challenge for community nurses: patients who cannot be labelled chronically sick but who have potential problems that can only be prevented by active interventions that may not be delivered by professionals.

The model of rehabilitation in Figure 35.1 can be applied here.

The background factors are independent variables or facts of life that have to be accepted for example:

- where someone was born
- type of family and job
- previous personality
- marital status
- age
- sex
- nature and extent of the functional impairments.

The contributory factors are those which it should be possible to alter.

Resources include:

- professional and lay carers
- aids
- adaptations
- environmental design.

Social support

- friends

- clubs
- mobility
- accessibility

Beliefs, attitudes and behaviour are modified by:

- education
- training
- the mass media
- legislation
- cultural developments.

Professional and political implications arise here. Many of the problems relate to human relationships, economics and bureaucracy, areas over which people perceive themselves to have little control.

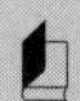

For further information see Beardshaw (1988).

Control has been a central concept in this chapter; people with disabilities are entitled to consultation and choice in all matters concerning their future. If they are to have reasonable quality of life their individually assessed needs must be identified and planned for. A holistic nursing assessment might group these needs into the following categories:

- personal care
- physical activity
- role fulfilment
- mental health status
- medical status
- economic productivity.

Personal care

The delivery of personal care may be in the hands of a mixture of family, friends, volunteers, neighbours, professionals and self-care. Standards must be maintained but needs will not be constant, for example, the normal care of pressure areas may be quite inadequate during a chest infection, and self-care in personal hygiene may be quite impossible outside the patient's specially adapted home. Respite care may make life at home, rather than in an institution, possible. The care givers' needs should be considered since they are a prime resource who should be cherished.

Physical activity

Physical activity is made possible by a sympathetic environment. Home adaptations may not be finished before discharge and situations that are acceptable for a short period become major causes of emotional trauma if they continue for a long-time. The local environment usually also presents some insurmountable barriers and it is not surprising that some people feel discriminated against. Some problems can be solved in personal ways, for example, a local landlord may provide ramped access to his public house, but in general terms it is a requirement of the 1970 Disabled Persons Act that no one should be denied access to a public building simply because of physical disability (see p. 953).

Role fulfilment

Role fulfilment depends on the breaking down of barriers between the able-bodied and the disabled; not just physical barriers but ignorance, prejudice and fear. People usually have many different roles, which enrich their lives. Being reduced to a single role and labelled 'disabled' diminishes the quality of life. Disability may mean that some roles are actually lost but new ones can be gained. Beethoven is one example. His prestige as a solo pianist was at its zenith when he became deaf but he subsequently poured more energy into composing. People may hold exaggerated notions of the degree to which disability limits them. The newly disabled must also decide whether or not to identify with other disabled people; for example, those who go deaf as adults may choose to suffer extreme isolation and curtailment of their social lives rather than learn sign language. Ideally, people should benefit from mutual support groups while enjoying integrated activities in other ways (see Case History 35.6).

Mental health status

All newly disabled people have to cope with stigma and find it is the task of the stigmatised to put others at their ease. Many need help in the early days if they are to be prevented from segregating themselves and becoming hermits. The truly fortunate receive sufficient empathetic encouragement from their families but the community nurse may be the only professional in a position to assess whether they need extra help or even psychiatric therapy.

Nurses must involve themselves actively in attempting to change social attitudes, as part of their educative role. However, problems are highly individual, and need to be handled as, and when, they occur.

? **35.12** Consider Case History 35.4. Discuss in your group whether B is exercising her rights of choice and personal control, or whether she is being grossly unfair to her caring husband and manifesting a negative mental health status that should be investigated and treated?

Case History 35.5 D

D, a 26-year-old woman, suffered a cervical fracture in a road-traffic accident. From early in her rehabilitation she stated her desire to go home as soon as possible.

Home for D was a semi-detached council house in a rural area, with her mother and adult brother, six cats, two parakeets and at least eight dogs. Home visits by the social worker and occupational therapist reported a very low standard of hygiene and housekeeping but an overwhelming feeling of warmth and love towards D, and a strong desire to have her home.

Accordingly, D was discharged, with all agencies alerted to the potential problems but respecting her wishes. Community nurses visit twice weekly, the general practitioner monthly, and the social worker on a regular basis. Readmission could be very promptly organised if necessary, but 9 months after discharge, all is well.

Case History 35.6 R

R, a 42-year-old man, married with two daughters, was involved in a road-traffic accident that caused paraplegia. He had to stay in his rehabilitation unit for 14 months because no suitable accommodation could be found in the town where he lived.

This inspired him to become active in fighting for the rights of disabled people and he has written books on both housing and sports for the disabled. A great fund raiser, he also set up many PHAB (physically handicapped and able bodied) clubs and would visit any newly spinal-injured person in his area to give support and encouragement.

Fiercely independent, he only recently had his first re-admission for treatment of a shoulder pain which was beginning to affect his lifestyle; the cost of an active life in pursuit of independence for himself and others over the last 20 years.

Medical status

Traditionally, medical status in the community is assessed by self-referral to a general practitioner when a problem already exists, or by checking into an out-patient department at intervals increasing in length and ranging from 3 months to 1 year, following discharge. This system does not allow for the early detection of potential problems.

Departments of rehabilitation have been given the task of breaking down barriers between hospital and primary health-care teams, so 'demonstration' centres have been created and resettlement or liaison nurses appointed. A demonstration centre should not only function as a centre of excellence but as a resource to the community, providing information, education, equipment and problem solving of many kinds. Changes in the medical status of patients can be reported and discussed on a day-to-day basis and, ideally, prompt interventions may avoid the need for readmission to hospital.

Economic productivity

The Tunbridge and Mair Reports in 1972 suggested that the DHSS should take over the work of industrial rehabilitation. However, the creation of the Manpower Services Commission has perpetuated the division between medical and industrial rehabilitation and therefore represents another area where collaboration is a necessary key to success.

Occupational therapy units may prepare the disabled for community life by teaching driving, computer, and other technical skills but the post-discharge picture for many is still quite bleak.

In 1987 Hudson surveyed 'disabled people who were on the dole'. Although the 1944 Disabled Persons (Employment) Act requires all firms employing more than 20 people to employ 3% of their labour force from the disabled persons register, it is not being implemented particularly well. He found three barriers to success:

- failure of the disabled person to register
- failure of firms to comply
- failure of Manpower Services Commission to enforce the Act.

In 1981 the Independent Living Movement described the ability to live productively, not only in terms of gainful employment, but also in terms of other contributions made to community and family life.

CONCLUSION

This chapter has shown that success in rehabilitation depends on many factors, social, political, economic, environmental and personal. Attitudes are crucial. The able bodied have been described as friends or foes, as allies of disabled people or as patronising oppressors. In their own words (Box 35.4) disabled people are presenting us, individually and collectively, with many challenges. Where do you stand: friend or foe?

? **35.13**

a. Investigate rehabilitation provision in the locality. Visit a Disabled Living Centre or an Employment Retraining Centre.
b. Study the role of several specialist rehabilitation nurses, for example:
   - mastectomy nurse
   - stoma nurse
   - spinal injury liaison nurse
   - neuro-rehabilitation nurse.
c. Study disability experientially, for example:
   - wear special lenses that simulate a visual impairment
   - go shopping in a wheelchair
   - eat, using only one hand — your left, if you are right-handed
   - try washing and dressing with only one hand.
d. Critically evaluate the patient-versus-client role.
e. Work with other professionals in the multidisciplinary team.
f. Attend a multidisciplinary team meeting.
g. Attend a care conference.
h. Secure a relationship with a family which contains a disabled member.
i. Lobby your MP or councillor about any handicapping situations that become apparent.
j. Read a biography of a severely disabled person, for example:
   - Hurley G (1983) Lucky break? Milestone Publications, Horndean
   - Hahn D (1984) The story of Margaret Price. Barker, London
   - Chevigny H (1962) My eyes have a cold nose. Yale University Press, New Haven

Box 35.4 Friend or foe? (Reproduced with kind permission from *New Internationalist* (1992) 233: 14–15)

Ask exactly what you can do if you want to help a disabled person — and listen to the reply. We know our needs best. Never help us without asking first whether your help is wanted. And don't expect us to be eternally grateful to you for the help you do offer . . .

Acknowledge our differences. For many disabled people our difference is an important part of our identity. Don't assume that our one wish in life is to be 'normal' or imagine that it is 'progressive' or 'liberal' to ignore our differences.

Respect our privacy and our need for independence. Don't assume that because we are disabled you can ask us more personal questions than you would a non-disabled person.

Think about the way society creates barriers for us. Take account of the social and economic context in which we experience our medical condition. But don't reduce us to our medical conditions. Why should it matter to you what our condition is called?

Challenge patronising attitudes towards us. We want your empathy not your pity. Putting us on a pedestal or telling us how 'wonderful' and 'heroic' we are does not help. This attitude often conceals the judgement that having an impairment is intolerable — which is very undermining for us.

Recognise our existence. A gaze can express recognition and warmth. Talk to us directly. Neither stare at us — nor immediately look away either. And never talk about us as if we weren't there.

Realise that we are sexual beings, with the same wishes, needs and desire for fulfilling relationships as non-disabled people. Don't assume that we will never have children. And if a disabled person has a non-disabled lover don't jump to the conclusion that the latter is either a saint or has an ulterior motive.

Appreciate the contribution that we make to society in the fields of work, politics and culture. We engage in these activities for the same reasons as you do — but we may have some different insights to offer. Don't assume that we are passive — or that our activities are a form of 'therapy' to take our mind off our disability. Most disabled people are financially hard up and so we may have a greater need to earn a living than you.

REFERENCES

Belanger L, Bolduc M, Noel M 1988 Relative importance of after effects, environment and socio-economic factors on the social integration of stroke victims. International Journal of Rehabilitation Research 11(3): 251–260

Black D (Chairman) 1980 Inequalities in health. HMSO, London

Blunkett D 1985 Partnership, participation and power: psychology and physical disability in the NHS. British Psychological Society, Leicester, Preface

Boore J R P 1978 Prescription for recovery. RCN, London

Brown C 1954 My left foot. Reprinted 1972 The childhood story of Christy Brown. Pan, London

Chamberlain M A 1989 Editorial: What is rehabilitation? British Journal of Hospital Medicine 41(4): 311

Chevigny H 1962 My eyes have a cold nose. Yale University Press, New Haven

Chow R, Harrison J, Dornan J 1989 Prevention and rehabilitation of osteoporosis program: exercise and osteoporosis. International Journal of Rehabilitation 12(1): 49–56

De Charms R 1968 Personal causation. New York Academic Press, New York

Disabled Persons (Employment) Act 1944 HMSO, London

Duckworth D 1982 The classification and measurement of disablement. HMSO, London

Engel G 1964 Grief and grieving. In: Schwartz L, Schwartz S (eds) The psychodynamics of patient care. Prentice Hall, New York

Evans C D 1982 Rehabilitation in multiple sclerosis. In: Capildeo R, Maxwell A (eds) Progress in rehabilitation. Macmillan, Basingstoke

Ewing G 1989 The nursing preparation of stoma patients for self-care. Journal of Advanced Nursing 14(5): 411–420

Fink S L 1967 Crisis and motivation: a theoretical model. Archives Physical Medicine and Rehabilitation 48(11): 592–597

Geddes J M L, Clayden A D, Chamberlain M A 1989 The Leeds Family Placement Scheme: an evaluation of its use as a rehabilitation resource. (In press)

Gibbon B 1991 A reassessment of nurses' attitudes towards stroke patients in general medical wards. Journal of Advanced Nursing 16(11): 1336–1342

Goffman E 1968 Stigma. Penguin, Harmondsworth

Gunther M S 1971 Psychiatric consultation in a rehabilitation hospital: a regression hypothesis. Comp. Psychiatry 12(6): 572–585

Guttman L 1976 Spinal cord injuries. Blackwell, Oxford

Hahn H 1983 Paternalism and public policy. Society (March–April): 36–46

Halstead L S, Grabois M (eds) 1985 Medical rehabilitation. Raven Press, New York

Hames A, Stirling E 1987 Choice aids recovery. Nursing Times 25 83(8) : 49–51

Hamilton Lady W M 1984 Am I living in the right place? The distribution of Health Care. The Harding Award. RADAR, London

Hayward J C 1975 Information: a prescription against pain. Royal College of Nursing, London

Henderson V 1966 Basic principles of nursing care. International Council of Nurses, Geneva

Henderson V, Nite G 1978 Principles and practice of nursing. Macmillan, London

Hirschberg G G, Lewis L, Vaughan P 1976 Rehabilitation p 5 Lippincott, Philadelphia

House R J 1971 A path goal theory of leader effectiveness. Administrative Science Quarterly 16(3)

Hudson B 1987 Disabled on the dole. Health Service Journal 97(5069): 1110–1111

Hurley G 1983 Lucky Break? Milestone, Horndean

Jennett B 1987 Decisions to limit treatment. Lancet 8562(2): 787–789

Kallio V 1982 Medical and social problems of the disabled. Euro Reports, WHO, Copenhagen

Kubler-Ross E 1974 Questions and answers on death and dying. Macmillan, New York

Lambert J 1985 Adjusting to tetraplegia. Nursing Times 981(6): 32–33

Lawes C 1984 Pressure sore readmission for spinal injured people. Care 4(2): 4–8

Maguire G P, Lee E G, Bevington D J, Küchemann C S, Crabtree R J & Cornell C E 1978 Psychiatric problems in the first year after mastectomy. British Medical Journal 1: 963–965

Mair A (Chairman) 1972 Medical rehabilitation: the pattern for the future. HMSO, Edinburgh

Maslow A H 1954 Motivation and personality. Harper & Row, New York

McColl I 1986 Physical disability, 1986 and beyond. Royal College of Physicians, London

Morris A The Chronically Sick and Disabled Act 1970 Private Member's Bill. HMSO, London

Nieuwenhuis R 1989 Breaking the speech barrier. Nursing Times 85(15): 34–36

Norton D, McLaren R, Exton-Smith A N 1975 An investigation of geriatric nursing problems in hospital. Churchill Livingstone, Edinburgh

Orem D E 1980 Nursing: concepts of practice. McGraw-Hill, New York

Parsons T 1951 The social system. The Free Press, Glencoe, Illinois

Pires M 1989 Ethical perspective: a nursing reaction to 'Tom's Story'. Rehabilitation Nursing 14(5): 255–256

Porter L W, Lawler E E 1968 Managerial attitudes and performance. Irwin-Dorsey, Illinois, p 16

Prince of Wales Advisory Group on Disability 1985. Living options. London

Richardson S A 1976 Attitudes and behaviour towards the physically handicapped. Birth Defects, Original Article Series 12: 15–34

Roy C W, Arthurs Y, Hunter J, Parker S & McLaren A 1988 Work of a rehabilitation medicine service. British Medical Journal 297: 601–604

Rubin Z, Peplau L 1975 Who believes in a just world? Journal of Social Issues 31: 65–89

Seligman M E P 1975 Helplessness. Freeman, San Francisco

Shearer A 1981 Disability: whose handicap? Blackwell, Oxford

Sutherland A T 1981 Disabled we stand. Souvenir Press, London

Tunbridge R (Chairman) 1972 Rehabilitation. HMSO, London

Waterlow J A 1985 Risk assessment card. Nursing Times, London

WHO 1980 International classification of impairments, disabilities and handicaps. WHO, Geneva

Wright J 1988 Trolley full of trouble. Nursing Times 84(9): 24–26

FURTHER READING

Beardshaw V 1988 Last on the list: community services for people with physical disabilities. King's Fund, London

Beardshaw V 1989 The Griffiths White Paper: hints to fill the gap. Health Service Journal, 99(5171): 1224

Bender A E, Brooks L J 1987 Body weight control. Churchill Livingstone, Edinburgh

Butler R J, Rosenthal G 1985 Behaviour and rehabilitation: behavioural treatment for long-stay patients. Wright, Bristol

Chevigny H My eyes have a cold nose. Yale University Press, New Haven

Coutts L C, Hardy L K 1985 Teaching for health: the nurse as health educator. Churchill Livingstone, Edinburgh

Dettenmeier P A 1990 Planning for successful home mechanical ventilation. Critical Care Nursing 1(2): 267–279

Ewles L, Simnett I 1991 Promoting health: a practical guide, 2nd edn. Wiley, Chichester

Gilbert S 1986 The psychology of eating: psychology and treatment. Routledge & Kegan Paul, London

Heslop A P, Bagnall P 1988 A study to evaluate the intervention of a nurse visiting patients with disabling chest disease in the community. Journal of Advanced Nursing 13(1): 71–77

Jamieson E M, McCall J M, Blythe R 1991 Guidelines for clinical nursing practices, 2nd edn. Churchill Livingstone, Edinburgh
Johnstone M 1987 Home care for the stroke patient. Churchill Livingstone, Edinburgh
Lake T, Acheson F 1988 Room to listen: a beginner's guide to analysis, therapy and counselling. Bedford Square Press, London
Newton T, Butler N M, Dawson J 1989 Engagement levels on a unit for people with a physical disability. Clinical Rehabilitation 3: 299–304
Oliver M 1988 Flexible services. Nursing Times 84(14): 25–29
Pentland B, Miller J D 1988 Head injury rehabilitation: 4-years experience in Edinburgh. British Journal of Neurosurgery 2(1): 61–65
Royal College of Nursing 1991 The role of the nurse in rehabilitation of elderly people. Scutari, London
Royal College of Nursing 1992 The guide to the handling of patients, 3rd edn. The National Back Pain Association in collaboration with the RCN, London
Shearer A 1981 Disability: whose handicap? Blackwell, Oxford
Vaughan R 1991 Manual handling of loads. Proposals for regulations and guidance. Health and Safety Executive, London
Waters K 1987 The role of nursing in rehabilitation care — science and practice. 5(3): 17–21

USEFUL ADDRESSES

Disabled Living Foundation
380–384 Harrow Road
London W9 2HU

Disability Rights Handbook
Disability Alliance ERA
25 Denmark St
London WC2H 8NJ

Holiday Care Service
2 Old Bank Chambers
Srahon Road
Horley
Surrey RH6 9HW

RADAR (Royal Association for Disability and Rehabilitation)
25 Mortimer St
London W1N 8AB

SPOD (Association to Promote the Sexual and Personal Relationships of People with Disabilities)
286 Camden Road
London N7 OBJ
Tel. 071 607 8851

CHAPTER 36

The older person

E. S. Farmer

CHAPTER CONTENTS

Introduction 959

Caring 959
Story-telling 960
Caring for older persons 961
A social problem? 961
Promoting health 961
A caring community? 962

Caring in action 963
Confusion and vulnerability 963
Commentary: Case History 36.1 963
Reducing vulnerability 963
'Taking care of patients' 963
Respect for persons 963
The right to independence 965
Commentary: Case History 36.2 965
The caring dilemma 965
Harmonising curing and caring 967
The challenge of severe disability 967
Commentary: Case History 36.3 967
Spiritual caring 968
Caring and the family 969
Commentary: Case History 36.4 969
Attitudes toward death 969
Family care-giving 969
The context of caring 969

Conclusion 969

References 971

Further reading 972

INTRODUCTION

For the complete life, the perfect pattern includes old age as well as youth and maturity. The beauty of the morning and the radiance of noon are good, but it would be a very silly person who drew the curtains and turned on the light in order to shut out the tranquillity of the evening. Old age has its pleasures, which, though different, are not less than the pleasures of youth. (W. Somerset Maugham, *The Summing Up*)

This chapter is based in the view that learning in nursing is a journey which starts with personal experiences of life and is facilitated by human caring. Teachers, therefore, need to be problem-posers, consultants, and nurturers of curiosity, inquiry, caring and interpretation (Bevis & Watson 1989). Students should not expect from this chapter a prescriptive account of how to nurse elderly people, for nursing care cannot be fully prescribed apart from the situation and the moment in which it is to be offered. It is, however, possible to identify likely *patterns* of caring and to describe these by means of narrative accounts of patients' experiences and of the nursing interventions taken in response to those experiences.

The first sections of the chapter set out the general principles of caring which inform holistic nursing practice. The second half of the chapter demonstrates through a series of Case Histories and accompanying commentaries how those principles might be applied. Throughout the chapter it is argued that the essential needs of elderly people are no different from those of any other group. But if the adoption of humanistic nursing practice seems a matter of particular urgency for elderly patients, perhaps it is because older people have typically been marginalised within a society that tends to view old age as an illness and to value cure above care.

CARING

Caring is the essence of holistic nursing practice. It implies relating to patients as complex persons with intrinsic worth, rather than as a collection of disorders and disabilities. The intention in this chapter is to focus on those aspects of nursing which have enormous healing power but which tend to be devalued in a society dominated by technology and economics. Love, hope, empathy, compassion, conscience, and commitment are some of the elements of holistic nursing which this chapter will try to highlight through accounts of caring in action.

Watson (1988) defines caring as:

the moral ideal of nursing whereby the end is protection, enhancement, and preservation of human dignity. Human caring involves values, a will, and a commitment to care, knowledge, caring actions, and consequences. All of human caring is related to intersubjective human response to health–illness; environmental–personal interaction; a knowledge of the nursing caring process, self knowledge, knowledge of one's power and transaction limitations.

According to Benner (1985), caring reflects interpersonal concern and liking so that the other person's plight and fate matters to the one who cares. Caring is possible only from an involved stance and sets up the conditions whereby significant details are noticed. Caring by its nature does not seek to control or master but to facilitate understanding and uncover possibilities inherent in the situation. Caring is thus contextual and empowering.

The disciplines of natural science reduce life to separate variables and processes, any of which can be studied apart from the others. Humanistic science, on the other hand, views life as a composite of multiple, inseparable realities that are irreducible and can only be studied holistically. Nursing practice synthesises natural and humanistic science in its response to human experiences. Carper (1978) supports this view through her argument that nurses need four types of knowledge, namely:

- scientific knowledge of human behaviour in health and illness
- the aesthetic perception of significant human experiences
- a personal understanding of the unique individuality of the self
- the capacity to make ethical choices within concrete situations involving particular moral judgements.

Nurses generally have no difficulty describing the biological components of their discipline, but often have trouble defining and describing the aesthetic, ethical and personal elements of nursing. Peplau (1988, p. 10) has described the blending of these components of nursing in the following way:

> Art is always an expressive response, a statement of what the artist sees, said in the artist's way, with great pride in the necessary craftmanship, and in the case of nursing, often for an audience of one. The unique blend of ideals, values, integrity, and commitment to the well-being of others, expressed in a nurse's self-presentation and responses to clients, makes each nurse a one-of-a-kind artist in nursing practice. Thus, the art of nursing is always pluralistic, characterized by great diversity and variety of nurse in action, and in this aspect is not replicable, from one situation to another, even by the same nurse.
>
> The art of nursing is highly personal, always imprecise, and nonscientific. Its language is behavior, ideally directed by the highest values of the human community, internally held by the nurse. Art is not bound by limits except for the nurse's conscience and the profession's ethics. A nomenclature to classify nursing's art is not possible. This aesthetic component is influenced by the style, taste, personality, and habits of both nurse and client and by the reactions of each to the expressions of the other.

Caring in nursing is concerned with relieving the vulnerability experienced by individuals as a consequence of illness, injury and disability (Gadow 1988, Leininger 1988, Watson 1988) as well as with promoting health. As Carper (1978) has suggested, the care which is provided should result from the sensitive blending of knowledge from both humanistic and natural science. Thus optimism, compassion and empathy can be called upon to moderate actions that might otherwise be based solely on empirical data or motivated by ritual adherence to idealised norms. To develop the 'artistic' and 'ethical' components of nursing demands, of course, the engagement of the nurse's *self* as expressed through body movement, tone of voice, eye contact, facial expression, and touch (Benner & Wrubel 1989, Watson 1988, Peplau 1988).

Gaut (1991, p. 5) argues that caring is a stance of respect for all living things that requires knowledge, trust, hope, honesty, and courage:

> If you define yourself as a caring person, then your responsibility is to develop your capacity to experience the other person and be receptive to that person's needs. Caring is a natural way to relate to another human being, and in that relating, both persons become more human.

Story-telling

Somerset Maugham's perspective on old age, expressed in the introductory quotation, points to a conception of life as a continuous narrative in which the meanings we attach to our experiences are crucial to how we exist in the world and to the effectiveness of the relationships we have with significant persons in our lives. In this view, life experiences are intelligible only in terms of the personal biography of the individual. As this living narrative unfolds, past and present experiences illuminate one another and give new meaning to the whole; thus, there can be no separation of persons into parts or of lives into stages. When this view is applied to holistic nursing practice, prediction and explanation do not *precede* caring, but *evolve from* the sensitive practice of nursing.

Human virtues (such as courage, strength and honesty) underpin every human activity, inquiry, and practice. These virtues dispose us to act and feel in particular ways within a given context, that is, within the flow of events — the enacted story — which constitutes every human life (Macintyre 1981). The virtues exhibited by an individual's character and actions constitute a complex moral unity which must be considered as a whole. They must also be considered within a wider sociocultural context: some qualities are prized more than others, depending upon culture and related social structures. Human behaviour cannot be characterised independently of the settings which make an individual's intentions intelligible both to himself and to others (Macintyre 1981).

We make sense of human experience by framing events and experiences in terms of a history or narrative. Narrative accounts of events are the chief means of moral education (Macintyre 1981) and are of critical importance for the interpretation of human behaviour. Sandelowski (1991) has argued that the current emphasis on story-telling in nursing marks a movement away from scientific reductionism, which views persons as no more than the sum of their parts, towards relativism and holism. In the context of health care provision this shift in perspective demands that the problems which patients encounter are no longer seen in the narrow terms of the biomedical model. From this shift also emerges an important distinction between *disease* and *illness*.

Disease refers to pathophysiological processes. Illness refers to the innately human experience of symptoms and suffering which are manifestations of disease. As Kleinman (1988, p. 6) notes:

> When chest pain can be reduced to a treatable acute lobar pneumonia, . . . biological reductionism is an enormous success. When chest pain is reduced to chronic artery disease for which calcium blockers and nitroglycerine are prescribed, while the patient's fear, the family's frustration, the job conflict, the sexual impotence, and the financial crisis go undiagnosed and unaddressed, [the biomedical model] is a failure.

An individual's experience of illness will, in part, be determined by culture. Within his social environment certain expectations will prevail as to how someone who is ill will or should behave. At the same time, the individual's responses will be shaped by his personal biography and by his unique character (Kleinman 1988).

Illness can be brief and minimally disruptive, or long-term and much more threatening. In either case, illness results in vulnerability and loss of control (Benner 1985). Nursing is concerned with reducing the patient's vulnerability, primarily through understanding the significance that his illness has for him and reducing the frustrating consequences of disability. This can be achieved through strengthening contact with social support, rekindling hope and aspirations, and enhancing independence (Roach 1987, Gadow 1988, Benner 1985, Kleinman 1988). This is particularly important in chronic illnesses which offer little or no hope of cure and challenge the individual to find new and satisfying ways of being in the world.

Our personal life histories influence our perceptions of situations, and give meaning and intelligibility to our experiences and our interactions with others. It is the nurse's task to be sensitive to the reality that has been created by each patient's personal biography, and to help him make sense of the experience of illness within his evolving view of the world.

Caring for older persons

An understanding of the lived experience of growing older is crucial to our ability to care for elderly patients. Lacking the direct experience of ageing herself, the student nurse may nonetheless gain invaluable insight by reading fictional accounts of old age. Wolf (1987) commends May Sarton's depiction of the experience of ageing in her novel *Kinds of Love*, which tells the story of a group of individuals facing the challenges of shared personal growth, creativity and mortality. One particularly sensitive passage describes a conversation between two elderly people, Christina and Eben. Eben declares that Christina 'grows more beautiful every day'; Christina, in response, says that she 'is getting to be a wrinkled old apple'. Christina's self-perception is not shared by Eben, who tells her, 'Don't look into mirrors, look into people's eyes. . . . After a certain age mirrors lie . . . they give the bare facts all right, but they leave out the poetry.'

In caring for older people the nurse must endeavour not to 'leave out the poetry'; she must always bear in mind that the frailty of the flesh is often at odds with the spirit underneath. As St Exupery's (1943) Little Prince learned, 'it is only with the heart that one sees rightly, what is essential is invisible to the eye'.

A social problem?

Census data show that there has been a gradual ageing of the United Kingdom population since the turn of the century. Decreased mortality and fertility rates are responsible for this change, which is in fact a feature of all Western societies. In the next decade, the number of elderly persons over 75 years of age is expected to increase significantly, while those in the age group 65–74 will be proportionately reduced (WHO/ICN 1988, Redfern 1991).

In the face of this demographic shift, there has been an unfortunate tendency in Western society to view its elderly population as a social problem rather than as an asset. Largely for economic reasons, society has attached chronological markers to the process of ageing, with old age being that part of the life cycle which begins at the statutory age of retirement. Age has become an important criterion for establishing social status and, implicitly, rights and obligations. Social status is defined largely by wealth, power and prestige (Yurick et al 1980). It has been argued that the close association between wealth and power means that elderly people have little impact on social trends and limited ability to control their own destinies and lifestyles (Victor 1987). Because the ability to work and to generate wealth is a major determinant of prestige, enforced retirement consigns elderly people to a low position in the social pecking order (Victor 1987).

The majority of elderly people in the UK are on low incomes, and it is unfortunate that the greatest material poverty is associated with extreme old age, a period when, paradoxically, expenses tend to be greatest (Evers 1991). The prevailing image of the elderly person is one of a dependent individual lacking social autonomy — a person who is powerless, unloved and neglected, and a burden on society because he consumes scarce resources but contributes nothing to the creation of wealth (Victor 1987, Redfern 1991). This view of old age as a period of stagnation and decline has been challenged by, among others, Altschul (1986), who decries the belief that elderly people are a burden on society. Rather, she argues, the current 'young elderly' provide a pool of unpaid carers for the oldest old, represent a large consumer group in commerce, travel, and education, and are the mainstay of many voluntary organisations. What would happen, Altschul asks, if the young elderly unpaid carers withdrew their charitable services and invested their time and energy campaigning for more rights and better pensions? Who would fill the gaps created by the unpaid labour force? How would a switch from voluntary to paid care be financed? What effect would increased spending power of elderly people have on health, welfare, and the economy? It is clear that prevailing notions of the 'dependent' status of the elderly population need to be re-examined.

The nurse should bear in mind that by stereotyping elderly people she will distort the professional–patient relationship and inhibit her ability to act therapeutically. She should also consider whether her attitudes toward elderly people reflect a personal fear of growing old. For many people, old age conjures up images of disease, disability, powerlessness, uselessness and death. Age need not, however, be a barrier to health and well-being. In spite of social and political discrimination, most elderly people live independent lives in the community.

Promoting health

In 1988, the World Health Organization (WHO) and the International Council of Nurses (ICN) produced a joint publication setting out programmes for nursing and health promotion for elderly people. In this document it was stressed that when the societies in which older people live have negative views about ageing and being old, the older people themselves are likely to have negative perceptions of themselves and their social roles. One of the main tasks of nursing is therefore to promote, primarily through caring, unconditional positive regard for elderly people.

The WHO/ICN report (1988) works from a definition of health as a state of complete physical, mental and social well-being rather than merely the absence of disease. It could be argued that if this definition were applied within the context of the biomedical model it would effectively mean that *no one* is healthy. It is important to appreciate that health is a relative concept and as such has personal meanings. The WHO/ICN report also tends to define the needs of elderly persons with reference to what they *cannot* do rather than what they *can* do. There is a danger that this approach will reinforce negative attitudes toward elderly people and overlook the potential for personal growth in old age.

Caution should also be exerted in any attempt to define health needs in elderly persons in terms of functional capacity using scales which aim to identify and measure deficits in physical and mental ability and the relationship of these to social functioning. In this approach norms are established for activities such as eating, dressing, walking, standing, and eliminating (e.g. Mahoney & Barthel 1965, Robinson et al 1986). Needs are assumed from the manifestation of certain behaviours relative to these norms. While this approach has some value in shifting the focus from disease to the impact of the disease on the person's lifestyle, it can have the effect of emphasising deficits rather than identifying possibilities for the enhancement of quality of life. Moreover, if an older person fails to perform at the expected level on a particular scale then he is described as disabled and is labelled accordingly. Diagnostic labels are often a means of identifying those individuals who are eligible for financial benefit. But labels can disempower individuals by implying that they occupy a marginal position within society and can therefore be given low priority in the provision of resources.

The requirements for well-being among older people are not necessarily different from those that apply to persons in other age groups. Family and community support, appropriate housing, adequate income, nutritious food in appropriate amounts, and screening and basic health services are identified in the joint WHO/ICN report (1988) as being of critical importance for health for everyone. The health of individuals within a society is in large measure determined by standards of, for example, nutrition, education, housing, and income. There is a prevailing notion, nonetheless, that the individual, not society, is responsible for health, that is, that illness is somehow a failure of the individual to stay well regardless of all the socioeconomic and environmental influences on his well-being (Gott & O'Brien 1990). Rather than regarding ill-health as a personal failure, however, it is more productive to assist individuals to attain or maintain good health through the provision of appropriate resources, including knowledge on how to achieve and maintain healthy lifestyles. Over the years, increasing emphasis has been placed on health promotion among older people through such means as individual counselling on diet and exercise, social clubs, keep-fit classes, art, dance, and drama classes, and further education programmes.

Health is contextual: it cannot be viewed solely as an individual achievement. Changing unhealthy lifestyles requires an examination of existing concerns, habits and skills within a social context in order to understand the relevant issues and any existing barriers to change. Health promotion also involves an exploration of the potential strengths and possibilities offered by the person's perspective on his own situation (Benner & Wrubel 1989).

Older people have essentially the same needs as others in society. Biological changes that occur with ageing may not of themselves be problematic; it may only be when disease is superimposed on such changes that vulnerability is experienced. Assessment of needs for nursing care should take account of these changes but they should be kept in their proper perspective; being old is neither a disease nor an illness.

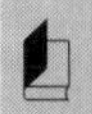

For descriptions of the changes associated with ageing see Redfern 1991 and Carnevali & Patrick 1979.

A caring community?

Community care is defined (Griffiths 1988) as providing the services and support which people who are affected by problems of ageing, mental illness, mental handicap or physical or sensory disability need to be able to live as independently as possible in their own homes, or in home-like settings in the community. The Government's community care proposals (Griffiths 1988) have six key objectives for service delivery:

- to promote the development of domiciliary day and respite services to enable people to live in their own homes wherever this is feasible and sensible
- to ensure that service providers make practical support for carers a high priority
- to make proper assessment of need and good case management the cornerstone of high quality care
- to promote the development of a flourishing independent sector alongside good quality public services
- to clarify the responsibilities of agencies and to make it easier to hold them to account for their performance
- to secure better value for taxpayers' money by introducing a new funding structure for social care.

? **36.1** While it would be difficult to argue against the principles implicit in the Griffiths report, questions need to be asked about how its objectives can best be met. Will the funds made available to implement the proposals be adequate? How is the assessment of need to be carried out, and by whom? What role will charitable organisations and families be expected to play in meeting any financial deficits? How is care provision to be monitored. Explore these issues with your colleagues, using the relevant texts from the Reference and Further Reading lists.

While stressing the importance of families in providing care for dependent elderly people, the WHO/ICN report (1988) highlights the fact that in Western societies families are small and often scattered. This means that responsibility for care will necessarily extend beyond family affiliations. In any case, as Dalley (1988) has argued, the familial mode of care may be somewhat idealistic. Divorce, marriage and cohabitation have produced many complex relationships and living arrangements. Dalley argues that there is a need for a societal alternative to the family unit which could provide care without self-sacrifice and would be flexible and responsive to individual needs. Dalley also argues that certain beliefs about the caring processes need to be re-examined in order to avoid major errors in policy and planning. In this connection, a distinction must be made between 'caring for' (tending another) and 'caring about' (having feelings for another). Dalley holds that these two processes are not necessarily equivalent. Caring *about* a dependent loved one does not necessarily imply a willingness to perform certain caring tasks for him. In support of this argument, Dalley refers to Ungerson's (1983) work which proposes that caring functions often require a transgressing of gender, age and sexual boundaries, creating tensions in relationships and disturbing the sensibilities of all involved.

According to Dalley (1988), the confusion of 'caring for' and 'caring about' may have devastating consequences. On the one hand, she argues, love often becomes fractured and distorted by feelings of obligation, burden and frustration. On the other, the assumption that kinship is a precondition for caring implies that professional carers are unable to 'care about' as well as to 'care for' dependent people.

? **36.2** Would you agree that Dalley's view (1988) runs counter to the humanistic philosophy of caring, which stresses connectedness, not individuality, and our moral obligation to care for one another? Why or why not?

CARING IN ACTION

The foregoing discussion provides a basis for the analysis of the examples of the nursing care of elderly people which follow. These Case Histories will illustrate the complexity of caring for older people who have been made vulnerable by chronic illness and highlight the need for the four types of knowledge described by Carper (1978; see p. 960) and others. At the beginning of this chapter, students were urged to view their learning as a journey. What has been provided here is barely a route map. The exploration which is part of the journey of learning to care for elderly people demands that students read widely as well as develop the skills of 'presencing' (see p. 965): sharing with elderly people their illness experience.

Confusion and vulnerability

Commentary: Case History 36.1

Reducing vulnerability

From a strictly biomedical perspective, the immediate concerns relating to Miss W.'s condition were:

- confusion
- alteration in the pattern of micturition
- altered mobility
- altered sleep patterns.

These problems resulted in maladaptive coping and in impairment of self-care responses and home management.

Confusion is a term which is often applied in nursing to describe patients whose behaviour does not conform to social expectations. In applying this term, however, the nurse should remember that behaviour can only be understood in context. It has been argued that confusion is a term which should be limited to the description of conditions which are temporary, have an identifiable cause, and are reversible (Open University 1988). The causes of confusion in older people are many and include brain injury, certain medications, sudden loss, environmental change, and system disorders such as respiratory infection, cardiac failure and renal disease. The distinction between acute and chronic confusional states is usually made in terms of time of onset. Acute confusion has a relatively sudden onset (days or weeks), whereas chronic confusional states develop more slowly (over months or even years).

In Miss W.'s situation the classification is difficult to apply and once more highlights the danger of labelling patients (see p. 962). The GP suspected dementia and responded with sedatives while awaiting expert advice. Dementia is a clinical syndrome in which there is acquired, persistent intellectual impairment with compromise in at least three of the following spheres of activity (Cummings 1980):

- language
- memory
- visuospatial skills
- personality / affect
- cognition (abstraction, judgement, mathematics etc.).

The emphasis on dementia as a clinical syndrome reinforces the idea that it is not a specific diagnosis but a constellation of signs of intellectual compromise that must be investigated to rule out irreversible as well as reversible causes (Shapira et al 1986). The two most common forms of dementia are Alzheimer-type (in which there is extensive brain cell loss, the causes of which are not yet known) and multiinfarct-type (which, as the name suggests, is caused by interruption of the blood supply resulting in multiple small infarcted areas of tissue throughout the cerebral cortex).

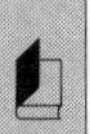
For a description of the care required by patients suffering from these disorders see Norman (1990) and Jacques (1988).

'Taking care of patients'

Since to give care to patients against their will is to commit the offence of battery, the time spent persuading Miss W. to stay and steering her away from the door has to be examined carefully. In their guidelines, the Mental Health Act (1983) Commissioners have tried to steer a middle course between the principle of the inviolable nature of the human body and the protection of the incompetent patient's interests. This position, however, is not at all clear-cut. Each situation needs to be judged as it arises by the professionals involved.

Hirsch & Harris (1988) have argued that respect for persons, which underpins nursing practice, has two dimensions, namely concern for the individual's welfare, and respect for his wishes. These two dimensions are usually complementary, but tension may arise between them, creating a dilemma. As Hirsch & Harris (1988, p. 41) see it, 'the problem for all who care about others is how to reconcile respect for the free choices of others with real concern for their welfare when their choices appear to be self-destructive or self-harming.' This emphasis on autonomy would be interpreted by Benner & Wrubel (1989) as extreme individualism posing a threat to health. This alternative view is based in the belief that the ultimate goal in human development is to care and feel cared for and that this caring implies involvement and interdependence.

The law is faced with the challenge of reconciling these opposing concerns for the autonomy of individuals on the one hand and for their protection on the other. In law, 'the fundamental principle, plain and incontestable, is that every person's body is inviolate' (Sullivan 1988, p. 37). The courts would disavow this principle only if they were satisfied that sufficient measures had been taken to protect the person's interests within the limits imposed by his incapability (Sullivan 1988). Common law is supplemented by statute law, which defines the circumstances under which consent for treatment, as defined in the Mental Health Act 1983, may be dispensed with. Murphy (1988) argues that the legalistic approach to the dilemmas of professional practice of caring for people judged to be incompetent gives no practical help in the day-to-day problems of treating incapable patients.

There are a number of important factors in Miss W.'s situation which influenced the giving of nursing care. In the first instance, fragmentation of services and poor communication among disciplines has left considerable gaps in knowledge of Miss W.'s life. The medical notes, containing only a brief introductory note from her GP, arrived in the ward only on the morning of admission. Only the briefest biographical history had been given to the ward sister by the niece, who made it clear that her mother was not fit to cope any longer and must have a rest. The niece's interpretation of Miss W.'s behaviour, and her subsequent actions, were based on the GP's provisional diagnosis of 'dementia'. Also, Miss W. had been told that she was going to the hairdresser. It is hardly surprising that she reacted as she did on arrival in the ward. Miss W.'s experience of hospitals can be inferred from her comments about the 'workhouse'. She perceived the situation as a threatening one, and in that context her behaviour could be considered quite reasonable.

Respect for persons

'Taking care' of people does not necessarily amount to genuine caring. In providing only physical care it is possible to view the

Case History 36.1

Miss W. is 76 years old and unmarried. She was admitted for respite care to a 30-bed ward in a continuing care unit for elderly people. Her admission had been arranged over the telephone by her general practitioner (GP) and the consultant physician in geriatric medicine. Miss W. had lived for a year with her widowed sister, who was 80 years old and had a married daughter living nearby, and a son living some 400 miles away. Miss W. had a history of hypertension which did not warrant medication and was prone to dizzy spells. She also suffered from osteoarthritis and walked with the aid of a stick. The arthritic pain was controlled through the administration of ibuprofen 400 mg 3 times daily.

Miss W. had gone to live with her sister because she was having difficulty getting out of the house and generally coping with the day-to-day activities of living. Increasingly in the 6 months prior to admission she had become verbally abusive towards her sister, had wandered about the house incessantly, was neglectful of her personal care, and had developed nocturnal urinary incontinence. (See Carnevali & Patrick 1979 and Redfern 1991 for discussions of these problems.) The GP prescribed night sedation, but this had little effect and appeared to increase the behavioural symptoms. Offers of community nursing services had been rejected.

Miss W. was driven to hospital by her niece. On arrival in the ward, she was verbally abusive and lashed out at the nurses with her stick. It very quickly became clear that she had not been told she was going to hospital for respite care. She thought she was only going to the hairdresser. The medical staff were summoned to the ward and, during discussions, Miss W.'s niece made it clear that she would not take her aunt home because of the adverse effect her behaviour was having on her mother's health. Consequently, it was decided that Miss W. should be persuaded to stay so that medical screening could be undertaken and to give her sister a much needed rest.

For some hours after admission, Miss W. walked up and down the ward looking for a way out and demanding that an ambulance take her home. The nurses gently steered her away from the doors, tried to engage her in conversation and offered refreshments to try to reduce her perception of threat. Some hours passed before Miss W. was finally persuaded to have a little food and drink, by which time darkness had fallen and Miss W. agreed to stay overnight. She slept through the night, apparently exhausted by the day's experiences.

Miss W. made it clear that she perceived her situation to be the consequence of a wicked deception. She believed she had been abandoned in what she referred to as the 'workhouse'. This perception was reinforced in her declaration that 'no matter what they [the nurses] do to me, I'll not do a hand's turn for them'. The nurses felt that the immediate need was to manage Miss W.'s aggression, primarily to reduce her energy demands. This was achieved by

- staying calm
- respecting Miss W.'s personal space
- keeping a safe distance and allowing Miss W. to remain in her position as long as her safety was not compromised
- encouraging Miss W. to express feelings, perceptions and fears
- being flexible and accepting, not rigid or rejecting
- communicating to Miss W. that staff members were accessible
- offering Miss W. alternative coping strategies.

In the immediate postadmission period, staff reinforced the reasons for Miss W.'s admission to hospital, engineered social activities so that although she did not initially participate she was at least exposed to them. They did ensure that she had her hair done: that was, after all, why she left home that fateful day.

Establishing trust

Three days passed before sufficient trust was established to enable Miss W.'s symptoms to be fully explored. There were two main aspects of nursing intervention: *organisation of care* through primary nursing, leading to *acceptance of physical care* through the expression of concern within the person-to-person relationship stressed in primary nursing. (See Pearson 1988. Primary nursing gives to designated, experienced, first-level nurses total responsibility for the planning, delivery and evaluation of care for a specific number of patients for the duration of their stay.) In view of the complexity of Miss W.'s situation, the ward sister took on the role of the primary nurse and selected associates from the nurses and nursing auxiliaries who would be continuously available for a few days following Miss W.'s admission. This meant that meaningful relationships could be established while the number of people involved in care, and hence the potential for confusion, was reduced.

By the end of the third day, Miss W. was lucid and well orientated, experiencing only minor lapses of short-term memory. She ate and drank well, was attentive to other patients and staff and attended to her personal hygiene without prompting, needing help only to get in and out of the bath. During the 2-week respite period, a toileting programme was developed which restored continence. Such a regime is described in Rooney 1987. This programme used the times of nocturnal wakefulness for bladder management, effectively turning a negative experience into a purposeful activity. A bond developed between Miss W. and the ward sister and in the course of many conversations it became clear that Miss W. resented having to give up her home and her friends because of 'memory lapses'. She was aware that on occasion she forgot to turn off the gas appliances and was finding shopping and cooking difficult because of her poor memory and the distance she had to go to the shops, and agreed that she needed someone to be with her most of the time. She and her sister had always been on good terms and it had seemed like the ideal solution for them to live together. However, they had never had to live together as adults, and the strain was 'getting to both of them'. Miss W. confessed to some jealousy over her sister's familial relationships and felt that she was looked upon as a visitor rather than as part of the family.

The challenge for the nursing team was to create a new perception of well-being for Miss W. in the context of her changed situation. This involved the significant people in Miss W.'s life — most importantly, her sister. Soon after Miss W.'s admission, the ward sister contacted the health visitor, who began addressing the needs of the carers. Following discussions with Miss W.'s sister and niece, arrangements were made for respite care for 2 weeks every 3 months and for day hospital care one day each week while Miss W. was at home. The offer of home-help services was rejected, as Miss W.'s sister could not reconcile herself to the idea of a 'stranger' in her home. The arrangement reached with Miss W.'s sister was communicated to the ward sister and through her to Miss W., who then had the opportunity to visit the day hospital while she was in respite care. These services were offered in the context of introducing new social contacts and creating new opportunities and new meanings in life for both Miss W. and her family.

Three years after the events described, Miss W. remains happily at home with her sister, enjoys her outings to the day hospital and looks forward to her regular 'holidays' in the ward where she has 'many friends'. Her sister is also content, feels that she is given adequate support, and is free of the guilt which she says she would have experienced had her sister remained permanently in care.

person as an object: 'the CVA', 'the coronary', 'the dementia'. Caring, on the other hand, involves 'presencing' as described by Marcel (cited in Reimen 1986, p. 88):

> When someone is present to me, I am unable to treat him as if he were merely placed in front of me: between him and me there arises a relationship which surpasses my awareness of him; he is not only before me, he is also with me.
>
> The person who is at my disposal is the one who is capable of being with me with the whole of himself when I am in need; while the one who is not at my disposal seems merely to offer me a temporary loan raised on his resources. For the one I am a *presence*; for the other I am an *object*.

The account of Miss W.'s care in Case History 36.1 illustrates that the nursing staff had respect for her as a person. In biomedical terms, Miss W. presented as 'confused', and if her behaviour had been separated from her life history she would have been 'taken care of' paternalistically by means of sedatives and permanent hospitalisation. This would have resulted in depersonalisation and learned helplessness. Paternalism claims a right to order the lives of others on the grounds that it is immoral to act against one's own general welfare (Hirsch & Harris 1988). In the first instance, a paternalistic approach was used by the ward sister, but only in order to ensure Miss W.'s safety and to buy time to get close enough to be 'present' for her. The ward sister knew from experience that she had to gain access to Miss W.'s world, to see things as she saw them. This is caring. Without shared meanings, the situation might have evolved into that which is sensitively described in the following poem:

Confused

If my confusion
Is your confusion
Then how confused you must be
For my confusion
Confuses me
To the point where I can't see
And if your confusion
Confuses me
As mine confuses you
Then the two of us
Must be confused
As to who's confusing who!

Fiona Sinclair (1991)

When there is no shared understanding, the potential for cruelty, however unintentioned, is enormous. The ward sister knew that Miss W. was not pathologically confused: she simply had no markers to help her to interpret a new experience.

Knowledge of persons requires openness, participation and empathy. Holistic caring is not possible otherwise. Miss W.'s usual lifestyle was compromised by disease (arthritis) and by a phenomenon of ageing (short-term memory lapse). This combination of factors produced anxiety, which can result in a withdrawal from the outside world (Yurick et al 1980). Thus, anxiety triggers a vicious circle of dulled memory and judgement, emotional lability, and impaired social psychological and physical reactions. Caring is not a fall-back position to be adopted when curing is not possible: caring is at all times primary. Through the caring relationship established between Miss W. and the ward sister it was possible to turn problems into possibilities and to establish new patterns. The use of nocturnal wakefulness to manage urinary incontinence is one example of this. Altered sleep patterns are not uncommon among older people but they can cause anxiety if they are not explained as a natural phenomenon. Imparting knowledge and offering explanations is part of health promotion. In Miss W.'s situation, the sleep disturbance which was originally perceived negatively became a new and purposeful pattern in her life: an opportunity to become continent was created. This is what Carper (1978) refers to as the artistic component of nursing.

Nursing care should be contextual, taking account of the person's environment and the way in which he perceives the situation which threatens his established patterns of living. Services should be well coordinated and supportive, and staffing levels must allow time and opportunity to implement and maintain the care plan negotiated with the person. Activities need to be purposeful and meaningful and to have some immediate goals. Thus, therapies should be built into activities of daily living. For example, stretching of limbs can be more easily encouraged by placing cutlery on a table at a slightly greater distance from the patient than would normally be expected, so encouraging him to reach out for it. The simplicity and regularity of such an exercise, the opportunity for increasing the degree of difficulty attached to the activity, and the immediacy and relevance of the goal is a formula much more likely to maintain flexibility of limbs than irregular programmes of apparently purposeless exercises requiring a degree of motivation. This is particularly important where there is cognitive impairment: activities have to be centred on the living skills which are retained. Similar observations have been made by McMahon (1988) with regard to reality orientation programmes. The traditional brief therapy sessions have been shown to have little effect on patients, and McMahon has argued that a 24-hour reality approach, in which orienting is part of every interaction, is more person-centred and respectful.

The nursing care provided for Miss W. required a skilful blending of the four types of knowledge identified by Carper (1978): scientific, aesthetic, personal and ethical (see p. 960). Through the understanding and dialogue implicit in caring, Miss W. and the significant persons in her life were able to establish different and meaningful lifestyles.

The right to independence

Commentary: Case History 36.2

The caring dilemma

The primary care team had agonised over the decision to try to support Mrs A. in her home as she wished. The health visitor described the whole experience as 'walking on eggshells'. When pressed to explain this statement, she described the feeling of being torn between wanting to provide safe and continuous care and recognising that these goals had to be reconciled with the patient's values. Whether or not this was achieved in the end is a matter for debate.

The disease-oriented model of care is dominant in the description of the care provided for Mrs A. This model views situations in terms of problems or deficits and, for Mrs A., identified a set of problems which included non-compliance with a drug regime, social withdrawal, impaired mobility worsened by excess weight, urinary incontinence, risk of injury, inability to attend to personal care independently, and impaired home management. This model assumes the dominance of the professionals concerned and confirms their problem-solving role. From the point of view of the patient,

Case History 36.2

Mrs A. was an 83-year-old widow who lived in a socially deprived urban area. She had no children and her nearest relatives lived on the other side of the city, visiting on average once a week. She lived in a one-bedroom flat in a four-storey building. Mrs A. was described in her medical record as arthritic, obese and reluctant to venture out of doors. She had an obliging neighbour who paid all her bills, collected her pension from the post office, and did all her shopping. Otherwise, Mrs A. managed her housework and her personal care independently.

Mrs A.'s local practice team of GP, health visitor and district nurse had a well-developed screening and support programme for the elderly people registered with the practice (as described, for example, in Littlewood & Scott 1990). This programme was based on agreed criteria for identifying those at risk. The programme worked well, with admissions to hospital or other care facilities being fairly low compared with patients with similar characteristics in other practices within the area.

During a particularly severe winter in which the threat of hypothermia intensified the visiting programme, Mrs A. appeared content and was coping well with her preferred lifestyle. She liked to be visited by people she knew but was reluctant to go out, partly because she found the stairs too much but mainly because she did not mix well with strangers. The health visitor offered to make arrangements for her to attend the local pensioners club but this was refused. Mrs A. got through the winter with no major problems and 6 months later was still coping well.

A further 6 months on, the health visitor found a different situation. She noted that the house was unkempt and that Mrs A.'s personal appearance had deteriorated. After much persuasion, Mrs A. agreed to have the district nurse visit weekly to give assistance with personal hygiene. Arrangements were also made for home-help services 3 days per week. The amount of persuasion needed to get Mrs A. to agree to a home-help prompted the health visitor to liaise with the home-help organiser more closely than usual in the hope of finding 'just the right person'. (Very often, a concerned relationship will develop between a client and home-help which usually means that more of the 'self' will be given than would be expected within the carefully prescribed job description of the home-help.) The 'right person' was duly found, Mrs A.'s situation improved 'practically overnight', and this new level was maintained for about 6 months, until the doctor was called because of Mrs A.'s increased breathlessness. A diuretic was prescribed which, while it relieved her breathlessness (diagnosed as cardiac failure), created a problem with urinary incontinence. Also, at this time, Mrs A.'s mobility deteriorated. Previously able to get about with a stick, she needed a Zimmer aid to get about her flat. Additionally, she had been found on the floor by her home-help on two occasions.

The GP, health visitor, and Mrs A.'s relatives combined forces to persuade her that a period in hospital was necessary to sort out her problems. She was subsequently admitted to an assessment unit for elderly people. This period of hospitalisation was described by the health visitor as a 'disaster' for Mrs A., who became confused and had great difficulty adjusting to her new drug regime of digoxin and long-acting, potassium-sparing diuretics (Royle & Walsh 1992). During the month in hospital Mrs A. was seen by a dietitian and subsequently commenced on a 1000-calorie diet. She agreed to this only because she thought it was expected of her. Physiotherapy was also introduced to try to improve her mobility, with no great success. Mrs A. was also seen by the occupational therapist, who assessed dressing and walking ability and the need for bathing aids and a commode for night use. Finally, the social worker was summoned to consider Mrs A.'s social circumstances to determine the capacity for independent living. Despite this well-intentioned care, the health visitor found Mrs A. confused, generally feeling helpless and hopeless, and pleading to be allowed home.

Mrs A. was, after much pleading, discharged home, whereupon she abandoned her diet and, it seems, her diuretics. Her home-help was recommenced and the district nurse called 3 times each week to attend to her personal hygiene. About one month after her discharge from the assessment unit, Mrs A. again became unwell and her GP suspected a cerebrovascular accident (CVA) because of left-sided weakness. Mrs A. refused to return to the assessment unit and after a great deal of persuasion was admitted to an acute medical ward where she stayed for 2 months. Compared with her previous time in hospital, this was a very positive experience. When asked what was different, Mrs A. said the nurses had let her be herself and did not make her do things she did not want to do. In particular, she had the same food as all the other patients, albeit in smaller portions.

Mrs A. made a full recovery from what appeared to have been a transient ischaemic attack. While in hospital it was put to her that she could no longer live safely at home and should consider a nursing home. With great reluctance, Mrs A. agreed to a 3-month trial in a local nursing home. During her time there, the health visitor called to see how she was settling in. On both occasions, she was described as 'weeping and miserable' and expressing a wish to die. Following a meeting with the GP and the district nurse, it was agreed, to Mrs A.'s delight, that she should go back home.

At home, the previous services were restored and a 'tuck-in' service was introduced whereby a nursing auxiliary visited in the evening to help Mrs A. get to bed safely. A commode was placed by her bed to avoid falls en route to the toilet and a supply of incontinence pads was provided to relieve the anxiety associated with possibly not making it to the toilet on time. In view of her previous reluctance to take her diuretics, (deemed necessary to control her heart failure), the health visitor explored further the reasons for Mrs A.'s non-compliance with her drug regime relative to the pattern of falls (occurring mainly at night) and the incontinence. The health visitor concluded that postural oedema developing during the day was being corrected through rest on retiring for the night, with a resulting improvement in diuresis. Consequently, the tuck-in service would not be as effective as it might be because Mrs A. would still need to get out of bed to use the commode, thus increasing the risk of falls. The health visitor therefore suggested that the patient should lie on her bed between 17.00 h and 19.00 h so that the improved diuresis would occur before the nursing auxiliary came to see her safely to bed at 20.30 h and she would be less likely to have to get up again to use the commode.

The strategy was very successful, and for about 3 months Mrs A. was happily maintained at home. Sadly, one morning, the home-help arrived to find that Mrs A. had died in bed sometime during the night.

however, it can create increased dependence and reinforce a feeling of powerlessness.

Conversely Kleinman (1988) has argued that the role of health professionals is to empower the persons for whom they care by helping them to assert what for them is important in their lives and their care. This view is expressed by Watson's (1979) identification of ten aspects of caring in nursing:

- formation of a humanistic–altruistic system of values
- instilling of faith/hope
- cultivation of sensitivity to one's self and others
- development of a helping/trusting relationship
- promotion and acceptance of the expression of positive and negative feelings
- systematic use of the scientific problem-solving method for decision-making

- promotion of interpersonal teaching/learning
- provision of a supportive, protective or corrective mental, physical, sociocultural and spiritual environment
- assistance with the gratification of human needs
- efforts to understand persons in concrete lived situations and moments, and the responses to these.

There is nothing in the NHS and Community Care Act (1990) which in principle prohibits sensitive caring. The difficulties arise primarily from practical limitations, such as the setting of predetermined cash limits as an incentive to obtaining value for money, disagreements on how best to assess needs, and fragmentation of services resulting in delays in intervention. One of the ways in which the government seeks to remove potential difficulties is through the case worker principle or brokerage. As this advocacy role has, in the context of community care, been given to the social worker, it is clear that social security policies must be aligned with community care policies if choice and adequacy of care are to be a reality.

Harmonising curing and caring

What can be identified from the account of Mrs A.'s care in Case History 36.2 is the importance of the patient's biographical details. During her first period of hospitalisation, the focus of treatment was on correcting Mrs A.'s heart failure. Unfortunately, the therapeutic regime implemented had an undesirable effect on Mrs A.'s mobility, continence, safety and general capacity for independent living. She was, not unnaturally, distressed and one wonders if the effects of the drug therapy had been explained to her in advance. Mrs A. expected to get better, not worse; given the amount of persuasion needed for her to accept hospitalisation, it would have been perfectly understandable if the bond of trust between the health visitor and the patient had been irreparably damaged by the fact that the latter's expectations were not immediately met.

Knowledge of the pathological effects of excess weight resulted in dietary restrictions which were not acceptable to the patient and clearly were not adhered to on discharge. Mrs A. was 83 years old and had an established dietary pattern. The medical aim was clearly to preserve life without regard to what would constitute an acceptable quality of life for Mrs A. Changes in the way in which a person leads his or her life can be made only if they are valued by that person.

Another contributing factor in Mrs A.'s distress in hospital was the fragmentation of care; she was not accustomed to this at home. It can be argued that there is a need for multicompetent practitioners to replace the host of specialists whose services have not been properly evaluated (Beachey 1988). If services are broken into a series of tasks it is unlikely that they will amount to genuinely holistic care. That said, however, increasing flexibility within the professions, cross-training, and the ability to perform duties in more than one discipline will not of themselves produce holistic care. What is needed is a shared view of the priorities of care for any given patient. Care plans need to be tailor-made in the light of the values, motivation and residual capacities of the patient. Thus, following Mrs A.'s second admission to hospital the goal of medical and nursing interventions was to enable her to be all she could be and not to make her what the medical model would consider 'normal'.

The short time in the nursing home was equally disastrous and again demonstrates the consequences of the dominance of professional goals which are not shared by patients. A residential home might have been a more acceptable alternative. On a positive note, what is perhaps most striking about the account of Mrs A.'s care is the sensitivity of the health visitor and her expert and skilful blending of the artistic and scientific elements of caring.

The challenge of severe disability

Commentary: Case History 36.3

The purpose of nursing is to reduce the vulnerability of persons who are facing particular challenges in their lives. If we are to help our patients to see new possibilities in otherwise hopeless situations, there needs to be commitment and involvement. The nursing team involved in Mrs R.'s care demonstrated this involvement by addressing her physical difficulties in a way that reflected an understanding of the implications of those problems for her social and emotional well-being. Good seating arrangements, for example, can enhance the individual's cognitive and communication skills and can influence for the better the attitudes and approaches of other people to the disabled person. The optimal sitting position for all persons is with the hips, knees and ankles flexed to 90°. Weight should be evenly distributed under the buttocks and thighs, with the feet firmly planted on the ground and forearms resting at elbow height on an armrest. In achieving proper positioning, attention should be directed first to the pelvis, followed in order by the buttocks and thighs, trunk and head (Fraser, Hensinger & Phelps 1987).

Optimal positioning remains the goal for all persons with multiple handicaps, even though its achievement is rarely possible. To even approximate this goal, seating systems need to be adapted to provide comfort and security, maximise function, prevent, minimise or delay contractures, inhibit abnormal reflex activity, and facilitate movement (e.g. from chair to bed). The careful use of positioning techniques in patients with athetoid movements may bring about some control in upper extremity movement and even provide a stable base for purposeful arm movements, however limited. When, as in the case of Mrs R., the problems of athetoid movements are compounded by tongue thrust, good positioning is absolutely essential if eating and drinking are to be assisted in a pleasurable, dignified manner. The critical factor is positioning of the head in flexion in a static midline position to give more control when assisting the patient to eat and drink (Fraser et al 1987).

In caring for people like Mrs R., nurses need to be sufficiently committed and involved to overcome enormous obstacles, not least of which is the cost of equipment. Additionally, in an era of cost containment and centralisation of services, central purchasing of equipment may militate against the provision of appropriate items for individual patients. Nurses must, therefore, insist on being involved in making choices to meet particular needs, especially when patients are themselves unable to communicate their preferences. To do this work effectively, nurses need to have some knowledge of ergonomics and anthropometrics, and often they will need to negotiate priorities with physiotherapists who may not perceive a patient's situation in quite the same way as they do.

Hobson & Molenbroek (1990) have highlighted the lack of anthropometric resource data appropriate for use with individuals with specific disabilities, and have identified important qualitative and quantitative factors influencing the design of seating and mobility devices for a specific segment of the population. The data generated by these authors is very different from that gathered from able-bodied subjects, which is generally used in the design of seating and other equipment which may be used by disabled people. This work clearly indicates the need for a resources data base specific to people with particular disabilities. Through observation and careful documentation of experiences, nurses could make a significant con-

Case History 36.3

A student nurse came on duty in a continuing care unit for elderly people. She learned that a patient she had been caring for had died during the night. The permanent members of staff were clearly saddened by the loss and the student nurse could not understand why. The patient, Mrs R., was 72 years old and had been a patient in the hospital for 6 years because of a CVA resulting in athetosis (see Ch. 9) with an accompanying spasticity and loss of verbal communication skills. Prior to her transfer to long-term care, Mrs R. had spent nearly one year in an acute care facility where she developed contractures of her hip and elbow joints. An additional complication was tongue thrust, a reflex pushing out of the tongue which makes eating and drinking difficult. (For information on tongue thrust and its management see Fraser et al 1987.)

Mrs R. had a devoted husband who visited every day. The couple had no children and friends had ceased to visit, largely because of her inability to communicate verbally and their feeling of awkwardness in trying to express their care. Consequently, her only other visitor was the minister of the church where Mrs R. had been an active member.

The ward in which Mrs R. was cared for was of the Nightingale style, and she was one of 30 patients with equally complex illnesses. Taking a problem-oriented view of Mrs R.'s situation, the challenges for nursing could be listed as follows:

- inability to communicate verbally
- impaired non-verbal communication
- disordered motor activity with potential for injury and total lack of purposeful movement
- eating disorder threatening her nutritional status
- inability to perform personal care
- uncontrolled voiding of urine and faeces
- imbalance between solitude and social interaction
- imbalance between activity and rest
- alteration in role
- potential alteration in perception and self-esteem
- possible pain of loss, loneliness, emptiness.

It was not possible even after multidisciplinary assessment to make a definitive statement about Mrs R.'s comprehension. She could make eye contact and turned toward sounds. Attempts to initiate eye signalling had all failed. Mrs R. was, in effect, wholly dependent on others for all aspects of living and the student nurse could not understand why the staff should mourn the passing of someone she would describe as a 'vegetable'.

The humanistic perspective taken by the ward sister, however, drew attention away from the deficits listed above toward the need for Mrs R. to find new meaning in life and to be empowered through the relationships and care offered by others. It is worth repeating that if a patient's situation is always viewed as a cluster of problems, opportunities for positive and healing interventions will be lost. The ward sister carefully explained to the student nurse the therapeutic use of self, by which she meant the ability to project oneself into a situation to achieve results no matter how small they may appear to be. In the first place, sister argued, Mrs R. did have some comprehension. In spite of her athetoid movements, Mrs R. followed with her eyes the significant persons in her life. Also, she would turn her head away from or towards people in rejection or approval of some act or comment.

Sister argued that Mrs R. knew she was cared for. Through the use of primary nursing, Mrs R. had her own, clearly identifiable, supporters who were sufficiently committed to act on her behalf. To care for Mrs R., each of her carers had to have a great breadth and depth of knowledge and a willingness to use this to help Mrs R. to find a way of being in the world. Sister gave the student the following examples of the challenges which the nurses had to meet in caring for Mrs R.

Mrs R. had very little physical mobility. She could not make purposeful or coordinated movements, had limb spasticity, and could not weight-bear or sit completely upright or unsupported. The challenge was to find a supported sitting position which would be comfortable and also fulfil certain other benefits such as facilitating cardiopulmonary and gastrointestinal function. Mrs R.'s care was complicated by limb contractures acquired in the acute care setting from which she was transferred. In addition to preventing pressure sores, the plan for Mrs R. was to try to control disturbing movements for energy conservation, aesthetic purposes, and, not least, for comfort. Good positioning was especially important at mealtimes. Mrs R.'s tongue thrust made it difficult for a spoon to be inserted into her mouth. This was accommodated by using slight downward pressure on the tongue with a spoon and the spout of a feeding cup to inhibit the tongue thrust and to encourage lip movement. Mrs R. had no teeth and had not worn dentures since the time of her stroke. The tongue thrust made it impossible to consider a prosthetic device of any kind, primarily for reasons of safety. This presented an additional challenge in the selection of food. Nonetheless, the sloppy soft diet that tends to be standard provision for patients who require assisted feeding was not resorted to. With good tongue and lip movements Mrs R. was able to manage most foods. She was particularly fond of fish and chips: this was confirmed by her husband and evidenced by the fact that she always cleared her plate!

The process of eating took into account Mrs R.'s social environment. She ate in the same area as the other patients and her need for assisted feeding gave her the individual attention of a nurse for about 45 minutes 3 times each day, in addition to 15 minutes every 2 hours for additional fluids.

Re-peopling Mrs R.'s world meant introducing her to all the other patients in the ward and sharing with her the general events affecting the lives of all the patients as well as the special things such as a new grandchild or a birthday. Much time was spent by the nurses with Mrs R.'s husband initially; they got to know his wife through him and subsequently involved him in the decisions affecting her life. In this way, clothing reflecting her personality and preferences could be selected. Consideration was also given to special needs such as slight oversizing of garments to accommodate contracted limbs, and selecting fibres that were warm, comfortable and helped to manage the excessive perspiration produced on occasion by the athetoid movements.

The hospital had large attractive grounds with patios and verandahs for those who were unable to make use of the gardens. These facilities were available to Mrs R., and the nurses believed she took pleasure from her time out of doors. Mrs R.'s husband became very much a part of the team and had daily opportunities to discuss his own feelings, hopes and desires. Thus, an extended caring role evolved.

tribution to the development of data bases for people with particular needs.

Caring should not focus on the pursuit of short- or long-term goals while disregarding the individual's state of mind in the present. To put this another way, interventions must support *being* as well as *becoming*. This may entail constructing imaginative and innovative ways of helping. Passant (1990), for example, has given a very sensitive account of her use of complementary therapies in the care of elderly people. Therapeutic touch, massage, aromatherapy and herbal remedies have brought great comfort and pleasure to many elderly people who were previously sad and unresponsive (Quinn 1988).

Spiritual caring

Before her illness, Mrs R. regularly attended church, yet no mention is made in Case History 36.3 of her spiritual needs. Simone Roach (1987) lists the characteristics of professional caring as compassion, competence, confidence, conscience, and commitment. In general, nurses may feel ill-equipped to enhance the spiritual well-being of patients. However, this aspect of caring does not depend upon religious belief per se. Creating space and quiet and using poetry and music are ways of nourishing the soul and replenishing the spirit. As nurses, we are not asked to enter into theological debate with patients but in caring we can demonstrate love in action and in so doing help to provide spiritual comfort and peace.

? **36.3** The ward sister believed that Mrs R. knew that she was loved, respected, and wanted. Does this, however, constitute an acceptable quality of life? Contemporary medicine goes to great lengths to keep people alive, sometimes even against their will. The moral and economic implications of this have put the subject of euthanasia on the legislative agenda of the Western world. In the majority of cases the motive for precipitating death is to end suffering and to preserve dignity. These motives must sit unhappily with the notion of caring as the essence of nursing. Discuss with your colleagues the following questions related to the debate on euthanasia:

- Can nurses reconcile mercy killing with their ethical codes (UKCC 1992), which are concerned with doing good and avoiding evil?
- How does the principle of the patient's autonomy operate in the context of withholding treatment?
- What happens to those who cannot communicate, or who are incapable of making decisions on their own?
- Is it likely that, in an era of increasing economic pressures, legalised euthanasia would be subject to grave abuse?

Caring and the family

Commentary: Case History 36.4

Attitudes toward death

Some nurses may be uncomfortable with the idea of death, seeing it as a failure, or as relief when life is perceived as meaningless. Patients' death wishes are seldom explored, and valuable insight into individuals' perspectives and values is lost as a result. The charge nurse did not, however, dismiss the issue of death but used the opportunity to help Mr F. discover new strengths and possibilities.

Benner & Wrubel (1989) have argued that ours is a future-oriented, death-denying society which is preoccupied more with achieving than with *being*. These authors further argue that one of the ways in which we cope with death is to identify it as a process with progressive stages and then turn the process into a developmental achievement. Kubler-Ross's (1970) work on death and dying identifies stages of denial, anger, rejection, bargaining and acceptance. This work has been cited by Benner & Wrubel as a prescription for a 'healthy way to die', and an example of society's obsession with goal-orientation even in dying.

Family care-giving

Larson & Dodd (1991) have defined caring as the intentional actions and attitudes that convey physical care and emotional concern and promote a sense of safeness and security in another. Mr F.'s age and chronic illness combined to classify him as being in need of continuing care. Hospitalisation was seen as the only response to this and, in the absence of more suitable accommodation, Mr F. found himself in a unit specialising in the care of elderly people. This is yet another example of the consequences of stereotyping. Mr F. did not consider himself as elderly, and indeed in terms of chronological age he was not. Persons with chronic illnesses and older people share an unenviably marginalised position in society.

The power of the professionals involved in Mr F.'s acute care to make decisions without consultation is evident in the description of the bewilderment of both Mr and Mrs F. and their ensuing anger and sense of hopelessness. Community nursing services might have been a more acceptable way of providing care in the post-acute phase of the illness and would at least have taken account of established family patterns of caring. Larson & Dodd (1991) have noted that though caring within a family may be inherently valuable, appropriate caring cannot always be given without support in a family during a crisis. It appeared to Mr and Mrs F. that the staff in the acute care setting did not care sufficiently to explore the possibility of alternative arrangements for caring. The emphasis of the professionals upon cure obscured the need for care.

By supporting the carers within a family, professionals can help to create a sense of togetherness, reciprocity and networking (Larson & Dodd 1991). Mr F.'s family had a well-established pattern of support and of physical caring which was disrupted and, in the acute area, apparently discounted. It would have been more helpful for the professionals concerned to investigate the established patterns by which Mr F.'s family functioned. The history of family relationships needs to be taken into account in helping patients and their families to establish new coping strategies when usual patterns are disrupted. Swimming against the tide of established caring practices is often counterproductive, if not futile. The artistry of the nurse is required in choosing interventions and approaches which are congruent with the family's perceived needs (Friedemann 1991).

The context of caring

Mr F. had been moved from a high-technology area in a modern, purpose-built hospital to a Victorian building which at first sight added to his sense of hopelessness. However Mr F. soon discovered that buildings were not the best indicators of the care which could be expected within. The account of Mr F.'s care in Case History 36.4 illustrates the establishment and effective use of a healing relationship in the context of nursing. There is clear indication of the use of dialogue and active listening to mobilise hope and to preserve personhood and dignity. Information was given to relieve anxiety and family care-giving was enhanced through emotional support and the mobilisation of collective strength, drive and desire. This approach helped to relieve Mr F.'s sense of alienation from the treatment and recovery process which was unwittingly created in the acute care setting. By being encouraged to set realistic and achievable goals, the family was helped to find a new but comfortable way of relating to one another in the context of caring.

CONCLUSION

In this chapter an attempt has been made to illustrate the use of the four types of knowledge identified by Carper (1978) — scientific, aesthetic, personal, and ethical — as being needed for the practice of nursing. Nursing practice synthesises subjective and objective data in the systematic study of human experiences of illness, injury or disease. A focus on a disease-oriented model can result in interventions based on idealised clinical norms which often bear little relation to the needs of individual persons.

The Case Histories focus on aspects of caring in nursing.

Case History 36.4

Mr F. is a 62-year-old previously self-employed timber merchant who for 3 years had suffered from motor neurone disease (characterised by spasticity and weakness of the limbs, loss of fine movements, and as the disease progresses, impaired speech, swallowing and respiration; see Royle & Walsh 1992). During the course of his illness, Mr F. had been cared for at home by his wife with support from his son and daughter, both of whom were married and jointly ran the family business. Mr F. developed a severe respiratory illness and had to be admitted to an acute care unit in a modern district general hospital, where he stayed for 3 weeks prior to his transfer to a continuing care hospital for elderly people. The charge nurse had been notified of his admission.

Mr F. arrived on the ward looking very apprehensive. He was accompanied by his wife, who explained that her husband had had a harrowing experience in hospital wherein he had gone from being a unique, dignified person to a dependent, dejected shell of his former self. Their well-established routines at home had been completely rejected and Mrs F.'s advice on ways of managing particular tasks was 'unwelcome'. The move to long-term care was seen as the last straw. The dilemma was that while it was felt that Mr F. was not well enough to be managed at home, he had no desire to remain in the acute setting, nor did he not want to be in a 'geriatric' ward. The beds in the acute care unit were needed, no option was given, and resentment and anger ensued.

The charge nurse welcomed Mr F. onto the ward. At first sight, he was pale, anxious, and breathless. He was settled in bed, and the charge nurse sat down beside the couple and, over a cup of tea, described the care that could be expected in the unit. It was clear that the patient had not fully recovered from the respiratory illness and, from the medical notes and the information provided largely by Mrs F., the following problems emerged:

- activity intolerance
- inefficient respiratory function
- impaired communication
- disrupted family relationships
- feelings of hopelessness
- fluid volume deficit
- constipation
- change from chronic to acute illness
- insufficient intake of nutrients
- alteration in the usual pattern of personal care
- urinary retention with overflow incontinence
- threat to skin integrity at pressure points.

Problems or possibilities?

Insofar as it reflected a deficit model of care, the above list could have obscured the possibilities for positive intervention. In view of Mr F.'s negative experience in the previous situation, and the complexity of his problems, the charge nurse decided to take the role of primary nurse. This was explained to Mr F. and his wife, who was encouraged to visit as and when she wished. It was also put to Mrs F. that while her need to satisfy herself about the standards of care her husband would receive was understood, she should also try to rest and share the visiting with her family. An alternative offer of visitor's accommodation was made.

Mr and Mrs F. were aware of the poor ultimate prognosis. They had a loving marital relationship and a fierce determination to protect and nurture one another. For Mrs F. the most upsetting part of the experience in the acute care unit had been her husband's expressed wish to die. Although they had from time to time spoken of separation, this had always been referred to as a distant event. These feelings were explored by the charge nurse, who discovered that the nature of the acute illness had not been fully explained to Mr F. Accordingly, arrangements were made for the couple to have an early meeting with the doctor. As a way of offering immediate support and comfort, the charge nurse explained that, with good care, there was every reason to believe that things would improve. He suggested that they start planning for discharge home and consider regular respite admissions to maintain optimum wellness. The idea that it was appropriate to make plans had a dramatic effect on the couple.

Mr F.'s value as a husband, father, grandfather and business adviser were explored in the context of his changed situation. In the process of the conversations, the charge nurse learned how the couple had coped with the illness thus far and used this information to structure the care plans so that no unnecessary disruption of routine occurred.

The charge nurse and Mr and Mrs F. agreed to set out a plan that would celebrate life and to work at this by devising acceptable ways of dealing with the difficulties of the immediate situation. Within 3 weeks of admission, Mr F. could transfer from bed to chair or chair to chair with the assistance of one person and could walk a few steps with the support of two people. His respiratory infection had resolved, his bowel function was restored to the previous pattern, he had gained weight, and fluid and electrolyte balance were maintained at appropriate levels. Mrs F. had regained her strength and vitality and felt she was ready to take her husband home. As planned, discharge was arranged with district nurse support for bathing, maintenance of the urinary catheter, controlling urinary retention, and general surveillance. It was arranged that respite care would be given for 2 weeks every 3 months.

Developing competencies is of course an important aspect of nursing practice and references for further reading have been provided to enable students to learn about the signs, symptoms and treatments associated with specific diseases. While the importance of disease phenomena cannot be denied, the concern in this chapter has been to stress the person- and situation-specific nature of the challenges to well-being created by illness experiences.

Growing old is not a disease. Social constructs tend to set older people apart and cause policy-makers to look upon them as a homogeneous group — which they clearly are not. Like any other person, the older individual is distinguished by a personal biography and by the meanings which he attaches to particular circumstances in his life at particular times. The introduction of the arts and the humanities in nursing education will perhaps help to create a balance between art and science in nursing. Of equal importance is the need for nurses, and others who are privileged to be with individuals in times of joy and sadness, to care for each other. Sheila Cassidy (1988, p. 3) writes:

> I have discovered that the world is not divided into the sick and those who care for them, but that we are all wounded and that we all contain within our hearts that love which is for the healing of the nations. What we lack is the courage to give it away.

It is hoped that this chapter will help to enrich the learning experiences of students, and to help create opportunities for shared personal growth for them as nurses and, especially, for the older persons whose worlds they must enter in order to care.

REFERENCES

Altschul A T 1986 The elderly make the world go round. Geriatric Nursing. March/April: 26–27

Beachey W 1988 Multicompetent health professionals: needs, combinations, and curriculum development. Journal of Allied Health 17(4): 319–329

Benner 1985 Preserving caring in an era of cost-containment, marketing and high technology. Yale Nurse August: 12–20

Benner P, Wrubel J 1989 The primacy of caring. Addison-Wesley, Menlo Park, CA

Bevis E O, Watson J 1989 Toward the caring curriculum: a new pedagogy for nursing. National League for Nursing, New York

Carper B A 1978 Fundamental patterns of knowing in nursing. Advances in Nursing Science. 1(1): 13–23

Cassidy S 1988 Sharing the darkness: the spirituality of caring. Darton, Longman & Todd, London

Cummings J L 1980 Reversible dementia. Journal of the American Medical Association. 243: 2434–2439

Dalley G 1988 Ideologies of caring. Macmillan Education, Philadelphia

Evers H K 1991 Care of the elderly sick in the UK. In: Redfern S (ed) Nursing elderly people, 2nd edn. Churchill Livingstone, Edinburgh, pp 417–436

Fraser B A, Hensinger R N, Phelps J A 1987 Physical management of multiple handicaps. Paul Brookes, Baltimore

Friedemann M-L 1991 Exploring culture and family caring patterns with the framework of systematic organization. In: Chinn P L (ed) Anthology on caring. National League for Nursing Press, New York

Gadow S 1988 Covenant without cure. In: Watson J, Ray M A (eds) The ethics of care and the ethics of cure. National League for Nursing Press, New York, pp 5–14

Gott M, O'Brien M 1990 The role of the nurse in health promotion. Unpublished paper, RCN Research Society Conference, University of Surrey

Griffiths Sir Roy 1988 Community care: agenda for action. A report to the Secretary of State for Social Services. HMSO, London

Gaut D A 1991 Caring and nursing: explorations in feminist perspectives. Introductory remarks. In: Neil R M & Watts R W (eds) Caring and nursing: explorations in feminist perspectives. National League for Nursing, New York

Hirsch S R, Harris J 1988 Consent and the incompetent patient: ethics, law and medicine. Gaskell, London

Hobson D A, Molenbroek JFM 1990 Anthropometry and design for the disabled: experiences with seating design for the cerebral palsy population. Applied Ergonomics 21(1): 43–54

Kleinman A 1988 The illness narratives: suffering, healing & the human condition. Basic Books, New York

Kubler-Ross E 1970 On death and dying. Tavistock, London

Larson P J, Dodd M J 1991 The cancer treatment experience: family patterns of caring. In: Gaut D A, Leininger M M (eds) Caring: the compassionate healer. National League for Nursing, New York, pp 61–78

Leininger M M (ed) 1988 Caring, the essence of nursing and health. Wayne State University Press, Detroit

Macintyre A C 1981 After virtue: a study of moral theory. Duckworth, London

Mahoney F I, Barthel D W 1965 Functional evaluation: the Barthel index. Maryland State Medical Journal 14: 61–65

Maugham W S 1938 The summing up. Garden City, New York, p 290

McMahon R 1988 The 24-hour reality orientation type approach to the confused elderly: a minimum standard for care. Journal of Advanced Nursing 13: 693–700

Mental Health Act 1983 HMSO, London

Murphy E 1988 Psychiatric implications. In: Hirsch S R, Harris J (eds) Consent and the incompetent patient: ethics, law, and medicine. Gaskell, London, pp 65–76

National Health Service and Community Care Act 1990. HMSO, London

Norman A 1991 Room for a view. Health Visitor 64(4): 103

Norman I F 1991 Mental health problems of elderly people: assessment and planning. In: Redfern S (ed) Nursing elderly people. Churchill Livingstone, Edinburgh, pp 309–340

Open University 1988 Handbook of mental disorders in old age. The Open University Press, Milton Keynes

Passant H 1990 A holistic approach in the ward. Nursing Times 86(4): 26–28

Pearson A (ed) 1988 Primary nursing: nursing in the Burford and Oxford nursing development units. Croom Helm, London

Peplau H E 1988 The art and science of nursing: similarities, differences, and relativities. Nursing Science Quarterly 1(1): 8–15

Quinn J F 1988 Building a body of knowledge: research on therapeutic touch 1974–1986. Journal of Holistic Nursing 6(1): 37–45

Roach S 1987 The human act of caring: a blueprint for the health professions. Canadian Hospital Association, Ottowa, Ontario

Redfern S J (ed) 1991 Nursing elderly people. Churchill Livingstone, Edinburgh

Reimen D 1986 The essential structure of a caring interaction: doing phenomenology. In: Munhall P, Oiler-Boyd C (eds) Nursing research: a qualitative perspective. Appleton-Century-Crofts, Norwalk, CT, pp 85–106

Robinson B, Lund C, Keller D, Cuervo C A 1986 Validation of a functional assessment inventory against a multidisciplinary home care team. Journal of the American Geriatric Society. 34: 851–854

Royle J A, Walsh M 1992 Watson's medical-surgical nursing and related physiology, 4th edn. Baillière Tindall, London

Sandelowski M 1991 Telling stories: narrative approaches in qualitative research. Image: Journal of Nursing Scholarship, 23(3): 161–166

Shapira J, Schlesinger R, Cummings J L 1986 Is it cortical or subcortical dementia? The answer makes a difference in nursing interventions. American Journal of Nursing. June: 699–702

Sinclair F 1991 To touch your heart. Clay Pot Publications, Edinburgh

Sullivan D 1988 The incapable patient and the law. In: Hirsch S R, Harris J (eds) Consent and the incompetent patient: ethics, law, and medicine, Gaskell, London, pp 1–8

St Exupery A de 1943 The little prince. Harcourt, Brace & World, New York

UKCC 1992 Code of professional conduct for the nurse, midwife and health visitor, 3rd edn. UKCC, London

Ungerson C 1983 Women and caring: skills, tasks and taboos. In: Gamarnikov E et al (eds) The public and the private. Heinemann, London

Victor C R 1987 Old age in modern society: a textbook of social gerontology. Croom Helm, London

Watson J 1979 The philosophy and science of caring. Little Brown, Boston

Watson J 1988 Nursing: human science and human care: a theory of nursing. National League for Nursing, New York

WHO/ICN 1988 The age of aging: implications for nursing. World Health Organization, Copenhagen

Wolf M A 1987 Human development, gerontology and self-development through the writings of May Sarton. Educational Gerontology 13(4): 289–95

Yurick A G, Robb S S, Spier B E, Ebert N J 1980 The aged person and the nursing process. Appleton-Century-Crofts, New York

FURTHER READING

Benner P 1984 From novice to expert. Addison-Wesley, Menlo Park, CA

Carnevali D L, Patrick M 1979 Nursing management for the elderly. Lippincott, Philadelphia

Chinn P L (ed) 1991 Anthology on caring. National League for Nursing Press, New York

Friere N 1970 Pedagogy of the oppressed. Herder & Herder, New York

Fromm E 1963 The art of loving. Bantam, New York

Jacques A 1988 Understanding dementia. Churchill Livingstone, Edinburgh

Lawler J 1991 Behind the screens. Churchill Livingstone, Edinburgh

Littlewood J, Scott R 1990 Screening the elderly. Health Visitor 63(8): 268–270

Morse J M, Johnson J L 1991 The illness experience: dimensions of suffering. Sage, London

Pirsig R M 1974 Zen and the art of motorcycle maintenance: an inquiry into values. Corgi, London

Rooney V M 1987 Toileting charts. Nursing 22: 827–830, Baillière Tindall, London

Veatch R M, Fry S T 1987 Case studies in nursing ethics. Lippincott, Philadelphia

Watson J, Ray M A (eds) 1988 The ethics of care and the ethics of cure. National League for Nursing, New York

Zarit S H (ed) 1982 Readings in aging and death: contemporary perspectives, 2nd edn. Harper & Row, New York

CHAPTER 37

The person with dependency problems

David B. Cooper

CHAPTER CONTENTS

Introduction 973
Definitions 974

A model for changing addictive behaviours 974

The role of the nurse 975
Identifying drug-related problems 976
Nurses and substance abuse 976
Approaching the patient with a suspected drug problem 977
Assessment 977
Prevention 978

Drug use and misuse: some facts 978
Legal substances 978
Tea and coffee 978
Tobacco 978
Alcohol 979
Tranquillisers 982
Solvents 983

Illegal substances 984
Rave culture 984
Opiates and opioids 984
Stimulants 984
Hallucinogens 985

Support agencies 986
Outreach workers 986
Voluntary and professional agencies 987

Conclusion 987

References 988

Further reading 988

Useful addresses 989

INTRODUCTION

?	**37.1** In preparation for reading this chapter, carry out the following exercise: a. List as many legal and illegal drugs as you can think of. Beside each, briefly write your feelings, positive or negative, relating to these substances. For example, are they acceptable? Attractive? Frightening? b. Write a brief description of your feeling in relation to: • illegal drug abuse and drug abusers • alcohol abuse and problem drinkers • tobacco use and smokers • legal drugs (e.g. prescribed medication, tea, coffee) and their users.

This chapter offers a basic introduction to drug misuse and drug-related problems, and outlines the important contribution that nurses can make to the care of people with drug dependencies. The term 'drug' is used to refer both to legal substances (i.e. alcohol, tea, coffee, tobacco and prescribed medications) and to illegal substances such as cannabis, cocaine, opiates and opioids. Throughout the chapter it is emphasised that whatever the nature of the dependency problem, it must be considered in the context of the individual's personal history and circumstances; stereotypes of the drug user must be abandoned in favour of a more individualised and holistic understanding of the *person*. As in all areas of nursing, interventions on behalf of patients with drug-related problems must be based on thorough assessment and should involve the individual to the greatest degree possible as a responsible partner in care.

Because dependency problems will have physical, mental, emotional, social and economic implications for the individual, a multidisciplinary approach to treatment will help to ensure that all dimensions of the patient's situation are considered as he makes the difficult adjustments necessary to overcoming an addiction. Prochaska & Di Clemente's (1986) integrative model of change is outlined as one which will be especially relevant to nurses working in this area of care.

The importance of early detection cannot be overstressed. To assist nurses in all fields in recognising the signs of drug abuse and in understanding the long-term effects of dependency, the second half of the chapter outlines the physical and psychological effects of a range of legal and illegal substances. Alcohol abuse is discussed at some length in recognition of the high prevalence of alchohol-related illness in the UK and in keeping with Dunne et al's (1989) observation that it is 'misleading to consider alcohol and drug misuse as separate entities', given the many similarities between their social, psychological and medical implications.

In view of the wide range of psychoactive drugs that can be obtained by legal or illegal means, and the wide range of therapies that are available to individuals who seek help, this chapter cannot hope to be comprehensive. The reader is urged to consult the Further Reading list as she pursues any topics of special relevance to her area of practice.

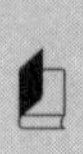

'Hooked', a six-part series introduced by S. Cosgrove and first aired on Granada Television in 1992, provides an excellent overview of dependency problems and helps to put drug use and misuse into perspective.

Definitions

Dependency and addiction

Drug dependency is described by the World Health Organization (WHO) as 'resulting from the interaction between a living organism and a drug, characterised by behavioural and other responses that always include compulsion to take the drug on a continuous or periodic basis in order to experience its psychic effects and sometimes avoid the discomfort of absence. Tolerance may or may not be present. A person may be dependent on more than one drug' (WHO 1969). Dependency may be psychological, physical, or both.

Psychological dependency is 'a condition in which a drug produces a feeling of satisfaction and a psychic drive that require periodic or continuous administration of the drug to produce pleasure or to avoid discomfort' (WHO 1974).

Physical dependency is 'an adaptive state that manifests itself by intense physical disturbances, i.e., the withdrawal or abstinence syndromes, which are made of specific arrays of symptoms and signs of a psychic and physical nature that are characteristic for each drug type' (WHO 1974).

Thus, dependency may develop when an individual becomes physically, socially or psychologically reliant on a drug such that life without it becomes intolerable. Dependency is not automatic. Any drug can be misused without the user becoming dependent on it. At the same time, dependence on a drug does not necessarily lead to drug abuse (Advisory Council on the Misuse of Drugs 1982).

During the 1960s many experts tried in vain to clarify the distinction between drug addiction and drug habituation. These two terms were subsequently abandoned in favour of drug dependence. It is therefore safe to assume that 'dependence' and 'addiction' refer to the same thing:

> The term 'addiction' is traditionally used to describe the situation when a person has to continue drug use to ward off withdrawal symptoms. This word has for some time been replaced by the term 'dependence'. (M A Plant 1987)

However, an increasing number of professionals working within the dependency field believe that such labels as dependence and addiction are at best unhelpful in the treatment setting.

Other terms

Drug. The WHO Expert Committee on Drug Dependence describe the word 'drug' as 'a term of varied usage'. As a medicinal product 'drug' can refer to 'any substance in a pharmaceutical product that is used to modify or explore physiological systems or pathological states for the benefit of the recipient' (WHO 1985). The term is also used to refer to substances of abuse, among which some people include alcohol, tobacco and caffeine.

Tolerance and cross-tolerance are generally understood in pharmacology as 'a decrease in response to a drug dose that occurs with continued use' and 'the development of tolerance to another substance, which the individual has not previously been exposed to, as a result of acute or chronic intake of a substance', respectively.

Drug abuse refers to the 'persistent or sporadic excessive use [of a drug] inconsistent with or unrelated to acceptable medical practice' (WHO 1969).

Detoxification. This is a process of removing from the body the substance on which the individual is physiologically dependent. During this process, medical treatment may be given and the patient is assisted in making adjustments to his lifestyle such that drugs are no longer needed. Detoxification is increasingly undertaken in the patient's home environment. Only severe cases in which complications have been identified require hospitalisation (Cooper 1993).

Withdrawal symptoms. These are best described as psychological and/or physiological reactions to the reduction or complete withdrawal of the substance of misuse. How long withdrawal lasts often depends on the previous use of the drug and on the nature and extent of both physiological and psychological dependence (Cooper 1993).

A MODEL FOR CHANGING ADDICTIVE BEHAVIOURS

As many as 250 different therapies are now available to individuals with dependency problems (Parloff 1980). In 1984, a conference held in Scotland aimed to 'develop a more comprehensive model of change for the treatment of addictive behaviours' (Prochaska & Di Clemente 1986). It was agreed that any model developed should apply to the broad range of ways people change, i.e. from those requiring maximum intervention (inpatient care) to those needing minimal intervention, as, for example, in the form of self-help manuals (Prochaska & Di Clemente 1986). This model had to apply to the variety of dependency behaviours that individuals wish to change, and, at the same time, to advance the understanding of *how* people change their behaviours, from the stage at which a problem is recognised to the point at which it is resolved.

Prochaska & Di Clemente proposed a model of change which is now widely accepted. This model provides a framework which can assist professionals in organising their knowledge, and in making case management decisions. Prochaska & Di Clemente felt that this model should take account of the person who self-changes as well as the individual progressing through therapy, and should be applicable to the wide range of dependency problems that exists. It should also help the therapist to synthesise the various treatment methods presently available.

The Prochaska & Di Clemente (1986) model is 'three-dimensional', integrating changes, processes and levels of change. The model comprises four stages — pre-contemplation, contemplation, action and maintenance — which may be conceived of as cyclical, thus allowing the individual to join or leave the process of change at any given stage (see Fig. 37.1). The Prochaska & Di Clemente model can be referred to as the integrative model of change or as the motivation to change model. Its stages may be described as follows.

Pre-contemplation stage

At this stage the individual is not aware of his dependency. This could be because of ambivalence, denial, or selective exposure to information. As the individual becomes aware of his problem progression to the next phase is made possible.

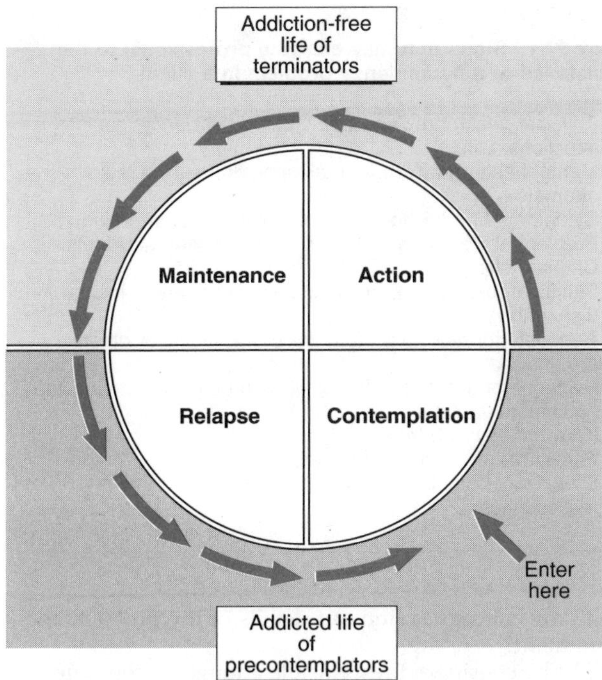

Fig 37.1 The integrative model of change (Prochaska and Di Clemente (1986)).

Contemplation stage
At this point the individual admits that something is wrong and begins to think seriously about changing his behaviour. This stage may last for a period ranging from a few weeks to many years, and some individuals never progress beyond this point.

Action stage
Here, the individual makes a commitment to alter his problematic behaviour. This is a brief stage, as when the decision has been made the individual progresses to the next stage.

Maintenance stage
At this point, new behaviour is strengthened and develops into self-efficiency, and the individual's feeling of being in control is maximised. This stage affords the exit point to termination.

At the maintenance stage, the individual may temporarily lapse as a result of the extreme effort required to maintain the change in behaviour. Occasionally this extends to relapse, in which case the individual often goes back to the pre-contemplation stage before rejoining the cycle. Prochaska & Di Clemente (1986) suggest that 84% of relapsers progress back into the contemplation stage. It would also appear that the typical self-changer makes three serious revolutions of the change cycle before exiting into a relatively dependency-free life (Prochaska & Di Clemente 1983, Schacter 1982). Some individuals do, however, become arrested at one particular stage.

It is essential that the individual and the professional are in agreement as to which stage of change is relevant at a given time. Any resistance to therapeutic interventions often comes as a direct result of the therapist and client working at different stages of the change process. Prochaska & Di Clemente (1986) explain the importance of this as follows:

> The more directive, action-orientated therapist would find a client who is at the contemplation stage to be highly resistive to therapy. From the client's perspective, however, the therapist may be seen as wanting to move too quickly . . . . A therapist who specialises in contemplating and understanding the causes of problems will tend to see the client who is ready for action as resistive to the insight aspect of therapy. The client would be warned against acting impulsively. From the client's perspective . . . the therapist might be warned against moving too slowly.

In giving the Prochaska–Di Clemente integrative model of change practical application in her interventions with drug-dependent patients the nurse should never hesitate to seek help and advice from more experienced or knowledgeable practitioners. At the same time, the nurse should strive to be well-informed about all aspects of substance abuse. Nurses of all levels and specialities have contact with people with dependency problems and therefore need to be aware of the physical, social, psychological and legal consequences of dependency and the implications of these for the individual, his family, and the nurse.

All nursing assessments should include investigations addressing substance use and abuse. While nurses become accustomed to asking about the most intimate details of bowel action or sexual function, many feel uncomfortable about broaching the subject of alcohol or drug use. This may reflect a lack of basic knowledge, as well as a need to make such questioning routine. The following section is devoted to the question of how nurses can enhance their ability to recognise drug-related problems and initiate appropriate interventions.

THE ROLE OF THE NURSE

Even though our understanding of dependency problems has improved in recent years, there is still a tendency for nurses and other professionals to shy away from individuals with drug- or alcohol-related problems as a client group. The 'Kessel' report (1979) is just one of many efforts to counter this tendency by encouraging primary intervention and responsibility. The DOH circular *Alcohol Misuse* (1989) called for all agencies to work together in an effort to supply effective interventions for those with drinking problems, and at a national symposium on 'Responding to Alcohol' in September 1989, Mr J Tate, Deputy Chief Nursing Officer, DOH, argued that 'Nurses should be at the forefront of services for problem drinkers and their care', adding that 'Nurses in basic education must receive alcohol education' and that 'this should be built upon in post-basic education'.

Unfortunately, nursing education in the area of dependency problems is still generally inadequate, making it difficult for some nurses to appreciate the difficulties experienced by drug users. One still hears nurses make comments such as these:

- 'It's not right her being here; it's different when people have to come in through no fault of their own.'
- 'He's always coming in and out; never changes.'
- 'They're all psychopaths.'

Such statements are often offered as justification for inaction. The following exercise might help the nurse to imagine herself in the substance-abuser's place.

> ? **37.2** For one week, stop using your favourite drug, e.g. tea, coffee, alcohol, chocolate, tobacco. At the end of the week, make a few notes on the following:
> a. How easy did you find it to live without your drug?
> b. Was your mood affected? If so, in what way? Did you experience cravings?
> c. What strategies did you use to avoid temptation?

In her interactions with individuals with a drug dependency, it is important for the nurse to realise that the substance abused forms only a small part of the problem. Each patient will present with a unique set of concerns which may have caused, contributed to, or interacted with the development of the problem.

Many drug-dependent individuals change their behaviour as a direct result of a major life event, such as a change in an important relationship, an accident or illness, redundancy, a birth or a death. Such events can curtail, neutralise or enhance the nurse's endeavours with an individual (Davidson 1991) and must be taken into account in the formulation of treatment programmes. Davidson (1991) argues for an eclectic approach to treatment, in which all relevant professionals should intervene as necessary.

In carrying out her own work with drug-dependent individuals the nurse should be prepared:

1. To identify the individual with a drug problem
2. To recognise the types of problems that are likely to be experienced by the individual
3. To assist the individual in the process of acknowledging, exploring and understanding the drug problem
4. To appreciate the individual's own perception of the problem
5. To consider with the individual the treatment options available
6. To facilitate the individual's achievement of his chosen goal(s)
7. To acquaint the individual with the services and facilities available to assist him
8. To act in a non-judgmental way
9. To provide nursing interventions in withdrawal
10. To provide understanding and support should relapse occur.

Identifying drug-related problems

Being aware of dependency problems and knowing when and how to seek advice can save valuable nursing time. Consider the example of a health visitor who is persistently requested to call on a mother and her crying baby. Each time, the mother is advised on feeding, comforting and how to rest while baby sleeps. Despite these reassurances the health visitor continues to receive requests to visit. Had the question of drug misuse been explored, it might have been realised that the woman's husband had a drug problem. The couple were behind on rent, had insufficient money to buy food, and the husband was resorting to theft to fund his drug use. The mother's resultant anxiety was being sensed by the baby and expressed in the only way it knew how, i.e. crying. This example is not meant to imply that all crying babies have substance-abusing parents, but simply that drug use is a potential contributing factor in a wide range of problems and therefore should be considered and explored in initial and subsequent assessment.

Box 37.1 lists various signs that can indicate the existence of a drug-related problem. The nurse should bear in mind, of course, that not every feature listed will apply to a given individual, nor does the existence of any one feature demonstrate conclusively that a dependency problem exists.

Nurses and substance abuse

It is equally important that nurses are aware of the high levels of stress that they experience in their professional lives and which can make them vulnerable to substance misuse. It is very hard for a nurse to broach this subject with a colleague whom she suspects of having drug-related problems. It is just as difficult for the nurse with a drug problem to come forward and ask for help. The nurse who is beginning to face up to a drug problem may find herself asking the following questions (Cooper & Faugier 1993):

Box 37.1 Signs that may alert the professional to the existence of a dependency problem in a client

- Physical health problem, e.g. vitamin deficiency, gastritis, infections, ulcers
- Mental health problem, e.g. anxiety, depression, suicide attempts
- Symptoms of addiction, e.g. tremor, shakes, sweating
- Problem at work, e.g. lateness, absenteeism, accidents
- Criminal offences
- Family problems, e.g. neglect, child disturbance, marital disharmony
- Requests for help, e.g. from the client, family or other professional
- Evidence of use of alcohol or other drugs, e.g. smell, used equipment
- Known history of drug problems
- Family history of drug problems
- Other: e.g. complaints of fatigue, lethargy, insomnia, restlessness

1. Will my colleagues find out details of my problem and treatment?
2. Will I be considered responsible enough to continue in my profession if I accept help?
3. If I cannot look after myself, how can others be entrusted to my care?
4. Will treatment for a drug problem be noted on my record and limit my professional development?
5. How will I relate to the nurses who are caring for me?
6. Will I be suspended, disciplined or asked to leave?
7. How will I convince others that I can be trusted to hold drug cupboard keys?
8. How can I impress on senior managers and nursing colleagues that any future time off from work is due to genuine illness and is not drug related?
9. How will I arrange regular time off to keep my counselling appointments?

How nurses can get help

The nurse who has acknowledged to herself that she has a drug-related problem should check to see if her Health Authority has an 'Alcohol (and Drug) in the Workplace' policy. If the problem has been brought into the open by a warning from an employer, then this policy will be invoked and the nurse referred to Occupational Health for further treatment. The nurse should make sure that the policy is duly followed. Although she will probably be under a contract by which improvement in work performance is required, the policy is usually in the nurse's favour, protecting her job security whilst she responds to agreed therapy and ensuring adequate time off to attend counselling and treatment sessions.

If the problem is one of alcohol use, the contract might not require the nurse to stop drinking altogether. However, if the problem is one of illegal drug misuse, total abstinence is the accepted outcome at the present time. The nurse will, however, not be rushed. It is normal procedure to refer an employee outside of the Health Authority which employs her for professional help in order to ensure confidentiality.

The nurse does not have to be referred to Occupational Health by her employer. It is possible for her to approach Occupational Health in confidence on her own. She will then be put in contact with a drug counselling agency. If the nurse has identified the problem herself, she may in fact wish to approach such an agency directly. Contact information can usually be found in the Yellow Pages or from Citizens' Advice

Bureaux. Again, whether the agency is voluntary or statutory, it is bound by rules of confidentiality. It will, however, make contact with the nurse's Occupational Health department, if she so requires.

If a nurse feels that she has a drug problem of any kind which is affecting her work, it is best for her to seek help before formal measures by her employer become necessary. Following assessment, treatment goals can be set. The nurse should be free to progress at her own pace without the worry of being 'found out' and losing her job. The nurse should not be considered weak at having to admit to a drug problem or to feeling unable to cope with the stresses of her work. On the contrary: it takes courage and determination to come forward and make the first, and possibly most difficult, step towards change.

If the nurse's colleagues have already suspected the existence of a problem because of little errors (or larger ones) she has made at work they may have already taken some responsibility away from her. As her improvement becomes apparent, their confidence will gradually be regained and responsibility will be handed back. It is important, however, that the nurse does not allow herself to be pushed into taking on more responsibility or a heavier workload than she feels ready for. Relapse is a real possibility and can be brought about by the nurse putting pressure on herself to make rapid change.

Approaching the patient with a suspected drug problem

If the nurse suspects that a patient has a dependency problem, she should be careful to raise the question of his drug use in a non-threatening manner. While the patient may be evasive or defensive at first, at least the nurse will have demonstrated her concern and made the first approach. The subject should not be belaboured at the initial stages, but the nurse should tactfully and sensitively try to progress at each contact. The nurse should remember that she is not a judge, but a facilitator, educator and carer.

Bedside conversations in large wards do not enhance confidentiality. Curtains round a bed do not block out sound. The nurse should consider where and how she would want to be approached if she were in the patient's situation and apply the same standards of confidentiality she would expect for herself in her interactions with others.

If the nurse feels unsure about how to proceed, she should seek advice and support and find out about local agencies that may be of benefit to her patient. The nurse should make contact with colleagues who have similar patients on their caseload, as mutual support is essential in all areas of nursing.

Assessment

Any intervention can be undertaken only following a full and systematic assessment of the needs of the patient and his family. If treatment is to have a favourable outcome, a complete picture of the patient's drug use must be obtained. Moreover, a clear understanding of the patient's own treatment goals is essential. Does he want to achieve a reduction in use, a change to a less harmful drug, controlled use, withdrawal, or total abstinence?

Many drug users 'sound out' a service before committing themselves to care. Therefore, any information given on treatment options should be clear and to the point, and should be communicated both verbally and in written form.

Assessment should include details of past and present drug abuse. In preparation, the patient could be asked to complete a diary similar to that shown in Figure 37.2. The following factors should always be considered in any assessment:

Day	Time drinking commenced and ended	Type and amount consumed	Mood prior	Mood after	Number of units consumed
Monday					
Tuesday					
Wednesday					
Thursday					
Friday					
Saturday					
Sunday					
Totals					

Fig. 37.2 Sample form for an alcohol use diary.

- psychological state
- work, social and cultural factors
- problematic effects of use
- motivation for treatment
- family psychodynamics
- relevant personal factors
- physical state and complications.

Prevention

Whether or not an individual develops a drug problem often depends on the social resources available to him. It is vital that the problems and experiences that can set the stage for drug abuse are recognised by the caring professions, and that the relevant agencies persevere in improving and developing preventive strategies both at the local and national level.

In recent years campaigns such as 'No Smoking Day' and 'Drinkwise Day' have had some effect. Most District Health Authorities now have community drug and alcohol teams, as well as a health promotion officer dealing with HIV/AIDS–related issues (see Ch. 38, p. 1001). The introduction of such initiatives as outreach programmes and needle exchange schemes has also proved valuable in the early identification of drug-related problems (see p. 986).

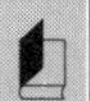
Readers with a special interest in the area of prevention are referred to Tether & Robinson (1986).

DRUG USE AND MISUSE: SOME FACTS

LEGAL SUBSTANCES

Tea and coffee

> The sufferer is tremulous and loses his self command; he is subject to fits of agitation and depression. He loses colour and has a haggard appearance. As with other agents, a renewed dose of the poison gives temporary relief, but at the cost of future misery. (Cited in Pickles 1991)

Coffee, tea, soft drinks such as Coca-Cola, and some analgesics contain caffeine, a drug which has a stimulating effect upon the central nervous system. Perhaps the reader will identify with some aspects of the above description of the effects of coffee-drinking, written anonymously in 1909.

In the UK, 70% of the adult population drink coffee, whilst 86% drink tea. The daily caffeine consumption for this group has been estimated at 440 mg per person (Cosgrove 1992). The existence of a caffeine withdrawal syndrome is now accepted. Silverman et al 1992 stated that 'Caffeine withdrawal can produce severe symptoms, and health care professionals should be aware of the problem'. They call for caffeine withdrawal to be included in the group of 'organic mental syndromes associated with psychoactive substances'. Participants in their double-blind study underwent physical and psychological tests during a period of normal diet followed by a period of caffeine-free diet. Half the group, who received a caffeine supplement during the second period, reported no significant change. The other half, who were given placebo drugs, recorded more headaches, increased use of analgesia and greater fatigue. Depression and anxiety scores were also abnormally high in this group.

Tobacco

It takes 7 seconds for the chemicals contained in tobacco smoke to produce an effect within the brain. These chemicals are stimulants, and assist in the maintenance of performance in cases of fatigue and monotony. They alleviate stress and anxiety by producing relaxation and stimulation. The rapid decline of these effects, however, encourages further use and dependence develops quickly. If tobacco use is stopped abruptly, depression, restlessness, irritability and craving may be experienced.

The United States Surgeon General's report for 1989 concludes that:

- cigarettes and other forms of tobacco are addictive
- nicotine is the drug in tobacco that causes addiction
- the pharmacological and behavioural processes that determine tobacco addiction are similar to those that determine addiction to drugs such as heroin and cocaine.

The Health Education Authority (1991) reports that smoking is the largest single cause of preventable and premature deaths in the UK. In excess of 111 000 people died in the UK in 1988 of tobacco-related illnesses at a cost of £400 million in NHS hospital services. It is estimated that each day as many as 500 children try smoking for the first time and that by the age of 19, 30% are regular smokers (HEA 1991).

Consequences for health

The high cost of tobacco use to the nation's health is clearly demonstrated in Box 37.2.

Tobacco use can also be a contributing factor in the development of pancreatic cancer, blood clots, lung infections, strokes, bronchitis, poor circulation, cancer of the mouth and throat, ischaemic heart disease, thrombosis and emphysema.

Women and smoking. In 1992 the DOH launched a 2-year national campaign aimed at women smokers, especially those who smoke during pregnancy. With a budget of over £1 million, this campaign includes national anti-smoking advertising and the financing of special training for midwives and community nurses. General practitioners, health visitors, family planning staff and other community workers will also receive 'cessation counselling' training (HEA 1991).

One in three women smoke during pregnancy, doubling the risk of underweight births, stillbirth and early infant deaths (HEA 1991). Krishna (1978) suggests that the health risks associated with tobacco use in women are increased in those 'who are poor, anaemic and have several children'. Fogelman (1988) also reported 'deficiencies in physical growth and intellectual development in children of women smokers'. It has been suggested that pregnant women who smoke run the risk of spontaneous abortion or of complications such as bleeding during pregnancy, premature detachment of the placenta and premature rupture of the membrane (Sidle 1982).

The HEA (1991) reports that nicotine has been found in breast milk and may be a causative factor in reduced production. The incidence of cancer of the cervix is high among women who smoke heavily (HEA 1991, Trevathan 1983), and women who smoke increase their risk of coronary heart disease, stroke, blood clots, pulmonary embolism, circulatory

Box 37.2 Incidence of tobacco-related disease in the UK, 1988 (Adapted from HEA 1991.)

32 300	lung cancer
32 100	coronary heart disease
22 000	chronic obstructive pulmonary disease (COPD)
11 300	other cancers: buccal cavity, oesophagus, larynx, bladder, kidneys and cervix
9 000	strokes
2 900	aortic aneurism and atherosclerotic peripheral disease
1 000	peptic ulcers

disease, and raised blood pressure and cholesterol levels (HEA 1991).

Passive smoking

As only 15% of tobacco smoke is inhaled by the smoker, the remaining 85% becomes environmental smoke which may be inhaled by others in the vicinity, who thus become 'passive smokers' (HEA 1991).

The effect of this 'passive smoking' is receiving increased attention. A report by the Independent Scientific Committee on Smoking and Health suggests that people who are subjected to the smoke of others have an increased risk (in the range of 10–30%) of developing lung cancer (ISCSH 1988). The Committee suggests that in view of the dangers of 'second-hand' smoke, 'nonsmoking should be regarded as the norm in enclosed areas frequented by the public or employees, special provision being made for smokers, rather than vice versa'.

The effects of tobacco smoke on nonsmokers can include nose, throat and chest irritations, breathing difficulties, coughing, red and runny eyes, headaches, dizziness, nausea, lack of concentration and decrease in lung function. Those with long-term health problems such as asthma, chronic bronchitis, allergies and heart problems are especially at risk. The WHO 'Charter Against Tobacco' (see Box 37.3) is in part an attempt to assert the right of non-smokers to a healthy environment.

Cessation aids

It has been suggested that the majority of smokers would like to stop (OPCS 1989). However, pharmacological and psychological dependence often prevents them from doing so. Some cessation aids contain nicotine, whilst others aim to reduce craving by producing an unpleasant taste when smoking takes place. It is not recommended that cigarette smokers switch to a pipe or cigars, as research has indicated that those who switch are more likely to inhale the smoke than those for whom these are the primary substance of use (Jarvis 1989).

Withdrawal symptoms experienced by smokers may last for a few weeks, although occasional cravings may occur for a few years after cessation.

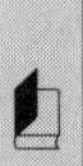

The Health Education Authority produces two booklets which nurses may find useful for themselves or their patients: *How to Stop Smoking for You and Your Baby*, and *A Smokers Guide to 'Giving Up'*.
Action on Smoking and Health (ASH) also produce a useful set of information sheets (see Useful Addresses, p. 989).

Box 37.3 WHO Charter Against Tobacco

- Fresh air, free from tobacco smoke, is an essential component of the right to a healthy and unpolluted environment.
- Every child and adolescent has the right to be protected from all tobacco promotion and to receive all necessary educational and other help to resist the temptation to start using tobacco in any form.
- All citizens have the right to smoke-free air in enclosed public places and transport.
- Every worker has the right to breath air in the workplace that is unpolluted by tobacco smoke.
- Every smoker has the right to receive encouragement and help to overcome the habit.
- Every citizen has the right to be informed of the unparalleled health risks of tobacco use.

Alcohol

I didn't really like the taste but the effect allowed me to be sophisticated and to feel good with others. I felt guilty at my unhappiness. I had a good husband, a nice house and healthy children. Everything I wanted really.

I suppose I drank because I couldn't cope with the reality of life. As my drinking progressed I blamed others for any problems I had. If I couldn't cope with a problem, I would blot it out with alcohol.

As my problems mounted I remembered as a teenager how alcohol took away my inhibitions, made me feel confident and able to converse. People liked me better then. (A problem drinker.)

? **37.3** For a one-week period keep a daily diary of your alcohol consumption, using the format given in Figure 37.2. When you have read the following section, refer to your diary as you discuss with your colleagues your reactions to and reflections on your own alcohol use.

Alcohol is the most popular psychoactive drug used in modern society and is consumed by approximately 90% of the adult population in the UK. When used in moderation, it does little more than act as a social 'lubricant', lowering inhibitions and facilitating social interaction. Excessive, heavy and prolonged use, however, can have serious consequences for health.

Alcoholic drinks are mainly comprised of water and ethanol (alcohol) and are produced by fermentation of fruits, vegetables or grain. Congeners are added to give the drink its distinctive flavour, taste and smell.

Units of alcohol

One unit of alcohol is that amount of a given drink which contains approximately 15 mg of pure ethanol. This is based on a standard pub measure of an average-strength drink, i.e. half a pint of beer, lager or cider, a single measure of spirits (e.g. whisky, gin, vodka), a standard glass of wine, a small glass of sherry, or a measure of vermouth (or aperitif). Therefore, if a total of 2 pints of average-strength lager and a small sherry were consumed, the total number of units consumed would be 5.

However, since many varieties of alcoholic drinks of varying strengths are available it can be very difficult to estimate how much alcohol one has consumed. Table 37.1 gives an approximate guide to the calculation of unit consumption for drinks of various strengths.

What is safe? It has been suggested that the following units represent maximum levels for 'safe' weekly consumption.

Table 37.1 Calculation of unit consumption for alcoholic drinks of various strengths (Adapted from HEA 1989.)

Type of drink	Measure	Number of units
Export beer	1 pint	2.5
	1 can*	2
Strong beer or lager	1 pint	4
	1 can*	3
Extra strong beer or lager	1 pint	5
	1 can*	4
Strong cider	1 pint	4
Spirits	1 bottle	30
Table wine	1 bottle	7
	1 L bottle	10
Sherry	1 bottle	13
Low-alcohol beers and lager	1 pint	⅔
Low-alcohol cider	1 pint	½

*1 can = ¾ pint

Consumption above this level can be expected to lead to health problems.

- For men: up to 21 units divided into 4 or 5 drinking occasions
- For women: up to 14 units divided into 4 or 5 drinking occasions.

Alcohol absorption and elimination

Alcohol is one of the quickest-acting orally administered drugs. It is a toxic substance and the only organ capable of eliminating it from the body is the liver.

Alcohol passes chemically unchanged from the stomach into the blood supply within 5 minutes. Adding carbonated drinks, alternating alcohol with carbonated drinks, drinking on an empty stomach and drinking quickly may speed up absorption.

It takes approximately 30 minutes for alcohol levels to peak in the blood and one hour for the liver to eliminate one unit. Any other alcohol taken during this time will accumulate in the blood, awaiting processing. Therefore, if 8 units are consumed (e.g. 4 pints of lager or 4 double spirits) the liver will take approximately 8–9 hours to eliminate all the alcohol.

Health consequences of excessive alcohol use

Alcohol abuse can lead to a wide range of health problems affecting virtually all parts of the body (see Fig. 37.3). In addition to the possible consequences of intoxication, excessive regular use and dependence (see Box 37.4), alcohol consumption (even at moderate levels) can interfere with the effects of many prescribed drugs such as oral contraceptives, antibiotics, anti-inflammatory agents, tranquillisers, antidepressants and diuretics. The habitual over-use of alcohol is associated with a number of psychosocial problems.

Long term use and withdrawal. Tolerance develops quickly with the regular use of alcohol. Physical as well as psychological dependence can occur. Sudden withdrawal after excessive use can be accompanied by unpleasant symptoms such as sweating, increased anxiety, tremor, headache, thirst, nausea and occasional vomiting. Full delirium tremens and convulsions may also be experienced.

Those who have suffered severe withdrawal symptoms in the past, or who following assessment appear to be at risk, will need a properly supervised withdrawal programme (Cooper 1993). Contrary to popular belief it *is* possible for someone with an alcohol problem to return to 'normal' social drinking or controlled drinking.

Teenage drinking

The issue of teenage drinking in the UK has given rise to a certain degree of public alarm. Newspaper articles condemn the behaviour of 'teenage lager louts' and demand that underage drinking be stopped. Yet there is little evidence to suggest that the majority of teenagers do anything other than drink sensibly, or, indeed, that heavy consumption at an early age leads to chronic alcohol abuse in later life.

Children in our society do, however, encounter alcohol at an early age. Plant (1982) found in one sample that 40% of 6-year-olds and 60% of 10-year-olds could identify alcoholic drinks by their smell. Cooper (1985) obtained similar results

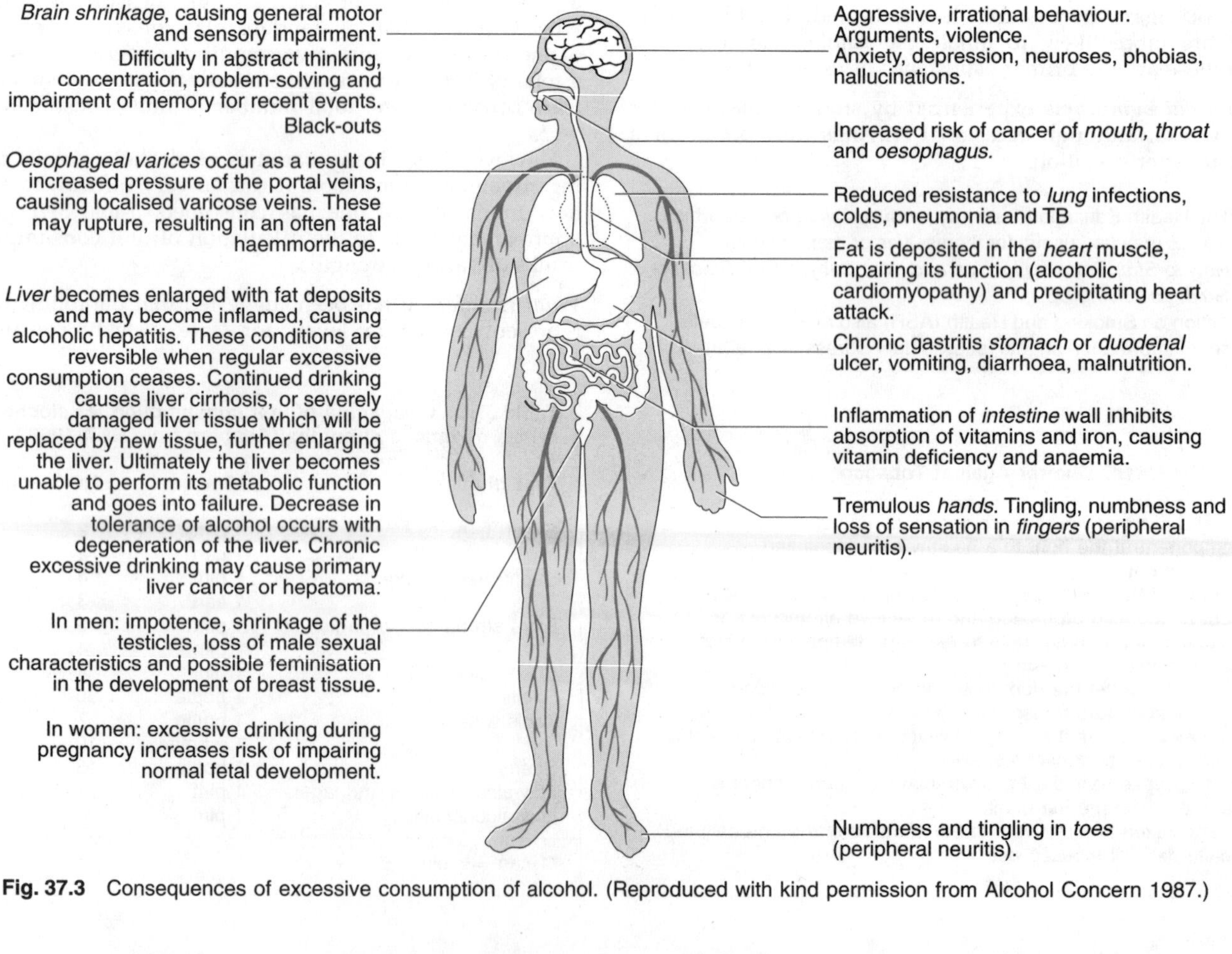

Brain shrinkage, causing general motor and sensory impairment.
Difficulty in abstract thinking, concentration, problem-solving and impairment of memory for recent events. Black-outs
Oesophageal varices occur as a result of increased pressure of the portal veins, causing localised varicose veins. These may rupture, resulting in an often fatal haemmorrhage.
Liver becomes enlarged with fat deposits and may become inflamed, causing alcoholic hepatitis. These conditions are reversible when regular excessive consumption ceases. Continued drinking causes liver cirrhosis, or severely damaged liver tissue which will be replaced by new tissue, further enlarging the liver. Ultimately the liver becomes unable to perform its metabolic function and goes into failure. Decrease in tolerance of alcohol occurs with degeneration of the liver. Chronic excessive drinking may cause primary liver cancer or hepatoma.
In men: impotence, shrinkage of the testicles, loss of male sexual characteristics and possible feminisation in the development of breast tissue.
In women: excessive drinking during pregnancy increases risk of impairing normal fetal development.
Aggressive, irrational behaviour. Arguments, violence.
Anxiety, depression, neuroses, phobias, hallucinations.
Increased risk of cancer of *mouth, throat* and *oesophagus*.
Reduced resistance to *lung* infections, colds, pneumonia and TB
Fat is deposited in the *heart* muscle, impairing its function (alcoholic cardiomyopathy) and precipitating heart attack.
Chronic gastritis *stomach* or *duodenal* ulcer, vomiting, diarrhoea, malnutrition.
Inflammation of *intestine* wall inhibits absorption of vitamins and iron, causing vitamin deficiency and anaemia.
Tremulous *hands*. Tingling, numbness and loss of sensation in *fingers* (peripheral neuritis).
Numbness and tingling in *toes* (peripheral neuritis).

Fig. 37.3 Consequences of excessive consumption of alcohol. (Reproduced with kind permission from Alcohol Concern 1987.)

Box 37.4 Alcohol misuse: associated harm

CONSEQUENCES OF INTOXICATION
- Accidents
- Acute poisoning
- Acute gastritis
- Drug overdose
- Epileptic-type seizures
- Head injury
- Suicidal behaviour

CONSEQUENCES OF EXCESSIVE REGULAR USE
- Anxiety
- Cancer of the mouth/throat
- Depression
- Fatty liver
- Liver cancer
- Liver cirrhosis
- Pancreatitis
- Peripheral neuritis
- Phobic illness
- Sexual impotence
- Stomach haemorrhage

CONSEQUENCES OF DEPENDENCE
- Alcoholic psychosis
- Anxiety
- Delirium tremens
- Depression
- Hallucination
- Paranoid states
- Polydrug abuse
- Withdrawal: epileptic seizures

in a survey of 14–16-year-olds. When asked about alcohol consumption 81% reported that they had consumed an alcoholic drink. However, most of this consumption was occasional in nature.

Young people tend to be introduced to alcohol by their parents. Most are primed from an early age to accept alcohol as part of everyday life. But while excessive alcohol use is a real problem for some teenagers, perhaps what is needed is not a demand for total abstinence among young people (since this would be unenforceable in practice anyway) but increased public education on the risks of alcohol misuse and its links with HIV/AIDS, promiscuous behaviour, drugs and smoking. Teenagers should be allowed to develop their own concepts about the appropriate use of alcohol in a straightforward and, most importantly, informed manner. A failure to be open in our approach to the subject of alcohol use may only serve to entice adolescents to explore this forbidden territory in a spirit of rebellion, without the benefit of adequate knowledge and experience.

?	37.4 Do you think that there is a widespread teenage drinking problem in the UK? If so, how could you as a nurse help to prevent drinking problems among young people?

Women and alcohol abuse

It is generally acknowledged that alcohol-related problems amongst women are increasing (Camberwell Council on Alcoholism 1986). However, this does not necessarily imply that women consume the same quantities of alcohol as men, since alcohol affects women in smaller quantities. M L Plant (1987) suggests: 'Important physical differences in the way in which women's bodies cope with alcohol and factors concerning their reproductive system which influence metabolism play an integral part in ARPs [alcohol-related problems] for this client group.'

Women present to caring agencies with the same alcohol-related problems as men, e.g. gastritis, duodenal ulcers, peripheral neuritis, cancer of the mouth, throat or oesophagus, amnesic episodes and suicidal behaviour. However, women who drink excessively have a greater risk of acute inflammation of the liver than men. Moreover, any damage to the liver in childbearing years may increase in severity even after cessation (M L Plant 1987).

Breeze (1985) records that the heaviest drinking among women occurs in those aged 25 years and under. Social factors such as marriage, a shortage of personal finance, responsibility for children and a lack of leisure time appear to moderate alcohol consumption (M A Plant 1987). In a survey of 15–16-year-olds, Plant et al (1985) report that 43% drank alcohol.

Society still views women with drug problems more critically than men and is quick to condemn women as weak, inadequate and as 'bad' mothers or wives when they have a dependency problem. Men appear to be generally less tolerant and supportive and more likely to leave a relationship than are women when their partner develops a dependency problem.

Women present to helping agencies with their own specific set of problems, which includes guilt, low self-esteem and depression. This requires sensitive nursing skills. The individual needs to feel sufficiently at ease with a professional to disclose her drug problem. In order to gain the patient's confidence the nurse must be non-judgmental, supportive and well-informed about appropriate sources of help.

Alcohol in pregnancy. The Royal College of Psychiatrists (1987) suggest that whilst there is a link between excessive alcohol consumption and birth deformities, 'it is a misuse of that evidence to preach hellfire to every woman who takes a glass of wine during pregnancy'. The main problem is that, as yet, no one knows how much alcohol it is 'safe' to drink during pregnancy.

There is, however, a recognised syndrome in babies of women who regularly consume large amounts of alcohol in pregnancy. Jones & Smith (1973) called this the 'fetal alcohol syndrome'. They recorded several features commonly found in babies of alcohol-dependent women, including growth deficiencies, delayed development, joint and heart abnormalities, microcephaly and fine motor dysfunction. Facial features included: asymmetrical ears, receding chin, receding forehead, and upturned nose and short palpebral fissure length.

(Plant 1985) has attempted to put the problem into perspective by suggesting that there are several social factors which may influence birth defects; these include tobacco and alcohol consumption and accommodation. Looking at specific levels of alcohol consumption during pregnancy, Plant found that 'Women who consumed 10 units of alcohol on a single occasion during pregnancy were more likely than other women to have damaged offspring'. She suggests that low levels of alcohol consumption are not associated with birth defects.

Alcohol Concern's (1992) advice to women is:

- drink in moderation
- avoid binge drinking
- cut down if you drink over 14 standard drinks per week; contact your GP, Alcohol Concern or your local alcohol advisory service
- take special care if you are pregnant.

? **37.5** Test your factual knowledge by answering the following questions. A

a. On average, how much (i) wine, (ii) spirits, (iii) beer, (iv) lager would you need to drink to be over the legal limit for driving?
b. Which parts of the body are affected by alcohol, and what are the effects?
c. What organ in the body breaks down alcohol?
d. After drinking 1 pint of ordinary beer, how long will it take before the alcohol in it is completely burned up by the body?
e. Which of these is an effective way of sobering up?
   - Drinking a cup of strong black coffee?
   - Taking fresh air?
   - Taking physical exercise?
   - Taking a cold shower?
   - Making yourself sick?
f. What level of daily consumption is considered to lead to the possibility of alcohol dependence?
   (i) 4 pints of beer?
   (ii) 8 glasses of wine?
   (iii) 2 single tots of whisky?
   (iv) 2 double tots of rum?
   (v) 6 glasses of fortified wine?
   (vi) 3 pints of lager?
g. Is the recommended safe limit of drinking for women lower, or higher, than that for men?
h. Equal amounts of alcohol have a greater effect on a young person than on the average adult male. Why is this?
i. What can speed up the effect of alcohol?

Alcohol and elderly people

As the body ages its ability to tolerate alcohol diminishes. The liver and kidneys become less efficient, and thus the elimination of alcohol from the body becomes slower. The effect of alcohol on reflexes, balance, self-control and judgement may compound existing health problems, increasing the risk of falls and other accidents. Equally, many older people take medication such as hypnotics, analgesics and anti-inflammatory drugs which, when mixed with alcohol, increase the risk of health problems.

Age can bring with it many difficulties such as financial hardship, loneliness, isolation, insomnia, pain, and susceptibility to cold. (**Note**: a 'hot toddy' will not warm a person up. Alcohol dilates the blood vessels, allowing heat to escape and increasing the risk of hypothermia.) Many older people eat unbalanced diets and have a poor appetite; some may sacrifice food for alcohol.

Alcohol may be used by some older people as a means of blocking out feelings of loneliness. Many of these individuals will find it hard to come forward for help, and it can sometimes be difficult for professionals to recognise alcohol-related problems among this client group. The relatives of an elderly person may dismiss his drinking as a minor foible or take the view that alcohol helps him to cope. Nurses working in this field may hear relatives and carers expressing sentiments such as 'It will do him no harm' or 'What else has he got to live for?'. Even GPs have been known to suggest alcohol as a remedy for insomnia in older people. This can be unwise, as the physical, social and psychological effects of alcohol are often felt among this client group at a relatively low level of consumption.

Treatment. Older people who have come forward for help or who have been identified as having a drink-related problem often feel guilt and shame. In many cases information on the sensible use of alcohol is all that is required to allay anxiety and enable the person to adopt healthier drinking habits. It is important to remember, however, that age does not make someone less able to make decisions about his own life. If the patient does not wish to reduce or modify his consumption, that is his choice. Professionals have a responsibility, nonetheless, to ensure that the individual has adequate information on which to base informed decisions. (See Research Abstract 37.1.)

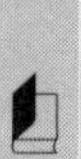

Alcohol Concern (see Useful Addresses, p. 989) has produced some useful booklets to promote safer drinking patterns among older people. These are: 'A DIY Guide for Older People', 'A Guide for Family, Relatives and Friends' and 'A Guide for Health and Social Services and Voluntary Group Workers', all published in 1988. Also recommended is Wesson (1992).

? **37.6** On the basis of the information given in this section, how would you define 'the sensible use of alcohol'? Can alcohol in any way be beneficial?

Tranquillisers

It is estimated that some 15% of the adult population of the UK have problems associated with prescribed medication: some 50 000 tranquillisers are swallowed daily, involving in excess of 3 million people, and £25 million of tranquillisers and sleeping tablets are prescribed each year (Cosgrove 1992). Among consumers of these drugs women form the largest group, although there is a steady increase in prescriptions for men which appears to be associated with unemployment and poor employment prospects. The most commonly prescribed tranquillisers are benzodiazepines (diazepam, temazepam). Ladar (1978) described these as the 'opium of the masses'.

Faugier (1992) suggests that 'withdrawal from tranquillisers is a process which carries with it serious physical and psychological risks'. Once addicted, it can be dangerous for the individual to cease abruptly. Therefore, it is essential that any withdrawal is gradual. Because the symptoms of withdrawal often mask the symptoms of the original complaint, dependence often goes unidentified until the drug is reduced or stopped or until tolerance develops. Symptoms are similar to phobic anxiety states and may include fear, agoraphobia, suicidal feelings and panic attacks.

Concern has been expressed over the lack of identification of those dependent on tranquillisers by members of the caring professions. Faugier (1992) claims that 'tranquilliser dependence has reached epidemic proportions, yet community nurses are not trained adequately to help those who are trying to cope with withdrawal'.

Many doctors have attempted to treat social problems with this group of drugs. Faugier (1992) remarks, however, that these drugs 'often produce quite disabling side effects which not only fail to solve the original problems, but, in fact, add to them significantly'.

Effects

The effects of tranquillisers commence within an hour of administration and last up to 12 hours. These effects include:

- relief from tension
- a sense of calm and relaxation
- decreased self-control, alertness, power of observation and level of dexterity
- control of anxiety
- short-term memory loss
- lowered inhibitions

Research Abstract 37.1 A study of the effectiveness of brief interventions for problem drinkers in acute hospital settings (Hazel E Watson)

A consecutive series of 998 patients who were admitted to general medical, surgical, orthopaedic and short-stay wards of a large teaching hospital were screened to identify potential problem drinkers.

The screening procedure consisted of recording a retrospective diary of the previous week's level of alcohol consumption, a structured interview to assess the frequency of experience of alcohol-related problems and blood samples to estimate levels of gamma-glutamyl transferase (GGT), aspartate transferase (AST) and mean cell volume (MCV).

Of those screened, 24.5% reported levels of alcohol consumption during the previous week as being in excess of the recommended 'sensible limits' as suggested by the Health Education Authority (1989). On further investigation it was found that 153 patients were regular consumers of alcohol who had not previously received treatment for an alcohol problem. These were patients who were receiving treatment for a wide variety of health problems which were not primarily alcohol-related.

The newly identified potential problem drinkers were assigned to one of four treatment groups as follows:

Group 1. Patients in this group were given a copy of the Health Education Authority booklet entitled 'That's the Limit: a Guide to sensible drinking'. This is a 14-page pamphlet which contains advice about the effects of alcohol and how to reduce consumption to within recommended sensible limits.

Group 2. Patients in this group were given brief advice in a one-to-one interpersonal interaction about the effects of alcohol consumption on health and about how to reduce consumption.

Group 3 were given both the booklet which was given to Group 1 and the advice as described for patients in Group 2.

Group 4 were given no intervention.

All the interventions were administered by a nurse.

One year later, 102 patients participated in follow-up interviews. It was found that the entire sample reported statistically highly significant reductions in the mean levels of alcohol consumption as recorded again by the diary method and also in the mean numbers of alcohol-related problems. These reductions were supported by statistically significant reductions in the mean levels of GGT and AST. Changes in mean cell volume, however, did not reach the levels of statistical significance.

The patients in all groups, including the control group (who had received no treatment) demonstrated improvements in each of the self-report measures and also in liver function tests. The extent of the improvement reported by the control group was not significantly different from any of the three treatment groups.

It is possible that the nurse's detailed inquiry into the level of alcohol consumption at a time when people are unwell and therefore perhaps more receptive to advice relating to health, was sufficient to cause them to consider their drinking habits and consequently reduce their consumption.

This does not require specialist experience of working with problem drinkers. The brief interventions described above are measures which can readily be carried out by nurses in a wide variety of health care settings. They are important because they have the potential to help nurses to recognise potential problem drinking at an early stage and, hopefully, prevent the development of alcohol dependence.

Watson H E 1993 Unpublished Ph.D. Thesis, University of Strathclyde, Glasgow

- release of aggression
- the onset of sleep.

With intoxication the individual may experience dysarthria, ataxia, nystagmus and emotional lability.

It is not clear how long it will take an individual to become dependent, though an increase in anxiety has been noted after 4 weeks' use. By 6 months, the risk of dependency is greatly increased. Psychological dependence is common.

Tolerance can develop in both therapeutic and non-therapeutic use and withdrawal symptoms may occur even with therapeutic doses (see Box 37.5). Whilst these are not potentially fatal, they can be very unpleasant and have been described by some as worse than those experienced in heroin withdrawal.

Support during withdrawal

As withdrawal symptoms commence even after a small reduction in tranquilliser dosage, the withdrawal process needs to be undertaken in slow steps. It may take several months or even some years for the patient to be able to live comfortably without the drug.

Support, whether given individually or in a group is essential. Nurses should be aware of the unpleasantness associated with tranquilliser withdrawal and the fear and emotional stress this process is likely to cause the individual and his family.

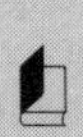

Useful information on the process of tranquilliser withdrawal can be found in Hammersley & Hamlin (1990) and in Trickett (1991).

Solvents

Many solvents, glues, gases and volatile substances are readily available in homes, shops, offices and factories. Under normal use, they are reasonably safe, but unfortunately they are sometimes inhaled specifically for their depressant effect on the central nervous system.

Ives (1990) describes three kinds of solvent abuse among young people:

- experimental: by those who want to know what it is like

Box 37.5 Common tranquilliser withdrawal symptoms

- Convulsions
- Dry retching
- Hand tremor
- Headaches
- Increased tension/anxiety
- Irritability
- Loss of feeling/emotion
- Mental confusion
- Muscle pain/stiffness
- Nausea
- Nightmares
- Palpitations
- Panic attacks
- Personality change
- Profuse sweating
- Rebound insomnia
- Weight loss

- recreational: by those who inhale solvents occasionally with friends
- dependent: regular, long-term abuse.

Re-Solv, the national charity devoted to this area of concern, has called for greater public awareness and vigilance. In their annual report for 1991 they record that, on average, 2 young people die in the UK each week as a consequence of solvent abuse, and that the total number of deaths in 1990 was 129.

The primary substances of abuse are adhesives, cleaning fluids, aerosols and fuels. The common street name for the misuse of these substances is 'huffing' or 'sniffing'. These substances are often inhaled in 'sniffing dens', which may be found by canals, in derelict buildings or on railway banks. They are relatively easy to obtain and offer a cheap alternative to alcohol and other drugs.

Effects of solvent inhalation

Effects commence within 7 seconds of inhalation and last for approximately 30 minutes. Continual sniffing maintains the effect. As the level of intoxication is reduced, the user experiences nausea and headache. With the repetition and deep inhalation overdose may result, causing loss of control, disorientation and unconsciousness. On cessation, recovery usually follows quickly. Concentration of the substance and intensification of effects can be achieved by placing a plastic bag over the head. This method brings with it the danger of asphyxiation.

It is not easy to identify abuse, as the presenting problems may appear to be of a piece with 'normal' adolescent behaviour e.g. moodiness, aggression, loss of appetite, disinterest, and aloofness. With regular use tolerance may develop. Whilst physical dependence does not appear to occur, psychological dependence has been suggested as a problem in a small number of users.

Dangers of excessive and frequent use. It is important for the abuser to avoid exertion, as some substances affect the function of the heart and increase sensitivity. Any exercise may lead to collapse and death. Other dangers include damage to the liver, lungs, kidneys, heart and central nervous system, as well as death by suffocation, accidents, direct toxic effect on the heart, and inhalation of vomit. Gas squirted directly into the mouth can cause suffocation.

Ives (1990) itemises the range of approaches that are taken to prevention and intervention in relation to solvent abuse:

- collecting information
- doing nothing
- using scare tactics
- policing
- providing information and education
- offering activity substitution: individual or group
- providing individual counselling or therapy
- encouraging parental education and involvement in treatment
- offering family counselling or therapy
- organising self-help groups for sniffers
- educating professionals
- organising community action.

> ? **37.7** As a nurse who may at some stage come into contact with solvent abusers, consider which method or combination of methods listed above would be most effective, and why? What other measures can you think of? How would you introduce them?

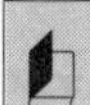

> For practical advice on this area of care the reader is referred to Ives (1990).

ILLEGAL SUBSTANCES

Rave culture

The Rave movement has become popular among some young people over the past years. It has been suggested that there is a strong link between the music played at a Rave and the youth drug culture. Case History 37.1 describes one teenager's brief flirtation with drugs, as recalled from diary entries.

Opiates and opioids

Opiates are derived from the sap of the opium poppy (*Papaver somniferum*). They are narcotic analgesics. Their synthetic equivalents are collectively known as opioids.

Heroin

Heroin ('H' or 'Smack'), a narcotic made from morphine, can be sniffed, injected ('shooting' or 'mainlining'), or smoked over tinfoil through a small tube ('chasing the dragon'). The purity of the drug is often unknown, and consequently accidental overdose can easily occur and may be lethal.

Heroin users who share needles and syringes ('works') are at risk of septicaemia, hepatitis and HIV/AIDS (see Ch. 38).

The effects of heroin include euphoria, drowsiness, a sense of well-being and raised self-esteem. Tolerance develops quickly, demanding increased intake to achieve the desired effect. Physical and psychological dependence may follow. Contamination of the drug often leads to severe allergic reactions, which may be exacerbated by poor diet and self-neglect. This degenerative process may lead to death if medical care is not available. Withdrawal is unpleasant, and is often described as being 'like a severe dose of flu'. Other problems include constipation and vomiting. Complaints of diarrhoea, abdominal cramps and muscle spasm are common. Although it has been suggested that withdrawal from heroin is easier than withdrawal from nicotine or methadone, it should be attempted gradually, using reducing doses of methadone as a heroin substitute.

Stimulants

Amphetamines

Amphetamines ('speed', 'amphs', 'whizz') are currently very popular. These drugs can be sniffed, injected or taken in tablet form. Initially introduced for the treatment of depression and as appetite suppressants, they are now rarely prescribed. Their main source of supply is therefore the illegal market.

The effects of these drugs can last for up to 5 hours and include an increase in pulse and respiration, reduced fatigue and increased muscular activity. The individual becomes restless and overtalkative. Weight loss and excessive body fluid loss are potential complications.

The user may complain of headache, tiredness and lack of social interest. During intoxication accidental injury and death may occur as a consequence of irrational behaviour. Amphetamine overdose may cause fever, paranoid psychosis, respiratory failure, hallucinations, seizures, coma, disorientation and cardiovascular collapse.

There are no specific withdrawal symptoms, although the user may complain of lethargy, prolonged sleep and excessive hunger. Psychological dependence is a major obstacle to successful withdrawal and much individual support and counselling will be needed.

Case History 37.1 G

G is an 18-year-old art student. His illegal use of drugs commenced when he was 16 years old, when he first smoked 'grass' at a sixth form party. He is a smoker (10–20 each day) and drinks alcohol, mainly for effect, i.e. to 'get merry'. His favoured drinks are 'Thunderbird' wine and 'Merrydown' cider, because they are cheap.

G's regular use of recreational 'Ganja' (cannabis) began when he commenced college in October 1990. He took his first dose of 'speed' (5 g) in July 1991. On the second occasion, G also 'took a trip' (i.e. on 'half a paper' of LSD). He recalled:

I felt very energetic and got the verbals. My arms and legs tingled and I kept getting head rushes when I stood up. These were very bad. I felt as if I had lost control. I knew where I was; it gave me a confidence boost. You can dance for ages at Raves without feeling tired.

In September 1991 I went to a college Rave; I took half a gram of speed and half an E [Ecstasy]. The effect depends on your mood. If you are in a thinking mood, it does your head in. I got very verbal that night.

In November my parents found out and we had a row. I went out to an all-nighter. I took 1 g of speed and also used Amily nitrate. If you sniff this it gives you an amazing head rush, it distorts noises and you see spots in front of your eyes and feel really light.

On Boxing Day I took a Triple X. It took 2 hours to work, then it started. I felt good and talked a lot. I had to keep on top of it, otherwise you get very confused, you don't know what to do — dance, talk, stand up, sit down. Sometimes it's enjoyable, sometimes it isn't. The music really scared me. It was hard core and got really deep in my head. I just had to sit down. If you use Vicks inhaler on your eyelids or the back of the neck, or sniff it, it brings on a rush. Certain songs can also bring on a rush.

Over the next 5 weeks G's drug intake increased. His diary extracts are as follows:

Jan 10th: Got 2 Es, white tablets, wasn't sure what they were. I did a lot of talking and got really worried. Real heavy head rushes; I started tripping badly. Curtains and carpets were moving in and out, a man was moving in and out of himself. I saw this picture, the eyes were moving, then a skeleton appeared and the hair grew. It was 26 hours before I could get to sleep. I was out of it, it got bad, I just wanted it to stop. I felt paranoid, as if everyone was talking about me, they didn't like me. I smoked Ganja to make me feel tired.

Jan 14th: Got 2 Es, £15 each, they must have been bad, I didn't get off.

Jan 11th: Took 1⅓ trip and went off on a mission.

Jan 18th: 1 g of speed.

Jan 25th: Had 2 Es, started in 20 minutes.

Feb 3rd: 1 g speed. I got caught in disco toilets and was made to leave.

I started to think what I was doing, making a mess of myself, getting in a mood with everyone. It seemed the night was all I was waiting for, I was getting off too often. When I first took them I swore it would be the only time, that I would never take E. Then only at Raves. I realised I was getting in deep. Everyone had realised except me.

If it were not for the drugs then there would be no Raves. They are made for people on them, the music entices you. If I had carried on it would have turned nasty. I just felt very depressed all the time, except when I took drugs.

I'm staying clear of the music. I think I'll be OK. Things actually got worse when my parents confronted me. I thought, mind your own business, you don't understand, it's my life, nothing to do with you.

Dealers spot you, they just walk around and ask as soon as you walk in. I buy my drugs then supplement them with Pro-plus. I'd take 10 tablets [Pro-plus] and 1 g speed, it does give you a buzz but not like the hard stuff.

I had offers to sell. It's OK taking them yourself, but not to give it to others. That's out of order. It's up to them.

I don't think I'm the strongest person mentally, I get easily led. I suppose as a one-off, it is worth it for the experience. But it's not worth doing it. I've seen my mates mess themselves up, all they talk about is drugs and Raves. It was a hard 5 weeks.

Cocaine

Cocaine ('coke', 'snow', or 'toot') is an alkaloid derived from the coca plant, a shrub native to South America. This white crystal-like powder is a powerful but short-acting stimulant. It can be sniffed ('snorted'), injected or smoked (in the form of 'crack'). Occasionally it is mixed with heroin to maximise the effect ('speedball'). When cocaine is treated with baking powder and water, it forms into tiny chalk-like lumps or 'rocks' and is referred to as 'crack'.

The effects of cocaine peak within 30 minutes and then gradually decrease. The user experiences a tremendous feeling of physical and mental power. This physiological arousal and euphoria lead to an indifference to pain and fatigue. Normal requirements for food are decreased. Large doses may lead to agitation, anxiety, hallucinations and erratic behaviour.

Dependence is usually psychological. The individual may complain of depression, fatigue and inability to cope. Chronic use may cause restlessness, nausea, sleeplessness, paranoid psychosis, hyperexcitability and severe depression. Repeated sniffing also leads to erosion of the nasal membrane.

Hallucinogens

Hallucinogens (psychedelics, psychotomimetics or psychotogens) include LSD (lysergic acid diethylamide), hallucinogenic mushrooms and cannabis. The prime effect of these drugs is the alteration of perceptual functions of the brain.

Cannabis

It is generally believed that, when used occasionally, cannabis has no long-lasting effects and is safer than alcohol. Cannabis, a preparation of the hemp plant, is available in three forms:

- 'grass', a dried leaf (marijuana)
- resin, a compact block ('hash')
- oil, the most highly concentrated form.

Cannabis is usually mixed with tobacco and smoked (as a 'joint'), although occasionally it is eaten or baked. The immediate effect is one of relaxation, talkativeness and hilarity. Intensification of sound and colour may also be experienced. There is a reduction in short-term memory function and in motor skill. Concentration is poor. These effects last up to one hour after social use.

High doses of cannabis can lead to confusion. However, the main health hazard appears to derive from the inhalation of tobacco smoke. The use of cannabis is often transient and it has been suggested that in order to experience the desired effects one has to be taught by a more competent user what to expect and how to inhale the smoke correctly to maximise effect and minimise the initial nausea (Becker 1987).

LSD

LSD is a derivative of ergot, a fungus commonly found on rye and other grasses. An exceedingly potent drug, only minute doses of LSD are required to achieve an hallucinogenic effect.

The short-term user experiences a 'trip', in which hallucinations, disturbance of perception, increase in awareness, disorientation and disassociation from the body may occur. These experiences commence within 30 minutes following ingestion and peak 2–6 hours later, gradually fading after 10 hours.

Excessive and long-term use can cause prolonged psychological reactions and re-experiencing of past 'trips' ('flashbacks'). However, LSD is not known to cause physical dependence.

'Magic' mushrooms

There are approximately 12 varieties of mushrooms which contain hallucinogenic chemicals. The most common of these is *Psilocybe semilanceata* ('liberty cap').

'Magic' mushrooms contain two active ingredients, psilocybin and psilocin. The mushrooms may be crushed, eaten fresh, brewed in a tea or cooked in a soup. The user experiences effects similar to those of LSD, along with euphoria, hilarity, increased heart rate and blood pressure, and dilated pupils. Commencing within 30 minutes, the effects peak at approximately 3 hours and last 4–10 hours.

Dependence, withdrawal and overdose are unlikely, the primary danger to health lying in the possibility that the individual may pick and consume a poisonous mushroom by mistake.

? **37.8** Consider the evidence for and against the main aspects of drug legislation. Discuss the following quotations. How convincing are the arguments? Should illegal drugs be legalised? Why or why not?

a. 'Legalising doesn't mean approval, it means control. It brings [the problem] into the open . . . [The legalisation of drugs would reduce drug-related problems by] saving money on law enforcement, unblocking courts and reducing prison overcrowding . . . [It would also] improve civil liberties and reduce the spread of AIDs.

[We should abolish] all offences related to cannabis. If this works it should be followed by other drugs. . . If consumption increases, [we should] stop and rethink the strategies. The sale of drugs to children should remain an offence, as it is with alcohol and tobacco. . . If someone becomes so addicted to a drug that he becomes a harm to others or his or her self, then the courts should be able to send him or her for treatment.' (Pickles 1991)

b. 'Drug problems will not be beaten out of society by yet harsher laws, lectured out of society by yet more hours of "health education", or treated out of society by yet more drug experts. There is a place, however, for legislation and education and treatment.' (Royal College of Psychiatrists 1987)

SUPPORT AGENCIES

Outreach workers

There are three main kinds of outreach worker in the field of drug rehabilitation. Some, mainly nurses or health promotion officers, are employed professionals. Others are unpaid or paid scripted users or ex-users. Whatever their background, the aim of these workers is to facilitate access to caring services for individuals who want to overcome a drug dependency. An example of how outreach work might be carried out is given in Box 37.6.

Box 37.6 Outreach work: an example

The outreach worker may go to a pub or Rave. During the evening he or she may meet up with an existing contact, who during the course of a conversation may introduce the worker to an associate who would like to talk (this form of contacting is often referred to as 'snowballing'). This individual may be experiencing drug-related problems or problems with his GP. In the case of a health care problem, the worker may be able to facilitate 'harm minimisation' (see below). For example, the user may be advised to go for a health check or for HIV/AIDS and hepatitis B testing, or he may be informed on how to obtain clean 'works'. In some cases the worker undertakes these tasks, dealing with the problem on street level.

As the user's trust develops, the worker may bring a colleague along to a meeting or encourage attendance at a clinic. This process gradually leads to a deeper level of care and involvement with the community drug team.

Professional outreach workers

These workers are usually nurses or health promotion officers; some in fact have dual qualifications. They work independently of the community drug team and their main function is to provide health education and health delivery at the 'grassroots' level. Advice on general care issues, drug use and safe practices is given with the aim of increasing the number of drug abusers coming forward to seek professional help.

Existing scripted users: unpaid

These outreach workers already live, work and socialise with other users. Their aim is to deliver a health promotion message, e.g. harm minimisation and HIV/AIDS advice, and to promote the idea that local agencies are 'user friendly'.

Ex-users and existing users: paid

In most cases employed by drug rehabilitation agencies, these individuals are detached youth workers dealing with all welfare aspects of drug use. Their aim is to increase levels of understanding, to give information on safer drug-taking practices and to encourage attendance at drug clinics for appropriate interventions.

Readers who would like to know more about this type of work are referred to Gilman (1992).

Harm minimisation

Harm minimisation is a form of intervention which has given rise to much controversy. It is a process by which drug users are advised on safe methods of drug use, rather than being urged to abstain. The user is offered blood tests and health checks, is given advice on safer drug-taking practices, and is supplied with clean 'works' and condoms. The underlying philosophy is that while it may be impossible to eradicate altogether the illegal use of drugs, it is nonetheless beneficial for individuals and society to make existing drug use as safe as possible (see Ch. 38, p. 1001).

Needle exchange schemes. Operated by either the community drug and alcohol team or by health promotion departments, the aim of these programmes is to distribute clean needles, syringes and containers with a view to preventing the sharing of equipment and thus reducing the spread of infection. These schemes allow for access to this equipment as well as to health promotion materials and advice, e.g. on cleaning equipment and on safe sexual practices.

Some pharmacists, GPs and community psychiatric nurses offer this service. The idea of a syringe-dispensing machine is presently being tested. Needle exchange schemes also facilitate the safe disposal of used equipment and help in maintaining the link between the abuser and helping agencies.

Voluntary and professional agencies

Local services

Most health districts have a community drug and alcohol team. These are usually staffed by specialist nurses, social workers and administrators; other professionals such as health promotion officers, occupational therapists, doctors/consultants and probation officers may also be attached to the team.

These teams offer help, advice, information, health education, treatment and counselling for the drug user and his family or close associates as well as for health care professionals. Some districts have a similar, voluntary service (e.g. an alcohol advisory service) staffed by trained counsellors. Contact with these agencies can be made via the Yellow Pages, Citizen's Advice Bureaux, community health councils or senior nurses and nurse teachers. Some regional alcohol and drug treatment units still operate, offering outpatient and inpatient treatment, usually on a 6-week basis. However, access to these may be difficult to obtain, and usually requires a doctor's recommendation.

National bodies

Technical information and advice relating to voluntary services may be obtained by making contact with the following organisations. (Relevant addresses are given on page 989.)

- The Association for Nurses in Substance Abuse (ANSA)
- Alcohol Concern
- RCN Substance Misuse Forum
- Standing Conference on Drug Abuse (SCODA)
- Re-Solv
- The Addictions Forum.

Support groups

District drug teams and voluntary services offer group therapy in a variety of formats. Membership in these groups may be open or closed, and may be for men only, women only, or mixed. Some aim for total abstinence, others for controlled use. Some groups are set up to provide support for family members.

'Drinkwatchers' is organised on lines similar to 'Weightwatchers'. Total abstinence is not a requirement. Alcoholics Anonymous (AA) and Narcotics Anonymous (NA) are self-help organisations offering individual and group support. Total abstinence is required. Al-Anon, Al-Ateen and Families Anonymous are run on similar lines to AA and NA groups to provide self-help for the families and friends of drug abusers. Tranquilliser support groups have also been established to offer support and encouragement to individuals during the often long and difficult process of withdrawal.

Additional programmes undertaken by drug teams may include group psychotherapy, social skills training, relaxation, family therapy, education and prevention, and telephone support. Most teams are able to access intensive residential courses, 'dry' hostels and other care facilities. Each of these offers a particular philosophy of care. Admission is usually agreed following assessment by the service provider.

? **37.9** The Kessel report (1979) suggests that all primary workers should have knowledge of the services and facilities available to them and how to access these. Produce your own 'resource catalogue' using the information and addresses contained within this chapter. In addition, to increase your familiarity with the services available in your own Health District carry out the following project:

a. Research all local resources which may assist you in the care of your patient, whether this would be with advice, help, information or statistics. Don't forget self-help groups and counselling services such as the Samaritans, as well as mother-and-toddler groups, which may provide much-needed support for a mother under stress.
b. Prepare a file card on each group, listing the contact name, address, phone number and type of help offered.

CONCLUSION

This chapter has attempted to provide an introduction for the nurse to the many issues surrounding the care of individuals with dependency problems. While work with this client group can constitute a specialism within nursing, the need for nurses in every field to be aware of the signs and the consequences of substance abuse cannot be overemphasised.

Dependency problems occur in every age group and social class. Within the family, a dependency problem will have serious implications not only for the individual directly affected, but for his or her spouse and children. Indeed, the nurse may first detect the existence of a dependency problem not through her contact with the substance abuser, but in her interactions with family members. It is vital that nursing interventions undertaken in response to drug-related problems are based on an assessment of not only the individual himself but also of his family circumstances.

As in many areas of nursing, prevention and education show the way forward. In averting or change from dependency, individuals must be given adequate information on which to base free and informed decisions. Nurses working with substance abusers may find that in order to be more responsive to the needs of their clients they must venture beyond traditional clinical settings into outreach work. In any event, rehabilitation will demand a holistic approach in which the unique identity of the individual is not lost sight of and in which all aspects of his physical, mental and social well-being are addressed by the cooperative efforts of a multidisciplinary team.

One might add that nurses are in a privileged position by virtue of their close and frequent contact with patients. They are often seen as the 'human face' of community and hospital health services, and are perceived to be 'on the patient's side' — practical, approachable, and down to earth. Nurses are well placed to listen to, support, advise and inform their patients. Dependency nursing can offer a particularly challenging and rewarding context for the practice of these invaluable skills.

? **37.10** Now that you have read through the chapter, repeat exercise 37.1, taking note of the following:

- Have your feelings changed? If so, in what way? What new information influenced this change?
- Are there any areas that you feel you need to investigate further? What are these, and what sources could you use?

REFERENCES

Advisory Committee on Alcoholism 1979 The pattern and range of services for problem drinkers. (Also referred to as the 'Kessel Report'.) HMSO, London

Advisory Council on the Misuse of Drugs 1982 Treatment and rehabilitation. HMSO, London

Alcohol Concern 1987 Teaching about alcohol problems. Tutor and student manual. Woodhead & Faulkner, Cambridge

Alcohol Concern 1992 A woman's guide to alcohol. Alcohol Concern, London

Becker H S 1987 Becoming a marijuana user. In: Heller T, Gott M, Jeffery C (eds). Drug use and misuse: a reader. Open University/HEA, Wiley, Chichester

Breeze E 1985 Women and drinking. HMSO, London

Camberwell Council on Alcoholism 1980 Women and alcohol. Tavistock, London

Cooper D B 1985 Teenage drinking: is there a potential problem? Paper presented to the 20th Scottish Alcohol Problems Research Symposium. Pitlochry, Scotland

Cooper D B, Faugier J 1993 Substance misuse. In: Wright H, Giddey M (eds) Mental health nursing – from first principle to professional practice. Chapman and Hall, London

Cooper D B 1993 Alcohol home detoxification and assessment. Radcliffe Medical Press, Oxford

Cosgrove S 1992 Hooked: facts and myths surrounding drugs. Video (6 parts), Granada Television

Davidson R 1991 Facilitating change in problem drinkers. In: Davidson R, Rollnick S, MacEwan I (eds) Counselling problem drinkers. Tavistock, London, pp. 3–20

Department of Health 1989 Alcohol misuse. Health circular HN (89) 4 DOH, London

Dunne F T, Paton A, Walker T 1989 Alcohol and drugs services: the case for combining. Alcohol and Alcoholism 2: 75–76

Faugier J 1992 What price tranquillity. Nursing Times 88(3)

Fogelman K R, Manor O 1988 Smoking in pregnancy and developing into adulthood. British Medical Journal November 297: 1233–36

Froggatt P 1988 Fourth report of the independent scientific committee on smoking and health. HMSO, London

Health Education Authority 1989 That's the limit. HEA, London

Health Education Authority 1991 The smoking epidemic: counting the cost in England. 14 regional volumes. HEA, London

Ives R 1990 Working with solvent sniffers. ISDD, London

Jarvis M 1989 Myths of cigar and pipes. Physician. February 8(2): 130

Jones K L, Smith D W 1973 Recognition of the fetal alcohol syndrome in early infancy. Lancet 2: 999–1001

Kennedy J, Faugier J 1989 Drugs and dependency nursing. Heinemann Nursing, Oxford

Krishna K 1978 Tobacco chewing in pregnancy. British Journal of Obstetrics and Gynaecology. October, 85(10): 726–28

Lader M 1978 Benzodiazepines: the opium of the masses. Neuroscience 3: 159–165

Office of population, census and survey 1989 National opinion poll survey. OPCS, London

Parloff M 1980 Psychotherapy and research: an anaclitic depression. Psychiatry 43: 279–293

Pickles Judge J 1991 A futile war. 'Byline', BBC 1

Plant M A 1982 Drinking and problem drinking. Junction, London

Plant M A 1987 Drugs in perspective. Hodder & Stoughton, London

Plant M A, Peck D F, Samuel E 1985 Alcohol, drugs and school leavers. Tavistock, London

Plant M L 1985 Women, drinking and pregnancy. Tavistock, London

Plant M L 1987 Alcohol and women. In: Alcohol Concern (comp.) Teaching about alcohol problems (tutor's manual), Ch. 9, pp. 89–95

Prochaska J O, Di Clemente C C 1983 Stages and process of self change of smoking: towards an integrative model of change. Journal of Consulting and Clinical Psychology 51(3): 390–395

Prochaska J O, Di Clemente C C 1986 Towards a comprehensive model of change. In: Miller W R, Heather N (eds) Treating addictive behaviours: processes of change. Plenum, London

Royal College of Psychiatrists 1987 Drug scenes: a report on drugs and drug dependency. Gaskell, Oxford

Schacter S 1982 Recidivism and self cure of smoking and obesity. American Psychologist 37: 436–444

Sidle N 1982 Smoking in pregnancy: a review. Spastic Society. Hera Unit, London

Silverman K, Evans S M, Stragin E C et al 1992 Withdrawal syndrome after the double-blind cessation of caffeine consumption. New England Journal of Medicine 327(16): 1109–1114

Trevathan E et al 1983 Journal of the American Medical Association 250: 499–501

US Department of Health and Human Services 1989 Reducing the health consequences of smoking: 25 years progress. A report of the Surgeon General U S Department of Health and Human Services, Public Health Services, Centre for Disease Control, Centre for Chronic Disease Prevention and Health Promotion, Office of Smoking and Health. DHHS Publication (CDC) 89: 8411

World Health Organization 1985 The use of essential drugs. Publication TRS722. WHO, Geneva

FURTHER READING

Alcohol Concern 1987 Teaching about alcohol problems: tutor's and student's manual. Woodhead & Faulkner, Cambridge

Alcohol Concern 1991/92 Alcohol services directory. Owen Wells, Ilkley

Campbell R H 1988 Overdose aid. ISDD, London

Cooper D B 1993 Alcohol home detoxification and assessment. Radcliffe Medical Press, Oxford

Drugs, Alcohol and Women Nationally (DAWN) 1980 Black women and dependency. ISDD, London

DOH 1991 Drug misuse and dependence: guidelines on clinical management. HMSO, London

DOH 1991 Solvents: a parent's guide. HMSO, London

Dorn N, Henderson S, South N (eds) 1991 AIDs: women, drugs and social care. Falmer Press, London

Gilman M 1992 Outreach. ISDD, London

Hammersley D, Hamlin M 1990 The benzodiazepine manual: a professional guide to withdrawal. ISDD, London

Heather N, Robertson I 1981 Controlled drinking. Methuen, London

Heller T, Gott M, Jeffery C 1987 (eds) Drug use and misuse. Open University/HEA, Wiley, Chichester

Institute for the Study of Drug Dependence 1991 So you've chosen drugs for your project. ISDD, London

Institute for the Study of Drug Dependence 1989 The misuse of drugs act explained. ISDD, London

Ives R 1990 Parents: what you need to know about solvent sniffing. ISDD, London

Ives R 1990 Working with solvent sniffers. ISDD, London

Kent R 1989 Say when: everything a woman needs to know about alcohol and drinking problems. ISDD, London

McVey J, Elsmore G (undated) Solvent and volatile substance abuse: national directory, 2nd edn. Re-Solv, Stone, Staffs

Miller W, Munoz R 1983 How to control your drinking. Sheldon Press, London

Miller W R, Heather N (eds) 1986 Treating addictive behaviours: processes of change. Plenum, London

Miller W R, Rollnick S 1991 Motivational interviewing — preparing people to change addictive behaviours. Guilford, New York

Ritson B (ed) 1988 A handbook for nurses, midwives and health visitors. The medical council on alcoholism, London

Stockwell T, Clement S 1987 Helping the problem drinker: new initiatives in community care. Croom Helm, London

Strang J, Farrell M 1992 Hepatitis. ISDD, London

Tether P, Robinson D 1986 Preventing alcohol problems: a guide to local action. Tavistock, London

Trickett S 1991 Coming off tranquillisers. Thorson, London

Wesson J 1992 The vintage years: older people and alcohol. Aquarius, Birmingham

USEFUL ADDRESSES

AA (Alcoholics Anonymous)
PO Box 1
Stonebow House
Stonebow
York YO1 2UL

The Addictions Forum
Membership secretary: Dr Martin Plant
Alcohol Research Group,
University of Edinburgh,
Morningside Park
Edinburgh EH10 5HF
031–447 2011 ext 4509

ADFAM (Aid for Addicts and Family)
Morelands House
80 Goswell Road
London EC1V 7DB

AIDS Helpline:
0800 567123
Minority languages:
071–992 5522
Hard of hearing:
0800 521361

Alcohol Concern
275 Gray's Inn Road
London WC1X 8QF
071–833 3471

Alcohol Recovery Project
68 Newington Causeway
London SE1 6DF
071–403 3369

ANSA (Association for Nurses in Substance Abuse)
Membership Secretary
CDTIC
Theatre Court
London Road
Northwich CW9 5HB
0606 49055

ASH (Action on Smoking and Health)
5–11 Mortimer Street
London W1N 7RH
071–637 9843

Council for Involuntary Tranquilliser Addiction
Cavendish House
Brighton Road
Waterloo
Liverpool L22 7NG

The Drink Crisis Centre
Women's House
PO Box 719
London SE5 8QB

Families Anonymous (FA)
5–7 Parsons Green
London SW6 4UL
071–731 8060

Health Education Authority
Hamilton House
Mabledon Place
London WC1H 9TX
071–383 3833

ISDD (Institute for the Study of Drug Dependence)
1 Hatton Place
Hatton Garden
London EC1N 8ND
071–430 1991

Narcotics Anonymous
PO Box 417
London SW10 0DP
071–351 6794

National Campaign Against Solvent Abuse
The Enterprise Centre
444 Brixton Road
London SW9 8EJ
071–733 7330

QUIT
102 Gloucester Place
London W1H 3DA
071–487 2858

Re-Solv (The Society for the Prevention of Solvent & Volatile Substance Abuse)
St Mary's Chambers
19 Station Road
Stone
Staffs ST15 8JP
0785 46097/817885

SCODA (Standing Conference on Drug Abuse)
1–4 Hatton Place
Hatton Garden
London EC1N 8ND
071–430 2341

Smokers' Quitline
071–323 0505
Cantonese 0800 181153
Silhetti 0800 181348

Terrence Higgins Trust
52–54 Gray's Inn Road
London WC1X 8JU
071–831 0330
Helpline: 071–242 1010

Women's Alcohol Centre
66a Drayton Park
London N5 1ND
071–226 4581

CHAPTER 38

The person with HIV/AIDS

John Atkinson

DEDICATION

Dedicated to Richard J Wells FRCN, clinical reviewer of this chapter, who died in January 1993.

CHAPTER CONTENTS

Introduction 991
Definitions 991

Viruses and normal immunology 993
Viruses 993

The human immunodeficiency virus 993
Modes of transmission 993
Stages of HIV infection 994

Political and social implications of HIV/AIDS 995
Political challenges 995
The impact of HIV/AIDS on health and social services 996
Philosophical issues for nurses 998

Testing and screening 999
Counselling 1000

Health education and promotion in HIV 1001
Elements of health promotion 1001

Clinical manifestations and management of HIV/AIDS 1002
Approaches to nursing care 1003

Conditions, treatments and specific nursing interventions 1003
Phases of HIV and AIDS 1003
Antiviral treatment 1007

Conclusion 1007

References 1008

Further reading 1009

Useful addresses 1009

INTRODUCTION

In June 1981 five young men in the USA were reported to have died of *Pneumocystis carinii* pneumonia (PCP), a rare infection. The only characteristics they had in common were their young age, their gender and the fact that they were homosexual (Youle et al 1988). Later that year a patient with similar symptoms died in a London hospital (Pratt 1991). The condition we now call acquired immune deficiency sydrome (AIDS) had arrived. In 1983–84 in France and the USA the causative agent, a virus from the family of retroviruses, (see p. 993) was isolated. This virus was found to infiltrate and destroy human helper T lymphocytes, which cooperate with B lymphocytes in the production of antibodies. To start with the retrovirus was called lymphadenopathy associated virus (LAV) by the French and human T-cell lymphotropic virus type III (HTLV-III) by the Americans, or HTLV-III/LAV by the world at large (Youle et al 1988). In May 1986 the International Committee on the Taxonomy of Viruses decided that the accepted name of the retrovirus would be: human immunodeficiency virus (HIV).

This chapter will present the main historical features of the advent of HIV/AIDS along with a profile of the retrovirus. It will address the social and economic implications of HIV/AIDS and the effect of the disease on patients and their carers. Testing will be highlighted together with concomitant ethical and practical dilemmas. The final sections of the chapter will consider the clinical manifestations of HIV/AIDS, giving details of the treatments currently available. The contribution of nurses to the care of individuals with HIV/AIDS will be discussed. Throughout, it should be remembered that the person with HIV/AIDS will spend most of his time at home, away from formal care.

By setting HIV/AIDS, at the outset, in a wide social context this chapter is intended to emphasise that HIV/AIDS is both a clinical *and* a sociopolitical issue. It is hoped that student nurses, armed with the information provided by this chapter, will be able to develop a knowledgeable and empathetic mode of practice with people who have HIV and related problems.

Definitions

In order for nurses to use the correct terminology relating to HIV/AIDS they need to understand how this terminology developed.

The syndrome

The only *clinical* factor linking the original patients with AIDS was the fact that they were so profoundly immunodepressed that they had contracted the rare infection PCP. Until that time this infection was seen only occasionally, in patients who were immunodepressed with diseases such as leukaemia or whose immunity was suppressed as a side-effect of medication. As no causative agent had been found to explain this new phenomenon it was called *acquired* (meaning the patient had not inherited the condition but had contracted it) *immune deficiency* (the main linking clinical factor) *syndrome* (a group of recognised clinical signs).

The retrovirus

The retrovirus, now called human immunodeficiency virus (HIV), was isolated and designated the causative agent of AIDS. A test was developed which could check an individual's blood for HIV antibodies. An individual who contracts the virus will respond by producing antibodies in a process known as seroconversion. When a person is found to have HIV antibodies he is said to be HIV antibody positive or, less correctly, HIV positive (HIV+) and is considered to have contracted HIV.

HIV 2

Since the discovery of HIV a second strain of the retrovirus, HIV 2, has been isolated. It has been found mainly in African countries but is seen elsewhere and appears to produce a more attenuated disease pattern. HIV 2 should not be confused with a longer known virus, HTLV-II, which is not connected with AIDS although it is in the same family of retroviruses.

AIDS diagnosis

A patient is diagnosed as having AIDS only if he is HIV antibody positive *and* has one of the designated infections or diseases associated with AIDS. The classification of these diseases devised by the Centers for Disease Control (CDC 1987) in the USA is used globally and will be adopted in this chapter. Also current but not yet formally ratified is the 'Interim Proposed World Health Organization Clinical Staging System for HIV Infection and Disease'. This system attempts to address some of the anomalies which the CDC system presented. A helpful explanation of the staging system is given in Pratt 1991, Appendix 2.

The CDC classification also includes a description of the disease process from the time an individual contracts HIV until he becomes ill. Some people who have contracted HIV go through a short 'flu-like illness during which they develop antibodies; this is called *acute seroconversion illness* (CDC Phase A; see Box 38.1). Many individuals will have the virus without knowing it for some time, and may be completely asymptomatic for several years (CDC Phase B–1: the asymptomatic or dormant phase).

It is important to understand the following relationship between HIV antibodies and AIDS: **Everybody who has AIDS is HIV antibody positive, but not everybody who is HIV antibody positive has got AIDS.** It should also be pointed out that an individual who has a positive HIV antibody status may become ill without being diagnosed as having AIDS. This may be because he has not yet contracted one of the classified list of infections and diseases but is ill with something else, or because he is experiencing side-effects of, for instance, antiretroviral treatment.

Nurses will meet many people who have at some earlier time been diagnosed as having AIDS but who are presently well. This is increasingly common as people with the syndrome survive longer. When the author began working in the field, death 18 months to 2 years after diagnosis was the 'norm'. Now one may meet individuals who have survived 4 to 6 years and sometimes longer. Thus the term *AIDS* can be unhelpful and even misleading because it does not necessarily reflect how the person is at a given moment. For nurses in particular the term has little relevance. More helpful is the term *HIV disease*, which conveys that someone is ill with one or a variety of conditions and is HIV antibody positive.

Issues surrounding terminology

HIV/AIDS has become a deeply politicised disease phenomenon. The nurse as educator and advocate must be sensitive to the sociopolitical issues surrounding HIV/AIDS and its description. The patient has the right to expect that nurse will use terminology which will promote well-being and not give offence.

Although the term AIDS has limited clinical usefulness it is

Box 38.1 The phases of HIV/AIDS and associated infections and conditions

PHASE A: ACUTE SEROCONVERSION ILLNESS

PHASE B: ANTIBODY POSITIVE PHASE

B-1:
asymptomatic HIV infection

B-2:
persistent generalised lymphadenopathy (PGL) or lymphadenopathy syndrome (LAS)

PHASE C: AIDS-RELATED COMPLEX (ARC)

PHASE D: AIDS

Constitutional disease; HIV wasting syndrome;

opportunistic infections

Protozoal infections
- Pneumocystis carinii pneumonia (PCP)
- cryptosporidiosis
- toxoplasmosis
- isosporiasis

Viral infections
- herpes simplex virus
- cytomegalovirus (CMV)
- progressive multifocal leukoencephalopathy (PML)

Bacterial infections
- mycobacterium tuberculosis (TB)
- salmonellosis
- mycobacterium avium complex (MAC)

Fungal infections
- Candidiasis (thrush)
- cryptococcus
- histoplasmosis
- coccidioidomycosis

Infestations

Secondary cancers (neoplasms)
- Kaposi's sarcoma (KS)
- Non-Hodgkin's lymphomas (B cell lymphomas, undifferentiated lymphomas)

Neurological disease; HIV encephalopathy

the one most commonly used by the media and the public. Also common are the terms 'the AIDS virus' and 'the HIV virus'. Neither is strictly correct and nurses should try to use simply 'HIV' instead.

It is now generally accepted that 'person with AIDS' is a more acceptable term than 'AIDS patient'. The latter term is inappropriate as an individual may live a normal life for long periods without recourse to medical or nursing care. Calling an individual a 'victim' raises questions of guilt or innocence and along with 'sufferer', implies that he is powerless to help himself.

VIRUSES AND NORMAL IMMUNOLOGY

The reader is referred to Ch. 16 for an outline of normal immunology.

Viruses

Viruses are not complete organisms. They can survive only as part of 'host' cells. Unlike bacteria, fungi, protozoa and other infective agents, all of which are complete and independently viable, viruses cannot replicate (multiply/reproduce) by themselves. They are also so small as to be insusceptible to filtration and cannot be seen by an ordinary microscope. Viruses are made up of a core of nucleic acid and are enveloped in a protein shell.

Retroviruses

These viruses, of which HIV and HIV 2 are two, contain RNA. They have the ability to infiltrate the DNA of the host cell and implant their genetic material there, after which the host cell will have the capability to reproduce the retrovirus instead of itself.

DNA is present in almost all organisms and cells. It plays a central part in heredity and because of its structure (two interwoven strands of nucleotides connected by hydrogen bonds) can replicate, carrying the genetic blueprint to the next generation of DNA. RNA is made up of a single strand of nucleotides and is involved in protein synthesis. It provides the genetic blueprint of some viruses, including HIV and HIV 2. The retrovirus HIV infects the helper T lymphocytes, which are its host cells, implanting them with its own genetic blueprint such that the helper T cells reproduce HIV instead of themselves.

The importance of this disruption of the T lymphocytes must be understood within the context of the normal immune response (see Ch. 16). The white blood cells (of which helper T, suppressor T and B lymphocytes are examples) have the function of seeking and destroying invading microorganisms (bacteria, viruses, protozoa, etc.) and malignant (cancer) cells. For a stage-by-stage summary of this process see Box 38.2. Given the essential role played by helper T cells in the immune system it is clear that their invasion and destruction by HIV will have devastating results.

THE HUMAN IMMUNODEFICIENCY VIRUS

Modes of transmission

The first stage of HIV infection occurs when the individual contracts the retrovirus HIV through any of the modes of transmission listed below. The essential criteria for successful transmission in *all* forms of contact is that there must be **an exchange of body fluids and/or blood between the infected individual and the recipient individual** (WHO 1989, p. 48). Sexual contact and blood-to-blood contact are known as 'horizontal' methods of transmission; that is, they move 'across' from one individual to another.

Box 38.2 The normal immune response (ENB 1989)

Warning
In response to the invading microorganism, helper T cells orchestrate defences by releasing chemicals which stimulate other cells of the immune system.

Preparation
Activated by these chemical signals, other kinds of T cells (cytotoxic cells and lymphokine producers) begin to proliferate, while B lymphocytes multiply and become plasma cells which start to manufacture antibodies.

Attack
Activated T cells and antibodies are released into the circulation, where they specifically target and destroy the invading organism.

Stand down
Once the foreign organism is routed and the infection is under control, the activity of the immune system is reduced, perhaps partly through the action of suppressor T lymphocytes.

Transmission through sexual contact

All forms of penetrative sexual contact have been recorded as having transmitted HIV. These are as follows:

1. Penis to vagina
2. Penis to anus
3. Penis to mouth
4. Vagina to mouth
5. Mouth to anus
6. Hand into vagina
7. Hand into rectum.

It is difficult to determine *absolutely* whether 3–7 transmit the virus as they do not often occur in isolation, but some individual cases have been reported. They are all considered to be 'high risk' activities.

There is much debate in the scientific and secular worlds about which of these activities is the most 'dangerous'. Until recently anal sex was considered to be most risky. Also, women were thought to be more at risk from penis/vagina sex than men. More recent findings are leading to a reexamination of these assumptions, and the scientific debate still rages. It is important to inform patients that they may be at risk from *any* of these forms of sexual contact.

Transmission through blood and blood products

Blood transfusions. The spread of HIV in Western countries with sophisticated blood transfusion services has been greatly reduced since the rigorous screening of donors has been instituted (1985 in most countries). In Britain it is now reckoned that there is a risk factor of something less than 1 transmission in a million units of blood. This works out at fewer than 3 transmissions a year.

The best-known recipients of blood products are haemophiliacs and those with other blood clotting disorders. Before 1985 many thousand haemophiliacs and others became infected through blood products. Since 1985 these products have been heat treated. The treatment is totally successful but reduces the efficacy of the products such that more of them are required.

Blood transmission through sharing of equipment. HIV

transmission can occur through the sharing of syringes, needles and other blood-giving equipment. In Western countries this is commonly through the illicit, intravenous use of drugs. Here the probability of infection is often increased by the user 'flushing' the syringe with his blood before injection. In poorer countries it is also seen where there is re-use of medical equipment and insufficient sterilising facilities. The mode of transmission is the same in both cases. Small amounts of infected blood remain in the equipment and are introduced straight into the bloodstream of the recipient. The recipient in fact receives a small and unintentional innoculation. So-called 'needlestick' injuries in which a used needle accidently stabs an individual are also dangerous. However, there have been very few proven cases of infection by this mode.

Transmission through skin piercing procedures. Transmission has been reported in a few cases from tattooing, ear piercing and skin grafting.

Transmission through other bodily fluids. Infection with HIV takes place only when there is sufficient concentration of the virus. (Infection through saliva, for instance, is therefore considered unlikely.) Worldwide retrospective studies have shown that the number of workers contracting the virus through urine, faeces, saliva, etc. has been extremely small (WHO 1989).

Mother-to-child transmission

This form of transmission is known as 'vertical' transmission, that is down 'from' an infected mother to her child in the womb or during delivery, when the mother's and child's blood become mixed. There is a possibility that transmission through amniotic fluid and ('horizontally') through breast milk can also take place.

From birth until 11–18 months the baby will carry his mother's HIV and other antibodies. Therefore all babies born to HIV infected mothers are found to be HIV antibody positive. At about 11–18 months the baby will lose the mother's antibodies and go on to *either* being HIV antibody negative (not carrying the virus) *or* developing his own antibodies (being infected in his own right). *A few* go on to become HIV antibody negative but positive to another test which isolates antigen (particles of the actual virus), so that they are carrying the virus but not the antibodies.

At the beginning of the HIV epidemic it appeared that about 50% of children born to HIV antibody positive mothers became infected in their own right.

In countries where there are good antenatal facilities and the mother remains well throughout pregnancy the rate of transmission from mother to child is dramatically lower. The babies still carry the mothers' antibodies but only about 20% appear to go on to be infected in their own right.

Stages of HIV infection

The dormant or asymptomatic stage

In HIV-related illness two main processes take place in the infected person's body:

1. The retrovirus destroys the helper T cells and replicates itself
2. The body's immunity is inexorably weakened and is attacked by other infections. The body becomes increasingly unable to fight off these attacks.

Since, unlike other microorganisms, viruses and retroviruses cannot multiply by themselves, they need to use the cell-building material of their host cells in order to reproduce themselves (see Fig. 38.1). When HIV enters the bloodstream it attaches itself to the outer cell membrane of the helper T lymphocyte. Following this it breaks into the cell and releases its genetic blueprint, which has the ability to replicate itself.

The disease process may then go no further for several months or even years. That is, the person *is* infected with HIV, and may or may not have produced antibodies (this may take 3 months or more). If he has seroconverted (started to produce antibodies) he may or may not have become ill.

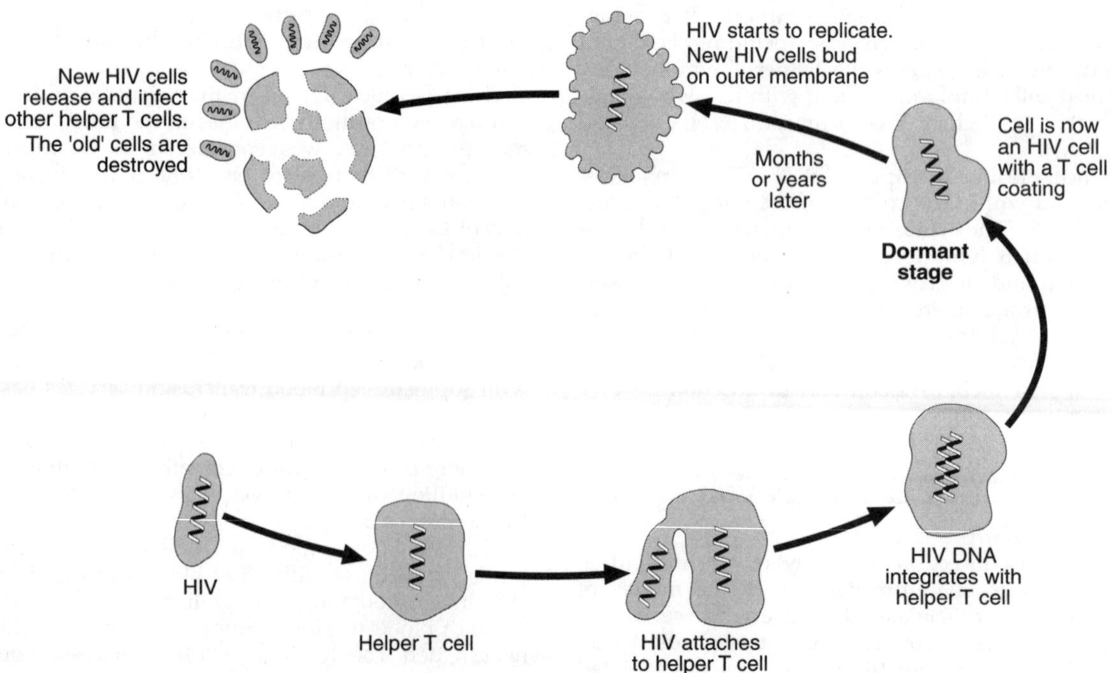

Fig. 38.1 The human immunodeficiency virus in action.

If he did become ill with acute seroconversion illness (CDC Phase A) the usually mild, 'flu-like symptoms were probably not recognised by the individual or his physician as a sign of HIV infection. The helper T lymphocyte blood count will still be normal and therefore the immune system will remain unaffected. The patient will continue to be well. This stage, often called the dormant stage, is referred to as 'Clinical stage one: 1. Asymptomatic' in the proposed WHO staging system (Pratt 1991).

Some time in the future the infected T cells will start to replicate new HIV retroviruses. It is unclear what triggers this process, however, it seems that if an individual keeps generally well and leads a healthy lifestyle the stage when HIV starts to replicate and destroys the T cells may be delayed. A clearer finding is that in conditions of deprivation and poor health the illness seems to progress faster.

The role of antibodies. Until quite recently it was thought that HIV antibodies had no effect whatsoever. However, more recent research in various countries is starting to suggest that the maligned HIV antibody may have some effect in delaying the onset of retrovirus replication and therefore the onset of HIV-related illness.

The replication stage

The first process. Some time after the retrovirus has been incorporated into the helper T lymphocyte it begins to replicate itself within the cell walls using the cell's own material. The new retroviruses gather within and start to break down the outer cell membrane. The new HIVs then break out of the helper T cell, encased in membrane stolen from the host cell and clinging onto the remnants of the cell. This is known as 'budding' (see Fig. 38.1). At this stage the host cell dies. The new HIVs then disperse throughout the bloodstream, infecting other helper T lymphocytes, and the process begins again.

The second process begins when other helper T cells have been infected and the level of normal, healthy helper T cells begins to drop. At this point the body's immunity to other infections will begin to be compromised. From the clinician's viewpoint this is a significant stage as the depletion of normal helper T cells can be measured in a blood sample with the 'CD4 T cell subsets' procedure (see Appendix 1).

Also significant is the ratio between the helper T lymphocytes and the suppressor T lymphocytes, which are reckoned to assist in the 'stand down' phase of the normal immune response (see Box 38.2). Normally the ratio is 1.5 helpers to 1.0 suppressors. As the number of healthy helper cells decreases this ratio is changed. This may have a detrimental effect on the immune system. It is also one of the diagnostic signs used to confirm the presence of HIV-related illness. In other forms of immune deficiency illnesses both helper and suppressor levels fall, and so the ratio between them remains roughly the same.

As the helper T cell level falls the body will become more susceptible to other infections. The individual may at first experience rather vague symptoms, progressing to debilitating but not life-threatening conditions and finally serious illness and death. (Information on the specific diseases which may appear is given later in the chapter.)

The illness profile represented in Figure 38.2 (p. 1004) is a very general description, only; how HIV/AIDS actually manifests itself will vary dramatically from one person to another. Many people with extremely low helper T cell counts will seem healthy; others with what should be a 'good' count will be extremely ill. The nurse must rely on her own observations of and discussions with the patient in assessing his condition, rather than on abstract clinical indicators alone (see p. 1003–1007).

POLITICAL AND SOCIAL IMPLICATIONS OF HIV/AIDS

AIDS has been compared to the great plagues of the past in that it appears to be spreading unchecked and has, as yet, no cure. Like other infectious diseases which have reached epidemic or pandemic proportions, HIV/AIDS has given rise to a great deal of fear and stigmatisation. In formulating health and social policies in response to AIDS, the Government has a duty not only to safeguard the health and well-being of the population as a whole but to protect the rights of those individuals affected by the disease.

The foundation for political and social responses to HIV/AIDS is provided by the work of epidemiologists, who define the disease, describe its typical progression and determine its national and international incidence. Also relevant is its prevalence, i.e. its incidence within particular groups. On the basis of these findings predictions are made as to the future impact of the disease (Barker & Rose 1990). Armed with this knowledge, nursing, medical and scientific practitioners, along with the individuals and groups affected, endeavour to raise awareness of HIV/AIDS and to lobby the Government to take appropriate action.

Although cases of HIV infection were known in 1981, it was not until two or three years later that HIV appeared *officially* to be recognised as a threat to the whole community. Various media campaigns were instigated from 1985 onwards and the first full debate was held in the House of Commons in November 1986 (Hansard 1986).

Some of the questions and issues raised by the epidemiology of HIV/AIDS are listed in Box 38.3.

Political challenges

The most intractable problem presented by HIV to policy makers is the length of time it takes for the disease to mani-

Box 38.3 Questions and issues raised by HIV/AIDS

- In the Third World, particularly Africa, HIV affects mainly heterosexual people. In the West, with some notable exceptions, the prevalence appears to be overwhelmingly among homosexual men and intravenous drug users. Why is the pattern so different, given that HIV is now present in all sections of the population in the West?
- In New York City the prevalence of HIV among young heterosexuals is rising dramatically. It is now the most common cause of death in this group. Will this happen everywhere?
- Given that there is no cure for AIDS, just how effective are education and prevention policies? Some countries, notably the USA, have strict entry laws. What is the case for stringent political action — for example, restricting the movements of known HIV positive individuals?
- Is there a case for testing as many people as possible anonymously to get a more accurate profile of what is going on so that policy makers are better able to provide proper services?
- Is the nurse's primary responsibility to the individual patient and to his confidentiality and wishes? If so, what responsibility does the nurse have to protect the public at large? Can she meet both responsibilities at the same time?

fest itself after an individual becomes infected. This has the following profound epidemiological implications:

- Most people who are infected are not aware of it until they become ill
- The government figures published regularly on people with AIDS do not reflect the prevalence of HIV at the present moment. *They give, at best, an idea of the prevalence 5–10 years ago*
- It is more difficult to gauge specifically *who* is at risk, although some 'high-risk' *activities* can be identified (e.g. intravenous drug use, unprotected sexual intercourse).

It is therefore vital that data on AIDS are as specific as possible. In the UK the following bodies collect, collate and distribute information on the incidence and prevalence of HIV and AIDS.

- Public Health Laboratory Services (PHLS), Colindale Avenue, London
- Communicable Diseases Surveillance Units (CDSUs)
- Department of Health, AIDS Unit, Blackfriars Road, London
- Health Boards and Authorities under the direction of the AIDS (Control) Act 1987.

Until January 1991 the number of reported AIDS cases was published monthly. The main figure quoted was the cumulative total, that is, the overall number known since reporting started. Since the implementation of the AIDS (Control) Act 1987 and other measures it has been possible to gather more specific, local, information from hospitals, clinics and health boards. There is now a yearly breakdown of HIV seropositive incidence, cases of AIDS, gender, high risk activity (e.g. drug use) and age. The Department of Health also produces a quarterly Press Release (DOH 1992). Internationally, data collection has been improved by the coordination of research projects and the collation of information. There is an annual global AIDS medical conference and recently the European Association for Nurses in AIDS Care has established conferences in both Western and Eastern countries. (A global organisation is also developing.)

The impact of HIV/AIDS on health and social services

Although qualified nurses tend to work exclusively either in a hospital or a community setting it is important to consider HIV in relation to the full range of services available to the (typically young) person living with HIV. The settings in which care may be given to individuals with HIV/AIDS may be categorised as follows (Atkinson 1989a):

A. Institutional/hospital
1. Ward: hospital/hospice
2. Day Care
3. Outpatients

B. Community
4. Treatment room: health centre/clinic
5. Home: with a district nurse, health visitor or other practitioner
6. Home: self-care or with family/partner/friends
7a. Outreach: residential (hostels, prisons, caravans)
7b. Outreach: non-residential (drop-in centres, street work).

Hospital care. HIV care was at first delivered almost exclusively in the ward setting. This was an expensive, labour-intensive and often 'patient-unfriendly' option. Individuals would spend many days or weeks in hospital per year, sometimes feeling relatively well but needing, say, intravenous therapy. The ward setting is now used for other purposes, including respite and day care. Day care units are now used extensively and often have flexible hours to facilitate patients' work commitments. Day care units and outpatients departments are used as places of treatment, monitoring, counselling and group work as well as of traditional consultation (Murphy & Atkinson 1990).

Community care. Most procedures, including continuous intravenous therapy, can now be performed in the patient's home. The author looked after a young person who having been in prison was frightened of being in hospital. Even though the patient lived in a very poor area in a crowded home with young children, a high standard of nursing care was possible, including the successful care of a gangrenous ulcer. This patient very rarely went into hospital.

Outreach care is a developing area of nursing particularly in relation to HIV and drug misuse. One health visitor describes setting up a drop-in centre for prostitutes (Thomson 1989). This facility is still in operation as a joint Social Work/Health Board project. It provides counselling, medical cover, family planning and antenatal care as well as direct access to the HIV unit when necessary.

HIV has an enormous social impact on the individual and his carers. In order to provide the best possible care it is essential to have an integrated, multidisciplinary service that addresses social as well as clinical concerns, particularly in discharge planning and follow-up (Pratt 1991).

Creating an environment which enables an effective but *confidential* service is difficult especially as more agencies become involved in care. The best principle to adopt is a 'need to know' policy of information disclosure involving the patient at every stage. This sometimes causes problems as many professionals, quite wrongly, think they have a 'blanket' right to know a patient's details.

Manpower implications

The two main effects which HIV has had on health service manpower have been:

- role change and extension of roles
- increased workloads and accompanying costs.

Role change has been seen in hospital and the community. By the 1970s it was felt that infectious disease nursing as a specialty was no longer needed and infectious diseases hospitals were increasingly used for other purposes. Now infectious disease hospitals and wards have been completely transformed by HIV. Special facilities have been built requiring a great number of new staff. To date there has been no audit of how many nurses in the UK have now been deployed in this field. However, each authority has to publish a yearly report on activities and services under the 1987 AIDS (Control) Act.

The National Audit Office has found that in some areas funds provided for AIDS care have not been taken up. All authorities have now been instructed that these monies *must* be used. The government has made a firm commitment to protect these resources for a period of three years (from 1992), during which time constant reevaluation will take place (Comptroller and Auditor General 1991, DOH 1991).

The ability of nurses to undertake more complex procedures has also had considerable effect on the services available to people with HIV-related illness. As patients have begun to receive more of their treatment and monitoring outside the ward setting the place of inpatient care has also changed.

Linked to this is the challenge of making sure that having gained the necessary skills, nurses are allowed to practice them. At present there are several initiatives to standardise procedures and to discover in how many areas, e.g. continuous i.v. care at home, nurses are practising (DOH AIDS Unit 1992, RCN Daphne Heald Research Unit/AVERT 1993).

Increased workloads. In the community HIV has had the effect of creating new fields of work for practitioners. District nurses, whose main workload lies in caring for elderly people, now have younger people with a variety of clinical needs on their caseloads. It has been estimated that 6 patients with HIV with varying levels of illness can make up a full-time caseload (Newbury 1988a–b). A district nurse, in normal circumstances, usually has 40–60 patients (Atkinson 1989b).

Community nurses are placed using such criteria as the Standard Mortality Ratio and the Jarman Deprivation Index. The national average is one district nurse to 2500–5000 of the population. In areas where there are few old people the ratio may be as low as one district nurse to 12 000 of the population. Unfortunately it is sometimes in just these areas, especially in conjunction with deprivation, where there is an HIV problem (SOHHD & GGHB 1992).

Increased input by social services is needed by most affected people at one stage or another as their situation changes. Typically the individual is young, independent and employed; he or she may be living alone (paying a mortgage or rent) and may have no regular partner. As the disease progresses these circumstances may change rapidly. In HIV units where there is no resident social worker the nurse may need to act as advisor and advocate in helping the patient to obtain benefits, housing, domestic assistance, meal supplements and other services. For such nurses the key to success is to identify the appropriate services (without divulging the patient's personal details) and then *with the patient* to approach them for help. Without careful management, this extension of the nursing role can result in staff being 'spread too thin'. Efficient and appropriate referral will be vital to the success of the shift toward community-based care.

As patient morbidity and mortality improves, people with HIV disease are requiring treatment for longer periods. At the same time, more types of treatment are becoming available to practitioners and patients. In countries such as the USA, where there is limited public medicine, who gets what treatment and for how long is becoming a major issue. In the UK the limitation of certain treatments on financial grounds is not overtly on the political agenda. Since each Health Authority has its own AIDS budget there is in theory no need to 'top slice' funds from other areas. The specific drugs used in HIV care (e.g. AZT, ddI see p. 1007) do not have to come out of a GP's budget and are underwritten at a central level. However, difficulty can arise when GPs' have several affected people on their caseload, many of whom will need long-term medication.

Cumulative totals of individuals with HIV and AIDS are given in Box 38.4. Although the largest proportion of people affected have been homosexual men, Virginia Bottomley, Minister for Health, has commented that the *most rapid increase is among heterosexuals* and that 'Regardless of where or how the infection is acquired, HIV is established in the UK and can be passed on' (DOH 1992). However, the reader should be cautioned that it is not good practice to multiply the figures *ad infinitum* to get projected numbers. At that rate, the whole world would eventually become infected. A more useful indicator is the number of new cases reported monthly and the increase (if any) in incidence that this represents.

Box 38.4 HIV and AIDS Statistics for the UK, December 1993 (with kind permission from the Communicable Diseases (Scotland) Unit)

People recorded as being HIV Antibody Positive
18 257 males
2 791 females
53 unknown
Total: 21 101

People recorded as having AIDS
7 850 males of whom 5 298 have died
679 females of whom 355 have died
Total: 8 529 of whom 5 653 have died

? **38.1** What are the current statistics on new AIDS cases?

Social implications

The social impact of HIV/AIDS is felt in two ways: on society as a whole, and on the individual as a social being. Here we will consider the wider societal implications first.

At least one American senator was heard to say 'somewhere along the way we are going to have quarantine'. (Connor & Kingman 1989.)

This quotation typifies the way in which epidemics are often viewed by the makers of social policy. When the management of an epidemic is seen as being analogous to the management of acute illnesses in clinical practice (Barker & Rose 1990) the following equation is made:

The organism + the individual = the disease + the population = the epidemic.

In this view an intervention must be made to prevent the transformation of 'organism' into 'epidemic'. Theoretically, the options are:

- to kill the organism
- to make the organism inoperative
- to ameliorate the effects of the organism on the individual
- to separate the individual from the organism
- to separate the individual from the population
- to separate affected groups from the rest of the population.

Looking at disease in this way the reader may see the role of antibiotics and disinfectants (killing the organism), immunisation (making the organism inoperative), symptom control (ameliorating the effects), infection control and health education (separating the individual from the organism), quarantine (separating the individual from the population) and banishment/leper colonies (separating groups from the population).

It may also be seen that HIV does not present many options. There is no antibiotic, no vaccine. As HIV takes a long time to manifest itself and has no very clear presenting features quarantine and isolation of potential and actual 'victims' is difficult. At present only the amelioration of the effects, health education and infection control (including in this case, the use of condoms) are available in the 'battle' against this epidemic.

These options may strike us as being very limited ones. And therein lies the key to public reaction to HIV and AIDS. In the eyes of society, those who have been appointed to protect the population from disease have not come up with a satisfactory solution for HIV/AIDS. This has led to a reaction of fear and to a willingness to stigmatise, and even make scapegoats of, those with HIV.

Fear. It is important for the nurse to appreciate the complex nature of fear. For example, the knowledge that one cannot catch HIV shaking hands may not be enough to dispel someone's fear of such contact, for along with the fear of actual physical contamination may be the fear of the very *idea* of the disease. HIV is particularly frightening because there are very few factors which separate an individual from the virus. This in itself may lead people to distinguish their own behaviour from that of individuals affected by HIV in the hope of confirming their own 'immunity', as in: 'I can't get HIV because I'm not homosexual'. At the same time, this implies that individuals with HIV/AIDS are themselves to blame, and that if everyone in society conformed to certain patterns of behaviour then everything would be all right. This process is often referred to as 'fear of moral contamination' and 'moral panic'. The reader is referred to Loney et al 1988 for a discussion of these and related issues.

Stigmatisation. Scapegoats are those chosen by society to take the blame for evil or misfortune. The selection of a scapegoat is either arbitrary or based in prejudice. This is clear in the case of HIV, which can infect anyone, particularly the sexually active. In the Western world, the virus happens to have affected large numbers of homosexual men first, followed by intravenous drug users. In other areas of the world its epidemiology has followed other patterns. In any event, the appearance of the virus among one group or another has been a matter of historical accident only and has no inherent moral significance. Nonetheless, people with HIV have been stigmatised officially (e.g. by being refused insurance, employment, or entry into certain countries) and unofficially (e.g. by physical and verbal abuse). Individuals affected often become isolated, and because they *expect* abuse start to avoid social interaction, thus compounding their isolation and stigmatisation.

Whether the person involved is a gay man, a drug user, a patient's mother or a child in the playground, fear and stigmatisation have devastating consequences. A thoughtful nurse often makes all the difference.

Effects on the individual. The psychological impact of HIV/AIDS is similar to that of other terminal illnesses. Many experts in oncology and palliative care have written about HIV and AIDS, most notably Kubler Ross (1987). For a fuller discussion of the psychological implications of terminal illness the reader is referred to Ch. 34. For further discussion on coping with an AIDS diagnosis the reader is referred to Miller & Bor (1988).

The sick role. Bond & Bond (1986, pp. 211–213) define 'the sick role' as 'the expectations of people in a society which defines the rights and duties of its members who are sick'. Thus, individuals diagnosed as being ill are implicitly or otherwise 'given permission' to behave in certain ways.

Conditions which are seen as 'self-inflicted' tend to elicit less sympathy than others. The author has worked with a patient who, while receiving treatment for a malignant illness became infected with HIV through a blood transfusion. The patient described to carers the shift in attitude that was then encountered. While the diagnosis was 'cancer' a great deal of sympathy was given. When the diagnosis became 'HIV' the sympathy was considerably less.

A patient who eventually becomes ill may think that he is to blame for not keeping fit enough and may feel guilty when he is forced to leave work or abandon his former social roles (Atkinson 1991).

The difficulties are compounded when the person, a young drug user who prostitutes, for example, has a disordered or chaotic lifestyle. Combined with all of his or her other problems a positive HIV diagnosis can be devastating.

It is often difficult for the patient to inform relatives of his diagnosis, thus cutting himself off from a potential source of support and practical help. The nurse can often help the patient and his family to achieve a mutually acceptable resolution. She must bear in mind that whereas a family caring for someone with, say, cancer may get support and practical help from neighbours and others, HIV often sets the scene for isolation, guilt, prejudice and despair. This can happen in any terminal illness, but is often a particularly acute problem in HIV.

Philosophical issues for nurses

The problems the patient experiences as a stigmatised member of society demand that nurses who seek to help are very clear about their own attitudes and professional philosophy. Central to any philosophy of nursing practice is the patient's right to 'quality health care in an atmosphere of human dignity without regard to age, ethnic or national origin, sex or sexual orientation, religion or presenting illness' (Pratt 1991, p. 191). Coupled with this is the duty of nurses to look after *all* patients: unlike other professionals nurses cannot choose whom they will look after.

Models of care

The so-called 'medical model' on which much of nursing practice is based tends not to provide a satisfactory approach to illnesses in which there is no cure. This model works best when the illness can be reduced to a few constituent parts which can then be treated, eliminated, or made ineffective. HIV and AIDS offer little scope for such an approach, although the search for a 'cure' continues. The reductionist medical model tends to be less effective with multifaceted problems, especially those such as AIDS which are heavily influenced by sociopolitical factors.

Western care systems are based on humanist and utilitarian philosophies by which the individual is respected and recognised as being capable of independent moral judgement and action. This respect is the basis for the quotation from Pratt above. While most people accept this sentiment, there is always difficulty in its application, for it tends to be put into practice only when the individual *asserts* his rights (Downie & Telfer 1980). Those who have difficulty expressing their rights or who are considered as less worthy than others to do so are often treated as second-class citizens. Many people with HIV fall into these categories. Moreover, professionals and society at large may impose what may be called 'existential assumptions' upon a situation. One patient who is thought to be 'going somewhere' or to have 'been someone' may be considered to be more 'worth while' than another patient who is 'going nowhere'. So the death of a 'promising' young pianist, say, is considered sadder than the death of a young prostitute. This attitude pervades care delivery as professionals prioritise their care using these value judgements as well as formal clinical signs (Boss 1979, Beauchamp & Perlin 1978).

Western models of care tend to hold that one person's rights and liberties must not impinge upon another's and that one may not interfere with a person, even for his own good, unless he is violating the rights of other people (Downie & Telfer 1980). In the case of people who are considered members of a 'minority' these principles often work against their right to high quality care.

Another possible reaction is for the professional to look at a patient in difficulty and say 'Who am I to interfere with this person's right to choose to live like this', as if the young, homeless, ill, drug user has made the same kind of choices and been afforded the same opportunities as for example, the nurse in training. This attitude is seen in specific cases where patients are 'left alone', and in general where whole groups of people are either ignored or given the minimum of care.

Finally, Western care models are structured on materialistic rationalism whereby only what is 'rational' is accepted as being 'real'. The reader is invited to consider how limiting this view is as an approach to someone whose mind, body and spirit are in turmoil. By being too rational the nurse may cut herself off from the patient's *real* lived experience.

Four research studies into nurses' knowledge and attitudes with regard to AIDS have been undertaken in the UK. Another is currently being undertaken with student nurses. Two were carried out in the community, the others in hospitals. These studies have shown that it is not enough for nurses to have *information* about AIDS. They must also have *confidence* in their knowledge and in their practice (Bond et al 1988a–b, Akinsanya 1991, Wells et al 1989, Aggleton & AVERT 1993).

TESTING AND SCREENING

AIDS/HIV testing involves analysis for HIV antibodies. Testing for the actual virus, i.e. testing for HIV core antigen (particles of the virus), is used for clinical prognosis and management, not generally for diagnostic purposes. Blood samples are used at present for all forms of testing, although urine and saliva tests are being developed, especially for use in screening.

Screening. The term 'screening' is generally used to refer to the process by which blood samples undergo laboratory analysis by enzyme-linked immunosorbent assay (ELISA). This procedure is carried out on several samples at once and is used to find out the prevalence of HIV antibodies in a batch of samples. The process may stop here, as in the case of anonymous prevalence surveys. The screening assay has a 'built-in' **false positive** rate which ensures that there are no **false negative** readings. The analysts know the percentage false positive rate of the assay and so when confronted with a batch of positive results can make a mathematical adjustment to get an accurate picture of the prevalence of HIV in the group.

Individual testing. While ELISA is an efficient method of mass screening it is far from satisfactory for testing an *individual*, for whom a false positive result would be devastating. Therefore in individual testing the sample first undergoes ELISA, and then immunoblotting or the Western blotting method (accurate to within thousandths of 1%) to confirm the diagnosis. This method is more complex and is available only in sophisticated laboratories. In poorer countries samples may undergo repeated ELISA procedures instead of Western blotting to achieve maximum accuracy in difficult circumstances. This method has an incidence level of less than 0.1% false positives (Green & McCreaner 1989).

Timing

Generally, HIV antibodies are produced between 3 weeks and 3 months after the individual becomes infected with HIV. This period can, however, be much longer — lapses of 2 years and more have been known. The timing of a diagnostic test is therefore important (Miller & Bor 1988). Individuals who have a test which proves negative are often advised to come back for repeat tests over a period of months. Because of this uncertainty and the personal impact of a positive result HIV antibody testing should take place only with pre- and post-test counselling.

Forms of testing

There are various forms of HIV testing, some of which have become controversial. All types are defined here so that the reader can differentiate between them and enter into the continuing debate over their efficacy, need and ethics.

Named voluntary testing with pre- and post-test counselling. This form occurs when an individual seeks a test following a specific high-risk activity or contact or when the individual, for reasons of his own, wants to know his sero status. It is available at genitourinary clinics and HIV units, and from some GPs and other community practitioners. People found to be positive are automatically referred to medical/nursing services. Professionals and others agree that this form is the most acceptable both practically and ethically.

Named voluntary testing with minimal or no counselling. Many people go for testing without being given the opportunity to discuss the implications of a positive or negative result. Many, on being found positive, are not referred to services. Others, on being found negative, think that they are 'safe' and need not worry or make behavioural changes.

Conditional named 'voluntary' testing. Increasingly, organisations, countries giving work permits, and insurance companies are asking applicants to have an HIV antibody test before gaining entry or obtaining services. The clinical value of these tests is doubtful as they are taken in isolation, often without counselling.

Patients on transplant and other medical waiting lists are often asked to be tested as a condition of entry onto the list. This is done mainly in a hospital setting.

Also increasing is the use of an HIV antibody test as part of a battery of tests seeking a diagnosis, especially for ill patients admitted with unusual or vague symptoms or for patients who appear to be from 'high-risk' groups. Nurses must be particularly careful in these cases. It is their legal duty, as well as the doctor's, to ensure that every patient gives his *informed consent* for the test. This may be difficult if the patient is very ill, but this does not change the nurse's legal and professional accountability.

Local anonymous HIV sero prevalence surveys. These surveys are carried out by hospital departments who use part of blood samples given for other purposes to screen for HIV seroprevalence in a given locality or patient group. This is perfectly legal as long as the patients are informed that this procedure may be carried out. The sample has to be made anonymous and the result is not given to the patient.

Controversy has arisen surrounding this form of testing, particularly when the results are published in medical journals and the media. This is because relatively small numbers of patients are highlighted. For example, 1000 or so pregnant women may be screened, of whom 15 are shown to be HIV antibody positive. Some publications may break this down even further and state that, of this 15, 8 came from Africa (for example). This narrows down the numbers so much that many people are of the opinion that it compromises anonymity. The Royal Colleges of Nursing and of Midwives have both strongly condemned the practice of publishing results in this manner (RCN Congress 1991).

National Anonymous Survey of the Seroprevalence of HIV. This is an ongoing survey directed by the DOH and organised by the Public Health Laboratory Service (PHLS). As in local surveys, surplus blood from patient samples is used. Again the patients do not have to give specific consent, but they must be informed that their blood may be used. This is done by a multilingual poster campaign and through the nursing and medical professions. The samples are made anonymous, but certain information such as gender, age and geographical area remains with the sample. The various governmental and professional organisations concerned, including nursing and midwifery, meet in a special forum to monitor and improve the project. The results are published nationally with a breakdown of regions and other groups. The UKCC have responded to HIV testing in various documents; particularly relevant to anonymous testing are UKCC 1989 and UKCC 1990. The Royal College of Nursing AIDS Nursing Forum has information on this and other related subjects, and the PHLS publishes guidelines on the Survey (PHLS 1991).

Advantages and disadvantages of anonymous testing

Voluntary, informed testing with counselling allows the HIV seropositive individual to be referred to the appropriate services. Ethically and practically this form is best for patient and professional carer alike. However, in the public perception the risk of HIV appears to centre around minority groups. Most people do not feel they are at risk. Of those that do feel some risk, most do not think they need to be tested.

Anonymous testing is the compromise that has emerged to satisfy, on the one hand, the need of professionals to find out how many people are, and are likely to be, affected and, on the other, the personal and civil liberties of individuals. Some professionals argue that not enough political effort has been made to increase the uptake of voluntary named testing. As HIV care improves it is becoming clearer that the earlier an individual knows the diagnosis and is referred into medical and nursing services the better.

This presents one of the ethical dilemmas of anonymous testing. As the number of anonymous positive samples increases it will become apparent that, for instance, X number of pregnant women and their babies are affected, but nothing can be done for them because they are unknown. Another objection made by some is that testing babies is an underhand way of testing mothers and that as the number of known but unnamed HIV positive babies increases the Government will be forced to establish Draconian measures such as mandatory testing for all mothers. Many professionals would argue, however, that the more we know about national and local prevalence, the more we can target services.

In these matters the rights of the individual must be balanced against the rights of the community. Nurses are bound to uphold the right of the individual, but also have a duty towards the community. These obligations are not mutually exclusive, but require that the issues are considered from every viewpoint. The professional bodies provide guidelines on many of the more contentious issues. It may be fair to say, however, that the nurse should generally 'err' on the side of the individual patient, for she is often his only advocate (UKCC 1992).

Targeted screening. Until the National Survey, screening took place almost exclusively in specialist areas and among particular groups who were considered 'high risk'. Whereas the information gleaned from this work was useful it was incomplete, yielding little knowledge about the population at large. Moreover HIV would always seem to affect mainly homosexuals or drug users if most of the samples continued to be taken from those groups. In Glasgow, for example, one area which had a higher proportion of known HIV positive drug users than other, similar deprived areas received a lot of research attention. Another similar area at the other side of the city had a 'lower' prevalence, but very few individuals had been tested (Ruchill Hospital 1989). When looking at research it is important to be aware of such factors which may distort results.

Counselling

While a comprehensive guide to counselling could hardly be presented here the following offers a few pointers to assist the nurse to meet the challenge of HIV-related counselling. The reader is also referred to Jones (1990), who was a student nurse at the time of writing her article, Burnard (1989) and, specifically in relation to HIV, Miller & Bor (1988).

- Counselling is a helpful tool, among other tools, which may be used to assist the patient. It is not an end in itself. One person with AIDS half jokingly remarked: 'Nurses are so keen to counsel me, it seems they forget I have practical needs. Sometimes I feel I'm being counselled to death!'
- Counselling is not advice-giving. Patients often ask, 'What would you do, nurse?' but the nurse must seriously consider the relevance of her reply. Advice of the 'If I were you . . .' type is rarely appropriate.
- Counselling is not about getting the patient to do the 'right' thing. A young, pregnant, HIV seropositive woman cannot be 'counselled' to have, or not to have, an abortion, for example.
- Counselling is about helping someone come to his own decisions.
- It is an exploration made by two people of issues and problems. The counsellor is an equal partner whose personal opinion is very often not relevant, although it may come up in the course of the conversation.
- It is difficult to counsel and do something else. On many occasions nurses gain the patient's confidence in the process of delivering clinical and personal services. This is a good entry into the counselling relationship, as is the provision of accurate information. To achieve the equality necessary it is advisable to be in a neutral place on an eye-to-eye level. This is difficult if the patient is lying down with few clothes on with the nurse standing over him!
- Good counselling does not have to take a long time. Some practitioners think counselling is rather fancy and too time-consuming for the busy clinical situation. This is not the case. Effective counselling can be achieved in half an hour or less, especially if the counsellor gives the individual her undivided attention.
- Know your limitations. During a session it may become apparent to the counsellor that she is getting into areas where one or both parties feel they cannot cope or are out of their depth. There is no shame in this. Seek appropriate help. No one is supposed to have all the answers.

Pre- and post-test counselling

Nurses are often asked to give pre- and post-test counselling. It is essential that the nurse is proficient before attempting this. Short courses are now available in many authorities. Counselling in other clinical areas especially oncology, genetics and terminal care can provide very good experience. The counsellor does not have to be an 'expert' on HIV, but she must have sound clinical knowledge, as she will often encounter unusual questions which are worrying the patient.

Pre-test counselling will involve the following:

- Establishing why the individual wants to be tested. Many

people come armed with erroneous conceptions. Clinical factors must also be established. A patient of the author's came seeking the test and a termination of pregnancy. She thought her partner was HIV positive and that her baby would die of AIDS. When she was investigated it was found that she was in fact not pregnant. Her partner's HIV status was not known. Because she had been worrying she had imagined the very worst.
- Exploring the pros and cons *for that individual* of having the test. Is it appropriate? Should he wait for 3–6 months? Has he been at risk?
- Considering the implications of a positive result. Most people come for a negative result, to be reassured.

Having decided to be tested the person usually has to wait about a week. Ideally the same counsellor should give the person the result, but in the hospital setting the result is often given by the doctor.

If the result is negative it is important that the individual knows how to avoid risk in the future and whether it is advisable to come back for a repeat test in, say, 6 months' and a year's time. If the result is positive the counsellor may want to be accompanied by a colleague who can be on hand to assist. There is no good way of divulging such devastating news. Experts in the field often say that every time they have to do it is different. Nor does it get easier.

> ? **38.2** When helping a person in distress with a condition such as HIV black and white answers seldom fit. Here are some true situations. How can you help?
> *Remember:* What *you* think is 'right' may not help you or the patient.
>
> a. A patient is found to be HIV positive. He understands the 'duty' he has to tell his partner but does not know how to do it and 'cannot go through with it'. How do you help him?
> b. A patient who is demonstrating signs of serious illness, has been advised to have the HIV test. She does not want to and asks you as the nurse to help her. What do you do?
> c. A colleague of yours receives a needlestick injury from a suspected drug user. There is pressure to test the drug user to see if he has HIV. What is your view of the matter?
> d. A patient with HIV tells you that he is scared of becoming ill and wants to die now. Is he depressed? Is there any hope? How do you cope when you can't say 'It'll be all right'?
> e. A patient tells you of a 'high-risk' activity he has engaged in. You want to help him. How do you reassure him without lying? On the other hand, how do you tell him the truth without panicking him or making him behave rashly?
>
> In all of these situations where do your 'loyalties' lie? To whom are you accountable or responsible — the patient, the public, the Government, yourself, your profession?

HEALTH EDUCATION AND PROMOTION IN HIV

Although treatment for AIDS is improving, it is still very limited. Health education must therefore take a central role in the fight against the disease. Caplan's (1961) model describes health education and promotion as having three parts:

- primary: preventing occurrence of the disease; providing education, raising awareness, giving information
- secondary: detecting disease early; screening, performing individual testing
- tertiary: preventing deterioration of individuals affected, giving support.

These general aims must be responsive to the physical, mental, emotional, spiritual and societal needs of the individual (Ewles & Simnett 1992).

Health promotion in HIV/AIDS entails more than raising general public awareness through mass media campaigns. It can also involve such activities as providing assertiveness training for individuals affected and helping them to learn self-care and nurturing skills. HIV awareness also has implications for the workplace, raising concerns about working practice and hiring policies. Legal and ethical issues must also be grappled with by nurses working with people who are involved in illicit drug use and prostitution and who consequently face particular difficulties.

To become equipped to operate on so many levels the reader is urged to read not only 'mainstream' publications on health promotion such as Ewles & Simnett (1992) but also books which take a particular perspective, such as Tatchell's (1990) book on AIDS, subtitled 'A radical self-help manual for understanding, preventing and fighting back'. Karpf's *Doctoring the Media* (1988), while not specifically on HIV education, may help the reader to take a more analytical view of large-scale media campaigns. For regular updating of information, the reader may refer to the Department of Health AIDS Unit's press releases, issued quarterly. The *Nursing Standard* also publishes a quarterly insert, 'AIDS Focus', which gives a research update and articles on both clinical and educational issues. In England and Wales nurses may obtain information from the National Health Education Authority and, in Scotland, from the Health Education Board. Help is also available locally from Health Promotion Departments and from professionals such as health visitors.

Elements of health promotion

Targeting the 'audience'

The way in which HIV educators convey their message sometimes seems to contradict that message itself. For example, the maxim that 'There are not high risk groups, there are only high risk activities' is generally 'targeted' at drug users, prostitutes, gay men, etc. Does this amount to ideological double talk?

The problem with labelling whole groups as being 'at risk' is that it is not precise. A gay man, for example, is not at risk if he refrains from unprotected sexual intercourse. An intravenous drug user who does not share injecting equipment is also not at risk. That is, these individuals are not at risk merely because they can be labelled 'gay' or 'drug user'. People are at risk if they undertake a high risk activity.

Advertisers and health educators, however, record that certain groups have certain behaviour patterns in common. It makes sense, therefore, to target these groups with certain services and messages, *always remembering* that general patterns will not fully reflect the complexity of individuals. In her work with prostitutes in Glasgow, Thomson (1989) found some of the general problems associated with drug use and prostitution but also encountered various other challenging issues.

The right medium and the right message

Leaflets are frequently used in various kinds of information campaigns because they are very simple to distribute. Most people can read in the UK, and by means of leaflets information can be placed unequivocally in the hands of the target audience. What could be better? Unfortunately, research over the years has shown that people tend not to read unsolicited leaflets. While they can be an excellent written adjunct to a spoken session, leaflets are of limited use 'cold' (AVERT 1992b).

The first public message from the UK government came in the form of an open letter, warning of the risks of HIV, from the Chief Medical Officer at the DOH. This message was published in all the national papers. Following this there was a leaflet drop to every household in the UK and a poster and television campaign. The commercials and posters carried the slogan 'Don't Die of Ignorance' but did not go into clinical detail. They were designed to raise awareness. A National AIDS Helpline was set up where people could (and still can) phone free to speak to a trained telephone counsellor.

Research subsequently showed that general messages warning of danger and giving non-specific information were of limited efficacy. Over the years mass media messages have therefore become much more specific, aiming at particular individuals and behaviour groups. Awareness and knowledge of HIV appear to be improving as a result (RCN Conference 1989, HEA 1991).

Although HIV education through the mass media has had some degree of effectiveness this kind of communication, no matter how expertly done, always has a high degree of 'wastage'. Even the most successful television advertising campaigns can only expect to 'reach', i.e. to elicit sales from, 2% of the adult population (Fletcher 1992a–b). But as long as this form of health promotion is successful in influencing the behaviour of some people for their own benefit and that of the larger community, mass media information campaigns must continue to constitute a vital part of the battle against HIV.

The nurse's role

Given the limitations of mass communications in influencing behaviour, the nurse must take every opportunity to make general messages relevant to the patients in her care. Nurses have always been involved in assisting patients to understand their treatment, and in answering their questions in terms that can be understood. In doing so they require sound clinical knowledge together with an understanding of the patient's needs, lifestyle and expectations, as obtained from the nursing assessment.

One of the nurse's greatest advantages as a health educator is that she is with the patient for long periods of time in a position of trust. Many other care professionals see the patient only during short visits and often have to work harder to establish a rapport. Nevertheless, the nurse may still experience some difficulty in discussing sexual matters and sexuality with her patients. Public campaigns are restricted by legislation and 'public taste', and it may be left to the nurse to provide more explicit information. Personal value judgements, embarrassment and questions of status may present obstacles. Answering questions on, say, oral sex from a person of a different sexual persuasion to oneself may be difficult. Speaking to an underage person who is sexually active may be embarrassing and raise ethical questions. Many practitioners become expert at putting up verbal and non-verbal barriers so that such discussions are avoided.

Despite this potential for awkwardness or discomfort it is clear, given the devastating effects of HIV, how important it is for nurses to fulfil their obligations as health educators. It is strongly suggested that the reader find an expert practitioner who can act as a role model and mentor. Attending an organised course may also help. It is *not* suggested that the nurse must *necessarily* change her mind about certain issues or that she must agree with what each patient has to say. However, her caring must be *unconditional*, answering to the patient's needs regardless of the nurse's personal judgement.

A mentor can also help the less experienced practitioner to deal with difficult ethical issues. Patients sometimes give the nurse information about past actions which places the nurse in a difficult position. In such cases nurses at all levels should seek advice, whilst ensuring that patient confidentiality is maintained. Under the UKCC guidelines the nurse is judged both on confidentiality and on the accounts she gives of her actions in a difficult situation (Pyne 1990). To give an example, the author once looked after an HIV antibody positive 15-year-old who was having penetrative sex with an underage partner who lived with her parents. The situation was discussed and acted upon, keeping the confidentiality of all parties. The 15-year-old was assisted to approach the partner and her parents accompanied by nursing staff. Although the medical consultant had in this case the power to make an approach without consent, sensitive work with the patient made this unnecessary and a good working relationship was maintained.

Health educators are sometimes faced with the dilemma that encouraging safe practice and encouraging someone to break the law seem to amount to the same thing. For example, nurses are now involved in giving drug users clean needles and syringes. This practice has Government and professional support. Is it correct, however, for the nurse to tell the patient how to inject safely or to use one form of drug instead of another? (see Ch. 37, p. 976). In the face of a bleak prognosis, the practitioner may see no option but to fall back on the pragmatic principle of 'harm reduction' rather than to insist upon an ideal. In such a situation the nurse should seek guidance and support from management.

Group work. Nurses are increasingly becoming involved in working with groups, particularly in the community. These may be self-help groups or people attending a clinic for a particular service. Whether the nurse sets the group up herself or 'piggy-backs' a service onto an existing group, the results can be dramatic. By speaking to a small number, answering questions *they* want to ask and offering individuals the opportunity to speak in private afterwards, the nurse can make health education messages *personally* relevant. Robertson, a health visitor in a deprived area in Glasgow, works from a health centre as a general community practitioner. She has described taking health education about HIV, safer sex, drug use, positive self-care and other related subjects to patients via group work with women, homeless teenagers and drug users (Robertson 1991). Ewles & Simnett (1992) describe the formal and informal intricacies of setting up groups, agendas and action plans.

CLINICAL MANIFESTATIONS AND MANAGEMENT OF HIV/AIDS

People with HIV disease rarely get all of the diseases associated with AIDS (see Box 38.1) and often those that do occur manifest one at a time. The precise course of the illness is virtually impossible to predict. A patient of the author's seemed so close to death in late 1987 that it seemed cruel to persist with his medication. In 1991 he was still alive. Another patient was reasonably well but then developed a B cell lymphoma and was dead in two months. Yet another, with the same diagnosis, became paralysed, got better and lived for two years.

The treatment of AIDS is a rapidly developing field in which modifications are being made all the time. This section will therefore present a matrix of current approaches that can be used by the nurse as a conceptual and practical framework as the medical and nursing management of HIV/AIDS advances.

Approaches to nursing care

Pratt (1991) and Flaskerud & Ungvarski (1992) provide detailed strategies and philosophies for ward and service management. The present author uses a process based on Roy's (1989) adaption model which takes into account the following aspects of the patient's illness experience:

- physiological adaptation: clinical signs, disease process
- self-concept adaptation: anxiety, aggression, grief, social belonging
- role function adaptation: (e.g. as a father, a partner, a worker) sense of failure, sense of conflict
- interdependency adaptation (loneliness, rejection, social interaction).

These four 'adaptive modes' are placed in the context of three 'stimuli':

- focal, e.g. the surrounding facilities, services available; other people
- contextual, e.g. space available, distance to toilet, room temperature
- residual, e.g. personal beliefs, prejudices, personal qualities (George 1985).

The nurse applying this model will, having identified a clinical problem (say, the patient's sudden inability to walk), consider not only his medication and treatment but also his ability to function and adapt. This is then put alongside the practicalities of the stimuli. Are the facilities at home suitable? How far is it to the toilet? Can the patient put up with a commode in his front room? Will he let his wife look after him?

Roy's model is also useful as it helps the nurse consider all the adaptations needed to make an individual service effective. Does the present service or nursing procedure need change? Does the environment suit the patient? Does the patient need to modify his lifestyle? How can the nurse help these factors come to fruition? The adaptation model encourages a flexible approach by nurse and patient using all the available hospital and community care settings.

People with HIV may present with seemingly minor problems which cannot always be diagnosed or predicted. For example, an individual may suffer weight loss, difficulty in swallowing, anorexia, night sweats, lethargy, mouth ulcers, diarrhoea, constipation and so on. In addition to this he may become depressed and desperate, for such conditions, even if not in themselves life-threatening, can be very distressing. A patient of the author's had, over two years, contracted two serious bouts of *Pneumocystis carinii* pneumonia. He had borne these very well. He became severely depressed, however, sometime later when he was back at work. Having contracted oral thrush he could not swallow properly and was losing weight. This made him feel powerless and he said it was worse than the 'serious' illnesses (Atkinson 1991). Such examples serve to remind the practitioner that the seriousness of a condition cannot be judged strictly by clinical criteria. Moreover, by taking notice of even the smallest signs and taking action nurses can help many patients remain alive. Many HIV-related conditions, if caught early, respond well to treatment.

Infection control

For general principles of infection control the reader is referred to Ch. 16. The essence of infection control with HIV is to use **universal precautions** and to **protect the patient**. Care should be taken with all body fluids, and gloves and aprons should be used for intimate procedures. Because of his damaged immune system the patient is quite often more at risk from the nurse than the other way round. However, there is no need for reverse barrier nursing.

In the home, basic hygiene is to be encouraged and clothes and bedding should be washed in a washing machine. Disposal of medical waste should be carried out in accordance with local nursing procedure. Needles and syringes found in the street are the responsibility of the Environmental Health Department, although health care professionals finding them have a duty to minimise the risk of injury to themselves and others where possible.

CONDITIONS, TREATMENTS AND SPECIFIC NURSING INTERVENTIONS

What follows is a description of the main presenting infections, conditions and treatments associated with HIV and AIDS (see Box 38.1). For further information, the following are recommended: Youle et al (1988) as a useful and compact guide; Pratt (1991) for discussion of nursing strategy; Flaskerud & Ungvarski (1992) for an American perspective. Adler (1991) has colour photographs and large illustrations. Sims & Moss (1991) from the Mildmay AIDS Hospice in London concentrate on terminal care. Articles relating to specific treatment and nursing care are referred to throughout the following sections.

At present there is no vaccine in general use against AIDS. Research is advancing and expectations of a vaccine to make people immune to HIV are cited by various establishments as being from 5 to 10 years away. Although there are various treatments which ameliorate the effects of viruses, there has never been anything in the nature of a broad-spectrum antibiotic which actually kills viruses. Antiviral agents which suppress HIV will be discussed later.

Possibilities for fighting and killing the virus are, therefore, limited. The best successes so far have been in the area of symptomatic control, i.e. stopping or slowing the associated diseases and conditions which can kill the patient. The other main aim of care is to improve the patient's quality of life. There is thus a similarity between AIDS nursing and oncology and terminal care. As medical treatment for AIDS is so limited, competent nursing care is at a premium.

At the beginning of the epidemic the life expectancy of someone diagnosed as having AIDS was anything from a few weeks to 2 years. Patients receiving care can now live for 5 or, very rarely, even 10 years. When one considers other life-threatening conditions, such as diabetes mellitus, which similarly depend on symptomatic control but in which there is a much longer life expectancy, it becomes apparent that the care of HIV-related illness is still at an early stage.

The general progress of HIV-related illness is represented in Figure 38.2.

Phases of HIV and AIDS

Phase A: acute seroconversion illness

In most individuals this illness is not recognised. It may be seen 2–6 weeks after exposure to HIV. Not everybody infected with HIV gets this 'flu or glandular fever like condition. It may be associated with joint pain and other non-specific signs. A

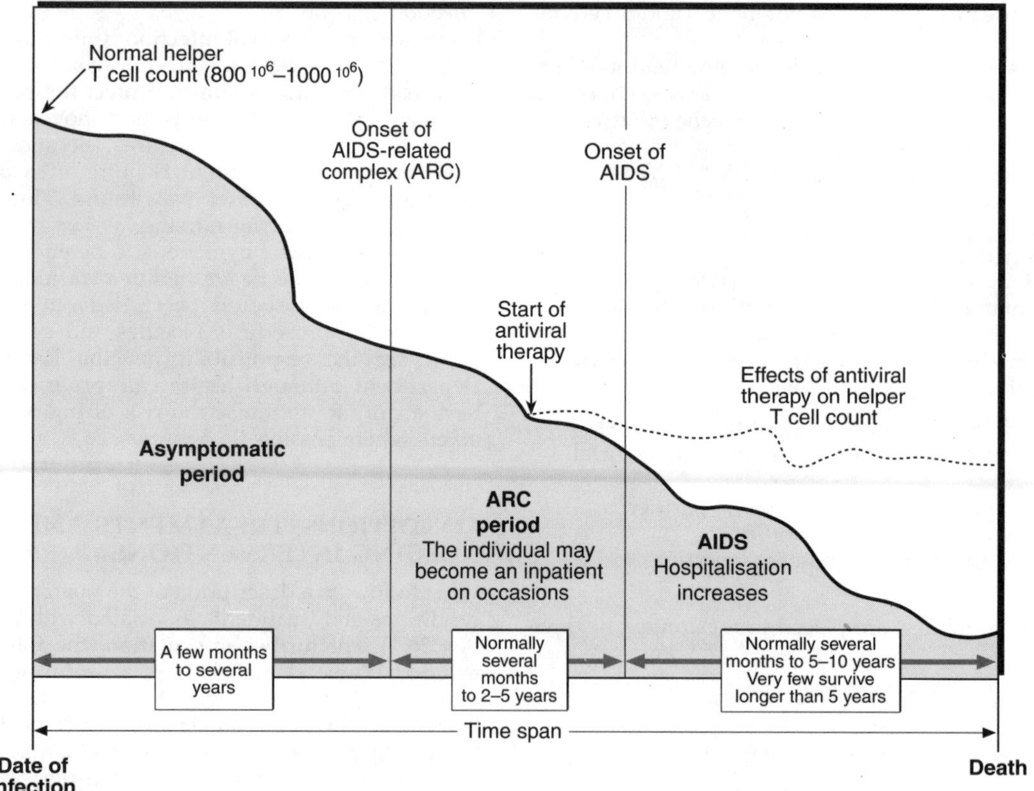

Fig. 38.2 Diagrammatic representation of the progress of HIV-related illness. Many people die when they get the first major opportunistic infection (onset of AIDS). It is very difficult to state when a person is going into the terminal stages of the disease. Many people make remarkable recoveries over a period of months or years.

skin rash is sometimes seen, as are swollen lymph glands (these usually reduce after some time). At this stage the body will be producing HIV antibodies (seroconversion). At this stage a few individuals may also show early signs of HIV affecting the central nervous system, particularly the layers of the brain (encephalopathy, meningitis; see Ch. 9).

Treatment of seroconversion illness is symptomatic and does not usually take place in hospital. For doctors and nurses on the alert the illness may be a useful diagnostic warning, rather as a thirst and boils suggest diabetes. However, the signs are very similar to those of many minor infections.

Phase B: antibody positive phase

B-1: asymptomatic HIV infection. As HIV has only been recognised for 13 years so far, one can only remark that the period between infection and the onset of clinical signs may be anything from a few weeks to 13 or more years. From this fact it may be seen that procedures such as contact tracing are not as simple or effective as in other sexually transmitted diseases as the asymptomatic period commonly covers much of an individual's sexually active life.

B-2: persistent generalised lymphadenopathy (PGL) or lymphadenopathy syndrome (LAS). This condition is sometimes the one which alerts medical services to investigate for HIV. The individual presents with swollen glands of more than 1 cm which persist for longer than 12 weeks. Although the individual may have swollen inguinal glands, he must also have other affected glands. Other reasons for swollen glands must be discounted before a diagnosis is given. As this is often the 'introductory' condition to HIV illness, monitoring of helper T cells and suppressor T cells (called the CD4 T cell subsets procedure; see Appendix 1) and other investigations may begin. It is at this stage that the individual may be tested for HIV for the first time.

Phase C: AIDS-related complex (ARC)

This phase refers to a period in an individual's illness career where he may contract a variety of well-known conditions, but *not* major, life-threatening, opportunistic infections or cancers. Common bacterial, viral and fungal infections frequently occur and are often marked by their persistence and virulence. Oral and genital herpes or athlete's foot are good examples. In a normally healthy person these conditions would resolve within a few days. When someone 'goes into' ARC the duration of the infection is lengthened and the whole foot, for instance, may become affected. Other conditions such as oral hairy leukoplakia are sometimes seen.

Loss of weight (up to 10% body mass) may be seen at this stage. This may be due to a specific mechanical problem, such as mouth ulcers, or from persistent low-grade attacks from infections. At this stage a significant drop may be seen in the helper T cells. In day-to-day practice nurses should bear in mind that young, healthy people should overcome common infections quickly without them becoming widespread. Any persistent condition (e.g. coughing, loss of weight) should be noted. While thrush *(Candida albicans)* is common in the vagina, it is very *uncommon* in the mouth of a young healthy person. Such an occurrence should immediately alert the practitioner that the individual may have an underlying condition such as HIV.

The nurse working with diagnosed patients should also be aware that since the positive diagnosis the individual will have been dreading the onset of illness. When weight loss, mouth ulcers or fungal infections occur he may become acutely anxious, considering himself to be in imminent danger of death or pain. Other professionals, such as clinical psychologists, can assist the patient during these periods. Involvement of the patient in all stages of decision-making and treatment right from the start will assist him to take control of his condition and reduce his feeling of helplessness.

Box 38.5 summarises treatments and medications used in various conditions associated with ARC.

Phase D: AIDS — constitutional disease, opportunistic infections, secondary cancers

Constitutional disease: HIV wasting syndrome. The diagnosis of AIDS depends on an individual being diagnosed as HIV antibody positive plus being diagnosed as having one of the life-threatening opportunistic infections or secondary cancers associated with HIV. Recently, a third criterion has come more to the fore, namely the constitutional or systemic condition known as HIV wasting syndrome. This has arisen from the experience in Africa, where AIDS is called 'slim disease'. In the West also it has become increasingly recognised that some individuals become extremely ill, losing extreme amounts of weight (more than 10% body mass) and suffering from morbid weakness and loss of function with or without having the 'label' of one of the listed conditions. In the USA 19% of adults with AIDS are diagnosed as having HIV wasting syndrome.

The causes of HIV wasting syndrome may be mechanical or systemic. As mentioned before, people lose weight if there are factors such as mouth ulcers and sickness which impede eating. Malabsorption may also be seen and may be due to the presence of a lesion such as Kaposi's sarcoma in the gut or to a more generalised dysfunction. In all these cases the patient is starved of nutrients.

Wasting may also occur as a result of metabolic changes. As in cancerous conditions, the body may go from its normal anabolic state into a catabolic crisis in which body mass is 'burnt up' at an increased and dangerous rate, often causing irreparable damage. These patients may recover some weight but they often do not recover muscle mass (Flaskerud & Ungvarski 1992).

Supervised nutritional rehabilitation is therefore necessary (Task Force on Nutrition Support in AIDS 1989). This may include nutritional supplements and more invasive therapy such as continuous or intermittent parenteral feeding. However, it is as well to remember that the nurse can play a life-saving role in the attention she pays to the ordinary nutritional service to the patient. MacCallum's research (1991) found that nutritionally compromised patients were often losing weight in hospital because of the meal and nutrition service. He concluded that nursing care and nutrition is as much about 'knives and forks' as it is about sophisticated tube feeding.

Opportunistic infections: protozoal. Some of the protozoal infections which may occur in AIDS are as follows.

Pneumocystis carinii pneumonia (PCP; pneumocystosis). About 60% of individuals contract PCP as the first AIDS-related infection. Because the vast majority of people diagnosed as having AIDS have been unaware of their HIV status, many people who have contracted PCP for the first time present not to specialist units but to A & E departments, GPs' offices and other non-specialist areas.

Although PCP is the most common cause of death in AIDS, the organism responsible, *Pneumocystis carinii*, can be found, quite normally, in most human beings. The immune system keeps the population of the organism at an acceptable level. When the immune system is compromised the level rises and causes severe, life-threatening pneumonia. The individual usually presents with a 2–5 week history of increasing shortness of breath, weakness and dry cough; cyanosis is often seen.

Treatment is by pentamidine isethionate i.v. Also used is co-trimoxazole, although some patients suffer from severe rashes with the high doses necessary. Pentamidine has side-effects

Box 38.5 Nursing care in ARC (Adler 1991, Flaskerud & Ungvarski 1992 and Pratt 1991)

Diarrhoea
Immediate monitoring should start with the help of a dietitian.

Weight loss
Measurements of muscle and fat loss should be included in care programme. Eating patterns should be discussed along with ways of increasing intake, for example taking frequent, smaller meals and perhaps supplementary feeds such as Ensure (Murphy & Atkinson 1990, MacCallum 1991).

Fluid and electrolyte replacement is essential. Codeine phosphate, loperamide hydrochloride and diphenoxylate hydrochloride may be useful, but it is emphasised that medication should always be given in combination with dietary monitoring and therapy. (See Chs 20 and 21.)

Herpes simplex
Acyclovir is used. Prophlactic doses may also be given.

Herpes zoster
Mouth and lip care is important to prevent cracking and secondary infection. Soothing lotions and loose clothing may be appropriate for attacks of shingles. Sleep, fluid intake and diet should be monitored.

Seborrhoeic dermatitis/skin care
Salicylic acid and tar-based lotions are used. Low-dose steroids and steroid/antibiotic/antifungal combinations (e.g. Trimovate) are sometimes used for short periods. Responding to the individual patient's discomfort is important. Giving attention to small details to alleviate the irritation of skin conditions is one of the most appreciated nursing services. (See Ch. 12.)

Tinea pedis
Miconazole and clotrimazole creams are used topically. Systemic griseofulvin is used if the infection is persistent. Keeping the feet dry and comfortable can be helped by such measures as drying with a cool hairdryer and leaving the end of the bed covers loose.

Oral candidiasis
Nystatin antifungal topical drops may be used. However, oral thrush is often persistent in HIV illness, in which case systemic fluconazole is used. Mouth care is vital, as is a high fluid intake. Some patients find mouth rinsing with benzydamide hydrochloride, which has anaesthetic properties, helpful. Others rinse with fizzy water or diet cola to relieve discomfort, although this is not research based. (See Ch. 12.)

Oral hairy leukoplakia
Acyclovir is used. Mouth care is again essential.

such as nephrotoxicity. Regular blood pressure observations and urinalysis are necessary. Diaminodiphenylsulfone is used as well as pyrimethamine; these also have side-effects. Aerosolised pentamidine is used as a treatment but is more commonly used as a prophylactic 2–4 weekly.

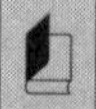

For more detail about PCP see Pratt (1991), Stevenson (1989), Atkinson (1989a) and Flaskerud & Ungvarski (1992).

Cryptosporidiosis. This condition has some notoriety in the specialist and the general care areas. It is caused by a protozoon which is present in small quantities in the water supply. In immunocompromised patients it rises to high levels in the gastrointestinal tract and causes diarrhoea. The loss of fluid can be as much as 10–20 litres a day, although less virulent attacks are also seen.

Cryptosporidiosis is generally seen only in patients who are already very ill and have suffered other infections. It is very difficult to manage this condition at home, as intravenous fluid replacement and constant bowel movements will need constant attention. For the patient this condition may mean hospitalisation and an extremely poor state of health. In its worst form it is an extremely distressing condition for the patient and his carers.

Treatments have varying success and are not well established (Adler 1991). Spiramycin and erythromycin are the main antibiotics used but combinations of others may be tried as well.

Another organism causes isosporiasis, which also leads to severe diarrhoea. Treatment is usually with cotrimoxazole.

Toxoplasmosis. The causative protozoon is sometimes heard mentioned in association with cats and raw meat, although it does not generally manifest itself as a disease in healthy people. Its most common manifestation is cerebral toxoplasmosis. The organism causes space-occupying lesions in the brain. These create cerebral oedema and intracranial pressure. The patient suffers the usual signs of these conditions: paralysis and unconsciousness. Toxoplasmosis is often fatal and treatment must be prolonged as relapses are almost inevitable. The main medication is pyrimethamine given with sulphadiazine. Dexamethazone is also used to reduce cerebral oedema. In the most serious cases constant nursing attention is needed as the patient's condition may deteriorate rapidly.

Opportunistic infections: viral. The most common of these are the following.

Herpes simplex virus. This condition has been mentioned in association with ARC, where it occurs in its less virulent forms. Sometimes seen are serious and life-threatening forms (e.g. encephalitis) affecting the central nervous system (Pratt 1991). Acyclovir is used in treatment.

Cytomegalovirus (CMV). This virus is encountered in general practice and in midwifery, where it is known to cause spontaneous abortion. In HIV-related illness it is most commonly seen causing CMV retinitis. Small 'cotton buds' are seen on the retina on examination. The patient may then rapidly become blind; the author has cared for people to whom this has happened over a few days. Treatment with gancyclovir i.v. is given; also used is trisodium phosphonoformate i.v. These may be given in the hospital setting but increasingly (especially gancyclovir) are given at home. Improvement with treatment is seen but relapse occurs in almost all cases.

CMV retinitis can have a devastating affect on the patient's morale and state of mind. Two of the author's patients decided to stop all treatment once they became blind, whereupon other illness and death followed quite quickly. This demonstrated to the author the vital importance of the patient's will to live when combating HIV-related illness.

Progressive multifocal leukoencephalopathy (PML). This unusual disease is caused by a Papovavirus and results in demyelination. Conditions most likely to be seen are blindness, hemiparesis, ataxia and aphasia (Adler 1991). No treatment is known for this crippling condition (Pratt 1991).

Opportunistic infections: bacterial. The following bacterial infections may be seen in people with AIDS.
(See also Ch. 16.)

Mycobacterium tuberculosis (TB). Tuberculosis is now increasingly seen in patients with HIV and is sometimes associated with poor social conditions. Work in prisons around the world has seen an increase in TB prevalence in some places where there is a high prevalence of HIV. Prisoners with HIV are affected, as are also other vulnerable inmates. Treatment is with rifampicin, ethambutol, isoniazid and pyrazinamide. TB in the general population, when treated, is not generally life threatening. Patients with HIV infected with TB, however, are often made even weaker by the condition.

Salmonellosis. As with other compromised and vulnerable individuals this infection, generally associated with food poisoning, poses a particular danger to people with HIV. Scrupulous care should be taken in food preparation and delivery. Patients should avoid undercooking foods such as eggs and poultry. Hand hygiene is also important. Treatment is with chloramphenicol, ampicillin or amoxycillin.

Mycobacterium avium complex (MAC). People in advanced stages of HIV illness are sometimes found to have atypical mycobacteria in their lungs. The effect of this on prognosis is still unclear although some minor clinical signs are associated with the condition. Treatment is not generally successful. Over the next few years this information may change.

Opportunistic infections: fungal. Candidiasis is sometimes seen in virulent manifestations in people with advanced HIV illness. Infection may extend from the mouth down into the alimentary tract. Vaginal candidiasis may be particularly persistent and distressing. Nystatin pessaries and other conventional treatments are used.

Cryptococcus is one of the systemic fungal conditions sometimes seen. Treatment is with amphotericin and fluconazole. Two others are histoplasmosis, which affects the lungs, liver and gastrointestinal tract, and coccidioidomycosis, which affects any organ, including the brain (Pratt 1991).

Infestation. Strictly speaking, infestation is not *associated* with HIV. However, it should be pointed out that if a patient with HIV happens to become infested with lice or scabies, particularly the variety known as Norwegian scabies, the infection may be particularly virulent, with several thousand times as many mites on the skin as in a patient who is not immunocompromised. Norwegian scabies occasionally strikes hospitals and institutions. Treatment is with gamma benzene hexachloride (Sims & Moss 1991).

Secondary cancers (neoplasms). The immune system has the function not only of fighting infection but also of fighting and inhibiting malignant cells. The following two forms of cancer are associated with HIV and an AIDS diagnosis.

Kaposi's sarcoma (KS). This purplish skin cancer was previously seen only in elderly men of certain races. With the advent of AIDS in the Western world it was one of the first manifestations of the condition. As with the opportunistic infections it is not seen in all patients. As a skin condition it is very disfiguring, particularly on the face. If it remains in small patches treatment is often confined to cosmetic camouflage, which the British Red Cross Society can provide. However, it sometimes forms into constricting bands on the skin (e.g. around the ankle). Internally it may also form gastrointestinal obstructions and it is sometimes found in the lungs and other internal organs. Irradiation treatment is sometimes used in these cases (Adler 1991).

Non-Hodgkin's lymphomas (B cell lymphomas, undifferentiated lymphomas). These cancers are seen in much higher numbers among people with AIDS than in the general population. They are found in the central nervous system, the bone marrow and the gastrointestinal tract. They are often rapidly fatal and treatment is often not successful. Various chemotherapies may be used (see Ch. 11).

Neurological disease; HIV encephalopathy. HIV neurological disease is *not* an opportunistic infection. It is the human immunodeficiency virus *directly* affecting the central nervous system, including the covering of the brain. It may manifest early on as peripheral neuropathy, in its many forms, and later progress to affect the individual's personality and lucidity. Eventually the person may become demented. One of the problems in diagnosing this condition is that changes in computerised tomograms (CT scans) do not necessarily accompany changes in behaviour; it is possible for a patient with a normal CT to be demented.

Nursing care of the various conditions associated with neurological disease and encephalopathy is often challenging. Caring for an active young person who suffers from cerebral dysfunction demands a flexible approach. Remissions can be experienced and there can be periods of despair for the individual. One of the author's patients, who refused to be cared for in hospital (he had spent long periods in prison and was afraid of institutions) was cared for at home. He began to suffer from forgetfulness, personality changes and eventually showed signs of dementia. This was distressing for him, as he often had insight into his condition, and he sometimes wanted to kill himself in these lucid periods.

On a more optimistic note, however, HIV neurological disease does appear to respond well to antiviral therapy. Many patients show a marked improvement as well as a slowing down of the advancement of the disease. The reader is referred to Weir-Hughes (1990) for more information on the neurological impact of AIDS.

ANTIVIRAL TREATMENT

Antiviral treatment of AIDS centres around two medications: azidothymidine (AZT, zidovudine) and dideoxyosine (ddI). **These treatments do not kill HIV**, but interrupt and inhibit the process of virus replication by interfering with the function of reverse transcriptase. Because the virus replication is slowed down the level of healthy helper T cells remains higher, giving the T cells a chance to recover and modestly increase.

When zidovudine first became available it was mainly used on people who were already in advanced stages of illness. Side-effects were considerable, nausea and depletion of red blood cells being the most damaging. Following worldwide double blind placebo controlled trials, it was found that zidovudine was more effective if given to people earlier on, after some drop in helper T cell level had occurred. Side-effects were less and recovery better. This remains the clinical view today. Because zidovudine therapy is now given earlier with encouraging results it has, some would say, strengthened the case for people to come forward, get tested and receive treatment.

Dideoxyosine (ddI) is a more recently developed antiviral agent which works in a similar way. Extensive clinical trials are being undertaken.

One of the main problems with antiviral treatment is that it appears to have limited efficacy over long periods of time. Some patients find a loss of effect after 18 months to 2 years. Side-effects are still seen. The one which may affect the individual most is the loss of red blood cells; some patients require blood transfusions every 5–8 weeks. During the intervening period the patient may need help adapting to the varying levels of energy and lethargy he may experience. Headaches and insomnia are also experienced by some (Adler 1991, AVERT 1992a).

CONCLUSION

Over the past few decades it has become the practice for nurses to become more involved with their patients and to be less aloof. More than ever before, nurses appreciate that they are privileged to be admitted into the trust of their patients. In the HIV field, as in other terminal care, nurses become very deeply involved in their patient's lives and in their experience of dying.

The nursing care of people with HIV has seen an explosion of innovative practice. Work with drug users, prisoners, prostitutes and other marginalised people has meant that nurses are increasingly working in non-traditional areas, using new procedures. Many myths have been shattered, particularly with regard to the amount of sophisticated equipment that was thought necessary to provide care. High-level nursing care is now given in the poorest areas and in the most difficult of circumstances (Thomson 1989, Mackay et al 1990).

Family recognition. People with HIV and AIDS have, like the rest of the population, a variety of domestic arrangements and relationships, and the nurse would do well to take the widest view of the terms 'family' and 'next of kin'. It is distressing to watch courtesy and kindness being shown to the 'official' family and next of kin, who may be estranged, while the patient's life-long partner and the people he chooses to spend every day with are pushed out of the picture. The author has seen this happen to both homosexual and heterosexual patients. In such matters the nurse should take the lead from the patient, not from the admission form.

Spirituality does not always manifest itself as the embracing of a formal religion. When an individual is seriously ill he may 'plug into the infinite' in many ways. One of my patients found solace in a trip to the opera (Atkinson 1989b). Another, who had gone blind, particularly loved sweet-smelling flowers. As an aspiring professional, I used to be rather contemptuous of what I considered sentimental or superstitious behaviour. Experience, however, has taught me greater wisdom and humility.

Grieving and the nurse

Over 40 of the patients I have cared for have now died. The oldest was 70, the youngest 18. I remember them all, and they have enhanced my practice. As I wrote this chapter their memory was close by, their faces very clear in my mind. I remember when each one died, and each time was an emotional experience. There is some debate as to whether it is a good thing to hang onto disturbing memories. My experience is that it is not a question of deliberately hanging on. When one becomes deeply involved in an individual's living and dying, his memory *will* live on. It is the nurse's role to bear witness to those memories *and* to the present experience of each patient alive today. This may be emotional sometimes, but it is not depressing. It is a positive attitude which improves care delivery.

One of my patients had a friend who during their working life together used to phone him in the morning. 'What news from the Rialto today, Bassanio?' he would quip. The two friends would then chat about their news, sometimes separated by the Atlantic, sometimes by a few streets. When my patient died a dedication appeared in a famous magazine. It sums up my feelings for all my patients: 'Farewell Bassanio, you are sadly missed'.

REFERENCES

Adler M (ed) 1991 ABC of AIDS, 2nd edn. British Medical Journal Publications, London

Aggleton P, AVERT 1993 A study of the attitudes of student nurses to HIV/AIDS. AIDS Education and Research Trust, Goldsmith College, London

Akinsanya J A 1991 Who will care: a survey of the knowledge and attitudes of hospital nurses to people with HIV/AIDS. Department of Health, Anglia Polytechnic, HMSO, London

Atkinson J 1989a Which care setting for pentamidine: a limited clinical trial. Nursing Standard/AIDS Focus 3(26): 26–28

Atkinson J 1989b A flexible friend. Community Outlook June: 4–6

Atkinson J 1991 Coping with the guilty ill. Nursing Standard 5(17): 42–43

AVERT 1992a A guide to the medical treatment of HIV related diseases, 2nd edn. AIDS Education and Research Trust, Horsham, West Sussex

AVERT 1992b HIV, AIDS and sex: information for young people. AIDS Education and Research Trust, Horsham, West Sussex

Barker D J P, Rose G 1990 Epidemiology in medical practice, 4th edn. Churchill Livingstone, Edinburgh

Beauchamp T, Perlin S 1978 Ethical issues in death and dying. Prentice-Hall, London

Blood Transfusion Service 1991 Information from leaflets and staff, London

Bond J, Bond S 1986 Sociology and health care. Churchill Livingstone, Edinburgh

Bond S, Rhodes T, Philips P, Setters J, Foy C, Bond J 1988a A national study of HIV infection. AIDS and community nursing staff in England. University of Newcastle, Health Care Resource Unit, Report No. 35

Bond S, Rhodes T, Philips P, Setters J, Foy C, Bond J 1988b A national study of HIV infection. AIDS and community nursing staff in Scotland. University of Newcastle, Health Care Resource Unit, Report No. 37

Boss M 1979 Existential foundations of medicine and psychology. Jason Aronson, New York

Caplan G 1961 An approach to community mental health. Tavistock, London

CDC 1987 A report by Council of State and Territorial Epidemiologists; AIDS Program, Centre for Infectious Diseases. Morbidity and Mortality Weekly Report Supplement 36 1S

Comptroller and Auditor General 1991 HIV and AIDS Related Health Services. (October) National Audit Office, London

Connor S, Kingman S 1989 The search for the virus. Penguin, Harmondsworth

Department of Health 1991 Information from staff, HMSO, London

Department of Health 1992 Quarterly AIDS Press Release (29 January) HMSO, London

Department of Health AIDS Unit 1992 Meeting of the regional nurses for HIV/AIDS. Unpublished. London

Downie R, Telfer E 1980 Caring and Curing. Methuen, London

ENB 1989 Meeting the challenge: a learning package. English National Board Publications, Sheffield

Ewles L, Simnett I 1992 Promoting health: a practical guide to health education, 2nd edn. Wiley, Chichester

Flaskerud J H, Ungvarski P J (eds) 1992 HIV/AIDS: a guide to nursing care, 2nd edn. Saunders, Pennsylvania

Fletcher W 1992a Hit and miss of mass marketing. The Guardian, Media Section (23 March): 29

Fletcher W 1992b A glittering haze. NTC Publications, London

George J 1985 Nursing theories: the base for professional practice, 2nd edn. Prentice Hall, London

Green J, McCreaner A 1989 Counselling in HIV infection and AIDS. Blackwell Scientific, London

Haemophilia Unit, Glasgow Royal Infirmary 1990 Information from staff, Glasgow

Hansard 1986 *Parliamentary Report on the Debate on HIV and AIDS.* House of Commons. November. London

HEA 1991 Information on the continuing mass media campaign. Health Education Authority, London

Kubler Ross E 1987 AIDS: the ultimate challenge. Macmillan, New York

MacCallum A 1991 Nutrition and the patient with HIV. Report on Research Project for MSc, Royal Free Hospital/Department of Nursing, King's College, Waterloo. Presented at Royal College of Nursing, AIDS Nursing Forum Conference, September

Mackay E, Robertson G, Atkinson J 1990 Own home, own bed, own life: terminal care of AIDS at home in a deprived area. Nursing Standard/Primary Health Care 4(43): 48–49

Miller R, Bor R 1988 AIDS: a guide to clinical counselling. Science Press, London

Murphy K, Atkinson J 1990 Nutritional support for the HIV positive patient: a practical approach. Nursing Standard 5(4): 54–56

Mok J 1988 HIV infection in infants and children. Medicine International 57: 2360–2363

Mok J 1991 Interview with author at the City Hospital, Edinburgh

Neal A 1989 Ring a ring o'roses. Nursing Times. 85(5): 49–50

Newbury J 1988a *Caring for the HIV positive patient in the community.* Paper presented to Professor C A Butterworth's Inaugural Conference. Monograph No. 1, 18 May, University of Manchester

Newbury J 1988b AIDS in the community. Community Outlook (November): 4–6

PHLS 1991 Proforma and guidance for the National Anonymous Survey of the Seroprevalence of HIV. Public Health Laboratory Service, London

Pratt R 1991 AIDS: a strategy for nursing care, 3rd edn. Edward Arnold, London

Pyne R 1990 Interview with Mr Pyne, Assistant Registrar, UKCC. September. London

RCN Conference 1989 AIDS Nursing Forum National Conference. Debate and discussion on the role, successes and failures of the continuing AIDS Health Education Campaign run by the Health Education Authority. Charing Cross Hospital, London.

RCN Congress 1991 Emergency Debate tabled by the Royal College of Nursing AIDS Nursing Forum on the practice of publishing results of local HIV prevalence screening. Harrogate

RCN Daphne Heald Research Unit/AVERT 1993 Research project examining clinical nursing practice in HIV care. Royal College of Nursing, London

Robertson M 1991 Group work by generic health visitors: HIV prevention and health promotion with young people, drug users, women, open days, needle exchange clinics. Report to Dr Laurence Gruer, AIDS Coordinator, Greater Glasgow Health Board. Possilpark Health Centre, Glasgow

Roy C 1989 The Roy adaption model. In: Reihl-Sisca J (ed) Conceptual models for nursing practice, 3rd edn. Appleton & Lange, Norwalk

Ruchill Hospital 1989 Collation of patient admissions and outpatients' visits, Glasgow
Sims R, Moss V 1991 Terminal care for people with AIDS. Edward Arnold, London
SOHHD and GGHB 1992 Information from Nursing Services Scottish Office Home and Health Department and Community Primary Care Unit Greater Glasgow Health Board
Stevenson S 1989 Administering pentamidine. Nursing Times 85(39): 30–32
Task Force on Nutrition Support in AIDS 1989 Guidelines for nutrition support. Nutrition (USA) 5(1): 39–45. Offprints available from: Task Force on Nutrition Support in AIDS c/o Wang Associates, 19 West 21st Street, New York, NY 10010
Thomson A 1989 Crisis on the streets. Community Outlook (January): 8
UKCC 1989 Anonymous testing for the prevalence of the human immunodeficiency virus. Circular PC/89/01. United Kingdom Central Council for Nurses, Midwives and Health Visitors, London
UKCC 1990 Anonymous testing for HIV. Register Journal of the United Kingdom Central Council for Nurses, Midwives and Health Visitors, London
UKCC 1992 Code of professional conduct for the nurse, midwife and health visitor. United Kingdom Central Council for Nurses, Midwives and Health Visitors, London
Weller B 1989 Children and HIV infection. Nursing Standard/AIDS Focus. 4(3): 50–52
Weller B 1990 HIV roundup. Nursing Standard/AIDS Focus 5(4): 50
Wells R, Nygaard M, Farrell M 1989 Spotlight on AIDS. Nursing Standard 4(7): 20–22
WHO 1989 Guidelines on Sexually Transmitted Diseases and AIDS for Family Planning Programmes. World Health Organization, Copenhagen
Youle M, Clarbour J, Wade P, Farthing C 1988 AIDS: therapeutics in HIV disease. Churchill Livingstone, Edinburgh

FURTHER READING

Abrams D 1992 Who's afraid of AIDS? SPA Journal (Spring): 43–46
AVERT 1991a Taking control of your diet if you are HIV positive. AIDS Education and Research Trust, Horsham, West Sussex
AVERT 1991b AIDS and childbirth. AIDS Education and Research Trust, Horsham, West Sussex
Burnard P 1989 Counselling skills for health professionals. Chapman & Hall, London
Dimond B 1990 AIDS and the law. Nursing Standard 4(7): 20–22
Expert Advisory Group on AIDS 1990 Guidance for clinical care workers: protection against infection with HIV and hepatitis viruses. HMSO, London
Gray J 1989 A testing dilemma. Nursing Standard 4(4): 20
Jones C 1990 All you ever wanted to know about counselling. Nursing Times 86(12): 55–58
Karpf A 1988 Doctoring the media: the reporting of health and medicine. Routledge, London
Loney M, Boswell D, Clarke J (eds) 1988 Social policy and social welfare. Open University Press, Milton Keynes
RCN AIDS Working Party 1986 Nursing guidelines on the management of patients in hospital and the community suffering from AIDS. Royal College of Nursing, London
Tatchell P 1990 AIDS: a guide to survival, 3rd edn. GMP Publications, London
Sontag S 1988 AIDS and its metaphors. Penguin, London
UKCC 1989 Statement on AIDS and HIV infection. Circular PC/89/02. United Kingdom Central Council for Nurses, Midwives and Health Visitors, London
Weir-Hughes D 1990 The neurological effects of AIDS. Nursing Standard/AIDS Focus 5(4): 51–53

USEFUL ADDRESSES & TELEPHONE HELPLINE

AVERT
AIDS Education and Research Trust
11 Denn Parade, Horsham
West Sussex RH12 1JD

Haemophilia Society
123 Westminster Bridge Road
London
SE1 7HR

National AIDS Helpline (24 hr)
Tel. 0800 567 123

Royal College of Nursing AIDS Nursing Forum
20 Cavendish Square
London
W1M OAB

Terence Higgins Trust
52/54 Gray's Inn Road
London
WC1X 8LT

Answers

CHAPTER 8

8.15 The following arrangements and interventions can make life easier for patients on dialysis.

- Transport can be arranged by the hospital, if necessary.
- Little can be done to avoid the 2 or 3 sessions a week away from home, but by involving the social worker it may be possible to assess and solve some home problems.
- Try and work out the times that will best fit in with the patient's job. Try also to provide a quiet environment that will allow him to rest and sleep.
- Discuss with the patient his fluid intake and come to some compromise that will prevent overload of fluid.
- Seek help from the dietitian. Involve the family in discussions about menus and permitted food.
- The social worker may be able to help with financial problems by informing the patient of help and benefits available, and also assisting in any form-filling requirements.
- The patient should have regular access to medical staff to address problems and assess medication.
- Give psychological help by listening to the patient's expressions of fears and hopes. Above all, always leave the patient with hope.
- Counselling the family as well as the patient will help keep stress to a minimum.

Patients can often gain a lot of support from other patients who are in a similar situation. They compare experiences and discuss their various problems and hopes between themselves. Do consider trying to treat patients who get on well together on the same shift.

CHAPTER 11

11.1 Liver, spinach, cauliflower, cabbage, peas.

11.2 In the small intestine, by commensal organisms.

11.3 Patients with:

- liver disease, because of reduced formation of clotting factors
- obstructive jaundice, because of reduced absorption due to lack of bile salts
- chronic diarrhoea.

11.4 a. Any healthy person aged 18–64 years.

b.
- complete health questionnaire to exclude any person who might transmit an infection. This includes having or contact with syphilis, malaria, other tropical diseases, HIV, AIDS, hepatitis (type A, B or C), infectious diseases and skin infections. Other categories excluded are a person who has had tooth extractions or oral surgery within 72 hours or been immunised with live attenuated vaccines (variable time limit).

  Other questions relate to the presence in donor's blood of antigens (e.g. allergies or asthma), or whether the patient has cancer, or the taking of any drugs.

  Other questions are to ensure the donor's health, e.g. recent donations, pregnancy and time of last meal.
- Health check including height, weight, temperature, pulse, blood pressure & haemoglobin level.

c. Important points include maintaining asepsis, the speed with which the unit of blood is withdrawn (1 pt over 15 min), the total amount each donation (1 pt), labelling of unit with donor's name, blood group and rhesus factor immediately it is withdrawn and each unit screened for hepatitis and HIV.

d. Care of donor includes explanation of the procedure, the donation being taken while donor is recumbent. After care includes the maintaining of recumbent position until donor is able to sit up and get up without feeling dizzy or faint, the recommendation to have a cup of tea and food and to wait another 15 minutes before leaving the centre, refraining from smoking (for 1 hr), drinking alcohol (3 hr), to increase fluid intake for 2 days and take a balanced diet for 2 weeks.

e. 4°C for 35 days.

11.6 a. Blood transfusion will increase blood volume and therefore stroke volume.

b. There may be a degree of cardiac failure because of lack of oxygen carrying capacity to the tissues, with a resultant increase in heart rate to compensate. For this the heart will also require adequate oxygen and if this is lacking it will fail.

11.7 a. Potential problems:

- compliance with taking medication
- balanced diet with adequate iron
- financial problems
- depression or loneliness
- inability to buy or cook

b. ways to resolve problems

- patient education about medication
- advice from the dietitian and nurses about balanced diet. Use menu choice card as a teaching aid.
- advice from the social worker about social services benefits and on budgeting.

- arrange attendance at day hospital or lunch club, or other social activity that appeals and is available in patient's area.
- assessment of necessary skills in OT department and home visit for possible adaptations, e.g. to gas taps or plugs.
- someone to shop for him.

c. community services: health visitor, social services for home help, meals on wheels, lunch clubs, outings, attendance at day hospital, OT, physiotherapy, possible rehousing or sheltered housing, contact with self-help group for bereavement e.g. Cruse, contract with local church.

11.8 The implications of this ongoing therapy might include:
- a need to understand the rationale for the treatment
- recurring anxiety about health and about the injections themselves
- disruption to social life. Where are the injections administered: GP surgery? health clinic? patient's home? Is transport available? Are there cost implications?
- a need to consider safety implications. How are needles and syringes stored and disposed of? Are there children in the home?

11.9 Green, leafy vegetables, liver, white fish, yeast extract (e.g. Marmite), fortified cornflakes.

11.10 By not overcooking foods.

11.13 a. Her fears and anxieties might relate to
- losing the protection of a sheltered environment and immediate access to specialist nursing and medical advice
- her perceived inability to cope at home.
- her future, e.g. her wedding, marriage and the possibility of having children
- the diagnosis, treatment and prognosis
- the prospect of meeting strangers, or friends who have not seen her since her admission.

b. By giving her advice about: wigs, turbans, hats or scarves to cover hair loss; make-up to disguise loss of eyebrows; jewellery and other fashionable accessories to distract attention from the alopecia.

c. Community support available could include: GP; clinical nurse specialist (if available); health visitor; self-help groups (e.g. Leukaemia Care Society, BACUP, Cancer Link); social worker; district nurse (if Hickman line catheter is in situ and the patient is unable to dress the exit site and heparinise the line herself); religious groups; DSS and/or Citizens' Advice Bureau.

d. How to take her own temperature and, if it is raised, whom to contact; general advice on reducing the possibility of infections, e.g. avoiding crowded places; ongoing mouth care and personal hygiene; care of Hickman line; details about medication; dietary advice; return to normal activity and work; advice about going away on holiday.

CHAPTER 18

18.6 a. Tachycardia is produced by an increase in sympathetic activity due to stressors such as fright, anxiety and pain. In the event of hypovolaemia the heart is required to work much more quickly to maintain the same cardiac output. Infection is usually associated with a pyrexia and an increase in the metabolic demands of the body, and hence with a faster heart rate. Arrhythmias are frequently observed following a myocardial infarction and in the patient with cardiogenic shock.

b. An increase of parasympathetic nervous activity produces a bradycardia. This finding is also associated with excessive vagal stimulation in the patient with spinal shock or myocardial infarction. A myocardial infarction may also cause an interruption in the heart's conducting mechanism and precipitate heart block and bradycardia. The traumatised and head-injured patient in shock frequently will have cerebral oedema, raised intracranial pressure and a reduced heart rate.

18.7 A low PAWP would indicate that the patient is depleted of fluid and needs rapid fluid replacement.

18.8 A high PAWP would indicate left ventricular failure, which if not corrected might lead to pulmonary oedema.

CHAPTER 24

24.13 a. Four situations in which catheterisation would be justified are:
- during operations on the lower abdomen
- for precise measurement of urinary output
- where the bladder fails to empty as in acute and chronic retention
- in case of intractable incontinence.

It may also be used for irrigation purposes, cytotoxic therapy and urodynamic investigations.

b. A Foley catheter is an indwelling flexible tube, retained in the bladder by a balloon, for the purpose of continuous drainage.

c. To aid haemostasis following prostatectomy.

d. For all catheterisation except that following prostatectomy, or where debris is a problem to drainage.

e. Four other features which should be considered are:
- catheter material
- tips
- eyes
- balloon size.

Also: shaft size and length.

f. PVC and plastic for in-and-out intermittent catheters and silicone, latex, Teflon and silicone elastomer or Hydrogel materials for indwelling catheters.

g. This type of catheter is called a Roberts catheter. It allows complete drainage of the bladder. It is not now available on prescription but may be available through the hospital service.

h. No: only sterile water can be used. Air would make the balloon float. Other substances may cause the introduction of crystals or debris into the inflation channel and block it. Some degree of osmosis occurs between the balloon and the bladder and harmful substances such as chlorhexidine are therefore not suitable. Prefilled balloons are available.

i. 10 ml. If only 5 ml are used then only the shaft would be filled; the balloon requires a further 5 ml.

j. Keep them on a shelf in strict date order in the boxes and packaging provided. Avoid sunlight and direct heat. Do not use rubber bands on the catheter or store in drawers. Avoid all contact with oil and spirit products such as petroleum jelly and paraffin based items.

24.14

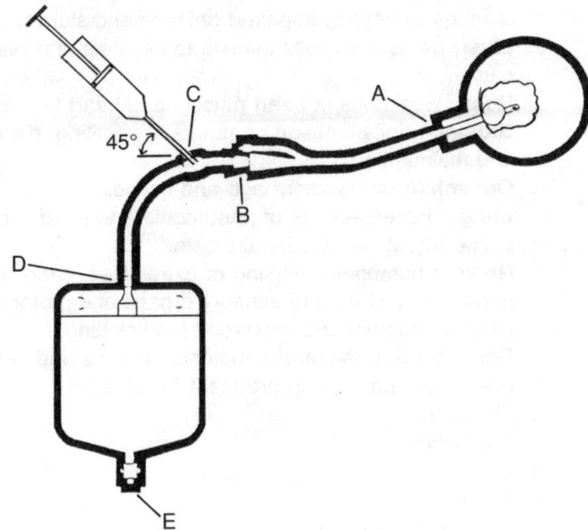

Fig. 24.7 Potential entry points for infection.

Key to diagram:
A — urethral meatus and around catheter
B — junction between catheter and connection tube
C — sample port
D — connection to drainage bag and reflux from bag to tubing
E — drainage outlet.

Procedures to prevent infection:

A. Water should be used for washing the area of the vulva or penis and may be more suitable than antiseptics (Bard 1984). Female-length catheters should be used for women to avoid the 'piston' effect.
B. Catheters should not be disconnected, expect when the bag is being changed. Add-on bags should be attached to leg bags for extra drainage through the night.
C. Samples of urine should be taken only by using the special sleeve on the urine bag tubing, which may be clamped or folded back to allow urine to collect.
D. Urine bags should always be kept at a level below the bladder, and tubing should be occluded by being folded or clamped, if movement across the bed is required.
E. Each time the bags are emptied this should be viewed as a separate procedure for each individual; multipurpose jugs and containers should never be used. Hands should be washed before and after emptying and the bag should be kept on its stand with the tap clear of the floor. Care should be taken when emptying leg bags that the tap does not come in contact with the toilet. The tap should be dried or wiped with an alcohol swab after emptying.

For further details of the care of catheters, the Bard pamphlets (1984, 1987) should be consulted.

CHAPTER 25

25.4 **Possible reasons**

- Postoperative pain:
  - at site of operation
  - backache
- Noise at night:
  - telephone
  - bedpan macerator
  - noisy shoes (nurses and doctors)
  - nurses giggling
  - IVI pump alarms
  - other patients snoring/crying out
  - ambulances driving past
- Uncomfortable beds:
  - hard mattresses
  - plastic covers on mattresses and pillows

Nursing interventions

- No unnecessary pain should be endured. Ensure that Mr B receives regular and careful assessment of pain, provision of analgesics and other comfort measures (positioning, support with pillows, etc) and monitor the effect of these interventions.
- Positive efforts should be made to keep noise to a minimum during the night. Telephones should be kept off the main ward where possible. Used papier maché bedpans should be rinsed and left until the next morning to be macerated. All ward staff should wear quiet shoes. Nurses should try to keep as quiet as possible while in the main ward. IVI pump alarms should be turned down (not off) where this is an option. Patients who snore should be positioned so that they are not on their backs (if appropriate to their care). Noisy patients and noise from outside the ward are more difficult to deal with. Mr B may find wax or silicone earplugs helpful, though not everyone finds these comfortable enough to use during sleep.
- The uncomfortable and unfamiliar beds found in hospital wards may take some adjusting to. A plastic drawsheet should not be left on Mr B's bed unless its presence is really necessary. Mr B is on an adjustable-height bed which should be left low during the night, so that he can get out with a minimum of assistance.

Expected outcomes

- Mr B's pain is well controlled throughout the night.
- The ward is as quiet as possible during the night.
- Mr B is as comfortable as possible in bed.
- Mr B is satisfied with his sleep.

CHAPTER 32

32.2 a. False. Some forms of cancer, such as testicular teratoma and Hodgkin's disease, are now curable. Many people with cancer are elderly and die from other causes.
b. False. Deaths due to cardiovascular disease are 3 times more prevalent than deaths due to cancer.
c. Partly true. The causes of cancer are not fully known. Epidemiological studies indicate that cancer may be a disease of lifestyle in the broadest sense. Social and environmental factors are as important as individual behaviour.
d. Partly true. Some forms of cancer, particularly those of childhood, are hereditary. A small number of other cancers have a high incidence in certain families. Daughters or sisters of women with breast cancer are 3 times more likely to develop the disease than are others.
e. False. There is no evidence to substantiate this claim. However, personality may affect the way a person copes with cancer, and may even have an influence on prognosis (Greer et al 1979).
f. False. Cancer cannot be 'caught'.
g. False. Many forms of cancer cause little or no change in physical appearance. Modern surgical techniques tend to be far more conservative and to achieve better cosmetic results than those used in the past.
h. True. For example, 96.8% of patients with skin cancer are

alive 5 years after diagnosis. In the case of breast cancer, 62% are still alive after 5 years (Cancer Research Campaign 1988).

i. False. Cancer cells are not alien or foreign to the body but derive from malignant changes in normal cells.

j. False. The side-effects of intensive radiotherapy and chemotherapy may be severe, but the manifestation of side-effects varies greatly between individuals. Some treatments, such as tamoxifen therapy for breast cancer, have little or no side-effects.

k. False. Approximately 60% of cancer patients develop pain. This is generally not until the later stages and is usually controllable (see Ch. 34 'The Terminally Ill Patient').

CHAPTER 37

37.5 a. (i) 5 glasses, (ii) 5 single measures, (iii) 2½ pints, (iv) 2½ pints.

b. **Brain:** aggression, irrational behaviour, arguments, violence, depression, nervousness, chronic anxiety, unknown fears, hallucination, serious mental health problems, epilepsy, dementia, memory loss, black-outs, damage to nerves, impaired balance and slurred speech.
Liver: damage to cells leading to cirrhosis and liver cancer.
Heart: weakness of heart muscle and heart failure.
Stomach: inflammation of stomach, vomiting, diarrhoea and malnutrition.
Oesophagus: haemorrhage and cancer.
Lungs: increased risk of pneumonia and tuberculosis.
Large intestine: duodenal ulcers.
Nerves: numbness, tingling of extremities, peripheral neuritis, impairment of sensory organs and motor control.
Blood: anaemia and impaired blood clotting.
Reproductive system: impotence in male and increased risk of fetal damage in pregnant females.

c. The liver.

d. 2–3 hours.

e. None.

f. (i) and (ii).

g. It is lower in women.

h. Lower body weight, lower tolerance level and the tendency to add carbonised mixers to alcohol.

i. An empty stomach, low body weight, adding carbonised drinks to alcoholic drinks, alternating carbonised and alcoholic drinks, drinking rapidly and low tolerance.

Appendices

APPENDIX 1
Tests and investigations 1017

APPENDIX 2
Normal values 1023

APPENDIX 1

Tests and investigations

The following tests and investigations should be seen as terms defined rather than processes described and are used to supplement and clarify reference made to them in the text.

Angiography
This involves the injection of contrast medium to outline blood vessels. The contrast is injected and rapid serial X-ray films are taken. The presence and location of aneurysms and other blood vessel anomalies such as stenosis are demonstrated. Angiography is not without risk and its performance may be delayed in the patient who is in a poor clinical condition.

Arteriography
A radio-opaque dye is injected into an artery and a series of X-rays taken to show the path of the dye in the arteries and pinpoint any obstruction to blood flow.

Arthroscopy
The direct examination of a joint by the surgical insertion of an arthroscope. The procedure can be performed on an out-patient basis and is used in the diagnosis of injuries. Although it is most commonly used for the knee joint, arthroscopic techniques can also be used for the hip, shoulder, wrist and ankle.

Barium studies
When plain radiography is inadequate to study an area of interest, contrast media can be used. Barium sulphate is an aqueous suspension, non irritant and radiodense. Administered orally or rectally, it allows the gastro-intestinal tract to stand out when viewed through a fluoroscope or on a radiograph. Barium studies of the gastro-intestinal tract can be used to visualise the tract and aid in the diagnosis of disorders such as peptic ulceration, malignant tumours, diverticulitis and colitis.

Blood count
Calculation of the number of red blood cells, white blood cells and platelets in a litre of blood. A differential blood count is the estimation of the relative proportion of the different white blood cells in the blood.

Blood film
Microscopic examination of the cellular components of the blood (that is, red and white blood cells and platelets).

Red cells

Size:
- microcytic — smaller than normal
- normocytic — normal size
- macrocytic — larger than normal
- anisocytic — inequality in size

Shape
- poikilocytic — marked irregularity in shape

Colour
- hypochromic — red cells contain less haemoglobin than normal, resulting in a pale colour
- normochromic — normal amount of haemoglobin in red blood cells and therefore normal colour

White cells

Size. Usually 10–15 micrometre in diameter.

Structure
- staining characteristics of granules are different for neutrophils, eosinophils and basophils
- excessive nuclear lobulation in neutrophils (indication of megaloblastic anaemia, iron deficiency, renal failure)

Cell differentiation between different granulocytes, lymphocytes and monocytes can be performed and commented on in the blood film report.

Platelets

Size. 2–4 micrometre in diameter.

Structure

Smaller or larger than average occur in certain haematological conditions, e.g. large platelets occur in thrombocytopenia due to platelet loss or destruction or post-splenectomy.

Cardiotocography

The simultaneous monitoring of the fetal heart rate and maternal uterine contractions as a means of monitoring fetal well-being.

Cholecystography

Radiological examination of the gallbladder using a radio-opaque contrast medium taken orally. A normal liver will normally remove the radio-opaque drugs from the blood stream and store and concentrate them in the gallbladder. Radiographs taken will show the dye-filled gallbladder as a dense shadow. Gallstones may be seen as filling defects. This technique will not outline the gallbladder when the serum bilirubin concentration is elevated (>34 μmols per litre), as insufficient contrast medium is excreted. Although oral cystography is a reliable means of detecting gallstones in non-jaundiced patients, it has been largely superseded by ultrasonography.

Computerised (axial) tomography (C(A)T scan)

The patient lies on a couch and the head is placed in an opening in the front of the scanner. A series of X-rays are beamed through the patient's head in trans-axial slices of various sizes and, depending upon the density of the tissue, are either transmitted or absorbed. Those that are transmitted are detected by a battery of sensitive crystals and this information is then fed to a computer, which creates an image of the scanned structures, e.g. brain tissue. Once one 'sweep' is complete, the machine moves through 1° until an 180° arc has been completed. CAT scanning may reveal alterations in tissue density, displacement of structures and abnormalities. Certain types of lesions are better demonstrated with the use of contrast enhancement; this involves the injection of an intravenous contrast and then scanning the patient as already described.

Coombs test

Test to detect antibodies to red blood cells.

Direct Coombs test detects those bound to the red blood cells.

Indirect Coombs test detects those not bound to the red blood cells but circulating in the serum.

Countercurrent immunoelectrophoresis (CCIE). A laboratory method for the detection of specific antibodies or antigens.

Culture (bacterial)

The specimen material is smeared onto a culture medium plate (containing nutrients and moisture), then incubated at 37°C to allow any bacteria present to grow and multiply. After 18–24 hours the culture plate is examined and bacteria can be identified.

Cystography/Cysto-urography

Via urinary catheter, the bladder is filled to capacity with a contrast medium and the bladder X-rayed. By so doing, bladder abnormalities may be revealed. The catheter is then removed to observe the function of the bladder and upper urethra during micturition — a cysto-urogram.

Cystometry

This investigation measures changes in the pressure in the bladder. A urinary catheter is inserted and the bladder drained. Water at body temperature is then introduced into the bladder at a slow and constant rate and, in response to the increasing volume, the bladder pressure is recorded using a pressure measuring device, a cystometrogram.

Cytology

Cytology is the study of the structure and function of cells, both normal and abnormal. Body cells may be collected by a variety of methods, e.g. from a specimen of urine or sputum, scraped from a skin lesion or from the cervix during a Papanicolau smear test, or from aspirate of a lump or the bone marrow. The cells are then examined microscopically for abnormalities.

Echocardiography

A non-invasive technique which uses pulses of high frequency sounds (ultrasound) emitted from a transducer to evaluate cardiac anatomy, pathology and function. The procedure involves an operator applying a lubricant to the skin surface of the chest wall and moving the transducer or probe back and forth by hand across the surface.

Electroencephalography (EEG)

A graphic recording of the electrical activity of the brain. Electrodes are attached to the scalp and the electrical activity is noted with a sensitive recorder. Some patients who are prone to seizures will demonstrate an abnormal waveform even while seizure-free.

Enzyme-linked immunosorbent assay (ELISA)

A laboratory method for the detection of specific antibodies or antigens.

Erythrocyte sedimentation rate (ESR)

Measurement of the height of red blood cells at the foot of a column of blood after the blood has been left standing in the narrow tube for 1 hour. (Normal value = <10 mm)

Evoked responses

In this test one of the sensory systems is artificially stimulated and the response noted with the use of appropriately placed electrodes, which detect disturbances of conduction. Visual evoked responses involve stimulating the patient by getting him to look at a reversing checkboard pattern or flashing lights. Electrodes placed on the scalp over the occipital lobes will detect if there is any delay in conduction along the optic pathway as may occur in the patient with multiple sclerosis.

Gonioscopy
Gonioscopy is performed to assess the angle of the eye, between the cornea and iris. A narrowed angle is indicative of closed-angled glaucoma.

The eye is anaesthetised with short-acting eye drops. A contact lens in which an angled mirror has been incorporated (gonioscope) is lubricated with methylcellulose eye drops and applied to the cornea. The eye is then examined through a slit lamp.

Haemoglobin estimation
Estimation of the amount of haemoglobin present in 100 ml of blood. (Normal values: men 14–18 g/100 ml; women 12–16 g/100 ml).

Haemostasis (clotting) tests

Kaolin cephalin clotting time (KCTT) or partial thromboplastin time (PTT): a coagulation test of the intrinsic clotting pathway. Kaolin is added to plasma and activation of Factors XI and XII. Cephalin reagent is added and the mixture recalcifies at 37°C. The clotting time depends on the presence of the components of the intrinsic pathway. Abnormalities in the test result from deficiencies of intrinsic pathway factors and final pathway factors. (Normal result: 40 seconds.)

Prothrombin clotting time (PCT). Tests the extrinsic pathway of blood coagulation. The test requires the presence of functional quantities of Factor VII and Vitamin K dependent facts 10. Result expressed as ratio of patient : control. (Normal result: clot forms in 13 seconds; normal result: 1.0–1.3.)

Thrombin clotting time (TT) tests the final reaction in the final pathway, i.e. fibrinogen converted to fibrin. (Normal value: about 10 seconds.)

Bleeding time. Time taken to stop bleeding after making a standardised superficial skin incision, e.g. with lancet. (Normal value: up to 9 minutes.)

Immunocoagglutination
A laboratory method for the detection of specific antibodies or antigens.

Immunodiffusion
A laboratory method for the detection of specific antibodies or antigens.

Immunoelectrophoresis
A laboratory method for the detection of specific antibodies or antigens.

Intravenous cholangiography
Contrast medium, given intravenously, is excreted into the biliary system. Serial radiographs are taken. However, this technique is less commonly used as results are often of poor quality, of no value in jaundiced patients and also carry a small but significant risk of an anaphylactic reaction to the contrast medium. As a result, methods that allow direct injection of the contrast into the biliary tree are preferred, for example, percutaneous transhepatic cholangiography (PTC), endoscopic retrograde cholangio-pancreatography (ERCP), operative cholangiography and T-tube cholangiography.

Intravenous fluorescein angiography
This technique is used as an aid in the diagnosis and treatment of many of the vascular disorders of the retina.

A 5 ml i.v. injection of 10% fluorescein sodium is given into an arm. A series of photographs are taken through a dilated pupil at timed intervals, using a fundal camera. Any defect in the retinal vessels will show up as a leakage of dye or occlusion of the vessel.

The patient may feel nauseated after the procedure. He should be informed that his sclera and skin will take on a yellow colour for about 24 h and that his urine will be greenish for 24–48 h as the dye is excreted through the kidneys.

Diabetic patients who carry out urine testing should be advised to test their blood sugar instead, as the dye can affect the results obtained by urine test strips.

Lymphangiogram
An X-ray of the lymphatic channels and lymph nodes, often used to diagnose lymphatic cancers or metastases. An oily radio-opaque medium is injected into a small lymph channel in the patient's foot. As this medium travels slowly upwards through the body, X-rays are taken at various stages. This involves the patient waiting in the X-ray department for several hours one day, and returning the following day. The small incision in the foot is sutured. The medium may cause temporary blue discolouration of the urine, and of the skin over the incision.

Lumbar puncture
This is the most common neurological investigation. It involves the insertion of a sterile needle and trocar between lumbar vertebrae 3 and 4, or 4 and 5, and the withdrawal of a quantity of CSF for analysis. The procedure is usually performed in the ward under local anaesthetic. The lumbar CSF pressure may also be measured prior to the removal of CSF. The normal constituents and their values of CSF may be altered in the presence of a disorder, e.g. the number of red blood cells in the CSF following subarachnoid haemorrhage will be markedly elevated.

Magnetic resonance imaging (MRI)
This investigation is based on the use of a magnetic field and radio pulse waves, instead of traditional irradiation. The patient lies on a couch and is then completely enclosed in a tunnel within the scanner. A strong magnetic field is applied and the nuclei within the tissues, which were previously spinning in a random fashion, line up in a north–south magnetic field orientation. A radio pulse wave is introduced at a right angle to the magnetic field and the nuclei are tipped out of alignment, causing uniform resonance. The pulse waves are stopped and the resonating nuclei will return to their previous state. Minute radiofrequency signals are given off as the nuclei enter this relaxed state and these are monitored by the scanner. By pre-programming the computer to simulate a non-uniform magnetic field, the positively charged particles in different parts of the the magnetic field will resonate at different speeds. Variable radio pulse waves result in differences in the emission of radio frequency data. The computer assimilates this data and constructs a tissue image.

This type of scanning has a particular use in detecting cerebral and spinal oedema, and cerebral and spinal blood-flow related disorders, such as infarction, haemorrhage and arteriovenous malformation.

Mean corpuscular haemoglobin concentrate (MCHC)
Is the average concentration of haemoglobin in a red blood cell.

$$\text{Calculation is } \frac{\text{Haemoglobin level}}{\text{PCV (see below)}}$$

(Normal range: 30–35 g/100 ml.)

Mean corpuscular or cell volume (MCV)
The average red cell volume. (Normal: 85 fl (75–95 fl.)

Microscopy
Direct visualisation of microorganisms using a light microscope or an electron microscope (uses a beam of electrons rather than light rays).

Myelography
This involves the injection of a water-soluble contrast into the subarachnoid space, usually via lumbar puncture. Cervical myelogram would require a cervical puncture. The patient is placed on a tilting table to encourage the contrast to flow up and down, thus highlighting the spinal cord and roots. X-ray pictures can then be taken at appropriate levels to detect blockage of, or interruption to, the flow of contrast, indicative of intraspinal pathology.

Magnetic resonance imaging of the spinal cord (magnetic myelography) has recently evolved and now provides greater detail of spinal pathology at less risk to the patient. Spinal CT scan may also be of some benefit.

Orthopantomogram (OPT)
Panoramic radiograph giving consistent image quality, usually of mandible or maxilla, for suspected neoplasia. Also in maxillofacial surgery for middle third fracture.

Packed cell volume (PCV) or Haematocrit
This list measures the relative red cell mass to plasma, i.e. the proportion of the blood sample composed of packed red blood cells to plasma. (Normal values; men 0.47; women 0.42.)

Paul–Bunnell (monospot) test
A method of determining the diagnosis of infectious mononucleosus (glandular fever), which may result from the Epstein-Barr virus (EBV). During the second week of the infection, specific EBV IgM antibodies indicate recent infection by the virus.

Precipitin test
A laboratory method for the detection of specific antibodies or antigens.

Radioisotope scanning
Radioisotope scans involve the use of small amounts of various radioactive substances, which are differentially taken up by normal and abnormal, or malignant, tissue. The most common radioisotope scans are those of the liver, brain and bones. The radioiostope is injected intravenously, and the scan occurs several hours later. The patient should be reassured that the radioactivity of their bodies during this waiting time is minimal and that they are not a danger to others.

Radio-allergosorbent test (RAST)
A laboratory method for the detection of specific antibodies or antigens.

Red cell mass
Estimation of the total volume of circulating red cells performed by labelling a sample of the patients own red blood cells with isotope ^{51}Cr or ^{99m}TC. A measured amount is re-injected and a sample is taken after specific period of time when the dilutation can be calculated. (Normal value: men 25–35 ml/kg; women 20–30 ml/kg.)

Radio-immunoassay (RIA)
A laboratory method for the detection of specific antibodies or antigens.

Renography
This is a radiological study to assess renal function. Some elements that the kidneys normally concentrate and excrete can be labelled with radioactive isotopes. These are administered intravenously and, by so doing, the function of the kidneys can be traced by recording the rate at which the isotopes are removed from the blood and passed into the urinary collecting system.

Reticulocyte count
The number of reticulocytes in the peripheral blood. (Normal range: 0.2–2.0% of RBC (red blood cells.))

Schilling test
Estimation of the gastrointestinal absorption of radioactive Vitamin B_{12} (Normal range >10% of administered oral dose in 24-hour urine sample.)

Sensitivity
A test used to determine which antibiotics will kill the bacteria in the specimen. It is done by placing antibiotic-impregnated discs over a film of cultured bacteria on a culture plate, and then reading the plate some hours later. A zone of inhibition around the disc indicates that the organism is sensitive to that antibiotic. If an organism is resistant, there will be growth right up to the disc.

Serology
The examination of blood serum, often to ascertain if infection is present by identifying antigen/antibody.

Sialogram
Radiograph following injection of contrast medium into salivary duct and gland.

Skeletal survey X-rays
A skeletal survey involves X-rays of the skull, spine, ribs, pelvis and the femoral and humeral heads. Primary bone tumours and bone metastases from other tumours may be detected in this way.

T-cell immunopheno typing (CD4 T-ceil subsets)
This procedure, used particularly for patients with HIV disease, shows the level of healthy T helper cells the patient has. This is a vital prognostic tool. The test uses a monoclonal antibody, which binds to a specific antigen on the T4 helper cells. The test counts these and presents them as a ratio of the total T cells.

Tonometry
Tonometric tests measure intraocular pressure (IOP). The normal range is 12–20 mmHg.

Applanation tonometry. Fluorescein and anaesthetic drops are instilled prior to this procedure. A prism attached to a slit lamp (or a portable Perkins' tonometer) is used to flatten a defined area of the cornea. The greater the force required to flatten the area, the higher the IOP.

Non-contact (air puff) tonometry uses a computerised instrument to direct a fine, high-pressure jet of air onto the cornea. The increase in force progresses linearly until the cornea becomes flat. At this point the cornea acts like a mirror and reflects light to a photoelectric sensor, which immediately shuts off the puff of air. The force required to flatten the cornea is recorded and converted into an IOP reading.

Tumour markers
Some malignant tumours produce substances that can be

detected in the blood, and that may serve as 'markers' of the presence or recurrence of the tumour, and sometimes as an indicator of its size and, therefore, response to treatment. For example, alpha-fetoprotein (AFP) and beta human chorionic gonadotrophin (BHCG) are produced by testicular tumours, and acid phosphatase by prostatic tumours.

Urinary flow rate
The voiding flow rate is measured using specially equipped facilities which allow the patient to void in privacy but where a machine can record the characteristics of the flow. The test will identify such things as peak flow, average flow, average flow and total flow time.

Urethroscopy
This is the endoscopic examination of the male urethra and prostate gland.

Videofluoroscopy
Video recording of swallowing mechanism, using fluorescent fluid.

Water depletion test (diabetes insipidus)
Fluids are withheld for 8–12 hours, or until 3% of the body weight has been lost. Regular measurements of plasma and urine are taken. The inability to increase urinary specific gravity and osmolality in response to water depletion is indicative of diabetes insipidus. The test must be closely supervised as the patient will experience excessive thirst. The test terminated if signs of tachycardia, hypotension or obvious dehydration occur.

APPENDIX 2

Normal values

Biochemical values 1023
Arterial blood analysis 1023
Cerebrospinal fluid 1023
Reference values in venous plasma 1024
Hormones 1025
Haematological values 1026

BIOCHEMICAL VALUES

Reference ranges are largely those used in the Department of Clinical Chemistry, the Royal Infirmary, University of Edinburgh. These can vary from laboratory to laboratory, depending on the assay method used and other factors; this is especially the case for the enzyme assays. Although the SI system of units is widely used in the UK, *units* of measurement can vary and lead to laboratory differences.

No details are given of the collection requirements which may be critical to obtaining a meaningful result.

Unless otherwise stated, reference ranges apply to adults; values in children may be different.

The values quoted for blood, except for Table A2.1, refer to plasma or serum. As far as possible, routine analyses are carried out on plasma, but serum is preferred for some analyses, especially certain hormones and electrophoretic studies.

Table A2.1 Arterial blood analysis

Analysis	Reference range	Units
Base excess	–4 to +4	mmol/l
Bicarbonate	21–27.5	mmol/l
Hydrogen ion	36–44	nmol/l
Pa_{CO2}	4.4–6.1	kPa
Pa_{O2}	12–15	kPa
Oxygen saturation	Normally >97	%

Table A2.2 Cerebrospinal fluid

Analysis	Reference range	Units
Cells	5 (all mononuclear)	cells/mm^3
Chloride	120–170	mmol/l
Glucose	2.5–4.0	mmol/l
Immunoglobulin G	20–50	mg/l
Total protein	100–400	mg/l

Table A2.3 Reference values in venous plasma for the more common analytes in adults

Analysis	Reference range	Units
α_1-Antitrypsin	1.7–3.2	g/l
Alanine aminotransferase (ALT)	10–40	U/l
Albumin	36–47	g/l
Alkaline phosphatase	40–100	U/l
Amylase	50–300	U/l
Aspartate aminotransferase (AST)	10–35	U/l
Bilirubin (total)	2–17	μmol/l
Calcium	2.12–2.62	mmol/l
Carboxyhaemoglobin	Not normally detectable Up to 1.5% in non-smokers	%
Ceruloplasmin	50–600	mg/l
Chloride	95–107	mmol/l
Cholesterol (total)	3.6–6.7	mmol/l
HDL-Cholesterol	0.5–1.6 (M) 0.6–1.9 (F)	
Copper	13–24	μmol/l
Creatine kinase (MB isoenzyme)	Normally <5% of total CK	
Creatine kinase (total)	30–200 (M) 30–150 (F)	U/l
Ethanol	Not normally detectable 65–87 (marked intoxication) 87–109 (stupor) >109 (coma)	mmol/l
Creatinine	55–150	μmol/l
Ferritin	15–350 (M) 8–300 (F)	μg/l
Gamma-glutamyl transferase (GGT)	10–55 (M) 5–35 (F)	U/l
Glucose (fasting)	3.6–5.8	mmol/l

Analysis	Reference range	Units
Glycated haemoglobin (HbA_1)	4.5–8	%
Immunoglobulin A	0.5–4.0	g/l
Immunoglobulin G	5.0–13.0	g/l
Immunoglobulin M	0.3–2.2 (M) 0.4–2.5 (F)	g/l
Iron	14–32 (M) 10–28 (F)	μmol/l
Iron binding capacity	45–72	μmol/l
Lactate	0.4–1.4	mmol/l
Lactate dehydrogenase (urea-stable)	100–300	U/l
Lead	<1.8	μmol/l
Magnesium	0.75–1.0	mmol/l
Osmolality	280–290	mmol/kg
Phosphate (fasting)	0.8–1.4	mmol/l
Potassium	3.3–4.7	mmol/l
Protein (total)	60–80	g/l
Sodium	132–144	mmol/l
Total CO_2	24–30	mmol/l
Transferrin	2.0–4.0	g/l
Triglycerides (fasting)	0.6–1.7	mmol/l
Urate	0.12–0.42 (M) 0.12–0.36 (F)	mmol/l
Urea	2.5–6.6	mmol/l
Zinc	9–29	μmol/l

Notes:

1. Values quoted are for venous plasma, but would also apply to serum.
2. For the definition of diabetes mellitus or impaired glucose tolerance, the following apply (WHO criteria for venous plasma):

	Glucose (mmol/l) (fasting)	Glucose (mmol/l) (2 h post 75 g glucose)
Diabetes mellitus	>8.0	>11.0
Impaired glucose tolerance	<8.0	>8.0 but <11.0

Table A2.4 Hormones

Hormone	Reference range	Units	Comments
Adrenocorticotrophic hormone (ACTH)	10–80 (at 08:00) <10 (at 22:00)	ng/l	Nycthemeral rhythm, so sampling time is critical. Avoid stress
Cortisol	160–565 (at 08:00) <205 (at 22:00)	nmol/l	Nycthemeral rhythm, so sampling time is critical. Avoid stress
Follicle-stimulating hormone (FHS) (Male)	1.5–9.0	U/l	
Follicle-stimulating hormone (FSH) (Female)	3.0–15 (early follicular) Up to 20 (mid-cycle) 30–115 (post-menopausal)	U/l	
Gastrin	60–200	pg/ml	Collect after overnight fasting
Growth hormone (GH)	Very variable, usually less than 2, but may be up to 50 with stress	mU/l	Avoid stress Stimulation and suppression tests required
Insulin	5–25 (variable)	mU/l	Inappropriate levels in relation to glucose should be assessed
Luteinizing hormone (LH) (Female)	2.5–9.0 (early follicular) Up to 30 (mid-cycle) 30–115 (post-menopausal)	U/l	
Luteinizing hormone (LH) (Male)	1.5–9.0	U/l	
Oestradiol-17β (Female)	110–180 (early follicular) 550–1650 (mid-cycle) 370–770 (luteal) <100 (post-menopausal)	pmol/l	
Oestradiol-17β (Male)	<200	pmol/l	
Parathyroid hormone (PTH)	10–55	ng/l	
Progesterone (Male)	<2.0	nmol/l	
Progesterone (Female)	<2.0 (follicular) >15 (Mid luteal) <2.0 (post-menopausal)	nmol/l	
Prolactin (PRL)	60–390	mU/l	Avoid stress
Testosterone (Male)	10–30	nmol/l	
Testosterone (Female)	0.8–2.8	nmol/l	
Thyroid stimulating hormone (TSH)	0.3–5.0	mU/l	
Thyroxine (free) (free T_4)	9–23	pmol/l	Reference range may change in pregnancy
Tri-iodothyronine (T_3)	1.1–2.8 (under 65) 0.5–2.2 (over 65)	nmol/l	
TSH receptor antibodies (TRAb)	<7	U/l	

Notes:

1. A number of hormones are unstable and collection details are critical to obtaining a meaningful result. Refer to the local handbook.
2. Values in the table are only a guideline; hormone levels can often only be meaningfully understood in relation to factors such as sex (e.g. testosterone). An (e.g. FSH in women), time of day (e.g. cortisol), or regulatory factors (e.g. insulin and glucose, PTH and $[Ca^{2+}]$). Also, reference ranges may be critically method-dependent.

HAEMATOLOGICAL VALUES

Table A2.5 Haematological values

	SI units	Other units
Bleeding time (Ivy)	Up to 11 min	
Body fluid (total)		50% (obese) – 70% (lean) of body weight
Intracellular		30–40% of body weight
Extracellular		20–30% of body weight
Blood volume		
Red cell mass – men	30 ± 5 ml/kg	
– women	25 ± 5 ml/kg	
Plasma volume (both sexes)	45 ± 5 ml/kg	
Total blood volume – men	75 ± 10 ml/kg	
– women	70 ± 10 ml/kg	
Erythrocyte sedimentation rate (Westergren) (Figures given are for patients under 60 years of age. Higher values in older persons are not necessarily abnormal)		0–6 mm in 1 h normal 7–20 mm in 1 h doubtful >20 mm in 1 h abnormal
Fibrinogen	1. –4.0 g/l	150–400 mg/dl
*Folate – serum	2–20 μg/l	2–20 ng/ml
– red cell	>100 μg/l	>100 ng/ml
Haemoglobin – men	130–180 g/l	13–18 g/dl;
– women	115–165 g/l	11.5–16.5 g/dl
Haptoglobin	0.3–2.0 g/l	30–200 mg/dl
Leucocytes – adults	4.0–11.0 × 10^9/l	4000–11 000 l/μ 4.0–11.0 × 10^3/mm^3
Differential white cell count		
Neutrophil granulocytes	2.5–7.5 × 10^9/l	40–75%
Lymphocytes	1.0–3.5 × 10^9/l	20–45%
Monocytes	0.2–0.8 × 10^9/l	2–10%
Eosinophil granulocytes	0.04–0.4 × 10^9/l	1–6%
Basophil granulocytes	0.01–0.1 × 10^9/l	0–1%
Mean corpuscular haemoglobin (MCH)	27–32 pg	27–32 μμg
Mean corpuscular haemoglobin concentration (MCHC)	30–35 g/dl	30–35%
Mean corpuscular volume (MCV)	78–98 fl	78–98 $μ^3$ or $μm^3$
Packed cell volume (PCV) or haematocrit – men	0.40–0.54	40–54%
– women	0.35–0.47	35–47%
Platelets	150–400 × 10^9/l	150 000–4000 000/μl or/mm^3
Prothrombin time	11–15 s	
Red cell count – men	4.5–6.5 × 10^{12}/l	4.5–6.5 × 10^6/μl or mm^3
– women	3.8–5.8 × 10^{12}/l	3.8–5.8 × 10^6/μl or mm^3
Red cell life span (mean)	120 days	
Red cell life span $T_{½}$ (^{51}Cr)	25–35 days	
Reticulocytes (adults)	10–100 × 10^9/l	0.2–2%
*Vitamin B_{12} (in serum as cyanocobalamin)	160–925 ng/l	160–925 pg/ml or μμg/ml

*Also measured by radioassay; normal range of reference values should be obtained from the laboratory carrying out the estimation.

Index

Page numbers in **bold** type indicate main discussions; those in *italics* refer to figures, tables or boxes. The alphabetical arrangement is letter-by-letter.

Index

A

A & E departments, *see* Accident and emergency departments
Abdominal hernia, *see* Hernia, abdominal
Abdominal injuries, 815
Abdominal pain
  acute cholecystitis, 121, 122
  appendicitis, 106, *107*
  ascites, 117
  diabetes mellitus, 157
  ectopic pregnancy, 246, 247
  inflammatory bowel disease, 102, 103
  liver disease, 114, 119
  pancreatic cancer, 128
  pancreatitis, 124, *125*, 127
  peptic ulcers, 96–97
  postoperative, *799*, 800
Abdominal paracentesis, *117*, 242
Abducens nerve, *330*
A-beta fibres, 619
ABO blood groups, 408–409
Abortion, **249–254**
  complications, 254
  incomplete, *250*, 252
  induced, 197–198, **253–254**
  inevitable, 250–251
  missed, *250*, 251
  recurrent, 252
  spontaneous (miscarriage), 251–252, 819
  threatened, 250
Abortion Act (1967), **252–253**
Abscess
  breast, 288
  cerebral, 363, 364
  extradural, 363
  pancreatic, 125, *126*
  peritonsillar (quinsy), **518–519**
  wound, *698*, 703
Absence seizures, *355*
Absorption, intestinal, 89–90
Acceptance, *925*
Accessory nerve, *330*, *523*
Accident and emergency (A & E) departments, **809–824**
  aggression and violence, 822–823
  burns injuries, 866
  death in, 818–819
  health promotion, 824
  major disasters, 823–824
  nursing process, 813
  reception of patients, 810–811
  resuscitation room, 811, 812
  workload, 810
  see also Trauma
Accidents, 810
  first-aid treatment, 384, *388*, 607, *608*
  involving infectious blood/body fluids, 564
  prevention, 824
  road traffic (RTAs), 335, 369, 531, 810
Accommodation (of eye), 469, 470
Acetylcholine, 746
Achalasia, 130
  of oesophagus, **92–93**, 667
Acid–base balance, **647–650**
  disorders, **649–650**
  hyperkalaemia and, 645
  shock, 599
  see also Acidosis; Alkalosis
Acidosis, **648**
  metabolic, *see* Metabolic acidosis
  respiratory, 648, **650**
Acids
  eye injuries, 488–489
  oesophageal injury, 95
Acne, **460–461**
Acne Support Group, 465
Acquired immune deficiency syndrome, *see* AIDS/HIV infection
Acromegaly, **139–140**, 220, *530*, 763
  amenorrhoea, 220
  oral signs, *530*
Acromioclavicular joint, fracture, *384*
ACTH, *see* Adrenocorticotrophic hormone
Actinomycosis, *529*
Action potential, cardiac, 11
Action on Smoking and Health (ASH), 66, 989
Activities of living (ALs), 657, 914–915
  factors influencing, 915–916
Activities of living model of nursing (Roper *et al*), 10
  cancer care, 898
  chronic illness and, **914–918**
  unconscious patients, 849–857
Activity, physical
  angina pectoris, 18
  epilepsy, 354–355
  heart failure, 40
  intraocular surgery and, 476
  mastectomy and, 275
  myocardial infarction, 27, 28–30
  see also Exercise; Mobility/mobilisation; Rest
Acupuncture, 631
Acute tubular necrosis (ATN), 319
ADA (adenosine deaminase) gene therapy, 189, *190*
Adaptation model of nursing, Roy's, *see* Roy's adaptation model of nursing
Addiction
  definition, 622, 974
  to narcotics, fear of, 622–623, 798
Addictions Forum, 987, 989
Addictive behaviour, model for changing, 974–975
Addisonian crisis, 149
Addison's disease, **149–150**
A-delta fibres, 617, 619
Adenomyosis, uterine, 222, 224
Adhesions, intra-abdominal, *107*
Adhesive strips, 819–821
Adipose tissue, brown (BAT), 685, 693
Adjuvant therapy, 904
  chemotherapy, 891
  radiotherapy, 887
Adrenal adenoma, 148
Adrenal carcinoma, 148
Adrenal cortex, 137
  chronic stress effects, 582
  disorders, **148–152**
  hormones, *see* Corticosteroids; Glucocorticoids; Mineralocorticoids
  stress response, 581–582
Adrenalectomy, 148, 149
Adrenal glands, *134*, **136–137**
  disorders, **147–152**
Adrenal hyperplasia, congenital (CAH), **151–152**
Adrenaline, 137, 156
  stress response, 581, 582, 599
  therapy, *78*, 559, 560, 607
Adrenal medulla, 137, 156
  dysfunction, **147–148**
  stress response, 581
Adrenocorticotrophic hormone (ACTH), *135*, 149
  blood glucose regulation, 155
  deficiency, *142*
  ectopic production, 148
  hypersecretion, **140**, *150*
  stress response, 581, 582
Adrenogenital syndrome, 220
Adriamycin (doxorubicin), 431, *892*, 893, *895*
Adult respiratory distress syndrome (ARDS), 62, 600, **613**
Advertising, tobacco, 66
Afferent nerve fibre/neurone, 326, 632
Afferent (sensory) pathways, 333–334, 617
Afterload, 13, *601*
Age
  body temperature and, 685
  breast cancer and, 266

Age (*contd*)
cancer and, 880
diabetes mellitus and, 158
scarring and, *702*
skin disorders and, 444
sleep and, 748–749
see also Children; Elderly
Aggression
A & E departments, **822–823**
defusing potential, 822
Agranulocytosis, **438–439**, *530*
Aid for Addicts and Family (ADFAM), 989
Aids/appliances
disabled, 947, 967–968
joint replacement patients, 399
see also Home aids/adaptations
AIDS Helpline, 989, 1009
AIDS/HIV infection, 544, 991–1008
acute seroconversion illness, 992, 1003–1004
antibody positive phase, 992, 1004
antiviral treatment, 1007
asymptomatic/dormant, 994–995, 1004
clinical manifestations/management, 1002–1003
constitutional disease, 1005
counselling, 999, 1000–1001
definitions/terminology, 991–993
diagnosis, 992
eye disorders, **494**
haemophilia patients, 203, 205, 993
health education and promotion, 1001–1002
impact on health and social services, 996–998
infection control, 551, 1003
neurological disease, 495, 1007
nursing interventions, 1003–1008
opportunistic infections, *992*, 1005–1006
oral manifestations, *529*, *1005*
phases, *992*, 1003–1007
philosophical issues for nurses, 998–999
political and social implications, 995–999
secondary cancers, *992*, 1006–1007
skin disorders, 463, *1005*
stages, 994–995
testing and screening, 999–1001
virus replication stage, *994*, 995
AIDS-related complex (ARC), 1004–1005
Air
composition, *63*
embolism, 674
pollution, 66, **67**
Airway management
burns patients, 867
emergency, **82**, *83*, *84*, 811
maxillofacial injuries, 533–534, 535
recovery from anaesthesia, 791
thyroidectomy patients, 141
tonsillectomy patients, 518
tracheostomy patients, 516
unconscious patients, 849–851
Airway obstruction, *513*, 516
burns, 865
speech problems, 762
Airways
artificial, **850**
obstructive disorders, **70–76**
suctioning, 515, 850–851
emergency, *84*
tracheostomy patients, 514, 515
unconscious patients, 850–851
Airways disease, chronic obstructive (COAD), **70**, 650, 911
Akinetic mutism, 844
Akinetic seizures, *355*
Al-Anon, 987
Alarm systems
machines in intensive care units, 830
nocturnal enuresis, 738
Al-Ateen, 987
Albumin, serum, 665, *666*
Alcohol, 658
absorption and elimination, 980
decontamination of surfaces, 553
parenteral infusion, 674
sleep and, 751, *754*
units, 979–980
Alcohol abuse, 973–974, **979–982**, *983*
burns and, 860
cancer and, 881
cirrhosis and, 116, 119–120
health impact, 980–982
by nurses, 976–977
nurse's role, 975–976
pancreatitis and, 124, 125, 126, 127
women, 981
young people, 980–981
Alcohol Concern, 987, 989
Alcohol consumption
angina, 19
elderly, 982
epilepsy, 354
head injuries and, 335
hypertension and, 44, 46
hypothermia and, 693
oesophageal carcinoma and, 93
oral cancer and, 537
safe, 979–980, 981
stroke and, 347
Alcoholic cirrhosis, 116, 119–120, *980*
Alcoholic hepatitis, **116**, *980*
Alcoholics Anonymous (AA), 987, 989
Alcohol Recovery Project, 989
Aldosterone, 137, 293, 294
functions, 14, 641, 645
shock, 599
Alienation, 926
Alkalis
eye injuries, 488–489
oesophageal injuries, 95
Alkalosis, **648**
metabolic, 648, **649**, 654
respiratory, 648, **649–650**
Alkylating agents, *892*, *895*
Alleles, 188
Allergic contact eczema, 452
Allergy
food, 454
surgery and, 789
to topical eye medication, **485**
Allodynia, 632
Allopurinol, 428
Alopecia, cancer patients, 431, *889*, 893
Alpha-adrenergic receptor blocking agents, 233
Alpha-adrenoceptors, 137
Alpha-antitrypsin deficiency, 70, 116
Alphafetoprotein (AFP)
amniotic fluid, 193
maternal serum (MSAFP), *197*
serum, 118, 229
Alpha particles, 886
Alternative/complementary therapies, 919
cancer, 896
chronic illness, 909
pain, 631–632
skin disorders, 451, 454
Alveolar ridges, 521
Alveolitis, extrinsic allergic (farmer's lung), **560**
AMBU bag resuscitator, *82*, *84*
Amenorrhoea, **219–221**
anorexia nervosa, 138, 220
pathological, 219–221
physiological, 219
primary, 219
secondary, 219
Ametropia, *470*
Amino acids, 660
parenteral solutions, 674, 797
Aminoglutethimide, 277–278
Amnesia, post-traumatic (PTA), 339, 534
Amniocentesis, 193
Amphetamines, 984
Amputation, limb, **388–391**
nursing priorities and management, 389–391
reasons for, 52, 388–389
sites, 389
Amylase, serum, 124
Anaemia, **411–425**
aplastic, **420–421**
blood loss causing, 412, **424–425**
causes, 405–406, 412
haemolytic, 412, **421–424**
iron deficiency, **414–416**, 424, *530*
leukaemia, *426*, 429–430
medical management, 412–413
megaloblastic, **416–420**
nursing priorities and management, 413–414
pathophysiology, 412
pernicious, *418*, *530*
sickle cell, 192, 421, **422–424**
transurethral resection of prostate and, 309–310
types, 411–412
Anaesthesia, **789–791**
myotonic dystrophy and, 206
recovery from, **791–792**
see also General anaesthesia; Local anaesthesia
Anaesthetic nurse, 786, *789*
Anaesthetist, 787, *789*, *798*
Anal fissure (fissure in ano), *112*, **113**, 733
Anal fistula (fistula in ano), **113**
Analgesia, 628
patient controlled (PCA), 629, 798, *800*
see also Pain relief
Analgesics, **628–629**
inadequate administration, 623–624
inadequate prescribing, 623
narcutic, *see* Narcotic analgesics
postoperative pain relief, 797–798
premenstrual syndrome, 227
routes of administration, 628–629
Anaphylactic shock, **559–560**, 604, 792
management/treatment, 559–560, 607
patients at risk, *605*
Anastomotic leaks, gastrointestinal, *798*
Androgens
syndrome of resistance, 152
testicular, 295
Anencephaly, *197*
Aneurysms, 15
aortic, *see* Aortic aneurysms
intracranial, 344, 346, *493*
ventricular, 34
Anger, *925*, 926
Angina pectoris, **15–22**, 46
anaemia, 412
chest pain, 15–16, 25
classification, *16*
medical management, 15–16

Angina pectoris (*contd*)
  nursing priorities and management, 16–22
  treatment, 16, *17*
Angioblastoma, intracranial, *351*
Angioedema, 559
Angiography
  cerebral, 346
  coronary, 16, *17*
Angioma, intracranial, 351
Angiotensin converting enzyme (ACE) inhibitors, 45
Angiotensin I, 14, 293
Angiotensin II, 14, 203–204
Ankle oedema, heart failure, 38, *39*
Ankle pressure index, 717, 718
Anorectal disorders, **111–113**
Anorexia
  anaemia, 412
  cancer, 899
  elderly, 528
  leukaemia, 432
  pancreatic cancer, 128–129
  terminally ill patients, 933
Anorexia nervosa, **137–139**, 220
Anosmia, 667
Antacids, 97, 649
Anterior chamber (AC), 469
  assessment, 471
  depth, 480
Anthropometry, 665
Antibiotics
  antitumour, *892*, *895*
CNS infections, 364, 365
  cystic fibrosis, 200, 201
  diabetic ketoacidosis, 166
  eczema, 453
  leukaemia, 427
  osteomyelitis, 391
  prophylactic, 789
  resistant organisms, 829
  toxic epidermal necrolysis, 459
Antibodies, 546
  antitumour, 894
Antibody-mediated immune response, 547–548
Anticholinergic, 741
Anticholinergic drugs, 360, 732, *786*
Anticholinesterase drugs, 561–562
Anticoagulants, 784
  angina, *17*
  cerebrovascular disease, 346
  dental treatment and, 526
  diabetic emergencies, 166, 170
  valvular heart disease, 43
Anticonvulsant drugs, 353, 354
Antidepressants, 589
Antidiuretic hormone, *see* Vasopressin
Anti-fibrinolytic agents, 346
Antihistamines, 453, 459, 519
Antimetabolites, *892*, *895*
Antinociceptive, 632
Antipyretics, *689*, 691
Antiseptics, wound care, 707
Antithyroid drugs, 144
Antiviral therapy, AIDS/HIV infection, **1007**
Antral lavage, 509
Antroscopy, 509, 519
Anus, 90
Anxiety
  anaemia and, 414
  aortic aneurysms, 48, 50
  attacks, **584**, 649–650
  bleeding oesophageal varices, 118
  blood transfusion, 417
  breast cancer screening, 269
  breast surgery and, 263
  diabetic ketoacidosis, 169
  drug therapy, 588–589
  ectopic pregnancy, 247
  enucleation of eye, 491
  eye injuries, 487–488, 489
  hysterectomy and, 237–238
  in vitro fertilisation and embryo transfer, 258
  intraocular surgery, 476, 479
  leukaemia, 431
  liver failure, 119
  myocardial infarction, 26
  orofacial trauma, 534, 535
  pain and, 620
  pancreatic cancer, 128
  preoperative, 781, 788
  renal colic, 303
  sleep problems and, 749–750
  total cystectomy and urinary diversion, 317
  transurethral resection of prostate and, 308
  see also Fear; Stress
Aortic aneurysms, **47–48**
  abdominal (AAA), 47
  dissecting, *25*, 47
  nursing care plan, 49–50
  ruptured, 47, 48
  thoracic, 47
Aortic incompetence, **44**
Aortic stenosis, 42, **43**
Aortic valve, *10*, 11, 12
Aphakic eye, postoperative care, 478
Aplastic anaemia, **420–421**
Apnoea, brain-stem death, 857
Apocrine glands, 446
  disorders, **460–461**
Appearance
  disorders affecting, 763
  non-verbal messages, 760
Appendicectomy, 106
Appendicitis, **105–106**, *107*, *108*
Appetite, loss of, *see* Anorexia
Appraisal, 577, **578**, 579–580, 594
  primary, 578
  secondary, 578
Aqueous humor, 469
Arachnoid mater, 329, *332*
Arch bar wiring, fractured mandible, 532
Arousal reaction, 840–841
Arrhenoblastoma, 220
Arrhythmias, cardiac, **34–37**
  atrial, 35–36
AV junctional, 36
  clinical features, 34–35
  myotonic dystrophy, 206
  pacemakers, 36–37
  sinus, 35
  ventricular, 36
Arterial blood gases (ABG), *63*, *64*, *65*
  asthma, *75*
  emphysema, 71–72
  normal results, *649*
  respiratory failure, 82
  sample handling, 72, 649, 815
  shock, 606, 613
Arterial bypass grafting, peripheral, 52
Arterial disease, peripheral, **48–53**
  clinical features, 48–52
  leg ulcers, *51*, **718**
  medical management, 51–52
  nursing priorities and management, 52–53
  pathophysiology, 48–51
Arterial lines
  blood pressure monitoring, 608–609, *610*
  insertion, 609
Arterial occlusion, peripheral, **48–53**
Arterial pressure, mean, 14
Arteries, 13
Arteriogram, 51, 55
Arterioles, 13
Arteriosclerosis obliterans, 48–52
Arteriovenous (AV) fistula, *322*
Arteriovenous malformations (AVM), cerebral, 344
Arthritis
  psoriatic, 448, 451
  rheumatoid, 370, **394–397**, *398*, *719*
  septic, **394**
Arthritis and Rheumatism Council, 397, 404
Arthritis Care, 404
Arthrodesis, 396, *398*
Arthrogram, *373*
Arthroplasty, 396, 398
Arthroscopy, *373*, 775
Ascites, 100, **116–117**
Asepsis
  eye disorders, 475
  operating theatre, 787–789
Aseptic technique, 553, *698*
  changing wound dressings, **708–710**
Aspartate transferase, serum, *24*
Aspermia, *256*
Aspiration
  nasogastric, *see* Nasogastric aspiration
  pneumonia, *671*, 784, 788
  tube feeding and, *671*
Aspirin, *17*, 96, 346, *689*
Assessment, nursing
  benign mammary dysplasia, 288
  breast cancer, 271, 278, 281, 283
  breast reconstruction, 279
  chronic illness, 916–917
  communication skills in, 766–767
  dependency problems, 975, 977–978
  diabetes mellitus, 178
  fluid and electrolyte status, 650
  leg ulcers, 717
  minor trauma, 819–821
  multiple trauma, 813–816
  musculoskeletal disorders, 373
  neurological status, 341
  preoperative, 781
  rehabilitation, 949
  sleep, **753**
  terminally ill patients, 929
  urinary incontinence, 729–731
  wound management, 704, 705–706
Association areas, brain, 327, *328*
Association for Continence Advice (ACA), 734, 741
Association for Nurses in Substance Abuse (ANSA), 987, 989
Association of Cystic Fibrosis Adults (UK), 210
Association of Teachers of Lip-reading for Adults (ATLA), 520
Association to Aid the Sexual and Personal Relationships of People with a Disability, *see* SPOD
Associative learning, insomnia, 755
Asteatotic eczema, 451–452
Asthma, 70, **73–76**
  acute severe, *60*, *76*, *77*, *78*
  extrinsic, 73
  intrinsic, 73
  medical management, 73–74
  nursing priorities and management, 74–76
  pathophysiology, 73
  self management, 64, *74*, 75–76, *78*

Astigmatism, *470*
Astrocytoma, 349, *350*
Asystole, 31, *33*
Atherosclerosis, **14–15**, 47, 48
  cerebrovascular, 344
  diabetes mellitus, **173**
  post-menopausal, **217**
Athlete's foot (tinea pedis), **454–455**, *1005*
Atkinson tube, 93, 95
Atonic seizures, *355*
Atopic eczema, 451
Atopy, 464, 559
Atria (heart), 10
Atrial arrhythmias, 35–36
Atrial fibrillation (AF), **35–36**, 41
Atrioventricular (AV) junction, 11, 12
Atrioventricular (AV) junctional arrhythmias, 36
Atrioventricular valves, *10*, 11
Atropine, *786*
Attachment, to patients, 940
Attending skills, **765–766**
Attico-antral disease, 504, 519
Audiomerry, *499*
Audiovisual materials, 761–762
Auditory tract, 858
Aura, 354, *355*
Auriscope, 519
Auspitz sign, 449
Autoclaving, 551
Autogenic training, 755
Autohalers, *75*
Autoimmune diseases, 544, **561–562**
Automatic cells, heart, 11
Autonomic dysreflexia, 385–386
Autonomic nervous system, 325, **336**, *337*, *337*
  blood pressure regulation, 14
  cardiac function regulation, 13
  see also Sympathetic nervous system
Autonomic neuropathies, diabetes, 175, *176*
Autonomy, *884*, 919, 963
Autoregulation, blood flow, 13
Autotransfusion, blood, 606
AVERT (AIDS Education and Research Trust), 1009
AVP, *see* Vasopressin
Axillary lymph node dissection, 264, 270, 271
  postoperative care, 273
  postoperative exercises, 275
Axillary lymph node metastases, *277*
Axillary lymph nodes, *266*
Axon, *326*
Azidothymidine (AZT), 1007

B

Backboards, 813
Back pain, **392–394**
  acute, 392
  myeloma, 437, 438
  postoperative, *798*
  prevention, 392, *393*
  recurrent, 392
  work-related, 369
Bacteria, **704**
  cell walls, 704
Bacterial infections, 563
AIDS/HIV infection, 1006
  keratitis, 484
  meningitis, 363, 364
  skin, **456–457**
  see also specific diseases
BACUP (British Association of Cancer Patients), 264, 290, 441, 904
Balance, 498
Balanitis, *232*, 305
Balanoposthitis, *232*, 305
Balloon tamponade, oesophageal varices, 117, 118
Balloon valvuloplasty, 42
Bandaging
  compression, 281, 717–718
  eczema, 453–454
Banding, oesophageal varices, 117
Band ligation, haemorrhoids, 111–112
Barbiturate overdose, 847
Bargaining, *925*
Baroreceptors, 14
Basal cell carcinoma (BCC), 537
Basal ganglia, 328
Basophils, *407*, 545
Bathing
Huntington's disease, 209
  preoperative, 785
  unconscious patients, 853
B cells, *see* B lymphocytes
BCG (Bacille Calmette-Guérin) vaccination, 70
Beard, facial burns and, 871
Becker muscular dystrophy, 205
Bed(s)
  getting in and out, 361
  pads, 735
  rolling over in, *361*
  special dermatological, 460
  special pressure-relieving, *936*
Bedrest
  bullous skin disorders, 459
  deep vein thrombosis, 54
  glomerulonephritis, 316–317
  prolapsed intervertebral disc, 395
  sleep problems and, 751
  see also Rest
Behavioural problems, head injury, 343
Behavioural thermoregulation, 681
Behaviour therapy, 631, 755
Bell's palsy, *529*, *763*
Beneficience, *884*
Benzodiazepines
  hypnotic, 753–754
  tranquillisers, 589, **982–983**
Benzydamine, 529
Bereavement, **938–939**
  nursing staff, 591–592, 939–940, 1007–1008
  sudden, **818–819**
  working through, 939
  see also Death; Grief
β2-agonists, *78*
Beta adrenoceptors, 137
Beta blockers, *17*, 45, 46
  topical eye therapy, *476*, 478
Beta (β) cells, pancreatic, 155, 157, 158
Beta-endorphin, 226, 581
Bicarbonate, sodium, 166
Bicarbonate ions, 648–649
Biguanides, 161
Bile, 89, 90–91
Bile duct
  cancer (cholangiocarcinoma), **124**, 130
  stenting, 128
  stones (choledocholithiasis), **123**, 130
T-tube insertion, 122, *123*
Biliary colic, 121, *123*
Biliary tract
  disorders, **120–124**
  tumours, **124**
Bioengineering, 370
Biofeedback, 741
  pain relief, 631
  stress incontinence, 731
Biological therapy, cancer, 894
Biopsy
  bladder tumours, *313*
  brain, 352
  breast, 270
  cervix, 235
  prostate gland, 312
  skin, 449, 452, 459
Biotin, *661*
Bladder, **294**
  disorders, **313–316**
    multiple sclerosis, 358
    stroke, *345*
    see also Urinary incontinence
  emptying, 295, 724
  innervation, 294, 724
  irrigation, 311, 800
  lavage (washout), **736–738**
  outflow obstruction, *306*, 320
  retraining, 731–732
  ruptured, 816
Bladder cancer, **313–316**
  medical management, 313–315
  nursing priorities and management, 315–316
  pathophysiology, 313
  staging, 313, *314*
  transurethral resection (TURT), 313, *314*
Bleeding
  episodes, haemophilia A, 204–205
  fungating breast tumours, 282, 283, **284–286**
  fungating wounds, 935
  uterine, *see* Uterine bleeding
  see also Haemorrhage
Bleeding tendency
  anaemia, 412
  leukaemia, 426, 428, 430
  liver failure, 120
  thrombocytopenia, 439, 440
Blindness
  diabetes mellitus, 173, 174
  incidence, 467–468
  registration, 473–474
Blisters
  bullous skin disorders, 458, 460
  burn wounds, 869
Blom Singer valve, *515*
Blood, **406–411**
  cellular components, 406–408
  coagulation, 408, *409*
  crossmatching, 411
  disease transmission by, 544, 993–994
  fresh whole, *410*
  functions, 406
  spillages, 553, *554*
  supply, wound healing and, 702
  universal precautions, **550**, *551*, 555, 563
  whole (stored), *410*
Blood brain barrier, 332
Blood count, 413
Blood disorders, **405–441**
  affecting mouth, *530*
  causes, 405–406
  nurse's role in treatment, 406
Blood film, 413
Blood flow
  peripheral arterial disease, *51*
  regulation, 13
Blood gases, arterial, *see* Arterial blood gases

Blood groups, **408–410**
Blood loss
  anaemia due to, 412, **424–425**
  chronic, 424
  fractures, 607
  see also Haemorrhage
Blood pressure, **13–14**
  arterial, 14
  burns, 867
  high, *see* Hypertension
  monitoring, shock, 608–610
  myocardial infarction, 25–26
  normal values, 14
  raised intracranial pressure, *331*, 341
  shock, 34, 608, 792
  unconscious patients, 846
Blood transfusion, **410–411**
  anaemia, 415–416, 417–418
  autotransfusion, 606
  HIV transmission, 993
  hypovolaemic shock, 606
  incompatible, 417
  Jehovah's witnesses, *416*
  leukaemia, 427
  nursing care plan, 417–418
  products available, *410*
  reactions, 409, 418, 560
Blood vessels
  anatomy and physiology, **13–14**
  tumour spread, 878
Blow-out fracture, orbital floor, *531*
B lymphocytes (B cells), *407*, 544, *545*, 546
  deficiency, 559
  immune responses, 547–548
Bodily contact, **761**, 763
  see also Touch
Body, viewing the, 818, 937
Body fluids, **638–640**
  cytotoxic chemotherapy and, *894*
HIV transmission, 993–994
  infectious, 564
  spillages, 553, *554*
  universal precautions, **550**, *551*, 555, 563
Body image
  cancer therapy and, 899–900
  enucleation of eye, 491
  leukaemia, 431–432
  mastectomy and, 272–273
  oral cancer area, 540
  orofacial trauma and, 535–536
  postoperative, **804**
  tracheostomy and, 516
  see also Self-image
Body language, *see* Communication, non-verbal
Body lice, **456**
Body mass index (BMI), 665
Body weight, *see* Weight, body
Bone, **370**
  healing, *371*
  tissue renewal, 370
  water, inaccessible, 638
Bone infections, **391**
Bone marrow, 406, 544, *545*
  aspiration, 413, 426
  failure, 420
  metastases, breast cancer, *277*
  suppression, 892–893
Bone pain, myeloma, 437
Bone tumours, **386–388**
  benign, 388
  malignant, 388
  medical management, 388
  metastatic, *277*, 312, 387, 388
  nursing priorities and management, 388
  pathophysiology, 387–388
Booklets, information, 782
Botulinum A neurotoxin, 486
Bowell–Webster risk assessment guide for identifying patients at risk of infection, *558*
Bowel preparation, preoperative, 315–316, 512, 785–786
Bowman's capsule, *292*
Brachial plexus nerve damage, 280
Brachytherapy, 887
Bradycardia, sinus, 35
Brain
  anatomy and physiology, **327–332**
  biopsy, 352
  blood supply, 331, *332*
  contusions, *340*
  damage, perinatal, 762
  diffuse injury, *340*
  injuries, *340*, 604
  lacerations, *340*
  pain pathways, 617–618
  space-occupying lesions, 762, 763
Brain stem, **329**, 746
Brain-stem death, **855–857**
Brain tumours, *see* Intracranial tumours
Bra(ssiere)
  benign mammary dysplasia, 288
  breast reconstruction and, 280
  fungating breast tumours, 286–287
  'mastectomy', *276*
Breast, **263–290**
  anatomy, **265**, *266*
  biopsy, 270
  fine-needle aspiration cytology, 269–270
  implants, 278, 279
  infections, 288
  malignant disorders, **266–287**
  phantom sensations, 275
  physiological changes, **265–266**
  prostheses, 275, *276*, 286–287
  quadrantectomy, 270
  self-examination, 267–268
  tissue expansion, 278–279, 280
  wide local excision, 264, 270
Breast cancer, **266–287**
  clinical features, 269
  fungating tumours, **282–287**
    medical management, 282–283
    nursing care plan, 284–286
    nursing priorities and management, 283–287
    pathophysiology, 282
  histology, 269
  incidence and mortality, 266, *877*
  informed consent, 264
  investigations, 269–270
  lymphoedema, 274, 275, **280–282**
  metastatic, **276–278**
    medical management, 277–278
    nursing priorities and management, 278
    pathophysiology, 276–277
  nursing priorities and management, **271–276**
    pre-treatment phase, 271
    treatment phase, 271–276
  patient education, 263–264, 271, 282, 286–287
  prevention, 267–269
  psychological impact, 263, 272–273
  risk factors, 266–267
  screening, 268–269, 883
  staging, *270*
  surgery, 264, 270
    breast reconstruction after, 278–280
    informed consent, 264
    nursing priorities and management, 271–276
    patient education, 264, 271
    psychological impact, 263
    see also Mastectomy
  treatment options, 264, 270–271
Breast Care and Mastectomy Association (BCMA), 264, 276, 279, 290
Breast care nurse specialist, 264, **265**, 269
Breast disease
  benign, **287–289**
  psychological impact, 263
Breast feeding, 219, 266
  see also Lactation
Breast lumpectomy, 263, *264*, 270
Breast milk, 266
Breast reconstruction, 264, **278–280**
  complications, 279
  medical management, 278–279
  nursing priorities and management, 279–280
Breathing
  angina pectoris, 18
  aortic aneurysms, 48, 50
  CNS infections, 364
  emphysema, 72–73
  exercises, 781
  heart failure, 39–40
  maintenance, *see* Airway management
  neurological control, 61, *62*
  paradoxical, *80*
  raised intracranial pressure, *331*, 342
  unconscious patients, 849–851
  valvular heart disease, 42
  see also Respiration; Respiratory disorders; Ventilation
Breathlessness, *see* Dyspnoea
British Association for Counsellors, 596
British Association of Cancer Patients (BACUP), 264, 290, 441, 904
British Association of the Hard of Hearing, 520
British Deaf Association, 520
British Dermatology Nursing Group, 465
British Diabetic Association (BDA), *181*, 184
British Epilepsy Association, 366
British Migraine Association, 596, 635
Broca's area, 759
Bromocriptine, 140, 227
Bronchiectasis, 70
Bronchitis
  acute, **68**
  chronic, 66, **70**
Bronchogenic (lung) cancer, 66, **78–79**
  epidemiology, *877*
  staging, *884*
Bronchopneumonia, **69**
Bronchoscopy, 78, 93
Brown adipose tissue (BAT), 685, 693
Buccal administration, analgesics, 629
Buchanan laryngectomy bib/protector, 514, 516, 519
Buerger's disease, 52
Buffers, **648–649**
Buildings, access by disabled, 953, 955
Build Up, 94–95
Bulbospongiosum, 741
Bulbourethral glands, 296
Bulimia nervosa, 139, *530*
Bullae, skin, 458, 460
Bullous skin disorders, **458–460**
Burn-out, 582
Burns, **859–873**
  assessing severity, 862–865, 867

Burns (*contd*)
causative agents, 860
complications, *868*
deep partial thickness, *863*, **864**, 870
depth classification, 863–865
extensive, **865–869**
early problems and nursing care, 865–868
post-shock phase, 868–869
extent, 862–863
face, 532, **870–871**
first-aid treatment, 607, 861–862
fluid losses, 643
full thickness, 863, **864**, 870
inhalation injury and, 865
metabolic rate, 682
predisposing factors, 860
prevention, 859–861
psychological effects, 872–873
superficial partial thickness, *863*, **864**, 870
Burns unit, regional, 866–868
Burn wounds, 720, 862, **869–872**
cleansing and debridement, 869
contraction, 871
dressing, 870
exposure treatment, 869–870
scar formation, 871–872
skin grafting, 870
special areas, 870–871
Burr hole, *341*
biopsy, 352
Buserelin, 227

C

Cachexia, cancer, 879–880, 899, 933
Caecum, 90
Caffeine, 751, *754*, 978
Calcitonin, 136, *137*
Calcium, **646–647**, 662
dietary requirements, *660*, *661*
myocardial contraction and, 12
regulation of plasma levels, 136, *137*
see also Hypercalcaemia; Hypocalcaemia
Calcium channel antagonists, *17*, 45, 647
Calculi, urinary, *see* Urinary stones
Calculus, dental, 526
Calories, 686
Campylobacter jejuni enteritis, *570–571*
Cancer, **875–904**
cachexia, 879–880, 899, 933
causes, 880–881
diagnosis, 883–885
disease process, 876–880
effects, 878–880
epidemiology, 876, *877*
medical intervention, 883–896
nursing care, 896–902
pain, **620–621**, 624, 720
psychosocial effects, 620–621
treatment, *621*, 624, *931*
prevention, 881–883
screening, 882–883
secondary, AIDS, *992*, 1006–1007
spread, 877–878, *879*
staging, 883–885, 904
stigma, *876*
terminally ill patients, 922, 925
treatment, **885–896**
aims, 885
new developments, 894–896
response to, 885
surgery, 885–886
see also Chemotherapy; Radiotherapy
wound management, **720**
see also specific types of cancer
Cancer & Leukaemia in Childhood Trust (CLIC), 441
CancerLink, 904, 923
Candidiasis (thrush; moniliasis), **455**
acute pseudomembranous, *529*, 530
AIDS patients, 1006
chronic atrophic, *529*
diabetes mellitus, 158
oesophageal, **91–92**
oral, 100, 455, *529*, **530**, 531
AIDS/HIV infection, 1004, *1005*
terminally ill patients, 929, *932*
vaginal, 455
Cannabis, 985
Capillaries, 13
fluid exchange across, 639
Capillary pressure, 639
Carbohydrate, 658, **659–660**
exchange system, 160
parenteral solutions, 674
Carbon dioxide (CO_2)
in air, *63*
exchange, 62–64
narcosis, *71*
partial pressure (PCO_2), shock, 613
transport, *61*
Carbonic acid–bicarbonate buffering system, 648–649
Carbonic anhydrase, 649
Carbon monoxide poisoning, 865
Carcinoembryonic antigen (CEA), 237
Carcinogenesis, 880
Carcinogens, 880, 881
Carcinoid tumours, 148
Carcinoma, *878*
Carcinoma in situ, 877
Cardiac arrest, 31–32
Cardiac arrhythmias, *see* Arrhythmias, cardiac
Cardiac catheterisation, 16, *17*, 20
Cardiac centre, 329
Cardiac cycle, **12–13**
Cardiac enzymes, 23, *24*
Cardiac failure, *see* Heart failure
Cardiac index, 13, *601*
Cardiac massage, external, 32
Cardiac monitoring, 25
Cardiac output, 12–13, *601*
monitoring, 610
thermodilution method of measuring, 610, *612*
Cardiac reserve, 38
Cardiac tamponade, 47
Cardiac valves, *10*, 11
incompetence and stenosis, 11, **43–44**
see also Valvular heart disease
Cardiogenic shock, **32–34**, 598, **600–601**
management/treatment, 34, 606, *607*
patients at risk, *605*
postoperative, 792
Cardiopulmonary resuscitation (CPR), **31–32**, *33*, 60
Cardiovascular centre, 13, 329
Cardiovascular disorders, 9–10, **14–57**
diabetes mellitus, 173
stress and, 582
terminal illness, 925
see also Cerebrovascular disease; Hypertension; Ischaemic heart disease; Peripheral vascular disease
Cardiovascular system, **9–58**
Cardioversion, *35*, 36
Carers
chronically ill patients, *912*
elderly, 961, 969
multiple sclerosis, *357*
pain and, 625
stroke patients, *349*
terminally ill patients, **936**
Caring, **959–962**
definition, 959–960
for older persons, 961
Carotid arteries, 331, *332*
Carotid endarterectomy, 346
Carriers
cystic fibrosis, 201
haemophilia A, 204
single-gene disorders, 192, 193, 197
Cartilage, 370
Cast cap splinting, 532
Casts, **376–378**
bracing, 377
Plaster of Paris (POP), 377
removal, 378
synthetic, 377
tibia and fibula fractures, 381
Casualty departments, *see* Accident and emergency departments
Catabolism, postoperative, 797
Cataplexy, 750
Cataracts, 467, 468, **477–478**
diabetes mellitus, 174
extraction and intraocular lens implantation, **477–478**
myotonic dystrophy, 206
Catecholamines, 156, 606
Catheterisation, urinary, *308*, *309*
benign prostatic hyperplasia, 307–308
clean intermittent self-, **732**
diabetic ketoacidosis, 166
long-term, **736–738**
multiple sclerosis, 358
Parkinson's disease, 362
postoperative, 800
hysterectomy, 239, 241
repair of uterine prolapse, 249
transurethral resection of prostate, 311
supplying equipment, 738
unconscious patients, 853
Causalgias, 632
CD4 T-cells, *see* Helper T lymphocytes
Celestin tube, 93
Cell architecture, 441
Ceil division, 188
Cell membrane, fluid movement across, 639
Cellulitis, 280–281, **457**
Central nervous system (CNS), 325, **327–335**
infections, **363–365**
medical management, 364
nursing priorities and management, 364–365
pathophysiology, 363
pain pathways, 617–618
Central venous cannulation
complications, 674–675
fluid therapy, 653
long-term (Hickman line), 427–428
parenteral nutrition, 673
Central venous pressure (CVP), *601*
monitoring, **611**, *613*
Cerebellum, **328**
Cerebral abscess, 363, 364
Cerebral angiography, 346
Cerebral cortex, 327, *328*
control of consciousness, 840–841
Cerebral embolus, 344

Cerebral haemorrhage, 344
Cerebral ischaemia, 346
Cerebral oedema, radiotherapy-induced, *889*
Cerebral thrombosis, 170, 344
Cerebrospinal fluid (CSF), **329–331**, *332*
  CNS infections, *364*
  functions, 329–331
  increased volume, *336*
  leakage, 343
  tumour spread, 878
Cerebrovascular accident (CVA), *see* Stroke
Cerebrovascular disease, **344–349**
  diabetes mellitus, 173
  medical management, 345–346
  nursing priorities and management, 346–349
  pathophysiology, 344–345
Cerebrum, 327, *328*
Cerumen (earwax) excess, **498–499**
Cervical carcinoma, **234–239**
  invasive, 236–237
  pathophysiology, 234
  pre-invasive, 235–236
  screening, 235, 883
Cervical collar, *401*
Cervical intraepithelial neoplasia (CIN), *235*
Cervical mucus, fertility and, *255*
Cervical smear test, 235, 245, 883
Cervical spine
  fractures/dislocations, 383
  traction, *387*
  whiplash injury, 383, *387*, 401
Cervico-vaginal prolapse, 247
Cervix
  biopsy, 235
  incompetent, 251–252
  partial stenosis, 224
Cetrimide, *708*
C fibres, 617, 619
Chair, rising from, *361*
Change, responses to, 924–925, *927*
Charcot's joints, diabetes mellitus, 176
Checks, preoperative, 786, *787*
Cheeks, 521
Cheilitis, angular, 415, *529*, 530
Chemicals
  burn injuries, 861
  carcinogenic, 881
  eye injuries, **488–489**
  hazardous, intensive care units, 829–830
  inhalation of toxic, **865**
Chemonucleolysis, intervertebral disc, 393
Chemoreceptors, 61, *62*
Chemosis, 471
Chemotaxis, *698*
Chemotherapy, 629, **891–894**, *896*
  adjuvant, 891
  administration, 892
  bladder cancer, 314–315
  breast cancer, **270**, 275–276, 277, 283
  choriocarcinoma, 243
  combination, 891–892
  endometrial carcinoma, 241
  intravesical, 314–315
  leukaemia, 427, 434
  liver rumours, *120*
  lymphoma, 435–436
  myeloma, 437
  non-cytotoxic, 894
  oral cancer, 538
  ovarian cancer, 242
  palliative, 891
  side-effects, *277*, 428–433, **892–893**, *895*
  testicular cancer, 230
Chest, Heart and Stroke Association, 349, 366
Chest drains, **80–81**, 811, 813
  insertion, 80
  lobectomy, 78–79
  pneumonectomy, 79
  removal, 81
  underwater seal, *81*
Chest infections, **68–69**
  leukaemia, 428
  postoperative, 317, **782–783**, 788
  see also Pneumonia
Chest injuries, **79–81**, 811, 813
Chest pain, *25*
  angina pectoris, 15–16, *25*
  aortic aneurysms, 47
  myocardial infarction, 22, *25*, 27
  oesophageal disorders, 91
Chest physiotherapy
  cystic fibrosis, 201, *202*
  emphysema, 73
  lobectomy, 78
  myotonic dystrophy, 206
  post-splenectomy, 130
  raised intracranial pressure, 342
  unconscious patients, 851
Chewing, 88, *522*, 523
  problems, 667
Cheyne–Stokes respiration, *849*
Chickenpox, *529*, 563, **569–570**
Childbirth, urinary incontinence and, 727
Childlessness, **254–260**
  see also Infertility/subfertility
Children
  acquiring continence, 724
  body temperature, 685
  burns injuries, 860, 863
  eczema, 451, 454
  febrile convulsions, *689*
  HIV transmission to, 994
  immunisation, 563
  nasal foreign bodies, 510–511
  secretory otitis media, 501–502
  speech problems, 762
  urinary incontinence, 726–727
  visiting patients in intensive care, 833
Chills, 689
Chinese herbalism, 454
Chiropractic, 631
Chlorhexidine, *708*
  mouthwashes, 528–529, *933*
Chloride, **644–645**, 662
Choking, Huntington's disease, 208
Cholangiocarcinoma, **124**, 130
Cholangiopancreatography, endoscopic retrograde (ERCP), *93*, 121, 123, 125, 128
Choleastoma, **501–502**
Cholecystectomy, 121, 125
  laparoscopic, 121, 123, 776
  open, **122**, 123
Cholecystitis
  acute, **121–122**, *123*
  chronic, **123**
Cholecystokinin, 89, 91
Choledocholithiasis, **123**, 130
Cholelithiasis (gallstones), **120–123**
  acute pancreatitis and, 124, 125
  pathophysiology, 121
Cholesterol, *19*, 347
  total serum, 18, *19*
Cholinergic crisis, 562
Chondrosarcoma, *388*
Chordoma, *351*
Choriocarcinoma, **243**
Chorionic gonadotrophin, human, *see* Human chorionic gonadotrophin
Chorionic villus sampling (CVS), 193–194, *199*
Choroid, 468
Choroiditis, 484
Choroid plexus, 329, *332*
Christmas disease, 202, 439
Chromosomal abnormalities, 188, **191**
  autosomal variations, 191
  sex, 191
  sexual differentiation disorders, **152**
  sources of tissue in diagnosis, *193*
Chromosomes, 188
Chronic illness, **905–918**
  experience, framework for understanding, 911
  features, 908–911
  location and organisation of care, 912
  nursing intervention, 912–916
  prevalence, 907–908
  Roper–Logan–Tierney model of nursing applied to, 916–918
  societal attitudes, 906–907
  terminology, 905–906
  urinary incontinence, 728
Chronic obstructive airways disease (COAD), **70**, 650, 911
Chvostek's sign, *147*
Chyme, 88, 89
Ciliary body, 468
Circadian rhythms, 743–744
  body temperature, **683–684**
  cortisol, *149*
  critical care units, 835
  disrupted normal, 744, *749*
Circle of Willis, 331, *333*
Circulating nurse, 787, *789*
Circulation
  maintenance, resuscitation, 811–812
  systemic, 13
Circumcision, 305–306
Cirrhosis, hepatic, **116**, 117
  alcoholic, 116, 119–120, *980*
Cisplatin, *885*, 893, *895*, 904
Claudication, intermittent, **51**, 53, *54*, 412
Clavicle, fractures, **383**, *384*
Cleaning, instruments and equipment, 553
Clean intermittent self-catheterisation, **732**
Cleansing
  burn wounds, **869**
  eyelids, 475
  wounds, **706–708**
Clean technique, changing dressings, 710
Cleft Lip and Palate Association (CLAPA), 524
Cleft lip/palate, 523–524, 666
Climacteric, **216–217**
Clips, wound, *799*, 802, *803*
Clomiphene citrate, 254, 257
Clonic seizures, *355*
Clostridium botulinum, 658
Clostridium tetani, 704, *817*
Clostridium welchii, 704
Clothing
  angina pectoris, 20
  burns and, 861
  fungating breast tumours and, 286–287
  Huntington's disease, 209
  laundering, 554, *555*
  nun-verbal messages, 760
  post-amputation, 390
  protective, 564, 867, 868–869
  rheumatoid arthritis, 397
  theatre staff, 788

Clothing (*contd*)
  trauma victims, 813, 817
  see also Dressing
Clotting factor disorders, **439**
CNS, *see* Central nervous system
Coagulation
  blood, 408, *409*
  disseminated intravascular (DIC), 599, **613–614**
Coagulation disorders, **439–440**
  missed abortion, 251
  see also Bleeding tendency
Coal tar ointments, 450
Cocaine, 985
Coccidioidomycosis, 1006
Cochlea, 498
Cocois ointment, 450
Coeliac disease, 101, *530*
Coffee, 978
Cognitive, 858
Cognitive–behavioural therapy, 631
Cognitive therapy
  insomnia, 755
  stress, **588**
Coitus, 296
Cold applications, pain, 631
Cold caloric testing, 857
Cold coagulation, pre-invasive cervical carcinoma, 235
Cold compresses, soft-tissue injuries, 402
Cold injuries, **693–694**
Cold sores (oral herpes simplex), 432, *529*, 563
Cold water, burns first-aid, 861–862
Colectomy, total, *111*
Colic
  biliary, 121, *123*
  renal, *see* Renal colic
Collaborative relationships, 919
Collagen, 446
  wound healing, *698*, 699, 700
Collagenase, *698*
Coiles' fracture, **383**
Colloid cyst of third ventricle, *351*
Colloid solutions, 605–606, 653
  combined with crystalloids, 606
Colon, 90
  reduced motility, *112*
Colorectal cancer, 101, **109–111**
  medical management, 110
  nursing priorities and management, 110–111
  pathophysiology, 109–110
Colostomy
  postoperative care, 793–795, 804
  preoperative preparation, *104*
  self-care, *948*
  terminally ill patients, 933, 935
Colour blindness, **472**
Colpoperineorrhaphy, posterior, 249
Colporrhaphy, anterior, 248–249
Colposcopy, 222–223, 235, 236
Colposuspension, 733
Coma, 843
  definition, 839
  epileptic seizures, *355*, 847
  hyperglycaemic hyperosmolar non-ketotic (HHNK), **167–171**
  hypoglycaemic, **171–172**, 847, *848*
  recovery from, 855
  see also Consciousness, impaired; Unconscious patients
COMAKIT, 851
Comedone, 464
Commensal microorganisms, 549
Communication, **757–771**
  angina pectoris, 20
  audiovisual materials, 761–762
  between colleagues, **767–769**
  cancer patients, 900–902
  critically ill patients, 832–833, 836
  disorders affecting, **762–763**, 914
    anaemia, 414
    CNS infections, 364–365
    head injury, 342
    hearing impairment, 500, 762
    Huntington's disease, 208–209
    laryngectomy, 513, 514, 762
    leukaemia, 433
    maxillofacial injuries, 535, 763
    multiple sclerosis, 356–357
    oral tumours, 541
    Parkinson's disease, 362, 763
    stroke, *345*, **347**, 762, 763
    visual impairment, 474
  effects of health care context, 764–765
  heart failure, 40–41
  myocardial infarction, 26
  non-verbal (body language), **760–761**, 765–766
    aggression and, 822
    disorders affecting, **763**
  nurse-to-nurse, 768–769
  in nursing practice, **764–765**
  patient education and, **769**
  rehabilitation and, 949–950
  role of mouth, 523
  setting, 761
  skills, **765–767**
    nurses', 764–765
    in practice, 766–767
    sleep assessment and, 753
  surgical patients, 802–803
  theories, **757–758**
  unconscious patients, 851
  verbal, **758–760**
    see also Speech
  written, readability, 761
  see also Information, giving
Community, nursing education in, 5–6
Community care, 4
  AIDS/HIV infection, 996
  bereaved relatives, 938
  bullous skin disorders, 460
  cancer, **896–897**
  chronic illness, 910–911, 912
  diabetes mellitus, 158, 181–182
  disabled, 954–956
  eczema, 454
  elderly, 962, 967
  epistaxis, 508
  eye injuries, 488, 489
  incontinence, 735, 738
  infectious diseases, **564**, 565
  leg ulcers, 715
  minor trauma, 821
  multiple sclerosis, 359–360
  myocardial infarction, 24
  oral cancer, 541
  respiratory disorders, 84
  stroke, 349
  terminally ill patients, 923, 936
  wounds, 706, 708–710
Community nurses
  AIDS/HIV infection and, 997
  breast cancer screening and, 269
  cancer care, 896–897
  death of patients, 938
  dental health and, *525*
  eye disorders and, 467, 473
  fractures of neck of humerus, 382
  fungating breast tumours, 283
  health education, 67
  hearing-impaired patients and, 500–501
  laryngectomy patients, 515
  minor trauma, 821
  palliative care, 923, 935
  postoperative care, 805
  prolapsed intervertebral disc and, 393, 395
  referral of patients, 778
  rehabilitation, 805
  respiratory disorders, *84*
  skin disorders and, 444
  see also District nurses; Macmillan nurses
Compartment syndrome, 375, *377*
Compassionate Friends, 819, 825
Complement, 546
  failure of activation, 559
Complementary therapies, *see* Alternative/complementary therapies
Compliance
  asthma therapy, *76*
  chronic renal failure, 321
  glaucoma therapy, 480
  lung, 61
Compression
  bandaging, 281, 717–718
  pumps, 281
  sequential pneumatic, 784
  sleeves, 281
  stockings, *see* Stockings, elastic support/compression
Computed tomography (CT scan), *373*
  bladder cancer, *313*
  neurological disorders, 207, 346, 352, 356, 364
Conducting system of heart, 11–12
Conduction, heat transfer by, *684*
Cone biopsy, 235–236
Cone cells, 468
Confidentiality, 557–558, *593*, 996, 1002
Confusion, 841–843, 845
  elderly, **963–965**
  terminally ill patients, 929, 931
  urinary incontinence and, 733
Congenital abnormalities
  mouth, **523–525**
  prenatal diagnosis, 193–194, *197*, *199*
  psychological impact, 197
Congenital adrenal hyperplasia (CAH), **151–152**
Coning (brain herniation), 337, **338–339**
Conjunctiva, 469
  assessment, 470–471
Conjunctivitis, 431, **485**
Consanguinity, 192
Consciousness
  anatomical and physiological basis, **840–841**
  clouding of, 841–843
  content, **841**
  definition, **839–840**
  impaired, **841–844**
    acute states, 841–843
    causes, *843*, **846–847**
    chronic states, 844
    CNS infections, 364
    diabetic ketoacidosis, 168
    hyperglycaemic hyperosmolar non-ketotic coma, 170
    raised intracranial pressure, *331*, 338, 339
    shock, 611
    stroke, *345*
  recovery, after anaesthesia, 791

Consciousness (*contd*)
  see also Coma; Unconscious patients
Consent, informed, *778*, **780**
  breast surgery, 264
  HIV antibody testing, 999
  hysterectomy, 238
  nurse's role, 780
  resolving dilemmas, 781
  transurethral resection of prostate, 308
Constipation, *112*, **739**
  enteral feeding causing, *672*
  haemorrhoids and, 111
  laryngectomy patients, 514
  Parkinson's disease, 362
  post-gastrectomy, 100
  prevention, *112*, 733
  relieving, 732–733
  terminally ill patients, 929, 931
  urinary incontinence and, 728, 732–733
Contact lenses, 473, *485*, *490*
Continence, **723–741**
  advisory services, **734**, 735
  definition, 724
  urinary, 723–739
    acquisition, 724
    delay in achieving, 726–727
    problem-solving approach to promotion, 728–734
    see also Urinary incontinence
Continence advisors, **734**
Continuous ambulatory peritoneal dialysis (CAPD), **321–322**
Contraception, 180, **249**
Contractility, myocardial, *601*
Contrecoup injury, *340*
Control
  critically ill patients, 835–836
  disability and, 946, 955
  locus of, 179
Contusions, brain, *340*
Convection, heat transfer by, 683, *684*
Convergence, 470
Conversion, *586*
Convulsions
  febrile, *689*
  see also Seizures
Coping, 577, **585–587**, 594
  indirect, *897*
  models, 585
  myocardial infarction, 28
  personality and, 585–586
  process model, 587
Copper, *661*
Cornea, 468
  assessment, 471
  foreign bodies, 489
  rust rings, *489*
Corneal abrasion, 489–490
Corneal grafting (keratoplasty), **481–482**, 489
Corneal reflex, 857
Coronary angiography, 16, *17*
Coronary angioplasty, percutaneous transluminal (PTCA), 20–21
Coronary artery bypass grafting (CABG), 21–22
Coronary blood supply, **10**, *11*
Coronary care units (CCUs), 24–26, 828, 829
Coronary heart disease, *see* Ischaemic heart disease
Corpus callosum, 327, *328*
Corpus luteum, 212–213, 215
Corrosive agents, *see* Acids; Alkalis
Corticobulbar tracts, *335*
Corticospinal tracts, *335*
Corticosteroids, 137, *138*
Corticosteroid (steroid) therapy
  adrenal cortex hypofunction, 149–150
  asthma, 73
  dental treatment and, 526
  eczema, 453
  eye drops/ointment, *476*
  intracranial tumours, 352, 931
  rheumatoid arthritis, 396
  temporal arteritis, 483
  toxic epidermal necrolysis, 459
Corticotrophin-releasing hormone (CRH), *135*, 581
Cortisol (hydrocortisone), 137, *138*
  blood glucose regulation, 155–156
  circadian rhythms, *149*
  replacement therapy, 142, 149–150
  shock, 599
  stress response, 581–582
Cost-effectiveness, wound-dressing materials, 712
Costs
  cardiovascular disease, 9
  chronic illness, 911
Council for Involuntary Tranquilliser Addiction, 989
Counselling, **767**
  A & E staff, 823–824
  AIDS/HIV infection, 999, **1000–1001**
  amputation of limb, 389
  cancer, 897
  genetic, *see* Genetic counselling
  infertility, 255–257, 259
  pre-vasectomy, 230–231
  rheumatoid arthritis, 397
  sexual, 739
  termination of pregnancy, 253
Cowper's (bulbourethral) glands, 296
Cox's man–environment interaction model, 578
Cranial arteritis, **483**
Cranial nerves, *330*, 336
  involved in swallowing, *523*
  motor responses, 857
Craniectomy, *341*
Craniopharyngioma, *351*
Craniotomy, *341*
Crash helmets, 813
Creams, *446*
Creatinine–height index (CHI), 665
Creatinine phosphokinase (CPK), *24*
Cretinism, 146
Cricoid pressure, *83*
Critical care units, *see* Intensive care units (ICUs)
Critically ill patients, **827–837**
  care of relatives/friends, 837
  environment, 828–833
  health, 833
  nursing care, 833–836
  oral hygiene, **528–529**
  the person, 827–828
Crockery, potentially infected, 564
Crohn's disease (CD), **102–104**, 113, *530*
  surgical intervention, 102–104, 778, *779*
Crossinfection, 549
Cross-tolerance, 974
CRUSE, 596, 819, 825
Cryoprecipitate, 203, *410*
Cryotherapy
  pre-invasive cervical carcinoma, 235
  retinal detachment, 480
Cryptococcus infections, 1006
Cryptomenorrhoea, **221–222**
Cryptorchidism, **227–228**, 229
Cryptosporidiosis, 1006
Crystalloids, 605, 653
  combined with colloids, 606
CSF, *see* Cerebrospinal fluid
CT scan, *see* Computed tomography
Culture, pain and, 616, 621–622
Curettage, 260
Cushing's disease, 140, 148, *352*
Cushing's syndrome, *143*, **148–149**, *150*, 220
  investigations, 148, *149*
  nursing care plan, 151
Cushing's triad, *339*
CVA, *see* Stroke
Cyanosis, central/peripheral, 72
Cyclophosphamide, *892*, *895*
Cystectomy, total, and urinary diversion, 314, **315–316**
  complications, *316*
  nursing care plan, 317
Cystic fibrosis (CF), 84, **199–202**
  case histories, *201*, *203*
  clinical features, 199–200
  medical management, 200–201
  nursing priorities and management, 201–202
Cystic fibrosis transmembrane regulatory (CFTR) gene, 200, 202
Cystine stones, *299*
Cystiris, 297, **298**, 738–739
  radiotherapy-induced, *890*
Cystocele, 247, 248
  repair, 248–249
Cystoscopy, *301*, *313*, 731
Cytokines, 689
Cytomegalovirus (CMV)
  AIDS/HIV infection, 1006
  retinitis, 495, 1006
Cytosine arabinoside (Ara C), 431, *895*
Cytotoxic chemotherapy, **891–893**, *894*, *895*
Cytotoxic T cells, 546, *548*

D

Danazol, 226–227
Day case surgery, 776, 804
DDAVP (desmopressin), *142*, 143, 738, 741
Deafness, **499–501**, 762
  conductive, 499
  nursing priorities and management, 500–501
  sensorineural, 499, 500
Death, **936–938**
  brain-stem, **855–857**
  cause of, in cancer, 880
  certificate, 938
  fear of, *see* Fear, of dying
  at home, 938
  nurses' attitudes, 969
  nurses' reactions, 591–592, 819, 939–940, 1007–1008
  patient with infectious disease, 564
  quality of, **925–926**
  sudden, 31–32, **818–819**
    care of relatives, 818–819
    organ donation, 818
    role of stress, 582
    spiritual needs, 818
    staff grief, 819
  unconscious patients, **855–857**
Debridement, *698*, 706, **707–708**
  burn wounds, **869**
  chemical, 707–708
  enzymatic agents, 708

Debridement (*contd*)
fungating breast tumours, 283
pressure sores, 713
surgical, 708
Defaecation, 90, 739
unconscious patients, 853
Defence mechanisms, *586*, **587**
Defibrillation (DC shock), 32, *33*
Dehiscence, *698*
Dehydration, **641**
diabetic ketoacidosis, 166
enteral feeding and, *672*
hyperglycaemic hyperosmolar non-ketotic coma, 170
wound healing and, 702
Delayed union, fractures, *382*
Deletions, chromosomal, 191
Delirium, 843
Delusions, 843
Dementia, 844, 925, 963
AIDS, 1007
urinary incontinence, 733
Demographic shift, 961
Demography, 919
Demonstration centres, 956
Dendritic ulcer, 484, 485
Denial, *586*, *925*
pain, 627
Dental caries, 525, 526, *890*
Dental disease, **526**
see also Orodental disease
Dental floss, 526
Dental health
changing patterns, 525
promotion, **525–526**, 528–529
Dental hygiene, 91, 525–526
see also Oral hygiene
Dental hygienist, 539
Dental plaque, 526
Dental surgery, 526, *527*
Dentist, 539
Dentition, constipation and, *112*
Dentures, 91, 528
Deodorisers, fungating breast tumours, 283
Dependence, drug, 622, 974
Dependence/independence continuum, 915
Dependency problems, **973–989**
approaching patient with suspected, 977
assessment, 977–978
definitions, 974
identifying, 976
illegal substances, 984–986
legal substances, 978–984
model for changing behaviour, 974–975
nurses in, 976–977
nurse's role, 975–978
prevention, 978
support agencies, 986–987
see also Alcohol abuse
Depilatory creams, 785
Depression, 582, **583–584**, *925*
after breast surgery, 263
drug therapy, 588–589
insomnia, 749–750
pain and, 620
terminally ill patients, 926
tinnitus and, *504*
Depressives Anonymous, 596
Dermatitis, *see* Eczema
Dermatome, 632
Dermis, 445–446
Dermoid cyst (cystic teratoma)
intracranial, *351*
ovarian, 242, **245**
Desmopressin (DDAVP), *142*, 143, 738, 741
Detoxification, 974
Dexamethasone suppression test, *149*
Dextran, 605–606
Dextrose solutions, 605
Diabetes insipidus, **143–144**, 643
nephrogenic, 142
Diabetes mellitus, **155–185**, *913*
achieving and maintaining normoglycaemia, 159–163
classification, 155
complications, 158, **165–177**, *530*, 909
acute metabolic, 165–172
chronic, 48, 53, 173–177, 347
Cushing's syndrome, *148*, 151
dental surgery, 526
eye disorders, **173–174**, 494
information sources/useful addresses, 184–185
insulin-dependent (IDDM; type I), 155, **157–158**, 173
aetiology, 157
insulin therapy, 161–163
pathophysiology, 157–158
management strategies, 159–182
maturity onset, of the young (MODY), 158
monitoring glycaemic control, 164–165
non-insulin-dependent (NIDDM; type II), 155, **158–159**, 167, 173
aetiology, 158
management, 160–161, 165
pathophysiology, 158–159
patient education, 171, **178**
primary, 155, **156–159**
psychological and social adjustment, 179–181
secondary, 127, 155, **159**
trends in health care provision, 181–182
Diabetic foot, **175–177**, *719*
Diabetic ketoacidosis (DKA), 157, 158, **165–167**
medical management, 166–167
nursing care plan, 168–169
nursing priorities and management, 167, 171
pathophysiology, 165–166
Diabetic maculopathy, 173
Diabetic nephropathy, **174–175**
Diabetic neuropathy, **175**, *176*
Diabetic nurse specialists, 178, 182
Diabetic retinopathy, **173–174**, **494**
background, 173, 494
proliferative, 173, 494
Dialect, 759–760
Dialysis, 174, **321–322**
Diamorphine, 25
Diarrhoea, **654**
AIDS/HIV infection, *1005*, 1006
enteral feeding causing, *672*, 853
faecal incontinence, 739
infectious, 565, *566*
inflammatory bowel disease, 102, 103
malabsorption syndrome, 101–102
oral rehydration therapy, 654
post-gastrectomy, 100
postoperative, 800
radiotherapy-induced, *890*
Diasrole, 12
Diastolic pressure, 14
Diathermy
bladder tumours, *314*
fungating breast tumours, 283
patient safety, *787*, 789
pre-invasive cervical carcinoma, 235
Diazepam, *786*
Diclofenac sodium, 300
Dideoxyosine (ddI), 1007
DIDMOAD syndrome, 159
Diencephalon, **328–329**
Diet
angina pectoris, 18–19
breast cancer, 286
bullous skin disorders, 459
cancer aetiology and, 109, 267, 881
cerebrovascular disease, 348
constipation and, *112*
dental health and, 525
diverticular disease and, 104
eczema, 454
gastrectomy patients, 100
head injury, 343
healthy, **658–659**
heart failure, 40
hypertension, 46
inflammatory bowel disease, 102
liver disease, 119
multiple sclerosis and, 359
myocardial infarction, 28, 31
peptic ulceration and, 96
peripheral arterial disease, 53
prolapsed intervertebral disc, 395
psoriasis, 451
renal disease, 318, 321
rheumatoid arthritis, 397
sleep and, 750–751
valvular heart disease, 42
venous disease, 55
weight-reducing, 663
see also Food(s); Nutrition
Dietary therapy, **662–664**
diabetes mellitus, **160**
Diet-induced thermogenesis (DIT), 686
Dietitians, 160, 433, 539
Differentiation, 904
Difflam (benzydamine), 529
Diffuse brain injury, *340*
Diffusion, *322*
Digestion, 88–89
Digestive tract, *see* Gastrointestinal system
Digoxin, 38, 647
1,25-Dihydroxycholecalciferol, *137*, 294
Dilatation and curettage, 222, 223–224, 252
Dilatation and evacuation of uterine contents, 253
Dining areas, 668
Dinner fork deformity, *383*
Diplopia, **486**
Dip-sticks, 164
Disability, **906**, 919, 944
disorders causing, *945*
elderly, **967–969**
further disease generated by, 909–910
nerve injuries, 402–103
psychology, **945–946**
rheumatoid arthritis, 397
social attitudes, 906–907
unemployment and, 906
see also Chronic illness; Physical handicap; Rehabilitation
Disability Rights Handbook, 950, 958
Disabled Living Foundation, 404, 958
Disablement Resettlement Officers, 947, 952
Disaster planning, 823
Disasters, major, **823–824**
Discharge
hospital–home liaison, *see* Liaison, hospital–home
minor trauma, 821–822
respiratory disorders, *84*
wound management and, 711

Discharge planning
amputation, 391
aplastic anaemia, 421
CNS infections, 365
colorectal cancer, 111
head injury, 344
hernia repair, 109
hysterectomy, 240
intracranial tumours, 353
intraocular surgery, 479
iron deficiency anaemia, 416
joint replacement, 399–401
laryngectomy, 515
leukaemia, 433
mastectomy patients, 275
multiple sclerosis, 359–360
myeloma, 438
myocardial infarction, 26–28
oral tumours, 540
orofacial trauma, 536
Parkinson's disease, 362–363
peptic ulcer surgery, 98
postoperative, **804–805**
terminally ill patients, 935
thrombocytopenia, 440
tonsillectomy, 518
total cystectomy and urinary diversion, 316
tracheostomy patients, 517
transurethral resection of prostate, 311
urinary stones, 302
uterine prolapse repair, 249
vascular surgery, 53, 57
Discogram, *373*
Disease, 4–5, 906, 960
cancer susceptibility and, 880
malnutrition and, 663–664
sleep problems and, 750
stress and, **582–585**
wound healing and, 702
Disfigurement, 763, 872
Disinfectants, chemical, 552–553, 565
Disinfection, **551–553**, *554*
policies, 564–565
Displacement, *586*
Disposal, safe, **553–554**
linen, 554, *555*
waste, 553–554, *555*, 1003
Disseminated disease, 904
Disseminated intravascular coagulation (DIC), 599, **613–614**
Disseminated sclerosis, *see* Multiple sclerosis
Distraction, 630
District nurses
AIDS/HIV infection and, 997
cancer care, 896–897
wound management, 710, 711
see also Community nurses
Dithranol, 450
Diuretics
angina pectoris, 20
ascites, 117
cardiogenic shock, 34
heart failure, 38, 40
hypertension, 45, 46
nephrotic syndrome, 319
premenstrual syndrome, 227
Diverticular disease, **104–105**
DNA, 188, 993
fingerprinting, 188, 189
linkage testing, *193*
recombinant (rDNA), 189
Dobutamine, 606
Documentation, *see* Records
Do-not-resuscitate (DNR) orders, 32, 833
Dopamine, 137, 360, 606
Dopexamine hydrochloride, 606
Doppler ultrasound, 51, 717, 718
Dorsal horn, 617
Dovonex, 450
Down's syndrome, 188, **199**
Down's Syndrome Association, 210
Doxorubicin (Adriamycin), 431, *892*, 893, *895*
Dressing (in clothes)
CNS infections, 365
disabled patients, 951
multiple sclerosis, 359
nerve injuries, 402
Parkinson's disease, 362
unconscious patients, 853
see also Clothing
Dressings, 706
breast reconstruction, 280
bullous skin disorders, 460
burn wounds, 862, **870**
cavity wounds, 705–706
changing
postoperative patients, *799*, 801, 802
techniques, **708–710**
characteristics of ideal, *707*
eye, 477
fungating breast tumours, 283, 284–286
mastectomy, 275
materials, 708, *709–710*
cost-effectiveness, 712
future, 708
provision in community, 711
odour-absorbing, 935
stump, 389, *390*
venous leg ulcers, 718
Drink Crisis Centre, 989
Drinking, *see* Eating/drinking
Drinkwatchers, 987
Driving
diabetes mellitus, 181
epilepsy, 354
valvular heart disease, 43
Drop foot, 375
Drowsing, 745
Drug(s)
definition, 974
dependence, 622, 974
overdose, **847**, *848*
self-administration by elderly, *29*
unconscious patients and, 854
Drug abuse, 974
Drug-induced disorders
blood disorders, 405–406
constipation, *112*
critically ill patients, 829–830
diabetes mellitus, 159
hearing loss, 500
hepatitis, *114*, 116
impaired wound healing, 703
sleep problems, 751, *754*
urinary incontinence, 728
Drug misuse/drug-related problems, *see* Dependency problems
Duchenne muscular dystrophy, 205
Dumping syndrome, 98
Duodenal ileus, *126*
Duodenal ulcer, *see* Peptic ulcer
Duodenum, 89
disorders, **96–100**
Dura mater, 329, *332*
Dying patients, *see* Terminally ill patients
Dysmenorrhoea, **223–225**
primary, 223–224
secondary, 223, 224–225
Dyspareunia, 260
Dyspepsia, 96
Dysphagia (swallowing problems), 91, 667
anaemia, 412, 415
Huntington's disease, 208
multiple sclerosis, 359
oesophageal disease, 93, **94–95**
Parkinson's disease, 362
radiotherapy-induced, *890*
stroke, 348
tracheostomy and, 517
Dyspnoea (breathlessness)
anaemia, 412, 414
heart failure, 39, 40
myocardial infarction, 26, 28
terminally ill patients, 932
valvular heart disease, 42
Dystrophic Epidermolysis Bullosa Research Association (DEBRA), 449, 465

E

Ear, **497–498**
external, 497
disorders, **498–499**
foreign bodies, **499**
inner, 498
disorders, **504–506**
middle, 497–498
disorders, **501–504**
oedema, facial burns, 871
syringing, 499
Ear, nose and throat (ENT) disorders, **497–520**
Earwax (cerumen) excess, **498–499**
Eating disorders, **137–139**
Eating/drinking, 657, **666–669**
aids, 667
assisting patients, 668–669
body temperature and, 686
cancer patients, 899
disabled patients, 950–951, 967, *968*
factors influencing, 666–667
head injury, 343
laryngectomy patients, 514
maxillofacial fractures and, 535
mealtime organisation and, 667–668
multiple sclerosis, 359
oral disease and, *536*
Parkinson's disease, 362
resumption after parenteral nutrition, 676
stroke, 348
terminally ill patients, 932–933
tonsillectomy patients, 518
unconscious patients, 852–853
visually impaired, 474
see also Diet; Nutrition
Eating out, diabetes mellitus, 181
ECG, *see* Electrocardlography
Echocardiogram, 55
Ectopic pregnancy, **246–247**
Ectropion, **492–493**
Eczema (dermatitis), **451–454**
allergic contact, 452
asteatotic, 451–452
atopic, 451
endogenous, 451
exogenous, 452
irritant, 452
medical management, 452–453
nursing priorities and management, 453–454
pathophysiology, 452

Eczema (*contd*)
  photo-contact, 461
  photosensitive/actinic reticuloid syndrome, 461, *462*
  pompholyx, 451
  seborrhoeic, AIDS/HIV infection, *1005*
  varicose, 452
Eczema herpeticum, 458
Edentulous patients, 91, 666
Education, health, *see* Health education
Education, patient, **769**
  aplastic anaemia, 421
  asthma, *74*, *76*, *78*
  benign mammary dysplasia, 288
  breast cancer, 263–264, 271, 282, 286–287
  breast reconstruction, 280
  diabetes mellitus, 171, **178**
  diabetic complications, 494
  disabled, 952–953
  emphysema, 73
  hepatitis B, *567*
  iron deficiency anaemia, 416
  leg ulcers, 719
  leukaemia, 433
  multiple sclerosis, 359
  myeloma, 438
  myocardial infarction, 27, *29*
  myotonic dystrophy, 206–207
  oral tumours, 541
  polycythaemia, 425–426
  postoperative, 804
  pressure sore prevention, 715
  respiratory disorders, *84*
  rheumatoid arthritis, 397
  salmonellosis, *566*
  stoma formation, *104*
  see also Information, giving
Education/training
  health professionals, pain management and, 621
  nurses, 5–6, 591
  role of genetic nurse specialist, 194–195
Eggs, *see* Oocytes
Ehlers–Danlos syndrome, 47
Eighth (vestibulo-cochlear) nerve, *330*
Ejaculation, 296
  disorders of, *256*
  retrograde, 308, *310*
Ejaculatory duct, *295*, *296*
Elastic cartilage, 370
Elastic garments, pressure therapy of burns, 872
Elastin, 446, *698*, *699*
Elastoplast kit, skin traction, *377*
Elderly, **959–970**
  alcohol consumption, 982
  body temperature, 685
  caring for, 961
  dental health promotion, 528
  disability, **967–969**
  eating/drinking problems, 666–667
  eye changes, 473
  eye disorders, 491–493
  femoral neck fractures, 380–381
  heart failure, 41
  hypothermia, *see* Hypothermia, elderly
  iron deficiency anaemia, 416
  nursing care, 963–970
  orofacial trauma, 536
  pain experience, 616
  rehabilitation, 805
  self-administration of medicines, *29*
  skin tumours, 444
  sleep, 744, 748–749
  surgery, 776
  terminal illness, 923
  urinary incontinence, 728, 733, 734, *964*, 965
  wound healing, 702
Electrical hazards, intensive care units, 830
Electrocardiography (ECG), **12**
  angina, 16
  heart failure, 38
  myocardial infarction, 23, 25
  shock, 608
Electroencephalography (EEG), 346
  sleep, 744–746
Electrolyte balance, **637–655**
  assessment, 650
  bullous skin disorders, 460
  diabetic ketoacidosis, 166–167, 168
  gastrointestinal disorders, **653–654**
  hyperglycaemic hyperosmolar non-ketotic coma, 170
  liver failure, 119
  myocardial infarction, 31
  nursing priorities and management, **650–653**
  postoperative, 655
  renal disease, 318, 320
  total cystectomy and urinary diversion, 317
  transurethral resection of prostate, 310
Electrolytes, **638–639**, **644–647**
  homeostasis, **640–641**
  parenteral nutrition, 674, *675*
  therapy, 651–653
  see also Calcium; Minerals; Potassium; Sodium
Electromechanical dissociation (EMD), 31, *33*, 55
Electromyography (EMG), 206, *373*
Electrons, 886
Electro-oculogram (EOG), 745
Electroretinography, 206
Eleventh (accessory) nerve, *330*, *523*
Elimination
  angina pectoris, 20
  aortic aneurysms and, 48
  disabled, 951
  habits, constipation and, *112*
  head injury, 343
  heart failure, 40
  hypertension, 46
  multiple sclerosis, 358–359
  myocardial infarction and, 31
  Parkinson's disease, 362
  rheumatoid arthritis, 397
  stroke, 348
  surgical patients, **800**
  terminally ill patients, 933–934
  unconscious patients, 853
Embolectomy, 52
Emboli, 15
  post-myocardial infarction, 34
  subacute bacterial endocarditis, **41**
Embolisation, hepatic tumours, *120*
Embolism, 55
  air, 674
  cerebral, 344
  fat, 379–380, *382*
  pulmonary, *see* Pulmonary embolism
Embryo research, **259**
Embryo transfer (ET), 247, 257, 258
Emergencies
  immediate treatment, **811–812**
  respiratory, **79–82**
Emergency surgery, 776, *779*
Emmetropia, *470*
Emollients, 450, 453, 464
Emotional deprivation, *143*
Emotional responses
  bereavement, 937–938
  cancer, 901
  loss and change, 924–925
  stroke patients, *345*, 347
  terminal illness, 925–926, 929
  see also Psychological impact
Emphysema
  alveolar, 70, *71*
  centrilobar, 70, 71
  pulmonary, 66, **70–73**
    medical management, 71
    nursing priorities and management, 71–73
    pathophysiology, 70–71
  surgical, 517
Employment
  amputation and, 391
  angina and, 18, 19
  chronic illness and, 906, 910
  diabetes mellitus, 181
  disabled, 952, 956
  epilepsy, 354
  heart failure, 40
  hypertension, 46
  laryngectomy patients, 515
  multiple sclerosis, 358
  nerve injuries, 403
  oral tumours and, 541
  peripheral vascular disease, 53, 55
  rheumatoid arthritis, 397
  valvular heart disease, 42–43
  visual impairment and, 473–474
Empyema, subdural, 363
Encephalitis, viral, 363
Endocarditis
  rheumatic, 41
  subacute bacterial (SBE), 41
Endocardium, 10
Endocrine disorders, 133–134, **137–152**
  affecting mouth, *530*
  amenorrhoea, 220
  see also specific disorders
Endocrine system, **133–153**
  anatomy and physiology, 134–137
Endocrine therapy, 629, 894
  breast cancer, 270–271, 276, 277–278, 283
  endometrial carcinoma, 241
  prostatic cancer, 312
Endometrial carcinoma (carcinoma of body of uterus), 222, **239–241**
Endometrial cycle, **215–216**
Endometrial polyps, 222, 224, **244**
Endometriosis, 222, 224, 254
Endometrium, 214
  disorders, *255*
  primary deficiency, 219
Endorphins, 226, 581
Endoscopes, disinfection, 553
Endoscopic retrograde cholangiopancreatography (ERCP), *93*, 121, 123, 125, 128
Endoscopic sphincterotomy, 121, 123
Endoscopy, gastrointestinal, *93*, 102
Endothelial cells, *699*
Endotoxins, 602, 704
Endotracheal (ET) tubes, 83, 811, **850**
  extubation, *83*
Endotracheal intubation, *83*
Energy, 659
  requirements, *660*
Enteral feeding, **669–672**
  burns, 868
  complications, 671–672, 852–853

Enteral feeding *(contd)*
indications, 669
infection control, 557
inflammatory bowel disease, 102
intermittent, bolus or continuous, 670–671
laryngectomy patients, 513–514
nasoenteral, 669–670
selection of feeds, 670
unconscious patients, 852–853
Enterocele, 248
Enterogastric reflex, 89
Enterogastrone, *89*
Enterostomies, 669
Entonox, 629, 790, 816
Entropion, **492**, 493
Enucleation, eye, 490, 491
Enuresis, 725
nocturnal, 725, 726–727, **738**
Enuresis Resource and Information Centre (ERIC), 738, 741
Enzymatic agents, debridement, 708
Eosinophils, *407*, 545
Ependymoma, *350*
Epidermis, 445
Epidermoid cyst, *351*
Epididymis, 295, *296*
disorders, *256*
Epididymo-orchitis, *232*
Epidural anaesthesia/analgesia, 790, *799*
Epilepsy, **353–356**, 847
case histories, *357*, *916*
medical management, 353
nursing priorities and management, 353–356
pathophysiology, 353
see also Seizures
Epilepsy Association, 355
Epispadias, **306**
Epistaxis, **506–508**, 509–510
medical management, 507
nursing priorities and management, 507–508
pathophysiology, 506–507
Epithalamus, 329
Epithelialisation, wounds, 699–700, 869
Epithelium, *698*
Epstein–Barr virus, 881
Equianalgesic, 632
Equipment
critical care units, 828–829, 830
disinfection, sterilisation and cleaning, **550–553**
resuscitation, organisation, 812
Ergometrine, 250, 251, 252, 253
Erythrocytes, *see* Red blood cells
Erythrocyte sedimentation rate (ESR), 23, 413, 483
Erythroderma, 452, 464
Erythropoietin, 294
Escharotomy, *864*
Escherichia coli, 549
Ethics
cardiopuimonary resuscitation, 32
genetic modification and gene therapy, 189–190
informing patients of cancer diagnosis, *884*
intensive therapy, 833
Ethinyloestradiol, *142*, 220
Ethnic differences
diabetes mellitus, 158
hypertension, 44
scarring, *702*
Etoposide, 893, *895*
Etretinate (Tigason), 451
Eugenics, 189
Euphemism, 759
European Wound Management Association, 722
Evaluation, nursing interventions, 918
Evaporation, heat transfer by, 683, *684*
Evening primrose oil, 226, 454
Evisceration, eye, 490
Examination under anaesthetic (EUA), 237
Excitation–contraction coupling, heart, 12
Excoriation, 464
Exenteration
eye, 490
pelvic, 237
Exercise
angina pectoris, 18
body temperature and, 685
constipation and, *112*
cystic fibrosis, 201
diabetes mellitus, *178*
multiple sclerosis, 358
myocardial infarction, 27, 29–30
Parkinson's disease, 361
post-hysterectomy, 238
rheumatoid arthritis, 396–397
sleep and, 749
stress and, 589–590
terminally ill patients, 934
valvular heart disease, 42
see also Activity, physical; Mobility/mobilisation
Exercises
active, 855
active-assistive, 855
after breast surgery, 275, 280
breathing, 781
head injury, 343
hyperglycaemic hyperosmolar non-ketotic coma, 171
isometric, 365
lymphoedema in breast cancer, 282
nerve injuries, 402
passive, 855
patients in plaster casts, *378*
pelvic floor, **731**
postoperative, 784
range-of-movement (ROM), 854–855
traction and, 375
venous leg ulcers, 718, *719*
see also Physiotherapy
Exercise tolerance test, 16
Exfoliation, 464
Expiratory reserve volume (ERV), 61, *63*
External fixation, **378–379**
maxillofacial fractures, 532–533, 535
tibia and fibula fractures, 381
Extracellular fluid (ECF), 638
exchange with intracellular fluid, 639
tissue–capillary fluid exchange, 639
volume
adjustments, 643
deficit, *see* Hypovolaemia
excess, *see* Fluid retention
regulation, **640–641**
Extracorporeal shock wave lithotripsy (ESWL), 300–301, 302
Extradural abscess, 363
Extradural haematoma, *340*
Extrapyramidal tracts, 334, *335*
Extravasation, cytotoxic agents, *893*, *894*
Exudate, *698*
burn wounds, 869
cavity wounds, 706
fungating wounds/tumours, 283, 720, 935
infection control precautions, 564
Eye, **468–470**
accessory structures, 469
age-related changes, 473
anatomy, 468–469
artificial, **490–492**, *491*
care, unconscious patients, 853
examination, **470–471**, 473, 475
after corneal grafting, 482
after retinal surgery, 481
perioperative, 476–477
foreign bodies in, 487
hot spoon bathing, *486*
irrigation, 475, *489*
opening, Glasgow Coma Scale, 844
padding, 475
physiology of vision, 469–470
red, **483–486**
surgical removal, **490–492**
Eye contact, **760**, 765–766
aggressive patients, 822
disorders affecting, 763
Eye disorders, 467–468, **474–495**
age-related, **492**
AIDS, 495
diabetes mellitus, **173–174**, **492–494**
general nursing procedures, 474–475
inflammatory, **490**
perioperative nursing care, 475–477
systemic diseases, **492–495**
Eye drops/ointment, 475, 480
Eye injuries, 473, **486–490**, 534
chemical burns, 489
minor, 489–490
penetrating, 487–488
radiation-induced, 489
Eyelet wiring, fractured mandible, 532
Eyelids, 469
assessment, 470, *471*
cleansing, 475
eversion, *490*
Eye testing charts, *471*
Eyewear, protective, *473*, 487, 489

F

Face
bones, 523, *524*
burns, 532, **870–871**
congenital deformities, 523–525
middle third fracture, *531*
soft tissue injuries, 531, 532
Face masks, burns, 872
Facial expression, 760
disorders affecting, 763
Facial injuries, *see* Orofacial trauma
Facial nerve, *330*, *523*
paralysis/palsy, 503, *529*, 763
Facial paralysis, stroke, *345*
Facioscapulohumeral dystrophy, 205
Factor IX, *410*
deficiency, 202
Factor VIII
deficiency, 202, 203
synthetic, 205
treatment, 204, 205
Faecal incontinence, **739**, 933–934
Fallopian tubes, *see* Uterine tubes
Falx cerebri, 329, *332*
Families Anonymous, 987, 989
Family
acute pancreatitis and, 127
AIDS patients, 1007

Family *(contd)*
bereaved, 818–819, 937–938
cancer patients, 898–899
critically ill patients, 833, 835, 837
diabetes mellitus and, 179–180
diabetic emergencies, 169, 171
disabled patients, 952
elderly, 969
epilepsy, 355–356
head-injured patients, 342, 343, 344
intracranial tumours and, 353
legal rights, 780
multiple trauma, **816–817**
myocardial infarction and, 26
oral cancer and, 539–540
pain and, 625
Parkinson's disease, 360
rheumatoid arthritis and, *398*
terminally ill patients, 857, 922, **936**
unconscious patients, 851–852, 857
see also Carers
Family planning, 180, **249**
Family trees, 194, *195*
Faradism, 731, 741
Farmer's lung, **560**
Fasting
postoperative, 797
preoperative, 664, **784–785**
Fat (adipose tissue), brown (BAT), 685, 693
Fat embolism, 379–380, *382*
Fatigue
anaemia, 412, 414
breast cancer therapy and, 275, 276
chronic renal failure, 321
diabetes mellitus, 157, 158
inflammatory bowel disease, 103
multiple sclerosis, 358
post-viral, 115, **585**
radiotherapy-induced, *889*
terminally ill patients, 934
Fats, *see* Lipids
Fatty acids, polyunsaturated (PUFA), *661*
Fear
AIDS/HIV infection, 998
of cancer, 881
of dying
cardiovascular disease, 19–20, 30–31, 48
nurses, 592
terminally ill patients, 926
Febrile convulsions, *689*
Feeding
patients, 668
symbolic, *936*
see also Eating/drinking; Nutrition
Female infertility, 254, *255*
Female reproductive system
anatomy and physiology, 211–217
disorders, **234–249**
post-menopausal changes, 216–217
Female sterilisation, 254, 260
Femoral hernia, 108, *109*
Femoral neck fractures, **380–381**
Femoral shaft fractures, **379–380**
Fertilisation, 296
Fetal alcohol syndrome, 981
Fetal blood sampling, 194
Fetal viability, 249, 260
Fever, *see* Pyrexia, **688–690**
Fibre, dietary, 658
constipation and, *112*, 733
diabetes mellitus and, 160
gastrointestinal disease and, 104, 109
Fibrin clot formation, 408
Fibroblasts, 699
Fibrocartilage, 370
Fibrocystic breast disease (mammary dysplasia), **287–288**
Fibromyomata, uterine, 222, 224, **244–245**
Fibronectin, 699
Fibrosis, around ureters, **304–305**
Fibula, fracture, **381**
Fifth (trigeminal) nerve, *330*, *523*
'Fight or flight' reaction, *see* Stress, response
Figure-of-eight bandage, **383**, *384*
Filtration, *322*
Financial aid
cancer, 898
incontinence, 735
Fine-needle aspiration cytology, breast, 269–270
Fingertip stimulation, 844, *845*
First-aid treatment
burns, 607, **861–862**
chest injuries, 80
shock, **607**, *608*
spinal injuries, 384, *388*
unconscious patients, *847*, *848*
First (olfactory) nerve, *330*, *523*
Fish oil capsules, 451
Fissure in ano (anal fissure), *112*, **113**, 733
Fissures, skin, 452
Fistula in ano, **113**
Fistulae
arteriovenous (AV), *322*
tracheo-oesophageal, *513*
upper GI tract, *669*
urinary, 297
vaginal, *779*, 804
Flail chest, **79–80**
Flaps, free, *540*
Fleas, **456**
Flexion contractures, post-amputation, 389
Fluid
compartments, **638**
exchange, **639**
extracellular (ECF), *see* Extracellular fluid
interstitial, 638, 639
intracellular (ICF), 638, 639
intravascular, 638
transcellular, 638
volume adjustments, 643
see also Body fluids; Water
Fluid balance, **637–655**
acute renal failure, 320
assessment, 650
bullous skin disorders, 460
charts, 651
CNS infections, 365
disorders, **641–643**
ectopic pregnancy, 247
gastrointestinal disorders, **653–654**
glomerulonephritis, 318
heart failure, 40
hysterectomy, 239
inflammatory bowel disease, 103
liver failure, 119
monitoring, **651**
myocardial infarction, 31
nursing priorities and management, **650–653**
postoperative, 655, **794–795**
psoriasis, 450
septicaemic shock, 603
total cystectomy a~d urinary diversion, 317
transurethral resection of prostate, 310
Fluid intake, 651–652
ascites, 117
burns, 868
chronic renal failure, 321
excessive, 643
head injury, 343
multiple sclerosis, 358–359
raised intracranial pressure, 340
terminally ill patients, 932–933
urinary stones, 299, 302
Fluid overload, 643
blood transfusion, 418
enteral feeding and, *672*
hyperglycaemic hyperosmolar non-ketotic coma, 170
Fluid retention (volume excess), *642*, **643**
heart failure, 38
premenstrual, 225
Fluid therapy, **651–653**
aims, 651
intravenous, *see* Intravenous (i.v.) fluid therapy
routes, 651–652
volume and content, 651
Fluoride, 526
5-Fluorouracil, *895*
Focal seizures, *355*
Folate, 416, *420*
deficiency, 416, 418, **419–420**, *659*
dietary requirements, *661*
supplements, 419
Folinic acid, *892*
Follicle-stimulating hormone (FSH), *135*, 257
deficiency, *142*
ovarian effects, 212, 213
Follicle-stimulating hormone releasing hormone (FSHRH), *see* Gonadotrophin-releasing hormone
Folliculitis, **456–457**
Food(s), 658
allergy, 454
carbohydrate values, 160
contaminants, 658
diabetic, 160
elemental, 670
enteral, **670**
groups, **659**, *661*
poisoning, 544, 565, 658
preparation, 666
presentation, 668
shopping for, 666
specific dynamic action (SDA), 686
supplementary oral/sip, 94–95, 668–669, 670, 899
see also Diet; Nutrition
Foot
athelete's (tinea pedis), **454–455**, *1005*
diabetic, **175–177**, *719*
drop, 375
Foot care, diabetes mellitus, *177*, *181*
Footwear, diabetes mellitus, *177*
Forced expiration technique (FET), 201, *202*
Forced expiratory volume (FEV), *63*
Foreign bodies
corneal, 489
ear, **499**
intraocular, 487
nose, **510–511**
oesophagus, 95
subtarsal, 489
Fornices, rodding of, *489*
Fothergill operation, 248
Fourth (trochlear) nerve, *330*
Fovea centralis, 468
Fractures, **373–386**
casts, 376–378
classification, 374
complications, *382*
first-aid treatment, 607

Fractures (*contd*)
fixation, 378–379
healing, 371
medical management, 374, 817
pathological, 373, 437
pathophysiology, 373
reduction, 374
splintage/reduced mobility, 374
stress, 373
traction, 374–376
Frank–Starling law of the heart, 13
Frohlich syndrome, 220
Frostbite, **693–694**
FSH, *see* Follicle-stimulating hormone
Functional residual capacity (FRC), 61, *63*
Funeral arrangements, 938
Fungal infections
AIDS/HIV infection, 1006
diabetes mellitus, 158
keratitis, 484–485
skin, **454–455**
see also Candidiasis
Fungating tumours/wounds, 720, 878, 935
breast cancer, **282–287**

G

Gag reflex, 857
Galen, 697
Gallbladder, 91
cancer, 124
Gallstones, *see* Cholelithiasis
Gamete intrafallopian transfer (GIFT), **258–259**
Gamma linolenic acid (GLA), 454
Gamma rays, 886
Gangrene, 51, *54*
Gaseous exchange, **62–63**, *64*
Gases, arterial blood, *see* Arterial blood gases
Gastrectomy
partial, *97*, *99*, *100*
proximal, *101*
total, *99*
Gastric carcinoma, **99–100**
Gastric juice, 88–89
Gastric ulcer, *see* Peptic ulcer
Gastric varices, 117
Gastrin, 89
Gastrinoma, 128
Gastritis, **96**
Gastrocolic reflex, 741
Gastrointestinal anastomotic leaks, *800*
Gastrointestinal (GI) disorders, 87–88, **91–113**
enteral feeding causing, *672*
fluid and electrolyte balance, **653–654**
nurse's role, 87
oral manifestations, *530*
postoperative, 49
total parenteral nutrition, 673
Gastrointestinal (GI) haemorrhage
acute pancreatitis, *126*
peptic ulcer, 98
portal hypertension, 117, 118
Gastrointestinal system, **87–131**
anatomy and physiology, 88–91
endoscopy, *93*, 102
fluid losses, 641–643
Gastrojejunostomy, *97*
Gastro-oesophageal reflux, **92**, *93*, *530*
Gastrostomy, 669
Gate control theory, **619**
Gaze, 760, 766
disorders affecting, 763
Gender
pain and, 616
sleep and, 749
Gene(s), 187, **188–189**
General Adaptation Syndrome, Selye's, **577**, 581
General anaesthesia, **790–791**
eye surgery, *490*
General practitioners (GPs), 778, 805, 810
care of bereaved, 939
stress management, 588
Gene therapy, **189–190**
ethics, 189–190
Genetic counselling, **194–198**, 424
appointments, 196
family follow-up, 196–197
pre-clinic visit/appointment, 196
preparation for, 196
procedure, 196–197
referral stage, 194
role of specialist genetic nurse, 194–195
special components, 195–196
team, 194
Genetic disorders, **187–210**, 405
categories, 191–192
classic, 198–209
diagnostic testing, 192
known, 194
Mendelian, *see* Single-gene disorders
multifactorial/polygenetic, 192
predictive/pre-symptomatic testing, 192–193
prenatal diagnosis, *see* Prenatal diagnosis
psychological impact of diagnosis, 197–198
respiratory system, 84
suspected, 194
testing for, 192–194
see also Chromosomal abnormalities
Genetic factors
breast cancer, 267
cancer, 880
diabetes mellitus, *157*, 158
hypertension, 44
obesity, 662
sleep and, 749
Genetic inheritance, *see* Inheritance
Genetic modification (engineering), **189–190**
Genetic nurse, specialist, **194–195**, 196
Genetic screening
cystic fibrosis carriers, 201
haemophilia A, 204
Huntington's disease, 208
myotonic dystrophy, 206
Genitalia, ambiguous, 151–152
Geographical variations
breast cancer, 266–267
cancer, 876
ischaemic heart disease, 9, 15
Germ cell tumours
ovarian, 242
pineal, *351*
testicular, 229
Gestures, 760–761
disorders affecting, 763
Giant cell arteritis, **482–483**
Gigantism, 139
Gingivae (gums), 521
Gingivitis, 526
acute ulcerative, 526
Girls
attitudes/knowledge of female health, *223*
termination of pregnancy, 253
Glasgow Coma Scale, 341, 841, *842*, **844–846**
Glaucoma, 467, **478–480**
diabetes mellitus, 174
primary closed-angle, **483–484**
primary open-angle (POAG), **478–480**, 481
Glial cells, 325–326
Glioblastoma multiforme, *350*
Glomerular filtration, 292–293
Glomerulonephritis, **316–318**
medical management, 318
nursing priorities and management, 318
pathophysiology, 316–318
Glossitis, 415
Glossopharyngeal nerve, *330*, *523*
Glucagon, 155, 156, 172
Glucocorticoids, 137
blood glucose regulation, 155–156
shock, 599
stress response, 581–582
therapy, *see* Corticosteroid therapy
Glucose
blood
acute pancreatitis, 124
diagnostic concentrations, *159*
monitoring, **164–165**
regulation, **155–156**
see also Hyperglycaemia; Hypoglycaemia
therapy, hypoglycaemia, 172
urinary, monitoring, 164
Glucose tolerance
impaired (IGT), 155, **159**
test, *149*
Glue ear (secretory otitis media), **501–502**
Glutamic oxaloacetic transaminase, serum (SGOT), *24*
Glutaraldehyde, 553
Glycaemic index of food, 160
Glycerine and thymol/lemon mouthwashes, 528, *933*
Glyceryl trinitrate (GTN), *17*, 18, 25, 27
Glycosuria, 157, 159, 164
Glycosylated protein estimation, **165**
Goeckerman regime, 450
Goitre
simple, 144, 145
toxic multinodular, 144
Go-lytely solution, 785
Gonadal development, abnormal, 152
Gonadotrophin-releasing hormone (GnRH; LHRH), *135*, 213
analogues, 227, 271, 277
Gonadotrophins
deficiency, 220
human menopausal (hMG), **257**
see also Follicle-stimulating hormone; Human chorionic gonadotrophin; Luteinising hormone
Goodpasture's syndrome, **561**
Government
AIDS/HIV policies, 995–996
community care initiatives, 4
policies on smoking, 66
Gram-negative bacteria, 602, *704*
Gram-positive bacteria, 602, *704*
Granulation (tissue), *698*, 701
excessive, 708
Granulocyte colony stimulating factor (GCSF), 894
Granulocytes, 407, *408*
Graves' disease, 144, *493*
Great cerebral vein, 331, *333*
Grief, 587, **924–925**, 937–938
amputation of limb, 389
anticipatory, 924–925
atypical, 925

Grief (*contd*)
ectopic pregnancy, 247
nurses/staff, 591–592, 819, 939–940, 1007–1008
sudden disability, 946
terminally ill patients, *927*
termination of pregnancy, 198
see also Bereavement; Death
Grommets, 501–502
Ground substance, *698*, 699
Group supervision, nurses, 593
Group work, AIDS/HIV infection, 1002
Growth delay
constitutional, *143*
systemic disease, *143*
Growth hormone (GH), *135*, *747*
blood glucose regulation, 155
deficiency, *142*, *143*
hypersecretion, 139
replacement therapy, 142
Growth hormone release-inhibiting hormone (GHIH), *135*, 139
Growth hormone releasing hormone (GHRH), *135*
Guedal airway, 850
Guide Dogs for the Blind Association, 496
Guilt reactions
diabetes mellitus, 179
termination of pregnancy, 198
Gums, 521
Gunning splint, 532, *533*
Gunshot wounds, 823
Gynaecological cancer, **234–243**
Gynaecomastia, 199, **288–289**

H

H_2 receptor antagonists, 96, 97
Haemangioblastoma, *351*
Haematocolpos, 221–222
Haematocrit, 413
Haematoma
after breast reconstruction, 279
intracranial, *340*
nasal septum, **510**, *531*
vaginal vault, 241
Haemoconcentration, burns, 866
Haemodialysis, 321, **322**
Haemodynamic status, monitoring, **608–610**
Haemoglobin, 406, 407
concentrations, anaemia, 412, 413
glycosylated, 165
sickle cell (HbS), 422
Haemoglobinuria, 867
Haemolysis, 441
Haemolytic anaemia, 412, **421–424**
Haemophilia, 439
HIV infection, 203, 205, 993
Haemophilia A, **202–205**
medical management, 204
nursing priorities and management, 204–205
pathophysiology, 202–203
Haemophilia B, 202, 439
Haemophilia Centre, 204, 205
Haemophilia Society, 210, 441, 1009
Haemopneumothorax, **80–81**
Haemorrhage
anaemia caused by, 424
cancer, 878
cerebral, 344
during surgery, 789
femoral shaft fractures, 379
fungating breast rumours, 282, 283, **284–286**
gastrointestinal, *see* Gastrointestinal haemorrhage
intra-abdominal, 815
leukaemia, 426, 428, 430
orofacial trauma, 534
postoperative, 792, 800–801
thyroidectomy, 141
tonsillectomy, 518
total cystectomy and urinary diversion, 317
transurethral resection of prostate, 309
shock due to, 600
see also Hypovolaemic shock
subarachnoid, *see* Subarachnoid haemorrhage
tracheostomy patients, 517
see also Bleeding; Blood loss
Haemorrhoidectomy, 112
Haemorrhoids, 111–113, 733
Haemosalpinx, 221
Haemostasis, 407–408, 441
Halitosis, 932
Hallucinations, 843
hypnagogic, 750
Hallucinogens, 985–986
Halo frame, 533
Hand(s)
burns, 871
gestures, 760–761
hygiene, **550**, 564
Handicap, **906**, 919, 944
see also Physical handicap
Hanging arm technique, 394, *395*
Harm minimisation, 986–987
Hartmann's solution (lactated Ringer), 605, 643
Hashimoto's thyroidiris, 145
HCG, *see* Human chorionic gonadotrophin
Headache
anaemia, 412
hypertension, 46
raised intracranial pressure, *331*, 339
subarachnoid haemorrhage, 345, 347
Head injury, **335–344**
communication problems, 342, 762
hearing loss, 500
medical management, 339–341
nursing priorities and management, 341–344
pathophysiology, 337–339
Head lice, **456**
Headway, 344, 366
Health
definition, 961–962
personality and, 586–587
responses to change in status, 924
Health belief model, 179, *180*, 882
Health education
AIDS/HIV infection, 1001–1002
asthma, 76
nurse's role, 66–67
orientations, *67*
orodental health, 525
preventing back strain, 392
Health Education Authority, 989
Health Education Board for Scotland, 769, 770
'Health of the Nation' (White Paper), 9–10, 66
Health professionals
biases in inferences of pain, 621–622
communication between, **767–769**
communication with patients, 764–765
Health promotion, 5
A & E departments, 824
AIDS/HIV infection, 1001–1002
cancer prevention, 881–882
cardiovascular disease, 10
elderly, 961–962
orodental health, 525
respiratory disease, **64–67**
Health visitors, *525*, 896
Hearing aids, 500, **501**
Hearing loss, **499–501**
noise-induced, 500
see also Deafness
Hearing tests, *499*
Heart
anatomy and physiology, **10–13**
autonomic regulation, 13
blood flow through, 12–13
conducting system, 11–12
excitation–contraction coupling, 12
Heart attack, *see* Myocardial infarction
Heart block, 36
Heartburn, 91, 92
Heart disease
ischaemic, *see* Ischaemic heart disease
rheumatic (RHD), 41
valvular, **41–44**, 526
Heart failure, **37–41**
cardiac causes, *37*
congestive (backward), 38, *39*, 40
death from, 925
forward, *39*
glomerulonephritis, *318*
medical management, 38
nursing priorities and management, 38–41
pathophysiology, 38, *39*
valvular heart disease, 41, 42
Heart–lung transplantation, 200, *201*
Heart rate
shock, 792
unconscious patients, 846
Heat
conservation, 681–682
disinfection, 551–552
loss
mechanisms, *682*, **683**, *684*, *692*
methods of increasing, 688
surgical patients, 791
production mechanisms, **682–683**, 692
Heat illness, *688*, **690**, *692*
Heat stroke, *688*, 690
Heat treatments, pain, 631
Height, 665
Helper T lymphocytes (CD4 T-cells), 546, *548*
HIV infection, 993, 994–995, 1004
Help for Health, 769, 770
Hemiplegia, 347
Heparin, 784
Hepatic artery ligation, *120*
Hepatic encephalopathy, 116, **118**, 120
Hepatic failure
fulminant, **115**
nursing care plan, 119–120
valvular heart disease, 42
Hepatitis, **114–116**
acute, 115, 116
alcoholic, 116, *980*
autoimmune chronic active, 116
chronic, 115–116
chronic active, 116
chronic persistent, 115–116
drug-induced, *114*, 116
non-A, non-B (NANB), 115

Hepatitis (*contd*)
  viral, 114–115
Hepatitis A (HAV), **114**
Hepatitis B (HBV), 114–115, **565–567**
  chronic, 116, 118, 881
  haemophilia, 205
  infection control precautions, 551, 553
  medical management, 114–115, 567
  nursing priorities and management, 567
  pathophysiology, 114, 566–567
Hepatitis C (HCV), **115**, 116, 118, 205
Hepatitis D (delta) virus, 115
Hepatitis E, 115
Hepatobiliary system, **90–91**
  disorders, **113–124**
Hepatocellular carcinoma, 118
Hepatomegaly, 130
Herbs
  Chinese, 454
  sleep-inducing, 754–755
Hermaphroditism, true, 152
Hernia
  abdominal, **106–109**, 279
    medical management, 108
    nursing priorities and management, 109
    pathophysiology, 108
    see also Inguinal hernia
  hiatus, **92**
  reducible/irreducible, 108
  strangulation, 108–109
Herniation, brain, 336, **337–338**
Herniorraphy, 108
Heroin, 984
Herpangina, *529*
Herpes simplex virus (HSV), **457–458**
  AIDS/HIV infection, *1005*, 1006
  cervical carcinoma and, 234
  encephalitis, 363
  keratitis, 484, 485
  oral (herpes labialis; cold sores), 432, *529*, 563
Herpes zoster (shingles), **458**, *529*, **569–570**
  AIDS/HIV infection, *1005*
  ophthalmicus, **485**
Hiatus hernia, **92**
Hickman line, 427–428
High-density lipoproteins (HDL), 18, *19*
Hip replacement, total, 399–401
Histaminase, plasma, 237
Histamine, 546
Histoplasmosis, 1006
HIV (human immunodeficiency virus), 992, **993–995**
  antibodies, 992, 995, 999
  disease, 992
  encephalopathy, 495, 1007
  infection, *see* AIDS/HIV infection
  modes of transmission, **993–994**
  retinopathy, 494
  seroprevalence surveys, 999–1000
  type 2 (HIV 2), 992
  vaccine, 1003
  wasting syndrome, 1005
Hoarseness, 511
Hodgkin's lymphoma, 434, 435–436
Holiday Care Service, 958
Home
  care at, *see* Community care
  carers, *see* Carers
  death at, 938
  professional–patient relationship, 765
  treatment, haemophilia A, 205
Home aids/adaptations, 910, 947, 955
  multiple sclerosis, 359–360
  rheumatoid arthritis, 397
Homeopathic medicines, **454**
Home visits, specialist genetic nurse, 196
Hordeolum (stye), **485**
Horlicks, 750–751
Hormonal therapy, *see* Endocrine therapy
Hormone replacement therapy (HRT), 217, **218**
Hormones, **134**
  cancer and, 880
  stress responses, **580–582**
  see also specific hormones
Hospice care, 353, 922, **923**
Hospice/palliative care teams, 629–630
Hospital, 4
  AIDS patients, 996
  discharge from, *see* Discharge
  nursing education in, 5–6
  palliative care, 922–923, 936
Hospital–home liaison, *see* Liaison, hospital–home
Hot flushes/flashes, **217**, *218*, *686*
Hot spoon bathing, eye, *494*
Human chorionic gonadotrophin (HCG)
  beta subunit, 229, 246
  choriocarcinoma, 243
  fertility therapy, 254, 257
  hydatidiform mole, 243
  pregnancy, 219
Human Fertilisation and Embryology Act (1990), 252, **259**
Human Fertilisation and Embryology Authority (HFEA), 257, 259
Human Genome Project (HGP), 189
Human immunodeficiency virus, *see* HIV
Human leucocyte antigens (HLA), *157*
Human menopausal gonadotrophin (hMG), 257
Human papilloma virus (HPV), 234, 881
Humerus, fracture of neck, **382**
Humidification of inspired air/oxygen, *68*
  laryngectomy patients, 514
  tracheostomy patients, 516, 517
  unconscious patients, 851
Huntington's disease (HD), *189*, 191, **207–209**
  medical management, 207–208
  nursing priorities and management, 208–209
  pathophysiology, 207
Huntington's Disease Association, 209, 210
Hyaline cartilage, 370
Hydatidiform mole, **242–244**
  medical management, 243
  nursing priorities and management, 243–244
  pathophysiology, 243
Hydration
  assessment of status, **650**
  burns, 868
Hydrocele, **228–229**
Hydrocephalus, 337, 346, *347*, 365
Hydrocolloids, 708, *710*
Hydrocortisone, *see* Cortisol
Hydrogels, 708, *710*
Hydrogen peroxide, *708*, *933*
Hydroxycobalamin, 418
21-Hydroxylase deficiency, 151
5-Hydroxytryptamine (5-HT; serotonin), 618, 746
Hygiene, personal
  angina pectoris, 20
  aortic aneurysms, 48
  bullous skin disorders, 459
  CNS infections, 365
  disabled patients, 951
  heart failure, 40
  multiple sclerosis, 359
  myocardial infarction and, 31
  nerve injuries, 402
  Parkinson's disease, 362
  peripheral arterial disease, 53
  postoperative, 247
  psoriasis, 450–451
  renal colic, 303
  terminally ill patients, 934–935
  total cystectomy and urinary diversion, 317
  unconscious patients, 853
  valvular heart disease, 42
  visual impairment and, 474
  see also Oral hygiene
Hymen, 215
Hyoscine, *786*
Hyperaemia
  blanching, 712
  non-blanching, 712
Hyperbilirubinaemia, *see* Jaundice
Hypercalcaemia, **146–147**, *647*, *648*
  malignant disease, 879
  myeloma, 437–438
Hyperglycaemia
  diabetes mellitus, 157, 173
  diabetic ketoacidosis, 166, 168
  enteral feeding and, *672*
  hyperglycaemic hyperosmolar non-ketotic coma, 167–169
  myocardial infarction and, 23
  postoperative, 798
Hyperglycaemic hyperosmolar non-ketotic coma (HHNK), **167–171**
  medical management, 170
  nursing priorities and management, 170–171
  pathophysiology, 167–170
Hyperkalaemia, 31, 320, **645–646**
  enteral feeding and, *672*
Hypermetropia, *470*
Hypernatraemia, 320, 641, 644
  hyperglycaemic hyperosmolar non-ketotic coma, 169–170
Hyperosmolar agents, 340
Hyperosmolarity, hyperglycaemic hyperosmolar non-ketotic coma, 169
Hyperparathyroidism
  primary, **146–147**
  secondary, **147**
  tertiary, **147**
Hyperpathia, 632
Hyperprolactinaemia, **140**
Hyperpyrexia, malignant, *688*
Hypersensitivity, **559–561**
  type I (anaphylactic; immediate), 559
  type II (antibody-dependent cytotoxic), 559
  type III (immune-complex mediated), 559
  type IV (cell-mediated; delayed), 559
Hypersplenism, **129–130**
Hypertension, **44–47**
  aortic aneurysms and, 47, 49
  associated factors, 44
  cerebrovascular disease and, 344, 347
  chronic renal failure, 321
  Cushing's syndrome, *148*, 151
  diabetes mellitus, 174
  epistaxis and, 508
  eye disorders, *493*, **495**
  malignant, 45
  medical management, 45
  mild, 45
  moderate, 45
  nursing priorities and management, 46

Hypertension (*contd*)
pathophysiology, 45
phaeochromocytoma, 147
portal, 116, **117–118**, 129
primary/essential, 45
secondary, 45
spinal injuries, 385
stress and, 45, 582
Hypertensive crisis, 46
Hyperthermia, 690
Hyperthyroidism (thyrotoxicosis), **144–145**, *493*
Hypertonic solutions, 653
Hypertrophy, 55
Hyperuricaemia, *299*, 431
Hyperventilation, 340
diabetes mellitus, 157
respiratory alkalosis, 649–650
shock, 599
Hyphaema, 471, 477, **486–487**
Hypnosis, 631
Hypnotic drugs, **753–754**
Hypocalcaemia, **147**, *647*, *648*
post-parathyroidectomy, 146–147
Hypochlorite solutions
disinfection, 553, *554*
wound cleaning, 707, *708*
Hypodermoclysis, 651
Hypoglossal nerve, *330*, *523*
Hypoglycaemia
awareness of symptoms, 172
exercise-induced, diabetics, *178*
insulin-induced, **171–172**
liver disease, 159
premenstrual syndrome and, 226
rebound, 172
sulphonylurea-induced, 161, 172
Hypoglycaemic coma, **171–172**, 847, *848*
Hypogonadism, hypogonadotrophic, 152
Hypokalaemia, 31, *645*, **646**
diabetic ketoacidosis, 166
Hyponatraemia, 320, 641, 644
enteral feeding and, *672*
Hypophosphataemia, *672*
Hypophysectomy, transsphenoidal, 139, 140, 148, *150*
Hypopituitarism, **140–142**, 220, *352*
Hypopyon, 471
Hypospadias, **306**
Hypotension
heart failure, *39*
shock, 598
Hypothalamopituitary–adrenal axis, stress response, 581
Hypothalamus, **134**, *135*, *136*, 213, 329
regulatory hormones, *135*
sleep–wake cycle and, 743
thermoregulation, 681
Hypothermia, **690–693**
accidental, causes, 691–693
elderly, 691–693
prevention, *685*, 693
rewarming, 693
rewarming methods, 693
Hypothyroidism, **145–146**
congenital, 146
endemic, 145–146
primary (myxoedema), 145, 146
Hypotonic solutions, 653
Hypovolaemia (fluid volume deficit), **641–643**
causes, *642*
ectopic pregnancy, 247
signs and symptoms, *642*
trauma, 811, 813–815, 816
see also Dehydration
Hypovolaemic shock, 598, **600**
aortic aneurysm repair, 49
burns, 866
management/treatment, 605–606, *607*
patients at risk, *605*
postoperative, 792–795
signs and symptoms, 600
Hypoxia
hypoxic, 72
stagnant, 72
Hypoxic drive, *71*
Hysterectomy, 222, 241, 243, 244
nursing care plan, 239–240
nursing priorities and management, **237–239**
postoperative care, **238–239**, 241, 245
preoperative care, 237–238
radical, 236–237

I

Identification
diabetic patients, 181
surgical patients, 238, *787*
Ileal conduit urinary diversion, 314, *315*
Ileoanal anastomosis, *103*
Ileorectal anastomosis, *111*
Ileostomy, 103–104, *111*, 935
Ileum, 89
Illness, 4–5, 906, 960–961
experiential aspects, 4–5
responses to, 924
Illusions, 843
Imagery, directed, 630–631
Immobilisation syndrome, 951–952
Immobility
after transurethral resection of prostate, 308
incontinence, 725
patients with fractures, *382*
see also Mobility/mobilisation
Immune response, **546–548**, *993*
antibody-mediated (humoral), 547–548
cell-mediated, 548
cells and chemicals involved, 545–546
non-specific/innate, 545, **546–547**
specific (natural immunity), 545, **547–548**
types, 545
Immune system, 543
anatomy and physiology, **544–548**
Immunisation
active, **548**, 563
passive, *547*
Immunocompromised patients, 543–544, 559
cancer, 880
infection control, 557
oral hygiene, 528
wound infections, 703
Immunodeficiency, **558–559**
primary, 558–559
secondary, 559
severe combined, *190*
Immunoglobulin(s), 546, *547*
therapy, *410*, *547*
Immunological disorders, **558–562**
epidemiology, 543–544
Immunosuppressive acid protein (IPA), 237
Immunotherapy, 894
Impairment, **906**, 919, 944
Impetigo, **456**
Implementation, nursing care plans, 917–918
Impotence, *51*, **232–234**
diabetes mellitus, 175
medical management, 233
nursing priorities and management, 233–234
pathophysiology, 232–233
total cystectomy and urinary diversion, 315
Incineration, waste, 554, *555*
Incisional hernia, 108
Incisions, surgical, *798*
Incontinence
faecal, **739**, 933–934
urinary, *see* Urinary incontinence
Independence
critically ill patients, 835–836
elderly, **965–967**
maintaining, 944
promoting, 944
Individualising nursing, 916
Industrial injuries/diseases, *see* Work-related disorders
Infantilism, 220
Infants, body temperature, 685
Infection control, **548–558**
AIDS/HIV infection, 551, 1003
burns, 868–869
confidentiality and, 557–558
critically ill patients, 829, 834–835
health and safety at work, 557
in patient care, 549
nursing process and, 556–557
policies, 549–550
safe working practice, 550–556
surgical patients, 789
Infections
acute pancreatitis, 125
agranulocytosis, 439
aortic aneurysm repair, 49
assessment of patients at risk, 556–557, *558*
bone, **391**
breast, 288
cancer, 878–879
central nervous system (CNS), **363–365**
Cushing's syndrome, 151
diabetes mellitus, 166, 168, 171, **177**
endogenous (self-infection), 557, 704
exogenous, 549, 704
fractures and, *382*
fungating breast tumours, 283
glomerulonephritis, 318
intravenous therapy and, *652*, 675, 853
isolation precautions, *see* Isolation precautions
leukaemia, 426, 427–428, 429
liver failure, 119
mouth, 100, **529–531**
non-specific barriers, 543, *544*, 546
opportunistic, AIDS, *992*, **1005–1006**
post-splenectomy, 130
respiratory tract, **68–70**
sickle cell disease, 422
skin, *see* Skin infections
tonsillectomy patients, 518
tracheostomy patients, 517
unconscious patients, 853–854
urinary tract, *see* Urinary tract infections
wound, *see* Wound infections
Infectious diseases, **563–570**
causes, 563
childhood, staff contact, *569*
epidemiology, 543–544
immunity to, 563
measures to prevent spread, 563–565
nurse's role, 544

Infectious diseases (*contd*)
  transmission, 563
Infertility/subfertility
  cystic fibrosis, 199
  cytotoxic chemotherapy inducing, 892
  ectopic pregnancy and, 247
  female, 254, *255*
  information and counselling, 255–257
Klinefelter syndrome, 199
  male, 254–255, *256*
  medical management, 254–255
  pathophysiology, 254
  see also In vitro fertilisation and embryo transfer
Infestation, 464
Inflammation, 700
Inflammatory bowel disease, 101, **102–104**
Influenza vaccination, 69
Information
  access to, by disabled, 950
  booklets, 782
  giving, **769**
    bereaved family, 938
    breast reconstruction, 279
    cancer, *884*, 900
    critically ill patients, 836
    ectopic pregnancy, 247
    family of trauma victims, 816–817
    hysterectomy and, 238
    incontinence aids/equipment, 735
    infertility, 255–257
    intraocular surgery, 476
    joint replacement, 399
    minor trauma, 821
    multiple sclerosis, 356–357
    myeloma, 438
    oral tumours, 539
    prostatectomy, *310*
    radiotherapy, 888, *892*
    surgical patients, *310*, 781–782
    terminal illness, *927*
    uterine prolapse repair, 249
    see also Education, patient
  withholding, 780
  see also Communication; Education, patient
Information agencies, 769
Informed consent, *see* Consent, informed
Infrared coagulation, haemorrhoids, 112
Infrared radiation
  eye injuries caused by, 489
  thermometer, 687
Ingram regime, 450
Inguinal hernia, 108, *109*, *777*
Inhalation anaesthetics, *791*
Inhalation analgesia, 629
Inhalation injuries, **865**, 867
Inhalations, 509
Inhalers, 75–76
Inheritance
  autosomal dominant, 191
  autosomal recessive, 192
  mechanics, **188–189**
  single-gene disorders, **191–192**
  X-linked, 192
Injuries, *see* Trauma
Inotropic agents, 34, 606
Insomnia, **749–752**
  liver failure, 119
  pharmacological treatments, **753–755**
  psychological/behavioural treatments, **755**
Inspiratory capacity, 61
Inspiratory reserve volume (IRV), 61, *63*
Institute for the Study of Drug Dependence (ISDD), 989
Institutionalised patients
  sleep patterns, *748*
  urinary incontinence, 733–734
Instrumentality model, 953–954
Instruments, **550–553**
  cleaning, 553
  disinfection, 551–553
  risk categories, 550–551
  sterilisation, 551
Insulin
  deficiency, 157
  functions, 155, *156*
  genetically engineered, 181, 189
  human, *161*
  intermediate- and long-acting, 162
  isophane, 162
  lente, 162
  mixing, 163
  resistance, 158
  short-acting, 161–162
  therapy, **161–163**
    diabetic emergencies, 166, 170, 171
    diabetic nephropathy, 174
    frequency, 162–163
    hyperkalaemia, 645–646
    injection sites, 163
    injection technique, 163
  types, 161–162
Insulinoma, 128
Insulin tolerance test, *149*
Insurance, diabetes mellitus, 181
Intellectual impairment
  dental health promotion, *525*, 528
  diagnosis in children, 197
Huntington's disease, 207, 209
  sex chromosome anomalies, 191
  urinary incontinence, 727
Intensive care (critical care) units (ICUs), *83*, **828–833**
  aortic aneurysms, 48
  hazards, 829–831
  human environment, 831–833
  physical environment and activity, 828–831
  sensory environment, 831
Intercalated discs, 11
Interferential therapy, 731, 741
Interferons, 189, 546, 894
Interleukin-1 (IL-1), 689
Interleukin-6 (IL-6), 689
Intermittent claudication, **51**, 53, *54*, 412
Internal capsule, 327, 328
Internal fixation, **379**
  maxillofacial fractures, 532–533
  tibia and fibula fractures, 381
International Glaucoma Association, 496
International Spinal Research Trust, 386
Interosseous plating, fractured mandible, 532
Intertrigo, 455
Intervertebral discs, 371
  chemonucleolysis, 393
  excision, 393
  prolapsed, **392–394**, 395
Interviews, nurse–patient, **766–767**
Intestinal obstruction, *110*
In Touch, 496
Intra-amniotic injection, 253
Intra-aortic balloon pump (IABP), 55, 606
Intracellular fluid (ICF), 638, 639
Intracerebral haematoma/haemorrhage, *340*, 344, 346
Intracranial aneurysms, 344, 346, *493*
Intracranial haematoma, *340*
Intracranial pressure (ICP), 337
  monitoring, 339, *340*
  raised, **335–344**, 346
    causes, 336–338
    nursing priorities and management, 341–344
    presenting features, 338, *339*
    terminally ill patients, 929, 931
    treatment, 339–341
Intracranial (brain) tumours, **349–353**, 762
  classification, 350–352
  medical management, 352
  metastatic, *277*, *351*, 929
  nursing priorities and management, 352–353
  pathophysiology, 349–352
Intramuscular (i.m.) injection, analgesics, 628–629, 798
Intraocular pressure (IOP), 469
  measurement, 480
  raised, 478, 480, 483
Intraocular surgery
  anaesthesia, *490*
  nursing care plan, 479
  perioperative care, **475–477**
Intrauterine contraceptive devices, 222
Intravenous anaesthetics, *791*
Intravenous (i.v.) fluids, 605–606, **653**
Intravenous (i.v.) fluid therapy, **652–653**
  burns, 867
  central lines, 653
  complications, 643, 652
  diabetic ketoacidosis, 166–167, 168
  hyperglycaemic hyperosmolar non-ketotic coma, 170
  hypovolaemic shock, 605–606, 794–795
  postoperative shock, 792–795
  selection of site, 652–653
  trauma, 811, 813–815
  unconscious patients, 852
Intravenous (i.v.) therapy
  analgesics, 629, 799
  complications, 652, 853
Intravenous urogram/pyelogram (IVU/IVP), *297*, *313*
Intrinsic factor deficiency, 418–419, **420**
Introjection, *586*
In vitro fertilisation and embryo transfer (IVF-ET), 247, **257–258**, 259
Iodine, 136
  deficiency, 145–146, *659*, 662
  dietary requirements, *661*
Iodine-131 (^{131}I) therapy, 144–145
Iodine preparations, wound cleaning, *708*
Iris, 468, 471
Iritis, 484
Iron
  deficiency, *659*, 662
  dietary requirements, 415, *660*, *661*, 662
  supplements, 415
Iron deficiency anaemia, **414–416**, 424, *530*
  medical management, 415
  nursing priorities and management, 415–416
  pathophysiology, 415
Irrigation
  bladder, 311, 800
  eye, 475, *488*
  wound, 706–707
Irritable bowel syndrome, **105**
Irritant eczema, 452
Irritant receptors, respiratory system, *62*
Ischaemia
  abdominal aortic aneurysms, 47
  cerebral, 346
  foot, diabetes mellitus, 177
  lower limb, 51, 718

Ischaemia (*contd*)
myocardial, **15**
Ischaemic heart disease, 9, **15–34**
diabetes mellitus, 173
expert nursing practice, 37
geographical variations, 9, 15
risk factors, 15, *16*
stress and, 582
see also Angina pectoris; Myocardial infarction
Ishihara colour plates, 472
Islet cell transplantation, 181
Islets of Langerhans, *134*, 155
Isolation (emotional), *586*
Isolation precautions, **555–556, 563–564**
body substance, 556
bullous skin disorders, 459
burns, 868
category-specific, 556
chickenpox/shingles, 570
choice of disinfectant, 564–565
disease-specific, 556
exudate, 564
home, 564
leukaemia, 427
patients not requiring, 556
quality of life of patients, 556
standard, 564
strict, 564
tuberculosis, 568
Isometric exercises, 365
Isosorbide mononitrate, *17*
Isosporiasis, 1006
Isotonic solutions, 653
Itching, *see* Pruritus

J

Jacksonian seizures, *355*
Jakob–Creutzfeldt disease, 363, 551
Jargon, 759
Jaundice, **114**
cholangiocarcinoma, 124
choledocholithiasis, 123
cholestatic (obstructive), 114
chronic pancreatitis, 127
haemolytic, 114
hepatitis, 115
hepatocellular, 114
pancreatic cancer, 128
Jehovah's witnesses, *416*
Jejunum, 89
Joint replacement surgery, 398–399
nursing priorities and management, 399–401
postoperative complications, 399
Joints
disorders, **391–401**
infection, **394**
postoperative pain/stiffness, *799*
synovial, 371–372
J receptors, *62*
Junctional tachycardia, 36

K

Kallman's syndrome, 152
Kaposi's sarcoma, 463, 495, *529*, 1006–1007
Karyotype, 188
Keep Fit Association, 596
Keloid scars, 701
Keratitis, **484–485**, *490*
Keratoplasty (corneal grafting), **481–482**, 489
Kernig's sign, 345
Ketoacidosis, diabetic, *see* Diabetic ketoacidosis
Ketonaemia, 157, 168
Ketonuria, 157
Kidneys, **291–294**
anatomy, 291–292
disorders, **318–322**
function, *see* Renal function
hormonal control, 293
water and sodium balance and, 293, 640, 641
Kilocalories, 686
Klinefelter syndrome, 152, **198–199**
Knee, *372*
ligament injuries, 401
meniscus lesions, **391–392**
Koilonychia, 415
Kussmaul's respiration, 157
KY jelly, 528

L

Labour, induction, 251
Lacerations, brain, *340*
Lacrimal apparatus, 469, *470*
Lactation, 266
amenorrhoea, 219
nutritional requirements, 659, *660, 661*
Lactic dehydrogenase (LDH), *24*
Lactose intolerance, 101
Lactulose, 118
Laminectomy, 393
Language, 759–760
failure of development, 762
sign, 761
Laparoscopic cholecystectomy, 121, 123, 776
Laparoscopy, 260, 775
ectopic pregnancy, 246
egg recovery for IVF, 257, 258
Laplace's law, 717, *718*
Large intestine, **90**
disorders, **101–111**
Large loop excision of transformation zone (LLETZ), 236
Laron dwarfism, *143*
Laryngeal carcinoma, **511–515**
medical management, 511–512
nursing priorities and management, 512–515
pathophysiology, 511
Laryngeal nerve damage, 141
Laryngectomy, total, **512–515**, 762
complications, *513*
nursing priorities and management, 512–515
Larynx, *506*, 511, 759
Lasers, eye injuries caused by, 489
Laser therapy, 775–776
cancer, 894–896
diabetic retinopathy, 493
glaucoma, 480, 481
oesophageal carcinoma, 93
pre-invasive cervical carcinoma, 235
Last offices, 937
Laundry
home, 554, 564
hospital, 554, *555*
incontinence and, 735
Learning, about pain, 616
Left bundle branch, 11, 12
Legs, *see* Lower limbs
Leg ulcers, 711, **715–719**
arterial, *51*, **718**
diabetic, 175, 177, *719*
epidemiology, 698
healing time, 698, *699*
measurement, 706
mixed arterial and venous, 718–719
vasculitic, *719*
see also Venous leg ulcers
Leisure, *see* Recreation/leisure
Lemniscal tract, 858
Lens(es)
contact, 473, *485, 490*
intraocular (IOL), 471
implantation, **477–478**
postoperative management, 478
Lethargy, *see* Fatigue
Leucocytes, *see* White blood cells
Leucopenia, *426*
Leukaemia, **426–434**, *878*, 881
acute, **426–433**, *530*
medical management, 426–428
nursing care plan, 429–432
nursing priorities and management, 428–433
pathophysiology, 426
aetiology, 426
chronic, 426, **434**
pathophysiology, 426
Leukaemia Care Society, 441
Leukaemia Research Fund, 441
Leukoencephalopathy, progressive multifocal (PML), 1006
Leukoplakia, oral, 537, *538, 1005*
Le Vant frame, 533
Levator ani, 731
LH, *see* Luteinising hormone
Liaison, hospital–home, **768**, 805, 821
cancer care, 896
rehabilitation, 950
respiratory disorders, *84*
Liaison nurses, 711, *768*, 805
Lice
body, **456**
head, **456**
Lichenification, 452
Lifespan, 915
Lifting techniques, 392, *393*
Ligament injuries, **401**
Limb
amputation, **388–391**
burn wounds, 871
movement in unconsciousness patients, 846
prostheses, 391
see also Lower limbs; Upper limbs
Limbic system, 332, 618
Linen laundering, **554**, *555*, 564
Linking, *84*
Lip(s), 521
cleft, 523–524, 666
oedema, facial burns, 871
tumours, **537**, *538*
Lipids (fats), 658, 659, **661–662**
dietary intake, 18, *19*
parenteral solutions, 674
Lipoproteins, *19*
high-density (HDL), 18, *19*
low-density (LDL), *19*
Listening
active, **766**
to aggressive patients, 822

Listening (*contd*)
therapeutic, 588, *589*
Lithium, 589
Lithotripsy, extracorporeal shock wave (ESWL), 300–301, 302
Little's area, *506*
Liver, **90–91**
blood glucose regulation, 156
Liver cancer, **118–120**
medical management, 118, *120*
nursing priorities and management, 118–120
primary, 118
secondary, 118, *277*
Liver disease, **113–120**, 159
clinical features, 113–114
Liver failure, *see* Hepatic failure
Lobectomy, postoperative care, **78–79**
Local anaesthesia, 629, **790**
eye surgery, *490*
postoperative, *799*
Local anaesthetics, eye, *476*
Locked-in syndrome, 844
Locus coeruleus, *617*, 618
Locus of control, diabetes mellitus, 179
London Hospital Pain Observation Chart, 625–627
Loop of Henle, *292*, 293
Loopogram, 316
Loss, **924–925**
terminally ill patients, 926
theories of, 924–925
see also Bereavement; Grief
Lotions, *446*
Low-density lipoproteins (LDL), *19*
Lower limbs, 371
arterial disease, 51, 718
elevation, 54, 55, 56
fractures, **379–381**
ulcers, *see* Leg ulcers
Lowthian's 24h turning clocks, *715*
LSD, 985–986
Lubricants, eye, *476*
Lumbar puncture, 346, 356, 364, 426
Lumbar spine disorders, **392–394**
acute back strain, 392
prolapsed intervertebral disc, 392–394
recurrent back strain, 392
Lumpectomy, breast, *263*, 264, 270
Lund and Browder burn chart, *863*
Lung, *60*
compliance, 61
effects of pollution, 66
expansion and recoil, 61–62
perfusion, 63
volumes, 61, *63*
Lung cancer, *see* Bronchogenic cancer
Lung function tests, 61, *63*, 71
asthma, 73, 75–76
Lupus erythematosus, systemic (SLE), **562**
Luteinising hormone (LH), *135*
deficiency, *142*
ovarian effects, 212, 213
recombinant, 189
Luteinising hormone releasing hormone (LHRH), *see* Gonadotrophin-releasing hormone
Lymphadenopathy syndrome (LAS), 1004
Lymphatic system, 639
tumour spread, 878
Lymph nodes, 544–545
Lymphocytes, 407, 544, *545*, **546**
development, *408*
immune response, 547–548
Lymphoedema, 639
breast cancer, 274, 275, **280–282**
terminally ill patients, 934
Lymphoid organs/tissues, **544–545**
disorders, **426–439**
primary, 544
secondary, 544–545
Lymphokines, 546, *548*
Lymphoma, **434–436**, *878*
AIDS patients, 1007
high-grade, 435, 436
low-grade, 435, 436
medical management, 435–436
nursing priorities and management, 436
pathophysiology, 434–435
Lymph vessels, skin, 446

M

Macmillan nurses, 95, 100, 540, 897, 923, 936
Macrophages, 445, **545**, 699
Macular degeneration, senile, **492**, *492*
Macules, 464
Maculopathy, diabetic, 173
Magic mushrooms, 986
Magnesium, *661*, 662
Magnetic resonance imaging (MRI), 356, *373*
Malabsorption syndrome, **101–102**, 127, 899
AIDS, 1005
Malar (zygomatic) bone, fractured, *531*, 533
Male infertility, 254–255, *256*
Male reproductive system
anatomy and physiology, **295–296**
disorders, **227–234**
Malignant disease, *see* Cancer
Malnutrition, **663–664**
cancer, 899
chronic pancreatitis, 128
liver failure, 119
protein-energy (PEM), *659*, *663*, 665
total parenteral nutrition, 673
wound healing and, 702
wound infection and, 703
see also Nutrition
Mal-union, fractures, *382*
Mammary dysplasia, benign, **287–288**
Mammography, 268–269, 883
Mammoplasty, reduction, 279
Manchester operation, 248
Mandible, fractured, *531*, 532
Manganese, *661*
Manic Depression Fellowship, 596
Mannitol, 340
Manpower Services Commission, 956
Mantoux skin test, 70, 559, 568
Marfan's disease, 47
Marie Curie home care nurses, 898, 923
Marriage Guidance Council (Relate), 359, 366, 596
Marsupial pants, 741
Masks, surgical, 788
Massage, 282, 631
MAST (medical antishock trousers), 606
Mast cells, 445, 545
Mastectomy
breast reconstruction after, 278–280
fungating breast tumours, 282
informed consent, 264
modified radical (Patey), 270
partial or segmental, 264, 270
breast augmentation after, 279
postoperative care, 271–275
psychological problems after, 263, 950
radical (Halsted's), 270
simple, 270
Mastication, *see* Chewing
Mastoidectomy, 504
Mastoiditis, acute, **504**
Maxilla, 521
fractured, *531*, 532–533
Maxillofacial fractures, 531, 763
medical management, 531–532
nursing priorities and management, 533–536
Maxillofacial technician, 539
McGill Pain Questionnaire (MPQ), 625
Mealtimes, **667–668**
Mean arterial pressure, 14
Mean corpuscular haemoglobin concentration (MCHC), 413
Mean corpuscular volume (MCV), 413
Measles, 544, *569*
Medical antishock trousers (MAST), 606
Meditative relaxation, *591*
Medroxyprogesterone, *142*, 241
Medulla oblongata, 13, **329**
Medulloblastoma, *350*
Megaloblastic anaemia, **416–420**
medical management, 418–419
nursing priorities and management, 419–420
pathophysiology, 416–418
Meiosis, 188
Melaena, 130
Melanoma, malignant, *463*, 537, 881
Melphalan, *895*
Memory cells, 545, 547, 548
Menarche, 216
Ménière's disease, **505–506**
Meninges, **329**, *332*
Meningioma, *351*
Meningism, 345
Meningitis
bacterial, 363, 364
meningococcal, 569
Meningitis Trust, 366
Meningococcal infection, **569**
Meniscectomy, arthroscopic, 391–392
Meniscus lesions, **391–392**
Menopause, **216–217**, 219
associated changes, 216–217
breast changes, 266
clinics, 218
disorders of, **217–218**
premature, chemotherapy-induced, 276, *891*
Menorrhagia, **222**
Menstrual cycle, **215–216**
body temperature and, 686
breast changes, 266
Menstruation, 215
attitudes of girls towards, *223*
chemotherapy and, 276
disorders, **218–227**
menopausal women, 217
Mental handicap, *see* Intellectual impairment
Mental Health Foundation, 596
Mesencephalon (midbrain), 329, 840, 858
Metabolic acidosis, 648, **649**
diabetic ketoacidosis, 157, 166
renal failure, 320
Metabolic alkalosis, 648, **649**, 654
Metabolic disorders, **133–153**, 750
cancer, 879
enteral feeding, *672*
postoperative patients, 797–798
total parenteral nutrition, *676*, 853
Metabolic rate, 682, **686**

Metabolic rate (*contd*)
basal (BMR), 686
Metastases, 877–878, *879*, 904
brain, 277, *351*, 929
breast cancer, **276–278**
liver, 118, *277*
Metformin, 161
Methotrexate, 451, *892*, *895*
Metronidazole, 935
Metrorrhagia, **222–223**
Microalbuminuria, 174, 175
Microorganisms, disease-producing, 549
Micturition, **295**, 724
Mid-arm circumference (MAC), 665
Mid-arm muscle circumference (MAMC), 665
Midbrain (mesencephalon), 329, 840, 858
Midwives, 67, *525*
Mifepristone, 251
Migraine, *493*, **582–583**
Migraine Trust, 596
Miles Laboratories Ltd, 184
MIND (National Association for Mental Health), 596
Mineralocorticoids, 137, 149
Minerals, 658, 659, **662**
dietary requirements, *660*, *661*
parenteral solutions, 674, *675*
see also Electrolytes; *specific minerals*
Miosis, 470
Miotics, *476*, 479
Miscarriage (spontaneous abortion), 251–252, 819
Misuse of Drugs Act (1971), 628
Mites, **456**
Mitosis, 188
Mitoxantrone, *895*
Mitral incompetence, **44**
Mitral stenosis, **43**, *53*
Mitral valve (left atrioventricular valve), *10*, 11, 12
prolapse, 34
MMR vaccination, 519
Mobility/mobilisation
aortic aneurysms, 48
CNS infections, 365
disabled patients, 951–952
eating and, 667
head injury, 343
heart failure, 40
ischaemic heart disease, 18, 28–30
maxillofacial injuries and, 535
multiple sclerosis, 358
myeloma, 438
Parkinson's disease, 361
peripheral vascular disease, 53, 55
postoperative, 50
amputation of limb, 389–390
hip replacement, 399
hysterectomy, 238, 240
prolapsed intervertebral disc, 393–394
rheumatoid arthritis, 396–397
soft tissue injuries, 402
spinal injuries and, 384–385
stroke, 547–348
terminally ill patients, 934
unconscious patients, 854–855
valvular heart disease, 42
visually impaired, 474
see also Activity, physical; Exercises; Immobility; Rest
Mobility officers, 473
Molluscum contagiosum, **457**
Moniliasis, *see* Candidiasis
Monitoring
asthma, 75
burns, 867–868
cardiac, 25
critically ill patients, 829
diabetic emergencies, 166, 170
fluid balance, **651**
glycaemic control in diabetes, **164–165**
hiatus hernia surgery, 92
inflammatory bowel disease, 103
leukaemia, 427–428
orofacial trauma, 534
pneumothorax, 80
raised intracranial pressure, 339, *340*, 341
shock, **608–613**
see also Observations of vital signs
Monoamine oxidase inhibitors (MAOIs), 589
Monocytes, 407, *408*, 545, 699
Mononeuropathies, diabetes mellitus, 175, *176*
Monosomy, 191
Mood changes, terminally ill patients, 926, *927*
Morphine, 95, *786*, *931*
Mortality, 919
Mosaicism, 191
Motherhood, surrogate, **259–260**
Mother-to-child transmission, HIV, 994
Motor deficits
raised intracranial pressure, *339*
stroke, *345*
Motor neurone disease, *970*
Motor neurones, 326
lower, 334, 335
upper, 334, 335
Motor pathways, spinal cord, 333, 334–335, *336*
Motor response, Glasgow Coma Scale, 845–846
Mouth, **521–541**
anatomy and physiology, **521–523**
assessment guide, *433*
congenital deformities, 523–525
disorders, 91, **523–541**
dry, 797
floor, tumours, 537
functions, **88**, *522*, **523**
hygiene, *see* Oral hygiene
infections/inflammatory conditions, 100, **529–531**
sore, *see* Stomatitis/sore mouth
Mouth tumours, **536–541**
medical management, 537–538
nursing priorities and management, 538–541
pathophysiology, 536–537
Mouthwashes/mouth rinses, 528, *933*
Movement abnormalities, Huntington's disease, 207
MPTP-induced parkinsonism, 360
Multiparity, menorrhagia and, 222
Multiple organ failure (MOF), 600
Multiple sclerosis, **356–360**, 909, 911
eye disorders, *493*
medical management, 356
nursing priorities and management, 356–360
pathophysiology, 326, 356
Multiple Sclerosis Society of Great Britain, 366
Multiple trauma, **813–818**
admission, 817–818
assessment and immediate treatment, 813–816
care of relatives, 816–817
diagnosis and further treatment, 817
Mumps, *232*, 537, *569*
Muscle, 372
atrophy/wasting, *51*, *148*, *382*
injuries, **401–402**
skeletal, glucose storage, 156
spasm, 401
weakness, 157, 561
Muscle relaxants, 790–791
Muscle spindles, *62*
Muscular dystrophies, 205
Muscular Dystrophy Group, 207, 210
Muscular system, 372
Musculoskeletal disorders
bioengineering and, 370
chronic, 908
epidemiology, 369–370
investigations, 373
principles of nursing management, *373*
Musculoskeletal system, **369–404**
anatomy and physiology, 370–373
assessment, 373
components, 373
Mutism, akinetic, 844
Myalgic encephalomyelitis, **585**
Myalgic Encephalomyelitis (ME) Association, 596
Myasthenia gravis, **561–562**, 763
Myasthenic (cholinergic) crisis, 562
Mycobacterium avium complex (MAC), 1006
Mycobacterium tuberculosis, 568, 1006
Mydriatics, *476*
Myelin, 326
Myelinated nerves, 326
Myelography, *373*, *394*
Myeloma, multiple (myeloma), **436–438**
medical management, 437
nursing priorities and management, 437–438
pathophysiology, 436–437
Myelosuppression, 892–893
Myocardial cells, 11
Myocardlal contractility, *601*
Myocardial depressant factor (MDF), 600, 601
Myocardial infarction, acute (AMI), 9, **22–34**
complications, 24, **31–34**, 601
fever in, 26, 689–690
medical management, 22–23
medical treatment, 23–24
nursing care plan, 27–28
nursing priorities and management, 24–31
immediate, 25–26
ongoing, 26–31
pathophysiology, 22
thrombolytic therapy, 24
Myocardial ischaemia, **15**
Myocardial rupture, post-infarction, 34
Myocardium, 10
dilatation, 38
hypertrophy, 38
Myoclonic seizures, *355*
Myoclonus, sleep-induced nocturnal, 750
Myocutaneous flaps, breast reconstruction 279, 280
Myofibroblasts, *699*
Myomectomy, 222, 244, 245
Myometrium, 214
Myopia, 470
Myosarcoma, **878**
Myotonic dystrophy, 191, **205–207**
medical management, 206
nursing priorities and management, 206–207
pathophysiology, 206
Myringotomy, 503
Myxoedema, 145, 146

N

Nappy rash, 455
Narcolepsy, 750
Narcotic analgesics, 628, *786*
  cancer pain, *931*
  fear of addiction, 622–623, 797
  myocardial infarction, 25
  postoperative pain relief, 799
  respiratory depression induced by, 623, 799
Narcotics Anonymous, 987, 989
Nasal obstruction, **510–511**
Nasal packs, 507, 508
Nasal polyps, **511**
Nasal septum
  deviation, **510**
  haematoma, **510**, *531*
  perforation, **510**
Nasal surgery, common problems, 510
Nasal tumours, **511**
Nasoduodenal tube, 669
Nasoenteral feeding, **669–670**
  see also Enteral feeding
Nasogastric aspiration
  diabetic ketoacidosis, 166
  hiatus hernia surgery, 92
  laryngectomy patients, 513
  peptic ulcer surgery, 97–98
Nasogastric (NG) tube, 669, *799*
  vomiting around, 654
Nasojejunal tube, 669
Nasopharynx, *506*, 511
National Association for Colitis and Crohn's disease (NACC), 103
National Association of Genetic Nurses and Social Workers, 195, 210
National Association of Laryngectomy Clubs, 520
National Asthma Campaign, 76, 86
National Back Pain Association, 635
National Campaign Against Solvent Abuse, 989
National Deaf Children's Society, 520
National Eczema Society, 465
National Hospice Council (NHC), 923, 942
National Meningitis Trust, 363
Natural killer (NK) cells, 546
Nausea, *see* Vomiting/nausea
Nebulisers, *74, 75*
Neck pain, postoperative, *800*
Nectotic tissue, *698*
  breast reconstruction, 279
  cavity wounds, 706
  fungating breast tumours, 283
Needie exchange schemes, 986–987
Needlestick injuries, 564, 566, 994
Neisseria meningitidis, 569
Neonatal death, 197
Neoplasm, 130, 877
Nephritis, *493*
Nephrogram, 302
Nephrolithotomy
  open, 302
  percutaneous (PCNL), 301–303
Nephron, 292
Nephrostomy, percutaneous, 300
Nephrostomy tube
  insertion, 300, 301–302
  postoperative management, 302, 303
Nephrotic syndrome, **318–319**
Nephrotoxicity, 904 ,
Nerve blocks, *790, 799*
Nerve cells, *see* Neurones
Nerve conduction velocities (NCVs), *373*
Nerve fibres, 326, *327*
Nerve impulse, **326–327**
Nerve injuries, **402–403**
Nervous system, **325–367**
  anatomy and physiology, 325–336
  autonomic, *see* Autonomic nervous system
  central, *see* Central nervous system
  peripheral (PNS), 325, **334–335**
  somatic, 325, 336
  tissue structure, 325–326
Neuralgias, 632
Neural tube defects, *197*
Neurilemmoma, *350*
Neurofibroma, *350*
Neurogenic shock, 604, *605*, 792
Neuroglia, 325–326
Neuroglycopenic symptoms, 172
Neurological deficits
  head injury, 343
  intracranial tumours, 349–352, 353
  reversible ischaemic, *345*
  stroke, *345*
Neurological Observation Chart, *842*, **844–846**
Neurological status, assessment, 341, **844–846**
Neuroma, *350*
Neurones, 325, **326**
  motor/efferent, *see* Motor neurones
  sensory/afferent, 326, 632
Neuropathic arthropathy (Charcot's joints), diabetes mellitus, 176
Neuropathic ulcers, diabetes mellitus, 175
Neuropathy, diabetic, **175**, *176*
Neurosurgery
  approaches, *341*
  cerebral abscess, 364
  complications, *342*
  head-injured patients, 340–341, 342
  intracranial tumours, 352
  subarachnoid haemorrhage, 346
Neurotransmitters, **327**, 746
Neurovascular complications, fractures, 375, 377–378, *382*
Neutropenia, 441, 558–559
Neutrophils (polymorphs), 407, 545, 699
Niacin, *659, 660, 661*
Nightingale, Florence, 948, *949*
Nightmares, 752
Night terrors, 752
Nikolsky's sign, 459
Ninth (glossopharyngeal) nerve, *330, 523*
Nipple
  areola reconstruction, 279
  Paget's disease, 269
Nitrates, *17*, 34
Nitrogen balance, 665
Nitroglycerine (glyceryl trinitrate; GTN), *17*, 18, 25, 27
Nitroprusside, 606
Nitrous oxide and oxygen (Entonox), 629, 790, 816
Nits, 456
Nociceptors, **616–617**, 632
Nocturia, 158, 725
Nocturnal enuresis, 725, 726–727, **738**
Nodules, 464
Noise
  intensive care units, **830**
  sleep and, 748, **752**
Noise-induced hearing loss, 500
Non-A, non-B hepatitis (NANB), 115
Non-Hodgkin's lymphoma, 434–435, 436, 1007
Non-shivering thermogenesis (NST), 683, 692
Non-steroidal anti-inflammatory drugs (NSAIDs), 96, *689*
Non-union, fractures, *382*
Noradrenaline, 137, 156
  sleep and, 746
  stress response, 581, 599
Norton risk scale, 712, 713
Nose
  anatomy and physiology, **506**
  care, facial burns, 871
  disorders, **506–511**
  foreign bodies, **510–511**
  injuries, **509–510**, *531*, 533
Nosebleeds, *see* Epistaxis
Novo Nordisk Pharmaceuticals Ltd, 184
NREM sleep, **745**, 746
Nulliparous, 741
Numerical rating scale (NRS), pain, 627
Nurse–patient interviews, **766–767**
Nurse–patient partnership, 5
Nurse–patient relationship, 5, 764–765
Nurse prescribing, 711
Nurses
  education, 5–6, 591
  preventing back injuries, 392, *393*
  substance abuse by, 976–977
  support and supervision, **592–593**, 939–940
  wearing of uniforms, 760
Nurse-to-nurse communication, 768–769
Nursing
  context, 3–6
  individualising, 916
  stress in, 541, **590–594**, *897*
Nursing assessment, *see* Assessment, nursing
Nursing homes, 912
Nursing process
A & E care, 813
  chronic illness and, 916–918
  infection control and, 556–557
Nutrients, 658, **659–662**
  energy values, *658*
  multiple reference values, 658, *661*
  recommended daily amounts (RDAs), 658, 659, *660*
Nutrition, **657–676**
  AIDS/HIV infection, 1005
  anaemia, 414
  angina pectoris, 18–19
  burns, 868
  cystic fibrosis, 201
  enteral, *see* Enteral feeding
  laryngectomy patients, 513–514
  leukaemia, 432
  maxillofacial fractures and, 535
  normal, 657–658
  oesophageal carcinoma, 94–95
  parenteral, *see* Parenteral nutrition
  postoperative, 797
  unconscious patients, 669, 852–853
  wound healing and, 702
  see also Diet; Eating/drinking; Food(s)
Nutritional assessment, **664–666**
  dietary and clinical history, 664–665
  laboratory tests, 665–666
  physical examination, 665
Nutritional deficiencies, 405, *530*
  clinical signs, *659*
  see also Malnutrition
Nystagmus, HIV encephalopathy, 495

O

Obesity, **662–663**
Cushing's syndrome, *148*

Cushing's syndrome (*contd*)
diabetes mellitus and, 158, 160, 165
hypertension and, 44
ischaemic heart disease and, 18
sleep apnoea syndrome, 752
stroke and, 347
Observations of vital signs
bullous skin disorders, 459–460
burns, 867–868
cardiogenic shock, 34
CNS infections, 364
myocardial infarction, 25–26
orofacial trauma, 534, 535
pneumothorax, 80
postoperative, 792
psoriasis, 450
see also Monitoring
Obturators, *538*
Occupation, colour vision and, 472
Occupational Health department, 976–977
Occupational health nurses, 67, 232, 370
dental health and, *525*
eye injuries and, 473, *488*
Occupational therapists, 348, 359, 433
Occupational therapy, 956
Octreotide, 139
Oculomotor nerve, *330*
Oculovestibular reflex, 857
Odour
body/wound, 763
fungating breast tumours, 283
terminally ill patients, 933–934, 935
Odynophagia, 667
Oedema, **639–640**
anaemia, 412
facial burns, 871
heart failure, 38, *39*, 40
management, 640
nasal, 510
nephrotic syndrome, 319
pitting, 639
pulmonary, *see* Pulmonary oedema
venous disease, *51*, 54
Oesophageal carcinoma, **93–95**
medical management, 93
nursing priorities and management, 93–95
pathophysiology, 93
Oesophageal perforation, 95–96
Oesophageal spasm, 91
Oesophageal speech, 513, 515
Oesophageal varices, 117–118, *980*
Oesophagectomy, *94*
Oesophagitis, 91, *890*
Oesophagus
achalasia, 92–93, 667
anatomy and physiology, **88**
disorders, **91–96**
traumatic disorders, 95–96
Oestradiol, 214
Oestrogens, 213–214
breast cancer and, 267
menstrual cycle, 215, 216
post-menopausal women, 216, 217
replacement therapy, 217, *218*
testicular cancer and, 229
Turner's syndrome, 220
Ointments, *446*
Older people, *see* Elderly
Olfactory nerve, *330*, *523*
Oligodendroglioma, *350*
Oligospermia, *256*
Oliguria, *39*, 320
Olive oil therapy, 450
Onchocerciasis, 468
Oncogenes, 877
Oncology, 876
Oncotic pressure, 639
Oocytes (eggs)
harvesting for IVF, 257, 258
production, 212–213
Oophorectomy, 220
Operant conditioning, 631
Ophthalmic artery, 469
Ophthalmitis, sympathetic, 487
Opiate analgesics, *see* Narcotic analgesics
Opiate/opioid abuse, 984
Opioids, endogenous, 618
Opportunistic infections, AIDS, *992*, **1005–1006**
Opticath fibreoptic catheter, 608
Optic chiasma, 134, 469
Optic nerve, *330*, 469
Optic nerve glioma, *350*
Oral administration
analgesics, 628, *798*
fluids, 651–652
Oral assessment guide, *433*
Oral cavity, *see* Mouth
Oral contraceptives
complications, 45, 55, 347
diabetes mellitus, 180
menorrhagia, 222
Oral hygiene, 91, **525–526**
congenital deformities of mouth, 525
Huntington's disease, 209
laryngectomy patients, 514
leukaemia, 428
oral tumours, 541
orofacial trauma, 534–535
special client groups, **528–529**
terminally ill patients, 932, *933*, *936*
unconscious patients, 853
Oral hypoglycaemic therapy, **160–161**, 171, 174
Oral rehydration therapy, 654
Oral surgery, 526, *527*
Oral tumours, *see* Mouth tumours
Orbital floor, blow-out fracture, *531*
Orchidectomy, 229, 312
Orchitis, *232*
Orem's self-care model of nursing, 10
asthma and, 64
chronic illness and, 913
menopause and, 218
palliative care and, 927–928, 929–935
rehabilitation and, 948
trauma and, 813
visual impairment and, 474
Organ donation, 818
Orientation, 844–845
Orodental disease, **525–529**
medical management, 526
nursing priorities and management, 526–529
Orofacial trauma, **531–536**, 763
causes, 531–532
medical management, 532–533
nursing priorities and management, 533–536
Oropharyngeal airways, 811, 850
Oropharynx, 511, 523
Orthognathic surgery, 524
Orthopnoea, valvular heart disease, 42
OSCAR (Organisation for Sickle Cell Anaemia Research), 441
Osmoreceptors, 640
Osmosis, *322*
Osmotic diuresis, 641, **643**
Ossicles, auditory, 497–498
Osteoarthritis, 370, **397–401**
fractures causing, *382*
medical management, 397–399
nursing priorities and management, 399–401
pathophysiology, 397
Osteochondroma, *388*
Osteoclastoma, *388*
Osteomalacia, **147**
Osteomyelitis, **391**
Osteopathy, 631
Osteophytes, *398*
Osteoporosis, 370
Cushing's syndrome, *148*, 151
post-menopausal, **217**
Osteosarcoma, 387, *388*
Osteotomy, 395, *398*
Otitis, external, **498**
Otitis media
acute suppurative (ASOM), **502–503**
chronic suppurative (CSOM), **503–504**
complications, **504**
secretory (glue ear), **501–502**
tube feeding causing, *671*
Otosclerosis, **502**
Ototoxicity, 904
Outreach workers, 986–987, 996
Ovarian cycle, 212, *213*
Ovarian follicles, 212, *213*
Ovarian tumours, 220
benign, **245**
malignant, **241–242**
Ovaries, *134*, 137, **212–214**
declining function, 216
failed development, 219–220
functions, 212–214
irradiation, 220, *891*
polycystic, 222
surgical removal, 220
Overdose, drug, **847**, *848*
Overflow incontinence, 725
Oviducts, *see* Uterine tubes
Ovulation, 212
disorders, *255*
Oxygen (O_2)
in air, *63*
exchange, 62–64
partial pressure (PO_2), shock, 613
saturation (SaO_2), shock, 608
toxicity, *68*
transport, *61*
Oxygen therapy, *68*
asthma, 73–74
cardiogenic shock, 606
emphysema, 71
at home, *72*
hyperbaric, *68*
lobectomy, 78
myocardial infarction, 26, 30
unconscious patients, 851
Oxytocin, 134, *135*, 266

P

Pacemakers, 36–37, 206
Packed ceil volume (PCV), 413
Paget's disease of the nipple, 269
Pain, **615–635**
abdominal, *see* Abdominal pain
acute, **619–620**
specialised services, 629
anatomy and physiology, 616–618
assessment, 622, **625–628**, 798, 834

Pain (*contd*)
content, 625–627
methods, 625
myths and misconceptions about, *623*
recording, 627–628
scales, 627
cancer, **620–621**, 624, 720, *931*
chest, *see* Chest pain
chronic, **620–621**, 630
non-malignant, **620**, 630
physiological effects, 620
psychosocial effects, 620–621
sleep problems, 750
clinics, 630
definition, 615
factors influencing, 616
fungating breast tumours, 286
intermittent claudication, 51, 53
ligament injuries, 401
management, **624–632**
factors affecting quality, 621–624
issues in, **621–624**
nurse's role, 624
patient's role, 624–625
role of family and carers, 625
see also Pain relief
nasal surgery, 510
orofacial trauma, 534
pathways, 617–618
phantom, 275, 389
postoperative, 620, **797–798**, *800*
sleep problems, 750, *751*
specialised services, 629
transurethral resection of prostate, 308
vascular surgery, 50, 56
referred, 621
sickle cell crisis, 422, 423
sleep problems, 750
terminally ill patients, 929, *931*, *934*
theories, **618–619**
threshold, 621
tolerance, 621, *623*
Painful stimuli, neurological assessment, 844, 845–846
Pain relief, **628–632**
acute cholecystitis, 121
aortic aneurysms, 48
attitudes and expectations about, 622–623
breast cancer, 280, 283, 286
bullous skin disorders, 459
burns, 867, 869
complementary methods, **630–632**
ectopic pregnancy, 247
femoral neck fractures, 381
head injury, 342
herpes zoster, 458
inadequate, 621, 623–624
minor trauma, 821
myocardial infarction, 23, 25
nerve injuries, 402
oesophageal carcinoma, 95
osteomyelitis, 391
pancreatic cancer, 128
pancreatitis, 125, 126, 127
peripheral vascular disease, 52–53, 55
postoperative, 791–792, **797–798**, *801*
adequacy, 621
breast reconstruction, 280
cholecystectomy, 122
ectopic pregnancy, 247
gastric surgery, 92, 99
hysterectomy, 239
mastectomy, 273–274, 275
pneumonectomy, 79
prolapsed intervertebral disc, 393
retinal detachment, 481
tonsillectomy, 518
total cystectomy and urinary diversion, 317
prostatic cancer, 312
renal colic, 300, 303
rheumatoid arthritis, 396
subarachnoid haemorrhage, 347
terminal illness, 931
withholding, A & E departments, 816
Pain services, specialised, 629–630
Palate
cleft, 523–524, 666
hard, 521
soft, 521
tumours, **537**
Palliative care, 278, 921, **926–935**
intracranial tumours, 352–353
organisation of services, 922–923
prostatic cancer, 312
teams, 629–630, 922, 928
see also Terminally ill patients
Palliative therapy, 885, 904
chemotherapy, 891
chronic illness, 909
gastric carcinoma, 99–100
radiotherapy, 887
Palpitations, anaemia, 412
Pancreas, **91**
disorders, **124–129**
endocrine, 91, *134*, 155
exocrine, 91
transplantation, 181
Pancreatectomy, distal, 127
Pancreatic abscess, 125, *126*
Pancreatic cancer, **128–129**, 159
Pancreatic enzymes, 89
supplements, 127, 128, 201
Pancreatic juice, 89, 91
Pancreatic necrosis, 125, *126*
Pancreatic pseudocyst, *126*, 130
Pancreatitis, **124–128**, 130, 159
acute, **124–126**
complications, *126*
nursing care plan, 126
chronic, 124, **127–128**
medical management, 127
nursing priorities and management, 127–128
pathophysiology, 127
Pancreatoduodenal resection (Whipple's procedure), 124, 124, 128
Pancreato-jejunustomy, 127
Pancuronium, *791*
Pancytopenia, 130, 420, 441
Panic attacks, **584**
Panproctocolectomy, *103*
Pantothenic acid, *661*
Papanicolaou (Pap) smear test, 235, 245, 883
Papaveretum, *786*
Papaverine, 233
Papillary muscle rupture, 34
Papilloedema, *331*
Papules, 464
Paracentesis, abdominal, *117*, 242
Paracetamol, *689*
Paradoxical breathing, *80*
Paradoxical intention, 755
Paraffin, soft yellow, 528
Paralysis agitans, *see* Parkinson's disease
Paralytic ileus, *110*
acute pancreatitis, *126*
postoperative, 317, *800*
Paranasal sinuses, **509**
Paraneoplastic disorders, 879–880
Paraphimosis, **306**
Paraplegia, 386, 934, *955*
Paraprotein, 436–437
Parasomnias, *749*, **752**
Parasympathetic nervous system, 13, 336, *338*
Parathormone (PTH), 136, 146
Parathyroidectomy, 141, 146–147
Parathyroid glands, *134*, **136**
disorders, **146–147**
Parenteral fluid therapy, *see* Intravenous (i.v.) fluid therapy
Parenteral nutrition, **672–676**
administration equipment, 673
burns, 868
nutritional assessment and monitoring, 673
total (TPN), **672–676**
complications, 674–676, 853
indications, 673
inflammatory bowel disease, 102
solutions for, 673–674, *675*
unconscious patients, 853
venous access, 673
Parkinson's disease, 328, **360–363**, 763
medical management, 360
nursing priorities and management, 360–363
pathophysiology, 360
Parkinson's Disease Society, 366
Paronychia, 455
Parotid gland, 521, 523
tumours, 537, *538*
Parous, 741
Partially sighted, registration, 473–474
Partially Sighted Society, 496
Partial pressure *(P)*, 63
Pastes, *446*
Patch testing, 452, 462
Paterson–Kelly (Plummer–Vinson) syndrome, 93, 130, 415
Pathogens, 549
Patient controlled analgesia (PCA), 629, 799, *800*
Patient Information Service, 771
Patients
effects of a death on other, 937
health needs, 5
image of, 5
lifting techniques, *393*
Patient's Charter, 776
Patulent, 741
Peak expiratory flow rate (PEFR), *63*, *75*
Pectoralis major muscle, 265, *266*
Pectoralis minor muscle, 265, *266*
Pediculosis capitis, **456**
Pediculosis corporis, **456**
Peer supervision, nurses, 593
Pelvic congestion, 224
Pelvic exenteration, 237
Pelvic floor
exercises, **731**
muscles, 731, *731*
reconstruction, 248
Pelvic inflammatory disease (PID), 224, 245
Pelvic injuries, 815–816
Pemphigoid, **459**, 460
Pemphigus, **458–459**, 460
Penile prosthesis (implant), 233–234
Penis, **296**
congenital disorders, **306**
disorders, **305–306**
revascularisation, 233
Penrose drains, 802, *803*
Pentamidine, 1005–1006

Peptic ulcer, **96–99**
complications, 98–99
medical management, 97
nursing priorities and management, 97–98
pathophysiology, 96
Percutaneous transluminal coronary angioplasty (PTCA), 20–21
Perfusion, lung, 63
Periaqueductal grey (PAG), *617*, 618
Pericarditis, *25*, 34
Pericardium, 10
Perineometer, 731, 741
Periodontal disease, **526**
Periodontitis, 526
Perioperative care, **786–792**
benign mammary dysplasia, 288
cholecystectomy, 122
colorectal cancer, 110–111
hypersplenism, 129–130
intraocular surgery, **475–477**
nasal surgery, 510
splenic injury, 129
transsphenoidal hypophysectomy, 140
see also Postoperative care; Preoperative care; Surgical patients
Peripheral nerve injuries, **402–403**
Peripheral nervous system (PNS), 325, **334–335**
Peripheral neuropathie
diabetic, 175, *176*
vitamin B_{12} deficiency, 416–418
Peripheral vascular disease, **48–55**, 389
Peripheral vascular resistance, 13–14, *601*
Peristalsis, oesophageal, 88
Peritoneal dialysis, *322*
continuous ambulatory (CAPD), **321–322**
Peritoneal lavage, *815*
Peritonitis, *106*
appendicitis, 106, *107*
perforated peptic ulcer, 98–99
Peritonsillar abscess (quinsy), **518–519**
Pernicious anaemia, *418*, *530*
Persistent generalised lymphadenopathy (PGL), 1004
Personal hygiene, *see* Hygiene, personal
Personality
coping and, **585–586**
health and, 586–587
pain and, 616
terminal illness and, *927*
type A, 582, **586**
Personal space, **761**, 763, 765
critically ill patients, 836
Person-centred therapy, **587–588**
Petechiae, 441
Pethidine, 300
pH
arterial blood, 647–648, *649*
plasma calcium and, 647
Phaeochromocytoma, **147–148**
Phagocytes, 545
primary impairment, 558–559
Phantom pain/sensations, 275, 389
Pharynx, *506*, 511
Phenomenological, 594
Phenomenological approach to stress, **578–580**
Phentolamine, 233
Phenylketonuria (PKU), 189
Phimosis, **305–306**
Phlebitis, 652
Phobias, 761
Phosphorus, *661*, 662
Phosphorus-32 (^{32}P) therapy, radioactive, 425
Photo-aggravated dermatoses, 461
Photochemotherapy (PUVA therapy), **447**, 449, 450
Photo-contact dermatitis, 461
Photodermatoses, **461–463**
Photographs, 818
Photophobia, 365
Photosensitive dermatitis/actinic reticuloid syndrome, 461, *462*
Phototesting, 462
Phototherapy, **447**, 449, 450
Phthisis bulbi, 487
Physical handicap
diagnosis, 197
oral hygiene, 528
urinary incontinence, 727
see also Disability
Physiotherapists, 348, 433, 539
Physiotherapy
chest, *see* Chest physiotherapy
psoriasis, 451
unconscious patients, 851
venous leg ulcers, 718
see also Exercises
Pia mater, 329, *332*
Piles (haemorrhoids), **111–113**, 733
Pilonidal sinus, **113**
Pinealoma, *351*
Pinprick sensation, burns injuries, 864
Piston effect, 741
Pituitary gland, **134**, *135*, 328
anterior, 134, *135*, *136*
hormones, *135*, *136*, 155
hypersecretion, **139–140**
hyposecretion, **140–142**, 220
negative feedback regulation, *134*
replacement therapy, *142*
ischaemic necrosis, 220
posterior, 134, *135*
Pituitary tumours (adenomas), *352*
functioning, 140, 148, *150*, 220
non-functioning, 140
Placebos, *623*, 628
Plan, nursing care, 917, 949
Plaque, 464
Plasma, 408, *409*
dried, *410*
fresh frozen, *410*
osmolality, regulation, 640–641
Plasma cells, 547
Plasmapheresis, 437
Plasma proteins
nutritional status and, **665–666**
tissue–capillary fluid exchange and, 639
Plasma volume, 638, 643
regulation, 640
Plaster of Paris (POP)
casts, 377
head cap, 533
Platelet(s), **407–408**
concentrate, *410*
disorders, **439–440**
transfusion, 427, 428
Pleura, 61
Plummer–Vinson syndrome, 93, 130, 415
Pluripotent cells, 441
Pneumatic post-amputation mobility aid (PPAM), 390
Pneumocystis carinii pneumonia (PCP), 991, 1005–1006
Pneumonectomy, 78, **79**
Pneumonia, **68–69**
aspiration, *671*, 784, 788
lobar, 69
Pneumocystis carinii (PCP), 991, 1005–1006
viral (primary atypical; PAP), 69
see also Chest infections
Pneumonitis, *890*
Pneumothorax, **80–81**, 674, 853
tension, 80
Police, 817, 822, 823
Pollution, respiratory disease and, 66, **67**
Polycystic ovaries, 222
Polycythaemia vera, **425–426**, *530*
Polydipsia, 157, 158
Polymenorrhagia, 222
Polymenorrhoea, 222
Polymorphic light eruption, 461
Polymorphonuclear leukocytes (neutrophils), 407, 545, 699
Polyneuropathies, diabetes mellitus, 175, *176*
Polyps
endometrial, 222, 224, **244**
nasal, **511**
Polysomnogram, 745
Polyuria, 157, 158, 643
Polyvinyl chloride (cling) film, 862
Pompholyx eczema, 451
Pons, 329
Portage, 741
Portal hypertension, 116, **117–118**, 129
Portosystemic shunting, transjugular intrahepatic (TIPS), 117
Positioning, patient
asthma, 75
emphysema, 72–73
head injury, 343
multiply handicapped patients, 967
postoperative
bronchogenic cancer, 78, 79
intraocular surgery, 476
prolapsed intervertebral disc, 393–394
retinal detachment, 480, 481
renal colic, 303
sleep problems and, 751
spinal injuries, 384–385
terminal illness, 935
unconscious patients, *847*, 850
Posterior column pathway, 333, *335*
Post-herpetic neuralgia, 458
Postoperative care, **792–805**
amputation of limb, 389–391
anorectal surgery, 113
aortic aneurysm repair, 49–50
breast reconstruction, 279–280
cholecystectomy, 122
corneal grafting, 482–483
ectopic pregnancy, 247
enucleation of eye, 490, *491*
gastrectomy, 99–100
grommet insertion, 502
hernia repair, 109
hiatus hernia surgery, 92
hysterectomy, **238–239**, 241, 245
inflammatory bowel disease, 103–104
joint replacement, 399
laryngectomy, 513–515
mastectomy, **271–275**
maxillofacial surgery, 535–536
neurosurgical patients, 342
nursing care plans, 239–240, 272–274, 793–796, 800–801
oral tumours, 539–541
peptic ulcer surgery, 97–98
pneumonectomy/lobectomy, **78–79**
prevention of deep vein thrombosis, 54, 783–784
prolapsed intervertebral disc, 393–394
retinal detachment, 480, 481
termination of pregnancy, 253–254

Postoperative care (*contd*)
thyroidectomy, 141
tonsillectomy, 518
total cystectomy and urinary diversion, 315–316
trabeculectomy, 480
tracheostomy, 516–517
transurethral resection of prostate, 309–311
tympanoplasty, 503–504
urinary stones, 302–304
uterine displacements, 249
vasectomy, 232
Post-traumatic stress disorder, **584–585, 823–824**
Postural drainage, 201, *202*, 206
Posture
disorders affecting, 763
non-aggressive, 822
non-verbal messages, 760, 765
Post-viral fatigue syndrome, 115, **585**
Potassium, **645–646**, 662
dietary intake, 645, *661*
postoperative monitoring, 797
supplements, 40, 46, 646
therapy, 166, 170
see also Hyperkalaemia; Hypokalaemia
Powerlessness, 926
Practice nurses, *67*, *525*
Practice profile, *84*
Prader–Willi syndrome, 137
Prealbumin, serum, 665, *666*
Preconception care, diabetes, 159, 180
Precordial thump, 32
Pregnancy
alcohol in, 981
amenorrhoea of, 219
breast changes, 266
cystic fibrosis females, 202
ectopic, **246–247**
multiple sclerosis, 359
nutritional requirements, 659, *660*
smoking in, 66, 978
termination, 197–198, **253–254**
urinary tract infections, 297
uterine bleeding during, 222
uterine fibroids and, 244–245
valvular heart disease, 43
venous disease, 55
see also Abortion
Pregnancy tests, 243, 246
Preload, 13, *601*
Premedication (premed), 785, *786*, 790
Premenstrual syndrome (PMS), **225–227**
medical management, 226–227
nursing priorities and management, 227
pathophysiology, 225–226
Prenatal diagnosis, 192, **193–194**, *197*, *199*
early embryos, 257
haemophilia A, 204
Preoperative care, **781–786**
amputation of limb, 389
anorectal surgery, 112–113
aortic aneurysms, 48
breast reconstruction, 279
ectopic pregnancy, 247
grommet insertion, 502
hernia repair, 109
hiatus hernia surgery, 92
hysterectomy, 237–238
laryngectomy, 512–513
nursing care plan, 788
oral tumours, 539
peptic ulcer surgery, 97
preventing postoperative complications, 782–785
stoma formation, 103, *104*
thyroidectomy, 144
total cystectomy and urinary diversion, 315–316
tracheostomy, 516
tympanoplasty, 503
uterine prolapse, 249
Presbycusis, 500
Presbyopia, *470*
Prescribing, nurse, 711
Pressure area care
anaemia, 414
critically ill patients, 830, 834
leukaemia, 432
multiple sclerosis, 358
postoperative patients, 240, 317, 514
shock, 606–607
terminally ill patients, 935, *936*
unconscious patients, 853
see also Skin care
Pressure sores, 711, **712–715**
aetiology, 712
assessment of risk, 712–713
classification, 712
definition, 712
epidemiology, 698–699
fractures and, 375, *382*
management, 713–715
measurement, 706
prevention, 713, *714*, *715*
Pressure therapy, burn wounds, 872
Presurgical care, **776–778**
Prevention
accidents, 824
back pain, 392, *393*
breast cancer, **267–269**
burns, 859–861
cancer, **881–883**
colorectal cancer, 111
constipation, *112*, 732–733
deep vein thrombosis/pulmonary embolism, 54, **783–784**, 788
dependency problems, 978
diabetic complications, 173–174, 175, 177
eye disorders, **473**
eye injuries, 473, 489
farmer's lung, 560
hypothermia in elderly, *685*, 693
infectious diseases, **563–565**
postoperative complications, 782–785, 802
pressure sores, 713, *714*, *715*
respiratory disease, **64–67**
salmonellosis, *566*
stroke, 346–347
tuberculosis, 70
Priapism, sickle cell disease, 424
Primary health care team, 768
PR interval, 12
Procidentia, uterine, 248
Proflavin cream, *708*
Progesterone, 214
menorrhagia, 222
menstrual cycle, 215, 216
pregnancy, 219
premenstrual syndrome and, 226
primary dysmenorrhoea, 223
recurrent abortion, 252
Progestogens, 214, 218, 226, 278
Prognosis, 904
cancer, 880
Progressive multifocal leukoencephalopathy (PML), 1006
'Project 2000', 6
Projection, *586*
Prolactin (PRL), *135*, 219, 266
hypersecretion, **140**
Prolactin-inhibiting hormone (PIH), *135*
Prolactinoma, 140, *352*
Prolactin-releasing hormone (PRH), *135*
Prolapse
anterior vaginal wall, 247–248
cervico-vaginal, 247
posterior vaginal wall, 248
utero-vaginal, 248–249
Prone, lying, 389
Proprioceptors, 858
Prostaglandins, 223, 225–226
Prostatectomy
open, 307
patient information, *310*
radical, 312
transurethral, *see* Prostate gland, transurethral resection
Prostate gland, 295–296
biopsy, 312
disorders, **306–312**
transurethral resection (TURP), **308–311**
complications, 307
indications, 307, 312, 733
informed consent, 308
postoperative care, 309–311
postoperative problems, 308
Prostatic cancer, **311–312**
Prostatic hyperplasia, benign, **306–311**, 733
medical management, 307
nursing priorities and management, 307–311
pathophysiology, 306–307
Prostatitis, *232*
Prosthodontist, 539
Protein(s), 658, 659, **660–661**
dietary requirements, *660*, *661*
plasma, *see* Plasma proteins
Protein-energy malnutrition (PEM), *659*, 663, 665
Proteinuria, 174, 318, 319, 730
Proteoglycans, 699
Proton pump inhibitors, 97
Protozoal infections, AIDS, 1005–1006
Pruritus (itching), 130, 464
eczema, 452
jaundice, 114
pancreatic cancer, 128
psoriasis, 448
Pseudocyst, 130
Pseudohypoparathyroidism, *143*
Pseudomonas aeruginosa, 704
Psoralen, 447
Psoriasis, **447–451**, 763
epidemiology, 447
erythrodermic, 448, 450
flexural, 447
guttate, 447
medical management, 447, 448–449
nursing priorities and management, 449–451
pathophysiology, 448
plaque, 447, *448*
pustular, 447–448, 450
social attitudes, *907*
Psoriasis Association, 449, 465
Psoriatic arthropathy, 448, 451
Psychological factors
cancer deaths, 880
impotence, 232–233
speech, 759
Psychological impact
burns, 872–873
cancer diagnosis, 884–885
deafness, 500

Psychological impact (*contd*)
  diagnosis of genetic disorders, 197–198
  see also Emotional responses
Psychological problems
  anorexia nervosa, 138
  breast cancer/mastectomy, 263, 272–273, 950
  chronic renal failure, 321
  Cushing's syndrome, *148*, 151
  diabetes mellitus, 179
  disabled, 945–946, 955
  enteral feeding, 672
  Huntington's disease, *207*, 208
  post-menopausal, 216
  see also Anxiety; Depression; Stress
Psychological support
  acromegaly, 139–140
  amputation of limb, 389
  aplastic anaemia, 421
  asthma, 74
  breast cancer, 271
  breast infections, 288
  breast reconstruction, 279, 280
  cancer, 885, 886, 888, 893, *896*, 901–902
  colorectal cancer, 110
  congenital adrenal hyperplasia, 152
  diabetes mellitus, 171
  ectopic pregnancy, 247
  eczema, 453
  emphysema, 71
  family, 936
  fungating wounds and, 935
  gastric carcinoma, 100
  gynaecomastia, 288–289
  hypopituitarism, 141–142
  intracranial tumours, 352
  Klinefelter syndrome, 198–199
  myotonic dystrophy, 206
  nerve injuries, 402
  oesophageal carcinoma, 95
  oral tumours, 541
  photodermatoses, 462–463
  premenstrual syndrome, 227
  psoriasis, 449
  rheumatoid arthritis, 397
  sexual differentiation disorders, 152
  termination of pregnancy, 197–198
  total cystectomy and urinary diversion, 315
Psychological therapy
  insomnia, 755
  stress, 587–588
Psychomotor seizures, *355*
Psychosis, amenorrhoea, 220
Psychosocial problems
  chronic pain, 620–621
  cystic fibrosis, 201–202, *203*
  parenteral nutrition, 676
  post-amputation, 391
  psoriasis, 449
  wound healing and, 703
  wounds, 720
Psychotherapy, impotence, 233
Puberty, breast changes, 265–266
Public awareness campaigns, chronic illness, 907
Pubococcygeus muscle, 731
Pulmonary artery catheters, 608, 610
Pulmonary artery pressure, monitoring, 609–610, *611*
Pulmonary artery (capillary) wedge pressure (PAWP; PCWP), *601*, 610, *611*
Pulmonary embolism, *25*, **783–784**
  post-myocardial infarction, 34
  prevention, 54, **783–784**, 788
  total cystectomy and urinary diversion, 317
Pulmonary oedema, **82**
  glomerulonephritis, *318*
  heart failure, 38, 39–40
  shock, 600
Pulmonary valve, *10*, 11, 12
Pulmonary vascular resistance, *601*
Pulse
  burns, 867
  myocardial infarction, 25
  peripheral arterial disease, 51
  raised intracranial pressure, *339*, 341
Pulse oximeters, 42, 608, 867
Pulse pressure, 14, 600
PULSES, 949
Pupils
  assessment, *339*, 471
  reaction to light, 846, 857
  size, 846
Purpura, 441
Pustules, 464
PUVA therapy (photochemotherapy), **447**, 449, 450
P wave, 12
Pyelolithotomy, 302, 303–304
Pyelonephritis, **297–298**
  acute, 297
  chronic, 298
Pyloric stenosis, 97, **99**
Pyloroplasty, *97*
Pyramidal tracts, 334, *336*
Pyrexia
  blood transfusion, 418
  CNS infections, 364
  myocardial infarction, 26, 689–690
  nursing care, 690, 691
  pathophysiology, 689
  septicaemic shock, 606
  sleep problems, 752
  unconscious patients, 855
  versus heat illness, 690
  wound healing and, 702
Pyridoxine (vitamin B_6), 226, *661*
Pyrogens, endogenous, 689

Q

QRS complex, 12
Quadriplegia, 386
Quality assurance, 741
Quality audit, 741
Quality of life
  disabled patients, 947, 954–956
  patients in isolation, 556
  terminally ill patients, **925–926**
Questioning, 766
Quinsy (peritonsillar abscess), **518–519**
QUIT, 989
Q wave, 12

R

Racial differences, *see* Ethnic differences
Radial artery cannulation, 609
Radiation
  cancer caused by, 881
  cellular effects, 886–887
  eye injuries caused by, **489**
  heat transfer by, 683, *684*
  intensive care units, 830–831
  ovarian effects, 220, *891*
  protection, 888
  sources, radiotherapy, 887
Radical radiotherapy, 887
Radical treatment, 885
Radioactive iodine (^{131}I) therapy, 144–145
Radioactivity, 886
Radioisotopes, 886
Radiotherapy, 629, **886–888**
  adjuvant, 887
  bladder cancer, 314
  breast cancer, 263, 270, 275, *276*, 277, 282–283
  cervical carcinoma, 237
  external beam, 887
  intracranial tumours, 352
  large field, 887
  lymphoma, 435, 436
  myeloma, 437
  myths and fears, 888
  oesophageal carcinoma, 93
  oral tumours, 538
  palliative, 887
  prostatic cancer, 312
  radical, 887
  side-effects, *276*, 888, *889–891*
  testicular cancer, 229
Raphe nuclei, *617*, 618
Rationalisation, *586*
Rave culture, 984, *985*
Raynaud's disease, 52, 694
Raynaud's phenomenon, 52, **694**
Reaction formation, *586*
Readability, written materials, 761
Reality orientation, 965
Records
  accessibility, 768
  genetic disorders, 195
  pain, 627–628
  personal medication, *29*, *30*
  respiratory disorders, *84*
  seizures, 354, 854
  shared, 769
  trauma, 813
  violent incidents, 822–823
  written, 769
Recovery position, *847*
Recovery room nurse, *789*, 791–792
Recreation/leisure
  disability, 947
  heart disease, 19, 40, 42–43
  hypertension, 46
Recrudescence, 464
Rectal administration, analgesics, 629
Rectocele, 248, 249
Rectum, 90
Red blood cells, **406–407**
  decreased production, 412
  disorders, **411–426**
  frozen, *410*
  leucocyte-poor, *410*
  overproduction, 425–426
  washed, *410*
Red cell concentrates, *410*
Red eye, **483–485**
Redivac drain, *803*
Re-epithelialisation, wounds, 699–700, 869
Referred pain, 621
Refuse, *see* Waste
Regional nerve blocks, 629
Rehabilitation, **943–956**
  aplastic anaemia, 421
  CNS infections, 365
  definition, 943–944

Rehabilitation (*contd*)
head injury, **343–344**
instrumentality model, 953–954
joint replacement, 399
laryngectomy patients, 514–515
model, *947*, 954–955
myocardial infarction, 26–28
nurse's role, 948
nursing activities in, 948–953
oral tumours, 541
patient–professional roles, 947–948
patients needing, 944, *945*
postoperative, 792, **805**
process, 946–947
research awareness and, 944–945
stroke, 348–349, *945*, 952, 954
units, 946, 948
see also Disability
Relate (National Marriage Guidance Council), 359, 366, 596
Relatives, *see* Family
Relaxation, **590, 630**
hypertension, 46
insomnia, 755
meditative, *591*
menstrual disorders, 221, 224
Religious advisors/ministers, 539, 857
Religious needs, *see* Spiritual needs
REM sleep, **745–746**
function, 747
neurological control, 746
Renal arteries, 292
Renal calculi, *see* Urinary stones
Renal colic, 299
medical management, 300–302
nursing care plan, 303
nursing priorities and management, 302–304
Renal disease, **316–322**
diabetes mellitus, 174–175
eye disorders, *493*
Renal failure
acute (ARF), *318*, **319–320**, 613
aortic aneurysm repair, 50
chronic, 318, **320–322**
medical management, 321
nursing priorities and management, 321–322
pathophysiology, 321
myeloma, 437–438
prostatic cancer, 312
Renal function, **292–294**
benign prostatic hyperplasia, 307–308
burns, 867
shock, 599–600, 611
Renal transplantation, 174, 321
Renal tubular necrosis, acute (ATN), 319
Renal tubules, 292
reabsorption, 293
secretion, 293
Renin, 14, 293
Renin–angiotensin–aldosterone system, 14, 641
Repression, *586*
Reproductive system, **211–262**
anatomy and physiology, 211–217
Research awareness, 944–945
Residential homes, 912, 922
Residual volume (RV), 61, *63*
Re-Solv, 984, 987, 989
Respect for persons, 963–964
Respiration
external, 60–63
internal (cellular), 60, 64
physiology, **60–64**
raised intracranial pressure, *341*
shock, 600, 603, 608
unconscious patients, 846
see also Breathing; Ventilation
Respiratory acidosis, 648, **650**
Respiratory alkalosis, 648, **649–650**
Respiratory centres, 61, *62*, 329
Respiratory depression, 623, 798
Respiratory disorders, 59, **67–85**
disabled, 950
genetic, 84
hypertension, 46
maxillofacial injuries, 533–534
myocardial infarction, 26, 28, 30
obstructive, 70–75
prevention and health education, 64–67
principles of nursing management, **64–67**
sleep and, 751
see also Breathing
Respiratory distress syndrome
adult (ARDS), 62, 600, **613**
infant, 62
Respiratory emergencies, **79–82**
Respiratory failure, **82**
Respiratory muscles, 61
Respiratory system, 59–86
anatomy and physiology, 60–64
burns-associated injury, **865**
speech production and, 759
Respiratory tract infections, **68–70**
cystic fibrosis, 201
see also Chest infections
Respolin inhaler, *75*
Response, 594
Rest
angina pectoris, 18, 19
aortic aneurysms, 48
eczema, 454
heart failure, 40
multiple sclerosis, 358
psoriasis, 451
unconscious patients, 852
see also Activity, physical; Bedrest
Resuscitation, **811–812**
cardiopulmonary (CPR), **31–32**, *33*, 60
facilities, organisation, 812
'neck breathing' patient, *513*
'not for', 32, 833
room, 811, 812
Reticular, 858
Reticular activating system (RAS), 746, **840–841**
Reticular formation, 329, *617*, 618, 746, **840–841**
Reticulocyte count, 406, 413
Retina, 468
assessment, 471
Retinal artery occlusion, central, **495**
Retinal detachment, 476, **480–482**
Retinol binding protein, serum, 665, *666*
Retinopathy
diabetic, **173–174, 493–494**
HIV, 494
hypertensive, 494
Retroperitoneal fibrosis, 304–305
Retroviruses, 993
Reversal, *586*
Rewarming methods, 693
Rhesus factor, 409–410
Rheumatic fever (RF), 41
Rheumatic heart disease (RHD), 41
Rheumatoid arthritis (RA), 370, **394–397**, *719*
family effects, *398*
medical management, 394–396
nursing priorities and management, 396–397
pathophysiology, 394
Rhinophyma, 461
Rhinorrhoea, cerebrospinal fluid, 343, 534
Riboflavin, *659, 660, 661*
Ribs, fractured, **79–80**
Rickets, **147**
Right bundle branch, 11, 12
Rigors, 689
Ringer's lactate (Hartmann's) solution, 605, 643
Rings, removal, 383
Ringworm, **455**
Risk factors
breast cancer, 266–267
cervical carcinoma, *234*
deep vein thrombosis, *783*
ischaemic heart disease, 15, *16*
stroke, 173, 347
RNA, 188, 993
Road traffic accidents (RTAs), 335, 369, 531, 810
Rod cells, 468
Rodding of fornices, *489*
Rodent ulcer, 537
Roger's crystal spray, 514, 519
Role fulfilment, disabled, 955
Roper–Logan–Tierney model of nursing, *see* Activities of living model of nursing
Rosacea, **461**
Royal Association for Disability and Rehabilitation (RADAR), 958
Royal College of General Practitioners, 184
Royal College of Midwives, 356, 366
Royal College of Nursing (RCN)
AIDS Nursing Forum, 1009
Orthopaedia Forum, 404
Substance Misuse Forum, 987
Royal Marsden Hospital, 264, 290
Royal National Institute for the Blind (RNIB), 174, 496
Royal National Institute for the Deaf, 520
Roy's adaptation model of nursing, 10, 898
AIDS/HIV infection and, 1003
chronic illness and, 913–914
Rubella, *569*
Rubrospinal tract, *335*
'Rule of Nines', 862–863
Rust rings, corneal, *490*
R wave, 12

S

Sacral oedema, heart failure, 38, *39*
Sadness, terminally ill patients, 926
Safety
cytotoxic chemotherapy, *894*
infection control and, 557
patient
anaemia, 414
aortic aneurysms, 48
CNS infections, 365
epilepsy, *355*
heart failure, 39
hysterectomy, 238
intensive care units, 829–831
ischaemic heart disease, 18, 25
multiple sclerosis, 357–358
perioperative, **786–792**
peripheral vascular disease, 52, 55
prolapsed intervertebral disc, 395
raised intracranial pressure, 342–343
rheumatoid arthritis, 397

Safety (*contd*)
stroke, 347
unconscious patients, 853–854
valvular heart disease, 43
visually impaired, 474
radiation, 888
staff, 822
theatre, 786, 788
Saline mouthwashes, 529
Saline solution, normal, 605, 643
Saliva, 88, 523
substitutes, 528
Salivary glands, 88, 523
tumours, **537**
Salmonellosis, **565**, *566*, 1006
Salpingectomy, 246–247
Salpingitis, **245–246**
Salpingolysis, 260
Salpingostomy, 260
Saltatory conduction, *327*, 365
Salt intake, *see* Sodium intake
Samaritans, 596
Sarcoidosis, **560–561**
Sarcoma, *878*
Scabies, **455**, *456*
Norwegian, 1006
Scalds, 607, 860
see also Burns
Scar tissue, 701, *702*
burn wounds, **871–872**
hypertrophic, 701, 871–872
Schiller test, 235
Schistosomiasis, urinary, 313
Schizophrenia, amenorrhoea, 220
Scholl (UK) Ltd, 185
School nurses, 67, 454, *525*
Schwann cells, 326
Schwannoma, *350*
Sclera, 468
Sclerotherapy, 130
haemorrhoids, 111
oesophageal varices, 117, 118
Scopolamine, *786*
Scottish Association for the Deaf, 520
Scottish Institute of Human Relations, 596
Scottish Partnership Agency for Palliative and Cancer Care (SPAPCC), 923, 942
Screening
AIDS/HIV infection, 999, 1000
breast cancer, **268–269**, 883
cancer, 882–883
cervical cancer, 235, 883
diabetic complications, 173, 175
genetic, *see* Genetic screening
glaucoma, 480, 484
testicular cancer, *229*
Scrotum, 296
Scrub nurse, 787, *789*
Seat belts, 336–337, 369
Sebaceous glands, 446
disorders, **460–461**
Second (optic) nerve, *330*, 469
Secretin, 89, 91
Sedatives, *786*
Seizures, 353, 847, 854
classification, *355*
CNS infections, 364
dealing with, 354, *854*
first-aid, *848*
generalised, *355*
glomerulonephritis, *318*
intracranial tumours, 352
nursing priorities and management, 353–356
partial, *355*
recording, 354, 854
subarachnoid haemorrhage, 346
triggers, 354
see also Epilepsy
Selective serotonin re-uptake inhibitors, 589
Selenium, *661*
Self-care
amputation of limb, 390–391
asthma, 64, *74*, 75–76, *78*
breast cancer, 282, 286
colostomy, *948*
diabetes mellitus, 171, **178**
disabled, 950–951
transurethral resection of prostate, 311
wound managment, 710–711
Self-concept, hysterectomy and, *238*
Self-esteem
critically ill patients, 835
terminally ill patients, 928
Self-help groups, *see* Support/self-help groups
Self-help in pain groups (SHIP), 635
Self-image
critically ill patients, 835
diabetes mellitus and, 179
Huntington's disease, 209
rheumatoid arthritis, 397
see also Body image
Selye's General Adaptation Syndrome, **577**, 581
Semen volume, *256*
Semicircular canals, 498
Semilunar valves, 11
Seminal vesicles, 295, *296*
Senile macular degeneration, **492**, *492*
Sensory deficits
stroke, *345*
unconscious patients, 854
Sensory deprivation, intensive care units, 831, *832*
Sensory neurone/nerve fibre, 326, 632
Sensory overload, intensive care units, 831, *832*
Sensory pathways, 333–334, 617
Sensory receptors
respiratory system, 61, *62*
skin, 446
Septicaemia, agranulocytosis, 438, 439
Septicaemic shock, **601–602**, 792
management/treatment, 606–607
nursing care plan, 603–604
pathophysiology, 602
patients at risk, *605*
Septic arthritis, **394**
Sequential pneumatic compression, 784
Seroma, after breast reconstruction, 279
Serotonin (5-hydroxytryptamine), 618, 746
Serotonin re-uptake inhibitors, selective, 589
Serum, 408
Serum proteins, *see* Plasma proteins
Serum sickness, 560
Servier Laboratories Ltd, 185
Seventh nerve, *see* Facial nerve
Sex, *see* Gender
Sex chromosome variations, **191**
Sex hormones, 137, 213–214, 295
Sexual activity
angina pectoris, 19
aortic aneurysms, 48
cancer patients, 899–900
cervical carcinoma and, 234
disabled patients, 952
heart failure, 41
hip replacement, 400–401
hypertension, 46
hysterectomy and, 238
leukaemia and, 432
multiple sclerosis, 359
myocardial infarction and, 28, 31
prostatectomy and, *310*
rheumatoid arthritis, 397
urinary tract infections and, 296, 297
valvular heart disease, 43
Sexual contact, HIV transmission, 993
Sexual counselling, 739
Sexual differentiation, disorders of, **152**
Sexually transmitted diseases, 544
Sexual problems
infertility, *255*, *256*
radiotherapy-induced, *891*
urinary incontinence, **738–739**
Sexual relationships
chronic illness, 910
diabetes mellitus, 180
Shared care, diabetes mellitus, 158, 182
Sharing, ad hoc, 593
Sharps disposal, 554, *555*
Shaving, preoperative, 703, 785
Shift-work, 744
Shingles, *see* Herpes zoster
Shirodker's procedure, 252
Shivering, 683, 692
Shock, 534, **597–614**
acute pancreatitis, 124, 125
anaphylactic, *see* Anaphylactic shock
burns, 865–866
cardiogenic, *see* Cardiogenic shock
compensatory stage, 598–599, 792–794, *792*
complications, 613–614
definitive/supportive therapy, 607
distributive, 598, **601–604**
ectopic pregnancy, 246
first aid treatment, 607, *608*
hypovolaemic, *see* Hypovolaemic shock
identifying patients at risk, *605*
management/treatment, 604–607
monitoring patient in, 608–613
neurogenic, 604, *605*, 792
pathophysiology, 597–600
postoperative, **792–795**
progressive stage (failing compensation), 599–600, 792, *792*
refractory stage, 600
septicaemic, *see* Septicaemic shock
spinal, **385, 604**, *605*
stages, 598–600
types, 600–604
Short stature, *143*
disproportionate, 143
hypopituitarism, 141, *142*
Shoulder
dislocated, **394**, *395*
exercises, after mastectomy, 275
Showers, preoperative, 785
Shunting, intrapulmonary, 63
Sickle cell anaemia, 192, 421, **422–424**
medical management, 422–423
nursing priorities and management, 423–424
pathophysiology, 422, *423*
Sickle cell crisis, 422, 423–424
Sickle Cell Society, 441
Sick role, 620, 910, 944, 998
Sign language, 761
Single-gene disorders, **191–192**
Sinoatrial (SA; sinus) node, 11, 12
Sinus arrhythmia (SA), 35
Sinus bradycardia, 35
Sinuses, paranasal, **509**

Sinusitis
  acute, **509**
  chronic, **509**
Sinus tachycardia, 35
Sixth (abducens) nerve, *330*
Skeletal disorders, **373–391**
Skeletal system, **370–372**
  appendicular, 371–372
  axial, 371
Skeletal traction, *374*, 375, *376*, *387*
Skin, **445–446**
  biopsy, 449, 452, 459
  cleaning, surgical patients, 789
  excessive fluid losses, 643
  functions, 446, *544*
  patch testing, 452, 462
  peripheral vascular disease, 51
  piercing, HIV transmission, 994
  preoperative preparation, **785**, 788
  scrapings, 452
  shock, 613
  structure, 445–446
  swabs, 449, 452, 459
  temperature, *see* Temperature, body, skin surface
Skin care
  AIDS/HIV infection, *1005*
  amputation stump, 390
  Cushing's syndrome, 151
  fractures of neck of humerus, 382
  fungating breast tumours, 286
  heart failure, 40
  Huntington's disease, 209
  hyperglycaemic hyperosmolar non-ketotic coma, 170
  liver failure, 119
  newly healed burn wounds, *871*
  peripheral arterial disease, 53
  rheumatoid arthritis, 397
  terminally ill patients, 934
  see also Pressure area care
Skin disorders, **443–465**, 763
  AIDS, 463
  bullous, 458–460
  cancer therapy inducing, *889*, *893*
  Cushing's syndrome, *148*
  epidemiology, **444**
  nurse's role, **444**
  principles of therapy, 446–447
  social attitudes, 443–444, *907*
Skinfold thickness, triceps (TSF), 665
Skin grafts, burn wounds, 870
Skin infections, **454–458**
  AIDS, 463
  diabetes mellitus, 158
Skin infestations, **455–456**, 1006
Skin traction, 375, *376*, *377*
Skin tumours, 444, **463**
Sleep, **743–755**
  angina pectoris, 19
  assessment, **752–753**
  deprivation, 747
  factors affecting, **747–749**
  functions, **746–747**
  heart failure, 40
  helping patients to, 753, *754*
  hypertension, 46
  myocardial infarction, 28, 30
  normal, **747–749**
  NREM, **745**, 746
  peripheral arterial disease, 53
  physiological control, **746**, 840–841
  positions, 751
  REM, **745–746**, 747
  rheumatoid arthritis, 397
  slow wave (SWS), 745, 746–747
  structure, **744–746**
  substances, 746
  surgical patients, 750, *751*, 799
  transurethral resection of prostate and, 308
  unconscious patients, 852
  valvular heart disease, 42
Sleep apnoea syndrome, 751–752
Sleep disorders, **749–752**
  of excessive somnolence (DOES), 749–750
  of initiating and maintaining (DIMS), *see* Insomnia
  parasomnias, *749*, **752**
  of sleep–wake cycle, *749*
Sleepiness, daytime, 750, 752
Sleep paralysis, 750
Sleep–wake cycle, **743–744**
  disrupted normal, 744, *749*
Sleepwalking, 752
Slit lamp examination, myotonic dystrophy, 206
Slough, *698*, 706
Small intestine, **89–90**
  disorders, **101–111**
Smell
  decreased sense of, 667
  see also Odour
Smoke detectors, 861
Smoke inhalation injuries, 865
Smokers' Quitline, 989
Smoking, **978–979**
  angina pectoris and, 18
  burns and, 860
  campaigns against, 881–882
  cancer and, 881
  cessation aids, 979
  diabetes mellitus and, 181
  and health, **66**, 978–979
  hernia repair and, 109
  hypertension and, 44, 46
  myocardial infarction, 30
  oesophageal carcinoma and, 93
  passive, 66, 979
  peptic ulceration and, 96
  peripheral arterial disease, 53
  preoperative cessation, 782
  respiratory disorders and, 64–66
  sleep and, *754*
  stroke and, 347
  withdrawal symptoms, 979
  women and, 978–979
  wound healing and, 702–703
Snellen test-type chart, *471*
Snoring, 751
Soaps, antibacterial, 550
Social activities
  chronic illness and, 910
  diabetes mellitus, 180
  rheumatoid arthritis, 397
  terminally ill patients, 934
Social attitudes
  AIDS/HIV infection, 997–998
  cancer, *876*
  chronic illness/disability, 906–907, 953
  elderly, 961
  incontinence, 724–725
  skin disorders, 443–444, *907*
Social impact, AIDS/HIV infection, 997–998
Social problems, *see* Psychosocial problems
Social services, AIDS/HIV infection and, 997
Social support
  breast cancer and, 271
  chronic illness, 910
  post-hysterectomy, *238*
Social workers, 433
  laryngectomy patients, 515
  oral tumours and, 539, 540
  visually impaired and, 473
Socioeconomic status
  anorexia nervosa and, 138
  breast cancer and, 267
  cardiovascular disease and, 9
  constipation and, *112*
  obesity and, 662–663
Sodium, **644**, *661*, 662
  balance, disorders of, **641–643**, 644
  regulation, 640–641
  see also Hypernatraemia; Hyponatraemia
Sodium chloride, 639
Sodium intake
  ascites, 117
  heart failure, 40
  hypertension and, 44, 46
Sodium–potassium pump, 639
Soft tissue injuries, *382*, **401–403**
  face, 531, 532
Solar urticaria, 461
Solutes, **638–639**
Solvent abuse, **983–984**
Somatostatin, *135*, 139
Somatotrophin, *see* Growth hormone
Sounds, 741
Space
  personal, *see* Personal space
  territorial, 761, 836
Space blanket, 166
Specific dynamic action (SDA) of foods, 686
Speech, **758–760**
  aids, *515*
  anatomy and physiology, 758–759
  oesophageal, 513, 515
  psychological factors affecting, 759
  tracheostomy and, 516
  use and interpretation, 759–760
Speech disorders, **762–763**
  Huntington's disease, *207*, 208–209
  management, 762–763
  multiple sclerosis, 357
  Parkinson's disease, 362
  stroke, *345*, **347**, 762, 763
Speech therapists, 763
  laryngectomy patients, 513, 515
  multiple sclerosis, 357
  oral tumours and, 539
  Parkinson's disease, 362
  stroke rehabilitation, 348
Speech therapy services, 762–763
Spermatic cords, 295, 296
Spermatozoa, 295
  agglutination, *256*
  treatment of poor quality, 257
Spider telangiectasia, 130
Spillages, 553, *554*
Spinal anaesthesia, 604, 790
Spinal anaesthetics/opioids, 629
Spinal cord, **332–335**
  injuries, 383, *386*, *404*
  motor pathways, 333, 334–335, *336*
  pain pathways, 617
  sensory pathways, 333–334
  structure, 333, *334*
  subacute combined degeneration, 419
Spinal injuries, **383–386**, 813, 816, 951
  medical management, 383
  nursing priorities and management, 384–386
  pathophysiology, 383
Spinal nerves, 333, *334*, **336**
Spinal shock, **385**, **604**, *605*

Spindle poisons, *892, 895*
Spine, 371
Spinex card, *385*
Spinocerebellar tracts, 333, *334*
Spinothalamic pathways, 334
Spinothalamic tract, 858
Spiritual needs
  AIDS patients, 1007
  cancer patients, 902
  critically ill patients, 836
  elderly, 968–969
  relatives of dying/deceased patients, 818
  terminally ill patients, *927*
Spirometry, *63*, 71
Spironolactone, 227
Spleen, **91**, 544
  disorders, **129–130**
  trauma/rupture, **129**, 815, 817
Splenectomy, 117, 129–130
Splintage
  Colles' fracture, 383
  fractures, 374
Splints
  joint, rheumatoid arthritis, *396*
  ligament injuries, 401
  nerve injuries, 402
  ureteroileal anastomosis, 316
SPOD (Association to Aid the Sexual Problems of the Disabled), 366, 397, 404, 739, 741, 958
Sporting injuries, 370, 532
Sports, for disabled, 947
Squamous cell carcinoma (SCC), oral, 537
Squint, 485–486
Staging, cancer, 883–885, 904
Staining agents, eye, *476*
Standing Conference on Drug Abuse (SCODA), 987, 989
Stapedectomy, 502
Staphylococcus aureus, 704
Staples, *799, 803*
Status asthmaticus, 73
Status epilepticus, 847
Statutory services
  chronic illness, 910–911
  rehabilitation, 946–947
Steatorrhoea, 101
Stem cells, 441
Stenting
  biliary tract, 128
  ureteric, 300, *301*, 302, 303–304
Sterilisation (instruments), 551
Sterilisation (operative), 260
  female, 254, 260
Sterility, 254, *891*
Steri-Strips, 819–821
Steroid therapy, *see* Corticosteroid therapy
Stigma, 761
  AIDS/HIV infection, 998
  cancer, *876*
  chronic illness, 906, *907*
  disability, 945–946, 955
Stillbirths, 197
Stimulant abuse, **984–985**
Stimulus, 594
Stimulus-based model of stress, **576**
Stockings, elastic support/compression
  prevention of deep vein thrombosis, 783–784
  venous insufficiency, 54, 55, 56
Stoma(s)
  colorectal cancer, 110–111
  inflammatory bowel disease, 103–104
  nurse, *104*, 316, 935
  terminally ill patients, 933, 935
  total cystectomy and urinary diversion, 314, 315–316
  see also Colostomy
Stomach
  anatomy and physiology, **88–89**
  carcinoma, **99–100**
  disorders, **96–100**
Stomatitis/sore mouth, 441, **530–531**
  anaemia, 412, 414
  cancer therapy inducing, *889*, 893
Story-telling, 960–961
Stress, **575–596**
  amenorrhoea and, 220, 221
  cancer and, 880
  chronic, pathophysiology, **582**
  depression and, 584
  disease and, **582–585**
  hypertension and, 45, 582
  irritable bowel syndrome and, 105
  management/treatment, **587–589**
    choosing therapeutic help, 588
    drug therapy, 588–589
    other methods, 589–590
    psychological therapies, 587–588
  migraine and, 583
  models, **576–580**
    phenomenological approach, 578–580
    response-based models, 576–577
    stimulus-based model, 576
    transactional models, 577–578
  newly disabled, 946
  nursing-related, 541, **590–594**, *897*
    nursing education and, 591
    sources, 590–591
    support and supervision, 592–593
    terminal care and, 591–592
  response
    acute, 580, **581–582**
    pain, 619–620
    physiological, 577, **580–582**
    shock, 599
    systems model, 576–577
  shock and, 599
Stress disorder, post-traumatic, **584–585, 823–824**
Stress fractures, 373
Stress incontinence, 725, 727
  treatment, 731, 733
Stressors, 576–577, 580
Stress ulceration, **96**
Stretch receptors, respiratory system, *62*
Stroke (cerebrovascular accident; CVA), **344–349**
  causes, 344
  communication problems, *345*, **347**, 762, 763
  completed, *345*
  effects, 345
  in evolution, *345*
  medical management, 345–346
  nursing care after, 347–348, 967–969
  nursing priorities and management, **346–349**
  prevention, 346–347
  rehabilitation, **348–349**, *945*, 952, 954
  risk factors, 173, 347
  visual deficits, *345*, 348, **494**
Stroke volume, 12, *601*
ST segment, 12
  changes, 16, *23*
Stump bandages, 389, 390–391
Stupor, 843
Stye, **486**
Subarachnoid haemorrhage, **344**
  causes, 344
  complications, 346
  medical management, 345, 346
  nursing care after, 347–348
  see also Stroke
Subcutaneous infusions
  analgesics, 629, *798*
  fluids and electrolytes, 651
Subdural empyema, 363
Subdural haematoma, *340*
Subfertility, *see* Infertility/subfertility
Sublingual administration, analgesics, 629, *798*
Sublingual gland, 523
Submandibular gland, 523
Substance abuse/misuse, *see* Dependency problems
Substance P, 617, 618
Substantia gelatinosa, 617, 619
Subtarsal foreign body, 489
Suction curettage, 253
Sudden death, *see* Death, sudden
Sudden infant death syndrome (SIDS), 818
Sugar, dietary intake, 525
Suicide, 208, 583
Sulphonylureas, **160–161**, 172
Sulphur, 662
Sunlight, 461, *463*
Sunscreens, 462
Superficial temporal–middle cerebral artery anastomosis (ST–MCA bypass), 346
Supervision, *see* Support and supervision
Support, psychological, *see* Psychological support
Support/self-help groups
  bereaved, 819
  cancer, 897–898
  dependency problems, 987
  pain sufferers, 632
  see also Voluntary agencies
Support services
  chronic illness, 910–911
  dependency problems, 986–987
  terminal illness, 923
Support and supervision, **592–593**, 594
  A & E staff, 823–824
  death of a patient and, 939–940
Supraclavicular lymph node metastases, *277*
Supraventricular tachycardia, 36
Surfaces, cleaning/disinfection, 553, *554*
Surfactant, 62, 865
Surgery
  cancer, 885–886
  changing patterns, 775–776
  classification, **776**
  complications, 802
  decision to operate, **778–780**
  elective, 776, *778*
  emergency, 776, *779*
  essential, 776, *778*
  incision lines, *798*
  pain-relieving, 629
  presenting for, **776–778**
  waiting times, 776
Surgical patients, **775–807**
  fluid and electrolyte balance, **655**
  informed decision-making, 778–781
  malnutrition, 663–664
  parenteral nutrition, 673
  perioperative care, **786–792**
  postoperative care, *see* Postoperative care
  preoperative care, *see* Preoperative care
  presurgical care, 776–778
  sleep problems, 750, *751*, 799
Surrogate motherhood, **259–260**
Suscard buccal, *17*

Sutured wounds, *see* Wound(s), sutured
Sutures, *799*, *803*
  removal, 719, 802, *803*
Suxamethonium, *791*
Swabs
  skin, 449, 452, 459
  throat, 449
  wounds, *705*, 867
Swallowing, 88, *522*, 523
  problems, *see* Dysphagia
Swan–Ganz catheter, 610
S wave, 12
Sweat glands, 446
Sweating
  excessive, 643
  heat loss by, 683, *684*, *692*
Swelling, soft tissue injuries, 402
Symbolic feeding, *936*
Sympathectomy, 52
Sympathetic nervous system, 336, *337*
  blood flow regulation, 13
  cardiac function regulation, 13
  hypoglycaemic symptoms and, 172
  shock, 598–599
Sympathetic ophthalmitis, 487
Synacthen test, short, 149
Synapse, 858
Synovectomy, 395
Synovial joints, 371–372
Syphilis, 41, 47, *529*
Syringing, ear, 499
Systemic lupus erythematosus (SLE), **562**
Systems model of human stress response, **576–577**
Systole, 12
Systolic pressure, 14

T

T_3 (tri-iodothyronine), 135, 136, 145
T_4, *see* Thyroxine
Tachycardia
  junctional, 36
  sinus, 35
  supraventricular, 36
  ventricular, 36
Taeniae coli, 90
Talking Newspaper Association of the UK (TNAUK), 496
Tamoxifen, 270–271, 276
Tamponade, cardiac, 47
Taste changes, 666–667, *890*, 899, 933
Tavistock Institute, 596
Tay–Sachs disease, 192
Tea, 978
Teaching, patient, *see* Education, patient
Team(s)
  community drug and alcohol, 987
  genetic counselling, 194
  multidisciplinary, **768–769**
  oral cancer care, 539
  palliative care, 629–630, 922, 928
  primary health care, 768
  rehabilitation and, 946, 950
Team supervision, nurses, 593
Tears, 469
Technology, high, 829
Tectospinal tract, *336*
Teenagers, *see* Young people
Teeth, 523
  impacted wisdom, 523, 527
Telangiectasia, 464
  haemorrhagic, 519
Teletherapy, 887
Temazepam, *786*
Temperature, ambient (room)
  intensive care units, 830
  sleep and, 752
Temperature, body, **679–694**
  axillary, *680*, *681*
  burns, 868
  CNS infections, 364
  core (deep), **680–681**
  disturbances, **687–694**
    see also Fever; Heat illness; Hypothermia
  head injury, 343
  measurement, 679, **686–687**
    elderly people at home, 693
    sites, *681*
    techniques, *681*, 687
    unconscious patients, 855
  monitoring, shock, 611–613
  myocardial infarction, 26
  normal range, 683–686
  oral, *681*
  rectal, 680, *681*
  regulation, 446, 679, **681–683**
    behavioural, 681
    heat conservation mechanisms, 681–682
    heat loss mechanisms, 683, *684*
    heat production mechanisms, 682–683, 686
  skin surface, **679–680**
    measurement, 687
    peripheral arterial disease, 52
  sleep and, 752
  unconscious patients, 846, 855
Temporal arteritis, **482–483**
Tendon injuries, **401–402**
Tensile (strength), *698*, 700
Tenth nerve, *see* Vagus nerve
Tentorium cerebri, 329
Teratoma
  ovarian, 242, **245**
  pineal, *351*
Terence Higgins Trust, 989, 1009
Terminally ill patients, **921–940**
  CNS infections, 364
  emotional responses, 925–926
  food presentation, *668*
  nursing issues, 921–922
  nursing management, 926–935
  organisation of services, 922–923
  physical symptoms, 925, 929–932
  quality of life, 925–926
  unconscious, 855–857
  see also Death; Palliative care
Termination of pregnancy, 197–198, **253–254**
Territorial space, 761, 836
Testes, *134*, 137, **295**, *296*
  disorders, *256*
  maldescent, **227–228**, 229
  self-examination, *230*, 232
  torsion, **228**
Testicular cancer, **229–230**, *884*, *885*
  vasectomy and, *232*
Testicular feminisation, 152
Testosterone, *142*, 295
Tetanus, 763
  immunoglobulin of human origin (HTIG), *817*
  toxoid vaccine, *817*, 821
Tetany, 141, *147*, 647, 763
Tetraplegia (quadriplegia), 386
Thalamus, 329, *617*, 840, 858
Thalassaemia, 192, 421
Theatre
  environmental safety, 787–789
  safety, 786, 788
Theatre nurse, 786–787
T-helper cells, *see* Helper T lymphocytes
Therapist–client relationship, 588
Thermodilution method, cardiac output measurement, 610, *612*
Thermogenesis
  chemical, 686
  diet-induced (DIT), 686
  non-shivering (NST), 683, 692
  shivering, 683, 692
Thermography, burns assessment, 864–865
Thermometers, **686–687**
  clinical, 686–687
  electronic, 687
  infrared radiation (tympanic membrane), 687
  liquid crystal, 687
Thermoregulation, *see* Temperature, body, regulation
Thiamme, *659*, *660*, *661*
Third (oculomotor) nerve, *330*
Third space fluid losses, 643
Thirst, 652
  excessive, 157, 158
  postoperative, 797
Thomas' splint, *376*
Throat
  anatomy and physiology, *506*, **511**
  benign tumours, 511
  disorders, **511–519**
  swabs, 449
Thromboangiitis obliterans, 52
Thrombocytes, *see* Platelet(s)
Thrombocytopenia, **439–440**, 441
  acquired, 439
  leukaemia, *426*
Thrombocytopenic purpura (TCP), **439–440**, *530*
  idiopathic, 439
Thrombolytic therapy, 24
Thrombophlebitis, 54, 55
Thrombosis, 15, 55
  cerebral, 170, 344
  deep vein (DVT), *see* Venous thrombosis, deep
Thrush, *see* Candidiasis
Thymus, 544, *545*
Thyroid adenoma, toxic (solitary nodule), 144
Thyroid carcinoma, **145**
Thyroid crisis, 141
Thyroidectomy
  near-total, 145
  nursing care plan, 141
  partial, 144, 145, 512
Thyroid gland, *134*, **135–136**
  disorders, **144–146**
Thyroid hormones, 135, 136
Thyrotoxicosis (hyperthyroidism), **144–145**, *493*
Thyrotrophic-stimulating hormone (TSH), *135*, *142*
Thyrotrophin-releasing hormone (TRH), *135*
Thyroxine (T_4), 135, 136
  replacement therapy, 142, 146
  shock, 599
Tibial fractures, **381**
Tidal volume (TV), 61, *63*
Tigason (etretinate), 451
Tinea, 454
Tinea corporis (ringworm), **455**
Tinea pedis (athelete's foot), **454–455**, *1005*

Tinnitus, **504–505**
Tiredness, *see* Fatigue
Tissue–capillary fluid exchange, 639
Tissue expansion, breast, 278–279, 280
Tissue necrosis, *see* Necrotic tissue
Tissue repair, 699–700
Tissue Viability Society, 722
T lymphocytes (T cells), *407*, 544, *545*, 546
  deficiency, 559
  helper, *see* Helper T lymphocytes
  immune response, 548
TNA (total nutrient admixture; triple mix), 674
TNM staging system, 883–884
Tobacco, **978–979**
  chewing, 537
  smoking, *see* Smoking
Toileting aids, 735
Tolerance
  drug, 622, 974
  hypnotic benzodiazepines, 754
  pain, 621, *623*
Tomograms, *373*
Tongue, 88, 91, 521–523
  smooth, 415
  thrust, *968*
  tumours, **537**, *538*
Tonic–clonic seizures, *355*
Tonic seizures, *355*
Tonometry, 480
Tonsillar tumours, 517–518
Tonsillectomy, 517, **518**
Tonsillitis, **517–518**
Toothbrushes, 526
Toothpaste, 526
Topical agents, wound cleansing, 707, *708*
Topical analgesia, *790*
Topical therapy
  bullous skin disorders, 460
  eczema, **453–454**
  eye, **475**, *476*
    allergy to, **485**
  glaucoma, 478, 480
  psoriasis, 449–450
  skin, **446–447**
Total lung capacity (TLC), 61, *63*
Total nutrient admixture (TNA; triple mix), 674
Touch, 761, 763
  head-injured patients, 342
  terminal illness and, 926
  therapeutic, 631
Toxic chemicals, *see* Chemicals
Toxic epidermal necrolysis, **459**, 460
Toxic multinodular goitre, 144
Toxoids, 548
Toxoplasmosis, 1006
Trabeculectomy, 480
Trace elements, 662
  parenteral solutions, 674, *675*
Tracheal mucosa, damage to, 517
Tracheal suction, *see* Airways, suctioning
Tracheobronchitis, acute, **68**
Tracheostomy, 514, **515–517**
  complications, *513*, 516–517
  indications, 515, *516*
  medical management, 515–516
  nursing priorities and management, 516–517, 541
  respiratory failure, 82
  tubes, 514, 516, 850
    blockage, 516
    changing, 517
    decannulation or removal, 517
    displacement, 517
  unconscious patients, 850
Trachoma, 467
Traction, **374–376**
  balanced/sliding, 374–375
  fixed, 375, *376*
  nursing management, 375–376
  prolapsed intervertebral disc, 393
  skeletal, *374*, 375, *376*, *387*
  skin, 375, *376*, *377*
Tranquillisers, 589, **982–983**
  withdrawal, 982, 983
Transactional, 594
Transactional models of stress, **577–578**
Transcutaneous electrical nerve stimulation (TENS), 631
Transferrin, serum, 665, *666*
Transfers
  burns patients, 862, 866
  disabled patients, 952
  surgical patients, 789
Transformation zone, cervical, 235
  large loop excision (LLETZ), 236
Transient ischaemic attacks (TIA), *345*, 346–347, 494
Transjugular intrahepatic portosystemic shunting (TIPS), 117
Translocations, 191
  balanced, 191
Trans-oral approach, *341*
Transport, patients with infectious diseases, 564
Transsphenoidal approach, *341*
Transurethral resection of prostate, *see* Prostate gland, transurethral resection
Trapezium pinch, 845–846
Trauma, **809–824**
  abdominal, 815
  amputation of limb, 389
  chest, **79–81**, 811, 813
  cold-induced, **693–694**
  death from, 818–819
  definition, 809
  discharge, 821–822
  epidemiology, 369–370
  eye, 473, **486–490**, 534
  head, *see* Head injury
  immediate treatment, 811–812
  minor, 819–822
    assessment and treatment, 819–821
    home care/community services and, 821
  multiple, *see* Multiple trauma
  nose, **509–510**, *531*, 533
  nursing process approach, 813
  oesophageal, 95–96
  orofacial, **531–536**, 763
  principles of nursing management, 373
  soft tissue, *see* Soft tissue injuries
  splenic, **129**
  wound management, 720
  see also Accident and Emergency (A & E) departments; Fractures
Travel
  bereaved relatives, 938
  diabetes mellitus, 181
  infectious diseases and, 544
Trazodone, 589
Triad model of supervision, 593
Triage, **810–811**
  ophthalmic, *486*
Triceps skinfold thickness (TSF), 665
Tricuspid incompetence, **44**
Tricuspid stenosis, **44**
Tricuspid valve (right atrioventricular valve), *10*, 11, 12
Tricyclic antidepressants, 589
Trigeminal nerve, *330*, *523*
Trigone, *294*
Tri-iodothyronine (T_3), 135, 136, 145
Trisomy, 191
Trochlear nerve, *330*
Trousseau's sign, *147*
Tryptophan, 751
T-suppressor cells, 546, 548
T-tube, 122, *123*
  management, *122*
Tubal pregnancy, 246–247
Tuberculosis, 544
  AIDS and, 1006
  bone, 391
  infection control, 551, 553
  oral, *529*
  pulmonary, **69–70**, **567–568**, *569*
    medical management, 69–70, 568
    nursing priorities and management, 70, 568
    pathophysiology, 69, 568
Tubocurarine, *791*
Tumour(s)
  benign, 877
  doubling time, 877
  fungating, *see* Fungating tumours
  histology, 877
  malignant, *see* Cancer
Tumour-associated antigen (TA-4), 237
Tumour lysis syndrome, 428, 431
Turner's syndrome, 152, 219–220
T wave, 12, 23
Twelfth (hypoglossal) nerve, *330*, *523*
Tympanoplasty, **503–504**
Type A behaviour, 582, **586**

U

UKCC Code of Professional Conduct, 781
Ulcerative colitis (UC), **102–104**
Ultrasound
  cholelithiasis, 121
  Doppler, 51, *717*, 718
  ectopic pregnancy, 246
  prenatal diagnosis, 193
Ultraviolet A (UVA), 447, 461
Ultraviolet B (UVB), 461
  phototherapy, 447, 449, 450
Ultraviolet radiation
  cancer and, 881
  eye injuries, 489
Umbilical hernia, 108, *109*
Unconscious patients, **839–858**
  emergency care, 847–849
  first aid, *847*
  medical management, 848–849
  neurological assessment, 844–846
  nursing management, 849–857
  nutrition, 669, 852–853
  see also Coma; Consciousness
Unemployment, disability and, 906
Uniforms, nurses', 760
Universal blood and body fluid precautions, **550**, *551*, 555, 563
Upper limbs, 371
  fractures, **382–383**
  lymphoedema in breast cancer, *see* Lymphoedema, breast cancer
Uraemia, 318, 320, *672*
Ureterolithotomy, 302, 303–304
Ureteroscopy, 300

Ureters, **294**
  fibrosis around, 304–305
  obstruction, 303
  stenting, 300, *301*, 302, 303–304
Urethra, **294–295**
  female, 295
  male, 294–295, *296*
    congenital disorders, **306**
    disorders, **305–306**
  trauma, 816
Urethral sphincters, 294–295
Urethral strictures, **304**
Urethrocele, 247–248
Urethroplasty, 304
Urethrotomy, 304
Urge incontinence, 725, 731–732
Urinals, for women, 735
Urinary catheterisation, *see* Catheterisation, urinary
Urinary diversion, and total cystectomy, *see* Cystectomy, total, and urinary diversion
Urinary fistulae, 297
Urinary incontinence, **723–739**
  aetiology, 726–728
  aids and equipment, 733, **735**
  assessment, 729–731
  attitudes towards, 724–725
  benign prostatic hyperplasia, 307
  elderly, 728, 733, 734, *964*, 965
  epidemiology, 725–726
  Huntington's disease, 209
  identifying patients, 726, *727*
  immobility, 725
  institutionalised patients, 733–734
  management of intractable, **734–739**
  multiple sclerosis, 358–359
  overflow, 725
  pads and pants, 735, 933
  Parkinson's disease, 362
  postmicturition, 733
  problem-solving approach, **728–734**
  referring patients, 733
  reflex, 725
  sexuality and, 738–739
  sociological factors in under-reporting, 726
  stress, *see* Stress incontinence
  stroke, 348
  terminally ill patients, 933–934
  treatment, 731–734
  types, 725
  urge, 725, 731–732
Urinary output, shock, 600, 611, 613, 792
Urinary retention
  acute, 307
  chronic, 307–308, 311, 312
  joint replacement, 399
  overflow incontinence, 725
  postoperative, *799*, 800
Urinary stones (calculi), **299–304**
  flush back, 300, 302
  medical management, 299–302
  nursing priorities and management, 302–304
  pathophysiology, 299
Urinary system, **291–323**
  anatomy and physiology, 291–296
  disorders, 291, **292–322**
Urinary tract infections, 174, **296–298**
  long-term catheterisation and, 736
  pathophysiology, 296–297
  post-prostatectomy, 311
  urinary stones, 303
Urinary tract obstruction, 296–297, **298–305**
Urine, 640
  excessive fluid losses, 643
  formation, 292–293
  midstream specimen (MSU), 297
  monitoring, burns, 867
  osmolarity, 611
  physical characteristics, *293*
  red, Adriamycin-induced, 431
  specific gravity, 611
Urodynamics, 730
Urticaria, 559
  solar, 461
Uterine bleeding
  abnormal, **222–223**
  dysfunctional, 222
  menopause and, 217
  pregnancy, 250–251, 252
  termination of pregnancy, 253
Uterine procidentia, **248**
Uterine (fallopian) tubes, *212, 213*, **215**
  disorders, *255*
  ligation, 222
  rupture, ectopic pregnancy, 246
  surgery, 254
Uterine tumours
  benign, **244–245**
  menorrhagia, 222
  see also Choriocarcinoma; Endometrial carcinoma
Utero-vaginal prolapse, **248**
  repair, 248–249
Uterus, *212, 213*, **214–215**
  adenomyosis, 222, 224
  anatomy, 214–215
  anteverted/anteflexed, 214, 247
  carcinoma of body, *see* Endometrial carcinoma
  congenital abnormalities, 219, 222
  congenital absence, 219
  displacements, **247–249**
  functions, 215
  retroverted, 214, 224, 247, *248*
Uveal tract, 468
Uveitis, **484**
U wave, 12

V

Vaccination, **548**, 563
Vaccines
  killed, 548
  live attenuated, 548
Vacuum aspiration, 253
Vacuum suction machine, impotence, 233
Vagina, *212*, **215**
  anterior wall prolapse, 247–248
  congenital absence, 219
  posterior wall prolapse, 248
Vaginal bleeding, *see* Uterine bleeding
Vaginal cones, 731
Vaginal dryness, urinary incontinence and, 728, 733
Vaginal fistula, *779*, 804
Vaginitis, urinary incontinence and, 728, 733
Vagotomy, *97*
Vagus nerve, 13, *330, 523*
Valerian, 754–755
Valsalva's manoeuvre, 81, 90
Valuables
  deceased patients, 938
  surgical patients, 786, *787*
  trauma victims, 817
Valvular heart disease, **41–44**, 526
  medical management, 41–42
  nursing priorities and management, 42–43
  pathophysiology, 41
Valvuloplasty, balloon, 42
Varicella (chickenpox), *529*, 563, **569–570**
Varices, oesophageal, 117–118, *980*
Varicocele, **229**
Varicose eczema, 452
Varicose veins, 54, **55**, *716*
  nursing care plan, 56–57
Vascular disease, peripheral, **48–55**, 389
Vascular resistance
  peripheral/systemic, 13–14, *601*
  pulmonary, *601*
Vasculitic leg ulcers, *719*
Vas deferens, 295, *296*
  disorders, *256*
Vasectomy, **230–232**, 249
  reversal, 231
  testicular tumours and, 232
Vasoconstriction, peripheral
  fever, 688
  heat conservation, 682, 690
  Raynaud's phenomenon, 694
  shock, 599–600, 792
Vasodilation, peripheral, 688, *692*
Vasomotor centre, 329
Vasopressin (AVP; antidiuretic hormone; ADH), 134, *135*, 293
  deficiency, *142*, 143–144
  disorders of secretion, **142–144**
  plasma osmolality and, **640–641**
  shock, 599
  syndrome of inappropriate secretion (SIADH), 144
Vegetarians, 659, *661*
Vegetative state, 844
Vein of Galen (great cerebral vein), 331, *333*
Veins, 13
  varicose, 54, **55**, 56–57, *716*
Venesection, polycythaemia vera, 425
Venous cannulation, central, *see* Central venous cannulation
Venous disease, *51*, **53–55**
Venous insufficiency, **53–55**
  chronic, 54
  nursing priorities and management, 55
  see also Venous leg ulcers
Venous leg ulcers, *51*, 54, **715–718**
  assessment, 717
  epidemiology, 698
  healing time, 698, *699*
  management, 717–718
  patient education, 719
Venous sinuses, brain, 331, *332*
Venous thrombosis, deep (DVT), **54**, 55, **783–784**
  joint replacement, 399
  prevention, 54, **783–784**, 788
  total cystectomy and urinary diversion, 317
Ventform kit, skin traction, *377*
Ventilation, **61–62**
  central control, 61, *62*
  mechanical, 32, *83*, 515, 811
  see also Breathing
Ventimask, 71, 72
Ventricles (heart), 10
Ventricular aneurysms, 34
Ventricular arrhythmias, 36
Ventricular assist device, 55
Ventricular conducting system, 11, 12
Ventricular fibrillation (VF), 31, 33, 36
Ventricular septal defects, post-infarction, 34

Ventricular system, brain, **329**, *332*
Ventricular tachycardia, 36
Ventriculo-peritoneal shunts, *347*
Ventro-suspension, 260
Venules, 13
Verbal rating scale (VRS), pain, 627
Verbal response, Glasgow Coma Scale, 844–845
Vertebrae, 371
Vertebral column, 371
Vertigo, **505**
Veruccae, *457*
Vesicles, **464**
Vesico-urethral reflux, 296
Vestibular apparatus, 498
Vestibule (mouth), 521
Vestibulo-cochlear nerve, *330*
Vestibulospinal tract, *335*
Viability, fetal, 249, 260
Videocystourethrography, 731
Villi, small intestine, 90
Vincristine, *892*, *895*
Violence, 810
  A & E departments, **822–823**
  domestic, 823
  orofacial trauma, 531
Viral encephalitis, 363
Viral infections, 563
  AIDS/HIV infection, 1006
  blood-borne, haemophilia A, 205
  diabetes mellitus and, 157
  hearing loss, 500
  hepatitis, **114–115**
  keratitis, 484
  pneumonia, 69
  skin, **457–458**
Virchow's triad, 783
Virilisation, 151, 152
Virilism, 220
Viruses, **993**
  cancer-causing, 881
Vision, **469–470**
  binocular, 472
  distance, 471–472
  double (diplopia), **485–486**
  near, 472
  painless loss, **477–483**
  preservation, **473**
  testing, **471–472**, 473, 475, 534
Visitors
  critically ill patients, 833
  isolated patients, 564
  mealtimes and, 668
Visual acuity (VA) testing, **471–472**
Visual analogue scale (VAS), pain, 627
Visual deficits, stroke, *345*, 348, 494
Visual display units (VDUs), 473
Visual evoked responses, 356
Visual field testing, **472**, 480
Visual impairment, **473–474**
  see also Blindness
Visual pathways, 469
Visual tract, 858
Vital capacity (VC), 61, *63*
Vitamin A, *659*, *660*, *661*
Vitamin B_6, 226, *661*
Vitamin B_{12}, 416, *419*
  deficiency, 416, 418–419, **420**
  dietary requirements, *661*
Vitamin B complex, deficiency, *659*
Vitamin C, *659*, *660*, *661*
Vitamin D, 136, *137*, 294, *661*
  deficiency, 147, *659*
  synthesis in skin, 446
Vitamin E, *661*
Vitamin K, 408
Vitamins, 658, 659, *662*
  parenteral solutions, 674, *675*
Vitrectomy, 476, 494
Vitreous chamber, 469
Vocal cords, 759
VOCAL (Voluntary Organisations Communication and Language), 763, 771
Voice
  production, 759
  tone of, 760
Volume–pressure relationship, intracranial pressure, 338, *339*
Voluntary agencies, 769
  bereavement and, 819
  chronic illness, 910–911
  dependency problems, 987
  disabled, 946–947
  incontinence, 735
  terminal care, 923
  see also Support/self-help groups
Vomiting/nausea, **653–654**
  chemotherapy-induced, 430, 893
  diabetes mellitus, 157
  enteral feeding causing, *672*
  gastrointestinal haemorrhage, 98
  nursing management, 654
  postoperative, 247, **799**
  radiotherapy-induced, *890*
  raised intracranial pressure, *331*, 339
  renal colic, 303
  terminally ill patients, 929, 931
  tracheostomy patients, 517
Von Willebrand's disease, 202, 439
Vulnerability, elderly, 963–965
Vulva, 215

W

Waiting times, for surgery, 776
Wakefulness, 745
Walking aids, 397
Warfarin, 43
Warts, **457**
Washbowls, cleaning, *552*
Waste
  clinical, 553, 554
  disposal, **553–554**, *555*, 564
  household/domestic, 553
  identification, 553–554
Water, 658, 659
  balance, *see* Fluid balance
  body, **638–640**
  cold, burns first-aid, 861–862
  homeostasis, **640–641**
  intoxication, 643
  renal reabsorption, 293
  total body (TBW), 638
Waterlow pressure sore prevention/treatment policy, 712–713, *714*
Weal, 464
Weight, body, 665
  burns patients, 867
  monitoring, diabetes mellitus, 165
  sleep and, 749
Weight loss
  AIDS/HIV infection, 1004, 1005
  cancer, 899
  diabetes mellitus, 157
  Huntington's disease, 208
  pancreatic cancer, 128–129
Westminster Pastoral Foundation, 596
Wheelchairs, 42, 358, *953*
Whiplash injury, cervical spine, 384, *387*, 401
Whipple's procedure, 124, *124*, 128
White blood cells, **407**, *410*, 545–546
  development, *408*
  disorders, **426–439**
Wilson's disease, 116, 130
Wisdom teeth, impacted, 523, 527
Withdrawal symptoms, 974
Women
  alcohol abuse, 981
  smoking, 978–979
Women's Alcohol Centre, 989
Work, *see* Employment
Work-related disorders
  cancer, 881
  eye injuries, 473, 489, 490
  farmer's lung, 560
  musculoskeletal injuries, 369–370
  orofacial injuries, 531–532
  respiratory tract, 67
World Health Organization (WHO), 5, 944, *979*
Wound(s)
  assessment, 705–706
  bed, appearance, 705
  burn, *see* Burn wounds
  cavity
    assessment, 705–706
    cleansing, 706–707
    excessive granulation, 708
  cleansing, **706–708**
  closure, 701–702
  debridement, *see* Debridement
  definition, **698**
  epidemiology, 698–699
  fungating, *see* Fungating tumours/wounds
  malignant, **720**
  measurement, 706
  odour, 763
  shape, 706
  size, 705–706
  sutured, 701–702, **719–720**
    assessment, 705
    management, 719–720
  swabs, *705*, 867
  traumatic, **720**
  types and classification, 698
  see also Leg ulcers; Pressure sores
Wound abscess, *698*, 703
Wound Care Society, 722
Wound drains, 703, *799*, 801–802, *803*
  cholecystectomy, 122
  hip replacement, 399
  mastectomy, 271–275
Wound healing, **697–722**
  burns, 869
  creating optimal environment for, **706–708**
  factors adversely affecting, 702–703, *802*
  physiology, 699–702
  by primary/first intention, **700–701**, 705, 802
  scarring and, 701, *702*
  by secondary intention, **701**, 702, 802
  sleep and, 746
  terminology, *698*
Wound infections, **703–704**, 705
  breast reconstruction, 279
  joint replacement, 399
  predisposing factors, 703
  risks after surgery, *802*
  skeletal traction sites, 375
  sources, 704

Wound infections (*contd*)
  total cystectomy and urinary diversion, 317
  venous leg ulcers, 718
Wound management, **704–712**
  assessment in, *704*, 705–706
  breast reconstruction, 279–280
  burns, *see* Burn wounds
  circumcision, 305–306
  conditions encouraging healing, 706–708
  dressing change techniques, 708–710
  expectations of outcome, 711–712
  fungating breast tumours, **283–286**
  inappropriate, 703
  leg ulcers, 717–718
  mastectomy, 271–275
  maxillofacial injuries, 535
  minor trauma, 819–821
  nurse prescribing, 711
  by patients, 710–711
  policies, 711
  postoperative, **801–802**
  pressure sores, 713–715
  provision of materials in community, 711
  sutured wounds, 719–720
  tracheostomy, 514, 516, 850
  traumatic injuries, 720
Written materials, readability, 761

X

Xanthine stones, *299*
X chromosome, *188*
Xeroderma pigmentosum, 464
Xerophthalmia, 468
Xerostomia, *890*
X-linked recessive disorders, 192
X-rays, *373*, 816, 831, 886

Y

Yoghurt, natural live, 283
Young people
  alcohol-related problems, 980–981
  contraceptive needs, 249
  solvent abuse, 983–984
  see also Girls

Z

Zeitgebers, 743, 744
Zidovudine (AZT), 1007
Zinc, *659*, *661*, 662
Zopiclone, 754
Zygomatic (malar) bone, fractures, *531*, 533

Dear Reader,

We would welcome your comments on this text, and would also be very pleased to hear from you with any suggestions you may have for new publications.

Do write to me at the following address:

Ellen Green
Commissioning Editor
Churchill Livingstone
1–3 Baxter's Place
Leith Walk
Edinburgh EH1 3AF

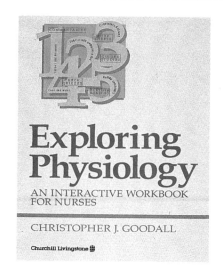

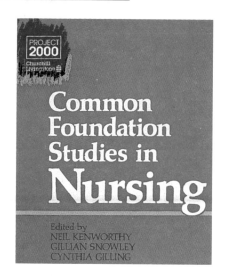

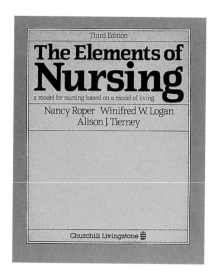

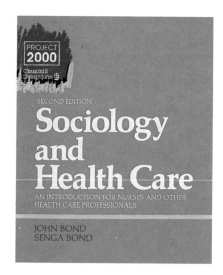

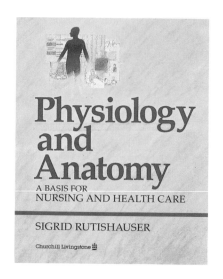

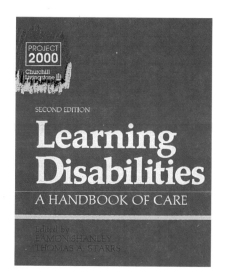